MW01196943

Youmans & Winn Neurological Surgery

VOLUME 1

Introduction and General Neurosurgery
William T. Couldwell, Basant K. Misra, Volker Seifert, and Ugur Türe

Basic and Clinical Sciences
Michel Kliot, Pierre J. Magistretti, Robert M. Friedlander, and Michael M. Haglund

Epilepsy
Guy M. McKhann II, Itzhak Fried, Andrew W. McEvoy, Steven V. Pacia, Dennis D. Spencer, and Nitin Tandon

Functional Neurosurgery
Ron L. Alterman, Andres M. Lozano, Joachim K. Krauss, and Takaomi Taira

VOLUME 2

Oncology
E. Antonio Chiocca, Henry Brem, Russell R. Lonser, Andrew T. Parsa, Zvi Ram, and Raymond Sawaya

Pain
Kim J. Burchiel, Feridun Acar, and Andrew C. Zacest

Pediatrics
Gerald A. Grant, James T. Rutka, Andrew H. Jea, James Tait Goodrich, Richard David Hayward, and Shenandoah Robinson

VOLUME 3

Peripheral Nerve
Aaron G. Filler, Allan J. Belzberg, Liang Chen, and Martijn J.A. Malessy

Radiation
Bruce E. Pollock, Dong Gyu Kim, and Jean Régis

Spine
Christopher I. Shaffrey, Sr., Michael G. Fehlings, Osmar José Santos de Moraes, Charles Kuntz IV, Praveen V. Mummaneni, Paul Santiago, and Daniel K. Resnick

VOLUME 4

Trauma
Geoffrey T. Manley, Peter J. Hutchinson, Andrew I.R. Maas, and Guy Rosenthal

Vascular
E. Sander Connolly, Jr., Gavin W. Britz, Kazuhiro Hongo, Michael T. Lawton, and Fredric B. Meyer

About the Cover Artist:
Dr. Kathryn Ko completed her neurosurgery training at Mount Sinai Medical Center in New York City and earned an MFA from the Academy of Art University in representational painting. Dr. Ko is the host of Art on Call, a series that deals with the intersection of art and medicine. Dr. Ko regards art as a necessary continuation of her surgical practice. The operating theater is her studio; the treatment of the subject begins with the scalpel and ends with the brush.

Youmans & Winn Neurological Surgery

SEVENTH EDITION

H. RICHARD WINN, MD
Professor of Neurosurgery
University of Iowa Carver College of Medicine
Iowa City, Iowa;
Professor of Neurosurgery and Neuroscience
Icahn School of Medicine at Mount Sinai
New York, New York

ELSEVIER

ELSEVIER

1600 John F. Kennedy Blvd.
Ste 1800
Philadelphia, PA 19103-2899

YOUMANS AND WINN NEUROLOGICAL SURGERY, SEVENTH EDITION ISBN: 978-0-323-28782-1

Notices

Knowledge and best practice in this field are constantly changing. As new research and experience broaden our understanding, changes in research methods, professional practices, or medical treatment may become necessary.

Practitioners and researchers must always rely on their own experience and knowledge in evaluating and using any information, methods, compounds, or experiments described herein. In using such information or methods they should be mindful of their own safety and the safety of others, including parties for whom they have a professional responsibility.

With respect to any drug or pharmaceutical products identified, readers are advised to check the most current information provided (i) on procedures featured or (ii) by the manufacturer of each product to be administered, to verify the recommended dose or formula, the method and duration of administration, and contraindications. It is the responsibility of practitioners, relying on their own experience and knowledge of their patients, to make diagnoses, to determine dosages and the best treatment for each individual patient, and to take all appropriate safety precautions.

To the fullest extent of the law, neither the Publisher nor the authors, contributors, or editors, assume any liability for any injury and/or damage to persons or property as a matter of products liability, negligence or otherwise, or from any use or operation of any methods, products, instructions, or ideas contained in the material herein.

Previous editions copyrighted 2011, 2004, 1996, 1990, 1982, and 1973.

Library of Congress Cataloging-in-Publication Data

Names: Winn, H. Richard, editor.
Title: Youmans and Winn neurological surgery / [edited by] H. Richard Winn.
Other titles: Youmans neurological surgery. | Neurological surgery
Description: Seventh edition. | Philadelphia, PA : Elsevier, [2017] | Preceded by: Youmans neurological surgery. 6th ed. c2011. | Includes bibliographical references and index.
Identifiers: LCCN 2016035901 | ISBN 9780323287821 (hardcover : alk. paper)
Subjects: | MESH: Neurosurgical Procedures | Nervous System Diseases–surgery | Neurosurgery–methods
Classification: LCC RD593 | NLM WL 368 | DDC 617.4/8–dc23 LC record available at https://lccn.loc.gov/2016035901

Senior Content Strategist: Charlotta Kryhl
Senior Content Development Specialist: Jennifer Shreiner
Publishing Services Manager: Catherine Jackson
Book Production Specialist: Kristine Feeherty
Design Direction: Julia Dummitt
Cover Art: Dr. Kathryn Ko

The artworks used on the cover from left to right are entitled:
The Unknown Human © Kathryn Ko, MD, MFA
Globus Pallidum © Kathryn Ko, MD, MFA
Lumbar Spine © Kathryn Ko, MD, MFA
Craniotomy in G Sharp © Kathryn Ko, MD, MFA

Printed in China

Last digit is the print number: 9 8 7 6 5 4 3 2 1

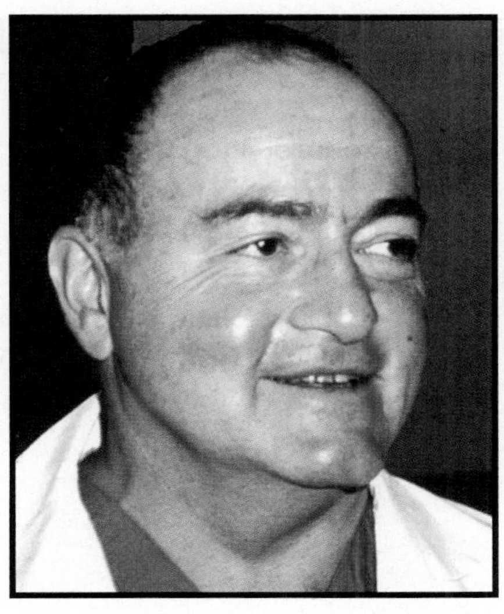

John A. Jane, Sr., MD, PhD, 1931-2015
Professor and Chair, Neurological Surgery
University of Virginia, Charlottesville, Virginia (1969-2006)
Editor-in-Chief of the *Journal of Neurosurgery* (1992-2013)

"Pigmaei gigantum humeris impositi plusquam ipsi gigantes vident."
(If I have seen further it is by standing on the shoulders of giants.) Issac Newton 1676[1]

"Though lives die, the life is not dead, and the memory of lives such as these will be reverently and forever shared not by a profession alone, not by a nation alone, but by the universal brotherhood of man." Andreas Vesalius 1543[2]

Dr. Jane was a giant whose shoulders were the foundation for advances in neurological surgery and for many generations of neurosurgeons. The department he fashioned at the University of Virginia was a fountainhead of originality, research, and advances in clinical care. Even more distinctively, he combined these efforts with a unique, compelling, and dominating focus on education. Dr. Jane united this scholarly emphasis with a warm and welcoming personality, an immense and eclectic intellect, and an ironic and unlimited sense of humor. Like Thomas Jefferson,[3] the founder of the University of Virginia, Dr. Jane sought to create an "academic village" that fostered curiosity, innovation, and intellectual rigor in a supportive milieu. With his personal involvement and encouragement, his students and trainees pursued careers and leadership positions in academic institutions throughout America and the world. These trainees and their descendants will affirm the validity of Vesalius's observation[2]: memories of John Jane's life and his "message"[4] will be shared with future generations of neurosurgeons.[5]

H. Richard Winn, MD
Resident in Neurological Surgery, University of Virginia (1970-1974)
Assistant, Associate, Professor and Vice Chair
Department of Neurological Surgery, University of Virginia (1976-1983)

REFERENCES

1. Turnbull HW, ed. *The Correspondence of Isaac Newton*. Vol. 1-7. New York: Cambridge University Press; 1960.
2. Rutka JT, Hoffman HJ. Medulloblastoma: a historical perspective and overview. *J Neurooncol*. 1996;29:1-7.
3. Boyd JP, Cullen CT, Catanzariti J, et al. *The Papers of Thomas Jefferson*. Princeton, NJ: Princeton University Press; 1950.
4. Hubbard E. *Message to Garcia*. The Philistine. 1899.
5. Dacey RG Jr. Obituary: John Anthony Jane Sr., MD, PhD, 1931-2015. *J Neurosurg*. 2016;124:1-4.

EDITOR-IN-CHIEF

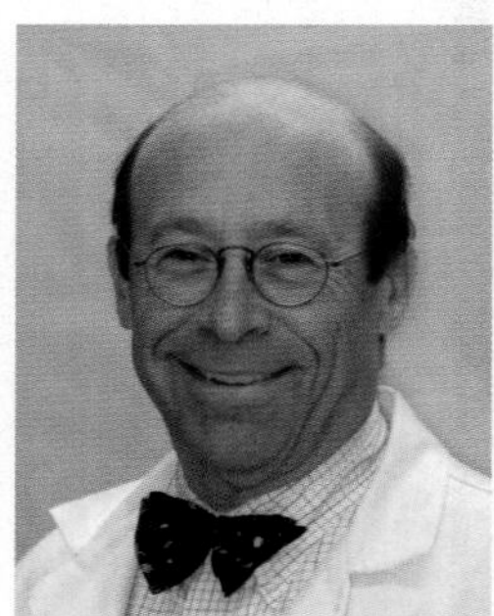

H. Richard Winn, MD
Professor of Neurosurgery
University of Iowa Carver College of Medicine
Iowa City, Iowa;
Professor of Neurosurgery and Neuroscience
Icahn School of Medicine at Mount Sinai
New York, New York

DEPUTY EDITORS-IN-CHIEF

Mitchel S. Berger, MD, MA
Professor and Berthold and Belle N. Guggenheim Endowed Chair
Department of Neurosurgery
Director, Brain Tumor Surgery Program
Director, Neurosurgical Research Centers, Brain Tumor Research Center
University of California, San Francisco
San Francisco, California

Kim J. Burchiel, MD, FACS
John Raaf Professor
Department of Neurological Surgery
Professor, Department of Anesthesiology and Perioperative Medicine
Oregon Health & Science University
Portland, Oregon

Ralph G. Dacey, Jr, MD
Henry G. and Edith R. Schwartz Professor and Chairman
Department of Neurological Surgery
Washington University School of Medicine in St. Louis
St. Louis, Missouri

M. Sean Grady, MD
Charles Harrison Frazier Professor and Chairman
Department of Neurosurgery
Perelman School of Medicine at the University of Pennsylvania
Philadelphia, Pennsylvania

Matthew A. Howard III, MD
Professor and Chair
Department of Neurosurgery
University of Iowa Carver College of Medicine
Iowa City, Iowa

Marc R. Mayberg, MD
Executive Director
Swedish Neuroscience Institute
Swedish Medical Center
Seattle, Washington

Section Editors

SECTION I. INTRODUCTION AND GENERAL NEUROSURGERY

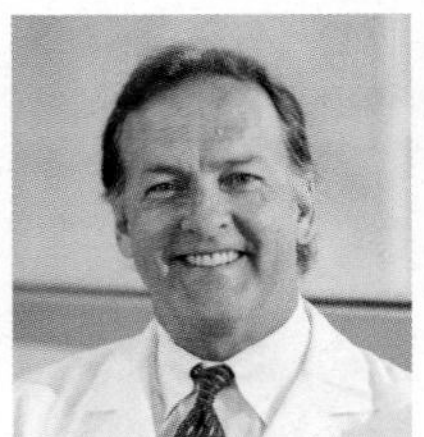

William T. Couldwell, MD, PhD
Professor and Chair
Department of Neurosurgery
University of Utah School of Medicine
Salt Lake City, Utah

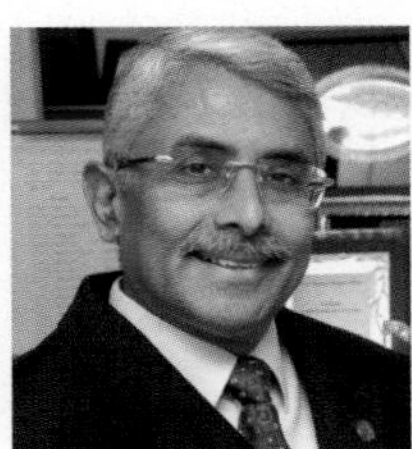

Basant K. Misra, MBBS, MS, MCh, Diplomate National Board
Chairman, Department of Neurosurgery and Gamma Knife Radiosurgery
PD Hinduja National Hospital & Medical Research Centre
Mumbai, India

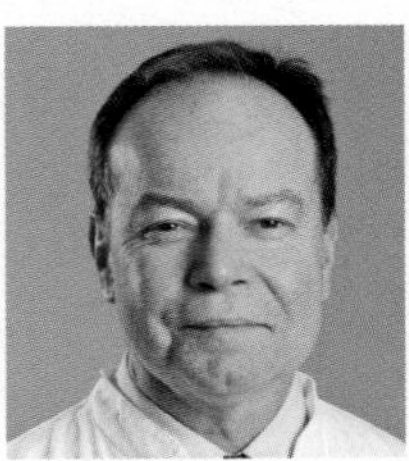

Volker Seifert, MD, PhD
Professor and Chairman
Department of Neurosurgery
Director, Center of Clinical Neurosciences
Johann Wolfgang Goethe-University Frankfurt am Main Germany
Frankfurt am Main, Germany

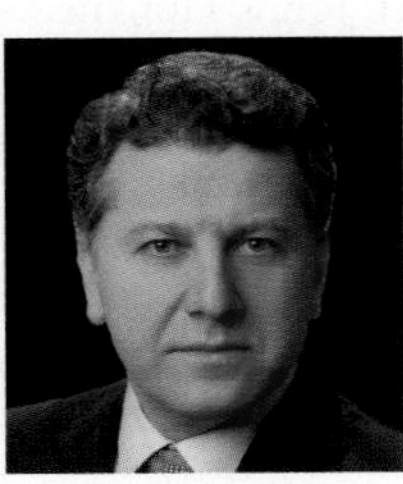

Ugur Türe, MD
Professor and Chair
Department of Neurosurgery
Hacettepe University School of Medicine
Ankara, Turkey

SECTION II. BASIC AND CLINICAL SCIENCES

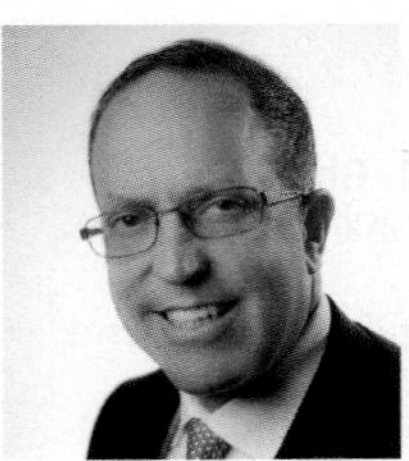

Michel Kliot, MD, MA
Professor and Interim Chair
Department of Neurological Surgery
Director, Peripheral Nerve Center
Northwestern University Feinberg School of Medicine
Chicago, Illinois

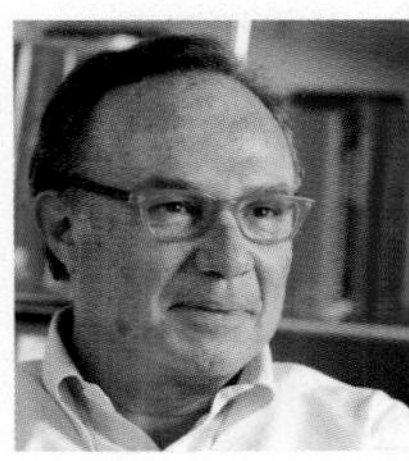

Pierre J. Magistretti, MD, PhD
Professor and Director
Brain Mind Institute
École Polytechnique Fédérale de Lausanne;
Director, Center for Psychiatric Neuroscience
Department of Psychiatry
Centre Hospitalier Universitaire Vaudois
Lausanne, Switzerland

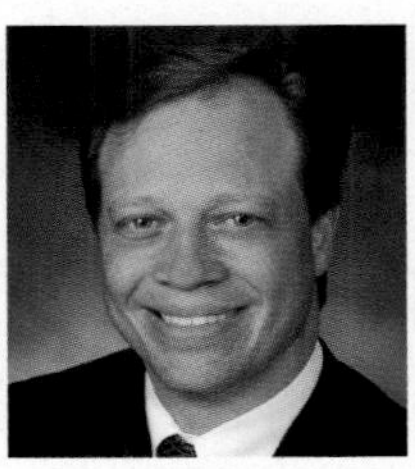

Robert M. Friedlander, MD, MA
Walter E. Dandy Professor and Chairman
Department of Neurological Surgery
University of Pittsburgh School of Medicine
Pittsburgh, Pennsylvania

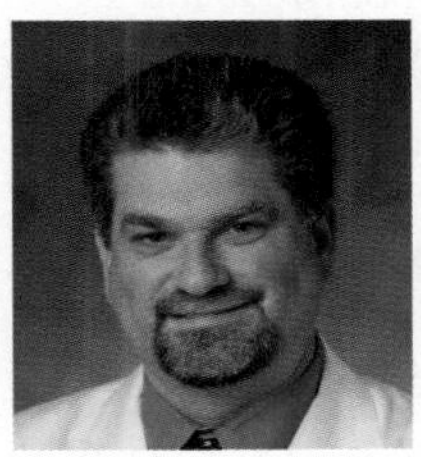

Michael M. Haglund, MD, PhD
Professor of Neurosurgery, Neurobiology, and Global Health
Department of Neurosurgery
Duke University School of Medicine
Durham, North Carolina

SECTION III. EPILEPSY

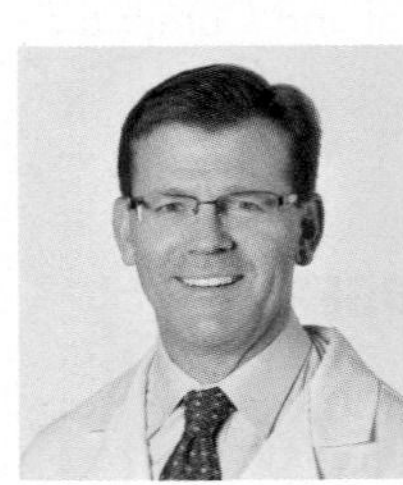

Guy M. McKhann II, MD
Florence Irving Associate Professor of Neurological Surgery
Columbia University College of Physicians and Surgeons;
Director, Epilepsy and Movement Disorder Surgery
Director, Adult Hydrocephalus Center
Director, Awake Brain Mapping for Tumors and Epilepsy
New York–Presbyterian Columbia University Medical Center
New York, New York

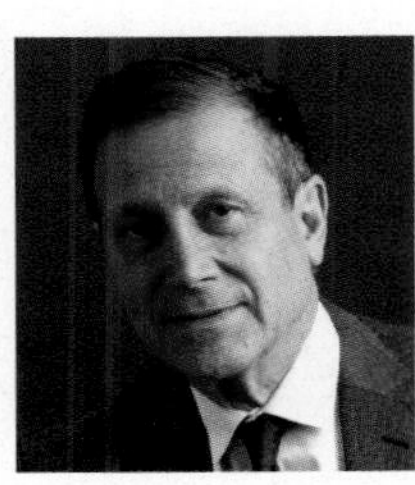

Itzhak Fried, MD, PhD
Professor of Surgery (Neurosurgery) and Psychiatry and Bio-behavioral Sciences
Director of Epilepsy Surgery
Department of Neurosurgery
David Geffen School of Medicine at UCLA
Co-Director, Seizure Disorder Center
UCLA Medical Center
Los Angeles, California;
Professor of Surgery (Neurosurgery)
Tel-Aviv Medical Center
Tel-Aviv, Israel

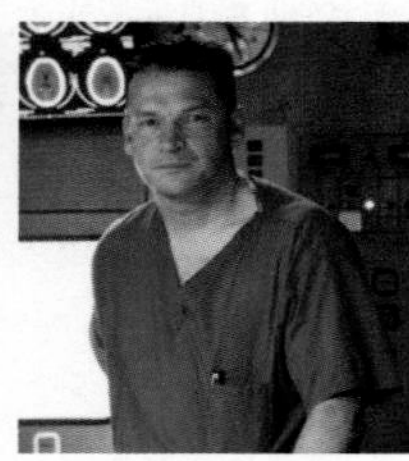

Andrew W. McEvoy, MBBS, MD, FRCS(Lond), FRCS(SN)
Consultant Neurosurgeon
National Hospital for Neurology and Neurosurgery
Institute of Neurology
University College London;
Honorary Consultant Neurosurgeon
Great Ormond Street Hospital for Children
London, United Kingdom

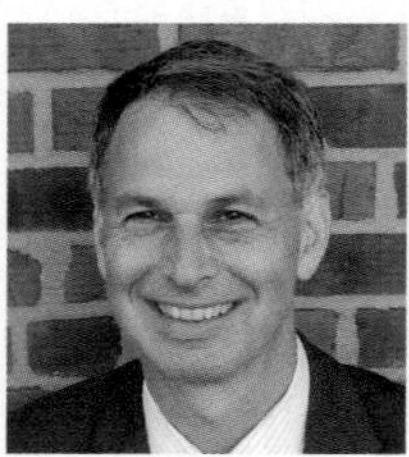

Steven V. Pacia, MD
Associate Professor of Neurology
New York University School of Medicine;
Director, Epilepsy Center
Lenox Hill Hospital
New York, New York

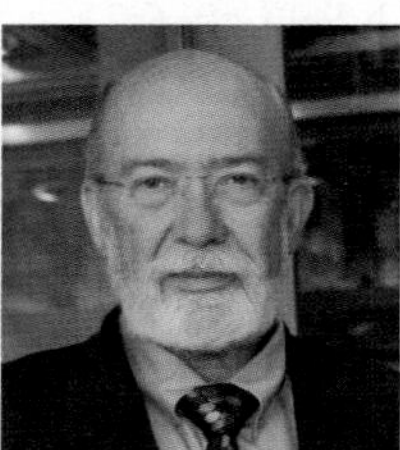

Dennis D. Spencer, MD
Harvey and Kate Cushing Professor of Surgery
Department of Neurosurgery
Director, Epilepsy Surgery Program
Yale University School of Medicine
New Haven, Connecticut

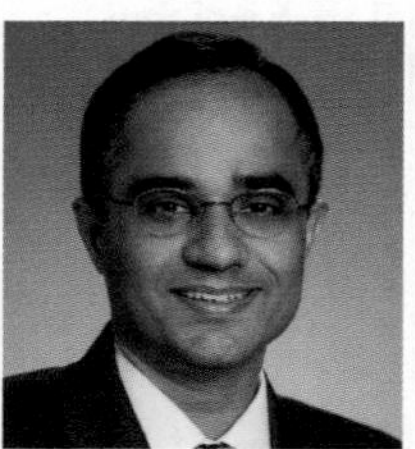

Nitin Tandon, MD, FAANS
Professor of Neurosurgery
University of Texas Health Science Center;
Director, Epilepsy Surgery
Memorial Hermann Hospital;
Adjunct Associate Professor
Department of Electrical and Computer Engineering
Rice University
Houston, Texas

SECTION IV. FUNCTIONAL NEUROSURGERY

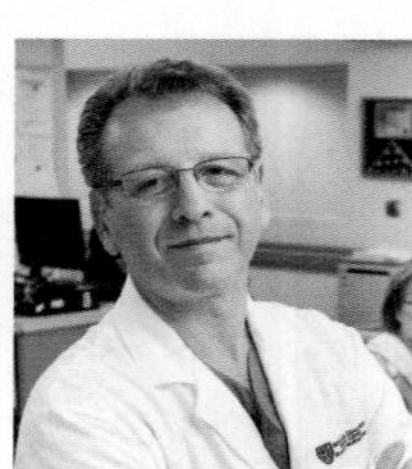

Ron L. Alterman, MD, MBA
Professor of Neurosurgery
Harvard Medical School;
Chief, Division of Neurosurgery
Beth Israel Deaconess Medical Center
Boston, Massachusetts

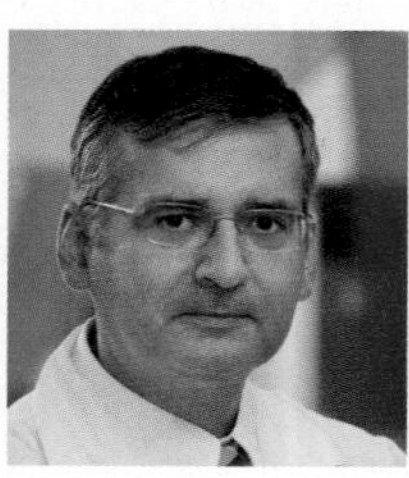

Andres M. Lozano, MD, PhD
Professor and Chairman
Division of Neurosurgery
University of Toronto Faculty of Medicine
Toronto, Ontario, Canada

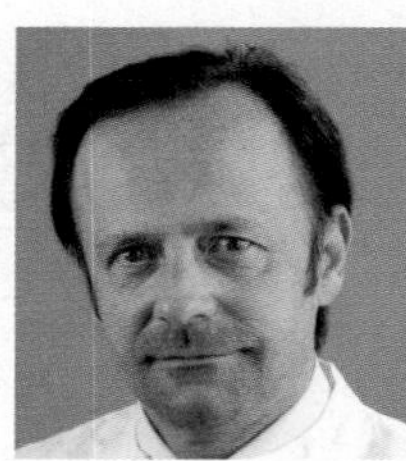

Joachim K. Krauss, Prof. Dr. med.
Chairman and Director
Department of Neurosurgery
Medical School Hannover, MHH
Hannover, Germany

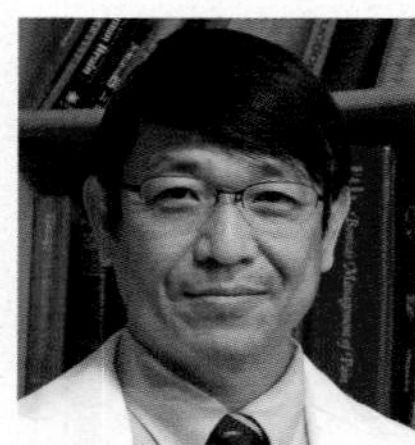

Takaomi Taira, MD, PhD
Professor
Department of Neurosurgery
Tokyo Women's Medical University
Tokyo, Japan

SECTION V. ONCOLOGY

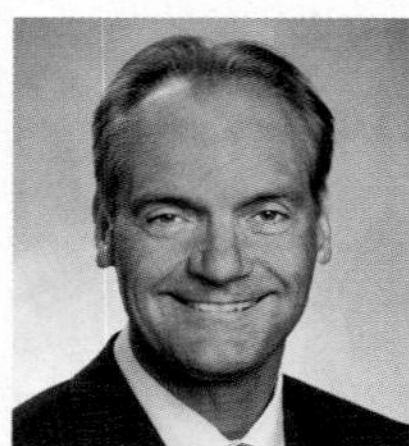

E. Antonio Chiocca, MD, PhD, FAANS
Harvey W. Cushing Professor of Neurosurgery
Harvard Medical School;
Neurosurgeon-in-Chief and Chair, Department of Neurosurgery
Co-Director, Institute for the Neurosciences
Brigham and Women's Hospital
Boston, Massachusetts

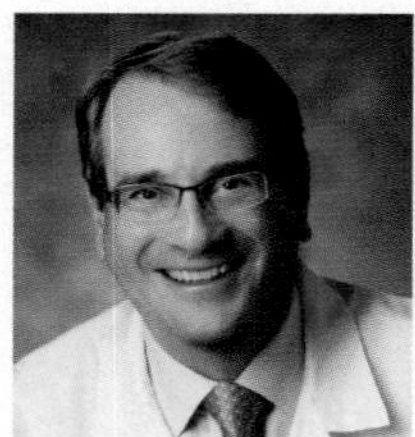

Henry Brem, MD
Harvey Cushing Professor and Director
Department of Neurosurgery
Professor of Neurosurgery, Ophthalmology, Oncology, and Biomedical Engineering
Johns Hopkins University School of Medicine;
Neurosurgeon-in-Chief, Johns Hopkins Medical Institutions
Director, Hunterian Neurosurgical Research Center
Baltimore, Maryland

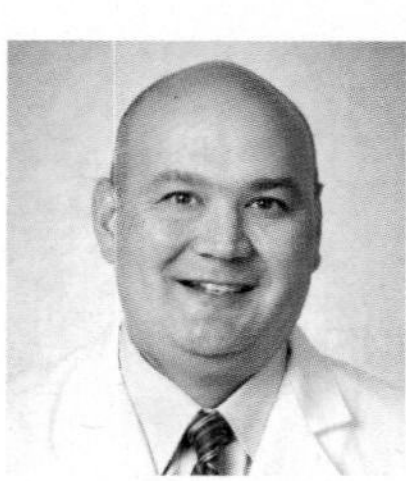

Russell R. Lonser, MD
Professor and Chairman
Department of Neurological Surgery
The Ohio State University Wexner Medical Center
Columbus, Ohio

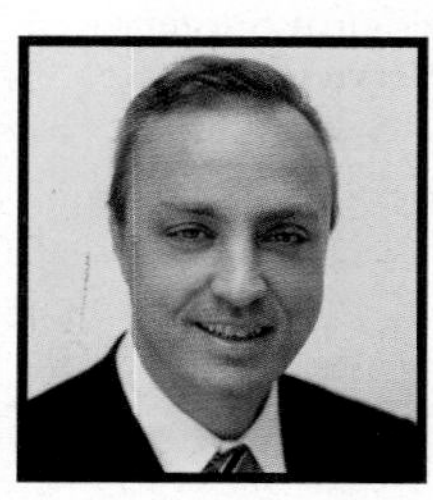

Andrew T. Parsa, MD, PhD[†]
Michael J. Marchese Chair in Neurosurgery
Professor in Neurological Surgery and Neurology
Northwestern University Feinberg School of Medicine
Chicago, Illinois

[†]Deceased.

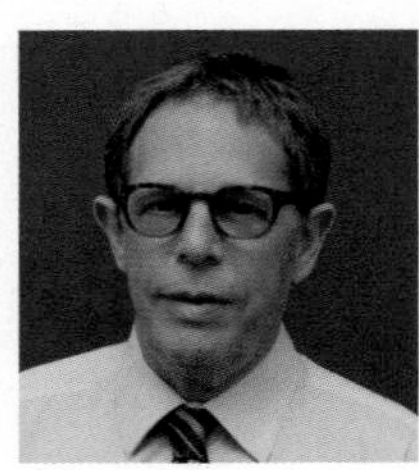

Zvi Ram, MD
Chairman
Department of Neurosurgery
Tel Aviv Medical Center
Tel Aviv, Israel

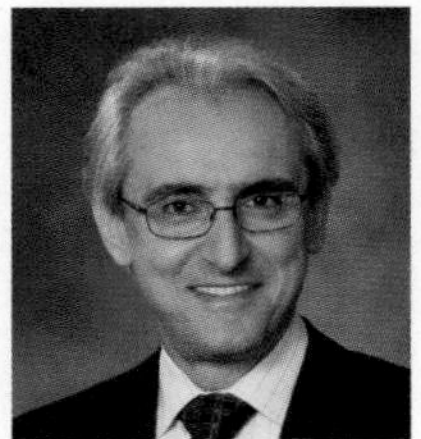

Raymond Sawaya, MD
Professor and Chair
Department of Neurosurgery
University of Texas MD Anderson Cancer Center
Houston, Texas

SECTION VI. PAIN

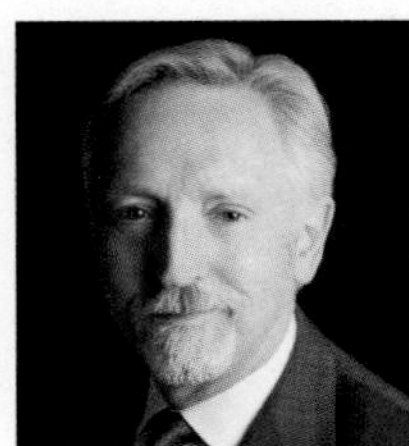

Kim J. Burchiel, MD, FACS
John Raaf Professor
Department of Neurological Surgery
Professor, Department of Anesthesiology and Perioperative Medicine
Oregon Health & Science University
Portland, Oregon

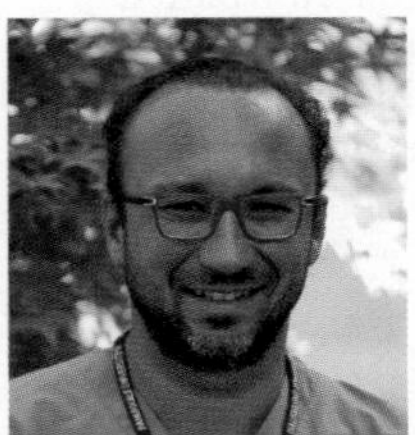

Feridun Acar, MD
Professor and Chair
Department of Neurosurgery
Pamukkale Üniversitesi
Denizli, Turkey

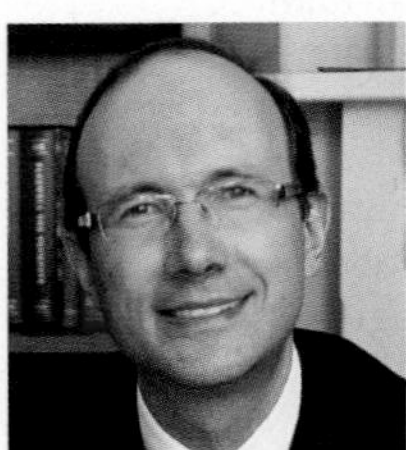

Andrew C. Zacest, MBBS, MS, FRACS, FFPMANZCA
Consultant Neurosurgeon
Royal Adelaide Hospital
Associate Clinical Professor of Neurosurgery and Pain Medicine
University of Adelaide
Adelaide, Australia

SECTION VII. PEDIATRICS

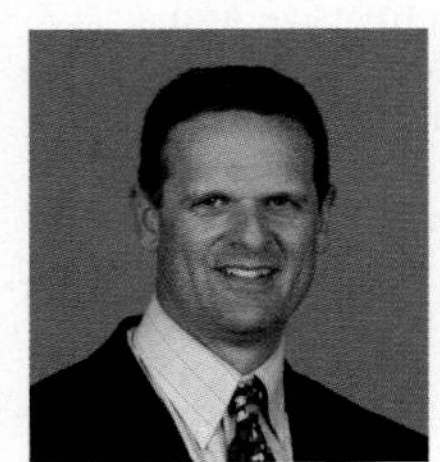

Gerald A. Grant, MD, FACS
Associate Professor of Neurosurgery
Arline and Pete Harman Endowed Faculty Scholar
Division Chief, Pediatric Neurosurgery
Stanford University School of Medicine
Stanford, California

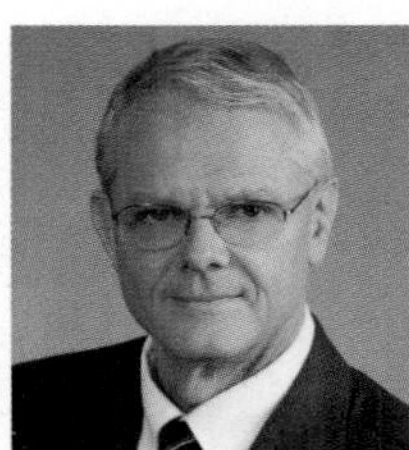

James T. Rutka, MD, PhD
Professor and R.S. McLaughlin Chair
Department of Surgery
University of Toronto Faculty of Medicine;
Director of the Arthur and Sonia Labatt Brain Tumour Research Centre
Division of Paediatric Neurosurgery
The Hospital for Sick Children
Toronto, Ontario, Canada

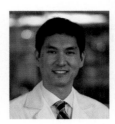

Andrew H. Jea, MD
Professor and Chief of Pediatric Neurosurgery
Indiana University School of Medicine;
Goodman Campbell Brain and Spine
Fellowship Program Director
Riley Hospital for Children
Indianapolis, Indiana

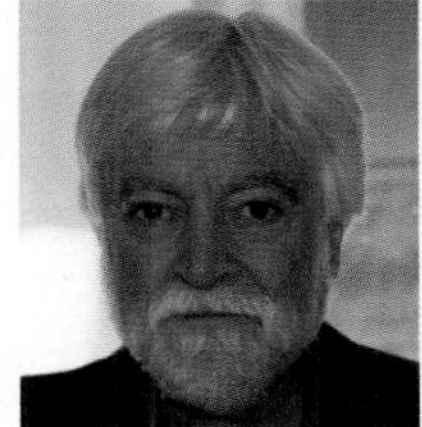

James Tait Goodrich, MD, PhD, DSci (Hon)
Professor of Clinical Neurosurgery, Pediatrics, Plastic and Reconstructive Surgery
Leo Davidoff Department of Neurosurgery
Director, Division of Pediatric Neurosurgery
Children's Hospital at Montefiore
Montefiore Medical Center
Albert Einstein College of Medicine
Bronx, New York

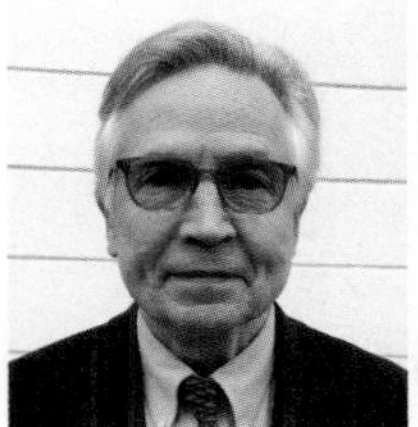

Richard David Hayward, MBBS, FRCS (Eng)
Professor
Department of Paediatric Neurosurgery
Great Ormond Street Hospital for Children
London, United Kingdom

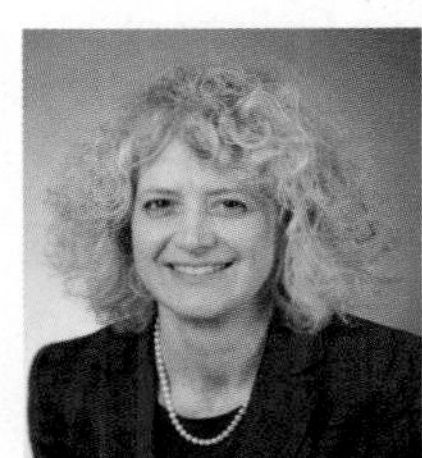

Shenandoah Robinson, MD, FAAP, FACS
Department of Pediatric Neurosurgery
Johns Hopkins University School of Medicine
Baltimore, Maryland

SECTION VIII. PERIPHERAL NERVE

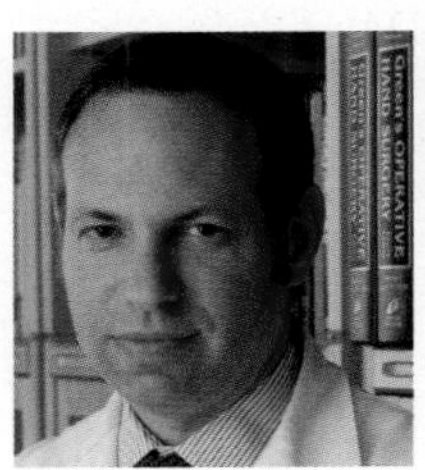

Aaron G. Filler, MD, PhD, JD, FRCS
Medical Director
Institute for Nerve Medicine
Santa Monica, California

Allan J. Belzberg, MD, FRCSC
George J. Heuer Professor of Neurosurgery
Johns Hopkins School of Medicine
Baltimore, Maryland

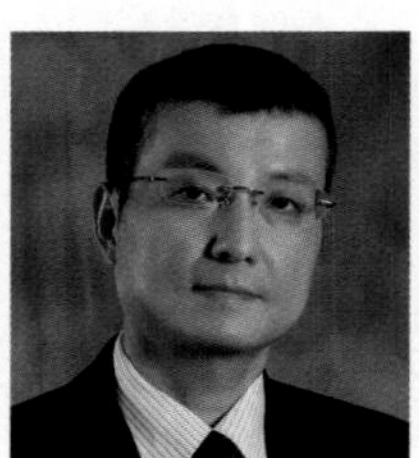

Liang Chen, MD, PhD
Professor
Hand Surgery Department
Huashan Hospital of Fudan University
Shanghai, China

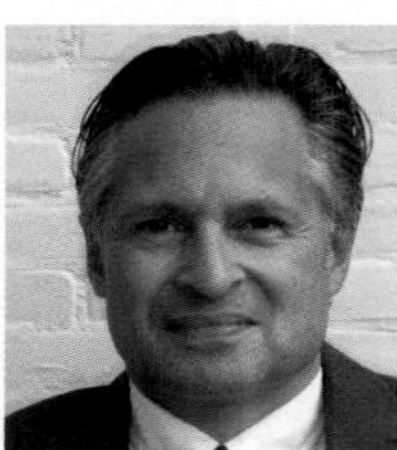

Martijn J.A. Malessy, MD, PhD
Professor of Nerve Surgery
Department of Neurosurgery
Leiden University Medical Center
Leiden, The Netherlands

SECTION IX. RADIATION

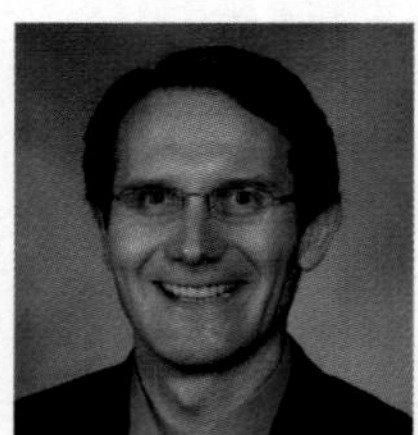

Bruce E. Pollock, MD
Professor of Neurological Surgery and Radiation Oncology
Mayo Clinic
Rochester, Minnesota

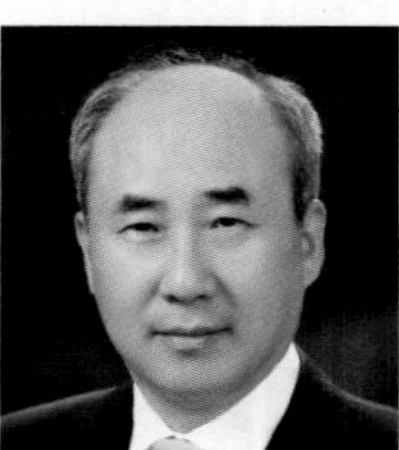

Dong Gyu Kim, MD, PhD
Professor
Department of Neurosurgery
Seoul National University College of Medicine
Seoul National University Hospital
Seoul, Republic of Korea

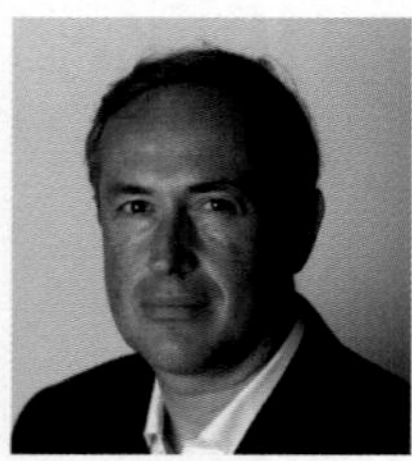

Jean Régis, MD
Professor of Neurosurgery
Head, Functional Neurosurgery Department
Aix-Marseille University
Timone Hospital APHM
Marseille, France

SECTION X. SPINE

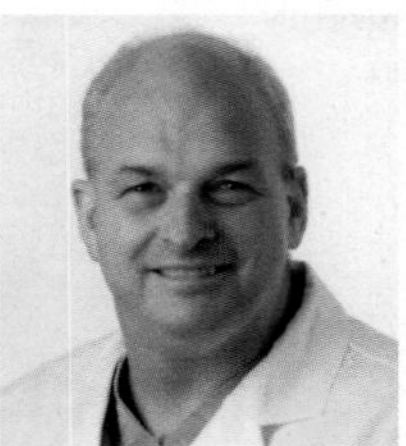

Christopher I. Shaffrey, Sr., MD
John A. Jane Professor
Departments of Neurological and Orthopaedic Surgery
University of Virginia Health System
Charlottesville, Virginia

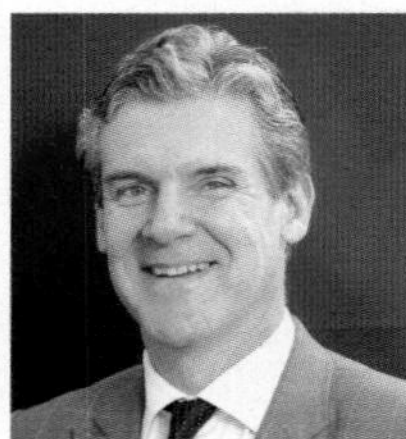

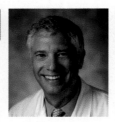

Michael G. Fehlings, MD, PhD, FRCSC, FACS
Professor of Neurosurgery;
Vice Chair, Research, Department of Surgery, University of Toronto Faculty of Medicine;
Co-Director of the University of Toronto Spine Program, Director of the Spinal Program at the Toronto Western Hospital;
Gerald and Tootsie Halbert Chair in Neural Repair and Regeneration, University Health Network;
Senior Scientist, Toronto Western Research Institute, University Health Network
Toronto, Ontario, Canada

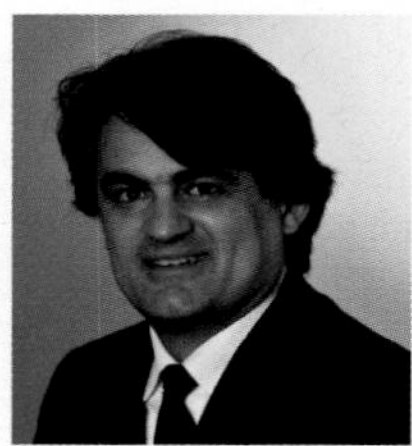

Osmar José Santos de Moraes, MD
Professor of Evidence Based Medicine
Santa Marcelina Medical School;
Head, Department of Neurosurgery
Santa Marcelina University Hospital
São Paulo, Brazil

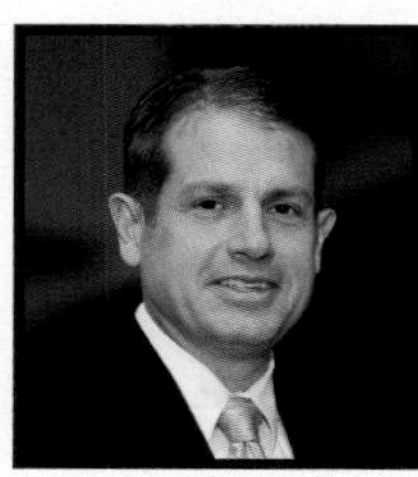

Charles Kuntz IV, MD[†]
Professor and Vice Chairman
Department of Neurosurgery
University of Cincinnati College of Medicine;
Director, Division of Spine and Peripheral Nerve Surgery
Mayfield Clinic
Cincinnati, Ohio

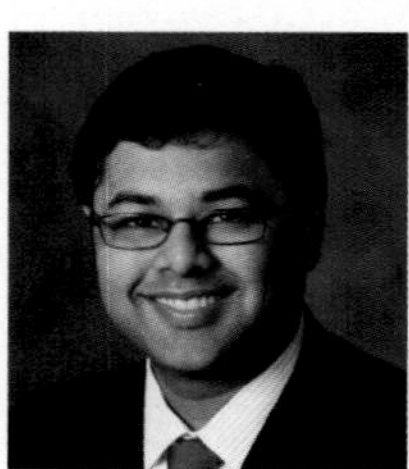

Praveen V. Mummaneni, MD
Professor and Vice Chair
Department of Neurological Surgery
Director of Minimally Invasive and Cervical Spine Surgery
Co-Director, Spinal Surgery
University of California, San Francisco
San Francisco, California

[†]Deceased.

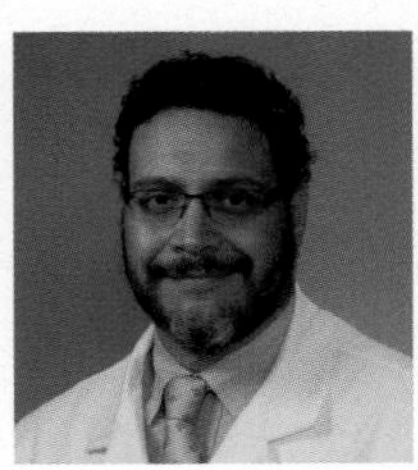

Paul Santiago, MD
Associate Professor
Departments of Neurological Surgery and Orthopedic Surgery
Washington University School of Medicine in St. Louis
St. Louis, Missouri

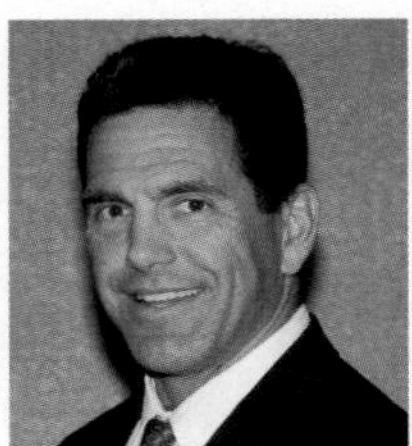

Daniel K. Resnick, MD, MS
Professor and Vice Chairman
Department of Neurosurgery
University of Wisconsin School of Medicine and Public Health
Madison, Wisconsin

SECTION XI. TRAUMA

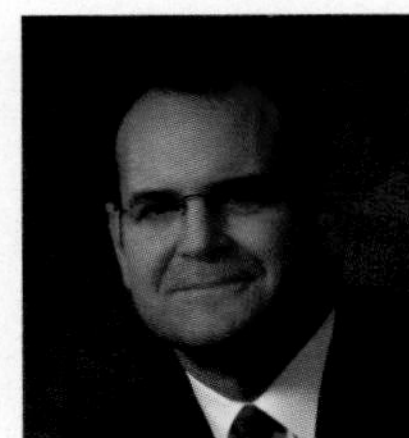

Geoffrey T. Manley, MD, PhD
Professor in Residence and Vice Chairman
Department of Neurological Surgery
Co-Director and Principal Investigator, Brain and Spinal Injury Center (BASIC)
University of California, San Francisco;
Chief of Neurosurgery
San Francisco General Hospital
San Francisco, California

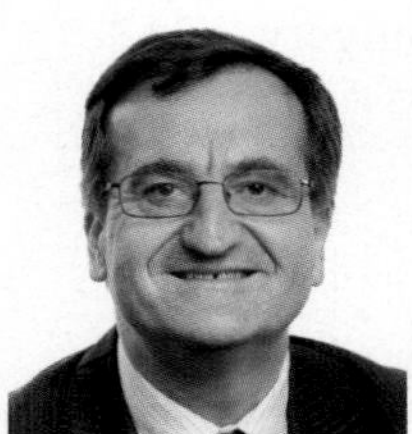

Peter J. Hutchinson, MBBS, PhD, FRCS (Surg Neurol)
Professor of Neurosurgery and NIHR Research Professor
Division of Neurosurgery, Department of Clinical Neurosciences
University of Cambridge
Addenbrooke's Hospital
Cambridge, United Kingdom

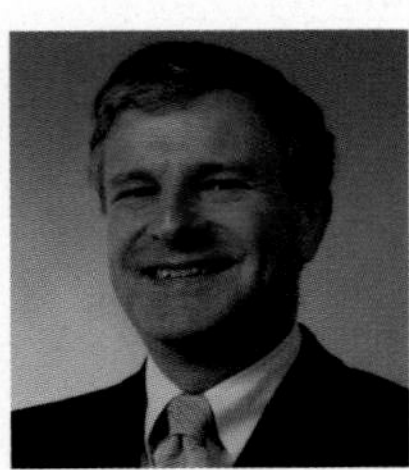

Andrew I.R. Maas, MD, PhD
Professor and Chair
Department of Neurosurgery
University Hospital Antwerp and University of Antwerp
Antwerp, Belgium

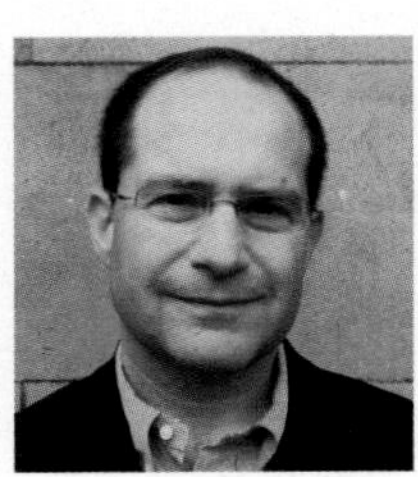

Guy Rosenthal, MD
Senior Staff
Department of Neurosurgery
Hadassah Medical Center
Jerusalem, Israel

SECTION XII. VASCULAR

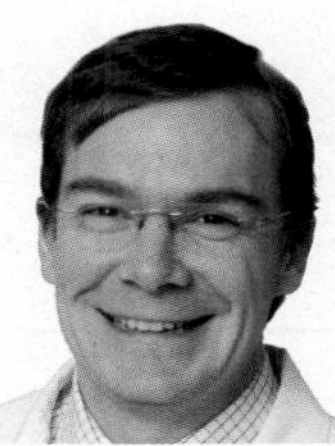

E. Sander Connolly, Jr., MD, FACS
Bennett M. Stein Professor of Neurological Surgery
Vice Chairman of Neurosurgery
Columbia University College of Physicians and Surgeons;
Director, Cerebrovascular Research Laboratory
Surgical Director, Neuro-Intensive Care Unit
New York–Presbyterian Columbia University Medical Center
New York, New York

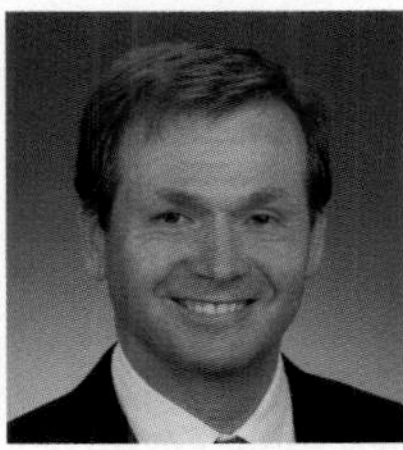

Gavin W. Britz, MD, MBBCh, MPH, MBA, FAANS
Professor and Chair
Department of Neurosurgery
Houston Methodist Hospital
Co-Director, Methodist Neurological Institute
Houston, Texas;
Professor of Neurological Surgery
Weill Cornell Medical College
Cornell University
New York, New York

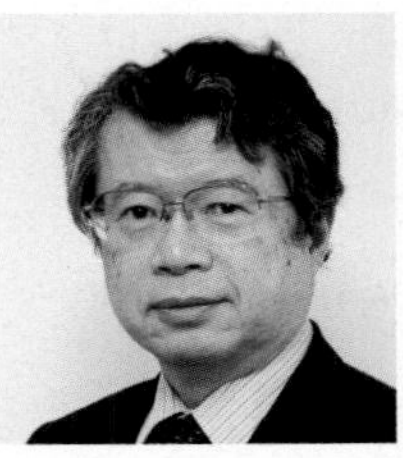

Kazuhiro Hongo, MD, PhD
Professor and Chair
Department of Neurosurgery
Shinshu University School of Medicine
Matsumoto, Japan

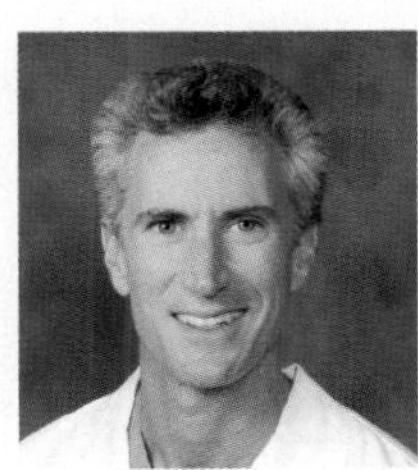

Michael T. Lawton, MD
Professor in Residence, Vice-Chairman, and Tong Po Kan Endowed Chair
Department of Neurological Surgery
Chief, Cerebrovascular and Skull Base Surgery Programs
Director, Cerebrovascular Disorders Program
Principal Investigator, Center for Cerebrovascular Research
University of California, San Francisco
San Francisco, California

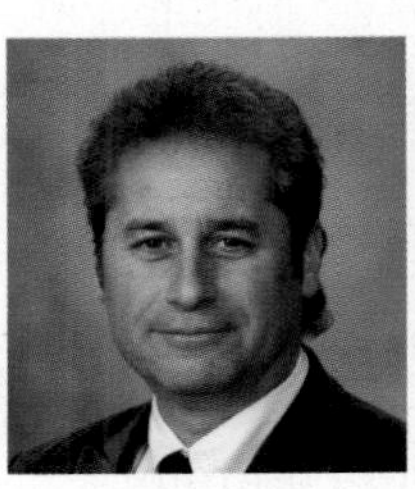

Fredric B. Meyer, MD
Professor and Chair
Department of Neurosurgery
Mayo Clinic
Rochester, Minnesota

Contents

VOLUME 1

†Deceased.

†Deceased.

†Deceased.

†Deceased.

†Deceased.

†Deceased.

SECTION IX
Radiation: Overview and Controversies, 2129

SECTION X
Spine: Overview and Controversies, 2255

†Deceased.

†Deceased.

---
†Deceased.

PART 10 Techniques for Spinal Procedures, 2622

VOLUME 4

SECTION XI Trauma: Overview and Controversies, 2743

Geoffrey T. Manley, Peter J. Hutchinson, Andrew I.R. Maas, Guy Rosenthal, Michael C. Huang, Hadie Adams, and Angelos G. Kolias

PART 1 Basic and Clinical Science, 2748

PART 2 Radiology in Traumatic Brain Surgery, 2819

PART 3 Management of Traumatic Brain Injury, 2843

Video Contents

Contributors

Bizhan Aarabi, MD
Professor of Neurosurgery
University of Maryland School of Medicine
Baltimore, Maryland
352: Traumatic and Penetrating Head Injuries

Rick Abbott, MD
Professor of Neurological Surgery
Albert Einstein College of Medicine
Montefiore Medical Center
Bronx, New York
236: Intraspinal Tumors in Children

Muhammad M. Abd-El-Barr, MD, PhD
Resident Neurosurgeon
Harvard Medical School
Brigham and Women's Hospital
Boston Children's Hospital
Boston, Massachusetts
192: Molecular Genetics and Priniciples of Craniosynostosis
215: Brainstem Gliomas

Taylor J. Abel, MD
Chief Resident
Department of Neurosurgery
University of Iowa Carver College of Medicine
Iowa City, Iowa
70: Investigation of Human Cognition in Epilepsy Surgery Patients

Todd A. Abruzzo, MD, FAHA
Professor
Departments of Neurosurgery, Radiology, and Biomedical Engineering
University of Cincinnati;
Chief of Pediatric Interventional Neuroradiology
Cincinnati Children's Hospital Medical Center
Mayfield Clinic
Cincinnati, Ohio
382: Endovascular Management of Cerebral Vasospasm

Feridun Acar, MD
Professor and Chair
Department of Neurosurgery
Pamukkale Üniversitesi
Denizli, Turkey
Overview and Controversies (Pain)
176: Evidence-Based Neurostimulation for Pain
180: Dorsal Rhizotomy and Dorsal Root Ganglionectomy

Rebecca L. Achey, BS
Cleveland Clinic Lerner College of Medicine
The Cleveland Clinic Foundation
Cleveland, Ohio
58: Electrophysiologic Properties of the Mammalian Central Nervous System

Paul D. Ackerman, MD
Attending Neurosurgeon
Northwestern Neurosurgical Associates
Chicago, Illinois
365: The Natural History and Medical Management of Carotid Occlusive Disease

Hadie Adams, MD
Research Fellow
Division of Neurosurgery
University of Cambridge and Cambridge University Hospitals NHS Foundation Trust
Cambridge, United Kingdom
Overview and Controversies (Trauma)

Nithin D. Adappa, MD
Assistant Professor of Otorhinolaryngology
Perelman School of Medicine at the University of Pennsylvania
Philadelphia, Pennsylvania
357: Traumatic Cerebrospinal Fluid Fistulas

P. David Adelson, MD, FACS, FAAP
Director, Barrow Neurological Institute at Phoenix Children's Hospital
Diane and Bruce Halle Chair of Pediatric Neurosciences
Chief, Pediatric Neurosurgery
Phoenix Children's Hospital
Phoenix, Arizona
224: Management of Head Injury: Special Considerations in Children

David H. Aguirre-Padilla, MD
Professor of Neurosurgery
Professor of Neuroanatomy and Neurophysiology
University of Chile Faculty of Medicine;
Chief, Division of Neurosurgery
Hospital Clínico San Borja Arriarán;
Attending Neurosurgeon
Emergency Department
Hospital de Urgencia Asistencia Pública
Santiago, Chile
92: Complication Avoidance in Deep Brain Stimulation Surgery

Raheel Ahmed, MD, PhD
Fellow, Division of Neurosurgery
The Hospital for Sick Children
University of Toronto
Toronto, Ontario, Canada
233: Developmental Anomalies of the Craniovertebral Junction and Surgical Management

Edward S. Ahn, MD
Associate Professor
Departments of Neurosurgery, Pediatrics, and Plastic Surgery
Johns Hopkins University School of Medicine
Baltimore, Maryland
234: Achondroplasia and Other Dwarfisms

Tamir T. Ailon, MD, MPH, FRCSC
Clinical Instructor
Department of Orthopaedics
University of British Columbia Faculty of Medicine;
Neurosurgeon
Vancouver Spine Surgery Institute
Vancouver, British Columbia, Canada
317: Evaluation and Treatment of Adult Scoliosis and Sagittal Plane Deformity

Michael C. Ain, MD
Associate Professor
Departments of Pediatrics and Orthopaedic Surgery
Johns Hopkins University School of Medicine
Baltimore, Maryland
234: Achondroplasia and Other Dwarfisms

Imoigele P. Aisiku, MD, MSCR, MBA, FCCP
Assistant Professor of Emergency Medicine
Harvard Medical School
Brigham and Women's Hospital
Boston, Massachusetts
349: Critical Care Management of Traumatic Brain Injury

Ali Alaraj, MD
Associate Professor
Department of Neurosurgery
University of Illinois at Chicago
Chicago, Illinois
364: Neurovascular Imaging
370: Extracranial Vertebral Artery Diseases

Amr AlBakry, MD, MSc
Assistant Lecturer
Neurological Surgery
Faculty of Medicine, Zagazig University
Zagazig, Egypt;
Functional and Stereotactic Fellow
Neurological Surgery
Oregon Health & Science University
Portland, Oregon
179: Evidence Base for Destructive Procedures

Felipe C. Albuquerque, MD
Endovascular Neurosurgeon
Department of Neurosurgery
Barrow Neurological Institute
St. Joseph's Hospital and Medical Center
Phoenix, Arizona
391: Endovascular Approaches to Narrow-Necked Intracranial Aneurysms
392: Endovascular Approaches to Wide-Necked Intracranial Aneurysms

Brian M. Alexander, MD, MPH
Associate Professor of Radiation Oncology
Harvard Medical School
Dana-Farber/Brigham and Women's Cancer Center
Boston, Massachusetts
265: Fractionated Radiotherapy for Brain Tumors

Michael J. Alexander, MD
Professor and Vice-Chairman
Department of Neurosurgery
Cedars-Sinai Medical Center
Los Angeles, California
369: Nonatherosclerotic Carotid Lesions

Andrei V. Alexandrov, MD
Professor of Neurology
Director, Division of Cerebrovascular Disease
Director, UAB Comprehensive Stroke Center
University of Alabama School of Medicine
Tuscaloosa, Alabama
363: Diagnostic and Therapeutic Neurosonology

Zarina S. Ali, MD
Assistant Professor of Neurosurgery
Perelman School of Medicine at the University of Pennsylvania
Philadelphia, Pennsylvania
249: Distal Entrapment Syndromes: Carpal Tunnel, Cubital Tunnel, Peroneal, and Tarsal Tunnel
357: Traumatic Cerebrospinal Fluid Fistulas

Kenan Al-Khalili, MD
Neurosurgery Resident
University of Arizona
Tucson, Arizona
157: Neoplasms of the Paranasal Sinuses

Ossama Al-Mefty, MD
Lecturer in Neurosurgery
Harvard Medical School;
Director, Skull Base Program
Department of Neurosurgery
Brigham and Women's Hospital
Boston, Massachusetts
147: Meningiomas

Kaith K. Almefty, MD
Assistant Professor
Department of Neurosurgery
Barrow Neurological Institute
Phoenix, Arizona
Overview and Controversies (Oncology)

Rami Almefty, MD
Clinical Fellow in Skull Base Surgery
Department of Neurosurgery
Harvard Medical School
Brigham and Women's Hospital
Boston, Massachusetts;
Resident Neurosurgeon
Barrow Neurological Institute
Phoenix, Arizona
147: Meningiomas

Ron L. Alterman, MD, MBA
Professor of Neurosurgery
Harvard Medical School;
Chief, Division of Neurosurgery
Beth Israel Deaconess Medical Center
Boston, Massachusetts
Overview and Controversies (Functional)
90: Deep Brain Stimulation for Dystonia
92: Complication Avoidance in Deep Brain Stimulation Surgery

Peter S. Amenta, MD
Assistant Professor
Co-Director of Cerebrovascular, Endovascular, and Skull Base Surgery
Department of Neurosurgery
Tulane University
New Orleans, Louisiana
375: Nonlesional Spontaneous Intracerebral Hemorrhage
414: Microsurgical Treatment of Spinal Vascular Malformations

Christopher P. Ames, MD
Professor of Clinical Neurological Surgery and Orthopaedic Surgery
Director of Spine Tumor and Spinal Deformity Surgery
Co-Director, Spinal Surgery and UCSF Spine Center
Director, Spinal Biomechanics Laboratory
University of California, San Francisco
San Francisco, California
317: Evaluation and Treatment of Adult Scoliosis and Sagittal Plane Deformity
318: Assessment and Treatment of Proximal Junctional Kyphosis

Sepideh Amin-Hanjani, MD
Professor and Program Director
Department of Neurosurgery
Co-Director, Neurovascular Surgery
University of Illinois at Chicago
Chicago, Illinois
370: Extracranial Vertebral Artery Diseases

Mario Ammirati, MD, MBA
Professor of Neurological Surgery and Radiation Oncology
Director, Skull Base Neurosurgery and Stereotactic Radiosurgery
Director, Dardinger Microneurosurgical Skull Base Laboratory
The Ohio State University Wexner Medical Center
Columbus, Ohio
154: Overview of Skull Base Tumors

Norberto Andaluz, MD
Associate Professor of Neurosurgery and Director of Neurotrauma
Department of Neurosurgery
University of Cincinnati, Mayfield Clinic
Cincinnati, Ohio
382: Endovascular Management of Cerebral Vasospasm

Richard C.E. Anderson, MD, FACS, FAAP
Associate Professor of Neurological Surgery
Columbia University College of Physicians and Surgeons
Division of Pediatric Neurosurgery
Morgan Stanley Children's Hospital of New York–Presbyterian
New York, New York
235: Surgical Management of the Pediatric Subaxial Cervical Spine

Pablo Andrade, MD, PhD
Neurosurgery Resident
Department of Stereotactic and Functional Neurosurgery
University Hospital of Cologne
Cologne, Germany
99: Surgery for Tourette's Syndrome

Peter D. Angevine, MD, MPH
Assistant Professor
Department of Neurological Surgery
Columbia University College of Physicians and Surgeons
New York, New York
21: Positioning for Spinal Surgery

Shaheryar F. Ansari, MD
Resident Neurosurgeon
Indiana University School of Medicine
Goodman Campbell Brain and Spine
Indianapolis, Indiana
239: Pediatric Vertebral Column and Spinal Cord Injuries

William J. Ares, MD
Resident Neurosurgeon
University of Pittsburgh Medical Center
Pittsburgh, Pennsylvania
361: Acute Surgical and Endovascular Management of Ischemic and Hemorrhagic Stroke

Jeffrey E. Arle, MD, PhD, FAANS
Associate Professor of Neurosurgery
Harvard Medical School;
Associate Chief, Division of Neurosurgery
Beth Israel Deaconess Medical Center
Boston, Massachusetts
93: Neurophysiologic Monitoring for Movement Disorders Surgery
106: Motor Cortex Stimulation for Pain and Movement Disorders

Rocco A. Armonda, MD
Associate Professor and Director
Department of Neurosurgery
Uniformed Services University of the Health Sciences
Bethesda, Maryland;
Director, Neuroendovascular Surgery
MedStar Washington Hospital Center and Georgetown University Hospital
Washington, DC
352: Traumatic and Penetrating Head Injuries

Omar Arnaout, MD
Chief Resident
Department of Neurosurgery
Northwestern Memorial Hospital
Chicago, Illinois
130: Basic Principles of Skull Base Surgery
149: Vestibular Schwannomas

Eric Arnaud, MD
Pediatric Neurosurgeon and Co-Director
Unité de Chirurgie Craniofaciale
Hôpital Necker Enfants Malades
Paris, France
194: Syndromic Craniosynostosis

Paul M. Arnold, MD, FACS
Professor of Neurosurgery
University of Kansas Medical Center;
Director, Spinal Cord Injury Center
University of Kansas Hospital
Kansas City, Kansas
305: Evaluation and Treatment of C2 (Axis) Fractures

Rachid Assina, RPh, MD
Assistant Professor
Department of Neurological Surgery
Rutgers New Jersey Medical School
Newark, New Jersey
24: Brain Retraction
334: Evaluation, Indications, and Techniques of Revision Spine Surgery

Oskar C. Aszmann, MD, PhD
Associate Professor of Plastic and Reconstructive Surgery
Director, Center of Extremity Reconstruction and Rehabilitation
Christian Doppler Laboratory for Restoration of Extremity Function
Medical University of Vienna
Vienna, Austria
260: Neuroelectronic Systems

Frank J. Attenello III, MD, MS
Clinical Instructor
Department Neurosurgery
Keck School of Medicine
University of Southern California
Los Angeles, California
18: Surgical Planning: An Overview

Jetan H. Badhiwala, MD
Resident Neurosurgeon
Department of Surgery
University of Toronto Faculty of Medicine
The Hospital for Sick Children
Toronto, Ontario, Canada
201: Ventricular Shunting Procedures

Joachim M. Baehring, MD, DSc
Associate Professor
Departments of Medicine (Medical Oncology), Neurology, and Neurosurgery
Yale School of Medicine
New Haven, Connecticut
139: Unusual Gliomas

Christopher D. Baggott, MD
Resident Neurosurgeon
University of Wisconsin Hospitals and Clinics
Madison, Wisconsin
307: Treatment of Cervicothoracic Junction Injuries

Anto Bagić, MD, PhD
Associate Professor of Neurology and Neurosurgery
Chief, Epilepsy Division
Director, University of Pittsburgh Comprehensive Epilepsy Center (UPCEC)
Director, UPMC MEG Epilepsy Program
Chief Scientific Advisor, MEG Research
Department of Neurology
University of Pittsburgh School of Medicine
Pittsburgh, Pennsylvania
66: Magnetoencephalography (MEG)/ Magnetic Source Imaging (MSI)

Diaa Bahgat, MD, MsSc, PhD
Department of Neurosurgery
University of Arkansas for Medical Sciences
Little Rock, Arkansas;
Lecturer in Neurosurgery
Fayoum University
El Fayoum, Egypt
169: Pharmacologic Treatment of Pain

Julian E. Bailes, MD
Clinical Professor of Medicine
University of Chicago Pritzker School of Medicine
Co-Director, NorthShore Neurological Institute
Evanston, Illinois
347: Mild Traumatic Brain Injury in Adults and Concussion in Sports

Mark Bain, MD, MS
Staff Neurosurgeon
Cerebrovascular Center
Cleveland Clinic
Cleveland, Ohio
393: Endovascular Flow Diversion for Intracranial Aneurysms

Perry A. Ball, MD
Professor
Departments of Surgery and Anesthesiology
Dartmouth-Hitchcock Medical Center
Lebanon, New Hampshire
16: Principles of Neurocritical Care

Gordon H. Baltuch, MD, PhD
Professor of Neurosurgery
Perelman School of Medicine at the University of Pennsylvania
Philadelphia, Pennsylvania
71: Intracranial Monitoring: Subdural Strip and Grid Recording

Scott C. Baraban, PhD
Professor of Neurological Surgery
William K. Bowes Jr. Endowed Chair in Neuroscience Research
Director, Epilepsy Research Laboratory
University of California, San Francisco School of Medicine
San Francisco, California
59: Animal Models of Epilepsy

Tanyeri Barak, MD
Associate Research Scientist
Department of Neurosurgery
Yale University
New Haven, Connecticut
376: Genetics of Intracranial Aneurysms

Igor J. Barani, MD
Associate Professor
Departments of Radiation Oncology and Neurological Surgery
University of California, San Francisco
San Francisco, California
265: Fractionated Radiotherapy for Brain Tumors

Giuseppe M.V. Barbagallo, MD
Associate Professor of Neurosurgery
Policlinico G. Rodolico University Hospital
Catania, Italy
323: Nucleoplasty and Posterior Dynamic Stabilization Systems

Nicholas M. Barbaro, MD
Betsey Barton Professor and Chair
Department of Neurological Surgery
Indiana University School of Medicine
Indianapolis, Indiana
78: Radiosurgical Treatment for Epilepsy

Frederick G. Barker II, MD
Associate Professor of Neurosurgery
Harvard Medical School;
Attending Neurosurgeon
Massachusetts General Hospital
Boston, Massachusetts
36: Postoperative Infections of the Head and Brain
57: Neurosurgical Epidemiology and Outcomes Assessment
126: Brain Tumor Outcome Studies: Design and Interpretation

Gene H. Barnett, MD, MBA
Professor and Vice-Chairman, Department of Neurological Surgery
The Rose Ella Burkhardt Chair in Neurosurgical Oncology
Director, The Rose Ella Burkhardt Brain Tumor and Neuro-Oncology Center
Associate Dean of Faculty Affairs
Cleveland Clinic Lerner College of Medicine of Case Western Reserve University
Cleveland, Ohio
132: Surgical Navigation for Brain Tumors

Constance M. Barone, MD, FACS
Barone's Cosmetic Surgery Center
San Antonio, Texas
195: Endoscopic Treatment of Craniosynostosis

Daniel Louis Barrow, MD
Pamel R. Rollins Professor and Chairman
Department of Neurosurgery
Emory University School of Medicine
Atlanta, Georgia
388: Surgical Management of Middle Cerebral Artery Aneurysms

Luigi Bassani, MD
Assistant Professor
Department of Neurosurgery
Rutgers New Jersey Medical School
Newark, New Jersey
204: Management and Prevention of Shunt Infections

Tracy T. Batchelor, MD, MPH
Giovanni Armenise-Harvard Professor of Neurology
Harvard Medical School;
Director, Division of Neuro-Oncology
Massachusetts General Hospital Cancer Center
Boston, Massachusetts
145: Primary Central Nervous System Lymphomas

Nuno Batista, MD, FEBOT
Consultant in Spinal Surgery
Oxford University Hospitals NHS Trust
Oxford, United Kingdom
293: Assessment and Treatment of Primary Malignant Tumors of the Axial Skeleton

H. Hunt Batjer, MD, FAANS, FACS
Professor and Chair
Department of Neurological Surgery
University of Texas Southwestern Medical School
Dallas, Texas
390: Microsurgery of Basilar Apex Aneurysms

Griffin R. Baum, MD
Resident
Department of Neurological Surgery
Emory University School of Medicine
Atlanta, Georgia
388: Surgical Management of Middle Cerebral Artery Aneurysms

Michael S. Beattie, PhD
Professor of Neurological Surgery
Director of Research, Department of Neurological Surgery
Brain and Spinal Injury Center
University of California, San Francisco School of Medicine
San Francisco, California
339: Animal Models of Traumatic Brain Injury

Andrew Beaumont, MD, PhD
Neurosurgeon and Clinical Director
Aspirus Spine & Neuroscience Department
Aspirus Wausau Hospital
Wausau, Wisconsin
52: Physiology of the Cerebrospinal Fluid and Intracranial Pressure

Danielle A. Becker, MD, MS
Assistant Professor of Clinical Neurology
Department of Neurology
Hospital of the University of Pennsylvania
Philadelphia, Pennsylvania
62: Antiepileptic Medications: Principles of Clinical Use

Joshua M. Beckman, MD
Resident Neurosurgeon
University of South Florida Morsani College of Medicine
Tampa, Florida
278: Electrophysiologic Studies and Monitoring

Tibor Becske, MD
Assistant Professor
Neuroendovascular Service
Neurosciences Division
Rochester Regional Health System
Rochester, New York
122: Endovascular Techniques for Tumor Embolization

Joshua B. Bederson, MD
Professor and Chairman
Department of Neurosurgery
Icahn School of Medicine at Mount Sinai
Mount Sinai Health System
New York, New York
19: Surgical Simulation and Robotic Surgery
396: Infectious Aneurysms

Rudolf W. Beisse, MD
Medical Director and Chief
Spine Center
Benedictus Krankenhaus
Tutzing am Starnberger See, Germany
27: Thorascopic Spine Surgery

Kimon Bekelis, MD
Chief Resident
Department of Neurosurgery
Dartmouth-Hitchcock Medical Center
Lebanon, New Hampshire
16: Principles of Neurocritical Care

Randy S. Bell, MD
Assistant Professor of Surgery
Department of Neurosurgery
Uniformed Services University of the Health Sciences
Bethesda, Maryland
352: Traumatic and Penetrating Head Injuries

Allan J. Belzberg, MD, FRCSC
George J. Heuer Professor of Neurosurgery
Johns Hopkins School of Medicine
Baltimore, Maryland
Overview and Controversies (PNS)
255: Early Management of Brachial Plexus Injuries
258: Benign and Malignant Tumors of the Peripheral Nerve

Eduardo E. Benarroch, MD, DSci
Professor and Consultant
Department of Neurology
Mayo Clinic
Rochester, Minnesota
359: Cerebral Blood Flow and Metabolism and Cerebral Ischemia

Bernard R. Bendok, MD
Professor and Chair
Department of Neurosurgery
Mayo Clinic
Rochester, Minnesota
390: Microsurgery of Basilar Apex Aneurysms

Arnau Benet, MD
Assistant Professor of Neurosurgery
Director, Skull Base & Cerebrovascular Laboratory
Department of Neurological Surgery
University of California, San Francisco
San Francisco, California
3: Surgical Anatomy of the Skull Base

Alejandro Berenstein, MD
Professor of Radiology, Neurosurgery and Pediatrics
Director, Pediatric Cerebrovascular Program
Icahn School of Medicine at Mount Sinai
New York, New York
221: Vein of Galen Aneurysmal Malformation

Mitchel S. Berger, MD, MA
Professor and Berthold and Belle N. Guggenhime Endowed Chair
Department of Neurosurgery
Director, Brain Tumor Surgery Program
Director, Neurosurgical Research Centers, Brain Tumor Research Center
University of California, San Francisco
San Francisco, California
3: Surgical Anatomy of the Skull Base
4: Improving Patient Safety
136: Low-Grade Gliomas: Astrocytomas, Oligodendrogliomas, and Mixed Gliomas

Marvin Bergsneider, MD
Professor of Neurosurgery
David Geffen School of Medicine at UCLA
Ronald Reagan UCLA Medical Center
Los Angeles, California
31: Shunting

Helmut Bertalanffy, MD, PhD
Professor of Neurosurgery
Director of Vascular Neurosurgery
International Neuroscience Institute
Hannover, Germany
153: Ventricular Tumors

Saurabha Bhatnagar, MD
Instructor in Physical Medical and Rehabilitation
Associate Residency Program Director
Chair, Clinical Competency Committee
Department of Physical Medicine and Rehabilitation
Harvard Medical School
Spaulding Rehabilitation Hospital
Massachusetts General Hospital
Boston, Massachusetts
358: Rehabilitation of Patients with Traumatic Brain Injury

Wenya Linda Bi, MD, PhD
Department of Neurosurgery
Brigham and Women's Hospital
Boston, Massachusetts
150: Pituitary Tumors: Functioning and Nonfunctioning
202: Neuroendoscopy

Harjus Singh Birk, BS
Medical Student
University of California, San Francisco School of Medicine
San Francisco, California
50: Cellular and Molecular Responses in the Peripheral and Central Nervous Systems: Similarities and Differences

Allen T. Bishop, MD
Professor of Orthopedic Surgery
Consultant, Division of Hand Surgery
Mayo Clinic
Rochester, Minnesota
256: Secondary Procedures for Brachial Plexus Injuries

Jaishri O. Blakeley, MD
Associate Professor
Departments of Neurology, Oncology and Neurosurgery
Johns Hopkins University School of Medicine
Baltimore, Maryland
124: Genetic Syndromes of Brain Tumors

Patric Blomstedt, MD, PhD
Professor of Stereotactic Functional Neurosurgery
Umeå University;
Consultant Neurosurgeon
University Hospital of Northern Sweden
Umeå, Sweden
87: Surgical Management of Tremor

Bryan D. Bolinger, DO
Department of Neurological Surgery
Geisinger Medical Center
Danville, Pennsylvania
308: Transient Quadriparesis and Athletic Injuries of the Cervical Spine

Phillip A. Bonney, MD
Resident Neurosurgeon
University of Southern California Keck School of Medicine
Los Angeles, California
133: Endoscopic Approaches to Brain Tumors

Zackary E. Boomsaad, MD
Interventional Pain Management Specialist
Southeastern Regional Medical Center
Newnan, Georgia
105: Treatment of Intractable Vertigo

Frederick A. Boop, MD
Professor and Chairman
Department of Neurosurgery
University of Tennessee Health Science Center;
Co-Director, Neuroscience Institute
LeBonheur Children's Hospital;
Chief, Pediatric Neurosurgery
Department of Neurosurgery
St. Jude Children's Research Hospital
Memphis, Tennessee
211: Pediatric Supratentorial Hemispheric Tumors

Nicholas Borg, MD
Department of Neurosurgery
Wessex Neurological Centre
Southampton General Hospital
Southampton, United Kingdom
34: Medical and Surgical Management of Chronic Subdural Hematomas

Bronek M. Boszczyk, Prof. Dr. med.
Consultant Spinal Surgeon
Centre for Spinal Studies and Surgery
Queen's Medical Centre
Nottingham University Hospitals NHS Trust
Nottingham, United Kingdom
297: Assessment and Treatment of Rheumatoid Arthritis and Inflammatory Spinal Diseases

Ricardo Vieira Botelho, MD, PhD
Spine Surgery Coordinator
Department of Neurosurgery
Hospital do Servidor Públido do Estado de São Paulo, e do Conjunto Hospitalar do Mandaqui;
Brazilian Guidelines Director
Brazilian Association of Neurological Surgeons
São Paulo, Brazil
280: Differential Diagnosis of Spinal Disease

Pascal Bou-Haidar, BMed, FRANZCR, MEngSc
Radiologist
St Vincent's Clinic Medical Imaging & Nuclear Medicine
Sydney, New South Wales, Australia
13: Physiologic Evaluation of the Brain with Magnetic Resonance Imaging

Susan M. Bowyer, PhD
Senior Scientist
Department of Neurology
Henry Ford Hospital
Assistant Professor of Neurology
Wayne State University School of Medicine
Detroit, Michigan;
Adjunct Professor
Department of Physics
Oakland University
Rochester, Michigan
66: Magnetoencephalography (MEG)/ Magnetic Source Imaging (MSI)

Taryn McFadden Bragg, MD, MS
Assistant Professor of Neurological Surgery
University of Wisconsin School of Medicine and Public Health
Madison, Wisconsin
230: Lipomyelomeningocele

Henry Brem, MD
Harvey Cushing Professor and Director
Department of Neurosurgery
Professor of Neurosurgery, Ophthalmology, Oncology, and Biomedical Engineering
Johns Hopkins University School of Medicine;
Neurosurgeon-in-Chief, Johns Hopkins Medical Institutions
Director, Hunterian Neurosurgical Research Center
Baltimore, Maryland
Overview and Controversies (Oncology)
129: Basic Principles of Cranial Surgery for Brain Tumors
137: Malignant Gliomas: Anaplastic Astrocytoma, Glioblastoma, Gliosarcoma, and Anaplastic Oligodendroglioma

Steven Brem, MD
Professor of Neurosurgery
Perelman School of Medicine at the University of Pennsylvania
Chief, Neurosurgical Oncology
Co-Director, Penn Brain Tumor Center
Abramson Cancer Center
Hospital of the University of Pennsylvania
Philadelphia, Pennsylvania
116: Angiogenesis and Brain Tumors: Scientific Principles, Current Therapy, and Future Directions

Jacqueline C. Bresnahan, PhD
Adjunct Professor of Neurological Surgery
Brain and Spinal Injury Center
University of California, San Francisco School of Medicine
San Francisco, California
339: Animal Models of Traumatic Brain Injury

Benjamin H. Brinkmann, PhD
Assistant Professor of Neurology
Mayo Clinic
Rochester, Minnesota
67: Single-Photon Emission Computed Tomography in Epilepsy Surgery Evaluation

Andrei Brînzeu, MD
Fellow in Functional Neurosurgery
Hôpital Neurologique Pierre Wertheimer Lyon
Lyon 1 University
Lyon, France;
Collaborator
Timisoara Medical University
Timisoara, Romania
182: Dorsal Root Entry Zone Lesions for Pain

Gavin W. Britz, MD, MBBCh, MPH, MBA, FAANS
Professor and Chair
Department of Neurosurgery
Houston Methodist Hospital
Co-Director, Methodist Neurological Institute
Houston, Texas;
Professor of Neurological Surgery
Weill Cornell Medical College
Cornell University
New York, New York
130: Basic Principles of Skull Base Surgery
Overview and Controversies (Vascular)
377: The Natural History of Cerebral Aneurysms
383: Surgical Approaches to Intracranial Aneurysms
399: Traumatic Cerebral Aneurysms Secondary to Penetrating Intracranial Injuries

Douglas L. Brockmeyer, MD, FAAP
Professor of Neurosurgery
Chief, Division of Pediatric Neurosurgery
University of Utah School of Medicine
Salt Lake City, Utah
235: Surgical Management of the Pediatric Subaxial Cervical Spine

Samuel R. Browd, MD, PhD
Assistant Professor of Neurological Surgery
University of Washington School of Medicine
Attending Neurosurgeon
Seattle Children's Hospital
Seattle, Washington
191: Craniopagus Twins

Desmond A. Brown, MD
Resident Neurosurgeon
Mayo Clinic
Rochester, Minnesota
359: Cerebral Blood Flow and Metabolism and Cerebral Ischemia

Martin Brown, PhD
Professor of Radiation Oncology
Stanford University School of Medicine
Stanford, California
262: Radiobiology of Radiotherapy and Radiosurgery

Matthew T. Brown, MD
Resident Neurosurgeon
University of Tennessee Health Sciences Center
Memphis, Tennessee
25: Visualization and Optics in Neurosurgery

Robert D. Brown, Jr., MD, MPH
John T. and Lillian Mathews Professor of Neuroscience
Department of Neurology
Mayo Clinic
Rochester, Minnesota
401: Epidemiology and Natural History of Intracranial Vascular Malformations

Jeffrey N. Bruce, MD
Edgar M. Housepian Professor of Neurological Surgery
Columbia University Medical Center
New York, New York
141: Pineal Tumors

Janice E. Brunstrom-Hernandez, MD
Director, 1 CP Place, PLLC
Plano, Texas;
Adjunct Professor of Neurology
Washington University School of Medicine in St. Louis
St. Louis, Missouri
241: Clinical Features and Management of Cerebral Palsy

Andrew Brunswick, MD
Neurosurgery Resident
New York University School of Medicine
NYU Langone Medical Center
New York, New York
217: Neurocutaneous Tumor Syndromes

Thomas J. Buell, MD
Resident Physician
Department of Neurosurgery
University of Virginia Health System
Charlottesville, Virginia
374: Cerebral Venous and Sinus Thrombosis

M. Ross Bullock, MD, PhD
Professor of Neurosurgery
University of Miami Miller School of Medicine
Miami, Florida
343: Therapeutic Strategies for Repair and Regeneration following Traumatic Brain Injury

Kim J. Burchiel, MD, FACS
John Raaf Professor
Department of Neurological Surgery
Professor, Department of Anesthesiology and Perioperative Medicine
Oregon Health & Science University
Portland, Oregon
Overview and Controversies (Pain)
172: Percutaneous Procedures for Trigeminal Neuralgia
174: Microvascular Decompression for Trigeminal Neuralgia
179: Evidence Base for Destructive Procedures
182: Dorsal Root Entry Zone Lesions for Pain

Anthony M. Burrows, MD
Resident Neurosurgeon
Mayo Clinic
Rochester, Minnesota
359: Cerebral Blood Flow and Metabolism and Cerebral Ischemia
398: Multimodality Treatments of Cerebrovascular Disorders

Mohamad Bydon, MD
Assistant Professor
Departments of Neurosurgery and Orthopedics
Mayo Clinic
Rochester, Minnesota
123: Brain Tumors during Pregnancy
292: Assessment and Treatment of Benign Tumors of the Axial Skeleton

Richard W. Byrne, MD
Professor of Neurosurgery
Rush University Medical Center
Chicago, Illinois
73: Surgical Techniques for Non–Temporal Lobe Epilepsy: Corpus Callosotomy, Multiple Subpial Transection, and Topectomy

Daniel P. Cahill, MD, PhD
Assistant Professor of Neurosurgery
Harvard Medical School
Massachusetts General Hospital
Dana-Farber/Harvard Cancer Center
Boston, Massachusetts
126: Brain Tumor Outcome Studies: Design and Interpretation

Kevin S. Cahill, MD, PhD, MPH
Carolina Neurosurgery and Spine Associates
Charlotte, North Carolina
330: Posterior, Transforaminal, and Anterior Lumbar Interbody Fusion: Techniques and Instrumentation

Maria Elisa Calcagnotto, MD, PhD
Professor
Biochemistry Department
Neurophysiology and Neurochemistry of Neuronal Excitability and Synaptic Plasticity Labotratory
Federal University of Rio Grande do Sul
Porto Alegre, Brazil
59: Animal Models of Epilepsy

Justin M. Caplan, MD
Resident
Department of Neurosurgery
Johns Hopkins University School of Medicine
Baltimore, Maryland
386: Microsurgery of Anterior Communicating Artery Aneurysms

Gregory D. Cascino, MD
Professor of Neurology
Mayo Clinic
Rochester, Minnesota
67: Single-Photon Emission Computed Tomography in Epilepsy Surgery Evaluation

Frederic Castinetti, MD, PhD
Assistant Professor of Endocrinology
Aix-Marseille University
Assistance Publique Hopitaux de Marseille
Marseille, France
268: Radiosurgery for Benign Intracranial Tumors

C. Michael Cawley, MD
Associate Professor
Department of Neurosurgery
Emory University School of Medicine
Atlanta, Georgia
408: Treatment of Other Intracranial Dural Arteriovenous Fistulas

Ibolja Cernak, MD, PhD, ME, MHS
Professor and Chair
Military and Veterans' Clinical Rehabilitation Research
Faculty of Rehabilitation Medicine
University of Alberta
Edmonton, Alberta, Canada
353: Blast-Induced Neurotrauma

Francesco Certo, MD
Neurosurgeon
Policlinico G. Rodolico University Hospital
Catania, Italy
323: Nucleoplasty and Posterior Dynamic Stabilization Systems

Justin S. Cetas, MD, PhD
Assistant Professor of Neurological Surgery
Oregon Health & Science University;
Chief of Neurosurgery, Operative Care Division
Portland VA Medical Center
Portland, Oregon
179: Evidence Base for Destructive Procedures

Michael D. Chan, MD
Associate Professor
Department of Radiation Oncology
Co-Director, Gamma Knife Program
Wake Forest School of Medicine
Winston-Salem, North Carolina
263: Radiation Therapy Technique

Amitabha Chanda, MBBS, MS, MCh (Neurosurgery)
Senior Consultant
Department of Neurosurgery
Fortis Hospitals
Kolkata, India
291: Evaluation and Treatment of Fungal and Tubercular Infections of the Spine

Edward F. Chang, MD
Associate Professor of Neurological Surgery
University of California, San Francisco School of Medicine
San Francisco, California
74: Surgery for Extratemporal Lobe Epilepsy

Steven D. Chang, MD
Robert C. and Jeannette Powell Professor
Department of Neurosurgery
Stanford School of Medicine
Stanford, California
272: Radiosurgery for Benign Spine Tumors and Vascular Malformations
406: Surgical and Radiosurgical Management of Grade IV and V Arteriovenous Malformations

Fady T. Charbel, MD
Professor and Head
Department of Neurosurgery
University of Illinois at Chicago
Chicago, Illinois
364: Neurovascular Imaging
370: Extracranial Vertebral Artery Diseases

Aswin Chari, MA, BMBCh, MRCS
Academic Foundation Trainee
Division of Neurosurgery, Department of Clinical Neuroscience
University of Cambridge
Addenbrooke's Hospital
Cambridge, United Kingdom
34: Medical and Surgical Management of Chronic Subdural Hematomas

Navjot Chaudhary, MD
Clinical Assistant Professor
Department of Neurosurgery
Stanford School of Medicine
Palo Alto, California
272: Radiosurgery for Benign Spine Tumors and Vascular Malformations

Patrick Chauvel, MD
Professor
Institut de Neurosciences des Systèmes
Aix-Marseille University
Marseille, France;
Epilepsy Center
Cleveland Clinic
Cleveland, Ohio
72: Intracranial Monitoring: Stereo-Electroencephalography Recording

Kevin S. Chen, MD
Resident Neurosurgeon
University of Michigan Health System
Ann Arbor, Michigan
246: Peripheral Neuropathies
288: Evaluation and Treatment of Degenerative Lumbar Spondylolisthesis
313: Evaluation and Treatment of Cervical Deformity

Liang Chen, MD, PhD
Professor
Hand Surgery Department
Huashan Hospital of Fudan University
Shanghai, China
Overview and Controversies (PNS)
252: Techniques in Nerve Reconstruction and Repair
253: Nerve Transfers

Joseph S. Cheng, MD, MS
Professor and Vice-Chair
Department of Neurosurgery
Yale School of Medicine
New Haven, Connecticut
275: Spinal Biomechanics and Basics of Spinal Instrumentation

Yuwei Cheng, MS, PhD
Department of Computational Biology and Bioinformatics
Yale University
New Haven, Connecticut
376: Genetics of Intracranial Aneurysms

Kenneth M.C. Cheung, MBBS(UK), MD(HK), FRCS, FHKCOS, FHKAM(Orth)
Jessie Ho Professor in Spine Surgery
Head, Department of Orthopaedics and Traumatology
The University of Hong Kong
Hong Kong
327: Anterior Thoracic Instrumentation

E. Antonio Chiocca, MD, PhD, FAANS
Harvey W. Cushing Professor of Neurosurgery
Harvard Medical School;
Neurosurgeon-in-Chief and Chair, Department of Neurosurgery
Co-Director, Institute for the Neurosciences
Brigham and Women's Hospital
Boston, Massachusetts
Overview and Controversies (Oncology)

Catherine Cho, MD, MSCR
Clinical Associate Professor
Departments of Neurology and Otolaryngology
NYU Langone Medical Center
New York, New York
85: Patient Selection Criteria for Deep Brain Stimulation in Movement Disorders

Dean Chou, MD
Professor of Neurosurgery
University of California, San Francisco
San Francisco, California
315: Evaluation and Treatment of Scheuermann's Kyphosis

Omar Choudhri, MD
Chief Resident
Department of Neurosurgery
Stanford University
Stanford, California
406: Surgical and Radiosurgical Management of Grade IV and V Arteriovenous Malformations

Cindy W. Christian, MD
Professor of Pediatrics
Perelman School of Medicine at the University of Pennsylvania
Chair, Child Abuse and Neglect Prevention
Children's Hospital of Philadelphia
Philadelphia, Pennsylvania
225: Inflicted Trauma (Child Abuse)

Jan Claassen, MD, PhD, FNCS
Associate Professor of Neurology and Neurosurgery
Head, Neurocritical Care
Medical Director, Neurological Intensive Care Unit
Columbia University College of Physicians and Surgeons
New York, New York
63: Continuous Electroencephalography in Neurological-Neurosurgical Intensive Care: Applications and Value

Elizabeth B. Claus, MD, PhD
Instructor
Department of Neurosurgery
Harvard Medical School
Brigham and Women's Hospital
Boston, Massachusetts
163: Scalp Tumors

Daniel R. Cleary, MD, PhD
Neurological Surgery Resident
University of California, San Diego
La Jolla, California
166: Anatomy and Physiology of Pain

Alan R. Cohen, MD, FACS, FAAP
Professor of Neurosurgery
Director of Pediatric Neurosurgery
Johns Hopkins University School of Medicine
Baltimore, Maryland
202: Neuroendoscopy

John Collins, MD, PhD
Assistant Professor of Radiology
University of Chicago Pritzker School of Medicine
Chicago, Illinois
41: Acquired Immunodeficiency Syndrome

E. Sander Connolly, Jr., MD, FACS
Bennett M. Stein Professor of Neurological Surgery
Vice Chairman of Neurosurgery
Columbia University College of Physicians and Surgeons;
Director, Cerebrovascular Research Laboratory
Surgical Director, Neuro-Intensive Care Unit
New York–Presbyterian Columbia University Medical Center
New York, New York
Overview and Controversies (Vascular)
387: Microsurgery of Distal Anterior Cerebral Artery Aneurysms

Jonathon Cooke, MD
Staff Neurosurgeon
U.S. Naval Hospital
Okinawa, Japan
365: The Natural History and Medical Management of Carotid Occlusive Disease

Jeroen R. Coppens, MD
Assistant Professor of Neurosurgery
Center for Cerebrovascular and Skull Base Surgery
St. Louis University School of Medicine
St. Louis, Missouri
26: Advantages and Limitations of Cranial Endoscopy

Daniel M. Corcos, PhD
Professor
Physical Therapy & Human Movement Sciences
Northwestern University
Chicago, Illinois
104: Management of Spasticity by Central Nervous System Infusion Techniques

Domagoj Coric, MD
Chief, Department of Neurosurgery
Carolinas Medical Center;
Carolina Neurosurgery and Spine Associates
Charlotte, North Carolina
330: Posterior, Transforaminal, and Anterior Lumbar Interbody Fusion: Techniques and Instrumentation

Erwin M.J. Cornips, MD
Pediatric Neurosurgeon
Department of Neurosurgery
Maastricht University Medical Center
Maastricht, The Netherlands
135: Intraoperative Magnetic Resonance Imaging

G. Rees Cosgrove, MD, FRCS(C)
Director, Epilepsy and Functional Neurosurgery
Brigham and Women's Hospital
Boston, Massachusetts
98: A History of Psychosurgery

William T. Couldwell, MD, PhD
Professor and Chair
Department of Neurosurgery
University of Utah School of Medicine
Salt Lake City, Utah
Overview and Controversies (General)
26: Advantages and Limitations of Cranial Endoscopy

Peter B. Crino, MD, PhD
Chair, Department of Neurology
University of Maryland School of Medicine
Baltimore, Maryland
60: Malformations of Cortical Development

Andrew Crofton, BA
Department of Pathology and Human Anatomy
Neurosurgery Center for Research, Training, and Education
Loma Linda University School of Medicine
Loma Linda, California
7: Coagulation for the Neurosurgeon

D. Kacy Cullen, PhD
Assistant Professor of Neurosurgery
Perelman School of Medicine at the University of Pennsylvania
Philadelphia, Pennsylvania
337: Biomechanical Basis of Traumatic Brain Injury

Brian P. Curry, MD
Resident Neurosurgeon
Walter Reed National Military Medical Center
Bethesda, Maryland
286: Evaluation and Treatment of Lumbar Disk Disease

Erasmo Barros da Silva, Jr., MD, MSc
Department of Neurosurgery
Instituto de Neurologia de Curitiba
Curitiba, Brazil
320: Bone Graft Options, Graft Substitutes, and Harvest Techniques

Andrew T. Dailey, MD
Associate Professor of Neurosurgery
University of Utah School of Medicine
Salt Lake City, Utah
37: Postoperative Infections of the Spine

Robert F. Dallapiazza, MD, PhD
Resident Neurosurgeon
Department of Neurosurgery
University of Virginia Medical Center
Charlottesville, Virginia
95: Transcranial Magnetic Resonance Imaging–Guided Focused Ultrasound Thalamotomy for Tremor

Richard Tyler Dalyai, MD
Neurosurgery Resident
Thomas Jefferson University Hospital
Philadelphia, Pennsylvania
17: The Neurosurgical Intensive Care Unit and the Unique Role of the Neurosurgeon

Deepa Danan, MD, MBA
Chief Resident
Department of Otolaryngology-Head and Neck Surgery
University of Virginia School of Medicine
Charlottesville, Virginia
181: Diagnosis and Management of Painful Neuromas

David J. Daniels, MD, PhD
Assistant Professor of Pediatric Neurosurgery
Assistant Professor of Pharmacology
Mayo Clinic
Rochester, Minnesota
211: Pediatric Supratentorial Hemispheric Tumors

Tim E. Darsaut, MD, MSc
Assistant Professor
Division of Neurosurgery, Department of Surgery
University of Alberta Hospital
Edmonton, Alberta, Canada
381: Medical Management of Cerebral Vasospasm

Alexander Dash
Undergraduate Research Assistant
Department of Oncology, Hematology, and Transplantation
University of Minnesota Medical Center
St. Paul, Minnesota
160: Juvenile Nasopharyngeal Angiofibromas

Matthew L. Dashnaw, MD, PharmD
Department of Neurosurgery
University of Rochester Medical Center
Rochester, New York
347: Mild Traumatic Brain Injury in Adults and Concussion in Sports

Carlos A. David, MD
Associate Professor
Department of Neurosurgery
Tufts University School of Medicine
Boston, Massachusetts;
Director, Cerebrovascular and Skull Base Surgery
Department of Neurosurgery
Lahey Clinic Hospital
Burlington, Massachusetts
371: Microsurgical Management of Intracranial Occlusion Disease

David J. David, MD, FRCSE, FRCS, FRACS, FRCST
Professor of Surgery
Australian Craniofacial Unit
Women's & Children's Hospital
North Adelaide, South Australia, Australia;
Faculty of Medicine and Health Science
Macquarie University
New South Wales, Australia;
Faculty of Health Science
University of Adelaide
Adelaide, South Australia, Australia
355: Craniofacial Injuries

Arthur L. Day, MD
Professor
Department of Neurosurgery
University of Texas Medical School at Houston
Houston, Texas
384: Microsurgery of Paraclinoid Aneurysms

Rafael De la Garza-Ramos, MD
Research Fellow in Neurosurgery
Johns Hopkins University School of Medicine
Baltimore, Maryland
292: Assessment and Treatment of Benign Tumors of the Axial Skeleton

Antonio A.F. De Salles, MD, PhD
Professor of Neurosurgery
University of California Los Angeles
David Geffen School of Medicine at UCLA
Los Angeles, California;
Chief, HCor Neuroscience
Hospital do Coração
São Paulo, Brazil
14: Molecular Imaging of the Brain with Positron Emission Tomography

Nicolas Dea, MD, MSc, FRCSC
Spinal Neurosurgeon
Assistant Professor
Department of Surgery
Université de Sherbrooke
Sherbrooke, Quebec, Canada
293: Assessment and Treatment of Primary Malignant Tumors of the Axial Skeleton

Matthew Decker, MD, MPH
Resident Neurosurgeon
University of Florida School of Medicine
Gainesville, Florida
279: Bone Metabolism and Osteoporosis

Oscar H. Del Brutto, MD
Director, The Atahualpa Project
Universidad Espiritu Santo School of Medicine
Guayaquil, Ecuador
42: Parasitic Infections

Bradley N. Delman, MD
Associate Professor of Radiology
Icahn School of Medicine at Mount Sinai
New York, New York
13: Physiologic Evaluation of the Brain with Magnetic Resonance Imaging

Mahlon R. DeLong, MD
W. P. Timmie Professor of Neurology
Emory University School of Medicine
Atlanta, Georgia
82: Rationale for Surgical Interventions in Movement Disorders

Franco DeMonte, MD, FRCSC, FACS
Mary Beth Pawelek Chair in Neurosurgery
Professor, Departments of Neurosurgery and Head and Neck Surgery
University of Texas MD Anderson Cancer Center
Houston, Texas
157: Neoplasms of the Paranasal Sinuses

Milind Deogaonkar, MBBS, MS, MCh
Associate Professor of Neurological Surgery
The Ohio State University;
Center for Neuromodulation
Wexner Medical Center
Columbus, Ohio
100: Surgery for Obsessive-Compulsive Disorder

Arati Desai, MD
Assistant Professor of Hematology-Oncology
Perelman School of Medicine at the University of Pennsylvania;
Co-Director, Penn Brain Tumor Center
Abramson Cancer Center
Hospital of the University of Pennsylvania
Philadelphia, Pennsylvania
116: Angiogenesis and Brain Tumors: Scientific Principles, Current Therapy, and Future Directions

Virendra R. Desai, MD
Resident Neurosurgeon
Houston Methodist Neurological Institute
Houston, Texas
383: Surgical Approaches to Intracranial Aneurysms

Federico Di Rocco, MD, PhD
Pediatric Neurosurgeon
Unité de Chirurgie Craniofaciale
Hôpital Necker Enfants Malades
Paris, France
194: Syndromic Craniosynostosis

Bassel G. Diebo, MD
Postdoctoral Fellow (Spine)
Hospital for Special Surgery
New York, New York
311: Classification of Spinal Deformity

Michael L. DiLuna, MD
Assistant Professor of Neurosurgery and Pediatrics
Yale School of Medicine
New Haven, Connecticut
139: Unusual Gliomas

Francesco DiMeco, MD
Chairman
Department of Neurosurgery
Fondazione Istituto Neurologico C. Besta
Milan, Italy;
Assistant Professor
Department of Neurological Surgery
Johns Hopkins University School of Medicine
Baltimore, Maryland
112: Brain Tumor Stem Cells

Peter Dirks, MD, PhD, FRCSC
Professor of Neurosurgery
University of Toronto Faculty of Medicine;
Staff Surgeon
Division of Neurosurgery
The Hospital for Sick Children
Toronto, Ontario, Canada
208: Thalamic Tumors

Brian J. Dlouhy, MD
Assistant Professor
Department of Neurosurgery
University of Iowa Hospitals and Clinics
Iowa City, Iowa
233: Developmental Anomalies of the Craniovertebral Junction and Surgical Management
243: Selective Dorsal Rhizotomy for Spastic Cerebral Palsy

Amish H. Doshi, MD
Assistant Professor of Radiology
Icahn School of Medicine at Mount Sinai
New York, New York
13: Physiologic Evaluation of the Brain with Magnetic Resonance Imaging

James M. Drake, MBBCh, MSc, FRCSC
Professor of Surgery
Harold Hoffman Shoppers Drug Mart Chair, Pediatric Neurosurgery
University of Toronto Faculty of Medicine;
Head, Department of Neurosurgery
The Hospital for Sick Children
Toronto, Ontario, Canada
32: The Role of Third Ventriculostomy in Adults and Children: A Critical Review
203: Cerebrospinal Fluid Devices

Alexander Drofa, MD, FRCSC
Cerebrovascular Neurosurgeon
Sanford Brain and Spine Center
Sanford Medical Center Fargo;
Clinical Instructor of Surgery
Department of Surgery
University of North Dakota
Fargo, North Dakota
393: Endovascular Flow Diversion for Intracranial Aneurysms

Andrew F. Ducruet, MD
Assistant Professor
Department of Neurosurgery
Barrow Neurological Institute
Phoenix, Arizona
361: Acute Surgical and Endovascular Management of Ischemic and Hemorrhagic Stroke

Hugues Duffau, MD, PhD
Professor and Chairman
Neurosurgery and INSERM 1051
Montpellier University Medical Center
Hôpital Gui de Chauliac
Montpellier, France
134: Awake Craniotomy and Intraoperative Mapping

Ann-Christine Duhaime, MD
Nicholas T. Zervas Professor of Neurosurgery
Harvard Medical School
Director, Pediatric Neurosurgery
Massachusetts General Hospital
Boston, Massachusetts
225: Inflicted Trauma (Child Abuse)

Aaron S. Dumont, MD
Charles B. Wilson Professor and Chair
Department of Neurosurgery
Tulane University School of Medicine
New Orleans, Louisiana
414: Microsurgical Treatment of Spinal Vascular Malformations

Gavin P. Dunn, MD, PhD
Assistant Professor
Departments of Neurological Surgery and Pathology and Immunology
Center for Human Immunology and Immunotherapy Programs
Washington University School of Medicine in St. Louis
St. Louis, Missouri
143: Intracranial Ependymomas in Adults

Ian F. Dunn, MD
Assistant Professor
Department of Neurosurgery
Harvard Medical School
Brigham and Women's Hospital
Boston, Massachusetts
143: Intracranial Ependymomas in Adults
150: Pituitary Tumors: Functioning and Nonfunctioning
202: Neuroendoscopy

Joshua R. Dusick, MD
Research Associate
Department of Neurosurgery
David Geffen School of Medicine at UCLA
Los Angeles, California
397: Revascularization Techniques for Complex Aneurysms and Skull Base Tumors

James H. Eberwine, PhD
Elmer Holmes Professor
Department of Systems Pharmacology and Experimental Therapeutics
Perelman School of Medicine at the University of Pennsylvania
Philadelphia, Pennsylvania
44: Molecular Biology and Genomics: A Primer for Neurosurgeons

Paula Eboli, MD
Fellow
Endovascular Neurosurgery
Cedars-Sinai Medical Center
Los Angeles, California
369: Nonatherosclerotic Carotid Lesions

Gerald W. Eckardt, MD
Global Neurosciences Institute
Capital Health Regional Medical Center
Trenton, New Jersey
326: Posterior Subaxial and Cervicothoracic Instrumentation

Michael S.B. Edwards, MD
Lucile Packard Endowed Professor of Neurosurgery and Pediatrics
Director of Pediatric Brain Tumor Center
Stanford University School of Medicine
Stanford, California
212: Ependymomas

Richard J. Edwards, MBBS, MD, FRCS (Neuro.Surg)
Consultant Neurosurgeon
Department of Pediatric Neurosurgery
Bristol Royal Hospital for Children and North Bristol NHS Trust;
Senior Clinical Lecturer in Neurosurgery
School of Clinical Sciences
University of Bristol Faculty of Biomedical Sciences
Bristol, United Kingdom
203: Cerebrospinal Fluid Devices

J. Bradley Elder, MD
Associate Professor
Department of Neurological Surgery
Director of Neurosurgical Oncology
The Ohio State University Wexner Medical Center
Columbus, Ohio
119: Local Therapies for Gliomas

Mohamed Samy A. Elhammady, MD
Associate Professor
Department of Neurological Surgery
University of Miami
Miami, Florida
405: Microsurgery of Arteriovenous Malformations

W. Jeffrey Elias, MD
Professor of Neurosurgery and Neurology
University of Virginia School of Medicine
Charlottesville, Virginia
95: Transcranial Magnetic Resonance Imaging–Guided Focused Ultrasound Thalamotomy for Tremor

Jason A. Ellis, MD
Chief Resident
Department of Neurological Surgery
Columbia University Medical Center
New York, New York
21: Positioning for Spinal Surgery
Overview and Controversies (Vascular)
387: Microsurgery of Distal Anterior Cerebral Artery Aneurysms
403: Adjuvant Endovascular Management of Brain Arteriovenous Malformations

Tarek M.I. Elmadhoun, MD, PhD, FICS
Clinical Fellow
Department of Clinical Neurosciences
University of Calgary Cumming School of Medicine;
Hotchkiss Brain Institute
Calgary, Alberta, Canada
245: Peripheral Nerve Examination, Evaluation, and Biopsy

Todd M. Emch, MD
Staff
Division of Neuroradiology, Imaging Institute
Cleveland Clinic
Cleveland, Ohio
12: Radiology of the Spine

Samuel Emerson, MD, PhD
Resident Neurosurgeon
University of Washington School of Medicine
Seattle, Washington
47: Stem Cell Biology in the Central Nervous System

Chibawanye Ene, MD, PhD
Resident
Department of Neurological Surgery
University of Washington School of Medicine
Seattle, Washington
113: Molecular Genetics and the Development of Targets for Glioma Therapy

Dario J. Englot, MD, PhD
Resident Neurosurgeon
University of California, San Francisco
San Francisco, California
340: Genetics of Traumatic Brain Injury

Ramin Eskandari, MD, MS
Assistant Professor of Neurosurgery
Director, Pediatric Neurosurgery
Medical University of South Carolina
Charleston, South Carolina
200: Experimental Hydrocephalus

Matthew G. Ewend, MD
Van L. Weatherspoon, Jr., Eminent Distinguished Professor and Chair
Department of Neurosurgery
University of North Carolina School of Medicine at Chapel Hill
UNC Chapel Hill Hospital
Chapel Hill, North Carolina
148: Meningeal Sarcomas and Hemangiopericytomas

Shayan Fakurnejad, BS
Department of Neurological Surgery
Northwestern University Feinberg School of Medicine
Chicago, Illinois
318: Assessment and Treatment of Proximal Junctional Kyphosis

Asdrubal Falavigna, MD, PhD
Professor of Neurosurgery
Dean, Medical School
University of Caxias do Sul
Caxias do Sul, Brazil
289: Treatment of Discitis and Epidural Abscess

Yi Fan, MD, PhD
Assistant Professor
Departments of Radiation Oncology and Neurosurgery
Perelman School of Medicine at the University of Pennsylvania
Philadelphia, Pennsylvania
116: Angiogenesis and Brain Tumors: Scientific Principles, Current Therapy, and Future Directions

Dario Farina, PhD
Professor and Chair
Department of Neurorehabilitation Engineering
Georg-August University;
Director, Institute for Neurorehabilitation Systems
Bernstein Focus Neurotechnology
University Medical Center Göttingen
Göttingen, Germany
260: Neuroelectronic Systems

Christopher J. Farrell, MD
Assistant Professor of Neurological Surgery
Thomas Jefferson University
Philadelphia, Pennsylvania
36: Postoperative Infections of the Head and Brain

Michael G. Fehlings, MD, PhD, FRCSC, FACS
Professor of Neurosurgery;
Vice Chair, Research, Department of Surgery, University of Toronto Faculty of Medicine;
Co-Director of the University of Toronto Spine Program, Director of the Spinal Program at the Toronto Western Hospital;
Gerald and Tootsie Halbert Chair in Neural Repair and Regeneration, University Health Network;
Senior Scientist, Toronto Western Research Institute, University Health Network
Toronto, Ontario, Canada
Overview and Controversies (Spine)
277: Pathophysiology and Treatment of Spinal Cord Injury
295: Assessment and Treatment of Metastatic Spinal Lesions
303: Medical Management of Spinal Cord Injury

Valery Feigin, MD, PhD, FAAN
Professor of Epidemiology and Neurology
Auckland University of Technology;
Director, National Institute for Stroke and Applied Neurosciences
Auckland, New Zealand
336: Epidemiology of Traumatic Brain Injury

Eva L. Feldman, MD, PhD
Russell N. DeJong Professor of Neurology
University of Michigan School of Medicine
Ann Arbor, Michigan
246: Peripheral Neuropathies

Neil Feldstein, MD, FACS
Associate Professor of Neurological Surgery
Director of Pediatric Neurosurgery
Columbia University Medical Center
New York, New York
229: Myelomeningocele and Myelocystocele

James E. Feng, BA
New York University School of Medicine
New York, New York
311: Classification of Spinal Deformity

Lief E. Fenno, PhD
Department of Neuroscience
Stanford School of Medicine
Stanford, California
45: Optogenetics and CLARITY

Sherise D. Ferguson, MD
Assistant Professor of Neurosurgery
University of Texas MD Anderson Cancer Center
Houston, Texas
40: Meningitis and Encephalitis

Matheus Fernandes de Oliveira, MD, MSci
Department of Neurosurgery
Hospital do Servidor Público Estadual de São Paulo;
Department of Neurosurgery
DFV Neuro
São Paulo, Brazil
280: Differential Diagnosis of Spinal Disease

Javier M. Figueroa, MD, PhD
Neurosurgery Resident
Neurosurgery
Barrow Neurological Institute
Phoenix, Arizona
136: Low-Grade Gliomas: Astrocytomas, Oligodendrogliomas, and Mixed Gliomas

Juan J. Figueroa, MD
Assistant Professor of Neurology
Medical College of Wisconsin
Milwaukee, Wisconsin
42: Parasitic Infections

Aaron G. Filler, MD, PhD, JD, FRCS
Medical Director
Institute for Nerve Medicine
Santa Monica, California
Overview and Controversies (PNS)
248: Imaging for Peripheral Nerve Disorders
250: Brachial Plexus Nerve Entrapments and Thoracic Outlet Syndromes
251: Piriformis Syndrome, Obturator Internus Syndrome, Pudendal Nerve Entrapment, and Other Pelvic Entrapments
257: Nerve Injuries of the Lower Extremity
259: Pain, Complications, and Iatrogenic Injury in Nerve Surgery

J. Max Findlay, MD, PhD
Department of Surgery
University of Alberta Hospital
Clinical Professor
Department of Medicine
University of Alberta
Edmonton, Alberta, Canada
381: Medical Management of Cerebral Vasospasm

Michael A. Finn, MD
Assistant Professor of Neurosurgery
University of Colorado School of Medicine
Denver, Colorado
37: Postoperative Infections of the Spine

Richard H. Finnell, MSc, PhD
Professor
Departments of Nutritional Sciences and Chemistry and Biochemistry
College of Natural Sciences
The University of Texas at Austin
Austin, Texas
186: Neuroembryology and Molecular Genetics of the Brain

Charles G. Fisher, MD, MHSc, FRCSC
Professor and Division Head, Spine Surgery
Department of Orthopaedic Surgery
University of British Columbia Faculty of Medicine;
Vancouver General Hospital
Vancouver Spine and Spinal Cord Institute
Vancouver, British Columbia, Canada
293: Assessment and Treatment of Primary Malignant Tumors of the Axial Skeleton

Eugene S. Flamm, MD
Chairman, Department of Neurosurgery
Leo Davidoff Department of Neurosurgery
Professor of Neurosurgery
Montefiore Medical Center
New York, New York;
Albert Einstein College of Medicine
Bronx, New York
1: Historical Overview of Neurosurgery

Kelly D. Flemming, MD
Neurologist
Department of Neurology
Mayo Clinic
Rochester, Minnesota
401: Epidemiology and Natural History of Intracranial Vascular Malformations

Laura Flores-Sarnat, MD
Research Professor
Department of Clinical Neurosciences
University of Calgary Faculty of Medicine
and Alberta Children's Hospital Research Institute
Calgary, Alberta, Canada
46: Neuroembryology

Kenneth A. Follett, MD, PhD
Professor and Chief
Division of Neurosurgery
University of Nebraska Medical Center
Omaha, Nebraska
175: Neurosurgical Management of Intractable Pain

Paul M. Foreman, MD
Resident Neurosurgeon
University of Alabama at Birmingham
Birmingham, Alabama
368: Blunt Cerebrovascular Injury

Kimberly A. Foster, MD
Pediatric Neurosurgery Fellow
Le Bonheur Children's Hospital
St. Jude Children's Research Hospital
Memphis, Tennessee
216: Intracranial Germ Cell Tumors

Benjamin S. Freeze, MD, PhD
Resident Physician
Department of Radiology
Weill Cornell Medical College
New York, New York
340: Genetics of Traumatic Brain Injury

Itzhak Fried, MD, PhD
Professor of Surgery (Neurosurgery) and Psychiatry and Bio-behavioral Sciences
Director of Epilepsy Surgery
Department of Neurosurgery
David Geffen School of Medicine at UCLA
Co-Director, Seizure Disorder Center
UCLA Medical Center
Los Angeles, California;
Professor of Surgery (Neurosurgery)
Tel-Aviv Medical Center
Tel-Aviv, Israel
Overview and Controversies (Epilepsy)

Robert M. Friedlander, MD, MA
Walter E. Dandy Professor and Chairman
Department of Neurological Surgery
University of Pittsburgh School of Medicine
Pittsburgh, Pennsylvania
Overview and Future Opportunities (Basic Science)

Donald E. Fry, MD
Adjunct Professor of Surgery
Northwestern University Feinberg School of Medicine
Chicago, Illinois;
Emeritus Professor of Surgery
University of New Mexico School of Medicine
Albuquerque, New Mexico
43: Surgical Risk of Transmittable Disease

Kai-Ming Gregory Fu, MD, PhD
Assistant Professor of Neurosurgery
Weill Cornell Medical College
New York, New York
273: Spinal Anatomy

Daniel H. Fulkerson, MD
Assistant Professor of Neurological Surgery
Indiana University School of Medicine
Goodman Campbell Brain and Spine
Indianapolis, Indiana
239: Pediatric Vertebral Column and Spinal Cord Injuries

Gregory N. Fuller, MD, PhD
Professor of Pathology
Chief, Section of Neuropathology
University of Texas MD Anderson Cancer Center
Houston, Texas
110: Brain Tumors: An Overview of Current Histopathologic and Genetic Classifications

Matthew R. Fusco, MD
Assistant Professor
Departments of Neurological Surgery and Radiology
Vanderbilt University Medical Center
Nashville, Tennessee
389: Microsurgery of Vertebral Artery and Posterior Inferior Cerebellar Artery Aneurysms

Adriana Galvan, PhD
Assistant Professor of Neurology
Emory University School of Medicine;
Yerkes National Primate Research Center
Emory University
Atlanta, Georgia
81: Anatomy and Synaptic Connectivity of the Basal Ganglia

Gurpreet S. Gandhoke, MD
Department of Neurological Surgery
University of Pittsburgh Medical Center
Pittsburgh, Pennsylvania
308: Transient Quadriparesis and Athletic Injuries of the Cervical Spine
332: Sacropelvic Fixation: Anterior and Posterior Options

Hector H. Garcia, MD, PhD
Head, Cysticercosis Unit
Instituto Nacional de Ciencias Neurologicas;
Director, Center for Global Health - Tumbes
Universidad Peruana Cayetano Heredia
Lima, Peru
42: Parasitic Infections

Paul A. Gardner, MD
Associate Professor of Neurological Surgery
University of Pittsburgh School of Medicine
Co-Director, Center for Cranial Base Surgery
University of Pittsburgh Medical Center
Pittsburgh, Pennsylvania
161: Tumors of the Orbit

Hugh Garton, MD, MHSc
Associate Professor
Department of Neurosurgery
University of Michigan School of Medicine
Ann Arbor, Michigan
57: Neurosurgical Epidemiology and Outcomes Assessment

Cormac G. Gavin, MB, BCh, BAO, FRCS(I), FRCS(SN)
Neurosurgeon
Victor Horsley Department of Neurosurgery
The National Hospital for Neurology and Neurosurgery
London, United Kingdom
400: Pathobiology of True Arteriovenous Malformations

Brandon G. Gaynor, MD
Resident
Department of Neurological Surgery
Jackson Memorial Hospital
Miami, Florida
405: Microsurgery of Arteriovenous Malformations

Timothy M. George, MD
Professor of Surgery
Dell Medical School
The University of Texas at Austin
Chief, Department of Pediatric Neurosurgery
Dell Children's Medical Center
Austin, Texas
186: Neuroembryology and Molecular Genetics of the Brain

George Georgoulis, MD
Neurosurgeon
Hôpital Neurologique Pierre Wertheimer
Lyon, France;
Medical School, University of Athens
Athens, Greece
103: Lesioning Surgery for Spasticity

Carter S. Gerard, MD
Resident Neurosurgeon
Rush University Medical Center
Chicago, Illinois
73: Surgical Techniques for Non–Temporal Lobe Epilepsy: Corpus Callosotomy, Multiple Subpial Transection, and Topectomy

Luke Gerke, MD
Assistant Professor of Radiology
Icahn School of Medicine at Mount Sinai
New York, New York
13: Physiologic Evaluation of the Brain with Magnetic Resonance Imaging

Massimo Gerosa, MD
Professor of Neurosurgery
University of Verona
University Hospital;
President, Verona Brain Research Foundation
Verona, Italy
156: Glomus Tumors

Kristina Gerszten, MD
Department of Radiation Oncology
Veteran's Administration of Pittsburgh Healthcare System
Pittsburgh, Pennsylvania
271: Radiosurgery for Malignant Spine Tumors

Peter C. Gerszten, MD, MPH, FACS
Peter E. Sheptak Professor
Departments of Neurological Surgery and Radiation Oncology
University of Pittsburgh Medical Center
Pittsburgh, Pennsylvania
271: Radiosurgery for Malignant Spine Tumors

Saadi Ghatan, MD
Associate Professor of Neurosurgery and Pediatrics
Icahn School of Medicine at Mount Sinai
Site Chair, Department of Neurosurgery
Mount Sinai West and Mount Sinai St. Luke's Medical Centers
Director of Pediatric Neurosurgery
Mount Sinai Health System
New York, New York
160: Juvenile Nasopharyngeal Angiofibromas
189: Arachnoid Cysts in Childhood
240: Pediatric Epilepsy Surgery

George M. Ghobrial, MD
Resident Neurosurgeon
Thomas Jefferson University Hospital
Philadelphia, Pennsylvania
309: Evaluation, Classification, and Treatment of Thoracolumbar Spine Injuries

Chaitali Ghosh, PhD
Assistant Professor of Molecular Medicine
Cleveland Clinic Lerner School of Medicine of Case Western Reserve University
Cleveland, Ohio
51: The Blood-Brain Barrier

Peter Giacobbe, MD, MSc, FRCPC
Assistant Professor
Department of Psychiatry
University of Toronto Faculty of Medicine;
Toronto, Ontario, Canada
101: Surgery for Major Depressive Disorder

Thomas J. Gianaris, MD
Resident Neurosurgeon
Indiana University School of Medicine
Indianapolis, Indiana
78: Radiosurgical Treatment for Epilepsy

Pierre Giglio, MD
Associate Professor
Division of Neuro-Oncology
The Ohio State University Comprehensive Cancer Center
Columbus, Ohio
120: Clinical Features: Neurology of Brain Tumor and Paraneoplastic Disorders

Ronit Gilad, MD
Assistant Professor of Neurosurgery
Icahn School of Medicine at Mount Sinai
New York, New York
6: Complication Avoidance in Neurosurgery

Albert H. Gjedde, MD, DSc
Professor
King Abdullah University of Science and Technology (KAUST)
Thuwal, Saudi Arabia;
Brain Mind Institute
Ecole Polytechnique Fédérale de Lausanne (EPFL)
Lausanne, Switzerland
49: Cellular Mechanisms of Brain Energy Metabolism

Selçuk Göçmen, MD
Department of Neurosurgery
Özel Denizli Cerrahi Hastanesi
Denizli, Turkey
176: Evidence-Based Neurostimulation for Pain
180: Dorsal Rhizotomy and Dorsal Root Ganglionectomy

Jakub Godzik, MD
Resident Neurosurgeon
Barrow Neurological Institute
St. Joseph's Hospital and Medical Center
Phoenix, Arizona
257: Nerve Injuries of the Lower Extremity

Atul Goel, M.Ch. (Neurosurgery)
Professor and Head
Department of Neurosurgery
Seth G. S. Medical College and K.E.M Hospital
Mumbai, India
324: Occiput, C1, and C2 Instrumentation

Steven L. Gogela, MD
Neurosurgery Resident
Mayfield Clinic
University of Cincinnati College of Medicine
Cincinnati, Ohio
188: Dandy-Walker Syndrome

Ziya L. Gokaslan, MD, FAANS, FACS
Gus Stoll, MD Professor and Chair
Department of Neurosurgery
The Warren Alpert Medical School of Brown University
Neurosurgeon-in-Chief
Rhode Island Hospital and The Miriam Hospital
Clinical Director, Norman Prince Neurosciences Institute
President, Brown Neurosurgery Foundation
Providence, Rhode Island
292: Assessment and Treatment of Benign Tumors of the Axial Skeleton

Hannah E. Goldstein, MD
Resident Neurosurgeon
Columbia University Medical Center
New York, New York
229: Myelomeningocele and Myelocystocele
235: Surgical Management of the Pediatric Subaxial Cervical Spine

John G. Golfinos, MD
Associate Professor and Chair
Department of Neurosurgery
New York University School of Medicine
NYU Langone Medical Center
New York, New York
20: Positioning for Cranial Surgery

Yakov Gologorsky, MD
Assistant Clinical Professor
Department of Neurosurgery
Mount Sinai Medical Center
New York, New York;
Attending Neurosurgeon
Department of Neurosurgery
Englewood Hospital and Medical Center
Englewood, New Jersey
413: Endovascular Treatment of Spinal Vascular Malformations

Kiarash Golshani, MD
Assistant Professor of Neurological Surgery
University of California, Irvine
Irvine, California
399: Traumatic Cerebral Aneurysms Secondary to Penetrating Intracranial Injuries

Nestor R. Gonzalez, MD, MSCR, FAANS, FAHA
Neurosurgeon
Cedars-Sinai Medical Center
Los Angeles, California
397: Revascularization Techniques for Complex Aneurysms and Skull Base Tumors

Jorge Gonzalez-Martinez, MD, PhD, FAANS
Staff
Epilepsy Center
Department of Neurological Surgery
Cleveland Clinic
Cleveland, Ohio
72: Intracranial Monitoring: Stereo-Electroencephalography Recording

John Goodden, MBBS (Lond), FRCS (Neuro, Surg.)
Consultant Neurosurgeon
Leeds General Infirmary
Leeds, West Yorkshire, United Kingdom
207: Optic Pathway Hypothalamic Gliomas

J. Clay Goodman, MD, FAAN
Professor of Pathology & Immunology, Neurosurgery and Neurology
Associate Dean of Foundational Sciences in Undergraduate Medical Education
Walter Henrick Moursund Endowed Chair of Neuropathology
Baylor College of Medicine
Houston, Texas
338: Neuropathology of Traumatic Brain Injury

James Tait Goodrich, MD, PhD, DSci (Hon)
Professor of Clinical Neurosurgery, Pediatrics, Plastic and Reconstructive Surgery
Leo Davidoff Department of Neurosurgery
Director, Division of Pediatric Neurosurgery
Children's Hospital at Montefiore
Montefiore Medical Center
Albert Einstein College of Medicine
Bronx, New York
1: Historical Overview of Neurosurgery
Overview and Controversies (Pediatrics)
187: Encephaloceles, Meningoceles, and Cranial Dermal Sinus Tracts
191: Craniopagus Twins

C. Rory Goodwin, MD, PhD
Resident Neurosurgeon
Johns Hopkins University School of Medicine
Baltimore, Maryland
123: Brain Tumors during Pregnancy
155: Chordomas and Chondrosarcomas

David S. Gordon, MD
Assistant Professor of Neurological Surgery and Radiology
Albert Einstein College of Medicine
Director, Vascular Neurosurgery
Montefiore Medical Center
Bronx, New York
396: Infectious Aneurysms

Alessandra Gorgulho, MD, MSc
Director of Research, Stereotactic Surgery Program
Adjunct Associate Professor of Neurosurgery
University of California Los Angeles
David Geffen School of Medicine at UCLA
Los Angeles, California;
Director of Clinical Affairs and Research
HCor Neurosurgery Program
Hospital do Coração
São Paulo, Brazil
14: Molecular Imaging of the Brain with Positron Emission Tomography

Liliana C. Goumnerova, MD
Associate Professor of Neurosurgery
Harvard Medical School
Director, Pediatric Neurosurgical Oncology
Boston Children's Hospital
Dana-Farber Cancer Institute
Boston, Massachusetts
215: Brainstem Gliomas

Anshit Goyal, MBBSc
Department of Neurosurgery
Johns Hopkins University
Baltimore, Maryland;
All India Institute of Medical Sciences
New Delhi, India
258: Benign and Malignant Tumors of the Peripheral Nerve

M. Sean Grady, MD
Charles Harrison Frazier Professor and Chairman
Department of Neurosurgery
Perelman School of Medicine at the University of Pennsylvania
Philadelphia, Pennsylvania
28: Cranioplasty
348: Initial Resuscitation, Prehospital Care, and Emergency Room Care in Traumatic Brain Injury
357: Traumatic Cerebrospinal Fluid Fistulas

Jordan H. Grafman, PhD
Chief, Cognitive Neuroscience Laboratory
Brain Injury Research Program
Rehabilitation Institute of Chicago;
Professor, Physical Medicine and Rehabilitation
Northwestern University Feinberg School of Medicine
Chicago, Illinois
56: Neuropsychological Testing

Cristian Gragnaniello, MD, PhD, MSurg, MAdvSurg
Neurosurgeon and Surgical Director
Harvey H. Ammerman Microsurgical Laboratory
Department of Neurosurgery
George Washington University
Washington, DC
177: Peripheral Nerve Stimulation for Neuropathic Pain

Andrew W. Grande, MD
Assistant Professor of Neurosurgery
Department of Neurosurgery
University of Minnesota
Minneapolis, Minnesota
25: Visualization and Optics in Neurosurgery
382: Endovascular Management of Cerebral Vasospasm

Gerald A. Grant, MD, FACS
Associate Professor of Neurosurgery
Arline and Pete Harman Endowed Faculty Scholar
Division Chief, Pediatric Neurosurgery
Stanford University School of Medicine
Stanford, California
7: Coagulation for the Neurosurgeon
51: The Blood-Brain Barrier
Overview and Controversies (Pediatrics)
206: General Approaches and Considerations for Pediatric Brain Tumors
214: Cerebellar Astrocytomas
224: Management of Head Injury: Special Considerations in Children

Ryan A. Grant, MD, MS
Neurosurgery Resident
Yale School of Medicine
New Haven, Connecticut
139: Unusual Gliomas

Christoph J. Griessenauer, MD
Clinical Fellow in Neurosurgery
Beth Israel Deaconess Medical Center
Boston, Massachusetts
368: Blunt Cerebrovascular Injury

Michael W. Groff, MD
Harvard Medical School
Director of Spinal Surgery
Brigham and Women's Hospital
Boston, Massachusetts
296: Assessment and Treatment of Malignant Primary Spinal Tumors

Robert E. Gross, MD, PhD
MBNA/Bowman Endowed Professor
Departments of Neurosurgery and Neurology
Emory University School of Medicine
Atlanta, Georgia
79: Electrical Stimulation for Epilepsy (VNS, DBS, and RNS)
88: Ablative Procedures for Parkinson's Disease

Jonathan A. Grossberg, MD
Assistant Professor
Department of Neurosurgery
Emory University School of Medicine
Atlanta, Georgia
408: Treatment of Other Intracranial Dural Arteriovenous Fistulas

Aaron W. Grossman, MD, PhD
Assistant Professor
Department of Neurology
Comprehensive Stroke Center at UC Neuroscience Institute
University of Cincinnati
Cincinnati, Ohio
382: Endovascular Management of Cerebral Vasospasm

Rachel Grossman, MD
Vice Chairman
Department of Neurosurgery
Tel-Aviv Medical Center
Tel-Aviv, Israel
Overview and Controversies (Oncology)
127: Neurocognition in Brain Tumor Patients

Mari L. Groves, MD
Assitant Professor
Department of Neurosurgery
Johns Hopkins University School of Medicine
Baltimore, Maryland
234: Achondroplasia and Other Dwarfisms

Marcelo Fernando Gruenberg, MD
Spine Surgeon
Orthopaedic Department
Hospital Italiano de Buenos Aires
Buenos Aires, Argentina
290: Treatment of Pyogenic Vertebral Spondylodiscitis

Jennifer Moliterno Gunel, MD
Assistant Professor of Neurosurgery
Yale School of Medicine
New Haven, Connecticut
139: Unusual Gliomas

Murat Günel, MD, FACS, FAHA
Nixdorff-German Professor of Neurosurgery
Professor of Genetics and of Neuroscience
Co-Director, Yale Program on Neurogenetics
Director, Neurovascular Surgery
Department of Neurosurgery
Yale School of Medicine
New Haven, Connecticut
376: Genetics of Intracranial Aneurysms
410: Genetics of Cerebral Cavernous Malformations

Nalin Gupta, MD, PhD
Professor
Departments of Neurological Surgery and Pediatrics
University of California, San Francisco;
Chief, Division of Pediatric Neurosurgery
UCSF Benioff Children's Hospital
San Francisco, California
209: Choroid Plexus Tumors

Georges F. Haddad, MD, FRCS(C)
Clinical Associate Professor of Neurosurgery
Department of Surgery
American University of Beirut
Beirut, Lebanon
147: Meningiomas

Michael M. Haglund, MD, PhD
Professor of Neurosurgery, Neurobiology, and Global Health
Department of Neurosurgery
Duke University School of Medicine
Durham, North Carolina
7: Coagulation for the Neurosurgeon
Overview and Future Opportunities (Basic Science)
69: Motor, Sensory, and Language Mapping and Monitoring for Cortical Resections

Stephen J. Haines, MD
Lyle A. French Chair
Professor and Head, Department of Neurosurgery
University of Minnesota School of Medicine
Minneapolis, Minnesota
38: The Use and Misuse of Antibiotics in Neurosurgery
57: Neurosurgical Epidemiology and Outcomes Assessment

Clayton L. Haldeman, MD, MHS
Resident Neurosurgeon
University of Wisconsin Hospitals and Clinics
Madison, Wisconsin
307: Treatment of Cervicothoracic Junction Injuries

Kyle G. Halvorson, MD
Chief Resident
Department of Neurosurgery
Duke University Medical Center
Durham, North Carolina
214: Cerebellar Astrocytomas

Marla J. Hamberger, PhD
Professor of Neuropsychology
Department of Neurology
Columbia University Medical Center
New York, New York
68: Wada Testing

Ihtsham U. Haq, MD
Associate Professor of Neurology
Wake Forest School of Medicine
Winston-Salem, North Carolina
84: Clinical Overview of Movement Disorders

Neil Haranhalli, MD
Resident Neurosurgeon
Albert Einstein College of Medicine
Montefiore Medical Center
Bronx, New York
236: Intraspinal Tumors in Children

Robert E. Harbaugh, MD, FAANS, FACS, FAHA
Director, Penn State Neuroscience Institute
Distinguished Professor and Chair, Department of Neurosurgery
Professor, Department of Engineering Science and Mechanics
Penn State Milton S. Hershey Medical Center
Hershey, Pennsylvania
365: The Natural History and Medical Management of Carotid Occlusive Disease

Marwan Hariz, MD, PhD
Simon Sainsbury Chair of Functional Neurosurgery
University College London Institute of Neurology;
Consultant Neurosurgeon
National Hospital for Neurology and Neurosurgery
London, United Kingdom;
Adjunct Professor of Stereotactic Neurosurgery
Department of Clinical Neuroscience
Umeå University
Umeå, Sweden
87: Surgical Management of Tremor

Mark R. Harrigan, MD
Associate Professor of Neurosurgery
Department of Neurosurgery
University of Alabama at Birmingham
Birmingham, Alabama
368: Blunt Cerebrovascular Injury

James S. Harrop, MD
Professor of Neurological Surgery and Orthopedics
Sidney Kimmel Medical College at Thomas Jefferson University
Section Chief, Division of Spine and Peripheral Nerve Disorders
Thomas Jefferson University Hospital
Philadelphia, Pennsylvania
309: Evaluation, Classification, and Treatment of Thoracolumbar Spine Injuries

Roger Härtl, MD
Professor of Neurological Surgery
Weill Cornell Medical College
New York–Presbyterian Hospital
New York, New York
329: Posterior Thoracic and Lumbar Instrumentation with Historical Overview
335: Minimally Invasive Techniques for Degenerative Disease

Daniel M. Harwell, MD
Resident Neurosurgeon
University of Cincinnati College of Medicine
Mayfield Clinic
Cincinnati, Ohio
131: Risks of Intrinsic Brain Tumor Surgery and Avoidance of Complications

David M. Hasan, MD
Associate Professor of Neurosurgery
University of Iowa Carver College of Medicine
Iowa City, Iowa
377: The Natural History of Cerebral Aneurysms

Rowshanak Hashemiyoon, PhD
Chief, Laboratory for Behavioral Neurophysiology and Computational Neuroscience
Department of Stereotactic and Functional Neurosurgery
University Hospital of Cologne
Cologne, Germany
99: Surgery for Tourette's Syndrome

Wael Hassaneen, MD, MSc, PhD
Neurosurgery Resident
Loyola University Medical Center
Maywood, Illinois
152: Epidermoid, Dermoid, and Neurenteric Cysts

Gregory W.J. Hawryluk, MD, PhD, FRCSC
Assistant Professor of Neurosurgery
Adjunct Assistant Professor of Neurology
Director of Neurosurgical Critical Care
University of Utah School of Medicine
Salt Lake City, Utah
277: Pathophysiology and Treatment of Spinal Cord Injury
341: Neurochemical Pathomechanisms in Traumatic Brain Injury

Richard David Hayward, MBBS, FRCS (Eng)
Professor
Department of Paediatric Neurosurgery
Great Ormond Street Hospital for Children
London, United Kingdom
Overview and Controversies (Pediatrics)

Lucy He, MD
Neurosurgery Resident
Vanderbilt University Medical Center
Nashville, Tennessee
232: Tethered Spinal Cord: Fatty Filum Terminale, Meningocele Manqué, and Dermal Sinus Tracts

Andrew T. Healy, MD
Resident Neurosurgeon
Cleveland Clinic
Cleveland, Ohio
117: Delivery of Therapy to Brain Tumors: Problems and Potentials

Robert F. Heary, MD
Professor of Neurosurgery
Rutgers New Jersey Medical School;
Director, Spine Center of New Jersey
Newark, New Jersey
334: Evaluation, Indications, and Techniques of Revision Spine Surgery

Amy B. Heimberger, MD
Professor of Neurosurgery
University of Texas MD Anderson Cancer Center
Houston, Texas
111: Brain Tumor Immunology and Immunotherapy

Paul F. Heini, Prof. Dr. med.
Spine Unit
Department of Orthopedic Surgery and Traumatology of the Musculoskeletal System
Sonnenhofspital
Bern, Switzerland
310: Evaluation and Treatment of Osteoporotic Fractures (Cement Augmentation)

Mary M. Heinricher, PhD
Professor
Departments of Neurological Surgery and Behavioral Neuroscience
Oregon Health & Science University
Portland, Oregon
166: Anatomy and Physiology of Pain

Karl J. Henrikson, MD
Resident Orthopaedic Neurosurgeon
University of Pittsburgh School of Medicine
Pittsburgh, Pennsylvania
276: Disk Degeneration and Regeneration

Roberto C. Heros, MD
Professor
Department of Neurosurgery
University of Miami
Miami, Florida
405: Microsurgery of Arteriovenous Malformations

Karl Herrup, PhD
Chair Professor and Head
Division of Life Science
Hong Kong University of Science and Technology
Clear Water Bay, Hong Kong
48: Neurons and Neuroglia

Shawn Hervey-Jumper, MD
Assistant Professor of Neurological Surgery
University of Michigan Medical School
Ann Arbor, Michigan
140: Primitive Neuroectodermal Tumors

Gregory G. Heuer, MD, PhD
Assistant Professor of Neurosurgery
Perelman School of Medicine at the University of Pennsylvania
Children's Hospital of Philadelphia
Philadelphia, Pennsylvania
60: Malformations of Cortical Development
71: Intracranial Monitoring: Subdural Strip and Grid Recording

Yoshinori Higuchi, MD, PhD
Associate Professor of Neurological Surgery
Chiba University Graduate School of Medicine
Chiba, Japan
267: Radiosurgery for Malignant Intracranial Tumors

Holly S. Gilmer Hill, MD
Associate Professor of Neurosurgery
Oakland University William Beaumont School of Medicine;
Chief, Division of Pediatric Neurosurgery
Beaumont Hospital
Royal Oak, Michigan
251: Piriformis Syndrome, Obturator Internus Syndrome, Pudendal Nerve Entrapment, and Other Pelvic Entrapments

Lawrence J. Hirsch, MD
Professor
Department of Neurology
Chief, Division of Epilepsy/EEG
Comprehensive Epilepsy Center
Yale School of Medicine
New Haven, Connecticut
61: Diagnosis and Classification of Seizures and Epilepsy

S. Alan Hoffer, MD
Assistant Professor of Neurological Surgery
Case Western Reserve University School of Medicine
University Hospitals Case Medical Center
Cleveland, Ohio
362: Intraoperative Cerebral Protection

Eric Holland, MD, PhD
Professor of Neurological Surgery
Director, Alvord Brain Tumor Center
University of Washington School of Medicine;
Director, Human Biology
Director, Solid Tumor Translational Research
Fred Hutchenson Cancer Research Center
Seattle, Washington
113: Molecular Genetics and the Development of Targets for Glioma Therapy

Ryan Holland, MDc
Department of Neurological Surgery
Rutgers New Jersey Medical School
Newark, New Jersey
24: Brain Retraction

Kazuhiro Hongo, MD, PhD
Professor and Chair
Department of Neurosurgery
Shinshu University School of Medicine
Matsumoto, Japan
Overview and Controversies (Vascular)

Shiro Horisawa, MD
Tokyo Women's Medical University
Tokyo, Japan
97: Thalamotomy for Focal Hand Dystonia

Philip J. Horner, PhD
Scientific Director, Center for Neuroregenerative Medicine
Co-Director, Center for Regenerative and Restorative Neurosurgery
Houston Methodist Research Institute
Houston, Texas
47: Stem Cell Biology in the Central Nervous System

Clifford M. Houseman, DO
Clinical Assistant Professor
Department of Osteopathic Surgical Specialties
Faculty Neurosurgeon
Michigan State University College of Osteopathic Medicine
Southfield, Michigan
275: Spinal Biomechanics and Basics of Spinal Instrumentation

Matthew A. Howard III, MD
Professor and Chair
Department of Neurosurgery
University of Iowa Carver College of Medicine
Iowa City, Iowa
70: Investigation of Human Cognition in Epilepsy Surgery Patients

Brian Hsueh, AB
Departments of Bioengineering and Neuroscience
Stanford University
Stanford, California
45: Optogenetics and CLARITY

Judy Huang, MD, FAANS
Professor of Neurosurgery
Director, Neurosurgery Residency Program
Fellowship Director, Cerebrovascular Neurosurgery
Johns Hopkins University School of Medicine
Baltimore, Maryland
386: Microsurgery of Anterior Communicating Artery Aneurysms

Michael C. Huang, MD
Assistant Clinical Professor
Department of Neurological Surgery
University of California, San Francisco
San Francisco, California
15: Intracranial Pressure Monitoring Overview and Controversies (Trauma)
351: Surgical Management of Traumatic Brain Injury

Raymond Y. Huang, MD, PhD
Instructor
Department of Radiology
Harvard Medical School
Brigham and Women's Hospital
Boston, Massachusetts
121: Radiologic Features of Central Nervous System Tumors

Eric Hudgins, MD, PhD
Resident Neurosurgeon
Hospital of the University of Pennsylvania
Philadelphia, Pennsylvania
348: Initial Resuscitation, Prehospital Care, and Emergency Room Care in Traumatic Brain Injury

Matthew A. Hunt, MD
Associate Professor
Department of Neurosurgery
University of Minnesota School of Medicine
Minneapolis, Minnesota
38: The Use and Misuse of Antibiotics in Neurosurgery

R. John Hurlbert, MD, PhD, FRCSC, FACS
Associate Professor of Clinical Neurosciences
University of Calgary Faculty of Medicine
Calgary, Alberta, Canada
281: Nonsurgical and Postsurgical Management of Low Back Pain

Peter J. Hutchinson, MBBS, PhD, FRCS (Surg Neurol)
Professor of Neurosurgery and NIHR Research Professor
Division of Neurosurgery, Department of Clinical Neurosciences
University of Cambridge
Addenbrooke's Hospital
Cambridge, United Kingdom
34: Medical and Surgical Management of Chronic Subdural Hematomas
Overview and Controversies (Trauma)

Anita Huttner, MD
Assistant Professor of Pathology
Yale School of Medicine
New Haven, Connecticut
139: Unusual Gliomas

Steven W. Hwang, MD
Assistant Professor of Neurosurgery
Chief, Pediatric Neurosurgery
Tufts University School of Medicine
Floating Hospital for Children at Tufts Medical Center
Boston, Massachusetts
237: Introduction to Spinal Deformities in Children
300: Adult Tethered Cord Syndrome
301: Adult Syringomyelia

Jeffrey J. Iliff, PhD
Assistant Professor of Anesthesiology and Perioperative Medicine
Oregon Health & Science University
Portland, Oregon
54: Extracellular Fluid Movement and Clearance in the Brain: The Glymphatic Pathway

Susan L. Ingram, PhD
Associate Professor
Department of Neurological Surgery
Oregon Health & Science University
Portland, Oregon
167: Molecular Basis of Nociception

Ioannis U. Isaias, MD
I.C.P. Parkinson Institute
Motion Analysis Laboratory
Department of Human Physiology
University of Milan
Milan, Italy
85: Patient Selection Criteria for Deep Brain Stimulation in Movement Disorders

Bermans J. Iskandar, MD
Professor of Neurosurgery and Pediatrics
Director, Pediatric Neurosurgery
University of Wisconsin School of Medicine and Public Health
Madison, Wisconsin
230: Lipomyelomeningocele

Aditya K. Iyer, MD, MEng
Resident Neurosurgeon
Stanford School of Medicine
Stanford, California
272: Radiosurgery for Benign Spine Tumors and Vascular Malformations

R. Patrick Jacob, MD, FACS
Chief, Neurosurgery Section
Malcolm Randall VA Hospital;
Adjunct Professor of Neurosurgery
University of Florida School of Medicine
Gainesville, Florida
279: Bone Metabolism and Osteoporosis

Ajit Jada, MD
Resident Neurosurgeon
Albert Einstein College of Medicine
Montefiore Medical Center
Bronx, New York
236: Intraspinal Tumors in Children

Ashutosh P. Jadhav, MD, PhD
Assistant Professor
Departments of Neurology and Neurological Surgery
University of Pittsburgh School of Medicine
Pittsburgh, Pennsylvania
361: Acute Surgical and Endovascular Management of Ischemic and Hemorrhagic Stroke

Hayder Jaffer, MD
Fellow in Pediatric Neurosurgery
Department of Neurosurgery
Cleveland Clinic Lerner School of Medicine of Case Western Reserve University
Cleveland, Ohio
199: Cerebrospinal Fluid Disorders and Transitional Neurosurgery

Regina I. Jakacki, MD
AstraZeneca
Gaithersburg, Maryland
216: Intracranial Germ Cell Tumors

George I. Jallo, MD
Professor of Neurosurgery, Pediatrics, and Oncology
Johns Hopkins University School of Medicine
Baltimore, Maryland
234: Achondroplasia and Other Dwarfisms

Jack I. Jallo, MD, PhD
Professor of Neurosurgery
Thomas Jefferson University and Hospitals
Philadelphia, Pennsylvania
17: The Neurosurgical Intensive Care Unit and the Unique Role of the Neurosurgeon

Osama Jamil, MD
Resident
Department of Neurosurgery
University of Utah School of Medicine
University of Utah Medical Center and Primary Children's Medical Center
Salt Lake City, Utah
197: Hydrocephalus in Children: Etiology and Overall Management

John A. Jane, Jr., MD
Professor of Neurosurgery and Pediatrics
Neurosurgery Residency Program Director
University of Virginia School of Medicine
Charlottesville, Virginia
193: Nonsyndromic Craniosynostosis: Introduction and Single-Suture Synostosis

John A. Jane, Sr., MD, PhD[†]
Professor of Neurosurgery
University of Virginia School of Medicine
Charlottesville, Virginia
193: Nonsyndromic Craniosynostosis: Introduction and Single-Suture Synostosis

Damir Janigro, PhD
Scientific Director
Flocel, Inc.;
Professor
Case Western Reserve University
Cleveland, Ohio
51: The Blood-Brain Barrier
58: Electrophysiologic Properties of the Mammalian Central Nervous System

Brian T. Jankowitz, MD
Assistant Professor of Neurosurgery
University of Pittsburgh School of Medicine
Pittsburgh, Pennsylvania
361: Acute Surgical and Endovascular Management of Ischemic and Hemorrhagic Stroke

Andrew H. Jea, MD
Professor and Chief of Pediatric Neurosurgery
Indiana University School of Medicine;
Goodman Campbell Brain and Spine
Fellowship Program Director
Riley Hospital for Children
Indianapolis, Indiana
Overview and Controversies (Pediatrics)

Owase Jeelani, MBBS, MBA, MPhil, FRCS(NeuroSurg)
Consultant Paediatric Neurosurgeon
Head of Clinical Services
Department of Neurosurgery
Great Ormond Street Hospital
London, United Kingdom
208: Thalamic Tumors

[†]Deceased.

Lara Jehi, MD
Epilepsy Center
Associate Program Director
Clinical Research Unit
Cleveland Clinic Lerner School of Medicine
Cleveland, Ohio
80: Epilepsy Surgery: Outcome and Complications

Kurt A. Jellinger, MD
Director
Institute of Clinical Neurobiology
Vienna, Austria
83: Neuropathology of Movement Disorders

Diana Jho, MD, MS
Department of Neurosurgery
Allegheny Health Network
Pittsburgh, Pennsylvania
107: Deep Brain Stimulation for Obesity

David F. Jimenez, MD, FACS
Professor and Chair
Department of Neurosurgery
The University of Texas at San Antonio Health Science Center
San Antonio, Texas
195: Endoscopic Treatment of Craniosynostosis

Jasmin T. Jo, MD
Fellow, Division of Neuro-Oncology
Dana-Farber Cancer Institute
Massachusetts General Hospital
Boston, Massachusetts
125: Principles of Chemotherapy

Conrad E. Johanson, PhD
Professor Emeritus of Neurosurgery
Alpert Medical School at Brown University
Providence, Rhode Island
29: Production and Flow of Cerebrospinal Fluid

Luke A. Johnson, PhD
Postdoctoral Associate
Department of Neurology
University of Minnesota Medical School
Minneapolis, Minnesota
91: Deep Brain Stimulation: Mechanisms of Action

Adrian C. Jones, MB, ChB, DM, FRCP
Physician
Rheumatology Unit
Queen's Medical Centre
Nottingham University Hospitals NHS Trust
Nottingham, United Kingdom
297: Assessment and Treatment of Rheumatoid Arthritis and Inflammatory Spinal Diseases

Kristen E. Jones, MD
Adjunct Assistant Professor
Department of Neurosurgery
University of Minnesota School of Medicine
Minneapolis, Minnesota
38: The Use and Misuse of Antibiotics in Neurosurgery

Jacob R. Joseph, MD
House Officer
Department of Neurosurgery
University of Michigan
Ann Arbor, Michigan
288: Evaluation and Treatment of Degenerative Lumbar Spondylolisthesis
313: Evaluation and Treatment of Cervical Deformity

Tudor G. Jovin, MD
Professor
Departments of Neurology and Neurological Surgery
Director, Stroke Institute and Neuroendovascular Therapy
University of Pittsburgh School of Medicine
Pittsburgh, Pennsylvania
361: Acute Surgical and Endovascular Management of Ischemic and Hemorrhagic Stroke

M. Yashar S. Kalani, MD, PhD
Assistant Professor
Department of Neurosurgery
Barrow Neurological Institute
St. Joseph's Hospital and Medical Center
Phoenix, Arizona
222: Pediatric Cerebral Aneurysms
409: Natural History of Cavernous Malformations

Paul S.A. Kalanithi, MD†
Department of Neurosurgery
Stanford University
Stanford, California
45: Optogenetics and CLARITY

Iain H. Kalfas, MD, FACS
Head, Section of Spinal Surgery
Department of Neurosurgery
Cleveland Clinic
Cleveland, Ohio
331: Image-Guided Spinal Navigation: Principles and Clinical Applications

Aleksandrs Uldis Kalnins, MD, MBA
Neuroradiology Fellow
Department of Radiology
Stanford University
Stanford, California
11: Computed Tomography and Magnetic Resonance Imaging of the Brain

Ricky Raj Singh Kalra, MD
Neurosurgery Resident
Department of Neurological Surgery
University of Utah School of Medicine
Salt Lake City, Utah
27: Thorascopic Spine Surgery

Ashwin A. Kamath, MD
Resident Neurosurgeon
Washington University School of Medicine in St. Louis;
Barnes-Jewish Hospital;
St. Louis Children's Hospital
St. Louis, Missouri
227: Neonatal Brain Injury

†Deceased.

Daniel G. Kang, MD
Assistant Professor of Orthopedic Surgery
Madigan Army Medical Center
Tacoma, Washington
314: Evaluation and Treatment of Adolescent Idiopathic Scoliosis

James D. Kang, MD
Professor of Orthopaedic Surgery
UPMC Endowed Chair in Spine Surgery
Harvard Medical School;
Chairman, Department of Orthopaedic Surgery
Brigham and Women's Hospital
Boston, Massachusetts
276: Disk Degeneration and Regeneration

Adam S. Kanter, MD, FAANS
Associate Professor of Neurological Surgery
Chief, Division of Spine Surgery
Director, Minimally Invasive Spine Program
Director, Neurosurgical Spine Fellowship Program
University of Pittsburgh Medical Center
Pittsburgh, Pennsylvania
308: Transient Quadriparesis and Athletic Injuries of the Cervical Spine
332: Sacropelvic Fixation: Anterior and Posterior Options

Michael G. Kaplitt, MD, PhD
Associate Professor of Neurological Surgery
Vice Chairman for Research
Director of Stereotactic and Functional Neurosurgery
Weill Cornell Medical College
New York, New York
94: Emerging and Experimental Neurosurgical Treatments for Parkinson's Disease

Reza J. Karimi, MD
Attending Neurosurgeon
Neurosurgery
Hackensack University Medical Center
Hackensack, New Jersey
334: Evaluation, Indications, and Techniques of Revision Spine Surgery

Manish K. Kasliwal, MD, MCh
Assistant Professor of Neurosurgery
University Hospitals Case Medical Center
Case Western Reserve University
Cleveland, Ohio
319: Treatment of High-Grade Spondylolisthesis

Hiroto Kawasaki, MD
Associate Professor of Neurosurgery
University of Iowa Carver College of Medicine
Iowa City, Iowa
70: Investigation of Human Cognition in Epilepsy Surgery Patients

John Paul Kelleher, MD
Assistant Professor of Neurosurgery
Pennsylvania State University School of Medicine
Penn State Milton S. Hershey Medical Center
Hershey, Pennsylvania
238: Thoracolumbar Spinal Disorders in Pediatric Patients
317: Evaluation and Treatment of Adult Scoliosis and Sagittal Plane Deformity

Christopher P. Kellner, MD
Fellow in Endovascular Neurosurgery
Icahn School of Medicine at Mount Sinai
New York, New York
394: Endovascular Hunterian Ligation
404: Endovascular Management of Arteriovenous Malformations for Cure

Andras A. Kemeny, MD, FRCS
Consultant Neurosurgeon
National Centre for Stereotactic Radiosurgery
Royal Hallamshire Hospital
Sheffield, United Kingdom
269: Radiosurgery of Intracranial Vascular Malformations

Benjamin C. Kennedy, MD
Resident Neurosurgeon
Columbia University College of Physicians and Surgeons
New York, New York
235: Surgical Management of the Pediatric Subaxial Cervical Spine

John R.W. Kestle, MD, FACS
Professor of Neurosurgery
Division of Pediatric Neurosurgery
University of Utah School of Medicine
Salt Lake City, Utah
197: Hydrocephalus in Children: Etiology and Overall Management

Imad Saeed Khan, MD
Resident
Department of Neurosurgery
Geisel School of Medicine at Dartmouth
Hanover, New Hampshire
16: Principles of Neurocritical Care

Nadia Khan, MD
Professor of Neurosurgery
Division of Pediatric Neurosurgery
Head, Moyamoya Center
University Children's Hospital
Zurich, Switzerland;
Consultant, Moyamoya and Revascularisation Surgery
Department of Neurosurgery
University Hospital Tübingen
Tübingen, Germany
373: Adult Moyamoya Disease

Vini G. Khurana, BScMed, MBBS, PhD, FRACS
Director, CNS Neurosurgery
Sydney, Australia
359: Cerebral Blood Flow and Metabolism and Cerebral Ischemia

Dong Gyu Kim, MD, PhD
Professor
Department of Neurosurgery
Seoul National University College of Medicine
Seoul National University Hospital
Seoul, Republic of Korea
Overview and Controversies (Radiation)
270: Radiosurgery for Functional Disorders

Dong H. Kim, MD
Professor and Chairman
Vivian L. Smith Department of Neurosurgery
The University of Texas at Houston
Houston, Texas
378: Pathobiology of Intracranial Aneurysms

Irene Kim, MD
New York University School of Medicine
NYU Langone Medical Center
New York, New York
20: Positioning for Cranial Surgery
151: Craniopharyngiomas in Adults
210: Pediatric Craniopharyngiomas

Jin Wook Kim, MD, PhD
Assistant Professor
Department of Neurosurgery
Seoul National University Hospital
Seoul, Republic of Korea
270: Radiosurgery for Functional Disorders

Louis J. Kim, MD
Professor
Department of Neurological Surgery
University of Washington School of Medicine
Seattle, Washington
412: Classification of Spinal Arteriovenous Lesions

Paul K. Kim, MD
Carolina Neurosurgery and Spine Associates
Charlotte, North Carolina
330: Posterior, Transforaminal, and Anterior Lumbar Interbody Fusion: Techniques and Instrumentation

Thomas Aquinas Kim, MD, MBA
Medical Director of Neuroimaging
Bronson Healthcare Group
Kalamazoo, Michigan;
Neuroradiologist
Advanced Radiology Services
Kalamazoo and Grand Rapids, Michigan
11: Computed Tomography and Magnetic Resonance Imaging of the Brain

Wolff Kirsch, MD
Professor of Neurological Surgery and Biochemistry
Director, Neurosurgery Center for Research, Training, and Education
Loma Linda University School of Medicine
Loma Linda, California
7: Coagulation for the Neurosurgeon

Neil D. Kitchen, MD, FRCS
Neurosurgeon
Victor Horsley Department of Neurosurgery
The National Hospital for Neurology and Neurosurgery
London, United Kingdom
400: Pathobiology of True Arteriovenous Malformations

James P. Klaas, MD
Assistant Professor of Neurology
Mayo Clinic
Rochester, Minnesota
359: Cerebral Blood Flow and Metabolism and Cerebral Ischemia

Joshua P. Klein, MD, PhD, FANA, FAAN
Associate Professor
Departments of Neurology and Radiology
Harvard Medical School;
Chief, Division of Hospital Neurology
Department of Neurology
Brigham and Women's Hospital
Boston, Massachusetts
165: Sarcoidosis, Tuberculosis, and Demyelinating Disease

Michel Kliot, MD, MA
Professor and Interim Chair
Department of Neurological Surgery
Director, Peripheral Nerve Center
Northwestern University Feinberg School of Medicine
Chicago, Illinois
3: Surgical Anatomy of the Skull Base
Overview and Future Opportunities (Basic Science)
50: Cellular and Molecular Responses in the Peripheral and Central Nervous Systems: Similarities and Differences

John J. Knightly, MD
Director of Neurosurgery
Morristown Memorial Hospital;
Atlantic Neurosurgical Specialists
Morristown, New Jersey
283: Evaluation and Treatment of Cervical Disk Herniations

Jared Knopman, MD
Assistant Professor of Neurological Surgery
New York–Presbyterian Hospital/Weill Cornell Medical Center
New York, New York
366: Carotid Endarterectomy

Andrew L. Ko, MD
Assistant Professor of Neurosurgery
University of Washington School of Medicine
Seattle, Washington
172: Percutaneous Procedures for Trigeminal Neuralgia

John D. Koerner, MD
Orthopaedic Spine Surgeon
Hackensack University Medical Center
Hackensack, New Jersey
306: Evaluation, Classification, and Treatment of Cervical (C3-C7) Injuries

Malgosia A. Kokoszka, PhD
Assistant Professor
Neurosurgery
Mount Sinai Health System
New York, New York
240: Pediatric Epilepsy Surgery

Angelos G. Kolias, BM, MSc, MRCS
Academic Clinical Registrar in Neurosurgery
Division of Neurosurgery, Department of Clinical Neurosciences
University of Cambridge
Addenbrooke's Hospital
Cambridge, United Kingdom
34: Medical and Surgical Management of Chronic Subdural Hematomas
Overview and Controversies (Trauma)

Miikka Korja, MD
Associate Professor
Department of Neurosurgery
Helsinki University Central Hospital
Helsinki, Finland
402: Therapeutic Decision Making in the Management of Arteriovenous Malformations of the Brain

Thomas Kosztowski, MD
Resident Neurosurgeon
Johns Hopkins Hospital
Baltimore, Maryland
123: Brain Tumors during Pregnancy

Joachim K. Krauss, Prof. Dr. med.
Chairman and Director
Department of Neurosurgery
Medical School Hannover, MHH
Hannover, Germany
Overview and Controversies (Functional)
96: Selective Peripheral Denervation for Cervical Dystonia

Chandan Krishna, MD
Department of Neurosurgery
Mayo Clinic
Scottsdale, Arizona
367: Carotid Artery Angioplasty and Stenting

Vibhor Krishna, MD
Assistant Professor of Neurosurgery
Center for Neuromodulation
The Ohio State University Wexner Medical Center
Columbus, Ohio
108: Deep Brain Stimulation for Alzheimer's Disease

Ajit A. Krishnaney, MD
Staff Surgeon
Department of Neurosurgery
Cleveland Clinic
Cleveland, Ohio
12: Radiology of the Spine

Pieter L. Kubben, MD, PhD
Neurosurgeon
Department of Neurosurgery
Maastricht University Medical Center
Maastricht, The Netherlands
135: Intraoperative Magnetic Resonance Imaging

Jens Kuhn, MD
Professor
Department of Psychiatry and Psychotherapy
University Hospital of Cologne
Cologne, Germany
99: Surgery for Tourette's Syndrome

Abhaya V. Kulkarni, MD, PhD, FRCSC
Associate Professor of Neurosurgery
Department of Surgery
University of Toronto Faculty of Medicine
The Hospital for Sick Children
Toronto, Ontario, Canada
201: Ventricular Shunting Procedures

Gomatam R. Vijay Kumar, MBBS, FRCS(Eng), FRCS(Neurosurgery)
Head of Neurosurgery
AMRI Hospitals
Salt Lake, Kolkata, India
291: Evaluation and Treatment of Fungal and Tubercular Infections of the Spine

Charles Kuntz IV, MD[†]
Professor and Vice Chairman
Department of Neurosurgery
University of Cincinnati College of Medicine;
Director, Division of Spine and Peripheral Nerve Surgery
Mayfield Clinic
Cincinnati, Ohio
Overview and Controversies (Spine)
280: Differential Diagnosis of Spinal Disease
312: Evaluation of Spinal Alignment

Jeffrey V. Kuo, MD
Professor of Radiation Oncology
University of California, Irvine
UC Irvine Medical Center
Orange, California
261: General and Historical Considerations of Radiotherapy and Radiosurgery

Kenny Kwan, BMBCh(Oxon), FRCSEd(Orth), FHKCOS, FHKAM(Orth)
Clinical Assistant Professor and Honorary Associate Consultant
Department of Orthopaedics and Traumatology
Queen Mary Hospital
The University of Hong Kong
Hong Kong
327: Anterior Thoracic Instrumentation

Frank La Marca, MD
Clinical Assistant Professor
Department of Neurosurgery
University of Michigan
Ann Arbor, Michigan
313: Evaluation and Treatment of Cervical Deformity

Nadia N. Issa Laack, MD, MS
Assistant Professor of Radiation Oncology
Mayo Clinic
Rochester, Minnesota
266: Fractionated Radiotherapy for Spine Tumors

Alim M. Ladha, MD
Department of Neurological Surgery
Midland Memorial Hospital
Odessa, Texas
148: Meningeal Sarcomas and Hemangiopericytomas

Virginie Lafage, PhD
Director, Spine Research
Hospital for Special Surgery
New York, New York
311: Classification of Spinal Deformity

Arthur M. Lam, MD, FRCPC, FNCS
Clinical Professor of Anesthesia and Pain Medicine
University of Washington School of Medicine;
Medical Director, Neuroanesthesia and Neurocritical Care
Swedish Neuroscience Institute
Swedish Medical Center
Seattle, Washington
5: Neuroanesthesia: Preoperative Evaluation

Tariq Lamki, MD
Fellow in Skull Base Neurosurgery and Radiosurgery
Department of Neurological Surgery
The Ohio State University Wexner Medical Center
Columbus, Ohio
154: Overview of Skull Base Tumors

Frederick F. Lang, MD
Professor of Neurosurgery
University of Texas MD Anderson Cancer Center
Houston, Texas
146: Metastatic Brain Tumors

Giuseppe Lanzino, MD
Professor of Neurological Surgery and Radiology
Department of Neurological Surgery
Mayo Clinic
Rochester, Minnesota
398: Multimodality Treatments of Cerebrovascular Disorders
407: Carotid-Cavernous Fistulas

[†]Deceased.

Paul Larson, MD
Associate Professor and Vice Chair
Department of Neurological Surgery
University of California, San Francisco
San Francisco, California
89: Deep Brain Stimulation for Parkinson's Disease

Catherine Y. Lau, MD
Assistant Clinical Professor
Department of Medicine
University of California, San Francisco
San Francisco, California
4: Improving Patient Safety

Darryl Lau, MD
Resident Neurosurgeon
University of California, San Francisco
San Francisco, California
315: Evaluation and Treatment of Scheuermann's Kyphosis

Sean D. Lavine, MD
Associate Professor of Neurological Surgery
Columbia University College of Physicians and Surgeons
New York, New York
394: Endovascular Hunterian Ligation

Sean E. Lawler, PhD
Assistant Professor of Neurosurgery
Harvard Medical School
Brigham and Women's Hospital
Boston, Massachusetts
115: Malignant Glioma Microenvironment

Edward R. Laws, Jr., MD
Professor of Neurosurgery
Harvard Medical School
Brigham and Women's Hospital
Boston, Massachusetts
150: Pituitary Tumors: Functioning and Nonfunctioning

Michael T. Lawton, MD
Professor in Residence, Vice-Chairman, and Tong Po Kan Endowed Chair
Department of Neurological Surgery
Chief, Cerebrovascular and Skull Base Surgery Programs
Director, Cerebrovascular Disorders Program
Principal Investigator, Center for Cerebrovascular Research
University of California, San Francisco
San Francisco, California
3: Surgical Anatomy of the Skull Base Overview and Controversies (Vascular)
395: Microsurgical Management of Giant Intracranial Aneurysms

Nealen G. Laxpati, MD, PhD
Department of Neurosurgery
Emory University School of Medicine;
Coulter Department of Biomedical Engineering
Georgia Institute of Technology
Atlanta, Georgia
79: Electrical Stimulation for Epilepsy (VNS, DBS, and RNS)

Joash T. Lazarus, MD
Movement Disorder Fellow
Department of Neurology
Emory University School of Medicine
Atlanta, Georgia
88: Ablative Procedures for Parkinson's Disease

Peter D. Le Roux, MD, FACS
Professor of Neurosurgery
Sidney Kimmel Medical College
Thomas Jefferson University
Philadelphia, Pennsylvania;
Co-Director, Brain and Spine Center
Lankenau Medical Center
Wynnewood, Pennsylvania
350: Physiologic Monitoring for Traumatic Brain Injury
379: Surgical Decision Making for the Treatment of Intracranial Aneurysms

Brett D. Lebed, MD
Attending Urologist
Department of Urologic Surgery
Urologic Associates of San Luis Obispo
San Luis Obispo, California
10: Neurourology

Cheng-Chia Lee, MD
Attending Physician and Clinical Lecturer
Department of Neurosurgery
Neurological Institute, Taipei Veterans General Hospital
Taipei, Taiwan;
Department of Surgery
Hsinchu Branch
Taipei Veterans General Hospital
Hsinchu, Taiwan
264: Radiosurgery Technique

Sangmi Lee, PhD
Research Scientist
Department of Neurological Surgery
Brain and Spinal Injury Center
University of California, San Francisco School of Medicine
San Francisco, California
339: Animal Models of Traumatic Brain Injury

Young M. Lee, MD
Department of Neurological Surgery
University of California, San Francisco
San Francisco, California
360: Acute Medical Management of Ischemic and Hemorrhagic Stroke
372: Endovascular Management of Intracranial Occlusion Disease

Ronald A. Lehman, Jr., MD
Professor of Orthopaedic Surgery
Columbia University College of Physicians and Surgeons
Chief, Degenerative and Minimally Invasive Spine Surgery
Director, Robotic Spine Surgery
Director, Athletes Spine Center
Co-Director, Spine Fellowship
Director, Clinical Spine Research
Co-Director, Orthopaedic Clinical Research
Advanced Pediatric and Adult Deformity Service
Columbia University Medical Center
New York, New York
314: Evaluation and Treatment of Adolescent Idiopathic Scoliosis

Lawrence G. Lenke, MD
Professor of Orthopaedic Surgery
Columbia University Medical Center;
Surgeon-in-Chief
The Spine Hospital at New York-Presbyterian/The Allen Hospital
Chief, Spine Division
Department of Orthopaedic Surgery
Chief, Spinal Deformity Surgery
Co-Director, Adult and Pediatric Comprehensive Spine Fellowship
New York, New York
314: Evaluation and Treatment of Adolescent Idiopathic Scoliosis

Eric C. Leuthardt, MD
Associate Professor
Departments of Neurosurgery, Biomedical Engineering, and Mechanical Engineering and Materials Science
Director, Center for Innovation in Neuroscience and Technology
Washington University School of Medicine in St. Louis
St. Louis, Missouri
109: Neuroprosthetics

Emily Lehmann Levin, MD
Assistant Professor of Neurosurgery
University of Michigan
Ann Arbor, Michigan
178: Spinal Cord Stimulation

Michael R. Levitt, MD
Assistant Professor
Department of Neurological Surgery
University of Washington
Assistant Professor
Department of Radiology
University of Washington
Adjunct Assistant Professor
Department of Mechanical Engineering
University of Washington
Seattle, Washington
392: Endovascular Approaches to Wide-Necked Intracranial Aneurysms

Evan M. Lewis, MD
Resident Neurosurgeon
University of Maryland School of Medicine
Baltimore, Maryland
282: Complication Avoidance in Spine Surgery

Dianyou Li, MD, PhD
Department of Stereotactic and Functional Neurosurgery
Shanghai Jiao Tong University
Rui Jin Hospital
Shanghai, China
102: Surgery for Anorexia Nervosa

Lydia J. Liang, BA
Research Assistant
Department of Neurosurgery
Johns Hopkins University School of Medicine
Baltimore, Maryland
155: Chordomas and Chondrosarcomas

Jason Liauw, MD
Resident Neurosurgeon
Johns Hopkins University School of Medicine
Baltimore, Maryland
128: Frame and Frameless Stereotactic Brain Biopsy

Roger Lichtenbaum, MD
Assistant Professor
Department of Neurosurgery
University of Illinois at Chicago
Chicago, Illinois
364: Neurovascular Imaging

David D. Limbrick, Jr., MD, PhD
Associate Professor
Chief, Division of Pediatric Neurosurgery
Departments of Neurological Surgery and Pediatrics
Washington University School of Medicine in St. Louis
St. Louis Children's Hospital
St. Louis, Missouri
200: Experimental Hydrocephalus
227: Neonatal Brain Injury

Kant Y. Lin, MD
Professor of Plastic Surgery and Pediatrics
University of Virginia School of Medicine
Charlottesville, Virginia
193: Nonsyndromic Craniosynostosis: Introduction and Single-Suture Synostosis

Hester F. Lingsma, PhD
Assistant Professor
Department of Public Health
Erasmus MC, University Medical Center
Rotterdam, The Netherlands
356: Prognosis after Traumatic Brain Injury

Mark E. Linskey, MD
Professor of Neurological Surgery
University of California, Irvine
UC Irvine Medical Center
Orange, California
171: Trigeminal Neuralgia: Diagnosis and Nonoperative Management
261: General and Historical Considerations of Radiotherapy and Radiosurgery

Nir Lipsman, MD, PhD
Resident Neurosurgeon
University of Toronto Faculty of Medicine
Toronto, Ontario, Canada
101: Surgery for Major Depressive Disorder
108: Deep Brain Stimulation for Alzheimer's Disease

Zachary N. Litvak, MD, MCR
Assistant Professor of Neurological Surgery and Surgery (Otolaryngology)
Director, Minimally Invasive Cranial Surgery
Co-Director, Endoscopic Pituitary and Skull Base Surgery Program
George Washington University
Washington, DC
231: Split Spinal Cord

James K. Liu, MD, FACS, FAANS
Associate Professor and Director
Center for Skull Base and Pituitary Surgery
Departments of Neurological Surgery and Otolaryngology-Head and Neck Surgery
Rutgers University New Jersey Medical School;
Neurological Institute of New Jersey
Newark, New Jersey
26: Advantages and Limitations of Cranial Endoscopy

Kenneth C. Liu, MD, FAANS
Associate Professor of Neurosurgery and Radiology
Co-Director, Cerebrovascular and Skull Base Surgery
Co-Director, University of Virginia Stroke Center
Department of Neurosurgery
University of Virginia
Charlottesville, Virginia
374: Cerebral Venous and Sinus Thrombosis

Wei Liu, MD, PhD
Department of Stereotactic and Functional Neurosurgery
Shanghai Jiao Tong University
Rui Jin Hospital
Shanghai, China
102: Surgery for Anorexia Nervosa

Karlo J. Lizarraga, MD, MS
Chief Resident
Neurology
Jackson Memorial Hospital/University of Miami Miller School of Medicine
Miami, Florida
14: Molecular Imaging of the Brain with Positron Emission Tomography

Robert M. Lober, MD, PhD
Assistant Clinical Professor of Pediatrics
Wright State University Boonshoft School of Medicine
Department of Pediatric Neurosurgery
Dayton Children's Hospital
Dayton, Ohio
214: Cerebellar Astrocytomas

Christopher M. Loftus, MD, Dr.h.c. (Hon.), FAANS
Professor and Chairman
Department of Neurosurgery
Loyola University Stritch School of Medicine
Maywood, Illinois
365: The Natural History and Medical Management of Carotid Occlusive Disease

Russell R. Lonser, MD
Professor and Chairman
Department of Neurological Surgery
The Ohio State University Wexner Medical Center
Columbus, Ohio
Overview and Controversies (Oncology)
119: Local Therapies for Gliomas
144: Hemangioblastomas

Angeliki Louvi, PhD
Associate Professor of Neurosurgery and of Neuroscience
Yale School of Medicine
New Haven, Connecticut
410: Genetics of Cerebral Cavernous Malformations

Andres M. Lozano, MD, PhD
Professor and Chairman
Division of Neurosurgery
University of Toronto Faculty of Medicine
Toronto, Ontario, Canada
Overview and Controversies (Functional)
101: Surgery for Major Depressive Disorder
108: Deep Brain Stimulation for Alzheimer's Disease

Mark G. Luciano, MD, PhD
Professor of Neurosurgery
Director, Cerebral Fluid Center
Johns Hopkins University School of Medicine
Baltimore, Maryland
199: Cerebrospinal Fluid Disorders and Transitional Neurosurgery

Rimas V. Lukas, MD
Associate Professor of Neurology
University of Chicago Pritzker School of Medicine
Chicago, Illinois
41: Acquired Immunodeficiency Syndrome

Teija Lund, MD, PhD
Helsinki University Hospital
Helsinki, Finland
287: Cervical, Thoracic, and Lumbar Stenosis

Lijun Ma, PhD
Professor of Radiation Oncology
University of California, San Francisco School of Medicine
San Francisco, California
262: Radiobiology of Radiotherapy and Radiosurgery

Tracy S. Ma, MD
Resident Neurosurgeon
Perelman School of Medicine at the University of Pennsylvania
Philadelphia, Pennsylvania
357: Traumatic Cerebrospinal Fluid Fistulas

Andrew I.R. Maas, MD, PhD
Professor and Chair
Department of Neurosurgery
University Hospital Antwerp and University of Antwerp
Antwerp, Belgium
Overview and Controversies (Trauma)
336: Epidemiology of Traumatic Brain Injury
356: Prognosis after Traumatic Brain Injury

R. Loch Macdonald, MD, PhD, FRCS(C), FACS, FAANS
Professor of Surgery and Keenan Endowed Chair in Surgery
Division of Neurosurgery
University of Toronto Faculty of Medicine;
Scientist, Labatt Family Centre of Excellence in Brain Injury and Trauma Research, Keenan Research Centre for Biomedical Science
St. Michael's Hospital
Toronto, Ontario, Canada
33: Pathophysiology of Chronic Subdural Hematomas
380: Perioperative Management of Subarachnoid Hemorrhage

Stephen C. Mack, PhD
Post-Doctoral Research Fellow
Cleveland Clinic Lerner Research Institute
Cleveland, Ohio
205: Genetics of Pediatric Brain Tumors

Lara S. MacLachlan, MD
Clinical Instructor
Department of Urology
Medical University of South Carolina
Charleston, South Carolina
10: Neurourology

Luke Macyszyn, MD, MA
Assistant Professor of Neurosurgery
Department of Neurosurgery
University of California, Los Angeles
Los Angeles, California
30: Clinical Evaluation of Adult Hydrocephalus

Jordan A. Magarik, MD, MS
Department of Neurological Surgery
Vanderbilt University Medical Center
Nashville, Tennessee
360: Acute Medical Management of Ischemic and Hemorrhagic Stroke
372: Endovascular Management of Intracranial Occlusion Disease

Dominic Maggio, MD, MBA
Resident Neurosurgeon
University of Virginia
Charlottesville, Virginia;
Physician
National Institute of Neurological Disorders and Stroke
National Institute of Health
Bethesda, Maryland
317: Evaluation and Treatment of Adult Scoliosis and Sagittal Plane Deformity

Pierre J. Magistretti, MD, PhD
Professor and Director
Brain Mind Institute
École Polytechnique Fédérale de Lausanne;
Director, Center for Psychiatric Neuroscience
Department of Psychiatry
Centre Hospitalier Universitaire Vaudois
Lausanne, Switzerland
Overview and Future Opportunities (Basic Science)
49: Cellular Mechanisms of Brain Energy Metabolism

Kelly B. Mahaney, MD, MS
Assistant Professor of Neurosurgery
University of Virginia School of Medicine
Charlottesville, Virginia
142: Medulloblastomas in Adults
213: Medulloblastomas

Cormac O. Maher, MD
Associate Professor of Neurosurgery
University of Michigan Medical School
Ann Arbor, Michigan
223: Pediatric Arteriovenous Malformations

Ramin Mahmoodi, MD, PhD
Clinical Fellow
Department of Neurosurgery
International Neuroscience Institute
Hannover, Germany
153: Ventricular Tumors

Babak Mahmoudi, PhD
Post-Doctoral Fellow
Department of Neurosurgery
Emory Neuromodulation and Technology Innovation Center
Emory University School of Medicine
Atlanta, Georgia
79: Electrical Stimulation for Epilepsy (VNS, DBS, and RNS)

Martijn J.A. Malessy, MD, PhD
Professor of Nerve Surgery
Department of Neurosurgery
Leiden University Medical Center
Leiden, The Netherlands
Overview and Controversies (PNS)
252: Techniques in Nerve Reconstruction and Repair
253: Nerve Transfers
255: Early Management of Brachial Plexus Injuries

Conor Mallucci, MBBS, FRCS
Consultant Paediatric Neurosurgeon
Alder Hey Childrens NHS Foundation Trust
Liverpool, United Kingdom
207: Optic Pathway Hypothalamic Gliomas

Francesco T. Mangano, DO, FACS, FACOS
Associate Professor of Neurosurgery
University of Cincinnati College of Medicine;
Chief, Division of Pediatric Neurosurgery
Cincinnati Children's Hospital and Medical Center
Cincinnati, Ohio
188: Dandy-Walker Syndrome

Allen H. Maniker, MD
Professor of Neurosurgery
Mount Sinai School of Medicine
Chief of Neurosurgery
Sinai Beth Israel Medical Center
New York, New York
22: Positioning for Peripheral Nerve Surgery
259: Pain, Complications, and Iatrogenic Injury in Nerve Surgery

Geoffrey T. Manley, MD, PhD
Professor in Residence and Vice Chairman
Department of Neurological Surgery
Co-Director and Principal Investigator, Brain and Spinal Injury Center (BASIC)
University of California, San Francisco;
Chief of Neurosurgery
San Francisco General Hospital
San Francisco, California
15: Intracranial Pressure Monitoring
Overview and Controversies (Trauma)
340: Genetics of Traumatic Brain Injury

Spiros Manolidis, MD
Associate Professor of Neurosurgery
Albert Einstein College of Medicine
Beth Israel Medical Center
New York, New York
160: Juvenile Nasopharyngeal Angiofibromas

Daniel Marchac, MD†
Professor
Chirurgie Plastique Reconstructrice et Esthétique
Chirurgie Cranio-Faciale
Collège de Médecine des Hôpitaux de Paris
Paris, France
194: Syndromic Craniosynostosis

Joseph Marchione, MD
Radiology Resident
Icahn School of Medicine at Mount Sinai
New York, New York
13: Physiologic Evaluation of the Brain with Magnetic Resonance Imaging

Joshua Marcus, MD
Postdoctoral Fellow in Endovascular Neurosurgery
and Interventional Neuroradiology
New York–Presbyterian Hospital/Weill Cornell Medical Center
New York, New York
366: Carotid Endarterectomy

Joseph C. Maroon, MD
Clinical Professor, Heindl Scholar in Neuroscience
Department of Neurological Surgery
University of Pittsburgh School of Medicine;
Vice Chair, Community Medicine
University of Pittsburgh Medical Center
Pittsburgh, Pennsylvania
161: Tumors of the Orbit

Alastair Martin, PhD
Adjunct Professor of Radiology
Co-Director, Image-Guided Surgery Specialized Resource Group
University of California, San Francisco
San Francisco, California
89: Deep Brain Stimulation for Parkinson's Disease

Neil A. Martin, MD
Professor and Chair
Department of Neurosurgery
David Geffen School of Medicine at UCLA
Los Angeles, California
397: Revascularization Techniques for Complex Aneurysms and Skull Base Tumors

Justin R. Mascitelli, MD
Resident
Department of Neurosurgery
Mount Sinai Health System
New York, New York
413: Endovascular Treatment of Spinal Vascular Malformations

Amit Mathur, MBBS, MD, MRCP (UK)
Professor of Pediatrics
Division of Newborn Medicine
Washington University School of Medicine in St. Louis;
St. Louis Children's Hospital
St. Louis, Missouri
227: Neonatal Brain Injury

Christopher M. Maulucci, MD
Neurosurgery Spine Fellow
Thomas Jefferson University Hospital
Philadelphia, Pennsylvania
309: Evaluation, Classification, and Treatment of Thoracolumbar Spine Injuries

Marcus D. Mazur, MD
Resident Neurosurgeon
Clinical Neurosciences Center
University of Utah School of Medicine
Salt Lake City, Utah
274: Assessment of Spinal Imaging

Nicole Mazwi, MD
Instructor in Physical Medicine and Rehabilitation
Harvard Medical School
Spaulding Rehabilitation Hospital
Boston, Massachusetts
358: Rehabilitation of Patients with Traumatic Brain Injury

James P. McAllister II, PhD
Professor of Neurosurgery
Washington University School of Medicine in St. Louis
St. Louis Children's Hospital
St. Louis, Missouri
200: Experimental Hydrocephalus

Craig D. McClain, MD, MPH
Assistant Professor
Department of Anesthesia, Critical Care and Pain Medicine
Harvard Medical School;
Associate in Anesthesia
Department of Anesthesiology, Perioperative and Pain Medicine
Boston Children's Hospital
Boston, Massachusetts
184: Neuroanesthesia in Children

Ian E. McCutcheon, MD
Professor of Neurosurgery
University of Texas MD Anderson Cancer Center
Houston, Texas
40: Meningitis and Encephalitis
162: Skull Tumors

Cameron G. McDougall, MD, FRCSC
Director of Endovascular Neurosurgery
Department of Neurosurgery
Barrow Neurological Institute
Phoenix, Arizona
391: Endovascular Approaches to Narrow-Necked Intracranial Aneurysms
392: Endovascular Approaches to Wide-Necked Intracranial Aneurysms

Andrew W. McEvoy, MBBS, MD, FRCS(Lond), FRCS(SN)
Consultant Neurosurgeon
National Hospital for Neurology and Neurosurgery
Institute of Neurology
University College London;
Honorary Consultant Neurosurgeon
Great Ormond Street Hospital for Children
London, United Kingdom
Overview and Controversies (Epilepsy)
65: Neuroradiologic Evaluation for Epilepsy Surgery: Magnetic Resonance Imaging

Patricia E. McGoldrick, NP, MPA, MSN
Instructor in Clinical Nursing
Columbia University College of Physicians and Surgeons
New York, New York
240: Pediatric Epilepsy Surgery

Robert A. McGovern III, MD
Chief Resident
Department of Neurological Surgery
New York–Presbyterian Columbia University Medical Center
New York, New York
Overview and Controversies (Epilepsy)
76: Selective Approaches to the Mesial Temporal Lobe

Guy M. McKhann II, MD
Florence Irving Associate Professor of Neurological Surgery
Columbia University College of Physicians and Surgeons;
Director, Epilepsy and Movement Disorder Surgery
Director, Adult Hydrocephalus Center
Director, Awake Brain Mapping for Tumors and Epilepsy
New York–Presbyterian Columbia University Medical Center
New York, New York
Overview and Controversies (Epilepsy)
58: Electrophysiologic Properties of the Mammalian Central Nervous System
76: Selective Approaches to the Mesial Temporal Lobe

David F. Meaney, PhD
Solomon R. Pollack Professor and Chair
Department of Bioengineering
University of Pennsylvania
Philadelphia, Pennsylvania
337: Biomechanical Basis of Traumatic Brain Injury

Ricky Medel, MD
Assistant Professor
Co-Director of Cerebrovascular, Endovascular, and Skull Base Surgery
Department of Neurosurgery
Tulane University
New Orleans, Louisiana
414: Microsurgical Treatment of Spinal Vascular Malformations

†Deceased.

Minesh P. Mehta, MbChB, FASTRO
Professor of Radiation Oncology
University of Maryland
Baltimore, Maryland;
Chief of Radiation Oncology and Deputy Director of Miami Cancer Institute
Miami, Florida
265: Fractionated Radiotherapy for Brain Tumors

William P. Melega, PhD
Professor of Molecular and Medical Pharmacology
University of California Los Angeles
David Geffen School of Medicine at UCLA
Los Angeles, California
14: Molecular Imaging of the Brain with Positron Emission Tomography

Arnold H. Menezes, MD
Professor and Vice Chairman
Department of Neurosurgery
University of Iowa Hospitals and Clinics
Iowa City, Iowa
233: Developmental Anomalies of the Craniovertebral Junction and Surgical Management

Patrick Mertens, MD, PhD
Head, Department of Neurosurgery
Hôpital Neurologique Pierre Wertheimer
Head, Department of Clinical Anatomy
Université Claude Bernard Lyon 1
Lyon, France
103: Lesioning Surgery for Spasticity

Fredric B. Meyer, MD
Professor and Chair
Department of Neurosurgery
Mayo Clinic
Rochester, Minnesota
Overview and Controversies (Vascular)
359: Cerebral Blood Flow and Metabolism and Cerebral Ischemia
398: Multimodality Treatments of Cerebrovascular Disorders

R. Michael Meyer IV, BS
F. Edward Hebert School of Medicine
Uniformed Services University of the Health Sciences
Bethesda, Maryland
352: Traumatic and Penetrating Head Injuries

Scott A. Meyer, MD
Director of Neurotrauma
Morristown Medical Center;
Atlantic Neurosurgical Specialists
Morristown, New Jersey
283: Evaluation and Treatment of Cervical Disk Herniations
396: Infectious Aneurysms

Emma Meyers, BS
Research Staff
Division of Critical Care Neurology
Department of Neurology
Columbia University College of Physicians and Surgeons
New York, New York
63: Continuous Electroencephalography in Neurological-Neurosurgical Intensive Care: Applications and Value

Philip M. Meyers, MD, FACR, FSIR, FAHA
Professor
Departments of Radiology and Neurological Surgery
Columbia University College of Physicians and Surgeons
Director
Department of Neuroendovascular Service
New York–Presbyterian Columbia Neurological Institute of New York
New York, New York;
Past President
Society of Neurointerventional Surgery
Fairfax, Virginia
403: Adjuvant Endovascular Management of Brain Arteriovenous Malformations
404: Endovascular Management of Arteriovenous Malformations for Cure

Rajiv Midha, MD, MSc, FRCSC, FAANS
Professor and Head
Department of Clinical Neurosciences
Calgary Zone
Alberta Health Services
University of Calgary Cumming School of Medicine;
Scientist, Hotchkiss Brain Institute
Calgary, Alberta, Canada
244: Pathophysiology of Surgical Nerve Disorders
245: Peripheral Nerve Examination, Evaluation, and Biopsy

Jerônimo Buzetti Milano, MD, PhD
Director, Spine Surgery Division
Department of Neurosurgery
Instituto de Neurologia de Curitiba
Curitiba, Paraná, Brazil
285: Evaluation and Treatment of Thoracic Disk Herniation
320: Bone Graft Options, Graft Substitutes, and Harvest Techniques

Catherine Miller, MD
Resident Neurosurgeon
University of Minnesota School of Medicine
Minneapolis, Minnesota
57: Neurosurgical Epidemiology and Outcomes Assessment

Charles A. Miller, MD
Neurosurgery Resident
National Capital Consortium
Walter Reed National Military Medical Center
Bethesda, Maryland
298: Assessment and Treatment of Ankylosing Spondylitis and Diffuse Idiopathic Skeletal Hyperostosis

Jonathan P. Miller, FAANS, FACS
Director, Functional and Restorative Neurosurgery Center
Associate Professor and Vice Chair for Educational Affairs
George R. and Constance P. Lincoln Endowed Chair
Department of Neurological Surgery
University Hospitals Case Medical Center
Case Western Reserve University School of Medicine
Cleveland, Ohio
174: Microvascular Decompression for Trigeminal Neuralgia

Neil R. Miller, MD
Frank B. Walsh Professor of Neuro-Ophthalmology
Professor
Departments of Ophthalmology, Neurology and Neurosurgery
Johns Hopkins University School of Medicine
Baltimore, Maryland
164: Pseudotumor Cerebri

Farhan A. Mirza, MBBS
Resident Neurosurgeon
University of Kentucky College of Medicine
Lexington, Kentucky
226: Growing Skull Fractures

Anna Miserocchi, MD
Consultant Neurosurgeon
Department of Clinical and Experimental Epilepsy
Institute of Neurology
University College London;
Department of Neurosurgery
National Hospital for Neurology and Neurosurgery
London, United Kingdom;
Epilepsy Society
MRI Unit
Chalfont St. Peter, United Kingdom
65: Neuroradiologic Evaluation for Epilepsy Surgery: Magnetic Resonance Imaging

Basant K. Misra, MBBS, MS, MCh, Diplomate National Board
Chairman, Department of Neurosurgery and Gamma Knife Radiosurgery
PD Hinduja National Hospital & Medical Research Centre
Mumbai, India
Overview and Controversies (General)

Symeon Missios, MD
Assistant Professor
Department of Neurosurgery
Louisiana State University
Shreveport, Louisana
132: Surgical Navigation for Brain Tumors

Kevin Y. Miyashiro, BA
Departments of Pharmacology and Psychiatry
Perelman School of Medicine at the University of Pennsylvania
Philadelphia, Pennsylvania
44: Molecular Biology and Genomics: A Primer for Neurosurgeons

Junichi Mizuno, MD, PhD
Director
Center for Minimally Invasive Spinal Surgery
Shin-Yurigaoka General Hospital
Kawasaki, Japan
284: Evaluation and Treatment of Ossification of the Posterior Longitudinal Ligament

J. Mocco, MD, MS
Professor and Vice Chair for Education
Department of Neurological Surgery
Director, Cerebrovascular Center
Icahn School of Medicine at Mount Sinai
New York, New York
360: Acute Medical Management of Ischemic and Hemorrhagic Stroke
372: Endovascular Management of Intracranial Occlusion Disease

Michael T. Modic, MD, FACR
Chairman
Neurological Institute
Cleveland Clinic
Cleveland, Ohio
12: Radiology of the Spine

Jeremy J. Moeller, MD, FRCPC
Assistant Professor
Department of Neurology
Yale School of Medicine
New Haven, Connecticut
61: Diagnosis and Classification of Seizures and Epilepsy

Maxim Mokin, MD, PhD
Assistant Professor of Neurology and Neurosurgery
University of South Florida College of Medicine
Tampa, Florida
367: Carotid Artery Angioplasty and Stenting

Stephen J. Monteith, MD
Cerebrovascular and Endovascular Neurosurgeon
Swedish Neuroscience Institute
Swedish Health System
Seattle, Washington
363: Diagnostic and Therapeutic Neurosonology

Karam Moon, MD
Neurosurgery Resident
Department of Neurosurgery
Barrow Neurological Institute
St. Joseph's Hospital and Medical Center
Phoenix, Arizona
392: Endovascular Approaches to Wide-Necked Intracranial Aneurysms

Saul F. Morales-Valero, MD
Resident
Department of Neurosurgery
University of Virginia
Charlottesville, Virginia
407: Carotid-Cavernous Fistulas

Jacques J. Morcos, MD, FRCS(Eng), FRCS(Ed), FAANS
Professor
Department of Neurological Surgery
University of Miami
Miami, Florida
375: Nonlesional Spontaneous Intracerebral Hemorrhage

Michael Kerin Morgan, MD, PhD (hons), MBBS, MMedEd, FRACS
Professor of Cerebrovascular Neurosurgery
Department of Clinical Medicine
Macquarie University
Sydney, New South Wales, Australia
402: Therapeutic Decision Making in the Management of Arteriovenous Malformations of the Brain

Ziev B. Moses, MD
Neurosurgery Resident
Harvard Medical School
Brigham and Women's Hospital
Boston, Massachusetts
215: Brainstem Gliomas

S. David Moss, MD
Associate Professor of Neurosurgery
Residency Pediatric Neurosurgery Training Director
University of Arizona School of Medicine
Tucson, Arizona;
Pediatric Neurosurgeon
Cardon Children's Medical Center
Mesa, Arizona
196: Nonsynostotic Plagiocephaly

Nelson Moussazadeh, MD
Resident Neurosurgeon
New York–Presbyterian Hospital/Weill Cornell Medical Center
New York, New York
273: Spinal Anatomy

J. Paul Muizelaar, MD, PhD
Professor of Neurosurgery
Marshall University School of Medicine
Huntington, West Virginia
346: Clinical Pathophysiology of Traumatic Brain Injury

Pratik Mukherjee, MD, PhD
Professor of Radiology
University of California, San Francisco;
Director, Center for Imaging of Neurodegenerative Disease
San Francisco VA Medical Center
San Francisco, California
340: Genetics of Traumatic Brain Injury
345: Advanced Structural and Functional Imaging of Traumatic Brain Injury

Srinivasan Mukundan, Jr., MD, PhD
Associate Professor of Radiology
Harvard Medical School
Section Head of Neuroradiology
Brigham and Women's Hospital
Boston, Massachusetts
121: Radiologic Features of Central Nervous System Tumors

Praveen V. Mummaneni, MD
Professor and Vice Chair
Department of Neurological Surgery
Director of Minimally Invasive and Cervical Spine Surgery
Co-Director, Spinal Surgery
University of California, San Francisco
San Francisco, California
Overview and Controversies (Spine)
321: Cervical Arthroplasty

Stephan A. Munich, MD
Neuroendovascular Fellow
Department of Neurosurgery
Jacobs School of Medicine and Biomedical Sciences
University at Buffalo, State University of New York
Buffalo, New York
367: Carotid Artery Angioplasty and Stenting

Karin Muraszko, MD
Chair and Julian T. Hoff Professor
Department of Neurosurgery
Professor of Pediatrics and Communicable Diseases and Plastic Surgery
University of Michigan Medical School
Ann Arbor, Michigan
140: Primitive Neuroectodermal Tumors

Gisela Murray-Ortiz, MD
Postdoctoral Fellow
Department of Neurosurgery and Brain Repair
University of South Florida College of Medicine
Tampa, Florida
328: Anterior and Lateral Lumbar Instrumentation

Antônio C.M. Mussi, MD
Attending Neurosurgeon
Hospital de Caridade
Florianópolis,
Santa Catarina, Brazil;
Former Research Fellow
Department of Neurological Surgery
University of Florida College of Medicine
Gainesville, Florida
2: Surgical Anatomy of the Brain

Sean J. Nagel, MD
Assistant Professor of Neurosurgery
Staff Neurosurgeon, Center for Neurological Restoration
Cleveland Clinic Lerner School of Medicine of Case Western Reserve University
Cleveland, Ohio
199: Cerebrospinal Fluid Disorders and Transitional Neurosurgery

Gábor Nagy, MD, PhD
Consultant Neurosurgeon
Department of Functional Neurosurgery
National Institute of Clinical Neurosciences
Budapest, Hungary
269: Radiosurgery of Intracranial Vascular Malformations

Imad M. Najm, MD
Director, Epilepsy Center
Vice Chair, Neurological Institute
Cleveland Clinic
Cleveland, Ohio
64: Evaluation of Patients for Epilepsy Surgery

Peter Nakaji, MD
Professor of Neurological Surgery
Barrow Neurological Institute
St. Joseph's Hospital and Medical Center
Phoenix, Arizona
222: Pediatric Cerebral Aneurysms

Takeshi Nakajima, MD, PhD
Assistant Professor
Department of Neurosurgery
Jichi Medical University
Shimotsuke, Tochigi, Japan
97: Thalamotomy for Focal Hand Dystonia

Hiroaki Nakashima, MD, PhD
Division of Neurosurgery
University of Toronto Faculty of Medicine
Toronto, Ontario, Canada;
Department of Orthopedic Surgery
Nagoya University Graduate School of Medicine
Nagoya, Japan
277: Pathophysiology and Treatment of Spinal Cord Injury

Anick Nater, MD
Resident Neurosurgeon
University of Toronto Faculty of Medicine
Toronto, Ontario, Canada
295: Assessment and Treatment of Metastatic Spinal Lesions

Rodrigo Navarro-Ramirez, MD, MSc
Spine Surgery Fellow
Weill Cornell Medical College
New York–Presbyterian Hospital
New York, New York
335: Minimally Invasive Techniques for Degenerative Disease

Edjah K. Nduom, MD
Staff Clinician
Surgical Neurology Branch
National Institute of Neurological Disorders and Stroke
Bethesda, Maryland
111: Brain Tumor Immunology and Immunotherapy

Taylor B. Nelp, BA
Department of Neurological Surgery
Columbia University College of Physicians and Surgeons
New York, New York
181: Diagnosis and Management of Painful Neuromas

John D. Nerva, MD
Chief Resident
Department of Neurological Surgery
University of Washington School of Medicine
Seattle, Washington
412: Classification of Spinal Arteriovenous Lesions

Breno Nery, MD
Resident Neurosurgeon
Hospital Heliópolis
São Paulo, Brazil
150: Pituitary Tumors: Functioning and Nonfunctioning

David W. Newell, MD
Cerebrovascular Surgery
Swedish Neuroscience Institute
Swedish Health System
Seattle, Washington
363: Diagnostic and Therapeutic Neurosonology

Angela Li Ching Ng, MBChB
Senior Resident Neurosurgeon
Neurosurgery Registrar
Royal Hobart Hospital
Hobart, Australia
177: Peripheral Nerve Stimulation for Neuropathic Pain

M. Kelly Nicholas, MD, PhD
Associate Professor of Clinical Medicine
Department of Neurology and Rehabilitation
University of Illinois College of Medicine at Chicago
Chicago, Illinois
41: Acquired Immunodeficiency Syndrome

Yasunari Niimi, MD
Director, Center for Neurological Diseases
Department of Neuroendovascular Therapy
St. Luke's International Hospital
Tokyo, Japan
221: Vein of Galen Aneurysmal Malformation

Shahid M. Nimjee, MD, PhD
Assistant Professor
Departments of Neurological Surgery, Radiology, and Neuroscience
The Ohio State University Wexner Medical Center
Columbus, Ohio
7: Coagulation for the Neurosurgeon
51: The Blood-Brain Barrier

Richard B. North, MD
Professor (ret.)
Departments of Neurosurgery, Anesthesiology and Critical Care Medicine
Johns Hopkins University School of Medicine;
President, Neuromodulation Foundation, Inc.
Baltimore, Maryland
175: Neurosurgical Management of Intractable Pain

Mark Nowell, MBBS, MA, MRCS
Clinical Research Fellow
Department of Experimental and Clinical Medicine
Institute of Neurology
University College London;
Department of Neurosurgery
National Hospital for Neurology and Neurosurgery
London, United Kingdom;
Epilepsy Society
MRI Unit
Chalfont St. Peter, United Kingdom
65: Neuroradiologic Evaluation for Epilepsy Surgery: Magnetic Resonance Imaging

Turo J. Nurmikko, MD, PhD
Professor in Pain Relief
Neuroscience Research Centre
The Walton Centre NHS Foundation Trust;
Professor of Pain Science (Hon.)
Faculty of Health and Life Sciences
University of Liverpool
Liverpool, United Kingdom
170: Evidence-Based Approach to the Treatment of Facial Pain

Marc R. Nuwer, MD, PhD
Professor and Vice Chair, Department of Neurology
David Geffen School of Medicine at UCLA;
Head, Department of Clinical Neurophysiology
Ronald Reagan UCLA Medical Center
Los Angeles, California
247: Monitoring of Neural Function: Electromyography, Nerve Conduction, and Evoked Potentials

W. Jerry Oakes, MD
Hendley Professor of Pediatric Neurosurgery
University of Alabama Birmingham School of Medicine
Children's of Alabama
Birmingham, Alabama
190: Chiari Malformations

Taku Ochiai, MD, PhD
Ochiai Neurological Clinic
Saitama, Japan
97: Thalamotomy for Focal Hand Dystonia

Christopher S. Ogilvy, MD
Professor of Neurosurgery
Harvard Medical School
Director, BIDMC Brain Aneurysm Institute
Director, Endovascular and Operative Neurovascular Surgery
Beth Israel Deaconess Medical Center
Boston, Massachusetts
389: Microsurgery of Vertebral Artery and Posterior Inferior Cerebellar Artery Aneurysms

Michael Y. Oh, MD
Vice Chair, Department of Neurosurgery
Program Director, Neurosurgery Residency Program
Chief, Division of Stereotactic and Functional Neurosurgery
Department of Neurosurgery
Allegheny Health Network
Pittsburgh, Pennsylvania
107: Deep Brain Stimulation for Obesity

Nathan Oh, DO
Resident Neurosurgeon
Loma Linda University Medical Center
Loma Linda, California
7: Coagulation for the Neurosurgeon

David O. Okonkwo, MD, PhD
Professor of Neurological Surgery
Executive Vice Chairman, Clinical Operations
Clinical Director, Brain Trauma Research Center
Chief, Division of Neurotrauma
University of Pittsburgh Medical Center
Pittsburgh, Pennsylvania
302: Assessment and Classification of Spinal Instability
332: Sacropelvic Fixation: Anterior and Posterior Options
342: Traumatic Brain Injury: Proteomic Biomarkers

Michael S. Okun, MD
Professor of Neurology
Center for Movement Disorders and Neurorestoration
University of Florida College of Medicine
Gainesville, Florida
84: Clinical Overview of Movement Disorders

Edward H. Oldfield, MD
Professor
Departments of Neurosurgery and Internal Medicine
University of Virginia School of Medicine
Charlottesville, Virginia
53: Cerebral Edema
144: Hemangioblastomas
414: Microsurgical Treatment of Spinal Vascular Malformations

Alessandro Olivi, MD
Professor and Chairman of Neurosurgery
Catholic University of the Sacred Heart
Agostino Gemelli Teaching Hospital
Rome, Italy
123: Brain Tumors during Pregnancy
128: Frame and Frameless Stereotactic Brain Biopsy

Francis O'Neill, PhD, MBChB, BDS
Clinical Senior Lecturer in Oral Surgery
Faculty of Life and Health Sciences
University of Liverpool
Liverpool, United Kingdom
170: Evidence-Based Approach to the Treatment of Facial Pain

Dennis P. Orgill, MD, PhD
Professor of Surgery
Harvard Medical School;
Medical Director, Wound Care Center
Vice Chairman for Quality Improvement
Department of Surgery
Brigham and Women's Hospital
Boston, Massachusetts
163: Scalp Tumors

Joshua W. Osbun, MD
Assistant Professor of Neurological Surgery
Washington University School of Medicine in St. Louis
St. Louis, Missouri
412: Classification of Spinal Arteriovenous Lesions

Koray Özduman, MD
Associate Professor
Department of Neurosurgery
Acibadem University School of Medicine
Istanbul, Turkey
159: Trigeminal Schwannomas

Steven V. Pacia, MD
Associate Professor of Neurology
New York University School of Medicine;
Director, Epilepsy Center
Lenox Hill Hospital
New York, New York
Overview and Controversies (Epilepsy)
62: Antiepileptic Medications: Principles of Clinical Use

Nikhil S. Pai, MD
Research Associate
Department of Neurosurgery
Houston Methodist Neurological Institute
Houston, Texas
383: Surgical Approaches to Intracranial Aneurysms

Margaret Pain, MD
Resident Neurosurgeon
Mount Sinai Hospital
New York, New York
160: Juvenile Nasopharyngeal Angiofibromas
189: Arachnoid Cysts in Childhood

Eva M. Palacios, PhD
Research Fellow in Neuroradiology
Department of Radiology
University of California, San Francisco
San Francisco, California
345: Advanced Structural and Functional Imaging of Traumatic Brain Injury

James N. Palmer, MD
Professor of Otorhinolaryngology
Perelman School of Medicine at the University of Pennsylvania
Philadelphia, Pennsylvania
357: Traumatic Cerebrospinal Fluid Fistulas

M. Necmettin Pamir, MD
Professor and Chair
Department of Neurosurgery
Acibadem University School of Medicine
Istanbul, Turkey
159: Trigeminal Schwannomas

Edward Pan, MD
Medical Director, Neuro-Oncology Program
Department of Neurology and Neurotherapeutics
University of Texas Southwestern Medical Center
Dallas, Texas
116: Angiogenesis and Brain Tumors: Scientific Principles, Current Therapy, and Future Directions

David M. Panczykowski, MD
Resident, Neurological Surgery
University of Pittsburgh Medical Center
Pittsburgh, Pennsylvania
302: Assessment and Classification of Spinal Instability
342: Traumatic Brain Injury: Proteomic Biomarkers

Fedor E. Panov, MD
Assistant Professor of Neurosurgery
Icahn School of Medicine at Mount Sinai
Associate Director of Adult Epilepsy
Mount Sinai Health System
New York, New York
89: Deep Brain Stimulation for Parkinson's Disease

Avelino Parajón, MD
Chief of Spine Section, Department of Neurosurgery
Hospital Universitario Ramon y Cajal
Madrid, Spain
329: Posterior Thoracic and Lumbar Instrumentation with Historical Overview

Srinivasan Paramasivam, MD, MCh, MRCS Ed, FINR
Assistant Professor of Neurosurgery
Center for Cerebrovascular Diseases
Icahn School of Medicine at Mount Sinai
New York, New York
221: Vein of Galen Aneurysmal Malformation

Andrew D. Parent, MD
Professor of Neurosurgery
University of Mississippi Medical Center
Jackson, Mississippi
219: Skull Lesions in Children: Dermoids, Langerhans Cell Histiocytosis, Fibrous Dysplasia, and Lipomas

Michael S. Park, MD
Resident Neurosurgeon
Department of Neurosurgery and Brain Repair
University of South Florida College of Medicine
Tampa, Florida
328: Anterior and Lateral Lumbar Instrumentation

Min S. Park, MD
Assistant Professor
Department of Neurosurgery
University of Utah Medical Center
Salt Lake City, Utah
391: Endovascular Approaches to Narrow-Necked Intracranial Aneurysms

Paul Park, MD
Associate Professor
Departments of Neurological and Orthopaedic Surgery
University of Michigan
Ann Arbor, Michigan
288: Evaluation and Treatment of Degenerative Lumbar Spondylolisthesis
313: Evaluation and Treatment of Cervical Deformity

T.S. Park, MD
Shi H. Huang Professor of Neurological Surgery
Washington University School of Medicine in St. Louis;
Neurosurgeon-in-Chief
Department of Neurosurgery
St. Louis Children's Hospital
St. Louis, Missouri
228: Birth Brachial Plexus Injury
243: Selective Dorsal Rhizotomy for Spastic Cerebral Palsy

Andrew T. Parsa, MD, PhD†
Michael J. Marchese Chair in Neurosurgery
Professor in Neurological Surgery and Neurology
Northwestern University Feinberg School of Medicine
Chicago, Illinois
Overview and Controversies (Oncology)
130: Basic Principles of Skull Base Surgery
149: Vestibular Schwannomas

Michael D. Partington, MD
Pediatric Neurosurgeon
Medical Director, Spina Bifida Services
Gillette Children's Specialty Healthcare
St. Paul, Minnesota
242: Intrathecal Baclofen Therapy for Cerebral Palsy

Akash J. Patel, MD
Assistant Professor of Neurosurgery
Baylor College of Medicine
Houston, Texas
146: Metastatic Brain Tumors

Aman B. Patel, MD
Attending Neurosurgeon
Department of Neurosurgery
Massachusetts General Hospital
Robert G. and Jean A. Ojemann Associate Professor
Department of Neurosurgery
Harvard Medical School
Boston, Massachusetts
413: Endovascular Treatment of Spinal Vascular Malformations

Vimal Patel, PhD
Clinician Researcher
University of Chicago Pritzker School of Medicine
NorthShore Neurological Institute
Evanston, Illinois
347: Mild Traumatic Brain Injury in Adults and Concussion in Sports

Parag G. Patil, MD, PhD
Associate Professor
Departments of Neurosurgery, Neurology, Anesthesiology, and Biomedical Engineering
University of Michigan Medical School
Ann Arbor, Michigan
105: Treatment of Intractable Vertigo

Russell Payne, MD
Resident Neurosurgeon
Penn State Milton S. Hershey Medical Center
Hershey, Pennsylvania
158: Esthesioneuroblastomas

Richard Deren Penn, MD
Professor of Neurosurgery
Rush Medical College
Chicago, Illinois
54: Extracellular Fluid Movement and Clearance in the Brain: The Glymphatic Pathway
104: Management of Spasticity by Central Nervous System Infusion Techniques

Brenton H. Pennicooke, MD, MS
Resident Neurosurgeon
New York–Presbyterian Hospital
Weill Cornell Medical College
New York, New York
218: Pediatric Intraventricular and Periventricular Tumors

Augustus J. Perez, MD
Resident Neurosurgeon
University of Mississippi Medical Center
Jackson, Mississippi
219: Skull Lesions in Children: Dermoids, Langerhans Cell Histiocytosis, Fibrous Dysplasia, and Lipomas

Alessandro Perin, MD, PhD
Consultant
Department of Neurosurgery
Fondazione IRCCS Istituto Neurologico Carlo Besta
Milano; Italy;
Adjunct Professor in Neuro-Oncology
Department of Life Sciences
University of Trieste
Trieste, Italy
112: Brain Tumor Stem Cells

Joel S. Perlmutter, MD
Elliot Stein Family Professor of Neurology
Professor of Radiology, Neuroscience, Occupational Therapy, and Physical Therapy
Head, Movement Disorders Section
Washington University School of Medicine in St. Louis
St. Louis, Missouri
86: Functional Imaging in Movement Disorders

John A. Persing, MD
Professor of Surgery
Chief, Section of Plastic Surgery
Yale School of Medicine
New Haven, Connecticut
23: Incisions and Closures
163: Scalp Tumors
193: Nonsyndromic Craniosynostosis: Introduction and Single-Suture Synostosis

Erika A. Petersen, MD
Associate Professor of Neurosurgery
University of Arkansas for Medical Sciences
Little Rock, Arkansas
169: Pharmacologic Treatment of Pain

†Deceased.

Eric C. Peterson, MD, MS
Assistant Professor
Department of Neurological Surgery
University of Miami Miller School of Medicine
Miami, Florida
405: Microsurgery of Arteriovenous Malformations

Anthony L. Petraglia, MD
Division of Neurosurgery
Rochester Regional Health
Rochester, New York
347: Mild Traumatic Brain Injury in Adults and Concussion in Sports

Martin Pham, MD
Resident Neurosurgeon
Keck School of Medicine
University of Southern California
Los Angeles, California
18: Surgical Planning: An Overview

Matthew A. Piazza, MD
Resident Neurosurgeon
Perelman School of Medicine at the University of Pennsylvania
Philadelphia, Pennsylvania
28: Cranioplasty

Joseph M. Piepmeier, MD
Nixdorff-German Professor of Neurosurgery
Vice Chair of Clinical Affairs, Neurosurgery
Section Chief, Neuro-Oncology
Yale School of Medicine
New Haven, Connecticut
139: Unusual Gliomas

Webster H. Pilcher, MD, PhD
Professor and Chair
Department of Neurosurgery
University of Rochester School of Medicine
Rochester, New York
80: Epilepsy Surgery: Outcome and Complications

Heather N. Pinckard-Dover, MD
Resident Neurosurgeon
University of Arkansas for Medical Sciences
Little Rock, Arkansas
169: Pharmacologic Treatment of Pain

José A. Pineda, MD, MSCI
Associate Professor
Departments of Pediatrics and Neurology
Washington University School of Medicine in St Louis;
Director, Neurocritical Care Program
St. Louis Children's Hospital
St. Louis, Missouri
185: Neurocritical Care in Children

Joseph D. Pinter, MD
Professor of Clinical Pediatrics
Institute on Development and Disability
Oregon Health & Science University
Portland, Oregon
46: Neuroembryology

Jared M. Pisapia, MD, MTR
Resident Neurosurgeon
Perelman School of Medicine at the University of Pennsylvania
Philadelphia, Pennsylvania
71: Intracranial Monitoring: Subdural Strip and Grid Recording

Mary L. Pisculli, MD, MPH
Division of Infectious Diseases
Brigham and Women's Hospital
Boston, Massachusetts
36: Postoperative Infections of the Head and Brain

Thomas Pittman, MD
Professor of Neurosurgery
University of Kentucky College of Medicine;
Kentucky Children's Hospital
Lexington, Kentucky
226: Growing Skull Fractures

Pedro H.I. Pohl, MD
Orthopaedic Spine Surgeon and Affiliated Professor
ABC Medical School
São Paulo, Brazil;
Research Fellow
Ferguson Laboratory for Orthopaedic and Spine Research
Department of Orthopaedic Surgery
University of Pittsburgh School of Medicine
Pittsburgh, Pennsylvania
276: Disk Degeneration and Regeneration

Ian F. Pollack, MD
Leland Albright Professor of Neurological Surgery
Vice-Chairman for Academic Affairs, Department of Neurological Surgery
Co-Director, UPCI Brain Tumor Program
Distinguished Professor of Neurosurgery
University of Pittsburgh School of Medicine;
Chief, Pediatric Neurosurgery
Children's Hospital of Pittsburgh
Pittsburgh, Pennsylvania
216: Intracranial Germ Cell Tumors

Bruce E. Pollock, MD
Professor of Neurological Surgery and Radiation Oncology
Mayo Clinic
Rochester, Minnesota
Overview and Controversies (Radiation)
269: Radiosurgery of Intracranial Vascular Malformations
398: Multimodality Treatments of Cerebrovascular Disorders

Kalmon D. Post, MD
Professor and Chairman Emeritus
Department of Neurosurgery
Professor of Medicine
Icahn School of Medicine at Mount Sinai
New York, New York
6: Complication Avoidance in Neurosurgery
149: Vestibular Schwannomas

Wyatt Potter, PhD
Epilepsy Research Laboratory
Department of Neurological Surgery
University of California, San Francisco School of Medicine
San Francisco, California
59: Animal Models of Epilepsy

Matthew B. Potts, MD
Assistant Professor
Departments of Neurological Surgery and Radiology
Northwestern University Feinberg School of Medicine
Chicago, Illinois
122: Endovascular Techniques for Tumor Embolization

Nader Pouratian, MD, PhD
Associate Professor of Neurosurgery
David Geffen School of Medicine at UCLA
Los Angeles, California
247: Monitoring of Neural Function: Electromyography, Nerve Conduction, and Evoked Potentials

Gustavo Pradilla, MD
Assistant Professor
Department of Neurological Surgery
Emory University School of Medicine;
Chief
Department of Neurosurgery Service
Grady Memorial Hospital
Atlanta, Georgia
388: Surgical Management of Middle Cerebral Artery Aneurysms

Briana C. Prager, BS
Cleveland Clinic Lerner College of Medicine of Case Western Reserve University
Cleveland, Ohio
51: The Blood-Brain Barrier

Charles J. Prestigiacomo, MD, FAANS, FACS
Professor of Neurological Surgery
University of Medicine and Dentistry of New Jersey
New Jersey Medical School
Newark, New Jersey
24: Brain Retraction

Mark R. Proctor, MD
Associate Professor of Neurosurgery
Harvard Medical School;
Boston Children's Hospital
Boston, Massachusetts
192: Molecular Genetics and Priniciples of Craniosynostosis

Laura M. Prolo, MD, PhD
Tashia and John Morgridge Scholar
Department of Neurological Surgery
Stanford University School of Medicine
Stanford, California
212: Ependymomas

Robert W. Prost, PhD
Associate Professor of Radiology
Froedtert Hospital;
Associate Professor of Biophysics
Biophysics Research Institute
Medical College of Wisconsin
Milwaukee, Wisconsin
11: Computed Tomography and Magnetic Resonance Imaging of the Brain

Vinay K. Puduvalli, MD
Professor and Director
Division of Neuro-Oncology
The Ohio State University Comprehensive Cancer Center
Columbus, Ohio
120: Clinical Features: Neurology of Brain Tumor and Paraneoplastic Disorders

David Purger, PhD
Departments of Neurosurgery and Neurology
Institute for Stem Cell Biology and Regenerative Medicine
Stanford University
Stanford, California
45: Optogenetics and CLARITY

Alfredo Quiñones-Hinojosa, MD, FAANS, FACS
Professor of Neurological Surgery and Oncology
Departments of Neuroscience and Cellular and Molecular Medicine
Johns Hopkins University School of Medicine
Baltimore, Maryland
112: Brain Tumor Stem Cells
137: Malignant Gliomas: Anaplastic Astrocytoma, Glioblastoma, Gliosarcoma, and Anaplastic Oligodendroglioma

Jason Pierce Rahal, MD
Neurological Surgeon
Department of Neurosurgery
Lahey Hospital
Burlington, Massachusetts
371: Microsurgical Management of Intracranial Occlusion Disease

Zvi Ram, MD
Chairman
Department of Neurosurgery
Tel Aviv Medical Center
Tel Aviv, Israel
Overview and Controversies (Oncology)
127: Neurocognition in Brain Tumor Patients

Nathan J. Ranalli, MD
Assistant Professor
Departments of Neurosurgery and Pediatrics
University of Florida Health Science Center Jacksonville
Jacksonville, Florida
228: Birth Brachial Plexus Injury

Leonardo Rangel-Castilla, MD
Cerebrovascular Fellow
Division of Neurological Surgery
Barrow Neurological Institute
St. Joseph's Hospital and Medical Center
Phoenix, Arizona
411: Microsurgery for Cerebral Cavernous Malformations

Daniel M.S. Raper, MBBS
Resident Physician
Department of Neurosurgery
University of Virginia Health System
Charlottesville, Virginia
238: Thoracolumbar Spinal Disorders in Pediatric Patients
374: Cerebral Venous and Sinus Thrombosis

Benjamin I. Rapoport, MD, PhD
Resident Neurosurgeon
Neurosurgery
Weill Cornell Medical College
New York, New York
94: Emerging and Experimental Neurosurgical Treatments for Parkinson's Disease

Jeffrey S. Raskin, MD, MS
Neurosurgery Resident
Oregon Health & Science University
Portland, Oregon
231: Split Spinal Cord

Ahmed M. Raslan, MD
Assistant Professor of Neurological Surgery
Oregon Health & Science University
Portland, Oregon
179: Evidence Base for Destructive Procedures
183: Percutaneous Cordotomy and Trigeminal Tractotomy-Nucleotomy

Peter Rasmussen, MD
Director
Cerebrovascular Center, Department of Neurosurgery
Cleveland Clinic
Cleveland, Ohio
393: Endovascular Flow Diversion for Intracranial Aneurysms

Jonathan Rasouli, MD
Neurosurgery Resident
Icahn School of Medicine at Mount Sinai
Mount Sinai Health System
New York, New York
19: Surgical Simulation and Robotic Surgery

Ali C. Ravanpay, MD, PhD
Chief Resident
Department of Neurological Surgery
University of Washington School of Medicine
Seattle, Washington
113: Molecular Genetics and the Development of Targets for Glioma Therapy

Vijay M. Ravindra, MD, MSPH
Resident Neurosurgeon
University of Utah School of Medicine
Salt Lake City, Utah
37: Postoperative Infections of the Spine

Wilson Z. Ray, MD
Assistant Professor
Department of Neurosurgery
Washington University School of Medicine in St. Louis
St. Louis, Missouri
109: Neuroprosthetics
257: Nerve Injuries of the Lower Extremity

Eytan Raz, MD
Assistant Professor
Department of Radiology
New York University School of Medicine
New York, New York
122: Endovascular Techniques for Tumor Embolization

Shaan M. Raza, MD
Assistant Professor of Neurosurgery
Skull Base Tumor Program
University of Texas MD Anderson Cancer Center
Houston, Texas
128: Frame and Frameless Stereotactic Brain Biopsy
157: Neoplasms of the Paranasal Sinuses

Jean Régis, MD
Professor of Neurosurgery
Head, Functional Neurosurgery Department
Aix-Marseille University
Timone Hospital APHM
Marseille, France
78: Radiosurgical Treatment for Epilepsy
Overview and Controversies (Radiation)
268: Radiosurgery for Benign Intracranial Tumors

Peter L. Reilly, MBBS, BMedSc(hons), MD, FRACS, FFPMANZCA
Professor of Neurosurgery
University of Adelaide School of Medical Sciences
Adelaide, Australia
355: Craniofacial Injuries

Florence C.M. Reith, MD
Department of Neurosurgery
University Hospital Antwerp and University of Antwerp
Edegem, Belgium
336: Epidemiology of Traumatic Brain Injury

Dominique Renier, MD
Pediatric Neurosurgeon
Unité de Chirurgie Craniofaciale
Hôpital Necker Enfants Malades
Paris, France
194: Syndromic Craniosynostosis

Daniel K. Resnick, MD, MS
Professor and Vice Chairman
Department of Neurosurgery
University of Wisconsin School of Medicine and Public Health
Madison, Wisconsin
Overview and Controversies (Spine)
307: Treatment of Cervicothoracic Junction Injuries

Renée Reynolds, MD
Assistant Professor of Neurosurgery
Division of Pediatric Neurosurgery
State University of New York University at Buffalo
Women and Children's Hospital of Buffalo
Buffalo, New York
206: General Approaches and Considerations for Pediatric Brain Tumors

Ali Rezai, MD
Professor and Stanley D. and Joan H. Ross Chair in Neuromodulation
Department of Neurosurgery;
Associate Dean and Director
Neuroscience Program;
Director, Center for Neuromodulation
The Ohio State University
Wexner Medical Center
Columbus, Ohio
100: Surgery for Obsessive-Compulsive Disorder

Laurence D. Rhines, MD
Professor of Neurosurgery
Director, Spine Program
University of Texas MD Anderson Cancer Center
Houston, Texas
294: Assessment and Treatment of Benign Intradural Extramedullary Tumors

Albert L. Rhoton, Jr., MD†
R.D. Keene Family Professor of Neurological Surgery
Department of Surgery
University of Florida College of Medicine;
Chairman Emeritus
Department of Neurological Surgery
Shands Hospital at the University of Florida
Gainesville, Florida
2: Surgical Anatomy of the Brain

Teresa Ribalta, MD, PhD
Chief, Department of Pathology
Scientific Director, Biobank
Sant Joan de Déu Barcelona Children's Hospital
Esplugues de Llobregat;
Professor of Pathology
Department of Fonaments Clínics
Faculty of Medicine, University of Barcelona;
Chief of Section
Department of Pathology: Neuropathology
Hospital Clinic of Barcelona
Barcelona, Spain
110: Brain Tumors: An Overview of Current Histopathologic and Genetic Classifications

Joseph A. Ricci, MD
Plastic Surgery Resident
Harvard Medical School
Brigham and Women's Hospital
Boston, Massachusetts
163: Scalp Tumors

R. Mark Richardson, MD, PhD, FAANS
Associate Professor of Neurological Surgery
Director, Epilepsy and Movement Disorders Surgery
University of Pittsburgh School of Medicine
Pittsburgh, Pennsylvania
343: Therapeutic Strategies for Repair and Regeneration following Traumatic Brain Injury

Callen J. Riggins
Department of Neurosurgery
Johns Hopkins University School of Medicine
Baltimore, Maryland
114: Genetic Origins of Brain Tumors

Gregory J. Riggins, MD, PhD
Professor of Neurosurgery and Oncology
Johns Hopkins University School of Medicine
Baltimore, Maryland
114: Genetic Origins of Brain Tumors

Howard A. Riina, MD, MPHI
Vice Chair and Director of the Neurosurgery Residency Training Program
Professor, Departments of Neurological Surgery, Neurology, and Radiology
New York University School of Medicine
New York, New York
122: Endovascular Techniques for Tumor Embolization

Jordina Rincon-Torroella, MD
Post-Doctoral Fellow
Department of Neurosurgery
Johns Hopkins University School of Medicine
Baltimore, Maryland
137: Malignant Gliomas: Anaplastic Astrocytoma, Glioblastoma, Gliosarcoma, and Anaplastic Oligodendroglioma

Andrew J. Ringer, MD
Professor of Neurosurgery and Director of Cerebrovascular Surgery
Department of Neurosurgery
Comprehensive Stroke Center at UC Neuroscience Institute
University of Cincinnati, Mayfield Clinic
Cincinnati, Ohio
382: Endovascular Management of Cerebral Vasospasm

Jay Riva-Cambrin, MD, MSc, FRCSC
Associate Professor
Division of Pediatric Neurosurgery
Department of Clinical Neuroscience,
University of Calgary Faculty of Medicine;
Alberta Children's Hospital
Calgary, Alberta, Canada
32: The Role of Third Ventriculostomy in Adults and Children: A Critical Review
204: Management and Prevention of Shunt Infections

Christopher D. Roark, MD, MS
Assistant Professor
Department of Neurosurgery
University of Colorado
Denver, Colorado
415: Pregnancy and the Vascular Lesion

David W. Roberts, MD
Professor of Surgery (Neurosurgery)
Geisel School of Medicine at Dartmouth
Hanover, New Hampshire
Chief, Section of Neurosurgery
Dartmouth-Hitchcock Medical Center
Lebanon, New Hampshire
74: Surgery for Extratemporal Lobe Epilepsy

Claudia S. Robertson, MD, FCCM
Professor of Neurosurgery
Baylor College of Medicine
Houston, Texas
349: Critical Care Management of Traumatic Brain Injury

Jon H. Robertson, MD
Professor of Neurosurgery
Semmes-Murphey Clinic
University of Tennessee College of Medicine
Memphis, Tennessee
25: Visualization and Optics in Neurosurgery

Shenandoah Robinson, MD, FAAP, FACS
Department of Pediatric Neurosurgery
Johns Hopkins University School of Medicine
Baltimore, Maryland
Overview and Controversies (Pediatrics)
198: Infantile Posthemorrhagic Hydrocephalus

†Deceased.

Aidan D. Roche, MBBS, PhD, BEng
Clinical Postdoctoral Research Fellow, Department of Surgery
Division of Plastic and Reconstructive Surgery
Christian Doppler Laboratory for Restoration of Extremity Function
Medical University of Vienna
Vienna, Austria;
Core Surgical Trainee
Department of Plastic and Reconstructive Surgery
North Bristol NHS Trust
Bristol, United Kingdom
260: Neuroelectronic Systems

Pierre-Hugues Roche, MD
Professor and Head
Department of Neurosurgery
Aix-Marseille University
Assistance Publique Hôpitaux de Marseille
Marseille, France
268: Radiosurgery for Benign Intracranial Tumors

Ana Rodríguez-Hernández, MD, PhD
Neurosurgeon, Attending
Department of Neurological Surgery
Vall d'Hebron University Hospital
Barcelona, Spain
395: Microsurgical Management of Giant Intracranial Aneurysms

Marie Roguski, MD, MPH
Resident Neurosurgeon
Tufts Medical Center
Boston, Massachusetts
300: Adult Tethered Cord Syndrome
301: Adult Syringomyelia

Jarod L. Roland, MD
Neurosurgery Resident
Washington University School of Medicine in St. Louis
St. Louis, Missouri
109: Neuroprosthetics

John D. Rolston, MD, PhD
Neurosurgery Resident
Department of Neurological Surgery
University of California, San Francisco
San Francisco, California
4: Improving Patient Safety

Brandon K. Root, MD
Resident
Department of Neurosurgery
Dartmouth-Hitchcock Medical Center
Lebanon, New Hampshire
16: Principles of Neurocritical Care

William S. Rosenberg, MD
Medical Director
Center for the Relief of Pain
Midwest Neuroscience Institute;
President, Cancer Pain Research Consortium
Kansas City, Missouri
175: Neurosurgical Management of Intractable Pain

Joshua M. Rosenow, MD, FAANS, FACS
Associate Professor of Neurosurgery, Neurology, and Physical Medicine and Rehabilitation
Northwestern University Feinberg School of Medicine;
Director of Functional Neurosurgery
Northwestern Memorial Hospital
Chicago, Illinois
168: Approach to the Patient with Chronic Pain

Guy Rosenthal, MD
Senior Staff
Department of Neurosurgery
Hadassah Medical Center
Jerusalem, Israel
Overview and Controversies (Trauma)
350: Physiologic Monitoring for Traumatic Brain Injury

Robert H. Rosenwasser, MD
Professor and Chair
Department of Neurological Surgery
Thomas Jefferson University and Hospitals
Philadelphia, Pennsylvania
17: The Neurosurgical Intensive Care Unit and the Unique Role of the Neurosurgeon

Michael K. Rosner, MD
Chief
Neurosurgery Service
Walter Reed National Military Medical Center
Bethesda, Maryland
286: Evaluation and Treatment of Lumbar Disk Disease
298: Assessment and Treatment of Ankylosing Spondylitis and Diffuse Idiopathic Skeletal Hyperostosis

Eric S. Rovner, MD
Professor
Department of Urology
Medical University of South Carolina
Charleston, South Carolina
10: Neurourology

Janet C. Rucker, MD
Bernard A. and Charlotte Marden Professor of Neurology
Associate Professor of Neurology
New York University School of Medicine
NYU Langone Medical Center
New York, New York
8: Neuro-ophthalmology

Stephen M. Russell, MD
Professor of Neurosurgery and Orthopaedic Surgery
New York University School of Medicine
NYU Langone Medical Center
New York, New York
259: Pain, Complications, and Iatrogenic Injury in Nerve Surgery

Jonathan J. Russin, MD
Cerebrovascular Fellow
Division of Neurological Surgery
Barrow Neurological Institute
St. Joseph's Hospital and Medical Center
Phoenix, Arizona
411: Microsurgery for Cerebral Cavernous Malformations

James T. Rutka, MD, PhD
Professor and R.S. McLaughlin Chair
Department of Surgery
University of Toronto Faculty of Medicine;
Director of the Arthur and Sonia Labatt Brain Tumour Research Centre
Division of Paediatric Neurosurgery
The Hospital for Sick Children
Toronto, Ontario, Canada
142: Medulloblastomas in Adults
Overview and Controversies (Pediatrics)
213: Medulloblastomas

Mina G. Safain, MD
Resident Neurosurgeon
Tufts Medical Center
Boston, Massachusetts
237: Introduction to Spinal Deformities in Children

Oren Sagher, MD
William Chandler Professor of Neurosurgery
University of Michigan
Ann Arbor, Michigan
178: Spinal Cord Stimulation

Arjun Sahgal, MD
Associate Professor of Radiation Oncology and Surgery
Deputy Chief, Department of Radiation Oncology
Sunnybrook Health Sciences Center
University of Toronto Faculty of Medicine
Toronto, Ontario, Canada
262: Radiobiology of Radiotherapy and Radiosurgery

Rajiv Saigal, MD, PhD
Assistant Professor of Neurosurgery
University of Washington
Seattle, Washington
50: Cellular and Molecular Responses in the Peripheral and Central Nervous Systems: Similarities and Differences
315: Evaluation and Treatment of Scheuermann's Kyphosis

Nobuhito Saito, MD, PhD
Professor of Neurosurgery
University of Tokyo Graduate School of Medicine
Tokyo, Japan
267: Radiosurgery for Malignant Intracranial Tumors

Stefan Salminger, MD
Christian Doppler Laboratory for Restoration of Extremity Function
Department of Surgery
Division of Plastic and Reconstructive Surgery
Medical University of Vienna
Vienna, Austria
260: Neuroelectronic Systems

Amer F. Samdani, MD
Chief of Surgery
Shriners Hospitals for Children
Philadelphia, Pennsylvania
237: Introduction to Spinal Deformities in Children
238: Thoracolumbar Spinal Disorders in Pediatric Patients
300: Adult Tethered Cord Syndrome
301: Adult Syringomyelia

Francesco Sammartino, MD
Division of Neurosurgery
University of Toronto Faculty of Medicine
Toronto Western Hospital
Toronto, Ontario, Canada
108: Deep Brain Stimulation for Alzheimer's Disease

Nader Sanai, MD
Director, Neurosurgical Oncology
Director, Barrow Brain Tumor Research Center
Barrow Neurological Institute
Phoenix, Arizona
136: Low-Grade Gliomas: Astrocytomas, Oligodendrogliomas, and Mixed Gliomas

Matthew R. Sanborn, MD
Neurological Surgeon
Department of Neurosurgery
Barrow Neurological Institute
St. Joseph's Hospital and Medical Center
Phoenix, Arizona
391: Endovascular Approaches to Narrow-Necked Intracranial Aneurysms

Adam L. Sandler, MD
Resident Neurosurgeon
Leo Davidoff Department of Neurological Surgery
Albert Einstein College of Medicine
Montefiore Medical Center
Bronx, New York
187: Encephaloceles, Meningoceles, and Cranial Dermal Sinus Tracts

Charles A. Sansur, MD, MHSc, FAANS
Associate Professor of Neurosurgery
Director of Spine Surgery
Assistant Program Director, Department of Neurosurgery
University of Maryland School of Medicine
Baltimore, Maryland
282: Complication Avoidance in Spine Surgery

Thomas Santarius, MD, PhD, FRCS (Surg Neurol)
Consultant Neurosurgeon
Division of Neurosurgery, Department of Clinical Neurosciences
University of Cambridge
Addenbrooke's Hospital
Cambridge, United Kingdom
34: Medical and Surgical Management of Chronic Subdural Hematomas

Paul Santiago, MD
Associate Professor
Departments of Neurological Surgery and Orthopedic Surgery
Washington University School of Medicine in St. Louis
St. Louis, Missouri
Overview and Controversies (Spine)
299: Adult Congenital Malformations of the Thoracic and Lumbar Spine

Teresa Santiago-Sim, PhD
Assistant Professor
Vivian L. Smith Department of Neurosurgery
University of Texas Health Science Center
Houston, Texas
378: Pathobiology of Intracranial Aneurysms

Osmar José Santos de Moraes, MD
Professor of Evidence Based Medicine
Santa Marcelina Medical School;
Head, Department of Neurosurgery
Santa Marcelina University Hospital
São Paulo, Brazil
Overview and Controversies (Spine)
285: Evaluation and Treatment of Thoracic Disk Herniation
287: Cervical, Thoracic, and Lumbar Stenosis
289: Treatment of Discitis and Epidural Abscess
320: Bone Graft Options, Graft Substitutes, and Harvest Techniques
322: Lumbar Arthroplasty

Christopher A. Sarkiss, MD
Neurosurgery Resident
Icahn School of Medicine at Mount Sinai
Mount Sinai Health System
New York, New York
19: Surgical Simulation and Robotic Surgery

Harvey B. Sarnat, MS, MD, FRCPC
Professor
Departments of Paediatrics, Pathology (Neuropathology), and Clinical Neurosciences
University of Calgary Faculty of Medicine
and Alberta Children's Hospital Research Institute
Calgary, Alberta, Canada
46: Neuroembryology

Christina Sarris, MD
Resident Neurosurgeon
Barrow Neurological Institute
Phoenix, Arizona;
Department of Neurosurgery
Rutgers New Jersey Medical School
Newark, New Jersey
24: Brain Retraction

Raymond Sawaya, MD
Professor and Chair
Department of Neurosurgery
University of Texas MD Anderson Cancer Center
Houston, Texas
Overview and Controversies (Oncology)
146: Metastatic Brain Tumors
152: Epidermoid, Dermoid, and Neurenteric Cysts

Justin K. Scheer, BS
School of Medicine
University of California, San Diego
La Jolla, California
318: Assessment and Treatment of Proximal Junctional Kyphosis

W. Michael Scheld, MD
Bayer-Gerald L. Mandell Professor of Internal Medicine
Clinical Professor of Neurosurgery
University of Virginia School of Medicine
Charlottesville, Virginia
35: Basic Science of Central Nervous System Infections
39: Brain Abscess

Nicholas D. Schiff, MD
Jerold B. Katz Professor of Neurology and Neuroscience
Professor of Medical Ethics in Medicine
Weill Cornell Medical College
New York, New York
55: Altered Consciousness

David J. Schlesinger, PhD
Associate Professor
Departments of Radiation Oncology and Neurological Surgery
University of Virginia
Charlottesville, Virginia
264: Radiosurgery Technique

Meic H. Schmidt, MD, MBA
Professor of Neurosurgery and Orthopedics
Ronald I. Apfelbaum, MD Endowed Chair in Spine Surgery
Vice Chair for Clinical Affairs
Department of Neurosurgery
University of Utah School of Medicine
Salt Lake City, Utah
27: Thorascopic Spine Surgery
37: Postoperative Infections of the Spine
274: Assessment of Spinal Imaging

Paul J. Schmitt, MD
Resident Physician
Department of Neurosurgery
University of Virginia Health System
Charlottesville, Virginia
374: Cerebral Venous and Sinus Thrombosis

Johannes Schramm, MD, PhD
Professor of Neurosurgery
Bonn University Faculty of Medicine
Bonn, Germany
77: Hemispheric Disconnection Procedures

Frank J. Schwab, MD
Professor of Clinical Orthopaedic Surgery
Weill Cornell Medical College
Chief, Spine Service
Hospital for Special Surgery
New York, New York
311: Classification of Spinal Deformity

Daniel M. Sciubba, MD
Associate Professor
Departments of Neurosurgery, Oncology, Orthopaedic Surgery, and Radiation Oncology
Director, Spine Tumor and Spine Deformity Research
Johns Hopkins University School of Medicine
Baltimore, Maryland
155: Chordomas and Chondrosarcomas

R. Michael Scott, MD
Neurosurgeon-in-Chief, Emeritus
Boston Children's Hospital;
Professor of Neurosurgery
Harvard Medical School
Boston, Massachusetts
220: Moyamoya Disease

Robert A. Scranton, MD
Resident Neurosurgeon
Department of Neurosurgery
Houston Methodist Neurological Institute
Houston, Texas
383: Surgical Approaches to Intracranial Aneurysms

Volker Seifert, MD, PhD
Professor and Chairman
Department of Neurosurgery
Director, Center of Clinical Neurosciences
Johann Wolfgang Goethe-University Frankfurt am Main Germany
Frankfurt am Main, Germany
Overview and Controversies (General)

Nathan R. Selden, MD, PhD, FACS, FAAP
Campagna Chair of Neurological Surgery
Residency Program Director
Department of Neurological Surgery
Oregon Health & Science University
Portland, Oregon
231: Split Spinal Cord

Jonathan N. Sellin, MD
Resident Neurosurgeon
Baylor College of Medicine
Houston, Texas
294: Assessment and Treatment of Benign Intradural Extramedullary Tumors

Warren R. Selman, MD
Harvey Huntington Brown, Jr. Professor and Chairman
Department of Neurological Surgery
Case Western Reserve University School of Medicine;
Director, The Neurological Institute
University Hospitals Case Medical Center
Cleveland, Ohio
19: Surgical Simulation and Robotic Surgery
362: Intraoperative Cerebral Protection

Sandra Serafini, PhD
Assistant Professor of Surgery
Duke University Medical Center
Durham, North Carolina
69: Motor, Sensory, and Language Mapping and Monitoring for Cortical Resections

Toru Serizawa, MD, PhD
President
Tokyo Gamma Unit Center
Tsukiji Neurological Clinic
Tokyo, Japan
267: Radiosurgery for Malignant Intracranial Tumors

Christopher I. Shaffrey, Sr., MD
John A. Jane Professor
Departments of Neurological and Orthopaedic Surgery
University of Virginia Health System
Charlottesville, Virginia
238: Thoracolumbar Spinal Disorders in Pediatric Patients
Overview and Controversies (Spine)
317: Evaluation and Treatment of Adult Scoliosis and Sagittal Plane Deformity
319: Treatment of High-Grade Spondylolisthesis

Kushal J. Shah, MD
Resident Neurosurgeon
University of Kansas Medical Center
Kansas City, Kansas
305: Evaluation and Treatment of C2 (Axis) Fractures

Lubdha M. Shah, MD
Associate Professor of Radiology
Clinical Neurosciences Center
University of Utah School of Medicine
Salt Lake City, Utah
274: Assessment of Spinal Imaging

Manish N. Shah, MD
Assistant Professor of Pediatric Surgery and Neurosurgery
The University of Texas Health Science Center at Houston
Houston, Texas
299: Adult Congenital Malformations of the Thoracic and Lumbar Spine

Kiarash Shahlaie, MD, PhD
Associate Professor of Neurological Surgery
University of California, Davis School of Medicine
Sacramento, California
346: Clinical Pathophysiology of Traumatic Brain Injury

Yuval Shapira, MD
Senior Neurosurgeon
Division of Peripheral Nerve Surgery
Department of Neurosurgery
Tel Aviv Medical Center and Tel Aviv University
Tel Aviv, Israel
244: Pathophysiology of Surgical Nerve Disorders

Maksim Shapiro, MD
Assistant Professor
Departments of Radiology and Neurology
New York University School of Medicine
New York, New York
122: Endovascular Techniques for Tumor Embolization

Deepak Sharma, MBBS, MD, DM
Professor of Anesthesiology and Pain Medicine
Division Chief, Neuroanesthesiology and Perioperative Neurosciences
University of Washington School of Medicine
Seattle, Washington
5: Neuroanesthesia: Preoperative Evaluation

Mayur Sharma, MD, MCh
Clinical Fellow
Center for Neuromodulation
The Ohio State University
Wexner Medical Center
Columbus, Ohio
100: Surgery for Obsessive-Compulsive Disorder

Mohan Raj Sharma, MD
Professor of Neurosurgery
Tribhuvan University Teaching Hospital
Kathmandu, Nepal
396: Infectious Aneurysms

Andrew Shaw, MD
Clinical Instructor House Staff
Department of Neurological Surgery
The Ohio State University
Wexner Medical Center
Columbus, Ohio
100: Surgery for Obsessive-Compulsive Disorder

Jason P. Sheehan, MD, PhD
Harrison Distinguished Professor and Vice Chair
Department of Neurological Surgery
University of Virginia
Charlottesville, Virginia
173: Stereotactic Radiosurgery for Trigeminal Neuralgia
264: Radiosurgery Technique

Jonas M. Sheehan, MD, FAANS, FACS
Professor of Neurosurgery
Penn State College of Medicine
Penn State Milton S. Hershey Medical Center
Director of Neuro-Oncology
Penn State Cancer Institute
Hershey, Pennsylvania
158: Esthesioneuroblastomas

James M. Shiflett, MD
Assistant Professor of Neurosurgery
University of Mississippi Medical Center
Jackson, Mississippi
219: Skull Lesions in Children: Dermoids, Langerhans Cell Histiocytosis, Fibrous Dysplasia, and Lipomas

Sushil Krishna Shilpakar, MD
Head of Neurosurgery
Tribhuvan University Teaching Hospital
Kathmandu, Nepal
396: Infectious Aneurysms

Jay L. Shils, PhD, D.ABNM, FASNM, FACNS
Associate Professor of Anesthesiology
Director of Intraoperative Neurophysiologic Monitoring
Rush University Medical Center
Chicago, Illinois
93: Neurophysiologic Monitoring for Movement Disorders Surgery
106: Motor Cortex Stimulation for Pain and Movement Disorders

Alexander Y. Shin, MD
Professor and Consultant
Department of Orthopedic Surgery
Mayo Clinic
Rochester, Minnesota
256: Secondary Procedures for Brachial Plexus Injuries

Samuel S. Shin, MD, PhD
Resident Neurosurgeon
University of Pittsburgh School of Medicine
Pittsburgh, Pennsylvania
343: Therapeutic Strategies for Repair and Regeneration following Traumatic Brain Injury

Adnan H. Siddiqui, MD, PhD
Professor of Neurosurgery and Radiology
Director, Toshiba Stroke and Vascular Research Center
Jacobs School of Medicine and Biomedical Sciences
University at Buffalo, State University of New York;
Director of Neuroendovascular Fellowship Program
Director of Research
Department of Neurosurgery
Gates Vascular Institute, Kaleida Health;
Director of Training and Education
Jacobs Institute
Buffalo, New York
367: Carotid Artery Angioplasty and Stenting

Mustafa S. Siddiqui, MD
Associate Professor of Neurology
Wake Forest School of Medicine
Winston-Salem, North Carolina
84: Clinical Overview of Movement Disorders

David M. Silvestri, MD, MBA
Resident Physician
Department of Emergency Medicine
Harvard Medical School
Brigham and Women's Hospital
Massachusetts General Hospital
Boston, Massachusetts
349: Critical Care Management of Traumatic Brain Injury

Marc Sindou, MD, DSc
Professor of Neurosurgery
Université Lyon 1
Hôpital Neurologique Pierre Wertheimer
Lyon, France
103: Lesioning Surgery for Spasticity
182: Dorsal Root Entry Zone Lesions for Pain

Robert J. Singer, MD
Associate Professor
Departments of Surgery and Radiology
Geisel School of Medicine at Dartmouth
Hanover, New Hampshire
16: Principles of Neurocritical Care

Jeffrey M. Singh, MD, MSc, FRCPC
Associate Professor of Medicine
University of Toronto Faculty of Medicine;
Medical Director, Intensive Care Unit
Toronto Western Hospital
Toronto, Ontario, Canada
303: Medical Management of Spinal Cord Injury

Manish K. Singh, MD
Assistant Professor
Department of Neurosurgery
Tulane University
New Orleans, Louisiana
414: Microsurgical Treatment of Spinal Vascular Malformations

Walavan Sivakumar, MD
Neurosurgery Resident
University of Utah School of Medicine
Salt Lake City, Utah
32: The Role of Third Ventriculostomy in Adults and Children: A Critical Review

Justin Slavin, MD
Spine Fellow
Brigham and Women's Hospital
Harvard Medical School
Boston, Massachusetts
282: Complication Avoidance in Spine Surgery

Edward R. Smith, MD
Associate Professor of Neurosurgery
Harvard Medical School;
Director, Pediatric Cerebrovascular Neurosurgery
Boston Children's Hospital
Boston, Massachusetts
220: Moyamoya Disease

Justin S. Smith, MD, PhD
Professor of Neurosurgery
University of Virginia Health System
Co-Director, UVA Spine Center
Charlottesville, Virginia
238: Thoracolumbar Spinal Disorders in Pediatric Patients
Overview and Controversies (Spine)
317: Evaluation and Treatment of Adult Scoliosis and Sagittal Plane Deformity
319: Treatment of High-Grade Spondylolisthesis

Timothy R. Smith, MD, PhD, MPH
Assistant Professor
Department of Neurosurgery
Harvard Medical School
Brigham and Women's Hospital
Boston, Massachusetts
150: Pituitary Tumors: Functioning and Nonfunctioning

Yoland Smith, PhD
Professor of Neurology
Emory University School of Medicine;
Yerkes National Primate Research Center
Emory University
Atlanta, Georgia
81: Anatomy and Synaptic Connectivity of the Basal Ganglia

Robert A. Solomon, MD
Byron Stookey Professor and Chairman
Department of Neurological Surgery
Columbia University College of Physicians and Surgeons
Director of Service
Department of Neurological Surgery
New York–Presbyterian Hospital
New York, New York
403: Adjuvant Endovascular Management of Brain Arteriovenous Malformations

Adam M. Sonabend, MD
Assistant Professor of Neurological Surgery
Department of Neurological Surgery
Columbia University College of Physicians and Surgeons
New York–Presbyterian Hospital
New York, New York
141: Pineal Tumors

Volker K.H. Sonntag, MD
Professor Emeritus of Neurological Surgery
Barrow Neurological Institute
St. Joseph's Hospital and Medical Center
Phoenix, Arizona
325: Anterior Cervical Instrumentation

Jeffrey M. Sorenson, MD
Associate Professor of Neurosurgery
Semmes-Murphey Clinic
University of Tennessee College of Medicine
Memphis, Tennessee
25: Visualization and Optics in Neurosurgery

Sulpicio G. Soriano, MD
Professor
Department of Anesthesia, Critical Care and Pain Medicine
Harvard Medical School;
Endowed Chair in Pediatric Neuroanesthesia
Boston Children's Hospital
Boston, Massachusetts
184: Neuroanesthesia in Children

Hector Soriano-Baron, MD
Postdoctoral Fellow in Spine Biomechanics
Department of Neurosurgery
Barrow Neurological Institute
Phoenix, Arizona
304: Classification and Treatment of O-C1 Craniocervical Injuries
325: Anterior Cervical Instrumentation

Mark M. Souweidane, MD, FACS, FAAP
Professor and Vice Chair
Department of Neurological Surgery
Weill Cornell Medical College;
Director, Pediatric Neurosurgery
New York–Presbyterian Hospital
Weill Cornell Medical Center
Memorial Sloan Kettering Cancer Center
New York, New York
218: Pediatric Intraventricular and Periventricular Tumors

Gwendolyn A. Sowa, MD, PhD
Associate Professor of Physical Medicine and Rehabilitation
University of Pittsburgh School of Medicine
Pittsburgh, Pennsylvania
276: Disk Degeneration and Regeneration

Giorgio Spatola, MD
Medical Doctor, Neurosurgeon
Departments of Neurosurgery and Radiosurgery
Ospedale San Raffaele
Milan, Italy
268: Radiosurgery for Benign Intracranial Tumors

Julian Spears, MD, SM, FRCSC, FACS
Assistant Professor of Neurosurgery and Medical Imaging
University of Toronto Faculty of Medicine;
Interim Head, Division of Neurosurgery
St. Michael's Hospital
Toronto, Ontario, Canada
380: Perioperative Management of Subarachnoid Hemorrhage

Dennis D. Spencer, MD
Harvey and Kate Cushing Professor of Surgery
Department of Neurosurgery
Director, Epilepsy Surgery Program
Yale University School of Medicine
New Haven, Connecticut
Overview and Controversies (Epilepsy)
75: Standard Temporal Lobectomy

Robert F. Spetzler, MD
Director and J.N. Harber Chair of Neurological Surgery
Barrow Neurological Institute
St. Joseph's Hospital and Medical Center
Phoenix, Arizona;
Professor of Neurosurgery
Department of Surgery
University of Arizona College of Medicine
Tucson, Arizona
222: Pediatric Cerebral Aneurysms
Overview and Controversies (Vascular)
411: Microsurgery for Cerebral Cavernous Malformations

Robert J. Spinner, MD
Chair, Department of Neurologic Surgery
Professor
Departments of Anatomy, Neurologic Surgery, and Orthopedic Surgery
Mayo Clinic
Rochester, Minnesota
256: Secondary Procedures for Brachial Plexus Injuries

Eric G. St. Clair, MD
Director of Neurosurgery
Cancer Treatment Centers of America at Eastern Regional Medical Center
Philadelphia, Pennsylvania
162: Skull Tumors

Robert M. Starke, MD, MSc
Assistant Professor of Clinical Neurosurgery and Radiology
Co-Director, Endovascular Neurosurgery JMH
Director of Neurovascular Research
Department of Neurological Surgery
University of Miami
Miami, Florida
374: Cerebral Venous and Sinus Thrombosis

Philip Starr, MD, PhD
Professor and Dolores Cakebread Endowed Chair
Department of Neurological Surgery
Co-Director, Functional Neurosurgery Program
University of California, San Francisco;
Surgical Director, Parkinson's Disease Research, Education and Care Center
San Francisco Veteran's Affairs Medical Center
San Francisco, California
89: Deep Brain Stimulation for Parkinson's Disease

S. Tonya Stefko, MD, FACS
Associate Professor of Ophthalmology, Otolaryngology and Neurological Surgery
University of Pittsburgh School of Medicine;
Director, Orbital, Oculoplastics and Aesthetic Surgery Service
University of Pittsburgh Medical Center
Pittsburgh, Pennsylvania
161: Tumors of the Orbit

Sherman C. Stein, MD
Clinical Professor
Department of Neurosurgery
Perelman School of Medicine at the University of Pennsylvania
Philadelphia, Pennsylvania
30: Clinical Evaluation of Adult Hydrocephalus

Gary K. Steinberg, MD, PhD
Bernard and Ronni Lacroute–William Randolph Hearst Professor of Neurosurgery and the Neurosciences
Chairman
Department of Neurosurgery
Stanford University School of Medicine
Chief
Department of Neurosurgery
Stanford Hospital and Clinics
Stanford, California
406: Surgical and Radiosurgical Management of Grade IV and V Arteriovenous Malformations

Bradley H. Stephens, MD, MPH
Resident Neurosurgeon
Washington University School of Medicine in St. Louis
St. Louis, Missouri
299: Adult Congenital Malformations of the Thoracic and Lumbar Spine

Frederick L. Stephens, MD
Madigan Army Medical Center
Tacoma, Washington
352: Traumatic and Penetrating Head Injuries

Matthew A. Stern, BS
Emory University School of Medicine
Atlanta, Georgia
88: Ablative Procedures for Parkinson's Disease

Ewout W. Steyerberg, PhD
Professor of Medical Decision Making
Department of Public Health
Erasmus MC, University Medical Center
Rotterdam, The Netherlands
356: Prognosis after Traumatic Brain Injury

Philip E. Stieg, MD, PhD
Chairman and Neurosurgeon-in-Chief
Professor of Neurological Surgery
New York–Presbyterian Hospital/Weill Cornell Medical Center
New York, New York
366: Carotid Endarterectomy

Scellig S.D. Stone, MD, PhD, FRCSC
Assistant Professor of Neurosurgery
Harvard Medical School;
Director, Movement Disorder Program
Boston Children's Hospital
Boston, Massachusetts
90: Deep Brain Stimulation for Dystonia

Russell G. Strom, MD
Department of Neurosurgery
NYU Langone Medical Center
New York, New York
20: Positioning for Cranial Surgery

Roy E. Strowd III, MD
Adjunct Assistant Professor
Department of Neurology
Johns Hopkins University School of Medicine
Baltimore, Maryland;
Assistant Professor
Departments of Neurology and Internal Medicine
Wake Forest School of Medicine
Winston-Salem, North Carolina
124: Genetic Syndromes of Brain Tumors

Michael E. Sughrue, MD
Associate Professor
Department of Neurosurgery
University of Oklahoma Health Sciences Center
Oklahoma City, Oklahoma
133: Endoscopic Approaches to Brain Tumors

John H. Suh, MD
Professor and Chairman
Department of Radiation Oncology
Cleveland Clinic
Cleveland, Ohio
262: Radiobiology of Radiotherapy and Radiosurgery

Dima Suki, PhD
Professor of Neurosurgery
University of Texas MD Anderson Cancer Center
Houston, Texas
146: Metastatic Brain Tumors

Wale A.R. Sulaiman, MD, PhD, FRCS(C)
System Chairman
Department of Neurosurgery
Medical Director, Spine Center
Ochsner Health Systems
New Orleans, Louisiana
254: Management of Acute Peripheral Nerve Injuries

Bomin Sun, MD, PhD
Director, Department of Stereotactic and Functional Neurosurgery
Shanghai Jiao Tong University
Rui Jin Hospital
Shanghai, China
102: Surgery for Anorexia Nervosa

Michele Tagliati, MD, FAAN
Associate Professor
Director of Movement Disorders
Department of Neurology
Cedars-Sinai Medical Center
Los Angeles, California
85: Patient Selection Criteria for Deep Brain Stimulation in Movement Disorders

Takaomi Taira, MD, PhD
Professor
Department of Neurosurgery
Tokyo Women's Medical University
Tokyo, Japan
Overview and Controversies (Functional)
97: Thalamotomy for Focal Hand Dystonia

Yasushi Takagi, MD, PhD
Associate Professor of Neurosurgery
Kyoto University Graduate School of Medicine
Kyoto, Japan
373: Adult Moyamoya Disease

Rafael J. Tamargo, MD, FACS
Walter E. Dandy Professor of Neurosurgery
Professor of Neurosurgery and Otolaryngology-Head and Neck Surgery
Director, Cerebrovascular Neurosurgery
Neurosurgical Co-Director, Neurocritical Care Unit
Johns Hopkins University School of Medicine
Baltimore, Maryland
386: Microsurgery of Anterior Communicating Artery Aneurysms

Shota Tanaka, MD
Assistant Professor of Neurosurgery
University of Tokyo Graduate School of Medicine
Tokyo, Japan
267: Radiosurgery for Malignant Intracranial Tumors

Nitin Tandon, MD, FAANS
Professor of Neurosurgery
University of Texas Health Science Center;
Director, Epilepsy Surgery
Memorial Hermann Hospital;
Adjunct Associate Professor
Department of Electrical and Computer Engineering
Rice University
Houston, Texas
Overview and Controversies (Epilepsy)

Omar Tanweer, MD
Resident Neurosurgeon
New York University School of Medicine
New York, New York
122: Endovascular Techniques for Tumor Embolization

Jessica A. Tate, MD
Assistant Professor of Neurology
Wake Forest School of Medicine
Winston-Salem, North Carolina
84: Clinical Overview of Movement Disorders

Matthew C. Tate, MD,PhD
Assistant Professor
Department of Neurological Surgery
Northwestern University Feinberg School of Medicine
Chicago, Illinois
134: Awake Craniotomy and Intraoperative Mapping

Claudio E. Tatsui, MD
Assistant Professor of Neurosurgery
University of Texas MD Anderson Cancer Center
Houston, Texas
294: Assessment and Treatment of Benign Intradural Extramedullary Tumors

Blake E.S. Taylor, BA, MDc
Resident
College of Physicians and Surgeons
Columbia University
New York, New York
404: Endovascular Management of Arteriovenous Malformations for Cure

Michael D. Taylor, MD, PhD, FRCS(C)
Associate Professor
Departments of Surgery and Laboratory Medicine and Pathobiology
University of Toronto
The Hospital for Sick Children
Toronto, Ontario, Canada
205: Genetics of Pediatric Brain Tumors

Steven A. Telian, MD
John L. Kemink Professor of Neurotology
Director, Division of Otology-Neurotology
Department of Otolaryngology-Head and Neck Surgery
University of Michigan Medical School
Ann Arbor, Michigan
105: Treatment of Intractable Vertigo

Zachary J. Tempel, MD
Resident Neurosurgeon and Spine Fellow
University of Pittsburgh Medical Center
Pittsburgh, Pennsylvania
332: Sacropelvic Fixation: Anterior and Posterior Options

Charles Teo, MBBS, FRACS
Conjoint Associate Professor
Department of Neurosurgery
University of New South Wales
Sydney, Australia;
Director, Center for Minimally Invasive Neurosurgery
Prince of Wales Private Hospital
Randwick, Australia
133: Endoscopic Approaches to Brain Tumors

Jeffrey M. Tessier, MD
Transplant Infectious Diseases
Texas Health Care, PLLC
Fort Worth, Texas
35: Basic Science of Central Nervous System Infections

Khoi D. Than, MD
Assistant Professor
Department of Neurosurgery
Oregon Health & Science University
Portland, Oregon
288: Evaluation and Treatment of Degenerative Lumbar Spondylolisthesis

Alice Theadom, PhD, MNZPSS, MIHP
Senior Research Fellow
National Institute for Stroke and Applied Neuroscience
Auckland University of Technology
Auckland, New Zealand
336: Epidemiology of Traumatic Brain Injury

Nicholas Theodore, MD, FACS, FAANS
Professor of Neurological Surgery
Chief, Spine Section
Director, Neurotrauma Program
Barrow Neurological Institute
Phoenix, Arizona
304: Classification and Treatment of O-C1 Craniocervical Injuries
325: Anterior Cervical Instrumentation

B. Gregory Thompson, Jr., MD
Professor and Program Director
Department of Neurosurgery
University of Michigan
Ann Arbor, Michigan
415: Pregnancy and the Vascular Lesion

Ann H. Tilton, MD
Professor of Neurology and Pediatrics
Section Chair, Child Neurology
Louisiana State Health Sciences Center;
Director, Children's Hospital Rehabilitation Center
Children's Hospital of New Orleans
New Orleans, Louisiana
241: Clinical Features and Management of Cerebral Palsy

Shelly D. Timmons, MD, PhD, FACS, FAANS
Professor of Neurosurgery
Vice Chair for Administration
Director of Neurotrauma
Penn State Milton S. Hershey Medical Center
Hershey, Pennsylvania
Danville, Pennsylvania
354: Indications and Techniques for Cranial Decompression after Traumatic Brain Injury

Nestor D. Tomycz, MD
Department of Neurosurgery
Allegheny Health Network
Pittsburgh, Pennsylvania
107: Deep Brain Stimulation for Obesity

Juan Torres-Reveron, MD, PhD
Assistant Clinical Professor
Functional and Epilepsy Surgery
Wright State University Boonshoft School of Medicine
Premier Health Clinical Neuroscience Institute
Dayton, Ohio
75: Standard Temporal Lobectomy

Gabor Toth, MD
Resident Physician
Cerebrovascular Center
Cleveland Clinic
Cleveland, Ohio
393: Endovascular Flow Diversion for Intracranial Aneurysms

Charles P. Toussaint, MD
Assistant Professor of Clinical Surgery
Department of Neurosurgery
University of South Carolina School of Medicine
Columbia, South Carolina
249: Distal Entrapment Syndromes: Carpal Tunnel, Cubital Tunnel, Peroneal, and Tarsal Tunnel

Duc A. Tran, MD, PhD
Assistant Professor of Physical Medicine and Rehabilitaton
Director of Traumatic Brain Injury Rehabilitation
Loma Linda University School of Medicine
Loma Linda, California
358: Rehabilitation of Patients with Traumatic Brain Injury

Bruce D. Trapp, PhD
Chairman
Department of Neurosciences
Cleveland Clinic
Cleveland, Ohio
48: Neurons and Neuroglia

R. Shane Tubbs, MS, PA-C, PhD
Chief Scientific Officer
Seattle Science Foundation
Seattle, Washington;
Adjunct Professor
University of Dundee
Dundee, United Kingdom
190: Chiari Malformations
232: Tethered Spinal Cord: Fatty Filum Terminale, Meningocele Manqué, and Dermal Sinus Tracts

Allan R. Tunkel, MD, PhD
Professor of Medicine and Medical Science
Associate Dean for Medical Education
Warren Alpert Medical School of Brown University
Providence, Rhode Island
39: Brain Abscess

Ugur Türe, MD
Professor and Chair
Department of Neurosurgery
Hacettepe University School of Medicine
Ankara, Turkey
Overview and Controversies (General)

Ali Hassoun Turkmani, MD
Resident Physician
Department of Neurosurgery
The University of Texas at Houston
Houston, Texas
384: Microsurgery of Paraclinoid Aneurysms

Juan S. Uribe, MD
Assistant Professor of Neurosurgery
Director, Cahill Spine Institute
University of South Florida Morsani College of Medicine
Tampa, Florida
278: Electrophysiologic Studies and Monitoring
328: Anterior and Lateral Lumbar Instrumentation

Mwiza Ushe, MD, MA
Assistant Professor of Neurology
Washington University School of Medicine in St. Louis
St. Louis, Missouri
86: Functional Imaging in Movement Disorders

Alexander R. Vaccaro, MD, PhD
Professor and Vice Chairman
Department of Orthopaedic Surgery
Thomas Jefferson University and Hospitals
Philadelphia, Pennsylvania
306: Evaluation, Classification, and Treatment of Cervical (C3-C7) Injuries

Martin J. van den Bent, MD
Professor of Neuro-Oncology
Erasmus MC Cancer Center
Rotterdam, The Netherlands
138: Radiologic and Clinical Criteria of Treatment Response

Jamie J. Van Gompel, MD
Associate Professor
Departments of Neurosurgery and Otolaryngology
Mayo Clinic
Rochester, Minnesota
67: Single-Photon Emission Computed Tomography in Epilepsy Surgery Evaluation

J.J. van Overbeeke, MD, PhD
Professor and Chair
Department of Neurosurgery
Maastricht University Medical Center
Maastricht, The Netherlands
135: Intraoperative Magnetic Resonance Imaging

Henk van Santbrink, MD, PhD
Neurosurgeon
Department of Neurosurgery
Maastricht University Medical Center
Maastricht and Heerlen, The Netherlands
135: Intraoperative Magnetic Resonance Imaging

Ciro Vasquez, MD
Resident Neurosurgeon
University of Minnesota School of Medicine
Minneapolis, Minnesota
38: The Use and Misuse of Antibiotics in Neurosurgery

Viren S. Vasudeva, MD
Resident Neurosurgeon
Harvard Medical School
Brigham and Women's Hospital
Boston Children's Hospital
Boston, Massachusetts
296: Assessment and Treatment of Malignant Primary Spinal Tumors

Ananth K. Vellimana, MD
Resident Neurosurgeon
Department of Neurological Surgery
Washington University School of Medicine in St. Louis
St. Louis, Missouri
143: Intracranial Ependymomas in Adults

Angela Verlicchi, MD
Unit of Neurology
Free University of Neuroscience Anemos
Reggio Emilia, Italy
156: Glomus Tumors

Emiliano Vialle, MD, MSc
Spinal Surgeon
Curitiba Spine Center
Hospital Universitário Cajuru
São Paulo, Brazil
322: Lumbar Arthroplasty

Mariano S. Viapiano, PhD
Assistant Professor of Neurosurgery
Harvard Medical School
Brigham and Women's Hospital
Boston, Massachusetts
115: Malignant Glioma Microenvironment

Shaleen Vira, MD
Resident Physician
Department of Orthopaedic Surgery
New York University Hospital for Joint Diseases
New York, New York
311: Classification of Spinal Deformity

Michael S. Virk, MD, PhD
Resident Neurosurgeon
Weill Cornell Medical College
New York–Presbyterian Hospital
New York, New York
335: Minimally Invasive Techniques for Degenerative Disease

Veerle Visser-Vandewalle, MD, PhD
Head, Department of Stereotactic and Functional Neurosurgery
University Hospital of Cologne
Cologne, Germany
99: Surgery for Tourette's Syndrome

Jerrold L. Vitek, MD, PhD
Professor and Chair
Department of Neurology
University of Minnesota Medical School
Minneapolis, Minnesota
91: Deep Brain Stimulation: Mechanisms of Action

Nam Vo, PhD
Assistant Professor of Orthopaedic Surgery
University of Pittsburgh School of Medicine
Pittsburgh, Pennsylvania
276: Disk Degeneration and Regeneration

Michael A. Vogelbaum, MD, PhD
Professor of Surgery (Neurosurgery)
Division of Neurosurgery
Director, Center for Translational Therapeutics
Associate Director, Brain Tumor and Neuro-Oncology Center
Neurological Institute
Cleveland Clinic
Cleveland, Ohio
117: Delivery of Therapy to Brain Tumors: Problems and Potentials

Matthew Volpini, BSc
Division of Neurosurgery
University of Toronto Faculty of Medicine;
Toronto, Ontario, Canada
101: Surgery for Major Depressive Disorder

P. Ashley Wackym, MD
Vice President of Research
Legacy Research Institute
Legacy Health;
President, Ear and Skull Base Center
Portland, Oregon
9: Neurotology

Rishi Wadhwa, MD
Assistant Clinical Professor
Complex and Minimally Invasive Spine Surgery
General Neurosurgery
Department of Neurosurgery-Marin
UCSF Spine Center-San Francisco
San Francisco, California
321: Cervical Arthroplasty

Mark S. Wainwright, MD, PhD
Founders' Board Chair in Neurocritical Care
Professor of Pediatrics and Neurology
Northwestern University Feinberg School of Medicine
Chicago, Illinois
185: Neurocritical Care in Children

Ben Waldau, MD
Assistant Professor of Neurological Surgery
University of California, Davis School of Medicine
Sacramento, California
69: Motor, Sensory, and Language Mapping and Monitoring for Cortical Resections

Marion L. Walker, MD
Professor of Neurosurgery
University of Utah School of Medicine
Salt Lake City, Utah
191: Craniopagus Twins

M. Christopher Wallace, MD, FACS, FRCS(C)
Professor of Surgery
Chair and Section Chief, Division of Neurosurgery
Queen's University School of Medicine
Kingston General Hospital
Kingston, Ontario, Canada
385: Intracranial Internal Carotid Artery Aneurysms

Scott A. Wallace, MD
Staff Pediatric Anesthesiologist
Naval Medical Center San Diego
San Diego, California
352: Traumatic and Penetrating Head Injuries

Kyle M. Walsh, PhD
Assistant Professor of Neurological Surgery
Division of Neuroepidemiology
University of California, San Francisco
San Francisco, California
118: Epidemiology of Brain Tumors

Huan Wang, MD, PhD
Associate Professor
Neurosurgery and Orthopedics
Department of Neurologic Surgery
Mayo Clinic
Rochester, Minnesota
256: Secondary Procedures for Brachial Plexus Injuries

Michael Y. Wang, MD, FACS
Professor of Neurological Surgery and Rehabilitation Medicine
University of Miami Miller School of Medicine
Miami, Florida
316: Minimally Invasive Treatment of Adult Scoliosis
333: Spinal Osteotomies

Shelly Wang, MD
Resident
Neurosurgery
University of Toronto Faculty of Medicine
Toronto,Ontario, Canada;
Student
Epidemiology and Biostatistics
Harvard School of Public Health
Boston, Massachusetts
303: Medical Management of Spinal Cord Injury

Tony R. Wang, MD
Resident Neurosurgeon
University of Virginia School of Medicine
Charlottesville, Virginia
95: Transcranial Magnetic Resonance Imaging–Guided Focused Ultrasound Thalamotomy for Tremor

Vincent Y. Wang, MD, PhD
Seton Brain and Spine Institute
Austin, Texas
15: Intracranial Pressure Monitoring

Xin Wang, BHSc
Departments of Neurosurgery and Laboratory Medicine and Pathobiology
University of Toronto
The Hospital for Sick Children
Toronto, Ontario, Canada
205: Genetics of Pediatric Brain Tumors

Ronald E. Warnick, MD
Professor of Neurosurgery
University of Cincinnati College of Medicine;
Director, Brain Tumor Center
University of Cincinnati Neuroscience Institute;
Neurosurgeon
Mayfield Clinic
Cincinnati, Ohio
131: Risks of Intrinsic Brain Tumor Surgery and Avoidance of Complications

Robert J. Weil, MD, FAANS, FACS
Chief Medical Executive
Geisinger Health System Northeast Region
System Associate Chief Scientific Officer and Medical Director
Geisinger Care Support Systems
Danville, Pennsylvania
53: Cerebral Edema

Howard L. Weiner, MD, FACS, FAAP
Professor of Neurosurgery
Baylor College of Medicine;
Chief of Neurosurgery
Texas Children's Hospital
Houston, Texas
217: Neurocutaneous Tumor Syndromes

Jon D. Weingart, MD
Professor of Neurosurgery
Johns Hopkins University School of Medicine
Baltimore, Maryland
128: Frame and Frameless Stereotactic Brain Biopsy
129: Basic Principles of Cranial Surgery for Brain Tumors

Martin H. Weiss, MD
Professor of Neurological Surgery and The Martin H. Weiss Chair in Neurological Surgery
Keck School of Medicine
University of Southern California
Los Angeles, California
18: Surgical Planning: An Overview

Nirit Weiss, MD
Assistant Professor of Neurosurgery
Icahn School of Medicine at Mount Sinai
New York, New York
6: Complication Avoidance in Neurosurgery

Michael Weller, MD
Professor and Chair
Department of Neurology
University Hospital Zurich
Zurich, Switzerland
111: Brain Tumor Immunology and Immunotherapy

John C. Wellons III, MD, MSPH
Professor of Neurological Surgery and Pediatrics
Chief, Division of Pediatric Neurosurgery
Vanderbilt University Medical Center
Nashville, Tennessee
232: Tethered Spinal Cord: Fatty Filum Terminale, Meningocele Manqué, and Dermal Sinus Tracts

Hung Tzu Wen, MD, PhD
Attending Neurosurgeon
Hospital das Clínicas
University of São Paulo College of Medicine
Hospital Samaritano
São Paulo, Brazil;
Former Co-Clinical Assistant Professor of Neurological Surgery
University of Florida College of Medicine
Gainesville, Florida
2: Surgical Anatomy of the Brain

Patrick Y. Wen, MD
Professor of Neurology
Harvard Medical School;
Director, Center for Neuro-Oncology
Dana-Farber Cancer Institute;
Director, Division of Neuro-Oncology
Department of Neurology
Brigham and Women's Hospital
Boston, Massachusetts
125: Principles of Chemotherapy

G. Alexander West, MD, PhD
Department of Neurosurgery
Houston Methodist Neurological Institute
Houston, Texas;
Assistant Professor of Clinical Neurological Surgery
Weill Cornell Medical Center
New York, New York
383: Surgical Approaches to Intracranial Aneurysms
399: Traumatic Cerebral Aneurysms Secondary to Penetrating Intracranial Injuries

Jonathan White, MD
Professor
Departments of Neurological Surgery and Radiology
University of Texas Southwestern Medical Center
Dallas, Texas
390: Microsurgery of Basilar Apex Aneurysms

Alexander C. Whiting, MD
Department of Neurosurgery
Barrow Neurological Institute
Phoenix, Arizona
107: Deep Brain Stimulation for Obesity

Donald M. Whiting, MD, MS
Chair, Department of Neurosurgery
Allegheny Health Network
Pittsburgh, Pennsylvania
107: Deep Brain Stimulation for Obesity

Thomas Wichmann, MD
Professor of Neurology
Emory University School of Medicine
Atlanta, Georgia
82: Rationale for Surgical Interventions in Movement Disorders

David M. Wildrick, PhD
Surgery Publications Program Manager
Department of Neurosurgery
University of Texas MD Anderson Cancer Center
Houston, Texas
110: Brain Tumors: An Overview of Current Histopathologic and Genetic Classifications
146: Metastatic Brain Tumors

D. Andrew Wilkinson, MD, MS
Resident Neurosurgeon
University of Michigan Medical School
Ann Arbor, Michigan
223: Pediatric Arteriovenous Malformations

Jesse L. Winer, MD
Department of Neurosurgery
Boston Children's Hospital
Boston, Massachusetts
198: Infantile Posthemorrhagic Hydrocephalus

Christopher J. Winfree, MD
Assistant Professor
Department of Neurological Surgery
Columbia University College of Physicians and Surgeons
New York, New York
181: Diagnosis and Management of Painful Neuromas

Ethan A. Winkler, MD, PhD
Resident Neurosurgeon
University of California, San Francisco
San Francisco, California
340: Genetics of Traumatic Brain Injury

H. Richard Winn, MD
Professor of Neurosurgery
University of Iowa Carver College of Medicine
Iowa City, Iowa;
Professor of Neurosurgery and Neuroscience
Icahn School of Medicine at Mount Sinai
New York, New York
Overview and Controversies (General)
39: Brain Abscess
377: The Natural History of Cerebral Aneurysms
379: Surgical Decision Making for the Treatment of Intracranial Aneurysms
396: Infectious Aneurysms

Jeffrey H. Wisoff, MD, FAANS, FAAP
Professor of Neurosurgery and Pediatrics
New York University School of Medicine
Director of Pediatric Neurosurgery
NYU Langone Medical Center
New York, New York
151: Craniopharyngiomas in Adults
210: Pediatric Craniopharyngiomas

Jens Witsch, MD
Research Fellow
Division of Critical Care Neurology
Department of Neurology
Columbia University College of Physicians and Surgeons
New York, New York
63: Continuous Electroencephalography in Neurological-Neurosurgical Intensive Care: Applications and Value

Steven M. Wolf, MD
Associate Professor
Departments of Neurology and Pediatrics
Icahn School of Medicine at Mount Sinai
New York, New York
240: Pediatric Epilepsy Surgery

Christopher E. Wolfla, MD
Professor of Neurosurgery
Medical College of Wisconsin
Milwaukee, Wisconsin
326: Posterior Subaxial and Cervicothoracic Instrumentation

Jean-Paul Wolinsky, MD
Professor of Neurosurgery
Director, Spine Program
Johns Hopkins University School of Medicine
Baltimore, Maryland
292: Assessment and Treatment of Benign Tumors of the Axial Skeleton

Cyrus C. Wong, MD
Neurological Surgery
North Texas Neurosurgical and Spine Center
Fort Worth, Texas
275: Spinal Biomechanics and Basics of Spinal Instrumentation

Eric T. Wong, MD
Associate Professor of Neurology
Harvard Medical School;
Director, Brain Tumor Center and Neuro-Oncology Unit
Beth Israel Deaconess Medical Center
Boston, Massachusetts
116: Angiogenesis and Brain Tumors: Scientific Principles, Current Therapy, and Future Directions

Margaret R. Wrensch, PhD
Professor and Virginia and Stanley Lewis Chair in Brain Tumor Research
Department of Neurological Surgery
University of California, San Francisco
San Francisco, California
118: Epidemiology of Brain Tumors

Jau-Ching Wu, MD, PhD
Assistant Professor
Department of Neurosurgery
Neurological Institute, Taipei Veterans General Hospital
National Yang-Ming University
Taipei, Taiwan
321: Cervical Arthroplasty

Linda Wei Xu, MD
Resident Neurosurgeon
Stanford University Hospital and Clinics
Palo Alto, California
224: Management of Head Injury: Special Considerations in Children

Zhiyuan Xu, MD, MSc
Clinical Instructor
Department of Neurological Surgery
University of Virginia
Charlottesville, Virginia
173: Stereotactic Radiosurgery for Trigeminal Neuralgia

Carol H. Yan, MD
Resident Physician
Department of Otorhinolaryngology
Perelman School of Medicine at the University of Pennsylvania
Philadelphia, Pennsylvania
357: Traumatic Cerebrospinal Fluid Fistulas

Edward Yap, MD
Resident Neurosurgeon
University of North Carolina School of Medicine at Chapel Hill
Chapel Hill, North Carolina
148: Meningeal Sarcomas and Hemangiopericytomas

Chester K. Yarbrough, MD, MPHS
Chief Resident
Department of Neurological Surgery
Washington University School of Medicine in St. Louis
St. Louis, Missouri
257: Nerve Injuries of the Lower Extremity

Katsuhito Yasuno, PhD
Research Scientist
Department of Neurosurgery
Yale University School of Medicine
New Haven, Connecticut
376: Genetics of Intracranial Aneurysms

Daniel Yavin, MD
Resident Neurosurgeon
Departments of Clinical Neurosciences and Community Health Sciences
University of Calgary Faculty of Medicine
Calgary, Alberta, Canada
281: Nonsurgical and Postsurgical Management of Low Back Pain

Ulaş Yener, MD
Assistant Professor
Department of Neurosurgery
Acibadem University School of Medicine
Istanbul, Turkey
159: Trigeminal Schwannomas

Yasuhiro Yonekawa, MD
Professor of Neurosurgery
Department of Neurosurgery
University Hospital Zurich
Zurich, Switzerland
373: Adult Moyamoya Disease

Timothy P. Young, MD
Instructor in Physical Medicine and Rehabilitation
Harvard Medical School
Spaulding Rehabilitation Hospital
Boston, Massachusetts
358: Rehabilitation of Patients with Traumatic Brain Injury

Mark W. Youngblood, MDc, PhDc
Department of Genetics
Yale University School of Medicine
New Haven, Connecticut
376: Genetics of Intracranial Aneurysms

Brett E. Youngerman, MD
Resident
Department of Neurological Surgery
Columbia University College of Physicians and Surgeons
New York, New York
181: Diagnosis and Management of Painful Neuromas

Jennifer S. Yu, MD, PhD
Assistant Professor
Departments of Radiation Oncology and Stem Cell Biology and Regenerative Medicine
Cleveland Clinic
Cleveland, Ohio
262: Radiobiology of Radiotherapy and Radiosurgery

John K. Yue, BA
Department of Neurological Surgery
University of California, San Francisco
San Francisco, California
340: Genetics of Traumatic Brain Injury

Esther L. Yuh, MD, PhD
Associate Professor
Departments of Radiology and Biomedical Imaging
University of California, San Francisco School of Medicine
San Francisco, California
344: Structural Imaging of Traumatic Brain Injury

Joseph M. Zabramski, MD
Professor
Department of Neurosurgery
Barrow Neurological Institute
Phoenix, Arizona
409: Natural History of Cavernous Malformations

Andrew C. Zacest, MBBS, MS, FRACS, FFPMANZCA
Consultant Neurosurgeon
Royal Adelaide Hospital
Associate Clinical Professor of Neurosurgery and Pain Medicine
University of Adelaide
Adelaide, Australia
Overview and Controversies (Pain)
177: Peripheral Nerve Stimulation for Neuropathic Pain

J. Christopher Zacko, MD, MS
Assistant Professor of Neurosurgery
Director, Neurotrauma and Neurocritical Care
Penn State Milton S. Hershey Medical Center
Hershey, Pennsylvania
341: Neurochemical Pathomechanisms in Traumatic Brain Injury

Gabriel Zada, MD, MS
Assistant Professor of Neurological Surgery
Director, Endoscopic Cranial Base Surgery
Keck School of Medicine
University of Southern California, Los Angeles
Los Angeles, California
18: Surgical Planning: An Overview

Eyal Zadicario, MSc
Vice President, Research and Development
Director, Neurosurgery Program
Insightec, Ltd.
Haifa, Israel
95: Transcranial Magnetic Resonance Imaging–Guided Focused Ultrasound Thalamotomy for Tremor

Patricia Leigh Zadnik, MD
Research Fellow
Department of Neurosurgery
Johns Hopkins University School of Medicine
Baltimore, Maryland
155: Chordomas and Chondrosarcomas

Ross D. Zafonte, DO
Ida S. Charlton Professor and Chair
Department of Physical Medicine and Rehabilitation
Harvard Medical School;
Vice President of Medical Affairs
Spaulding Rehabilitation Hospital;
Chief of Physical Medicine and Rehabilitation
Massachusetts General Hospital
Brigham and Women's Hospital
Boston, Massachusetts
358: Rehabilitation of Patients with Traumatic Brain Injury

Eric L. Zager, MD
Professor of Neurosurgery
Perelman School of Medicine at the University of Pennsylvania
Philadelphia, Pennsylvania
249: Distal Entrapment Syndromes: Carpal Tunnel, Cubital Tunnel, Peroneal, and Tarsal Tunnel

Bruno Zanotti, MD, PhD
Unit of Neurosurgery
Neuroscience Department
S.M. della Misericordia University Hospital
Udine, Italy
156: Glomus Tumors

Elizabeth G. Zellner, MD
Resident Surgeon
Section of Plastic Surgery
Yale School of Medicine
New Haven, Connecticut
23: Incisions and Closures

Shikun Zhan, MD, PhD
Department of Stereotactic and Functional Neurosurgery
Shanghai Jiao Tong University
Rui Jin Hospital
Shanghai, China
102: Surgery for Anorexia Nervosa

Chencheng Zhang, MD
Department of Stereotactic and Functional Neurosurgery
Shanghai Jiao Tong University
Rui Jin Hospital
Shanghai, China
102: Surgery for Anorexia Nervosa

Xiaoxiao Zhang, MD
Department of Stereotactic and Functional Neurosurgery
Shanghai Jiao Tong University
Rui Jin Hospital
Shanghai, China
102: Surgery for Anorexia Nervosa

Y. Jonathan Zhang, MD
Department of Neurosurgery
Houston Methodist Neurological Institute
Houston, Texas;
Assistant Professor of Clinical Neurological Surgery
Weill Cornell Medical Center
New York, New York
383: Surgical Approaches to Intracranial Aneurysms

Athanasios K. Zisakis, MSc, MBBS, MD, PhD
Senior Fellow in Functional and Stereotactic Neurosurgery
Department of Neurosurgery
Pamukkale University
Denizli, Turkey
176: Evidence-Based Neurostimulation for Pain
180: Dorsal Rhizotomy and Dorsal Root Ganglionectomy

Scott L. Zuckerman, MD
Resident Neurosurgeon
Vanderbilt University Medical Center
Nashville, Tennessee
275: Spinal Biomechanics and Basics of Spinal Instrumentation

Daniel W. Zumofen, MD
Clinical Instructor, Department of Radiology
Neurointerventional Section
New York University School of Medicine
New York, New York;
Attending Physician
Klinik und Poliklinik fuer Neurochirurgie und Abteilung fuer Diagnostische und Interventionelle
Universitaetsspital Basel
Basel, Switzerland
122: Endovascular Techniques for Tumor Embolization

Marike Zwienenberg-Lee, MD
Assistant Clinical Professor
Department of Neurological Surgery
University of California, Davis School of Medicine
Sacramento, California
346: Clinical Pathophysiology of Traumatic Brain Injury

Foreword

The human brain, it has often been observed, is the most complicated object in the known universe. The sheer size and scale of *Youmans and Winn Neurological Surgery*, now in its seventh edition and surely the Bible of our craft, is testament to that. It is, however, a salutary thought that despite immense strides in neuroscience in the last few decades, we still understand remarkably little about how our brains really work. We are like Newton, who described himself as a boy, standing on the seashore, playing with pebbles, while "the great ocean of truth lay all undiscovered" before him.

Despite all the science, technology, and clinical knowledge with which, as neurosurgeons, we must remain conversant at all stages of our careers, and which this great textbook embodies so well, the fundamental purpose of everything we do is to help our patients. Neurosurgery has the justifiable reputation of being difficult, and many people (especially neurosurgeons!) consider it to be the acme of surgery. Yet once we have mastered all the intricacies of operating and acquired an understanding of the brain, both in health and disease, most neurosurgeons come to understand that the greatest difficulty of their work is not so much in the technicalities of operating (which for most of us is a joy, albeit at times a painful one) but instead in the decision-making—when to operate and especially when not to operate. Neurosurgical procedures, despite all the recent technological advances, are still very dangerous because the brain is so complex, delicate, and vital to all that makes life worth living. Our patients are very vulnerable. To make the right decisions and to give our patients the best advice, we depend not just on our own experience but on the experience and accumulated knowledge of the thousands of surgeons and scientists who have gone before us or who are continually carrying the specialty forward with new research. It can be a daunting experience to open a textbook as massive as *Youmans and Winn*, edited so expertly for many years by H. Richard Winn. It can fill you with both amazement and alarm that there is so much you do not know but feel that you should. No neurosurgeon can hope—or should try—to assimilate all of it. Besides, in this age of increasing specialization, it is unlikely to be necessary. Nevertheless, here in one place, we can find all that we need to know to remain fully grounded and up-to-date in the science and craft of neurological surgery, the practice of which for most of us is more than just a career and instead something that fills us with the deepest awe and love.

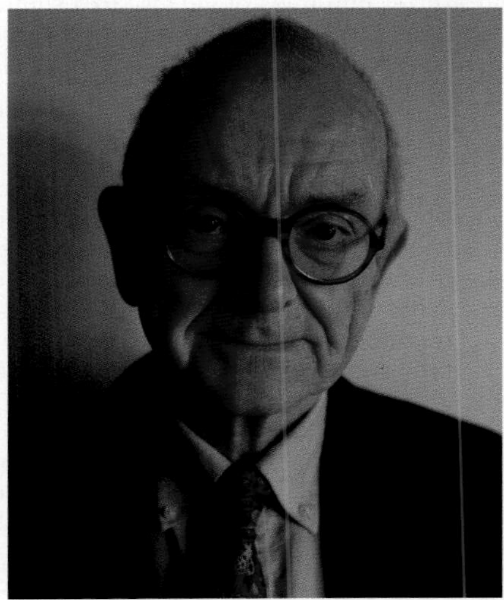

Henry T. Marsh, CBE, FRCS
St. George's Hospital
London

Henry T. Marsh was the senior neurosurgeon at Atkinson Morley Hospital/St. George's, University of London until he retired in 2015. He was made Commander of the British Empire (CBE) by Queen Elizabeth II for his contributions to British and international neurosurgery in 2010. Dr. Marsh has worked as a neurosurgeon in many countries as noted in the documentary film, *The English Surgeon* (2009). He is the author of two widely acclaimed books about neurosurgery and neurosurgeons: *Do No Harm* (2014) and *Admission* (2016).

Preface

The seventh edition of *Youmans and Winn Neurological Surgery* reflects the dynamic and expansive nature of neurosurgery in the second decade of the 21st century and endeavors to provide an encyclopedic overview of neurological surgery for both the experienced and nascent clinician. Time alone will not convert the latter to the former; the acquisition of knowledge and judgment are essential for this transformation.

This edition is larger than its predecessor, introduces more than 50 new topics and chapters, has both printed and Web-based content, and utilizes hundreds of videos. To a significant extent, we have redesigned the entire book with every illustration, photograph, chart, and table now in color. Some of the changes are described as follows.

- A totally new feature is the addition of introductory chapters for each of the 12 sections. These introductory chapters, written by the subspecialty section editors, are composed of two components: a review of the contents of the section and a thoughtful evaluation of ongoing controversies related to the subspecialty. Thus, each introduction discusses multiple unresolved questions that neurosurgeons, irrespective of their level of training and years of experience, may need to address in dealing with patients.
- The vast majority of chapters now contain videos to supplement the written text. In addition, we have upgraded the quality and added audio commentary. These electronic features are designed to facilitate understanding of the complexities of neurological procedures. The seventh edition also includes videos on perioperative techniques such as patient positioning. For example, Chapter 22 contains 18 different videos on positioning for peripheral nerve surgery. These videos, however, are not restricted to the operating room but are critical components of chapters focused on basic sciences and clinical topics. For example, the 36 videos in Chapter 2, "Surgical Anatomy of the Brain," by Rhoton and his colleagues, provide a broad yet in-depth educational supplement.
- An example of electronic enhancement in the clinical realm is Chapter 8, which deals with ophthalmology and contains many videos demonstrating multiple eye movement disorders associated with cranial nerve dysfunction. Written descriptions of such disorders can be confusing, whereas these videos quickly and more clearly convey the neurological abnormalities.
- We extensively revised and totally rewrote all retained chapters. References were likewise rigorously updated. Retention of previous topics and chapters required a clear indication of relevance and importance to neurosurgical education and practice.
- Because of the dynamic nature of fundamental research, all the basic science chapters have been extensively revised to provide cutting-edge information. In addition, several new topics have been added: examples include "Optogenetics and Clarity" (Chapter 45) and "Extracellular Fluid Movement and Clearance in the Brain" (Chapter 54). The latter has been termed the "glymphatic pathway" and may have a significant impact on patient disorders.
- We have extensively expanded our focus on anatomy by adding a new chapter, "Surgical Anatomy of the Skull Base" (Chapter 3), which complements Rhoton's chapter, "Surgical Anatomy of the Brain" (Chapter 2). In addition, each subspecialty section contains a chapter focused on the relevant anatomy pertinent to the subspecialty topics.
- Radiology, especially magnetic resonance imaging, is the technique by which neurosurgeons study anatomy in the 21st century. Accordingly and reflecting our approach to anatomy, we have expanded the radiology components in the seventh edition. There are initial introductory overviews of brain and spine radiology, including physiologic techniques, and then more highly focused radiology chapters contained within each subspecialty section.
- Patient safety must be of paramount concern for neurosurgeons, and consequently we added new chapters on this topic: "Improving Patient Safety" (Chapter 4) and "Coagulation for the Neurosurgeon" (Chapter 7). In addition, we upgraded several chapters that deal with complication avoidance, which is covered broadly in the initial section and more narrowly in each subspecialty section.
- Cutting-edge practice of neurosurgery demands the knowledge of new technologies, many of which have been added in the seventh edition (e.g., see Chapter 25, "Visualization and Optics in Neurosurgery"). Even new twists on older methods are contained in new chapters such as Chapter 24 ("Brain Retraction").
- Because advances in the neurosciences and neurological surgery are not limited by national boundaries, we have significantly broadened our international authorship to reflect this global basis of knowledge.

The first edition of *Neurological Surgery* by Julian Youmans appeared in 1973 and contained 112 chapters and 2024 pages. Now, almost five decades later, the seventh edition, with much larger pages and resultant 30% increase in the number of words per page, has expanded to 415 chapters and almost 5000 pages. By comparing each section of the first and seventh editions, one can easily see how much has changed in the knowledge base of neuroscience and neurosurgery and the breadth and practice of neurosurgery. Consequently, the neurosurgery trainee of today (and tomorrow) must master considerably more information and techniques while simultaneously assimilating the existing knowledge base. Not to be forgotten are the historical precedents responsible for present-day neurosurgery practice, which are reviewed in detail in the first chapter of the seventh edition.

It should be self-evident that the provision of this knowledge in the seventh edition represents the diligent work of many individual experts. I enthusiastically express my appreciation to the stellar and thoughtful authors of the 415 chapters. Their work represents the essential building blocks for the practice of neurological surgery.

The creation of this multi-authored textbook required hard work and discipline by the section editors, to whom I offer much gratitude. If the individual authors are the building blocks, then the following section editors represent the mortar:

Introduction and General Neurosurgery Section

- William T. Couldwell, MD, PhD
- Basant K. Misra, MBBS, MS, MCh, Diplomate National Board
- Volker Seifert, MD, PhD
- Ugur Türe, MD

Basic and Clinical Sciences Section
- Michel Kliot, MD, MA
- Pierre J. Magistretti, MD, PhD
- Robert M. Friedlander, MD, MA
- Michael M. Haglund, MD, PhD

Epilepsy Section
- Guy M. McKhann II, MD
- Itzhak Fried, MD, PhD
- Andrew W. McEvoy, MBBS, MD, FRCS(Lond), FRCS(SN)
- Steven V. Pacia, MD
- Dennis D. Spencer, MD
- Nitin Tandon, MD, FAANS

Functional Neurosurgery Section
- Ron L. Alterman, MD, MBA
- Andres M. Lozano, MD, PhD
- Joachim K. Krauss, Prof. Dr. med.
- Takaomi Taira, MD, PhD

Oncology Section
- E. Antonio Chiocca, MD, PhD, FAANS
- Henry Brem, MD
- Russell R. Lonser, MD
- Andrew T. Parsa, MD, PhD[†]
- Zvi Ram, MD
- Raymond Sawaya, MD

Pain Section
- Kim J. Burchiel, MD, FACS
- Feridun Acar, MD
- Andrew C. Zacest, MBBS, MS, FRACS, FFPMANZCA

Pediatrics Section
- Gerald A. Grant, MD, FACS
- James T. Rutka, MD, PhD
- Andrew H. Jea, MD
- James Tait Goodrich, MD, PhD, DSci (Hon)
- Richard David Hayward, MBBS, FRCS (Eng)
- Shenandoah Robinson, MD, FAAP, FACS

Peripheral Nerve Section
- Aaron G. Filler, MD, PhD, JD, FRCS
- Allan J. Belzberg, MD, FRCSC
- Liang Chen, MD, PhD
- Martijn J.A. Malessy, MD, PhD

Radiation Section
- Bruce E. Pollock, MD
- Dong Gyu Kim, MD, PhD
- Jean Régis, MD

Spine Section
- Christopher I. Shaffrey, Sr., MD
- Michael G. Fehlings, MD, PhD, FRCSC, FACS

[†]Deceased.

- Osmar José Santos de Moraes, MD
- Charles Kuntz IV, MD[†]
- Praveen V. Mummaneni, MD
- Paul Santiago, MD
- Daniel K. Resnick, MD, MS

Trauma Section
- Geoffrey T. Manley, MD, PhD
- Peter J. Hutchinson, MBBS, PhD, FRCS (Surg Neurol)
- Andrew I.R. Maas, MD, PhD
- Guy Rosenthal, MD

Vascular Section
- E. Sander Connolly, Jr., MD, FACS
- Gavin W. Britz, MD, MBBCh, MPH, MBA, FAANS
- Kazuhiro Hongo, MD, PhD
- Michael T. Lawton, MD
- Fredric B. Meyer, MD

I thank my long-time associates, Mitchel S. Berger, MD, MA; Kim J. Burchiel, MD, FACS; Ralph G. Dacey, Jr., MD; M. Sean Grady, MD; Matthew A. Howard III, MD; and Marc R. Mayberg, MD, for their creative input. These deputy editors-in-chief were critical architects in helping with the intellectual design of the seventh edition. And I thank my former laboratory postdoc and neurosurgical colleague, Kathryn Ko, MD, MFA, for allowing her insightful paintings to grace the cover of the seventh edition.

To bring to fruition a work of this magnitude requires a highly professional editorial effort, and for this, I thank the members of the Elsevier global team. Firstly, I thank Senior Content Development Specialist Jennifer Shreiner in Philadelphia, Pennsylvania, who was indispensable on a daily basis in the hard work of organizing chapters and prodding the authors, section editors, and me; Book Production Specialist Kristine Feeherty in St. Louis, Missouri, who masterfully oversaw copyediting, proofreading, and conversion of manuscripts into printed proofs; and lastly, Senior Content Strategist Charlotta Kryhl in London, England, for her long-term advice, input, and patience. The seventh edition would not have been brought to fruition without the assistance of Mss. Shreiner, Feeherty, and Kryhl.

A personal note of gratitude goes to my wife, Debbie, for her sustaining support and editorial assistance; our son, Randy, and his wife, Tamara; our daughter, Allison, and her husband, Adam; and Campbell, Mia, Amelia, Lexi, and Charlie for being here.

H. Richard Winn

[†]Deceased.

Overview and Controversies

William T. Couldwell, Basant K. Misra, Volker Seifert, Ugur Türe, and H. Richard Winn

The "Introduction and General Neurosurgery" section is composed of 43 chapters that are divided into seven subparts: "History and Background"; "Related Systems"; "Overview of Radiology"; "Intensive Care"; "The Operating Room"; "Geriatric Neurosurgery"; and "Infections." We designed the "Introduction and General Neurosurgery" section with the goal of providing neurosurgeons in practice and those still in training with comprehensive, up-to-date information on a broad scope of topics central for the mastery of neurosurgery. In this introduction, the section editors initially review the topics contained in the "Introduction and General Neurosurgery" section and then present a series of essays about controversies and unresolved questions related to these topics.

OVERVIEW

The first part of this section opens with a superb chapter on an important topic: the history of neurosurgery. Neurosurgeons have shown an increasing interest in the history of their discipline, as demonstrated by the expanding history section of the American Association of Neurological Surgeons. Neurosurgeons should remember George Santayana's[1] warning that "those who cannot remember the past are condemned to repeat it." The next two chapters comprehensively review the anatomy of the brain and skull base. Chapter 2, by Rhoton and colleagues, contains 35 videos, and Chapter 3 is a totally new entity in which bony cranial and brain landmarks are correlated. Each of the subsequent chapters in the "History and Background" part discusses a subject that is critical for patient care: improving patient safety (Chapter 4), preoperative evaluation for neuroanesthesia (Chapter 5), and complication avoidance (Chapter 6). The final chapter in this part, "Coagulation for the Neurosurgeon," is another new topic and succinctly contains vital insights.

The second part of this section, "Related Systems," focuses on the related topics and systems of neuro-ophthalmology (Chapter 8), neurotology (Chapter 9), and neurourology (Chapter 10). Neurosurgeons have many patients whose problems involve these systems; consequently, they work closely and consult frequently with colleagues in these fields. These chapters are highly focused on the essential information that allows neurosurgeons to knowledgeably provide care and seek appropriate and timely consultation.

The third part of this section, "Overview of Radiology," comprehensively covers basic neuroradiology with separate chapters on computed tomography (CT) and magnetic resonance imaging (MRI) of the brain (Chapter 11) and spine (Chapter 12) and then intensive chapters on physiologic analysis involving the use of MRI (Chapter 13) and positron emission tomography (PET; Chapter 14). This entire part on neuroradiology and imaging serves as a cornerstone for multiple individual neuroradiologic chapters that appear in the specialty sections (e.g., "Oncology" [Section V], "Pediatrics" [Section VII], and "Vascular" [Section XII]) later in the book.

The fourth part of this section, "Intensive Care," begins with Chapter 15, in which the scientific basis of intracranial pressure is reviewed and the various approaches to monitoring intracranial pressure are described. Separate chapters then deal with principles of intensive care unit (ICU) treatment (Chapter 16) and the unique role of neurosurgeons in providing care in the neurosurgical ICU (Chapter 17).

The fifth part of this section, "The Operating Room," opens with Chapter 18, an overview of surgical planning. Surgical simulation and surgical robotics, a new and emerging field with the potential for a major influence on neurosurgery, is then explored in Chapter 19. Positioning is a critical component of neurosurgery and is covered in separate chapters related to cranial, spinal, and peripheral nerve surgery. All these positioning chapters contain illustrative and extensive videos. For example, Chapter 22 ("Positioning for Peripheral Nerve Surgery") contains 18 separate videos. Although incisions and closings are seemingly routine, many difficulties can arise when they are performed. We thus included Chapter 23, which deals with these two topics. Chapter 24, a new topic, provides insights on a technique "routinely" used but not frequently discussed in neurosurgery: retraction. Continuing the "insights" theme, Chapter 25 covers visualization and optics. Chapter 26 explores the advantages and disadvantages of endoscopic surgery. With this background, the reader is then presented with Chapter 27, which focuses on thoracic endoscopic surgery. "The Operating Room" part of this section then concludes with Chapter 28, about another "routine" procedure that necessitates attention to detail to achieve success: cranioplasty.

Because of the aging population throughout the world, the sixth part of this section, "Geriatric Neurosurgery," concentrates on two topics: normal-pressure hydrocephalus (NPH) and chronic subdural hematomas. For each of these entities, we provide chapters describing the relevant basic science and pathophysiologic features, patient evaluation, and treatment options, including a critical review of third ventricular ventriculostomy (Chapter 32).

The seventh part of this section, "Infections," covers this important topic broadly, starting with Chapter 35, a very comprehensive discussion of the basic science of central nervous system (CNS) infections. Separate chapters (36 and 37) deal with postoperative infections of the brain (and head) and the spine. Next, the important topic of antibiotic usage is explored in Chapter 38. Specific types of infections affecting the CNS are then discussed in separate chapters: brain abscess (Chapter 39), meningitis and encephalitis (Chapter 40), acquired immunodeficiency syndrome (Chapter 41), and parasitic infections (Chapter 42). This section closes with an increasingly important topic for surgeons: surgical risk of transmittable diseases (Chapter 43).

CONTROVERSIES AND UNRESOLVED QUESTIONS

In this part of the introduction, we discuss a number of important and controversial topics in modern neurosurgery: treatment of hydrocephalus; coagulation for the neurosurgeon; the proper treatment of chronic subdural hematomas; the use of endoscopy with transfacial surgery; technical advances involving robotic surgery, visualization and optics, and brain retraction; the glymphatic system; the role of the neurosurgeon in neurointensive care; and education and training of neurosurgeons. Although perhaps we do not offer definitive answers, our goal is to focus attention, raise awareness, provide context, and perhaps point the way to answering unresolved questions.

Question 1: Adult and Pediatric Hydrocephalus: The Role of Third Ventriculostomy and Choroid Plexus Cauterization

Endoscopic third ventriculostomy (ETV) has been increasingly used for treating both adult and pediatric hydrocephalus since the early 2000s (see Chapter 32). This procedure has much inherent appeal, in that avoiding or removing an indwelling ventricular shunt—which condemns the patient to probable lifelong dependency on a device with a high failure rate over time—is a laudable goal. Rates of success with ETV vary from 50% to 90%. The indications for this procedure are in evolution. It is clear that the success of the procedure is highly dependent on the cause of the hydrocephalus. Patient selection is the key to achieving clinical success.

In the adult population, late-onset idiopathic aqueductal stenosis is the indication for which the implantation of a shunt has the highest success rate. In addition, lesional obstructive hydrocephalus (secondary obstructive hydrocephalus) remains an intuitively appealing indication for which shunt implantation has a high success rate. Perhaps more surprisingly, NPH, long believed to be a disorder of cerebrospinal fluid (CSF) dynamics and absorption, is an emerging indication. The published rates of success with ETVs in patients with NPH have been variable, ranging from 21% in a study of 14 patients[1a] to 87% in a study of 15 patients with 27 months of follow-up.[2] Gangemi and colleagues[3] had a success rate of 69% in their series of 110 patients with NPH treated with ETVs at four centers and monitored for a minimum of 2 years. Potential predictors of success included a shorter duration of symptoms and milder symptoms; patient age was not predictive of response. In adult patients with shunts, conversion to ETV and removal of the shunt has been successful in 70% at a median follow-up of 36 months. This population represents a considerable opportunity.

The success rate of ETV in children with hydrocephalus secondary to tectal gliomas is high (close to 90%), whereas ETVs performed in the context of intraventricular hemorrhage associated with prematurity succeed in only a third or fewer of cases. Young age (<6 months) is associated with a lower success rate, independent of cause; however, this age effect either plateaus or diminishes after the age of 2 years, perhaps because of cranial maturation.[4,5] The literature indicates that the rate of success with ETV is high in patients older than 2 years in whom noncommunicating hydrocephalus is caused by aqueductal stenosis, tectal glioma, and posterior fossa tumors.

With regard to the question of whether a choroid plexus coagulation should be added to the ETV procedure, data suggest that in the infant population (<2 years old) with noninfectious hydrocephalus, adding choroid plexus coagulation may further bolster the success rates of this procedure. ETV with choroid plexus coagulation is now routinely performed at children's hospitals around the world and has resulted in an approximately 30% decrease in the placement of new ventricular shunts in the pediatric age group in selected institutions (W.T. Couldwell, personal communication, University of Utah Department of Neurosurgery).

Question 2: Clotting and the Neurosurgeon

The imperative in neurosurgery, as in other fields of surgery, is to critically balance the risks of bleeding against thrombosis in patients. The assessment of the coagulation system is vital in preoperative management, as well as in the determination of any deleterious effects of medications used by the patient. In this regard, there is a paucity of high-level evidence concerning the effects of antiplatelet agents and anticoagulants on patients with neurosurgical conditions.

Currently, more than 1% of the general population is receiving some form of oral anticoagulation for various cardiovascular conditions. These problems are further confounded by the increasingly common use of dual antiplatelet agents in patients with cardiac, peripheral vascular, and intracranial stents. The management of such patients after neurotrauma represents a controversial area in neurosurgery (see Chapter 7). Although some investigators have focused on the management and outcome of patients with trauma who receive anticoagulants or antiplatelet therapy, there are no strict guidelines (and a lack of class I evidence). Several questions have been raised about testing of antiplatelet and anticoagulation effects on patients at hospital admission, reversal of the pharmacologic effects of these agents to mitigate against neurological deterioration, and the timing of reinstitution of therapy. Patients taking oral anticoagulation medication are considered to be at high risk for neurological deterioration, and more prospective and comparative effectiveness research is necessary to answer these important questions.

Another related dilemma is posed by the use of contemporary anticoagulants for the management of cardiovascular conditions. Several small compounds that specifically block activated coagulation factor X (FXa) or thrombin (FIIa) have become popular alternatives to vitamin K antagonist compounds. As opposed to vitamin K antagonists, direct oral anticoagulants (DOACs) target a specific coagulation factor. Such direct oral anticoagulants include dabigatran etexilate (thrombin inhibitor) and edoxaban and rivaroxaban (inhibitors of FXa). These agents have become popular for venous prophylaxis or treatment of thromboembolism and for prevention of neurological events associated with atrial fibrillation. With regard to intracranial hemorrhage, the safety profile of the DOACs has been shown to be poorer than that of vitamin K antagonists. The difficulty arises with the use of these agents when intracranial hemorrhage occurs, either spontaneously or in relation to trauma.[6-8] The development of reversal agents has lagged behind the introduction of these agents for therapeutic benefit for common cardiovascular problems; as a result, difficulty arises when bleeding events occur, especially in relation to the CNS. Because most DOACs have a short half-life, time is an efficient way to eliminate the anticoagulant effect if waiting is possible; however, devastating neurological outcomes have been reported with the use of these agents.[9] New agents are currently being developed that should reduce this problem over time.[10,11]

Question 3: Correct Surgical Management of Chronic Subdural Hematomas: Do Surgeons Now Have the Definitive Answer?

Chronic subdural hematoma, for which the mean age at occurrence is in the eighth decade, represents a growing problem in much of the developed world as the population ages. This demographic shift, together with the increasing use of anticoagulants and antiplatelet agents in older patients, complicates the management of these patients.

Treatment for chronic subdural hematoma remains surgical; observation is recommended for affected patients with minimal or no symptoms. The three options for surgical drainage are burhole drainage (which can be performed with the patient under local or general anesthesia, usually in the operating room), twist-drill craniostomy (which is usually performed with the patient under local anesthesia, at the patient's bedside), or open craniotomy (in the operating room). The results of these options, compared in a contemporary meta-analysis, were that craniotomy was associated with a lower rate of recurrence (usually less than 10%), but rates of morbidity and mortality may be higher with this procedure. Twist-drill craniostomy produces the least morbidity, but it is associated with a higher recurrence rate (exceeding 30% in some studies). Thus the compromise option, bur-hole drainage, remains the most commonly used because its morbidity and recurrence rates are balanced.[12,13] There is high-quality evidence that drains reduce the incidence of recurrence and should be used.[14]

The technical controversies in the use of bur-hole drainage are related to the number of bur holes and the type of drain to be used (external drain, subperiosteal, or subgaleal). There appears to be little consensus in the literature on these points.

Furthermore, the recurrence rates between studies are remarkably variable. In studies since the 1990s, the reoperation rate has been reduced to a range of 10% to 20%.[12] This probably indicates that although chronic subdural hematoma is treated as a single entity, it is not advisable to perform procedures without tailoring treatment according to individual hematoma characteristics. Experienced surgeons define treatment on the basis of the patient's age, comorbid conditions present, and imaging characteristics of the hematoma. In studies, researchers have not stratified data for such factors to provide strong evidence-based conclusions for treatment in this nuanced manner.

In addition, the role of adjuvant therapies such as steroids needs to be better defined. Because the burden of chronic subdural hematoma is likely to rise, outcomes for this common neurosurgical condition must be improved.

Question 4: Endoscopy: When Should Transfacial Endoscopy or Traditional Open Microsurgery Be Used in Skull Base Surgery?

Since the 1990s, neurosurgeons have been increasingly interested in approaching various tumors of the base of the skull by using a transfacial (transnasal or transmaxillary) corridor. This has been the result of enhanced endoscopic techniques primarily developed and used by and with otolaryngologists to address sinus disease and is an extension of the transsphenoidal approach to approach other lesions besides traditional pituitary tumors (see Chapter 26).

The use of an endoscopic approach to a pituitary tumor was first documented by Guiot and associates[15] in Paris in 1962. Although Bushe and Halves[16] reported the first use of the endoscope for pituitary tumors in the literature in 1978, the endoscope was not used widely until the mid-1990s, when endoscopic sinus surgery was universally adopted by otolaryngologists. Neurosurgeons were attracted to its use by the increased visualization of the surgical site and began to explore the possibilities in transsphenoidal surgery. Jho and Carrau[17] reported on a series of 50 patients who underwent endoscopic endonasal transsphenoidal surgery, with encouraging results. Thereafter, the endoscopic approach to transsphenoidal surgery for resection of pituitary macroadenomas was adopted rapidly by neurosurgeons.

With the expansion of the transsphenoidal approach to other tumors of the skull base,[18] the endoscope was an ideal tool to apply to these approaches because it offers wide-angle and side-angle visualization, a capability that is not possible with the microscope from below. In addition, there are several advantages to approaching anterior skull base lesions from below. For example, an anterior endoscopic endonasal transcribriform or transplanum approach may confer advantages to anterior skull base management for certain meningiomas, depending on size and location. Complete resection of hyperostotic bone of the olfactory groove, planum sphenoidale, and tuberculum sellae is more easily accomplished, and manipulation of neurovascular structures and brain retraction on the frontal lobes to increase exposure is avoided. In an endoscopic approach, the craniotomy through the anterior skull base is made directly over the basal dural attachment at the anterior skull base. The meningioma can be devascularized early in the operation to decrease blood loss and facilitate tumor removal. Complete removal of all bone that has become hyperostotic from tumor infiltration facilitates a Simpson grade I resection. The endoscopic approach may be suitable for an anterior skull base meningioma that has recurred or extends into the paranasal sinuses.

Disadvantages of the endonasal endoscopic approach stem from the inherent limitations of its midline exposure. Tumors that have extended beyond the medial orbital wall or over the superior orbital roof and those with dural attachments extending lateral to the optic canal or into the sphenoid wing are difficult to access from a midline endonasal approach and may be better approached via an open transcranial technique. Cranial nerves and vascular structures are identified later in the dissection during an endonasal endoscopic technique and may be prone to injury if manipulated. Tumors encasing the internal carotid arteries or anterior cerebral arteries should be approached by an open technique for more complete visualization and to avoid vascular injury. High-quality studies of the extent of resection, recurrence rates, and complications of each approach are lacking.

CSF leaks that necessitate endonasal exploration to repair may be more common with endoscopic surgery. The osteodural defect is larger when created by an approach from below than when created by a Simpson grade I resection with a transcranial approach from above. Approaching a meningioma in the olfactory groove may necessitate resection of bone and dura extending from the posterior wall of the frontal sinus to the planum sphenoidale. Resection of the hyperostotic endonasal bones and entering the paranasal sinuses further increase the risk of a CSF leak.

Modern surgical techniques, such as the use of vascularized nasoseptal mucosal flaps or allogenic acellular dermal allograft (AlloDerm; LifeCell Corporation, Bridgewater, NJ), may decrease the rate of CSF leaks without the need for lumbar drainage and may grant surgeons the confidence to perform a more complete surgical resection; however, prospective trials in which the effectiveness of these newer techniques are evaluated have not yet been published.

Question 5: Technical Advances: Revolutionary or Evolutionary?

Several new chapters deal with innovation and technical advances in operative neurosurgery: simulation and robotics (Chapter 19), brain retraction (Chapter 24), and visualization and optics (Chapter 25). In those chapters, the authors endeavor to place these advances in context, evaluate whether they truly deserve to be termed "revolutionary," and attempt to address what effect these advances will have on the future of neurosurgery (Fig. I-1).

With regard to the terms *revolutionary* and *evolutionary*, many investigators make claims for the former but rarely for the latter. *Revolutionary* means a complete or fundamental change. It therefore follows that the majority of innovations contributing to advances in neurosurgery are evolutionary. Gordon[19] reviewed examples of revolutionary changes that transformed the 20th century: the internal combustion engine, distribution of electricity, and public health advances. The internal combustion engine evolved into the automobile and the airplane; distribution of electricity enabled the development of household and business devices such as the refrigerator and, later, the computer; and public health advances led to the delivery of potable drinking water and sanitary collection of sewage. According to Gordon's line of reasoning, a major revolutionary change in neurosurgery was Wilhelm Röntgen's discovery of x-rays, and all subsequent events and discoveries were evolutionary, including Walter Dandy's description of ventriculography and

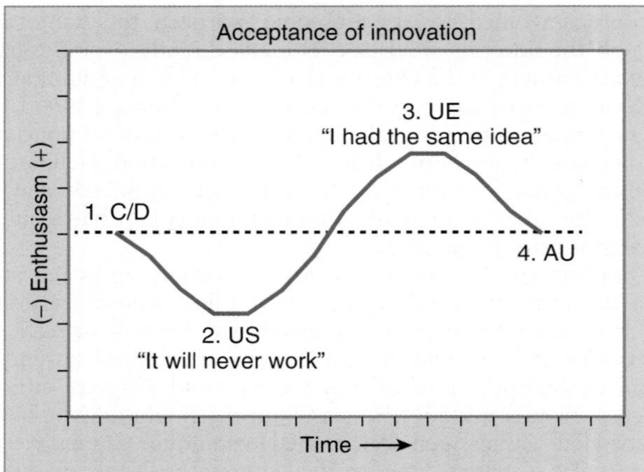

Figure I-1. Four phases of acceptance of innovation. Phase 1: Creation/Development, (C/D). Phase 2: Unrestricted Skepticism (US). Phase 3: Unrestricted Enthusiasm (UE). Phase 4: Appropriate Utilization (AU). The duration of each phase is highly variable. With medical innovation, the transition from phase 3 to phase 4 may be prolonged, or phase 4 potentially may never be achieved.

pneumoencephalography (1918/1919), António Egas Moniz's achieving opacification of the carotid artery (1927), and Sir Godfrey Hounsfield's development of the CT scanner (1973).

Before physicians attempt to predict the future, it would be wise to remember that "rational prediction of future developments is, to some degree, an oxymoron. Predictive accuracy would probably be higher with Isaac Asimov* and other science-fiction writers than with academics limited by conditioned skepticism."[21] It would also be prudent to remember Bergland's 1973 article "Neurosurgery May Die," published in the *New England Journal of Medicine*.[22] Unlike Bergland, modern neurosurgeons can use the "retrospectoscope" to see that almost simultaneously with the publication of Bergland's article predicting the demise of this specialty, Hounsfield and James Ambrose were in the midst of perfecting the CT scanner. The CT scanner and MRI, while evolutionary only from a technology perspective, nevertheless had a revolutionary effect on neurosurgical practice. These devices profoundly expanded the scope of neurosurgery and prevented its demise. However, Bergland based his prediction on the failure of neurosurgical education and, as will be discussed later, he may be correct about future difficulties ahead for neurosurgery.

Simulation and Robotic Surgery

In 1921, Karel Capek, a Czech playwright, introduced the term *robots*, using it to mean forced labor; today this term applies to tools that can perform a variety of tasks under the direction of a human or computer. The first robotic application in the realm of surgery was in 1988 in neurosurgery—for needle biopsy.[23] Since then, robotics have been applied widely in radiosurgery and, to a lesser extent, in spinal and cranial surgery. However, few studies have demonstrated a clear advantage to robot-assisted surgery across the breadth of surgery.

Instead of surgery itself, perhaps the major application for robotics in the near term will be in simulation and training, as noted in Chapter 19; however, neurosurgeons and engineers need to make significant progress before virtual operations simulate actual conditions in the operating theater. Advances in virtual reality technology are transforming the gaming and other industries and will soon be applied to simulation of neurosurgical procedures. Such advances will not only affect patient safety (see Chapter 4) but will probably also have a major positive effect on neurosurgery training, at a time when education is being eroded (see later discussion).

Should neurosurgeons be concerned about the steady march toward the mechanized and robotic future, or do such concerns represent the reflex protestations against progress by a generation of Luddites who are unfamiliar with emerging technology? Without question, potential losses and negative consequence lie ahead. In the absence of robotics, surgery is at the end of a spectrum that begins with the individual surgeon's knowledge, mental visualization of the neuroanatomy in three dimensions, correlation of the anatomy and imaging, and then activation of personal executive function to create a surgical plan. Robotic surgery in the future may allow bypass of these important intellectual tasks; therefore, when technology fails, surgeons will be left poorly equipped to handle certain situations.

We are mindful, however, of how the introduction of the CT scanner and MRI, while changing the practice of neurosurgery, has had a secondary effect on neurosurgical education and neuroanatomy. Before the development of CT and MRI, the popularity of neuroanatomy was in decline, considered a nice bit of knowledge to acquire (comparable to knowing the distinction between Doric, Ionic, and Corinthian columns), but not thought to be essential to the practice of neurosurgery. The "imaging studies" before CT were pneumoencephalography and ventriculography. These techniques required some knowledge of the cerebral ventricles and, in general terms, what could displace them, but knowledge about the brain outside of the ventricles was still sparse. With the introduction of CT and MRI, knowledge of neuroanatomy became a necessity, not a luxury, and led to a vastly increased emphasis on neuroanatomy teaching and research. This is reflected in the expansion of chapters devoted to anatomy in the 7th edition of *Youmans and Winn Neurological Surgery*.

Visualization and Optics

Most neurosurgical procedures on the brain, spine, or peripheral nerves as of the second decade of the 21st century remain "open" surgeries involving direct vision and similar to those performed by Harvey Cushing in the second decade of the 20th century. Ted Kurze's introduction of the microscope into the neurosurgery operating room, as well as subsequent refinements by Raymond M.P. Donaghy, Gazi Yaşargil, Albert L. Rhoton, and other innovative pioneers, fundamentally expanded the neurosurgical operative universe. Less well recognized and documented is the role that illumination has played in advancing microneurosurgery.

In their insightful Chapter 25, on visualization and optics, Sorenson and colleagues correct this deficit in recognition by reviewing the development and current status of lighting for microsurgery; they also review the past and current status of optics. Obviously, without adequate light, microscopic neurosurgery would be impossible. Similarly, lack of light initially impaired the widespread use of endoscopes (see the earlier section "Question 4: Endoscopy").

According to the analysis of Sorenson and colleagues, lighting, rather than optics, is rate limiting for the development of magnification more powerful than what is used today, which is based primarily on human vision. Increasing the power of illumination has limitations related to effects on tissue and the inability to discriminate difference in contrasts. Sorenson and colleagues believe that the use of digital technology and high dynamic range (HDR) imaging will replace the current optical systems. Such tools could ensure superb illumination and focus that will exceed today's optic systems, which are dependent on human vision

*A famous science fiction writer who popularized the term *robotics* in 1941.[20]

alone. In addition, they envision the development of systems that will allow the neurosurgeon to "see through the brain," truly "image"-guided surgery, and they even foresee the introduction of detached remote visual techniques. Such developments, like the effect of digital cameras on photography, are destined to expand the current microsurgical world.

Brain Retraction

Is old technology with staying power no longer critical in today's "micro"/"endo" world of neurosurgery? Improvements in visualization may have a secondary effect by altering the degree of and even the need for brain retraction (see Chapter 24). As with the case of illumination, the development of retractors specialized for neurosurgery contributed to the expansion of microsurgery. As outlined in Chapter 24, replacing handheld retraction with self-retaining systems increased the surgeon's manual options. One- or three-handed surgery was expanded to two- or four-handed procedures and undoubtedly increased patient safety. The neurosurgery literature has largely ignored the contribution of self-retaining retractors to patient safety.

Although retractors are universally used in neurosurgery, the science of brain retraction and the causes of retraction injury are not as well studied. Few laboratory-based studies have documented the pressure/duration limits of neural tissue or biologic strategies designed to decrease retraction injuries. Mechanical and engineering advances have been made in retractor design, but on-line pressure-sensing retractors remain primitive. The increasing advocacy for minimal retracting techniques may reflect the acknowledgment and underreporting of the frequency of retraction injuries. Minimal retraction methods may also be related to more radical skull base dissection and advances in anesthesia methods to maximize brain relaxation.

The correct, rational, step-by-step application of retractors is based on achieving appropriate exposure with minimal risk to neural tissue while simultaneously enabling operating surgeons' access. Success or failure may depend on initial placement of the head holder and subsequent stabilization of the flexible arms. These seemingly minor steps can optimize surgical access or, if retraction is incorrectly applied, result in significant neural injury. An infrequently recognized truth is that brain retraction does indeed involve an art, as well as a science.

In summary, historic and more recent technical advances in neurosurgery have been impressive, but in the current and future environment, there remains the risk of overreliance on technology. As with humans, technology can fail and, at some point, the individual neurosurgeon must recognize this failure. For example, as reported in the *Daily Mail*,[24] a woman, planning to drive to a railroad station 38 miles from home, instead drove 900 miles over 2 days because she slavishly followed the incorrect directions provided by her global positioning system (GPS) device (Fig. I-2). The ability to recognize technology-related errors is dependent on previous training and education, as well as common sense. As indicated previously and discussed in detail subsequently, training and educational exposure are being constrained. The combination of increased dependency on technology and constriction in clinical training may be a lethal mixture.

Question 6: Advances in Basic Sciences: New Information and Possible Clinical Implications

As noted previously in the preceding discussion, revolutionary changes occur infrequently in neurosciences and neurosurgery; evolutionary changes are more common. We would describe Chapter 45 ("Optogenetics and Clarity," by Fenno, Hsueh, Purger, and Kalanithi) and Chapter 54 ("Extracellular Fluid Movement and Clearance in the Brain: The Glymphatic Pathway," by Iliff and Penn) as having revolutionary content that has

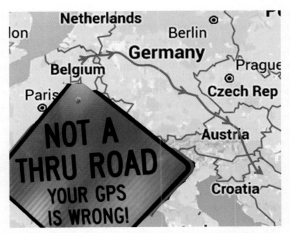

Figure I-2. Drive of 38 miles to a local train station became a 900-mile, 2-day journey *(red arrows)* because of the driver's adherence to erroneous directions by a global positioning system (GPS).

potential clinical application. Optogenetics is a laboratory tool that involves the expression of light with cellular activation and allows real-time insights into the basic physiologic mechanisms of neural networks in the brain.

The glymphatic system is a network of perivascular pathways throughout the brain along which CSF recirculates through the brain parenchyma and interstitial fluid (ISF) solutes are cleared to CSF. This novel concept may help explain physiologic activities such as memory acquisition and has profound implications about several clinical entities such as Alzheimer's disease, brain edema, and hydrocephalus.[25,26] Accordingly, we think it is important to draw neurosurgeons' attention to the glymphatic system.

Because the brain and spinal cord lack a conventional lymphatic vasculature, classical lymphatic functions such as interstitial protein homeostasis and immune surveillance are thought to occur through the interactions between the CNS extracellular fluid compartment and the CSF compartments. According to the "CSF sink hypothesis," articulated by Oldendorf and Davson[27] in the middle of the 20th century, interstitial wastes from CNS were eliminated through the exchange of ISF with CSF and the subsequent reabsorption of CSF into the bloodstream. However, more recent data by Iliff (who began his investigatory career in a neurosurgery laboratory right after high school[28]) and his collaborators have mandated revision of the basic elements of this classical model of CSF-ISF exchange.[29,30] The characterization of classical lymphatic vessels associated with dural sinuses and vasculature on the margins of the CNS suggests that waste clearance and immune surveillance may be taking place in a much more complex manner than previously believed. These data have demonstrated that the process of CSF-ISF exchange is both more organized and more functionally consequential than previously realized.

Using dynamic imaging approaches in rodents, researchers have demonstrated that, contrary to the conventional view of CSF circulation and reabsorption, a substantial proportion of CSF from the subarachnoid compartment recirculates back into and through the brain parenchyma along perivascular spaces surrounding penetrating cerebral arteries, rapidly exchanging with surrounding ISF. Interstitial solutes, in turn, are cleared from the brain along a distinct set of perivascular pathways surrounding large-caliber draining veins, including the internal cerebral vein. The exchange of CSF and ISF along these perivascular pathways, driven in part by arterial pulsation, supports the clearance of interstitial solutes, including metabolic wastes and pathologic substrates such as amyloid β peptide and tau protein.

Perivascular spaces therefore function as a crossroads in the CNS, in which, in proximity to the blood-brain barrier, the extracellular compartment of the CNS interacts with the peripherally communicating CSF. Fluid exchange along these perivascular pathways is supported by astrocytic water transport. Astrocytes express large amounts of the water channel aquaporin-4 in perivascular end-feet that ensheathe the cerebral vasculature, which helps organize water movement within the CNS along the axis of the cerebral vasculature, in a manner similar to the way that water diffusion organizes along axons in white matter tracks. Disruption of aquaporin-4, or its perivascular localization, slows perivascular CSF-ISF exchange and impairs the clearance of interstitial solutes from brain tissue.

Researchers have also shown that glymphatic function is a feature primarily of the sleeping brain, inasmuch as perivascular CSF-ISF exchange and the clearance of interstitial solutes, including amyloid β peptide, are dramatically slower in the awake brain than in the sleeping brain. In an intriguing finding, electrophysiologic measurements suggested that during slow-wave sleep, the brain extracellular space increases in volume, facilitating more rapid solute diffusion and perivascular exchange. These findings suggest that the clearance of extracellular wastes may be one of the physiologic bases of the restorative functions of sleep.

From a physiologic perspective, the clearance of extracellular wastes and the reabsorption of interstitial proteins are basic and essential elements of organ function. Within the CNS, with its high rate of metabolic activity and neural cells' sensitivity to changes in extracellular environment, the glymphatic pathway is probably a key contributor to basic brain function. In addition to facilitating the efflux of solutes that cannot be locally degraded or cross the blood-brain barrier, the glymphatic system probably provides a route along which signaling molecules, such as trophic factors, neuropeptides, and neuromodulators, are distributed through different brain regions. The association of the choroid plexus and dural vasculature—known nodes of peripheral immune cell trafficking—with the CSF and perivascular spaces of the glymphatic system suggests that these anatomic features constitute an integrated system that facilitates peripheral immune surveillance of the brain without breaching the relative "immune privilege" of the CNS.

Because glymphatic function underlies basic elements of brain function, it is likely that its dysfunction contributes to the development or progression of many different pathologic states. Glymphatic function, including the clearance of interstitial amyloid β peptide, slows in the aging brain, which suggests that age-related decline in its function may underlie the vulnerability of the aging brain to neurodegenerative disease characterized by misaggregation of different protein species, including amyloid β peptide and tau protein in Alzheimer's disease or α-synuclein in Parkinson's disease and Lewy body dementia. Similarly, glymphatic function is impaired in the young brain after traumatic brain injury, which may promote the development of neurodegeneration, including Alzheimer's disease or chronic traumatic encephalopathy, in the decades after traumatic injury.

In addition to its impairment after traumatic brain injury, glymphatic function is compromised after cerebral ischemia and subarachnoid hemorrhage, according to the results of several experimental studies. The failure of interstitial solute and fluid efflux in the setting of blood-brain barrier disruption may support the formation and persistence of cerebral edema after neurovascular injury. Conversely, the creation of an oncotic sink within edematous brain tissue may disrupt wider glymphatic pathway function, exacerbating the local effects of brain injury.

The emerging understanding of the glymphatic system and interactions between the CSF and ISF compartments along perivascular pathways has important implications in neurosurgery. Many different kinds of brain disease can interfere with fluid movement. For example, cerebral edema probably affects the dimensions of extracellular pathways, whereby the dimensions of the extracellular compartment are increased by vasogenic extracellular edema and decreased by neurotoxic edema with cellular swelling. In hydrocephalus, tissue edema around the ventricles and tissue compression of the cortex also change these flow patterns. Likewise, brain tumors change the pattern of flow because of tissue compression and breakdown of the blood-brain barrier. Successful therapeutic interventions, such as delivering medicines to gliomas, are highly dependent on flow patterns.

Convection within the extracellular compartment must be considered for effective delivery of therapeutic molecules to CNS targets through the CSF via intracerebroventricular or intrathecal infusion, directly within CNS tissue by convection-enhanced delivery, or across the blood-brain barrier. Perivascular solute flux is a key determinant of therapeutic distribution through CSF compartments. Thus a greater understanding of the mechanics and determinants of perivascular fluid movement will help surgeons optimize therapeutic delivery. A better understanding of the effects that aging, brain injury, or other pathologic processes have on these dynamics will enable more accurate drug delivery. In principle, drug delivery methods could be adapted to the individual patients once the dynamics of CSF and ISF flow are known.

Question 7: What Should Be the Neurosurgical Involvement in the Critical Care Management of Neurosurgical Patients?

Critical care medicine has developed as a specialty to diagnose, treat, and prevent life-threatening illnesses that necessitate invasive monitoring, as well as pharmacologic and mechanical organ support. Since the era of Harvey Cushing, neurosurgeons have been integrally involved in the delivery of critical care to their patients. Since 2000, interest in the management of neurosurgical patients in the ICU has intensified in several specialties. These units are now referred to as "neurocritical care units" but were previously referred to as "neurosurgical ICUs," which represented the predominance of the patients that occupied the beds. In North America, several professional associations in neurology established a certification council as a mechanism to codify subspecialties, accredit training programs, and certify physicians—all laudable goals. They defined neurocritical care as such a subspecialty.

This career path represents a significant opportunity for neurosurgical trainees. With the accreditation from the Committee on Advanced Subspecialty Training (CAST) of the Society of Neurological Surgeons, neurosurgery has a comparable mechanism for accreditation of programs and certification of trainees. About one critical care position is created by the business generated by four practicing neurosurgeons: a considerable opportunity for neurosurgery as a specialty.

Within neurosurgical residency in the United States, critical care training is now formally included within the curriculum, and competency is monitored by the residency program director and tested in certification examinations (both written and oral) by the American Board of Neurological Surgery. This has been a concerted effort on behalf of neurosurgery organizations to emphasize the importance of critical care management in the training of a contemporary neurosurgeon. With the parallel effort of other specialties, such as neurology and anesthesia, it is yet unclear whether these units will be staffed by multidisciplinary groups or primarily by neurosurgeons. What is also unresolved is whether such an interest in critical care training for neurosurgery residents will be embraced in other countries. The neurosurgeon has a unique responsibility and necessary role in managing and coordinating care for patients in the neurocritical care unit, which should not be abrogated.

Question 8: Neurosurgical Education and Training: Have Duty Hour Restrictions Accomplished the Goals Envisioned by Those Who Advocated for Changes in Neurosurgery Training?

One of the most important goals of the 7th edition of *Youmans and Winn Neurological Surgery* and of this section is educational: to provide comprehensive, up-to-date, neurosurgically relevant information to neurosurgeons in practice and in training. Time alone will not convert those in training to those in practice. This transformation requires what constitutes "training": the acquisition of knowledge, judgment, and technical skill.

Historically, training in neurosurgery grew out of general surgery, as did the discipline as a whole. In the Cushing and post-Cushing era, full training in general surgery preceded a 1- to 2-year experience in neurosurgery with the educational mode akin to an apprenticeship. Before and after World War II, specialty-specific residency training evolved into a more organized educational experience with a specified number of years in duration. Daily work hours were not constrained except by the duration of a day.

As residencies evolved, so did organizations designed to provide oversight and regulation of postgraduate training. As a result of a tragic case in the mid-1980s, the state of New York investigated working conditions and supervision of house officers and, through subsequent legislation, limited work hours of house officers to 80 hours per week. Adding to the general public concern was a study issued in 2000 by the U.S. Institute of Medicine titled *To Err Is Human: Building a Safer Health System.*[31] This study suggested that 50,000 to 100,000 hospital-based deaths occurred in the United States each year in relation to errors. In 2003, the Accreditation Council for Graduate Medical Education (ACGME) enacted (and, in 2011, modified) duty hour restrictions (DHRs) that affected all medical residencies in the United States. These DHRs were not unique to the United States, inasmuch as similar but more constraining regulations were instituted in Europe and the United Kingdom. The changes mandated by the ACGME were envisioned as decreasing patient-related errors and improving resident well-being without compromising resident education and training; however, as outlined as follows, those advocating for change in duty hours appear to be incorrect in their underlying assumptions:

- The ACGME assumed that mastering different disciplines was identical to training required for postresidency work. Common sense would dictate otherwise, and yet DHRs were identical for disparate specialties such as dermatology and neurosurgery. In the nonmedical world, no one questions that training differs according to the task; whether for the Bolshoi Ballet or a baseball team.
- As in specialties, differences exist among individuals in their ability to tolerate sleep deprivation, a trait that may be related to adenosine receptor sensitivity.[32] Individuals choosing to enter specialties known to require long hours and conditions in which sleep deprivation is common may self-select a career in neurosurgery. Moreover, substantial human and animal data demonstrate that individuals can expand their ability to tolerate sleep deprivation. Training in neurosurgery should focus on development of coping skills related to sleep deprivation. After all, neurosurgery training is not an abstract concept; in essence, the goal is to prepare the individual for the practice of neurosurgery, an environment in which hour restrictions currently do not apply.
- Furthermore, many advocates predicated the need for DHRs on the assumption that fatigue, caused by sleep deprivation, compromised patient care; they assumed that DHRs would improve patient safety. These advocates ignored the existing data derived from two decades of DHRs in the state of New York and the lack of improvement in hospital errors. Furthermore, a study from 1995 on surgical residents failed to demonstrate that fatigue affected patient errors or outcome,[33] and these results were further supported by a later study of neurosurgery residents and manual skills.[34] After 2003, when the ACGME instituted DHRs, the preponderance of studies across many disciplines have failed to demonstrate the hoped-for improvement in patient care,[35] even with modification of the DHRs.[36] In contrast, in several neurosurgical studies, DHRs have had a negative effect on patient care.[37-42] For example, in a novel study, Dumont and associates[41] evaluated meningioma resection before and after implementation of DHRs and demonstrated an increase in complication rates in academic units, but not in nonteaching institutions in which DHRs were not in effect.
- Another promised benefit of DHRs was that residents would have more time for education and research. The opposite has occurred because limitation on hours applies to time spent both in teaching and in patient care.[42] In neurosurgery, surveys of faculty members yielded uniformly negative responses about the influence of DHRs on teaching both inside and outside the operating room.[42] An objective measurement of the effect of DHRs is the decrease in residents' performance on in-service examinations for self-assessment, administered by the American Board of Neurological Surgery.[42,43] In addition, many neurosurgery residencies restricted their research exposure for residents, with the resultant decrease in the number of resident-presentations at national neurosurgery meetings.[42]
- House officers have high rates of depression, suicides, and job burnout. Consequently, another motivation for the introduction of DHRs was the concern for the well-being of residents. However, studies have uniformly failed to demonstrate an improvement in psychological difficulties or job burnout in house staff after institution of DHRs.[44,45]

In summary, DHRs have failed to achieve the intended goals of improving patient care or the well-being of house staff. Over the long term, in neurosurgery and perhaps other specialties, compromised inpatient care will potentially continue, and society will come late to recognize that organized medicine failed to anticipate the unintended adverse effect of DHRs. Specifically for neurosurgery education, the implementation of DHRs has had three negative effects: diminution in the overall educational emphasis, constraint on flexibility of individual training, and a deemphasis on research. These three negative effects echo the concerns that Bergland[22] raised in his 1973 article.

See a full reference list on ExpertConsult.com

1 Historical Overview of Neurosurgery

James Tait Goodrich and Eugene S. Flamm

Neurosurgery, as a subspecialty in general surgery, is a very recent development, having occurred only in the latter half of the 19th century. Three critical developments and concepts had to occur for neurosurgery to become a specialized subspecialty: anesthesia, antisepsis, and cerebral localization. All three of these developments occurred over less than 40 years (the 1840s to the 1870s). In this chapter, the underlying theme is that neurosurgery advanced as surgeons obtained a better understanding of the anatomy and pathophysiology of the nervous system, a goal that continues to be followed today.

This concept was clearly provided in 1602 by **William Clowes,**[1] a leading surgeon of the Elizabethan age. Clowes invoked a challenge that neurosurgeons must still overcome, even in the age of computerized imaging, microsurgery, and functional neurosurgery:

> Those which are Masters and Professors chosen to performe the like operation, ought indeede to have a Lyons heart, a Ladies hand, and a Haukes eye, for that it is a worke of no small importance.

Hippocrates, the father of medicine, had even further detailed this concept when he stated, "Nullum capitis vulnus contemnendum est": no head injury should be considered trivial.[2]

NEUROSURGERY IN THE PREHISTORIC PERIOD

Neurosurgery is, in many ways, one of the most ancient of professions. Early humans clearly recognized that to bring down an enemy, a blow to the head was the quickest means. To accomplish this goal, a number of weapons and, in particular, clubs were fashioned to inflict these injuries. Numerous anthropologic collections around the world include examples of skulls with head injuries; more remarkable are a number of skulls with successful trephinations: that is, the patient clearly survived the surgical opening of the skull.[3-5] From some cultures, such as early Peruvian communities, there exist many skulls that show evidence of trephinations, in most cases for reasons that remain unknown. Paul Broca (1824-1880) in the mid-19th century was one of the first to speculate that this procedure was performed for religious or medical reasons, but there is no documentation for why these procedures were done. It has become apparent that the surgical skill for performing a trephination was worldwide; there are examples from virtually every major civilization, some dating back approximately 12,000 years. There are three common methods for performing a trephination: (1) scraping away the bone, (2) drilling a series of small holes and connecting them, and (3) making cross-hatch cuts in the bone and connecting them to remove a rectangular piece of bone. A trephine skull on which the scraping technique was used, from the early Chimu culture in Peru, and two examples of the typical tool used to perform the scraping (called a *tumi*) are illustrated in Figure 1-1.

ANCIENT EGYPTIAN NEUROSURGERY

The earliest known written documents that relate to early neurosurgery date from the ancient Egyptian period. During this period, which covered approximately 30 successive dynasties, the earliest known practicing physician and Egyptian polymath lived: **Imhotep,** or **Ii-em-Hotep** (c. 2650-2600 BC). So powerful was Imhotep's influence that he was given divine status after his death. This period of history has provided the earliest known existing medical and surgical writings. Three Egyptian papyri that have relevance to medicine still exist: the Ebers, Hearst, and Edwin Smith papyri.[6-8]

According to these Egyptian papyri, the practice of medicine was based largely on magic and superstition. Medical and surgical treatment relied on simple principles, whereby nature provided restoration of health with little intervention and mostly observation with simple mendicants. Of interest to modern neurosurgeons is the concept that the Egyptians realized that immobilization in a neck or back injury was important in reducing further injury. These early physicians commonly prescribed and applied splints for treatments.

The oldest medical text dates from this early civilization and was written in the 16th century BC, approximately 300 years after Hammurabi. This text, now called the *Ebers papyrus,* includes more than 100 pages of hieratic writing and is of interest for its extensive discussions of contemporary surgical practice. Included are discussions of the removal of tumors, along with recommendations for the surgical drainage of abscesses.[6]

The oldest work that deals extensively with medical and surgical techniques to deal with traumatic injuries is the *Edwin Smith papyrus.* Edwin Smith was from New York but had moved to Luxor, Egypt, to become an antiquities dealer; he acquired this papyrus in 1862. Smith spent considerable time translating the document into English. This didactic work appears to have been intended to be a surgical textbook. It was originally written during the time of the New Kingdom. This papyrus scroll is 15 feet in length and 1 foot in width and is written in a cursive hieratic script. The surviving text consists solely of a list of 48 cases, including 22 cases of injuries to the spine and cranium. There is even a case of a cranioplasty (Case 9), discussed along with what might be the earliest reported case of neurofibromatosis (Case 45). Each case is discussed with a diagnosis, followed by a formulated prognosis. As a result of scholarly research by Professor James Henry Breasted, this papyrus was translated again in 1930 from the original hieratic script. More recently (2012), a neurosurgeon (Gonzalo M. Sanchez) and a hieratic script expert (Edmund S. Meltzer) collaborated on reinterpreting the document and provided a more detailed medical/surgical explanation of the various cases. The papyrus is now in possession of the New York Academy of Medicine.[8-10] The following two cases show the insight and some of the techniques illustrated in this early historical papyrus[9]:

> <u>Case Two</u>
>
> **Title:** Instructions concerning a gaping wound in his head, penetrating to the bone.
>
> **Examination:** If thou examinest a man having a gaping wound in his head, penetrating to the bone, thou shouldst lay thy hand upon it and thou shouldst palpate his wound. If thou findest his skull uninjured, not having a perforation in it....
>
> **Diagnosis:** Thou shouldst say regarding him: "One having a gaping wound in his head. An ailment which I will treat."
>
> **Treatment:** Thou shouldst bind fresh meat upon it the first day; thou shouldst apply for him two strips of linen, and treat

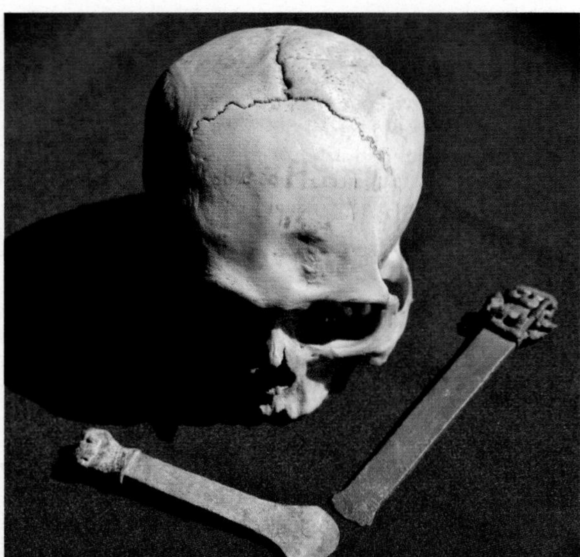

Figure 1-1. A skull from Peru with a left frontal trephination accomplished by the "scraping" technique. The surgeon would use the two hand-held Peruvian tumis, positioned in front of the skull. These tumis, made of a copper/bronze mix, date from the period 800-1100 AD. The patient survived the procedure, as indicated by evidence of healed bone regeneration at the site. *(Courtesy James Tait Goodrich, MD, PhD.)*

afterward with grease, honey, and lint every day until he recovers.

Gloss: As for: "Two strips of linen," it means two bands of linen which one applies upon the two lips of the gaping wound in order to cause that one join to the other.

Case Five

Title: Instructions concerning a gaping wound in his head, smashing his skull.

Examination: If thou examinest a man having a gaping wound in his head, penetrating to the bone, and smashing his skull; thou shouldst palpate his wound. Shouldst thou find that smash which is in his skull deep and sunken under thy fingers, while the swelling which is over it protrudes, he discharges blood from both his nostrils and both his ears, and he suffers with stiffness in his neck, so that he is unable to look at his two shoulders and his breast…

Diagnosis: Thou shouldst say regarding him: "One having a gaping wound in his head, penetrating to the bone, and smashing his skull, while he suffers with stiffness in his neck. An ailment not to be treated."

Treatment: Thou shalt not bind him but moor him at his mooring stakes, until the period of his injury passes by….

Other than the isolated cases, these remaining papyri provide little information about the actual practice of neurosurgery.[9,10] It is evident from these writings that Egyptian physicians recognized head injury and would elevate a skull fracture if necessary. At the same time, if the injury appeared to be too severe, then no treatment was advocated. Both the management and the codification of head injury were not formalized until the development of the Greek schools of medicine (c. 460 BC), by individuals such as Hippocrates.

CLASSICAL PERIOD: GREEK AND BYZANTINE NEUROSURGERY

Hippocratic School

The intellectual evolution of neurological surgery originated in the golden age of Greece with the founding of the Alexandrian School in 300 BC. For the first time, open anatomic dissection was incorporated into formal lectures.[11] The concept of a surgeon performing surgery on the head and spine also became formalized for the first time. Because of sporting injuries, particularly gladiator injuries, and wars, head injuries were clearly plentiful and provided ample opportunities to develop the early skills of neurosurgery.

The earliest medical writings from this period are those of **Hippocrates** (c. 460-370 BC), the most celebrated of the Asclepiadae.[12-14] Classical philologists consider that many of the writings attributed to Hippocrates were in reality composed by members of the Hippocratic School. The Hippocratic collection includes clinical cases based mainly on observation, and in most cases, only the simplest of theories are offered. The many neurological cases within the Hippocratic corpus reveal that the understanding of head injury was rather sophisticated. Hippocrates was the first to describe a number of neurological injuries, most resulting from battlefield injuries. The vulnerability of the brain to injury was categorized by location in the brain, from lesser to greater, with injury to the bregma being represented as a higher risk than one to the temporal region, which, in turn, was more dangerous than an injury to the occipital region.[14-16] Hippocrates devoted a full chapter to injuries of the head, *De capitis vulneribus*, which deals with the diagnosis and management of head injuries and is the first systematic work devoted to head injuries. He divided head injuries into five categories that were based on the details of the skull fracture. Five types of fractures are described: linear fracture, contusion, depressed fracture, hedra (or dent) occurring with and without fracture, and contrecoup fracture.[14] The neurological condition of the patient was not thought to have any bearing on the surgical indications. Surgery was advised according to the type of fracture. The greater the injury to the skull, the less was the need for trephination. The technical aspects of the process of trephination are presented in a curious mixture of sound advice and incomprehensible admonitions (Fig. 1-2).

The Hippocratic writings contain numerous anatomic descriptions, even though human dissection appears not to have been routinely practiced. The Greeks also were without an anatomic vocabulary, not to be introduced until Galen standardized the use of the Latin language in medicine. These deficiencies combined to limit any standardized anatomic procedures or the practice of surgery. Despite these drawbacks, the Hippocratic writings contain a number of interesting neurological case studies that reflect a view of the early practice of neurosurgery (Fig. 1-3).

One of the earliest descriptions of subarachnoid hemorrhage appears in the *Aphorisms*[17,18]:

> When persons in good health are suddenly seized with pains in the head, and straightway are laid down speechless, and breathe with stertor, they die in seven days, unless fever comes on.

Hippocrates and his followers also warned against incising the brain, as convulsions can occur on the opposite side and render the prognosis especially serious. Hippocrates advised against making an incision over the temporal artery, because this could also lead to contralateral convulsions. The writings of Hippocratic schools demonstrate the simple concepts of cerebral localization. Also well understood was the concept of a potential critical prognosis in head injury and that sometimes it was best not to operate. In this early era of medicine, the risk of infection, lack of antiseptic technique, and minimal anesthesia all precluded any serious or aggressive surgical intervention in head injury.

Herophilus of Chalcedon

From the region of the Bosporus, among the crowded schools of Alexandria, came **Herophilus (Herophilos)** (335-280 BC), a student of Praxagoras and Chrysippus and a member of the educated dynasty of Ptolemies. According to his writing, Herophilus performed dissection on humans and not on animals as was the common practice then.[19-21] The work of Herophilus, along with that of Galen later, was key in the task of developing an anatomic nomenclature and in forming a much-needed language of anatomy. In examinations of the nervous system, Herophilus's neurological contributions included following the origin of nerves to the spinal cord anatomically. He was the first to recognize the difference in the motor and sensory tracts. Furthermore, he differentiated between nerves and tendons, thereby correcting a common earlier error. Herophilus was first to detail the anatomy of the brain ventricles and venous sinuses. The description of the "confluence of the sinuses," or *torcular herophili* (Λανοζ = wine press), comes from his early investigations. Herophilus provided the first description and naming of the choroid plexus *(plexus choroides)*, so named because of its resemblance to the vascular membrane (chorion) of the fetus. Herophilus also provided the first detailed account of the fourth ventricle and that peculiar arrangement at its base that he called the *calamus scriptorius* (Αναγλυφη τχ χαλαμχ), which he described as "resembles a pen in writing." Among his many other contributions was his recognition of the brain as the central organ of the nervous system and the seat of intelligence.[20]

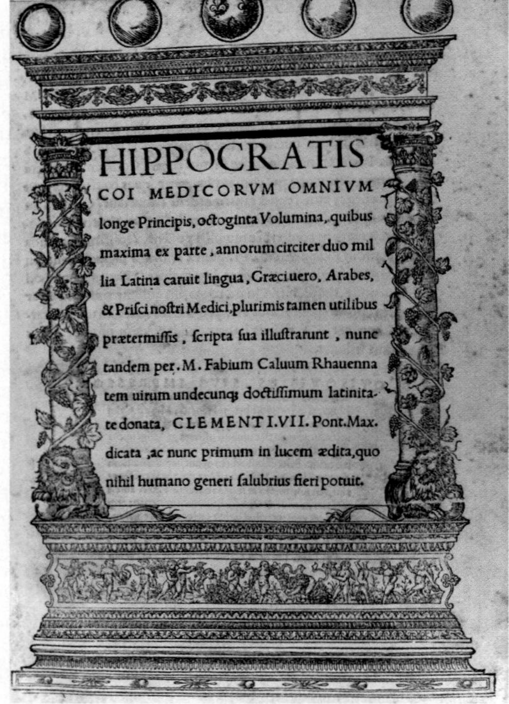

HIPPOCRATIS
COI MEDICORVM OMNIVM
longe Principis, octoginta Volumina, quibus
maxima ex parte, annorum circiter duo mil
lia Latina caruit lingua, Græci uero, Arabes,
& Priſci noſtri Medici, plurimis tamen utilibus
prætermiſſis, ſcripta ſua illuſtrarunt, nunc
tandem per M. Fabium Caluum Rhauenna
tem uirum undecunq; doctiſſimum latinita-
te donata, CLEMENTI.VII. Pont.Max.
dicata, ac nunc primum in lucem ædita, quo
nihil humano generi ſalubrius fieri potuit.

Figure 1-2. Title page from the first printed edition of the writings of Hippocrates, in 1525. *(From Hippocrates.* Coi Medicorum Omnium Longe Principis, Octoginta Volumina, Quibus Maxima ex Parte, Annorum Circiter Duo Millia Latina Catruit Lingua, Gaecivero, Arabes & Prisci Nostri, Scripta sua Illustrarunt....Latuita te Donata, Clementi. LVII. Pont. Max. Dictata.... *Rome: Franciscus Minutius Calvus; 1525. Courtesy James Tait Goodrich, MD, PhD.)*

Herophilus's writings were not free of errors. An anatomic error that remained in vogue for nearly 1800 years was his introduction into the anatomic literature of the *rete mirabile*, a structure present in ungulates but notably lacking in higher primates. In ungulates this structure acts as an anastomotic network at the base of the brain, a structure that the Greeks incorporated into the early physiologic theories of brain function.[22] In the 2nd century AD, the *rete mirabile* was later further detailed and elaborated on by Galen of Pergamon. The concept of this structure became entrenched in the anatomic literature, having been codified by the Byzantine Islamic and later European medieval writers, until the 16th century, when it was finally challenged in the anatomic accounts of Andreas Vesalius (1514-1564) and Jacopo Berengario da Carpi (1460-1530).[23-25] Both of these anatomists, who performed their own human dissections, clearly recognized that the *rete mirabile* did not exist in humans. It is possible that the human cavernous sinus confused the early writers and they in turn thought that this represented the *rete mirable*.

Aulus Aurelius Cornelius Celsus

Celsus (25 BC-50 AD) was neither a physician nor a surgeon, nor was he a bedside practitioner; rather, he was an intellectual patrician and a medical encyclopedist who attempted to compile all of the important writings of his time. His writings had an important early influence on medicine and surgery. His medical writings were mostly a compilation of the writings from the schools

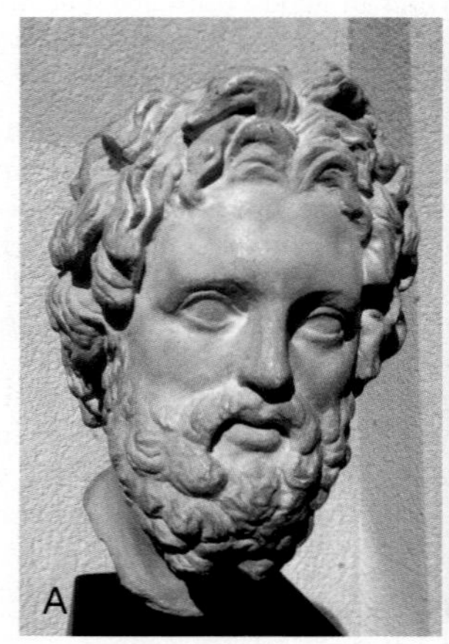

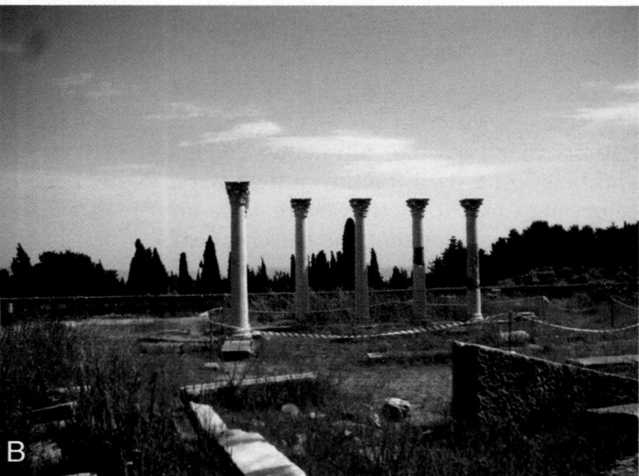

Figure 1-3. A, Bust of Asclepius (Aesculapius). **B,** Temple of Asclepius on the island of Kos, Greece. Kos is the birthplace of Hippocrates and the Hippocratic schools of medicine. *(Courtesy James Tait Goodrich, MD, PhD.)*

of Hippocrates and the Asclepiadae and from the Alexandrian schools. Celsus lived during the height of the Roman Empire. As counselor to the emperors Tiberius Caesar and Caligula, Celsus was held in great esteem. His book on medicine, titled *De Re Medicina*,[26,27] is now considered one of the most important early medical documents after the Hippocratic writings. Because this work was originally lost, Celsus was one of the few major authors whose works were not transcribed by the Islamic/Arabic writers. In 1443, an early Celsus manuscript was uncovered by Thomas of Sarzanne (later Pope Nicolas V) and reintroduced to the medical community. With the introduction of printing and moveable type, Celsus's manuscript became the first medical writing to be printed (1478), before even the writings of Hippocrates and Galen. In the *De Re Medicina*, Book IV, Chapter 10, his classic description of inflammation appears: "Notae vero inflammationes sunt quattuor, rubor, et tumor, cum calore et dolore [There are four signs of an inflammation: redness, swelling, heat, and pain]."

Celsus made a number of interesting early observations in the field of neurosurgery. Celsus believed that all surgeons should be ambidextrous. Book VIII, Chapter 4, contains one of the earliest descriptions of an epidural hematoma resulting from a ruptured middle meningeal artery.[27] For head-injured patients, Celsus recommended that the surgeon always operate on the side of greater pain. Celsus was a strong advocate for use of the trephine in head injuries. He noted that the trephine should always be placed at the point where the pain is best localized. Celsus described a technique for a craniectomy that involved drilling a number of holes and then connecting them with a hammer and chisel. The chisel had a protective blade, which separated the dura from the bone and prevented injury to it during the surgical dissection. However, he regarded the operation of trephination as the *ultimum refugium*, to be used only when all conservative measures had been exhausted (Fig. 1-4).

Several interesting neurological conditions are described in the *De Re Medicina*, including accurate descriptions of hydrocephalus and facial neuralgia. In accordance with earlier writings, Celsus clearly recognized that a high cervical spine fracture could lead to vomiting and difficulty in breathing. Injury to the lower lumbar spine could cause weakness or paralysis of the legs, as well as urinary retention or incontinence.

Galen of Pergamon

Galen of Pergamon (129-200 AD), whose name comes from *galenos*, meaning "calm" or "serene," is remembered as a powerful personality and an original investigator, as well as a leading proponent of the doctrines of Hippocrates and the Alexandrian school. Galen began his writing career at the age of 13 and continued to add to the literature of medicine, philosophy, mathematics, and grammar until his death at the age of 70. His writings remained the most extensive in early antiquity in size, scope, and influence. Galen's prodigious output still accounts for more than 80% of all the surviving medical writings of antiquity.[28] Many of his writings and manuscripts, however, were lost in a fire at the Temple of Peace in Rome (Figs. 1-5 and 1-6).

Galen's life and activity occurred during the reigns of two of the greatest Roman emperors: Antoninus Pius (86-161 AD; reigned 138-161 AD) and Marcus Aurelius (121-180 AD; reigned 161-180 AD). Galen became the physician to the gladiators of Pergamon and, as a result, saw and treated many traumatic injuries. Drawing from both his surgical experiences and anatomic studies, he made a number of contributions to the fields of neurology, neurosurgery, and neuroanatomy. In his writings, Galen differentiated between the pia mater and the dura mater and gave one of the earliest accurate descriptions of the corpus callosum, the ventricular system, the pineal and pituitary glands, the infundibulum, and what is now called the *aqueduct of Sylvius.* Nearly 1600 years before the Scottish anatomist Alexander Monro *secundus* (1733-1817), Galen also described the structure now called the *foramen of Monro.* He performed a number of anatomic experiments, including early studies on the effects of transection of the spinal cord.[29,30] From these studies, Galen was able to describe the specific loss of function below the level of the transection. In a now classic experiment, he sectioned the recurrent laryngeal nerve in dogs and described the hoarseness

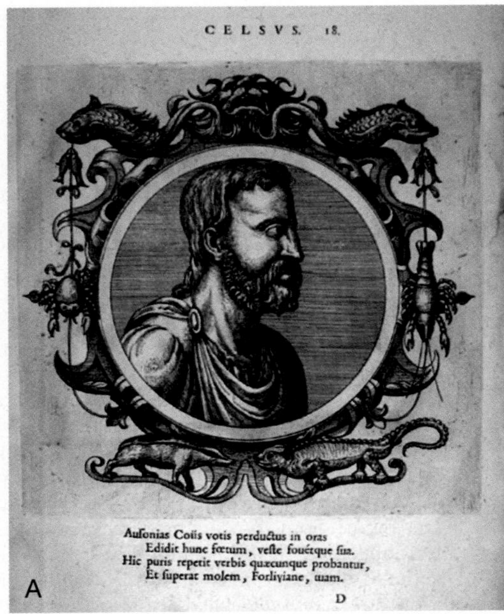
CELSVS. 18.
Aufonias Coiis votis perductus in oras
Edidit hunc fœtum, vefte fouétque fua.
Hic puris repetit verbis quæcunque probantur,
Et fuperat molem, Forliviane, tuam.
D
A

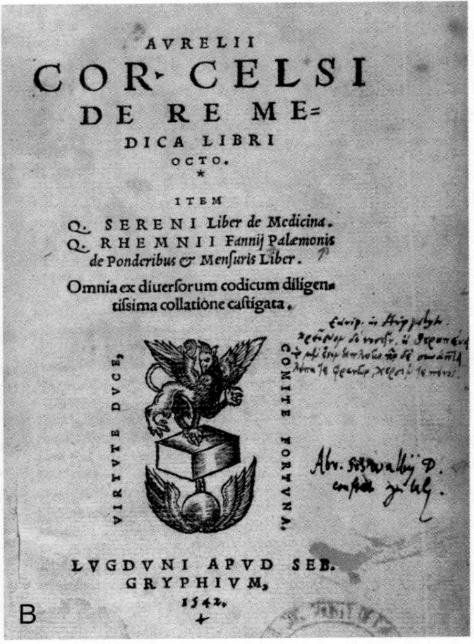
AVRELII
COR. CELSI
DE RE ME=
DICA LIBRI
OCTO.
*
ITEM
Q. SERENI Liber de Medicina.
Q. RHEMNII Fannij Palæmonis
de Ponderibus & Menfuris Liber.
Omnia ex diuerforum codicum diligen=
tifsima collatione caftigata.
VIRTVTE DVCE, COMITE FORTVNA.
LVGDVNI APVD SEB.
GRYPHIVM,
1542.
B

Figure 1-4. A, Portrait of Celsus. **B,** Title page from a 1542 edition of Celsus's writings. *(Courtesy James Tait Goodrich, MD, PhD.)*

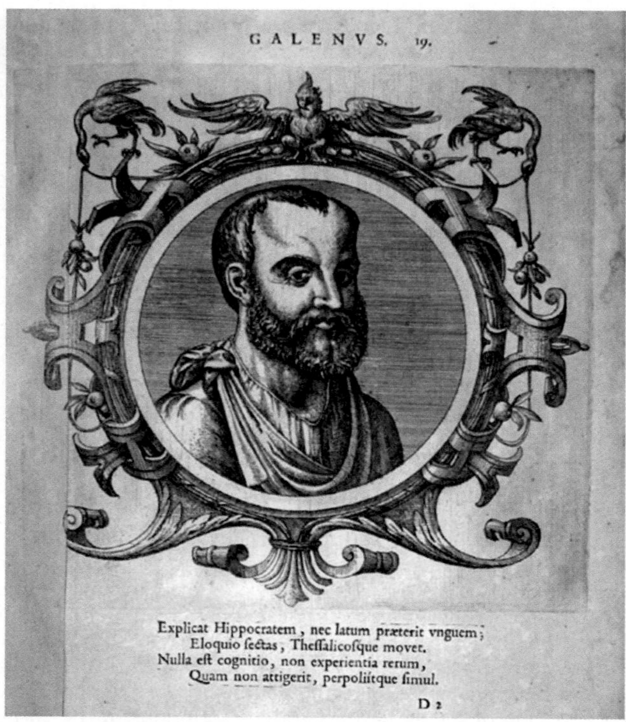
GALENVS. 19.
Explicat Hippocratem, nec latum præterit vnguem;
Eloquio ſectas, Theſſalicoſque movet.
Nulla eſt cognitio, non experientia rerum,
Quam non attigerit, perpoliitque ſimul.
D 2

Figure 1-5. Portrait of Galen of Pergamon. *(Courtesy James Tait Goodrich, MD, PhD.)*

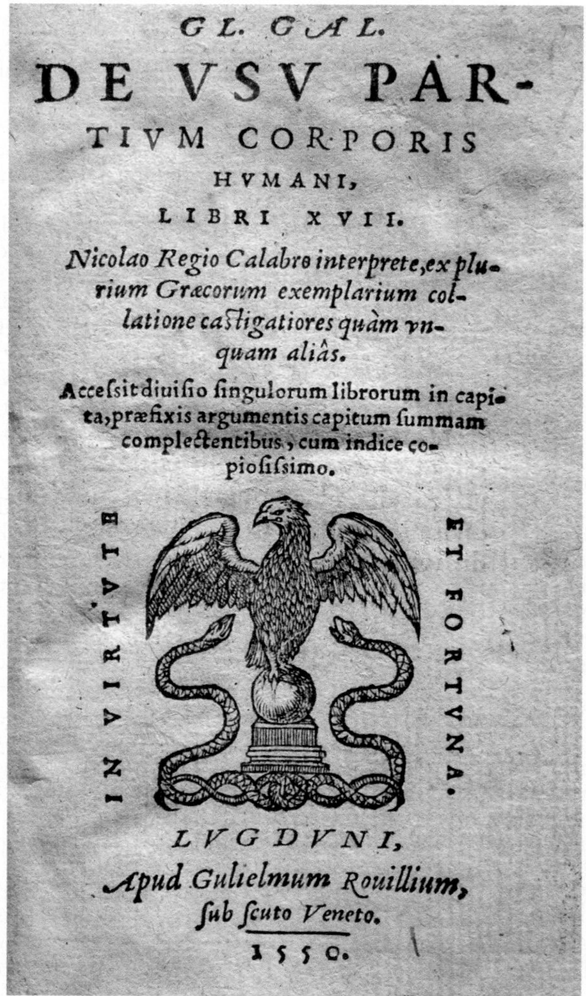
GL. GAL.

DE VSV PAR-
TIVM CORPORIS
HVMANI,
LIBRI XVII.

Nicolao Regio Calabro interprete, ex plu-
rium Græcorum exemplarium col-
latione caſtigatiores quàm vn-
quam aliâs.

Acceſsit diuiſio ſingulorum librorum in capita, præfixis argumentis capitum ſummam
complectentibus, cum indice co-
pioſiſsimo.

IN VIRTVTE ET FORTVNA.

LVGDVNI,
Apud Gulielmum Rouillium,
ſub ſcuto Veneto.
1550.

Figure 1-6. Title page of one of Galen's important writings on the anatomy and physiology of human anatomy. *(From Galen of Pergamon.* De Usu Partium Corporis Humani, Libri XVII. Nicolao Regio Calabra Interprete.... *Lugduni [Lyons]: Apud Gulielmum Roullium; 1550. Courtesy James Tait Goodrich, MD, PhD.)*

that occurred (discussed further in Chapter 7; see also *De usu partium corporis humani*, Book VII, Chapters 11-18).[29]

Galen was the first to provide an early classification of the cranial nerves. In his original classification, he described 11 of the 12 cranial nerves, but because he combined several, he thought the total was only 7. In his descriptions, Galen regarded the olfactory nerve as merely a prolongation of the brain and hence did not consider it as a cranial nerve.[29] Galen published a number of interesting views on higher cortical functions, embracing views that the brain was responsible for intelligence, fantasy, memory, and judgment. In studying muscle contractions, Galen made the observation that the stimulus originated in the brain and the impulse was carried to the muscle by nerves. These views were original and represented an important departure from the cardiocentric teachings of the earlier medical and philosophical schools such as Aristotle's. Galen challenged the Hippocratic view that that the brain was only a gland and instead attributed to the brain the powers of voluntary action and sensation (encephalocentric), this last being a remarkable advance in thinking for the period.

From a series of anatomic studies, Galen provided some of the earliest observations on cervical spine injury and the resulting disturbance in arm function. Further study of spinal cord injury led to his elegant description of what is now called the *Brown-Séquard syndrome*, a hemiplegia with contralateral sensory loss that results from a hemisection of the cord.[30] Galen provided one of the earliest clinical descriptions of hydrocephalus and clearly recognized the poor prognosis in affected individuals. Using his extensive experience in head injuries, he provided some innovative arguments for elevation of depressed skull fractures, fractures with hematomas, and comminuted fractures. Galen was more aggressive in his treatment by recommending the removal of bone fragments, particularly those pressing into the brain. In describing surgical techniques, Galen detailed a safer and more reliable use of the trephine and argued particularly for continuous irrigation to a trephine to avoid delivering excessive heat and causing injury to the underlying brain. Galen, following or adapting earlier Hippocratic views, reiterated the concept that the dura should never be violated by the trephine.

Galen was clearly a brilliant physician, surgeon, and early innovator in medicine. Unfortunately, Galen's writings contained a number of errors, but the historical world, particularly the Byzantine world, later accepted Galen's writings as the only true authority. As a result, Galen's writings obtained the status of unchallengeable medical dogma. Galen's work on neurology and neuroanatomy also remained essentially unchallenged for the next 1500 years. For all practical purposes, any relevant new investigations ceased altogether from Galen's death until the Renaissance. Some writers have pointed out that Galen was literally idolized by Arabic/Islamic writers and, later, the physicians of the Middle Ages. As a result, Galen's errors (e.g., writings about the *rete mirabile*) also remained part of the anatomic literature. Each of these errors or incorrect beliefs were carefully repeated and scribed by subsequent Arabic/Islamic and medieval physicians and surgeons. Because of the strength of Galen's views and those of subsequent writers, no one was willing to challenge what were clearly anatomic and scientific errors, which had a stultifying effect on science and medicine for approximately 1500 years.

Paulus Aegineta (Paul of Aegina)

Paulus Aegineta (625-c. 6) was a brilliant Byzantine Greek physician and surgeon who also trained in the Alexandrian school. He was an influential compiler of works in both the Latin and Greek schools; his writings, especially *The Seven Books of Paul of Aegineta*, were being consulted until well into the 17th century; the *Compendium* was translated into English in the 19th century.[31,32] His skill as a surgeon, described in the sixth book of the *Compendium*, clearly reflected an unusual understanding of surgical principles. His skills became legendary, causing patients from far away to consult him. Although Paulus venerated the teachings of the ancients as tradition required, he also introduced his own techniques with good results. His classic work, *The Seven Books of Paul of Aegineta*, contains an excellent section on head injury and the use of the trephine.[31,32] Paulus classified skull fractures in several categories: fissure, incision, expression, depression, arched fracture, and, in infants, dent (what is now called a *ping pong fracture*). In dealing with fractures, he used an interesting skin incision: two incisions intersecting one another at right angles, forming the Greek letter X, one leg of the X incorporating the scalp wound. For the comfort of the patient undergoing a trephination, he would stuff the patient's ear with wool so that the noise of the trephine would not cause undue distress (see *The Seven Books of Paul of Aegineta*, Book VI, Section XC[32]) (Fig. 1-7).

In a contemporary discussion on hydrocephalus, Paul of Aegina introduced the intriguing concept that traumatic birth delivery and intraventricular hemorrhage were related; he appears to have been the first to suggest the possibility that an intraventricular hemorrhage and its "inert fluid" might actually cause hydrocephalus:

> The hydrocephalic affection…occurs in infants, owing to their heads being improperly squeezed by midwives during parturition, or from some other obscure cause; or from the rupture of a vessel or vessels, and the extravasated blood being converted into an inert fluid….
>
> **(Book VI, Section 3, page 250[32])**

One of the reasons for Paulus's longstanding influence was that several of his manuscripts survived and were continuously recopied by amanuenses over the centuries. These manuscripts depict a number of surgical instruments that he designed specifically for neurosurgical procedures; these include elevators, raspatories, and bone biters. He also introduced trephine bits with conical styles to reduce the risk of plunging, along with different biting edges. Because of his sophisticated wound management, he probably had better-than-average surgical outcomes. He made use of wine-soaked dressings (helpful in antisepsis, although a concept then unknown), and he stressed that dressings should be applied with no compression to the brain itself.

The Greek and Byzantine periods were eras of intense scholarship and original investigation in medicine and surgery and produced physicians and surgeons who were intensely interested in the better management of their patients. As discussed, individuals such as Galen of Pergamon, Paulus Aegineta, Herophilus of Chalcedon, and members of the Hippocratic school all attempted to improve management in head injuries and at the same time uncover some of the principles of brain function. Unfortunately, as discussed in the next section, further neurological investigation and the development of new surgical techniques were seriously impaired because of scholarly reverence of these earlier writers. Although there were some exceptions to this trend, they were distinctly uncommon.

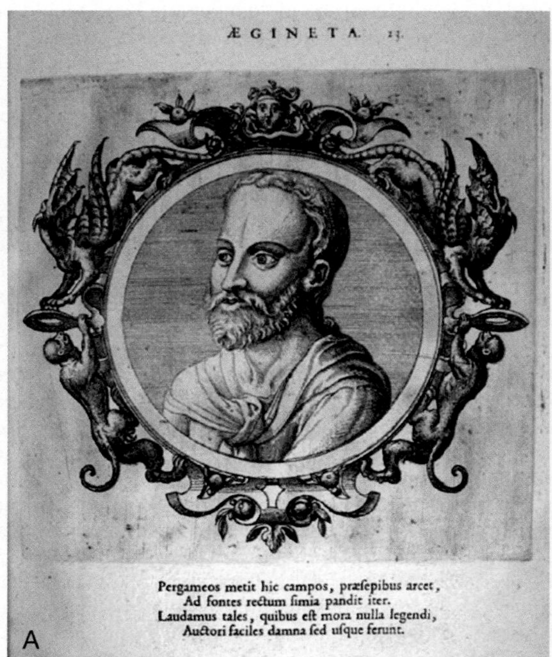
ÆGINETA.
Pergameos metit hic campos, præſepibus arcet,
Ad fontes rectum ſimia pandit iter.
Laudamus tales, quibus eſt mora nulla legendi,
Auctori faciles damna ſed uſque ferunt.
A

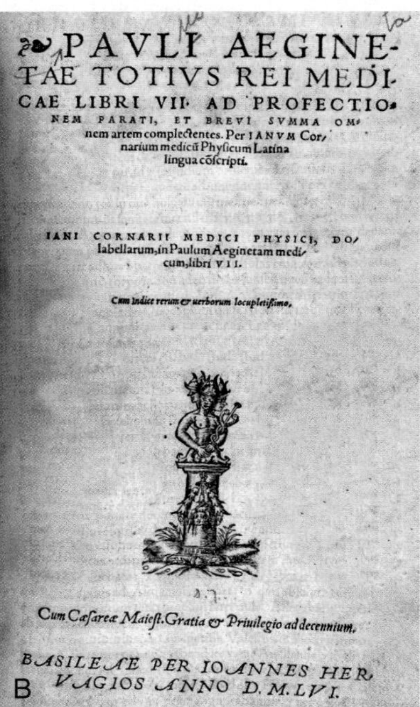
PAVLI AEGINETAE TOTIVS REI MEDICAE LIBRI VII. AD PROFECTIONEM PARATI, ET BREVI SVMMA OMNEM ARTEM COMPLECTENTES. Per IANVM Cornarium medicũ Phyſicum Latina lingua cõſcripti.

IANI CORNARII MEDICI PHYSICI, DOlabellarum, in Paulum Aeginetam medicum, libri VII.

Cum Indice rerum & uerborum locupletiſſimo.

Cum Cæſareæ Maieſt. Gratia & Priuilegio ad decennium.

BASILEAE PER IOANNES HERVAGIOS ANNO D.M.LVI.

B

Figure 1-7. A, Portrait of Paulus Aegineta. **B,** Title page of the collected works of Paulus Aegineta. *(Courtesy James Tait Goodrich, MD, PhD.)*

ISLAMIC/ARABIC MEDICINE: PRESCHOLASTIC PERIOD

After the great Greek and Roman periods of medicine, the intellectual centers of this discipline shifted to the Islamic/Arabic and Byzantine cultures. This era, "The Golden Age of Islamic Medicine," had an influence that lasted from approximately AD 750 until 1200, when the medievalist era began and the influential schools of medicine shifted to Europe. Interestingly, this period in Europe was intellectually quiescent and unimaginative because this area of the world had been overrun and ruled by barbarians (Huns, Goths, and Norsemen), individuals not concerned with high scholarship. Unfortunately for neurosurgery, this was a dormant period; the dormancy prevailed in all facets of surgery. The Islamic/Arabic schools were satisfied to codify the surviving manuscripts from the Greek and Roman period. Remarkable insights were offered, but this was a rather rare phenomenon. However, thanks to the zeal of the Arabic amanuenses, the best of Greek medicine was made available to Arabic readers by the end of the ninth century and remained available into the Middle Ages.

Unfortunately, a rigid scholastic dogmatism became characteristic of these learning centers. Rather than offering innovation, the "writers" became copyists of the great works of antiquities. As a result of their efforts, an amazing number of manuscripts were translated from Latin, Greek, and Hebrew into Arabic, and knowledge that could have been easily lost into antiquity was systemized. Unfortunately, as copyists, these writers frequently added their own "favorite" or contemporary view of the manuscript, and some of the originality was consequently lost in translation. In fairness to these early copyists, they rendered the service of preserving knowledge; in Europe at this time, having been overrun by barbarians, scholarly pursuit remained at a standstill.

A number of modern writers have offered the view that it was the religious influence of the Koran that caused the absence of originality and progress in Islamic/Arabic medicine. It has often been commented on that the Koran forbade dissection; this is only partially correct. Some dissection was allowed and reported on by writers of this time. However, as a practical consideration, the climate in this part of the world was hot, which caused rapid putrefaction of cadavers and made anatomic dissection undesirable. The opinion of these schools was that the Greeks had already accomplished most of the anatomic studies of interest, and so Islamic students of medicine felt no need to duplicate these earlier and more superior efforts. There were some rare exceptions that are discussed as follows.

In Islamic/Arabic medicine, the concept of a physician doubling as a surgeon was rarely acceptable. The more typical practice for a physician was to confine himself to writing learnedly and assign the "menial" tasks of surgery to an individual of a lower class, most typically an apprentice surgeon. As a result of this "demotion" of the surgeon to a mere plebian, the advances in surgery and anatomy developed by the great Alexandrians, among others, were essentially ignored or lost. Fortunately, the writings of physicians such as Galen of Pergamon and Paulus Aegineta were saved and translated into Arabic, but few new techniques or concepts were added.

The dominant period for Islamic scholarship in medicine was the 10th through 12th centuries. Several medical scholars rose to prominence during this period; among the most illustrious were Avicenna (980-1037), Rhazes (865-925), Avenzoar (d. 1162), Albucasis (1013-1106), and Averroës (1126-1198). The writings of these great physicians reveal an extraordinary effort to canonize the writings of their Greek and Roman predecessors. Rather than innovation, these Islamic/Arab scholars and physicians became the guardians and academics of Hippocratic, Greek, and Galenic writings, which now became dogma.

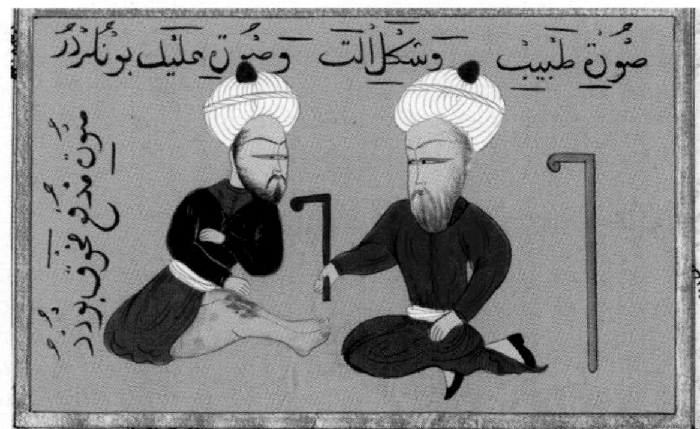

Figure 1-8. Image from a later copy of a manuscript by Avicenna. A physician is depicted applying "red-hot" cautery to a patient's leg. *(Courtesy James Tait Goodrich, MD, PhD.)*

One of the most beneficial teaching methods, and quite modern, did arise during the Islamic/Arabic period: the concept of bedside medical care and teaching. The relative paucity or lack of regular anatomic dissection, along with the prevalent view that surgery was performed only by individuals of inferior status, inevitably reduced any preoccupation with surgical art. Another unfortunate surgical practice that occurred during this period was the reintroduction of the Egyptian technique of using the hot cautery for control of bleeding. In addition, hot cautery was also employed in lieu of the scalpel to create a surgical incision, the results of which often proved unfortunate for surgical patients (Fig. 1-8).

One of the significant scholars of this period was **Rhazes (Abu Bakr Muhammad Ibn Zakariya)** (865-925). Rhazes was a scholarly physician, learned in diagnosis, and a review of his writings reveals him to be loyal exclusively to Hippocratic teachings. Rhazes developed a considerable reputation that led him to become a court physician. Rhazes was not a surgeon, although he did write on surgical topics.[33] Rhazes introduced the use of animal gut as a suture material. Rhazes was an early believer in the concept of "concussion" and would advocate surgery for penetrating injuries of the skull—this in a period when these types of surgical outcomes were almost always fatal. Rhazes believed that head injuries were among the most devastating of all injuries. Because skull fractures could be permanently damaging to the patient as a result of the compression of the brain, his surgical advice would be to elevate these depressed areas of the fractured skull.

Among the most influential physicians of this period was **Avicenna** (980-1037), physician and philosopher of Baghdad, also known as the chief or "second doctor," the first being Aristotle. Avicenna's writings and translations clearly extended the original Greek influence with a force so persuasive and durable that it remained the dominant scholarship until well into the 18th century. His greatest contribution must be judged to have been the detailed translation of Galen's collected works, the *Opera Omnia*. Avicenna's major work, *Canon Medicinae*, was an encyclopedic effort clearly based on the writings of Galen and Hippocrates.[34] The Greek word *canon* refers to a straight rod, a carpenter rule, or standard of measurement. Accordingly, Avicenna's *Canon* became the "rule," the codification of Galen's and Greek medicine. The *Canon* contains a number of interesting neurological discussions. Avicenna provided an early and accurate clinical understanding of epilepsy, for which his treatment consisted of administering various medicants and herbals with described good results. Avicenna apparently conducted anatomic studies, although he did not discuss this directly. He gave a correct anatomic commentary on the vermis of the cerebellum

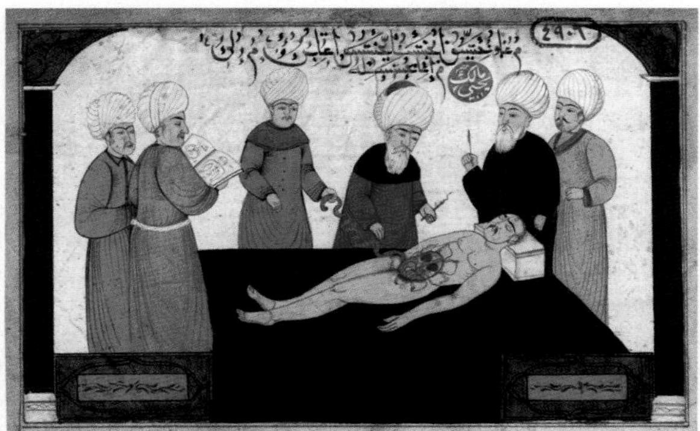

Figure 1-9. Unpublished manuscript leaf from a later collection of works of Avicenna. Avicenna is depicted participating in an anatomic dissection. *(Courtesy James Tait Goodrich, MD, PhD.)*

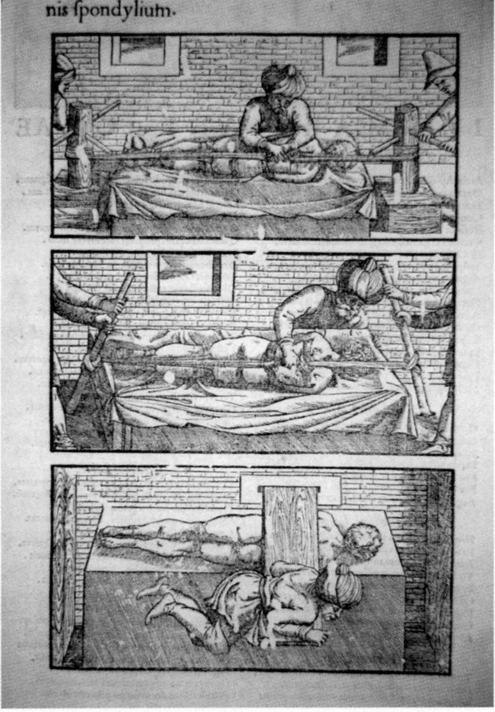

Figure 1-10. An illustration from Avicenna's *Libor Canonis.* Pictured is a "rack" device for dealing with fractures and injuries to the spine. *(From Avicenna.* Liber Canonis, de Medicinis Cordialibus, et Cantica. *Basel: Joannes Heruagios; 1556. Courtesy James Tait Goodrich, MD, PhD.)*

and the "tailed nucleus," now known as the *caudate nucleus.* Avicenna's writings on the treatment of spine injuries and stabilization reveal remarkably modern views for this area[35-37] (Figs. 1-9 and 1-10; see also Fig. 1-8).

Whereas Avicenna was clearly the "second doctor," **Albucasis (Abu Al-Qasim or Al-Zahrawi)** (936-1013), a learned Islamic Moorish Spaniard, was clearly the best surgeon of the times. In the Islamic tradition, Albucasis was both a great compiler and a serious scholar whose writings (≈30 volumes) were focused mainly on surgery, dietetics, and materia medica. Albucasis's insights into the importance of surgery are clearly revealed in his introduction to the collected works.[38,39] In his introduction, Albucasis provides an interesting discussion about why Arabs had made so little progress in surgery. Albucasis attributed this lack of progress to a lack of anatomic study and inadequate knowledge of the classics. Albucasis clearly believed that anatomic studies were the key to learning and certainly key in performing any surgical interventions. Although his thoughts on anatomic studies were excellent, Albucasis unfortunately popularized the frequent use of emetics as prophylaxis against disease, a form of medical treatment that survived in the form of "purging" and a medical practice that continued until well into the 19th century. So influential were Albucasis's surgical writings that they remained in use in the schools of Salerno and Montpellier for approximately 500 years and had an enormous influence on medicine in the Middle Ages (Fig. 1-11).

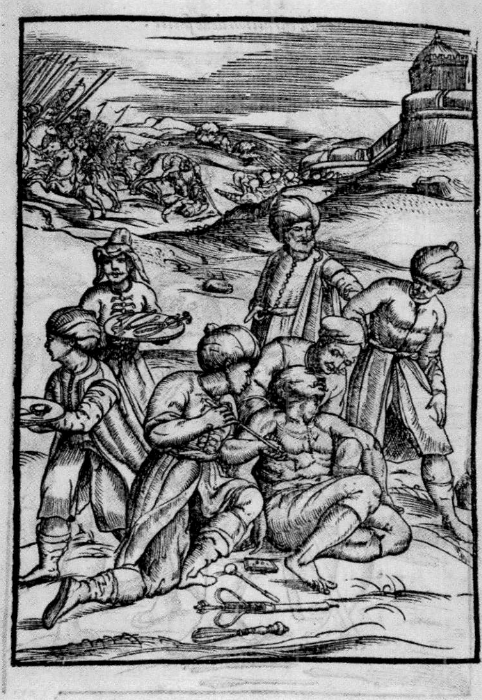

Figure 1-11. An allegorical scene of Albucasis operating in the field on an injured soldier. Albucasis is shown removing an arrow from a patient's chest. Described in the 17th-century Scultetus monograph on surgery. *(From Scultetus J.* Χειροπλοθηκη [Cheiroplothiki]. Armamentarium Chirurgicum XLIII. *Ulm, Germany: Balthasar Kühnen; 1655. Courtesy James Tait Goodrich, MD, PhD.)*

The final section of the *Compendium* contains a lengthy summary of contemporary surgical practice.[38-40] Also included in this part of Albucasis's work is a unique collection of illustrations of surgical instruments. These illustrations became a long-lasting influence, inasmuch as his style of instrument was used extensively in the schools of Salerno and Montpellier and later became an important influence in the medieval period. Many of the instruments illustrated were probably designed by Albucasis. In the text, he clearly described their design, along with technical aspects of their use. Following up on the earlier writings of the Greeks, he provided a novel design for a "nonsinking" trephine. The design for this instrument and others became classic and formed the template for many later such instruments. An early and apparently unique technical innovation involved placing a collar on the trephine in a circular manner, a further and rather ingenious design to prevent the trephine from plunging into the brain. Some of the instruments were clearly copied from those described earlier by Paulus Aegineta, but their practical use was further enhanced by their inclusion in the *Compendium.*

Albucasis's treatise on surgery is an extraordinary work in so many ways. The text is rational, comprehensive, well illustrated, and designed with the intent to educate the surgeon on details of each treatment, neglecting not even the types of wound dressings to be used. Albucasis's techniques of brain surgery, however, were extremely crude. In fact, modern readers can only wonder how patients would allow themselves to undergo some of his surgical practices. For chronic headache, he applied a hot cautery to the occiput, burning through the skin but not the bone. Another headache treatment he described required hooking the temporal artery, twisting it, placing ligatures, and then, in essence, ripping it out.

For neurosurgeons, Albucasis identified and described various types of spinal injury. Albucasis recognized the seriousness of spinal injury, particularly dislocation of the vertebrae. In cases of total subluxation, he appreciated that the prognosis was essentially terminal because affected patients demonstrated involuntary activity (passing urine and stool), along with flaccid limbs. He was quite innovative in dealing with the lesser spinal injuries. In his surgical writings, Albucasis described and illustrated some of the methods and splints he used for reduction of such injuries. To modern readers, some of these techniques might seem to be dangerous in design, especially stabilizations that required an aggressive combination of spars and winches, as well as a "stretching" of the spinal column. Following earlier Greek and Byzantine views, Albucasis believed that bone fragments in the spinal canal should be removed. In reviewing skull fractures, Albucasis has an elegant discussion of the pediatric "ping-pong" fracture of the skull[38]:

> This is a fracture due to a fall or a blow from a stone and the like, making a dent in the surface of the bone and a hollow at the site as occurs in a bronze bowl when a blow falls on it and a portion of it is pushed in. This mostly occurs in heads whose bones are soft, as those of children.

The treatment of hydrocephalus was a vexing problem for surgeons and physicians because its outcome was almost always fatal. Albucasis recommended drainage of cerebrospinal fluid in hydrocephalus via a series of drains and wicks. He designed a lenticular shaped surgical tool to make the puncture, which was performed over the anterior fontanelle. Having detailed the technique well, he then noted the outcome is almost always fatal. Of interest is that the surgery was not the issue; rather, he attributed the poor outcomes to "paralysis" of the brain from relaxation. Albucasis cleverly pointed out that the physician must pick the site for drainage carefully and must never cut over an artery because the potential hemorrhage can rapidly lead to death. Some 20th century authors have advocated the treatment of hydrocephalus by binding the head with tight wraps. Albucasis was advocating this form of treatment more than 1000 years ago. For a child with hydrocephalus, he would bind the head with a wrap and then put the child on a "dry diet" with limited fluid intake to help dehydrate the child. In retrospect, this was a rather progressive and reasonable treatment plan for this disorder.[38,39]

MIDDLE AGES: THE AGE OF MEDIEVAL MEDICAL SCHOLASTICISM

In the early Middle Ages, the influence of the Islamic/Arabic schools on medicine was beginning to lessen, along with a geographic switch in which intellectual centers for medicine were forming in Europe. With the advent of medieval scholasticism, a new school of thought developed in which philosophical and metaphysical explanations and dialectic interpretations became prominent in medical schools. One of the preeminent schools proposing this view was the School of Salerno in what is now Italy.[41,42] In much of Europe, the barbarians were still in control, but despite that, physicians were being trained, and libraries were being built and expanded. Throughout Europe, new medical schools were being established at a steady rate.

At the School of Salerno, an early leader in developing medical scholasticism was **Constantinus Africanus** (1020-1087), *magister orientis et occidentis*.[42] Constantine provided an important bridge in medicine by introducing the scholarship of Islamic/Arabic medicine at Salerno and eventually to all of Europe. Constantine received his medical education in Baghdad, learning the prevalent views of Islamic medicine. He moved to a monastery at Monte Cassino, where, in the tradition of this period, he translated Arabic manuscripts into Latin. Modern scholars believe that his translations were somewhat inaccurate and, as a result, introduced errors in the subsequent medical literature. In reviewing some studies, modern historians considered Constantine to be mostly a plagiarist and an unreliable translator. However, his translation of texts from Arabic to Latin were the earliest transfer of Arabic/Islamic medical literature into Europe, which was valuable. Nonetheless, because the original Greek texts had been translated into Arabic, and Constantinus translated the Arabic works into Latin, the legacy of Galen and other early writers remained firmly entrenched as dogma. Rather than providing or developing new ideas, the classical texts in medicine merely propounded medical dogma. How much medical and surgical knowledge was lost or distorted by inaccuracies in these successive translations is unimaginable.

Constantine did make a key contribution to medieval medicine when he reintroduced anatomic dissection with an annual dissection of a pig. Of interest is that as the dissection progressed, the findings were compared with those recorded in the Greek classics. If the dissector's findings did not match those of the ancient texts, they were simply ignored! Constantine was clearly a learned scholar, but his style of teaching became typical of the Medical Ages. Extensive compilations and translations were undertaken, but original thought or advance in knowledge was notably lacking. In the Middle Ages, the School of Salerno did lead the way and was subsequently followed by the great medical schools at Naples, Bologna, Paris, and Montpellier, the early pillars of medieval medicine (Figs. 1-12 and 1-13).

An unusual and remarkable book was produced during this period: *Regimen Sanitatis Salernitum* [*Salernitan Rule of Health*], a work that first appeared in the 12th century and was later republished in approximately 140 different editions extending well into the 19th century.[41,42] This book summaries the Salernitan school directions for medical maintenance and care of patients. In Europe, a strong educational system was being developed, but the treatment of health care remained cloaked in the literature of classical Greeks and Islamic writing; for the most part, surgical

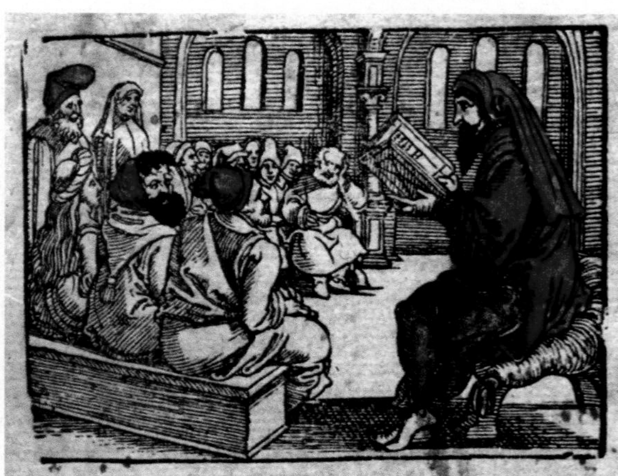

Figure 1-12. An illustration of Constantine the African lecturing at the School of Salerno. *(Courtesy James Tait Goodrich, MD, PhD.)*

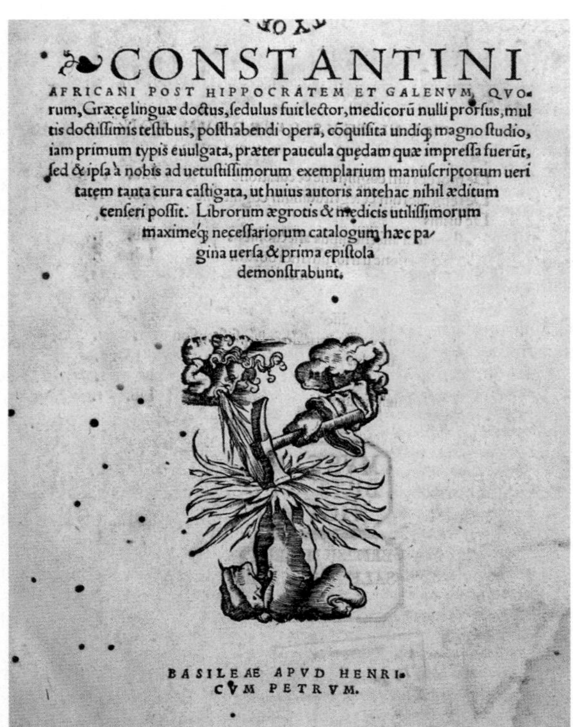

CONSTANTINI

AFRICANI POST HIPPOCRATEM ET GALENVM, QVOrum, Græcę linguæ doctus, sedulus fuit lector, medicorū nulli prorsus, multis doctissimis testibus, posthabendi opera, cōquisita undiq; magno studio, iam primum typis euulgata, præter paucula quędam quæ impressa fuerūt, sed & ipsa à nobis ad uetustissimorum exemplarium manuscriptorum ueritatem tanta cura castigata, ut huius autoris antehac nihil æditum censeri possit. Librorum ægrotis & medicis utilissimorum maximeq; necessariorum catalogum hæc pagina uersa & prima epistola demonstrabunt.

BASILEÆ APVD HENRICVM PETRVM.

Figure 1-13. Title page from a collection of works of Constantine the African, 1536. *(From Constantinus Africanus.* Constantini Africani Post Hippocratem et Galenum. *Basel: Henricus Petrus; 1536. Courtesy James Tait Goodrich, MD, PhD.)*

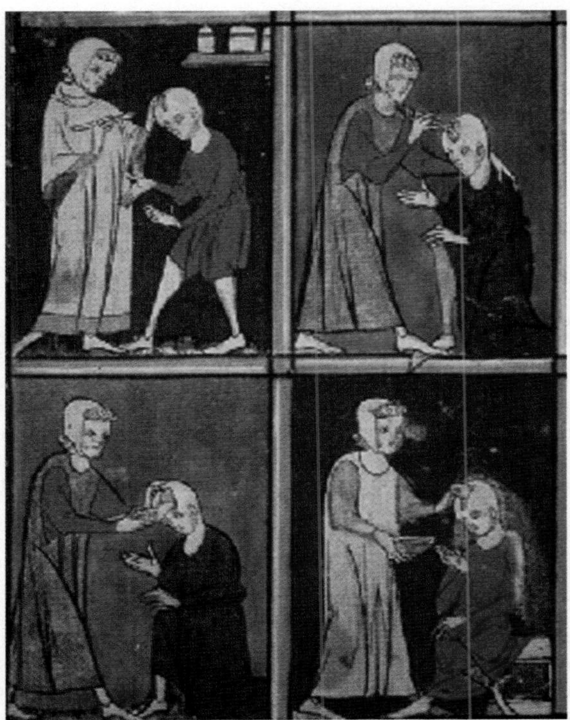

Figure 1-14. Illustrations of Roger of Salerno demonstrating brain and skull surgery. *(From the Sloane manuscript 1977. Courtesy British Library Board.)*

education and surgical practice continued to be an avocation limited to uneducated barber-surgeons and apprentices. Nonetheless, there were a few exceptionally talented surgeons who developed some original surgical works and practices.

Roger of Salerno (Ruggiero Frugardi) (fl. 1170) is considered the first learned medieval European writer on surgery (Figs. 1-14 and 1-15). Roger was educated in the Salerno tradition and followed many of its teachings. His book on surgical practice, *Practica Chirurgiae*,[43] offers several interesting surgical techniques of interest to neurosurgeons. An example was his technique for checking for a tear of the dura and leakage of cerebrospinal fluid in a patient with a skull fracture. To detect a leak, Roger would have the patient hold his or her breath and strain (i.e., the Valsalva maneuver) and then look for air bubbles around the fracture site, this being a clear sign of a leak. Roger was a pioneer in the techniques of managing peripheral nerve injury. For a severed nerve, he argued for reanastomosis of the nerve ends with close attention paid to their alignment. In dealing with the large bleeding veins of the neck, he urged direct ligation with a suture rather than cautery. For neurosurgeons, several chapters of his text are devoted to the treatment of skull fractures. Much of the described technique mirrors views of earlier classical writers, but the style is clearer and more succinct. This style is exemplified in this short description of management of various skull fractures[43,44]:

> When a fracture occurs it is accompanied by various wounds and contusions. If the contusion of the flesh is small but that of the bone great, the flesh should be divided by a cruciate incision down to the bone and everywhere elevated from the bone. Then a piece of light, old cloth is inserted for a day, and if there are fragments of the bone present, they are to be thoroughly removed. If the bone is unbroken on one side, it is left in place, and if necessary elevated with a flat sound (spatumile) and the bone is perforated by chipping with the spatumile so that clotted blood may be

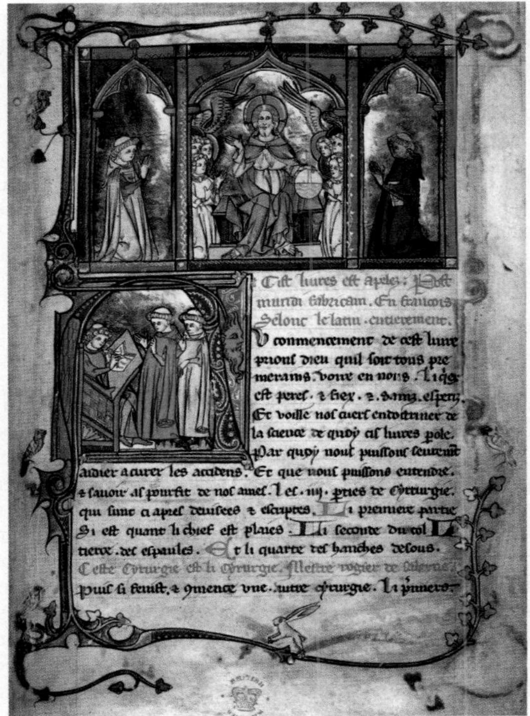

Figure 1-15. Medieval manuscript on the writings of Roger of Salerno. The lower left image is a gilt-scribed image of Roger lecturing. *(From the Sloane manuscript 1977. Courtesy British Library Board.)*

soaked up with a wad of wool and feathers. When it has consolidated, we apply lint and then, if it is necessary (but not until after the whole wound has become level with the skin), the patient may be bathed. After he leaves the bath, we apply a thin cooling plaster made of wormwood with rose water and egg.

A 12th-century manuscript owned by Harvey Cushing and attributed to Roger of Salerno contains an early description of a soporific for pain relief, for use in surgery. The soporific consisted of bark of mandragora (mandrake), hyoscyamus (henbane), and levisticum (lovage) seed, all of which were mixed together and ground and then applied wet to the forehead of the patient.[44] In view of the ingredients, it was unlikely that this soporific was able to achieve any real pain relief. In Roger's writings on surgical anatomy, many of the old errors persisted because of his recapitulating earlier anatomic treatises. Roger was particularly fond of citing the writings of Albucasis and Paulus Aegineta. He strongly favored therapeutic plasters and salves but was not a strong advocate of the popular treatment of application of grease to injuries of the dura. Interestingly, Roger advocated the use of trephination in the surgical treatment of epilepsy, although he did not indicate why this technique would work. Chapters (capita) 1 to 13 are of particular interest to neurosurgeons because they detail contemporary surgical treatment of scalp wounds and fractures of the skull. One of Roger's most significant errors in surgical practice was the concept that provoking pus suppuration in a wound encouraged healing. The concept of "laudable pus" in wound healing was introduced here and seriously hampered wound care until the time of Sir Joseph Lister and 19th-century antisepsis.

An unusually talented and inventive medieval surgeon from Bologna was **Theodoric of Cervia (Borgognoni)** (1205-1298). In comparison with Roger of Salerno, Theodoric was a pioneer in the use of aseptic technique: not the "clean" aseptic technique of today, but rather a method based on avoidance of "laudable pus." Theodoric believed that he had found the ideal conditions for good wound healing, which included control of bleeding, removal of contaminated or necrotic material, avoidance of dead space, and careful application of a wound dressing bathed in wine, the last providing a degree of antisepsis. He also argued for primary closure of all wounds when possible and avoiding "laudable pus"[45,46]:

For it is not necessary, as Roger and Roland have written, as many of their disciples teach, and as all modern surgeons profess, that pus should be generated in wounds. No error can be greater than this. Such a practice is indeed to hinder nature, to prolong the disease, and to prevent the conglutination and consolidation of the wound.

Theodoric's surgical work was first written in 1267, and it is one of the best reviews of contemporary medieval surgery.[45] He is also remembered as one of the earliest writers to include illustrations of his techniques in his book. Theodoric surgical technique called for meticulous (almost Halstedian) techniques, with gentle handling of surgical tissues being key. Theodoric believed that aspiring surgeons should train only under competent masters. In the field of head injury, Theodoric argued that parts of the brain could be removed through a wound with little effect on the patient. In the treatment of skull fractures, he strongly argued for elevating depressed fractures. Theodoric advocated avoiding any punctures of the dura because these could lead to abscess and convulsions, thereby resulting in adverse outcomes. For pain relief during surgery, he developed his own "soporific sponge," containing opium, mandragora, hemlock, and other less important ingredients, which he applied to the patient's nostrils; once the patient fell asleep, Theodoric began surgery. Opium was probably the key ingredient in this recipe.

William of Saliceto (Guglielo da Saliceto) (1210-1277) was a uniquely skilled Italian surgeon and a professor at the University of Bologna. William's book on surgery, *Chirurgia* (or *Cyrurgia*), completed in 1275, contained some highly original concepts that were not totally based on previous classical writings but in which the influence of Galen and Avicenna is clear.[47] This book was written by William for his son Bernardino. The text is mostly original and based on his own observations. Rarely did William quote other writers. Book IV contains the earliest known treatise on surgical and regional anatomy. His most significant contribution during this era was his decision to discard the surgical technique of burning with cautery and use instead the surgical knife[47]:

De anathomia in communi et de formis membrorum et figures que sunt considerande in incision et cauterizatione.

[The anatomy of the members and the figures concerning the forms of which are to be considered in general and in the incision and cauterization.]

William's writings contain some interesting and unique techniques for a primary peripheral nerve suture repair. In this pre-Harveian era, he was able to distinguish arterial bleeding from venous bleeding by the "spurting" of blood. William's views on the brain were also unique by contemporary standards, inasmuch as he put forth some interesting neurological concepts that the cerebrum governs voluntary motion and the cerebellum involuntary function.

Leonardo of Bertapaglia (ca. 1380-1460) was a prominent 15th-century Italian surgeon and writer. Leonardo established an extensive and lucrative practice in the area of Padua and in neighboring Venice. At a time when anatomic dissection was rarely practiced in Europe, Leonardo became one of the earliest proponents of the study of anatomy. In 1429 he offered a course of surgery that included the dissection of an executed criminal. Leonardo devoted one third of his book to surgery of the nervous system and head injuries.[48,49] He considered the brain the most precious of organs, regarding it as the source of voluntary and involuntary functions. In his treatment of skull fractures, he always avoided materials that might generate pus. Leonardo argued for never placing a compressive dressing that might drive bone into the brain; if a piece of bone pierced the brain, the surgeon was to remove it.

Leonardo put together a set of rules to guide the practice of a 15th-century surgeon that are still applicable five centuries later[49]:

To…be the perfect surgeon, you must always bear in mind these eight notations, and remembering them you will be preferred to others.

The first task…to become a good surgeon should be to use his eyes….

Second, you must accompany and observe the qualified physician, seeing him work before you yourself practice….

Third, you must command the most gentle touch in operating and treating lest you cause pain to the patient….

Fourth, you must insure that your instruments be sharp and unrusted whenever you cut anywhere….

Fifth, you must be courageous in operating and cutting but timid to cut in the vicinity of nerves, sinews and arteries, and, so as not to commit error, you should study anatomy, which is the mother of this art…perform your surgery cleverly and never operate on human flesh as if you were working on wood or leather….

Sixth, you must be kind and sympathetic to the poor, for piety and humility greatly augment your reputation and the sick will more freely commit themselves to your care.

Seventh, you must never refuse anything brought you as a fee, for the sick will respect you more.

Eighth, you must never argue about fees with the sick, or indeed demand anything unless it be previously agreed upon, for avarice is the most ignoble of vices and should you be so inflicted, you will never achieve the reputation of a good doctor.

Lanfranchi (Lanfranc) of Milan (c. 1250-1306) was a pupil of William of Saliceto and was often referred to as the father of French surgery. Lanfranchi also advocated his teacher's use of the knife in place of the burning cautery. Although born and educated in Italy, he had to leave Italy for France to avoid political strife. His *Cyrugia Parva* details a number of interesting surgical techniques. Lanfranchi perfected the use of the suture for primary wound repairs.[50] He was among the first to associate the direct effect of head injury on brain function. Hippocrates had been the first to articulate the concept of *commotio cerebri*, but Lanfranchi provided the first modern characterization of what is now known as a cerebral concussion. For surgeons, he developed a series of guidelines for trephination in skull fractures and "release of irritation" of dura. Because of the dangers of skull surgery, Lanfranchi argued for employing the trephine only when absolutely necessary; for other cases, he invoked the skills of the "Holy Ghost" to provide the cure. Among his innovative surgical techniques was the development of esophageal intubation during surgery, a technique not commonly practiced until the 19th century. As an educated surgeon and a "surgeon of the long robe" (i.e., academic), he attempted to elevate the art and science of surgery above the mediocre level of the menial barber-surgeon ("surgeons of the short robe"). Lanfranchi also argued against the separation of surgery and medicine, advocated since the time of Avicenna, believing that a good surgeon should also be a good physician (Fig. 1-16).

Another important person in the history of French medicine and surgery was **Henri de Mondeville** (c. 1260-1317). Educated in Paris and Montpellier, Henri later went on to become a professor at Montpellier. Henri was strongly motivated to elevate the profession of surgeon, and he clearly detested the barber-surgeons, stating, "Most of them were illiterates, debauchees, cheats, forgers, alchemists, courtesans, procuresses, etc."[51]

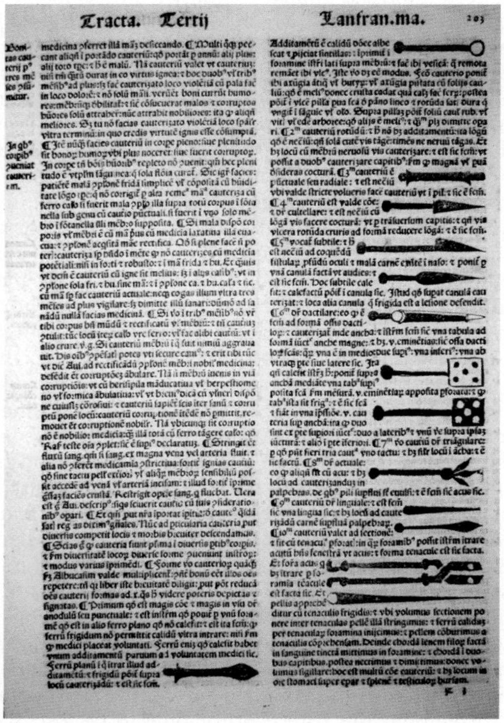

Figure 1-16. Surgical instruments designed by Lanfranchi of Milan. This illustration appeared in this early 1519 book. *(From Lanfranchi of Milan. Chirurgia. In:* Cyrurgia Guidonis de Cauliaco et Cyrurgia Bruni, Teodorici, Rolandi, Lanfranci, Rogerii, Bertapalie. *Venice: Bernardinus Venetus de Vitalibus; 1519. Courtesy James Tait Goodrich, MD, PhD.)*

In 1306 Henri undertook the task of developing a new treatise on surgery for the education of his students at Montpellier. Unfortunately, because of tuberculosis and general ill health, he never completed the manuscript; the edited portions were not published until 1892, when Professor Julius Pagel of Berlin completed the task.[52] Henri adopted and followed a number of the views of Lanfranchi. He was a believer in clean wounds and avoiding "laudable pus." Unfortunately, Henri would be the last surgeon in this era to argue for avoiding "laudable pus." Subsequent surgeons returned to the older belief that the development of pus in a wound was a good sign of healing. Henri offered some originality in wound management by advocating for healing by primary intention: *modus novus noster*. In surgical treatment of wounds, he encouraged the removal of foreign bodies and the use of wine dressings in wound care, the wine acting as an antiseptic and providing better healing. Henri's designs of a number of surgical instruments were clever. He is remembered for the design of a needle holder and also a forceps-type instrument for extraction of arrowheads. Henri was a bit more conservative than his predecessors in dealing with head injuries. He argued against elevating skull fractures if there was no injury to the overlying soft tissues, believing that nature would do a better job of healing the fracture by natural union. It was his opinion that unnecessary exploration and probing of the wound would only cause more injury than natural healing: in retrospect, such an insight into wound care was brilliant.[51]

No history of surgery can be complete without a discussion of the contributions of **Guy de Chauliac** (1300-1368).[53] He was clearly the most influential European surgeon of the 14th and 15th centuries. He was so highly respected that he became physician to three popes at Avignon (Clement VI, Innocent VI, and Urban V) and leading surgeon and educator at the school of Montpellier. Guy was educated in Toulouse, Paris, Montpellier, and Bologna. He was an early proponent of anatomic dissection of a human cadaver. He stated, "In these two ways we must teach anatomy on the bodies of men, apes, swine, and divers other animals, and not from pictures, as did Henri de Mondeville who had thirteen pictures for demonstration of anatomy."[51] His writings were popular and continued to exert an influence on surgery until well into the 17th century. His principal didactic surgical text, scribed in 1363, was titled the *Collectorium Cyrurgie*.[53,54] There are 34 known manuscripts of this work; the first printed edition appeared in 1478, and more than seventy editions have been published since (Fig. 1-17).

In promoting surgeons as individuals more skilled than "mechanics" (i.e., barber-surgeons), he stated four conditions that must be satisfied for a practitioner to be a good surgeon: (1) the surgeon should be learned; (2) he should be expert; (3) he must be ingenious; and (4) he should be able to adapt himself (from the introduction of *Ars Chirurgica*). Guy devised interesting techniques for the treatment of head injuries. For example, before the beginning of surgery, he recommended shaving the patient's head so as to prevent hair from getting into the wound and interfering with primary healing. For depressed skull fractures, Guy preferred to put wine-soaked cloths into the injured site to assist healing. He categorized head injuries into seven types and discussed the management of each in detail. He believed that scalp wounds required only cleaning and débridement but that a compound depressed skull fracture must be treated by means of trephination and elevation. Skin closure was done by primary repair, for which he claimed good results. To help control excessive bleeding and provide hemostasis, he used egg albumin. For reasons that are not at all clear, Guy set back good surgical healing by readopting the views of "laudable pus" as being good for wound healing. "Laudable pus" remained part of surgical

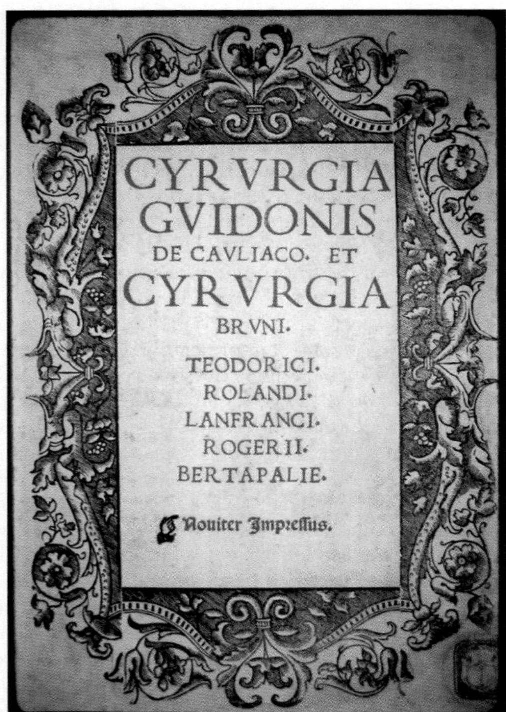

Figure 1-17. Title page from a collected works dealing with the surgical writings of a number of medieval surgeons, including Guy de Chauliac. *(From Guy de Chauliac. Chirurgia magna. In:* Cyrurgia Guidonis de Cauliaco et Cyrurgia Bruni, Teodorici, Rolandi, Lanfranci, Rogerii, Bertapali. *Venice, Bernardinus Venetus de Vitalibus, 1519. See also Leonardo RA:* History of Surgery. *New York: Froben Press; 1943:116. Courtesy James Tait Goodrich, MD, PhD.)*

practice and was not to be corrected until the works of Sir Joseph Lister nearly 500 years later.

As England was moving away from the period of barbarian invasions and into the Middle Ages, university education in England began to become comparable with the European model. The leading surgeon of this period in England was **John Arderne (Arden)** (1307-1380), who trained as a military surgeon and had much war experience. In 1370 he came to London and joined the Guild of Military Surgeons. He characterized himself as *chirurgus inter medicos* (a surgeon among physicians). His manuscript on surgery was written circa 1412. This manuscript, *De Arte Phisicali et de Cirurgia*, translated into English by D'Arcy Power in 1922, was a valuable addition to the English literature on early surgery.[55] John Arderne was evidently a very skilled surgeon with a number of practical insights into what could or could not be done surgically. He believed firmly in clean hands and well-shaped nails for surgery, although some writers have thought that this was more for social reasons than surgery.[56] In addition, he would bathe his open wounds with an irrigation that contained turpentine, a useful surgical antiseptic for keeping wounds clean. Of most importance, John Arderne was a firm believer in education and learning. In addition, he wrote that the surgeon must "always be sober during any surgery as drunkenness destroys all virtue and brings it to naught."[56-58]

The late Byzantine/Islamic and medieval periods were an era of great misguided intellectual activity and of unoriginality of thought. Clearly the educators had more faith in the teachings of antiquity. From the fall of the Roman Empire to the beginning of the 16th century, anatomy and the practice of surgery, with only rare exceptions, remained stagnant, guided by a staunch Galenic and Hippocratic orthodoxy. The translation of medical manuscripts from Latin, Greek, and Hebrew into Arabic and back into Latin resulted in many errors of translation and interpretation. The combination of a lack of anatomic knowledge and poor surgical outcomes naturally led physicians to recommend against operating on the brain, except in simple cases. A review of the work done by the surgical physicians just described reveals that despite a period of intellectual paralysis, a number of prominent physicians did make some advances. It is clear that monastic recluses in often-inaccessible mountain retreats carefully guarded medical knowledge, but despite this state of affairs, some surgeons clearly succeeded in mastering their art in the midst of intellectual darkness[58]:

> The history of medicine consists of a successive series of intellectual movements proceeding from different centers and each engulfing its predecessor.

ORIGINS OF NEUROSURGICAL PRACTICE IN THE RENAISSANCE

With the Renaissance came interesting innovations in surgical concepts and techniques. Beginning in the mid-15th century, physicians and surgeons introduced basic investigative techniques to learn human anatomy and physiology. Of enormous significance was the introduction of routine anatomic dissection in medical schools. Moving away from subservience to the medievalists, great physicians such as Leonardo da Vinci, Jacopo Berengario da Carpi, Nicholas Massa, and Andreas Vesalius explored the human body without being encumbered by the erroneous writings of earlier authors. Codified anatomic errors, many ensconced since the Greco-Roman era, were being corrected. A better understanding of human anatomy led to a change of epistemiologic presuppositions, which led to a great surge of interest in surgery. Putting the teachings of antiquity aside, surgeons began, with great vigor and enthusiasm, to investigate medical mysteries. As a result of this shift from the somber and somnolent medieval period to the enlightened, radically inventive Renaissance, the early foundations of modern neurosurgery were laid.

Any discussion of Renaissance surgery and anatomy has to begin with **Leonardo da Vinci** (1452-1519), the quintessential Renaissance man. Multitalented, recognized as an artist, an anatomist, and a scientist, da Vinci used the dissection table to better understand surface anatomy and its relationship to art and sculpture. From his studies, da Vinci is now recognized as the founder of iconographic and physiologic anatomy.[59-62] He provided the earliest, albeit crude, diagrams of the cranial nerves, the optic chiasm, and the brachial and lumbar plexi. He developed a wax casting technique that allowed him to work out and understand the anatomy of the ventricular system. To do this, he took a fresh brain and poured a liquid wax into the ventricles and placed a hollow tube to allow egress of the air. His experimental studies included sectioning a digital nerve in a living person and noting that the affected finger no longer had sensation, even when placed in a fire. Da Vinci was not a surgeon, but he gave an important impetus to the study of anatomy and the defining of correct anatomic relationships—vital concepts for any surgeon. Unfortunately, he died before he could finish his great opus on anatomy, which was to be published in approximately 120 volumes.[59] His anatomic manuscripts did circulate among the artist community in Italy throughout the 16th century, only to be lost; then they were rediscovered in the 18th century by William Hunter (1718-1783). These anatomic works had a profound influence on artists and physicians and subsequently on the development of modern anatomic studies. Da Vinci, as a founder of modern anatomy, provided a creative spark to reexplore the human body by hands-on dissection (Figs. 1-18 to 1-20).

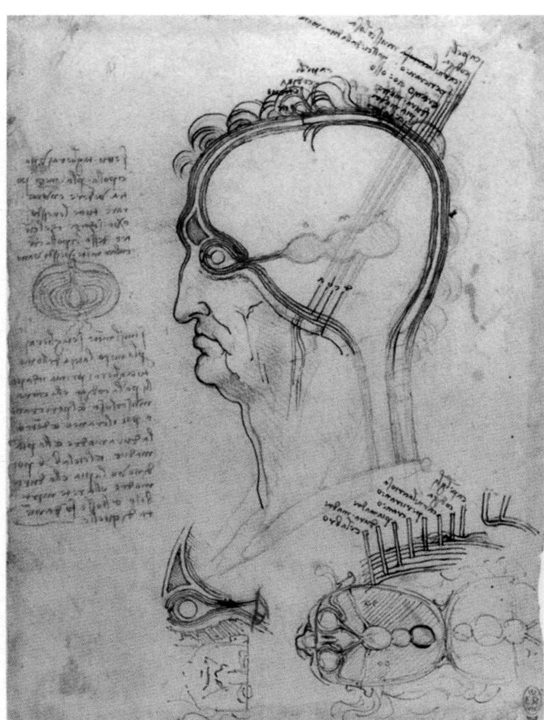

Figure 1-18. Leonardo da Vinci's drawing of the ventricular system and also the "cell doctrine" theory, a belief that the functions of the brain arose from the ventricular system and not the brain itself. *(Courtesy Royal Collection Trust; copyright Her Majesty Queen Elizabeth II, 2015.)*

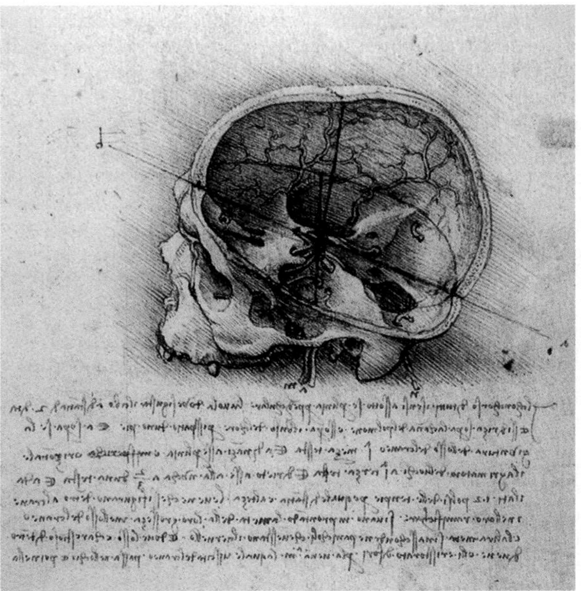

Figure 1-19. Leonardo da Vinci's three-dimensional drawing of skull anatomy. *(Courtesy of the Royal Collection Trust; copyright Her Majesty Queen Elizabeth II, 2015.)*

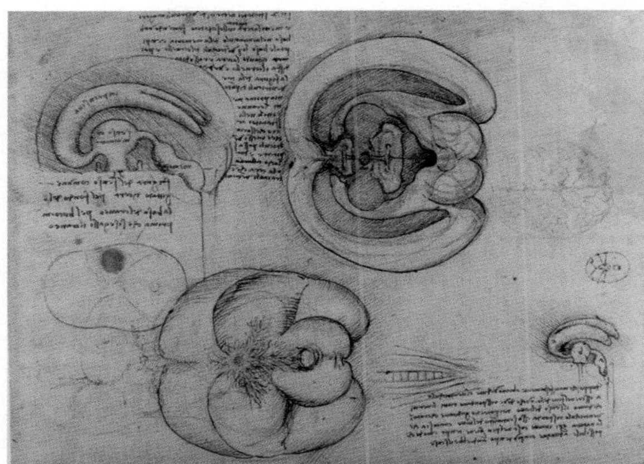

Figure 1-20. Leonardo da Vinci's wax casting modeling of the ventricular system. *(Courtesy of the Royal Collection Trust; copyright Her Majesty Queen Elizabeth II, 2015.)*

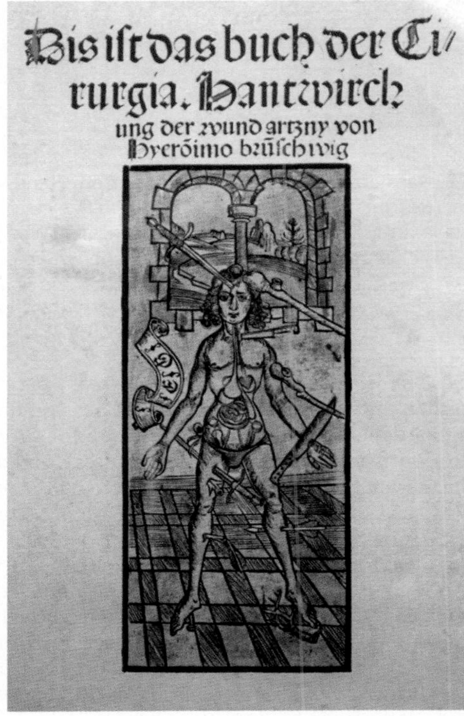

Dis ist das buch der Ci/
rurgia. Hantwirch
ung der wund artzny von
Hyerõimo brũschwig

Figure 1-21. Title page from the first edition of an important work in surgery showing a "wound man" figure with the various injuries a surgeon could expect to treat. *(From Brunschwig H.* Dis Ist das Buch der Cirurgia. *Strasbourg, France: J Grüninger; 1497. Courtesy James Tait Goodrich, MD, PhD.)*

The earliest printed surgical work to contain illustrations was *Dis Ist das Buch der Cirurgia*, authored by **Hieronymus Brunschwig** (ca. 1450-1512) and published in Strasbourg in 1497.[63] Although the images have nothing to do with specific surgical procedures, the book is the first to discuss the management of gunshot wounds; gunpowder had only just recently been introduced in weapons of war. This work was considered to be valuable enough to be plagiarized and published in a pirated edition the same year and appeared in many other editions throughout the 16th century. In the 1513 edition, the first illustration of a patient with a head injury undergoing treatment was added to the work (Fig. 1-21).

One of the early Renaissance surgeons who incorporated some of the recently revealed anatomic concepts was **Hans von Gersdorff** (1455-1529). In his surgical book *Feldtbüch der Wundartzney*, published in 1517, are some of the earliest illustrations on surgical technique.[64] Gersdorff was a military surgeon and,

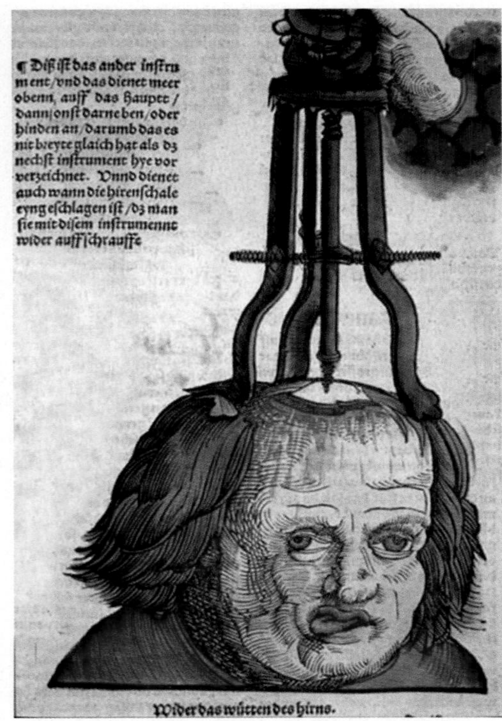

Figure 1-22. Rare colored trephination plate from Hans von Gersdorff's 1517 manual on surgery. The victim has clear evidence of a third nerve palsy caused by a depressed skull fracture. *(From Gersdorff HF.* Feldtbüch der Wundartzney. *Strasbourg, France: J Schott; 1517. See also Flamm ES: The dilated pupil and head trauma.* Med Hist. *1972;16:194-199. Courtesy Reynolds-Finley Historical Library, the University of Alabama at Birmingham.)*

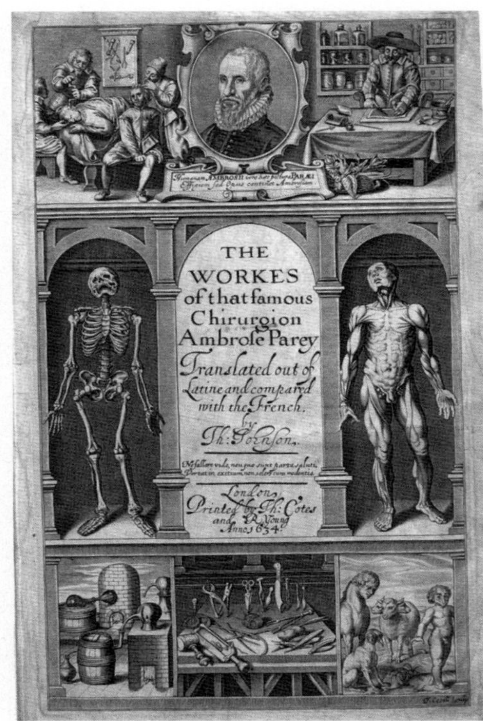

Figure 1-23. Title page of the English publication of Ambroise Paré's collected works on surgery. *(From Johnson T, Trans.* The Workes of That Famous Chirurgion Ambroise Parey. *London: Richard Coates; 1649. Courtesy James Tait Goodrich, MD, PhD.)*

with more than 40 years of war experience, became quite adept at handling battlefield injuries. This handbook for surgeons was divided into four parts: anatomy, surgery, leprosy, and a glossary of anatomic terms, diseases, and medications. The section on anatomy was based on his own extensive experience, and he used the earlier writings of the Islamic physicians and the works of Guy de Chauliac. The surgical portion deals with military surgery, mostly on how to extract foreign objects, tourniquet techniques to control bleeding, and amputation techniques. Several woodcuts dealing with surgical technique and surgical instrumentation are of interest to modern neurosurgeons; one woodcut clearly illustrated a third nerve palsy on the side of the depressed skull fracture and a facial paralysis on the opposite side. Included in this work is also the first plate showing a dissection of the human brain. This surgical work became very popular and was published in several editions; this was because of both its practical presentation of surgery and the illustrations in the text (Fig. 1-22).

One of the greatest physicians in the history of surgery remains **Ambroise Paré** (1510-1590), a poorly educated, humble Huguenot, an individual whom many historians have considered the father of modern surgery. After extensive military surgical experience, Paré was able to organize and publish a great deal of practical knowledge, along with innovative instrument designs. At this time, most physicians and surgeons published their writings in Latin; Paré preferred to publish in French instead.[65-68] Paré's books therefore were more widely disseminated and appreciated. As his reputation grew, Paré became a valued surgeon to the European royal courts. One of Paré's most famous cases was a head injury sustained by Henri II of France. Paré (and also Andreas Vesalius) attended the king and was also present at the autopsy. Henri II had suffered penetrating right orbital injury and a subdural hematoma after a joust during the celebration of the marriage of his daughter, Elizabeth of France, to Philip, King of Spain. When Paré described the clinical findings in Henri II, he noted that the patient complained of a headache and blurred vision. Henri II went on to develop vomiting, lethargy, and ominous signs of decreased respiration, and he died 11 days after the injury. Paré postulated that the injury was caused by a tear in one of the bridging cortical veins, and he was clearly describing signs of increased intracranial pressure. Paré's remarkable clinical observations and clinical history were confirmed at autopsy. Thus, despite humble beginnings, Paré became one of the most celebrated physicians in this formative period of surgery (Figs. 1-23 and 1-24).

Paré commented on the "surgeon's duties":

> Five things are proper to the duty of a Chirurgeon: To take away that which is superfluous; to restore to those places such things as are displaced; to separate those things which are joyned together; to joyn those which are separated and to supply the defects of nature. Thou shalt far more easily and happily attain to the knowledge of these things by long use and much exercise, than by much reading of Books, or daily hearing of Teachers. For speech, how perspicuous and elegant soever it be, cannot so vively express anything, as that which is subjected to the faithfull eyes and hands.

Among Paré's surgical works, his writings on the brain remain the most remarkable.[67,68] Book X is devoted to the diagnosis and management of skull fractures. Although it was not an original idea, Paré popularized the interesting technique of elevating a depressed skull fracture through the use of the Valsalva maneuver[66]:

> …for a breath driven forth of the chest and prohibited passage forth, swells and lifts the substance of the brain and meninges where upon the frothing humidity and sanies sweat forth.

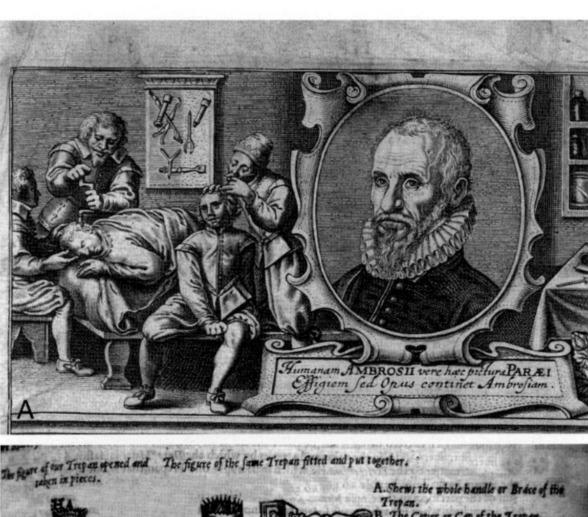
Humanam AMBROSII vere hæc pictura PARÆI
Effigiem ſed Opus continet Ambroſiam.
A

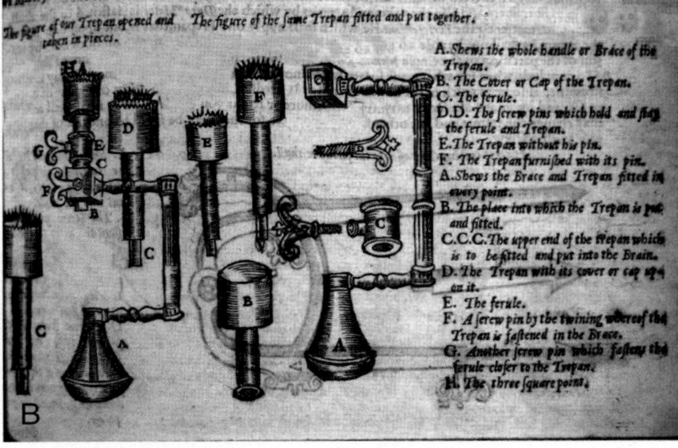

Figure 1-24. Trephination plate **(A)** and neurosurgical tools **(B)** from Ambroise Paré's surgical works. *(From Johnson T, Trans.* The Workes of That Famous Chirurgion Ambroise Parey. *London: Richard Coates; 1649. Courtesy James Tait Goodrich, MD, PhD.)*

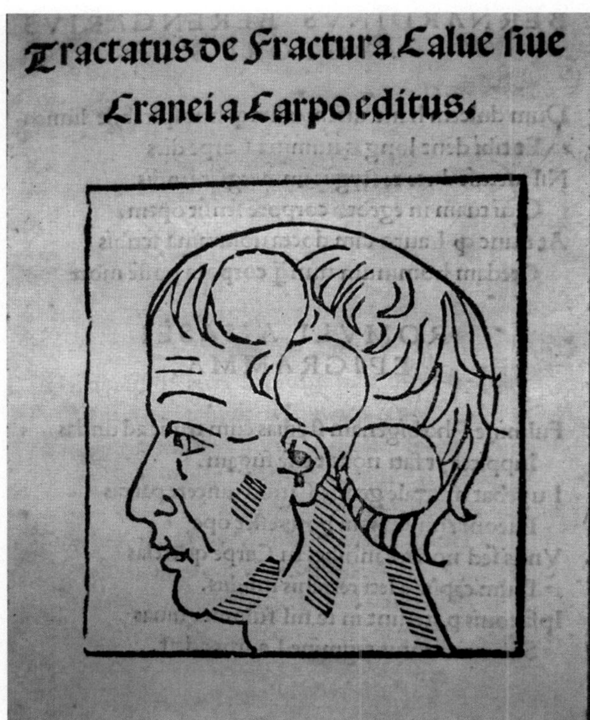
Tractatus de Fractura Calue siue Cranei a Carpo editus.

Figure 1-25. Title page from Jacopo Berengario da Carpi's treatise on head injury. *(From Berengario da Carpi J.* Tractatus de Fractura Calvae Sive Cranei. *Bologna, Italy: Hieronymus de Benedictus; 1518. Courtesy James Tait Goodrich, MD, PhD.)*

Through this method, both blood and pus can be expelled from the fracture site.

Paré's surgical techniques demonstrated some unusual and unique advances over those of previous writers. Paré provides extensive discussion on the use of trephines, shavers, and scrapers. He was skilled at removal of osteomyelitic bone, incising the dura and evacuating blood clots and pus, procedures that surgeons had previously performed only with a great deal of trepidation. He advocated débridement of wounds for good healing, emphasizing that foreign bodies must be removed from injury sites. Paré's most significant change in contemporary surgical practice was the serendipitous discovery that boiling oil should not be used in gunshot wounds, contrary to common surgical practice; instead, a dressing of egg yolk, rose oil, and turpentine provided for much improved wound healing and in turn led to a dramatic reduction in morbidity and mortality. Paré also discarded the older Islamic technique of hot cautery for control of bleeding, substituting instead the use of ligatures, which enhanced healing and reduced blood loss.[67] The improvement in his results was a source of wonder to Paré and gave rise to his famous aphorism[67]:

> Je le pansay, Dieu le guarit.
> [I took care of him, but God cured him.]

Among the Renaissance "giants" of anatomy and surgery was the great Italian surgeon and anatomist **Jacopo Berengario da Carpi** (1470-1550). In 1518, Berengario wrote the second monograph devoted solely to treating injuries of the head[69] (the first being that of Hippocrates). This book was motivated by Berengario's successful treatment of a serious head injury in Lorenzo dé Medici, Duke of Urbino. Shortly after he had treated the duke, Berengario dreamed that he was visited by a man wearing a cap adorned with a rooster feather and golden-winged sandals (i.e., Hermes Trismegistus, or the Third Mercury), who encouraged Berengario to write a treatise on skull fractures and head injuries. The result was a marvelous *tractatus*, the first printed work devoted solely to injuries of the head. In the text, original surgical techniques are discussed, along with the earliest illustrations of cranial instruments designed for surgical treatment of head injury. As an anatomist, Berengario, like Leonardo da Vinci, provided one of the earliest and most complete discussions of the ventricular system. Berengario presented some of the earliest descriptions of the pineal gland, choroid plexus, and lateral ventricles.[70] His anatomic illustrations are among the first published from actual anatomic dissections. He was a firm believer in anatomic dissection because that was the only way to learn the anatomy; he believed that the written word alone was useless, and he observed that the earlier writings were full of anatomic errors. His anatomic writings were among the first to challenge the medieval dogmatic writings of Galen and others (Figs. 1-25 to 1-27).

A less known writer and anatomist of the Renaissance was a Marburg professor by the name of **Johannes Dryander (Johann Eichmann)** (1500-1560). In 1536, Dryander published an illustrated work (expanded in 1537) on the brain and skull.[71,72] Within this most remarkable work are 16 plates of the brain, showing successive layered dissections of the scalp, dural coverings, and the brain itself. The drawings of the anatomy of the cerebellum and the posterior fossa are particularly striking. There are inaccuracies in the text because of the prevailing influence of Galen and medieval scholasticism; nonetheless, this book can be considered the first textbook of neuroanatomy. Despite Dryander's allegiance to Galen's teaching, he advocated public anatomic

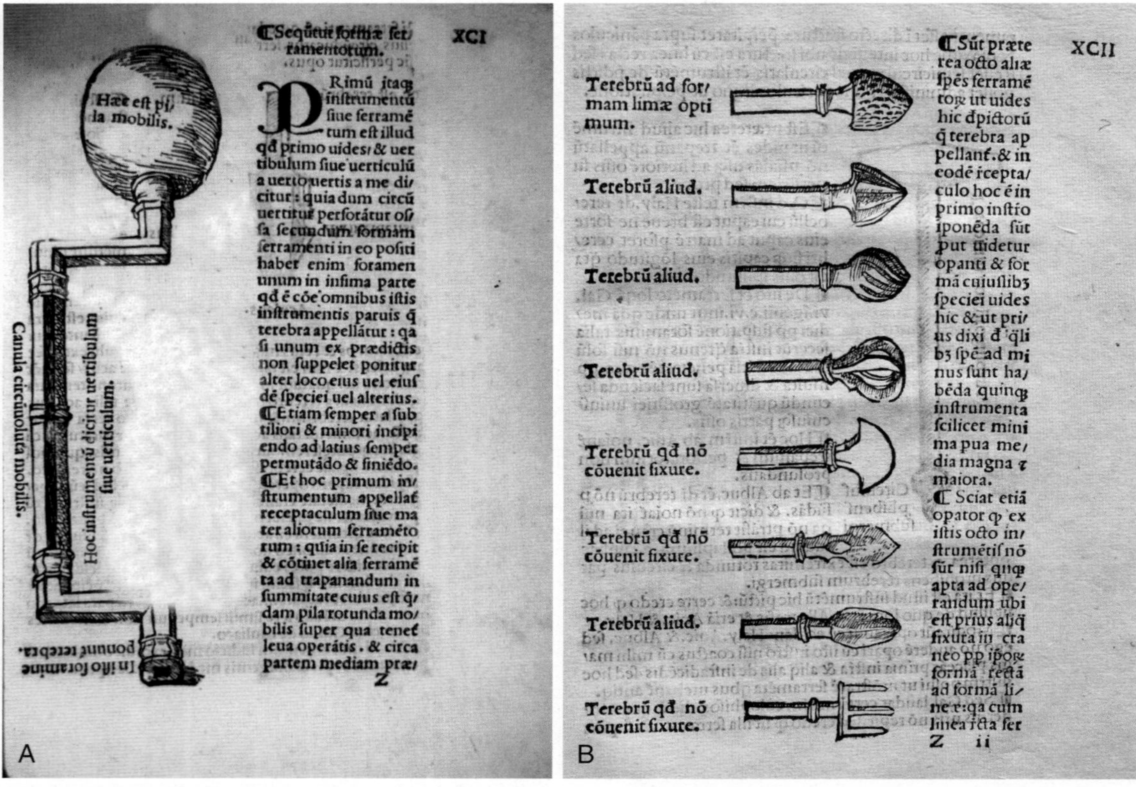
A

Hæc est pi-la mobilis.

Canula circiuoluta mobilis.

Hoc instrumentũ dicitur uertibulum siue uerticulum.

In fine foramine pounct terebra.

¶ Sequitur formæ ferramentorum.

XCI

PRimũ itaq; instrumentũ siue ferramẽtum est illud qđ primo uides, & uertibulum siue uerticulũ a uerto uertis a me dicitur: quia dum circũuertitur perforatur ossa secundum formam ferramenti in eo positi habet enim foramen unum in infima parte qđ ẽ cõe omnibus istis instrumentis paruis q̄ terebra appellãtur: qa si unum ex prædictis non suppelet ponitur alter loco eius uel eius dẽ speciei uel alterius. ¶ Etiam semper a subtiliori & minori incipiendo ad latius semper permutãdo & finiẽdo. ¶ Et hoc primum instrumentum appellat receptaculum siue mater aliorum ferramẽtorum: quia in se recipit & cõtinet alia ferramẽta ad trapanandum in summitate cuius est q̄dam pila rotunda mobilis super qua tenet leua operãtis. & circa partem mediam præ

Z

B

XCII

Terebrũ ad formam limæ optimum.

Terebrũ aliud.

Terebrũ aliud.

Terebrũ aliud.

Terebrũ qđ nõ cõuenit fixure.

Terebrũ qđ nõ cõuenit fixure.

Terebrũ aliud.

Terebrũ qđ nõ cõuenit fixure.

¶ Sũt præterea octo aliæ spẽs ferramẽtoꝝ ut uides hic đpictorũ q̄ terebra appellant. & in eodẽ rcepta culo hoc ẽ in primo instro iponẽda sũt put uidetur opanti & formã cuiuslib; speciei uides hic & ut prius dixi đ q̄libz spẽ ad minus sunt habẽda quinq; instrumenta scilicet minima pua media magna ⁊ maiora. ¶ Sciat etiã opator q ex istis octo instrumẽtis nõ sũt nisi quaq; apta ad operandum ubi est prius aliq̄ fixura in craneo pp ipoꝝ formã rectã ad formã lineę: qa cum linea rcta ser

Z ii

Figure 1-26. **A,** Neurosurgical trephine (hand brace) designed by Jacopo Berengario da Carpi, very similar to what we call a Hudson brace today. **B,** Berengario designed a series of very imaginative trephine bits for making bur holes and craniectomies. To prevent plunging, the bits are designed with a conical shape. *(From Berengario da Carpi J.* Tractatus de Fractura Calvae Sive Cranei. *Bologna, Italy: Hieronymus de Benedictus; 1518. Courtesy James Tait Goodrich, MD, PhD.)*

dissections, the results of which included these remarkable neuroanatomic drawings (Figs. 1-28 and 1-29).

Military surgery has always been a great educator of surgeons, and one of those particularly influenced by his military service was **Volcher Coiter** (1534-1576). Coiter was an army surgeon and city physician in Nuremberg who had the good fortune to study under several contemporary experts, including Gabriele Fallopius, Bartolomeo Eustachius, and Ulisse Aldrovandi. As a result of their teachings and education, Coiter was able to undertake unique and original anatomic and physiologic investigations.[73] Among his anatomic descriptions are the first anatomically correct details of the anterior and posterior spinal roots. He was the first to distinguish gray from white matter in the spinal cord. Coiter had a particularly strong interest in the spine, which led him to conduct a number of anatomic and pathologic studies of the spinal cord, including an early model of decerebrate posturing. Coiter also provided a number of details on how to trephine skulls of birds, lambs, goats, and dogs.[73] He was the first to associate the pulsation of the brain with the arterial pulse. As an early neurosurgeon and investigator, he reported on opening the brain and removing parts of it with no ill effects noted: an early, surprising precursor attempt at cerebral localization.

One of the most skilled of Renaissance surgeons was a Venetian, **Giovanni Andrea della Croce** (c. 1509-1580). Della Croce was a follower of Paré and adopted many of his techniques and beliefs. A combination of surgical skill and a Renaissance flair for design led della Croce to produce a remarkable book on surgery in 1573.[74] Within this monograph are some of the most beautifully engraved scenes of neurosurgical operations. As was typical for the period, surgical operations were performed in family homes, typically in the bedroom (with the occasional dog lying at the foot of the bed). Della Croce verbally, and in drawings, described the techniques for performing trephinations. Several illustrations show the various types of arrows, spears, and bullets used in warfare, and the techniques for their removal are detailed. An additional series of plates shows his instrument designs for performing neurosurgical procedures. One illustration is of a bloody trephination being performed with minimal anesthesia—a concept considered horrific by modern readers—in a beautifully appointed nobleman's bedroom (Figs. 1-30 and 1-31).

Della Croce illustrated a number of trephination instruments in this monograph, some of which were an improvement on their predecessors. Della Croce's trephination drill was rotated by means of an attached bow, in the manner of a carpenter's drill. Various trephine bits are proposed and illustrated, many surprisingly modern, with conical designs to avoid plunging. The illustrations of surgical instruments include Penfield-style elevators for lifting depressed skull bone.

An expert in surgery and anatomy whose work typifies the great strides of learning in the Renaissance was **Andreas Vesalius** (1514-1564). Vesalius was educated at Louvain, Montpellier, and Paris, all staunch schools of Galenic orthodox teaching. Rejecting the views of his Galen-enthralled professors, Vesalius provided an innovative and dramatic approach to anatomic dissection (Figs. 1-32 and 1-33). Following up on the theme of the earlier 16th century anatomists such as Leonardo da Vinci and Jacopo Berengario da Carpi, Vesalius argued that anatomic dissections had to be performed by the teacher, not by an ignorant prosector being guided by a professor who sat at the lectern reading from a Galenic monograph on anatomy.

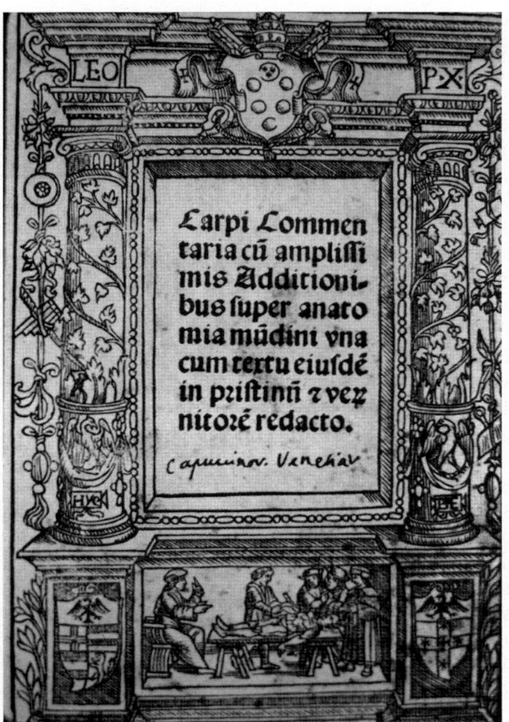

LEO P·X

Carpi Commen
taria cũ amplissi
mis Additioni-
bus super anato
mia mũdini vna
cum textu eiusdé
in pristinũ ꝛ ve-
nitoꝛé redacto.

Figure 1-27. Title page with an allegorical anatomic dissection scene from Jacopo Berengario da Carpi's 1522 work on anatomy. *(From Berengario da Carpi J.* Isagoge Breves: Perlucide ac Ubertine in Anatomia Humani Corporis: A Co[m]muni Medicorum Academia Usitatam.... *Bononiae, Italy: B. Hectoris; 1522. Courtesy James Tait Goodrich, MD, PhD.)*

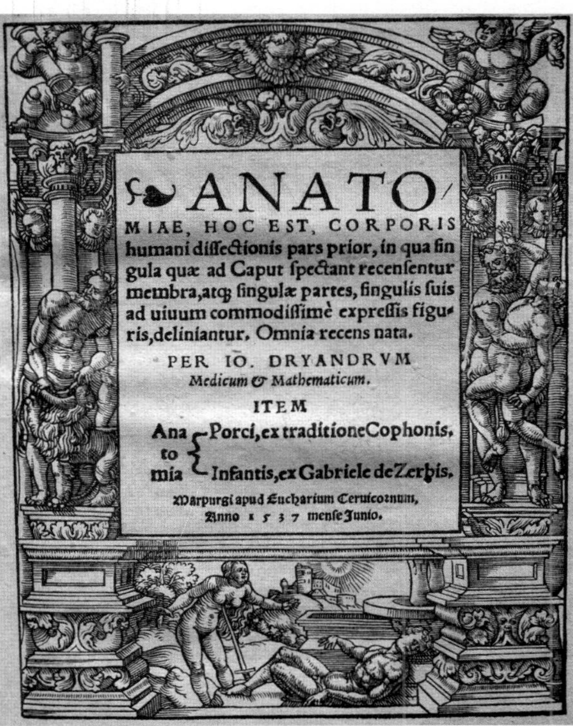

ANATO-
MIAE, HOC EST, CORPORIS
humani dissectionis pars prior, in qua sin
gula quæ ad Caput spectant recensentur
membra, atq; singulæ partes, singulis suis
ad uiuum commodissimè expressis figu-
ris, deliniantur. Omnia recens nata.

PER IO. DRYANDRVM
Medicum & Mathematicum.

ITEM

Ana- Porci, ex traditione Cophonis.
to-
mia Infantis, ex Gabriele de Zerbis.

Marpurgi apud Eucharium Ceruicoꝛnum,
Anno 1 5 3 7 mense Iunio.

Figure 1-28. Title page from Johannes Dryander's work on the anatomy of the human brain. This work included the earliest realistic illustrations of brain anatomy. *(From Dryander J.* Anatomiae. *Marburg, Germany: Eucharius Cervicornus; 1537. Courtesy James Tait Goodrich, MD, PhD.)*

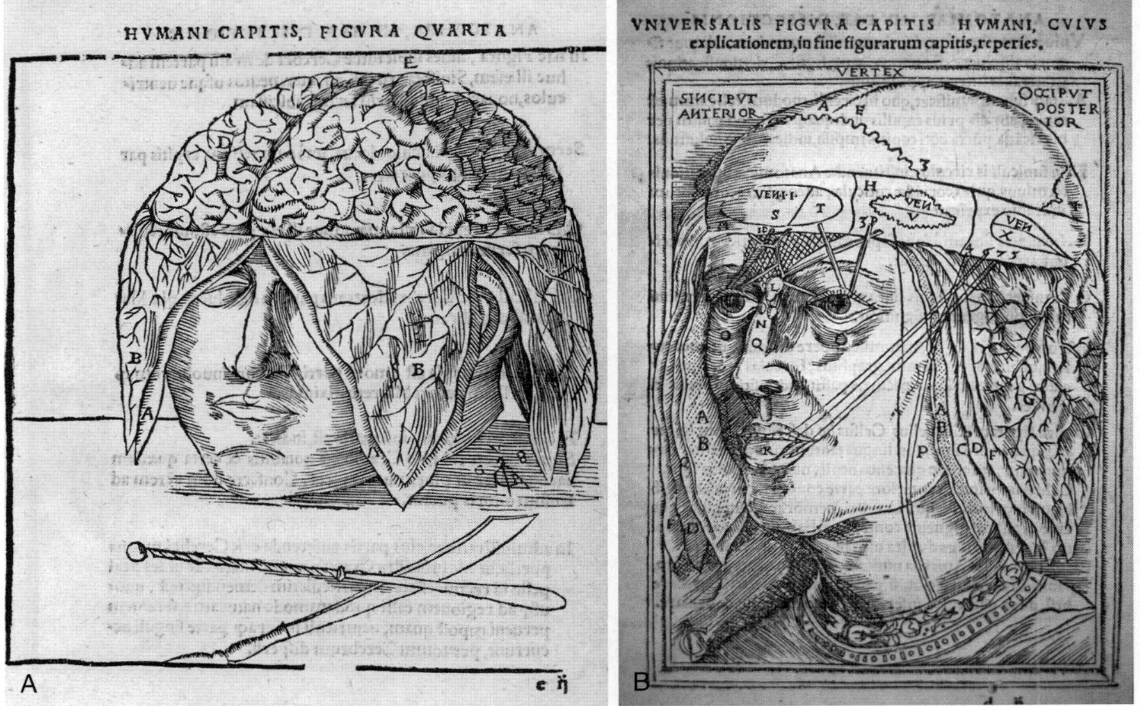

Figure 1-29. A, Johannes Dryander's illustrations of scalp and skull dissection, revealing the dura and brain in layers. **B,** "Cell doctrine" theory within the ventricular system, as illustrated by Dryander. *(From Dryander J.* Anatomiae. *Marburg, Germany: Eucharius Cervicornus; 1537. Courtesy James Tait Goodrich, MD, PhD.)*

Vesalius was appointed professor of anatomy at Padua at the young age of 23. At the age of 28, in 1543, Vesalius produced his great work, *De Humani Corporis Fabrica.*[75] Book VII is an extensive discussion on the anatomy of the brain.[76] Included in the chapter are detailed anatomic discussions with excellent illustrations. Following up on his anatomic caveats, Vesalius noted the "heads of beheaded men are the most suitable [for study] since they can be obtained immediately after execution with the friendly help of judges and prefects."[76]

Vesalius was also trained as a surgeon. The *Fabrica* contains a section of text on the brain and the dural coverings in which Vesalius discussed mechanisms of brain injury and how the various membranes and bone have been designed to protect the brain. In his second edition of *Fabrica* (1555), Vesalius provided an early and interesting case of a child with hydrocephalus and remarked on the condition as originating from cerebrospinal fluid; however, Vesalius was unable to offer any surgical treatment: "…in ipsius cerebri cavitate, adeoque in dextro sinistroque illius ventriculis: quorum cavitas amplitudoque ita increverat, ipsumque cerebrum ita extensum fuerat, ut novem fere aquae libras…continuerint" ["In the same brain cavity, the right and left ventricles' cavity space thus increased, and the brain was so spread out; nearly nine pounds of water…was contained"].[77] Of interest is that several of the initial letters in the text are illustrated with little cherubs performing trephinations!

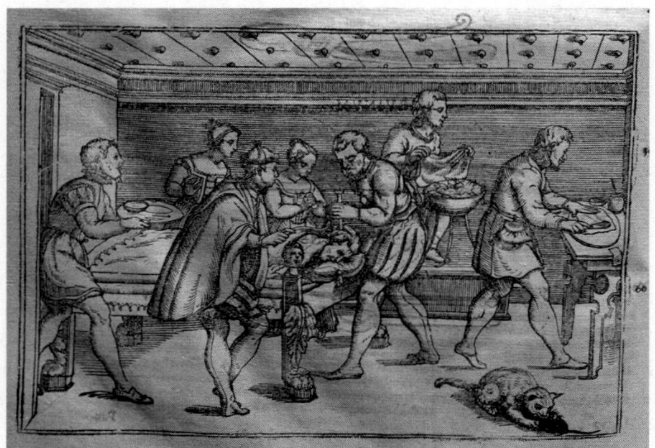

Figure 1-30. An elegant drawing from Giovanni Andrea della Croce's work of trephination being performed in a nobleman's bedchamber. The patient is in bed, in the prone position; servants are around the room serving and dealing with the instruments. While the surgeon is performing the trephination, a cat is seen in the foreground chewing on a rat on the floor. *(From della Croce GA.* Chirurgiae Libri Septem. *Venice: Jordanus Zilettus; 1573. Courtesy James Tait Goodrich, MD, PhD.)*

A contemporary of Vesalius and another leader in Renaissance anatomic studies was a Parisian anatomist, **Charles Estienne** (1504-1564). His book on anatomy, *De Dissectione Partium Corporis Humani Libri Tres,*[78] was actually completed in 1539, thereby predating Vesalius's work by 4 years, but legal problems delayed its publication until 1546. This book is most notable for a wealth of beautiful anatomic plates dealing with neuroanatomy. It contains representations of a series of anatomic figures with the subjects posed against sumptuous and imaginative Renaissance backgrounds. In the text, the anatomic details are not as original as Vesalius's anatomic treatise. In addition, many of the errors introduced by Galen and his followers are repeated in Estienne's text descriptions. However, the plates on the nervous system are quite graphic and among the most illustrative of this period. An important work, albeit with errors, it does detail the anatomy of the skull and brain more accurately than did previous works (Figs. 1-34 and 1-35).

In view of the contributions of the aforementioned physicians and their works, advances made in the Renaissance were clearly remarkable. Back in vogue was originality in anatomic research, replacing the ex cathedra writings of Galen and the classicists. No surgeon could explore the human body without an accurate understanding of the underlying anatomy. In addition, during the Renaissance, important events included the introduction of the printed book and the production of accurate anatomic illustrations.

The Hippocratic emphasis on the skull fracture continued to dominate the management of head injuries, as it had for the preceding 2000 years. With developments in anatomic knowledge now well under way, the next era was an understanding of

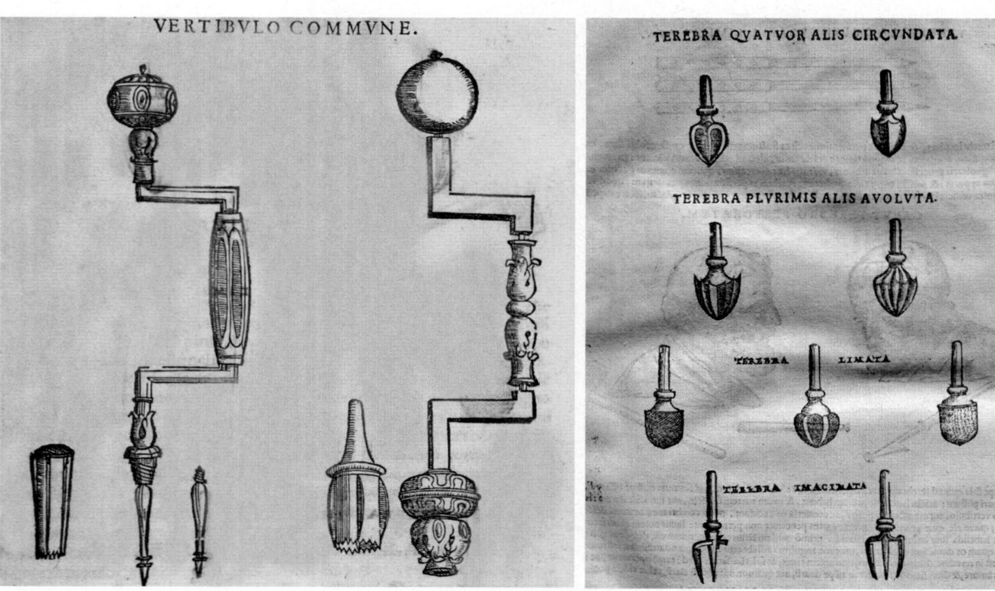

Figure 1-31. Neurosurgical instruments designed and illustrated by Giovanni Andrea della Croce. *(From della Croce GA.* Chirurgiae Libri Septem. *Venice: Jordanus Zilettus; 1573. Courtesy James Tait Goodrich, MD, PhD.)*

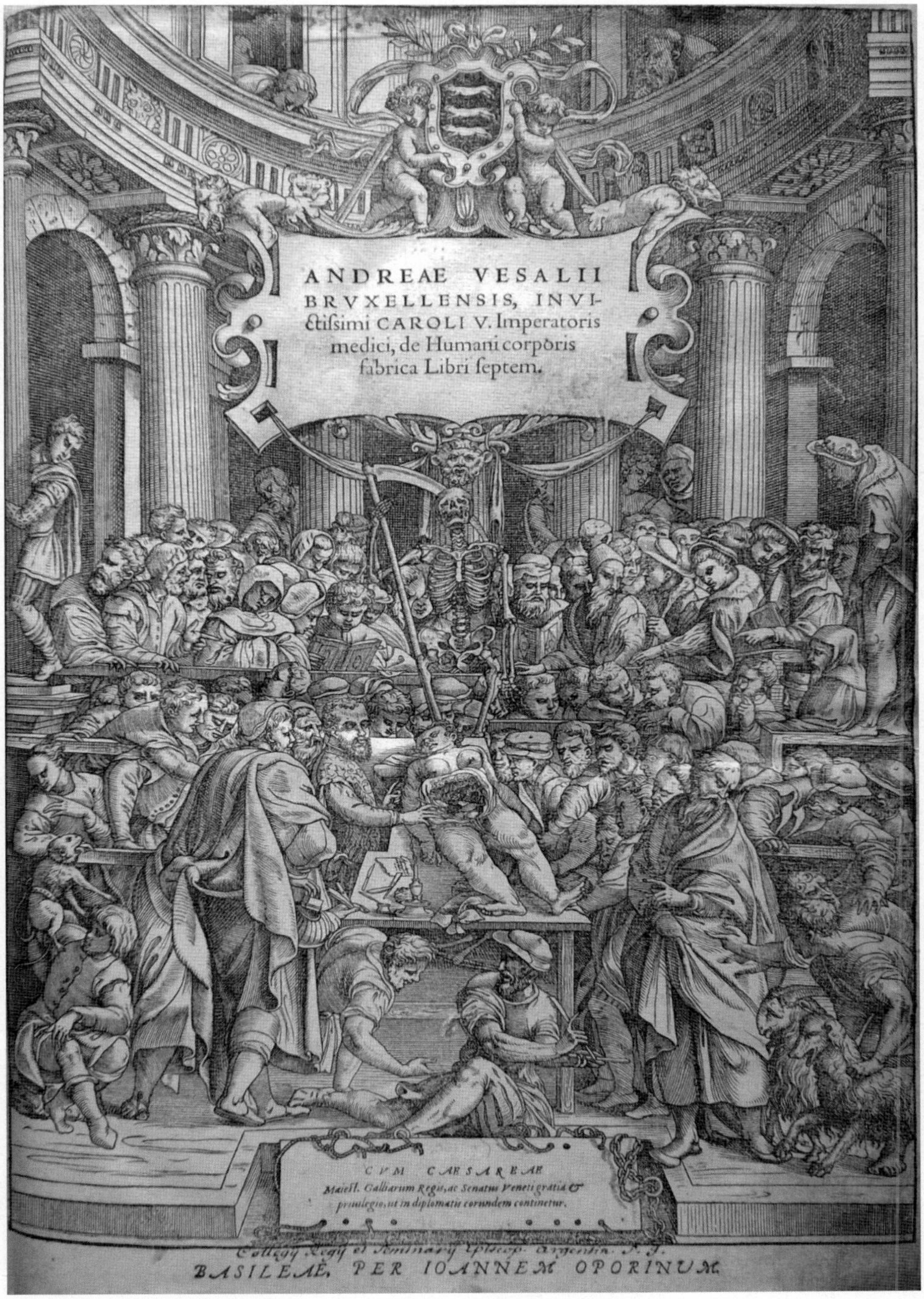

Figure 1-32. Frontispiece from Vesalius's 1555 (second edition) magnum opus on anatomy. Vesalius is depicted in the center, posed over a cadaver and performing a hands-on anatomic dissection. *(From Vesalius A.* De Humani Corporis Fabrica, Libri Septem. *Basel: Johannes Oporinus; 1555. Courtesy James Tait Goodrich, MD, PhD.)*

physiology of the human body: the major theme of the 17th century.

SURGEONS OF THE INSURGENCY: SEVENTEENTH CENTURY

Sixteenth-century medicine and the influence of the Renaissance clearly changed the direction of education and surgical practice for those interested in operating on the brain and spinal cord. The 17th century, the so-called insurgent century, carried these themes even further with significant achievements in science and medicine. Some historical "giants" produced their scientific contributions during this century: Isaac Newton (1642-1727), Francis Bacon (1561-1625), William Harvey (1578-1657), and Robert Boyle (1627-1691) contributed their ideas and innovation in the introduction of physics, experimental design, discovery of the circulation of blood, and physiologic chemistry. Another critical advance was the formation of scientific societies, with the first

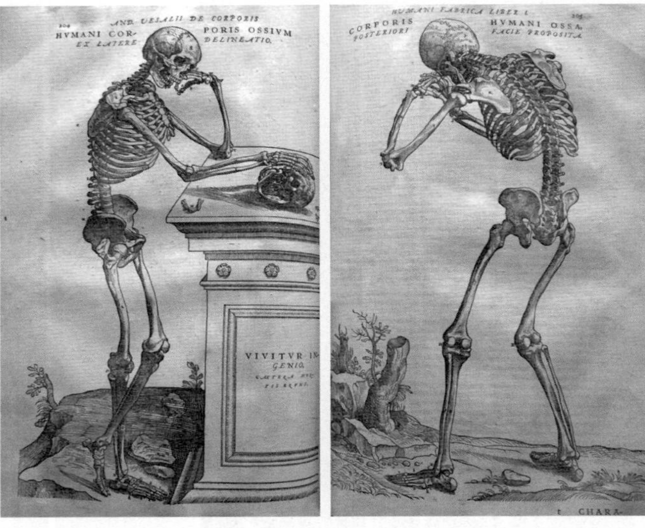

Figure 1-33. Two anatomic views of skeletal anatomy in Vesalius's book. The artistic skill and details represent an enormous improvement over previous anatomic texts. *(From Vesalius A.* De Humani Corporis Fabrica, Libri Septem. *Basel: Johannes Oporinus; 1543. Courtesy James Tait Goodrich, MD, PhD.)*

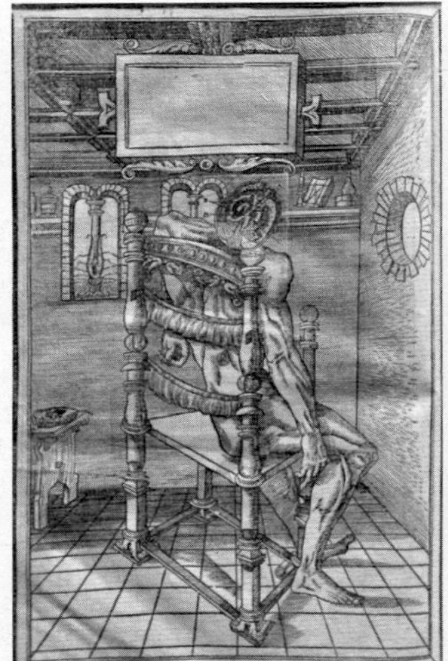

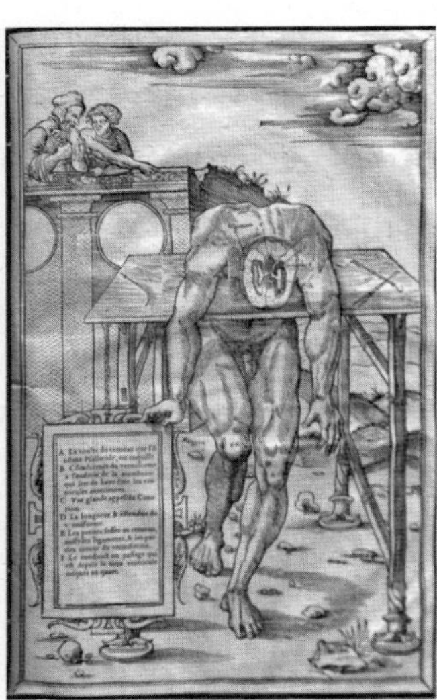

Figure 1-35. Charles Estienne's discussion of the anatomy of the brain, showing a cross section of the head and the ventricular system. *(From Estienne C.* De Dissectione Partium Corporis Humani Libri Tres. *Paris: Simon Colinaeus; 1546. Courtesy James Tait Goodrich, MD, PhD.)*

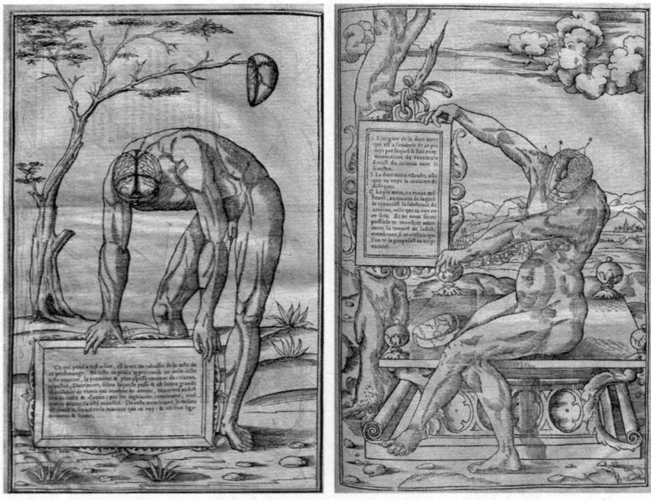

Figure 1-34. Charles Estienne's discussion of the anatomy of the brain and skull. Note the skull hanging from a tree limb on the left and at the knee on the right. *(From Estienne C.* De Dissectione Partium Corporis Humani Libri Tres. *Paris: Simon Colinaeus; 1546. Courtesy James Tait Goodrich, MD, PhD.)*

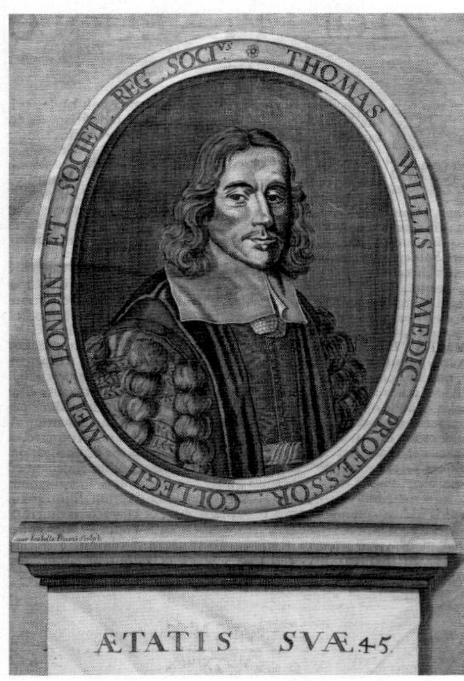

Figure 1-36. Portrait of Sir Thomas Willis at the age of 45. *(Courtesy James Tait Goodrich, MD, PhD.)*

open public presentations of scientific ideas. Among the most important societies were the Royal Society of London, the Académie Des Sciences in Paris, and the Gesellschaft Naturforschender Aerzte in Germany. Thus scientific education and exchange of information were advanced. For the first time, scientific ideas and information could be distributed publicly, and their merits discussed, in open dialogue.

A distinctive scholar of this period in the early understanding of the brain was **Thomas Willis** (1621-1675), an early describer of the eponymous circle of Willis, familiar to every physician. Willis was educated at Oxford and became a fashionable London physician (Fig. 1-36). Willis published a number of important monographs, but the one that stands out is his *Cerebri Anatomie*, published in London in 1664.[79,80] With methodic attention to detail, this book became the most accurate anatomic study of the brain to date. Willis was assisted in this work by **Richard Lower** (1631-1691) in demonstrating that when parts of the "circle" were tied off, the anastomotic network still provided blood to the brain. The superb and anatomically accurate engravings of the brain (Fig. 1-37) were produced by Sir Christopher Wren (1632-1723).

Willis introduced the concept of *neurology*, or the doctrine of neurons. Willis used the term in a purely anatomic sense, inasmuch as the concept of "neurological" disease had not yet been

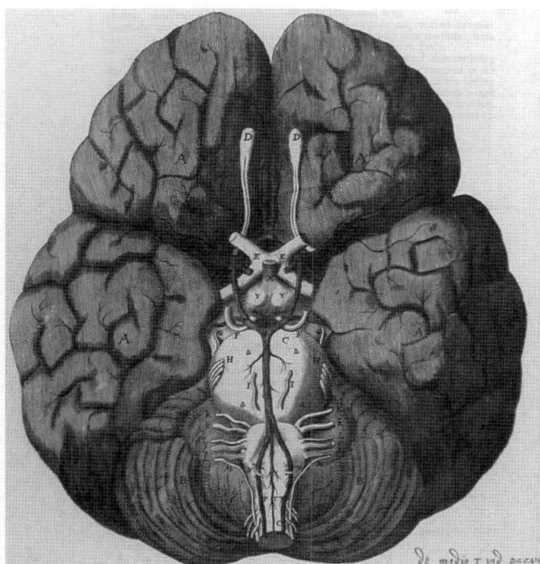

Figure 1-37. The circle of Willis as described by Thomas Willis and drawn by Sir Christopher Wren. *(From Willis T.* Cerebri Anatome: Cui Accessit Nervorum Descriptio et Usus. *London: J Flesher; 1664. Courtesy James Tait Goodrich, MD, PhD.)*

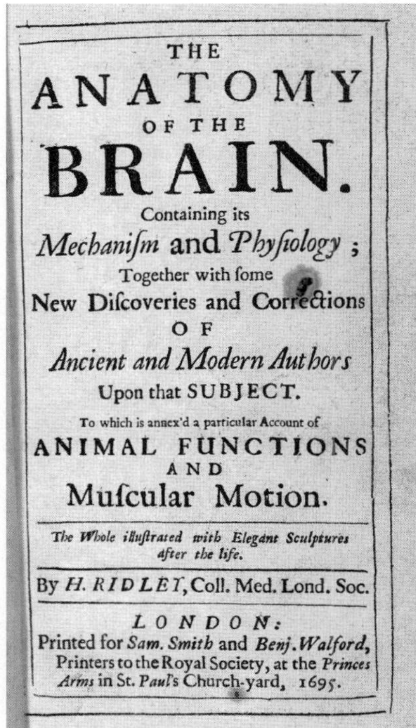

THE
ANATOMY
OF THE
BRAIN.
Containing its
Mechaniſm and *Phyſiology*;
Together with ſome
New Diſcoveries and Corrections
OF
Ancient and Modern Authors
Upon that SUBJECT.
To which is annex'd a particular Account of
ANIMAL FUNCTIONS
AND
Muſcular Motion.
The Whole illuſtrated with Elegant Sculptures after the life.
By *H. RIDLEY*, Coll. Med. Lond. Soc.
LONDON:
Printed for *Sam. Smith* and *Benj. Walford*, Printers to the Royal Society, at the *Princes Arms* in St. *Paul's* Church-yard, 1695.

Figure 1-38. The title page from Humphrey Ridley's work on brain anatomy. *(From Ridley H.* The Anatomy of the Brain, Containing Its Mechanisms and Physiology: Together With Some New Discoveries and Corrections of Ancient and Modern Authors Upon That Subject. *London: Samuel Smith; 1695. Courtesy James Tait Goodrich, MD, PhD.)*

introduced. *Neurology* as a noun did not enter general use until Samuel Johnson (1709-1784) defined it in his dictionary of 1765.[81] At this point, neurology came to be understood as the entire field encompassing anatomy, function, and physiology. It is also worth noting that the circle of Willis was not described uniquely by Willis; other anatomic descriptions of this circle were provided in several contemporary anatomic publications (the reader is referred to the writings of Vesling,[82] Casserius,[83] Fallopius,[84] and Ridley[85]).

A prominent anatomist at this time and one often overlooked by contemporary writers was **Humphry Ridley** (1653-1708). Ridley was educated at Merton College, Oxford, and at the University of Leyden, where he received his doctorate in medicine in 1679. Ridley produced an important anatomic work on the brain, *The Anatomy of the Brain*, written in English, which became widely circulated and influential (Figs. 1-38 and 1-39).

The Anatomy of the Brain was published in London in 1695.[85] At the time his work on the brain appeared, many of the classic Greek views of the brain were in vogue. Seventeenth-century anatomy and medicine moved away from the earlier "cell doctrine" theory (in which brain function was considered to reside within the ventricles); anatomists had begun to recognize the brain as a distinct anatomic entity. In contrast to the "cell doctrine," cerebral function came to be viewed as a property of the brain.[86,87]

Ridley recorded a number of original observations. Ridley's description of the circle of Willis was even more accurate in details than Willis's and included a more complete anatomic description of both the posterior cerebral artery and the superior cerebellar artery, defined as separate entities. Ridley provided a better demonstration of the principle of anastomotic flow and better elucidated the anastomotic principle of this network with his anatomic studies. To conduct his studies, Ridley had access to recently executed criminals. The method of execution was typically hanging, which caused vascular engorgement of the brain and thus facilitated identification of the vascular anatomy. Ridley's understanding of the deep nuclei of the cerebellum, particularly the anatomy of the posterior fossa, was superior to Willis's. Ridley also provided one of the earliest descriptions of the arachnoid membrane. Of note, Ridley still believed in the *rete mirabile*, a tenacious holdover from Galenic times. To Ridley this was a legitimate anatomic structure, and he provided a strong argument for its existence in this monograph. In addition, Ridley provided the first accurate description of the fornix and its pathways in this monograph. This volume and the work by Willis presented the first scientific anatomic studies of the brain and thereby provided an essential anatomic foundation for future neurosurgeons.

A surgical expert often overlooked in neurosurgical history is **Wilhelm Fabricius von Hilden** (1560-1634). Although Fabricius (also known as Fabry) had received a classical education in his youth, family misfortune did not allow him to go on to a formal medical education. He went on to study in the "lesser field" of surgery, being educated in the apprentice system then prevalent. Fortunately, the teachers who trained him were among the finest wound surgeons of the day. Lacking a formal university education and excelling with a surgical apprentice education, he went on to develop a distinguished career in surgery.

Fabricius produced one of the most important surgical works of the 17th century: *Observationum et Curationum*, a monograph that included more than 600 surgical cases, along with a number of important and original observations on the brain.[88] Fabricius's observations on the brain and surgery included descriptions of a number of congenital malformations, skull fractures, and techniques for bullet extraction, along with original designs for field surgical instruments. He described operations for intracranial hemorrhage (with cure of insanity), vertebral displacement, congenital hydrocephalus, and an occipital tumor in the newborn (probably an encephalocele). Fabricius carried out trephinations for treatment of a brain abscess and cure of a longstanding

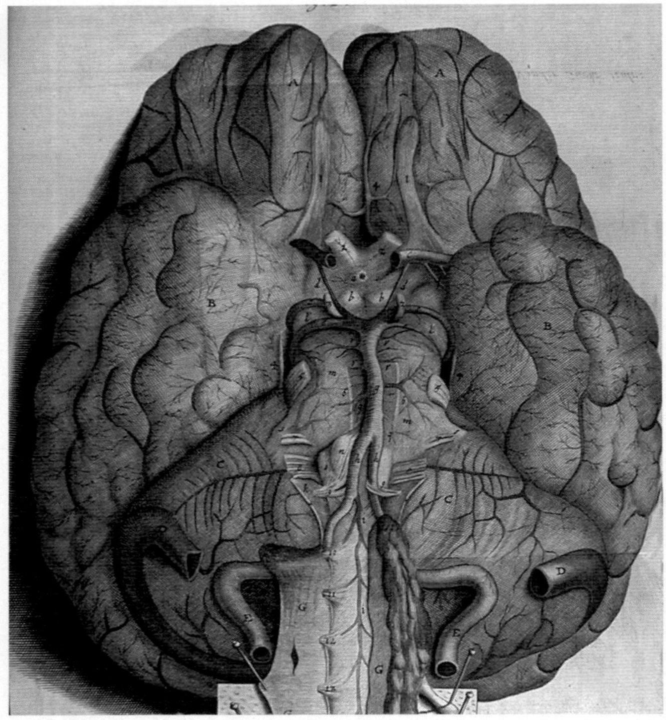

Figure 1-39. Humphrey Ridley's illustration of the anastomotic network at the base of the brain: the circle of Willis. Ridley's anatomic details are better than Willis's and include a more complete anatomic description of both the posterior cerebral artery and the superior cerebellar artery, here described as separate entities. *(From Ridley H.* The Anatomy of the Brain, Containing Its Mechanisms and Physiology: Together With Some New Discoveries and Corrections of Ancient and Modern Authors Upon That Subject. *London: Samuel Smith; 1695. Courtesy James Tait Goodrich, MD, PhD.)*

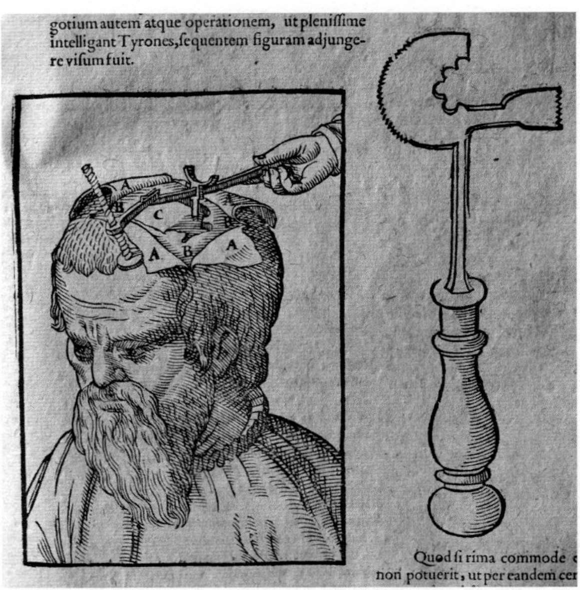

Figure 1-40. A "lever and screw" device, used to elevate a depressed skull fracture. To the right is a saw used to make a series of rectangular cuts for performing a craniectomy. This style of instrument became known later as a Hey saw. *(From Fabricius W.* Observationum et Curationum Chirurgicarum Centuriae. *Lugduni [Lyons]: I. A. Huguetan; 1606-1641. A number of neurosurgical cases are also contained in a later publication of collected works: Fabricius W.* Opera Observationum et Curationum. *Frankfurt: Joannis Beyer; 1646. Courtesy James Tait Goodrich, MD, PhD.)*

aphasia. He even removed a splinter of metal from an eye by using a magnet, a cure that only enhanced his reputation (Figs. 1-40 and 1-41).

Some early and skillfully designed neurosurgical instruments are illustrated in a work by **Johann Scultetus (Schultes)** (1595-1645) of Ulm, titled *Armamentarium Chirurgicum XLIII*.[89] Scultetus provided unique and graphic details of neurosurgical instruments, clearly the finest to appear since those published by Berengario in 1518 and della Croce in 1573. The illustrations graphically reveal surgical techniques for treating fractures and dislocations, along with a variety of bandaging techniques for dealing with wounds. This surgical work was so popular that it was translated into many languages, including English, and it exerted a considerable influence on surgery throughout Europe for more than two centuries. The surgical plates and descriptions of various operations contain exacting details, including concepts from antiquity to the present. Of interest is that many of the instruments illustrated by Scultetus remain in use today. Scultetus's details of surgical operations for injury of the skull and brain are remarkable plebiscite (Figs. 1-42 and 1-43).

Neurosurgical practice continued to evolve in the 17th century. A surgeon who offered some interesting technical advice on developing neurosurgical operating skills was **John Woodall** (c. 1556-1643). Woodall was a military surgeon by training and surgeon-general to the East India Company. For surgeons of the East India Company, he compiled a surgical monograph titled *The Surgeon's Mate* (1617).[90] In his collected works, published in 1639, Woodall provided a list of surgical instruments and sound

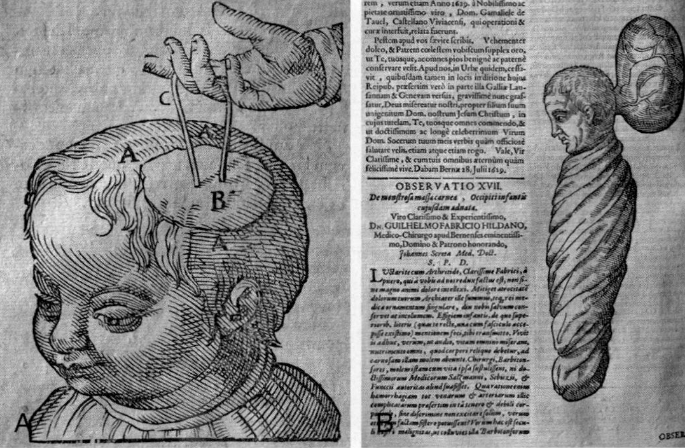

Figure 1-41. A, Wilhelm Fabricius von Hilden's technique for elevating a depressed skull (ping pong) fracture in a child. Two small holes were made, and a leather strap was passed through and pulled up to elevate the depressed fracture. **B,** A very early illustrated example of an occipital encephalocele. Fabricius discussed a case of a child with a large "swelling" in the occipital region that was full of clear fluid. *(From Fabricius W.* Observationum et Curationum Chirurgicarum Centuriae. *Lugduni [Lyons]: I. A. Huguetan; 1606-1641. A number of neurosurgical cases are also contained in a later publication of collected works: Fabricius W.* Opera Observationum et Curationum. *Frankfurt: Joannis Beyer; 1646. Courtesy James Tait Goodrich, MD, PhD.)*

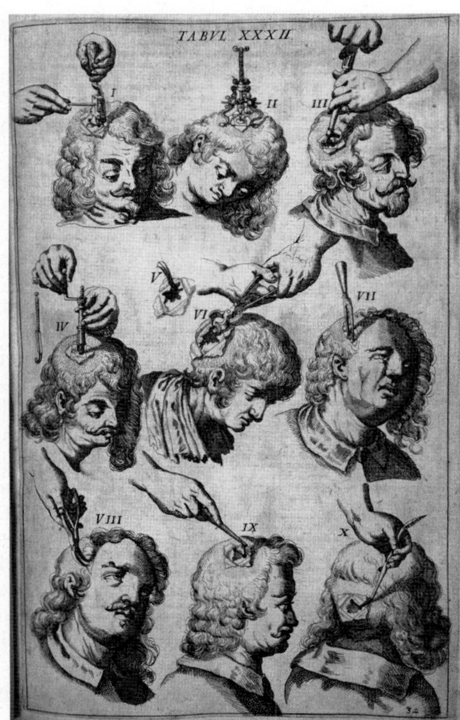

Figure 1-42. Surgical techniques and instruments designed by Johann Scultetus for trephining the skull and dealing with skull fractures. *(From Scultetus J:* Χειροπλοθηκη [Cheiroplothiki]. Armamentarium Chirurgicum XLIII. *Ulm, Germany: Balthasar Kühnen; 1655. Courtesy James Tait Goodrich, MD, PhD.)*

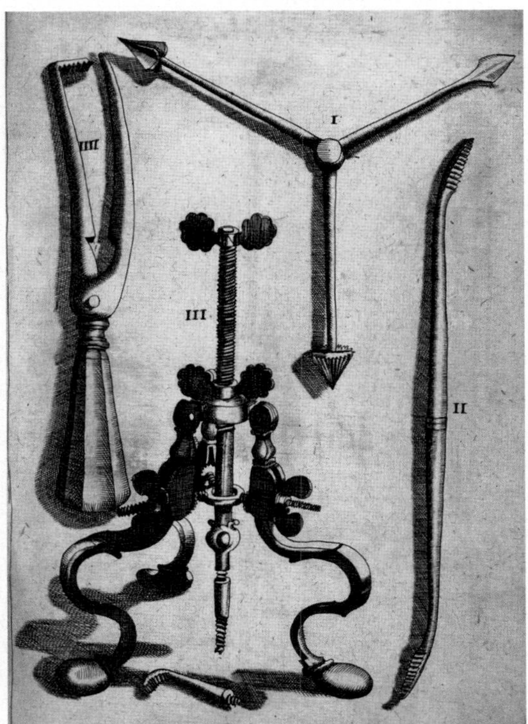

Figure 1-43. Scultetus's tripod-style trephine, with a center pin for elevation. Illustrated also are an elevator (right), a corkscrew type elevator (top), and bone rongeur (left). *(From Scultetus J:* Χειροπλοθηκη [Cheiroplothiki]. Armamentarium Chirurgicum XLIII. *Ulm, Germany: Balthasar Kühnen; 1655. Courtesy James Tait Goodrich, MD, PhD.)*

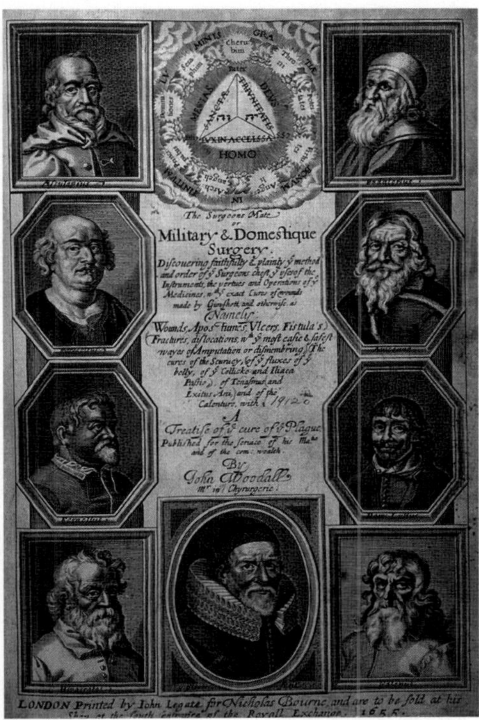

Figure 1-44. Title page from John Woodall's book on military and domestic surgery. *(From Woodall J:* The Surgeon's Mate, or Military and Domestique Surgery Discouering Faithfully & Plainly ye Method and Order of the Surgeon's Chest…. *London: Rob. Young for Nicholas Bourne; 1639. Courtesy James Tait Goodrich, MD, PhD.)*

advice for a surgical practice.[91] Woodall fabricated a trephine with a then-unique design of a crown that included a center pin; this innovation prevented the crown from slipping on a bloody skull. A brace was added to this trephine, which could be placed against the surgeon's chest for additional support and driving force. This innovative design allowed the surgeon to drive the trephine with one hand while the other held the head, all of which could be accomplished on a rolling ship's deck. Woodall, recognizing the ignorance of his contemporary German surgeons, believed that a surgeon should practice trephining on sheep or calf skulls first before performing one on a human head (Figs. 1-44 and 1-45):

> "The Germane Surgeons use no Trapan, that ever I could see my eight years living among them, though they both speak and write of it. But for as much as it is apparent, the work of a Trapan is very good, I therefore would advise a young Artist to make some experience first upon a calves head, or a sheep's head, till he can well and easily take out a piece of the bone; so shall he the more safely do it to a man without error when occasion is."
>
> **(J. Woodall, *The Surgeon's Mate,*[91] p 4)**

An Englishman and Plymouth naval surgeon, **James Yonge** (1646-1721), was among the first to argue emphatically that "wounds of the brain are curable"; Galen had earlier announced, "I have seen the wounded brain heal."[28] Yonge's first surgical text was a small monograph titled *Wounds of the Brain Proved Curable.*[92] Yonge provided a surgical account of a brain operation on a child of 4 with extensive compound fractures of the skull from which brain tissue issued forth. The surgery was successful, with the child surviving, and this inspired Yonge to publish the account. Yonge also reported on more than 60 cases in which brain wounds were cured that he was able to locate in the older literature,

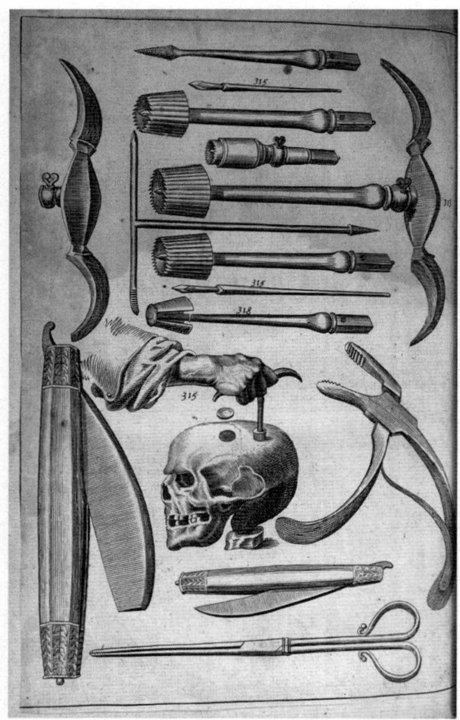

Figure 1-45. John Woodall designed a hand trephine with a series of interchangeable burs, along with bone rongeurs. The trephine center pin design was especially useful on a rolling ship deck when applied to a bloody skull. *(From Woodall J:* The Surgeon's Mate, or Military and Domestique Surgery Discouering Faithfully & Plainly ye Method and Order of the Surgeon's Chest…. *London: Rob. Young for Nicholas Bourne; 1639. Courtesy James Tait Goodrich, MD, PhD.)*

beginning with Galen. The bibliography records the earlier cases that he was able to locate. Yonge commented that this work was written in defense of surgery on the skull and the brain. From the preface[92]:

> I had the good fortune to be a successful chirurgeon to the child, whose case is contained in the following narrative: but I had scarcely wiped my instruments, and put up my plaister-box, before a physician of this town, sneakingly and maliciously endeavor to stifle…[my] reputation…insinuating that it was impossible to [cure brain wounds …because Wounds of the brain were *absolutely mortal*….

Yonge was clearly a proponent of trephination and operating on the skull and brain, and he proved that both could be done safely.

Other technical innovations for treating head injuries occurred in this period. **Augustin Belloste** (1654-1730) described a technique for repairing "holes in the head," from trauma or trephination, with the use of lead plates. Keeping the brain from being exposed to "corrupt air" led to better outcomes in brain surgery.[93] Belloste provided a case discussion of what is now called the "syndrome of the trephined" (sinking skin flap syndrome): a situation in which the cranial defects are left unrepaired, foreign implants are placed to cover the defects, and affected patients become very sensitive to temperature and atmospheric changes.

The 17th century, the insurgent century, clearly brought a number of advances to the field of brain surgery. Neuroanatomy became an area of intense investigation. Physiologic experimentation, along with the scientific societies, allowed wide dissemination of the new investigations and also allowed scholarly disagreement. The surgeons of that time with adventurous personalities realized that in certain cases, brain surgery could be performed safely; not all patients died if the dura mater was opened.

EIGHTEENTH CENTURY: AN ENLIGHTENED PERIOD FOR NEUROSURGERY

The 17th century clearly provided a sound scientific and anatomic basis for neurosurgery and neurosciences. The 18th century continued this trend and was a period of intense activity in the medical and scientific world. Chemistry as a true science was being propelled forward in the works of Joseph Priestley (1733-1804), Antoine Lavoisier (1743-1794), Alessandro Volta (1745-1827), James Watt (1736-1819), and others. Clinical bedside medicine, essentially lost since the Byzantine and Islamic era, was reintroduced by Thomas Sydenham (1624-1689), William Cullen (1710-1790), and Herman Boerhaave (1668-1738). With bedside examination came a number of original and new diagnostic examination tools. Of particular note are the contributions of Leopold Auenbrugger (1722-1809) and his introduction of percussion of the chest; William Withering (1741-1799) and his pharmacologic introduction of the use of digitalis for cardiac problems; and Edward Jenner (1749-1823), who helped eliminate a world scourge by inventing the vaccine against smallpox. In the emerging field of neurosurgery, a number of surgeons were trying to bring some sense to the management of head injury. For the first time, the focus for the surgeon was switching from the skull to the brain. This new direction and change in the neurological status of the patient marked a major paradigm shift that represented a very important step toward the origins of a separate surgical discipline of neurosurgery[94]:

> Judgment in distinguishing, and ability in treating diseases, are not to be attained by a transient cursory view of them; merely running round an Hospital for a few months, or reading a general system of surgery, will not form a compleat practitioner: the man, who aims at that character, must take notice of many little things, which the inattentive pass over, and which cannot be remarked by writers; he must accustom himself to see, and to think for himself; and must regard the rules laid down by authors, as the outlines only of a piece, which he is to fill up and finish: books may give general ideas, but practice, and medication, must make him adroit and discerning; without these, his reading may possibly keep him clear of very gross blunders, but he will still remain injudicious, and inexpert.

In this period, one of the most accomplished physicians was clearly **Percivall Pott** (1714-1788), considered by many historians to be the greatest English surgeon of the 18th century. His list of contributions, several of which apply to neurosurgery, is enormous. In his work *Remarks on That Kind of Palsy of the Lower Limbs Found to Accompany a Curvature of the Spine*, he described the disease entity now known as Pott's disease (i.e., tuberculous caries of the spine).[95] His clinical descriptions clearly describe the gibbus and tuberculous infection of the spine. Surprisingly, Pott failed to associate the relationship between the deformity and paralysis. An osteomyelitic infection of the scalp and skull in which pus collects under the pericranium is now called *Pott's puffy tumor*. Pott strongly argued that these lesions should be opened and drained (Fig. 1-46).

Eighteenth-century surgeons generated much discussion over the surgical practice of trephination. Pott was a strong proponent of intervention. In his classic work on head injury, he clearly appreciated the observation that clinical findings of head injury resulted from injury of the brain and not of the skull.[94] Pott studied head injuries and began to differentiate between compression and concussion injuries of the brain. The following

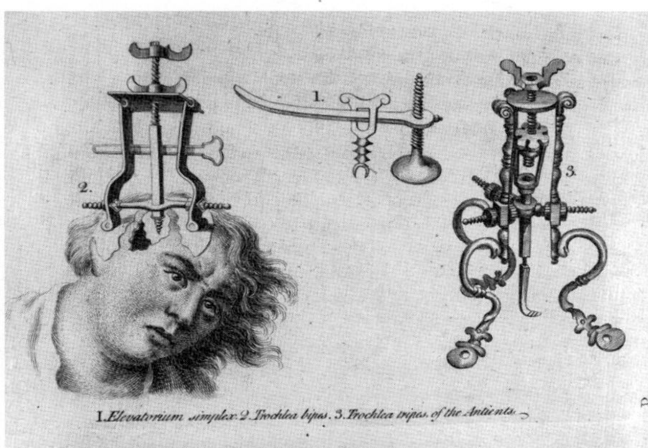

Figure 1-46. Trephination instrumentation as designed by Percivall Pott. The left and right illustrations are of the tripod-style instrument, with a center pin that could be driven into the fracture. The legs were often quite ornate in style. The center illustration is of a lever and screw–style instrument. The screw was driven into the fracture, and the lever arm was used to elevate the depressed bone. *(From Pott P.* Observations on the Nature and Consequences of Wounds and Contusions of the Head, Fractures of the Skull, Concussions of the Brain. *London: C. Hitch and L. Hawes; 1760:x-xi. Courtesy James Tait Goodrich, MD, PhD.)*

clinical description from his book on head injury[95] outlines some of his views:

> The reasons for trepanning in these cases are, first, the immediate relief of present symptoms arising from pressure of extravasated fluid; or second, the discharge of matter formed between the skull and dura mater, in consequence of inflammation; or third, the prevention of such mischief, as experience has shown may most probably be expected from such kind of violence offered to the last mentioned membrane….
>
> In the…mere fracture without depression of bone, or the appearance of such symptoms as indicate commotion, extravasation, or inflammation, it is used as a preventative, and therefore is a matter of choice, more than immediate necessity.

Pott clearly developed his outstanding reputation by his astute clinical observations and bedside treatment. Because of his aggressive management of head injuries, he is considered the first of the modern neurosurgeons. His caveats, presented in the preface to his work on head injury, are still pertinent today.

The most significant development in 18th-century writings on neurosurgical topics was the gradual recognition of the effects of trauma on brain function in addition to the skull. Several French surgeons drew a clear-cut distinction between the loss of consciousness accompanying a blow to the head and the drowsiness that appeared later. The former came to be recognized as a direct result of cerebral concussion, and the latter, after a lucid interval, came to be accepted as being caused by a collection of blood that produced compression of the brain. This idea was introduced by **Jean Louis Petit** (1674-1750), the leading surgeon in Paris in the first half of the 18th century, in a series of lectures that he gave in Paris.[97] The realization that a delayed loss of consciousness could serve as an indication for surgical intervention is one of the epochal events that mark the origins of neurosurgery as a discipline that deals with alterations in brain function and not just superficial injuries to the skull. It was a major conceptual change in the approach that had been followed for 2000 years and marks an important turning point in surgical thinking.

One of the earliest descriptions of the "lucid interval" in head injury was provided by **Henri François Le Dran** (1685-1770). Le Dran was both an anatomist and a surgeon who developed a large surgical experience by serving as the chief surgeon to the French Army. Le Dran established a very popular school of anatomy in Paris, attracting students from all over Europe. His text *Observations de Chirurgie*[98] reveals a skilled surgeon with a wide variety of surgical talents. This work became Le Dran's most popular surgical text, being reprinted several times and translated into English in 1749.[99] It contained a broad review of surgery, but of most importance to neurosurgeons are his views on surgery of the head. Le Dran detailed the concept of the "lucid interval" after a head injury and then attributed its aftermath most commonly to epidural hematomas (Fig. 1-47).

A remarkable and talented physician in English medicine and surgery and a student of Percivall Pott was **John Hunter** (1728-1793). Many writers consider Hunter equally as skilled as Pott, but his additional work in anatomy, pathology, physiology, and surgery helped him make a number of important contributions.[100] Hunter, often referred to as the founder of experimental and surgical pathology, spent the main part of his career at St. George's Hospital in London. Hunter was trained in the apprentice style of learning and had minimal formal education. He began his training under his older brother, William Hunter (1718-1783), and spent time with William Cheselden (1688-1752), two clearly talented teachers. As a surgeon, Hunter was clearly atypical for his time in that he approached the field of surgery in a more practical manner and at the same time added a benchside experimental touch. His *A Treatise on the Blood, Inflammation, and Gun-Shot Wounds*[101] was based on his years of military experience and was an important work on management of gunshot wounds.

Hunter did not offer much on neurosurgery; the section on skull fractures took up only one paragraph and is quite limited. In understanding vascular disorders, however, Hunter was insightful and innovative by describing the concept of collateral circulation. These circulation studies were conducted on a buck whose carotid artery he tied off to see the effect on the antler; no ill effect was noted, and the response was development of collateral circulation. Hunter later applied these concepts to the treatment of popliteal aneurysms, previously treated by amputation; he tied off the artery and realized that collateral circulation would develop. In Hunter's view, a patient's leaving the operating room a "cripple" was clearly not a good outcome. Hunter was adroit at posing questions raised by his clinical experiences, performing animal experiments to answer the questions and integrating his clinical and scientific results into the best available treatment. Hunter anatomically dissected an interesting case of craniopagus parasiticus, a set of twins from India of whom one child was fully formed and the other twin's body consisted of only the head. The incomplete twin would express emotion and move the lips and mouth during eating (Fig. 1-48).[102]

Hunter is also remembered as a devoted student of anatomic curiosities and would go to great lengths, sometimes nefariously, to obtain specimens. The most famous case was the Irish giant Charles Byrne, whom Harvey Cushing (1869-1939) later determined had acromegaly. Byrne knew of Hunter's interest in him and went to great lengths to avoid his laboratory after death. Byrne was not successful; his skeleton became part of the Hunterian museum, which contains more than 13,000 specimens and is now part of the Royal College of Surgeons pathologic collection, a direct donation by Hunter.

A student of Hunter was **John Abernethy** (1764-1831), also a talented anatomist and surgeon. Abernethy is remembered for publishing the first book in America devoted to a neurosurgical topic.[103] So popular was Abernethy as a lecturer that the governors of St. Bartholomew's Hospital built an anatomic theatre for him, a place of training sought out by brilliant students of the period. Abernethy eventually went back to Scotland, his country of birth, and settled in Edinburgh to establish a general practice. He continued to develop a large apprenticeship program, which

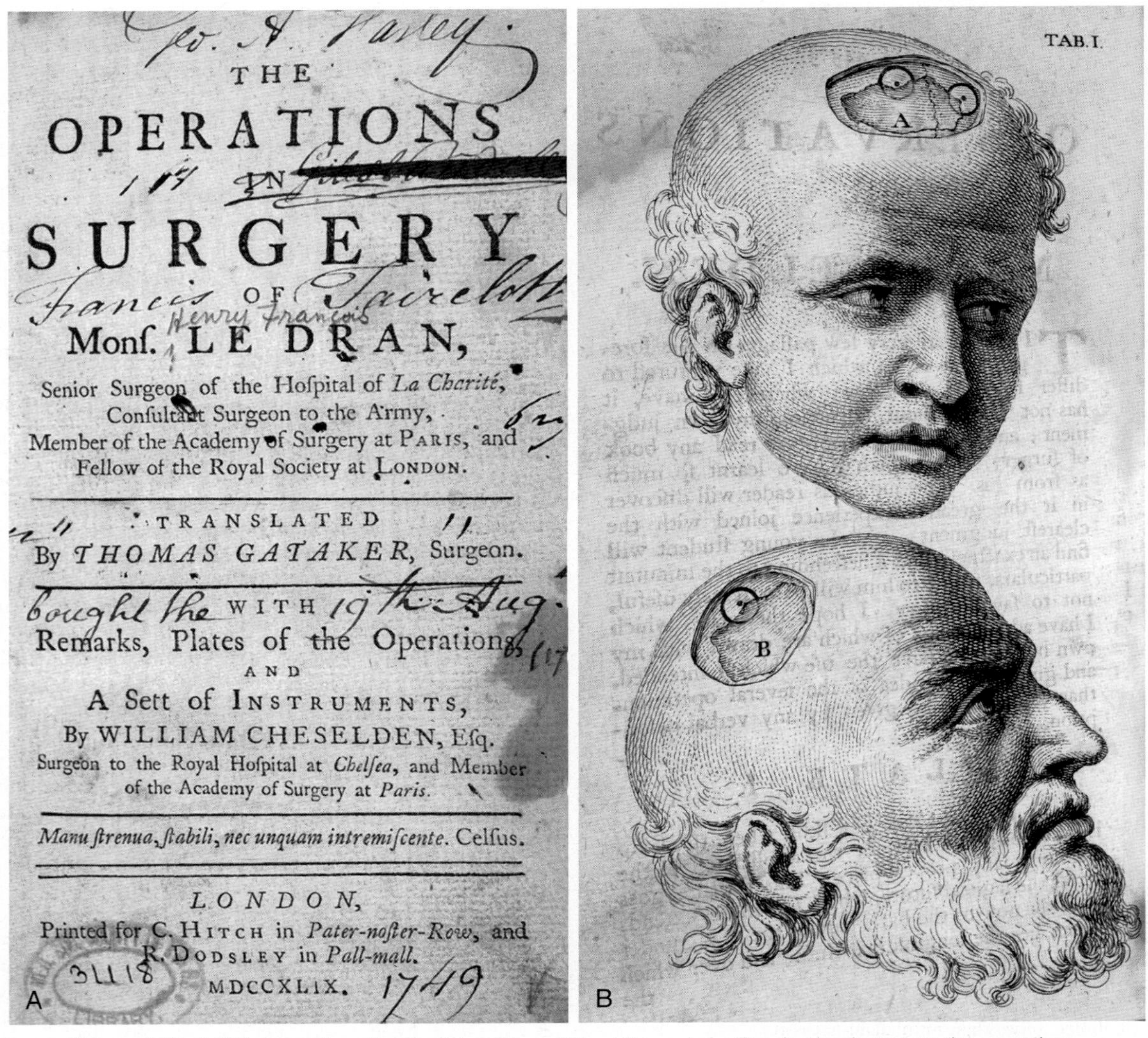

THE

OPERATIONS

IN

SURGERY

OF

Monſ. LE DRAN,

Senior Surgeon of the Hoſpital of *La Charité*,
Conſultant Surgeon to the Army,
Member of the Academy of Surgery at PARIS, and
Fellow of the Royal Society at LONDON.

TRANSLATED

By *THOMAS GATAKER*, Surgeon.

WITH

Remarks, Plates of the Operations,

AND

A Sett of INSTRUMENTS,

By WILLIAM CHESELDEN, Eſq.
Surgeon to the Royal Hoſpital at *Chelſea*, and Member
of the Academy of Surgery at *Paris*.

Manu ſtrenua, ſtabili, nec unquam intremiſcente. Celſus.

LONDON,
Printed for C. HITCH in *Pater-noſter-Row*, and
R. DODSLEY in *Pall-mall*.
MDCCXLIX.

Figure 1-47. A, Title page from the English edition of Henri François Le Dran's classic text on the operations for surgery. **B,** A surgical illustration from Le Dran, demonstrating trephination techniques for elevating skull fractures. In this case, it was a combination of bur holes with a "scraping" technique to remove the fracture. *(From Le Dran HF:* The Operations in Surgery of Mons. Le Dran, Senior Surgeon of the Hospital La Charité, Consultant Surgeon to the Army…Translated by Thomas Gataker…. *London: C. Hitch and R. Dodsley; 1749. Courtesy James Tait Goodrich, MD, PhD.)*

attracted students from far and wide. His contributions to neurosurgery included one of the earliest treatments of neuralgia of the arm; he performed a neurectomy in 1793, which provided instant relief to the patient.[104] Later the patient went on to regain sensation in the hand, which showed that there had been successful reunion of the nerve. Abernethy was an early advocate of ligating the common carotid artery for a cerebral hemorrhage. He later published his writings on the brain in an important work called *Pathological and Practical Researches on Diseases of the Brain and Spinal Cord.*[105] This work contains more than 150 cases of various neurological and neuropathologic conditions that affected, the brain, spinal cord, and peripheral nerves (Figs. 1-49 and 1-50).

A contemporary of Abernethy was **Benjamin Bell** (1749-1806), among the most prominent and successful surgeons in 18th-century Edinburgh. Bell was a compassionate surgeon and among the first to emphasize the importance of reducing pain during surgery. Bell published a popular textbook of surgery, *A System of Surgery.*[106] This book was widely read because of its clarity and precision in style of writing. The section on head injury contains an interesting and important discussion on the differentiation of concussion, compression, and inflammation of the brain, each necessitating different modes of treatment.[107] Bell was a remarkably aggressive surgeon for conditions of the brain; he stresses the importance of relieving compression (i.e., trephination) of the brain, whether it is caused by a depressed skull fracture or by pus or blood. The concept of an epidural hematoma and its symptoms were appreciated by Bell; he argued for a rapid and prompt evacuation:

> Affections of the Brain from external violence, often induce a very complicated set of symptoms; are attended with imminent danger, and give much embarrassment to practitioners: Accordingly, both with respect to the hazard with which they are attended, and the difficulty that we meet with in the cure, there is perhaps no class of diseases to be compared with them. Wounds and bruises of the head, which at first exhibit no marks of danger, often induce a train of symptoms which elude the skill of the most experienced practitioner; and, without admitting of any mitigation, proceed to a fatal period, ending only the death of the patient.
>
> ***A System of Surgery*, Volume 3, Chapter X, Section I**[108]

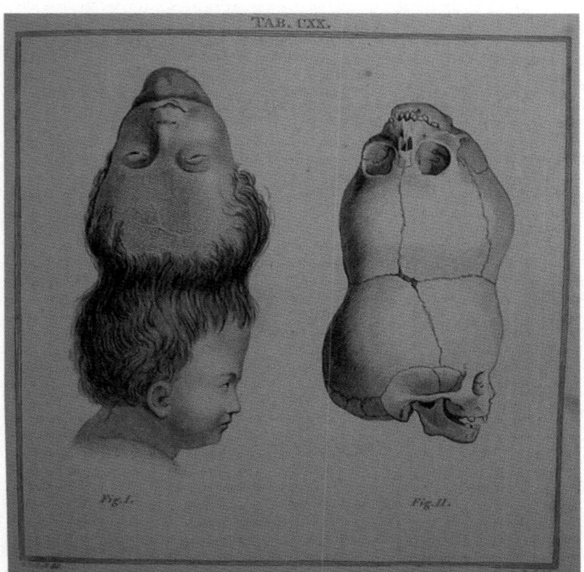

Figure 1-48. An illustration of craniopagus parasiticus twins originally described by John Hunter in manuscript and later published in Evard Home's collected work. These twins were from India. The parasitic twin expressed some emotion and moved the face when the other twin was eating. They died after a venomous snakebite at the age of 4. *(From Home E.* Lectures on Comparative Anatomy; in Which Are Explained the Preparations in the Hunterian Collection. *London, G. & W. Nichol, 1814-1828; Courtesy James Tait Goodrich, MD, PhD.)*

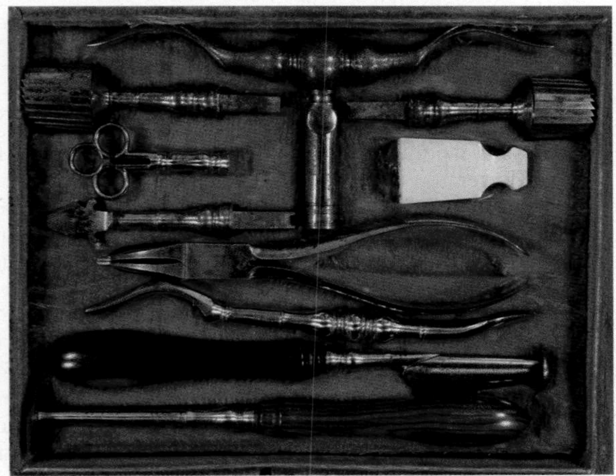

Figure 1-49. An 18th-century hand trephine set designed by Samuel Sharp (1709-1778) with interchangeable bits, elevators, and a bone brush to remove the accumulated bone dust. A "gull-wing" handle was designed for a better grip. The trephines are of two different sizes: one for pediatric patients and one for adult patients. *(Courtesy James Tait Goodrich, MD, PhD.)*

His description of the symptoms of brain compression from external violence is classic:

> A great variety of symptoms…indicating a compressed state of the brain [with]…the most frequent, as well as the most remarkable, are the following: Giddiness; dimness of sight; stupefaction; lots of voluntary motion; vomiting; an apoplectic stertor in the breathing; convulsive tremors in different muscles; a dilated state of the pupils, even when the eyes are exposed to a clear light; paralysis of different parts, especially of the side of the body opposite to the injured part of the head; involuntary evacuation of the urine and faeces; an oppressed, and in many case an irregular pulse….
>
> ***A System of Surgery*, Volume 3, Chapter X, Section III**[109]

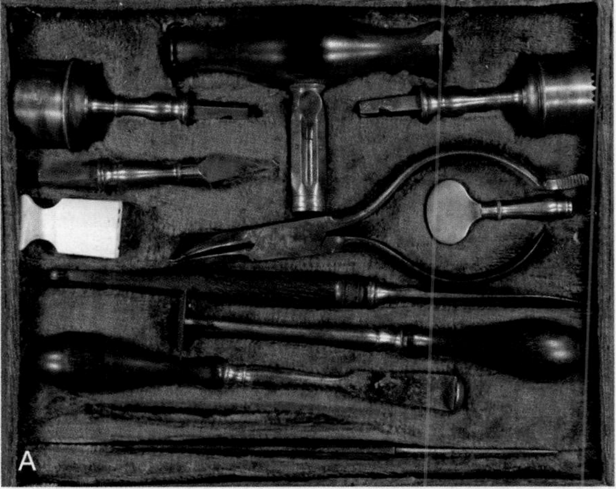

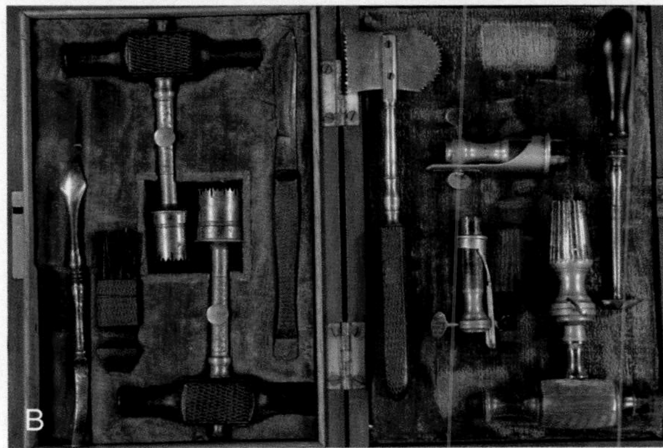

Figure 1-50. Nineteenth-century traveling trephine sets. A, An example of an early 19th-century traveling trephine set. This set was designed to be compact and easy to carry with changeable burrs of different sizes. This trephine set shows considerable use. **B,** Another example of a mid-19th-century traveling trephine set, in this case with additional different styles of hand trephines. On the right side is a Hey saw used for making craniectomies. The trephine bits on the right are a bit more elaborate, with adjustable center pins. *(Courtesy James Tait Goodrich, MD, PhD.)*

Bell was among the first to note that hydrocephalus was often associated with spina bifida. His treatment of a myelomeningocele involved placing a ligature around the base of the myelomeningocele sac and slowly cinching it down until it was allowed to slough off. Bell also noted that outcomes in these cases were almost always poor. The thoroughness and clarity of Bell's writings on the brain demonstrate why it was one of the most important and popular surgical works in this era.

In 1709 a small and now rare monograph was authored by **Daniel Turner** (1667-1741)[110]: A Remarkable Case in Surgery: *Wherein an Account Is Given of an Uncommon Fracture and Depression of the Skull, in a Child About Six Years Old; Accompanied with a Large Abscess or Aposteme upon the Brain….* This monograph provides a contemporary view of an 18th-century surgeon and the concerns of trephining the brain (Fig. 1-51).

Turner's case is most disturbing to read because it is written in the frank and somewhat verbose style of this period. Turner was " …called in much hast, to a Child about the Age of Six Years,…wounded by a Catstick (thrown by a youth who missed

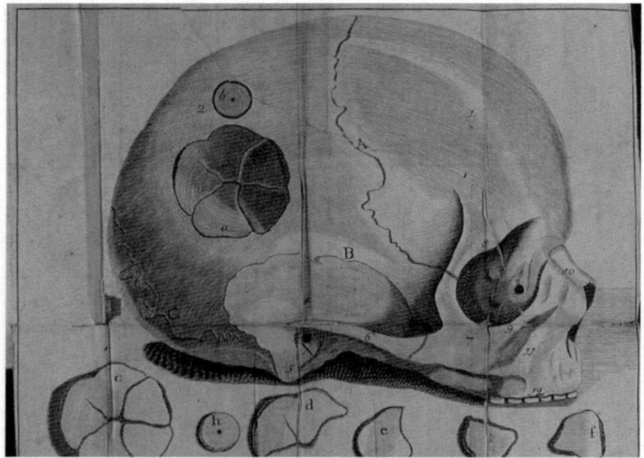

Figure 1-51. An illustration from Daniel Turner's book, *A Remarkable Case in Surgery….* In this book, Turner demonstrated the skull fracture and the elevation of the injury as described in the text. *(From Turner D.* A Remarkable Case in Surgery: Wherein an Account Is Given of an Uncommon Fracture and Depression of the Skull, in a Child About Six Years Old; Accompanied with a Large Abscess or Aposteme upon the Brain. With Other Practical Observations and Useful Reflections Thereupon. Also an exact Draught of the Case, Annex'd. And for the Entertainment of the Senior, but Instruction of the Junior Practitioners, Communicated. *London: R. Parker; 1709 [see p. 52 in Turner[110] for quotation]. Courtesy James Tait Goodrich, MD, PhD.)*

his aim) unfortunately struck the Child over the Head, and knock'd him down. He was taken up for dead and continued speechless for some time." On examination of the head, Turner found a considerable depression and believed that the child was in great danger. He sent for the barber to shave the child's head; while waiting for the barber, he performed a common practice by opening a vein in the arm to bleed the child, taking about 6 oz. The patient regained consciousness, complaining of a headache, and vomited. With this good response, Turner decided to delay surgery. The next day, he found the child still vomiting, restless, and feverish, and so he decided on an exploration of the wound. Through a typical X-shaped incision, he found bone driven into the brain:—"the Bones were beat thro' both meninges into the substance of the brain." Upon elevating the bone he found "a cavity sufficient to contain near two Ounces of Liquor." Postoperatively, the patient was awake with "a quick pulse, thirst and headache…but no vomiting. He was very sensible." Turner visited the child the following day and found him still feverish but without other symptoms. He removed the dressings and realized the extent of the fracture, which he now realized had been only partially elevated. Turner pulled out a trephine, surveyed the situation, and decided where it was safest to trephine. He removed what bone he thought was safe to remove and applied a clyster. The next day Turner called in a consultant, a Mr. Warden Herenden, to whom he showed the wound and the magnitude of the operation. Herenden was impressed with the extent of surgery and the condition of the wound, noting that despite all this, the patient complained only of a headache and was able "to walk about the Chamber."

This child was to go on and have several explorations for removal and drainage of pus. Surgical cannulas were placed for drainage, and the wound was carefully attended to; despite all this, the patient nonetheless died: "Thus did this little Hero, of truly Manly Courage, who had struggled under, and got thro' so many Difficulties,…at last decease, after Fourscore and four days"

This poignant little treatise perhaps gives the best example of an 18th-century effort at dealing with a head injury. Turner concluded "That wounds of the brain, are not always mortal" (see page 52 in Turner[110]).

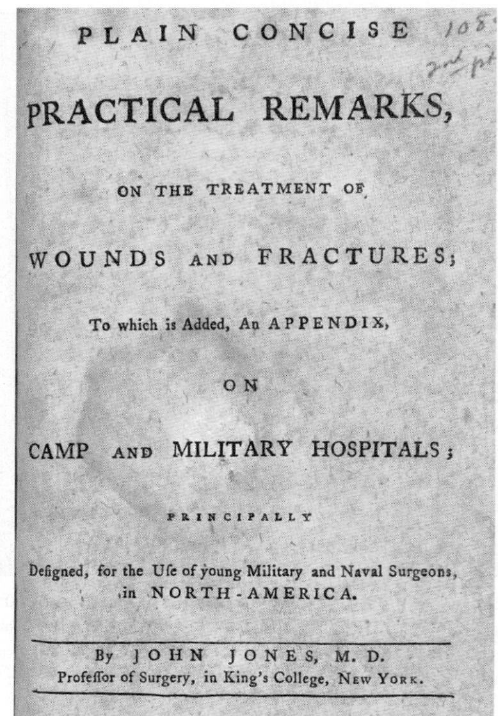

PLAIN CONCISE

PRACTICAL REMARKS,

ON THE TREATMENT OF

WOUNDS AND FRACTURES;

To which is Added, An APPENDIX,

ON

CAMP AND MILITARY HOSPITALS;

PRINCIPALLY

Deſigned, for the Uſe of young Military and Naval Surgeons, in NORTH-AMERICA.

By JOHN JONES, M. D.

Profeſſor of Surgery, in King's College, NEW YORK.

Figure 1-52. The title page from the first American textbook printed on surgery in the American Colonies. This book became the handbook for American Revolutionary War surgeons. *(From Jones J.* Plain Concise Practical Remarks, on the Treatment of Wounds and Fractures; to Which Is Added, an Appendix, on Camp and Military Hospitals; Principally Designed, for the Use of Young Military and Naval Surgeons, in North-America. *Philadelphia: Robert Bell; 1776 [Original work published 1775]. Courtesy James Tait Goodrich, MD, PhD.)*

An American surgeon who made an interesting contribution to neurosurgery was **John Jones** (1729-1791). In what is now a rare monograph, published in New York in 1776, this Revolutionary War–era surgeon provided the first American textbook on surgery.[111] Jones was educated in Europe; studied under Pott, Hunter, Alexander Monro, Petit, and Le Dran; and carried this education back to the United States. Jones was among the physicians to form the first medical school in America, the University of Pennsylvania, in Philadelphia. Jones was also one of the founders of New York Hospital. Jones's monograph on surgery became the handbook of surgery for Revolutionary War surgeons. His views and techniques on trephination clearly reflect the views of his European teachers, especially Pott, Le Dran, and Petit (Fig. 1-52).

In Europe, a number of important people were refining the art and skills of surgery. These physicians were important in leading surgical treatment away from the more common itinerant charlatan and barber-surgeon, most of whom were ignorant charm and relic dispensers. One of the most popular surgical textbooks of this century was published by a German surgeon, **Lorenz Heister** (1683-1758). Heister was educated as both a surgeon and an anatomist, which is now common. Heister began his lectures in Latin, but because his students were so uneducated, he changed to German. Heister went on to publish his first textbook in German.[112] The text was so popular that it was subsequently translated into a number of languages, including English, and circulated widely in Europe and England.[113] Because it

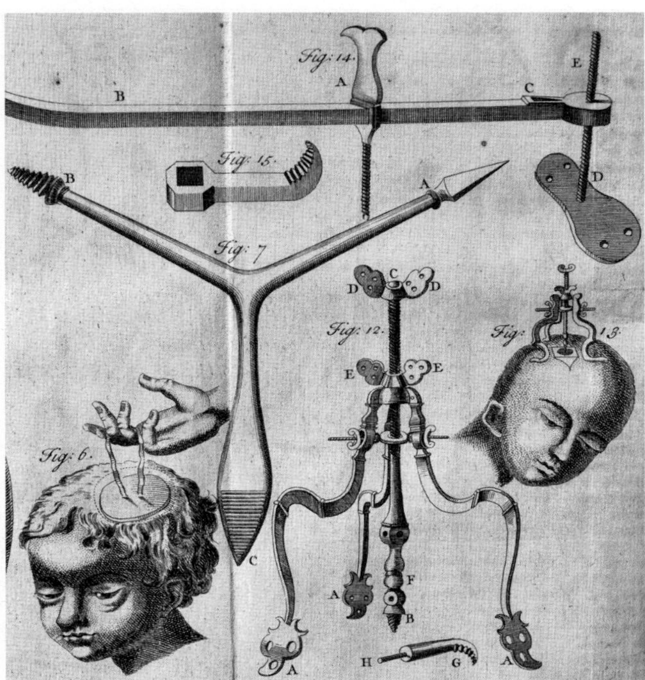

Figure 1-53. Some trephination instruments and tools for elevating depressed skull fractures. Text illustration from Heister's popular 18th-century textbook on surgery. *(From Heister L.* A General System of Surgery in Three Parts. *London: W. Innys; 1743. Courtesy James Tait Goodrich, MD, PhD.)*

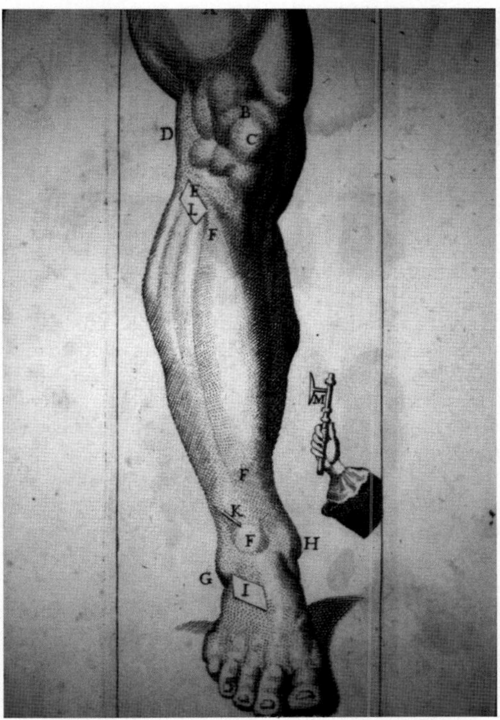

Figure 1-54. Illustration by Domenico Cotugno outlining the origins of sciatica. Cotugno was the first to describe cerebrospinal fluid and the first to demonstrate the "nervous" origins of sciatica, differentiating it from the then-common view that sciatica was secondary to arthritis. *(From Cotugno D.* De Ischiade Nervosa Commentarius. *Neapoli, Italy: Apud Fratres Simonios; 1764. Courtesy James Tait Goodrich, MD, PhD.)*

communicated a wide range of surgical knowledge and contained many practical surgical illustrations, bandaging techniques, and surgical techniques, this informative surgical text was widely used.

Heister would treat a head injury, but philosophically he remained conservative with regard to trephination. Following the earlier, more conservative views, he thought that trephination should be restricted to cases of skull fracture associated with depression. In wounds involving only concussion and contusion, he believed that trephination was too dangerous. Inasmuch as Heister was practicing during the pre-Listerian era, a period of very high risk of infection and injury to the brain, his convictions might have been pragmatic (Fig. 1-53):

> XXVII. But when the Cranium is so depressed, whether in Adults or Infants, as to suffer a Fracture, or Division of its Parts, it must instantly be relieved. The Part depressed, which adheres, after cleansing the Wound, must be restored to its Place; what is separated must be removed, and the extravasated Blood be drawn off through the Aperture…. [With regard to the use of "sneezing" (i.e. the Valsalva maneuver) in elevating depressed fractures] …the ill Consequences that attend this Practice are so grievous, that in my Opinion it ought to be rejected.
>
> **Book I, Chapter XIV, page 100**[114]

Heister popularized a number of techniques that proved helpful to contemporary surgeons. To control scalp hemorrhage, he used a "crooked needle and thread" that was weaved in and out of the scalp and then drawn tight. An astute observer, Heister pointed out that when the assistant applied pressure to the skin edge, bleeding could be markedly reduced. Heister's management of spinal injuries was aggressive: he would operate, expose the fractured vertebra, and then remove the fragments that had damaged the spinal marrow; he recognized that grave outcomes of such attempts were not uncommon and that the surgeon should be prepared for that.

An early and successful treatment of a brain abscess was accomplished by **Sauveur-François Morand** (1697-1773). Morand's patient, a monk, developed an otitis and subsequently mastoiditis, which led to a temporal brain abscess.[115] Morand trephined over the carious bone and discovered pus. He then placed a catgut wick into the open surgical wound, but it continued to drain. He reopened the wound, this time performing a very adventurous maneuver of opening the dura through a cruciate incision, and found a brain abscess. He explored the abscess with his finger, removing as much of the contents as he could, and then instilled balsam and turpentine into the cavity. He placed a silver tube for drainage, and as the wound healed, he slowly withdrew the tube. The abscess healed, the patient survived, and Morand reported this case as a successful treatment of a brain abscess.

The Neapolitan physician **Domenico Cotugno** (1736-1822) published a monograph of only 100 pages, *De Ischiade Nervosa Commentarius*, which contains the first classic descriptions of cerebrospinal fluid and sciatica.[116] Cotugno performed a number of experiments on the cadavers of approximately 20 adults. Using a lumbar puncture technique, he was able to demonstrate the characteristics of cerebrospinal fluid. In *De Ischiade Nervosa Commentarius*, Cotugno demonstrated the "nervous" origin of sciatica, differentiating it from arthritis, which was the explanation prevalent at that time. Cotugno discovered the pathways of cerebrospinal fluid, showing that it circulated in the pia-arachnoid interstices and flowed throughout the brain and spinal cord via the aqueduct and convexities. Cotugno also described hydrocephalus ex vacuo, the type of hydrocephalus that occurs in cerebral atrophy (Fig. 1-54).

A popular and skilled French military surgeon was **Louis Sébastien Saucerotte** (1741-1814) (also listed as Nicolas). Saucerotte was at one time surgeon to the King of Poland and then a military surgeon in various French Army units. As has often been the case in the history of neurological surgery, the occasion to deal with war injuries provided the most training and insight into the management of head injury. Saucerotte reintroduced the concept of the contrecoup injury, lost since antiquity. In his surgical textbook *Mélanges de Chirurgie*,[117] he described a series of intracranial injuries and their symptoms, including compression of brain as a result of blood clot. Saucerotte described a classic case of ataxia caused by a cerebellar lesion, whose symptoms included opisthotonus and rolling of the eyes. Saucerotte divided the brain into "areas" of injury, pointing out that injury at the base of the brain produces the most severe debilitation, whereas injuries of the forebrain are the best tolerated. Saucerotte also contributed one of the earliest clinical descriptions of acromegaly.

The close of the 18th century brought some remarkable change in philosophy about surgery of the brain. Surgeons' management of head injury became much more aggressive. Clinical symptoms associated with brain injury were better recognized. Anatomic concepts such as the circulation of cerebrospinal fluid were better understood. What surgeons still lacked was a better understanding of cerebral localization, methods to treat surgical infection, and the ability to provide insensibility to pain during surgery. The role of trephination for head injuries was being fiercely debated in the surgical literature. There was a backlash because of the inability of surgeons to distinguish between the lack of efficacy of the operation and the introduction of infection by a surgical procedure. As a result of iatrogenic infection, the outcomes often seemed better without surgery than with intervention, especially if a surgical infection developed. The developments of the 19th century included cerebral localization, anesthesia, and antisepsis, all critical in the origins of modern neurosurgery.

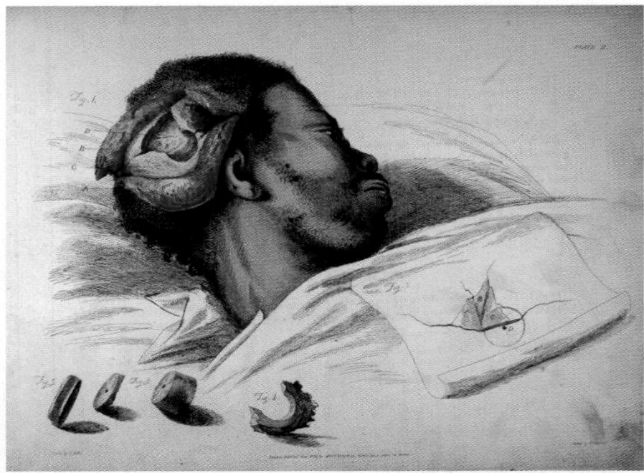

Figure 1-55. Hand-drawn illustration by Sir Charles Bell of a severe open head injury with a depressed skull fracture. A series of trephinations have been performed, and the bone fragments can be seen in the lower left of the image. *(From Bell C.* Illustrations of the Great Operations of Surgery…. *London: Printed for Longman, et al; 1821:iv. Courtesy James Tait Goodrich, MD, PhD.)*

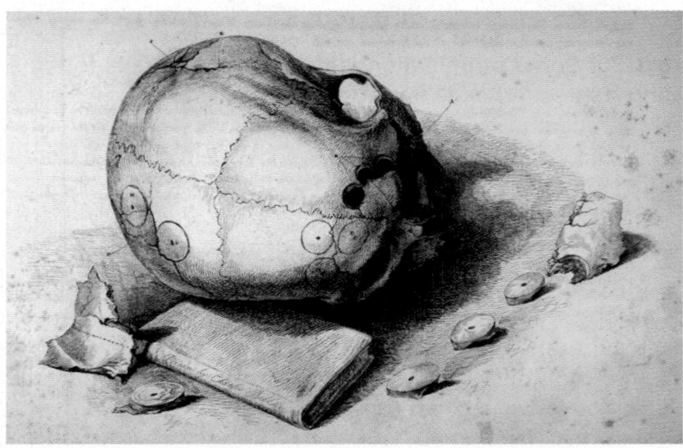

Figure 1-56. Sir Charles Bell's illustrations of "safe" areas of the skull. Bell believed that there were areas in which use of the trephine was safe and areas in which it was quite dangerous. In this skull, Bell outlined areas that are safe; of further interest is that the opinions offered here differ little from those in Hippocrates' original writings. *(From Bell C.* Illustrations of the Great Operations of Surgery…. *London: Printed for Longman, et al; 1821:iv. Courtesy James Tait Goodrich, MD, PhD.)*

NINETEENTH CENTURY: INCUNABULA PERIOD OF MODERN NEUROSURGERY

Modern neurosurgery began with three important developments that occurred in the 19th century. The first was the introduction of anesthesia, which provided patients freedom from pain during surgery. The second was the introduction of cerebral localization (neurological signs and symptoms), which helped surgeons establish diagnoses and plan their operative approach. The third was the introduction of antisepsis and aseptic technique, which enabled the surgeon to operate with a reduced risk of perioperative complications resulting from infection.

A noted medical and surgical expert in this period was **Sir Charles Bell** (1774-1842), a Scottish surgeon and anatomist. Bell was educated at the University of Edinburgh and spent most of his professional career in practice in London. Bell is remembered for his many contributions to the neurosciences, including the differentiation of the motor and sensory component of the spinal root. Bell wrote a number of works on surgery, many of which were illustrated with his own drawings. These surgical drawings remain unrivaled in detail, accuracy, and beauty (Figs. 1-55 and 1-56)[118]:

> If a drawing of all that we see in an operation, be an imperfect demonstration, so is the lesson of an operation performed on the dead body imperfect, for the circumstances most essential to know, cannot be presented there: so is the actual operation on the living body an imperfect demonstration, from the partial and rapid view which the spectator obtains. And, finally, as to description, words alone will never inform the young Surgeon of the things most necessary to a safe operation.

Bell provided a skillful contemporary account[119] of a trephination technique as practiced in 1821:

> Let the bed or couch on which the patient is lying be turned to the light—have the head shaved—put a wax-cloth on the pillow—let the pillow be firm, to support the patient's head. Put tow [sic] or sponge by the side of the head—let there be a stout assistant to hold the patient's head firmly, and let others put their hands on his arms and knees.
>
> The surgeon will expect the instruments to be handed to him in this succession—the scalpel; the rasparatory; the trephine; the brush, the quill, and probe, from time to time; the elevator, the forceps, the lenticular.

Combined with his detailed description of trephination is a discussion of techniques and pitfalls to avoid. The hand-colored illustrations that accompany the text are quite dramatic in detail and are designed to assist the surgeon in mastering the technique.

Bell's work is an important work in providing illustrations of detailed neurosurgical technique.

Over the previous centuries, surgeons had tried various methods of reducing sensibility to pain, with minimal success. Mandrake, *Cannabis*, opium and other narcotics, the "soporific sponge" (saturated with opium), and alcohol had all been tried. In 1844, **Horace Wells** (1815-1848), a dentist in Hartford, Connecticut, introduced the use of nitrous oxide in dental procedures, and for the first time, a good anesthetic result was achieved.[120] Unfortunately, the death of one of his patients from what was probably an overdose of the anesthetic stopped him from investigating further. In Boston, another early investigator, **William T. G. Morton** (1819-1868), also a dentist and an early collaborator with Wells, persuaded a surgeon, **Dr. John C. Warren** (1778-1856), to use ether to induce anesthesia. On October 16, 1846, Warren did so and produced a state of insensibility in a patient, during which a vascular tumor of the submaxillary region was removed.[121]

In the United Kingdom another surgeon, **James Young Simpson** (1811-1870), was using another agent called chloroform that had just been introduced in 1847 as an anesthetic agent.[122] The contemporary literature was full of arguments then being pursued regarding the issue of which was the best agent. Morton turned out to be quite bold by patenting the ether technique and then asking the U.S. Congress for compensation for his discovery of ether and its use in surgery. Politics aside, the result of all of this research was the first opportunity for a surgeon to operate on a patient without the need for heavy restraints on the patient or for the physician to operate at unsafe speed. As a result, patients gained freedom from pain during the procedure, along with a new lack of fear of surgery—developments whose importance cannot be underestimated in a surgery practice and particularly in the treatment of brain lesions.

Early surgeons approached either a skull or brain injury with great trepidation. Even with the best of surgical technique, patients often died postoperatively of suppuration and infection. Fevers, purulent material, brain abscess, and draining wounds all defeated the best surgeons. No surgeon could hope to invade or open the dura mater without inviting disaster until the risk of operative infection could be reduced. The first significant change came about when **Sir Joseph Lister** (1827-1912), using concepts developed by medical practitioners, introduced antisepsis in the operating room.[123,124] In a different operating arena, **Oliver Wendell Holmes, Sr.** (1809-1894), and **Ignaz G. Semmelweis** (1818-1865) first showed that it was the contaminated hands of the obstetrician that spread puerperal fever, a devastating infection for women during delivery.[125,126] Holmes and Semmelweiss strongly argued for hand washing between cases, a concept that became bitterly debated at the time. To provide a contrast, it is beneficial to understand the typical conditions in which mid-19th century obstetricians worked. The obstetrician typically entered an operating room wearing a black cloth coat, soaked in old blood and grime from his many deliveries. The table on which the soon-to-be-born baby was to be delivered was rarely cleaned, much less sterilized. These conditions easily led to the spread of multiple organisms on hands, instruments, and table surfaces, and many women died in childbirth of puerperal fever. The infection and contagion concepts developed by **Louis Pasteur** (1822-1895) and **Robert Koch** (1843-1910) and their introduction to antisepsis and aseptic technique revolutionized surgery. By using an aseptic technique in a clean operating theater, a surgeon operating on the brain or skull could complete the surgery with a significant reduction in surgical infection.

Diagnosing a brain lesion or localizing a brain injury was not meaningful until the concept of neurological localization was formulated. In the 1860s, several investigators, including **Gustav T. Fritsch** (1838-1927) and **Eduard Hitzig** (1838-1907), as well as **Paul Broca** (1824-1880), first introduced the concept that each part of the brain corresponded to a particular function.[127-129] In 1861, during the autopsy of a patient with an expressive aphasia, Broca clarified within the brain the area of speech localization.[128] Later **Carl Wernicke** (1848-1905) identified a different area of the brain in which speech was associated with conduction defects.[130] These studies led to an explosion of research on the brain, with further investigations involving electrical stimulation in work pioneered by **David Ferrier** (1843-1928) and **John Hughlings Jackson** (1835-1911). Jackson is now considered the founder of modern neurology.[131,132] Both physicians demonstrated important areas of brain function by means of electrical studies and developed an understanding of epilepsy. The study of neurology received its greatest impetus in this period. The neurological examination now became a rigorous study designed to uncover subtle anatomic and physiologic findings, which in turn provided a surgical map for the surgeon to plan incision and exploration.

The surgical luminaries of the 19th century were quite varied and talented. Until the end of the 19th century, neurosurgery was still not specialized; such operations were still performed by general surgeons. By the middle of the 19th century, the distinction between brain concussion and compression was accepted. In 1841, **William Sharp** (1805-1896), a homeopathic physician, published a short monograph titled *Practical Observations on Injuries of the Head*.[133] He provided a modern definition of concussion as "a loss of function without change in structure." Sharp advised against trephining in concussion because there was no extravasated blood to remove and the procedure would not prevent inflammation. He notes that the middle meningeal artery is the usual source of an epidural hematoma and concluded his monograph with an interesting review of Percivall Pott's earlier surgical experience of head injuries. In Pott's 43 reported cases, 29 underwent surgery, of whom 17 recovered and 12 died. Of the 14 patients who did not undergo surgery, 2 recovered and 12 died.

Sir Jonathan Hutchinson (1828-1913) provided an important chapter in the acceptance of neurological signs and symptoms as indicators for surgical intervention. In 1867, the same year that Lister published his first papers on the role of antisepsis in surgery, Hutchinson published a series of papers on brain compression that introduced a new diagnostic sign for head injury.[134] His recognition of third nerve paralysis remains one of the most useful signs for head injury and increased intracranial pressure. Coupled with the recognition of a lucid interval after head trauma, it provided an important neurological sign to enable surgeons to recognize the need for trephining. Hutchinson also argued that a pupil that was fixed and dilated was likely to indicate the side of the hematoma. For the first time in 350 years, since a 16th century artist (Gerzdorf, 1517[64]) recorded this observation, the mechanism and significance of this finding was established. Hutchinson wrote as follows[134]:

> ...from the position of the clot there can be little doubt that the third nerve is compressed and thus, the dilatation of the pupil is explained. These two cases, so exactly parallel, seem to supply us with a new and very valuable symptom indicative of effusion of blood in this situation.

He went on modestly to note,

> ...nor can we boast of having learnt much which may aid us in the diagnosis of future cases, with the one exception of having discovered the meaning of the one dilated pupil. This point we will store up carefully for future use."[134]

Sir Rickman J. Godlee (1849-1925) performed one of the most celebrated of operations, the removal of a brain tumor, the first to be successfully diagnosed by cerebral localization in 1885.[135] The patient had suffered for 3 years from focal motor seizures. They started as focal seizures of the face and proceeded to involve the arm and then the leg. In the 3 months before

CASE OF CEREBRAL TUMOUR.

BY

A. HUGHES BENNETT, M.D., F.R.C.P.,

PHYSICIAN TO THE HOSPITAL FOR EPILEPSY AND PARALYSIS, AND ASSISTANT PHYSICIAN TO THE WESTMINSTER HOSPITAL.

THE SURGICAL TREATMENT

BY

RICKMAN J. GODLEE, M.S., F.R.C.S.,

SURGEON TO UNIVERSITY COLLEGE HOSPITAL.

Received January 13th—Read May 12th, 1885.

THE chief features of interest in the case, to which the attention of the Society is directed, are, that during life the existence of a tumour was diagnosed in the brain, and its situation localised, entirely by the signs and symptoms exhibited, without any external manifestations on the surface of the skull. This growth was removed without any immediate injurious effects on the intelligence and general condition of the patient. Although he died four weeks after the operation, the fatal termination was due, not to any special effects on the nervous centres, but to a secondary surgical complication. The case, moreover, teaches some important physiological, pathological, and clinical lessons, and suggests practical reflections which may prove useful to future medicine and surgery.

Figure 1-57. A celebrated case in the history of neurosurgery. In this publication, Sir Rickman J. Godlee, a neurologist, described cerebral localization techniques used to determine where the tumor might lie in the brain. Under the direction of the neurologist, a prominent British surgeon performed the craniectomy, located the tumor, and successfully removed it—an important landmark in neurosurgery. *(From Bennett AH, Godlee RJ. Case of cerebral tumor.* Med Chir Trans. *1885;68:243-245. Courtesy James Tait Goodrich, MD, PhD.)*

A CASE

OF

TUMOUR OF THE SPINAL CORD.

REMOVAL; RECOVERY.

BY

W. R. GOWERS, M.D., F.R.S.,

AND

VICTOR HORSLEY, B.S., F.R.S.

Received March 8th—Read June 12th, 1888.

Medical History of the Case, by Dr. GOWERS.

CAPT. G—, æt. 42, had good health until the year 1884. There was no history of syphilis. During 1883 and 1884 he endured much mental anxiety, and in the latter year he had a considerable mental shock—his wife was knocked down and run over in his presence, and he was able to save himself from a similar fate only by suddenly throwing himself backwards. Soon afterwards he began to suffer from a dull pain across the lower part of the back, which he thought was due to the strain of the accident. This pain passed away in the course of a few weeks and did not return. In June, 1884, he first felt a peculiar pain that was the most

Figure 1-58. William R. Gowers and Victor Horsley described the first diagnosis, localization, and then successful removal of a spinal cord tumor in 1888. *(From Gowers WR, Horsley V. A case of tumour of the spinal cord. Removal, recovery.* Med Chir Trans. *1888;71:377-428. Courtesy James Tait Goodrich, MD, PhD.)*

surgery, the patient also developed weakness and eventually had to give up his work. Working with a neurologist, Alexander H. Bennett (1848-1901), Godlee was able to localize the tumor and remove it. This case was an important landmark in neurosurgery. For the first time a neurologist, basing his conclusions on the findings from a neurological examination, localized a brain tumor and enabled it to be removed surgically. Godlee made an incision over the Rolandic area, and through a small cortical incision, the tumor was removed. The patient survived the surgery with some mild weakness and did well, only to die 1 month after surgery from a wound infection. Added to the importance of the surgery itself was the presence in the operating room of three important scholars: A. Hughes Bennett, a prominent English physician, and the two neurologists J. Hughlings Jackson and David Ferrier. These men were extremely interested in whether the cerebral localization studies were to provide good results in the operating theatre. This operation was the impetus that truly moved neurosurgery forward (Fig. 1-57).

Three years later, in 1888, **Victor Horsley** (1857-1916) performed the first removal of a spinal cord tumor that had been diagnosed and localized by **William R. Gowers** (1845-1915).[136] Horsley performed a laminectomy on Gowers's patient, Captain Golby. Golby was slowly losing function in his legs as the result of a spinal cord tumor. Gowers localized the tumor by examination and suggested to Horsley where to operate; the tumor was successfully removed. A postoperative photograph of the patient with a healed midline thoracic scar is included in the original paper (Fig. 1-58).

William R. Gowers was one of an extraordinary group of English neurologists of that era. Using some of the recently developed techniques in physiology and pathology, he made great strides in refining the concept of cerebral localization. Gowers was noted for the clarity and organization of his writing, works that remain classics in the field.[137,138] Studies such as these allowed surgeons to consider operating on the central nervous system for nonheroic reasons. Godlee and Horsley were trained general surgeons who had both the ambition and fortitude to consider surgically exploring the central nervous system now that our neurology colleagues could localize the tumors.

The successful removal of a spinal tumor brought Horsley to the forefront in the development of neurosurgery during its birthing period. Horsley began his experimental studies on the brain in the early 1880s, at the height of the cerebral localization controversies. Using faradic stimulation, he worked with Sir Edward A. Sharpey-Schafer (1850-1935) in analyzing and localizing motor functions in the cerebral cortex, internal capsule, and spinal cord of primates.[139] In a classic study (Croonian Lectures 1891)[140] performed with his brother-in-law, Francis Gotch (1853-1913), Horsley, using a string galvanometer, showed that electrical currents originate in the brain. These electrical currents were propagated from the brain out through the nerves.[140] These intraoperative experimental studies showed Horsley that localization was possible and that operations on the brain could be conducted safely with techniques adapted from general surgery (Fig. 1-59).

Horsley was a very fast and deft surgeon, typically performing the most complex surgeries in less than 40 minutes. He carried

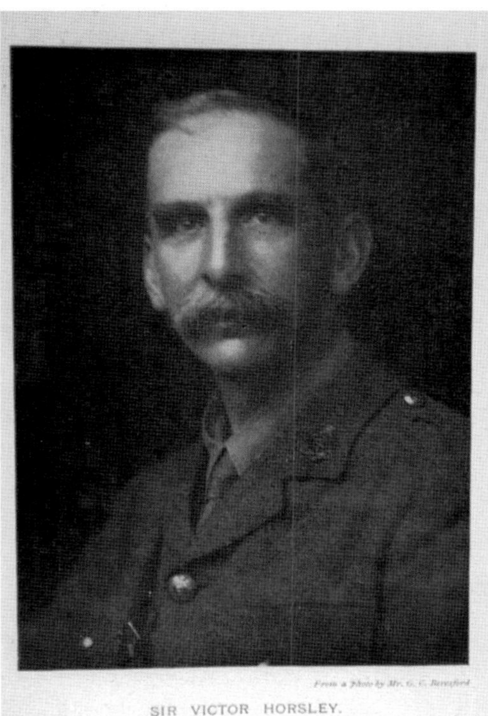

Figure 1-59. Victor Horsley. This photograph dates from his World War I military experience and was taken shortly before he died during the war from severe hyperpyrexia. *(Courtesy James Tait Goodrich, MD, PhD.)*

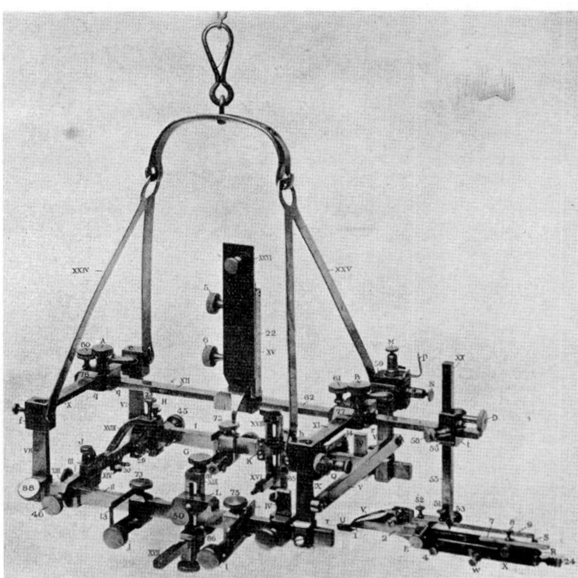

Figure 1-60. Stereotactic frame for performing localized brain lesions in animals. Victor Horsley provided a number of original scientific contributions to our literature. Horsley and Robert H. Clarke were the first to develop a stereotactic frame for performing localized brain lesions in animals. Although this frame was never used on humans or for human studies, it did serve as a prototype for the stereotactic frames developed in the 1940s for humans. *(From Horsley V, Clarke RH. The structure and functions of the cerebellum examined by a new method.* Brain. *18;31:45-124. Courtesy James Tait Goodrich, MD, PhD.)*

a trunk full of surgical instruments, sterilized the night before at his home. The surgery was often performed in the bedroom of the patient.

Horsley made a number of technical contributions to neurosurgery, including the use of beeswax to stop bone bleeding.[141,142] He performed one of the earliest operations for craniostenosis and relief of increased intracranial pressure. The patient, a child, had a premature closure of the anterior fontanelle. The child survived and went on to serve in World War I. For trigeminal neuralgia, Horsley pioneered the technique of sectioning the posterior root of the trigeminal nerve for pain relief, the first effective treatment for this relentless condition.[143] Using his technical gifts, he helped Robert H. Clarke (1850-1926), a physiologist, design the first useful stereotaxic apparatus for brain surgery. The apparatus was designed to localize a series of numerical coordinates (three-dimensional cartesian coordinates) associated with specific areas of the brain. In the original description, the authors coined the term *stereotaxis*, which is derived from the Greek *steros*, meaning "three-dimensional," and *taxis*, which refers to an "an order or arrangement." Although this apparatus was used only on animals, the Horsley-Clark stereotaxic frame remains the standard concept on which all subsequent stereotactic designs/frames have been based[144] (Fig. 1-60).

At the age of 59, with the onset of World War I, Horsley was sent to Amara, Mesopotamia (Iraq), to help develop hygienic procedures in a desert outpost. Ironically, he died within 2 days of arrival after contracting a severe desert fever (reported outside temperature, 120° F), an early tragic loss of a brilliant mind and surgeon. Horsley was one of those talented scholars who were able to combine experimental research with clinical practice and in turn provided remarkable advances in neurosurgery.

William Macewen (1848-1924), a Scottish surgeon and pioneer in the field of neurosurgery, successfully accomplished one of the early brain operations on July 29, 1879.[145] Macewen operated on a 14-year-old patient, removing a periosteal tumor over the right eye. Using meticulous technique and the recently developed neurological examination, he localized the tumor and removed it. The patient lived 8 years afterwards, only to die of Bright's disease; at autopsy, no tumor was detected. By 1888, Macewen had operated on 21 neurosurgical cases with only 3 deaths and 18 successful recoveries: a remarkable turnabout from earlier studies. Macewen's monograph, published in 1893, on pyogenic infections of the brain and their surgical treatment represented a revolution in neurosurgery.[146] This monograph was the earliest to deal with the successful treatment of brain abscess. His morbidity and mortality statistics, reflecting the application of localization techniques and effective antisepsis, were not inferior to those in any series reported today. Without good surgical results, neurologists of that era were hesitant to recommend surgery; Macewen helped immensely to make the case for soundly conducted operations on the brain (Figs. 1-61 and 1-62):

> Though not sharing the hopelessness of the opinion expressed in 1883 by a distinguished neurologist as to the inutility of operations on the brain undertaken for abscess, the author was then inclined to take a more sombre view of the prospects of recovery from such operations than his subsequent experience has proven to be necessary. He now regards an uncomplicated cerebral abscess, early recognized, accurately localized, and promptly operated on, as one of the most satisfactory of all intracranial lesions, the patient being at once relieved from a perilous condition, and usually restored to sound health
>
> **—from the Preface to Pyogenic Infections**[146]

The concept of "early recognized, accurately localized, and promptly operated on" is still a fundamental concept for neurosurgeons.

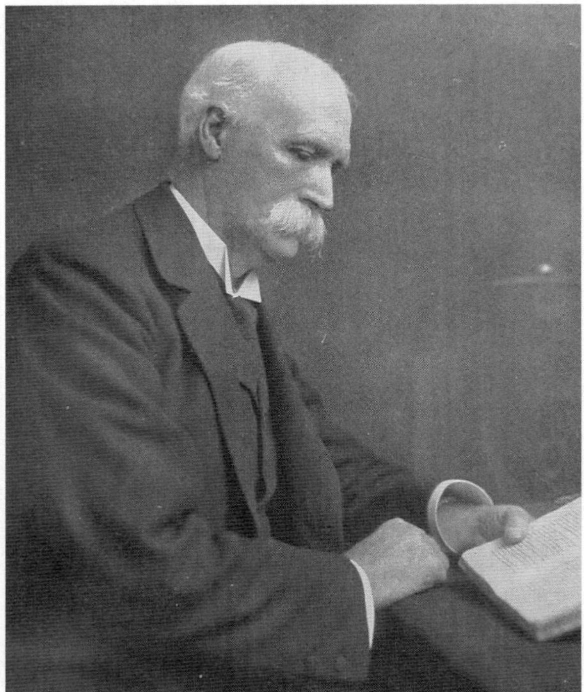

Figure 1-61. William Macewen. Macewen developed sterile surgical techniques that remained among the best in the literature for nearly 50 years. *(Courtesy James Tait Goodrich, MD, PhD.)*

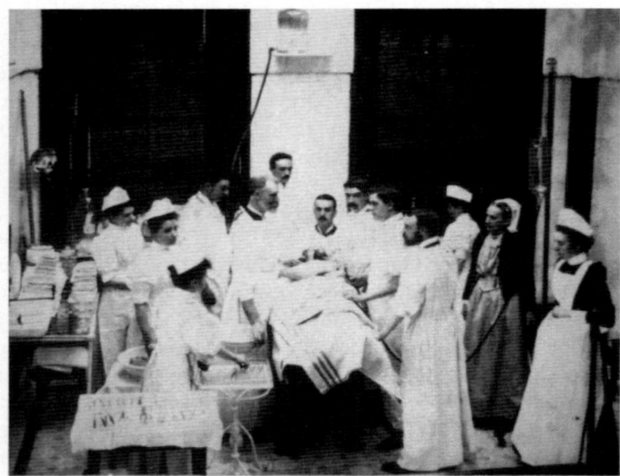

Figure 1-62. William Macewen in the operating room. He is the bearded gentleman on the patient's right side, surrounded by his staff. Although not gloved and masked, they were using sterile principles in the operating room, including the Lister carbolic sprayer, clean gowns, and clean hands. *(Courtesy James Tait Goodrich, MD, PhD.)*

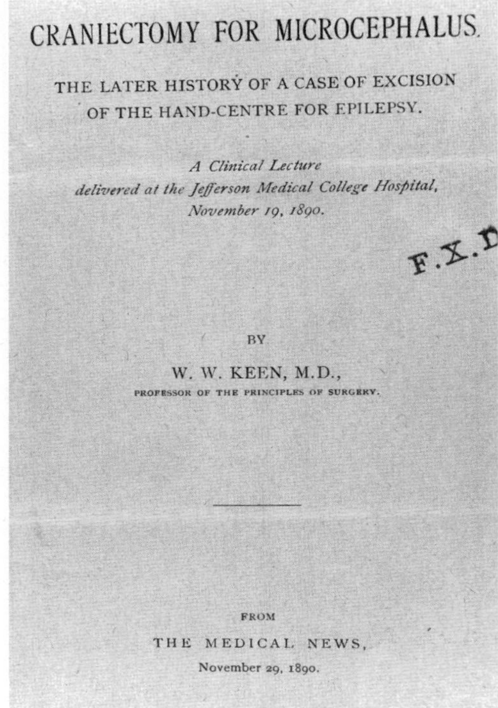

CRANIECTOMY FOR MICROCEPHALUS.

THE LATER HISTORY OF A CASE OF EXCISION OF THE HAND-CENTRE FOR EPILEPSY.

A Clinical Lecture delivered at the Jefferson Medical College Hospital, November 19, 1890.

F.X.D

BY

W. W. KEEN, M.D.,

PROFESSOR OF THE PRINCIPLES OF SURGERY.

FROM

THE MEDICAL NEWS,

November 29, 1890.

Figure 1-63. Title page of William W. Keen's paper on the treatment of microcephaly. Keen was one of the great pioneers in early American neurosurgery and is little recognized today. An early advocate of Listerian aseptic techniques, he made some important contributions to surgery, particularly in neurosurgery. One of the earliest techniques developed for multisuture craniosynostosis is discussed in this paper. *(From Keen WW.* Linear Craniotomy. *Philadelphia: Lea Bros. and Co.; 1891 [Original work published 1890]. Courtesy James Tait Goodrich, MD, PhD.)*

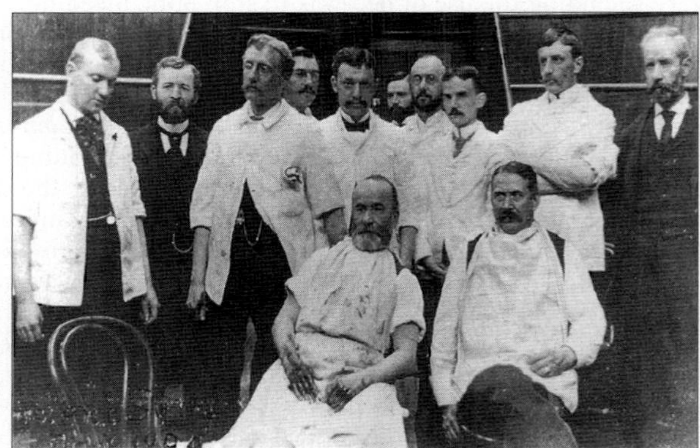

Figure 1-64. William W. Keen in the operating room with his surgical team. Note Keen's "bloody" ungloved hands and the lack of mask and head covering. *(Courtesy James Tait Goodrich, MD, PhD.)*

In the United States, among the earliest pioneers in neurosurgery was **William W. Keen** (1837-1932), professor of surgery at Jefferson Medical College in Philadelphia. Keen was one of the strongest American advocates for the use of the recently introduced Listerian antiseptic techniques in surgery. The concept of surgical bacteriology, along with those of asepsis and antisepsis, was aggressively discussed in his writings.[147] One of the earliest American monographs on neurosurgery was prepared by Keen, a book called *Linear Craniotomy*.[148] He developed a technique for treatment of spastic torticollis by division of spinal accessory nerve and posterior roots of the first, second, and third spinal nerves.[149] For treatment of the excoriating pain associated with trigeminal neuralgia, he devised a technique for resection of the gasserian ganglion.[150] Keen exercised a rare inventiveness in surgical technique: he used bent spoons from his kitchen to act as brain retractors. Keen was also the first to introduce the Gigli saw to American surgeons, an important technical advance in performing a craniotomy[151] (Figs. 1-63 and 1-64).

A professor of surgery in Berlin, **Fedor Krause** (1857-1937), was a general surgeon who developed a keen interest in neurosurgery. Krause's three-volume atlas on neurosurgery,[152] published in the first decade of the 20th century, was among the first surgical textbooks to provide detailed illustrated techniques of neurosurgery. Digital extirpation of a meningioma is graphically described. A number of neurosurgical techniques are reviewed, including resection of scar tissue for treatment of epilepsy. Krause was an early pioneer in the extradural approach to the gasserian ganglion for treatment of trigeminal neuralgia (Figs. 1-65 and 1-66).

The first American monograph devoted solely to brain surgery was written, not by a neurosurgeon, but by a New York neurologist, **Moses Allen Starr** (1854-1932).[153] Starr was Professor of Nervous Diseases at Columbia and an American leader in the field of neurology. He trained in Europe, working in the laboratories of Wilhelm Erb, Friedrich Schultze, Theodor Meynert, Hermann Nothnagel, Jean-Marie Charcot, and Sigmund Freud. These experiences provided him with a strong foundation in neurological diagnosis (Fig. 1-67). Starr was present at the 1888 Congress of American Physicians and Surgeons when David Ferrier and Victor Horsley presented a symposium dealing with recent findings on the cerebral localization of brain function. In the late 1880s, Starr began working closely with Charles McBurney (1845-1913), a general surgeon in New York City,[154,155] and the two became important collaborators. Starr realized quickly that brain surgery not only could be performed safely but was clearly necessary in treatment of certain neurological problems. Before this collaboration, the only brain surgeries being performed in New York were cases of visible tumors and injuries of the scalp and skull, such as a fungating tumor of the skull or a depressed skull fracture. Of interest is that McBurney performed the first antiseptic surgical procedure in the United States at the Presbyterian Hospital in New York City in 1876. Starr's book describes cases involving epilepsy, hemorrhage, abscess, and tumors (see Fig. 1-67).

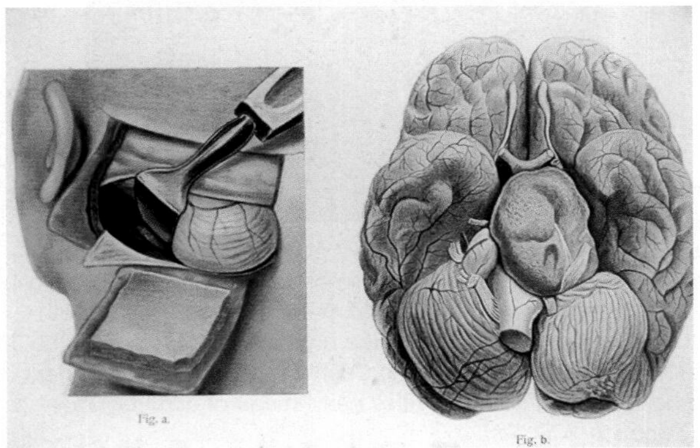

Figure 1-65. One of the earliest cerebellopontine angle approaches for removing an acoustic neuroma. Both the surgical approach and the anatomy of the tumor in relation to the seventh and eighth cranial nerves are clearly outlined in the image on the right. *(From Krause F.* Surgery of the Brain and Spinal Cord Based on Personal Experiences *[Haubold H, M. Thorek M, Trans.]. New York: Rebman Co.; 19-1912. Courtesy James Tait Goodrich, MD, PhD.)*

Starr summarized his views in the preface of his book on *Brain Surgery*[153]:

> Brain surgery is at present a subject both novel and interesting. It is within the past five years only that operations for the relief of epilepsy and of imbecility, for the removal of clots from the brain, for the opening of abscesses, for the excision of tumors, and the relief of intra-cranial pressure have been generally attempted.... Brain surgery has as its essential basis the accurate diagnosis of cerebral lesions, which was impossible until the localization of cerebral functions had been determined. And this diagnosis must be made by the physician before the surgeon is called in to remove the disease. It is the object of this book to state clearly those facts regarding the essential features of brain disease which will enable the reader to determine in any case both the nature and situation of the pathological process in progress, to settle the question whether the disease can be removed by surgical interference, and to estimate the safety and probability of success by operation. The facts have been reached by a careful study of the literature of the subject and by a considerable personal experience.... It is my hope that this work may aid the physician to diagnosticate brain diseases with more accuracy, and to select such cases as are properly open to surgical treatment by trephining, and also that may enable the surgeon to perform his delicate task with more precision and with a fuller knowledge of those principles of local diagnosis which should form this constant guide.

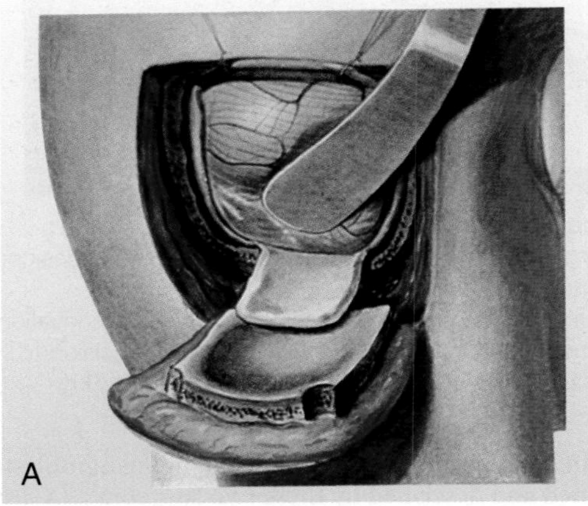

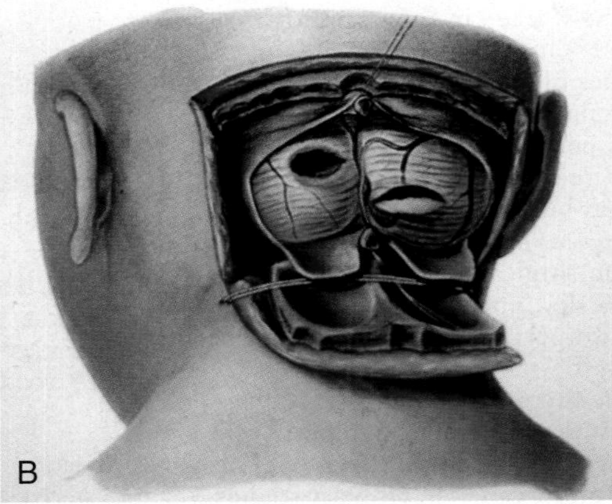

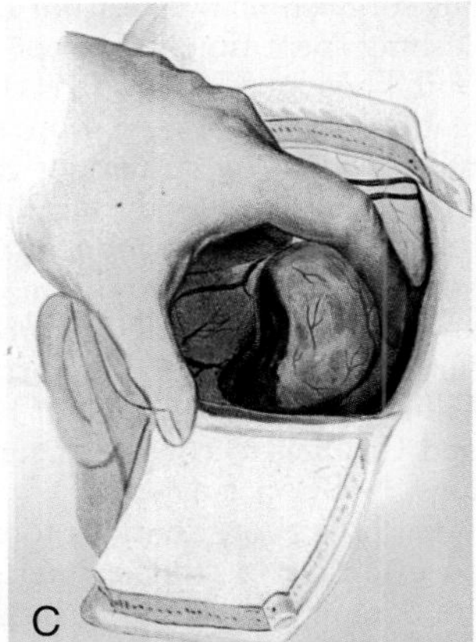

Figure 1-66. Fedor Krause's "osteoplastic" flap technique. Krause was a firm advocate of this technique, in which the craniotomy was elevated with the overlying muscle and scalp. Krause performed a unilateral craniotomy to expose the cerebellum **(A** and **B)**. On reaching the tumor, Krause removed it **(C)** by taking his index finger and scooping the tumor out. *(From Krause F.* Surgery of the Brain and Spinal Cord Based on Personal Experiences *[Haubold H, Thorek M, Trans.]. New York: Rebman Co.; 19-1912. Courtesy James Tait Goodrich, MD, PhD.)*

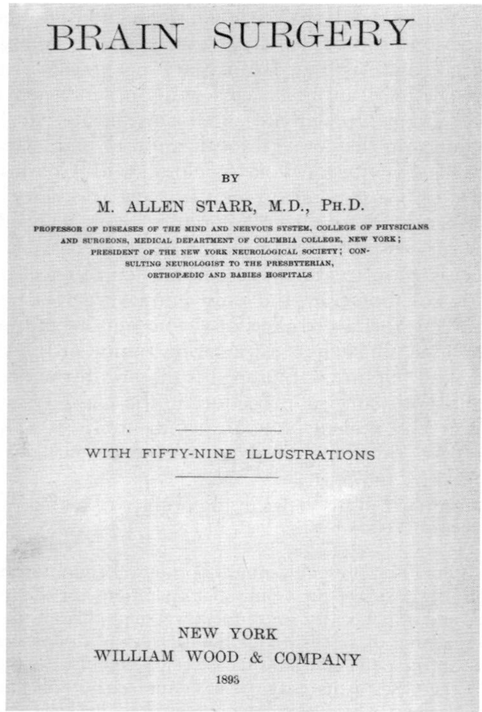

BRAIN SURGERY

BY

M. ALLEN STARR, M.D., PH.D.

PROFESSOR OF DISEASES OF THE MIND AND NERVOUS SYSTEM, COLLEGE OF PHYSICIANS AND SURGEONS, MEDICAL DEPARTMENT OF COLUMBIA COLLEGE, NEW YORK; PRESIDENT OF THE NEW YORK NEUROLOGICAL SOCIETY; CONSULTING NEUROLOGIST TO THE PRESBYTERIAN, ORTHOPÆDIC AND BABIES HOSPITALS

WITH FIFTY-NINE ILLUSTRATIONS

NEW YORK
WILLIAM WOOD & COMPANY
1893

Figure 1-67. Title page of Moses Allen Starr's 1893 publication. The first monograph on brain surgery to be published in the United States was authored by a neurologist, not a neurosurgeon. Starr, a neurologist at the New York Neurological Institute, could have easily been a neurosurgeon as he was one of the earliest and strongest advocates of exploring of the brain on the basis of a thorough neurological examination at the patient's bedside. *(From Starr MA.* Brain Surgery. *New York: William Wood and Co.; 1893. Courtesy James Tait Goodrich, MD, PhD.)*

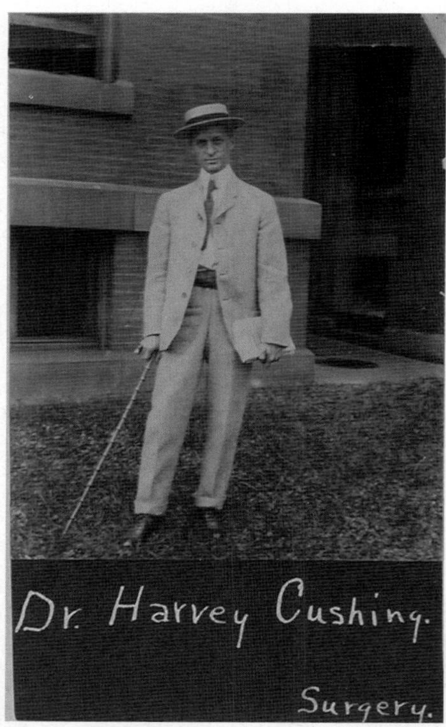

Figure 1-68. Harvey Cushing. This photo of a young, dapper Cushing was taken during his early period at Johns Hopkins Hospital. It comes from a rare album, issued in the early part of the 20th century, that illustrated some of the prominent physicians of the Johns Hopkins University and Hospital. Cushing's personality is evident in both his pose and posture in this early image of him. *(Courtesy James Tait Goodrich, MD, PhD.)*

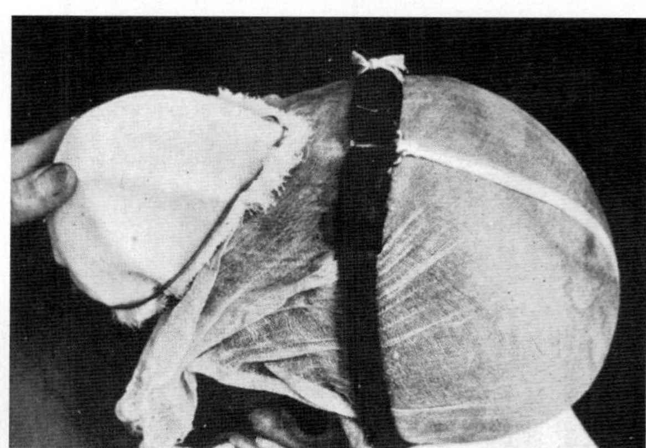

Figure 1-69. Pneumatic tourniquet. A key to Harvey Cushing's success as a surgeon was a number of inventive techniques designed to reduce both morbidity and mortality during neurosurgical procedures. Illustrated here is one of Cushing's numerous innovations, a pneumatic tourniquet, placed on the scalp before skin incision to reduce blood loss. *(Courtesy James Tait Goodrich, MD, PhD.)*

Harvey William Cushing (1869-1939) was the founder of American neurosurgery. Cushing had the good fortune to be alive and in training during the formative years of neurosurgery. Trained at Johns Hopkins Hospital by one of the premier general surgeons, William Halsted (1852-1922), Cushing learned meticulous surgical technique from his mentor. As was standard then, Cushing spent time in Europe; he worked in the laboratories of Emil Theodor Kocher (1841-1917) in Bern, Switzerland, investigating the physiologic properties of cerebrospinal fluid. These studies led to his important monograph in 1926 on the third circulation.[156] It was during this period of experimentation that the cerebral phenomenon of increased intracranial pressure in association with hypertension and bradycardia was defined; it is now referred to as *Cushing's phenomenon*. While traveling through Europe, he met several important surgical luminaries, including William Macewen and Victor Horsley. These individuals encouraged Cushing to consider neurosurgery as a full-time endeavor (Figs. 1-68 and 1-69).

Cushing's contributions to the literature of neurosurgery are too extensive for this chapter. Among his most significant is a monograph on pituitary surgery, published in 1912.[157] This monograph was to inaugurate a sterling career in pituitary studies. Cushing's syndrome was defined in his final monograph on the pituitary gland, published in 1932.[158] In a 1926 monograph written in collaboration with an early resident named Percival Bailey (1892-1973), Cushing brought the first rational approach to the classification of brain tumors. Before this volume, classifications of brain tumors were in a complete state of disarray and confusion.[159] The tumors medulloblastoma and hemiangioblastomas were classified and described by these two surgeons.[157] Cushing's monograph on meningioma, written in 1938 with Louise Eisenhardt (1891-1967), a collaborator and neuropathologist, set an extraordinarily high standard for the profession.[160]

Cushing retired as Moseley Professor of Surgery at Harvard in 1932. By the time he completed his 2000th brain tumor operation, he had unquestionably made one of the most important contributions to the field of neurosurgery: a contribution comprising meticulous, innovative surgical techniques and a career-long attempt to understand brain function from both physiologic and pathologic points of view.[161] An ardent bibliophile, Cushing spent his final years in retirement as Sterling Professor of Neurology at Yale, where he wrote his extraordinary monograph on Andreas Vesalius.[162] Cushing's life was faithfully recorded by his close friend and colleague, John F. Fulton (1899-1960),[163] and in a more recent biography by Michael Bliss.[164]

If Harvey Cushing was the father of American neurosurgery, his prodigal son was **Walter Dandy** (1886-1946). Dandy trained under Cushing at the Johns Hopkins Hospital. He made a number of important contributions to neurosurgery. Using the serendipitous finding of Luckett,[165] the presence of air in the ventricles after a skull fracture, Dandy developed the technique of pneumoencephalography (PEG).[166,167] The introduction of PEG provided the neurosurgeon, for the first time, the opportunity to localize a tumor by analyzing the displacement of air in the ventricles.[168] Dandy was an innovative neurosurgeon, considerably more aggressive in style and technique than Cushing. Dandy was the first to show that acoustic neuromas could be removed in their totality.[169a,169b] The publication of this technique led to some significant and vehement clashes between Cushing and Dandy. Cushing believed that a subcapsular resection was safer and produced less morbidity (Fig. 1-70).

Dandy was a pioneer in the diagnosis and treatment of hydrocephalus.[168-171] Dandy developed the technique of ablating and removing the choroid plexus to reduce the production of cerebrospinal fluid.[172] Dandy was among the first to treat cerebral aneurysms surgically by obliterating them through the use of snare ligatures or metal clips.[173] The concept of a postoperative "recovery room" with a specialized "brain team" originated with Dandy. This is now the accepted standard; before Dandy's time, this was not case.

In the field of textbooks, Dandy provided some brilliantly illustrated monographs on the brain with illustrations by Dorcas H. Padget (1906-1973), a largely self-taught illustrator. Dandy's monograph on the third ventricle and its anatomy is still a textbook standard to this day, with illustrations that remain among the finest illustrations ever produced[174] (Fig. 1-71).

In the field of spinal surgery, one important American in the first quarter of the 20th century was **Charles H. Frazier** (1870-1936), Professor of Surgery at the University of Pennsylvania. Work published by James L. Corning (1855-1923) in 1885 proved that lumbar puncture in both dogs and humans could be safely performed.[175] Corning was injecting cocaine into the epidural space and providing local anesthetic via an epidural block. This procedure was popularized by Heinrich Irenaeus Quincke (1842-1922), who used it in the treatment of hydrocephalus; from this procedure, spinal surgery developed.[176,177] When Charles Frazier's book on spinal surgery appeared in 1918, it was recognized as the most comprehensive work on spinal surgery written and an important prescient work in spine surgery that set a new standard.[178] In this work and the bibliography, Frazier summarized much of the spinal surgery literature up to the time of publication. Frazier firmly established that spinal surgery could be performed with minimal morbidity and mortality. Frazier's

Figure 1-70. Pneumoencephalograms. One of the landmark contributions to neurosurgery was Walter Dandy's (and Kenneth Blackfan's) introduction of pneumoencephalography, a technique in which air was introduced into the ventricles and radiography was then used to image the ventricular system in outline. *(Courtesy James Tait Goodrich, MD, PhD.)*

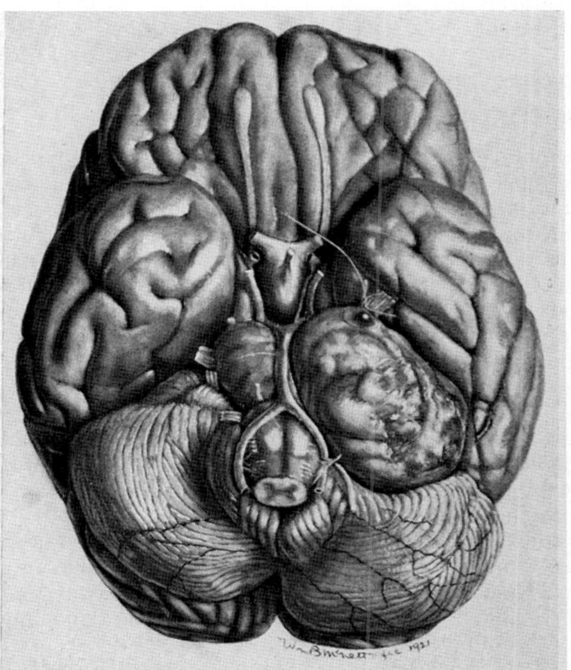

Fig. 1. An example of the characteristic cerebellopontile tumor showing the extent to which the brain-stem is excavated by the neoplasm. The intimate relationship with the medulla and pons explains the great danger which has attended all efforts at removal.

Figure 1-71. An illustration by Dorcas H. Padgett for Walter Dandy's work on acoustic tumors. *(Dandy WE. An operation for the total extirpation of tumors in the cerebellopontine angle. A preliminary report.* Bull Johns Hopkins Hosp. *1925;33:344-345; and Dande WE. An operation for the total removal of cerebello-pontine (acoustic) tumors.* Surg Gyn Obstet. *1922;41:129-148. Courtesy James Tait Goodrich, MD, PhD.)*

experience in World War I led him to devote his career to neurosurgery. Frazier was considered a gracious individual who followed a heavy work schedule. His staff reported that it was not uncommon for Frazier to sweep the operating room at the completion of a case. He apparently did this to relax his shoulder muscles, after which he then started a discussion with his colleagues of the operation that had just been completed.

Charles Elsberg (1871-1948), professor of neurosurgery at the New York Neurological Institute and a New York City pioneer in spinal surgery, is described as having surgical techniques that both were impeccable and consistently led to excellent outcomes. In 1912, Elsberg published a landmark paper in which he reported on a series of 43 laminectomies.[179] In 1916, Elsberg published the first of what were to be three monographs on surgery of the spine.[180] One of Elsberg's seminal contributions was a staged technique to allow the extrusion of an intramedullary spinal cord tumor.[179] Elsberg's technique consisted of first a myelotomy, which in theory allowed an intramedullary tumor to extrude over time into the laminectomy. At a later stage second operation, the tumor, having extruded through the myelotomy, could be removed. Elsberg was known as a driven worker who approached the practice of neurosurgery with a fierce intensity, always looking for new techniques. Working with Cornelius G. Dyke (1900-1943), a neuroradiologist at the New York Neurological Institute, Elsberg treated spinal glioblastomas with directed radiation in the operating room after the tumor had been exposed. Procedures such as these were performed with the patients receiving only local anesthesia. During the half-hour therapy, while the radiation was being delivered, the surgeon and assistants stood off in the distance behind a glass shield.[181]

FURTHER ADVANCES IN NEUROSURGERY: TWENTIETH CENTURY

The 19th century brought the introduction of anesthesia, antisepsis, and cerebral localization. In the latter half of the 19th century, certain surgeons were adventurous enough to perform surgery on the formidable cranial vault and spine. In the first half of the 20th century, the field of neurosurgery was formalized. Besides the pioneering techniques of Horsley, Macewen, Krause, Dandy, Cushing, and others, a number of diagnostic techniques were introduced that enabled the neurosurgeon to localize the lesions. One such technique, myelography, in which opaque substances were used, was promoted by **Jean Athanase Sicard** (1872-1929).[182] With the use of radiopaque iodized oil, the spinal cord and its elements could be outlined on radiographs. **Antonio Caetano de Abreu Freire Egas Moniz** (1874-1955), professor of neurology in Lisbon, perfected arterial catheterization techniques and cerebral angiography in animal studies.[183,184] This procedure, viewed in combination with PEG, offered neurosurgeons a more detailed view of the intracranial contents. Egas Moniz was awarded the Nobel Prize in Physiology or Medicine in 1949 for his work on prefrontal leucotomy (lobotomy) for treatment of psychiatric disorders.

In 1929, **Sir Alexander Fleming** (1881-1955) published a report on the first observation of a substance that blocked a bacterium from growing in tissue culture.[185] This substance, identified as penicillin, introduced a wholly new era of medicine and surgery. With the World War II experience, antibiotics were perfected in the treatment of bacterial infection, reducing even further the risk of infection during brain and spine surgery.

CONCLUDING THOUGHTS

Three scientific innovations had a dramatic effect on neurosurgery: the computer, the use of Röntgen rays (x-rays), and the computed tomographic (CT) scanner.

Charles Babbage and the Concept of the Computer

If asked when the computer was invented, few individuals today would even comprehend that the origins of this technology date back approximately 200 years. The term *computer* was first coined in 1613, and it was used to describe a person who performed calculations or computations. In 1822, **Charles Babbage** (1791-1871) began developing a model of a programmable computer, but it existed only on paper. Babbage called his machine a "difference engine." Babbage was a true polymath, skilled in mathematics, philosophy, and mechanical engineering. The machine design was created to calculate a series of values automatically through the use of computable polynomial functions. Despite superb intellectual skills, Babbage had great difficulty in landing a university position, having been turned down for academic positions a number of times. In 1828 he finally became Lucasian Professor of Mathematics at Cambridge (Trinity College), this after having been rejected for the position three times previously. Ironically, Babbage lacked interest in lecturing and teaching students and did not deliver a single lecture as a professor.

Babbage was awarded a Gold Medal by the Astronomical Society in 1824 for "his invention of an engine for calculating mathematical and astronomical tables." The computer that Babbage proposed on paper was not to be built until 1991, when the London Science Museum constructed a functioning model from his drawings. The computer in the final design turned out to be a large and heavy machine. His basic design was a forerunner of and very similar to a modern computer. In Babbage's design, the data and program memory were housed separately. The binary concept is not as modern people might think, inasmuch as Babbage constructed his machine with this very same computational design (Fig. 1-72). The London Museum of the

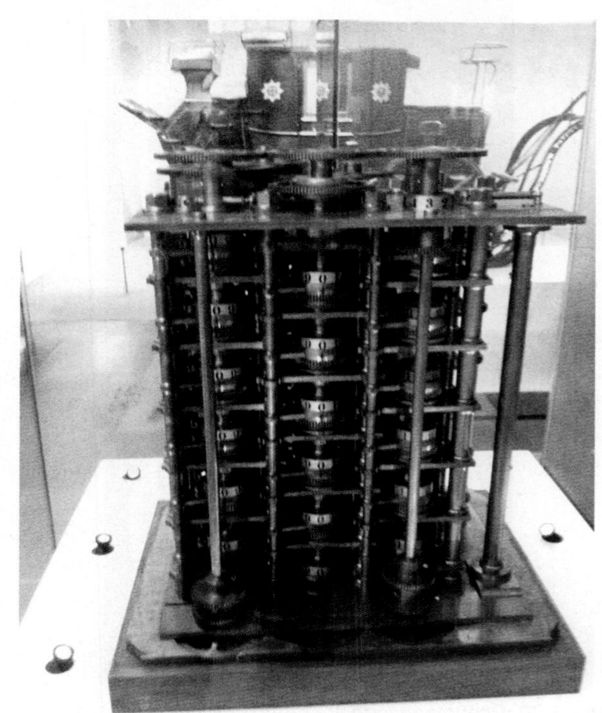

Figure 1-72. A model of Charles Babbage's computer, built by the Science Museum in London. The "0" and "1" can be seen etched into the revolving balls.

History of Science has calculated that Babbage's first difference engine would have been composed of about 25,000 parts with a weight of 15 tons (>13,600 kg). When the machine was completed and tested, the first calculation returned results to 31 digits. There is a project under way in the United Kingdom to build from Babbage's plans his "analytical engine": when complete, it will have the equivalent of 675 bytes of memory and run at a clock speed of 7 Hz. This chapter was written on a computer with a clock speed of 1.7 GHz and a hard drive storage of 512 GB; it weighed 3 lb (1361 g) and fit inside of a 9 × 12 inch (23 × 30.5 cm) manila envelope.

Upon Babbage's death, his brain was divided into two parts; one part is now in the Science Museum in London, and the other part is housed at the Hunterian Museum at the Royal College of Surgeons, London (Fig. 1-73).

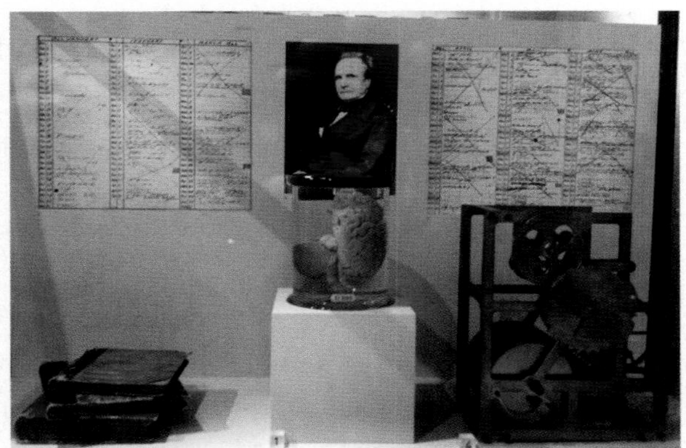

Figure 1-73. Container housing half of Charles Babbage's brain. *(From the Charles Babbage exhibit at the Science Museum in London.)*

Wilhelm Röntgen and the X-Ray

Wilhelm Röntgen (1845-1923), a German mechanical engineer and physicist by training, discovered on November 8, 1895, what he would call the "x-ray."[186] Röntgen was chair of the physics department at the University of Würzburg. Of interest is that at one point, he accepted an appointment at Columbia University, but the beginning of World War I prevented his coming. Röntgen was interested in the external effects of various types of vacuum tube devices. Using a cathode ray and a coil that generated an electrostatic charge, he was able to generate an x-ray image on a barium platinocyanide screen. For two intensive weeks in November 1895, Röntgen rarely left his laboratory; he performed various experiments, perfecting what he called the "x-ray." The very first radiographs were images of the hand of his wife, Anna Bertha. Röntgen then published in rapid sequence three papers on the x-ray in 1895 and 1896. Röntgen titled his papers *Über Eine Neue Art von Strahlen [On a New Kind of Rays]* (Fig. 1-74).[186] Röntgen is considered the father of diagnostic radiology and for his efforts was awarded the Nobel Prize in Physics in 1901. Use of x-rays was rapidly adopted in medicine and science throughout the world. Röntgen died in 1923 from an intestinal carcinoma. Because he used lead shields routinely, it is not thought this carcinoma was caused by the radiation experiments. The effect of radiography on medicine and science was immediate, and it is now used for many different purposes, from diagnosis to medical therapeutics.

Computed Tomography

Sir Godfrey Newbold Hounsfield (1919-2004), a computer expert and engineer working at the Central Research Laboratories of EMI, developed the first computed tomographic (CT) scanner. Hounsfield initially conceptualized the use of x-rays coming from multiple directions to reconstruct the internal structure of objects being imaged. Like Charles Babbage, he

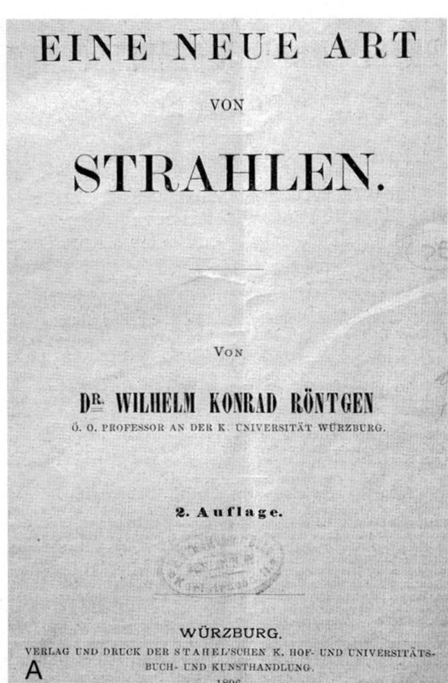

EINE NEUE ART

VON

STRAHLEN.

VON

DR. WILHELM KONRAD RÖNTGEN

Ö. O. PROFESSOR AN DER K. UNIVERSITÄT WÜRZBURG.

2. Auflage.

WÜRZBURG.

VERLAG UND DRUCK DER STAHEL'SCHEN K. HOF- UND UNIVERSITÄTS-BUCH- UND KUNSTHANDLUNG.

1896.

A

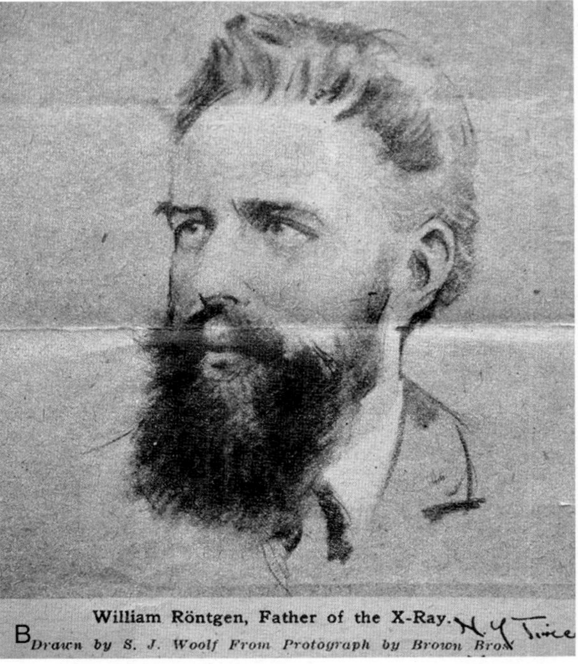

B
William Röntgen, Father of the X-Ray.
Drawn by S. J. Woolf From Protograph by Brown Bro

Figure 1-74. A, An offprint of Wilhelm Röntgen's seminal paper on the discovery of the x-ray. **B,** A 1922 drawing of Röntgen, showing this scientist at the age of 50, when he was doing his seminal work on the x-ray. *(Courtesy James Tait Goodrich, MD, PhD.)*

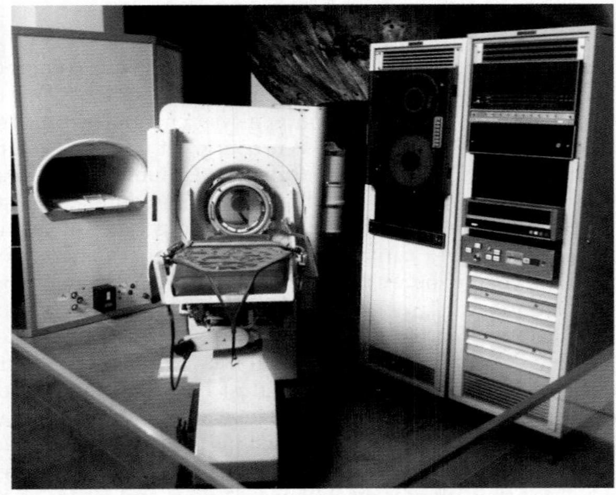

Figure 1-75. An early prototype of the EMI computed tomographic scanner developed by Housfield. This scanner is on display at the Science Museum in London.

realized he would need a computer with mathematical calculating ability that would need to be combined with the x-ray source to scan and construct the image. Housfield had no medical background training, and so this task was an enormous one. He initially developed the concept of the "slice" and of then building up a series of slices to make an image. His original machine design took 9 days to produce a single image. The first images were of "kosher-killed" beef brains. By changing the source of x-rays, he was able to develop a more efficient machine, but the image production was still extremely slow, with only a single image in a day. Work on human subjects began in 1970 at the Atkinson Morley's Hospital in Wimbledon, England. By 1971, Hounsfield was able to produce a single scan in 4 minutes, meaning that a total study (10 scans) took 40 minutes. By converting to a more powerful computing language (FORTRAN), he was able to reduce scan times to 20 minutes. Since then, computers with better resolution and scan times have been introduced[187,188] (Fig. 1-75).

As a result of their surgical forebears, neurosurgeons can now complete a neurosurgical procedure with minimal pain to the patient, along with a marked reduction in infections. The 19th-century surgeons pioneered techniques in cerebral localization, and modern neurosurgeons are even more fortunate with the introduction of frameless guidance systems. The surgical fear of operating on the wrong area should no longer be an issue, thanks to the efforts and studies of the surgical pioneers and the specialty called neurosurgery.

SUGGESTED READINGS

Bakay L. *An Early History of Craniotomy. From Antiquity to the Napoleonic Era*. Springfield, Ill: Charles C Thomas; 1985.

Bakay L. *Neurosurgeons of the Past*. Springfield, III: Charles C Thomas; 1987.

Castiglioni AA. *History of Medicine*, revised and enlarged, 2nd ed [Krubhaar EB, Trans. and ed]. New York: A.A. Knopf; 1947.

Clarke ES, Dewhurst K. *An Illustrated History of Brain Function*. San Francisco: Norman Publishing; 1992 [Original work published 1972].

Clarke E, O'Malley CD. *The Human Brain and Spinal Cord. A Historical Study Illustrated by Writings from Antiquity to the Twentieth Century*. San Francisco: Norman Publishing; 1992 [Original work published 1968].

DeJong RN. *A History of American Neurology*. New York: Raven Press; 1982.

Garrison FH. *An Introduction to the History of Medicine*, revised and enlarged, 4th ed. Philadelphia: W.B. Saunders; 1929.

Gurdjian ES. *Head Injury from Antiquity to the Present with Special Reference to Penetrating Head Injury*. Springfield, III: Charles C Thomas; 1973.

Haymaker W, Schiller F. *The Founders of Neurology*. 2nd ed. Springfield, Ill: Charles C Thomas; 1970.

Leonardo RA. *History of Surgery*. New York: Froben Press; 1943.

McHenry LC. *Garrison's History of Neurology Revised and Enlarged with a Bibliography of Classical, Original and Standard Works in Neurology*. Springfield, III: Charles C Thomas; 1969.

Mettler CC, ed. *History of Medicine. A Correlative Text, Arranged According to Subjects*. Philadelphia: Blakiston; 1947.

Meyer A. *Historical Aspects of Cerebral Anatomy*. London: Oxford University Press; 1971.

Norman JM, ed. *Norton's Medical Bibliography*. 5th ed. Cambridge, U.K.: Scholar Press; 1991.

Poynter FNL, ed. *The History and Philosophy of Knowledge of the Brain and Its Functions*. Springfield, Ill: Charles C Thomas; 1958.

Rose FC, Bynum WF. *Historical Aspects of the Neurosciences. A Festschrift for Macdonald Critchley*. New York: Raven Press; 1982.

Sachs E. *The History and Development of Neurological Surgery*. New York: Paul Hoeber; 1952.

Soury J. *Le Système Nerveux Centrale Structure et Fonctions. Histoire Critique des Théories et des Doctrines*. Paris: Georges Carré & Naud; 1899.

Spillane JD. *The Doctrine of the Nerves. Chapters in the History of Neurology*. London: Oxford University Press; 1981.

Walker AE. *A History of Neurological Surgery*. Baltimore: Williams & Wilkins; 1951.

Wilkins RH. *Neurosurgical Classics*. New York: Johnson Reprint Co; 1965.

See a full reference list on ExpertConsult.com

2 Surgical Anatomy of the Brain

Hung Tzu Wen, Albert L. Rhoton, Jr.,† and Antônio C.M. Mussi

We believe that a successful microneurosurgery is based on six solid foundations: (1) anatomic knowledge; (2) an understanding of the information provided by imaging and the correlation of that information with anatomy; (3) a planned surgical strategy based on an understanding of that anatomic and radiologic correlation; (4) a focus on bringing together the anatomy, imaging, and presurgical planning during surgery; (5) the practice of fine surgical skill through extensive training and experience; and (6) a good anesthesiologist and proper instruments.

An understanding of the anatomy of the brain from different angles is the key to assembling an authentic tridimensional knowledge. Knowledge of the surface anatomy and the anatomy of the deeply located structures is as important as the establishment of the correlation between them. This correlation will empower us to have "x-ray vision," enabling us to see the depths of the brain through its surface.

In this chapter, the surgical anatomy of the neural and vascular structures of both the cerebrum and the cerebellum are reviewed as stepwise dissection following the logical sequence based on the three surfaces that each one of them presents.

CEREBRUM

Lateral Surface: Neural Structures

Superficial Anatomy

The cerebrum is arbitrarily divided into five lobes: frontal, parietal, temporal, occipital, and the hidden insula. On the lateral surface, they are limited by the central sulcus, the posterior ramus of the sylvian fissure, the lateral parietotemporal line (from the impression of the parieto-occipital sulcus to the preoccipital notch), and the temporo-occipital line (from the posterior end of the posterior ramus of the sylvian fissure to the midpoint of the lateral parietotemporal line). The cerebrum presents four main sulci that are 100% continuous: the sylvian fissure, the callosal, the parieto-occipital, and the collateral sulci; and it presents two almost continuous (92%) sulci, the central and the calcarine sulci. There are two 100% interrupted sulci: the precentral and the inferior temporal sulci.[1] The central sulcus starts from the medial surface of the hemisphere above the cingulate sulcus and extends on the lateral surface of the hemisphere from medial to lateral, superior to inferior, and posterior to anterior. It usually does not intercept the posterior ramus of the sylvian fissure and leaves a bridge connecting the precentral gyrus to the postcentral gyrus known as *pli de passage frontoparietal inferior*, *opercule rolandique*, or *subcentral gyrus* (Fig. 2-1A).

Frontal Lobe. The two main sulci are the superior and the inferior frontal sulci, which are anteroposteriorly oriented and extend from the precentral sulcus to the frontal pole. At their posterior end, these two sulci are intercepted perpendicularly by the precentral sulcus, which has a direction very similar to that of the central sulcus. The precentral sulcus forms the anterior limit of the precentral gyrus. These two frontal sulci divide the lateral surface of the frontal lobe into three gyri: the superior, the middle, and the inferior frontal gyri (see Fig. 2-1A). The anterior horizontal, the anterior ascending, and the posterior rami of the sylvian fissure divide the inferior frontal gyrus into three parts: pars orbitalis, triangularis, and opercularis. The apex of the pars triangularis is usually retracted superiorly, leaving a space in the sylvian fissure that is usually the largest space in the superficial compartment of the sylvian fissure. The apex of the pars triangularis is directed inferiorly toward the junction of three rami of the sylvian fissure; this junctional point coincides with the anterior limiting sulcus of the insula in the depth of the sylvian fissure. It marks the anterior limit of the basal ganglia and the location of the anterior horn of the lateral ventricle. At the intercepting point between the superior frontal and the precentral sulci, the precentral gyrus often presents the morphology of the Greek letter Ω (omega) with its convexity pointing posteriorly. This is the most easily identifiable landmark of the motor strip and corresponds to the hand area (Fig. 2-1B; Videos 2-1 and 2-2).

Parietal Lobe. The parietal lobe is limited anteriorly by the central sulcus, medially by the interhemispheric fissure, inferolaterally by the sylvian fissure and the temporo-occipital line, and posteriorly by the lateral parietotemporal line. Its two main sulci are the postcentral and the intraparietal sulci. The postcentral sulcus is very similar to the central sulcus except for its variable continuity. The postcentral sulcus is the posterior limit of the postcentral gyrus, and in some individuals, it is double. The intraparietal sulcus starts at the postcentral sulcus and is directed posteriorly and inferiorly toward the occipital pole; its direction is often parallel and is 2 to 3 cm lateral to the midline. The bottom of the intraparietal sulcus is related to both the roof of the atrium and the occipital horn. The intraparietal sulcus divides the lateral surface of the parietal lobe into two parts: the superior and inferior parietal lobules. The superior parietal lobule, the superomedial and smaller part, continues as precuneus in the medial surface of the parietal lobe. The inferior parietal lobule is constituted by the supramarginal and the angular gyri. The supramarginal gyrus is the posterior continuation of the superior temporal gyrus and turns around the posterior ascending ramus of the sylvian fissure. The angular gyrus is the posterior continuation of the middle temporal gyrus and turns superiorly and medially behind the posterior ramus of the sylvian fissure up to the intraparietal sulcus; in some individuals, it is limited between the two posterior terminations of the superior temporal sulcus: the angular and anterior occipital rami (Fig. 2-1C).

The postcentral and intraparietal sulci and the superior parietal lobule are a mirror image of the precentral and superior frontal sulci and the superior frontal gyrus, with the central sulcus as the "mirror" (Video 2-3).

Temporal Lobe. The temporal lobe is limited superiorly by the posterior ramus of the sylvian fissure and posteriorly by the temporo-occipital and lateral parietotemporal lines. It presents two main sulci, the superior and inferior temporal sulci, which divide the lateral surface of the temporal lobe into three gyri, the superior, middle, and inferior temporal gyri. The inferior temporal gyrus occupies the lateral and basal surfaces of the cerebrum. The superior and inferior temporal gyri converge anteriorly to form the temporal pole (see Fig. 2-1A; Video 2-4).

Occipital Lobe. The occipital lobe is located behind the lateral parieto-temporal line and is composed of a number of irregular convolutions that are divided by a short horizontal sulcus, the lateral occipital sulcus, into the superior and inferior occipital gyri (Video 2-5). The "x-ray vision" concept can be demonstrated

†Deceased.

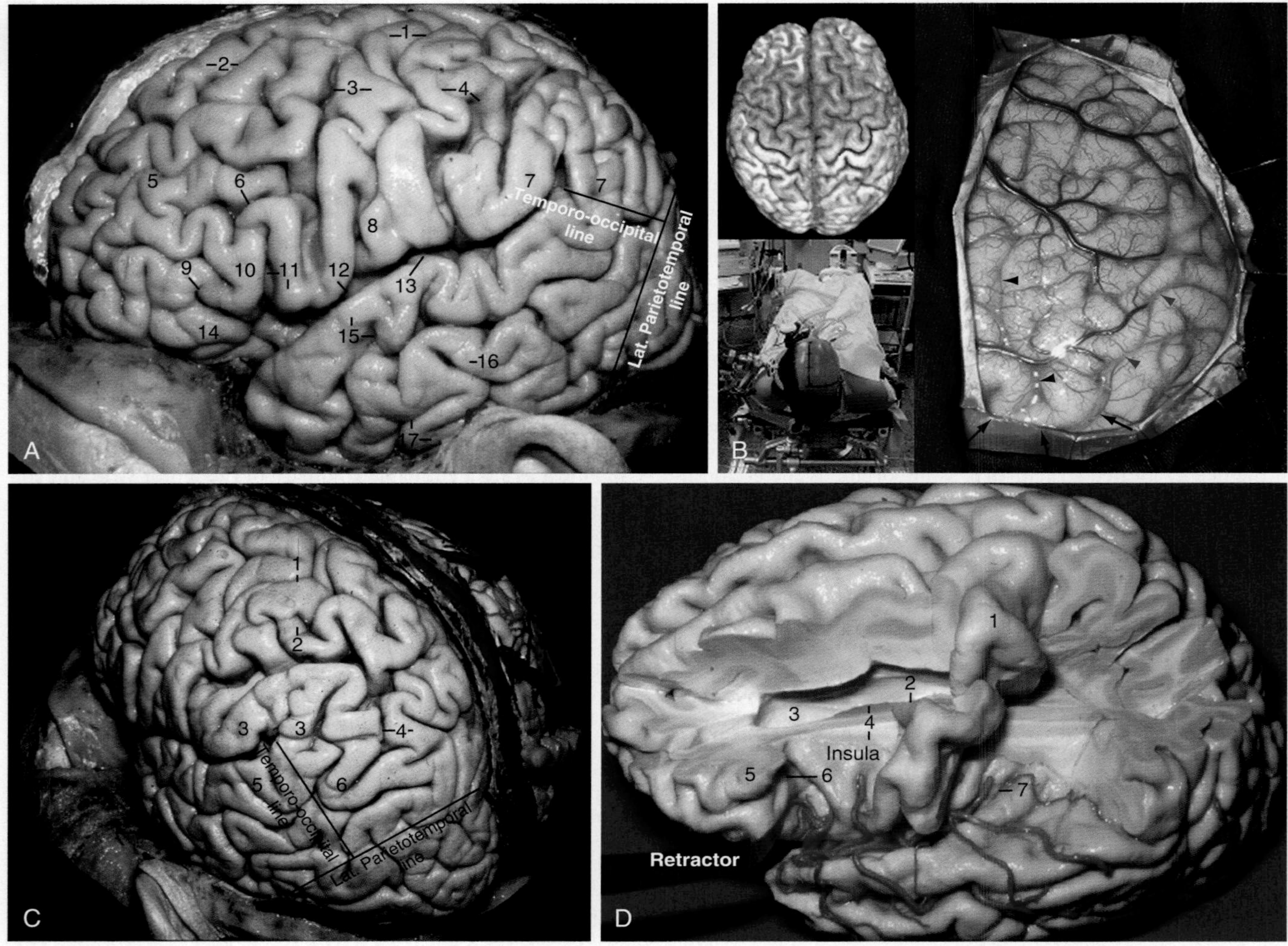

Figure 2-1. A, Lateral view of the left hemisphere. 1, Omega (motor hand area) and the central sulcus; 2, superior frontal sulcus and gyrus; 3, precentral sulcus and gyrus; 4, postcentral sulcus and gyrus; 5, middle frontal gyrus; 6, inferior frontal sulcus; 7, supramarginal gyrus; 8, pli de passage; 9, anterior horizontal ramus; 10, pars triangularis; 11, ascending ramus and pars opercularis; 12, posterior ramus; 13, Heschl's gyrus; 14, pars orbitalis; 15, superior temporal gyrus and sulcus; 16, middle temporal gyrus; 17, inferior temporal sulcus and gyrus. **B,** *Upper left,* The "omega" sign. *Lower left,* Surgical positioning. *Right, Black arrows* indicate omega; *black arrowheads* indicate the superior frontal sulcus; *blue arrowheads* indicate the central sulcus. **C,** Posterolateral view of left hemisphere. 1, Central sulcus; 2, postcentral gyrus and sulcus; 3, supramarginal gyrus; 4, intraparietal sulcus and superior parietal lobule; 5, superior temporal gyrus; 6, angular gyrus. **D,** Superolateral view of left hemisphere. 1, Precentral gyrus; 2 foramen of Monro; 3, frontal horn; 4, head of caudate nucleus and superior limiting sulcus (insula); 5, pars orbitalis; 6, anterior limiting sulcus (insula); 7, inferior limiting sulcus (insula).

by the precentral gyrus, which begins on the medial surface of the cerebrum, above the level of the splenium of the corpus callosum, and passes above the body of the lateral ventricle, thalamus, posterior limb of the internal capsule, and posterior part of the lentiform nucleus to reach the sylvian fissure approximately midway between the anterior and posterior limits of the insula (Fig. 2-1D).

Sylvian Fissure. The sylvian fissure is the space between the frontal, parietal, and temporal opercula and the insula and extends from the basal to the lateral surface of the brain. It is constituted by a superficial part and a deep part. The superficial part presents a stem (on the basal surface) and three rami (on the lateral surface); the stem extends medially from the semilunar gyrus of the uncus to the level of the tip of pars triangularis, where the stem divides into anterior horizontal, anterior ascending, and posterior rami (see Fig. 2-1A). The transition between the basal and lateral parts of the superficial sylvian fissure can therefore be considered as located at the level of the pars triangularis. The deep part is divided into an anterior operculoinsular compartment (on the basal surface) and a lateral operculoinsular compartment (on the lateral surface). The anterior operculoinsular compartment consists of an anterior opercular compartment and an anterior insular compartment. The anterior opercular compartment is located between the opercular portions of the lateral and posterior orbital gyri on the frontal side and the upper part of the anterior portion of the planum polare on the temporal side. The anterior insular compartment is not restricted only to the narrow space posterior to the sphenoid ridge between the frontal and temporal lobes, in front of the insular pole (sphenoidal compartment), but also extends upward over the anterior surface of the insula, between the posterior surfaces of the lateral, posterior, and medial orbital gyri anteriorly and the anterior surface of the insula posteriorly (see Fig. 2-4E, later). The anterior insular compartment communicates medially with the carotid cistern, also called *sylvian vallecula*[2] (see Fig. 2-4D, later). The lateral operculoinsular compartment is formed by two narrow clefts: the opercular cleft between the opposing lips of the frontoparietal and the temporal opercula and the insular cleft, which has a superior limb between the insula and the frontoparietal opercula and an inferior limb between the insula and the temporal operculum[3] (Fig. 2-2A). The gyri that constitute the frontal and parietal opercula of the sylvian fissure are, posteriorly to anteriorly: the supramarginal, postcentral, and precentral gyri; pars opercularis; triangularis; and orbitalis (see Fig. 2-1A). The gyri that constitute the temporal operculum of the sylvian fissure are, posteriorly to anteriorly: the planum temporale, Heschl's gyrus, and planum polare (Fig. 2-2B, *left*). Each gyrus of the frontoparietal opercula is related to its counterpart on the temporal side: the supramarginal gyrus is in contact with the planum temporale; the postcentral gyrus is related to Heschl's gyrus; and the precentral gyrus, pars opercularis, triangularis, and orbitalis are related to the planum polare.[4] The site on the posterior ramus of the sylvian fissure where the postcentral gyrus meets Heschl's gyrus is projected in the same coronal plane of the external acoustic meatus. The medial wall of the lateral insular compartment is the insula or island of Reil, which can only be seen when the lips of the sylvian fissure are widely separated (Video 2-6).

Insula. The insula has the shape of a pyramid with its apex directed inferiorly and presents an anterior surface and a lateral surface. The anterior surface presents a triangular shape and is constituted by the transverse and accessory gyri and the insular pole. The medial portion of the insular pole is marked by an arched ridge of variable prominence, the limen insulae, which is composed of fibers of uncinate fasciculus covered by a thin layer of gray matter that extends from the anterior end of the long

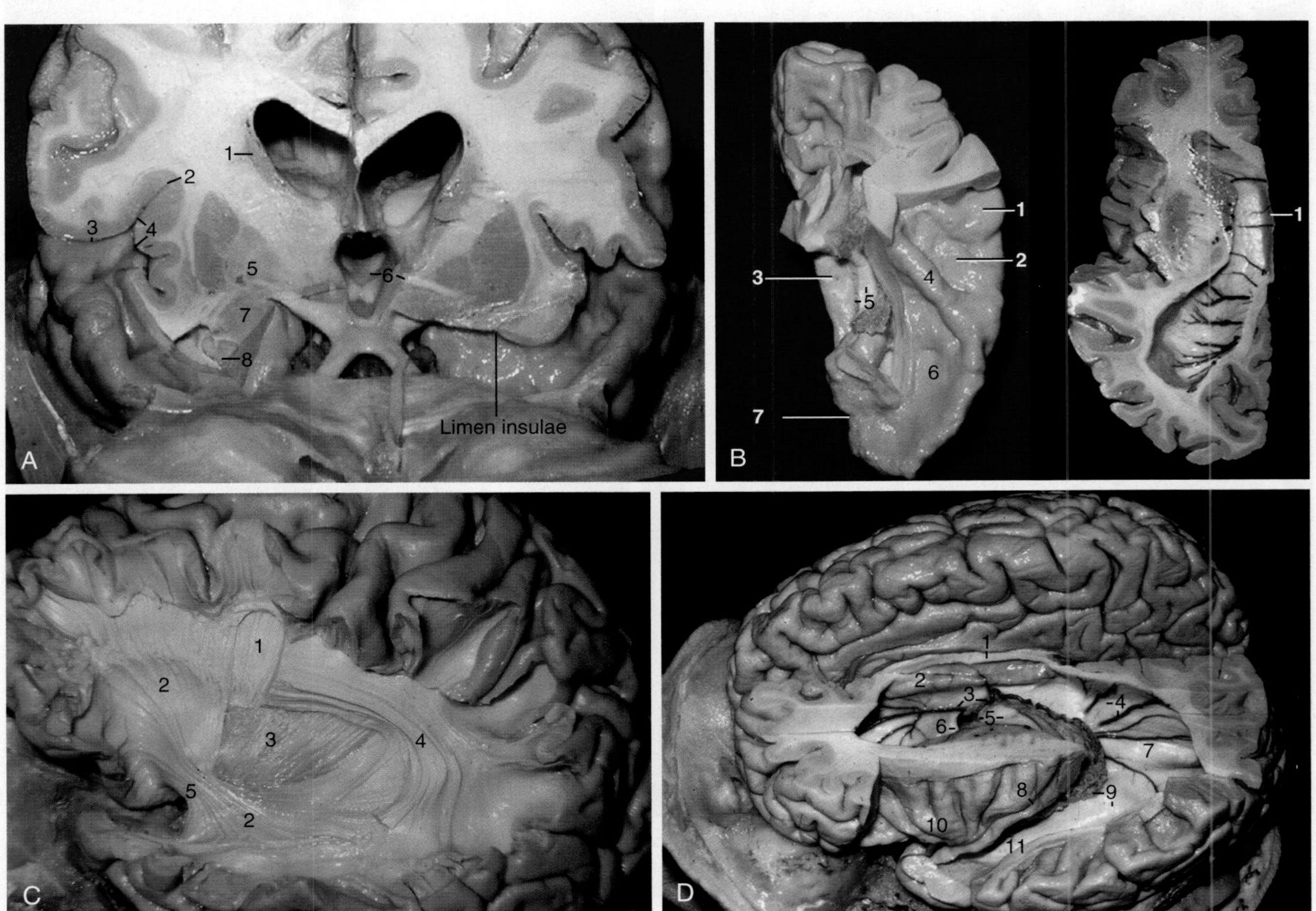

Figure 2-2. A, Coronal view. 1, Body of caudate nucleus; 2, superior limiting sulcus; 3, opercular compartment; 4, insular compartment; 5, globus pallidus; 6, floor of third ventricle and anterior commissure; 7, amygdala; 8, head of hippocampus. **B,** *Left,* Anterosuperior view of left temporal lobe. 1, Posterior transverse temporal gyrus; 2, middle transverse temporal gyrus; 3, parahippocampal gyrus; 4, Heschl's gyrus; 5, fornix and dentate gyrus; 6, planum polare; 7, rhinal incisura. *Right,* Basal view of roof of lateral ventricle. 1, Septum pellucidum. The veins of the roof of the lateral ventricle drain toward the midline. **C,** Fiber dissection of left hemisphere. 1, Corona radiata; 2, inferior occipitofrontal fascicle; 3, putamen; 4, superior longitudinal fascicle; 5, uncinate fascicle. **D,** Lateral view of left lateral ventricle. 1, Corpus callosum; 2, septum pellucidum; 3, anterior septal and superior choroidal veins; 4, bulb of callosum and medial atrial vein; 5, thalamostriate vein and thalamus (anterior tubercle); 6, column of fornix and foramen of Monro; 7, calcar avis; 8, central sulcus of insula; 9, choroid plexus and atrium; 10, apex of insula; 11, temporal horn.

gyrus, passes through the medial part of the insular pole, and ends at the middle of the posterior orbital gyrus. *Limen* means "threshold," and the limen insulae is the threshold between the carotid cistern medially and the sylvian fissure laterally (see Fig. 2-2A). The insula is encircled and separated from the opercula by a deep furrow called the *circular* or *limiting sulcus of the insula,* which presents three parts, the superior, anterior, and inferior parts (see Fig. 2-1D). From the limen insulae, the sulci and gyri of the insula are directed superiorly in a radial manner. The deepest sulcus, the central sulcus of the insula, is a constant sulcus that extends upward and backward across the insula in the general line of the central sulcus of the cerebrum. It divides the lateral surface of the insula into a large anterior zone that is divided by several shallow sulci into three to five short gyri and a posterior zone that is formed by anterior and posterior long gyri (Fig. 2-2D). From microsurgical and radiologic viewpoints, the insula represents the external covering of the central core, constituted by the extreme, external, and internal capsules, the claustrum, basal ganglia, and thalamus (see Figs. 2-2A and 2-3A, *left*). The anterior, inferior, and posterior limits of the insula on the lateral projection correspond to anterior, inferior, and posterior limits of the central core. The upper limit of the central core (caudate nucleus) is higher than the upper limit of the insula (see Fig. 2-2A; Videos 2-7 to 2-9).

Association Fibers of the Cerebrum. The association fibers are tracts of myelinated fibers that connect cortical areas in the same hemisphere; they may be divided into short- and long-association fibers. Short-association fibers connect adjacent gyri,

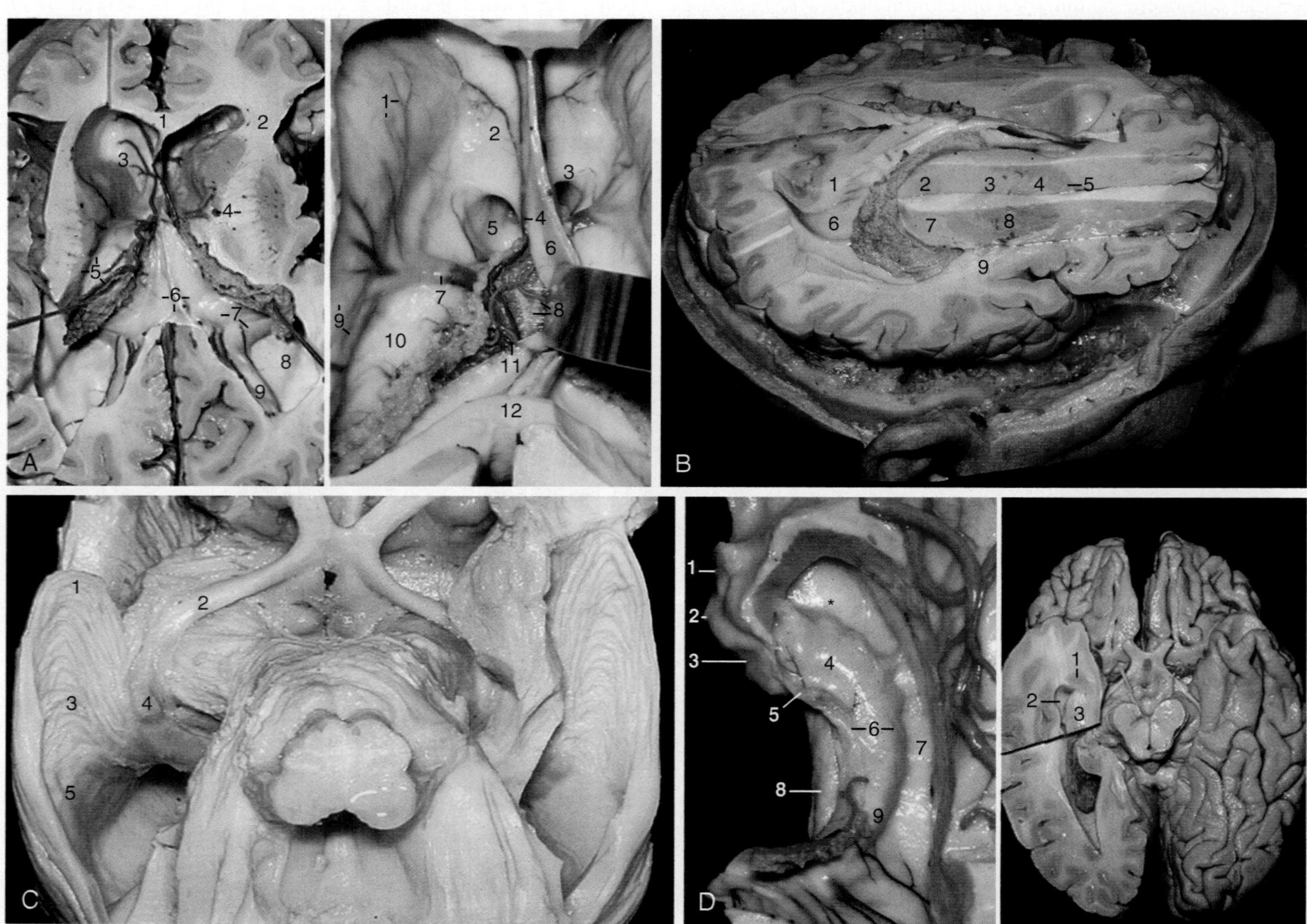

Figure 2-3. A, *Left,* Superior view. 1, Genu of corpus callosum; 2, anterior limb of internal capsule; 3, frontal horn; 4, genu of internal capsule and thalamostriate vein; 5, striothalamic sulcus, thalamus, and the superior choroidal vein; 6, bodies of fornix and hippocampal commissure; 7, crus of fornix and tail of hippocampus; 8, collateral trigone; 9, calcar avis. *Right,* Roof of third ventricle through transchoroidal approach. 1, Head of caudate nucleus and anterior caudate vein; 2, rostrum of corpus callosum; 3, column of fornix; 4, anterior septal vein; 5, foramen of Monro; 6, body of fornix; 7, thalamostriate vein; 8, inferior membrane of tela choroidea and choroid plexus of third ventricle (the superior membrane of the tela has been removed); 9, body of caudate nucleus and thalamostriate vein; 10, dorsal surface of thalamus; 11, internal cerebral vein and medial posterior choroidal artery; 12, splenium of corpus callosum. **B,** Superolateral view of right hemisphere. 1, Bulb of callosum; 2, thalamus; 3, internal capsule (genu); 4, internal capsule (anterior limb); 5, caudate nucleus; 6, calcar avis, 7, internal capsule (retrolenticular portion); 8, lentiform nucleus; 9, internal capsule (sublenticular portion). **C,** Basal view of optic radiation. 1, Meyer's loop; 2, optic tract; 3, middle part; 4, lateral geniculate body; 5, posterior part. **D,** *Left,* Superior view of floor of right temporal horn. 1, Uncus (anterior segment); 2, uncus (apex); 3, uncus (posterior segment); 4, head of hippocampus; 5, inferior choroidal point; 6, body of hippocampus and fimbria; 7, collateral eminence; 8, parahippocampal gyrus; 9, tail of hippocampus. *, Uncal recess. *Right,* Basal view. 1, Amygdala; 2, temporal horn; 3, hippocampus.

and long-association fibers (fasciculi) connect distant gyri. The long-association fibers form distinct, compact bundles. The main fasciculi are the superior longitudinal, uncinate, inferior occipitofrontal, and cingulum. The superior longitudinal fasciculus is the largest of these; it arches around the insula and connects parts of the frontal, parietal, and temporal lobes. The uncinate fasciculus lies in the depth of the limen insulae and presents a marked curvature; it connects the basal parts of the frontal lobe with the temporal lobe. The inferior occipitofrontal fasciculus connects the frontal and occipital lobes, and it also connects with the posterior part of the temporal and parietal lobes; these fibers converge from the frontal lobe as a single bundle that runs lateral to the lentiform nucleus, where they are closely associated with the uncinate fasciculus (Fig. 2-2C). Cingulum fibers lie within the cingulate gyrus from below the rostrum of the corpus callosum to the parahippocampal gyrus.

Lateral Ventricles. Wrapping around the central core of the hemisphere are the lateral ventricles (see Fig. 2-2D). Each ventricle has five components: frontal horn, body, atrium, occipital, and temporal horns.[5] The frontal horn is located in front of the foramen of Monro and presents a roof, a floor, and anterior, lateral, medial, and posterior walls. The transition between the genu and the body of the corpus callosum forms the roof, the rostrum of the corpus callosum forms the narrow floor, the septum pellucidum forms the medial wall, and the thalamus forms the posterior wall. The head of the caudate nucleus forms most of the lateral wall, but the most anterior part is constituted by the most anterior part of the anterior limb of the internal capsule, and it is in close relation to the anterior limiting sulcus of the insula. The body of the lateral ventricle is located behind the foramen of Monro and extends to the point where the septum pellucidum, corpus callosum, and fornix meet. It presents roof, floor, and lateral and medial walls. The body of the corpus callosum forms the roof, the septum pellucidum above and the body of the fornix below form the medial wall, the body of the caudate nucleus forms the lateral wall, and the thalamus forms the floor. The caudate nucleus and the thalamus are separated by the striothalamic sulcus, the groove in which the stria terminalis and the thalamostriate vein course. The atrium has a roof, a floor, and anterior, medial, and lateral walls. The roof is formed by the body, splenium, and tapetum of the corpus callosum; the floor is formed by the collateral trigone, a triangular area that bulges upward over the posterior end of the collateral sulcus. The medial wall is formed by two roughly horizontal prominences: the upper prominence, the bulb of the callosum, is formed by the large bundle of fibers called the *forceps major* that connects the two occipital lobes; the lower prominence, the calcar avis, overlies the deepest part of the calcarine sulcus. The lateral wall has an anterior part formed by the caudate nucleus as it wraps the lateral margin of the pulvinar and a posterior part formed by the fibers of the tapetum as they sweep anteroinferiorly along the lateral margin of the ventricle and separate the ventricular cavity from the optic radiation. The anterior wall has a medial part composed of the crus of the fornix as it wraps the posterior part of the pulvinar and a lateral part formed by the pulvinar of the thalamus. The occipital horn extends posteriorly into the occipital lobe from the atrium. It varies from being absent to extending far posteriorly in the occipital lobe. The bulb of the callosum and the calcar avis form its medial wall; the tapetum forms the roof and the lateral wall; and the collateral trigone forms the floor (see Fig. 2-3A and B).[5] The temporal horn extends forward and inferiorly from the atrium into the medial part of the temporal lobe and presents roof, floor, and anterior, lateral, and medial walls. The tapetum, the tail of the caudate nucleus, part of the retrolentiform and sublentiform components of the internal capsule, and the amygdaloid nucleus form the roof. The retrolentiform component is the posterior thalamic radiation that includes the optic radiation (Fig. 2-3C); the sublentiform component is formed mainly by the acoustic radiation. The amygdaloid nucleus constitutes the most anterior part of the roof of the temporal horn and is located above and in front of the head of the hippocampus (Fig. 2-3D, *right*), anterior to the inferior choroidal point, which is the most anterior site of attachment of the choroid plexus in the temporal horn.[6] There is no clear separation between the roof of the temporal horn and the thalamus because all fibers of the optic radiation come from the lateral geniculate body. Therefore, it is reasonable to consider the roof of the temporal horn as a lateral extension of the thalamus.[6] The attachment site of the choroid plexus can be a surgical landmark to separate the thalamus from the roof of the temporal horn (see Fig. 2-6D, *right*, later). The tapetum and the optic radiation form the lateral wall; the amygdaloid body forms the anterior wall; the head of the hippocampus forms the anterior one third of the medial wall; and the choroidal fissure forms the posterior two thirds.[6] The floor is formed medially by the hippocampus and laterally by the collateral eminence (Fig. 2-3D, *left*). The temporal horn is projected onto the middle temporal gyrus on the lateral view.

The structures related to the lateral ventricle are the foramen of Monro, internal capsule, corpus callosum, fornix, thalamus, caudate nucleus, hippocampus, temporal amygdala, and choroidal fissure (Videos 2-10 and 2-11).

Foramen of Monro. The foramen of Monro communicates the lateral ventricle to the third ventricle. It usually presents a crescent shape and is bounded anteriorly and superiorly by the columns of the fornix and posteriorly by the thalamus.[7] The elements that run close to the foramen of Monro are the anterior septal vein superiorly and medially, the choroidal plexus posteriorly and medially, and the thalamostriate vein laterally and posteriorly (see Figs. 2-2D and 2-3A).

Internal Capsule

The internal capsule has five parts: the anterior and posterior limbs, the genu, the retrolentiform, and the sublentiform parts. The anterior limb is located between the head of the caudate nucleus and the anterior half of the lentiform nucleus and contains frontopontine fibers; the posterior limb is located between the thalamus and the posterior half of the lentiform nucleus and contains the corticospinal tract, frontopontine, and corticorubral fibers and fibers of the superior thalamic radiation (somaesthetic radiation). The genu comes to the ventricular surface immediately lateral to the foramen of Monro in the interval between the caudate nucleus and the thalamus, where the thalamostriate vein usually drains into the internal cerebral vein; the genu contains corticonuclear fibers and anterior fibers of the superior thalamic radiation. The retrolentiform part is located posteriorly to the lentiform nucleus and contains mainly parietopontine, occipitopontine, occipitocollicular, and occipitotectal fibers and the posterior thalamic radiation that includes the optic radiation. The sublentiform part is located below the lentiform nucleus and contains temporopontine and parietopontine fibers and acoustic radiation from the medial geniculate body to the superior temporal gyrus and to the transverse temporal gyri (see Figs. 2-3A, *left*, and 2-3B).

Corpus Callosum. The corpus callosum is the largest transverse commissure connecting the cerebral hemispheres. It contributes to the wall of each of the five parts of the lateral ventricle (Fig. 2-2B, *right*). The corpus callosum is divided into four parts: rostrum, genu, body, and splenium. The rostrum is the floor of the frontal horn. The genu gives rise to a large fiber tract, the forceps minor, which forms the anterior wall of the frontal horn, and the genu connects the frontal lobes. The splenium gives rise to a large tract, the forceps major, which forms a prominence called the *bulb of callosum* in the upper part of the medial wall of the atrium and occipital horn as it sweeps posteriorly to connect the occipital lobes. Another fiber tract, the tapetum, arises in the posterior part of the body and splenium and sweeps laterally and inferiorly to form the roof and lateral wall of the atrium and the temporal and occipital horns (Video 2-12).

Optic Radiation. The optic radiation is a bundle of fibers that extend from the lateral geniculate body to the visual area in the occipital lobe. The optic radiation may be divided into three parts: anterior, middle, and posterior. In the anterior part, the fibers initially take an anterior direction along the roof of the temporal horn, usually reaching as far anteriorly as the tip of the temporal horn, and then loop backward in the lateral and inferior aspects of the atrium and the occipital horn to end in the lower lip of the calcarine fissure; this anterior loop is called *Meyer's loop*. The anterior part represents the upper quadrants of the visual field. In the middle part, the fibers take a lateral direction initially, coursing along the roof of the temporal horn, and then proceed posteriorly along the lateral wall of the atrium and the occipital horn; the middle part contains the macular fibers. The fibers of the posterior part course directly backward along the lateral wall of the atrium and the occipital horn to end in the upper lip of the calcarine fissure; these fibers are responsible for the lower quadrants of the visual field (see Fig. 2-3C).

Fornix. The fornix is a C-shaped structure that wraps around the thalamus in the wall of the lateral ventricle. The initial portion of the fornix, the fimbria, arises from the alveus, which is the subcortical white matter of the hippocampal allocortex, and thickens along the medial edge of the hippocampus, separated from the dentate gyrus by the fimbrodentate sulcus. The fimbria then passes posteriorly to become the crus of the fornix representing the subcortical radiation of the hippocampal allocortex. In the atrium, the crus wraps around the posterior surface of the pulvinar of the thalamus and arches superomedially toward the lower surface of the splenium of the corpus callosum; at the junction between the atrium and the body of the lateral ventricle, the paired crura meet to form the body of the fornix. At the anterior margin of the thalamus, the body of the fornix separates into two columns that arch along the superior and anterior margins of the foramen of Monro. The columns of the fornix then split, passing predominantly posterior to the anterior commissure, and are directed inferiorly and posteriorly through the lateral wall of the third ventricle to reach the mammillary bodies at the floor of the third ventricle. In the area below the splenium, the two crura of the fornix are united by the hippocampal commissure (see Figs. 2-3A, 2-3D, *left*, and 2-4A).

Basal Ganglia. Although macroscopically fused and gathered into a "core" that is covered laterally by the insula, the basal ganglia and the thalamus are embryologically and functionally distinct structures. The basal ganglia are telencephalic structures, and the thalamus is a diencephalic structure. The basal ganglia consist of four nuclei: the striatum (caudate nucleus, putamen, and the nucleus accumbens), globus pallidus, substantia nigra, and subthalamic nucleus.

The caudate nucleus is a C-shaped structure that wraps around the thalamus; it has a head, body, and tail. The head and body are lateral walls of the frontal horn and body of the lateral ventricle. The tail extends from the atrium into the roof of the temporal horn and is continuous with the amygdaloid nucleus (see Figs. 2-2A and D and 2-3A).

Thalamus. The thalamus is located in the center of the lateral ventricle. Each lateral ventricle wraps around the superior, inferior, and posterior surfaces of the thalamus. The anterior tubercle of the thalamus is the posterior limit of the foramen of Monro; the posterior part, called the *pulvinar* (pillow) *of the thalamus*, is the wall of three compartments in the cerebrum: the posterolateral part of the pulvinar is the lateral half of the anterior wall of the atrium; the posteromedial part is covered by the crus of the fornix and is part of the superolateral wall of the quadrigeminal cistern; the inferolateral part of the pulvinar is the roof of the wing of the ambient cistern. The medial part of the thalamus is the lateral wall of the third ventricle (see Figs. 2-3A and 2-4B; see Fig. 2-9B, later).

Hippocampus. The hippocampus occupies the medial part of the floor of the temporal horn and is divided into three parts: the head, body, and tail. The head of the hippocampus, the anterior and largest part, is directed anteriorly and inferiorly and then medially. At the medial end of the tip of the temporal horn, it turns up vertically and bends over laterally, forming the medial wall of the tip of the temporal horn ahead of the choroidal fissure. The head of the hippocampus is free of choroid plexus and is characterized by three or four hippocampal digitations; its overall shape resembles a feline paw, and it is directed toward the posterior segment of the uncus. Its posterior limit is characterized by the initial segment of the fimbria and the choroidal fissure. Superiorly, the head of the hippocampus is related to the posteroinferior portion of the amygdala. Anteriorly, it is related to the uncal recess of the temporal horn, which is the anterior continuation of the collateral eminence. The emergence of the choroid plexus, the fimbria, and the choroidal fissure marks the beginning of the body of the hippocampus. The body of the hippocampus has an anteroposterior and inferosuperior direction and narrows as it approaches the atrium of the lateral ventricle. Posterior to the head of the hippocampus, the medial wall of the temporal horn is the choroidal fissure. At the atrium of the lateral ventricle, the body of the hippocampus changes direction and has its longitudinal axis oriented transversely to become the tail of the hippocampus. The tail of the hippocampus is slender and constitutes the medial part of the floor of the atrium; medially, the tail of the hippocampus fuses with the calcar avis. Histologically, the terminal segment of the hippocampal tail continues as the subsplenial gyrus, which covers the inferior splenial surface (see Figs. 2-3D, *left*, and 2-4A).

Amygdala. The amygdala and the hippocampus constitute the core of the limbic system. The temporal amygdala is composed of a series of gray matter nuclei classified into three main groups: basolateral, corticomedial, and central. From the neurosurgical viewpoint, the temporal amygdala can be considered as being entirely located within the boundaries of the uncus: superiorly, the amygdala blends into the globus pallidus; inferiorly, the temporal amygdala bulges inferiorly into the most anterior portion of the roof of the temporal horn above the hippocampal head and the uncal recess; medially, it is related to the anterior and posterior segments of the uncus. The amygdala also constitutes the anterior wall of the temporal horn (see Figs. 2-2A, 2-3D, *right*, and 2-4A).

Choroidal Fissure. The choroidal fissure is a cleft located between the thalamus and the fornix. It is the site of attachment of the choroid plexus in the lateral ventricle. It is a C-shaped arc that extends from the foramen of Monro through the body and atrium to the temporal horn.[8] The body part of the choroidal fissure is between the body of the fornix and the thalamus[9]; the atrial part is between the crus of the fornix and the pulvinar of the thalamus (see Fig. 2-3A); the temporal part is between the fimbria of the fornix and the stria terminalis of the thalamus. The choroid plexus is attached to the fornix and to the thalamus by ependymal coverings called the *taenia fornicis* and *taenia choroidea*, respectively; in the temporal part, the taenia fimbriae attaches the choroidal plexus to the fimbria. The choroidal fissure is one of the most important landmarks in microneurosurgeries involving the temporal lobe: it separates temporal structures that can be

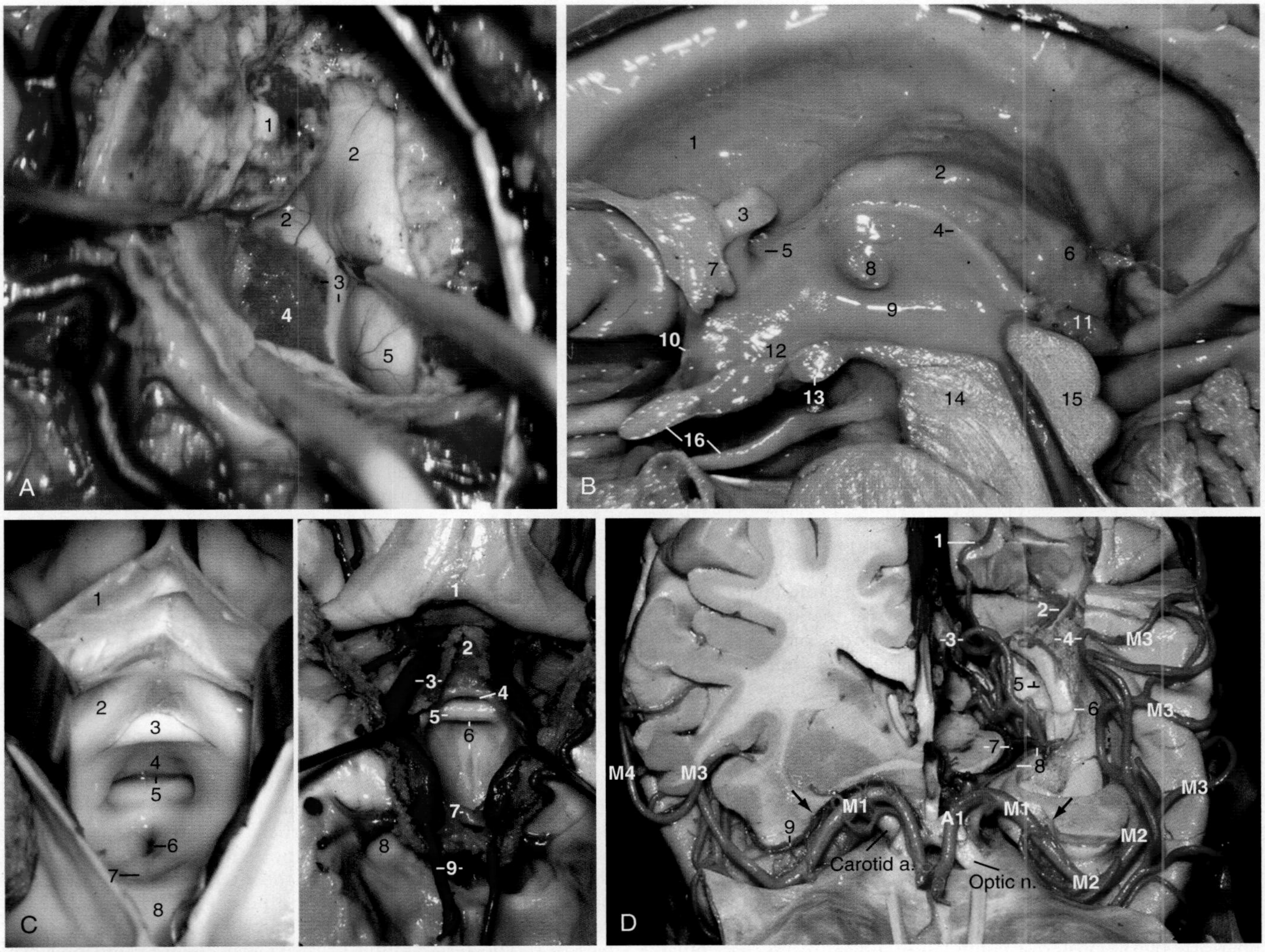

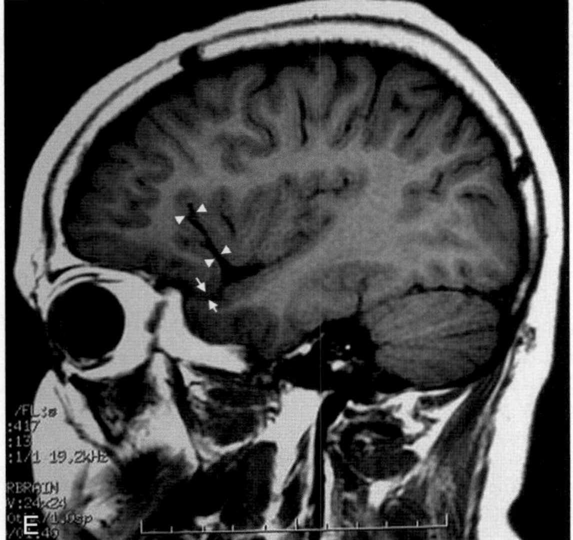

Figure 2-4. A, Intraoperative view of right temporal horn. 1, Amygdala; 2, head of hippocampus; 3, fimbria and taenia fimbriae; 4, choroid plexus; 5, body of hippocampus. **B,** Medial view of right thalamus. 1, Caudate nucleus; 2, thalamus (dorsal surface); 3, fornix (column); 4, taenia thalami; 5, foramen of Monro; 6, thalamus (pulvinar); 7, anterior commissure; 8, massa intermedia; 9, hypothalamic sulcus; 10, lamina terminalis; 11, pineal gland; 12, hypothalamus; 13, mammillary body; 14, midbrain; 15, quadrigeminal plate; 16, optic nerve and oculomotor nerve. **C,** *Left,* Posterosuperior view of anterior wall and floor of third ventricle. 1, Fornix (column); 2, fornix (column); 3, anterior commissure; 4, lamina terminalis; 5, optic recess; 6, infundibular recess; 7, tuber cinereum; 8, midbrain. *Right,* Anterosuperior view of posterior wall of third ventricle. 1, Fornix (reflected); 2, suprapineal recess and pineal gland; 3, internal cerebral vein and choroid plexus; 4, habenular commissure; 5, posterior commissure; 6, aqueduct and midbrain; 7, massa intermedia; 8, thalamostriate vein; 9, anterior septal vein. **D,** Frontal view. 1, Parieto-occipital artery; 2, calcarine artery; 3, vein of Galen and P3; 4, sylvian point and atrium; 5, parahippocampal and dentate gyri; 6, lateral posterior choroidal artery; 7, crus cerebri and basal vein; 8, anterior choroidal artery and inferior ventricular vein; 9, deep middle cerebral vein. *Black arrows* indicate limen insulae. **E,** Sagittal magnetic resonance imaging. The *arrows* indicate the anterior opercular compartment of the sylvian fissure, located between the posterior portion of the orbital gyri and the planum polare. The *arrowheads* indicate the anterior insular compartment of the sylvian fissure.

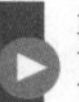
removed from thalamic structures that should be preserved (see Fig. 2-4A; Video 2-13).

Third Ventricle

The third ventricle is a narrow, funnel-shaped, unilocular, midline cavity. It communicates at its anterosuperior margin with each lateral ventricle through the foramen of Monro and posteriorly with the fourth ventricle through the aqueduct of Sylvius (see Fig. 2-4B). It has a roof, a floor, and anterior, posterior, and two lateral walls.[10] The roof extends from the foramen of Monro anteriorly to the suprapineal recess posteriorly and is constituted superiorly to inferiorly by five layers (see Fig. 2-3A). The first layer is the fornix; the body of the fornix is the anterior part of the roof of the third ventricle, and the crura and the hippocampal commissure are the roof of the posterior portion. The second layer is the superior membrane of the tela choroidea, which passes thorough the forniceal side of the choroidal fissure to cover the choroid plexus of the lateral ventricle. The third layer is the vascular layer located in a space between the superior and inferior membranes of the tela choroidea called the *velum interpositum*, which contains internal cerebral veins and branches of the medial posterior choroidal arteries. The fourth layer is the inferior membrane of the tela choroidea, which forms the floor of the velum interpositum. It is attached anterolaterally to the taenia thalami, a small ridge on the free edge of a fiber tract, the striae medullaris thalami, which extends along the superomedial border of the thalamus from the foramen of Monro to the habenular commissure (see Fig. 2-4B). The posterior part of the inferior membrane of the tela choroidea is attached to the superior surface of the pineal body. The fifth layer is the choroidal plexus of the third ventricle, usually represented by two parallel strands of choroid plexus projecting backward on each side of the midline. The floor extends from the optic chiasm anteriorly to the orifice of the aqueduct of Sylvius posteriorly; it is constituted anteriorly to posteriorly by the optic and infundibular recesses, tuber cinereum, mammillary bodies, posterior perforated substance, midbrain, and aqueduct (see Fig. 2-4B). The anterior wall is constituted by the lamina terminalis, and the posterior wall is represented inferiorly to superiorly by the posterior commissure, pineal recess, habenular commissure, pineal gland, and suprapineal recess (Fig. 2-4C). At the inner angle formed by the roof and the anterior wall is the anterior commissure. Frequently, there is another commissure in the cavity of the third ventricle located posteriorly to the foramen of Monro called *massa intermedia*, which connects both thalami. The lateral wall of the third ventricle is constituted by thalamus above and hypothalamus below, separated by hypothalamic sulcus, a shallow groove extending from the foramen of Monro to the aqueduct. The hypothalamic sulcus is the rostral continuation of the sulcus limitans of the brainstem (see Fig. 2-4B; Video 2-14). The thalamus is located above the midbrain and extends laterally above the oculomotor nerve and the parahippocampal gyrus. The floor of the frontal horn is located above the optic nerve and the planum sphenoidale. The head of the caudate nucleus is located above the bifurcation of the carotid artery, anterior clinoid process, and anterior perforated substance. The globus pallidus is located above the temporal amygdala and uncus. The splenium of the corpus callosum is located above the vein of Galen, and the pineal gland is located just anterior to the inferior surface of the vein of Galen. These structures are therefore related to the region of the tentorial incisura.[11]

Lateral Surface: Arterial Relationships

The *middle cerebral artery* (MCA)[12,13] is divided into four segments, M1 through M4. The *M1* or *sphenoidal segment* extends from the bifurcation of the internal carotid artery (ICA) to the limen insulae and will be discussed later in the section on the basal surface. The *M2* or *insular segment* extends from the limen insulae to the superior and inferior circular sulci of insula; it runs in the insular compartment of the sylvian fissure and is constituted by the superior and the inferior trunks and their branches. After reaching the superior or inferior circular sulcus of insula, the M2 branches enter the opercular compartment and are called the *M3 segment*. The *M3* or *opercular segment* runs in the opercular compartment and is related to the frontal and parietal opercula superiorly and to the temporal operculum inferiorly. The loop of the most posterior M3 segment branch that exits from the sylvian fissure is called the *M point* or *sylvian point*.[14] Anatomically, the sylvian point is located behind the insula, above the medial end of Heschl's gyrus (Fig. 2-4D). The angiographic sylvian point or M point displays the location of the medial end of Heschl's gyrus, the posterior end of the insula, and the central core, atrium, and pulvinar of the thalamus (Fig. 2-5A). On lateral projection, the M2 and M3 segments form the sylvian triangle that depicts the shape of the insula and the anterior, inferior, and posterior limits of the central core (Fig. 2-5B). The caudate nucleus is projected above the superior level of the sylvian triangle on lateral projection (Fig. 2-6A). The fourth segment is the *M4* or *cortical segment*, which extends from the sylvian fissure to the lateral surface of the cerebrum (Videos 2-15 and 2-16).

Lateral Surface: Venous Relationships

The superficial venous system drains the superficial one fifth of the thickness of the cerebrum, whereas the deep venous system drains the other four fifths of the depth of the cerebrum. On the lateral surface of the cerebrum, the superficial venous drainage system is accomplished by venous channels adjacent to the lobes. On the frontal and parietal lobes, the venous drainage can direct superiorly toward the superior sagittal sinus or inferiorly toward the superficial sylvian vein; on the temporal lobe, the veins can drain superiorly toward the superficial sylvian vein or inferiorly toward the dural sinuses below the temporal lobe.[15] There are three main anastomotic veins on the lateral surface of the cerebrum: the superficial sylvian vein, the vein of Trolard, and the vein of Labbé. The *superficial sylvian vein* begins at the posterior part of the posterior ramus of the sylvian fissure, runs inferiorly and anteriorly along the fissure, and commonly anastomoses with veins of Trolard and Labbé. It may arise as two trunks or present several variations. In the region of the pterion, it enters the dura and runs along the lesser wing of the sphenoid, in the sphenoparietal sinus or sinus of the lesser wing of the sphenoid, to enter the anterior end of the cavernous sinus through the medial end of the superior orbital fissure, then drains into the basilar sinus and the inferior petrosal sinus. The *vein of Trolard*, or superior anastomotic vein, is the largest anastomotic vein crossing the lateral surface of the brain between the superior sagittal sinus and the sylvian fissure. It is more frequently located at the parietal lobe. The *vein of Labbé*, or inferior anastomotic vein, is the largest anastomotic vein that crosses the temporal lobe between the sylvian fissure and the transverse sinus. It usually arises from the middle portion of the sylvian fissure and is directed posteriorly and inferiorly toward the anterior part of the transverse sinus at the level of the preoccipital notch (Fig. 2-6B).

The deep part of the sylvian fissure is related to the deep sylvian or middle cerebral vein and its tributaries. The tributaries of the deep sylvian vein come mainly from the sulci of the insula. The *deep middle cerebral vein* begins as a vein in the central sulcus of the insula and runs anteriorly and inferiorly toward the limen insulae, where it joins other insular veins to form a common trunk (see Fig. 2-6B).[16]

The deep venous system is divided into ventricular and cisternal groups; the cisternal group will be discussed in the basal surface section later. The ventricular veins are named mainly according to the locations they course, as follows, respectively:

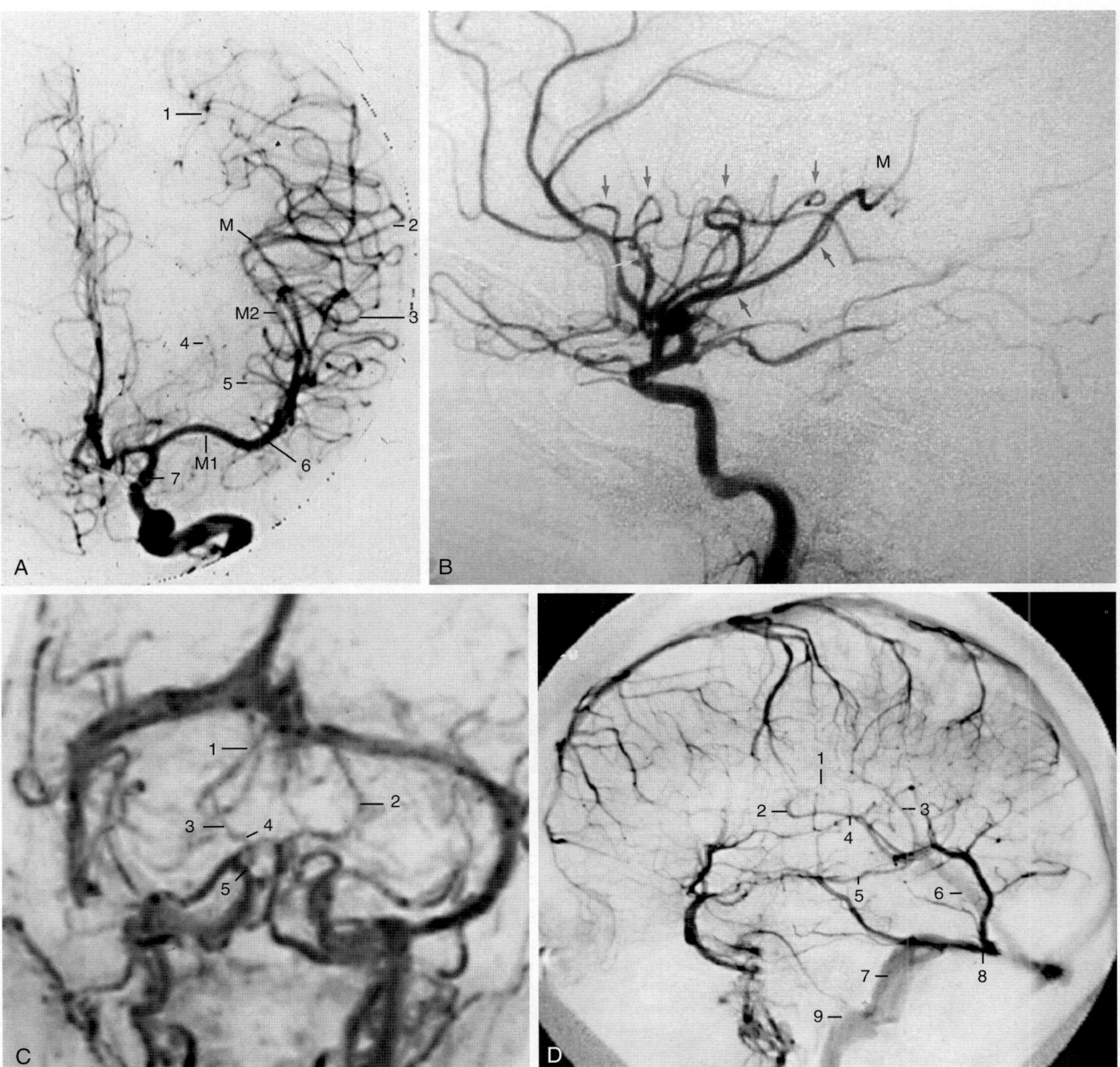

Figure 2-5. A, Frontal view of left carotid angiography. 1, Intraparietal sulcus; 2, M3 branches on planum temporale; 3, M3 branches in central sulcus region; 4, lateral lenticulostriate arteries; 5, M3 branches in anterior limiting sulcus of insula; 6, genu of middle cerebral artery; 7, internal carotid artery (supraclinoid segment). M, M point or sylvian point. **B,** Lateral view of carotid angiography. The *blue arrows* indicate the superior limiting sulcus of the insula; the *red arrows* indicate the inferior limiting sulcus of the insula; the *yellow arrow* indicates the anterior limiting sulcus of the insula. **C,** Frontal view of venous angiographic magnetic resonance imaging to display the basal vein. 1, "Thigh" (posterior mesencephalic segment); 2, "knee" (junction between anterior and posterior peduncular segments); 3, "leg" (anterior peduncular segment); 4, "ankle" (junction between striate and peduncular segments); 5, "foot" (striate segment). **D,** Lateral view of venous angiography. 1, Thalamostriate vein; 2, venous angle; 3, inferior sagittal sinus; 4, internal cerebral vein; 5, basal vein; 6, straight sinus; 7, sigmoid sinus; 8, transverse sinus and vein of Labbé complex; 9, bulb of jugular vein.

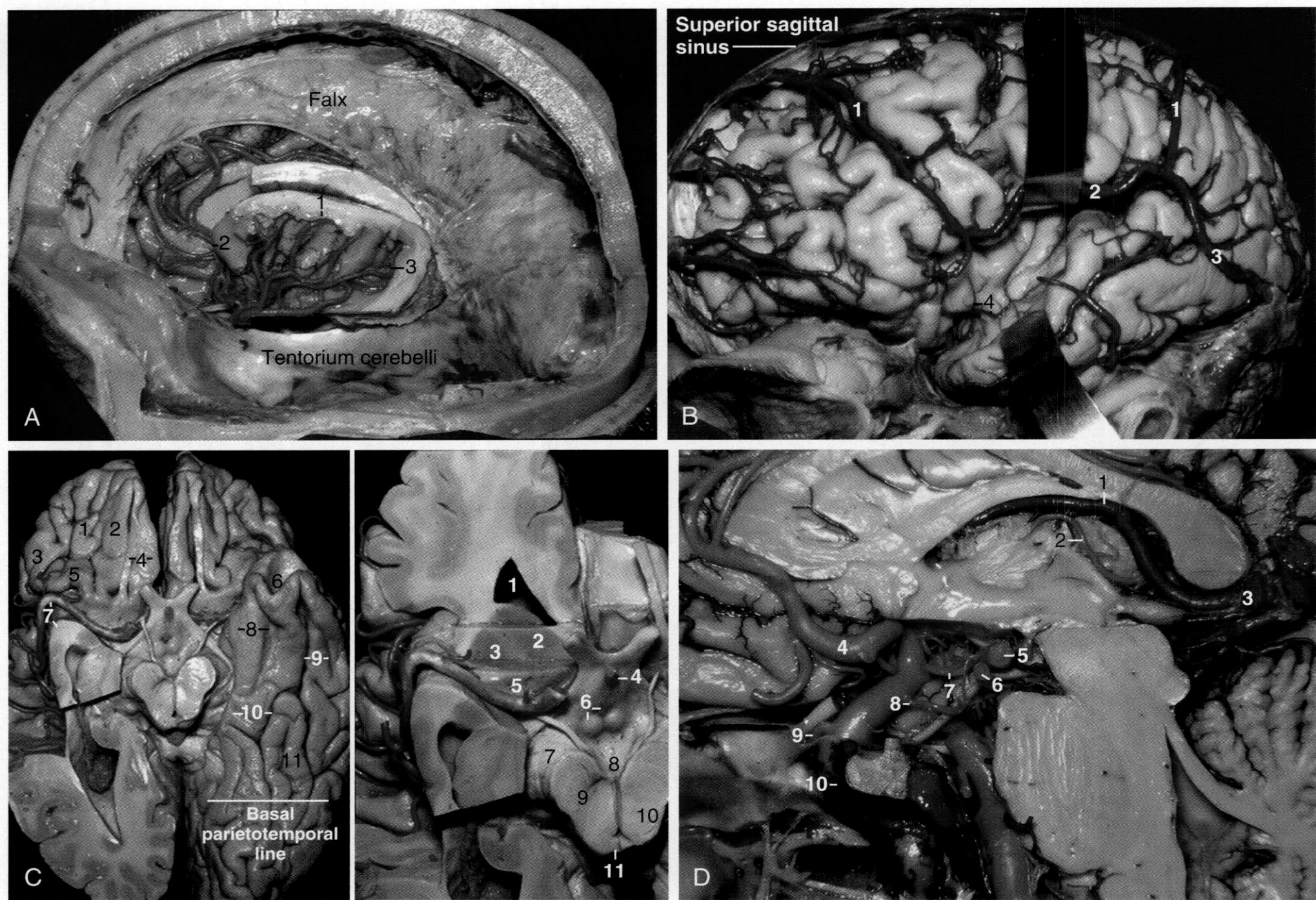

Figure 2-6. A, Lateral view of M2 branches over left insula. 1, Superior limiting sulcus; 2, anterior limiting sulcus; 3, inferior limiting sulcus. **B,** Lateral view. 1, Superior anastomotic vein; 2, superficial sylvian vein; 3, vein of Labbé; 4, insular veins. **C,** Basal view. Left. 1, Anterior orbital gyrus; 2, medial orbital gyrus; 3, lateral orbital gyrus; 4, rectus gyrus and olfactory tract; 5, posterior orbital gyrus; 6, temporal pole; 7, genu of middle cerebral artery and insular pole; 8, uncus and rhinal sulcus; 9, occipitotemporal sulcus and inferior temporal gyrus; 10, parahippocampal gyrus and collateral sulcus; 11, fusiform gyrus. Right. 1, Frontal horn; 2, caudate nucleus (head); 3, lentiform nucleus; 4, pituitary stalk; 5, anterior perforated substance; 6, tuber cinereum and mammillary body; 7, crus cerebri; 8, posterior perforated substance; 9, substantia nigra; 10, tegmentum; 11, tectum. **D,** Medial view. 1, Internal cerebral vein; 2, medial posterior choroidal artery; 3, vein of Galen; 4, anterior cerebral artery; 5, P2A; 6, superior cerebellar artery; 7, anterior choroidal artery; 8, posterior communicating artery; 9, ophthalmic artery and optic nerve; 10, intracavernous carotid artery.

the *frontal horn* by the anterior caudate and anterior septal veins; *body of the lateral ventricle* by the thalamostriate, thalamocaudate veins, posterior caudate, and posterior septal veins; *atrium* and *occipital horn* by medial and lateral atrial veins; *temporal horn* by inferior ventricular, amygdalar, and transverse hippocampal veins; *deep thalamic area* by anterior and superior thalamic veins; *superficial thalamic area* by anterior, superior, and posterior superficial thalamic veins; and *choroidal veins*—superior and inferior.[16]

Basal Surface: Neural Relationships

The basal surface is composed of frontal, temporal, and occipital lobes. The olfactory tract and sulcus divide the basal surface of the *frontal lobe* in two uneven parts: a smaller and medial part is the rectus gyrus; and a larger and lateral part, the orbital surface, is located above the orbit and composed of orbital gyri. The orbital surface is divided by the orbital sulcus, a complex sulcus that presents a rough configuration of the letter "H," into four quadrants: anterior, medial, posterior, and lateral orbital gyri. The pars orbitalis of the inferior frontal gyrus is continuous with the posterior part of the lateral orbital gyrus and with the lateral part of the posterior orbital gyrus. The *temporal lobe* is separated posteriorly from the occipital lobe by the basal parietotemporal line (from the preoccipital notch to the junction between the parieto-occipital and calcarine fissures) and presents, laterally to medially, the inferior temporal gyrus, occipitotemporal sulcus, fusiform gyrus, collateral sulcus, and parahippocampal gyrus (Fig. 2-6C, *left*). The collateral sulcus is an inferior-to-superior, medially to laterally oriented sulcus that bulges into the lateral part of the floor of the temporal horn (collateral eminence) and the atrium (collateral trigone). The collateral sulcus separates medially the allocortical parahippocampal gyrus from the mesocortical fusiform gyrus laterally. These gyri are kept separated anteriorly by the rhinal sulcus that separates the uncus medially from the temporal pole laterally. The rhinal sulcus can be considered an anterior continuation of the collateral sulcus, and it continues superiorly on the surface of the planum polare to separate this from the uncus medially (see Fig. 2-6C).

The *interpeduncular region* is determined by two oculomotor nerves, the posteromedial surface, and the apex of the uncus laterally; the diencephalic membrane of the Liliequist membrane (the membrane that extends from the dorsum sellae to the mammillary bodies), the pituitary stalk, and the dorsum sellae anteriorly; the tuber cinereum, mammillary bodies, and posterior perforated substance superiorly; and the inner surface of both crura cerebri posteriorly. The prepontine cistern forms the inferior limit of the interpeduncular fossa (see Fig. 2-6C and D).

Anterior Perforated Substance

The anterior perforated substance (APS) is the entry site for the perforating arteries from the internal carotid, the anterior choroidal, and the anterior and middle cerebral arteries to the basal ganglia, the anterior portion of the thalamus, the genu, and the anterior and posterior limbs of the internal capsule. It is also the exit site for the inferior striate veins. The APS is a convex cavity extending upward at the posterior end of the basal surface of the frontal lobe, bounded anteriorly by the lateral and medial olfactory striae; it is bounded posteromedially by the optic tract and posterolaterally by the anteromedial surface of the uncus; it is bounded laterally by the limen insulae. Medially, the APS extends above the optic chiasm to the interhemispheric fissure. The APS and the carotid bifurcation can be identified intraoperatively by following the olfactory tract posteriorly. The APS can be considered the floor of the anterior half of the basal ganglia (Fig. 2-6C, *right*).

Basal Surface: Arterial Relationships

The *internal carotid artery* is divided into five parts: cervical, petrous, cavernous, clinoid, and supraclinoid. The supraclinoid portion has been divided into three segments based on the origin of its major branches: the *ophthalmic segment* extends from the origin of the ophthalmic artery to the origin of the posterior communicating artery (PComA); the *communicating segment* extends from the origin of the PComA to the origin of the anterior choroidal artery (AChA); and the *choroidal segment* extends from the origin of the AChA to the bifurcation of the ICA (see Fig. 2-6D). The *ophthalmic artery* arises under the optic nerve, usually from the medial one third of the superior surface of the ICA, then it passes anteriorly and laterally to become superolateral to the carotid to enter the optic canal and the orbit. The perforating arteries from this segment arise from the posterior or medial or posteromedial aspect of the ICA and are distributed to the stalk of the pituitary gland, the optic chiasm, and less commonly the optic nerve, the premammillary portion of the floor of the third ventricle, and the optic tract. The *superior hypophyseal arteries*, which can range from 1 to 5 in number, pass medially to supply the pituitary stalk and the anterior lobe of the pituitary gland. The inferior hypophyseal artery from the meningohypophyseal trunk of the cavernous ICA supplies the posterior lobe. The *infundibular arteries* are another group of arteries that arise from the PComA and supply the same area as the superior hypophyseal artery (Video 2-17). The *posterior communicating artery* arises from the posteromedial or the posterior or the posterolateral aspect of the ICA and passes posteromedially to join the posterior cerebral artery (PCA) (Fig. 2-7A, *left*). In the embryo, the PComA continues as the PCA, but in an adult, the PCA becomes part of the basilar system. If the PComA remains the major origin of the PCA, the configuration of the PComA is termed *fetal* (Fig. 2-7A, *right*). In 60% of individuals, there are no perforating arteries arising from the communicating segment of the ICA; when present, the perforating arteries from the PComA range from 4 to 14 in number, arising predominantly from the proximal half of the artery, course superiorly, and terminate in the floor of the third ventricle. The largest branch from the PComA is the *premammillary artery*, or *anterior thalamoperforating artery* (Fig. 2-7B; Video 2-18). The *anterior choroidal artery* arises either from the posterolateral or the posterior aspect of the ICA. The AChA courses posteriorly below the optic tract toward the temporal horn by passing through the choroidal fissure (see Fig. 2-7A, *left*). The AChA sends off branches to the optic tract, crus cerebri, lateral geniculate body, and uncus and supplies the optic radiation, globus pallidus, midbrain, thalamus, and retrolenticular and posterior portions of the posterior limb of the internal capsule.

The choroidal segment of the ICA is the most frequent site of perforating arteries, ranging in number from 1 to 9, arising from the posterior aspect of the ICA. They terminate in the posterior half of the central region of the APS, optic tract, and uncus[17] (Videos 2-19 through 2-23).

The *anterior perforating arteries* are those arising from the ICA, MCA, AChA, and anterior cerebral arteries; they enter the brain through the APS (see Fig. 2-7B).

The M1 or *sphenoidal segment* of the MCA extends from the bifurcation of the ICA to the limen insulae. It courses first in the carotid cistern, then continues in the sphenoidal compartment. The proximal half of the M1 is related posteriorly and inferiorly to the anteromedial surface of the uncus, anteriorly to the lesser wing of sphenoid, and superiorly to the APS; the distal half is related inferiorly to the planum polare, anteriorly to the lesser wing of sphenoid, and superiorly and posteriorly to the insular pole. The M1 presents two types of branches: the lateral lenticulostriate arteries, which arise mostly from the superior or posterosuperior aspect of the M1 and penetrate the middle and posterior portions of the lateral half of APS, and the early branches, which course toward the temporal lobe to supply the temporal pole. The bifurcation of the MCA occurs before the limen of insulae in 86% of individuals (see Figs. 2-4D, 2-6C, and 2-7B).[3]

Embryologically, the *posterior cerebral artery*[18] arises as a branch of the ICA, but up to birth, its most common origin is the basilar artery. The PCA is classified into four segments: P1, P2A, P2P, and P3. The *P1* segment extends from the basilar bifurcation to the site where the PComA joins the PCA. The *P2* segment extends from the PComA to the posterior aspect of the midbrain. P2 is further divided into P2A (anterior) and P2P (posterior) segments. P2A begins at the PComA and courses around the crus cerebri, inferiorly to the optic tract, AChA, and basal vein and medially to the posteromedial surface of the uncus, up to the posterior margin of the crus cerebri. P2P begins at the posterior margin of the crus cerebri and runs laterally to the tegmentum of the midbrain within the ambient cistern, parallel and inferiorly to the basal vein, inferolaterally to the geniculate bodies and pulvinar, and medially to the parahippocampal gyrus to enter the quadrigeminal cistern. P3 begins under the posterior part of the pulvinar in the lateral aspect of the quadrigeminal cistern and ends at the anterior limit of the anterior calcarine sulcus. P3 is often divided into its major terminal branches, the calcarine and parieto-occipital arteries, before reaching the anterior limit of the anterior calcarine sulcus. The point where the PCAs from each side are closer to each other is called the *collicular* or *quadrigeminal point*. It marks the posterior limit of the midbrain on angiograms (see Fig. 2-14A, later). The P4 segment is composed of the cortical branches of the PCA (Fig. 2-7C).

The main branches arising from the PCA are the posterior thalamoperforating, direct perforating, short and long circumflex, thalamogeniculate, medial and lateral posterior choroidal, inferior temporal, parieto-occipital, calcarine, and posterior pericallosal arteries. The *posterior thalamoperforating arteries*, which arise from P1 and enter the brain through the posterior perforated substance, interpeduncular fossa, and medial crus cerebri, supply the anterior and part of the posterior thalamus, hypothalamus, subthalamus, substantia nigra, red nucleus, oculomotor and trochlear nuclei, oculomotor nerve, mesencephalic reticular formation, pretectum, rostromedial floor of the third ventricle, and posterior portion of the internal capsule. The *direct perforating arteries* to the crus cerebri arise mainly from the P2A segment

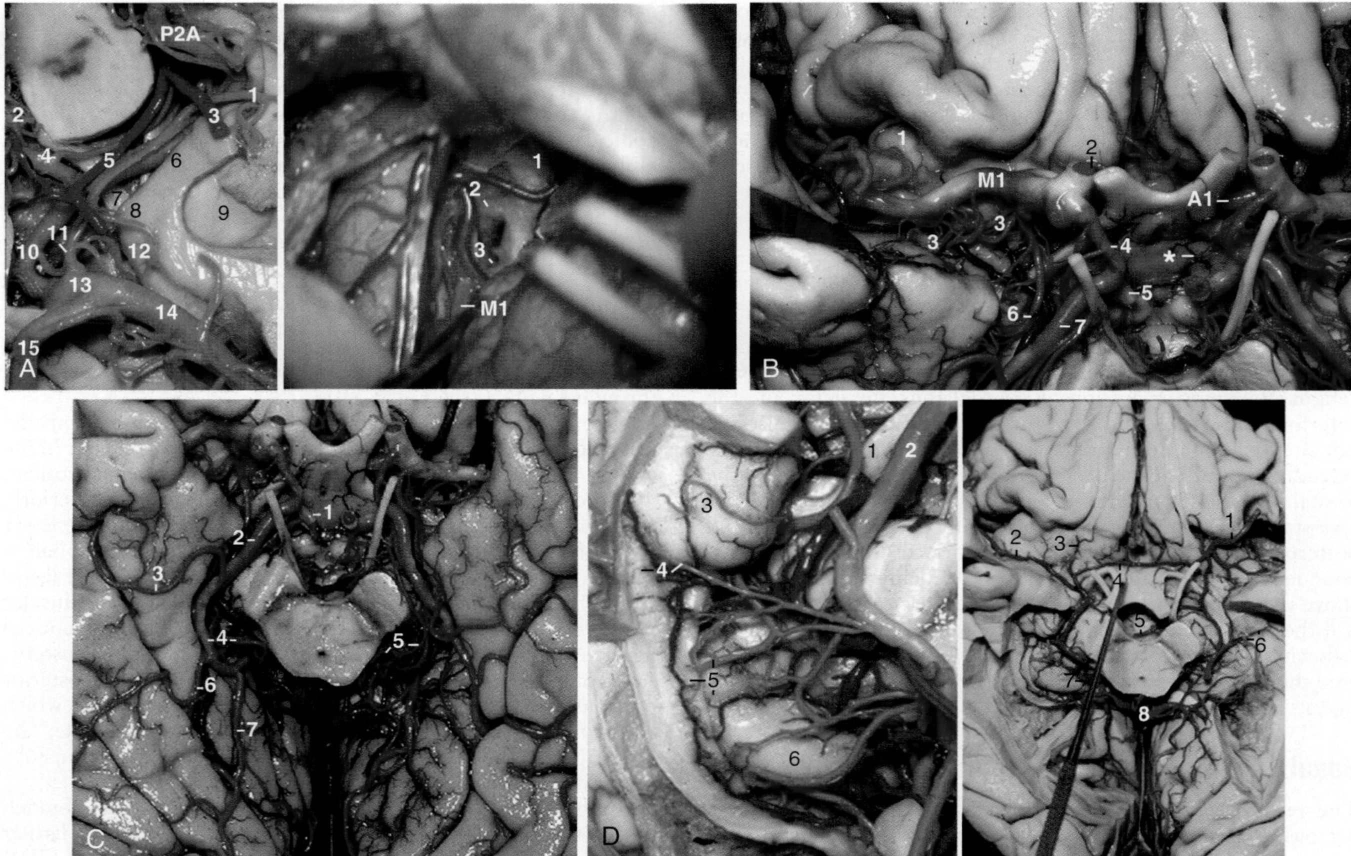

Figure 2-7. A, *Left.* 1, Inferior choroidal point; 2, posterior perforating arteries; 3, inferior ventricular vein; 4, P1 and medial posterior choroidal artery; 5, basal vein; 6, uncus (posterior segment); 7, oculomotor nerve; 8, uncus (apex); 9, hippocampus (head); 10, posterior communicating artery (PComA); 11, anterior choroidal artery (AChA); 12, uncus (anterior segment); 13, internal carotid artery; 14, M1; 15, A1. *Right,* Left transsylvian approach. 1, Supraclinoid carotid artery; 2, fetal PComA; 3, AChA. **B,** Basal view. 1, Insula; 2, supraclinoid carotid artery; 3, lateral lenticulostriate arteries; 4, PComA; 5, P1; 6, AChA; 7, P2A. *, Premammillary artery. **C,** Basal view. 1, P1; 2, P2A; 3, anterior inferior temporal artery; 4, P2P and long circumflex arteries; 5, short circumflex arteries; 6, middle inferior temporal artery; 7, posterior inferior temporal artery. **D,** Basal view. *Left.* 1, Optic tract; 2, P2A; 3, uncus (inferior surface); 4, hippocampal artery and dentate gyrus; 5, lateral posterior choroidal artery, fornix, and lateral geniculate body; 6, thalamus (pulvinar). Basal view. *Right.* 1, Fronto-orbital vein; 2, deep middle cerebral vein; 3, olfactory vein; 4, anterior cerebral vein; 5, peduncular vein; 6, inferior ventricular vein and inferior choroidal point; 7, posterior mesencephalic segment; 8, vein of Galen. The choroids plexus separates the roof of the temporal horn from the thalamus.

and supply the crus cerebri. The *short* and *long circumflex arteries* to the brainstem arise mainly from the P1 and less frequently from the P2A; the short circumflex artery courses around the midbrain and terminates at the geniculate bodies; the long circumflex artery courses around the midbrain and reaches the colliculi. The *thalamogeniculate arteries* arise equally from the P2A or P2P segment, perforate the inferior surface of the geniculate bodies, and supply the posterior half of the lateral thalamus, posterior limb of the internal capsule, and optic tract (see Fig. 2-7C). The *medial posterior choroidal arteries* (MPChAs) arise mainly from the P2A and less frequently from the P2P and P1 segments and course around the midbrain, medial to the main trunk of the PCA; turn around the pulvinar of the thalamus to proceed superiorly at the lateral side of colliculi and pineal gland to enter the roof of the third ventricle through the velum interpositum; and finally course through the foramen of Monro to enter the choroid plexus in the lateral ventricle (see Figs. 2-3A, *right*, and 2-6D). The MPChA supplies the crus cerebri, tegmentum, geniculate bodies (mainly the medial), colliculi, pulvinar, pineal gland, and medial thalamus. Angiographically on lateral projection, the MPChA describes the shape of the number 3. The inferior curve of the "3" is when it turns around the pulvinar, and the superior curve is where it contours the colliculi before entering the roof of the third ventricle (see Fig. 2-14B, later). The *lateral posterior choroidal arteries* (LPChAs) arise mainly from the P2P and less frequently from the P2A segment and pass laterally to enter the ventricular cavity directly through the choroidal fissure to supply the choroid plexus in the atrium and the temporal horn. They anastomose with the AChA (see Figs. 2-4D and 2-14B). The *inferior temporal arteries* are distributed to the basal surface of the temporal and occipital lobes. They include the hippocampal artery and three groups of temporal arteries, namely, the anterior, middle, and posterior temporal arteries (see Fig. 2-7C and D, *left*). The anterior temporal artery arises mainly from the P2A, whereas the middle and posterior temporal arteries arise mainly from the P2P segment. *Parieto-occipital and calcarine arteries* are usually terminal branches of the PCA; they arise predominantly from P3; however, they may also arise from the P2P segment and course respectively in the parieto-occipital fissure and the calcarine fissure. As the calcarine fissure reaches laterally to bulge into the medial wall of the atrium and the occipital horn, the calcarine artery also follows laterally into the depth of the calcarine fissure (see Fig. 2-4D). The *splenial* or *posterior pericallosal artery* supplies the splenium of the corpus callosum and arises from the parieto-occipital artery in 62% of individuals, but it also can arise from the calcarine artery, MPChA, posterior temporal artery, P2P, P3, and LPChA.

Basal Surface: Venous Relationships

The inferior frontal veins drain the basal surface of the *frontal lobe*, either anteriorly to the superior sagittal sinus (anterior group) or posteriorly to join the deep sylvian vein in the sylvian fissure (posterior group). The *anterior group* is composed of anterior fronto-orbital and frontopolar veins; the *posterior group* is composed of olfactory and posterior fronto-orbital veins. The inferior temporal veins drain the *temporal lobe*; they are divided into a lateral group that drains into the sinuses in the anterolateral part of the tentorium and a medial group that empties into the basal vein. The *lateral group* is composed of the anterior, middle, and posterior temporobasal veins. The temporobasal veins appear to radiate from the preoccipital notch across the inferior surface of the temporal lobe. The *occipital lobe* is drained by the *occipitobasal vein* that courses anterolaterally toward the preoccipital notch and frequently joins the posterior temporobasal vein before emptying into the lateral tentorial sinus.

The most important deep venous channel on the basal surface is the basal vein of Rosenthal. The *basal vein* originates below the APS and is divided into three segments (Fig. 2-7D, *right*): the *first*, or *anterior* or *striate*, *segment* originates from the junction of the anterior cerebral, inferior striate, and olfactory, fronto-orbital, and deep middle cerebral veins under the APS and runs posteriorly under the optic tract, medially to the anterior portion of the crus cerebri. This point corresponds to the most medial (before its termination into the vein of Galen) and usually most inferior part of the basal vein. This point indicates laterally the location of the apex of the uncus. The *second*, or *middle* or *peduncular*, *segment* starts from the most medial point in the course of the basal vein, usually correspondent to the site where the peduncular vein joins the basal vein. It runs laterally between the upper part of the posteromedial surface of the uncus and the upper part of the crus cerebri, and under the optic tract to reach the most lateral part of the crus cerebri, which corresponds to the most lateral point of the vein as it turns around the crus cerebri, usually where the inferior ventricular vein joins the basal vein; this is called the *anterior peduncular segment* by Huang and Wolf.[19] It then turns medially, superiorly, and posteriorly to the plane of the lateral mesencephalic sulcus behind the crus cerebri to constitute the posterior peduncular segment. The main tributaries of the second segment are the peduncular or interpeduncular, inferior ventricular, inferior choroidal, hippocampal, and anterior hippocampal veins. The *third*, or *posterior* or *posterior mesencephalic*, *segment* runs medially, superiorly, and posteriorly from the lateral mesencephalic sulcus and under the pulvinar of the thalamus to penetrate the quadrigeminal cistern and generally drain into the vein of Galen. The main tributaries of the third segment are the lateral mesencephalic, posterior thalamic, posterior longitudinal hippocampal, medial temporal, and medial occipital veins. In some individuals, the precentral cerebellar, superior vermian, internal occipital, splenial, medial atrial, and direct lateral and lateral atrial subependymal veins drain into the third segment of the basal vein. In the angiographic frontal view, the overall shape of both basal veins resembles the legs of a frog lying on its back with its toes directed anterolaterally. The foot corresponds to the striate segment and is related superiorly to the APS, laterally to the anterior segment of the uncus, medially to the optic tract, and inferiorly to the contents of the carotid cistern. The ankle corresponds posteriorly to the anterior aspect of the crus cerebri, laterally to the apex of the uncus, and superiorly to the optic tract. The leg corresponds to the anterior peduncular segment and is related superiorly to the optic tract, laterally to the upper portion of the posteromedial surface of the uncus, and medially to the upper portion of the crus cerebri. The knee corresponds to the most lateral aspect of the crus cerebri and to the posterior edge of the posterior segment of the uncus. It is related laterally to the inferior choroidal point, superiorly to the optic tract just before it reaches the lateral geniculate body, and inferiorly to the contents of the ambient cistern. The thigh, which includes the posterior peduncular and posterior mesencephalic segments, is related medially to the tegmentum of the midbrain, laterally to the parahippocampal gyrus, superiorly to the medial aspect of the pulvinar of the thalamus, which is the roof of the wing of the ambient cistern, and inferiorly to the contents of the wing of the ambient cistern (see Fig. 2-5C).[18] In the angiographic lateral view, the basal and internal cerebral veins delimit the thalamus and the hypothalamus (see Fig. 2-5D; see Fig. 2-8A, later).

Medial Surface: Neural Relationships

The medial surface of the cerebrum is composed of the sulci and gyri of the frontal, parietal, occipital, and temporal lobes. The general organization of the gyri of the frontal, parietal, and occipital lobes on this surface can be compared to that of a three-layer roll: the inner layer is represented by the corpus callosum, the intermediate layer by the cingulate gyrus, and the outer layer by the medial frontal gyrus, paracentral lobule, precuneus, cuneus, and lingual gyrus. The cingulate gyrus is separated inferiorly from the corpus callosum by the callosal sulcus and superiorly from the outer layer by the cingulate sulcus. Several secondary rami ascend from the cingulate sulcus in a radial pattern and divide the outer layer into several sections. There are two secondary rami of particular importance: the *paracentral ramus*, which ascends from the cingulate sulcus at the level of the midpoint of the corpus callosum and separates the medial frontal gyrus anteriorly from the paracentral lobule posteriorly, and the *marginal ramus*, which ascends from the cingulate sulcus at the level of the splenium of the corpus callosum and separates the paracentral lobule anteriorly from the precuneus posteriorly. The *marginal ramus* intercepts the postcentral gyrus in almost 100% of individuals, and it is an important landmark to determine the location of the sensory or motor areas in the lateral convexity through midsagittal magnetic resonance imaging (MRI). The parieto-occipital sulcus separates the precuneus superiorly from the cuneus inferiorly, and the calcarine sulcus separates the cuneus superiorly from the lingual gyrus inferiorly. The paracentral ramus, along with the marginal ramus, determines the *paracentral lobule*, which is concerned with movements of the contralateral lower limb and perineal region and is involved in voluntary control over defecation and micturition. The paracentral lobule is composed of the anterior part of the postcentral and precentral gyri and the posterior portion of the superior frontal gyrus. The *precuneus* and the part of the paracentral lobule behind the central sulcus form the medial part of the parietal lobe; the precuneus corresponds to the superior parietal lobule on the lateral surface. The precuneus consists of the *subparietal sulcus*, a vaguely H-shaped sulcus whereby the vertical arm of the H tends to align with the marginal ramus, and the parieto-occipital sulcus, which separates the precuneus above from the cingulated gyrus below (Fig. 2-8A). The parieto-occipital and calcarine sulci determine the *cuneus*; the cuneus and the medial part of the lingual gyrus make up the medial portion of the occipital lobe (Video 2-24). The *calcarine sulcus* starts at the occipital pole and directs anteriorly, presenting a slightly curved course with its characteristic

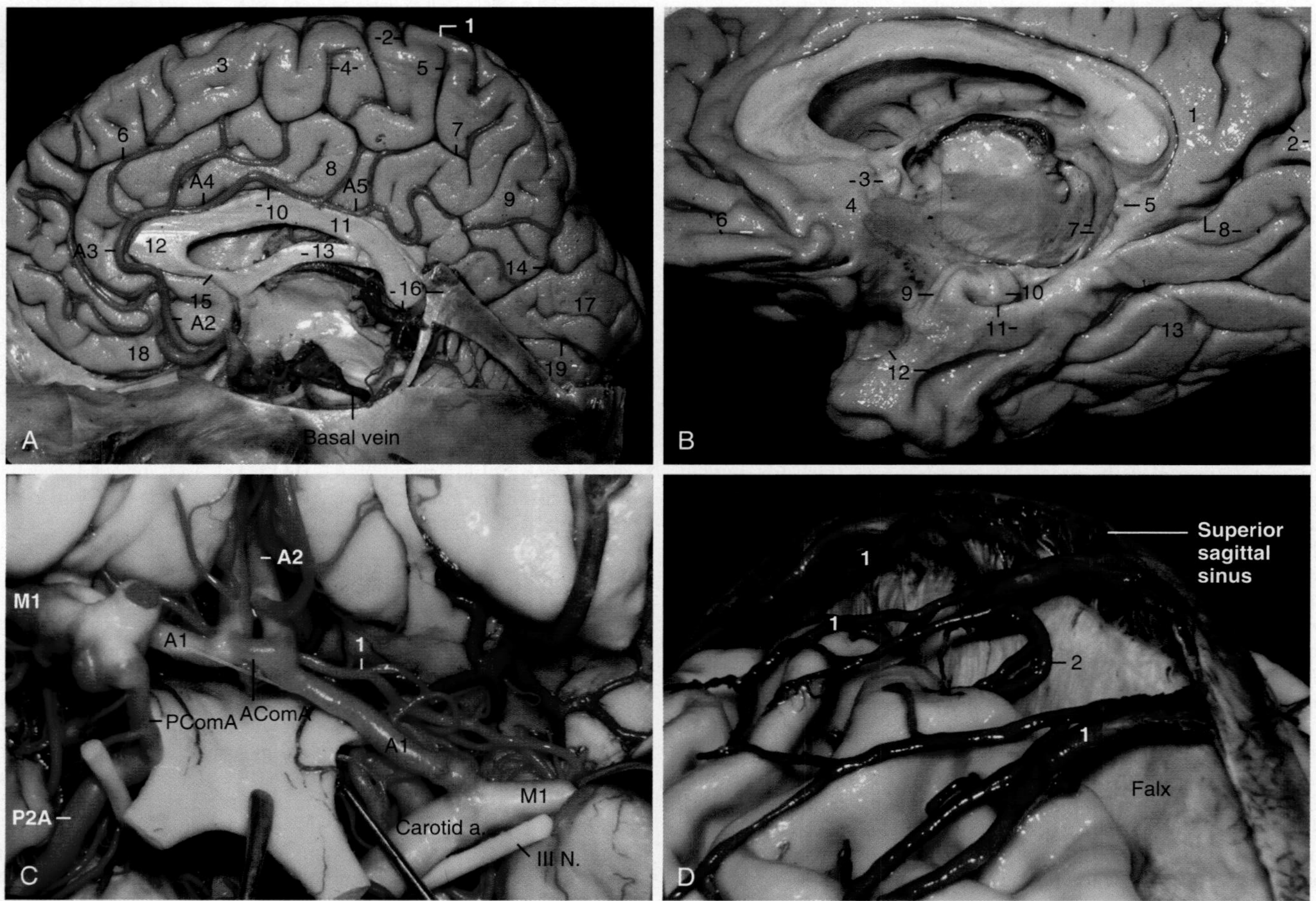

Figure 2-8. A, Medial view. 1, Postcentral gyrus; 2, precentral gyrus and central sulcus; 3, medial frontal gyrus; 4, paracentral ramus and paracentral lobule; 5, marginal ramus; 6, cingulate sulcus; 7, intraparietal sulcus; 8, cingulate gyrus; 9, precuneus; 10, corpus callosum (body) and callosal sulcus; 11, corpus callosum (isthmus); 12, corpus callosum (genu); 13, fornix and internal cerebral vein; 14, parieto-occipital sulcus; 15, corpus callosum (rostrum); 16, corpus callosum (splenium), vein of Galen, and straight sinus; 17, cuneus; 18, rectus gyrus; 19, posterior calcarine sulcus and lingual gyrus. **B,** Medial view. 1, Cingulate gyrus (isthmus); 2, parieto-occipital sulcus and cuneus; 3, anterior commissure and subcallosal area; 4, paraterminal gyrus; 5, dentate gyrus; 6, superior and inferior rostral sulci; 7, choroidal fissure and fornix; 8, anterior calcarine sulcus and lingual gyrus; 9, uncus (anterior segment); 10, uncus (posterior segment); 11, uncal notch; 12, rhinal incisura and rhinal sulcus; 13, fusiform gyrus. **C,** Basal view. 1, Recurrent artery. AComA, anterior communicating artery; PComA, posterior communicating artery. **D,** Anterolateral view of right parasagittal area. 1, Vein from lateral surface; 2, vein from medial surface.

upward convexity. The calcarine sulcus joins the parieto-occipital sulcus (only superficially) at an acute angle behind the isthmus of the cingulate gyrus and continues anteriorly to intercept the isthmus of the cingulate gyrus. The portion of the calcarine sulcus anterior to the junction is called the *anterior calcarine sulcus*; it is crossed by a buried *anterior cuneolingual gyrus* and bulges into the medial wall of the atrium of the lateral ventricle as the calcar avis. It contains the visual cortex only on its lower lip. The part of the calcarine sulcus posterior to the union is called the *posterior calcarine sulcus* and contains striate (visual) cortex on its upper and lower lips (see Fig. 2-9C, later). Anteriorly, the cingulate and the medial frontal gyri wrap around the genu and the rostrum of the corpus callosum. At the inferior end of these two gyri, under the rostrum of the corpus callosum and in front of the lamina terminalis, is a narrow triangle of gray matter, the *paraterminal gyrus*, separated from the rest of the cortex by a shallow *posterior paraolfactory sulcus*. Slightly anterior to this sulcus, a short vertical sulcus may occur, the *anterior paraolfactory sulcus*; the cortex between the posterior and anterior paraolfactory sulci is the *subcallosal area* or paraolfactory gyrus. Frequently, two anteroposteriorly directed sulci, the *superior* and *inferior rostral sulci*, which are parallel to the floor of the anterior fossa, divide the inferior portion of the medial frontal gyrus into three parts. Posteriorly, the cingulate gyrus continues inferiorly with the parahippocampal gyrus through the isthmus of the cingulate gyrus. The *mesial portion of the temporal lobe* presents intraventricular and extraventricular elements. The intraventricular elements are the hippocampus, fimbria, amygdala, and choroidal fissure; the extraventricular elements are the parahippocampal gyrus, uncus, and dentate gyrus. The *parahippocampal gyrus* extends anteriorly to posteriorly and, at its anterior extremity, deviates medially and bends posteriorly to constitute the uncus. Posteriorly, just bellow the splenium of the corpus callosum, the parahippocampal gyrus is often intersected by the anterior calcarine sulcus, which divides the posterior portion of the parahippocampal gyrus into the isthmus of the cingulate gyrus superiorly and the parahippocampal gyrus inferiorly and which continues posteriorly as the lingual gyrus. Superiorly, the parahippocampal gyrus is separated from the dentate gyrus by the hippocampal sulcus. Laterally, the parahippocampal gyrus is limited by the collateral sulcus posteriorly and the rhinal sulcus anteriorly. The rhinal sulcus marks the lateral limit of the entorhinal area of the parahippocampal gyrus; the parahippocampal gyrus is separated from the inferior surface of the posterior segment of the uncus by the *uncal notch*. Medially, the parahippocampal gyrus is related to the tentorium edge and to the contents of the ambient cistern. The various components of the parahippocampal gyrus are the subiculum, presubiculum, parasubiculum, and entorhinal area, the subiculum being its medial round edge. The name *uncus* means "hook." It is formed by the anterior portion of the parahippocampal gyrus, which has deviated medially and folded posteriorly. Inferiorly, the uncus is separated from the parahippocampal gyrus by the uncal notch. Anteriorly, the uncus continues with the anterior portion of the parahippocampal gyrus without a sharp limit; superiorly, the uncus is continuous with the globus pallidus. At the basal surface, the uncus is separated laterally from the temporal pole by the rhinal sulcus, and its medial part is normally herniated medially to the tentorial edge. When viewed from its basal surface, the uncus presents the shape of an arrowhead with its apex pointing medially, featuring an apex, an anterior segment, and a posterior segment (see Fig. 2-3D). The anterior segment of the uncus presents one surface, the anteromedial, and the posterior segment presents two surfaces, the posteromedial and the inferior. The two segments converge superiorly to the junction between the amygdala and the globus pallidus. The uncus is composed of five small gyri and a small part of the entorhinal area, which occupies the anterior part of the anteromedial surface. The *anterior segment* or *anteromedial surface* belongs to the parahippocampal gyrus and consists of the semilunar and ambient gyri. The semilunar gyrus occupies the superior portion of the anteromedial surface and is bordered inferiorly by the sulcus annularis; the ambient gyrus is medial and inferior to the semilunar gyrus; the anteroinferior area of this surface is occupied by the entorhinal area, which continues anteriorly and inferiorly with the entorhinal area of the parahippocampal gyrus (Fig. 2-8B). The anteromedial surface is related to the proximal sylvian fissure and carotid cistern and is the posterolateral limit of the APS. The *posterior segment* is related to the hippocampus and has two surfaces, a posteromedial surface and an inferior surface (see Fig. 2-3D, *left*). The posterior segment is occupied by three small gyri; from anterior to posterior, they are the uncinate gyrus, the band of Giacomini, and the intralimbic gyrus. The superior and inferior portions of the posteromedial surface of the uncus are related, respectively, to the crural and ambient cisterns. Posteriorly and superiorly to the uncus is the inferior choroidal point, where the choroid plexus of the temporal horn begins. The inferior choroidal point corresponds to the site where the AChA enters and the inferior ventricular vein leaves the temporal horn through the choroidal fissure (see Figs. 2-7A to D, *right*). The inferior surface is the superior lip of the uncal notch, and it is visible only from below when the parahippocampal gyrus is removed. The *dentate gyrus* bears this name because of its characteristic toothlike elevations; the margo denticulatus is prominent mainly in its anterior and middle portions. The dentate gyrus continues anteriorly with the band of Giacomini, also called the *tail of the dentate gyrus*, and continues posteriorly with the fasciolar gyrus, a smooth, grayish band that is located posterior to the splenium of the corpus callosum; the fasciolar gyrus continues above the corpus callosum as the indusium griseum to end as the paraterminal gyrus. The fimbrodentate and hippocampal sulci separate the dentate gyrus, respectively, from the fimbria superiorly and the parahippocampal gyrus inferiorly (see Fig. 2-8B).

The extraventricular and intraventricular structures of the mesial temporal lobe are intimately related. The anterior segment of the uncus is related to M1, the carotid artery, and the amygdala. The apex of the uncus passes above the oculomotor nerve and is related to the uncal recess and the amygdala laterally (see Figs. 2-6D and 2-7A); the posterior segment is related to the head of the hippocampus and the amygdala laterally, to the P2A inferomedially, and to the AChA superomedially (Videos 2-13 and 2-25).

Medial Surface: Arterial Relationships

The *anterior cerebral artery* (ACA) is classified into five segments, A1 through A5. The *A1 segment* extends from the bifurcation of the ICA to the anterior communicating artery (AComA). The *A2 segment* extends from the AComA to the junction between the rostrum and the genu of the corpus callosum. The *A3 segment* extends from the genu of the corpus callosum to the point where the artery turns sharply and posteriorly above the genu of the corpus callosum. The A2 and A3 segments together are also called the *ascending segment*. The *A4* and *A5 segments* extend above the corpus callosum, from the genu to the splenium. These two segments together are also called the *horizontal segment*, and the point bisected in the lateral view close behind the coronal suture separates them. The segment of the ACA distal to the AComA (A2 to A5) has also been called the *pericallosal artery* (see Fig. 2-8A). The junction of the AComA with the A1 segment occurs above the chiasm in 70% and above the nerve in 30% of individuals. The shorter A1 segments are usually stretched tightly over the chiasm; the longer ones pass anteriorly over the optic nerve, can be elongated and tortuous, and reach either the tuberculum sellae or the planum sphenoidale (see Fig. 2-8A). The medial lenticulostriate perforators, ranging from 1 to 11 branches (average 6.4), arise from the superior, posterior, or posterosuperior aspect of the proximal half of the A1 segment and pursue a direct posterior and superior course to enter the medial half of the APS.[20] Embryologically, the AComA develops from a multichanneled vascular network that coalesces to a variable degree by the time of birth.[20] In only 20% of individuals does the AComA communicate two A1 segments of equal size. The AComA complex probably exists as a single channel in about 75% of individuals.[20] The perforators from AComA, ranging from 0 to 4 (average, 1.6), usually arise from its posteroinferior aspect to supply the infundibulum, APS, optic chiasm, subcallosal area, and preoptic areas of the hypothalamus. The *recurrent artery of Heubner* of the ACA arises in 78% of individuals from the proximal A2, and it doubles back on its parent vessel, courses anteriorly to the A1 segment in 60% of individuals, and can be seen by elevating the frontal lobe before the visualization of the A1 segment; it is the largest and longest branch directed to the APS. After its origin, it passes above the carotid bifurcation and accompanies the M1 into the medial part of the sylvian fissure before entering the anterior and middle portions of the full mediolateral extent of the APS (Fig. 2-8C). The *A2 segment* is also the source of the central or the basal perforating arteries, which pass posteriorly to enter the optic chiasm, lamina terminalis, and anterior forebrain, below the corpus callosum. The two first cortical branches of the ACA supplying the medial surface, the *orbitofrontal* and the *frontopolar* arteries, usually arise from the A2 segment. Segments A3 to A5 give rise to other cortical branches to supply the medial surface of the hemisphere. All the cortical branches arise more frequently from the pericallosal than from the callosomarginal artery (Videos 2-26 and 2-27).

Medial Surface: Venous Relationships

The *medial frontal veins* drain the medial surface of the *frontal lobe*. They can empty either superiorly into the superior sagittal sinus or inferiorly into the inferior sagittal sinus, or into the veins that pass around the corpus callosum to drain into the anterior end of the basal vein. The medial parietal veins drain the medial surface of the *parietal lobe*. They can either empty superiorly into the superior sagittal sinus or course around the splenium of the corpus callosum and drain inferiorly into the vein of Galen or its tributaries. On both lobes, the veins commonly curve over the superior margin of the hemisphere onto the upper part of the lateral surface, where they join the terminal end of the veins from the lateral surface before emptying into the superior sagittal sinus (Fig. 2-8D). The *posterior pericallosal veins*, one on each side, arise from tributaries that drain the posterior part of the cingulate gyrus and the precuneus, and they course side by side around the splenium of the corpus callosum to terminate in either the vein of Galen or the internal cerebral vein. The anterior and posterior calcarine veins drain the *occipital lobe*. The *anterior calcarine* or *internal occipital vein* arises from tributaries that drain the anterior portion of the cuneus and lingual gyrus and passes forward to join the posterior pericallosal vein near the splenium before terminating in either the internal cerebral vein or in the vein of Galen. The *posterior calcarine vein* arises from tributaries that drain the area bordering the posterior part of the calcarine fissure and then curves sharply upward on the cuneus to reach the superior sagittal sinus.

The deep venous system of the *mesial temporal region* drains into the basal vein of Rosenthal.

Arachnoid Membrane

The arachnoid membrane covers the whole surface of the brain, including the sulci, arteries, and veins, and it also follows each sulcus and folds into the depth of each sulcus and cistern; the arachnoid membrane separates two adjacent gyri and entraps the veins and arteries inside the sulcus or cistern. It can constitute an important tool for the surgeon to establish a dissection plane by opening the sulcus either to reach a lesion located in the depth of a sulcus or to perform a subpial resection preserving the arteries and veins inside the sulcus.

Gray Matter and White Matter

It is important for the surgeon to be familiar with the consistency, color, and vasculature of the normal gray and white matter because it plays a major role in tumor, vascular malformation, and cortical dysplasia surgeries, and the surgeon has to distinguish the abnormal tissue that has to be removed from the normal brain tissue that has to be preserved. Sometimes, this distinction is not as easy as we might imagine (Video 2-28).

POSTERIOR FOSSA

The posterior fossa is characterized by the "rule of three" whereby the brainstem presents three parts (midbrain, pons, and medulla) and the cerebellum presents three surfaces (petrosal, tentorial, and suboccipital), three cerebellar peduncles (superior, middle, and inferior), three fissures (cerebellomesencephalic, cerebellopontine, and cerebellomedullary), three main arteries (superior cerebellar artery [SCA], anterior inferior cerebellar artery [AICA], and posterior inferior cerebellar artery [PICA]), and three main venous draining groups (petrosal, galenic, and tentorial).

Brainstem

The brainstem is divided into three parts: midbrain, pons, and medulla.

The *midbrain* is divided by a midline sagittal plane into two cerebral peduncles. Each peduncle is further divided into three parts: an anterior part consisting of the crus cerebri or basis pedunculi; an intermediate part, the tegmentum; and a posterior part located behind the aqueduct, the tectum. The substantia nigra and the lateral mesencephalic sulcus separate the crus cerebri from the tegmentum. The oculomotor nerves emerge from the medial side of the crura cerebri in the interpeduncular fossa (see Fig. 2-6C, *right*). The pontomesencephalic sulcus, which separates the midbrain from the pons, originates in the depth of the interpeduncular fossa and runs around the inferior margin of the crus cerebri to join the lateral mesencephalic sulcus behind the crus cerebri. The posterior aspect of the midbrain presents superior and inferior colliculi (quadrigeminal plate). The trochlear nerve exits the brainstem below the inferior colliculus.

The *pons* or *protuberance* presents a prominent anterior surface that is considerably convex from side to side, and it consists of transverse fibers that cross the median plane and converge on each side to form the middle cerebellar peduncles. The basilar sulcus is a shallow median groove on the anterior surface of the pons and usually lodges the basilar artery; this sulcus is bounded on each side by an eminence caused by the descent of the corticospinal fibers through the substance of the pons. The *middle cerebellar peduncle* is separated from the belly of the pons by a vertical shallow groove, the lateral pontine sulcus. Just lateral to the lateral pontine sulcus is the emergence of the trigeminal nerve, with its smaller superomedial motor root and a larger inferolateral sensory root. From the microneurosurgical standpoint, the apparent origin of the trigeminal nerve can be considered as the limit between the pons and the middle cerebellar peduncle. Posteriorly, the pons constitutes the upper portion of the floor of the fourth ventricle (Video 2-29).

The *medulla* presents at its anterior aspect three longitudinal fissures: one median and two paramedian. The median one is the anterior median fissure, which continues inferiorly as the anterior median fissure of the spinal cord. The paramedian sulci of the anterior aspect of the medulla are the anterolateral sulci. At the medulla, the anterolateral sulcus is located medially to the olive and is also called the *preolivary sulcus*. The preolivary sulcus is the upper continuation of the anterolateral sulcus of the spinal cord. The rootlets of the hypoglossal nerve that exit from the preolivary sulcus are analogous to the ventral motor rootlets that exit from the anterolateral sulcus of the spinal cord. The pyramid characterizes the *anterior region*, located between the anterior median fissure and the preolivary sulcus.

The rootlets of the accessory, vagus, and glossopharyngeal nerves exit from the postolivary sulcus, the continuation of the posterolateral sulcus of the spinal cord in the medulla; therefore, these cranial nerve rootlets are analogous to the dorsal spinal rootlets. These rootlets emerge from the brainstem and extend almost straight laterally to the jugular foramen. The pontomedullary sulcus separates the pons from the medulla, and its junction with the preolivary sulcus marks the apparent origin of the abducent nerve.

The *supraolivary fossette* is a triangular depression located behind and above the olive, anteromedial to the flocculus, and corresponds to the junction of the pons, the medulla, and the middle and inferior cerebellar peduncles. It is limited superiorly by the inferior aspect of the pons and the middle cerebellar peduncle and posteriorly by the inferior cerebellar peduncle. The fossette resembles a right-angled triangle with its right angle located between the superior pole of the olive and the inferior aspect of the pons; the superior catheti corresponds to the inferior border of the pons and the middle cerebellar peduncle; the vertical catheti corresponds to the posterior border of the olive; and the hypotenuse corresponds to the inferior cerebellar peduncle. The VI, VII, VIII nerves exit the brainstem at the superior catheti, and the IX, X, XI nerves exit the brainstem at the hypotenuse (Fig. 2-9A; Video 2-30).

Cerebellum

The cerebellum presents three surfaces: petrosal, tentorial, and suboccipital. The petrosal surface is related anteriorly to the petrous part of the temporal bone; the tentorial surface is related superiorly to the tentorium cerebelli and inferiorly to the upper part of the roof of the fourth ventricle; the suboccipital surface is related inferiorly to the squamosal part of the occipital bone

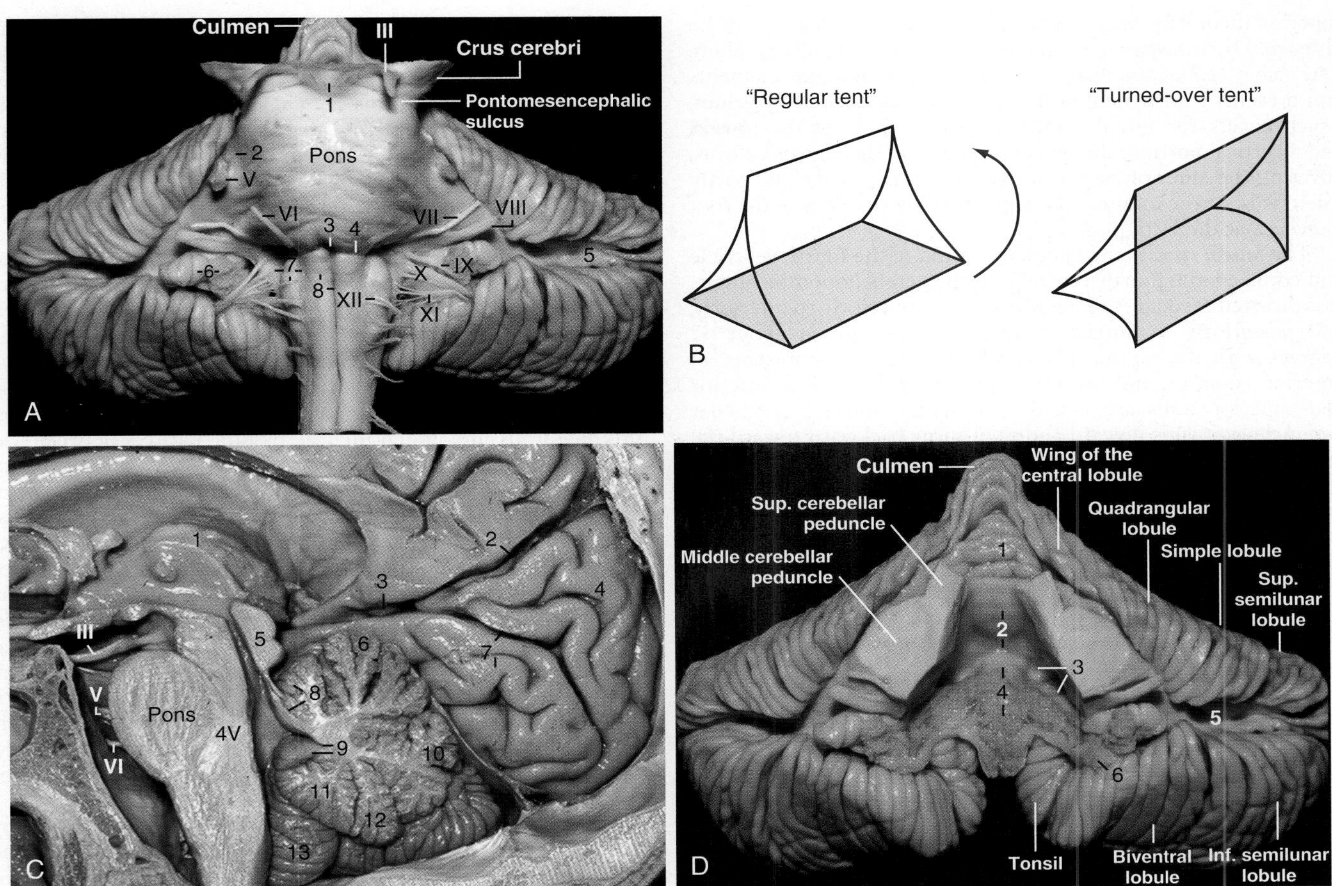

Figure 2-9. A, Frontal view. 1, Interpeduncular fossa; 2, lateral pontine sulcus; 3, inferior foramen caecum; 4, pontomedullary sulcus; 5, great horizontal or petrosal fissure; 6, flocculus and choroid plexus; 7, supraolivary fossette, olive, and anterolateral sulcus; 8, pyramid and anterior median fissure. **B,** A regular tent is shown on the left, with its floor in *yellow* and the two portions of the roof transparent. The fourth ventricle resembles a turned-over tent with its floor facing forward. **C,** Sagittal view. 1, Thalamus; 2, parieto-occipital sulcus; 3, anterior calcarine sulcus; 4, cuneus; 5, quadrigeminal plate; 6, culmen; 7, posterior calcarine sulcus and lingual gyrus; 8, lingula and central lobule; 9, fastigium and nodule; 10, folium; 11, uvula; 12, pyramid; 13, tonsil. **D,** Frontal view. The brainstem has been removed to display the roof of the fourth ventricle. 1, Central lobule; 2, superior medullary velum (overlying lingula) and fastigium; 3, superolateral recess and inferior medullary velum (overlying tonsil); 4, inferior medullary velum (overlying nodule), choroid plexus, and tela choroidea; 5, petrosal fissure; 6, rhomboid lip.

and anteriorly to the inferior part of the roof of the fourth ventricle. Because the fourth ventricle and the cerebellum are closely related, their anatomy will be considered together.

The *fourth ventricle* is often described as a tent-shaped midline structure surrounded mainly by the vermian components of the cerebellum. A regular tent has a roof that is divided into halves, a floor and two lateral walls; the fourth ventricle resembles a turned-over tent with its base facing forward and two open lateral walls. The floor is represented by the pons and medulla; the superior cerebellar peduncles, the superior medullary velum, and the adjacent lingula constitute the superior part of the roof; the inferior part of the roof is composed of the inferior medullary velum, tela choroidea, choroid plexus, uvula, and nodule; the two open lateral walls are represented by the lateral recesses that communicate the fourth ventricle with the cerebellopontine angle (Figs. 2-9B and C).

Petrosal Surface of the Cerebellum and Fourth Ventricle

Each half of the petrosal surface is intersected by the great horizontal fissure, or petrosal fissure, that circumscribes the cerebellum.[21] At the level of the flocculus, the petrosal fissure bifurcates into a larger suprafloccular portion and a smaller infrafloccular portion of the *posterolateral fissure*, which separates the flocculonodule lobule from the rest of the cerebellum and communicates with the cerebellomedullary fissure at the cerebellopontine angle. The folia that constitute the upper half of the petrosal surface are those of the tentorial surface that have folded over the middle cerebellar peduncle and over the core of the cerebellum. Those folia are the wing of the central lobule, the quadrangular, simple, and superior semilunar lobules. The folia that constitute the lower half of the petrosal surface are from the suboccipital surface that have folded over the inferior cerebellar peduncle and over the core of the cerebellum and correspond to the inferior semilunar and biventral lobules (see Fig. 2-9A and D).

The choroid plexus and the rhomboid lip of the foramen of Luschka are located anteriorly and inferiorly to the flocculus. The glossopharyngeal nerve is the most superior rootlet; a single nerve, it is located immediately in front of the choroid plexus. The flocculus is located below the lateral extension of the pontomedullary sulcus, and it is the hemispheric correspondent of the nodule.

The *upper half of the roof* of the fourth ventricle is constituted by neural elements: the superior cerebellar peduncles, the superior medullary velum, and the lingula. The lingula can be visualized by transparency behind the superior medullary velum. The *lower half of the roof* is composed of nonneural elements and presents a horizontal portion, the inferior medullary velum, which covers the nodule and the superior pole of the tonsils, and a vertical portion, the tela choroidea and the choroid plexus, covering the anterior aspect of the nodule, the uvula, and partly the tonsils. At the midline, the upper and lower halves of the roof converge at the fastigium.

The *lateral recess* is the lateral extension of the fourth ventricle and connects the fourth ventricle to the cerebellopontine angle. It is directed medially to laterally, slightly superiorly to inferiorly, and posteriorly to anteriorly, forming an angle of about 45 degrees with the sagittal plane. The lateral recess presents an anterior, superior, and posterior wall and a floor. The anterior and superior walls are constituted by the inferior cerebellar peduncle as it runs upward and then turns backward toward the cerebellum. The floor of the lateral recess is constituted by the tela choroidea anteriorly, the choroid plexus in the middle, and the inferior medullary velum posteriorly; at the foramen of Luschka, the inferior medullary velum becomes thicker and is called the *peduncle of the flocculus* and constitutes the posterior wall of the foramen of Luschka. The *superolateral recess* is the space in the fourth ventricle limited medially by the nodule and inferiorly by the superior pole of the tonsil covered by the inferior medullary velum. Above the superolateral recess, the superior cerebellar peduncle presents a prominence, the dentate tubercle, where the dentate nucleus comes to the surface (see Fig. 2-9D).

The morphology of the choroid plexus of the fourth ventricle resembles the letter "T" with two vertical bars. The horizontal part of the choroid plexus that starts from the fourth ventricle and protrudes into the cerebellopontine angle resembles the horns of a bull. The vertical part and the proximal half of the horizontal part of the choroid plexus of the fourth ventricle are usually supplied by PICA; the lateral half of the horizontal part and the choroid plexus located at the cerebellopontine angle are generally supplied by AICA.[22]

The *tonsils* are two riniform structures that are hemispheric components of the uvula and are attached to the cerebellum through the peduncles of the tonsil, located at the superolateral aspect of each tonsil. The superior, medial, anterior, posterior, and most of the lateral surfaces of the tonsils are free. The spaces around the tonsils are as follows: between its superior pole and the inferior medullary velum is the supratonsillar space; between the medial surfaces of the two tonsils is the vallecula; between the anterior surface of the tonsil and the medulla is the cerebellomedullary fissure; between the posterior surface of the tonsil and the adjacent vermis is the retrotonsillar space, constituted by the furrowed band of Reil, which connects the uvula to the tonsil, and by the copula pyramidis, which connects the pyramid to the biventral lobule (Fig. 2-10A). The copular point is an angiographic landmark at which the retrotonsillar veins unite to form the inferior vermian vein; the copular point denotes the location of the copula pyramidis. The copular point can also be defined as the lowest part of the inferior vermian artery, the vermian branch of PICA surrounding copula pyramidis.

Tentorial Surface of the Cerebellum and Fourth Ventricle

The tentorial surface faces the tentorium and consists of two cerebellar incisurae, three margins, and two angles. The cerebellar incisurae are the anterior and posterior cerebellar incisurae; the brainstem fits into the *anterior cerebellar incisura*, and the falx cerebelli fits into the *posterior cerebellar incisura*. The margins are the *anterosuperior margin*, the posterior wall of the cerebellomesencephalic fissure that extends from the top of the culmen downward, forward, and laterally to reach a point above and behind the middle cerebellar peduncle; the *anterolateral margin*, which separates the tentorial from the petrosal surfaces; and the *posterolateral margin*, which separates the tentorial from the suboccipital surfaces. The junction between the anterosuperior and the anterolateral margins forms the *anterior angle*, and the junction between the anterolateral and the posterolateral margins forms the *lateral angle* (see Figs. 2-12C and 2-14D, later). Angiographically on the lateral projection, the lateral angle is located just below the knee between the transverse and sigmoid sinuses, and the outer portion of the anterolateral margin runs somewhat below the superior petrosal sinus (see Fig. 2-15A, later). The vermis and the hemispheric counterpart of the tentorial surface are, anteriorly to posteriorly, the lingula (without hemispheric correspondent), central lobule (wing of the central lobule), culmen (quadrangular lobule), declive (simple lobule), and folium (part of the superior semilunar lobule), which is the primary fissure between the quadrangular and simple lobule, and the most prominent fissure, the postclival fissure, located between the simple and the superior semilunar lobules. The tentorial surface presents the *cerebellomesencephalic* or *precentral cerebellar fissure*, which is located between the cerebellum and the midbrain. Posteriorly, it is limited by the culmen and quadrangular lobule above and the central lobule and its wing below. Anteriorly, it is limited from the midline to laterally by the lingula and the superior and middle cerebellar peduncles. The *interpeduncular* or *interbrachial sulcus*, which separates the superior from the middle cerebellar peduncles, ascends from the bottom of the cerebellomesencephalic fissure toward the lateral aspect of the pons, where it is joined by the pontomesencephalic sulcus to proceed superiorly as the lateral mesencephalic sulcus to the medial geniculate body; the *lateral mesencephalic sulcus* separates the crus cerebri from the tegmentum (Fig. 2-10B).

Among the cerebellar nuclei (fastigial, globose, emboliform, and dentate), the *dentate nucleus* is the most laterally located and the largest. Because most of the fibers that constitute the superior cerebellar peduncle arise from the dentate nucleus, this nucleus is located at the posterior projection of the superior cerebellar peduncle. The dentate nucleus can be considered the roof of the superolateral recess. The superior pole of the tonsils, covered by the inferior medullary velum, is the floor of the superolateral recess.

Suboccipital Surface of the Cerebellum and Fourth Ventricle

The suboccipital surface is located below the transverse and sigmoid sinuses, and its surface faces inferiorly, almost parallel to the ground; therefore, for a better visualization of this surface either in surgery or for anatomic studies, the head has to be bent forward.

The suboccipital surface consists of the posterior cerebellar incisura and the vermohemispheric or paravermian fissure, which separates the inferior vermis from the cerebellar hemisphere. The components of the inferior vermis and its hemispheric correspondents are the folium (superior semilunar lobule), tuber (inferior semilunar lobule), pyramid (biventral lobule), uvula (tonsil), and nodule (flocculus). In the anatomic position, the most inferior part of the inferior vermis is the pyramid. The most prominent fissure on the suboccipital surface is the *great horizontal fissure*, which is a circumferential fissure that begins in the posterior cerebellar notch between the folium and the tuber and runs forward and slightly downward on the suboccipital surface, between the superior and inferior semilunar lobules, and then onto the petrosal surface as the petrosal fissure. The *secondary fissure* is located between the tonsils and the biventral lobule (Fig. 2-10C).

After the removal of the tonsils, the inferior portion of the roof of the fourth ventricle comes into view (Fig. 2-10D). After the removal of the inferior portion of the roof of the fourth ventricle, the floor of the fourth ventricle is exposed.

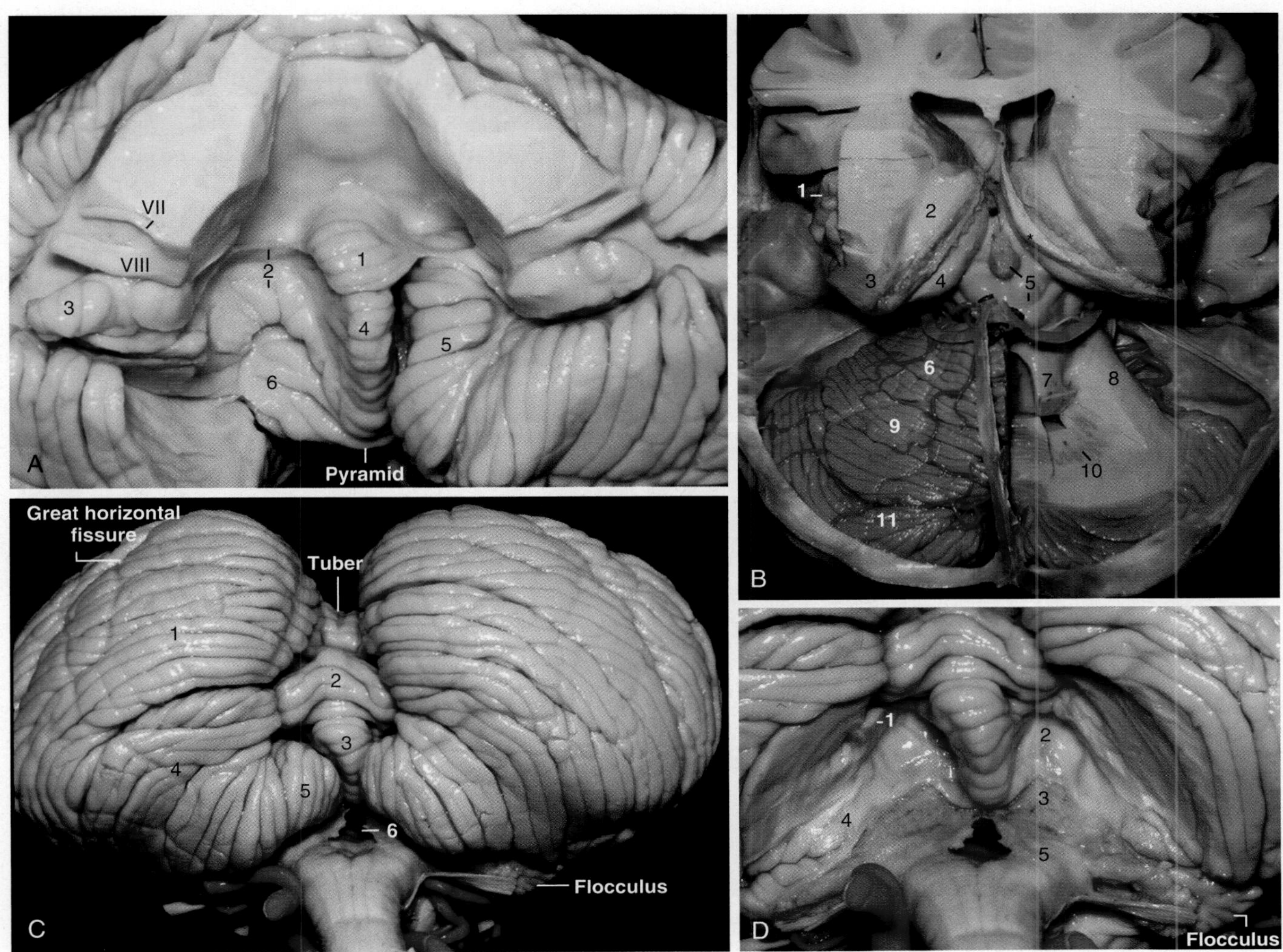

Figure 2-10. A, Frontal view of roof of fourth ventricle. The right tonsil has been removed to display the retrotonsillar space. 1, Nodule; 2, inferior medullary velum and furrowed band of Reil; 3, flocculus; 4, uvula; 5, tonsil; 6, copula pyramidis. **B,** Posterosuperior view. 1, Insula; 2, thalamus (dorsal surface); 3, thalamus (pulvinar, atrial surface); 4, thalamus (pulvinar, cisternal surface); 5, pineal gland and superior colliculus; 6, quadrangular lobule; 7, superior cerebellar peduncle; 8, middle cerebellar peduncle; 9, simple lobule; 10, dentate nucleus; 11, superior semilunar lobule. *, Fornix. **C,** Suboccipital view. 1, Inferior semilunar lobule; 2, pyramid; 3, uvula; 4, biventral lobule; 5, tonsil; 6, foramen of Magendie. **D,** Suboccipital view. The tonsils and the biventral lobules have been removed to display the inferior portion of the roof of the fourth ventricle. 1, Peduncle of tonsil; 2, inferior medullary velum; 3, tela choroidea and choroid plexus; 4, peduncle of flocculus; 5, inferior cerebellar peduncle.

The *floor of the fourth ventricle* has a rhomboid shape and presents a strip between the lower margin of the cerebellar peduncles and the site of attachment of the tela choroidea; this strip, called the *junctional part*, is characterized by the striae medullary that extends into the lateral recesses. The junctional part divides the floor of the fourth ventricle into two unequal triangles; the superior and larger one, with its apex directed to the aqueduct, is the pontine part, and the inferior and smaller one, with its apex directed toward the obex, is the medullary part of the floor. These three parts of the floor are also divided longitudinally into symmetrical halves by the median sulcus. The sulcus limitans, another longitudinal sulcus, divides each half of the floor into a raised median strip called the *median eminence* and a lateral strip called the *area vestibular.* The motor nuclei of the cranial nerves are located medial to the sulcus limitans, and the sensory nuclei are located lateral to it. The pontine part is characterized by two rounded prominences, the *facial colliculi*, located on the median eminence, one on each side of the median sulcus. The facial colliculi is limited laterally by the superior fovea, a dimple formed by the sulcus limitans. The medullary part presents the configuration of a feather, or pen nib, called the *calamus scriptorius*, with three triangular areas overlying the hypoglossal and vagus nuclei (hypoglossal and vagal trigones), and the area postrema; just lateral to the hypoglossal trigone, the sulcus limitans sulcus presents another dimple called the *inferior fovea*. At the junctional part, the sulcus limitans is discontinuous (Fig. 2-11A; Videos 2-31 and 2-32A, B, and C).

Veins of the Posterior Fossa

The posterior fossa venous system is divided into three groups: the anterior or petrosal group that drains into the superior and inferior petrosal sinuses; the superior or galenic group that drains into the vein of Galen; and the posterior or tentorial group that

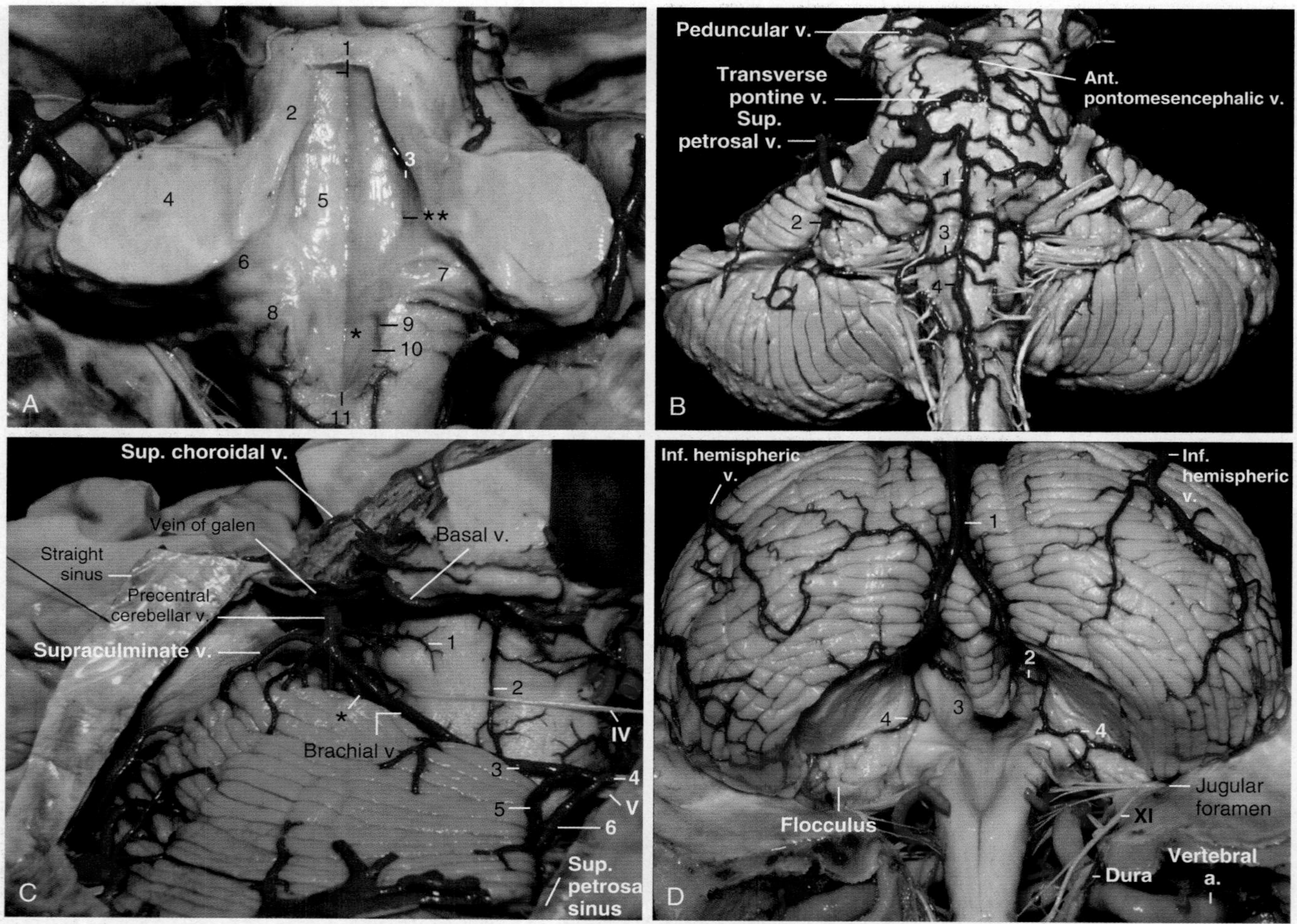

Figure 2-11. **A,** Floor of fourth ventricle. 1, Median sulcus and median eminence; 2, superior cerebellar peduncle; 3, sulcus limitans and vestibular area; 4, middle cerebellar peduncle; 5, facial colliculus; 6, cochlear area; 7, striae medullary; 8, inferior cerebellar peduncle; 9, inferior fovea; 10, vagal trigone; 11, obex and area postrema. *, Hypoglossal trigone; **, superior fovea. **B,** Frontal view. 1, Anterior pontomesencephalic vein; 2, vein of great horizontal fissure; 3, transverse medullary vein; 4, anterior medullary vein. **C,** Right posterolateral view of the tentorial surface. 1, Tectal veins; 2, lateral mesencephalic vein; 3, pontotrigeminal vein; 4, superior petrosal vein; 5, superior hemispheric vein; 6, vein of great horizontal fissure. *, Vein of cerebellomesencephalic fissure. **D,** Suboccipital view. 1, Inferior vermian vein; 2, superior retrotonsillar vein; 3, superior cerebellar peduncle; 4, vein of lateral recess of fourth ventricle.

drains into the sinuses near the torcula.[23] There is a tendency for the veins to drain into the nearest draining system.

The veins running on the *petrosal surface* of the cerebellum and the anterior surface of the brainstem tend to drain into the petrosal sinuses through the superior petrosal vein except those veins running on the surface of the midbrain that drain to the galenic system. The superior petrosal vein usually is formed by the junction of the transverse pontine, the pontotrigeminal (brachial) veins, and the vein of the cerebellopontine fissure (great horizontal fissure) (Fig. 2-11B).

The *tentorial surface* and the posterior aspect of the brainstem are enclosed within three draining systems; the midline portion of the cerebellomesencephalic fissure, the veins near the central lobule and culmen (superior vermian veins), and the veins draining the intermediate portion of the wing of the central lobule and the quadrangular lobule (superior hemispheric veins, anterior group) tend to drain into the vein of Galen. The veins draining the lateral portion of the wing of the central, quadrangular, and simple lobules and the tentorial part of the superior semilunar lobule (superior hemispheric veins lateral group) tend to drain into the superior petrosal sinus. The veins draining the declive, folium (declival vein), and intermediate portion of the simple and superior semilunar lobules (superior hemispheric veins, posterior group) tend to drain into the torcula or transverse sinus or tentorial sinus in the tentorium cerebelli (Fig. 2-11C).

The posterior inferior hemispheric veins drain the cerebellar hemispheres of the *suboccipital surface*. The inferior vermis is drained by the inferior vermian veins formed by the junction of the superior and the inferior retrotonsillar veins that run in the retrotonsillar space (Fig. 2-11D).

The inferior portion of the roof of the fourth ventricle and the lateral recess are drained by the vein of the lateral recess of the fourth ventricle, also called the *vein of the cerebellomedullary fissure*. It courses laterally under the lateral recess toward the cerebellopontine angle, then passes above or below the flocculus and joins the vein of the middle cerebellar peduncle or the vein of the cerebellopontine fissure to finally empty into the superior petrosal sinus through the superior petrosal vein. The vein of the lateral recess of the fourth ventricle also can anastomose with the retrotonsillar veins at the retrotonsillar space, establishing a communication between the petrosal and tentorial groups of venous drainage (see Fig. 2-11D).

The brachial veins running in the cerebellomesencephalic fissure can also establish a communication between the petrosal and galenic groups through the pontotrigeminal and precentral cerebellar veins (see Fig. 2-11C).

The veins of the posterior fossa can be differentiated into the petrosal group, the superior or galenic group, and the posterior or tentorial group (see Figs. 2-14D and 2-15A to C, later).

The *petrosal group* may be divided into (1) veins related to the anterior aspect of the brainstem, the anterior pontomesencephalic, transverse pontine, lateral pontine, anterior medullary, and parenchymal perforating veins; (2) veins in the wing of the precentral cerebellar fissure, the brachial veins; (3) veins on the superior and inferior surfaces of the cerebellar hemispheres, the superior and inferior hemispheric veins, including the veins of the great horizontal fissure; (4) veins on the cerebellar side (the medial tonsillar vein); (5) veins on the medullary side (the retro-olivary vein and vein of the inferior cerebellar peduncle of the cerebellomedullary fissure); and (6) the vein of the lateral recess of the fourth ventricle.

The *superior* or *galenic group* includes (1) mesencephalic tributaries—the median anterior pontomesencephalic, lateral anterior pontomesencephalic, lateral pontomesencephalic, lateral mesencephalic, peduncular, posterior mesencephalic, and tectal veins; and (2) cerebellar tributaries—the precentral cerebellar vein and its variants and the superior vermian vein.

The *posterior* or *tentorial group* includes the inferior vermian vein and its superior and inferior retrotonsillar tributaries and the superior and inferior hemispheric veins.

Arteries of the Posterior Fossa

The *vertebral artery* (VA) arises from the subclavian arteries, then enters the transverse foramen of the C6 and ascends through the transverse foramina of the upper cervical vertebrae up to the C2. After exiting the transverse foramen of the C2, the VA deviates laterally to enter the laterally placed transverse foramen of C1. The VA then turns behind the lateral mass and above the posterior arch of the C1 to course medially and superiorly to pierce the dura at the foramen magnum. At this level, the VA usually originates posterior spinal and posterior meningeal arteries. The intradural segment of the VA is divided into lateral medullary and anterior medullary segments before joining its contralateral mate to form the basilar artery (see Fig. 2-11D; see Figs. 2-12B and 2-13B, later).

The lateral medullary segment of the VA extends from its entrance into the posterior fossa to the preolivary sulcus. From its entrance, the VA courses anteriorly, medially, and superiorly through the lower cranial nerve rootlets, laterally to the medulla to reach the preolivary sulcus. The anterior medullary segment begins at the preolivary sulcus, courses in front of or between the hypoglossal rootlets, and crosses the pyramid to join the other VA at or near the pontomedullary sulcus to form the basilar artery. The main branches of the VA are the posterior spinal, anterior spinal, PICA, and anterior and posterior meningeal arteries. The VA also sends off branches to supply the lateral and anterior parts of the medulla along its way around the medulla (Figs. 2-12B, 2-13B, and 2-14A).

The *posterior inferior cerebellar artery* arises from the VA and supplies the medulla, inferior vermis, inferior portion of the fourth ventricle, tonsils, and inferior aspect of the cerebellum. The "regular" PICA has the most complex and variable course of the cerebellar arteries and is divided into five segments.[24] The *anterior medullary segment* lies in front of the medulla and extends from the origin to the level of the inferior olive. The *lateral medullary segment* courses beside the medulla and extends from the inferior olive to the origin of the glossopharyngeal, vagus, and accessory nerves. The *tonsillomedullary* or *posterior medullary segment* begins at the level of the nerves and loops below the inferior pole of the cerebellar tonsil and upward along the medial surface of the tonsil toward the inferior medullary velum (caudal loop). The *telovelotonsillar* or *supratonsillar segment* courses in the cleft between the tela choroidea and the inferior medullary velum rostrally and the superior pole of the cerebellar tonsil caudally. This segment begins below the fastigium, where the PICA turns posteriorly over the medial side of the superior pole of the tonsil, and forms the cranial loop. In some individuals, this segment passes posteriorly before reaching the superior pole of the tonsil, thus giving the cranial loop a variable relationship to the fastigium. The junction of the posterior medullary and supratonsillar segments is called the *choroidal point*. The *cortical segment* begins after a short distance distal to the apex of the cranial loop, the PICA continues posteriorly downward in the retrotonsillar fissure, where it usually bifurcates into the tonsillohemispheric branch that supplies the under aspect of the cerebellar hemisphere and the inferior vermian branch, which lies on the lower aspect of the inferior vermis, and forms a loop convex around the copula pyramidis (pyramidal loop). The most anterior point of the pyramidal loop is called the *copular point*. The terminal portion of the vermian branch curves around the tuber in the posterior cerebellar notch (Figs. 2-12A, B, and D, *left*, 2-13A, 2-14A, 2-15C and D, and 2-16A and B; Videos 2-33 and 2-34).

The *anterior inferior cerebellar artery* and PICA are defined according to their origins rather than by the portions of cerebellum they supply. The AICA arises more frequently from the lower third and less frequently from the middle third of the basilar artery. It courses posteriorly, laterally, and usually downward on the belly of the pons, in contact with either the superior or inferior aspect of the abducent nerve. In this course, it supplies the lateral aspect of the lower two thirds of the pons and the upper medulla. Either immediately before or after crossing the roots of the facial, intermedius, and acoustic nerves within the cerebellopontine angle, the AICA bifurcates into its two major branches: the *rostrolateral* and *caudomedial* arteries. The main trunk, or the *rostrolateral trunk*, has been divided into three segments according to their relationships to the seventh and eighth nerves[25]: the premeatal, meatal, and postmeatal segments. The *premeatal segment* begins at the basilar artery and courses around the brainstem to reach VII and VIII and the region of the meatus, usually anteroinferiorly to the nerves. Seventy-seven percent of the internal auditory arteries and 49% of the recurrent perforating arteries to the brainstem arise from this segment. The *meatal segment* is located in the vicinity of the internal auditory meatus, where the nerve-related vessels turn toward the brainstem; this segment often forms a laterally convex loop, the meatal loop, directed toward or through the meatus. It usually stays medial to the meatus, but in some patients it protrudes into the canal. The *postmeatal segment* begins distal to the nerves and courses medially to supply the brainstem and the cerebellum. The subarcuate artery usually arises from this segment (see Figs. 2-12B and D, *right*, 2-13B, 2-14A and C, 2-15C, and 2-16A and B).

The *caudomedial artery* originates on the lateral aspect of the pons in the vicinity of the sixth nerve and courses posterosuperiorly toward the pontomedullary sulcus to describe its own caudal loop on the lateral aspect of the pons and medulla. This lateral loop can course on the anteroinferolateral aspect of the flocculus or on the petrosal aspect of the biventral lobule. Multiple small arteries to the choroid plexus of the lateral recess often arise from the inner aspect of this lateral loop. Distal to the loop, the biventral segment turns posteroinferiorly on the lateral edge of inferior aspects of the biventral lobule or within the cerebellomedullary fissure to reach the posterior surface of the cerebellum to anastomose with branches of the PICA (see Fig. 2-13B).

The *superior cerebellar artery* is the most rostral of the infratentorial vessels, and it arises near the apex of the basilar artery and

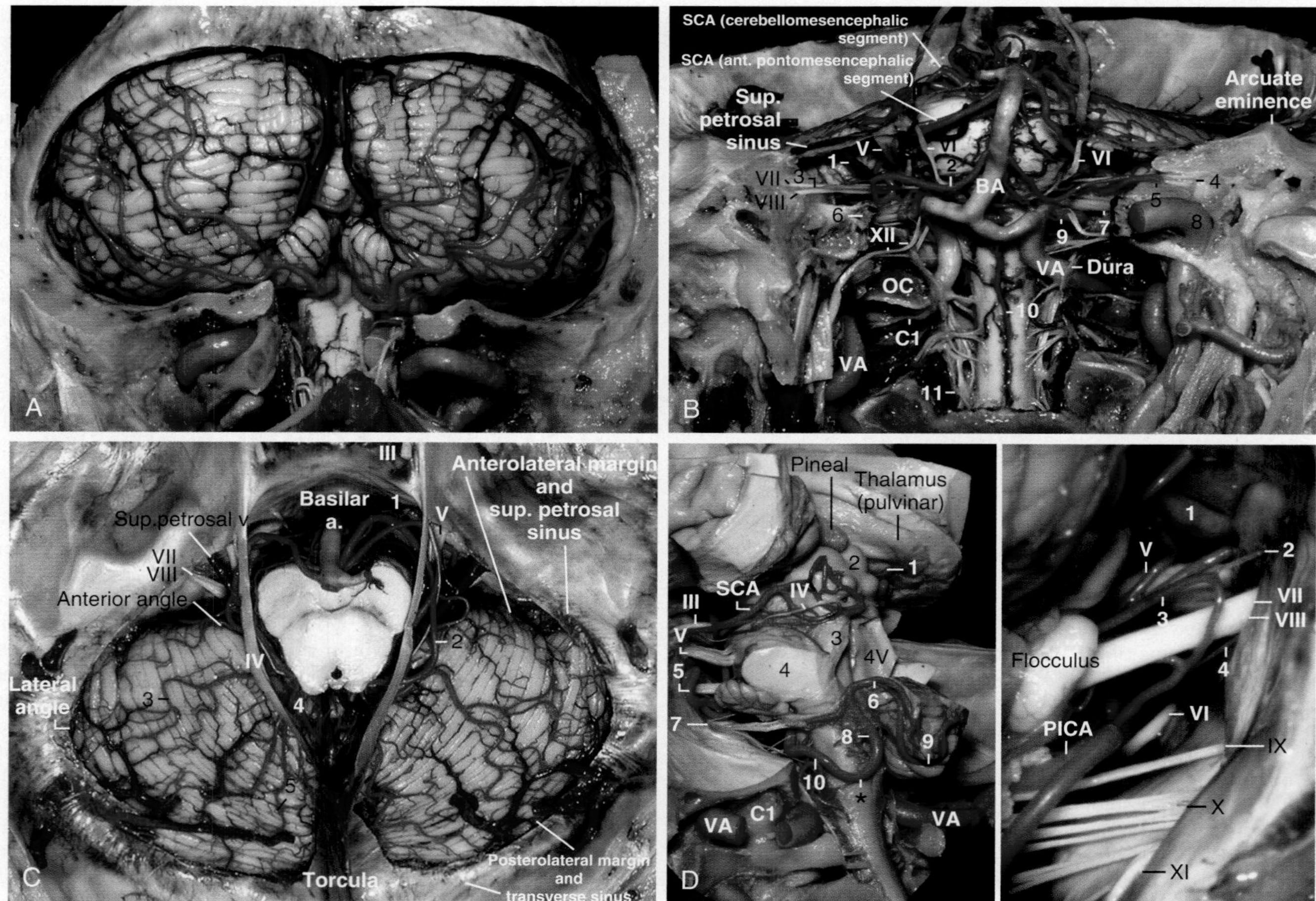

Figure 2-12. A, Suboccipital view to display the cortical branches of PICA. **B,** Frontal view. 1, Superior petrosal vein; 2, anterior inferior cerebellar artery (AICA); 3, internal auditory artery; 4, internal acoustic meatus; 5, meatal loop of AICA; 6, inferior petrosal sinus; 7, vagus nerve; 8, petrous carotid artery; 9, posterior inferior cerebellar artery (PICA); 10, anterior spinal artery; 11, triangular process of dentate ligament. BA, basilar artery; OC, occipital condyle; SCA, superior cerebellar artery; VA, vertebral artery. **C,** Superior view of tentorial surface. 1, Anterior pontomesencephalic segment of SCA; 2, lateral pontomesencephalic segment of SCA; 3, superior hemispheric branches of SCA; 4, cerebellomesencephalic segment of SCA; 5, superior hemispheric branches of SCA. **D,** *Left,* Posterolateral view. 1, Medial geniculate body; 2, superior colliculi; 3, superior cerebellar peduncle; 4, middle cerebellar peduncle; 5, AICA, VII, and VIII; 6, PICA (supratonsillar segment); 7, jugular foramen; 8, PICA (retrotonsillar segment); 9, PICA (pyramidal loop); 10, PICA (lateral medullary segment). *, Caudal loop. *Right,* Retromastoid view of cerebellopontine angle. 1, Superior petrosal vein; 2, subarcuate artery (AICA); 3, AICA; 4, internal auditory artery.

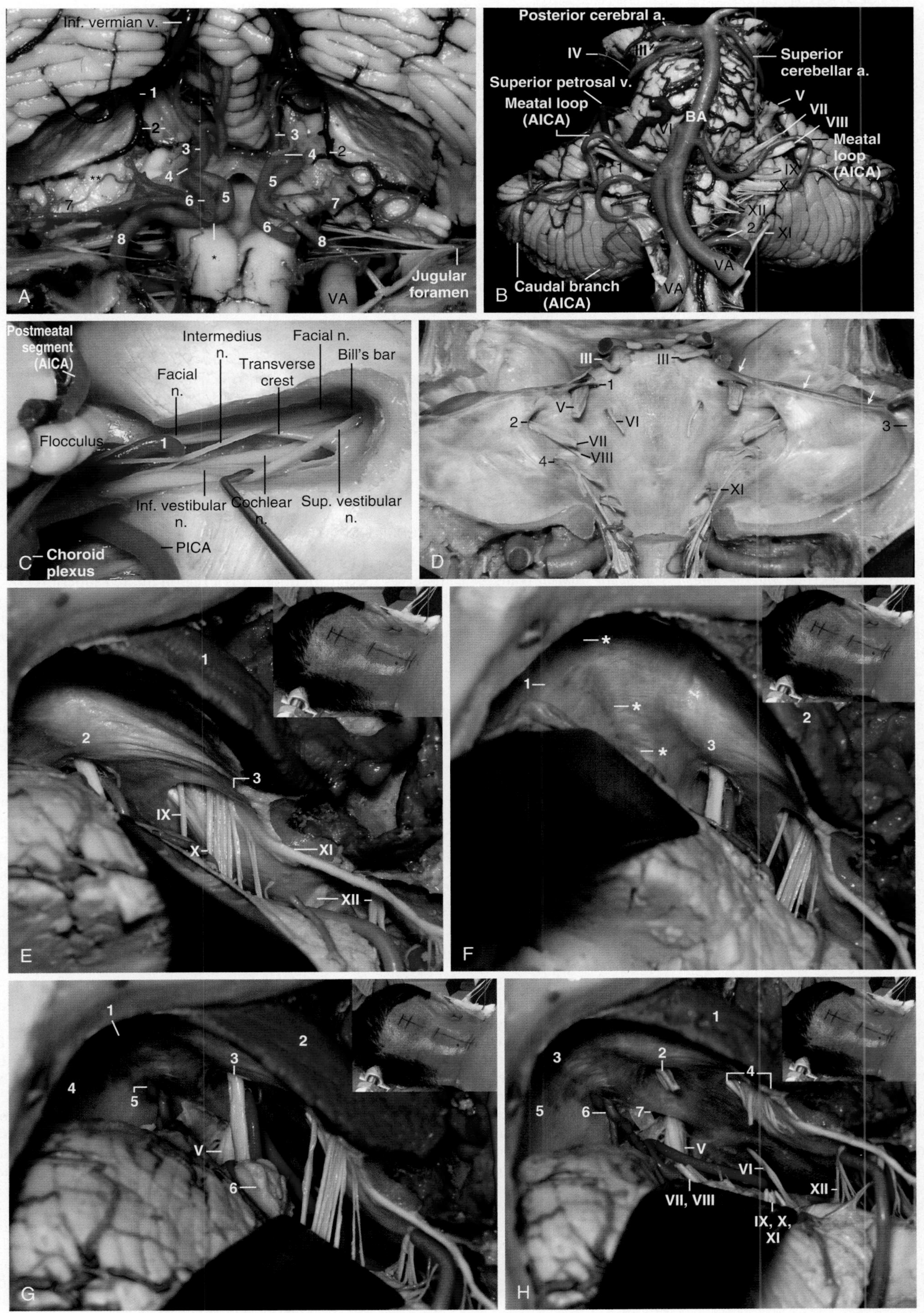
Inf. vermian v.
1
2
3
4
5
6
7
8
**
*
VA
Jugular foramen
A
Posterior cerebral a.
IV
III
Superior cerebellar a.
Superior petrosal v.
Meatal loop (AICA)
BA
VI
V
VII
VIII
Meatal loop (AICA)
IX
X
XII
XI
VA
Caudal branch (AICA)
B
Postmeatal segment (AICA)
Intermedius n.
Facial n.
Bill's bar
Facial n.
Transverse crest
Flocculus
Inf. vestibular n.
Cochlear n.
Sup. vestibular n.
PICA
Choroid plexus
C
III
V
VI
VII
VIII
XI
D
IX
X
XI
XII
E
F
V
G
V
VI
VII, VIII
IX, X, XI
XII
H

Figure 2-13. A, Suboccipital view. The tonsils and the biventral lobule have been removed. 1, Superior retrotonsillar vein; 2, vein of lateral recess of fourth ventricle and inferior medullary velum; 3, posterior inferior cerebellar artery (PICA) (vermian branch); 4, PICA (supratonsillar segment, cranial loop); 5, PICA (posterior medullary segment); 6, PICA (tonsillohemispheric branch); 7, PICA (choroidal branches); 8, PICA (lateral medullary segment); VA, vertebral artery; *, caudal loop; **, peduncle of flocculus. **B,** Anterior view. 1, Flocculus; 2, PICA (anterior medullary segment). AICA, anterior inferior cerebellar artery; BA, basilar artery. **C,** Posterior view of contents of right internal acoustic meatus. 1, AICA (meatal segment). **D,** Posterior view of the posterior fossa.1, Trigeminal porus; 2, internal acoustic meatus; 3, sigmoid sinus; 4, jugular foramen. *Arrows* indicate the superior petrosal sinus. **E,** Anatomic dissection of the right cerebellopontine (CP) angle as when the patient is in park bench position *(inset).* In some patients, there are curved creases in the dura just posterior to the jugular foramen; they curve toward the posterior wall of the internal acoustic meatus. 1, Sigmoid sinus; 2, posterior wall of the internal acoustic meatus; 3, posterior edge of the jugular foramen. **F,** Anatomic dissection of the right CP angle as when the patient is in the three-quarter prone position *(inset).* 1, Tentorium; 2, sigmoid sinus; 3, posterior wall of the internal acoustic meatus. *, Superior petrosal sinus. **G,** Anatomic dissection of the right CP angle as when the patient is in the three-quarter prone position *(inset).* 1, Superior petrosal sinus; 2, sigmoid sinus; 3, internal acoustic meatus; 4, tentorium; 5, superior petrosal vein; 6, flocculus. **H,** Anatomic dissection of the right CP angle as when the patient is in the three-quarter prone position *(inset).* The VII, VIII, IX, X, and XI nerves have been cut to display the VI nerve. The superior petrosal sinus is located at the edge between the tentorium and the petrous temporal bone. 1, Sigmoid sinus; 2, internal acoustic meatus and VII and VIII nerves; 3, superior petrosal sinus; 4, jugular foramen and IX, X, and XI nerves; 5, tentorium; 6, superior petrosal vein; 7, trigeminal porus.

encircles the pons and the lower midbrain. It supplies the tentorial surface of the cerebellum, the upper brainstem, the deep cerebellar nuclei, and the inferior colliculi. The SCA is divided in four segments. The *anterior pontomesencephalic segment* courses laterally under the oculomotor nerve, on the anterior aspect of the upper pons, often in an arcuate curve convex inferiorly; the configuration of the anterior pontomesencephalic segment is related to the height of the basilar bifurcation. With a low basilar bifurcation (anterior to the pons), this segment tends to pass upward, whereas with a high basilar bifurcation (anterior to the midbrain), this segment presents an anterior and inferior course. The *lateral pontomesencephalic segment* begins at the anterolateral margin of the brainstem and follows caudally onto the lateral side of the upper pons in the infratentorial portion of the ambient cistern to terminate at the anterior margin of the cerebellomesencephalic fissure. It is related medially to the brainstem, laterally to the wing of the central lobule, and inferiorly to the middle cerebellar peduncle. The anterior part of this segment is often visible above the free edge of the tentorium, whereas its caudal loop projects toward and often reaches the root entry zone of the trigeminal nerve. The bifurcation of the SCA into its rostral and caudal trunks often occurs in this segment; the rostral trunk supplies the vermis and a variable portion of the adjacent tentorial surface, and the caudal trunk supplies the surface lateral to the area supplied by the rostral trunk. The *cerebellomesencephalic segment* courses in the cerebellomesencephalic fissure through a series of hairpin curves, then passes upward to reach the anterosuperior margin of the cerebellum. Inside the cerebellomesencephalic fissure, the rostral and caudal trunks send off small precentral branches. Those precentral branches arising from the rostral trunk supply the inferior colliculi (the superior colliculi are supplied by PCA) and superior medullary velum, and those arising from the caudal trunk supply the deep cerebellar nuclei. The *cortical segment* is represented by the hemispheric and vermian branches to supply the tentorial surface of the cerebellum. Among these cortical branches, the *marginal* or *lateral branch* deserves special attention: it is present in 62% of individuals; it is the first large cortical branch of the SCA; and it arises from the lateral pontomesencephalic segment to course anteriorly and laterally to reach the anterolateral margin of the cerebellum. It is an important arteriographic landmark to locate the anterolateral margin and anterior angle of the cerebellum (see Figs. 2-12B and C, 2-14A, 2-15C, and 2-16A and B).

Cerebellopontine Angle Region

Because of its surgical importance, the cerebellopontine angle deserves special attention: it is a region limited superiorly by the infratentorial portion of the ambient cistern (SCA, IV nerve), medially by the prepontine cistern (basilar artery, VI nerve, origin of the AICA and transverse pontine vein), inferiorly by the lateral cerebellomedullary cistern (IX, X, XI, and XII nerves, VA, and first segment of the PICA), and laterally by the petrous portion of the temporal bone. The cerebellopontine angle is composed of the V, VII, and VIII nerves, AICA, auditory artery, branches of the petrosal vein and the vein of the middle cerebellar peduncle, vein of the lateral recess of the fourth ventricle, and the transverse pontine vein.

After their origin from the brainstem, the facial and intermedius nerves pass anterolaterally with the vestibulocochlear nerve; in this location, the facial nerve is in an anterosuperior groove on the vestibulocochlear nerve, with the intermedius nerve between them. At the lateral end of the internal acoustic meatus, the vertical Bill's bar and the transverse crest divide the fundus of the meatus into four quadrants: the facial nerve in the anterosuperior quadrant, the cochlear nerve in the anteroinferior quadrant, the superior vestibular nerve in the posterosuperior quadrant, and the inferior vestibular nerve in the posteroinferior quadrant (Fig. 2-13C).

The early identification of the cranial nerves, either at the brainstem or at their respective foramina, is a key step in cerebellopontine angle surgery, especially in tumor surgery, where the normal trajectory of the cranial nerves is usually distorted. The normal arrangement of the cranial nerves in the cerebellopontine angle can be seen in Figure 2-12D, *right.* The jugular foramen is the most inferior and can be identified by following the IX, X, and XI cranial nerves and the sigmoid sinus that converge to it. The internal acoustic meatus is slightly anterior and approximately 6 to 7 mm superior to the jugular foramen and contains VII, VIII, and intermedius nerves (Fig. 2-13D). In some individuals, there are short curved creases in the dura just posterior to the jugular foramen; they curve toward the posterior edge of the internal acoustic meatus (Fig. 2-13E). The trigeminal porus is anterior and medial to the petrous apex and is approximately 7 to 8 mm anterior to the anterior wall of the internal acoustic meatus; the trigeminal porus is inferior to the superior petrosal sinus (see Fig. 2-13D and H). The arrangement of the neural,

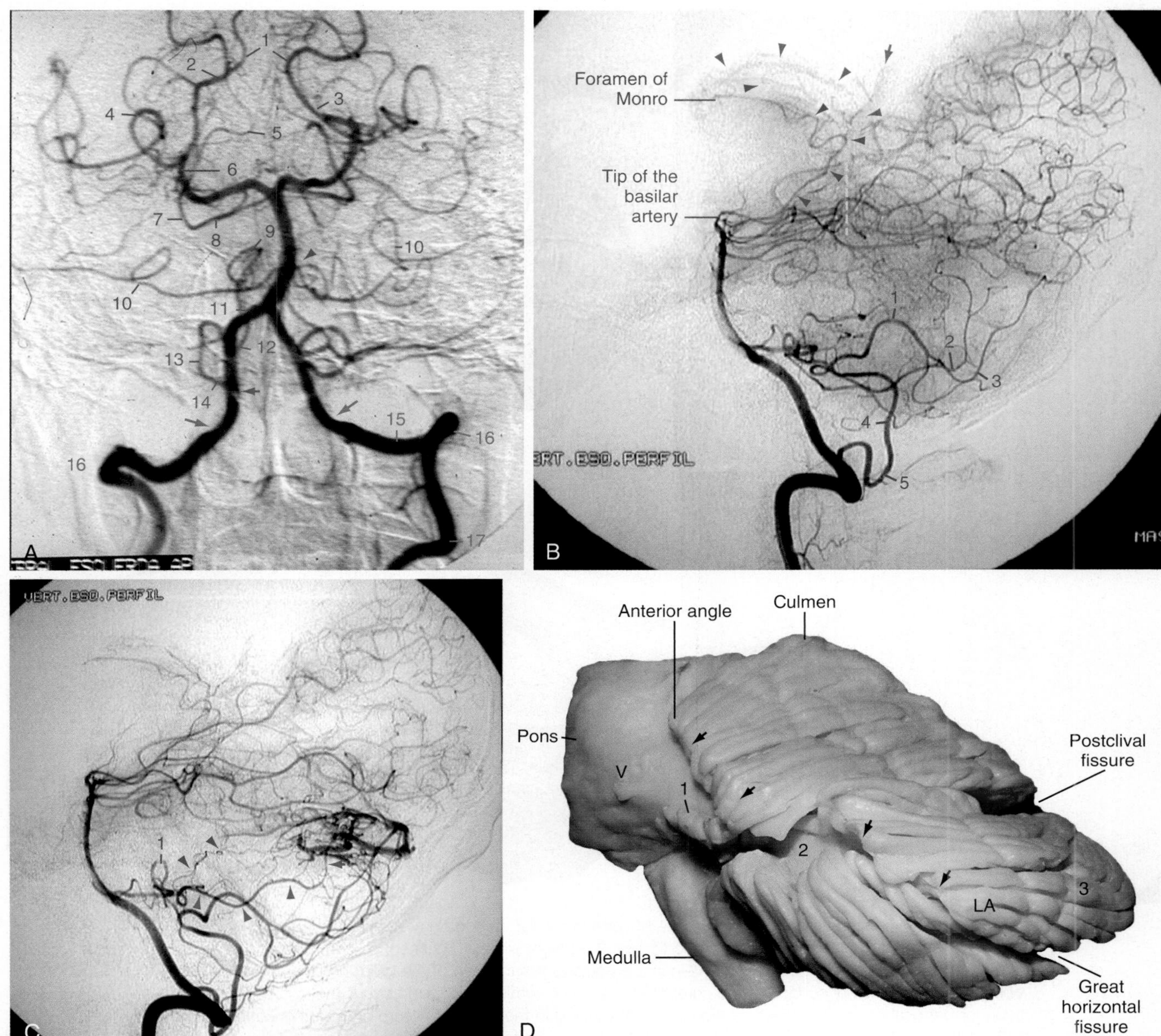

Figure 2-14. A, Frontal view of vertebrobasilar angiography. 1, Collicular or quadrigeminal point; 2, P3 segment; 3, beginning of P2P segment; 4, collateral sulcus; 5, beginning of cerebellomesencephalic segment of superior cerebellar artery (SCA); 6, P2A segment; 7, lateral pontomesencephalic segment of SCA; 8, anterior pontomesencephalic segment of SCA; 9, supratonsillar segment of posterior inferior cerebellar artery (PICA) (cranial loop); 10, meatal loop of anterior inferior cerebellar artery (AICA); 11, posterior medullary segment of PICA; 12, caudal loop of PICA; 13, lateral medullary segment of PICA; 14, anterior medullary segment of PICA; 15, extradural vertebral artery behind lateral mass of C1; 16, vertebral artery in foramen transversarium of C1; 17, vertebral artery in foramen transversarium of C2. *Blue arrowhead* indicates the origin of AICA from the basilar artery; *red arrow* indicates the origin of PICA from the vertebral artery; *green arrows* indicate the probable transition between the extradural and intradural segments of the vertebral artery. Note the constriction in the vertebral artery. **B,** Lateral view of late arterial phase of vertebrobasilar angiography. 1, Cranial loop of posterior inferior cerebellar artery (PICA); 2, vermian division of PICA (pyramidal loop); 3, hemispheric branch of PICA; 4, posterior medullary segment of PICA; 5, caudal loop of PICA. The *red arrowheads* indicate the lateral posterior choroidal arteries in the lateral ventricle (indicate the location of the posterior wall of the pulvinar of the thalamus); the *green arrowhead* indicates the posterior pericallosal artery; the *blue arrowheads* indicate the medial posterior choroidal artery (MPChA). The most posterior point of the trajectory of the MPChA indicates the posterior limit of the quadrigeminal plate and consequently the posterior limit of the brainstem of the lateral view *(yellow dotted line)*. For the anatomic location of the lateral posterior choroidal artery and MPChA please refer to Figures 2-4D and 2-6D. Note that the foramen of Monro is located above the tip of the basilar artery (in the same coronal plane). **C,** Lateral view of arterial phase of vertebrobasilar angiography. 1, Meatal loop of AICA. The *blue arrowheads* indicate the small branches to the lateral recess of the fourth ventricle through the foramen of Luschka; the *red arrowheads* indicate the main trunk of AICA in the great horizontal fissure to supply an arteriovenous malformation located in the superior semilunar lobule. **D,** Lateral view of cerebellum. This figure correlates with Figures 2-14B and C and 2-15A. 1, Flocculus; 2, petrosal fissure or great horizontal fissure; 3, superior semilunar lobule. *Black arrowheads* indicate the anterolateral margin. LA, lateral angle.

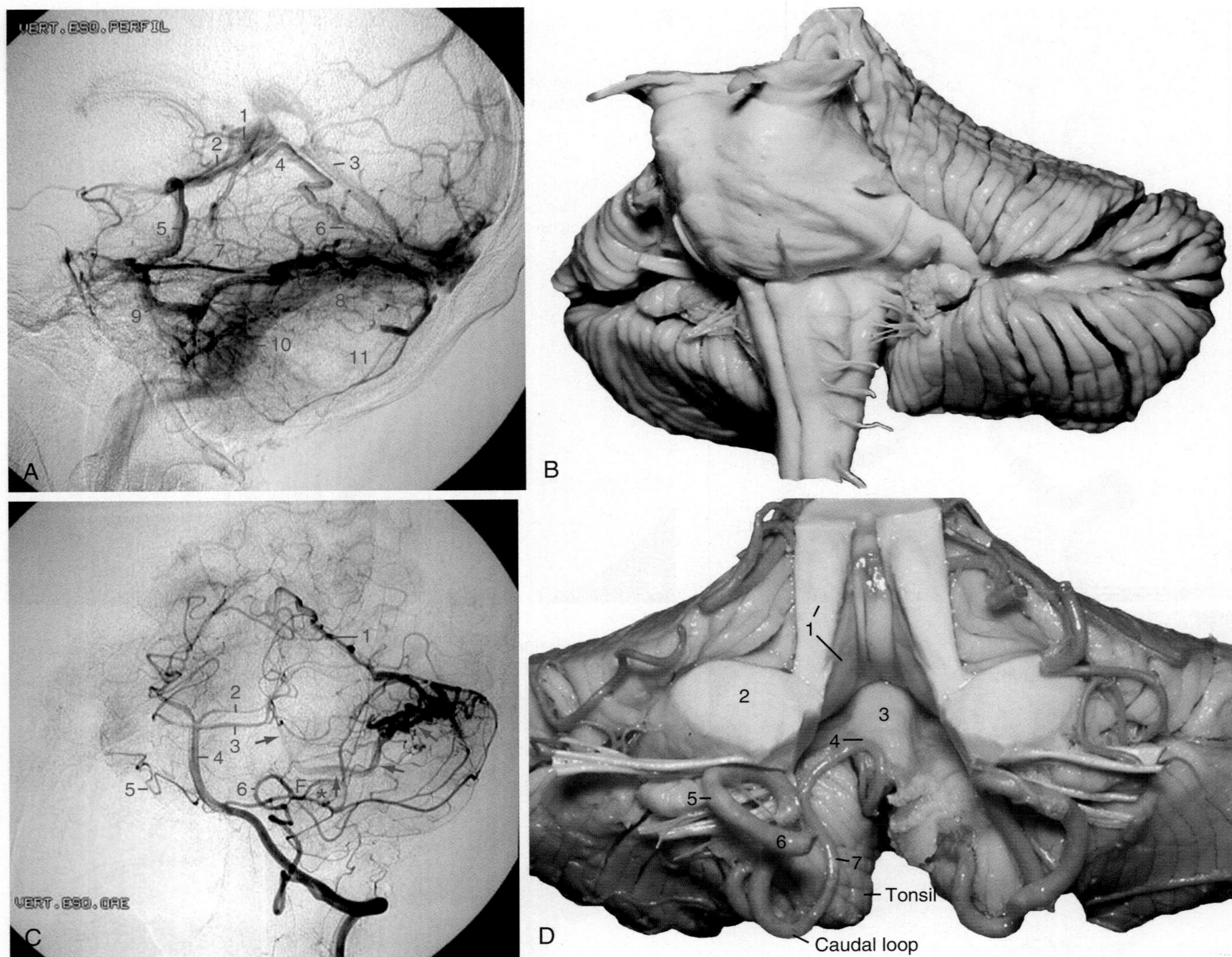

Figure 2-15. A, Lateral view of venous phase of vertebrobasilar angiography. Correlated with Figure 2-14D. 1, Vein of Galen; 2, cerebellomesencephalic fissure; 3, straight sinus; 4, culmen; 5, vein running on middle cerebral peduncle that continues with a vein in the petrosal fissure (vein of the great horizontal fissure) (9); 6, vein running on tentorial surface of the cerebellum (superior hemispheric vein) toward the vein of Galen; 7, superior petrosal sinus; 8, transverse sinus; 9, vein running in the petrosal fissure or great horizontal fissure (vein of the great horizontal fissure); 10, sigmoid sinus; 11, suboccipital surface of the cerebellum. *, A superior hemispheric vein that drains the arteriovenous malformation, which runs on the tentorial surface and descends toward the petrosal surface to join the vein of the great horizontal fissure. **B,** Left anterior oblique view of cerebellum and brainstem. This figure correlates with Figure 2-15C. **C,** Left anterior oblique view of venous vertebrobasilar angiography. 1, Vein running on the tentorial surface toward the vein of Galen (superior hemispheric vein); 2, posterior cerebral artery; 3, superior cerebellar artery; 4, basilar artery; 5, meatal loop of anterior inferior cerebellar artery (AICA); 6, posterior inferior cerebellar artery (PICA). The *arrows* indicate the vein shown in Figure 2-15A that originates from the tentorial surface (superior hemispheric vein) and descends toward the petrosal surface to join the vein in the great horizontal fissure. F, Approximate location of the flocculus; it was estimated by the location meatal loop of the AICA (*). **D,** Anterior view of PICA and roof of fourth ventricle. This figure correlates with Figure 2-14A. 1, Superior cerebellar peduncle; 2, middle cerebellar peduncle; 3, nodule (covered by the inferior medullary velum); 4, supratonsillar segment of PICA (cranial loop); 5, lateral medullary segment of PICA; 6, anterior medullary segment of PICA; 7, posterior medullary segment of PICA.

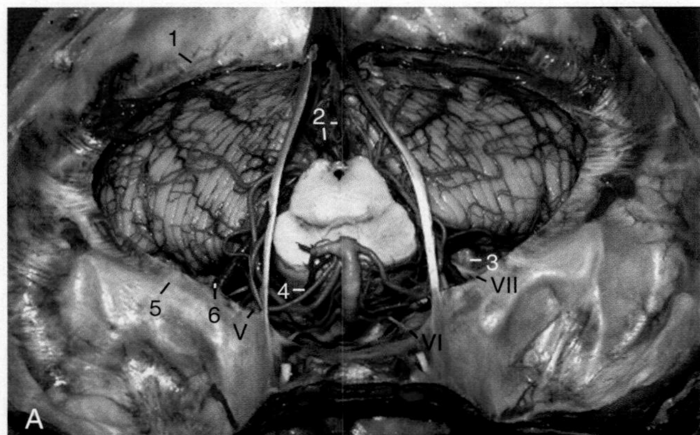

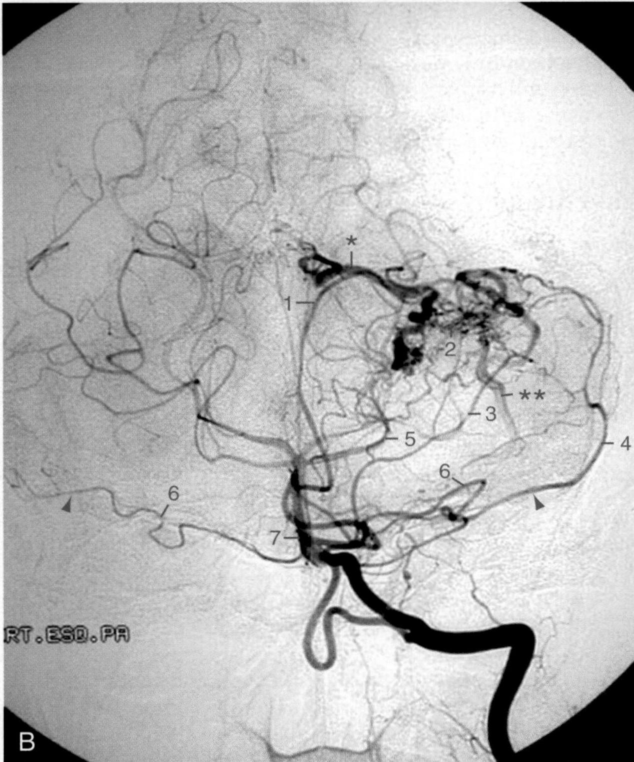

Figure 2-16. A, Anterosuperior (Towne) view of posterior fossa. This figure correlates with Figure 2-16B. 1, Transverse sinus; 2, precentral cerebellar vein and cerebellomesencephalic fissure; 3, flocculus; 4, superior cerebellar artery (SCA); 5, superior petrosal sinus; 6, superior petrosal vein. **B,** Towne view of vertebrobasilar angiography. This figure correlates with Figure 2-16A. 1, Vermian branch of posterior inferior cerebellar artery (PICA); 2, arteriovenous malformation located at the superior semilunar lobule; 3, inferior hemispheric branch from PICA; 4, branch from anterior inferior cerebellar artery (AICA) in great horizontal fissure; 5, lateral pontomesencephalic segment of SCA; 6, meatal loop of AICA; 7, basilar artery. The *arrowheads* indicate the location of the great horizontal fissure or petrosal fissure. *, A superior hemispheric vein draining toward the vein of Galen; **, a superior hemispheric vein coursing initially on the tentorial surface then descending to the great horizontal fissure on the petrosal surface of the cerebellum.

dural, and vascular elements of the cerebellopontine angle with the patient positioned in the three-quarter prone position can be seen in Figure 2-13E to H; in that surgical position, the site where the abducent nerve pierces the dura of the clivus can be visualized between the VII and VIII, and the IX, X, and XI cranial nerves (see Fig. 2-13H).

SUGGESTED READINGS

Matsushima T, Rhoton AL Jr, Lenkey C. Microsurgery of the fourth ventricle: Part 1: microsurgical anatomy. *Neurosurgery*. 1982;11: 631-667.

Ono M, Kubik S, Abernathey CD. *Atlas of the Cerebral Sulci*. Stuttgart: Georg Thieme Verlag; 1990.

Timurkaynak E, Rhoton AL Jr, Barry M. Microsurgical anatomy and operative approaches to the lateral ventricles. *Neurosurgery*. 1986; 19:685-723.

Wen HT, Rhoton AL Jr, de Oliveira E. Transchoroidal approach to the third ventricle: An anatomic study of the choroidal fissure and its clinical application. *Neurosurgery*. 1998;42:1205-1219.

Wen HT, Rhoton AL Jr, de Oliveira E, et al. Microsurgical anatomy of the temporal lobe: Part 1 Mesial Temporal Lobe and Its Vascular Relationship as Applied to Amygdalohippocampectomy. *Neurosurgery*. 1999;45(3):549-592.

Wen HT, Rhoton AL Jr, de Oliveira E, et al. Microsurgical anatomy of the temporal lobe: Part 2—Sylvian fissure region and its clinical application. *Neurosurgery*. 2009;65(suppl 6):1-36.

Yasargil MG. *Microneurosurgery: Microsurgical anatomy of the basal cisterns and vessels of the brain*. Vol. 1. Stuttgart: Georg Thieme Verlag; 1984.

See a full reference list on ExpertConsult.com 

3 Surgical Anatomy of the Skull Base

Arnau Benet, Michael T. Lawton, Michel Kliot, and Mitchel S. Berger

The skull base is a beautiful landscape of compartments, bony ridges and prominences, winding sutures, scattered foramina, and dural folds. This exquisite complexity is multiplied by relationships with cranial nerves, brainstem surfaces, posterior circulation arteries, and veins. It is difficult to put anatomy to words; inspection and direct handling are imperative. There is no substitute for time spent in the cadaver laboratory with a scalpel, drill, and microscissors, peering through an operating microscope at the magnified and illuminated landscape of the brainstem. Repeating this exercise many times over transforms learning into mastery.

Our collective knowledge of skull base anatomy appears to be dwindling in this era of digital learning, surgical subspecialization, and minimally invasive surgery. Computer-generated atlases and three-dimensional videos are replacing cadaver laboratories and eliminating hands-on dissection. Neurosurgeons are partnering with neurotologists who make the temporal bone and all of its complex anatomy their domain. While this partnership enhances the expertise of the skull base team, it diminishes neurosurgical familiarity with this anatomy. Endoscopy is changing neurosurgical management of skull base lesions and decreasing *classical* skull base operations. Advances in stereotactic radiosurgery and endovascular intervention are similarly reducing case volumes of tumors, arteriovenous malformations, and aneurysms. The end result is diminished expertise in skull base surgery and diminished knowledge of skull base anatomy. It is easy to wonder if skull base anatomy is clinically relevant to modern neurosurgical practice.

We think that knowledge of skull base anatomy is a cornerstone of neurosurgery. Many consider manual dexterity to be the most important quality in a skillful neurosurgeon, but knowledge of anatomy guides the hands and gives the neurosurgeon the confidence to explore the surgical field. Mastery of anatomy is the cognitive skill that informs the neurosurgeon where to work, what to see, how to maneuver better, and what to protect. Comfort in the anatomic arena around the skull base translates to confidence in executing the surgical strategy designed for the patient's pathology. Analyzing anatomic relationships, practicing surgical steps, and committing learning mistakes in bloodless cadavers translate to better surgery on live patients.

In this chapter, we review the anatomy of the skull base as it relates to five approaches used frequently in skull base surgery: the far lateral approach, the retrosigmoid approach, the transpetrosal approaches, the orbitozygomatic approach, and the endoscopic endonasal approach. We present the bone anatomy, surgical technique, and important anatomy encountered within the surgical corridor. This information is intended to facilitate, rather than replace, hands-on learning in cadaveric dissection and will be more valuable if read in this context.

THE FAR LATERAL APPROACH

Surgical Targets

The far lateral approach and its variants (trans-, supra-, and paracondylar) use a posterior trajectory to reach the cerebellomedullary and premedullary cisterns through different corridors between the lower cranial nerves. The retrosigmoid and endoscopic endonasal approaches are the two surgical options most directly related to the far lateral approach. For complex lesions with large invasion of the ventral compartment of the posterior fossa, a combined far lateral–endoscopic endonasal "far medial" approach could provide an efficient and safe surgical option. Likewise, lesions with infra- and supratentorial components might benefit from combining a far lateral with a retrosigmoid, translabyrinthine, and middle fossa approach. Therefore, the far lateral approach might be used as a stand-alone standardized approach or in combination with other skull base approaches for complex lesions. Knowledge of the full surgical potential of the far lateral and its related approaches will enable the neurosurgeon to find the most efficient and safe treatment for each lesion of the posterior cranial fossa.

Bone Anatomy

The far lateral approach uses a posterior trajectory to access the posterior fossa. Therefore, thorough knowledge of the anatomy of the occipital bone is the key to a safe and efficient execution of the far lateral approach. Additionally, if the transcondylar, supracondylar, and paracondylar extensions of the far lateral approach are planned, the anatomy of the atlas (C1) and petrous part of the temporal bone become relevant as well.

The occipital bone can be divided into three parts: (1) the squamous part, which forms the posterior wall of the posterior fossa; (2) the basilar part, which forms the anterior wall of the posterior fossa together with the dorsum sellae of the sphenoid bone; and (3) the condylar part, which attaches to the petrous part of the temporal bone to form the lateral walls of the posterior fossa. Only the squamous and condylar parts of the occipital bone are directly related to the far lateral approach and are discussed in this section.

The squamous part of the occipital bone has a concave surface that accommodates and protects the occipital lobes, cerebellar hemispheres, and transverse and superior sagittal sinuses (Fig. 3-1A). The external occipital protuberance, called the inion, is an evident osseous structure that stands at the center of the squamous part. The inion serves as a reliable landmark to infer the position of the torcula—the confluence of the superior sagittal, straight, and transverse sinuses, which is located 1 cm superior to the inion at the endocranial surface (Fig. 3-1B).

Two osseous crests arise from the inion and extend horizontally; the superior nuchal line extends inferiorly and the highest (also known as supreme) nuchal line extends superiorly. The superior nuchal line is shaped by the tendinous insertion of the nuchal muscles (sternocleidomastoid, trapezius, splenius capitis, and semispinalis capitis). Therefore, the superior nuchal line is an important landmark for the muscular incision during the far lateral approach. The highest nuchal line is less evident and corresponds to the insertion of the occipitofrontal muscle. Both the superior and the highest nuchal lines may be used to infer the position of the tentorium during the craniotomy design. If the superior nuchal line is followed laterally, the asterion (a confluence of the lambdoid, parietomastoid, and occipitomastoid sutures) is found.

The asterion is a reliable landmark for the exocranial inference of the position of the transverse sinus as it becomes the sigmoid sinus. Inferiorly is a slight bone furrow parallel to the occipitomastoid suture that typically corresponds to the trajectory of the occipital artery. Anterior to the occipitomastoid suture is a groove carved by the posterior belly of the digastric muscle (digastric groove). The digastric groove belongs mostly to the mastoid part of the temporal bone but may serve as a landmark to identify the mastoid and the sigmoid sinus in the supracondylar extension, and the facial nerve in the stylomastoid foramen in the paracondylar extension, during the far lateral craniectomy.

Between the superior nuchal line and the foramen magnum is the inferior nuchal line. The inferior nuchal line corresponds to the insertion of the suboccipital muscles, the identification of which is very important during the muscular dissection of the far lateral approach (discussed below). The occipital crest is a vertical ridge that extends superiorly from the opisthion—midpoint on the posterior margin of the foramen magnum—to the inion. The occipital crest is a useful landmark to infer the position of the falx cerebelli in the intracranial space and to reference the midline during the design of the craniotomy.

The condylar part of the occipital bone is formed by the occipital condyle, the condylar fossa, and the jugular tubercle. The condylar fossa is an osseous depression between the squamous part of the occipital bone and the occipital condyle in the base of the skull. In most cases, the condylar fossa becomes relevant during a far lateral approach because it often contains a rich venous channel: the posterior condylar emissary vein. When present, the posterior condylar emissary vein serves as a connection between the vertebral venous sinus and the sigmoid sinus. It is important to identify the posterior condylar emissary vein surgically, because its bleeding can be profuse and it may be confused with bleeding from the hypoglossal venous plexus, which could misguide the next surgical steps.

The occipital condyle is an oval-shaped structure at the base of the skull that articulates with the superior articular facet of the atlas to form the atlanto-occipital joint. Understanding the size and orientation of the occipital condyle is key to preventing craniocervical instability and the need for cervical fusion after a transcondylar extension of the far lateral approach. Just above the occipital condyle is the hypoglossal canal, which crosses the occipital bone at 45 degrees in an anterolateral trajectory. It contains the hypoglossal nerve (cranial nerve [CN] XII) and its venous plexus. The trajectory of the hypoglossal canal plays an important role in the transcondylar extension of the far lateral approach. While drilling into the occipital condyle from the far lateral perspective, the hypoglossal canal is encountered first in the medial aspect of the exposure and is exposed progressively laterally when the drilling is continued anteriorly.

The hypoglossal canal and nerve divide the condylar part of the occipital bone into the condylar compartment (below the hypoglossal canal) and the jugular tubercle compartment (above the hypoglossal canal). If drilling of the condylar compartment is directed medially, the lower third of the clivus is accessed. In contrast, if the jugular tubercle compartment is drilled, the jugular foramen and the lateral and anterior medullary spaces are exposed. The jugular tubercle serves as both the roof of the hypoglossal canal and the floor of the jugular foramen. The jugular foramen, however, belongs to both the occipital bone inferiorly and the petrous part of the temporal bone superiorly.

The richness in anatomic detail and complexity of the jugular foramen may be interpreted as an advantage to the neurosurgeon because it provides several valuable landmarks (Fig. 3-1C and D). The jugular foramen, although described as a single orifice, has three compartments: sigmoid, neural, and petrous. When the jugular foramen is studied in a dry skull, a central bony spur in the jugular surface of the temporal bone becomes evident. This bony spur, referred to as the superior intrajugular process, is continued by a dural fold to the jugular tubercle. In some cases, the attachment of this dural fold creates a small promontory in the jugular tubercle, known as the inferior intrajugular process. The superior and inferior intrajugular processes, together with the dural fold that unites them, create a posterior space within the jugular foramen: the sigmoid compartment. The sigmoid compartment is used by the sigmoid sinus, the jugular bulb, and the meningeal branches of the ascending pharyngeal, vertebral, or occipital arteries. The sigmoid compartment is the first structure encountered during the drilling of the jugular tubercle in a supracondylar extension of the far lateral approach. The accessory (CN XI), vagus (CN X), and glossopharyngeal (CN IX) nerves are immediately anterior to the sigmoid compartment, embedded in dural and connective tissue. This space formed by the dura is called the neural compartment (also known as intermediate portion).

The neural compartment is further divided into the glossopharyngeal meatus (anterior) and the vagal meatus (posterior) by a dural septum. The glossopharyngeal meatus contains the glossopharyngeal nerve and its tympanic branch (also called Jacobson's nerve). The vagal meatus contains the vagus nerve and its auricular branch (also called Arnold's nerve) and the accessory nerve. The most anterior space of the jugular foramen is the petrous compartment, limited posteriorly by the neural compartment and anteriorly by the petroclival synchondrosis. The petrous compartment contains the inferior petrosal sinus.

The atlas (C1 vertebra) becomes relevant to the far lateral approach if caudal spinal exposure is required or if the third segment of the vertebral artery loops superiorly toward the occipital bone, becoming a risk for lesion during the suboccipital craniotomy. The atlas is an extraordinary vertebra in that it is the first of the spine (C1), has a ring shape, and lacks a vertebral body and spinous process. The main functions of the atlas are to hold the skull, provide support for the occipital and spinal muscles, and transmit multiple force vectors to the spine. The atlas consists of an anterior and a posterior arch and two lateral masses. Only the posterior arch and lateral masses are relevant to the far lateral approach and are briefly discussed in this section.

The lateral masses are a pair of rounded osseous protuberances on each side of the atlas. Their main function is to support and transmit the weight and motion forces applied by the occipital condyles of the skull to the axis (C2). Each lateral mass has two articular surfaces. The superior articular facet is an oval, concave surface that matches the inferior surface of the occipital condyle. During the drilling phase of the transcondylar extension, it is very important to identify the atlanto-occipital joint and preserve it to prevent neck instability and to ensure a proper anteromedial trajectory. The inferior articular facet of the lateral mass has a slightly less concave surface to match the superior articular facet of C2.

Lateral to the lateral masses are the transverse foramen and the transverse process. The transverse foramen of the atlas anchors the vertebral artery before it loops medially above the posterior arch of the atlas. The transverse foramen may be opened during a far lateral approach to free the vertebral artery and mobilize it laterally away from the surgical field. The transverse process provides the anterior, lateral, and posterior aspects of the transverse foramen and also contains the attachments for several suboccipital and cervical muscles.

The posterior arch is the most surgically relevant part of the atlas during the far lateral approach. It is a wide, semicircular flat bone that contains two depressions (one in each side) each carved by the third segment of the vertebral artery. In addition to the vertebral artery, the first cervical (C1) nerve also runs through the superior surface of the posterior arch of the atlas, embedded in the vertebral venous plexus and connective tissue, which puts it at risk of inadvertent lesioning during vertebral artery manipulation. The posterior arch of the atlas may be completely or partially removed to gain access to the spinal cord and upper cervical nerves during a far lateral approach.

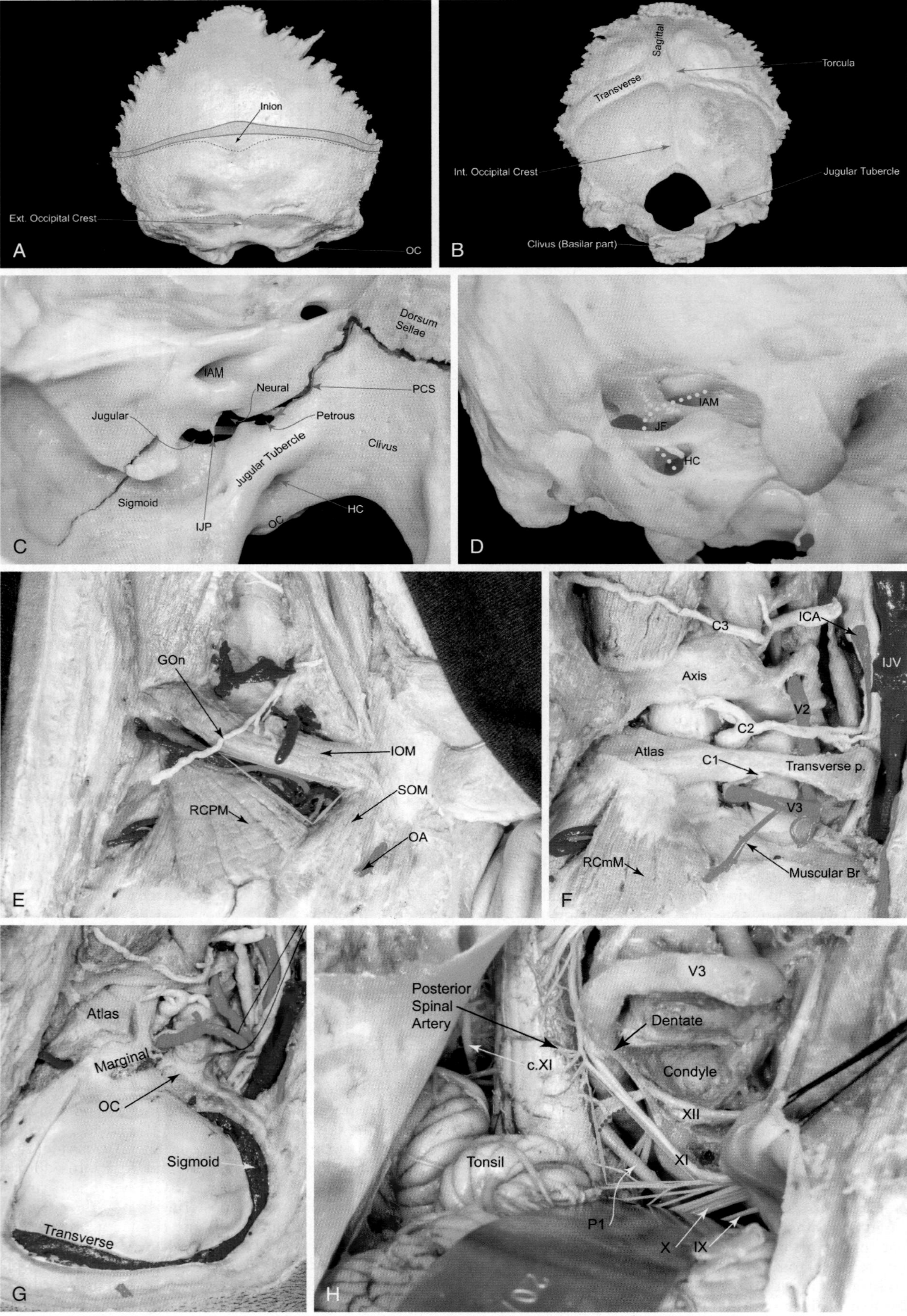
Inion
Ext. Occipital Crest
OC
A
Sagittal
Torcula
Transverse
Int. Occipital Crest
Jugular Tubercle
Clivus (Basilar part)
B
Dorsum Sellae
IAM
Neural
PCS
Jugular
Petrous
Clivus
Jugular Tubercle
Sigmoid
IJP
OC
HC
C
IAM
JF
HC
D
GOn
IOM
SOM
RCPM
OA
E
ICA
C3
IJV
Axis
V2
C2
Atlas
C1
Transverse p.
V3
RCmM
Muscular Br
F
Atlas
Marginal
OC
Sigmoid
Transverse
G
V3
Posterior Spinal Artery
Dentate
c.XI
Condyle
XII
Tonsil
XI
P1
X
IX
H

Figure 3-1. Bone anatomy and surgical landmarks relevant to the far lateral approach. A, Squamous part of the occipital bone showing the location of the inion, external occipital crest (Ext. Occipital Crest), and occipital condyle (OC). *Blue dotted line,* superior nuchal line; *blue line,* transverse sinus; *brown dotted line,* inferior nuchal line. **B,** Location of the torcula and the jugular tubercle. Int. Occipital Crest, internal occipital crest. **C,** The three compartments (sigmoid, neural, and petrous) of the jugular foramen. The intrajugular septum *(blue rectangle)* divides the jugular part from the neural part. HC, hypoglossal canal; IAM, internal acoustic meatus; IJP, intrajugular process; OC, occipital condyle; PCS, petroclival synchondrosis. **D,** Relationship of the hypoglossal canal (HC), internal acoustic meatus (IAM), and jugular foramen (JF). **E,** Exposure of the suboccipital triangle *(yellow triangle),* formed by the superior oblique muscle (SOM), the inferior oblique muscle (IOM), and the rectus capitis posterior major muscle (RCPM). GOn, greater occipital nerve; OA, occipital artery. **F,** The vertebral venous plexus within the suboccipital triangle, including the muscular branches (Muscular Br) of the vertebral artery (V2 and V3) and the first, second, and third cervical nerves (C1, C2, and C3). ICA, internal carotid artery; IJV, internal jugular vein; RCmM, rectus capitis posterior minor muscle; Transverse p, transverse process. **G,** Exposure of dura after suboccipital craniotomy, showing the marginal, sigmoid, and transverse sinuses. OC, occipital condyle. **H,** The cisterna magna and the ipsilateral cerebellar hemisphere. *Green dotted line,* limit between the supra- and infra-hypoglossal corridors; *yellow triangle,* vagoaccessory triangle. c.XI, contralateral cranial nerve XI; IX-XII, cranial nerves IX through XII; P1, first segment (anterior medullary) of the posterior inferior cerebellar artery; V3, third segment of the vertebral artery. *(Published with permission of the University of California San Francisco's Skull Base & Cerebrovascular Laboratory.)*

Surgical Anatomy

Positioning

The key for optimal patient positioning in any skull base procedure is to orient the head in a way that, while safe for the patient, allows the best final working corridor to expose the target. In many instances, both objectives are fulfilled if the position of the head takes into account the effect of gravity on the brain being exposed. The park bench, or three-quarter prone, position allows for natural retraction of the cerebellar hemisphere away from the surgical corridor. The park bench position requires positioning the patient at a 45-degree angle from a completely prone position with the head rotated 45 degrees away from the lesion and flexed laterally toward the floor. At the end of the positioning, the neurosurgeon should be able to effortlessly palpate the mastoid tip, the inion, and the spinous processes of the upper vertebrae while standing above the patient.

Skin Incision

An optimal skin incision for the far lateral approach takes into consideration the location of the lesion, which determines the surgical exposure, the surgical time (longer skin incisions may generate more bleeding and increased surgical time), and aesthetics. Two valid skin incisions are widely used for the far lateral approach: the inverted hockey stick and the lazy "S." The inverted hockey stick incision starts 2 cm below the tip of the mastoid process, continues straight superiorly until above the superior nuchal line, where it turns medially toward the level of the inion. It then turns inferiorly until the level of the C2 or C3 vertebra. The benefit of the inverted hockey stick incision is that it provides wide exposure of the ipsilateral suboccipital musculature, allows access to the lateral aspect of the occipital condyle and transverse process of the atlas, and uses an avascular plane along the midline over the suboccipital space and spinous processes in the neck. Although it provides exceptional, wide exposure, drawbacks of the inverted hockey stick incision include a longer surgical time, potentially more blood loss, and suboptimal cosmesis compared with the lazy "S." A lazy S-shaped incision uses a diagonal trajectory from the asterion to the foramen magnum and then curves medially toward the spinous process of the axis (C2). This incision provides space enough for a basic far lateral approach and its trans- and supracondylar variants. However, complete exposure of the transverse process of the atlas, if necessary, may be limited for a paracondylar variant of the far lateral approach.

Muscular Layer

It is generally agreed that the optimal muscular flap is that which creates the least distortion of the muscular structure while providing sufficient bone exposure. Multiple-layer dissection during the muscular phase can prompt dehiscence, loss of function, or ischemic atrophy and is typically avoided. However, the far lateral approach requires that all efforts be made to protect the vertebral artery, and this is best accomplished if the muscular phase is divided into two stages: the nuchal and the suboccipital. The nuchal muscles are anatomically contained between the superior and inferior nuchal lines. The nuchal muscular flap is obtained en bloc from 1 cm inferior to the superior nuchal line. The nuchal muscular flap contains the sternocleidomastoideus, trapezius, longissimus capitis, and splenius and semispinalis capitis muscles. The posterior belly of the digastric muscle along with the occipital artery, which runs on the medial surface of it, may be spared if transmastoid access is not needed in the final exposure. After the nuchal muscular flap is reflected inferiorly and laterally, the suboccipital triangle is exposed (Fig. 3-1E). The suboccipital triangle is formed by the superior oblique (superior and lateral), the inferior oblique (inferior and lateral), and the rectus capitis (posterior) major muscles. Identifying the suboccipital triangle is key to avoid both copious venous bleeding and damage to the third segment of the vertebral artery. The dorsal ramus of the C1 cervical nerve and the posterior arch of the atlas may be exposed if the suboccipital triangle is dissected.

The vertebral venous plexus is a complex of tangled and densely anastomosed veins that fills the suboccipital triangle and connects to the sigmoid sinus and jugular bulb via the posterior condylar emissary vein. Embedded in this venous plexus are the muscular branches of the vertebral artery and the dorsal roots of the C1 cervical nerves. In some cases, the third segment of the vertebral artery loops higher than normal, being at special risk of inadvertent injury if the venous plexus is not dissected with extreme caution. Although rare, both the posterior spinal and the posterior inferior cerebellar arteries can take off at this segment of the vertebral artery and be mistaken for a muscular branch. After the muscles forming the suboccipital triangle are reflected, three additional muscles become relevant. At the superior aspect of the C1 transverse process, deep below the superior oblique muscle, is the rectus capitis lateralis. The rectus capitis lateralis is a short muscle that attaches to the jugular process at the posterior edge of the jugular tubercle. Although very small, this muscle is of extraordinary value in guiding the paracondylar dissection toward the jugular foramen. In the same axis as this muscle, but inferior to the transverse process of the atlas, is the levator scapulae muscle. Early identification of the levator scapulae muscle during the cervical dissection of the far lateral approach is advisable. This muscle provides an invaluable landmark to safely expose the second segment of the vertebral artery (medial to the muscle) and protect the carotid compartment of the parapharyngeal space (lateral to the muscle). Finally, the rectus capitis posterior minor muscle is reflected medially for a complete exposure of the atlanto-occipital membrane (Fig. 3-1F).

Craniotomy

A fundamental rule in skull base surgery is to gain maximal surgical exposure through bone removal. Therefore, there is an optimal craniotomy, or combination of craniotomy and craniectomy, for each lesion. However, for educational purposes, the far lateral approach can be standardized into a basic lateral suboccipital craniotomy with three different extensions: transcondylar, supracondylar, and paracondylar. The lateral suboccipital craniotomy opens a window in the squamous part of the occipital bone. It is limited superiorly by the transverse sinus and laterally by the sigmoid sinus and the occipital condyle (Fig. 3-1G). In most cases, the suboccipital craniotomy includes the condylar fossa and its posterior condylar vein. The asterion is a useful landmark to design the craniotomy in relation to the sigmoid sinus. The superior nuchal line may also be used to limit the cranial extension of the craniotomy so as to avoid the transverse sinus and the torcula. The medial extent of the suboccipital craniotomy may be guided with the external occipital crest and can be extended widely beyond it if the lesion occupies the majority of the cisterna magna. Although there is no anatomic boundary, the medial margin of the suboccipital craniotomy usually does not cross the occipital crest, providing enough room for cerebellar distention.

The standard suboccipital craniotomy can be accompanied by the removal of the ipsilateral half of the posterior arch of the atlas. The first and most important step in the preparation for the removal of the posterior arch of the atlas is dissecting the vertebral artery from its connective sheath. Next, the root of the C2 spinal nerve can be identified medial to the atlantoaxial joint and protected with the muscular flap. Two cuts are placed to elevate the ipsilateral half of the posterior arch of the atlas in one piece. The first cut is placed in the midline, medial to the rectus capitis posterior minor muscle. The second cut divides the lateral mass from the posterior arch. After the completion of the two cuts, the posterior arch is elevated in one piece and the vertebral artery is freed from the transverse foramen after unroofing the foramen transversarium. At this point, the vertebral artery can be displaced laterally to gain access to both the posterior fossa and the occipital condyle.

Of the three main types of craniectomy that can follow the suboccipital craniotomy, the transcondylar extension is the most used. The posterior third of the occipital condyle is removed uniformly until a change in bone consistency and color is noticed. The cancellous body of the condyle becomes the solid posterior wall of the hypoglossal canal. The hypoglossal canal contains a venous plexus, which adds a dark blue color to its wall. The hypoglossal canal should be preserved if there is no lesion involving it, yet the condylectomy can advance below and medial to the hypoglossal canal en route to the clivus. The transcondylar approach provides direct access to the intracranial segment of the vertebral artery and a wide access to the anterior medullary zone and lower clivus. However, if the lesion infiltrates the condyle or its vicinity, a complete condylectomy may be necessary.

If access to the jugular foramen or upper medulla is required, the supracondylar extension may be performed. The supracondylar craniectomy requires removing the posterior aspect of the jugular tubercle in a narrow window limited inferiorly by the hypoglossal canal, superiorly by the sigmoid sinus, and laterally by the jugular bulb. It is imperative that the drilling of the jugular tubercle be done with a diamond bur and using extreme caution at the medial (dural) limit of the drilling, because the spinal rootlets of the accessory nerve travel alongside and in contact with the dura at this region. The accessory, vagus, and glossopharyngeal nerves are exposed at the neural compartment of the jugular foramen. The supracondylar approach allows maneuvering above the vagus nerve, the petroclival junction, and the midclivus.

Lesions involving the jugular bulb, the lower sigmoid sinus, and the meatal segment of the glossopharyngeal, vagus, and accessory nerves can be accessed through the paracondylar variant of the far lateral approach. This craniectomy is directed to the superior and lateral aspect of the occipital condyle, the exocranial aspect of the jugular foramen, and the posterior aspect of the mastoid process. A more lateral muscular flap must be raised, which may also include the posterior belly of the digastric muscle. The digastric groove should be identified because it provides an excellent landmark to the position of the stylomastoid foramen, where the facial nerve exits the mastoid process. Drilling around the exocranial aspect of the jugular foramen must be carried out with a diamond bur and constant electrophysiologic monitoring of the glossopharyngeal, vagus, accessory, and hypoglossal nerves. The bone removal is mainly directed to the jugular process, an osseous protuberance at the posterior aspect of the jugular foramen. At the end of the craniectomy, the lower part of the sigmoid sinus, the jugular bulb, and jugular vein are exposed together with the neural compartment of the jugular foramen and the pharyngeal segment of the internal carotid artery.

These variants of the far lateral approach could be combined with different levels of mastoidectomy (retro- or translabyrinthine approach) and a supratentorial craniotomy for full access to the lateral and anterolateral zones of the brainstem.

Dural Opening

The dura exposed after a suboccipital craniotomy is limited superiorly by the transverse sinus, laterally by the sigmoid sinus, and inferiorly by the marginal sinus—all potential sources of bleeding (see Fig. 3-1G). Other potential sources of bleeding include the posterior meningeal artery, which in some rare cases originates from the intradural segment of the vertebral artery; the posterior spinal artery, which may take off from the vertebral artery at its dural cuff; and the meningeal branch of the ascending pharyngeal artery in cases in which the dural incision extends to the lateral margin of the bone opening (especially after a supracondylar extension). Each dural flap may be customized to adapt to the features of each patient. However, many, if not all, include long midline and superior incisions to reflect the dural flap laterally. The dural opening should always be designed according to the lesion location and size and should create a surgical window that allows all anticipated surgical trajectories. In the case of the far lateral approach, a wide dural flap eases cerebellar retraction and access to the superior spinal region. In addition, if the lesion extends to the cerebellopontine angle, the dura should be opened close to the transition between the transverse and sigmoid sinuses, leaving a margin for safe closure. After the dura is opened, the cisterna magna is incised, and the cerebrospinal fluid is evacuated to allow atraumatic retraction of the cerebellar hemispheres and maximize the effect of gravity.

Intradural Anatomy

The intradural phase of the far lateral approach provides wide access to the dorsolateral compartment of the posterior fossa and limited access to the ventromedial compartment, including the petroclival region and the lateral aspect of the middle and lower thirds of the clivus (see Fig. 3-1D). Like most skull base approaches, the number and exposure of structures accessed through the far lateral approach increases proportionally to the progressive bone removal of its three variants (i.e., trans-, supra-, and paracondylar craniectomies). The suboccipital craniotomy allows complete access to the cisterna magna and the ipsilateral cerebellar hemisphere (Fig. 3-1H). In the cisterna magna, the inferomedial aspect of the cerebellar hemisphere, the cerebellar tonsil, and the lower medulla coexist. The obex (inferior angle of the fourth ventricle) is also viewed upon arachnoidal dissection and points toward the fourth ventricle in the foramen of Magendie. Opening the cisterna magna also exposes the vertebral artery. The vertebral artery transitions from its third segment (V3, over the posterior arch of the atlas) to its intradural segment around the inferomedial aspect of the occipital condyle. At this point it is anchored to the craniocervical junction by the dentate ligament.

After the vertebral artery becomes intradural, it travels through the cerebellomedullary and premedullary cisterns in an anteromedial trajectory toward the clivus, where it joins the contralateral vertebral artery to form the vertebrobasilar junction. In the majority of individuals, the posterior inferior cerebellar artery (PICA) takes off from the vertebral artery at the premedullary cistern close to the inferior olive (anterior medullary segment). After a short course, the PICA crosses the rootlets of the vagus and accessory nerves (CNs X and XI) toward the cerebellomedullary cistern below the cerebellar hemisphere (lateral medullary segment). It then turns medially and upward around the cerebellar tonsil (tonsillomedullary segment). Following this, the PICA runs between the cerebellum and the posterior wall of the fourth ventricle (telovelomedullary segment) away from the surgical exposure obtained with the far lateral approach. It finally turns superficial (cortical segment) to feed the posterior aspect of the cerebellar hemisphere. Another critical branch of the vertebral artery is the posterior spinal artery. The neurosurgeon dissecting the arachnoid space in the cisterna magna should identify this artery early and protect it.

The accessory nerve comes into view at the lateral aspect of the cisterna magna. The accessory nerve has a long cisternal segment, which receives rootlets from both the upper spine and the lower aspect of the posterolateral sulcus in the medulla. It has a superolateral trajectory from its spinal origin toward the jugular foramen. At the jugular foramen, the accessory nerve joins the vagus nerve, which has a straight pathway from its origin at the posterolateral sulcus of the medulla. The accessory and vagus nerves form the vagoaccessory triangle, the main surgical corridor to access the ventromedial compartment of the posterior fossa (see Fig. 3-1H, yellow triangle). The superior aspect of the vagoaccessory triangle is formed by the vagus and medullary rootlets of the accessory nerve; it is limited laterally by the body of the accessory nerve and medially by the medulla oblongata. The vagoaccessory triangle is further divided by the hypoglossal nerve into supra- and infra-hypoglossal windows (see Fig. 3-1H, green line). As it transitions to the intracranial space, the accessory nerve is intimately related to the dentate ligament and the vertebral artery. The relationship between the accessory nerve and the dentate ligament is surgically relevant. At the spine, the dentate ligament is anterior to the rootlets of the accessory nerve. However, as these structures ascend, they cross each other as the dentate ligament anchors to the dural cuff of the vertebral artery, and the accessory nerve runs in an anterosuperior trajectory toward the posterior aspect of the jugular foramen (in the neural compartment). Therefore, any mobilization or manipulation of the dentate ligament (e.g., transposition of the vertebral artery) should be done with continuous visual contact with the accessory nerve. The vertebral artery, after piercing the dura and passing the dentate ligament, runs anterior to the accessory nerve. This leaves an unobstructed space between the accessory nerve and the lateral aspect of the medulla that is of surgical relevance. The suboccipital craniotomy also provides direct access to the inferior vermian and hemispheric veins draining the ipsilateral cerebellum to the torcula and the transverse and tentorial sinuses.

The transcondylar craniectomy allows access to the cisternal, canalicular, and cervical segments of the hypoglossal nerve. Additionally, this extra window allows for an increased angle of attack and surgical exposure of both the intradural portion of the vertebral artery and the inferior half of the cerebellomedullary and premedullary cisterns. The exposure of the cerebellomedullary cistern allows for manipulation of the medullary rootlets of IX-XII, the lateral aspect of the medulla, and the lateral medullary segment of the PICA. The transcondylar variant of the far lateral approach maximizes the infra-hypoglossal window of the vagoaccessory triangle.

As the craniectomy is progressed through the jugular tubercle via a supracondylar extension, access to the superior aspect of the premedullary and cerebellomedullary cisterns increases. These cisterns can be widely accessed after a combined trans- and supracondylar craniectomy. The supracondylar approach provides the optimal bone opening for maximal access through the vagoaccessory triangle. Working through its supra- and infra-hypoglossal windows, the vertebral artery, vertebrobasilar junction, and lower basilar artery may be accessed. If the drilling of the jugular tubercle is continued anteriorly, the petroclival junction and medial aspect of the clivus can be accessed. The number and magnitude of the neurovascular structures and lesions accessible through the far lateral approach is highly dependent on the angulation of the microscope and the positioning of the retraction blades. If the jugular tubercle is removed and retraction is applied at the midportion of the cerebellar hemisphere, the hypoglossal canal, jugular foramen, internal acoustic meatus, and inferior surface of the tentorium may be accessible. This brings a broad spectrum of both anatomic landmarks and surgical lesions that can be explored from a single approach. If the microscope is angled toward the petrous bone, the distal anterior inferior cerebellar artery (AICA), the facial and vestibulocochlear nerves (CNs VII and VIII), the foramen of Lushka, and the trigeminal nerve may be explored. The three working corridors from this perspective are: (1) the space formed between the vestibulocochlear and glossopharyngeal nerves (CNs VIII and IX), (2) the space between the trigeminal nerve and the facial-vestibulocochlear nerve (CN VII-VIII) bundle, and (3) the space between the trigeminal nerve and the tentorium. However, if the microscope is angled toward the brainstem, access to the pons in the cerebellopontine cistern, the lateral aspect of the pontomedullary sulcus, and the medulla in the premedullary and cerebellomedullary cisterns may be possible.

When used during a far lateral approach, the endoscope allows further exploration of the ventromedial compartment of the posterior fossa. The main advantage of the endoscope, used in combination with the microscope, is that the point of view and light can be brought beyond the limits of microsurgery. This is especially relevant when angled scopes are used. A 30-degree endoscope passed through the vagoaccessory triangle allows exploration of the medial portion of the medulla and the abducens nerve (CN VI) at the pontomedullary sulcus medially, and the floor and medial aspect of the jugular foramen laterally. Additionally, if the angled endoscope is advanced through the space between the vestibulocochlear and glossopharyngeal nerves, the origin of the trigeminal nerve, the prepontine cistern, the proximal segment of the AICA, and the cisternal segment of the abducens nerve can be explored medially and the internal acoustic meatus can be completely explored in the cerebellopontine angle laterally. However, the expanded view provided by the endoscope carries significant surgical limitations; the instrumentation is limited, the corridors are lengthy, and there is no visual control over the external surface of the endoscope, potentially making it difficult to be aware of retraction damage caused by the rod of the endoscope.

THE RETROSIGMOID APPROACH

Surgical Targets

The retrosigmoid approach is a variation of the suboccipital craniotomy that is designed to provide optimal access to the cerebellopontine and cerebellomedullary cisterns and the posterior aspect of the cerebellopontine angle (Fig. 3-2A). The retrosigmoid approach uses a lateral suboccipital craniotomy combined with a partial mastoidectomy to enter the superior aspect of the posterior fossa in the dorsolateral compartment. This approach is best used to access tumors of the cerebellopontine angle, which, while having their epicenters posterior to the lower cranial nerves, may infiltrate superiorly to the middle incisural space, laterally to the internal acoustic meatus, or medially to the lateral aspect of the pons or into the cerebellar hemisphere. It also provides an exposure to aneurysms of the AICA, the proximal segment of the PICA, the basilar trunk, and vascular compression of the trigeminal nerve. When planning the surgical strategy for a particular case, the retrosigmoid approach may be weighed against the far lateral, the endoscopic endonasal, and the transmastoid approaches.

A useful rule to maximize extent of resection while staying in the safe zone is to design the surgical strategy around the concept of "not crossing the nerves." Consequently, the neurosurgeon should consider all the surgical approaches that may be used for a particular lesion and their potential combinations (360-degree approach to the lesion).

Bone Anatomy

The bone anatomy relevant to the retrosigmoid approach belongs to the squamous part of the occipital bone and the mastoid and petrous parts of the temporal bone. The inion (external occipital protuberance) is a prominent landmark that may be easily identified by palpating the occiput and may be used to infer the position of the transverse sinus and the tentorium. The transverse sinus generally runs just above the superior nuchal line (which extends laterally from the inion), in the endocranial surface of the squamous part of the occipital bone.

Although the retrosigmoid craniotomy uses a bone window primarily based at the occipital bone, there are several features of the temporal bone that are critical to safety and efficiency. The temporal line is the posterior projection of the axis of the zygomatic process (and also the zygomatic arc) to the squamous and mastoid parts. The temporal line may be used to infer both the floor of the middle fossa (tegmen of the temporal bone) and the inferior limit of the temporal muscle.

In the mastoid part of the temporal bone, there are two structures relevant to the retrosigmoid approach: the digastric groove and the mastoid emissary foramen. The digastric groove is an osseous depression carved by the posterior belly of the digastric muscle. It starts as a bone groove in the posterior aspect of the mastoid process and becomes a deep furrow as it progresses anteriorly, medial to the mastoid tip, toward the stylomastoid foramen. Therefore, the digastric groove may be used to infer the extracranial segment of the facial nerve if the approach requires inferior and anterior exposure (e.g., to the jugular bulb). In addition, the posterior belly of the digastric muscle and its groove may be used to infer the position of the vertical segment of the sigmoid sinus (Fig. 3-2B). In many cases, the posterior aspect of the mastoid process presents an opening: the mastoid emissary foramen. When present, the mastoid emissary foramen is located 3.5 cm posterior to the center of the external acoustic meatus and 1.5 cm inferior to the temporal line. The mastoid emissary foramen is used by the mastoid emissary vein, which drains to the sigmoid sinus. Early identification of this emissary vein is critical because it may cause substantial bleeding (and be a source for air embolism) during the retrosigmoid craniectomy in some patients.

In the lateral view of the skull, the occipital bone attaches to the mastoid process through the occipitomastoid suture, and to the parietal bone through the lambdoid suture. In the same view, the temporal bone attaches to the parietal bone through the squamous suture (between the squamous part of the temporal bone and the parietal bone) and the parietomastoid suture (between the mastoid process and the parietal bone). The lambdoid, parietomastoid, and occipitomastoid sutures merge together to form the asterion. The asterion is located an average of 4.5 cm posterior to the external acoustic meatus and 1 cm below the temporal line. An easy rule to infer the location of the asterion during the skin incision is to project a line between the temporal line and the inion and intersect it with a line along the posterior edge of the mastoid process (see Fig. 3-2B, purple lines). When identified surgically, the asterion may be used to infer the posterior edge of the angle formed by the transverse and sigmoid sinuses. The asterion is also used to start the lateral suboccipital craniotomy. The occipitomastoid suture is typically used as the anterior boundary of the retrosigmoid craniotomy because it may be close to the posterior edge of the sigmoid sinus in many patients.

Understanding the surface of the petrous bone that forms the lateral wall of the posterior fossa (Fig. 3-2C and D) is essential to safely access the internal acoustic meatus during the intradural phase of a retrosigmoid approach (e.g., resection of the canalicular portion of a vestibular schwannoma). The sigmoid sulcus is an osseous depression carved by the sigmoid sinus, which runs approximately 5 to 15 mm anterior to the occipitomastoid suture. Anterior to the sigmoid sulcus, in the petrous bone, there is a narrow osseous depression impressed by the endolymphatic sac (see Fig. 3-2D). The endolymphatic sac is connected to the vestibular system via the vestibular aqueduct. In some individuals, the vestibular aqueduct may be larger than normal, which could be asymptomatic or a feature of Pendred's syndrome. The medial border of the endolymphatic sac may be used to infer the position of the common crus. Additionally, the osseous protuberance on the roof of the vestibular aqueduct may be used to set the surgical trajectory to the internal acoustic meatus because it lines up with the meatus when viewed under the microscope through the retrosigmoid approach. The internal acoustic meatus, located at the middle third of the petrous bone in its posterior fossa surface, is divided into a superior and an inferior space by the transverse crest (see Fig. 3-2C, lower left). The inferior space is used by the cochlear (anterior) and inferior vestibular (posterior) nerves. The superior division of the internal acoustic meatus is further divided by the vertical crest (also known as Bill's bar) into an anterior compartment, which contains the facial nerve, and a posterior compartment, which is used by the superior vestibular nerve. Between the internal acoustic meatus and the tentorium is the suprameatal tubercle, an osseous protuberance that may be drilled away during the retrosigmoid approach.

Posterior to the internal acoustic meatus and anterior to the vestibular aqueduct are the subarcuate fossa and foramen. The subarcuate foramen is located at the same coronal plane as the arcuate eminence (protuberance of the superior semicircular canal at the tegmen of the temporal bone) (see Fig. 3-2C). The subarcuate artery, which enters the foramen it is named after, runs through the center of the superior semicircular canal in the petrous bone. This artery, which nourishes the petrous bone and part of the semicircular canals, can be sacrificed during the retrosigmoid approach. The subarcuate artery is a distal branch of the AICA, which is the main artery encountered during the intradural phase of the retrosigmoid approach.

Surgical Anatomy

Positioning

The optimal patient positioning for the retrosigmoid approach is that which exposes the lesion in the center of the surgical corridor, uses gravity as means of cerebellar retraction, and entails minimal overall risk for the patient. Many positions have been described to prepare the patient for the retrosigmoid approach. The sitting and lateral decubitus positions have been the most widely used. Whereas the sitting position provides an anatomic view of the structures encountered throughout the approach and remains the simplest, it entails more risk for air embolism (especially if a large mastoid emissary vein is present), the surgical corridor depends on active cerebellar retraction, and it is less ergonomic to the surgeon.

The lateral decubitus position seems to overcome all these limitations and provide better surgical exposure for the majority of lesions approached through the retrosigmoid trajectory. In the lateral decubitus, the patient rests on the side contralateral to the lesion (lesion side up). An inverse Trendelenburg position is used to decrease venous congestion. The head is tilted to the ground and flexed so that the chin is two fingerwidths from the sternum. Head flexion brings the mastoid process away from the ipsilateral shoulder, which provides more room for the surgeon's hand. Finally, the head is turned to the side contralateral to the lesion to set the surgical target in line of sight of the retrosigmoid corridor, between the cerebellar hemisphere and the petrous bone. However, if the lesion requires exposure of the cerebellar flocculus and the foramen of Lushka, a sitting position may be more advantageous.

Skin Incision

Visualizing the venous sinuses and the asterion is essential to the correct design of the skin incision during a retrosigmoid approach. Three topographic (palpable) landmarks may guide the surgical incision: the inion, the tip and posterior edge of the mastoid process, and the zygomatic arch (see Fig. 3-2B). The zygomatic arch and its posterior projection (temporal line) are connected to the inion. The temporal line allows inferring the lower margin of the transverse sinus (posterior to the mastoid process) and the tegmen of the temporal bone (above the mastoid process). Then the tip of the mastoid process is identified and the posterior margin of the mastoid, which forms a vertical line, is palpated and used to infer the posterior margin of the sigmoid sinus. The intersection of the two lines approximates the asterion, which is used both to infer the transition between the transverse and sigmoid sinuses and to start the craniotomy. The typical lateral suboccipital craniotomy is 3 to 4 cm in diameter, is started immediately posterior to the sigmoid sinus, and includes the asterion.

A *C-shaped* skin incision is started 2 cm above the pinna, curved posteriorly to include the planned craniotomy area and stopped below the tip of the mastoid process, depending on the inferior extent of the surgical target (Fig. 3-2E). It is particularly important to include the margins of the planned craniotomy in the skin flap because it is difficult to retract the posterior lip of the incision posteriorly. The skin incision should be superficial to identify and preserve the lesser occipital nerve and the greater auricular nerves, running through the inferior and posterior borders of the skin incision over the sternocleidomastoid muscle. Preserving these nerves may reduce postoperative headache and dysesthesia, and they may serve as autologous neural grafts to repair cranial nerve damage.

Muscular Layer

The superficial myocutaneous flap, including the posterior auricular and sternocleidomastoid muscles, is elevated and reflected anteriorly toward the ear. The accessory nerve crosses the sternocleidomastoid muscle 5 cm below the mastoid tip, which allows safe manipulation of the muscle at this stage of the procedure. The posterior third of the temporalis muscle is spared along with its fascia and periosteum if no supratentorial access is needed. Upon retraction of the myocutaneous flap, the mastoid process is exposed. The longissimus capitis and digastric muscles are identified in the posterior aspect of the mastoid process, and the longissimus capitis muscle is reflected inferiorly. At this point, the occipital artery is exposed. The occipital artery takes off from the external carotid artery at the margin of the mandible and turns posteriorly under the posterior belly of the digastric muscle (see Fig. 3-2E). Then it turns upward and becomes superficial to the longissimus capitis and ascends to the scalp across the superior nuchal line. The main distal territory of the occipital artery is the scalp, which is very rich in anastomoses, a factor that favors safe ligation of the artery during a retrosigmoid approach. However, in some individuals the occipital artery gives rise to a large artery distally, which may be critical for nourishing the hypoglossal nerve extracranially. The superior nuchal muscular aponeurosis is incised and the nuchal muscles are reflected inferiorly and medially, leaving a muscle cuff for reapproximation. The superior oblique muscle and part of the inferior oblique muscle are exposed if access to the jugular bulb is required. Use of cautery may be limited around the suboccipital triangle because an aberrant loop of the vertebral artery may be at risk of inadvertent transection.

Craniotomy

A lateral suboccipital craniotomy and an additional posterior mastoidectomy maximize surgical exposure and minimize retraction during a retrosigmoid approach (Fig. 3-2F). This strategy provides extra space anterior to the craniotomy by exposing and collapsing the sigmoid sinus. The bone removal is started with a bur hole at the posterior edge of the transition from the transverse sinus to the sigmoid sinus (typically the asterion). The transverse sinus superiorly and the occipitomastoid suture anteriorly are the craniotomy boundaries. After removing the bone flap, the posterior mastoidectomy is started by drilling anteriorly over the temporal line until the entire width of the superior portion of the sigmoid sinus is revealed. The sigmoid sinus is completely exposed from the transverse junction to the jugular bulb. In most cases, a mastoid emissary vein may be encountered at the lateral aspect of the sigmoid sinus. Bleeding from the mastoid emissary vein can be managed with bone wax. Finally, an additional craniectomy at the inferior aspect of the craniotomy may be necessary to expose the foramen magnum and jugular foramen.

Dural Opening

There are two main designs for the dural incision: semicircular and cruciate. For the semicircular incision, a dural flap is raised in a semicircular fashion in the same orientation as the skin flap (see Fig. 3-2F). However, the cruciate incision, which bases two of its four facets on the transverse and sigmoid sinuses, allows for accessing the lateral supracerebellar space for lesions expanding toward the posterior incisural space. The dural flap is then retracted anteriorly with sutures until the sigmoid sinus is flattened to the mastoid process. Potential sources of bleeding at the dural incision are the distal meningeal branches of both the ascending pharyngeal and occipital arteries. Upon dural opening, the surgeon must be ready to evacuate cerebrospinal fluid (CSF)

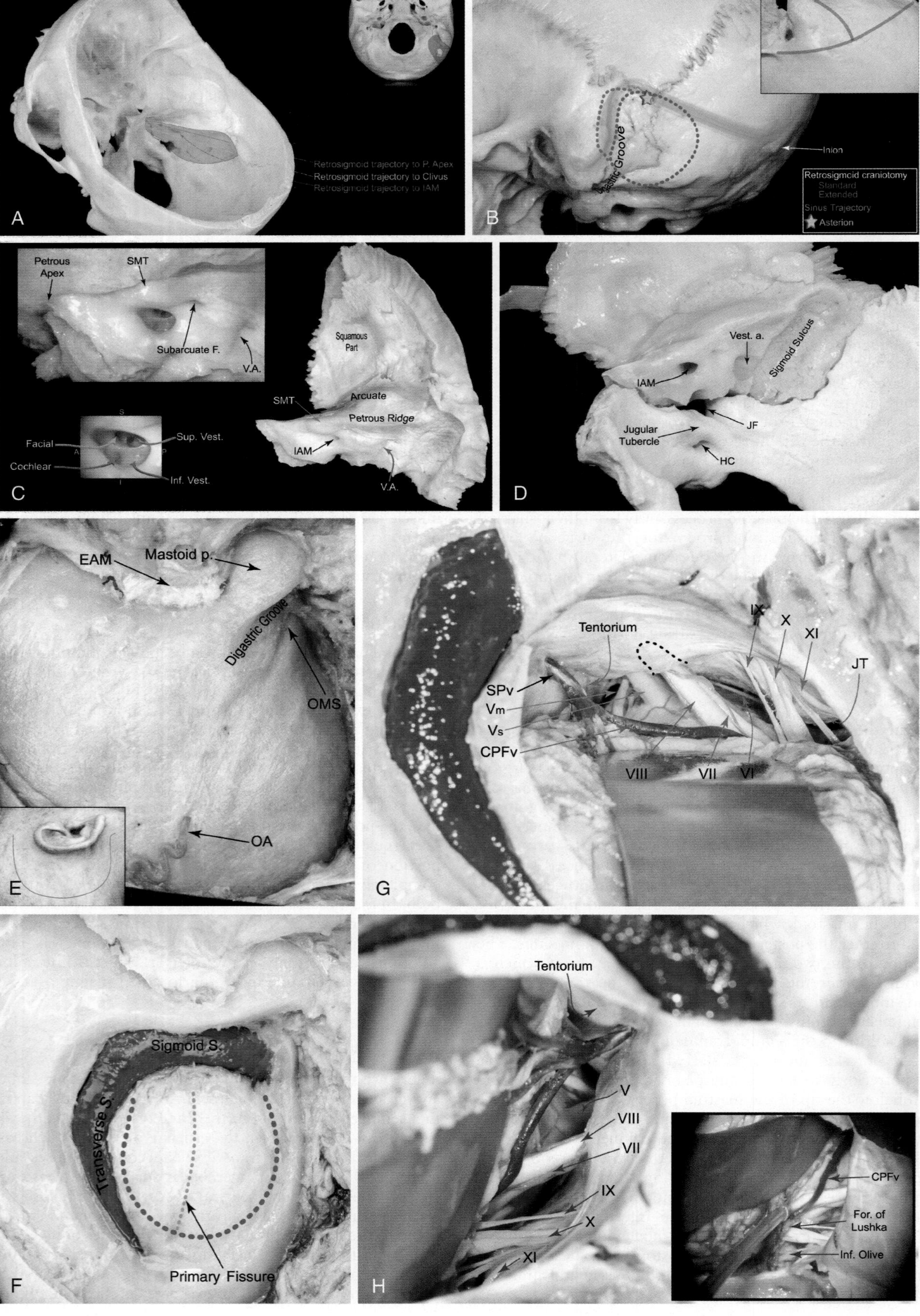
Retrosigmoid trajectory to P. Apex
Retrosigmoid trajectory to Clivus
Retrosigmoid trajectory to IAM
A
Digastric Groove
Inion
Retrosigmoid craniotomy
Standard
Extended
Sinus Trajectory
Asterion
B
Petrous Apex
SMT
Subarcuate F.
V.A.
Squamous Part
SMT
Arcuate
Petrous Ridge
IAM
V.A.
S
Facial
Sup. Vest.
Cochlear
Inf. Vest.
C
Vest. a.
Sigmoid Sulcus
IAM
JF
Jugular Tubercle
HC
D
EAM
Mastoid p.
Digastric Groove
OMS
OA
E
Tentorium
IX
X
XI
JT
SPv
Vm
Vs
CPFv
VIII
VII
VI
G
Sigmoid S.
Transverse S.
Primary Fissure
F
Tentorium
V
VIII
VII
IX
X
XI
CPFv
For. of Lushka
Inf. Olive
H

Figure 3-2. Bone anatomy and surgical landmarks relevant to the retrosigmoid approach. A, Surgical corridor of *(green areas)* and dissection trajectories available during *(lines)* the retrosigmoid approach; *yellow arrow* shows the line of view from the surgeon's perspective. IAM, internal acoustic meatus; P. Apex, petrous apex. **B,** Lateral suboccipital (classic) craniotomy *(green dotted circle)* and extended transmastoid retrosigmoid craniectomy *(red dotted line); star,* asterion. Venous flow through the transverse (horizontal portion) and sigmoid ("S" portion) sinuses is shown by the *blue line. Upper right,* Inferred location of the asterion during the skin incision *(purple lines).* **C,** *Right,* The internal acoustic meatus (IAM) is located at the middle third of the petrous bone in its posterior fossa surface, between the suprameatal tubercle (SMT) and the vestibular aqueduct (V.A.). *Upper left,* closeup view showing the relationship of the IAM to the SMT and the subarcuate foramen (Subarcuate F.). *Lower left,* Locations of the facial, superior vestibular (Sup. Vest.), cochlear, and inferior vestibular (Inf. Vest.) nerves. **D,** The jugular tubercle serves as both the roof of the hypoglossal canal (HC) and the floor of the jugular foramen (JF). IAM, internal acoustic meatus; Vest. a., vestibular aqueduct. **E,** C-shaped skin incision *(red line, lower left)* includes the planned craniotomy area and stops below the tip of the mastoid process (Mastoid p.). EAM, external acoustic meatus; OA, occipital artery; OMS, occipitomastoid suture. **F,** For the semicircular dural incision *(green dotted arc),* a dural flap is raised in a semicircular fashion in the same orientation as the skin flap. Bone removal is started at the posterior edge of the transition from the transverse sinus *(Transverse S.)* to the sigmoid sinus *(Sigmoid S.).* **G,** Dissection of the cerebellopontine cistern exposes the motor (Vm) and sensory (Vs) roots of cranial nerve V, as well as cranial nerves VI through XI, the cerebellopontine fissure vein (CPFv), the jugular tubercle (JT), and the superior petrosal vein (SPv, also called Dandy's vein). *Dotted line,* drilling area for accessing the internal acoustic canal. **H,** The cerebellomedullary cistern provides access to cranial nerves V, VII, VIII, and IX to XI. *Lower right,* The inferior olive (Inf. Olive) and the foramen of Lushka (For. of Lushka) are exposed near the cerebellopontine fissure vein (CPFv). *(Published with permission of the University of California San Francisco's Skull Base & Cerebrovascular Laboratory.)*

because the cerebellar hemisphere may protrude to the craniotomy. The safest and most efficient CSF drainage is obtained from opening the cisterna magna at the lowest margin of the craniotomy. Additional CSF drainage points may include the superior cerebellar and the cerebellopontine cisterns.

Intradural Anatomy

The retrosigmoid is an excellent approach to the majority of lesions of the cerebellopontine angle. Using a surgical corridor limited posteriorly by the petrosal surface of the cerebellum and anteriorly by the petrous bone, the retrosigmoid approach provides optimal exposure of the cerebellopontine and cerebellomedullary cisterns, and limited exposure of the inferior portion of the ambiens cistern and lateral aspect of both the prepontine and premedullary cisterns.

Thorough anatomic knowledge of the arachnoid cisterns allows the neurosurgeon to navigate the intracranial space safely and efficiently. Therefore, in this section the surgical anatomy of the intradural phase of the retrosigmoid approach is described according to the arachnoid cisterns to which it is related (outlined above). After CSF is evacuated, the cerebellar hemisphere is retracted medially, which creates a natural corridor. This natural corridor corresponds to the lateral aspect of the cerebellopontine cistern, where the arachnoid dissection is started. The cerebellopontine cistern is limited inferiorly by the lateral pontomedullary membrane, a thick arachnoid band that divides the subarachnoid space into the cerebellopontine cistern superiorly and the cerebellomedullary cistern inferiorly. The lateral pontomedullary membrane also divides the space between the vestibulocochlear and the glossopharyngeal nerves. Medially, the cerebellopontine cistern is limited by the prepontine cistern, which is medial to the cisternal segment of cranial nerve VI. Superiorly, the cerebellopontine cistern is limited by the ambiens cistern, which contains cranial nerve IV and the posterior cerebral artery. As arachnoid dissection progresses, the cerebellar hemisphere is then displaced posteriorly, which allows exposure of the facial-vestibulocochlear nerve (CN VII-VIII) bundle. The retrosigmoid approach provides a posterior trajectory to the CN VII-VIII bundle in which manipulation of the vestibulocochlear nerve is required to expose the facial nerve (Fig. 3-2G).

Some lesions, such as an intracanalicular extension of a vestibular schwannoma, require exposure of the internal acoustic meatus (also known as transcanalicular extension). In such instances, all available bone landmarks may be used to guide a safe and direct drilling of the posterior wall of the internal acoustic meatus. In brief, the osseous protuberance above the vestibular aqueduct is used to approximate the floor of the internal acoustic meatus, the medial border of the lymphatic sac serves as the surface landmark for the common crus, and the subarcuate artery points to the center of the superior semicircular canal. Upon exposure of the luminal aspect of the internal acoustic meatus, the superior and inferior vestibular nerves are exposed. Hearing preservation is one of the main advantages of the retrosigmoid approach. To preserve hearing, it is important to preserve the labyrinthine artery (branch of the AICA) and the cochlear nerve, as well as the vestibular apparatus, during the drilling of the petrous bone.

The AICA takes off from the inferior third of the basilar artery, near the abducens nerve. After a short distance in the prepontine and premedullary cisterns (anterior pontine segment), the AICA turns laterally toward the cerebellopontine angle (lateral pontine segment) to reach the internal acoustic meatus. In the lateral pontine segment, the AICA is further divided into premeatal, meatal, and postmeatal portions in relation to the internal acoustic meatus. At this segment, the AICA gives rise to the labyrinthine artery, which supplies the facial and vestibulocochlear nerves; the recurrent perforating arteries, which turn around and supply the brainstem; and the subarcuate artery (described above). The subarcuate artery is typically sacrificed during the transcanalicular approach because it anchors the AICA to the petrous bone, blocking access to the internal acoustic meatus through the retrosigmoid trajectory. In a small subgroup of individuals, the premeatal division of the AICA loops into the petrous bone (subarcuate segment), which requires skilled bone drilling to free it from its osseous ring. It is imperative to protect the labyrinthine artery to preserve hearing and facial motility, as well as the recurrent perforating arteries to prevent pontine ischemic strokes. The AICA continues its pathway toward the flocculus (flocculopeduncular segment) and ends at the petrosal surface of the cerebellum. In cases in which the PICA is absent, the AICA may also feed the suboccipital cerebellar surface (cortical segment). If the arachnoid dissection is continued superiorly, the trigeminal nerve is exposed. The postmeatal segment of the AICA inferiorly and the superior cerebellar artery superiorly can present tortuous pathways and be a potential cause for vascular compression of the trigeminal nerve. Additionally, the trigeminal nerve is surrounded by the superior petrosal venous plexus and vein. The superior petrosal vein drains venous blood from the lateral surface of the pons and the cerebellopontine fissure to the superior petrosal sinus. It is important to protect the superior petrosal vein from excessive coagulation and overtension caused by excessive cerebellar retraction because it is the main output of venous blood of the cerebellopontine angle. The suprameatal extension of the retrosigmoid approach may be used to increase exposure of the cisternal segment of the trigeminal nerve by removing the suprameatal tubercle. If arachnoid dissection is continued along the axis of the trigeminal nerve, Meckel's cave, the superior petrosal sinus, and the petrous apex can be explored. If the microscope is angled superiorly, the inferior aspect of the ambiens cistern can be explored as well. The ambiens segment of the cisternal segment of the trochlear nerve may be accessed in the middle incisural space at this point.

The cerebellomedullary cistern offers a working space limited superiorly by the pontomedullary membrane, medially by the premedullary cistern, and inferiorly by the foramen magnum (Fig. 3-2H). Wide exposure of the cerebellomedullary cistern requires an additional craniectomy to enlarge the lateral suboccipital craniotomy inferiorly and anteriorly. The jugular foramen and glossopharyngeal, vagus, and accessory nerves (CNs IX through XI) are in the center of the cerebellomedullary cistern. In the neural compartment of the jugular foramen, the glossopharyngeal nerve exits the intracranial space, separated from the vagus and accessory nerves by a dural septum. In some cases, the space between the rootlets of the glossopharyngeal and vagus nerves is used by the PICA as it transitions from the premedullary cistern (anterior medullary segment) to the cerebellomedullary cistern (lateral medullary segment). The accessory nerve can be followed inferiorly to the foramen magnum. If the microscope is angled inferiorly, the rootlets of the hypoglossal nerve and the inferior olive can be viewed through the windows existing between the medullary rootlets of the accessory nerve. The flocculus and foramen of Lushka remain in the cerebellar side of the approach and are typically obstructed by the retraction blade. However, gentle dynamic retraction of the cerebellar hemisphere at this level may expose the flocculus immediately lateral to the vestibulocochlear nerve and the foramen of Lushka between the vestibulocochlear and glossopharyngeal nerves.

Overall, the retrosigmoid approach provides wide access to both the cerebellopontine and cerebellomedullary cisterns. If the arachnoid space of both cisterns is completely dissected, the cisternal segments of the trigeminal nerve; the facial-vestibulocochlear nerve bundle; and the glossopharyngeal, vagus, and accessory nerves are optimally exposed. In situations in which the lesion distorts the normal anatomy of the cerebellopontine angle, the bone anatomy may guide the surgeon to identify the posterior fossa foramina because the hypoglossal canal, the jugular foramen, the internal acoustic meatus, and Meckel's cave are almost aligned. Furthermore, there are multiple neural corridors to structures or lesions medial to these nerves. The corridor between the ambiens segment of the trochlear nerve, the tentorium, and the trigeminal nerve may be used to access the middle incisural space, the petrous apex, and the superior aspect of the pons. The corridor between the trigeminal and vestibulocochlear nerves allows access to the inferior portion of Meckel's cave. The corridor between the vestibulocochlear and glossopharyngeal nerves (CN VIII-IX corridor) provides sufficient space to access the lower pons, the pontomedullary sulcus, the cisternal segment of the abducens nerve and its entrance into the dura, and the proximal segment of the AICA. Although the space between the glossopharyngeal and vagus nerves and the rootlets of the accessory nerve is very narrow in the normal brain, lesions that provoke mass effect may enlarge such spaces, converting them into useful corridors.

The use of the endoscope during the retrosigmoid approach provides the surgeon with an extraordinary advantage to navigate, identify, and manipulate beyond the cerebellopontine and cerebellomedullary cisterns. The endoscope brings light and point of view (lens) within a few millimeters of the surgical target. These unique features of endoscopic surgery allow an unobstructed, close view of structures situated deep within the surgical corridor. Furthermore, the use of angled lenses allows the surgeon to see structures outside the view of the microscope. During the retrosigmoid approach, the endoscope may be used to navigate beyond each neural corridor. If passed through the corridor above the trigeminal nerve, the quadrigeminal and ambiens segments of the cisternal segment of the trochlear nerve, as well as its entrance to the tentorium, can be explored. If the endoscope is navigated through the corridor between the trigeminal and vestibulocochlear nerves, the prepontine cistern and the lower aspect of the interpeduncular cistern may be explored, including the basilar trunk, proximal segment of the superior cerebellar artery, and transverse pontine vein. Navigating the endoscope through the CN VIII-IX corridor allows a direct view of the proximal segments of both the abducens nerve and the pontomedullary sulcus. It also provides an unobstructed view of the vertebrobasilar junction and the upper medulla in many cases. If the endoscope is angled inferiorly, the lower portion of the cerebellomedullary cistern can be explored. The cisternal segment of the hypoglossal nerve and the craniocervical transition of the spinal nerve at the foramen magnum may be explored as well. Additionally, if combined with appropriate positioning of the retraction blades, the foramen of Lushka may be completely exposed. The excellent features of the endoscope during a retrosigmoid approach are tempered by the risk inherent to the lack of visual control of the interaction between the endoscope rod and the surrounding anatomy, and the limited margin for maneuvering in the depth of the corridor, which may be insufficient to handle an arterial rupture.

THE TRANSPETROSAL APPROACHES

Surgical Targets

Thorough knowledge of the temporal bone anatomy is critical to performing the transpetrosal approaches safely and efficiently. Consequently, the anatomy of the temporal bone is reviewed in this section (Fig. 3-3A-C). In the surgical anatomy section below, landmarks relevant to transpetrosal approaches are discussed (Fig. 3-3D-H).

The approaches through the mastoid process and the petrous part of the temporal bone open a surgical route to the center of the skull and the anterolateral aspect of the brainstem. We categorize the surgical approaches through the mastoid process into three variations: retrolabyrinthine, translabyrinthine, and transcochlear (see Fig. 3-3D). Although each variation has its own surgical indications and characteristics, the transmastoid and transpetrosal dissections should be understood as a continuous progression in which each step provides an increase of skull base exposure, as well as gradual sacrifice in function. In brief, the retrolabyrinthine approach uses the window resulting from removing the bone between the sigmoid sinus (posteriorly) and the semicircular canals (anteriorly). The surgical access obtained through the retrolabyrinthine approach is limited to the anterior aspect of the cerebellar hemisphere, the cerebellopontine fissure, and the roots of the facial and vestibulocochlear nerves (CNs VII and VIII). As dissection progresses, the translabyrinthine approach removes the semicircular canals and vestibule to add access to the internal acoustic meatus and the canalicular segment of the facial and vestibulocochlear nerves, as well as the cisternal segment of the trigeminal nerve (CN V) and the posterior half of the incisural space. However, by opening the semicircular canals, the translabyrinthine approach sacrifices hearing. The transcochlear approach provides access to the petrous apex and lateral clivus and maximal access to the brainstem. However, drilling around the cochlea and farther anterior requires transposing the tympanic and mastoid portions of the facial nerve, which often adds facial palsy to hearing loss (from the translabyrinthine approach).

While the transmastoid and transpetrosal approaches are very effective in accessing both the internal acoustic meatus and the anterolateral aspect of the brainstem, they may work even better when combined with either a lateral suboccipital craniotomy (retrosigmoid or far lateral approaches) to gain access to the cerebellomedullary cistern and its contents, or a supratentorial craniotomy (temporal or extended pterional approach) to expose the incisural space and the supratentorial region around the dorsum sellae, petrous apex, or midbrain. Finally an extended supra- and infratentorial approach, which combines a far lateral approach, a temporal bone approach, and a supratentorial craniotomy, may be designed for well-selected lesions that require exposure from the dorsum sellae to the foramen magnum. Therefore, all the skull base surgical routes and corridors can be at any point integrated and combined so that a customized approach is designed for optimal treatment of each patient's lesion.

Bone Anatomy

The temporal is a remarkable bone because it plays a critical role in shaping the intracranial space, contains sensory function, and protects the transcranial segments of both the internal carotid artery and the facial nerve. The temporal bone shapes the intracranial space by providing most of the osseous floor and lateral wall of the middle fossa and the lateral wall of the posterior fossa, which is continued inferiorly by the occipital bone. It also protects the lateral and inferior surfaces of the temporal lobe of the brain and the lateral aspect of the pons and upper medulla. Another feature that makes the temporal a unique bone is that it forms the osseous structure for the vestibular and acoustic apparatus. The magnificent osseous design of the semicircular canals and vestibule is the essence of vestibular function. The shapes of the ossicles and the cochlea are fundamental to acoustic function. Moreover, the temporal bone serves as the osseous tunnel for both the petrous segment of the internal carotid artery and the canalicular, labyrinthine (also called petrous), and mastoid segments of the facial nerve.

The temporal bone is divided into squamous, petrous, tympanic, and mastoid parts (see Fig. 3-3A). The squamous part arises vertically from the temporal bone to join the parietal and sphenoid bones in the lateral aspect of the skull. At the extracranial surface, the squamous part serves as an attachment surface for the temporalis muscle. The attachment of the temporalis muscle shapes the superior temporal line in the lateral aspect of the skull, including the squamous part of the temporal bone. At the base of the extracranial aspect of the squamous part, the temporal bone projects anteriorly to form the zygomatic arch. The zygomatic arch is formed by the fusion of the zygomatic process of the temporal bone to the posterior process of the zygoma. The zygomatic process of the temporal bone is continued posteriorly by a linear bone elevation (temporal line) and the supramastoid crest (projecting posteriorly) (see Fig. 3-3C). The temporal line and supramastoid crest are reliable landmarks to infer the level of the tegmen of the temporal bone (also called the tegmen tympani) and the tentorium, which is essential to the design and extent of the craniotomy. At the root of the zygomatic process, the squamous part forms the roof of the mandibular fossa (anteriorly) and the superior aspect of the external acoustic meatus (posteriorly). Below the temporal line and posterior to the external acoustic meatus is the spine of Henle, an important landmark for inferring the location of the lateral semicircular canal during a mastoidectomy. The temporal line, external acoustic meatus, and spine of Henle may be connected to form the suprameatal triangle (also known as Macewen's triangle). Although not a real osseous shape, the suprameatal triangle may be used as a reliable landmark to infer the location of the mastoid antrum (the largest mastoid air cell). At the endocranial surface, the squamous part has a flat shape that relates to the temporal lobe of the brain in the intradural space. Inferiorly, the squamous part fuses with the petrous part, forming the lateral angle of the tegmen tympani.

The petrous part is the core of the temporal bone and contains the petrous segment of the internal carotid artery and the labyrinthine segment of the facial nerve (CN VII) and the acoustic and vestibular apparatuses. The petrous part of the temporal bone has a pyramidal shape with an apex, superior facet (i.e., the tegmen of the temporal bone), medial facet (i.e., the lateral wall of the posterior fossa), and inferior facet (i.e., extracranial surface). The superior facet of the petrous part is a relatively flat surface with an osseous protuberance, the arcuate eminence, at the center. In most cases, the arcuate eminence corresponds to the superior semicircular canal protruding to the tegmen of the temporal bone. Anterior to the arcuate eminence is a bone orifice that corresponds to the geniculate ganglion of the facial nerve. This osseous orifice is continued anteriorly as a furrow for the greater superficial petrosal nerve, which takes off at the geniculate ganglion and runs below the gasserian ganglion toward the pterygoid foramen at the base of the pterygoid plate. Using the greater superficial petrosal nerve as a reference, the anterior portion of the petrous bone can be further divided into a lateral compartment, which corresponds to the posterolateral (Glasscock's) triangle of the middle fossa, and a medial compartment, which corresponds to the posteromedial (Kawase's) triangle of the middle fossa. The posteromedial triangle is limited by the internal acoustic meatus and the cochlea posteriorly. The proximal aspect of the greater superficial petrosal nerve and, if visible, the geniculate ganglion may be used to infer the position of the cochlea, which sits approximately 5 mm medial to them. The anterior portion of the posteromedial triangle contains an osseous depression known as the trigeminal impression. Lateral and anterior to the trigeminal impression is the foramen lacerum, a space at the skull base between the petrous part of the temporal bone and the greater wing of the sphenoid bone. The foramen lacerum contains a fibrous and dense connective tissue band that serves as a base for the lacerum segment of the internal carotid artery as it transitions from the petrous bone to the cavernous sinus. The petrous apex is the most anterior part of the temporal bone, which attaches to the body of the sphenoid bone (at the clival part) through the petroclival (also called petro-sphenoidal) or Gruber's ligament. Gruber's ligament is a dense band of connective tissue that forms the roof of Dorello's canal, a narrow opening between the clivus and the petrous apex used by the abducens nerve to enter the cavernous sinus. Below Dorello's canal is the petroclival synchondrosis, which corresponds to the anterior edge of the medial facet of the petrous bone. The petroclival synchondrosis leaves a space used by the inferior petrosal sinus. At the petrous apex, the inferior petrosal sinus merges with the superior petrosal sinus (running at the edge of the petrous bone), the basilar sinus (draining the dura of the clivus), the cavernous sinus (draining the superficial sylvian vein, sphenoparietal sinus, ophthalmic veins, and vein of foramen ovale), and the circular sinus (draining the pituitary fossa) to form the sphenopetroclival venous gulf.

When viewed from in front, the petrous apex reveals very important relationships and structures (see Fig. 3-3B). Starting medially, the petrous canal of the internal carotid artery is the largest and most inferior cavity of the petrous bone. Interestingly,

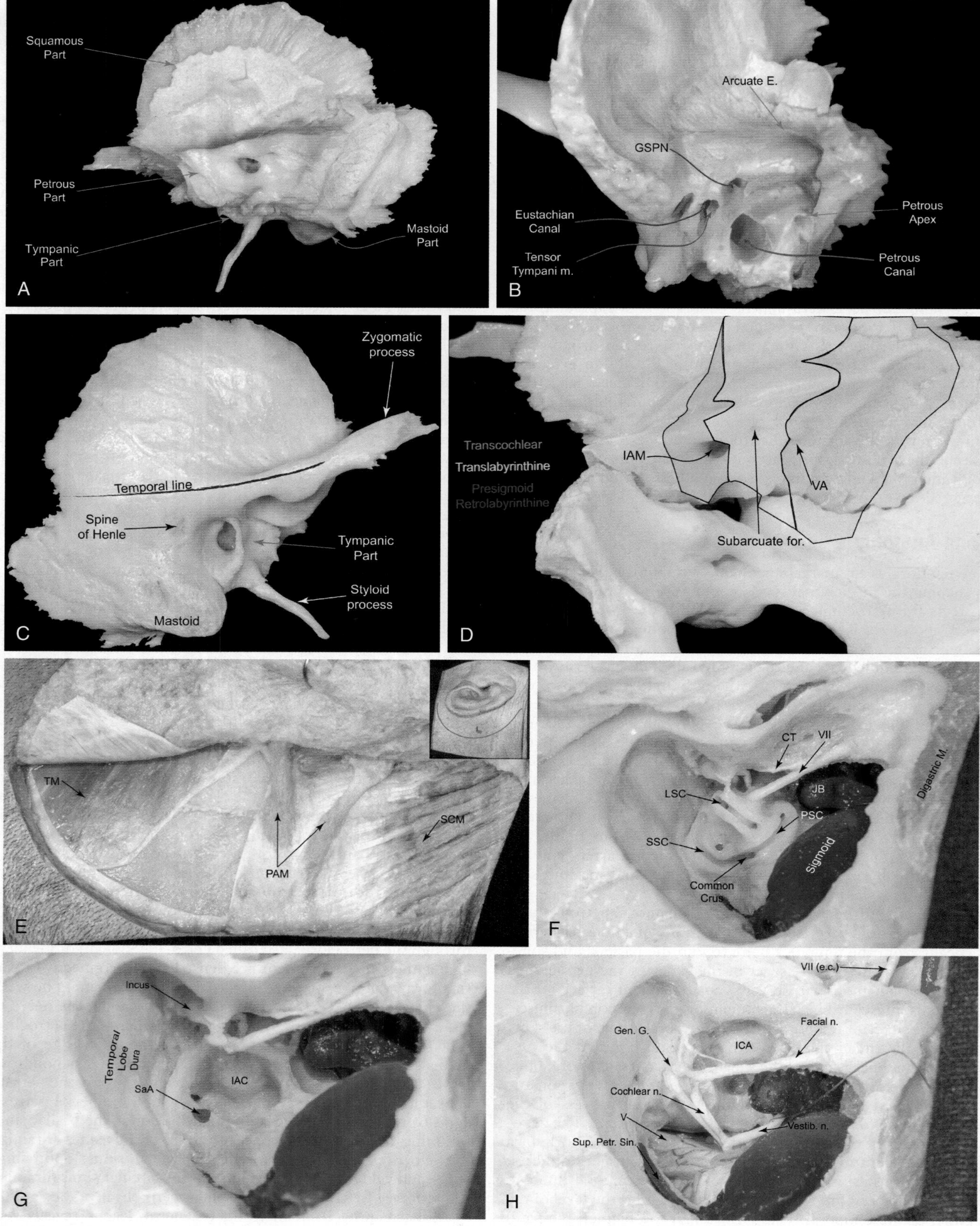

Squamous Part
Petrous Part
Tympanic Part
Mastoid Part
A
Arcuate E.
GSPN
Eustachian Canal
Tensor Tympani m.
Petrous Apex
Petrous Canal
B
Zygomatic process
Temporal line
Spine of Henle
Tympanic Part
Styloid process
Mastoid
C
Transcochlear
Translabyrinthine
Presigmoid
Retrolabyrinthine
IAM
VA
Subarcuate for.
D
TM
PAM
SCM
E
CT
VII
Digastric M.
LSC
JB
PSC
SSC
Sigmoid
Common Crus
F
Incus
Temporal Lobe Dura
SaA
IAC
G
VII (e.c.)
Gen. G.
Facial n.
ICA
Cochlear n.
V
Vestib. n.
Sup. Petr. Sin.
H

Figure 3-3. Bone anatomy and surgical landmarks relevant to the approaches through the temporal bone. A, The squamous, petrous, tympanic, and mastoid parts of the temporal bone. **B,** The petrous apex reveals very important relationships and structures, including the petrous canal, the eustachian canal, the arcuate eminence (Arcuate E.), the greater superficial petrosal nerve (GSPN), and the tensor muscle of the tympanic membrane (Tensor Tympani m.). **C,** The tympanic part of the temporal bone is the smallest, containing the zygomatic process and the temporal line (a linear bone elevation). The mastoid part contains the spine of Henle. **D,** Three surgical approaches through the mastoid process: transcochlear (green), translabyrinthine (yellow), and presigmoid/retrolabyrinthine (pink). IAM, internal acoustic meatus; Subarcuate for., subarcuate foramen; VA, vestibular aqueduct. **E,** The musculocutaneous flap contains part of the posterior third of the temporalis muscle (TM), the two bellies of the posterior auricular muscle (PAM), and the sternocleidomastoid muscle (SCM). *Upper right,* C-shaped skin incision *(red line)* for the transmastoid approaches; *yellow arrow* indicates the surgical trajectory. **F,** The retrolabyrinthine approach removes the mastoid part of the temporal bone, which contains the facial nerve (VII), sigmoid sinus, and jugular bulb (JB) and surrounds the lateral (LSC), posterior (PSC), and superior (SSC) semicircular canals. CT, chorda tympani; Digastric M., digastric muscle. **G,** The translabyrinthine approach removes the semicircular canals and vestibule to add access to the internal auditory canal (IAC) and the subarcuate artery (SaA). **H,** The transcochlear approach provides access to the petrous apex and lateral clivus and maximal access to the brainstem. Cochlear n., cochlear nerve; Gen. G., geniculate ganglion; ICA, internal carotid artery; Sup. Petr. Sin., superior petrosal sinus; VII (e.c.), cranial nerve VII, extracranial segment; Vestib. n., vestibular nerve. *(Published with permission of the University of California San Francisco's Skull Base & Cerebrovascular Laboratory.)*

the petrous segment of the internal carotid artery lies just below the groove formed by the greater superficial petrosal nerve, which may be used as guidance to the artery during any middle fossa approach and especially during the anterior petrosectomy. Lateral and deep to the groove of the greater superficial petrosal nerve is a tunnel with two compartments: the tensor tympani muscle medially and the osseous portion of the eustachian tube laterally. Both structures are revealed during an approach to the posterolateral (Glasscock's) triangle of the middle fossa. The medial facet of the petrous bone faces the lower mesencephalon, lateral aspect of the pons, and upper medulla at the cerebellopontine angle. It fuses to the clivus anteriorly and to the occipital bone inferiorly. It has an angulation such that the posterior fossa becomes wider posteriorly to accommodate the cerebellar hemispheres. The medial facet of the petrous part contains the internal acoustic meatus at the center and forms the jugular foramen together with the occipital bone. It contains numerous osseous features that have been described earlier in this chapter.

When the skull is viewed from below, the temporal bone sits between the occipital and sphenoid bones. The inferior portion of the petrous part provides most of the important structures that define the skull base and its surgical approaches. In a dry skull, the foramen lacerum becomes very obvious between the petrous apex and the posterior margin of the foramen ovale. Posterior to the foramina ovale and lacerum is the osseous portion of the eustachian tube, which is immediately lateral to the basilar part of the occipital bone. The eustachian tube has an angulation of 30 degrees from the midline and becomes progressively lateral from its origin at the nasopharynx toward the middle ear. The carotid canal is just posterior to the eustachian tube. The relationship between the eustachian tube and the carotid canal is critical when the posterior fossa is accessed from the endonasal corridor because the pharyngeal segment of the internal carotid artery may be inadvertently reached after lateral transposition or transection of the eustachian tube. The carotid canal is a few millimeters in front of the jugular foramen. An osseous ridge divides the carotid canal from the jugular foramen. A microscopic foramen at the center of this ridge (tympanic canaliculus) is used by the tympanic branch of the glossopharyngeal nerve to enter the temporal bone and reach the tympanic plexus. Also, at the lateral wall of the jugular foramen there is another microscopic foramen, the mastoid canaliculus, which is used by the auricular branch of the vagus nerve (CN X).

Lateral to both the carotid canal and jugular foramen is the tympanic part of the temporal bone, forming the posterior wall of the mandibular fossa. The styloid process arises medial to the tympanic part and lateral to the jugular foramen. At the medial aspect of the styloid process, the petrous, tympanic, and mastoid parts of the temporal bone merge. The stylomastoid foramen, which is the cranial opening for the facial nerve, can be found between the base of the styloid process and the mastoid part.

The osseous features on the surface of the petrous part of the temporal bone that have just been described may help orient the neurosurgeon accessing the floor of the middle fossa or the posterior fossa. However, thorough knowledge of the contents of the petrous part is essential to preserve function and safety when performing a transpetrosal approach. The petrous part contains the bony labyrinth, which gives shape to the cochlea, vestibule, and semicircular canals. Opening any portion of the bony labyrinth may cause hearing loss, which is one of the main risks related to using this bone as a surgical corridor. The internal acoustic meatus divides the labyrinth into anterior and posterior compartments in relation to the configuration of the nerves within the canal. The cochlear nerve runs below the facial nerve in the anterior half of the fundus of the internal acoustic meatus. Therefore, the cochlea sits anterior to the meatus in the depth of the tegmen of the temporal bone, where it receives the cochlear nerve. Also, the cochlea is medial and slightly posterior to the first genu of the internal carotid artery, where it turns horizontal after a short ascending portion. The vestibule is the central part of the labyrinth and serves as the confluence of all semicircular canals. The vestibule is located posterior to the cochlea, in line with the fundus of the internal acoustic meatus, superior to the jugular bulb, and medial to the lateral semicircular canal. All these relationships are very important during a translabyrinthine approach. The height of the jugular bulb determines the surgical corridor and final exposure of the internal acoustic meatus. If the bone removal is progressed anteriorly from the vestibule, the cochlea, anterior to it, will be exposed next. However, if the drilling is advanced medially, the fundus of the internal acoustic meatus is exposed. The posterior half of the internal acoustic meatus contains the vestibular nerves. Above the transverse crest, the superior vestibular nerve turns posterior at the fundus and innervates the superior and lateral semicircular canals. Below the transverse crest, the inferior vestibular nerve divides into the singular nerve, which innervates the posterior semicircular canal; the saccular nerve; and the utricular nerve.

There are three semicircular canals: lateral, superior, and posterior. The semicircular canals are located in the petrous part of the temporal bone, posterior to the internal acoustic meatus (and the vestibule) and surrounded by cancellous bone. The superior semicircular canal starts at the vestibule, loops superiorly to the tegmen of the temporal bone (sometimes shaping the arcuate eminence), and ends posteriorly at the common crus. The subarcuate artery is located in the middle of the superior semicircular canal and may be used as a landmark during a translabyrinthine approach. The posterior semicircular canal connects the vestibule and the common crus posteriorly, where it contacts the superior semicircular canal. The common crus, or confluence of the superior and posterior semicircular canals, sits lateral to the entrance of the subarcuate artery. The posterior semicircular canal is adjacent to the endolymphatic sac, which contacts its medial aspect before exiting the petrous bone through the vestibular aqueduct. Therefore, both the vestibular aqueduct and the endolymphatic sac may be used as landmarks to infer the position of the posterior semicircular canal during a posterior fossa approach. Finally, the lateral semicircular canal arises from the vestibule perpendicular to the surface of the mastoid, which puts it at risk during a general mastoidectomy. The lateral semicircular canal has a key relationship with the facial nerve, which runs medial and inferior to it. The facial nerve comes from the tympanic space—and segment—and turns inferiorly to become the mastoid segment exactly at the lateral semicircular canal. This relationship is widely used to ensure preservation of the facial nerve while cautiously drilling around this area.

The tympanic part of the temporal bone is the smallest and is important in shaping the tympanic cavity, forming the majority of the eustachian tube and the external acoustic meatus (see Fig. 3-3C). When the extracranial (lateral) aspect of the temporal bone is observed, the tympanic part can be identified forming the anterior, inferior, and part of the posterior walls of the external acoustic meatus. The anterior wall of the external acoustic meatus also serves as the posterior wall of the mandibular fossa, which is greatly shaped by the tympanic bone. The medial aspect of the tympanic part fuses to the petrous part through the petrotympanic suture. The anterior portion of the petrotympanic suture provides the opening through which the chorda tympani exits the temporal bone. Inferiorly, the tympanic part forms the base from which the styloid process projects inferiorly. The styloid process provides attachment to the stylopharyngeus, stylohyoid, and styloglossus muscles and also helps with surgical exposure of the stylomastoid foramen, posterior to it, where the facial nerve becomes extracranial. In some individuals, the styloid process is more than 3 cm long and may impinge on the carotid compartment of the pharynx, which may result in Eagle's syndrome.

The mastoid part of the temporal bone is a highly pneumatized bone that shapes the middle ear (mastoid cavity); contains the facial nerve, sigmoid sinus, and jugular bulb; and surrounds the semicircular canals (see Fig. 3-3C and F). The mastoid part is the inferior prolongation of the squamous part behind the ear, as well as the posterior projection of the petrous part up to the occipitomastoid suture. Extracranially, the mastoid part has a triangular shape with its apex pointing inferiorly close to the external acoustic meatus. It contains the spine of Henle, which forms Macewen's triangle together with the temporal line of the squamous part. It forms the upper two thirds of the posterior wall of the external acoustic meatus, which is completed inferiorly by the tympanic part. The mastoid part serves as an attachment for the sternocleidomastoid muscle, the splenius capitis muscle, the longissimus capitis muscle, and the posterior belly of the digastric muscle (from superficial to deep). The size of the extracranial aspect of the mastoid part is largely related to the size of the sternocleidomastoid and splenius capitis muscles and their traction during childhood, which are responsible for the variety of shapes and sizes of the mastoid process.

The most surgically relevant muscular relationship of the mastoid part is to the posterior belly of the digastric muscle and the groove it carves into the mastoid process. The digastric groove is a linear osseous furrow that the digastric muscle carves into the medial and posterior aspect of the mastoid. The surgical relevance of the digastric groove is that it points to the stylomastoid foramen and therefore to the exit of the facial nerve. Also, the anterior aspect of the posterior belly of the digastric muscle may be used to infer the course of the sigmoid sinus, inside the mastoid. After transitioning from the transverse sinus at the asterion, the sigmoid sinus turns inferiorly, along the posterior edge of the mastoid toward its base, where it enters the jugular foramen and forms the jugular bulb. The jugular bulb protrudes into the cancellous bone of the mastoid toward the vestibule. The facial nerve, which is reviewed later in this section, also transitions through the anterior aspect of the mastoid process. Understanding the mastoid process and its cavities is essential to a safe mastoidectomy, especially if hearing is to be preserved (retrolabyrinthine or transcrural approaches).

The mastoid antrum is the largest pneumatized mastoid cell. It is located beyond Macewen's triangle and is easily exposed during the first stages of a mastoidectomy (see Fig. 3-3F). The mastoid antrum is slightly posterior and superior to the mastoid segment of the facial nerve. In its anterior wall, the mastoid antrum connects to the tegmen tympani (roof of the middle ear) through a narrow opening called an aditus. The epitympanum (also called the epitympanic space) forms the superior and posterior walls of the middle ear and contains the head of the malleus and the body of the incus. At the epitympanum, the bone around the incus forms a larger air cell known as the fossa incudis, which is of surgical relevance during the translabyrinthine approach. The anterior wall of the middle ear is formed by the eustachian tube and the tensor tympani muscle and its tendon, which attaches to the handle of the malleus. Also, a thin bony lamina separates the anterior wall of the middle ear from the internal carotid artery as it transitions from the pharyngeal to the petrous segment (first genu). The lateral wall of the middle ear is formed by the tympanic membrane and the chorda tympani. The floor of the middle ear is formed by the temporal part of the jugular foramen. Therefore, if surgically opened, the floor of the middle ear provides access to the jugular bulb and the neural compartment of the jugular foramen. The posterior wall of the middle ear contains the anterior portion of the lateral semicircular canal, which is in close contact with the facial nerve, and the mastoid antrum aditus superiorly. The medial wall of the middle ear contains the promontory, the oval and round windows, and the vestibular apparatus. The tympanic nerve plexus protrudes over the promontory in the middle ear. The center of the middle ear is occupied by the ossicular chain, which facilitates mechanical transmission from the vibrations of the tympanic membrane to the oval window. The ossicles are, from the tympanic membrane to the oval window, the malleus (Latin for *hammer*), the incus (Latin for *anvil*), and the stapes (Latin for *stirrup*). Each ossicle has several stabilizing ligaments that radiate from the ossicle's surface to the middle ear walls. There are two important muscles that control the tension of the ossicular chain and therefore modulate its mechanical behavior as part of the acoustic (tympanic) reflex: the tensor tympani and the stapedius muscles. The tensor tympani muscle travels parallel to the eustachian tube in the petrous bone and anchors to the lower aspect of the malleus. The tensor tympani is innervated by the medial pterygoid nerve (a branch of the mandibular nerve, the third division of the trigeminal nerve [V3]) and reacts to peaks of loud sound diminishing the mechanical transmission from the tympanic membrane to the cochlea. The stapedius muscle attaches to the stapes in the posterior wall of the middle ear. The stapedius is the smallest muscle in the body and modulates the transmission between the stapes and the oval window; it is innervated by the facial nerve.

The facial nerve is the most relevant structure in the mastoid process and one of the most important causes of iatrogenic injury during any transmastoid approach. Preservation of the facial nerve requires thorough knowledge of both its trajectory and the different key anatomic relationships in each of its segments. Because the course of the facial nerve is complex and its anatomic relationships are multiple, it is very advantageous to subdivide its path into several segments and study them thoroughly. The facial nerve is grossly divided into two main portions: the intracranial (from its exit at the brainstem until the stylomastoid foramen) and the extracranial (from the stylomastoid foramen until the facial muscles). These two portions have different segments, which correspond to different anatomic spaces.

The facial nerve exits the brainstem at the lateral margin of the pontomedullary sulcus. It courses through the cerebellopontine cistern medial to the vestibulocochlear nerve (CN VIII) in the cerebellopontine angle (cisternal segment). In the cisternal segment, the facial nerve is in contact with the AICA and the labyrinthine artery (also called the internal auditory artery) and the cerebellopontine fissure vein. The facial nerve enters the internal acoustic meatus medial to the vestibulocochlear nerve and pierces the fundus of the canal superior to the transverse crest and anterior to Bill's bar (canalicular segment). In the canalicular segment, the facial nerve is easily identified through the middle fossa approach, whereas its exposure requires mobilizing the superior vestibular nerve when approached through the translabyrinthine approach. The facial nerve pierces the fundus of the acoustic canal in the petrous part of the temporal bone, surrounded by the labyrinth, and forms the geniculate ganglion (labyrinthine segment). The geniculate ganglion serves as the main parasympathetic output of the facial nerve, which gives rise to the greater superficial petrosal nerve (anteriorly), the lesser superficial petrosal nerve (inferiorly), and a branch of the tympanic plexus (inferiorly and posteriorly). After its labyrinthine segment, the facial nerve turns posterior and lateral and runs for a short distance through the middle ear (tympanic segment). Within the tympanic segment, the facial nerve runs below the anterior margin of the lateral semicircular canal (of surgical relevance during the translabyrinthine approach) and posterior to the stapes and oval window, where the stapedius nerve takes off. Finally, the facial nerve turns inferiorly for a vertical course through the mastoid process (mastoid segment). Within the mastoid process, the facial nerve is covered by the fallopian canal, a solid osseous canal that contains the facial nerve and its feeding arteries. Before exiting the skull through the stylomastoid foramen, the facial nerve gives rise to the chorda tympani (Latin for *tympanic string*, for its relationship with the tympanic membrane in the tympanic space). The chorda tympani, a small but very important branch of the facial nerve, exits at the inferior third of the fallopian canal and runs anteriorly and superiorly to the center of the middle ear, where it runs in contact with the body of the incus, the handle of the malleus, and the inner and superior aspect of the tympanic membrane (see Fig. 3-3H). It then exits the middle ear through the petrotympanic suture to merge with the lingual nerve (a branch of the mandibular nerve, V3) until its final destination in the anterior two thirds of the tongue.

In the extracranial portion, the facial nerve is in close proximity to the styloid process and the posterior belly of the digastric muscle (digastric or paravertebral segment). After a short, straight paravertebral segment, the facial nerve pierces the parotid gland and splits into two trunks, superior and inferior (parotid segment). The superior trunk runs above the anterior third of the zygomatic arch and the body of the zygoma and splits into the temporal branches, which supply the frontalis, orbicularis oculi, and corrugator supercilii muscles; the zygomatic branches, which supply the lateral margin of the orbicularis oculi and merge with the temporal branches; and the buccal branches, which innervate the buccinator and orbicularis oris muscles. The inferior trunk gives rise to the marginal mandibular nerve, which supplies the muscles at the angle of the mouth and at the lips and the mentalis muscle, and the cervical branch, which primarily supplies the platysma.

Surgical Anatomy

Positioning

Positioning the patient for a transmastoid transpetrosal approach is fairly straightforward. The angle of the patient's head should allow access to Trautmann's triangle for the presigmoid and transcrural approach; the internal acoustic meatus for the translabyrinthine approach; and the prepontine and premedullary cisterns and lateral pons for the complete petrosectomy (transcochlear approach). To achieve the required trajectories and provide a comfortable, ergonomic positioning of the surgeon, the patient is set in a lateral position, with the head slightly flexed and the nose either in a neutral position or slightly to the ipsilateral side to set the surface of the mastoid process perpendicular to the surgeon's line of sight. Although simple, positioning for a transmastoid approach is very important because this approach requires prolonged drilling, which becomes more complex and requires more skill and precision toward the end of the bone removal. Good drilling skills and optimal positioning of the patient, including adjusting the operating table, are two of the most important factors to increase safety and efficiency in the more complex phases of the transpetrous approach at the end of the procedure.

Skin Incision

The skin incision for the transmastoid approaches is a "C" shape extending from above the vertex of the pinna to at least 1 cm below the pinna at the belly of the sternocleidomastoid muscle. The superior extension of the skin incision may be customized depending on the location of the target. If the internal acoustic canal is the final target, a C-shaped skin incision with its superior extension around the pinna may be optimal. If the lesion has both supra- and infratentorial components, and a combined supra-infratentorial approach is considered, the superior aspect of the skin incision may be extended 2 cm above the pinna to expose the squamous part of the temporal bone superiorly.

Muscular Layer

The musculocutaneous flap contains part of the posterior third of the temporalis muscle, the posterior auricular muscle, and the sternocleidomastoid muscle, which are reflected en bloc anteriorly toward the ear (see Fig. 3-3E). After exposing the bone of the lateral surface of the mastoid process, the splenius and longissimus capitis muscles are reflected inferiorly with care to protect the occipital artery, which loops around the longissimus capitis muscle. At this time, the posterior belly of the digastric muscle and the posterior edge of the mastoid process become accessible.

Craniectomy

Drilling the mastoid process is much like paleontology, where revealing the important structures requires meticulous study of the ground and constant and judicious inference of the location of the target beyond the field. Safely exposing the critical structures of the mastoid process (sigmoid sinus) and the petrous bone (vestibular apparatus, facial and vestibulocochlear nerves, and internal carotid artery) requires understanding changes in bone consistency and color, as well as constant anticipation of critical structures using landmarks exposed in earlier steps.

When the surface of the mastoid process and squamous part of the temporal bone are exposed, the surgeon should use all landmarks available to locate the position of the critical structures to be preserved during the mastoidectomy: the transverse and sigmoid sinuses; the tegmen of the temporal bone, which corresponds to the tentorium and the level of the supratentorial space; and the lateral semicircular canal, which is the first canal exposed through this approach. Several landmarks are very valuable to infer the position of the sinuses. The superior nuchal line, which may be identified surgically at the insertion of the trapezius muscle or by projecting the main axis of the zygomatic arch to the inion, may be used to infer the base of the transverse sinus. The asterion may also be used to infer the transition between the transverse and the sigmoid sinuses. Also, a presigmoid point, located at the convergence between the squamous and parietomastoid sutures, may be used to infer the anterior aspect of the transverse sinus–to–sigmoid sinus transition, which will correspond to the sinodural (Citelli's) angle later in the approach. Finally, the location of the sigmoid sinus in the mastoid process can be inferred by following the most anterior aspect of the posterior belly of the digastric muscle. The temporal line and its posterior projection (the supramastoid crest) may be easily identified at this point to infer the tegmen of the temporal bone and therefore design the supratentorial extent of the bone opening.

The mastoidectomy is started by drilling the cortical bone layer of the mastoid process. In some cases, the dense cortical bone layer may be raised as a bone flap for closure, especially if the surgical approach is limited to the mastoid process. The cancellous mastoid bone should be drilled evenly throughout the field. This technique serves two purposes: to reveal as many surface landmarks as possible and to prevent inadvertent drilling into the sinuses, the facial nerve, or the semicircular canals. The limits of the mastoidectomy are the posterior wall of the external acoustic meatus and spine of Henle, the sigmoid sinus, and the supramastoid crest (if the approach is intended to be only infratentorial). The first relevant structure (most superficial) that will be revealed is the sigmoid sinus, because the cancellous bone over the anterior aspect of the digastric muscle turns bluish and dense. As the mastoidectomy progresses medially, the spine of Henle and Macewen's triangle are used as reference to infer the position of the lateral semicircular canal (posterior—deep—to the spine of Henle and the mastoid antrum, deep to Macewen's triangle). While the lateral semicircular canal (and the whole labyrinth) are typically anticipated by sensing the transition from cancellous to hard bone, cases exist in which there is a septum of hard bone superficial to the lateral semicircular canal, which can lead to disorientation. This Körner's septum, typically found at the level of the lateral edge of the sigmoid sinus, is part of the squamopetrosal suture (dense thick bone) transitioning into the mastoid process and should be drilled away en route to the lateral semicircular canal. While drilling around the bony labyrinth, cancellous mastoid bone becomes hard petrous bone. At this point, the spine of Henle could be used to infer the position of the lateral semicircular canal, which becomes evident if the blue line (the lumen of the lateral semicircular canal seen through a fine translucent layer of bone) is exposed. The blue line or the bony labyrinth is the deepest limit of the presigmoid, retrolabyrinthine approach.

To finish the retrolabyrinthine approach, Trautmann's triangle must be widely exposed, which requires extending the mastoidectomy posterior to the mastoid portion of the facial nerve and the bony labyrinth. The mastoid segment of the facial nerve may be safely exposed using two landmarks: the lateral semicircular canal and the digastric groove (see Fig. 3-3F). If the blue line of the lateral semicircular canal is exposed, the facial nerve may be exposed entering the fallopian canal perpendicular to the canal and inferior to it. Also the digastric groove, in the depth of the digastric muscle, may be followed anteriorly and medially to expose the extracranial part of the facial nerve at the stylomastoid foramen. The space posterior to the facial nerve is the retrofacial recess, which contains the endolymphatic sac (toward the sigmoid sinus) and the jugular tubercle (deep to the facial nerve). The endolymphatic sac is relevant to the labyrinth and acoustic function. The endolymphatic sac comes in many shapes and sizes, and, if very large, may be related to a genetic condition known as Pendred's syndrome. Efficient identification and anticipation of the location of the endolymphatic sac is achieved by projecting a line from the blue line of lateral semicircular canal to the sigmoid sinus and by widely opening the retrofacial recess. To complete the retrolabyrinthine exposure, Trautmann's triangle is widened superiorly by exposing the sinodural angle, between the temporal lobe dura and the superior portion of the sigmoid sinus, and drilling the tegmen of the temporal bone superior to the blue line of the superior semicircular canal until the superior petrosal sinus is reached. The retrolabyrinthine approach may be expanded anteriorly by drilling the common crus (confluence between the posterior and superior semicircular canals), which may increase the working window to the lateral aspect of the pons and the incisural space. While respecting the integrity of the semicircular canals is key to preserve auditory function, it is very important to know their location and shape as seen through the transmastoid approach in order to maximize the surgical corridor and freedom of maneuverability during the retrolabyrinthine approach.

After completing the retrolabyrinthine approach, the translabyrinthine (posterior transpetrosal) approach may begin (see Fig. 3-3G). The translabyrinthine approach provides optimal exposure of the posterior half of the internal acoustic meatus, the middle ear, and the epitympanum and their respective contents at a remarkable cost: ipsilateral hearing loss. Exposing the lumen of the semicircular canals (opening all three blue lines) is advantageous at this point because they provide orientation and landmarks for exposing the posterior wall of the internal acoustic meatus and adjacent structures. Drilling into the body of the superior semicircular canal (from its lumen toward the lateral semicircular canal) exposes the subarcuate artery, which might be used to infer the roof of the internal acoustic meatus in the depth of the canal. However, the most accurate way to anticipate the location of the roof of the internal acoustic meatus through this surgical route is by projecting a line from the ampulla of the superior semicircular canal (at the anterior end of the canal) to the sinodural (Citelli's) angle. Drilling the semicircular canals exposes the vestibule (in the center) and the ampulla of the posterior semicircular canal inferiorly (see Fig. 3-3G). The ampulla of the posterior semicircular canal may be used to infer the level of the floor of the internal acoustic canal. Drilling through the vestibule will allow access to the posterior wall of the internal acoustic canal, from its fundus to its foramen.

Opening the dura of the meatus must be done carefully because the course of the labyrinthine artery (also called the internal auditory artery) is variable and sometimes adjacent to the dura at this level. The superior and inferior vestibular nerves are encountered first, divided by the transverse crest. If the bone removal is continued inferior to the floor of the internal acoustic meatus, within the retrofacial recess, the jugular bulb is exposed. The height of the jugular bulb is somewhat variable and its size and geometry greatly impact the final surgical corridor obtained through the translabyrinthine approach. In individuals with short, small jugular bulbs, the surgical access to the cerebellomedullary cistern is greater, which sometimes allows exposure of the glossopharyngeal nerve. This exposure can be maximized by transposing the facial nerve anteriorly. If the superior vestibular nerve is detached and transposed posteriorly, the vertical crest (also called Bill's bar) is exposed. If Bill's bar is removed, the labyrinthine segment of the facial nerve is revealed. Exposing the tympanic segment of the facial nerve requires exploring the middle ear and epitympanum. To optimally explore the middle ear through the translabyrinthine approach, the posterior wall of the external acoustic meatus may be removed (a technique known as *wall-down*). The incus is the first bone observed, with its body protruding into the mastoid antrum above the external acoustic meatus (fossa incudis). Below the incus and posterior to the tympanic membrane is the stapes. A few millimeters below the stapes, in the fallopian canal, the chorda tympani enters the bone for a short path toward the tympanic membrane. Exposing the chorda tympani requires a very advanced drilling technique, which consists of using a microscopic diamond bur and drilling superficially (movement similar to that of shaving) starting lateral, then posterior, and finally anterior to the chorda tympani until it is completely exposed.

Once the chorda tympani is freed, the facial nerve can be fully transposed anteriorly toward the middle ear or posteriorly toward the sigmoid sinus to maximize access to the cochlea and the petrous bone medial to the internal carotid artery. If the tympanic membrane is sectioned across the external acoustic meatus, the malleus may be completely exposed, as well as the promontory of the cochlea. The tympanic or Jacobson's nerve (a branch of the glossopharyngeal nerve [CN IX]) forms a plexus (tympanic plexus) at the surface of the promontory. Medial to the tympanic membrane in the depth of the operative field, the eustachian canal and the tensor tympani become visible. At this point, the transcochlear (also called transotic) approach can begin (see Fig. 3-3H). Drilling the promontory exposes the cochlea. If the drilling is angled medially to the cochlea, the fibers of the cochlear nerve are exposed entering the modiolus, which is further limited superiorly by the transverse crest. Transposing the facial nerve anteriorly allows completion of the transcochlear approach anteriorly, which requires removing the cochlea, exposing the first (petrous) genu of the internal carotid artery, and continuing the anterior petrosectomy medial to it.

Dural Opening

The dura can be opened in many ways and in different sizes according to the progression of the drilling (retrolabyrinthine, translabyrinthine, transcochlear). It is key to preserve the integrity of the dura until the drilling is completed, to limit the bone dust entering the cisternal space, and to prevent injury to the facial and vestibulocochlear nerves (CNs VII and VIII), the AICA, and the labyrinthine artery. The basic dural opening is based on Trautmann's triangle and can be progressively expanded to the dura over the suprameatal tubercle, the internal acoustic meatus, and the petrous apex. Superiorly, the dural opening can be extended to the supratentorial space by dividing the superior petrosal sinus along the tentorium, and also by opening the dura of the temporal lobe.

Intradural Anatomy

Like the retrosigmoid approach, the transpetrosal approaches use a trajectory tangential to the anterior aspect of the cerebellar hemisphere. In all the presigmoid approaches, the lateral, superior, and posterior aspects of the cerebellar hemisphere are not exposed. As the bone removal progresses, access to the cerebellopontine and prepontine cisterns is widened, providing a workable window between the facial and trigeminal nerves (CNs VII and V) parallel to the petrous apex, which may be used to access the abducens nerve (CN VI) (see Fig. 3-3H). While advancing within the arachnoid cisterns, the AICA may be found looping between the facial and vestibulocochlear nerves and the lateral trunk of the superior cerebellar artery above the trigeminal nerve. After the transcochlear approach, the intracranial portion of the facial nerve is completely exposed, including the geniculate ganglion, the stapedial nerve, and the chorda tympani. The glossopharyngeal nerve may be also exposed both in the cerebellomedullary cistern and in the neural part of the jugular foramen (if the jugular bulb is small or retracted inferiorly).

THE ORBITOZYGOMATIC APPROACH

Surgical Targets

One of the main features of the pterional approach and its variants is that all cranial fossae may be accessed through one craniotomy. With excellent exposure of the lateral aspect of the sphenoid bone, the pterional approach allows direct exposure of the cavernous sinus, pituitary fossa, petroclival region, middle fossa, and sphenoid ridge and planum. Also, the lateral surface of the frontal, temporal, parietal, and insular lobes may be exposed through a pterional approach, which exposes the sylvian fissure at the center of the surgical field. The pterional approach is a workhorse for cerebrovascular surgery too, because it provides continued longitudinal access to the entire middle cerebral artery, basilar apex, and posterior cerebral artery, and to the internal carotid artery from its petrous to its intradural segment. The maximal surgical access to the intracranial space is accomplished by adding an orbitozygomatic osteotomy to the pterional approach (orbitozygomatic approach). The orbitozygomatic approach allows reflecting the temporalis muscle lower than the pterional approach, and also allows a steep angle of attack along the base of the middle fossa and the roof of the orbit to the basal surface of the brain.

In this section the surgical anatomy of the sphenoid bone, pituitary fossa, and cavernous sinus is discussed in the context of the orbitozygomatic approach.

Bone Anatomy

The lateral surface of the skull is formed by the frontal, parietal, temporal, sphenoid, and zygomatic bones (Fig. 3-4A). The frontal bone attaches posteriorly to the parietal bone through the coronal suture. Inferiorly, the frontal bone attaches to the greater wing of the sphenoid bone through the frontosphenoid suture and to the frontal process of the zygomatic bone through the frontozygomatic suture. The frontosphenoid suture may be used to infer the position of the sylvian fissure, which at this level relates to the pars orbitalis and orbitofrontal cortex superiorly and the temporal pole inferiorly. The frontosphenoid suture is also very relevant for the correct placement of McCarty's keyhole, which may be started over the anterior portion of this suture (Fig. 3-4B). Anteriorly, the frontal bone attaches to the frontal process of the zygomatic bone through the frontozygomatic suture and forms the orbital rim. The posterior edge of the zygomatic process of the frontal bone serves as the attachment surface for the anterior portion of the temporalis muscle. The traction force caused by the tendon of the temporalis muscle forms the superior temporal line, which is used to place Dandy's (pterional) keyhole. The frontozygomatic suture is typically identified during an orbitozygomatic approach and may be used to infer the correct placement of McCarty's keyhole, approximately 1 cm posterior to it (1 ± 0.4 cm), over the frontosphenoid suture. Medially, the anterior (orbital) part of the frontal bone contains the supraorbital foramen, which anchors the supraorbital neurovascular bundle. However, in some individuals, the supraorbital foramen may be only a notch, which eases the detachment of the periorbita without damaging the supraorbital nerve and artery. The frontal sinus sits above the orbital rim, and its volume and shape are very variable.

The parietal bone covers the posterior portion of the frontal lobe (precentral gyrus and premotor cortex) and the parietal lobe (superior and inferior parietal lobules).

The parts of the temporal bone relevant to the anterolateral skull base approaches are the squamous (extracranially) and petrous (intracranially) (Fig. 3-4C). The squamous part of the temporal bone attaches anteriorly to the greater wing of the sphenoid bone through the sphenosquamous suture and superiorly to the parietal bone through the squamous suture. It contains the superior and middle temporal gyri, as well as part of the inferior temporal gyrus. The squamous suture, and specifically its horizontal segment, may be used as a landmark to infer the level of the sylvian fissure. The temporal bone has a lateral protrusion, the zygotic process, that attaches to the temporal process of the zygoma through the temporozygomatic suture. Together, the temporal and zygomatic bones form the zygomatic arch, which contains the temporalis muscle.

The body of the zygoma is a flat, square surface that gives shape to the malar eminence of the face. The zygomaticofacial foramen is located at the center of the body of the zygoma and is the natural passage for the zygomaticofacial nerves, distal branches of the maxillary division of the trigeminal nerve (V2) that provide the neurovascular bundle responsible for sensation over the cheek. Three processes arise from the body of the zygoma: temporal, frontal, and maxillary. The maxillary process forms the lower margin of the orbit and attaches to the orbital process of the maxillary bone. The infraorbital foramen, at the zygomaticomaxillary suture, is the natural opening for the infraorbital nerve (a branch of V2). The temporal process emerges posteriorly to form the zygomatic arch with the temporal bone. The superior trunk and distal branches of the facial nerve run over the lateral (superficial) surface of the temporal process of the zygoma (anterior two thirds of the zygomatic arch). The frontal process attaches to the frontal bone through the frontozygomatic suture at the orbital rim and to the greater wing of the sphenoid bone through a shallow bone lamina, which forms the anterior part of the lateral wall of the orbit. In the orbital cavity, the angle between the frontal and maxillary processes of the zygoma forms the anterior limit of the inferior orbital fissure, which continues posteriorly within the floor of the orbit between the greater wing of the sphenoid and the maxillary bones.

The sphenoid bone is not only the core of the skull base but also a structure with exquisite anatomic detail that may be used to navigate safely to the pituitary, middle, and posterior fossae. Extracranially, the sphenoid bone is related posteriorly to the

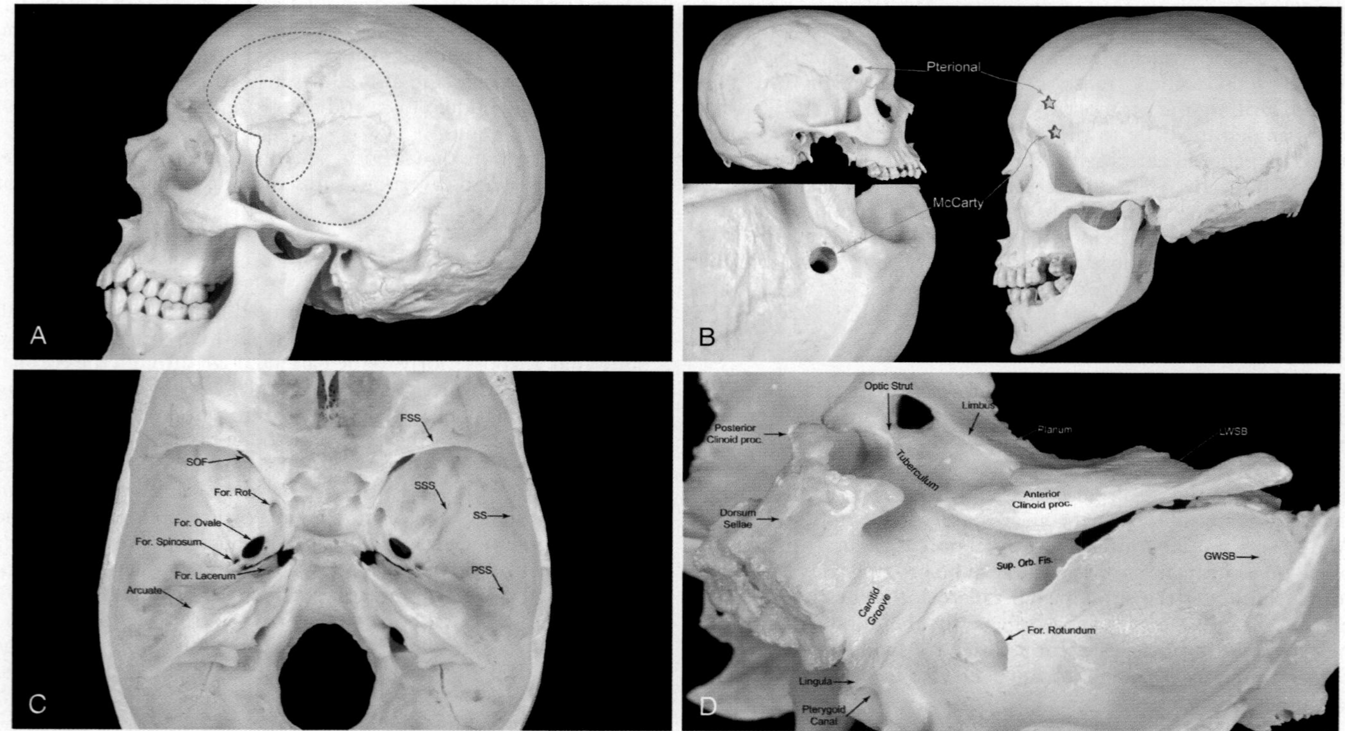

Figure 3-4. Bone anatomy and surgical landmarks relevant to the pterional and orbitozygomatic approaches. A, Locations on the lateral surface of the skull for the standard pterional craniotomy for middle fossa, cavernous sinus, pituitary fossa, posterior fossa, and anterior fossa access *(green dotted circle),*; and for the mini–pterional craniotomy for access to the sylvian fissure, sphenoid bone, and pituitary fossa *(red dotted circle).* **B,** Correct placement of pterional craniotomy *(upper star)* and of McCarty's keyhole *(lower star),* which may be started over the anterior portion of the frontosphenoid suture. **C,** The body of the sphenoid bone contains the pituitary fossa, the upper clivus, and the sphenoid sinus. For., foramen; For. Rot, foramen rotundum; FSS, frontosphenoid suture; PSS, petrosquamous suture; SOF, superior orbital fissure; SS, squamous suture; SSS, sphenosquamous suture. **D,** The anterior aspect of the pituitary fossa is formed by the limbus, which corresponds to the edge of the planum, the chiasmatic sulcus, and the tuberculum sellae. Anterior Clinoid proc., anterior clinoid process; For. rotundum, foramen rotundum; GWSB, greater wing of the sphenoid bone; LWSB, lesser wing of the sphenoid bone; Posterior Clinoid proc., posterior clinoid process; Sup. Orb. Fis., superior orbital fissure.

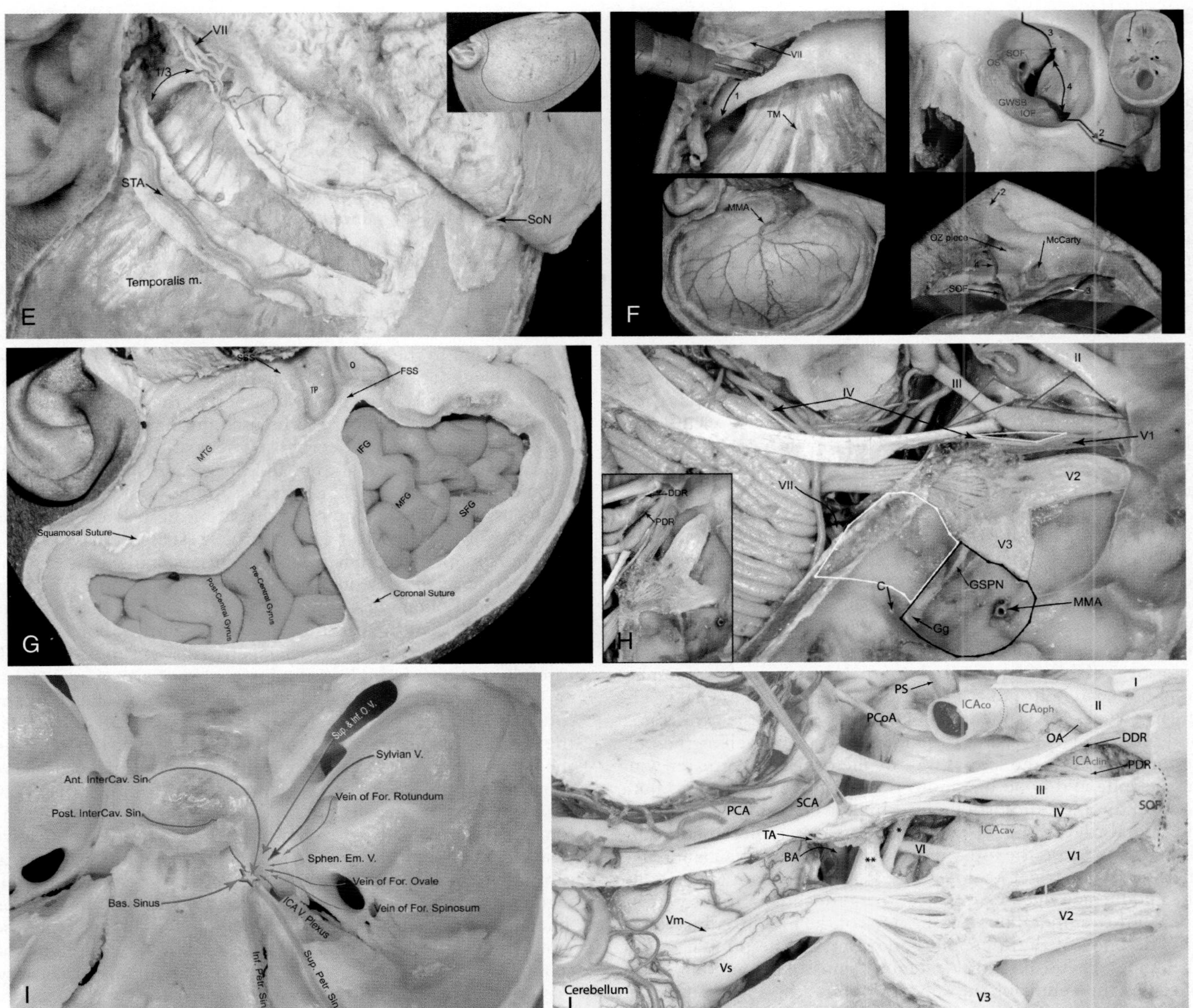

Figure 3-4, cont'd. E, A question mark skin incision *(red line, upper right)* is preferred for the extended pterional/orbitozygomatic approach. The facial nerve (VII) intersects the zygomatic arch approximately one third anterior to the posterior margin of the arch *(1/3).* SoN, supraorbital nerve; STA, superficial temporal artery; Temporalis m., temporalis muscle. **F,** The orbitozygomatic craniotomy consists of a series of bone cuts *(1-4)* to detach both the lateral surface of the cranial vault and the superolateral margin of the orbit from the skull. *Upper left,* TM, temporalis muscle; VII, facial nerve. *Lower left,* MMA, middle meningeal artery. *Upper right,* GWSB, greater wing of the sphenoid bone; IOF, inferior orbital fissure; OS, optic strut; SOF, superior orbital fissure. *Lower right,* McCarty, McCarty's keyhole; OZ piece, orbitozygomatic piece; SOF, superior orbital fissure. **G,** Opening the dura exposes the parietal lobe *(blue)* through the parietal window of the pterional craniotomy, the frontal lobe *(green)* through the frontal (anterior) and parietal (posterior) bone windows, and the temporal lobe *(yellow)* through the temporal bone; red *dotted line,* central sulcus. FSS, frontosphenoid suture; IFG, inferior frontal gyrus; MFG, middle frontal gyrus; MTG, middle temporal gyrus; O, orbit; SFG, superior frontal gyrus; SSS, sphenosquamous suture; TP, temporal pole. **H,** The oculomotor (III), trochlear (IV), ophthalmic (V1), and maxillary (V2) nerves run close to the lateral wall of the cavernous sinus. The oculomotor nerve (III) enters the cavernous sinus between the posterior clinoid process and the edge of the tentorium, over the posterior petroclinoid ligament, in the oculomotor (Hakuba's) triangle *(purple).* Other triangles of the cavernous sinus are the posterolateral (Glasscock's) triangle *(black),* clinoidal (anteromedial) triangle *(blue),* anterolateral triangle *(brown),* anteromedial (Mullan's) triangle *(green),* infratrochlear (Parkinson's) triangle *(red),* posteromedial (Kawase's) triangle *(white),* and supratrochlear (paramedian) triangle *(yellow).* The geniculate ganglion (Gg) of the facial nerve (VII) may be used to infer the anterior margin of the fundus of the internal acoustic canal. *Lower left,* If the anterior clinoid is removed, two dural bands encircling the internal carotid artery are revealed: the proximal (PDR) and distal dural rings (DDR). C, cochlea; GSPN, greater superficial petrosal nerve; II, optic nerve; MMA, middle meningeal artery; V3, mandibular nerve. **I,** The venous drainage of the middle cranial fossa is both very interesting and rich in anastomoses. While the cavernous sinus is the center for venous drainage of the middle fossa, it mainly acts as a relay and funnel for the sphenopetroclival venous gulf *(star),* which is the critical intracranial venous drainage pathway for the skull base. Ant. InterCav. Sin., anterior intercavernous sinus; Bas. Sinus, basilar sinus; ICA V. Plexus, internal carotid artery venous plexus; Inf. Petr. Sin., inferior petrous sinus; Post. InterCav. Sin., posterior intercavernous sinus; Sphen. Em. V., sphenoid emissary vein; Sup. & Inf. O. V., superior and inferior orbital vein; Sup. Petr. Sin., superior petrous sinus; Sylvian V., sylvian vein; Vein of For. Ovale, vein of foramen ovale; Vein of For. Rotundum, vein of foramen rutundum. **J,** When fully exposed, the cavernous sinus is a beautiful landscape formed by the internal carotid artery medially, and cranial nerves III-VI laterally as they run into the superior orbital fissure. BA, basilar artery; ICAcav, cavernous segment; ICAclin, clinoid segment; ICAoph, ophthalmic segment; ICAco, communicant segment; PCA, posterior cerebral artery; PCoA, posterior communicant artery; PS, pituitary stalk; SCA, superior cerebellar artery; TA, tentorial (Bernasconi-Cassinari) artery; Vm, motor root of CNV; Vs, sensory root of CNV; * petrosphenoidal (petroclival or Gruber's) ligament; **, posterior petroclinoid ligament. *(Published with permission of the University of California San Francisco's Skull Base & Cerebrovascular Laboratory.)*

temporal bone through the sphenosquamous suture; superiorly to the frontal bone through the frontosphenoid suture and the parietal bone through the sphenoparietal suture; and anteriorly to the zygoma through the sphenozygomatic suture. The sphenozygomatic suture may be followed inferiorly to find the inferior orbital fissure. Superiorly, the greater wing of the sphenoid bone is intersected by the coronal suture and forms the pterion. The middle meningeal artery runs within the inner table of the greater wing of the sphenoid bone, which exposes it to inadvertent damage during a pterional craniotomy. Extracranially, the greater wing of the sphenoid bone may be used to infer the intracranial position of the temporal pole and the sphenoparietal sinus. At its base, the sphenoid bone projects inferiorly toward the nasal cavity in the form of the pterygoid plates. The pterygoid plates contain the pterygoid canal (for the vidian nerve) and form the lateral wall of the choana medially, the pterygopalatine fossa (where V2 exits the skull) at the center, and the pterygomaxillary fissure laterally.

Intracranially, the lesser wing of the sphenoid bone (or sphenoid ridge) is a triangular structure that forms the posterior edge of the anterior cranial fossa (Fig. 3-4C and D). Laterally, the lesser wing of the sphenoid bone merges with the greater wing of the sphenoid bone at the lateral surface of the cranial vault. Medially, the lesser wing of the sphenoid bone attaches to the body of the sphenoid through the optic strut and the planum. Inferior to the lesser wing are both the greater wing of the sphenoid bone laterally and the superior orbital fissure medially. The greater wing of the sphenoid bone shapes part of the extracranial and intracranial surfaces of the middle fossa, as well as the posterior portion of the lateral wall of the orbit. The greater wing of the sphenoid bone fuses into the body of the sphenoid bone to form the anterior portion of the middle cranial fossa, including the lateral edge of the superior orbital fissure and foramen rotundum. It also forms the foramina ovale (passage for the mandibular division of the trigeminal nerve, V3) and spinosum (passage for the middle meningeal artery) near to its attachment to the petrous apex of the temporal bone at the floor of the middle cranial fossa.

The body of the sphenoid bone contains the pituitary fossa, the upper clivus, and the sphenoid sinus. The pituitary fossa occupies the center of the sphenoid bone (see Fig. 3-4C). The anterior aspect of the pituitary fossa is formed by the limbus, which corresponds to the edge of the planum, the chiasmatic sulcus, and the tuberculum sellae (see Fig. 3-4D). The relationship between the optic chiasm and its sulcus and the limbus may be of great value when selecting the optimal approach (endonasal versus open transcranial) for lesions in the suprasellar space. The tuberculum sellae is an osseous protuberance that sets the limit between the dura of the pituitary gland and the optic chiasm. Posteriorly, the pituitary fossa is limited by the dorsum sellae and the superior portion of the clivus. The anterior and posterior clinoid processes and their interclinoid ligaments form the lateral boundaries of the pituitary fossa. The optic canal is formed by the limbus and chiasmatic sulcus medially and anteriorly, the proximal part of the lesser wing of the sphenoid superiorly, the anterior clinoid process posteriorly, and the optic strut inferiorly. The optic strut, which anchors the anterior clinoid process to the body of the sphenoid bone, also divides the optic canal from the carotid groove. The relationship between the optic strut and both the internal carotid artery (clinoid segment) and the optic nerve is critical when performing an extradural anterior clinoidectomy.

At the base of the dorsum sellae, the petrous apex anchors to the sphenoid bone through both sutures and ligaments (see Fig. 3-4C). The petrosphenoidal fissure brings together the anterior petrous edge of the temporal bone with the greater wing of the sphenoid bone, immediately posterior to the foramina spinosum and ovale. The petrous apex and the clivus are attached through the petroclival synchondrosis, which also forms a furrow used by the inferior petrosal sinus. The temporal bone also attaches to the greater wing of the sphenoid bone through the sphenosquamous suture, which is visible exocranially. Three ligaments are relevant for the approaches to the middle fossa: the petroclival, petrolingual, and anterior and posterior petroclinoid ligaments.

The petroclival ligament (also called Gruber's ligament or the petrosphenoidal ligament) arises from the vertex of the petrous apex, travels within the cavernous sinus above the petroclival synchondrosis, and attaches to the body of the sphenoid bone. The petroclival ligament forms the roof of Dorello's canal, which is the space used by the abducens nerve to enter the cavernous sinus. Lateral to the petroclival ligament is the petrolingual ligament, a band of periosteum and connective tissue connecting the sphenoid lingula and the posterior aspect of the foramen lacerum. The petrolingual ligament can be used during surgery to anticipate the position of the lacerum segment of the internal carotid artery inferior and medial to it, and the greater superficial petrosal nerve superior to it. The anterior and posterior petroclinoid ligaments connect the anterior portion of the petrous bone and the anterior and posterior clinoid processes, respectively.

The foramen lacerum is an osseous opening between the lateral edge of the petrous apex medially, the carotid groove of the sphenoid bone anteriorly, the greater wing of the sphenoid bone laterally, and the carotid canal of the petrous bone and the groove of the greater superficial petrosal nerve posteriorly. If carefully examined, the lateral margin of the carotid groove has an osseous spur, the sphenoidal lingula, that protrudes into the foramen lacerum. The sphenoidal lingula is very useful to infer the position of the pterygoid (or vidian) canal inferior to it, and the proximal part of the cavernous segment of the abducens nerve superior and medial to it (see Fig. 3-4D). The foramen lacerum is patent only in the dry skull. When explored surgically, the foramen lacerum is a horizontal canal with a thick connective tissue at its inferior edge that serves as a bed to hold the internal carotid artery transitioning from its petrous to its cavernous segment. Lateral to the foramen lacerum is the foramen ovale. The foramen ovale contains the mandibular branch and the motor root of the trigeminal nerve (CN V). It also is used by the vein of the foramen ovale and by the accessory meningeal artery. Posterior and lateral to the foramen ovale is the foramen spinosum, which is the natural opening for the middle meningeal artery and vein to enter the intracranial space. The anatomic features at the surface of the petrous bone, detailed earlier in this chapter, become critical to guide the middle fossa approach. Relevant to the middle fossa approach are the groove of the greater superficial petrosal nerve, the trigeminal impression, the arcuate eminence, and (if visible) the cave of the geniculate ganglion of the facial nerve.

Surgical Anatomy

Positioning

The patient is positioned supine and the head is turned 20 to 30 degrees away from the lesion. The neck is extended and the vertex of the head is tilted inferiorly until the body of the zygoma (malar eminence) becomes the highest point of the head, from the surgeon's view. The degree of tilt to be applied to the vertex of the head is relevant for lesions involving the sylvian fissure and especially the deep sylvian cistern.

Skin Incision

In general, a "question mark" skin incision is preferred when performing an orbitozygomatic approach (Fig. 3-4E). The question mark skin incision is started behind the hairline of the forehead near the midline and arched back to approximately the level of the external acoustic meatus, and then continued as a vertical line until the zygomatic process of the temporal bone. The inferior portion of the skin incision may be placed either 1 cm anterior to the tragus, to prevent inadvertent damage to the main trunk of the superficial temporal artery, or along the posterior edge of the tragus for optimal cosmetic results.

Mastering the anatomy of the extracranial part of the facial nerve is fundamental during the musculocutaneous dissection of the orbitozygomatic approach. After dividing into superior and inferior trunks within the parotid gland, the facial nerve becomes progressively superficial. The superior trunk of the facial nerve is directed anteriorly and superiorly and leaves the parotid gland near the inferior edge of the zygomatic arch (see Fig. 3-4E). The facial nerve intersects the zygomatic arch at its middle third and runs superficial to the temporal fascia. The temporal fascia is a layer of connective tissue that attaches to the superior temporal line, the posterior edge of the zygoma, and the superior edge of the zygomatic arch. At the superior edge of the zygomatic arch, the temporal fascia is divided into two laminae—superficial and deep—that contain the superficial temporal fat pad. Below the deeper lamina of the temporal fascia, and superficial to the temporalis muscle, the deep temporal fat pad is thicker and continues inferiorly to the parapharyngeal space. The orbitozygomatic approach requires detaching the temporal fascia (with the facial nerve running superficial to it) and the masseter tendon. To protect the facial nerve, the superficial lamina of the temporalis fascia must be preserved. Two techniques exist to raise a facial nerve flap: interfascial and subfascial. The interfascial dissection is done between the two laminae of the temporal fascia. It creates a flap of the superficial lamina of the temporal fascia, leaving the superficial temporal fat pad attached to the deep lamina of the temporal fascia. For the subfascial dissection, both laminae of the temporal fascia are transected and reflected together, exposing the temporalis muscle and protecting the facial nerve in between them. The frontal branch of the facial nerve is the most superior and runs over the posterior margin of the superior belly of the orbicularis oculi. If the orbital rim needs to be completely exposed, a secondary flap known as the omega incision is raised to protect the supraorbital neurovascular bundle.

The superficial temporal artery runs at the root of the zygomatic process of the temporal bone. The superficial temporal artery splits into the frontal (anterior) and parietal (posterior) branches approximately 4 to 5 cm superior to the zygomatic arch. Preserving the superficial temporal artery should be encouraged in every case because it may be used as a donor artery for an extracranial-intracranial bypass if needed.

Muscular Layer

The temporalis muscle attaches to the superior temporal line and converges to its distal attachment at the coronoid process of the mandible. The main vascular supply for the temporalis muscle comes from the deep temporal arteries (branches of the maxillary artery), running underneath the temporalis muscle, and from perforating arteries branching from the middle meningeal artery, running within the inner table of the skull. The temporalis muscle is typically detached from the skull and reflected either inferiorly and posteriorly (during the orbitozygomatic approach) or inferiorly and anteriorly (during a pterional approach).

Craniotomy

The orbitozygomatic craniotomy consists of a series of bone cuts to detach both the lateral surface of the cranial vault and the superolateral margin of the orbit from the skull (Fig. 3-4F). The orbitozygomatic craniotomy may be performed in one or two pieces. The two-piece orbitozygomatic craniotomy uses a standard pterional bone flap to gain access to the intracranial space and to complete the cuts of the roof and lateral wall of the orbit from the intracranial space. In brief, the pterional bone flap is obtained by placing a bur hole a few millimeters inferior and posterior to the anterior margin of the superior temporal line (pterional keyhole) and sawing a bone flap as close to the floor of the middle fossa as possible. Next, the orbitozygomatic piece is removed en bloc by cutting the root of the zygomatic arch, cutting the body of the zygoma (from the inferior edge of the body of the zygoma to the inferior orbital fissure), sawing the roof of the orbit from the intracranial space (from the orbital rim to the superior orbital fissure), and finally connecting the inferior and superior orbital fissures. The one-piece craniotomy, however, requires simultaneous access to both the intraorbital and intracranial (McCarty's keyhole) spaces because the intracranial space is not accessed until the craniotomy is finished.

Three additional craniectomies may be considered to complement the orbitozygomatic craniotomy: anterior clinoidectomy, posterior clinoidectomy with partial removal of the dorsum sellae, and anterior petrosectomy. Removing the anterior clinoid process reveals the clinoid segment of the internal carotid artery, the optic canal, and the origin of the ophthalmic artery. It may be used in combination with the transcavernous approach for ophthalmic aneurysms and sphenoid wing meningiomas invading the cavernous sinus. The anterior clinoid process may be removed extradurally or intradurally.

The posterior clinoid process and part of the dorsum sellae also may be removed during the orbitozygomatic approach if access to the interpeduncular fossa is necessary. The posterior clinoid is exposed through the oculomotor triangle, after gentle retraction of the temporal lobe. The interclinoid and posterior petroclinoid ligaments may be cut to expose the bone of the dorsum sellae. Anterior to the dorsum sellae are the diaphragm of the pituitary fossa and the posterior intercavernous sinus. The basilar apex, the thalamostriate arteries (perforators), the precommunicating segment (P1) of the posterior cerebral artery, and the cisternal segment of the oculomotor nerve (CN III) may be accessed through this route.

Dural Opening

The dura is incised following the shape of the pterional bone flap, and a pedicle is based at the sphenoid ridge. The dural flap is then reflected toward the lesser wing of the sphenoid bone. If the middle meningeal artery was preserved during the craniotomy, the pedicle of the dural flap may be enlarged inferiorly to contain the artery. Care should be taken to preserve the periorbita if intraconal access is not required.

Intradural Anatomy

Opening the dura exposes the lateral surface of the brain (Fig. 3-4G). Splitting the sylvian fissure requires skilled dissection of the cortical, opercular, and insular arteries, as well as the superficial and deep sylvian veins within the superficial and deep sylvian cisterns. Splitting the sylvian fissure during a skull base approach may be advantageous if the lesion sits deep in the supraclinoid segment of the internal carotid artery or around the dorsum sellae, because it untethers the temporal lobe from the frontal operculum and the adhesions to the greater wing of the sphenoid bone.

Access to the cavernous sinus may be accomplished by positioning the retraction blades over the temporal pole for a pretemporal corridor, or at the base of the temporal lobe for a subtemporal corridor. The pretemporal corridor offers access to the majority of the cavernous sinus, with direct exposure of the sphenoid ridge and lateral aspect of the pituitary fossa. The subtemporal corridor may be advantageous when access to the posterior aspect of the cavernous sinus, the petroclival region, and the incisural space is required.

The cavernous sinus is a dural space on either side of the pituitary fossa and the base of the greater wing of the sphenoid bone (Fig. 3-4H). Anteriorly, the cavernous sinus is limited by the lesser and greater wings of the sphenoid bone (sphenoid ridge). Medially, the dura of the cavernous sinus is continuous with the dura of the floor of the pituitary gland, the sellar diaphragm, and the interclinoid ligament. The posteromedial boundary of the cavernous sinus is formed by the dura over the dorsum sellae and clivus, as well as the tentorium. At its posterior medial region, the cavernous sinus merges with the sphenopetroclival venous gulf, which also contains Gruber's ligament. Laterally, the cavernous sinus joins the dense connective tissue of the foramen lacerum and the dura over Meckel's cave.

The venous drainage of the middle cranial fossa is both very interesting and rich in anastomoses (Fig. 3-4I). It is formed by different sinuses, draining veins, and venous plexuses, which shunt at the sphenopetroclival area (around the petrous apex) and communicate with the extracranial venous drainage (through the foramina of the greater sphenoid wing). The cavernous sinus is the main venous complex in the middle fossa. Posteriorly, the cavernous sinus receives inflow from the carotid venous plexus at the foramen lacerum. Adjacent to the foramen lacerum, the sphenobasal sinus, at the base of the sphenoid and petrous apex, is connected to both the cavernous sinus and the tentorial sinus. Posterior and lateral to the sphenobasal sinus are the veins of the foramina ovale and spinosum, which shunt the cavernous sinus and the sphenobasal sinus to the pterygoid venous plexus in the infratemporal space (intracranial-extracranial venous shunt). Running through the parietal aspect of the greater wing of the sphenoid bone is the sphenoparietal sinus, which receives the superficial sylvian vein and the temporopolar vein and drains to the cavernous sinus. The tributaries of the sphenoparietal sinus run together with the middle meningeal artery and converge around the lesser wing of the sphenoid bone. Inferior and medial to the sphenoparietal sinus is the vein of the foramen rotundum, which shunts the cavernous sinus to the sphenopalatine fossa and the pterygoid venous plexus. Also, at the base of the greater wing of the sphenoid bone, the sphenoid emissary vein provides a straight shunt inferiorly to the pterygoid venous plexus, much like a sinkhole at the bottom of the cavernous sinus. Anteriorly, the superior and inferior ophthalmic veins use the superior orbital fissure to drain the contents of the orbit, including the vein for the center of the retina. Medially, the cavernous sinus receives the venous drainage from the pituitary fossa, which comes in two different patterns: the anterior and posterior intercavernous sinuses independently or, if they merge around the pituitary diaphragm, the circular sinus.

While the cavernous sinus is the center for venous drainage of the middle fossa, it mainly acts as a relay and funnel for the sphenopetroclival venous gulf, which is the critical intracranial venous drainage pathway for the skull base (see Fig. 3-4I, star). The sphenopetroclival venous gulf is a high-flow confluence of the cavernous sinus anteriorly, the superior petrosal sinus posteriorly, the inferior petrosal sinus inferiorly, and the basilar sinus medially. The sphenopetroclival venous gulf sits at the petrous apex and contains Gruber's ligament, Dorello's canal, and the abducens nerve transitioning from its transdural to its cavernous segment.

The oculomotor (CN III), trochlear (CN IV), ophthalmic (first division of the trigeminal nerve, V1), and maxillary (second division of the trigeminal nerve, V2) nerves run close to the lateral wall of the cavernous sinus, whereas the abducens nerve (CN VI) runs over the inferior layer (periosteal) close to the body of the sphenoid bone and the internal carotid artery. Whereas mastering the course and relationships of each cranial nerve running within the cavernous sinus is critical, the spaces between the nerves (the middle fossa and cavernous sinus triangles) may be used to infer the structures beyond the dissection plane and design optimal dissection windows (Table 3-1). The oculomotor nerve enters the cavernous sinus between the posterior clinoid process and the edge of the tentorium, over the posterior petroclinoid ligament (oculomotor triangle) (see Fig. 3-4H). After piercing the cavernous sinus, the oculomotor nerve runs at the top of the cavernous sinus lateral to the cavernous segment of the internal carotid artery and immediately inferior to the anterior clinoid process. Approximately 5 to 10 mm before entering the superior orbital fissure, the oculomotor nerve is crossed by the trochlear nerve, which becomes superior and medial to it. The trochlear nerve transitions from its tentorial to its cavernous segment at the top of the sphenopetroclival venous gulf, over the petrous apex. The trochlear nerve runs underneath the lateral wall of the cavernous sinus (first nerve encountered through the transcranial approaches). The trochlear nerve follows a superior, anterior, and medial straight path toward the superior orbital fissure. During its course, the trochlear nerve relates to the oculomotor nerve medially (supratrochlear triangle) and V1 inferiorly (infratrochlear triangle). When the trochlear nerve reaches the root of the anterior clinoid process, it crosses the oculomotor nerve to reach the superior oblique muscle in the orbit.

The trigeminal nerve sets the lateral limits of the surgical corridors to the cavernous sinus. Medially, the medial edge of the main trunk, gasserian ganglion, and V1 form the lateral limit of the infratrochlear triangle. V1 runs straight to the superior orbital fissure inferior to the trochlear nerve. If the cavernous sinus is dissected transcranially, V1 obstructs the view of the abducens nerve. The abducens nerve enters the cavernous sinus at Dorello's canal (below the petroclival ligament). It runs medial and inferior to V1 and lateral to the posterior (also called medial) bend of the internal carotid artery in a straight trajectory toward the superior orbital fissure. The maxillary branch of the trigeminal nerve exits the gasserian ganglion at its center and runs for a short distance to the foramen rotundum, which is the lateral limit of the cavernous sinus. The space between V1 and V2 is called the anteromedial triangle (Mullan's triangle). The sympathetic nerve fibers of the cavernous sinus originate at the superior cervical ganglion and travel through the parapharyngeal space around the internal carotid artery. At the lacerum segment of the internal carotid artery, the nerve fibers from the sympathetic plexus split and follow either the abducens nerve (deep petrosal nerve) or the greater superficial petrosal nerve. The sympathetic fibers that gather around the abducens nerve at Dorello's canal travel with it for a short distance in the cavernous sinus. When the abducens nerve approaches V1, approximately 60% of the sympathetic fibers cross over V1 and continue toward the superior orbital fissure to provide sympathetic input to the orbit. The sympathetic fibers that do not cross over V1 (40%) continue with the abducens nerve through the superior orbital fissure.

The anterolateral triangle is the space posterior to V2 and anterior to the mandibular division of the trigeminal nerve (V3). If the anterolateral triangle is entered anteriorly, the lateral recess of the sphenoid sinus and the base of the lateral pterygoid plate may be exposed. However, a perpendicular trajectory through the anterolateral triangle enters the infratemporal space, where the internal maxillary artery may be exposed. The posterolateral triangle (also called Glasscock's triangle) is limited by the posterior margin of V3 anteriorly, the greater superficial petrosal nerve medially, and the arch connecting the foramen ovale, the foramen spinosum, and the proximal part of the greater superficial petrosal nerve. Drilling through the posterolateral triangle reveals the eustachian canal and the tensor tympani muscle laterally and the petrous segment of the internal carotid artery medially. If the petrosectomy is continued posterior to the posterolateral triangle, the middle ear and epitympanic space are opened. The greater superficial petrosal nerve serves as a superficial boundary between the posterolateral and the posteromedial triangles. The posteromedial triangle (also called Kawase's triangle) is limited

TABLE 3-1 Skull Base Triangles of the Middle Fossa and Cavernous Sinus

Triangle	Anatomic Limits	Targets
Oculomotor (Hakuba's)	• Anterior clinoid process • Posterior clinoid process • Petrous apex	• Horizontal portion of cavernous ICA • Interpeduncular fossa
Clinoidal (anteromedial)	• Optic nerve (CN II) • Oculomotor nerve (CN III) • Edge of the tentorium	• Clinoidal segment of ICA • Proximal and distal dural rings
Supratrochlear (paramedian)	• Oculomotor nerve (CN III) • Trochlear nerve (CN IV) • Tentorial edge	• Capsular artery of McConnell • Horizontal segment of cavernous ICA • Rarely, meningohypophysial trunk
Infratrochlear (Parkinson's)	• Trochlear nerve (CN IV) • Ophthalmic nerve (V1) • Petrous bone ridge	• Abducens nerve (at Dorello's canal) • Sphenopetroclival venous gulf • Gruber's ligament • Meningohypophysial trunk • Inferolateral trunk
Anteromedial middle fossa (Mullan's)	• Ophthalmic nerve (V1) • Maxillary nerve (V2) • Line between superior orbital fissure and foramen rotundum	• Ophthalmic vein • Sphenoid sinus • Abducens nerve
Anterolateral middle fossa	• Maxillary nerve (V2) • Mandibular nerve (V3) • Line between foramina rotundum and ovale	• Lateral recess of sphenoid sinus • Sphenoid emissary vein • Veins of foramina rotundum and ovale • Infratemporal fossa
Posterolateral middle fossa (Glasscock's)	• Mandibular nerve (V3) • Greater superficial petrosal nerve • Line between foramen ovale and geniculate ganglion	• Eustachian tube and canal • Tensor tympani muscle • Petrous segment and posterior loop of ICA • Middle meningeal artery (foramen spinosum) • Infratemporal fossa
Posteromedial middle fossa (Kawase's)	• Greater superficial petrosal nerve • Mandibular nerve (V3) and trigeminal nerve (CN V) • Petrous bone ridge	• Petrous apex • Internal acoustic meatus • Vertebrobasilar junction • Trunk of basilar artery • Anterolateral brainstem
Inferolateral paraclival	• Line between dural entry points of CN IV and abducens nerve (CN IV and VI) • Line between dural entry point of CN VI and superior petrosal vein • Line between dural entry point of CN IV and superior petrosal vein	• Meckel's cave • Superior petrosal sinus • Medial surface of Kawase's triangle
Inferomedial paraclival	• Line between dural entry point of CN VI and posterior clinoid process • Line between dural entry point of CN IV and CN VI • Line between dural entry point of CN IV and posterior clinoid process	• Lateral edge of dorsum sellae • Dorello's canal • Medial edge of sphenopetroclival venous gulf

CN, cranial nerve; ICA, inferior carotid artery; V1-V3, first, second, and third divisions of the trigeminal nerve (cranial nerve V).

anteriorly by the posterior edge of the trigeminal nerve, the gasserian ganglion, and V3. Its lateral limit is the greater superficial petrosal nerve (at the surface) and the petrous segment of the internal carotid artery (deep). The medial limit of the posteromedial triangle is formed by the superior petrosal sinus running at the petrous ridge and the inferior petrosal sinus running within the petroclival synchondrosis. The posterior limit of the posteromedial triangle is formed by the cochlea and the anterior wall of the internal acoustic canal in the depth of the petrous bone.

Anticipating the location of the cochlea is critical to preserve audition, which is lost when the cochlea is opened. The cochlea is medial to the geniculate ganglion, which is visible either on the surface of the petrous bone or just posterior to the proximal end of the greater superficial petrosal nerve. The geniculate ganglion, when visible, also may be used to infer the anterior margin of the fundus of the internal acoustic canal (see Fig. 3-4H). If the petrous bone is removed along the posterior margin of Kawase's triangle, the internal acoustic canal is opened and the facial (superior) and cochlear (inferior) nerves are encountered first. Extremely careful maneuvering is necessary around the petroclival region during Kawase's approach to prevent damage to the abducens nerve at Dorello's canal or the trochlear nerve transitioning from the tentorium to the lateral wall of the cavernous sinus. The anterior petrosectomy may be combined with a transtentorial trajectory to widen access to the anterior and middle incisural space. At the posterior aspect of the cisternal segment of the trigeminal nerve, the superior petrosal (also called Dandy's) vein enters the superior petrosal sinus. It is advisable to preserve the outflow of the superior petrosal vein, either to the transverse sinus or the sphenopetroclival venous gulf, because it drains the lateral pons, cerebellopontine fissure, and upper medulla.

The anatomy of the internal carotid artery and its branches is very relevant to understanding both the anatomy of and surgical approaches to the cavernous sinus. The internal carotid artery becomes intracranial at the carotid canal. After entering the carotid canal, it runs in a vertical segment for a short distance and turns anteriorly (posterior loop) for a horizontal segment at the floor of the middle fossa (petrous segment). Within the petrous segment, the internal carotid artery is related to the middle ear posteriorly, the geniculate ganglion and cochlea at the posterior loop, and the greater superficial petrosal nerve, gasserian ganglion, tensor tympani, and eustachian tube within the horizontal segment (see earlier discussion of temporal bone). At the floor of the middle crania fossa, the petrous segment of the internal carotid artery runs inferior to the gasserian ganglion, sometimes without bony cover. At the transition from the petrous to the lacerum segment, the internal carotid artery is anchored by a dense fibrous band known as the lateral ring. For a short distance the internal carotid artery transitions over the foramen lacerum (lacerum segment) and turns superiorly (medial loop) to reach the carotid groove at the body of the sphenoid bone. At the lacerum segment, the internal carotid artery is related superiorly to the abducens nerve, laterally to the vidian nerve and the sphenoid lingula, and medially to the posterior clinoid process. Within the cavernous segment, the internal carotid artery has a horizontal portion, where the artery runs medial to V1 and the abducens nerve, and an anterior loop, where the artery makes a sudden posterior turn at the root of the anterior clinoid process.

While transitioning through the cavernous sinus, the internal carotid artery gives rise to two important trunks: meningohypophysial and inferolateral. The meningohypophysial trunk arises from the ventral portion of the medial loop of the internal carotid artery, medial to the abducens nerve, and trifurcates into the inferior hypophysial artery, supplying the adenohypophysis and floor of the sella; the tentorial artery (also called the artery of Bernasconi and Cassinari), nourishing the tentorial segment of the trochlear nerve; and the dorsal meningeal artery, which supplies both the abducens nerve at Dorello's canal and the dura over the clivus. Distal to the meningohypophysial trunk is the inferolateral trunk, which gives four branches: the anteromedial branch, which supplies the oculomotor, trochlear, and abducens nerves and V1; the anterolateral branch, which runs parallel to V2 and exits through the foramen rotundum, where it anastomoses with the branches of the internal maxillary artery at the pterygopalatine fossa; the posterior branch, which follows V3 to the foramen ovale; and the superior branch, responsible for supplying the trochlear nerve. Although rare, the ophthalmic artery may arise from the anterior loop of the internal carotid artery.

After the anterior loop, the internal carotid artery remains inferior and slightly medial to the anterior clinoid process (clinoid segment). If the anterior clinoid is removed, two dural bands encircling the internal carotid artery are revealed: the proximal and distal dural rings (see Fig. 3-4H). The proximal dural ring (also called the carotico-oculomotor membrane) is a thin dural band at the root of the anterior clinoid process and contains the oculomotor nerve, the internal carotid artery, and the anterior clinoid process. The distal dural ring is a strong band of connective tissue that fuses to the tunica externa of the internal carotid artery and extends to the falciform ligament, planum sphenoidale, diaphragma sellae, and anterior clinoid process. After exiting the distal dural ring, the internal carotid artery enters the carotid cistern in the intradural space (ophthalmic or supraclinoid segment). In the ophthalmic segment, the internal carotid artery gives rise to the ophthalmic artery, proximal to the optic nerve, and the superior hypophysial artery, which supplies the neurohypophysis, pituitary stalk, and optic chiasm.

THE ENDOSCOPIC ENDONASAL APPROACH

Surgical Targets

At present, there are many surgical variants of the endoscopic endonasal approach that can be successfully used for treatment of lesions involving most areas of the ventral skull base. The focus of the present section is to provide the reader with useful anatomic landmarks and knowledge regarding the surgical steps common to all endoscopic endonasal approaches.

The endoscopic endonasal approach, and all its variants, expose the neurovascular structures of the skull base from the ventral perspective (viewed from below and medial). Although the endonasal corridor deals with the same anatomic structures encountered during a classic transcranial approach, their spatial relationships and the order in which they are surgically exposed changes dramatically.

Bone Anatomy

The nasal cavity is a rectangular space divided by the septum into two cavities—left and right. The nasal cavity could be conceptualized as a geometric space similar to that of a rectangular cuboid, enlarged in its anterior-posterior axis. We follow this concept and describe the anatomy relevant to its six facets.

The anterior facet of the nasal cavity is a triangular space formed laterally by the frontal processes and inferiorly by the palatine processes of both maxillary bones (Fig. 3-5A). After entering this triangle, the anterior nasal spine of the maxillary bone articulates with the vomer to form the bony portion of the nasal septum (Fig. 3-5B).

The medial facet of the nasal cavity is the nasal septum. The nasal septum is formed superiorly by the vomer and its articulation with the perpendicular plate of the ethmoid, inferiorly by the palatine process and the nasal crest of both the maxillary and palatine bones, and posteriorly by the rostrum of the sphenoid bone (Fig. 3-5B and C).

The inferior facet of the nasal cavity is formed by the palatine process of the maxillary bone (anteriorly) and the horizontal plate of the palatine bone (posteriorly), which merge to form the maxillary plane. The maxillary plane is the horizontal axis along the hard palate, which can be identified preoperatively on a computed tomography scan and used to evaluate the inferior limit of the trajectory of the endonasal approach in relation to the target.

The turbinates shape the lateral facet of the nasal cavity into superior, medial, and inferior meatuses, which have different anatomic structures and relationships as the endoscope is advanced through (Fig. 3-5B-D). In the inferior meatus, the lateral wall is formed by the perpendicular plate of the palatine bone posteriorly, the medial wall of the maxillary sinus in the middle and anteriorly. The inferior turbinate attaches to the maxillary and palatine bones at their conchal crest. The inferior turbinate is shaped like a jet turbine with its tail projecting to the choana.

The lateral wall of the middle meatus can be divided as well into posterior, medial, and anterior thirds. In the posterior third of the middle meatus, the perpendicular plate of the ethmoid articulates with both medial and lateral pterygoid plates of the sphenoid bone and contains the sphenopalatine notch, which is named after the artery that runs through it. In the center of the middle meatus, the medial wall of the maxillary sinus (inferiorly) and the ethmoid bulla (superiorly) coexist (see Fig. 3-5C). Anterior to the bulla, the uncinate process arises from the ethmoid, leaving an effective space—the hiatus semilunaris—between the bulla and the uncinate process. The uncinate process can be further divided into a superior half that, if opened, exposes the floor of the orbit, and an inferior half that corresponds to the medial wall and ostium of the maxillary sinus. The anterior third of the middle meatus contains both the ethmoid crest and sometimes the frontal process of the maxillary bone.

The middle and superior turbinates arise from the core of the ethmoid bone very close to one another. When explored surgically, the middle turbinate becomes evident and divides the middle meatus from the superior. The superior turbinate sits above and posterior to the middle turbinate.

The cribriform plate of the ethmoid bone mainly forms the superior facet (roof) of the nasal cavity. Anteriorly, the cribriform plate and the perpendicular plate of the ethmoid bone attach to the nasal part of the frontal bone. Posteriorly, the ethmoid articulates with the planum or jugum of the sphenoid bone. Also, when viewed through the endonasal perspective, the posterior aspect of the superior meatus is continuous with the superior portion of the sphenoid rostrum.

The posterior facet of the nasal cavity is divided into the sphenoid rostrum superiorly and the choana inferiorly (Fig. 3-5D and E). The sphenoid bone is the main structure in the posterior facet

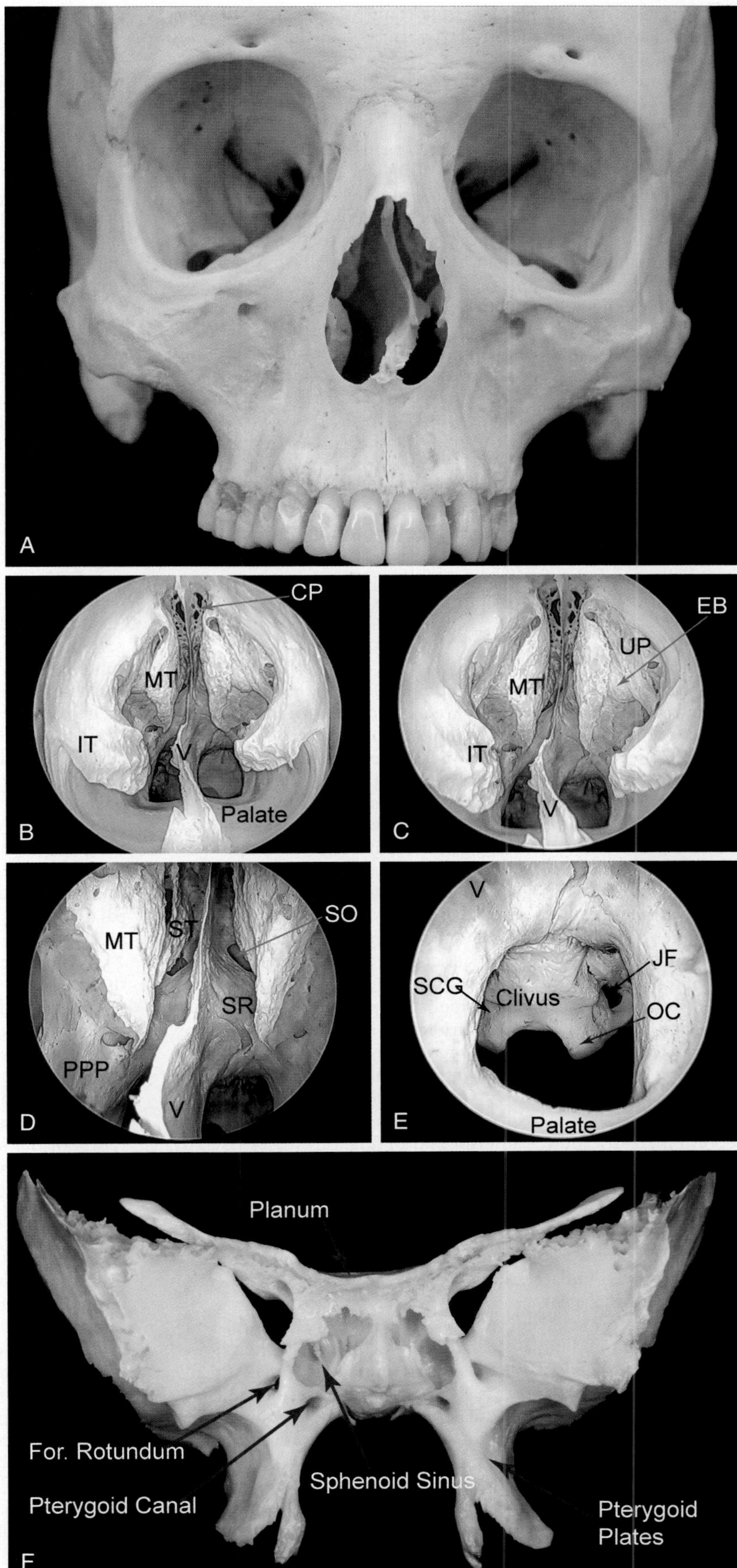

Figure 3-5. Bone anatomy relevant to the endoscopic endonasal approach. A, The anterior facet of the nasal cavity is a triangular space formed laterally by the frontal processes and inferiorly by the palatine processes of both maxillary bones. **B,** The anterior nasal spine of the maxillary bone articulates with the vomer (V) to form the bony portion of the nasal septum. *Green circle,* choana. CP, cribriform plate; IT, inferior turbinate; MT, middle turbinate. **C,** In the center of the middle meatus, the medial wall of the maxillary sinus (inferiorly) and the ethmoid bulla (EB) (superiorly) coexist. MT, middle turbinate; UP, uncinate process; V, vomer. **D,** The turbinates shape the lateral facet of the nasal cavity into superior, medial, and inferior meatuses. MT, middle turbinate; PPP, perpendicular plate of the palatine bone; SO, sphenoid ostium; SR, sphenoid rostrum; ST, superior turbinate; V, vomer. **E,** The posterior facet of the nasal cavity is divided into the sphenoid rostrum and the choana. JF, jugular foramen; OC, occipital condyle; SCG, supracondylar groove; V, vomer. **F,** Between the base of the lateral pterygoid plate and the greater wing of the sphenoid bone, the foramen rotundum (For. Rotundum) connects Meckel's cave to the pterygopalatine fossa for the maxillary nerve to reach the nasal pharynx. *(Published with permission of the University of California San Francisco's Skull Base & Cerebrovascular Laboratory.)*

of the nasal cavity and plays an important role in the endoscopic endonasal approach to the pituitary fossa and any of its variations. When studied from the endonasal perspective, the sphenoid bone presents the rostrum in the center with two bony projections at each side—the pterygoid plates. The sphenoid rostrum articulates with the body of the vomer and the posterior aspect of the ethmoid bone. The rostrum has two ostia—one in each side—that are natural draining openings of the sphenoid sinus. In well-pneumatized patients, the sphenoid sinus may present a lateral recess that extends to the base of the pterygoid plates. When the rostrum (body) of the sphenoid transitions to the base of the pterygoid plates, two foramina are found. Medially, in the base of the pterygoid plate, the pterygoid canal exits to the pterygopalatine fossa for the vidian nerve to pierce the pterygopalatine ganglion. Nearby, between the base of the lateral pterygoid plate and the greater wing of the sphenoid bone, the foramen rotundum connects Meckel's cave to the pterygopalatine fossa for the maxillary nerve to reach the nasal pharynx (Fig. 3-5F). The inferior border of the sphenoid rostrum fuses with the base of the pterygoid plate (laterally), and the body of the vomer (medially) to form the choana. The choana is the natural opening of the posterior facet of the nasal cavity to the nasopharynx and oropharynx, which, if transected, reveals the clivus. When the endoscope is passed through the choana, the basilar portion of the occipital bone (occipital clivus) is completely exposed together with the occipital condyles and the apex of the petrous bone, with the jugular foramen as the lateral limit of the exposure.

Surgical Anatomy

The patient positioning and the equipment used during an endoscopic endonasal approach require an operating room setup different from that of the classic skull base procedures. For optimal surgical trajectory, the patient is positioned supine with the neck slightly extended (10 to 20 degrees) and the head turned 5 to 15 degrees toward the surgeon. The surgeon stands by the side of the surgical table with direct access to the nostrils of the patient, which will be the only working corridor throughout the approach. For a complex endoscopic endonasal procedure, a skull base team consisting of a neurosurgeon and an ear, nose, and throat surgeon works simultaneously.

The endoscopic endonasal approach to skull base lesions has two well-defined stages: the nasal-pharyngeal dissection (Fig. 3-6) and the intradural exposure (Fig. 3-7). At present, the endoscopic endonasal approach is widely accepted and used for treating lesions located in the pituitary fossa. Therefore, the anatomy relevant to the endoscopic endonasal access to the pituitary fossa is the center of this discussion, with special focus on the skull base dissection.

An early endonasal inspection through one nostril exposes the septum medially and the inferior and middle turbinates laterally, which divide the space into inferior, middle, and superior meatuses (Fig. 3-6A). The vast majority of the endoscopic endonasal approaches to the skull base use the middle meatus to pass the endoscope and instruments. Therefore, the middle turbinate, which limits access to the skull base, will either be fractured laterally or removed unilaterally depending on the size and location of the surgical target.

After gentle medial retraction or fracture of the middle turbinate, the ethmoid bulla—a characteristic pneumatized ethmoid cell—is exposed (Fig. 3-6B). Using an angled view, it is possible to expose the uncinate process anterior to the bulla. The uncinate process is an important landmark to expose the maxillary sinus ostia and can be used as a key landmark to expose either the maxillary sinus (inferior half) or the medial part of the orbit (superior half). Using backbiting rongeurs introduced into the semilunar hiatus, the uncinate process can be removed superiorly to access the orbit or inferiorly (together with the inferior turbinate) to expose the maxillary sinus (Fig. 3-6C). If directed superiorly, the lamina papyracea—a shallow bony wall to the orbit—can be removed very carefully to protect the orbital contents. However, if the inferior half of the uncinate process is opened, the maxillary sinus is exposed. The portion of the maxillary bone that forms the roof of the maxillary sinus is often translucent enough to see the infraorbital nerve. Next, the dissection can be extended posteriorly to the sphenopalatine fossa after removing the posterior wall of the maxilla and the lateral pterygoid plate (Fig. 3-6D). Care should be taken to preserve the superior alveolar nerves in the former and the greater palatine nerve and artery in the latter. Further dissection through the pterygopalatine fossa will expose the lateral pterygoid muscle, foramen rotundum (passage for the maxillary division of the trigeminal nerve, V2), and foramen ovale (passage for the mandibular division of the trigeminal nerve, V3).

In contrast, if the middle turbinate is lateralized, the ipsilateral choana and sphenoid rostrum are exposed and can be accessed. Before passing beyond the mucosa over the sphenoid rostrum, the sphenopalatine artery should be identified and preserved. The sphenopalatine artery is a distal branch of the maxillary artery that originates in the sphenopalatine fossa, crosses the rostrum of the sphenoid approximately 5 mm superior to the choana, and turns anteriorly to feed the nasal septum—mucosa, periosteum, and perichondrium (Fig. 3-6E and F). If the middle turbinate is removed for an expanded endonasal approach, the posterior extension of the turbinate root can be used effectively to locate the sphenopalatine artery at the sphenopalatine foramen of the palatine bone. As the reader might anticipate, preserving the sphenopalatine artery is of critical importance to the survival of the nasoseptal flap for closure. Once the sphenopalatine artery is identified, the vidian nerve may also be identified, because it is a key landmark to infer the location of the internal carotid artery and preserve it if the approach requires transclival drilling. The vidian nerve can be located using two landmarks: the palatovaginal neurovascular bundle and morphometric references to the choana. If the mucosa of the roof of the choana is sharply incised, the palatovaginal bundle can be identified running through the suture between the body of the sphenoid and the vomer, toward the sphenopalatine ganglion. If followed to the ganglion, the palatovaginal bundle points to the vidian nerve as it exits the pterygoid canal. Also, the vidian nerve can be located roughly 1 cm superior to the choana and 5 mm lateral to the midline of the choana.

Opening the sphenoid sinus is common to the majority of endonasal skull base approaches (Fig. 3-7A and B). In patients with well-pneumatized sinuses, the sella turcica can be completely exposed. To safely open the sphenoid sinus, the sphenoid ostia must be first identified. Then the ostia are widened until the sphenoid rostrum is completely opened. In some cases, a lateral recess of the sphenoid sinus is present and its exposure requires different degrees of pterygoid plate removal. In extremely pneumatized sinuses, both the pterygoid canal (vidian nerve) and V2 can be readily exposed after opening the sinus cavity. After removing the rostrum, one or more septae might be present. It is critical not to use these structures as midline reference without presurgical assessment because they typically lead to one of the internal carotid arteries. The septae and sinus mucosa are removed next to expose the anterior wall of the sella turcica and clival process of the sphenoid bone.

A successful transsphenoidal approach is highly dependent on the ability to navigate safely through the sphenoid sinus, which, for the most part, relates to the wise use of the bony landmarks identified during surgery. The posterior wall of the sphenoid sinus is greatly shaped by the neurovascular structures beyond the bone (i.e., internal carotid artery, optic nerve, and pituitary gland), which can sometimes be seen through a very shallow bone. There are two important landmarks that should always be

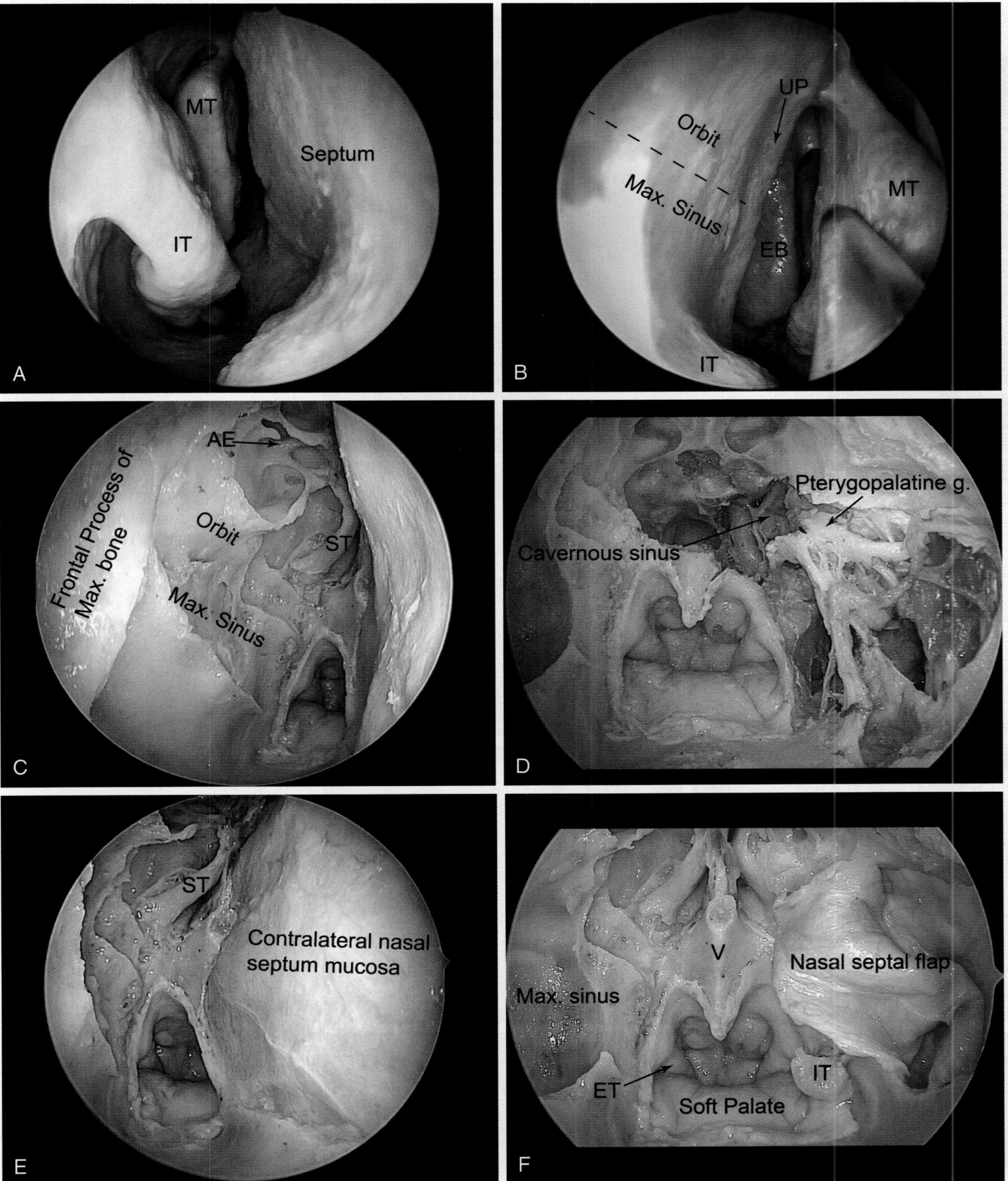

Figure 3-6. Nasal dissection landmarks relevant to the endoscopic endonasal approach. A, Endonasal inspection through one nostril exposes the septum and the inferior turbinate (IT) and middle turbinate (MT). **B,** Gentle medial retraction or fracture of the middle turbinate (MT) exposes the ethmoid bulla (EB). IT, inferior turbinate; Max. Sinus, maxillary sinus; UP, uncinate process. **C,** The uncinate process can be removed superiorly to access the orbit or inferiorly to expose the maxillary sinus (Max. Sinus). AE, anterior ethmoid; Max. bone, maxillary bone; ST, superior turbinate. **D,** Posterior extension of the dissection to the sphenopalatine fossa after removing the posterior wall of the maxilla and the lateral pterygoid plate. Pterygopalatine g., pterygopalatine ganglion. **E,** If the middle turbinate is lateralized, the ipsilateral choana and sphenoid rostrum are exposed and can be accessed. ST, superior turbinate. **F,** Before transgressing the mucosa over the sphenoid rostrum, the sphenopalatine artery, which is of critical importance to the survival of the nasoseptal flap for closure, should be identified and preserved. ET, eustachian tube; IT, inferior turbinate; Max. Sinus, maxillary sinus; V, vomer. *(Published with permission of the University of California San Francisco's Skull Base & Cerebrovascular Laboratory.)*

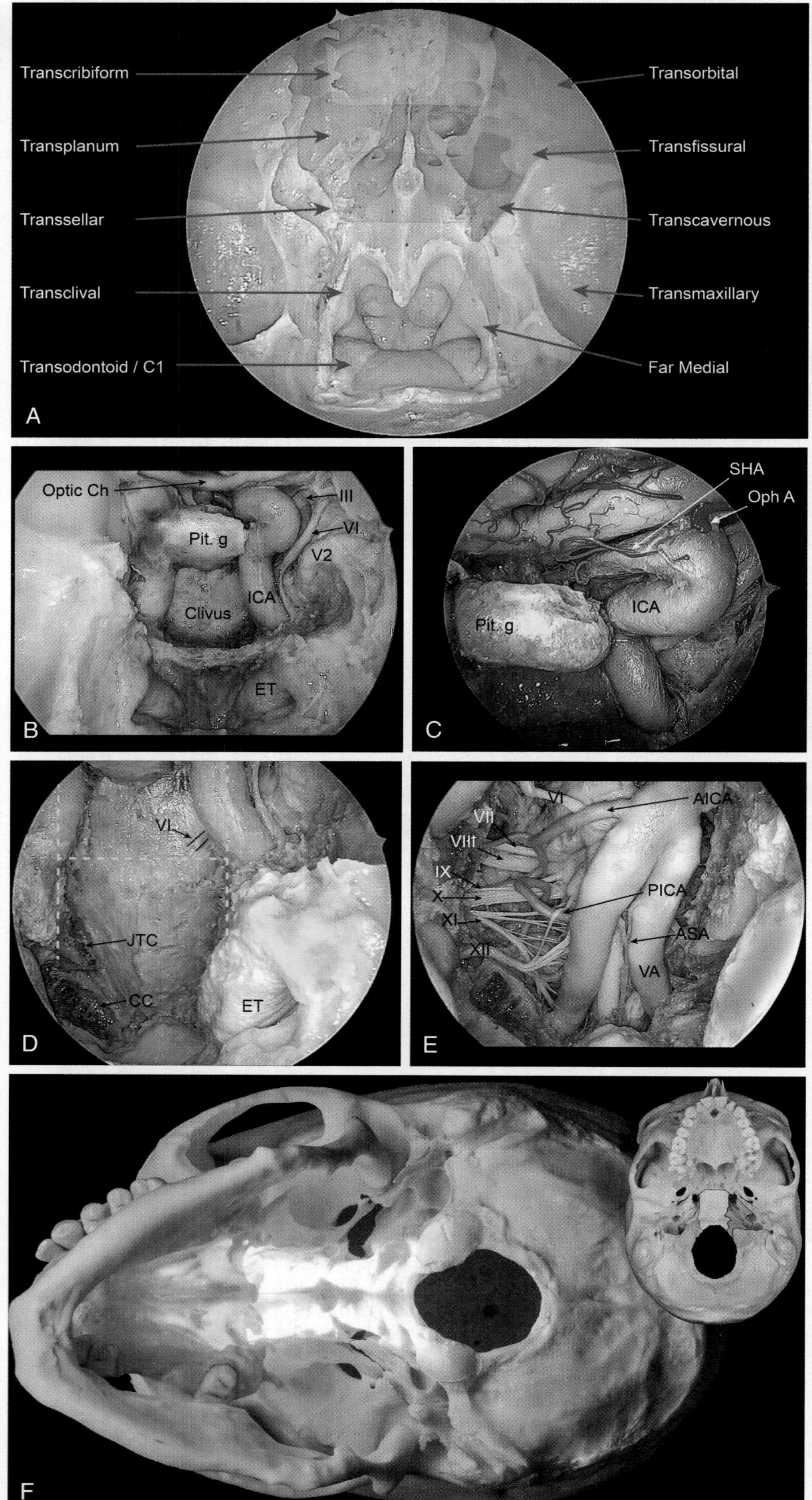

Figure 3-7. Skull base anatomy relevant to the endoscopic endonasal approach. **A,** Opening the sphenoid sinus is common to the majority of endonasal skull base approaches. C1, atlas. **B,** The posterior wall of the sphenoid sinus is shaped by the internal carotid artery (ICA), optic nerve, and pituitary gland (Pit. g). ET, eustachian tube; III, IV, cranial nerves III and IV; Optic Ch, optic chiasm; V2, second segment of the vertebral artery. **C,** The suprasellar dissection toward the sphenoid tuberculum and planum requires an extensive posterior ethmoidectomy. ICA, internal carotid artery; Oph A, ophthalmic artery; Pit. g, pituitary gland; SHA, superior hypophyseal artery. **D,** The natural limits of the transclival approach are typically the floor of the soft palate inferiorly, the internal carotid arteries and eustachian tubes (ET) laterally, and the pituitary gland superiorly. The abducens nerve (VI) pierces the dura and runs transdurally in the upper portion of the "H" *(yellow dashed lines).* CC, condylar compartment; JTC, jugular tubercle compartment. **E,** Opening the dura after an expanded endoscopic transclival approach provides direct, unobstructed access to the ventral compartment of the posterior fossa. AICA, anterior inferior cerebellar artery; ASA, anterior spinal artery; PICA, posterior inferior cerebellar artery; VI-XII, cranial nerves VI through XII; VA, vertebral artery. **F,** The transclival approach *(white rectangle)* exposes the midline aspect of the pons, the cisternal and transdural segments of cranial nerve VI, and the pyramids and cranial nerve XII at the preolivary sulcus. However, the coronal expansion at this level (the "far medial" approach, *blue region*) will reveal the cisternal segments of cranial nerves IX to XII, as well as the inferior petrosal sinus entering the jugular foramen. *(Published with permission of the University of California San Francisco's Skull Base & Cerebrovascular Laboratory.)*

identified: the medial opticocarotid recess (MOCR), which gives access to the pituitary fossa and suprasellar region, and the lateral opticocarotid recess (LOCR), which points to the parasellar space and cavernous sinus. The MOCR is located in the inferomedial angle formed between the internal carotid artery and the optic nerve. If opened, the MOCR provides access to the adenohypophysis, optic chiasm, and tuberculum sellae. In contrast, the LOCR is located in the superolateral angle between the internal carotid artery and the optic nerve, which directs the dissection laterally to the optic strut toward the oculomotor nerve, the cavernous sinus, and Meckel's cave. Further lateral dissection anterior to the cavernous sinus exposes the superior orbital fissure and apex of the orbit. Dissection through the MOCR gives access to the pituitary fossa and the anterior intercavernous sinus between both internal carotid arteries. At this point, the dissection can be directed either cranially or caudally.

The suprasellar dissection toward the sphenoid tuberculum and planum requires an extensive posterior ethmoidectomy (Fig. 3-7C). At this point, the optic chiasm posteriorly and the posterior ethmoid artery anteriorly are the major anatomic features of this region. If the surgical approach requires wide exposure of the anterior cranial fossa, a complete ethmoidectomy may be required, including the middle and superior turbinates, perpendicular lamina, and air cells. The extradural exposure of the endoscopic endonasal approach to the anterior cranial fossa exposes the anterior ethmoid arteries, the cribriform plate and olfactory bulb and tracts, the base of the crista galli, and the posterior wall of the frontal sinus. There is general consensus that access to lesions invading the frontal sinus and its anterior wall through the endoscopic endonasal approach is technologically severely limited and therefore discouraged.

To access the posterior fossa, the transsphenoidal approach is extended caudally to the clivus. The extracranial shape of the clivus is flat, with a slight posterior slope—away from the surgeon—as it reaches the anterior arch of the atlas (see Fig. 3-5E). For an optimal transclival exposure, the nasopharynx should be completely exposed. To that end, the choanae may be exposed completely following a posterior septectomy. The natural limits of the transclival approach are typically the floor of the soft palate inferiorly, the internal carotid arteries and eustachian tubes laterally, and the pituitary gland superiorly (Fig. 3-7D). To expose the clivus, both the nasopharyngeal mucosa and pharyngobasilar fascia are incised and dissected away. Inferiorly, the clivus is covered by the longus capitis and rectus capitis anterior muscles and deeper by the atlanto-occipital ligaments, which anchor the clivus and occipital condyles to the spine. This inner muscular-connective layer is also transected and removed to expose the clivus, occipital condyles, dens of the axis, and anterior arch of the atlas.

Three key landmarks will guide a safe dissection during the transclival approach: the vidian nerve, the supracondylar groove, and the foramina lacerum. The clivus should be drilled applying low pressure and uniformly, while controlling bleeding from the basilar venous plexus, which occasionally may be copious. The clivectomy should start with the identification of the vidian nerve in the pterygopalatine fossa (see Fig. 3-6D). It is important to mention that the vidian nerve points to the internal carotid artery as it turns up at the foramen lacerum (lacerum segment). Specifically, the vidian nerve has been proven to be a safe landmark to use to infer the position of the internal carotid artery throughout the clivectomy. With the vidian nerve in the center of an imaginary clock, drilling should proceed first from 3 o'clock to 6 o'clock in the right side. When the depth of the foramen lacerum and the genu of the internal carotid artery are understood, drilling can proceed from 3 o'clock to 9 o'clock counterclockwise (in the same side). If complete clivectomy is required, care should be taken when drilling around the occipital condyle because it encases the hypoglossal nerve. A key landmark to infer the location of the hypoglossal canal before starting the inferior clivectomy is the supracondylar groove. The supracondylar groove exists roughly 1 cm above the basion bilaterally and lateral to the pharyngeal tubercle. It points directly to the hypoglossal canal in the depth and provides a reference to design a customized craniectomy.

Once the clivectomy is completed, the dura mater is exposed from the dorsum sellae to the anterior arch of the atlas (C1). At this point, the structures limiting the exposure laterally are the internal carotid arteries superiorly and the eustachian tubes and craniovertebral junction inferiorly (Fig. 3-7D). Two very delicate structures dictate the safest dural opening: the abducens and hypoglossal nerves. The abducens nerve takes off near the midline at the pontomedullary sulcus, has a straight cisternal segment and pierces the dura for a short distance—the transdural segment—toward Dorello's canal, and finally enters the cavernous sinus. Hence, the abducens nerve is at risk when opening the dura during the endonasal approaches. Fortunately there is a simple reference to save the abducens nerve when opening the dura during a transclival approach. If the long axis of the paraclival (cavernous) segment of the internal carotid artery is projected inferiorly to the occipital condyle and a line is traced between both foramina lacerum, an "H" or football goal shape is obtained. The abducens nerve always pierces the dura and runs transdurally in the upper portion of the "H" (i.e., *the abducens nerve scores a goal*) (see Fig. 3-7D, yellow lines). More precisely, the abducens nerve pierces the dura, on average, along the line between the upper walls of the lacerum segment of the internal carotid artery, as it turns in the foramen lacerum, and approximately 5 mm medial to the paraclival internal carotid artery. The main trajectory of the transdural segment of the abducens nerve is around the internal carotid artery posteriorly, and ascending through the cavernous sinus to reach the superior orbital fissure.

If the lesion is located in the ventromedial compartment of the posterior fossa, with a lateral extension to the hypoglossal nerve, the far medial or lateral expansion of the transclival approach should be considered. In this region, the hypoglossal nerve divides the lower third of the clivus into condylar (inferior) and jugular tubercle (superior) compartments. Whereas drilling into the condylar compartment may be straightforward to the skilled skull base surgeon, drilling into the tubercular compartment requires experience and mastering the anatomic relationships of the jugular foramen, which contains critical neurovascular structures. Drilling of the jugular tubercle also requires skilled navigation of the endoscope and a wide septectomy and ethmoidectomy to allow for a steep angle of attack through the nasal cavity. While working around the hypoglossal canal, the use of a fine diamond bur is critical to respect both the dura and hypoglossal venous plexus and the limits of the craniocervical junction. The lateral expansion (coronal plane modules) of the lower half of the clivus involves two vascular structures: the petrous and lacerum segments of the internal carotid artery around the petrous apex, and the inferior petrosal sinus running in the petroclival synchondrosis. Between the inferior petrosal sinus (superiorly) and the hypoglossal canal (inferiorly) is the jugular tubercle. Further lateral exposure becomes available to the petrous apex and the venous compartment of the jugular foramen if the ipsilateral eustachian tube and pterygoid plates are removed early in the nasopharyngeal dissection.

Opening the dura after an expanded endoscopic transclival approach provides direct, unobstructed access to the ventral compartment of the posterior fossa (Fig. 3-7E). The vertebral arteries are exposed from their entrance into the arachnoid space until the vertebrobasilar junction (segment 4 of the vertebral artery). In this segment, the vertebral artery gives rise to the anterior spinal artery medially and the PICA in its lateral surface. The first segment of the PICA (anterior medullary), which may be difficult to reach through the open approaches, now becomes accessible. The anterior medullary segment of the PICA is intimately related to the hypoglossal nerve (CN XII) and the vagoaccessory triangle, which is the posterior limit of the endonasal approach at this level. The basilar artery is entirely exposed. The AICA may arise at the vertebrobasilar junction or at the lower third of the basilar artery and is consistently related to the cisternal segment of the abducens nerve (CN VI). Many pontine perforators arise from the posterior and lateral edges of the trunk of the basilar artery. Superiorly, the basilar artery gives rise to the superior cerebellar arteries and posterior cerebral arteries. In some individuals, the superior cerebellar artery may be duplicated, which may correspond to the cranial and caudal trunks of the superior cerebellar artery. In the interpeduncular fossa, the cisternal segment of the oculomotor nerve (CN III) is intimately related to both the precommunicating segment (P1) of the posterior cerebral artery, the posterior communicating artery, and the superior cerebellar artery. The basilar apex corresponds to the bifurcation of the basilar artery into both posterior communicating arteries (left and right). The posterior edges of both the basilar apex and P1 are densely populated by the thalamostriate arteries (perforators). Access to the postcommunicating segment (P2) of the posterior cerebral artery is severely limited from the endonasal route.

The anatomy of the internal carotid artery is very relevant to the endonasal approaches. The endoscopic endonasal approach to the sella is limited laterally by the anterior genu of the internal carotid artery (cavernous and clinoid segments). If the cavernous segment of the internal carotid artery is exposed through the endonasal corridor, the proximal and distal dural rings are revealed, as well as the ophthalmic artery branching off from its superomedial aspect. Although the origin of the ophthalmic artery is variable, its trajectory under the optic nerve is relevant and accessible through the endonasal approach. The cavernous segment of the internal carotid artery is also the lateral boundary of the transclival approach. In the literature, the segment of the internal carotid artery lateral to the clivus may be labeled as paraclival or cavernous.

The endoscopic endonasal approaches lateral to the cavernous segment of the internal carotid artery (coronal modules) often target the cavernous sinus, Meckel's cave, and the petrous apex. When the cavernous sinus is exposed through the endonasal corridor, the abducens nerve is revealed first. The oculomotor nerve is superior to the abducens nerve, and the ophthalmic division of the trigeminal nerve (V1) is inferior and lateral to the abducens nerve. The trochlear nerve runs on top of the cavernous sinus and its exposure requires manipulation of the abducens and oculomotor nerves. If the exposure is continued inferiorly and anteriorly, the superior orbital fissure, as well as the foramen rotundum, may be opened. At this point V2 may be exposed at the floor of Meckel's cave, as well as the anteromedial triangle of the middle fossa and the petrous apex. Upon completion of the endoscopic anterior petrosectomy, the root of the trigeminal nerve (CN V), and the cisternal segments of the facial and vestibulocochlear nerves (CNs VII and VIII) in the cerebellopontine fissure may be exposed.

The endoscopic endonasal approach to the lower third of the clivus opens a bony widow to the lower pons and the medulla, below the foramen lacerum. The transclival approach exposes the midline aspect of the pons, the cisternal and transdural segments of the abducens nerve, and the pyramids and the hypoglossal nerve at the preolivary sulcus. However, coronal expansion at this level (the *far medial* approach) will reveal the cisternal segments of CNs IX to XII and the inferior petrosal sinus entering the jugular foramen (Fig. 3-7E and F). Although visible, the neurovascular structures sitting in the dorsolateral compartment of the posterior fossa (i.e., cerebellar hemisphere, choroid plexus and foramen of Lushka, flocculus and second and third segments of the PICA) are blocked to the endonasal corridor by the cisternal segments of CNs VII to XII. The pharyngeal segments of the internal carotid artery, along with CNs IX to XII, may be exposed by dissecting the parapharyngeal space, lateral to the occipital condyle and posterior to the eustachian tube. This maneuver may require angled scopes and aggressive resection of the nasopharynx.

Acknowledgment

The authors acknowledge and are grateful for the contribution of Dr. Ali Tayebi Meybodi in this chapter.

SUGGESTED READINGS

Benet A, Prevedello DM, Carrau RL, et al. Comparative analysis of the transcranial "far lateral" and endoscopic endonasal "far medial" approaches: surgical anatomy and clinical illustration. *World Neurosurg.* 2014;81:385-396.

de Notaris M, Cavallo LM, Prats-Galino A, et al. Endoscopic endonasal transclival approach and retrosigmoid approach to the clival and petroclival regions. *Neurosurgery.* 2009;65(suppl 6):42-50; discussion 50-52.

Figueiredo EG, Deshmukh V, Nakaji P, et al. An anatomical evaluation of the mini-supraorbital approach and comparison with standard craniotomies. *Neurosurgery.* 2006;59(4 suppl 2):ONS212-220; discussion ONS220.

Gonzalez LF, Amin-Hanjani S, Bambakidis NC, et al. Skull base approaches to the basilar artery. *Neurosurg Focus.* 2005;19(2):E3.

Hsu FP, Clatterbuck RE, Spetzler RF. Orbitozygomatic approach to basilar apex aneurysms. *Neurosurgery.* 2005;56(suppl 1):172-177; discussion 172-177.

Iaconetta G, de Notaris M, Benet A, et al. The trochlear nerve: microanatomic and endoscopic study. *Neurosurg Rev.* 2013;36:227-237; discussion 237-238.

Kassam A, Snyderman CH, Mintz A, et al. Expanded endonasal approach: the rostrocaudal axis. Part I. Crista galli to the sella turcica. *Neurosurg Focus.* 2005;19(1):E3.

Kassam A, Snyderman CH, Mintz A, et al. Expanded endonasal approach: the rostrocaudal axis. Part II. Posterior clinoids to the foramen magnum. *Neurosurg Focus.* 2005;19(1):E4.

Kassam AB, Gardner P, Snyderman C, et al. Expanded endonasal approach: fully endoscopic, completely transnasal approach to the middle third of the clivus, petrous bone, middle cranial fossa, and infratemporal fossa. *Neurosurg Focus.* 2005;19(1):E6.

Kassam AB, Prevedello DM, Carrau RL, et al. The front door to Meckel's cave: an anteromedial corridor via expanded endoscopic endonasal approach—technical considerations and clinical series. *Neurosurgery.* 2009;64(suppl 3):ONS71-82; discussion ONS82-83.

Labib MA, Prevedello DM, Fernandez-Miranda JC, et al. The medial opticocarotid recess: an anatomic study of an endoscopic "key landmark" for the ventral cranial base. *Neurosurgery.* 2013;72(1 Suppl Operative):66-76; discussion 76.

Lanzino G, Paolini S, Spetzler RF. Far-lateral approach to the craniocervical junction. *Neurosurgery.* 2005;57(suppl 4):367-71; discussion 367-71.

Osawa S, Rhoton AL Jr, Tanriover N, et al. Microsurgical anatomy and surgical exposure of the petrous segment of the internal carotid artery. *Neurosurgery.* 2008;63(4 suppl 2):210-238; discussion 239.

Quiñones-Hinojosa A, Chang EF, Lawton MT. The extended retrosigmoid approach: an alternative to radical cranial base approaches for posterior fossa lesions. *Neurosurgery.* 2006;58(4 suppl 2):ONS208-214; discussion ONS-214.

Rhoton AL Jr. The far-lateral approach and its transcondylar, supracondylar, and paracondylar extensions. *Neurosurgery.* 2000;47(suppl 3): S195-209.

Rhoton AL Jr. The temporal bone and transtemporal approaches. *Neurosurgery.* 2000;47(suppl 3):S211-265.

Safavi-Abbasi S, de Oliveira JG, Deshmukh P, et al. The craniocaudal extension of posterolateral approaches and their combination: a quantitative anatomic and clinical analysis. *Neurosurgery.* 2010;66(3 Suppl Operative):54-64.

Snyderman CH, Carrau RL, Kassam AB, et al. Endoscopic skull base surgery: principles of endonasal oncological surgery. *J Surg Oncol.* 2008;97:658-664.

Stippler M, Gardner PA, Snyderman CH, et al. Endoscopic endonasal approach for clival chordomas. *Neurosurgery.* 2009;64:268-277; discussion 277-278.

Tedeschi H, Rhoton AL Jr. Lateral approaches to the petroclival region. *Surg Neurol.* 1994;41:180-216.

Zabramski JM, Kiris T, Sankhla SK, et al. Orbitozygomatic craniotomy. Technical note. *J Neurosurg.* 1998;89:336-341.

4 Improving Patient Safety

John D. Rolston, Catherine Y. Lau, and Mitchel S. Berger

Physicians routinely dedicate their time, skills, and expertise to their patients, helping to prevent illness and restore health. Despite the best efforts of health care workers, however, many patients are unintentionally injured by the very medical system from which they seek help. Understanding why these injuries happen, how they happen, and how we can prevent them from happening forms the core of the patient safety movement in contemporary medicine.

EPIDEMIOLOGY OF PATIENT SAFETY

The modern patient safety movement arguably coalesced in the wake of the 2000 publication of *To Err is Human*, by the National Academy of Medicine (formerly the Institute of Medicine).[1,2] This decidedly influential report drew on the 1991 Harvard Medical Practice Study,[3] and estimated that between 44,000 and 98,000 Americans were killed yearly by medical errors. This shockingly high figure spawned the evocative "jumbo jet" analogy—deaths caused by medical errors were numerically equivalent to one passenger jet crashing daily. More recent studies, following the Harvard Medical Practice Study, have adjusted the estimate of those killed by errors even higher, at 210,000 to 440,000.[4]

The early report by the National Academy of Medicine stoked renewed national interest in patient safety, and a large contingent of researchers, physicians, nurses, and administrators have invested heavily in identifying and preventing such errors.[2] Medication errors have been reduced through computerized provider order entry,[5] an increase in clinical pharmacists,[6-9] medication reconciliation,[10-12] and bar-code scanning.[13-15] Hospital-acquired infections have been reduced though standardized protocols for central line placement,[16-18] daily "sedation vacations" to reduce ventilator-associated pneumonia,[19,20] and timely use of perioperative antibiotics to prevent surgical site infections (SSIs).[21,22] Surgical errors are reduced by "time-out" procedures,[23,24] instrument counts,[25,26] site marking,[27] and other standardized procedures.[28-32]

Yet the size and impact of these errors remains vast. Medication errors are perhaps the best documented. By some estimates, 5% of all hospital admissions are due to adverse events related to medications,[2] and at least 5% of all hospitalized patients suffer at least one adverse drug event.[33] Cost estimates place ambulatory medication errors at $5 billion yearly[34] and inpatient errors at $16.4 billion yearly.[2,35]

Surgical adverse events are also unfortunately common. An estimated 3% of all surgical patients suffer an adverse event in the perioperative period, half of which are preventable.[36] In neurosurgical patients specifically, 14.3% suffer at least one complication.[37] Roughly 1 in every 100,000 operations involves the wrong site or wrong patient, and the wrong side is operated on in 2.2 of every 10,000 craniotomies.[38] A recent poll of neurosurgeons revealed that 25% reported making an incision on the wrong side of the head, and 35% reported wrong-level lumbar surgery during their career.[39] Retained instruments and sponges occur in about 1 in every 5500 to 10,000 operations.[2] The economic cost of these errors is high. Analysis of the National Practitioner Data Bank shows $1.3 billion in settlements alone between 1990 and 2010.[40] This does not include the 90% of patients who do not receive payments and are not included in the database. A single wrong-site surgery has an average payout of $127,159 and that for a retained foreign body is $86,247.[41] More troubling, the number of these events appears to be increasing over time.[42]

Infections are another source of preventable harm. As many as 1 in 10 patients will suffer from an iatrogenic infection, according to the Centers for Disease Control and Prevention.[2,43] Some estimates place the number of resulting deaths from iatrogenic infections at 100,000 annually, with costs of around $40 billion.[2,43]

ERRORS AND ADVERSE EVENTS

As seen above, there are many ways in which the medical field can inadvertently harm patients. The taxonomy below was developed to categorize these types of events[2] (Fig. 4-1).

Adverse events are inadvertent injuries resulting from medical care, or the failure to deliver appropriate care. The Institute for Healthcare Improvement (IHI) further defines adverse events as "unintended physical injury resulting from or contributed to by medical care (including the absence of indicated medical treatment) that requires additional monitoring, treatment, or hospitalization, or that results in death."[2]

Adverse events can further be split into *preventable adverse events* and *nonpreventable adverse events*. *Nonpreventable* adverse events include accepted surgical complications, such as the risk of hemorrhage with external ventricular drain placement, and some medication side effects, such as the increased risk of hyperglycemia with high-dose dexamethasone. *Preventable* adverse events, on the other hand, include harm caused by clear errors, such as wrong-side and wrong-level surgery, or failure to offer standard treatment, such as neglected deep venous thromboembolism prophylaxis in surgical patients.

Complications, a common term in surgical specialties, are less well defined but are probably best understood as including all adverse events, both preventable and nonpreventable, but also including harm directly related to the disease rather than from medical care associated with the disease. An example of a complication would include an intracranial hemorrhage associated with a brain tumor, even if it happened outside the hospital and without medical care contributing at all to its occurrence (i.e., an inevitable "complication" of the disease).

Errors are acts or omissions that lead to undesirable outcomes or have a high potential for such an outcome. Thus errors overlap with preventable adverse events but crucially include events that cause no harm (so-called near misses or close calls). That is, some errors by health care workers are detected by the health care system and prevented from injuring the patient, such as incorrectly ordered medication doses or medication cross-reactions caught by computerized provider order entry systems or clinical pharmacists.

Errors can be further broken down into *active errors* (or "sharp end" errors) and *latent errors* (or "blunt end" errors) (Table 4-1). Active errors are errors that occur when the patient is in contact with health care personnel, are usually readily apparent, and almost always involve a health care worker on the front line. Latent errors refer to less apparent failures of the organization or design that allow harm to come to patients. An example is chemotherapy being infused at the wrong rate. The active error would be a nurse programming the wrong rate into the intravenous (IV) pump. A latent error would be the health care system

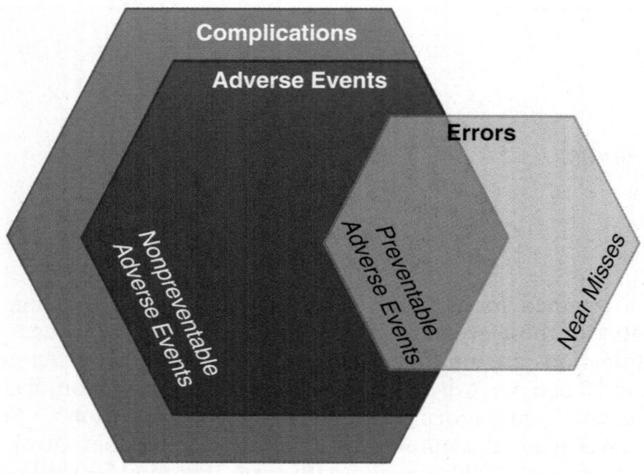

Figure 4-1. Diagram depicting patient safety terminology.

TABLE 4-1 Systems View for Sources of Errors

Level	Examples
Governmental	• Federal laws and regulations (e.g., EMTALA, Affordable Care Act) • U.S. Food and Drug Administration requirements and reporting • Centers for Disease Control and Prevention reporting • The Joint Commission regulations • Occupational Safety and Health Administration regulations
Institutional	• Medication formulary decisions • Hiring and staff sizes • Shift length and timing policies
Infrastructure	• Electronic medical record system • Building and facility layout • Equipment and facility maintenance
Team	• Ease of physical communication (pager, phone, e-mail, etc.) • Frequency of interactions • Formalized procedures for information exchange (e.g., SBAR) • Hierarchy and ability to question plans
Individual health care worker	• Medical knowledge base • Physical and mental health • Institutional knowledge base (i.e., ability to navigate the current system)
Individual patient	• Complexity of case • Language and communication barriers • Social or personality barriers • Health literacy

Errors can be latent or active (see text). Latent errors occur at a variety of levels, from governmental regulations to hospital policies that increase the risk of a patient experiencing an adverse event. Active errors occur at the system's "sharp end," where a health care worker makes a slip or mistake. However, most active errors occur in a background of latent errors. Latent errors are a major contributor to adverse events, and arguably have more impact in protecting patients than individual practitioners.

EMTALA, Emergency Medical Treatment and Active Labor Act; SBAR, situation, background, assessment, and recommendation.

or organization using multiple types of IV pumps, thus leading to increased nursing confusion and the increased probability of an adverse event occurring.

Active errors have been extensively studied in psychology, and many subdivisions have been proposed to further delineate errors and identify common mechanisms. Examples are James Reasons' classification of active errors into *slips* and *mistakes*.[44] Slips occur when an intended action is carried out imperfectly—as in literally slipping with a scalpel when operating and damaging uninvolved tissue. Thus slips occur as a result of lapses of concentration or failures of schematic behaviors, and can happen in the face of competing distractions, fatigue, and stress. Mistakes occur when the wrong action is selected, even if carried out perfectly. Thus mistakes are failures of active problem solving resulting from incorrect judgment, lack of knowledge or skills, or intentional failure to adhere to common standards. A classic example is wrong-side or wrong-level surgery.

More complex divisions of errors include the classification by the National Coordinating Council (NCC) for Medication Error Reporting and Prevention, which divides errors into nine classes (A through I) determined by how much harm, if any, was caused.[2] The NCC classification is notable, however, for dividing errors by their effects, as compared to Reasons' classification, which focuses on mechanisms.

SYSTEMS THINKING

Adverse events and medical errors are costly and common. What is the source of these errors? When prospectively analyzing errors in neurosurgical procedures, only 23.7% to 27.8% were related to the technical skills of the surgeon.[45] The remainder, roughly 75%, involved various other participants in the patient's care—for example, nurses, anesthetists, and equipment technicians.[45]

It is crucial for the surgeon to acknowledge that many errors arise from factors outside his or her direct control. Such observations, which abound across medical specialties, make it clear that improving patient safety requires an analysis of the entire health care system to which a patient is exposed. Thus *systems thinking* is critical.[2,46] Even if a surgeon performs his or her procedure perfectly, only a quarter of errors might be prevented.

Systems thinking has been advocated for patient safety since the publication of *To Err is Human*. Essentially, a complex system such as medicine produces errors not only through technical mistakes and slips, but also via cultural, social, and organizational problems.[47] All of these domains feed into each other and are interrelated (Fig. 4-2). Systems thinking acknowledges that all humans will make mistakes, and these mistakes will occur throughout the health care system. To prevent these inevitable errors from harming patients, the system should be robustly designed to catch these errors and mitigate their harm, which has long been the case in other industries concerned with safety, such as nuclear power and air transportation.[2]

In order to rationally develop processes to address patient safety, two main steps are involved. First, errors and adverse events must be reliably identified and documented. Only when the problem scope is known can limited resources be directed to the most pressing areas. Second, solutions can be proposed to prevent or mitigate adverse events across the extent of the health care system (see Table 4-1). In line with systems thinking, these solutions are not restricted to the "sharp end" of the system—that is, surgeons and other providers directly interacting with the patient—but also can be applied at the "blunt end"—the management, regulations, facilities, and other entities that influence patient care in sometimes dangerous ways.[2]

TOOLS FOR IMPROVING PATIENT SAFETY

A large variety of tools have arisen to improve patient safety, often targeted to a single previously identified problem (e.g., surgical checklists, site marking). Yet even identifying threats to patient safety in the first place remains challenging. Many strategies exist, such as the Global Trigger Tool, chart reviews, incident reports, and claims data, and all offer tradeoffs between expense, sensitivity, and specificity.

The Patient Safety Ecosystem

Healthcare as a complex adaptive system

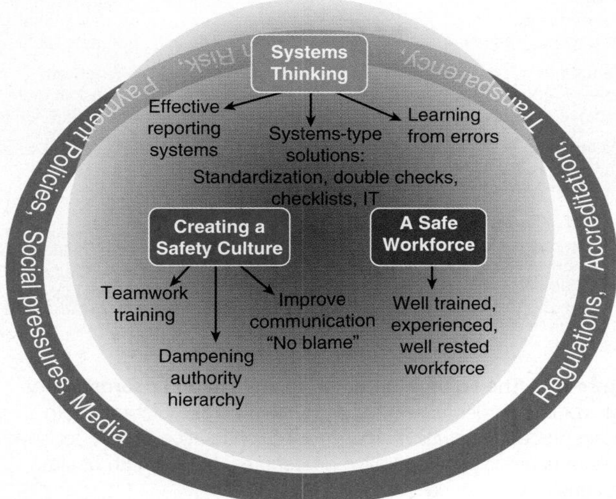

Figure 4-2. The "Patient Safety Ecosystem" consists of systems-based approaches to avoid errors, a culture in which open communication is valued, and a well-trained and well-rested workforce. These are created and influenced by a variety of external forces.

Finding Errors and Complications

The IHI *Global Trigger Tool* relies on a variety of events that are likely associated with adverse events and errors, such as return to the operating room, intraoperative death, transfer to a higher level of care, readmission to the emergency department after discharge, or naloxone use. Each case that produced one of these events (and set off the "trigger") is then manually analyzed for errors and adverse events. This process is laborious and currently impractical with large patient volumes. However, the sensitivity and specificity are superb, estimated at 94.9% and 100%, respectively.[48]

Incident reports are generally unstructured event reports by nurses, physicians, and other health care workers via a paper or, increasingly, a computerized hospital-based system. Such reports are not standardized, for example, in that different workers harbor different thresholds for reporting events. Furthermore, the unrewarded effort in generating reports and frequent failure to "close the loop" and visibly act on reports by the hospital lowers the incentive for reporting. Hospital-wide cultures also play a role, with few physicians generally taking part in these systems[49] and large variances existing between floors and even units within floors.

Morbidity and mortality conferences are a well-established method of identifying errors and complications in the neurosurgical field.[35,50,51] Benefits include a relatively low-cost method of surveillance that has educational relevance and importance and that allows for self and group reflection on performance. A major limitation to morbidity and mortality conferences is that they traditionally involve physicians focused on individual (and sometimes team) performance. As discussed earlier, there needs to be less of a focus on individual blame and more of a discussion on systems issues and the latent errors that result from these systems-based problems. That being said, individual accountability should also remain important because patient safety is also compromised if there is a lack of individual accountability.

Automated reports in electronic medical records may also be used to find errors and complications. This is an active form of surveillance because the user can specify what types of events to look for over what time period. Another advantage is that, once these reports are built, little manpower is needed to run these automated reports. Drawbacks to this method of surveillance include a heavy reliance on what is documented in the electronic medical record, thus leading to high rates of false positives that may require manual chart review to validate each event or error. This leads to large amounts of data that must be manually sorted in order to improve the specificity of these reports.

Claims data are perhaps the most widely used form of complication detection and reporting in the neurosurgical literature. Many databases exist, such as the Nationwide Inpatient Sample, that are easily obtainable and codify patient complications with International Classification of Diseases, 9th and 10th Revisions (ICD-9, ICD-10) or Current Procedural Terminology (CPT) codes. However, this information is rarely complete (especially with regard to demographic data), and there are serious concerns about the accuracy of this coding, which is rarely done by physicians or health care workers who have physically seen the patient or taken part in the patient's care. Use of structured Agency for Healthcare Research and Quality indicators, which include events such as retained foreign bodies, postoperative wound dehiscence, and postoperative sepsis, was shown to have a high specificity of 98.5% but an abysmal sensitivity of 5.8%, showing that many adverse events are going underreported in such systems.[48]

Prospective databases and registries are increasingly used as methods for tracking adverse events associated with medical care. In surgery, the American College of Surgeons National Surgical Quality Improvement Program (NSQIP) database began tracking patients in 2005, and includes data from over 300 participating hospitals.[52,53] Cases are followed for a set of defined complications such as urinary tract infections, strokes, and thromboembolic events. The specially trained personnel responsible for entering data are frequently audited to ensure uniformity and accuracy. In neurosurgical patients, the NSQIP records complications in 14.3% of cases, with cranial patients 2.6 times more likely than spine patients to suffer a complication.[37] However, because the NSQIP addresses all surgical specialties, it fails to account for some complications specific to neurosurgery (e.g., spinal fluid leaks). Therefore, several databases dedicated solely to neurosurgery have been created, such as the National Neurosurgery Quality and Outcomes Database[54] and the International Spine Study Group,[55,56] which focuses on spinal deformity research. While these databases are successful in tracking complications and adverse events, they do not track errors, which is a major limitation.

Preventing Specific Errors and Complications

One standard method of not only identifying but also preventing subsequent specific errors and complications is through a root cause analysis (RCA). RCAs are typically performed by an interdisciplinary team, and are deliberate and comprehensive dissections of an error in a protected environment to discover all relevant facts to determine the underlying "root causes" of an error. RCA teams also design and implement risk reduction strategies to prevent subsequent similar errors from happening in the future. Lastly, effective RCA teams evaluate their changes over time and communicate the results of such change to the affected providers.

In addition, many other processes have been developed to address frequent and dangerous medical errors, such as adverse medication events and central line–associated infections. For neurosurgery in particular, three main areas of improvement are notable: preventing wrong-site, wrong-side, and wrong–spinal level surgeries; preventing postoperative infections; and examining volume-outcome relationships.

Wrong-Site Surgery and Checklists

Neurosurgery is the third most likely specialty to perform a wrong-site or wrong-level surgery, after orthopedic and general surgery,[38] with an estimated incidence of 2.2 wrong-side surgeries per 10,000 craniotomies.[39] Wrong-side and wrong-level surgeries are classified as "sentinel events" by The Joint Commission (formerly "never events"), and are reportable to the state in which they occur. When such events occur, they garner serious public scrutiny, cause severe patient harm, and often lead to costly litigation or settlements. The etiology of these adverse events in neurosurgery appears to stem largely from communication breakdown,[38] helping to bolster the argument for formalized time-out procedures and surgical checklists.

In response to similar worries across multiple surgical disciplines, the World Health Organization (WHO) developed a Surgical Safety Checklist in 2008 to improve team communication and ensure that critical preoperative steps were carried out.[30,31] The hypothesis was that the WHO formalized protocol would not only prevent wrong-site surgeries but also contribute to the reduction of other surgical complications, such as SSI, ventilator-associated pneumonia, and unplanned returns to the operating room. A multisite pilot study using the WHO checklist found a 4% reduction in complications and 0.7% reduction in mortality.[31] Subsequently, many neurosurgical programs have adopted similar checklists and time-out procedures[57] and have reported a consequent reduction in wrong-site surgeries.[58] The ability to prevent complications other than wrong-site surgery by using checklists has not been directly investigated in neurosurgical procedures, but strong evidence exists across multiple studies involving diverse surgical disciplines.[59] An important lesson of these processes is that the most successful method to prevent wrong-site surgeries is not solely under the control of the surgeon. An entire surgical team must be involved and leveraged to prevent these mistakes, an example of systems thinking. That is, while the surgeon is ultimately responsible for carrying out the wrong-site operation, the best way to prevent these errors in the future is by stepping back to understand the whole system in which the surgeon operates, rather than simply placing all the focus on the system's "sharp end," the surgeon.

Surgical Site Infections

SSIs are another costly adverse event suffered by neurosurgical patients, occurring in around 1% of cases and more frequently in spine than cranial cases.[37] Many techniques have been proposed to help prevent such infections. Preoperative antibiotics have long been shown to lower the risk of subsequent infection, as long as they are administered in a timely fashion.[60] This likely explains why preoperative checklists (see above) lead to reduced SSIs, because they act as reminders for this critical step. Other researchers have looked at techniques such as instilling vancomycin powder into wounds, particularly in spine cases. Meta-analyses suggest that vancomycin powder can reduce the odds of postoperative infection in spine surgery to 0.19 compared to surgeries without,[61,62] although these analyses compile nonrandomized trials and so will require further verification. Other techniques include substituting cyanoacrylate glue for staples,[63] negative pressure wound therapy,[64] irrigation with saline[65] or antibiotics,[66] and careful control of medical comorbidities such as diabetes.[60,65] Again, SSIs, like wrong-site surgeries, are best controlled through a systems approach. Checklists, operative techniques, and management of outpatient diseases such as diabetes all contribute to the prevention of disease.

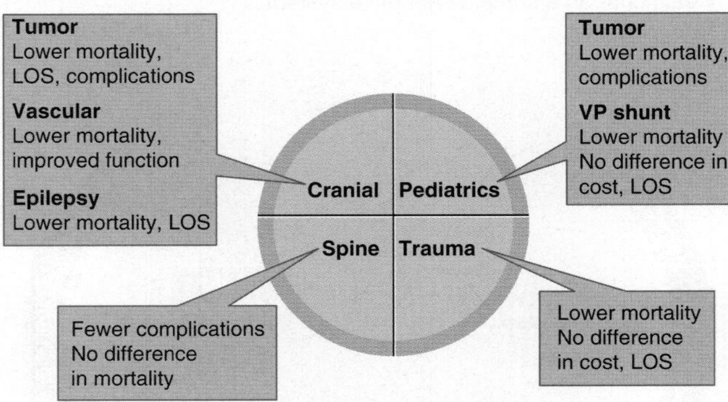

Figure 4-3. The volume-outcome relationship in neurosurgery. High-volume surgeons and hospitals have better outcomes with certain procedures, which argues for regionalization of care for several types of neurosurgical operative procedures. LOS, length of stay; VP, ventriculoperitoneal.

Volume-Outcome Relationships

Volume-outcome relationships refer to the often-noted effect of reduced morbidity and mortality at centers with high procedural volumes, at least when compared to low-volume centers. This effect has been observed in epilepsy surgery,[67] transsphenoidal surgery,[68] aneurysm surgery,[69] endovascular therapy,[70] carotid endarterectomy,[71] and spine surgery[72,73] (Fig. 4-3). The cause is frequently attributed to surgical provider practice, and evidence exists for such learning curves. For example, surgeons performing laparoscopic cholecystectomies have a 1.7% chance of causing an injury on their first surgery, compared to a 0.17% chance on their 50th.[74] Evidence for such learning curve effects exists in recent studies of neurosurgical procedures, such as vestibular schwannoma surgery,[75] transsphenoidal surgery,[76] and transforaminal lumbar interbody fusions.[77] However, another aspect of improving outcomes with higher volumes is dependent on the surrounding system—specialized anesthesia, nursing, hospital policies, scrub technicians, and the like. Again, it is the system as a whole that cares for the patient. To improve the patient's outcome, the entire system must be improved.

CONCLUSION

Medical errors contribute to an alarming number of deaths each year, and neurosurgery is not exempt from this. However, it is not enough for the surgeon to improve his or her technical skills, striving for perfection—nearly three quarters of neurosurgical errors are due to factors involving the health care system at large. Systems thinking is essential to enhancing patient safety. To improve patient safety, we must first document where errors and adverse events arise, through registries, incident reports, and global trigger tools, and then develop systems-level solutions to help prevent errors and mitigate them as they inevitably occur. As has been acknowledged in numerous other safety-conscious industries, humans will make mistakes. Blaming and shaming such practitioners does little to prevent these errors from recurring. Solutions must come from the system itself, targeting the entire organizational span of surgical practice, to truly improve patient safety.

SUGGESTED READINGS

Borchard A, Schwappach DL, Barbir A, et al. A systematic review of the effectiveness, compliance, and critical factors for implementation of safety checklists in surgery. *Ann Surg*. 2012;256:925-933.

Haynes AB, Weiser TG, Berry WR, et al. A surgical safety checklist to reduce morbidity and mortality in a global population. *N Engl J Med*. 2009;360:491-499.

Kohn LT, Corrigan J, Donaldson MS. *To Err is Human: Building a Safer Health System*. Washington, DC: National Academy Press; 2000.

McGirt MJ, Speroff T, Dittus RS, et al. The National Neurosurgery Quality and Outcomes Database (N2QOD): general overview and pilot-year project description. *Neurosurg Focus*. 2013;34:E6.

Mehtsun WT, Ibrahim AM, Diener-West M, et al. Surgical never events in the United States. *Surgery*. 2013;153:465-472.

Neily J, Mills PD, Young-Xu Y, et al. Association between implementation of a medical team training program and surgical mortality. *JAMA*. 2010;304:1693-1700.

Reason JT. *Human Error*. New York: Cambridge University Press; 1990.

Wachter RM. *Understanding Patient Safety*. 2nd ed. New York: McGraw Hill Medical; 2012.

See a full reference list on ExpertConsult.com

5 Neuroanesthesia: Preoperative Evaluation

Deepak Sharma and Arthur M. Lam

The preanesthetic evaluation is defined as the clinical assessment that precedes the delivery of anesthesia care for surgical and nonsurgical procedures.[1] The primary aim of preanesthetic evaluation is to minimize the overall patient morbidity associated with surgery and anesthesia. This aim is achieved by assessing the patient's medical condition and the balance between the anesthetic risk and surgical benefit, optimizing the medical condition within limitations of the surgical circumstances, and formulating the best possible anesthetic plan. Other benefits are improved safety of perioperative care, optimal resource utilization, and better outcomes and patient satisfaction.[1] With the changes in the health care delivery environment in the United States of America, the American Society of Anesthesiologists (ASA) has adopted the model of the Perioperative Surgical Home—a patient-centered, physician-led system of coordinated care striving for better health, better health care, and reduced costs of care (see Fig. 5-1).[2] The goal of this model is to create a better patient experience and make surgical care safer, more efficient, and more aligned in order to promote a better medical outcome at a lower cost. Appropriate preoperative evaluation of patients by anesthesiologists is a critical component of this model, which incorporates, among other things, efforts to reduce unnecessary interventions that do not have potential to benefit patients (e.g., routine preoperative laboratory studies) as well as efforts to reduce cancellations and the length of postoperative hospital stays.[3] Preoperative consultation with an anesthesiologist has, in fact, become increasingly common and has shown some clear benefit in perioperative care and outcomes[4]; it has the potential to further decrease the cost of unnecessary routine "medical consultations," which are driven by highly variable clinical and nonclinical factors.[5] The preanesthetic evaluation, therefore, is critical and its broad objectives include the following:

1. Establishment of rapport with the patient and immediate family members/significant others in order to minimize their anxiety and to have a cooperative and relaxed patient.
2. Provision of information to the patient and family regarding anesthetic techniques and procedures and the associated risks and benefits, postoperative management issues including pain control, and the possible need for postoperative mechanical ventilation in major procedure.
3. Complete review of medical, surgical, and anesthetic history and current medications, thus establishing a baseline profile.
4. Review of relevant personal, family, and social history and history of allergies.
5. General physical examination, including recording of vital signs and examination of individual systems, particularly the nervous and cardiopulmonary systems.
6. Interpretation of relevant laboratory data, arrangements for further investigations and consultations if deemed necessary, and elimination of unnecessary preoperative standing "screening tests," to limit investigations to only appropriate ones.
7. Optimization of the patient's physiologic condition.
8. Stratification of patient risk regarding morbidity and mortality based on the preceding considerations.
9. Formulation of an anesthetic plan, organization of resources for perioperative care, and postoperative recovery.
10. Documentation of informed consent for the proposed anesthetic technique and procedures.

The preanesthetic evaluation may be performed well in advance of the planned surgery for most elective procedures during a visit to the preanesthetic evaluation clinics. It may be performed at the bedside in the hospital ward or intensive care unit the "night before" for inpatients. For urgent and emergency procedures, a brief, focused preanesthetic evaluation is performed just before surgery. The consensus of the ASA Task Force on Preanesthesia Evaluation is that an initial record review, patient interview, and physical examination should be performed prior to the day of surgery for patients with high severity of disease.[1] Of the patients with low severity of disease, those undergoing procedures with high surgical invasiveness should have the interview and physical examination prior to the day of surgery; those undergoing procedures with medium or low surgical invasiveness may be interviewed and examined on or before the day of surgery.[1] Although the task force cautions that timing of such assessments may not be practical with the limitation of resources, it recommends that at a minimum, the preanesthetic examination should include an assessment of the airway, lungs, and heart, with documentation of vital signs.[1]

These preanesthetic evaluation clinics have been shown to improve operating room efficiency and minimize unexpected delays and cancellations due to poorly prepared patients.[6,7] It has been shown that the preoperative conditions of patients predict their postoperative mortality and morbidity.[8-11] In one study, the preoperative evaluation of patients led to a change in the proposed anesthetic plan in up to 15% of healthy individuals and 20% of ill patients.[12] In a study from Stanford University, implementation of the preanesthetic evaluation clinic produced an 87.9% reduction in day-of-surgery cancellations.[7] It is estimated that \$30 to \$40 billion is spent annually on preoperative testing and subsequent follow-up in North America alone, of which 50% could be saved by the appropriate and selective ordering of tests.[13] In one study, implementation of the preoperative evaluation clinic, in which the ordering of tests was at the anesthesiologist's request, resulted in a savings of \$112.09 per patient. This figure was equated with an annual potential saving of more than \$1.01 million at one institution.[7] As the concept of Perioperative Surgical Home evolves (Fig. 5-1), and anesthesiologists assumes the role of perioperative physicians, the preanesthetic evaluation constitutes an importance process of the perioperative continuum. In short, the preanesthetic evaluation is critical to ensure patient safety, good surgical outcomes, patient satisfaction, and reduction of health care costs. It is crucial, therefore, that a timely preanesthetic evaluation be planned for all neurosurgical patients.

GENERAL PREANESTHETIC EVALUATION

During the preanesthetic evaluation, the effects of anesthesia, positioning, surgery, and postoperative pain must be considered in relation to the individual patient's surgical state and medications. The patient's preexisting medical condition, which may be unrelated to the proposed surgical procedure, may require more intense scrutiny than the pathologic process being treated. The ASA classification of physical status is a universally accepted system used for stratification of the patient's preexisting health status (Table 5-1). Although it does not take into account the surgical risk and is not primarily designed for outcome prediction, this system's classifications correlate with perioperative morbidity and mortality.[14-16] In fact, ASA physical status classes 3

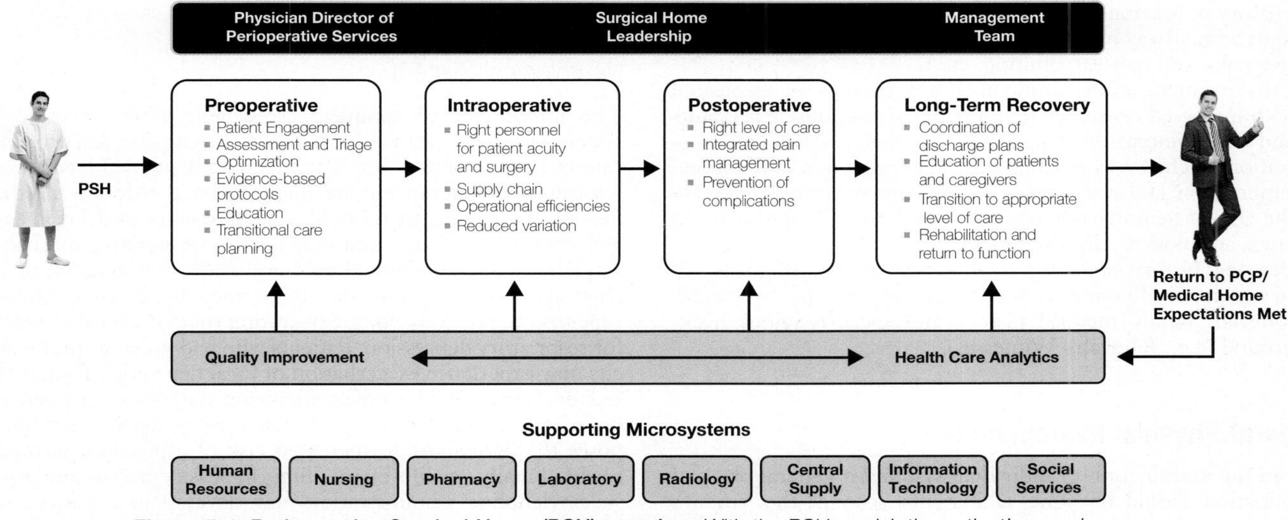

Figure 5-1. Perioperative Surgical Home (PSH) overview. With the PSH model, the patient's experience of care is coordinated by a director of perioperative services, additional surgical home leadership, and supportive personnel, all of whom constitute an interdisciplinary team. The expected metrics include improved operational efficiencies, decreased resource utilization, a reduction in length of stay and readmission, and a decrease in complications and mortality—resulting in a better patient experience of care. PCP, primary care provider. *(Figure developed by Dr. Daniel J. Cole, UCLA David Geffen School of Medicine for the American Society of Anesthesiologists, 1061 American Lane, Schaumburg, IL 60173-4973 or online at https://www.asahq.org/psh. © ASA.)*

TABLE 5-1 American Society of Anesthesiologists (ASA) Classification of Physical Status

ASA Physical Status Classification	Definition	Examples (Including but Not Limited to)
1	A normal healthy patient	Healthy, nonsmoking, no or minimal alcohol use
2	A patient with mild systemic disease	Mild diseases only without substantive functional limitations. Examples include (but not limited to) current smoker, social alcohol drinker, pregnancy, obesity (30 < BMI < 40), well-controlled DM/HTN, mild lung disease.
3	A patient with severe systemic disease	Substantive functional limitations; one or more moderate to severe diseases. Examples include (but not limited to) poorly controlled DM or HTN, COPD, morbid obesity (BMI ≥40), active hepatitis, alcohol dependence or abuse, implanted pacemaker, moderate reduction of ejection fraction, ESRD undergoing regularly scheduled dialysis, premature infant PCA <60 wk, history (>3 mo) of MI, CVA, TIA, or CAD/stents.
4	A patient with severe systemic disease that is a constant threat to life	Examples include (but not limited to) recent (<3 mo) MI, CVA, TIA, or CAD/stents, ongoing cardiac ischemia or severe valve dysfunction, severe reduction of ejection fraction, sepsis, DIC, ARDS, or ESRD not undergoing regularly scheduled dialysis.
5	A moribund patient who is not expected to survive without the operation	Examples include (but not limited to) ruptured abdominal/thoracic aneurysm, massive trauma, intracranial bleed with mass effect, ischemic bowel in the face of significant cardiac pathology or multiple organ/system dysfunction.
6	A patient who has been declared brain-dead and whose organs are being removed for donor purposes	

Excerpted from the *Relative Value Guide 2016* of the American Society of Anesthesiologists. A copy of the full text can be obtained from ASA, 1061 American Lane, Schaumburg, IL 60173-4973 or online at www.asahq.org.

ARDS, acute respiratory distress syndrome; BMI, body mass index; CAD, coronary artery disease; COPD, chronic obstructive pulmonary disease; CVA, cerebrovascular accident (stroke); DIC, disseminated intravascular coagulation; DM, diabetes mellitus; ESRD, end-stage renal disease; HTN, hypertension; MI, myocardial infarction; PCA, postconceptional age; TIA, transient ischemic attack.

through 5 independently predict perioperative cardiovascular complications in patients undergoing intracranial surgery and are also risk factors for perioperative mortality.[11]

Careful evaluation of the patient rates the severity of medical problems as well as detects risks for asymptomatic disease. A good starting point is the primary disease process requiring surgical intervention, which may alert the anesthesiologist to potential problems, such as trauma and a full stomach, head injury and the development of coagulopathy, and intracranial aneurysm and the need for blood pressure control. Thereafter, the evaluation should focus on each system. The specific neurosurgical aspects are discussed separately later in this chapter. The general approach is summarized here.

Medical History

The medical history part of the preanesthetic evaluation involves the following areas:

1. Medical history related to intended surgical procedure and other constitutional diseases that may or may not have a bearing on the intended procedure.

2. History of previous surgery and anesthesia (insight into problems with airway management, intravenous access, postoperative pain, and nausea/vomiting, etc.).
3. Current medications (anticonvulsant therapy is associated with increased resistance to nondepolarizing muscle relaxants and hence, increased requirement for them; steroid administration might be associated with hyperglycemia and adrenal suppression; and antiplatelets or anticoagulants would increase the risk of hemorrhagic complications) and allergies (e.g., to latex, antibiotics, adhesive tape).
4. Personal history (smoking, alcohol, recreational drug use—all of which have bearing on anesthesia and intraoperative care).
5. Relevant family medical history and social/religious background (e.g., Jehovah's Witnesses).

General Physical Examination

Before the examination of individual systems, a general physical examination should be done, taking into account the patient's level of consciousness, mental status, build, nutrition, and vital parameters. Patients with malignant tumors and those with high cervical lesions might be emaciated with significantly reduced muscle mass. On the other hand, obesity might be coexisting in many patients. Obese individuals have increased likelihood of associated diabetes, hypertension, coronary artery disease, restrictive lung disease, sleep apnea, and gastroesophageal reflux, which might warrant alteration in anesthetic plan. Difficulty in tracheal intubation may be encountered more frequently in obese than in lean individuals,[17] and the pharmacologic profile of anesthetic agents may also be altered.[18] Some neurosurgical patients might be dehydrated owing to reduced intake of fluids (because of impaired consciousness) or vomiting, or because of the use of diuretics and contrast agents. Correction of significant dehydration before induction of anesthesia can prevent post-induction hypotension in such patients. Significant blood loss is a possibility in surgery for intracranial aneurysms, arteriovenous malformations, vascular tumors, craniosynostoses, and extensive spine procedures. Preanesthetic evaluation should look for preexisting anemia and target to correct it preoperatively or arrange for intraoperative transfusion on a case-by-case basis. Recording of preoperative vital parameters (heart rate, blood pressure) provides baseline values for intraoperative management, this being particularly important in procedures requiring strict hemodynamic control (e.g., in aneurysms and arteriovenous malformations).

Perhaps the most crucial aspect of general examination is assessment of the patient's airway. Inadequate management of the airway may adversely affect the neurological outcome. Routine maneuvers used for airway management may worsen spinal instability in patients with cervical lesions and may lead to increased intracranial pressure with potentially devastating consequence in patients with decreased intracranial compliance. Hence, the patient's airway should be assessed carefully for ease of ventilation and difficulty in tracheal intubation, in consideration with specific surgical needs such as hemodynamic stability and spinal immobilization. Mallampati scoring,[19] thyromental distance, presence of overbite or underbite, and neck flexion and extension collectively provide an estimate of the risk of difficult intubation.[20] Some specific patients in whom difficult airway should be anticipated include patients with recent supratentorial craniotomy, in whom the mouth opening might be significantly reduced secondary to ankylosis of temporomandibular joint,[21] acromegalic patients undergoing pituitary surgery,[22] and patients with cervical spine lesions. Recognition of potential airway difficulty allows proper planning with accessory equipment and resources as well as formulation of backup plans, leading to improved patient safety and efficient use of operating time.

Assessment of System Functions

Neurological System

The importance of complete assessment of the neurological system of a patient scheduled for a major neurosurgical procedure cannot be overemphasized. Patients with depressed level of consciousness preoperatively are likely to have reduced anesthetic need for induction, are more likely to have slow or delayed emergence from anesthesia, and may need postoperative mechanical ventilation. Such patients should not receive any sedative or narcotic agent as premedication unless they are under continuous supervision, preferably in the operating room itself with vigilance for respiratory depression. Patients who had previous motor deficits may experience exacerbation of focal neurological signs after sedative doses of benzodiazepines and narcotics.[23] Presence of brainstem lesions and/or lower cranial nerve dysfunction predisposes the patient to an increased risk of aspiration postoperatively. Finally, a life-threatening hyperkalemia secondary to succinylcholine administration may develop in a patient with preexisting motor deficits.[24] Succinylcholine has also been reported to cause hyperkalemia in patients with ruptured cerebral aneurysms independent of the presence of motor nerve disturbances,[25] although this event appears to be uncommon. Elevated intracranial pressure often manifests as headache with nausea and vomiting but can also lead to olfactory nerve dysfunction with loss of sense of smell. Unilateral uncal herniation would result in a dilated unresponsive ipsilateral pupil, which should be distinguished from incidental anisocoria and from unilateral third nerve palsy due to compression by a space-occupying lesion. Limitations of the field of vision in patients with pituitary and other suprasellar tumors should be documented for postoperative comparison. Dysfunction of the trigeminal nerve or facial nerve may interfere with mask ventilation and tracheal intubation. A patient with a damaged vagus nerve may present with a hoarse voice secondary to vocal cord paralysis and may be at increased risk of airway obstruction.

The patient with a history of recent stroke presents a challenging problem. With the exception of a patient scheduled for emergency carotid endarterectomy or carotid stenting to prevent an impending stroke, patients with recent stroke are generally advised to wait for 60 days for an elective surgical procedure (an approach similar to that used after a recent myocardial infarction). However, a recent observational population study suggests that the risk of cardiovascular morbidity and mortality does not plateau until 9 months after a stroke.[26] For urgent but not emergency neurological procedures, the risks and benefits must be weighed carefully together with patient input for determination of the optimal time for surgery.

Respiratory System

The risk of perioperative respiratory complications is increased in the presence of preexisting obstructive or restrictive pulmonary disease. Perioperative hypoxemia or hypercapnia is more likely to occur and can aggravate an already compromised cardiorespiratory status. The patient with associated pulmonary disease requires an assessment of baseline status, and any element of potential reversibility should be addressed.[27-29] Smoking is a common important risk factor for both cardiovascular disease and pulmonary disease and is associated with a threefold increase in perioperative morbidity. Cessation of smoking for 6 to 8 weeks before surgery is recommended for reactivation of mucociliary clearance, but cessation for as little as 24 hours can reduce the carboxyhemoglobin levels and improve oxygenation.[29] The presence of reactive airway disease indicates an increased risk of bronchospasm with airway manipulation and tracheal extubation as well as an increased risk of coughing and laryngospasm during emergence from anesthesia. In patients with symptomatic obstructive pulmonary disease, preoperative pulmonary function testing before and after bronchodilators and arterial blood gas sampling allow assessment of reversibility and determination of optimal preparation. Abnormally high $Paco_2$ or low Po_2 before surgery is predictive of postoperative respiratory complications and may warrant elective postoperative mechanical ventilation after a major neurosurgical procedure. In the patient with sleep apnea who is using a continuous positive airway pressure (CPAP) device at home, it is important to ensure that the same device is available in the recovery area and afterward.

Preoperative management of upper respiratory tract infection in children is controversial because the effects of the infection on the airway last for 2 to 4 weeks after clinical resolution. The patient is at increased risk of perioperative respiratory morbidity during this period.[30] Postponement of elective surgery must be balanced against the risk of progressive neurological disability or the occurrence of a potentially catastrophic complication during the waiting period.

Patients with decreased levels of consciousness due to intracranial pathology and those with high spinal lesion or lower cranial nerve paralysis might have preexisting, preoperative atelectasis, which puts them at increased risk of requiring postoperative mechanical ventilation. Aspiration pneumonitis and/or superimposed pneumonia can also occur. A restrictive pattern of lung disease often occurs in patients with preoperative craniovertebral junction anomalies that persists in the postoperative period.[31] In their systematic review of preoperative pulmonary risk stratification for noncardiothoracic surgery for the American College of Physicians, Smetana and colleagues found good evidence to support the following patient-related risk factors as predictive of postoperative pulmonary complications: advanced age, ASA class 2 or higher, functional dependence, chronic obstructive pulmonary disease (COPD), and congestive heart failure.[32] They also found fair evidence indicating increases in risk with the presence of impaired sensorium, abnormal findings on chest examination, cigarette use, alcohol use, and weight loss.[32] Although asthma is not a risk factor if well controlled, the perioperative risk may be increased the disease it is poorly controlled.[32] Important procedure-related risk factors include neurosurgery, emergency surgery, and prolonged surgery.[32] The value of preoperative testing to estimate pulmonary risk is controversial. An abnormal chest radiograph does indicate an increased risk for postoperative pulmonary complications and spirometry may provide some risk stratification, but among potential laboratory tests to stratify risk, a serum albumin level less than 35 g/L is the most powerful predictor.[32]

Cardiovascular System

Hemodynamic stability is important to avoid adverse neurological effects in neurosurgical patients. The presence of cardiovascular disease significantly increases anesthesia risk and optimizing the patient's condition can significantly improve outcome. Major adverse cardiac event (MACE) after noncardiac surgery is often associated with prior coronary artery disease (CAD). The stability and timing of a recent myocardial infarction (MI) affect the incidence of perioperative morbidity and mortality. The rate of postoperative MI and 30-day mortality decrease substantially as the length of time from first MI to operation increases. Most data indicate that 60 days or more should elapse after an MI before noncardiac surgery, in the absence of a preoperative coronary intervention.

Patients with hypertension often have reduced plasma volume, making them more susceptible to the systemic vasodilatory effects of anesthetic agents, so cardiovascular instability and labile blood pressure occur intraoperatively. Moreover, in chronic hypertension, increased cerebrovascular resistance causes the lower and upper limits of cerebral blood flow (CBF) autoregulation to shift to higher pressure levels, leading to poor tolerance of acute hypotension.[33,34] However, adaptive hypertensive changes in CBF autoregulation may be reversible with adequate control of blood pressure.[33,34]

Left ventricular dysfunction with symptoms of cardiac failure indicates significantly reduced cardiac output, which can worsen with general anesthesia. In fact, patients with heart failure may have a higher 30-day postoperative mortality rate than those with atrial fibrillation or coronary artery disease (CAD).[35] Mannitol must be used carefully and judiciously or not at all in the presence of left ventricular failure. Patients on long-term beta blocker therapy who are to undergo surgery should continue taking the agents.[35,36] Particular attention should be paid to the need to modify or temporarily discontinue beta blockers as clinical circumstances (e.g., hypotension, bradycardia, bleeding) dictate.[35,36] In patients in whom intermediate- or high-risk MI is noted in preoperative risk stratification tests, it may be reasonable to begin perioperative beta blockers. However, beta blocker therapy should not be started on the day of surgery.[35] The overall risk for a cardiac patient undergoing a noncardiac procedure is assessed with the Revised Cardiac Risk Index (RCRI).[8] According to this index, the presence of three or more of the following factors is associated with a major cardiac event risk of 11%: (1) high-risk surgery, (2) history of ischemic heart disease, (3) history of congestive heart failure, (4) history of cerebrovascular disease, (5) preoperative treatment with insulin, and (6) preoperative serum creatinine value greater than 2.0 mg/dL.[8]

Preoperative cardiac evaluation must be carefully tailored to the circumstances and nature of the surgical illness. The 2014 update of the American College of Cardiology/American Heart Association (ACC/AHA) guidelines on perioperative cardiovascular evaluation and care for noncardiac surgery defines urgency of surgery in the context of perioperative risk.[35] An *emergency* procedure is one in which life or limb is threatened if the patient is not in the operating room and the time for clinical evaluation is limited, typically less than 6 hours. For an *urgent* procedure, 6 to 24 hours may be available for a limited clinical evaluation. A *time-sensitive* procedure is one in which a delay of more than 1 week to 6 weeks to allow for an evaluation and significant changes in management would negatively affect outcome. An *elective* procedure is one that could be delayed for up to 1 year. A *low-risk* procedure is one in which the combined surgical and patient characteristics predict the risk of a MACE such as death or MI to be less than 1%. Procedures with a risk of MACE of 1% or more are considered to have an *elevated risk*. Moreover, new tools have been created by the American College of Surgeons, which prospectively collected data on operations performed in more than 525 participating hospitals in the United States and data on more than 1 million operations to create the risk calculators (www.riskcalculator.facs.org or www.surgicalriskcalculator.com). Importantly, anesthesia and surgery are increasingly becoming safer, and this development affects the subjective "readiness" of a patient with cardiac disease for noncardiac surgery, including neurosurgery. For instance, the cardiac risk for patients with significant aortic stenosis (AS) in undergoing noncardiac surgery has substantially declined. Consequently, according to the current recommendations, it is reasonable to perform elevated-risk elective noncardiac surgery with use of appropriate intraoperative and postoperative hemodynamic monitoring in patients with asymptomatic severe AS.[35] Likewise, elevated-risk elective noncardiac surgery with use of appropriate intraoperative and postoperative hemodynamic monitoring is now considered reasonable in asymptomatic patients with severe mitral stenosis if valve morphology is not favorable for percutaneous mitral balloon commissurotomy.[35]

Functional status is a reliable predictor of cardiac events, both perioperatively and over the long term. Patients with reduced preoperative functional status are at increased risk of complications. Conversely, those with good preoperative functional status are at lower risk. Moreover, in highly functional asymptomatic patients, it is often appropriate to proceed with planned surgery without further cardiovascular testing. If a patient has not had a recent exercise test before noncardiac surgery, functional status can usually be estimated from activities of daily living, often expressed in terms of metabolic equivalents (METs).[35] Perioperative cardiac and long-term risks are increased in patients unable to perform 4 METs of work during daily activities.[35] Examples of activities associated with more than 4 METs are climbing a flight of stairs or walking up a hill, walking on level ground at 4 mph, and performing heavy work around the house. In an acute surgical emergency, preoperative evaluation might have to be limited to simple and critical tests (like rapid clinical assessment, hematocrit, electrolytes, renal function, and electrocardiogram [ECG]), with a more extensive evaluation conducted after surgery. In patients in whom coronary revascularization is not an option, it is often not necessary to perform a noninvasive stress test. In general, preoperative tests are recommended only if the information obtained will result in a change in the surgical procedure performed, a change in medical therapy or monitoring during or after surgery, or a postponement of surgery until the cardiac condition can be corrected or stabilized. A cardiologist consultation should be sought if deemed necessary and if surgical circumstances allow. Preoperative evaluation by the cardiologist may involve changes in medication, additional preoperative tests or procedures, or recommendations for higher levels of postoperative care.

On the basis of the available evidence and expert opinion, the 2014 ACC/AHA guidelines recommend an algorithmic approach to perioperative cardiac assessment, which may be conveniently described in the following steps[35]:

Step 1: In patients scheduled for surgery with known CAD or risk factors for it, the urgency of surgery should be determined. If emergency, surgery should proceed with appropriate monitoring and management strategies.

Step 2: If the surgery is urgent or elective, determine whether the patient has an acute coronary syndrome. If yes, the patient should be referred for cardiology evaluation and management.

Step 3: If the patient has risk factors for stable CAD, the perioperative risk of a MACE is estimated on the basis of the combined clinical/surgical risk using the American College of Surgeons risk calculator or incorporating the RCRI.

Step 4: If the patient has less than a 1% risk of a MACE, no further testing is needed and surgery may proceed.

Step 5: If the patient is at elevated risk of a MACE, functional capacity is determined. If the functional capacity is 4 METs or higher, surgery can proceed without further evaluation.

Step 6: If the patient's functional capacity, is less than 4 METs or is unknown, the need for further testing depends on the possibility that the test results will affect patient decision making (e.g., decision to have original surgery or willingness to undergo cardiac intervention, depending on the results of the test). In patients with unknown functional capacity, it may be reasonable to perform exercise stress testing. If the result is abnormal, cardiac intervention may have to be considered prior to either the planned surgery or to an alternative noninvasive treatment of the indication for surgery (e.g., radiation therapy). If the result is normal, surgery should proceed.

Step 7: If testing is unlikely to impact decision making, surgery should proceed or alternative noninvasive treatment of the indication for surgery may be considered.

The guidelines also recommend that elective noncardiac surgery should be delayed 14 days after balloon angioplasty, 30 days after bare metal stent implantation, and 365 days after drug-eluting stent implantation (but may be considered after 180 days of implantation of a drug-eluting stent if the risk of further delay is greater than the expected risks of ischemia and stent thrombosis).[35] In patients undergoing urgent noncardiac surgery during the first 4 to 6 weeks after bare metal or drug-eluting stent implantation, dual antiplatelet therapy should be continued unless the relative risk of bleeding outweighs the benefit of preventing stent thrombosis.[35] In patients undergoing surgical procedures that mandate the discontinuation of platelet receptor–inhibitor therapy, it is recommended that aspirin therapy be continued if possible.[35] In patients undergoing nonemergency or nonurgent noncardiac surgery who have not had previous coronary stenting, it may be reasonable to continue aspirin therapy when the risk of potential increased cardiac events outweighs the risk of increased bleeding.

Gastrointestinal System

Patients at risk of aspiration include those with full stomachs, bowel obstruction, and gastroesophageal reflux. Patients with dysfunction involving the 9th or the 10th cranial nerve as well as those with decreased level of consciousness are also at risk if they have not been fasting. In these patients, general anesthesia should be induced via a rapid sequence with cricoid pressure to minimize the risk of aspiration. Morbidly obese patients also have a higher incidence of hiatal hernia and/or gastroesophageal reflux and of larger volume of residual gastric volume despite fasting.

Renal System

Patients presenting for neurosurgical intervention sometimes have coexistent renal dysfunction, which might be acute or chronic. Patients with renal disease pose an anesthetic challenge because they may have autonomic neuropathy, encephalopathy, fluid retention (congestive heart failure, pleural effusion, ascites) and yet intravascular volume depletion, hypertension, metabolic acidosis, electrolyte imbalances (hyperkalemia, hyponatremia, hypocalcemia), anemia, and delayed gastric emptying, among other manifestations. The generalized effects of azotemia mandate a thorough evaluation of the patient in renal failure. Signs of fluid overload or hypovolemia should be sought. Hematocrit, serum electrolytes, coagulation studies, blood urea nitrogen (BUN), and creatinine measurements are advisable. A chest radiograph and arterial blood gas analysis might be required in patients with breathlessness, and an ECG should be examined for signs of hyperkalemia or hypocalcemia as well as ischemia and conduction blocks. Severely anemic patients may require preoperative red blood cell transfusions. Preoperative drug therapy should be carefully reviewed for drugs with significant renal elimination. Dosage adjustments and measurements of blood levels are sometimes necessary to prevent drug toxicity.

Intravascular volume depletion, contrast dye injections, aminoglycoside antibiotics, angiotensin-converting enzyme inhibitors, and nonsteroidal antiinflammatory drugs (NSAIDs) are risk factors for an acute deterioration in renal function and must be avoided. Hypovolemia appears to be a particularly important factor in the development of acute postoperative renal failure. The emphasis in management of patients with these risk factors is on prevention because of the high mortality associated with postoperative renal failure. Optimal management may require preoperative dialysis in select situations, the usual indications being severe acidosis or volume overload, hyperkalemia, metabolic encephalopathy, and drug toxicity. Volume status is often difficult to assess and may necessitate invasive monitoring, including placement of intra-arterial and central venous pressure catheters. Neuromuscular blocking agents not dependent on renal function for their elimination should be selected. Mannitol is contraindicated in anuric patients. Postoperative mechanical ventilation is sometimes required in patients with renal failure because inadequate spontaneous ventilation with progressive hypercapnia can result in respiratory acidosis that may exacerbate preexisting acidosis, lead to potentially severe circulatory depression, and dangerously increase serum potassium concentration.

Hematologic System

Intracranial hemorrhage is a potentially lethal catastrophe. Thus, any bleeding tendency should be investigated thoroughly and corrected preoperatively. If deemed necessary, appropriate clotting factors and platelets should be made available at the time of surgery.[37] Patients taking NSAIDs such as aspirin should stop their medications for a week before intracranial surgery.[38] This decision may have to be modified in patients with transient ischemic attacks, in whom the risks of discontinuation may exceed the benefits.

Endocrine System

Patients with diabetes mellitus presenting for surgery require special attention because hyperglycemia is associated with hyperosmolarity, infection, and poor wound healing. More importantly, it may worsen neurological outcome after an episode of cerebral ischemia. Nonetheless, hypoglycemia is also detrimental because the brain depends on glucose for its energy supply. Close perioperative monitoring of glucose is therefore essential, and treatment with insulin is often required to maintain euglycemia, although sulfonylureas and metformin should not be used for 24 to 48 hours before surgery because of their long half-lives. The perioperative morbidity of diabetic patients is related to preoperative end-organ damage. Hence, the pulmonary, cardiovascular, and renal systems should be carefully examined. Diabetic patients have an increased incidence of ST segment and T-wave segment abnormalities on ECG, and myocardial ischemia may be evident despite a negative history (silent myocardial ischemia). Diabetic autonomic neuropathy may predispose patients to cardiovascular instability and even sudden cardiac death. Furthermore, autonomic dysfunction contributes to gastroparesis, which may require preoperative treatment with histamine-2 (H_2) blockers and/or metoclopramide. Chronic hyperglycemia can lead to glycosylation of tissue proteins and a stiff joint syndrome. Diabetic patients, especially those with type I diabetes, should be routinely evaluated preoperatively for adequate temporomandibular joint and cervical spine mobility to help anticipate difficult intubations.[39]

Glucocorticoid excess (Cushing's syndrome) in the neurosurgical setting may be exogenous (due to administration of steroid hormones) or endogenous (due to hypersecretion by a pituitary adenoma; Cushing's disease); it is characterized by muscle wasting and weakness, osteoporosis, truncal obesity, abdominal striae, glucose intolerance, hypertension, and mental status changes. Patients with Cushing's syndrome tend to be volume overloaded and have hypokalemic metabolic alkalosis resulting from the mineralocorticoid activity of glucocorticoids, which should be corrected preoperatively. Patients with osteoporosis are at risk for fractures during positioning, whereas preoperative weakness may indicate an increased sensitivity to neuromuscular blocking agents. On the other hand, acute adrenal insufficiency can be triggered in steroid-dependent patients who do not receive supplemental doses during the perioperative period.

Elective neurosurgical procedures should be undertaken in the patient with hyperthyroidism or hypothyroidism when the patient is clinically and chemically euthyroid with medical treatment. However, mild to moderate hypothyroidism is not an absolute contraindication to surgery. Antithyroid medications and beta blockers are continued through the morning of surgery in hyperthyroid patients and thyroid hormone supplements in hypothyroid patients (though most thyroid preparations have long half-lives). If emergency surgery must proceed in a hyperthyroid patient, the hyperdynamic circulation can be controlled by titration of esmolol infusion. Possibility of associated myopathies and myasthenia gravis should be considered in hyperthyroid patients. Hypothyroid patients, on the other hand, are very prone to drug-induced respiratory depression and usually do not require much preoperative sedation. Premedication with H_2 antagonists and metoclopramide may be considered because of delayed gastric-emptying times. Other potential problems with hypothyroidism include hypoglycemia, anemia, hyponatremia, difficult intubation due to a large tongue, and hypothermia from a low basal metabolic rate. Emergence from anesthesia may be delayed in hypothyroid patients because of hypothermia, respiratory depression, or slowed drug biotransformation.

Laboratory Investigations

According to the ASA Task Force on Preanesthesia Evaluation,[1] preoperative tests may be ordered, required, or performed selectively on the basis of clinical characteristics for purposes of guiding or optimizing perioperative management. Preoperative resting 12-lead ECG is reasonable for patients with known coronary heart disease, significant arrhythmia, peripheral arterial disease, cerebrovascular disease, or other significant structural heart disease, except for those undergoing low-risk surgery. Routine preoperative resting 12-lead ECG is not useful for asymptomatic patients.[1,35] Chest radiographs may be required in smokers and in patients with recent upper respiratory infection, chronic obstructive pulmonary disease, or cardiac disease.[1] Measurements of hemoglobin or hematocrit and of serum glucose and electrolytes as well as coagulation studies are indicated in most neurosurgical patients, and blood levels of phenytoin may sometimes be required. For all intracranial procedures, blood should be typed and crossmatched; for minor neurosurgical procedures, blood should be at least typed and screened.

Hormone assays are often ordered in patients with endocrinopathies. Urinalysis is not indicated when urinary tract symptoms are absent. Pregnancy testing should be considered for all female patients of childbearing age, especially when pregnancy history is not clear or is suggestive of current pregnancy.[1] The ASA Task Force suggests that test results obtained from the medical record that have been performed within 6 months of surgery are generally acceptable if the patient's medical history has not changed substantially, but that more recent test results may be desirable when the medical history has changed or when test results may play a role in the selection of a specific anesthetic technique.[1] Patients with dyspnea of unknown origin and patients with heart failure with worsening dyspnea or other change in clinical status may need preoperative evaluation of left ventricular function.[35]

CONSIDERATION OF SPECIFIC NEUROLOGICAL DISORDERS

The principles of general assessment of neurosurgical patient have been summarized previously. In this section specific considerations of distinct neurological disorders and procedures are discussed. There is a considerable overlap among these situations and so a discussion pertinent to all neurosurgical patients is followed by a procedure-specific summary.

General Principles and Normal Cerebrovascular Physiology

The normal brain is a metabolically active organ that receives 14% of cardiac output while consuming 20% of the oxygen intake. Its blood flow is coupled to metabolic needs, both globally and regionally. The homeostatic mechanism of autoregulation keeps the CBF relatively constant at approximately 50 mL/100 g/min over a wide range of cerebral perfusion pressures (CPPs) (50 to 150 mm Hg), although the actual limits of autoregulation vary among healthy individuals.[40] The CPP is related to both mean arterial pressure and intracranial pressure (ICP). The latter depends on cerebral blood volume (CBV), brain mass, cerebrospinal fluid (CSF) volume, and central venous pressure. CBF is profoundly influenced by $Paco_2$ and, to a smaller extent, Pao_2. Within the physiologic range of 20 to 60 mm Hg, CBF changes by 3% to 4% per mm Hg change in CO_2 tension, with an accompanying decrease in CBV. The CO_2 reactivity is brisk and occurs within seconds of the change in arterial $PaCO_2$.

Thus, acute hyperventilation can reduce both CBV and ICP. However, excessive hyperventilation may cause iatrogenic ischemia. Prolonged change in systemic CO_2 tension is accompanied by active transport of bicarbonate in or out of CSF to restore a normal acid-base balance. Therefore, the effects of hyperventilation on CBF are not sustained beyond 24 hours. Hypoxemia causes vasodilation of the cerebral vessels and an increase in CBF, but this does not occur until the Pao_2 is less than 50 mm Hg. Neurosurgical patients may have one or more impaired homeostatic mechanisms. Cerebral metabolism is depressed in a patient with altered level of consciousness, ICP may be elevated, cerebral blood flow–cerebral metabolic rate (CBF-CMR) coupling may be lost, autoregulation may be impaired, and the blood-brain barrier may be disrupted. Except in severe injury, CO_2 reactivity is usually preserved.

Anesthetic techniques also affect cerebral physiology. Intravenous anesthetic agents, including thiopental and propofol,[41] are indirect cerebral vasoconstrictors, reducing cerebral metabolism and causing a corresponding reduction in CBF. Both autoregulation[42] and CO_2 reactivity[41] are preserved. Ketamine is a weak noncompetitive NMDA (*N*-methyl-D-aspartate) antagonist that has sympathomimetic properties. Its cerebral effects are complex and are partly dependent on the action of other concurrently administered drugs. For example, concurrent administration of benzodiazapines[43] or inhalation anesthetics[44] would eliminate any cerebrostimulatory or vasodilatory actions. Etomidate lowers the cerebral metabolic rate, CBF, and ICP. At the same time, because of minimal cardiovascular effects, CPP is well maintained. Although changes on electroencephalography (EEG) caused by etomidate resemble those associated with barbiturates, etomidate enhances somatosensory evoked potentials[45] and causes less reduction of motor evoked potential amplitudes than thiopental or propofol.[46] However, it may reduce brain tissue oxygen tension. Dexmedetomidine is a highly selective α_2-adrenoreceptor agonist that achieves sedation without causing respiratory depression, does not interfere with electrophysiologic mapping except when used in higher doses, and provides hemodynamic stability. It has been found to be particularly useful for implantation of deep brain stimulators in patients with Parkinson's disease[47] and for awake craniotomies,[48] when sophisticated neurologic testing is required. CBF-CMR coupling is preserved during dexmedetomidine administration in human volunteers.[49]

The cerebral effects of inhaled anesthetics are twofold; they are intrinsic cerebral vasodilators, but their vasodilatory actions are partly opposed by CBF-CMR coupling–mediated vasoconstriction secondary to reduction in CMR.[50] The overall effect is unchanged flow during low-dose inhalation anesthesia but increased flow with high doses. With the exception of sevoflurane, which appears to preserve autoregulation at all clinically relevant doses,[51-53] the inhalational agents impair autoregulation in a dose-dependent manner.[42] Opioids can cause increased ICP from hypercapnia secondary to respiratory depression if ventilation is not well controlled. In patients with decreased intracranial compliance, systemic hypotension can also lead to secondary increase in ICP from compensatory vasodilatation.[54] There is no evidence of direct opiate-mediated cerebral vasodilatory action.[55] Muscle relaxants generally have negligible or clinically insignificant effects on ICP.

Specific Neurosurgical Categories

Intracranial Tumors

The preoperative evaluation of patients with intracranial tumors should include assessment of the patient's neurological and general states and of current treatment as described previously. In addition, any intracranial hypertension and the extent to which it is controlled preoperatively with medical therapy, should be evaluated. Although a slowly growing tumor may reach a considerable size before ICP starts rising, a rapidly growing tumor may manifest as higher ICP even if its mass is smaller because compensatory mechanisms are not effective. The signs and symptoms of elevated ICP include headache, nausea and vomiting, altered mental status, decreased level of consciousness, diplopia, visual disturbances, and systemic hypertension. Seizures and hemiparesis secondary to direct mass effect can also occur.

Unilateral cortical lesions generally do not result in coma, except when there is brainstem herniation. Patients with such lesions may be exquisitely sensitive to the actions of sedatives and opioids, both direct and indirect. The decreased level of consciousness makes them sensitive to the hypnotic actions of sedatives, whereas poor intracranial compliance makes them susceptible to the respiratory depressant effects of opioids and CO_2-mediated increase in ICP. However, in anxious patients with no signs or symptoms of raised ICP, mild anxiolytics administered under supervision might be warranted.

Preoperative steroid administration helps control ICP by reducing peritumoral edema but the anesthesiologist should remain cognizant of the possibility of perioperative intracranial hypertension. In patients receiving steroids for long periods with the possibility of suppression of pituitary axis, stress coverage with supplemental steroids should be provided. H_2 blockers and prokinetics may be considered to protect against the reduced gastric emptying and greater acid secretion associated with increased ICP and steroid treatment. Diuretics—mannitol and furosemide—administered preoperatively may also be effective in reducing ICP, but the neuroanesthesiologist should assess the volume status of the patient as well because excessive diuresis without adequate fluid replacement may lead to hypotension during anesthesia. Phenytoin and other anticonvulsants should be continued in the perioperative period, and due consideration should be given to their interactions with anesthetic drugs. A loading dose of phenytoin or levetiracetam is often administered during anesthesia.

In patients with pituitary adenomas, the visual field and the endocrine functions need careful evaluation. Presence of Cushing's disease should alert the neuroanesthesiologist to the risk of sleep apnea (which occurs in one third of patients with the disease) in addition to other metabolic effects previously described. The incidence of difficult laryngoscopy and intubation in acromegalic patients is higher than in normal patients, and conventional methods of assessment of airway may not predict the difficulty.[56] Diabetes mellitus, hypertension, and cardiomyopathy might be associated with acromegaly, and the presence of carpal tunnel syndrome as a result of hypertrophic ligaments may make radial artery cannulation more hazardous if ulnar flow is already compromised.[57]

Computed tomography (CT) scans and magnetic resonance (MR) images should be examined for the size, location, and vascularity of the tumor and the signs of elevated ICP. The degree of midline shift and a diagnosis of glioblastoma multiforme or metastasis are independent predictors of brain swelling,[58] as is

TABLE 5-2 The Mayo Clinic Preoperative Classification of Risk*

Grade	Neurological Findings	Medical Findings	Angiographic Findings	Risk of Myocardial Infarction/Stroke
1	Stable	No defined risk	No major risk	1%
2	Stable	No defined risk	Significant risk	2%
3	Stable	Major risk	With or without risk	7%
4	Unstable	With or without risk	With or without risk	10%

*Medical risk: angina, myocardial infarction (<6 months), congestive heart failure, severe hypertension (blood pressure 180 mm Hg systolic/110 mm Hg diastolic), chronic obstructive lung disease, age ≥70 years, severe obesity. Neurologic risk: progressing deficit, new deficit (<24 hours), frequent daily transient ischemic attacks, multiple cerebral infarcts. Angiographic risk: contralateral carotid artery occlusion, internal carotid artery siphon stenosis, proximal or distal plaque extension, high carotid bifurcation, presence of soft thrombus.

peritumoral edema.[59] Small increases in intracranial volume in patients with signs of elevated ICP may lead to brain swelling and further disproportionate increase in ICP or herniation. Supratentorial meningiomas are vascular tumors that may occur in surgically difficult locations (e.g., near the sagittal sinus, optic nerve sheath) but are generally curable with complete surgical excision. When dealing with such a tumor, the neuroanesthesiologist should anticipate blood loss with need for transfusion and sometimes long, technically difficult surgery requiring maximal brain relaxation.

Although most commonly used anesthetic regimens have been shown to be acceptable in patients undergoing elective supratentorial surgery, because short-term outcomes are not affected,[60] lower subdural ICP and better brain relaxation have been observed during anesthesia maintained with propofol than with isoflurane or sevoflurane.[61] Hence, intravenous anesthetics may be preferable over inhaled agents in patients in whom intraoperative brain swelling is suspected. On the other hand, a recent multicenter trial did not find anesthetic regimen to affect brain bulk assessment or ICP but did find that hyperventilation reduced the risk of increased brain bulk.[62]

Vascular Diseases

Ischemic Cerebrovascular Disease. Patients with arteriosclerotic carotid disease often present for carotid endarterectomy (CEA) and less frequently for extracranial/intracranial revascularization. This cerebrovascular disease is but one manifestation of the underlying disorder of generalized atherosclerosis. Patients who undergo CEA commonly have significant CAD, arterial hypertension, peripheral vascular disease, chronic obstructive pulmonary disease, diabetes mellitus, or renal insufficiency.[63] The predominant symptoms and any neurological deficits should be recorded because neurologically unstable patients are more likely to have perioperative stroke. The Mayo Clinic classification of preoperative risk according to neurological, medical, and angiographic findings is widely used (Table 5-2).[64]

Data from the North American Symptomatic Carotid Endarterectomy Trial (NASCET) suggest that increased surgical risk is associated with the following five baseline variables: (1) hemispheric versus retinal transient ischemic attack as the qualifying event, (2) left-sided procedure, (3) contralateral carotid occlusion, (4) ipsilateral ischemic lesion found on CT, and (5) irregular or ulcerated ipsilateral plaque.[65] A review of medical, non–stroke-related complications among patients enrolled in the NASCET reported cardiac complications to be the most common cause of postoperative morbidity and to be responsible for all fatalities.[66] The NASCET results indicated that a history of MI or unstable angina and hypertension are independent risk factors for medical complications after surgery. On the other hand, aggressive blood pressure control in patients undergoing CEA, including preoperative treatment of hypertension, has been associated with improved outcome, emphasizing the effectiveness of preoperative treatment of high blood pressure.[67] Routine coronary angiography before CEA is sometimes advised despite the lack of evidence to suggest that it improves cardiac outcome. A prudent approach is to assume that all patients scheduled for CEA have associated atherosclerotic heart disease and to assess perioperative risk and the need for further investigation and intervention on the basis of the patients' functional status. Although diabetes mellitus was not an independent risk factor for medical complications in NASCET patients,[65] it does increase the risk of perioperative stroke or death.[68] Because hyperglycemia adversely affects outcome following temporary focal or global ischemia, it is best to optimize blood glucose levels preoperatively, and to manage them carefully in the perioperative period to avoid both hyperglycemia and hypoglycemia.

TABLE 5-3 Modified Hunt and Hess Clinical Grades of Aneurysm*

Grade	Criteria
0	Unruptured aneurysm
I	Asymptomatic or minimal headache and slight nuchal rigidity
II	Moderate to severe headache, nuchal rigidity, but no neurological deficit other than cranial nerve palsy
III	Drowsiness, confusion, or mild focal deficit
IV	Stupor, mild or severe hemiparesis, possible early decerebrate rigidity, vegetative disturbance
V	Deep coma, decerebrate rigidity, moribund appearance

Modified from Hunt WE, Hess RM. Surgical risk as related to time of intervention in the repair of intracranial aneurysm. *J Neurosurg.* 1968;28:14-20.

*Serious systemic disease such as hypertension, diabetes, severe arteriosclerosis, chronic pulmonary disease, and severe vasospasm seen on arteriography result in the placement of the patient in the next less favorable category.

Aneurysmal Subarachnoid Hemorrhage. The most important aspect of preoperative evaluation of patients with intracranial aneurysms is assessment of the patient's neurological status and grading of subarachnoid hemorrhage (SAH). Classically, SAH is graded with the Hunt and Hess scale (Table 5-3).[69] This grading system has prognostic importance because patients with higher grades of SAH have higher morbidity and mortality. However, higher grades are also more likely to be associated with vasospasm, elevated ICP,[70] impaired cerebral autoregulation,[71,72] and impaired cerebrovascular reactivity to CO_2.[71] A worse clinical grade is also associated with a higher incidence of cardiac arrhythmia and myocardial dysfunction,[73] hypovolemia, and hyponatremia.[74,75] All of these observations are crucial and have impact on the anesthetic management of patients with intracranial hemorrhage.

An alternative scale for grading severity of SAH is that of the World Federation of Neurological Surgeons, which is based on Glasgow Coma Scale score and presence or absence of motor deficit (Table 5-4).[76] The Fisher Scale and its modification are based on the amount of subarachnoid blood seen on CT scan, which correlates with the risk for development of vasospasm (Tables 5-5 and 5-6).[77,78] While examining the CT scan, the neuroanesthesiologist can also assess the degree of mass effect, midline shift, cerebral edema, and hydrocephalus, which can help anticipate intraoperative brain swelling.

A variety of medical conditions are known to be associated with the development of cerebral aneurysms and SAH. The preoperative evaluation should look for any of these associated conditions, which include hypertension, coarctation of the aorta, polycystic kidney disease, and fibromuscular dysplasia as well as history of smoking, and should take into consideration the specific anesthetic concerns for any of these conditions present in a given patient.[79]

Patients with SAH frequently have contracted intravascular volume, which may be caused by multiple factors, as follows: altered sensorium associated with reduced fluid intake, use of diuretics and radiographic contrast agents (for diagnostic imaging), bed rest, supine diuresis, negative nitrogen balance, decreased erythropoiesis, and iatrogenic blood loss. In some patients, hypovolemia may be associated paradoxically with hyponatremia, secondary to increased release of atrial natriuretic peptide (cerebral salt-wasting syndrome),[80] and may be related to the subsequent development of vasospasm.[81] Erroneous attribution of hyponatremia to syndrome of inappropriate antidiuretic hormone secretion (SIADH) may lead to treatment with fluid restriction, raising the risk of delayed cerebral ischemia and infarction.[82] Hypertonic or isotonic saline should be used judiciously to correct hyponatremia from SAH.[83] Other significant electrolyte abnormalities include hypokalemia and hypocalcemia. Preoperative treatment should be aimed at correcting electrolyte abnormality while maintaining normal intravascular status.

ECG changes, primarily involving ST-segment changes or T-wave inversion, are common, occurring in 40% to 60% of patients with SAH.[84] Three etiologies could account for the ECG abnormalities in these patients: coincidental MI, SAH-induced MI, and ECG changes without infarction. The ECG changes, however, usually correlate with the neurological dysfunction, being more prevalent in patients with poor-grade SAH,[85,86] and do not affect surgical morbidity or mortality.[87] They do not necessarily correlate with ventricular dysfunction, although the presence of symmetrical inverted T waves and severe QTc (corrected QT) interval prolongation on serial ECG readings has been shown to be indicative of ventricular dysfunction.[88] Echocardiographic ventricular dysfunction can occur in 10% to 20% of patients and is also more prevalent in patients with high-grade SAH.[73,89] It is of note that neurogenic stress cardiomyopathy, including Takotsubo's myopathy, has been well described in SAH and is associated with increased morbidity and poor clinical outcome.[90] Acute ST-segment elevation is rare with SAH and should prompt suspicion of MI. Cardiac enzymes and echocardiography are required to rule out MI and to ascertain degree of ventricular dysfunction in patients with these findings,[85] and elevations of troponin and brain natriuretic peptide (BNP) are associated with poor prognosis.[91] Although the anesthetic risk is increased if MI has occurred, this risk must be balanced against the risk of rebleeding if surgery is postponed. Unless the patient is hemodynamically unstable and/or has poor ventricular function (ejection fraction < 30%) or is clinically diagnosed as being in heart failure, surgery should proceed with appropriate hemodynamic monitoring.[92] On the other hand, in the patient with poor ventricular function refractory to medical management, it would be prudent to defer surgery until the patient is hemodynamically stable; alternatively, endovascular treatment of aneurysm might have to be considered. Table 5-7 shows the various ECG changes seen in patients with SAH and their possible implications.[93]

Patients often suffer transient loss of consciousness with the initial SAH. Pulmonary aspiration can occur during or after this event, leading to impaired gas exchange. Neurogenic pulmonary edema can also occur owing to intense sympathetic discharge. Patients who continue to remain in stupor may have shallow breathing and can experience atelectasis. Supplemental oxygen may often be required. Premedication should be carefully planned

TABLE 5-4 World Federation of Neurological Surgeons (WFNS) Grading Scale

WFNS Grade	Glasgow Coma Scale Score	Motor Deficit
I	15	Absent
II	14-13	Absent
III	14-13	Present
IV	12-7	Absent or present
V	6-3	Absent or present

From Drake C. Report of World Federation of Neurological Surgeons Committee on a universal subarachnoid haemorrhage grading scale. *J Neurosurg.* 1988;68:985-986.

TABLE 5-5 Fisher Grading of Computed Tomography (CT) Scan Findings in Subarachnoid Hemorrhage

Grade	CT Scan Finding
1	No blood detected
2	Diffuse thin layer of subarachnoid blood (vertical layers < 1 mm thick)
3	Localized clot or thick layer of subarachnoid blood (vertical layers ≥ 1 mm thick)
4	Intracerebral or intraventricular blood with diffuse or no subarachnoid blood

From Fisher C, Kistler J, Davis J. Relation of cerebral vasospasm to subarachnoid hemorrhage visualized by computerized tomographic scanning. *Neurosurgery.* 1980;6:1-9.

TABLE 5-6 Modified Fisher Grading of Computed Tomography (CT) Scan Findings in Subarachnoid Hemorrhage

Grade	CT Scan Finding				Description
	No SAH	Focal or Diffuse Thin SAH	Focal or Diffuse Thick SAH	IVH	
0	+	–	–	–	No SAH; no intraventricular blood
1	–	+	–	–	Thin diffuse or focal subarachnoid blood, but no intraventricular blood
2	–	+	–	+	Thin focal or diffuse subarachnoid blood with intraventricular blood
3	–	–	+	–	Thick focal or diffuse subarachnoid blood, but no intraventricular blood
4	–	–	+	+	Thick focal or diffuse subarachnoid blood with intraventricular blood

From Frontera JA, Claassen J, Schmidt JM, et al. Prediction of symptomatic vasospasm after subarachnoid hemorrhage: the modified Fisher Scale. *Neurosurgery.* 2006;59:21-27.
IVH, intraventricular hemorrhage; SAH, subarachnoid hemorrhage.

TABLE 5-7 Electrocardiographic and Myocardial Dysfunction Seen in Subarachnoid Hemorrhage

Benign changes	Sinus bradycardia
	Sinus tachycardia
	Atrioventricular dissociation
	Premature ventricular contractions
	Nonspecific ST depression
	T-wave inversion
	U wave
Possible wall motion abnormality	Symmetrical T-wave inversion
	Prolonged QT interval (>500 msec)
	ST-segment elevation
Possible myocardial injury	Q wave
	ST-segment elevation
	Elevated myocardial enzymes
	Elevated troponin I

TABLE 5-8 Grading System of Spetzler and Martin for Arteriovenous Malformations (AVMs)*

Graded Feature	Point(s) Assigned
AVM SIZE (DIAMETER)	
Small (<3 cm)	1
Medium (3-6 cm)	2
Large (>6 cm)	3
ELOQUENCE OF ADJACENT BRAIN	
Noneloquent	0
Eloquent	1
PATTERN OF VENOUS DRAINAGE	
Superficial only	0
Deep	1

Based on Spetzler RF, Martin NA. A proposed grading system for arteriovenous malformations. *J Neurosurg.* 1986;65:476-483.
*Grade = size + eloquence + venous drainage.

depending on the patients' level of consciousness or anxiety, respiratory status, and blood pressure.

Arteriovenous Malformations. Treatment options for patients with intracranial arteriovenous malformations (AVMs) include surgical resection, endovascular embolization, and stereotactic radiosurgery. The usual indications for intervention are spontaneous intracranial hemorrhage, intractable seizures, and progressive neurologic deficits. Surgical risk for AVM resection is classically estimated according to the grading system of Spetzler and Martin (Table 5-8).[94] In general, patients with Spetzler-Martin scores of 1 through 3 have a lower risk of permanent neurological deficit following surgery in comparison with patients with higher scores.

The preoperative evaluation of the patient with an AVM should focus on the patient's age, presenting symptoms of the AVM, grading, and planned intervention (surgical excision/endovascular procedure/radiosurgery). Of particular concern are preexisting symptoms of cerebral ischemia and mass effect with elevated ICP resulting either from the AVM itself or the bleed. History of seizure should be sought, and prescribed anticonvulsants should be continued. It is not uncommon for the patient to present for interval surgical resection of an AVM after endovascular embolization. Fluid and electrolyte status need special attention in such patients because of the possibility of diuresis induced by a radiographic contrast agent. Although preoperative embolization has dramatically changed the surgical demands of AVM resection, the residua remain highly vascular and may lead to significant blood loss during resection, with the need for transfusion. Moreover, intraoperative coagulopathy may develop in these patients. Hence preoperative crossmatching of compatible blood is needed. The AVM is a low-pressure, high-flow system, and hypertension does not usually lead to AVM hemorrhage. However, documentation of preoperative blood pressure is important to establish a "baseline" to facilitate postoperative control of blood pressure and prevent "normal perfusion pressure breakthrough" syndrome. Preoperative imaging studies should be examined for assessment of AVM location, midline shift, and any associated aneurysms. Patients with vein of Galen malformation can present as neonates with intractable congestive heart failure, as infants with hydrocephalus and seizures, or as older children with spontaneous intracranial hemorrhage. Infants presenting with heart failure may require optimization and are frequently receiving inotropic support preoperatively, which is continued during anesthesia.

Posterior Fossa Procedures

The posterior cranial fossa is a tight anatomic space that contains vital structures including the brainstem with cranial nerves III through XII, cerebellar hemispheres, and the vertebrobasilar vascular system. A variety of lesions and vascular malformations can occur in the posterior fossa, and the surgical exposure is complex, requiring any of the variety of surgical positions. Lateral position is usually required for surgery on cerebellopontine angle tumors, cerebellar hemispheric lesions, and lesions involving the clivus, petrous ridge, and anterior and lateral foramen magnum. Midline and fourth ventricular lesions can be operated in the prone or sitting position, and the park-bench (or three-quarter prone) position allows rapid positioning with quick access to cerebellar hemispheres.

Preoperative evaluation of the patient undergoing a posterior fossa procedure should highlight the patient's physical status, especially cardiopulmonary status, because positioning can exert extra demands on the cardiorespiratory system. Although the sitting position offers considerable advantages to the neurosurgeon in terms of an optimal operating field (gravity-assisted drainage of blood and CSF), reduced cerebellar retraction, and easier anatomic localization with improved postoperative cranial nerve function, it can be associated with serious complications, including venous air embolism (VAE) and paradoxical air embolism (PAE), hypotension (leading to cerebral/cervical ischemia), pneumocephalus, lingual and laryngeal trauma, and, rarely, quadriplegia or paraplegia (midcervical flexion myelopathy). Despite several studies substantiating relative safety of the sitting position,[95,96] its use is diminishing largely because of the potential for serious complications and malpractice liability claims. VAE is the most common complication and because 20% to 25% of the general population has a probe-patent foramen ovale,[97] a reversal of the right-left atrial pressure gradient can lead to PAE with devastating complications. Hence probe-patent foramen ovale is considered a relative contraindication to the sitting position, and preoperative or intraoperative echocardiography should be performed before this position is selected.[98] Other contraindications to sitting position include patent ventriculoatrial shunt, severe hypovolemia, cachexia, severe cardiovascular disease, and postural hypotension, which should be ruled out preoperatively.

The preoperative evaluation should include assessment of neurological status, encompassing any evidence of raised ICP or signs of brainstem compression (ipsilateral cranial nerve and contralateral sensorimotor deficits, chronic aspiration syndromes, respiratory pattern, cardiovascular instability). Hemangioblastoma may occur as a part of von Hippel-Lindau syndrome, and polycythemia may be associated, whereas acoustic neuroma may be associated with neurofibromatosis type 2. Patients with previous CSF shunting procedures may be at increased risk of postoperative pneumocephalus following surgery in head-up position. Narcotics and sedatives for premedication are best avoided in

BOX 5-1 Causes of Secondary Insults to the Injured Brain

SYSTEMIC CAUSES

Hypoxemia
Hypercapnia
Hypotension or hypertension
Hypo-osmolality or hyperosmolality
Hyperglycemia or hypoglycemia
Shivering, fever

INTRACRANIAL CAUSES

Increased intracranial pressure
Seizures
Cerebral vasospasm

patients with tumors and obstructive hydrocephalus, although small titrated doses given under continuous supervision may be ordered for very anxious patients. In the preoperative work-up, the risks and benefits of positioning and anesthetic interventions should be explained to the patient or next-of-kin.

Traumatic Brain Injury (TBI)

Patients with traumatic brain injury (TBI) usually present for emergency surgery. Hence, a full preoperative history and physical examination are often difficult, if not impossible. A brief history pertaining to time and mode of injury and associated extracranial injuries may be obtained quickly. The neuroanesthesiologist's goal is to prevent secondary injury to the injured brain (listed in Box 5-1) and to facilitate early surgery, providing optimal operating conditions while continuing cerebral protection.

The preoperative assessment often involves ongoing resuscitation and management of other injuries. Care being given preoperatively according to the guidelines of Advanced Trauma Life Support should be continued. As in all resuscitation situations, the priorities are establishment of airway, breathing, and circulation, and the neuroanesthesiologist should first of all ensure adequacy of ventilation and oxygenation. If the patient is already intubated and mechanically ventilated, the anesthesiologist should reconfirm correct position of the endotracheal tube and its patency and should note the ventilator settings to ensure good ventilation while avoiding hypoxemia and hypercapnia. If the patient is not intubated, the anesthesiologist should quickly decide whether or not the patient needs immediate intubation. Tracheal intubation can be challenging in the patient with an "uncleared" cervical spine (in which injury and fracture have not been ruled out). The decision making regarding the technique of airway management is based on the urgency of the situation and the neuroanesthesiologist's personal expertise. Fiberoptic intubation may not be possible because of either the urgency of situation or bleeding in the airway. In such situations, direct or video laryngoscopy with manual in-line stabilization should be performed. Pharmacologic measures (opioids, lidocaine, beta blockers, or intravenous anesthetics) may be used to prevent ICP increase in response to laryngoscopy and intubation. After the airway is secured, ventilation should be adjusted, as already mentioned, to avoid both hypercapnia and profound hypocapnia.

During preoperative evaluation and continuing into anesthetic care, maintenance of adequate systemic blood pressure and cerebral perfusion pressure is vital. Repeated studies have shown that even transient hypotension is associated with poor outcome in patients with TBI.[99] In adults, systemic hypotension as a manifestation of isolated head trauma is rare in the absence of brainstem injury. When present, it is often associated with an extracranial source of bleeding, from thoracic, abdominal, long

BOX 5-2 Major Multisystem Sequelae of Acute Head Injury

RESPIRATORY SYSTEM

Airway obstruction
Irregular breathing
Adult respiratory distress syndrome (ARDS)
Neurogenic pulmonary edema
Aspiration pneumonia
Diaphragmatic paralysis

CARDIOVASCULAR SYSTEM

Hypotension/shock
Electrocardiographic changes, cardiac arrhythmias
Fat embolism

HEMATOLOGIC SYSTEM

Coagulopathy
Disseminated intravascular coagulation

GASTROINTESTINAL SYSTEM

Cushing's ulcers

ENDOCRINE SYSTEM

Syndrome of inappropriate antidiuretic hormone secretion (SIADH)
Diabetes insipidus (DI)
Anterior pituitary insufficiency

METABOLIC

Hyperglycemia
Water and electrolyte imbalances

bone or spinal cord injuries all of which should be quickly ruled out. Aggressive fluid resuscitation with or without vasopressors should be continued. In order to avoid delay in surgery, quick examination should focus on Glasgow Coma Scale score, gross motor deficits, and pupillary abnormalities in addition to assessment of extracranial injuries. If ICP is being monitored, it should be noted and any therapeutic modalities being used to control elevated ICP (e.g., mannitol) should be continued. Cerebral perfusion pressure should be maintained between 50 and 70 mm Hg.[100] There may be multisystem sequelae of TBI in addition to coexisting injuries (Box 5-2). As part of preoperative work-up, only the most important laboratory tests are required: measurements of hemoglobin and blood glucose, and a coagulation profile. Blood must be crossmatched, and blood products should be available.

Spinal Surgery

Patients with spinal disorders may present electively or emergently, with or without neurological symptoms. Patients undergoing elective spinal surgery may present with acquired or congenital defects. The latter include spina bifida, meningocele, and tethered cord. These defects are often part of a syndrome, and other organ systems should be closely inspected for evidence of associated abnormalities. Scoliosis can also be congenital, and patients with it can present for surgery at any age. Respiratory compromise is common with scoliosis, the severity of which increases with increasing bony deformity. Total lung capacity is affected by the inefficient muscle contraction brought on by rotation of the spine and rib cage. This occurs at spinal curvatures greater than 60 degrees. Once the curvature is more than 90 degrees, vital capacity is reduced and right ventricular hypertrophy may develop secondary to pulmonary hypertension. Lung function should be carefully assessed, as should be any increased risk of difficult tracheal intubation and airway control. Acquired spinal lesions include herniated disks, spinal stenosis, tumor, infection, and trauma. Patients with them may present with neurological symptoms, the severity of which must be carefully evaluated preoperatively. Their presence indicates that the spinal cord is at risk, either directly from pressure (slipped disk, tumor) or from hypoperfusion. Efforts are made to prevent further cord damage, maintain adequate blood flow, and avoid secondary insults. Patients who present emergently after spinal injury usually have actual cord compromise from trauma or instability, and up to 20% may have concurrent injury to other organ systems.

Certain procedures may require intraoperative "wake-up" tests, indicating the use of a rapid-offset anesthetic technique. Informing the patient and reassurance are important aspects of the preoperative visit for a procedure involving such tests. In other patients, somatosensory and motor evoked potentials may be monitored, and the anesthetic technique has to be planned accordingly so that it does not interfere with the monitoring. Preoperatively, the neurological assessment should note both the present symptoms and their response to movement. Patients who report worsening of symptoms with motion and who are lucid and cooperative may be candidates for awake fiberoptic intubation of the trachea. In fact, patients with cervical spine pathology may require awake fiberoptic intubation even in the absence of symptoms. In patients who are intoxicated or otherwise uncooperative, rapid sequence anesthesia induction followed by direct laryngoscopy with manual in-line stabilization is indicated. Succinylcholine is a quick-onset, short-acting neuromuscular blocking agent ideally suited for urgent tracheal intubation. However, in patients with denervation injury, it can cause an acute elevation in serum potassium, leading to cardiac standstill. Proliferation and development of the extrajunctional receptors responsible for this potentially lethal complication develop over time, so it is safe to use succinylcholine in first 48 hours after the injury. Beyond this point, it is best to avoid succinylcholine in patients with significant denervation injury and to use alternative quick-onset nondepolarizing muscle relaxants such as rocuronium.

Patients with spinal cord injury are often started on methylprednisolone therapy, which should be continued through the intraoperative period, although this practice is no longer recommended in current guidelines.[101] The prone position necessitates a firmly secured airway and the placement of adequate intravenous and arterial lines before the patient is turned. The preoperative interview should include providing the patient information about possible complications of the prone position, including orbital edema, facial swelling, and airway swelling, which may warrant elective postoperative ventilation, as well as the potential of postoperative visual loss.[102] Patients with a history of coronary artery bypass may have increased risk of myocardial ischemia because of compression of the graft against the chest wall. Adequate ventilatory effort depends on the integrity of the phrenic nerve (C3-C5) and the innervation of the intercostal muscles. The patient with a spinal cord injury above C3 will be ventilator dependent.[103] Such a patient's inability to cough and clear secretions increases the risk of respiratory insufficiency and occurs with loss of intercostal muscle action and chest wall excursion. Elective tracheal intubation and ventilation may be required postoperatively, as indicated by the parameters listed in Box 5-3.

BOX 5-3 Indications for Tracheal Intubation in the Patient with Spinal Cord Injury

Maximum expiratory force < +20 cm H_2O
Maximum inspiratory force < −20 cm H_2O
Vital capacity < 15 mL/kg or 1 L
PaO_2/FiO_2 < 250
Severe atelectasis on chest radiograph

Cardiovascular collapse is common after acute cervical cord trauma. Immediately at the time of trauma there is sympathetic activation, leading to a slight increase in cardiac contractility as well as in mean arterial pressure and systemic vascular resistance. In some patients this intense sympathetic discharge can result in neurogenic pulmonary edema. This development is followed by the onset of spinal shock, which is characterized by bradycardia and hypotension with reduced contractility.[104] The spinal shock can last from 1 to 4 weeks. During this period there is complete vasoparalysis. Vasoconstriction cannot occur to maintain cardiac filling pressure, and fluid resuscitation is required to correct the relative hypovolemia and restore the cardiac output. Because the contractility is also reduced, inotropic support may be required. Invasive hemodynamic monitoring with placement of a central venous or pulmonary artery catheter might facilitate the management of the patient with cervical cord trauma during the acute period.[105]

Epilepsy Disorders

Epileptic patients can present to the neuroanesthesiologist for a number of reasons, including resection of epileptic focus, recording of electrocorticography, diagnostic radiologic procedures, non-epilepsy surgery, and management of status epilepticus. Surgery for epilepsy can be done with the patient under general anesthesia or under local anesthesia with minimum intravenous sedation. A sleep-awake-sleep technique is frequently used, with or without an artificial airway.[106,107] Awake craniotomy allows the surgeon to communicate with a sedated yet cooperative patient and precisely map the location and extent of resection. An important part of preanesthetic evaluation is to counsel patients regarding the procedure and to allay their fears and anxiety. With the introduction of propofol, it is now possible to introduce short periods of "deep anesthesia" during the painful period to maximize patient comfort without sacrificing the subsequent need for lucidity and cooperation.[106] Intraoperative electrocorticography has shown that high-dose propofol does not cause seizure[108] and that, provided that the infusion is suspended for 15 minutes before recording, it does not interfere with mapping.[109] A good preoperative rapport with the patient nevertheless facilitates this process. In some centers patient-controlled sedation has been used with some success.[110]

The newer anesthetic drugs have minimal effects on the electrocorticogram and do not interfere with mapping, and hence, general anesthesia with controlled ventilation can be safely selected for patients with increased ICP or impaired cerebral autoregulation, in order to prevent intraoperative brain swelling due to carbon dioxide retention, with spontaneous breathing under sedation alone. For all epileptic patients, it is important to note that the use of phenytoin makes them more resistant to nondepolarizing neuromuscular blocking drugs,[111] and these patients may also have increased requirement for opioids.[112] The placement of a stereotactic frame is a potential airway concern for the anesthesiologist. Ventilation by mask can be difficult, and direct laryngoscopy can be impossible with use of a frame. If tracheal intubation is required, fiberoptic laryngoscopy or use of an intubating laryngeal mask airway may be required and must be readily available.[113] Any sedation technique has the potential risk of overmedication, with the accompanied loss of protective airway reflexes and/or onset of severe respiratory depression. Thus, during the preoperative evaluation of patients with epilepsy, special attention should be paid to airway assessment and the need for airway adjuncts.

Neuroradiology

With the exception of very young children, most diagnostic neuroradiologic procedures are performed on sedated patients under local anesthesia. Anesthetic assistance is requested usually for children, uncooperative adults, and debilitated patients at high risk. Monitored sedation may be adequate even in children.[114] The aim is to provide a calm, comfortable, and cooperative patient. The technique of patient-controlled sedation with propofol has also been used successfully for interventional radiologic procedures.[115] However, patients with mass lesions and intracranial hypertension, who would benefit from avoidance of sedation-induced hypercapnia, need general anesthesia with controlled ventilation. General anesthesia and complete immobility are also desirable for embolization of AVMs and intraluminal balloon angioplasty for cerebral vasospasm. For patients undergoing endovascular treatment of acute ischemic stroke, existing evidence increasingly suggests that conscious sedation may be associated with better outcome than general anesthesia,[116] yet sedation alone is not appropriate for every patient. The preoperative assessment therefore must take into consideration both the nature of the neuroradiologic procedure and the medical and psychological condition of the patient. Added to the anesthetic challenge is the fact that the procedure is performed in an area remote from the familiar operating room environment, where technical and expert assistance are more readily available. For this reason, the preoperative evaluation must include anticipation of the complications and formulation of backup plans. All necessary drugs and equipment must be immediately available. For procedures in the MR suite, anesthetic and monitoring equipment must be MRI compatible.

CONCLUSION

Although the general principles governing the intracranial hemodynamics and function are the same, patients undergoing different surgical procedures for different pathologic conditions can have vastly different anesthetic and monitoring requirements. The successful intraoperative management of these challenging patients requires a basic understanding of the pathophysiology and surgical demand of the procedure, which starts with a thorough preoperative evaluation and preparation of the patient.

SUGGESTED READINGS

Akavipat P, Ittichaikulthol W, Tuchinda L, et al. The Thai Anesthesia Incidents (THAI Study) of anesthetic risk factors related to perioperative death and perioperative cardiovascular complications in intracranial surgery. *J Med Assoc Thai*. 2007;90:1565-1572.

Brain Trauma Foundation; American Association of Neurological Surgeons; Congress of Neurological Surgeons; Joint Section on Neurotrauma and Critical Care, AANS/CNS, Bratton SL, Chestnut RM, Ghajar J, et al. Guidelines for the management of severe traumatic brain injury. IX. Cerebral perfusion thresholds. *J Neurotrauma*. 2007; 24(suppl 1):S59-S64.

Dernbach PD, Little JR, Jones SC, et al. Altered cerebral autoregulation and CO_2 reactivity after aneurysmal subarachnoid hemorrhage. *Neurosurgery*. 1988;22:822-826.

Dexter F, Wachtel RE. Strategies for net cost reductions with the expanded role and expertise of anesthesiologists in the perioperative surgical home. *Anesth Analg*. 2014;118:1062-1071.

Diringer MN, Lim JS, Kirsch JR, et al. Suprasellar and intraventricular blood predict elevated plasma atrial natriuretic factor in subarachnoid hemorrhage. *Stroke*. 1991;22:577-581.

Drummond JC, Dao AV, Roth DM, et al. Effect of dexmedetomidine on cerebral blood flow velocity, cerebral metabolic rate, and carbon dioxide response in normal humans. *Anesthesiology*. 2008;108: 225-232.

Fleisher LA, Fleischmann KE, Auerbach AD, et al. 2014 ACC/AHA guideline on perioperative cardiovascular evaluation and management of patients undergoing noncardiac surgery: a report of the American College of Cardiology/American Heart Association Task Force on practice guidelines. *J Am Coll Cardiol*. 2014;64:e77-e137.

Gelb AW, Craen RA, Rao GS, et al. Does hyperventilation improve operating condition during supratentorial craniotomy? A multicenter randomized crossover trial. *Anesth Analg*. 2008;106:585-594.

Gronert GA, Theye RA. Pathophysiology of hyperkalemia induced by succinylcholine. *Anesthesiology*. 1975;43:89-99.

Holt NF. Trends in healthcare and the role of the anesthesiologist in the perioperative surgical home—the US perspective. *Curr Opin Anaesthesiol*. 2014;27(3):371-376.

Hunt WE, Hess RM. Surgical risk as related to time of intervention in the repair of intracranial aneurysms. *J Neurosurg*. 1968;28:14-20.

Lee LA, Roth S, Posner KL, et al. The American Society of Anesthesiologists Postoperative Visual Loss Registry: analysis of 93 spine surgery cases with postoperative visual loss. *Anesthesiology*. 2006;105:652-659.

Lee TH, Marcantonio ER, Mangione CM, et al. Derivation and prospective validation of a simple index for prediction of cardiac risk of major noncardiac surgery. *Circulation*. 1999;100:1043-1049.

Mallampati SR, Gatt SP, Gugino LD, et al. A clinical sign to predict difficult tracheal intubation: a prospective study. *Can Anaesth Soc J*. 1985;32:429-434.

Paciaroni M, Eliasziw M, Kappelle LJ, et al. Medical complications associated with carotid endarterectomy. North American Symptomatic Carotid Endarterectomy Trial (NASCET). *Stroke* 1999;30:1759-1763.

Petersen KD, Landsfeldt U, Cold GE, et al. Intracranial pressure and cerebral hemodynamic in patients with cerebral tumors: a randomized prospective study of patients subjected to craniotomy in propofol-fentanyl, isoflurane-fentanyl, or sevoflurane-fentanyl anesthesia. *Anesthesiology*. 2003;98:329-336.

Practice advisory for preanesthesia evaluation: an updated report by the American Society of Anesthesiologists Task Force on Preanesthesia evaluation. *Anesthesiology*. 2012;116(3):522-538.

Rasmussen M, Bundgaard H, Cold GE. Craniotomy for supratentorial brain tumors: risk factors for brain swelling after opening the dura mater. *J Neurosurg*. 2004;101:621-626.

Rozet I, Vavilala MS, Lindley AM, et al. Cerebral autoregulation and CO_2 reactivity in anterior and posterior cerebral circulation during sevoflurane anesthesia. *Anesth Analg*. 2006;102:560-564.

Skucas AP, Artru AA. Anesthetic complications of awake craniotomies for epilepsy surgery. *Anesth Analg*. 2006;102:882-887.

Smetana GW, Lawrence VA, Cornell JE; American College of Physicians. Preoperative pulmonary risk stratification for noncardiothoracic surgery: systematic review for the American College of Physicians. *Ann Intern Med*. 2006;144:581-595.

Thal GD, Szabo MD, Lopez-Bresnahan M, et al. Exacerbation or unmasking of focal neurologic deficits by sedatives. *Anesthesiology*. 1996;85:21-25.

Van der Bilt IA, Hasan D, Vandertop WP, et al. Impact of cardiac complications on outcome after aneurysmal subarachnoid hemorrhage: a meta-analysis. *Neurology*. 2009;72:635-642.

Wijeysundera DN, Duncan D, Nkonde-Price C, et al. Perioperative beta blockade in noncardiac surgery: a systematic review for the 2014 ACC/AHA guideline on perioperative cardiovascular evaluation and management of patients undergoing noncardiac surgery: a report of the American College of Cardiology/American Heart Association Task Force on practice guidelines. *Circulation*. 2014;130:2246-2264.

Wolters U, Wolf T, Stützer H, et al. ASA classification and perioperative variables as predictors of postoperative outcome. *Br J Anaesth*. 1996;77: 217-222.

See a full reference list on ExpertConsult.com

6 Complication Avoidance in Neurosurgery

Nirit Weiss, Ronit Gilad, and Kalmon D. Post

As with all neurosurgical procedures, avoidance of complications is as important as treatment of disease. In general, avoidance of surgical complications requires attention to making the correct diagnosis, choosing the appropriate surgery, and correctly selecting patients. This chapter is intended to review how to prevent complications of neurosurgical procedures in general, with additional emphasis placed on the specific complications that might be encountered in particular approaches to the spine and brain. Avoidance of complications in neurosurgery begins with the correct selection of patients who are likely to benefit from the surgical intervention planned. When possible, patients with nonmedical issues that have a known association with poor outcomes, such as workers' compensation claims or pending lawsuits, should be investigated further to determine the patient's motivation for recovery.[1-7] Taking the time to explain the probable risks and benefits of the procedure allows the patient to make an informed decision and protects the surgeon in the event of an adverse outcome from claims of inadequate consent. The remainder of this chapter focuses on prevention of complications once the patient has arrived in the operating room. Intraoperative complications may be related to anesthetic issues, positioning of the patient, or technical or anatomic aspects of the specific surgery selected.

Before induction of anesthesia, the surgeon and anesthesiologist must discuss the case in detail and review what is likely to happen and the possible risks. Ideally, an experienced neuroanesthesiologist should be available for neurosurgical procedures. Adequate venous access, placement of a single- or double-lumen tube as required by the surgical approach, and insertion of an intracardiac central venous pressure line to potentially remove air emboli must be planned in advance. The presence of blood products in proximity to the operating room and notification of the blood bank that more may be required depend on the scope of the surgical procedure. Antibiotics should be administered within 1 hour before incisions to ensure therapeutic blood levels.[8] In addition, during long cases, antibiotics should be readministered at regular intervals.[9,10]

COMPLICATIONS RELATED TO PATIENT POSITIONING

After the anesthesiologist has determined that the airway has been adequately secured and that all lines and monitoring equipment are in place, the patient is ready to be positioned. Several common positioning errors can lead to complications,[11-23] but most can be prevented with meticulous positioning protocols.

Supine Positioning

Exposure, bleeding, and complications such as air embolism depend on the angle of the head relative to the operative site and the patient's heart. Overflexing the neck may lead to kinking of the endotracheal tube in the pharynx or obstruction of the jugular vein, which may increase venous pressure in the head and cause increased bleeding or decreased perfusion. The heels, gluteal area, shoulders, and head need to be sufficiently padded. Preferably, rolls are placed under both knees so that they are slightly flexed, and the feet should be suspended by padding under the calves. This position prevents heel pressure ulcers and compression on the Achilles tendon. If the arms are to be secured at the patient's side, adequate padding of the elbow and wrist and any points of contact with monitoring devices need to be verified before the procedure starts.

Prone Positioning

Nerve palsies and compression injuries are the most frequent complications seen and the most easily preventable. Radial and ulnar neuropathies can occur as a result of positioning the patient in the prone position with the arms extended if padding is inadequate or an inappropriate position is used. Keeping the arms in a mildly flexed position prevents excessive traction in either direction. Padding may be in the form of sheets or blankets placed under the elbows and forearms, or egg-crate foam padding can be used. Brachial plexus injuries can occur with rostral or caudal traction on the shoulders[24] and frequently occur with the prone position when the arms are extended in the cruciate position or too far above the head. Downward traction, such as when the shoulders need to be pulled down for x-ray localization in the low cervical or cervicothoracic junction, can also cause brachial plexus injury. If possible, any tension placed on the patient's shoulders during radiography should be removed after the x-ray film has been obtained. There are newer traction devices available that can be fastened to the patient during positioning and apply traction only during fluoroscopy use.[25] Neurophysiologic monitoring of the ulnar nerve with somatosensory evoked potentials during spinal procedures has been shown to be effective in correcting and preventing position-related stretch injuries to the brachial plexus.[26,27] Another common peripheral neuropathy associated with the prone position is the result of inadequate padding of the anterior superior iliac crest, which can lead to pain or numbness in the distribution of the lateral femoral cutaneous nerve.[28] A rare complication is obstruction of the external iliac artery or femoral artery from prolonged compression in the inguinal region.[29,30]

Starting at the top, the face and head should be gently suspended without any compression on any one area (discussed later in the chapter in further detail). If the patient is being placed on chest rolls or chest bolsters, the ideal position is to have the shoulders slightly overhanging the chest rolls. Breasts should be tucked between the two rolls to prevent excessive pressure. Prone positioning on a spinal table (e.g., Jackson table, Orthopedic Systems, Inc., Union City, CA) requires placement of the hip pads (of a size appropriate for the patient) so that the top of the pads is at the anterior superior iliac crest. The thigh pads are placed just below the hip pads. The ankles should be allowed to dangle off the edge of the leg supports, if possible. Inadequate padding of the anterior superior iliac crest can cause pressure necrosis of the overlying skin. Male genitalia should be examined to verify that they are not being compressed between the thighs or gluteal folds and that a Foley catheter, if present, is not causing undue traction on the penis. The knees need to be padded, and a padded roll should be placed underneath the ankles so that the feet hang suspended.

The abdomen should be hanging suspended to prevent venous compression and improve venous return to the heart. This point is critical because excessive venous compression can lead to significant intraoperative bleeding secondary to epidural venous hypertension. If the abdomen cannot be adequately suspended, the three-quarter prone position can be used instead (discussed later), particularly in morbidly obese patients, who may not fit on any chest bolstering system, such as the Kamden frame, the four-post Relton frame, or chest rolls. This position allows the abdomen to remain free while the surgeon works from behind, but the position also makes intraoperative radiography very difficult.

Another difficulty with positioning for spine surgery is the difference between the ideal position for a decompressive procedure, with the spine and hips flexed, and that for spinal fusion, with the spine in a more lordotic position and the hips and spine in neutral positions. Many patients have been subjected to iatrogenic flat-back syndrome because of improper position during a fusion procedure.[31]

Surgeons must be aware of the potential for unilateral or bilateral blindness after prolonged prone surgery. Causes have been hypothesized to be occlusion of the retinal artery or vein, direct trauma, orbital compartment syndrome, and ischemic optic neuropathy. Although rare, devastating complications have been described even when no direct trauma occurred, and therefore patients' eyes should be checked frequently during the procedure. Minimizing blood loss and hypotensive episodes and maintaining a slightly elevated head of the bed may reduce the chance for this complication. If orbital compartment syndrome is suspected, emergency orbital decompression is the best chance for recovery.[32-37]

Lateral Positioning

The lateral or three-quarters lateral decubitus position carries with it specific risks for peripheral nerve injuries. Stretch on the brachial plexus can be prevented by placement of an axillary roll slightly thicker than the diameter of the upper part of the arm. This roll should be placed approximately four fingerbreadths below the armpit to prevent compression of the long thoracic nerve. Failure to place an adequately sized roll may lead to excessive stretch of the brachial plexus, with the greatest effects on the C5 and C6 nerve roots. The upper extremities need to be supported in relatively neutral positions to prevent ulnar neuropathies. Horner's syndrome can occur when the head is inadequately padded and allowed to hang laterally in such a manner that excessive tension is placed on the superior cervical ganglion.[38] Excessive traction on the lateral femoral cutaneous nerve can be caused by undue extension of the upper part of the leg at the hip while bending the dependent leg. Compression of the common peroneal nerve can occur as a result of inadequate padding laterally under the knee.

Intraoperative Monitoring

Various electrophysiologic modalities can be used to detect subtle signs of neurological compromise before they become fixed deficits. The use of intraoperative monitoring can reduce the likelihood of significant neurological deficits in the appropriate circumstances. Some positioning complications can be avoided with the concomitant use of intraoperative monitoring.[11,39-43] At our institution, we use motor evoked potentials or somatosensory evoked potentials before and after positioning that may result in injury to the cervical cord. We have found excellent correlation between the lack of changes in evoked potentials and patient outcome. Monitoring is not necessary or indicated in all cases because it is time-consuming, can cause inappropriate movement of the patient, results in bleeding, and has the potential for needlestick injury to the operating room staff. However, in procedures with a potential for significant risk to the cord or neural structures, neurological monitoring is a helpful adjunct to the surgeon. Electrophysiologic neurological monitoring can consist of somatosensory evoked potentials, motor evoked potentials, intraoperative electromyographic responses, nerve action potential monitoring, direct spinal cord stimulation, and other methods.[40,41,44-48] The information gleaned from these modalities can be used to determine whether manipulation of the neural elements is compromising conduction. Numerous authors have published series in which the surgeon has changed some portion of the procedure as a reaction to changes in electrophysiologic monitoring.[11,39-43,47-52] Changes in ulnar nerve somatosensory evoked potentials can also indicate traction injury to the brachial plexus and are increasingly being used to monitor positioning, even with lumbar and thoracic procedures.[26,27,49]

Although not appropriate to monitor for position-related changes, direct epidural electrode motor evoked potential monitoring provides real-time evaluation of the spinal motor tracts and allows quantification of the measured output. This technique may be used during intramedullary spinal cord tumor resection and has been suggested to be helpful in minimizing injury during intramedullary resection.[54]

Cranial Fixation Complications

Positioning of the head for cranial fixation is a frequent source of complications. In sacral, lumbar, and midthoracic surgery performed with the patient in the prone position, the head does not need to remain immobile, nor does the cervical spine need to be kept straight. In these circumstances, the head is positioned on loose foam padding (with a cutout for the airway and no compression on the eyes), or the head is turned to the side on loose padding. The objective is to prevent compression on the eyes, face, and forehead. However, for many types of cranial, craniocervical, cervical, or cervicothoracic surgery, it is necessary to firmly immobilize the head and prevent unwanted motion of the neck. Several devices can be used to immobilize the head, the most effective of which is the Mayfield head clamp. This clamp involves three-point pin fixation into the skull so that the skull and neck are rigid relative to the table and, assuming that the body is adequately secured to the table, rigid relative to the body. Because it is more difficult to correct spine deformities after the head is secured in this manner, if part of the goal is to reconstitute cervical lordosis, this issue needs to be considered when positioning. Placing the patient in traction with Gardner-Wells tongs, for example, may be more appropriate for this situation. Pin site complications include lacerations,[55] skull fractures, associated intracranial hemorrhage (i.e., epidural, subdural, or subarachnoid hemorrhages), and infections that can lead to osteomyelitis.[56-61] Lacerations can be prevented by making sure that the two-pin arm swivels freely so that the force is evenly distributed between the two pins without one pin being shielded from tension, which can potentially result in pivoting on the other pin. If the pins are placed into muscle, it is wise to recheck tension on the single pin to make sure that the muscle has not settled and reduced the pressure. The three pins should be placed slightly below the center of gravity of the head when it is in final position to prevent gravity or personnel from pulling the head down and out of the pins. Ideally, the pins should not be placed directly into the coronal suture or temporal squamosal bone because these bones are most prone to fracture.[62-64] Pins should be tightened to 60 to 80 pounds in adults and 40 to 60 pounds in children younger than 15 years. In general, pins are avoided in children younger than 2 years; however, some skull clamp systems do exist for these patients for procedures in which they are required.[65] Pivoting within the pins by one of these methods or by inadequately locking the clamp before positioning the patient can result in changes in neck position (which can cause cervical spinal cord injury), lacerations, or compression on the eyes and subsequent blindness. These complications can also occur with Gardner-Wells–type tong traction.

Other forms of head support include the horseshoe headrest and the four-cup headrest. Because the horseshoe headrest is not a rigid form of fixation, the head may shift during the procedure, and thus it is imperative that the anesthesiologist continuously observe for any signs of movement. The four-cup headrest is an excellent alternative to the horseshoe, although blindness, skin and scalp compression, and abnormal cervical motion are possible with either support. Alopecia has been reported as a result of scalp compression.[66-72]

Dependent Edema

One complication associated with the prone position is the development of orofacial edema when the head is dependent. This complication occurs more frequently with longer procedures and when the spine is more flexed for facilitation of the surgical approach. Such edema can be prevented by minimizing the amount of fluid given by the anesthesiologist and by placing the patient slightly more in a reverse-Trendelenburg position to elevate the head relative to the heart. Facial edema can result in lingual or laryngeal edema and resultant airway obstruction. If obstruction occurs, the patient should be kept intubated until the edema has improved or resolved. Premature attempts at extubation can result in hypoxia and may necessitate emergency tracheotomy.

CATASTROPHIC MEDICAL COMPLICATIONS

Venous Air Embolism

In positioning patients for neurosurgical procedures, the anesthesia team and the surgeons must be aware of the gradient between the patient's head and the right atrium. Venous air embolism (VAE) is most often encountered with the patient in the seated position for posterior fossa surgery or cervical spine surgery.[73-78] It has also been described in patients who have undergone procedures in the prone, supine, and lateral positions.[73,76-82] Dehydration or blood loss leading to decreased central venous pressure may potentiate the risk for VAE. Patients with a patent foramen ovale or a known right-to-left shunt should be given special consideration before the seated position is used because the risk for paradoxical air embolism after VAE appears to be higher.

Most VAEs are thought to be caused by air entering noncollapsible veins, dural sinuses, or diploic veins. They also have arisen from central venous lines and pulmonary artery catheters. Air travels from the head down the venous system to the heart and eventually to the lungs, where pulmonary constriction and pulmonary hypertension ensue, or in patients with a right-to-left heart shunt, paradoxical air embolism may occur. Peripheral resistance decreases, and cardiac output initially increases to compensate and maintain blood pressure. Later, as the volume of air infused increases, cardiac output drops, as does blood pressure. Without intervention, cardiac arrest may occur.

Given the dangers of VAE, early detection of the embolus is paramount in reducing the severity of this complication. Monitoring methods and devices used to detect emboli include precordial Doppler ultrasonography, capnography or mass spectrometry, transesophageal echocardiography, transcutaneous oxygen, esophageal stethoscope, and right heart catheter.[73,74,76-79,82] The most sensitive are transesophageal echocardiography and Doppler, followed by expired nitrogen and end-tidal carbon dioxide. Electrocardiographic changes, hypotension, and heart murmurs are late signs. Because no single monitor is completely reliable, two or more should be used simultaneously. In awake patients, the presence of a cough may be the earliest sign of VAE, and it can be treated before the VAE becomes hemodynamically significant.[83] Detection of VAE has increased over the past several decades, but serious morbidity and mortality have decreased. Its incidence varies from 1.2% to 60%, with morbidity and mortality rates of less than 3% in most series.

Treatment of VAE includes aspiration of air through a right atrial catheter, discontinuation of nitrous oxide because it may enlarge the air bubble, and administration of pure oxygen. Surgeons should immediately seal the portals of entry with bone wax, electrocautery, and full-field irrigation. Arrhythmias, hypotension, and hypoxemia should be corrected quickly. Repositioning the patient in the left lateral decubitus position may facilitate removal of air from the right atrium. Stabilization of the patient's hemodynamic status becomes the first priority, and the procedure may have to be prematurely terminated if hemodynamic stabilization cannot be achieved easily.

Deep Venous Thrombosis and Pulmonary Embolism

Deep venous thrombosis (DVT) and pulmonary embolism are major contributors to morbidity and mortality in postoperative neurosurgical patients. The incidence of DVT, as measured by the labeled fibrinogen technique, ranges from 29% to 43%. It can be as high as 60% in patients with malignant intracranial neoplasms.[84-97] Most DVTs are asymptomatic and never come to medical attention. Pulmonary embolism, however, is thought to subsequently occur in 15% of such patients.[85,89,94,98,99] Significant thrombi are thought to arise from the popliteal and iliofemoral veins. Risk factors include prolonged surgery and immobilization, previous DVT, malignancy, direct lower extremity trauma, limb weakness, use of oral contraceptives, gram-negative sepsis, advanced age, hypercoagulability, pregnancy, and congestive heart failure.[84,86,88-94,98-106]

A diagnosis of DVT made by clinical examination is generally unreliable. Ankle swelling, calf pain, calf tightness, and a positive Homans sign may all be absent, even in the presence of significant DVT. Doppler ultrasonography and impedance plethysmography are useful in detecting proximal venous thrombosis and are the mainstay of diagnosis, with sensitivities exceeding 90%. When Doppler results are equivocal, extremity venography can be used to diagnose distal and proximal DVTs.

Because of the often-fatal result of pulmonary embolism, prophylaxis against DVT is of major importance in neurosurgery. Many studies have confirmed the usefulness of sequential pneumatic leg compression devices in preventing DVT.[85,86,88,89,94,95,107,108] These devices are placed on the patient preoperatively and should be continued until the patient is ambulatory. Early mobilization of postoperative patients is important in preventing thrombus formation. The prophylactic use of low-dose ("mini-dose") subcutaneous heparin (e.g., 5000 IU twice daily) has been well studied over the past 25 years and has been demonstrated to be efficacious in preventing DVT.[91,106-113] However, some studies have shown an increase in the rate of postoperative intracranial bleeding with mini-dose administration of heparin.[108,109] Low-molecular-weight heparin (LMWH) has more recently been used for DVT prophylaxis in surgical patients. Several meta-analyses have been conducted, but it remains unclear whether unfractionated heparin or LMWH is superior for DVT prophylaxis in neurosurgical patients or whether increased efficacy correlates with increased hemorrhagic complications.[114-117]

Accordingly, in patients with brain neoplasms, there are no clear guidelines as to when pharmacologic prophylaxis should be started. In general, those with hemorrhagic tumors as well as multiple metastasis from known hemorrhagic primary tumors (thyroid, renal cell, choriocarcinoma, and melanoma) should not receive pharmacologic prophylaxis. After surgery, safe prophylaxis has been reported as early as 12 hours. In addition, enoxaparin and heparin have been shown to be equally safe and effective.[97] For intracranial hemorrhages and subarachnoid hemorrhages, American Stroke Association (ASA) guidelines recommend mechanical prophylaxis and consideration of pharmacologic prophylaxis with heparin after documentation of cessation of growth of the hemorrhage. In subarachnoid hemorrhage patients, aneurysms should be secured before initiation of pharmacologic prophylaxis. LMWH may be used safely after elective neurosurgical procedures as early as postoperative day 1.[97,118]

Despite the use of such prophylactic methods, thrombi inevitably develop in one or both lower extremities in some patients. Management options include full-dose heparinization or inferior vena cava interruption. In the immediate and early postoperative period, many neurosurgeons believe that neurosurgical patients with documented DVT should undergo transvenous Greenfield filter placement.[85,86,88,89,93,94,104,108] There appears to be a general consensus that full anticoagulation is acceptable 1 to 3 weeks after surgery; our institution uses the 1-week rule. Treatment with intravenous heparin (target partial thromboplastin time of 45 to 60 seconds) is followed by oral warfarin sulfate (target international normalized ratio of 2) when not contraindicated. Anticoagulation should be continued for 6 weeks to 3 months in uncomplicated cases. Gastrointestinal bleeding is the most common serious complication encountered.

Patients experiencing pulmonary embolism complain of pleuritic chest pain, hemoptysis, and dyspnea. Jugular venous distention, fever, rales, tachypnea, hypotension, and altered mental status may be found on physical examination. Arterial blood gas determination reveals a Po_2 of less than 80 mm Hg in 85% of patients, accompanied by a widened alveolar-arterial gradient. The level of fibrin degradation products is elevated in most cases. In patients with massive embolism, right axis deviation, right ventricular strain, or right bundle branch block may be identified on electrocardiography. Chest radiography demonstrates an effusion or infiltrate in 90% of cases. A nuclear medicine ventilation-perfusion scan is sensitive in detecting pulmonary embolism but is not specific. The entire clinical scenario, including patient examination, laboratory results, and radiographic evaluation, leads to the diagnosis.[85,89,94,99,119-123] Spiral computed tomography (CT) has become the preferred diagnostic study for pulmonary embolism.[124] However, pulmonary angiography is the "gold standard" and may be necessary to confirm the diagnosis in as many as half of patients.

Guidelines similar to those discussed for treatment of DVT should be used for the treatment of pulmonary embolism. Patients with a massive, life-threatening embolus, however, should be fully anticoagulated despite the risk for intracranial hemorrhage. This subset of patients usually requires ventilatory support and vasopressor therapy to ensure adequate oxygenation and blood pressure. Because thrombolytic therapy with urokinase or streptokinase has a higher risk for complications than does treatment with heparin, with no significant improvement in outcome, these modes of therapy have largely been abandoned. When all else fails, pulmonary embolectomy may be performed as a lifesaving measure.

Hemorrhagic and Transfusion-Related Issues

Two significant and somewhat similar complications related to bleeding are diffuse intravascular coagulation and transfusion reactions. Both are a consequence of excessive bleeding and transfusions. The first results in a consumptive coagulopathy and further paradoxical bleeding. The other is a reaction to incompatible blood and can result in fever, rash, or shock. Both can be prevented by meticulous hemostasis. When bone is bleeding in an area where the need for fusion precludes the use of bone wax, thrombin-soaked Gelfoam can be rubbed on the bleeding bone surfaces and acts in much the same way as bone wax. When hemostasis alone is not enough to minimize transfusion requirements, as with some long spinal procedures, autologous blood salvage (e.g., Cell Saver) can be used to recycle the patient's own blood. Other modalities to minimize allogeneic transfusions include autologous blood donation (with or without the use of preoperative erythropoietin), hemodilution, or induced hypotension. Patients about to undergo neurosurgery should, when medically suitable, avoid the use of aspirin products in the week before surgery and other nonsteroidal anti-inflammatory agents on the day before surgery.

Wound Complications

Because of the vascularity of the scalp, most cranial wounds heal well. Postoperative pseudomeningocele formation from persistent leakage of cerebrospinal fluid (CSF) is more common when the normal CSF reabsorption pathways are impaired, as with hydrocephalus, subarachnoid hemorrhage, and meningitis. CSF finds the path of exit of least resistance from the head.

Several potential problems related to the wound area and wound closure can be anticipated and prevented. The first category is postoperative blood collections, or hematomas. Ideally, postoperative hematomas can be prevented by meticulous hemostasis during the procedure, but such is not always the case. The use of postoperative drainage devices (e.g., Hemovac, Jackson-Pratt drain) in wounds for which hemostasis was difficult to achieve before closure can reduce the incidence of postoperative hematoma. Postoperative drainage may also be advantageous in patients in whom postoperative anticoagulation may be required because some of these patients have slightly delayed hematoma formation.[125] An obese patient undergoing spine surgery may have significant serous exudation that can continue for up to 5 days or longer postoperatively. It is best to keep a drain in the submuscular space during this time to prevent a postoperative seroma that can become infected. Recent guidelines for infection prevention recommend prophylactic antibiotics 1 hour before incision and 24 hours postoperatively. However, there is no consensus as to whether antibiotics should be continued until a wound drain is removed. For ventriculostomy drains, antibiotic-coated catheters have been shown to be more effective than prophylactic antibiotic use in preventing infection.[126-128]

Several factors can predispose to loss of wound integrity. Prolonged steroid use, irradiation or chemotherapy, reoperations, and malnutrition can predispose patients to poor wound healing. With the increasing use of bevacizumab, a vascular endothelial growth factor (VEGF) inhibitor, for malignant brain tumors, one may consider using a plastic closure for the scalp.[129-131] Patients who are likely to lie on their incisions because of an inability to move or the location of an incision are also likely to experience wound breakdown because of pressure-related ischemia and failure to heal adequately. Known or unknown intraoperative violations of sterility may lead to subcutaneous infection and resultant loss of wound integrity. Failure to use perioperative antibiotics can also lead to local infection and failure of the incision line. Maintenance of a dry, sterile wound area results in better wound healing, and if a dressing becomes significantly stained or wet, it must be changed immediately. One way to prevent wound breakdown in a compromised host is the use of an incision that avoids the impaired area. Craniotomies may require a larger incision, such as a bicoronal or larger curvilinear incision that avoids a focused radiation area. In spine surgery, this means use of a paramedian incision. Through removal of the incision from the avascular midline plane and creation of a vascularized myocutaneous flap, patients with cancer or severe malnutrition can have wound-healing rates that are the same as or better than those in healthy patients. If the incision is made off the midline, the pressure is also not directly on the wound and the instrumentation.

Other modalities being investigated include the use of cultured keratinocytes or fibroblasts injected back into the wound area, supplemental or hyperbaric oxygen therapy for several days after surgery, and injection of various growth factors into the wounds.

RISK FACTORS RELATED TO ANATOMY OR TECHNIQUE IN SPECIFIC SURGERIES

Cranial Surgery

Postoperative Seizures

The risk for postoperative seizures within the first week after supratentorial procedures has been well described in the literature.[132-145] The underlying cause of these seizures may be metabolic derangements, cerebral hypoxia, preoperative structural defects, stroke and vascular abnormalities, or congenital seizure disorder. Manipulation of brain tissue, postoperative edema, and hematoma formation are common causes of surgically induced seizures. The overall incidence of immediate and early seizures after craniotomy is 4% to 19%. It is important to identify any risk factors that may contribute to the development of seizures postoperatively. Lesions of the supratentorial intracranial compartment are responsible for seizures after craniotomy in most situations; seizures after infratentorial procedures are attributed to the resultant retraction or movement of supratentorial structures.[132,133,137-142,144,146-149] Brain abscesses, hematomas, intra-axial and extra-axial tumors, aneurysms, arteriovenous malformations, and shunts have been reported to be epileptogenic.[141,149-162] Patients with a preoperative history of epilepsy are at a higher risk for seizures postoperatively. Patients with subtherapeutic levels of prophylactic agents are also at a higher risk for immediate and early postoperative seizures.[139,142,147,163-166]

All types of seizures can occur after neurosurgery. The diagnosis of a postoperative epileptic event is usually obvious. Multiple episodes are more common than single episodes, but status epilepticus is relatively uncommon. Seizures can occur in unconscious, comatose patients and may manifest as nonconvulsive status epilepticus. An electroencephalogram may be useful in these situations. The consequences of seizures are neurological and systemic and include neuronal damage, increased cerebral blood flow, and increased intracranial pressure (ICP). Metabolic acidosis, hyperazotemia, hyperkalemia, hypoglycemia, hyperthermia, and hypoxia may develop and exacerbate the situation, thereby leading to further seizure activity.

Preventing a seizure is preferable to treating one that has already begun. Adequate preoperative loading of parenteral or oral phenytoin has definitively been shown to decrease the incidence of postoperative seizures.[167-169] In patients unable to tolerate phenytoin, phenobarbital or carbamazepine may be substituted. It follows that therapeutic preoperative levels should be measured in patients undergoing supratentorial procedures whenever possible. Administration of the anticonvulsant should continue through the acute and early postoperative period. Electrolyte abnormalities should be corrected immediately in the postoperative period to further reduce the chance for a seizure.[170,171] Most seizures in neurosurgical patients are self-limited and last between 2 and 4 minutes. A chemistry profile should be obtained and any abnormalities corrected. Blood levels of antiseizure medications should also be verified and brought into the therapeutic range. Multiple seizures or any seizure lasting longer than 5 minutes should be aggressively treated rather than waiting 30 minutes to fulfill the criteria for status epilepticus. Treatment may entail the administration of lorazepam, diazepam, or midazolam, followed by fosphenytoin. Cardiorespiratory support measures may need to be initiated as well. For refractory cases, reintubation followed by phenobarbital coma or general anesthesia may be necessary. In most cases, it is probably best to image the patient postoperatively after the seizure episode has been treated. The possibility of intracranial hemorrhage, edema, infarction, or pneumocephalus must be entertained and the appropriate surgical or medical management initiated as soon as possible.

Reports have called into question the routine practice of phenytoin prophylaxis for patients without a history of seizures.[139,165,172]

Electrocorticography has recently been studied in patients preoperatively as a way to predict whether a patient is at risk of seizures after supratentorial procedures.[170,171,173] However, in our institution, all patients undergo seizure prophylaxis for 1 week after supratentorial procedures. In patients who have a history of seizures preoperatively, antiepileptics are continued for 3 to 6 months after surgery.

Postoperative Edema and Increased Intracranial Pressure

Neurosurgical procedures involving direct manipulation of brain tissue may lead to postoperative swelling. The amount of edema is related to many factors. The duration and force of tissue retraction on central nervous system tissue are directly related to the amount of postoperative swelling in the supratentorial and infratentorial compartments. Bipolar coagulation can further contribute to this edema when cortical bleeding is caused by retraction. The edema may be worsened if venous drainage is impaired and results in local congestion. Sustained venous hypertension may cause infarction and petechial hemorrhage, often with disastrous consequences. Noncompliance of the cranium then leads to increased ICP. Cerebral perfusion is limited, and neurological dysfunction ensues. In severe cases, herniation follows.

For lengthy procedures or when significant brain retraction is necessary, the use of a rigid, self-retaining retractor system combined with rigid head fixation can help limit the damage caused by tissue manipulation. Preservation of the cerebral vasculature during surgery, with limited coagulation and careful tissue handling, can reduce the occurrence of severe edema postoperatively.

The neurological deficits caused by brain swelling may be permanent or transient, and the severity of the deficit depends on the patient. Edema usually begins within 5 hours after the procedure and reaches its maximum approximately 48 to 72 hours later.[174-182] Altered mental status, cranial nerve deficits, and motor or sensory dysfunction can all occur. The diagnosis may be confirmed with non–contrast-enhanced CT, and hemorrhage, hydrocephalus, and pneumocephalus may be ruled out. Cerebral hypodensity, sulcal effacement, midline shift, loss of the gray-white matter interface, and small lateral ventricles are the hallmarks of postoperative edema. If impaired venous drainage secondary to the incompetence of venous sinuses is suspected, conventional venous-phase angiography or magnetic resonance venography may be helpful in diagnosing the location and severity of the occlusion. Appropriate surgical and medical measures may then be instituted.

The goal of treatment of increased ICP is to maintain cerebral perfusion pressure (CPP) at greater than 55 to 60 mm Hg while reducing the amount of cerebral edema.[182-189] This entails measuring arterial blood pressure and ICP continuously. Induction of arterial hypertension with vasopressors may be necessary to achieve the desired CPP. Short-term hyperventilation to a Pco_2 of 30 mm Hg can reduce ICP effectively. High-dose dexamethasone should be given to patients with vasogenic edema to alleviate tumor-related swelling. Increasing the head of the bed to 30 to 45 degrees can assist in venous return, and maintaining a neutral midline head position and administering diuretics such as furosemide and mannitol can further reduce ICP. When using diuretics, it is important that serum chemistries and osmolalities be monitored to ensure that the patient does not become severely dehydrated. Hypertonic saline solutions are now increasingly being used with success for the treatment of vasogenic edema.[190,191] In refractory cases, sedation may be used to suppress cerebral metabolism and paralysis may be induced to reduce

TABLE 6-1 Morbidity and Mortality Rates for Cranial Parenchymal Tumors

Study	Patients	Medical Morbidity (%)	Neurological Morbidity (%)	Mortality (%)
Fadul et al,[192] 1988	104	12	19.7	3.3
Cabantog and Bernstein,[193] 1994	207	8.2	17	2.4
Sawaya et al,[194] 1998	327	5	8.5	1.7
Taylor and Bernstein,[195] 1999	200	3.5	13	1

TABLE 6-2 Neurological Complications in Intraparenchymal Tumor Surgery

Complication	Rate (%)
Motor or sensory deficit	7.5
Aphasia	0.5
Visual field deficit	0.5

From Sawaya R, Hammoud M, Schoppa D. Neurosurgical outcomes in a modern series of 400 craniotomies for treatment of parenchymal tumors. *Neurosurgery.* 1998;42:1044-1055.

ICP by limiting agitation and muscle exertion. As a final resort, barbiturate coma with mild hypothermia or temporal lobectomy may be used to control ICP and maintain CPP.

Specific Cranial Disorders

Supratentorial Craniotomy. Numerous lesions may be approached via supratentorial craniotomy. In low-grade gliomas, long-term control and cure are possible. Because high-grade gliomas are not curable by surgery, surgery represents a palliative treatment aimed at reducing tumor bulk and maximizing quality of life. Patients with metastatic brain lesions can have a significant improvement in their survival by removal of brain metastases. It is therefore incumbent on neurosurgeons to minimize complications when patients are in the early stages of their disease and their clinical condition is best. The decision about whether surgery is warranted involves carefully weighing the possible surgical complications against the potential benefits. Studies have shown that craniotomies for intraparenchymal lesions typically result in mortality rates of 2.2% and morbidity rates of 15% (Table 6-1).[192-195]

Tumors located in eloquent or deep brain areas are more difficult to surgically debulk and carry a higher risk for neurological morbidity. Surgery on gliomas typically results in more morbidity and mortality than does surgery on brain metastases.[194] Surgical outcome is closely tied to the patient's age and preoperative neurological status as measured by the Karnofsky performance status score.[192-194] Patients are at risk for general complications of craniotomies, including complications related to positioning, anesthesia, infection, seizures, hemorrhage, and neurological compromise. Neurological compromise may result from resection or retraction of normal functional brain tissue or compromise of the vascular supply. Neurological morbidities usually consist of motor or sensory deficits or aphasias (Table 6-2). Occasionally, visual field deficits can occur.

Gliomas lack a well-defined boundary between abnormal and normal tissue. Pathologic analysis demonstrates tumor cells in grossly normal-appearing tissue. The result is a tradeoff between radical tumor resection and risk for resection of functional brain tissue and subsequent neurological deterioration. Avoidance of vascular compromise involves meticulous attention to detail and preservation of all significant vasculature seen to supply normal brain tissue. If significant vessels are taken during surgery, postoperative CT or magnetic resonance imaging (MRI) can reveal the evolution of an infarction in the vessel's vascular distribution.

Computer-assisted stereotactic systems enhance the ability of the surgeon to delineate between normal brain and tumor. Stereotactic systems also facilitate targeting of tumors that cannot be visualized at the brain's surface. Intraoperative functional mapping helps identify and avoid injury to eloquent cortex. Craniotomy performed while the patient is awake is particularly helpful in resecting lesions surrounding the speech centers. Using an awake craniotomy technique, Taylor and Bernstein reported an overall complication rate of 16.5% and a mortality rate of 1%.[195] New postoperative neurological deficits were seen in 13% of patients, but they were permanent in just 4.5%. Increasingly, functional imaging is being applied intraoperatively, with evidence suggesting that it allows more complete resection while minimizing the risk for deficits. Functional MRI and diffusion-weighted imaging can be integrated with most neuronavigation systems to allow identification and protection of motor tracts.[196-199]

Eyupoglu and colleagues reported using fluorescence-guided surgery with 5-aminolevulinic acid (5-ALA) and intraoperative MRI with integrated functional neuronavigation to resect malignant gliomas in a small series of patients. By using these modalities, they were able to improve extent of resection by 15% without incurring postoperative neurological deficit.[200]

Hemorrhage into the postoperative tumor bed is a serious complication that may require reoperation for evacuation of hematoma. Prevention begins with checking preoperative coagulation studies and ensuring that the patient has not been taking an aspirin-containing product. Intraoperatively, meticulous hemostasis must be achieved with a variety of hemostatic agents and bipolar electrocautery. The tumor cavity may be lined with hemostatic agents such as Surgicel. Tight blood pressure control during extubation and in the postoperative period is important. Rarely, distal intracerebral or intracerebellar hemorrhages can occur, although their cause is unexplained.[201]

All patients undergoing surgery have a risk for thromboembolic events, but those with malignant gliomas are at significantly increased risk. Prophylaxis with low-dose heparin and external pneumatic leg muscle compression must be initiated promptly. The neurosurgical staff must maintain a high index of suspicion for phlebitis and pulmonary embolism so that treatment can be initiated early. Inferior vena cava filters may be placed to prevent the occurrence of pulmonary embolism. Full anticoagulation is preferable in patients seen more than 3 weeks after surgery.[95,202] Wound infection and wound dehiscence occur rarely with craniotomies and develop in less than 1% of patients.[194] The routine use of steroids in patients with intraparenchymal tumors apparently has little effect on overall wound healing. However, prolonged high-dose steroid use does increase the risk of wound-healing problems and infection.[129]

Surgery for gliomas is rarely curative, and many patients with recurrences are subject to reoperation. However, studies have demonstrated that reoperation does not necessarily predispose patients to a greater complication rate.[192,194,203]

More important, carmustine (BCNU) wafer implantation, adjuvant chemotherapeutic agents, and radiation increase the rates of wound complications significantly. Preparations for such complications should be made in advance if the patient is anticipated to receive these treatments.[130,131]

TABLE 6-3 Meningiomas and Seizure Frequency

Study	Preoperative Seizure Frequency (%)	Postoperative Seizure Frequency (%)	First Seizure Occurring Postoperatively (%)
Ramamurthi et al,[204] 1980	29	25	17
Chan and Thompson,[205] 1984	—	36	19
Pertuiset et al,[206] 1985	50	32	20
Chozick et al,[132] 1996	40	20	9

Meningiomas differ from parenchymal tumors in that they are often associated with venous sinuses, and thus venous infarction or injury to the sinuses is an additional risk. These tumors can invade the wall of sinuses and eventually narrow and obliterate the sinus lumen. When meningiomas are located in proximity to a sinus, preoperative venous angiography, magnetic resonance angiography, or magnetic resonance venography is essential to avoid complications. Entering a patent sinus can result in difficult bleeding that may require surgical reconstruction or bypass of the sinus. Sacrifice of a major venous sinus should be avoided. Complications associated with sacrificing a major venous sinus include increased ICP as a result of brain edema and venous hemorrhagic infarction. Obtundation and seizures can develop in such patients (Table 6-3). Aggressive ICP management is essential in controlling this complication. Prudent surgical management may necessitate leaving a portion of the tumor adherent to the sinus and using adjuvant therapy or observation with surveillance MRI.[207] Postoperative seizures are seen with convexity and parasagittal meningiomas.[205] Sacrifice of a significant vein can result in venous infarction and an increased risk for seizures. The mortality rate for craniotomies performed for convexity and parasagittal meningiomas is 3.7% to 13%.[205,208-215]

Posterior Fossa Craniotomy. Infratentorial craniotomies carry many of the same risks as do supratentorial craniotomies. However, some risks are more pronounced when operating in the posterior fossa.

Positioning-related risks have already been described—air embolism, for example—and are particularly commonly encountered when performing surgery with the patient in the sitting position. Most surgeons choose to operate with the patient in a lateral, park bench, or prone position instead.

Leakage of CSF is seen frequently after a posterior fossa craniotomy and occurs in 3% to 15% of patients.[216-218] Leakage can occur from the wound or can manifest as rhinorrhea or otorrhea. Openings into the mastoid air cells and air cells in the vicinity of the meatus can lead to otorrhea. Fluid can drain into the nasopharynx through the eustachian tube. Packing the mastoid air cells with bone wax can prevent CSF leakage. Aggressive drilling of the porus acusticus and larger tumor size have been associated with an increasing risk for CSF leaks.[219] To minimize the risk for postoperative rhinorrhea, we apply bone wax aggressively to all mastoid air cells exposed during the craniectomy, as well as fibrin glue before closure. However, unroofing of air cells within the internal auditory canal can lead to persistent leakage, and we routinely apply a muscle plug, Gelfoam, and fibrin glue in this region to minimize the risk for leakage. In addition, routine prophylactic high-volume lumbar puncture may be performed daily for 3 days postoperatively to minimize the risk for leakage. When leakage occurs, management typically involves placement of a spinal drain. Operative repair may be necessary in patients in whom a trial of spinal drainage fails. Early recognition plus treatment of CSF leaks is imperative because CSF leakage places patients at risk for meningitis.[218] Meningitis occurs in about 1% of patients, and early treatment with appropriate antibiotics is essential. Aseptic meningitis also occurs infrequently after surgery. Patients may have some elements of ataxia postoperatively, but these symptoms are usually limited and resolve within a few days.

TABLE 6-4 Common Complication Rates in Transsphenoidal Surgery

Complication	Rate (%)
Mortality	0-1.75
Nasal septum perforation	1-3
Sinusitis	1-4
Epistaxis	2-4
Visual disturbances	0.6-1.6
Transient diabetes insipidus	10-60
Permanent diabetes insipidus	0.5-5
Anterior pituitary insufficiency	1-10
Cerebrospinal fluid leakage	1-4
Meningitis	0-1.75

Significant headaches occur in half of patients postoperatively, and 25% complain of headaches persisting for more than a year after surgery.[220]

Mortality from infratentorial surgery is generally higher than that seen with supratentorial procedures. Compromise of the anterior inferior cerebellar artery and the resultant lateral pontine infarction are implicated in a third of postoperative deaths.[221] The second biggest contributor to postoperative mortality is aspiration pneumonia resulting from lower cranial nerve deficits. Patients may require placement of a feeding tube and a tracheostomy to prevent aspiration pneumonia. Cerebellar contusions or hematomas can occur as a result of overaggressive retraction. Distant supratentorial hemorrhages occasionally occur for unclear reasons.[222] Surgeons must be prepared to place an occipital ventricular catheter intraoperatively on an emergency basis if acute hydrocephalus results.

Transsphenoidal Surgery. Transsphenoidal surgery is commonly used to reach tumors in the sellar region. This procedure can be performed with extremely low mortality and low morbidity. Deaths have occurred in 0% to 1.75% of patients (Table 6-4). Laws[223] reported seven deaths in 786 procedures (0.9%), and Wilson[224] reported two deaths (0.2%) in a series of 1000 patients. At our institution, two deaths occurred in 1800 procedures. Morbidities associated with the transsphenoidal approach are distinct from general neurosurgical complications because the approach is quite different from most transcranial approaches.

Avoidance of complications begins with appropriate patient selection. Patients with sphenoid sinus infections should not undergo transsphenoidal surgery because of the risk for meningitis. Tumor morphology may also dictate the operative approach. Tumors located eccentrically may not be accessible transsphenoidally and instead might require a transcranial approach. In tumors with dumbbell morphology, a constrictive diaphragma sellae may limit adequate tumor decompression. Tumor consistency also influences the surgical outcome. Most adenomas have a soft consistency and are easily and safely removed with curets and suction. Firm tumors, seen in 5% of patients, can be difficult to remove transsphenoidally. Adequate preoperative radiologic evaluation is essential because of the wide range of pathologies that are found in the sella. For example, misdiagnosis of an aneurysm as an adenoma can result in a potentially fatal complication. Any vascular anomalies in the sellar region may be a contraindication to the transsphenoidal approach.

Anesthetic complications in transsphenoidal surgery are rare. Acromegalic patients exhibit cardiomyopathy and macroglossia, which may complicate airway management. Patients with pituitary lesions are often deficient in one or more pituitary hormones. A comprehensive preoperative endocrine analysis is essential, and adequate stress doses of steroids should be administered. Postoperatively, the patient's endocrine status should be carefully monitored. Other medical complications are relatively rare and are commensurate with complications in other elective procedures.

Several complications can arise as a consequence of the transsphenoidal approach. If a sublabial incision is used, anesthesia of the upper lip and anterior maxillary teeth can occur, although this condition is usually transient.[225] Removal of the superior cartilaginous septum may result in a saddle nose deformity.[226] Perforation of the nasal septum occurs in 1% to 3% of patients and is more likely with reoperations.[223] Postoperative sinusitis can occur in 1% to 4% of patients and may be reduced by postoperative antibiotics.[227] Opening the speculum can result in diastasis of the maxilla or fracture of the medial orbital wall.[223,228] Damage to the optic nerve or the carotid arteries can occur if the speculum is advanced too far. Inadequate removal of mucosa in the sphenoid sinus can lead to the postoperative formation of a mucocele.[229]

Vascular injuries represent serious morbidities and can lead to death. Intraoperative mucosal bleeding and delayed postoperative bleeding from the mucosal branch of the sphenopalatine artery can occur. If postoperative epistaxis persists, embolization of the internal maxillary artery may be necessary.[230] Damage to the carotid arteries can occur in the sphenoid sinus or in the sella. Maintaining a midline trajectory is vital to avoid the carotid artery, and preoperative radiologic studies are essential in localizing the carotids. There are significant variations in the carotid's parasellar course, and the distance between the two arteries may be as little as 4 mm.[225] Frameless stereotaxis can be used to maintain a midline approach and may be especially useful in reoperations.[231] Endoscopy is increasingly being used to minimize tissue trauma and to obtain more expansive views than those provided by microscopic visualization alone.[232,233] Excessive arterial bleeding signals intraoperative injury to the carotid artery, and the only treatment involves packing the operative field.[230] Other maneuvers are limited by the exposure, although if packing fails, ligation of the carotid may be required. Carotid artery injury can result in subarachnoid hemorrhage, vasospasm, false aneurysms, and carotid cavernous fistulas. A postoperative cerebral angiogram is essential to identify any of these complications.[234] About 25% of deaths occurring during transsphenoidal operations are attributable to vascular injuries.[23,230] Visual disturbances are also possible because of the close association of the chiasm, optic nerve, and pituitary. Damage can occur as a result of direct trauma, traction injury, or vascular compromise. Visual disturbances are more likely after reoperations because of adhesion formation between the chiasm and sella. Adhesions predispose the chiasm, optic nerve, and hypothalamus to traction injuries. In general, visual disturbances occur in 0.6% to 1.6% of patients.[235] Postoperative visual loss can also signal the formation of a hematoma in the tumor bed. Such hematomas can be prevented by meticulous hemostasis. They can occur in 0.3% to 1.2% of cases.[223,227,229] Injuries to the hypothalamus can also take place and potentially result in death.[230] These patients are comatose and exhibit hyperthermia. Hypothalamic injury is the most common cause of death in patients undergoing transsphenoidal operations.[230]

Several complications can be anticipated in the postoperative period, and early recognition and appropriate treatment can circumvent catastrophic results. Patients should be closely monitored for diabetes insipidus (DI) with frequent serum sodium evaluations and careful accounting of patients' fluid intake and urine output. An elevated serum sodium level or urine output may indicate DI. Temporary postoperative DI can occur in 10% to 60% of patients.[227,236] Permanent DI is much less common and occurs in just 0.5% to 5% of patients.[227] Delayed onset of the syndrome of inappropriate antidiuretic hormone secretion can also occur about a week postoperatively.[230]

Postoperative anterior pituitary insufficiency is one of the most commonly seen postoperative complications. Its incidence varies from 1% to 10%.[223,224] Postoperative steroid therapy should be used in all postoperative patients until a thorough endocrine evaluation is complete. Adrenal insufficiency is a potentially serious complication if adequate steroid replacement therapy is not initiated.

CSF rhinorrhea is another commonly encountered complication of the transsphenoidal approach and occurs in 1% to 4% of patients.[223,230] Intraoperatively, penetration of the arachnoid membrane can result in a gush of CSF into the operative field and the potential for postoperative CSF rhinorrhea. Packing the sella intraoperatively with an autologous fat graft and bone from the removed vomer can help prevent CSF leakage. Care must be taken to not overpack the sella, which may lead to compression of the chiasm.[229] Patients in whom CSF rhinorrhea develops are first treated by spinal drainage for several days. Failure to close a CSF fistula with spinal drainage may indicate the need for reoperation and repacking of the sella. Early recognition and treatment of CSF rhinorrhea are important because a CSF leak can lead to meningitis. The incidence of meningitis in patients undergoing transsphenoidal surgery has been reported to be 0% to 1.75%.[227,229,237] Patients with diabetes mellitus are at greater risk for the development of meningitis.

Cranial Base Surgery. Cranial base lesions represent a heterogeneous group of pathologies associated with the cranial base bony structures. Although once considered inaccessible, advances in microsurgery and neurodiagnostics have extended the neurosurgeon's reach into the cranial base. The surgical approaches for cranial base surgery are challenging, and minimizing surgical morbidity is essential to achieve good outcomes. Complications are usually related to the lesion's location and the surgical approach necessary for exposure.

The surgical approaches often call for brain retraction to adequately expose the lesion. Overly aggressive retraction can lead to tissue damage and infarction, with postoperative swelling resulting in increased ICP. Several maneuvers, including adequate bone removal, CSF drainage, and diuretics, can aid in achieving adequate exposure without excessive brain retraction. Resection of noneloquent brain tissue may be required to prevent contusions and possible postoperative herniation occurring from retraction injuries. Retraction can also compromise or injure venous outflow and result in venous stasis and hemorrhagic infarctions. This is especially important with regard to the vein of Labbé. Excessive retraction of the posterior temporal lobe can lead to tearing of the vein of Labbé and severe hemorrhagic temporal lobe edema.[238]

Postoperative hematomas can also develop. Prevention involves meticulous hemostasis, tight blood pressure control in the postoperative period, and prompt correction of any coagulopathy. Early recognition involves having a high index of suspicion and performing early postoperative CT. Treatment usually involves operative evacuation of the hematoma.

CSF leakage is one of the most common postoperative complications in cranial base surgery. The surgery often creates a communication between the CSF space and the facial sinuses. The sphenoid sinus is most commonly involved because of its association with the clivus and cavernous sinus.[239] CSF leaks occur in about 8% of patients undergoing cranial base operations.[239] However, newer endoscopic repair techniques have been reported with CSF leak rates as low as 3.2%.[240] A persistent CSF fistula may develop. Leaks generally occur in the immediate postoperative period, or they rarely develop months after surgery.[239] CSF leaks manifest clinically as clear spinal fluid draining from the nose, ear, or wound. The fluid can be collected on a pledget, and the presence of β2-transferrin confirms the discharge as CSF. Confirmatory radiographic examinations can be performed. Radioisotopic cisternography with cotton pledgets in the nasal cavity can corroborate the presence of a CSF leak. CT cisternography with intrathecal metrizamide or magnetic resonance cisternography can be used to localize the leak.[241]

A watertight dural closure can prevent CSF leaks, but invasion of the dura by tumor or anatomic considerations often make closing the dura impossible. If watertight closure cannot be achieved, the cranial base should be reconstructed with muscle, fat, and fascia packing. Spinal fluid drainage can divert CSF and allow the dura or reconstruction to seal. Initial treatment of a postoperative CSF leak is a trial period of lumbar spinal drainage. CSF leaks that fail to resolve or CT demonstrating progressive increases in intracranial air necessitate surgical repair. A leak that recurs after spinal drainage is stopped necessitates reexploration with repacking and reconstruction of the cranial base. Early recognition of hydrocephalus is important because increased ICP can predispose a patient to a CSF leak, and correction of hydrocephalus may prevent a CSF leak.

Pneumocephalus is another postoperative complication frequently encountered in cranial base surgery. Air may be found in the extradural or intradural spaces. Intracranial air can produce alterations in a patient's mental status that result in lethargy or agitation. Some degree of pneumocephalus is commonly found on postoperative CT, and the air is usually reabsorbed quickly. Patients operated on in the sitting position have a higher incidence of pneumocephalus.[242] Increasing amounts of intracranial air signal the presence of a communication between the subarachnoid space and air sinuses and imply an undetected CSF leak. Having patients lie flat in bed and discontinuing external spinal drainage can facilitate the absorption of intracranial air. Passing a spinal needle through the bur-hole site into the air pocket can decompress the subdural air in the event of a tension pneumocephalus.[239]

Infection-related complications are relatively rare in cranial base neurosurgery, but they are of concern because of the communication established by surgery between the paranasal sinuses and the brain. Prevention involves standard sterile techniques and the administration of broad-spectrum antibiotics in the operating room and in the immediate postoperative period. Meningitis can occur, and early diagnosis, isolation of the causative agent, and appropriate antibiotic treatment are essential. CSF leaks predispose patients to meningitis, so repair of the CSF leak must be performed promptly. Epidural and parenchymal brain abscesses can also occur and are treated by operative drainage and appropriate antibiotics.

Skull base lesions often involve the cranial blood vessels. Tumors can encase or displace these vessels, and adequate tumor removal may require sacrifice of vessels. The neurosurgeon must know the consequences of sacrificing cranial base blood vessels to minimize morbidity. Sacrifice of vessels can result in ischemic neurological deficits and infarctions in a vascular territory or watershed distribution. Preoperatively, balloon occlusion testing and xenon-enhanced CT cerebral blood flow testing can determine whether patients can tolerate sacrificing a blood vessel. Patients in whom neurological deficits develop with the balloon occlusion test or who have cerebral blood flow of less than 35 mL/100 g per minute cannot tolerate vessel sacrifice and may require a bypass graft.[243]

Cranial nerve morbidity is commonly encountered with cranial base surgery, and the dysfunction may be temporary or permanent. Accurate preoperative cranial nerve examination is important because postoperative dysfunction is more likely in patients with preoperative deficits. Neurophysiologic monitoring is an important adjuvant for localizing cranial nerves and preventing injury. Cranial nerve VII may be monitored via continuous facial electromyographic responses. A nerve stimulator can help locate the facial nerve. Cranial nerve VIII can be monitored using brainstem auditory evoked potentials. New devices that attach to the cuff of the endotracheal tube can be placed such that they make contact with the posterior pharyngeal wall. These devices are useful in monitoring cranial nerves IX and X, and continuous monitoring of these nerves has been shown to help reduce swallowing difficulties postoperatively.[244] Cranial nerve XI can be localized with a nerve stimulator and observation of shoulder twitching.[215]

Cranial nerve injury can occur as a result of nerve retraction or direct injury during tumor dissection. Cranial nerves may also be injured by compromise of the nerves' blood supply during surgical dissection distant from the nerves. Damage to the cranial nerves is especially significant during surgery in the cavernous sinus. Optic nerve damage occurs in 0% to 6% of patients.[214,245] Permanent damage involving extraocular nerve function (i.e., cranial nerves III, IV, and VI) occurs in 20% to 30% of patients.[213,214] The incidence of V1 neuropathy is 8% to 20%.[213,214,245]

Certain cranial nerves are more susceptible to injury than others. Cranial nerves I, II, and VIII are very sensitive to injury. Minimal manipulation can result in profound deficits, and the loss of function is often irreversible. Cranial nerves III, IV, and VI are less sensitive to manipulation, and some recovery typically occurs postoperatively if the nerve's continuity is maintained. Injury to these nerves results in diplopia. Loss of cranial nerve IV function can be corrected by tilting the head or using prism glasses. Oculoplastic procedures may be necessary to correct persistent diplopia caused by injury to cranial nerve III or VI. Cranial nerve V damage is generally well tolerated, with the exception of damage to the V1 segments, which mediate the corneal reflex. Damage to the V1 division results in corneal sensory dysfunction, and patients must have meticulous eye care to prevent corneal abrasions and loss of vision in the desensitized eye.[239]

Damage to cranial nerve VII results in significant cosmetic morbidity as a consequence of facial paralysis and functional loss because of an inability to close the eye effectively. Damage can occur from direct injury to the nerve, injury to the geniculate ganglion, or nerve traction. Traction can occur during retraction of the greater superficial petrosal nerve or caudal retraction of the mandible after dislocation of the temporomandibular joint (TMJ). Maintaining nerve continuity offers the best chance of functional recovery. Direct end-to-end anastomosis can be performed, or a cable graft using a sural nerve graft may be necessary. Other options include XII-VII or XI-VII anastomoses. Tarsorrhaphy or insertion of a gold weight implant in the upper eyelid may be necessary if eye closure is not adequate. In the immediate postoperative period, eye care with artificial tears and eye lubricants is essential to prevent keratitis.

Cranial nerves IX and X are usually injured together. Unilateral, slowly developing lesions are usually well tolerated because of the patient's compensatory mechanisms. Acute lesions result in difficulty swallowing, inability to protect the airway, and unilateral vocal cord paralysis. Long-term dysfunction requires treatment with a tracheostomy and placement of a gastrostomy tube. Tracheostomies and feeding tubes may be removed if patients recover function sufficiently or compensatory mechanisms develop. Failure to initiate such measures can lead to malnutrition and aspiration pneumonia.

Unilateral injury to cranial nerve XII is generally well tolerated. When combined with other cranial nerve injuries, such as injury to cranial nerves VII, IX, or X, significant dysarthria can occur. Bilateral cranial nerve XII injury results in severe functional limitation and ultimately requires a tracheostomy and placement of a feeding tube.[239]

Cranial base surgery can cause morbidity from TMJ manipulation. Dislocation of the TMJ can result in postoperative trismus. Resection of the mandibular condyle may be preferred because it avoids retraction of the mandible and associated postoperative trismus. Resection of the condyle leads to a contralateral jaw deviation but no functional loss.[239]

Complications of Stereotactic Brain Surgery

Advances in medical technology have resulted in a host of neurosurgical procedures using three-dimensional stereotactic guidance systems. Many procedures involve the use of stereotactic guidance in performing conventional craniotomies or other operations. This section deals with complications related to stereotactic procedures performed through small bur holes or using focused radiation (i.e., Gamma Knife). Such procedures include brain biopsy, cyst aspiration, functional lesioning, and stereotactic radiosurgery.

A stereotactic frame is applied to the patient, and CT or MRI is performed. The most commonly used frames are the Leksell (Elektra Instruments, Atlanta, GA) and the Brown-Roberts-Wells (Radionics, Burlington, MA) systems.[246] The fiducial markers on the frame are registered into the system and allow accurate three-dimensional navigation and localization in reference to the neuroimaging. Proper application of the stereotactic frame and precise registration are essential to achieve accurate results. Frameless systems that use cutaneous fiducial markers are available, as well as some that use surface landmarks alone, with no need to place cutaneous fiducial markers.

One of the most commonly performed stereotactic procedures is brain biopsy. Brain biopsies are safe and effective procedures. The procedure can usually be performed under monitored anesthesia care and can avoid the complications associated with general anesthesia. CT or MRI is used to stereotactically guide biopsy of a lesion through a small bur hole. Possible complications include hemorrhage, neurological deficits, seizures, and infections.[246] The mortality rate in several large series has been less than 1%, and complication rates vary from 0% to 7% (Table 6-5).[246-253] Seizures and infections are rare during brain biopsy. The most serious complication usually involves postoperative hematoma formation. Properly performed brain biopsies are more than 90% effective in establishing a tissue diagnosis in patients with radiographic lesions.[246]

Recent studies have demonstrated no significant difference in the accuracy and the retrieval of diagnostic tissue between frame-based and frameless stereotactic biopsy. The use of frozen section is critical in confirming the retrieval of diagnostic tissue.[254,255]

Preventing complications related to brain biopsy requires adequate preoperative planning. Only patients in whom the results of brain biopsy may change medical management should undergo biopsy. Because thrombocytopenia or coagulopathies predispose patients to intracranial hemorrhage, all candidates should have normal coagulation profiles and platelet counts. Preoperative radiographic imaging is essential to rule out vascular lesions that may result in serious hemorrhage when biopsied. The planned trajectory must avoid vessels and important structures. Intraoperative hypertension may predispose patients to hemorrhage.[246]

When bleeding is discovered during a brain biopsy, allowing the blood to drain out of the needle may prevent the formation of a hematoma.[246] Craniotomy may be required to control persistent hemorrhage. Instillation of thrombin through the biopsy cannula has been used to control hemorrhage.[256] Routine postoperative CT can be performed to rule out hematoma formation, and asymptomatic hematomas are often discovered postoperatively. Neurological deficits develop in about 10% of patients with asymptomatic postoperative hematomas.[257] Most postoperative hematomas are managed by observation and serial CT.

Brain biopsies are increasingly being performed on patients infected with human immunodeficiency virus (HIV), who may be subject to several central nervous system infections or neoplasms. Biopsies in patients with acquired immunodeficiency syndrome have higher complication rates. Skolasky and coworkers reviewed 435 HIV-positive patients undergoing biopsy and determined that the morbidity rate was 8.4% and the mortality rate was 2.9%.[258] Complications were associated with preoperative poor functional status and thrombocytopenia. It is not clear whether the presence of HIV infection predisposes to higher complication rates.

Stereotactic Radiosurgery

Stereotactic radiosurgery is a safe and effective treatment modality for vascular malformations, brain tumors, and in some cases, functional surgery. Stereotactically applied radiation provides precise delivery of high-dose radiation to a well-defined target. Complications in radiosurgery are related to the effects of radiation on the brain and structures in proximity to the lesion. Significant early complications rarely occur but can include seizures or worsening neurological deficits. Approximately a third of patients experience mild transitory symptoms, including headaches, nausea, and dizziness.[259] This is thought to be secondary to transient swelling 12 to 48 hours after therapy. A course of steroids may help alleviate some of these symptoms.[260] Late complications develop 6 to 9 months after the procedure and can include facial palsy, trigeminal neuropathy, and visual symptoms.[246] Exposure of the optic nerve to more than 8 to 10 Gy of radiation leads to visual deterioration and optic neuropathy.[238,261] Patients may become symptomatic from radiation necrosis or local brain edema. In a review of 1600 patients undergoing radiosurgery with at least a 3-year follow-up, the rate of significant morbidity was 1.9%.[245] The risk for carcinogenesis secondary to radiosurgery is estimated to be less than 1 in 1000.[262]

Gamma Knife radiosurgery has been applied effectively to the treatment of acoustic neuromas. The complications associated with acoustic neuroma radiosurgery are related to exposure of cranial nerves to radiation. The rate of facial nerve paresis after 5-year follow-up has been 21%, and the rate of trigeminal

TABLE 6-5 Complications of Stereotactic Brain Biopsy

Series	No. of Cases	Hemorrhage (%)	Nonhemorrhage Deficit (%)	Seizure (%)	Infection (%)	Death (%)
Ostertag et al,[247] 1980	302	2.9	1	—	—	2.3
Lunsford and Martinez,[248] 1984	102	2	0	1	1	0
Apuzzo,[249] 1987	500	0.4	0.2	0.2	0.2	1
Kelly,[250] 1991	547	0.9	0.9	1.1	—	0.3
Voges et al,[251] 1993	338	2.4	0.3	0.6	0	0.6
Bernstein and Parrent,[252] 1994	300	4.7	0	0	0	1.7
Kondziolka et al,[246] 1998	367	0.3	0.3	0	0	0
Hall,[253] 1998	134	0.7	0.7	0	0	0

dysfunction has been 27%. Hearing was preserved in 51% of patients undergoing radiosurgery for acoustic neuromas.[263,264] Peritumoral edema after radiosurgery has occasionally led to hydrocephalus.[265] There is a significant increase in mass effect and tumor size, approximately 43%, after high-dose Gamma Knife radiosurgery for vestibular schwannomas that correlates with deterioration of facial and trigeminal function. The effect is much smaller at lower doses.[266] Because tumor control is greater with larger doses of radiation, fractionated stereotactic radiosurgery is usually performed to allow increased control of growth while minimizing risk to the facial, cochlear, and trigeminal nerves.[267] Intracanalicular tumors may be associated with higher cranial nerve morbidity when treated with radiosurgery.[268] Improvements in target imaging and reduction in doses have led to lower cranial nerve morbidity.[263,265]

Radiosurgery has also been applied to cranial base meningiomas. The morbidity rate is about 5% to 8%.[260,261,269,270] Most complications involve transient cranial nerve palsies and occur 3 to 31 months after surgery. High radiation doses applied to Meckel's cave increase risk for the development of trigeminal neuropathy.[261] Radiosurgery is also used to treat gliomas and brain metastasis. Preliminary reports indicate a morbidity rate of about 10% and a mortality rate of 1%.[271] However, newer studies are reporting a morbidity of up to 40% for treatment of multiple metastatic lesions.[272] Early complications can involve increased ICP, which may lead to death.[273] Radiotherapy for brain parenchymal lesions can result in seizure complications. Patients with lesions in the motor cortex are especially susceptible to seizures after radiosurgery.[274] Gamma Knife radiosurgery for trigeminal neuralgia is generally well tolerated and associated with minimal morbidity. Loss of facial sensation has been reported infrequently.[275]

Spine Surgery

Cerebrospinal Fluid Leak or Pseudomeningocele Formation

Prevention of CSF leakage is critical for optimizing wound healing, for preventing neural elements from herniating through the defect in the dura and leading to pain syndromes or neurological deficits, and for eliminating positional headaches. It is generally accepted that reduction of intraspinal CSF pressure facilitates healing of a dural defect. This can be achieved by maintenance of strict bed rest or by placement of a CSF diversion drain, such as a lumbar drain. The use of spinal subarachnoid drains after a CSF leak is supported as an adjunct.[276-280] One treatment element that seems to be accepted almost uniformly as being beneficial is the use of fibrin glue sealants.[281-286] The sealant can be prepared autologously in the operating room, from cryoprecipitate obtained from the blood bank, or from commercial kits made from donated blood products. Regardless of the cause, fibrin glue sealants, when applied in the area of the dural repair, dramatically increase the rate of healing. The use of dural replacements is more controversial. Repair with fascia, AlloDerm, DuraGen, or other techniques is more a matter of choice than evidence-based medicine.

Primary repair of a dural violation, when possible, is clearly indicated. Multiple surgeons have documented increased infection rates and decreased fusion rates associated with CSF leaks.[278,285-288] In addition to CSF leaking from the durotomy, nerve roots have been known to herniate into the durotomy and result in painful syndromes.[289]

A tight, multilayer closure is critical to prevent local CSF collections from leaking outward to the skin. If a CSF leak exists, organisms have a portal of entry and may cause meningitis. Any CSF leak should be treated immediately by oversewing of the wound and institution of some form of CSF pressure–reducing strategy. The decision to revise a wound rather than treat conservatively depends on several factors, including the tightness of the dural and fascial closure, the presence of and size of the subfascial collection, and the patient's underlying ability to heal a wound spontaneously. A CSF pseudomeningocele, even in the absence of an external leak, can increase the likelihood of local infection.

Instrumentation-Related Risks

Instrumentation has increased the incidence of complications in all series that have compared the results of instrumented with noninstrumented fusions.[290-293] This finding is not surprising in that instrumentation adds time, complexity, and an implanted foreign body to the operative procedure. Fusion rates are uniformly higher in instrumented cases, and most experienced spine surgeons believe that the risks are outweighed by the benefits of rigid segmental fixation. However, each surgeon must feel confident and comfortable with any technique because morbidity rates vary from surgeon to surgeon.[291,294-312]

Identification of the correct level is critical for most spine operations. Whether preoperative or intraoperative, the use of radiography or fluoroscopy to adequately identify the level in question is vital for medical and legal documentation. Surgical operations at the wrong level can be prevented by identifying landmarks with radiographs, but surface and deeper landmarks must be correlated. One common problem is failure to take into account the downward projection of the spinous process; for example, a needle placed on one spinous process but in front of the next lower body may lead to confusion about the level. Obvious bony landmarks (e.g., loss of a pedicle or a fracture seen on the localizing film) can facilitate identifying the surgical site. Subtle findings, such as the location of unique osteophytes or compression fractures, can assist in localization when obvious findings are absent. The use of a tangible marker, such as a bite from bone with a rongeur or placement of a stitch into a spinous process, reduces ambiguity later in the procedure.

The use of intraoperative imaging has grown dramatically. Ultrasonography as an intraoperative localizing device can help verify the correct level and locate hidden, deep lesions within the spinal cord.[313-316] More medical centers are using portable and dedicated MRI and CT scanners for determination of the adequacy of procedures for resection of tumor or osteophytes, placement of instrumentation, or other needs of the surgeon. Stand-alone MRI scanners have been developed that function in an operating room or even as an operating room.[317] Some of these modalities require specialized equipment that is compatible with the modality (e.g., nonmagnetic instruments for intraoperative MRI). Each has its advantages and limitations, and the use of these devices depends on the needs of the surgeon and the institution. Intraoperative CT scanners are available, as are fluoroscopy-based systems that create three-dimensional reconstructions resembling CT scans. These modalities can be useful in confirming the adequacy of decompression or screw placement before leaving the operating room.

Stereotactic navigational adjuncts have increasingly been used in spine surgery.[317-321] The accuracy of stereotaxis depends on the quality of the scan used, the position of the patient intraoperatively and in the scanner, performance of the stereotactic portion of the procedure before any resection or opening that would distort the landmarks used for calibration, and user-dependent variables. Currently, numerous intraoperative navigation techniques are available that rely on preoperative CT, intraoperative three-dimensional reconstruction from planar fluoroscopy, or three-dimensional reconstruction using intraoperative isocentric circumferential fluoroscopy. All appear to provide accuracy with respect to screw placement.[322-326] Although each system has its pros and cons, there is no evidence that one system is clearly superior to another.[324] Miniature robotic systems are also being developed to improve the accuracy of targeting and screw placement.[325,326] Navigational techniques are increasing being applied to spinal arthroplasty procedures, as well as fusion procedures.[327]

Complications of Bracing and Halo Use

No intervention is without risk for complications, and the use of external orthoses is no exception. Problems are related to improper placement, to proper placement but brace limitations, and to the brace itself. Improper placement of cervical collars can result in skin and spinal cord injuries. The skin can be abraded if the chin falls inside the jaw support. Use of a properly fitted collar and instruction to the patient that the chin is not supposed to slide under the chin support can significantly reduce this risk. Spinal cord injury can occur when an unstable spine is moved as a result of placement of a brace. A brace should be applied in such a way that the spine is not moved, and this includes not reducing a deformity. One common situation is a patient with ankylosing spondylitis and a fixed kyphotic deformity who sustains a transdiscal fracture.[328-337] A well-intentioned first responder may place this patient in neutral alignment and cause a spinal cord injury. It is critical to obtain a history from the patient or family before reduction, if possible, and to keep the patient in the baseline position, not just what "looks right." Many spinal cord injuries occur after the patient has been placed in a collar. Injury may also result because no external orthotic device limits movement completely.[338-340] The range of motion in a given device varies but is easily quantifiable. Wearing a brace of any kind can trap moisture and impede dressing changes, thereby leading to wound maceration and cellulitis. A brace that does not contour the patient's anatomy can cause pressure, pain, necrosis, and wound breakdown.

Use of a halo vest orthotic, which has less range of motion than nonfixed devices, is complicated by several factors, including local pin site complications, problems with the vest device, movement despite the halo, and issues related to the size, bulk, and location of the device.[56-61,311,337,341-350]

Local complications range from the mundane, such as cellulitis at the skin insertion site, to deeper complications related to the point at which the pin enters the skull.[57,58,61,351,352] Pin-related complications also include the development of epidural hematoma or epidural or subdural abscess at the placement site. These complications are insidious because they cannot be seen directly. Loosening of the pin in the outer table may result in a catastrophic loss of tension, which leads to loss of fixation, scalp laceration, and in rare instances, oculofacial trauma. Fracture of the outer table can also lead to fracture of the inner table and intracranial injury.[344,349,351] The halo is large, unwieldy, and for many frail or slender patients, heavy. It raises the center of gravity for the patient and challenges the coordination skills of many patients, especially those already neurologically impaired.

Anterior Cervical Approach

Anterior cervical approaches include the transoral, ventromedian, and ventrolateral approaches for vertebrectomy or odontoidectomy, diskectomy, and instrumentation. Each has a particular complication pattern, and there are steps to minimize them.

The transoral approach, because of passage through the oral cavity, is associated with a significant incidence of wound infection and healing problems.[353-355] They can be diminished by judicious minimization of steroids, care on opening to not destroy tissue planes and the mucosa, and the perioperative use of antibiotics. Unfortunately, many patients requiring a transoral approach are metabolically or nutritionally challenged to begin with, and they may not heal well. Palate injury is also a significant potential problem. The palate (soft and hard) may need to be split for adequate exposure, and it does not always heal well afterward. The assistance of an ear, nose, and throat surgeon for the approach and closure can help a surgeon who is not familiar with the management of these tissues. The potential neurological morbidities related to the transoral approach to the dens and anterior rostral spinal cord are related to the approach, the use of rongeurs instead of drilling, and the adequacy of exposure.

Anterior ventromedian cervical approaches carry with them risks related to the structures nearby, including the esophagus, carotid and jugular branches, and nerves such as the vagus and recurrent laryngeal. Care in the approach includes remaining in an avascular plane and making sure that the prevertebral fascia is dissected inferiorly with a peanut to prevent direct injury to these structures.

Esophageal injury can result from the dissection or from manipulation during the procedure after the retractors are in place. Migration of the retractors may tear the esophagus directly, or the esophagus may creep into the surgical field and then be injured by a wayward instrument. Injury can be prevented by the surgeon remaining constantly aware of the position of the retractors and the esophagus. After the procedure but before closure, the entire length of the exposed esophagus should be inspected for tears because an unnoticed tear can allow spillage of contents into the surgical bed and lead to infection, pseudarthrosis, or osteomyelitis. The esophagus can be repaired directly with a muscle patch from the sternocleidomastoid (as a vascularized pedicle of the manubrial head or as a free segment) or with a direct external drain and an esophagostomy.[356-360] If the surgeon does not have experience with such a repair, an ear, nose, and throat surgeon should be called in to perform the restoration. Reoperations are frequently associated with problems related to scarring of the esophagus at the old surgical site, especially with instrumentation. If there is a question about difficult planes of dissection, an ear, nose, and throat surgeon should obtain exposure. The incidence of acute or subacute esophageal tears ranges from 0% to 1.9% and averages less than 1% in most series.[361] Delayed perforation has been described and may occur a decade after the surgery. Whether this represents an injury at the time of surgery or a delayed injury caused by erosion from the anterior plate or screws is unclear. Every attempt should be made to place the anterior plate as flush along the spine as possible.[362] Esophageal perforations appear to occur most commonly at C5-C6 because the wall of the esophagus is thinnest at this level.[362] Some surgeons prefer to place a nasogastric tube at the beginning of the procedure to serve as a palpable landmark for the esophagus in an effort to avoid injuring it.

Dysphagia without direct esophageal perforation is far more common in patients after anterior cervical spine surgery. Reports range from rates of 10% to 60%. When carefully studied, there appears to be a 13.6% rate of dysphagia in patients 2 years after surgery.[363] Dysphagia was more common in women, after revision surgery, and in patients undergoing multilevel surgeries. Minimizing retraction and retraction time and avoiding injury to the upper pharyngeal nerves are recommended. There are reports that placement of newer stand-alone devices, cages with inherent screws, have no profile from a plate and result in lower incidences of dysphagia.[364]

Recurrent laryngeal nerve (RLN) injury is a well-described risk with this anterior cervical approach. It leads to hoarseness and other changes in voice quality. The incidence is generally reported to be 2% to 3%.[365] RLN injury appears to be less likely when the spine is approached through a left-sided exposure because of anatomic differences in the right and left RLNs. There does not appear to be a clear benefit from endotracheal tube cuff deflation.[366] When considering the choice of approach for a revision anterior cervical procedure, preoperative laryngoscopy should be performed to look for evidence of existing unilateral RLN palsy.[367] If this is identified, the approach should be through the ipsilateral side to prevent bilateral RLN palsy and the need for emergency tracheostomy. Continuous RLN electromyographic monitoring during surgery is practiced by some surgeons in an attempt to minimize the risk for injury.[368,369]

The risk of graft movement (i.e., migration in toward the cord or ventrally out of the disk space) can be reduced with use of a plate to buttress the graft ventrally or by drilling an adequate ledge to prevent the graft from moving dorsally. Use of a graft slightly longer than the space available (requiring some distraction but maintenance of tension and compression on the graft) can maintain adequate tension such that the graft is unlikely to move. This force needs to be balanced against too much tension, which may lead to telescoping of the graft into the bodies above or below or to overdistraction, which may result in cord or root injury.

One of the most feared complications in the anterior cervical approach is injury to the vertebral artery. The incidence of this injury during anterior cervical approaches is less than 0.2%.[370,371] When such an injury occurs, packing of the vessel to obtain hemostasis should be followed by angiography and consideration of endovascular vessel occlusion. The risk for vertebral artery injury can be minimized by an understanding of the anatomy of the transverse foramen to the vertebral bodies and careful evaluation of preoperative CT and MRI scans.[372]

Postoperative formation of a hematoma in the operative field can have devastating consequences.[373-377] It may lead to a retropharyngeal hematoma or an epidural hematoma. It can initially manifest as dysphagia or pain but may result in stridor and airway obstruction. Immediate surgical evacuation and reestablishment of hemostasis must be instituted if there is any chance of significant size of the hematoma. It may be able to be prevented with the use of a drain leading from the vertebral surface (bone edges are often the source of the bleeding), although removal of the drain sometimes promotes bleeding.

Complications related specifically to corpectomies rather than diskectomies include C5 traction injuries, collapse of the fusion segment, dislodgement of the implant, and a higher incidence of CSF leaks as a result of the more extensive involvement, especially in patients with ossification of the posterior longitudinal ligament.[378-386] The C5 nerve root is especially at risk because of the short length of the root and its tendency to be injured when overdistraction takes place.[380,385,387] By limiting the distraction and width of the decompression, this risk can be minimized.

The longer a fusion segment, the greater impact collapse or telescoping has on alignment of the spine. With graft settling, loss of lordosis and frank kyphosis can lead to pain, instability, and compromise of the canal. This problem can be prevented by not overdrilling the end plates above or below and by choosing a graft that is as wide as possible to decrease the pressure (i.e., force per unit area) of the graft into the adjacent bodies.

The approach for placing an odontoid screw is similar to that for anterior cervical diskectomy and fusion. This method has all the risks of complication as the other anterior cervical approaches, with additional risks related to capture of the odontoid tip. Risks include failure to maintain the correct lateral angle and missing the tip of the dens and the potential for spinal cord injury from migration of the dens or a poorly placed drill or screw.[298,388-390] Risks can be minimized by wide exposure of the C2-C3 interspace to demonstrate the uncovertebral joints bilaterally and determine the midline more accurately. Patients should be selected in whom the dens is aligned with the C2 body and not significantly displaced. Screw fracture, because of the long moment arm and high torque on the odontoid screw, can be prevented by using a tapered thread (i.e., the screw is thicker at the end), which strengthens the screw at the point where the force is greatest. Dens capture is easier with threaded lag screws because they reduce the likelihood of the screw pushing the fragment instead of threading into it.

Posterior Cervical Approach

Posterior cervical surgical procedures carry risks different from those of anterior procedures. The prototypical procedure is cervical laminectomy, which is performed for numerous indications, from Chiari decompression to cervical stenosis to intramedullary tumor exposure. The primary risks associated with cervical laminectomy are similar to those of laminectomy at other levels and include cord injury, dural injury, and nerve root injury. The simplest way to minimize injury to these elements is to judiciously and minimally use monopolar cautery when down to the lamina and dura, use neurosurgical cotton patties (Cottonoid; Codman Neuro, Raynham, MA) to retract the dura away from the ligamentum flavum and lamina, and take care in preventing overly aggressive use of rongeurs, which can result in fragments being twisted into the dura or nerve roots. Even with no evidence of direct trauma to the roots, transient C5 palsy can be seen in approximately 5% to 15% of patients undergoing posterior cervical decompression, with or without instrumentation.[391,392] This injury manifests as a deltoid muscle weakness. Although some authors recommend intraoperative monitoring with motor evoked potentials and deltoid electromyographic recording, C5 root injury may occur in the absence of intraoperative findings.[391,393]

The risk for injury to vascular elements is primarily limited to the vertebral artery, which runs laterally in the vertebral canal until its exit from the C2 body. At this point, the artery becomes most vulnerable to injury because the vessel turns from a lateral course and moves dorsally before entering the dura adjacent to the C1 lamina. Frequently, injury to the venous plexus is initially confused with injury to the vertebral artery, but the consequences are not nearly as significant. As with most venous bleeding, it can be controlled easily by tamponade with Gelfoam or Surgicel and a neurosurgical cotton patty. Injury to the vertebral artery may require opening the dura and ligating or performing a bypass or end-to-end anastomosis, depending on the nature of the injury and its location. Injury to the vertebral artery during posterior cervical procedures occurs more frequently than during anterior procedures, with a rate of up to 1.9%.[371]

Complications associated with posterior subaxial cervical spinal procedures are related to the degree of exposure, the neural elements exposed, and the use of instrumentation. Risks related to the decompression procedures laminotomy and laminectomy are similar, regardless of location, and consist primarily of injury to surrounding neural elements, injury to bony elements, and excessive bleeding. CSF leakage from an unintended durotomy may be minimized if care is taken to not leave any sharp bone spicules that may point downward into the thecal sac. Additional care should be taken with placement of a Kerrison rongeur to exclude dura within the teeth of the instrument. A small neurosurgical cotton patty can be gently passed underneath the bony edge and used to bluntly dissect the dura away while protecting it from the rongeur. Generous and temporary use of thrombin-soaked Gelfoam along the lateral aspects of the bony opening assists in obtaining hemostasis at Batson's plexus.

Lateral mass screws require precise localization of the entry point and angle with respect to the lateral and rostrocaudal planes. The orientation of the facet joints is an angle oblique to the coronal plane, and to avoid injury to the vertebral artery when anteromedial to the entry point, the screws need to be aimed significantly laterally. One rule of thumb is that if the drill guide is not leaning on the spinous process of the caudal vertebra, the surgeon is not aiming laterally enough. It is easier to understand the angle in the coronal plane if the dissection is taken widely enough that the lateral aspect of the facet joints' angle can be visualized directly. The angle should be parallel to the facet joints. Failure to angle upward sufficiently may result in the screw leaving the lateral mass and pinching the nerve root distal to the

6

pedicle. As with the use of anterior plates, overtightening a screw results in fracture of the threads and loss of pullout integrity. If this complication occurs, a rescue screw should be used, or methyl methacrylate should be injected into the screw hole and the screw replaced. Use of a screw that is a little too long (1 to 2 mm), if in the correct orientation, is not likely to cause significant morbidity and can achieve bicortical purchase. Screws that are too long and in the inappropriate orientation are potentially dangerous.

Thoracic Spinal Procedures

Thoracic spinal procedures, because of the surrounding organs, carry risks different from those of cervical spine procedures. Anterior approaches, such as the transthoracic, endoscopic, and retropleural approaches, put major arteries, veins, and organs such as the heart, lungs, and diaphragm at risk for injury.[296,394-404] Posterior approaches, such as laminectomy, costotransversectomy, and transpedicular approaches, have fewer risks but can still injure the ventral organs and vessels if reaching too far forward.[85,296,405-408] All approaches can result in complications involving neural elements, CSF leakage, and infection. Some complications are related to the exposure, whereas others are related to the procedure being performed.

Thoracic laminectomy has long been performed for many procedures, including repair of intramedullary, intradural, and epidural lesions. Risks are similar to those for the subaxial cervical spine, and it is important to keep the lateral exposure to the minimum that can provide the necessary exposure. Too wide an exposure risks taking down the costotransverse ligaments and even risks pneumothorax. For tumor patients in whom the wound has been or will be irradiated, a curvilinear incision with a myocutaneous flap should be used to maintain vascular supply to the skin and reduce the risk for infection and tissue breakdown.[409,410]

Thoracic pedicle screw instrumentation can be performed safely by experienced surgeons using freehand techniques.[411-413] However, many of the intraoperative navigation systems previously discussed were designed specifically to increase safety in thoracic instrumentation.

Thoracoscopic procedures need smaller incisions to approach the spine and thus reduce the likelihood of significant wound breakdown and postoperative incisional pain, but because of the multiple ports used and the limited sight angles, the potential for injury to structures such as vessels and organs remains significant.[394,397,414-416] Conversion to open thoracotomy should be performed if there is a significant problem because trying to fix a large injury through a small opening will probably provide greater challenges.

Anterior Lumbar Procedures

Anterior lumbar procedures can be subdivided into three main categories: transperitoneal open, endoscopic transperitoneal, and retroperitoneal approaches. Potential morbidities are associated more with the approach than with the individual procedure, and when the spinal procedures differ, they are discussed separately. Anterior procedures are performed to augment spinal stability by bone fusion or instrumentation or to perform arthroplasty. The choice of approach depends on the exposure needs of the procedure, the type of instrumentation being performed, and preferences of the surgeon and patient.

The transperitoneal open procedure is performed through a laparotomy, usually through a midline incision, although a Pfannenstiel bathing suit line incision can also be performed. The procedure calls for mobilization of the abdominal viscera with a midline anterior approach to the spine after mobilization of the various branches of the aorta, inferior vena cava, or iliac vessels. This approach has a higher risk than the retroperitoneal approach for postoperative complications such as injury to the major vessels, adhesions, and adynamic ileus.[417-422] Injury to other structures, including the ureter and pelvic contents, is rare but of significant consequence.

Anterior endoscopic procedures are performed through multiple small incisions and with the use of multiple ports.[423,424] The smaller incisions are thought to heal better than a single, large incision of the same total length. The approach is essentially the same as an anterior transperitoneal approach in terms of mobilization of the abdominal viscera and major vessels, although because of the port size and the use of endoscopic techniques, mobilization is more difficult. The assistance of a general surgeon with significant endoscopic experience in performing the exposures is recommended for neurosurgeons who are not comfortable with the management of injury to the structures being mobilized. Other possible complications include hypercapnia if carbon dioxide insufflation is used and delay in converting to an open procedure if bleeding or another major complication occurs. Lost time in gaining control of a difficult situation can lead to greater morbidity from blood loss.

The retroperitoneal approach can be used in two ways. It can be performed with a wide exposure to allow extensive instrumentation,[421,425,426] or it can be used with a short incision for placement of an interbody fusion construct (e.g., mini–anterior lumbar interbody fusion [mini-ALIF]). The main risks are vascular, although entry into the peritoneum or sigmoid colon is possible. Previous surgery in this area distorts the anatomy and leads to scarring. The primary risk with this approach is tearing segmental arteries and veins that may be under tension and difficult to visualize as retraction for the exposure proceeds. This exposure may be extended up to the diaphragm, with further mobilization of the kidney and, if necessary, the spleen and liver. The approach is usually done from the left side because of the smaller size of the liver on the left. Because of the retroperitoneal exposure, the ureter is less subject to injury in the lower levels than with a transperitoneal approach. The location of the ureter should be anticipated to reduce the chance for injury.

Anterior interbody fusions can be performed with the use of interbody threaded cages, interbody square cages, interbody threaded bone dowels, femoral ring allografts, and autograft bone. Fusion can be performed from a straight anterior transperitoneal or a lateral retroperitoneal approach, depending on the technique and device used. Whether an endoscopic or open procedure is used depends on the body habitus of the patient, the preference of the surgeon and patient, and the availability of equipment and assistance.

One significant risk related to the anterior approach is retrograde ejaculation in male patients undergoing L5-S1 fusion.[427] The incidence of this complication was initially reported to be about 5%, but the later literature has reported an incidence as high as 20%. There is a 10-fold higher incidence of retrograde ejaculation with a transperitoneal approach than with a retroperitoneal approach to L4-L5 and L5-S1.[428] This is thought to result from the fact that the superior hypogastric sympathetic plexus lies midline over the disk spaces at L4-L5 and L5-S1. When approaching from a retroperitoneal trajectory, the plexus is mobilized off the disk spaces along with the posterior peritoneum to protect it from injury. When the approach is via a midline transperitoneal route, the plexus itself is directly injured. This may play a role in the choice of approach in men. Minimal use of electrocautery in this region is also recommended. If a transperitoneal approach is required, dissecting the plexus off the right-sided iliac vessels and mobilizing the fascia toward the left may protect the plexus and prevent this complication.[429]

Other major risks associated with anterior interbody procedures include the possibility of neurological injury or CSF leakage from the anterior diskectomy, pushing of disk fragments dorsally as the cage is advanced, and misdirection or misplacement of the fusion construct. The best way to reduce the chance of neurological injury is to remove the disk under fluoroscopic guidance. If the surgeon can visualize just how deep each pass of the pituitary rongeur goes, there is less chance of going too deep, passing the annulus, and biting the dura or nerve roots. Continuous use of fluoroscopy allows evaluation of each step of the reaming and tapping, thereby allowing the surgeon to correct any misalignment before it becomes irreversible and leads to instability of the construct. One way to reduce the chance that the cage or bone graft will push disk fragments posteriorly is to ensure that the diskectomy is adequately performed and that no residual disk remains in the path of the construct.

Vertebrectomies are best performed through the retroperitoneal approach because the screws can be placed along the long axis of the bodies and achieve better purchase. The exposure can be carried up or down multiple levels without significant risk to structures that cross the midline and only minimal risk to structures that cross the exposure (primarily the radicular arteries and veins). The chance of causing a significant injury to the artery of Adamkiewicz and resulting in ischemia of the lower cord can be reduced by avoiding sacrificing the radicular artery too far distal from the aorta. The location of the radicular vessels in the middle of the bodies makes it nearly impossible to save them at the level above or below if a plate or other instrumentation is applied. To prevent unnecessary blood loss, it is best to isolate the vessels, sacrifice them cleanly with ties or hemoclips, and then cut them under direct vision. This technique prevents avulsion and retraction of the vessels into surrounding soft tissue or, worse, avulsion at their insertion into the aorta or vena cava.

Posterior Lumbar Procedures

Dorsal lumbar procedures are primarily used for laminectomy, laminotomy, and fusions, with or without instrumentation, and they are the oldest and most commonly performed procedures for spine surgery.

Hemilaminotomies can be performed for small exposure of intraspinal epidural lesions such as disk herniations, synovial cyst herniations, and ligamentous or bony hypertrophy as a result of degenerative disk disease. Minimal exposure (i.e., unilateral muscle and bone dissection) results in reduced pain, decreased length of hospital stay, and reduced operative time for most patients. However, the reduced exposure carries several risks. Retraction of the muscles laterally is often performed with a Taylor retractor. If retraction is performed too aggressively or in the wrong location, a facet fracture can occur. This risk can be minimized with the use of a retractor that spreads the tissue without digging lateral to the facet joint. Use of such a retractor, however, carries with it the risk of spinous process fracture, so careful use of any retractor is recommended. Fracture of the facet can also occur if the medial facetectomy is carried too far laterally. The usual landmark for completion of bone removal laterally is the medial border of the pedicle below, which is located right under the root of the ascending facet. Going beyond this point confers a greater chance of fracture of the ascending or descending facet and, consequently, pain on movement postoperatively. At least half the width of the pars interarticularis should be preserved to prevent postoperative pars fracture and spondylolisthesis.

Prevention of postoperative epidural scarring after dorsal procedures is a challenge that does not have a simple answer. Several techniques are available, such as placement of a fat graft, Gelfoam sponge, or artificial adhesion barrier.[430-433] None is without complications or is universally effective.[434-437]

Postoperative reherniation of disk fragments occurs in approximately 10% of cases.[438-446] Differentiating reherniation from scar requires a contrast-enhanced scan (unless it is in the first week or two after surgery); the scar enhances, and the disk usually enhances only in the periphery of a fragment.[277,431,447-450] Injury to the nerve root can occur in several ways. The nerve root can be unintentionally cut during opening of the annulus if the root has not been adequately identified and retracted. Frequently, overly aggressive retraction can result in transient weakness or sensory changes in a root that has not been cut. This injury tends to respond to steroids and physical therapy, although it is better avoided by careful dissection. Failure to recognize a redundant nerve root may lead to injury to the root, even after presumed protection of one of the branches.

Cauda equina syndrome as an immediate or delayed result of lumbar diskectomy is a catastrophic neurological complication. It can occur as a result of injury to the nerve roots from epidural hematoma after closure, from infection of the arachnoid or epidural space, from retraction of neural elements against a calcified herniated fragment, or from extrusion of disk or end-plate fragments postoperatively.[451-457] The mechanism usually determines the time frame for the onset of symptoms.

Catastrophic injury to the organs or vessels of the abdomen and pelvis can result from diskectomy.[417,458-465] Injury can occur from placement of any sharp instrument into the disk space that passes through the annulus and anterior longitudinal ligament. Bleeding, which may or may not well up into the surgical field, is not responsive to attempts to arrest it. The patient may become tachycardic or hypotensive. The onset of symptoms may be more insidious and not appear until the patient is in recovery, or in the case of bowel injury, symptoms can develop after discharge. Management of life-threatening vascular injury requires termination of the neurosurgical procedure, turning the patient over, and performing an exploratory laparotomy and vascular repair of some kind. Ignoring the problem, failing to obtain a vascular surgical consultation, or simply transfusing the patient can result in catastrophic blood loss and perhaps death.

Minimally invasive techniques for the treatment of lumbar disease include chemonucleosis, thermal or laser coagulation, and automated percutaneous diskectomy.[466-483] These procedures are performed using local anesthesia with fluoroscopic guidance, and their aim is internal decompression of the disk and the affected nerve roots. One benefit of the absence of regional or global anesthesia is that any irritation or compression of the nerve root can be felt, and the surgeon is able to change whatever it was that triggered the response. The entry point is from the side of the disk, and it may be difficult to enter the L5-S1 space directly because of the position of the iliac crest relative to the disk space. Up to 10% of patients are unable to have percutaneous instruments placed into this disk space. Causalgia, injury to the thecal sac or nerve roots, injury to the end plate, fracture of an instrument, injury to a hollow viscus, injury to a vessel, and hematoma of the psoas muscle are all acute complications of percutaneous diskectomy.[467-471,474,481,484-486] Delayed complications include diskitis and progression of the degenerative processes.[487,488] Success rates for percutaneous treatment are in the range of 60% to 80%,[466-471,484,488,489] much lower than those for microdiskectomy but without the attendant risks associated with general or regional anesthesia.

The risks related to posterior lumbar interbody fusion (PLIF) are similar to those for posterior decompression but are amplified by the additional manipulation required to distract the two end plates, retract the neural elements, and implant bone wedges or segments.[290,299,490-501] Overdistraction can lead to neurapraxia of one of the nerve roots and may tear adherent dura. Blood loss is greater with PLIF than with laminectomy or diskectomy because of the extra removal of the end plate and osteophytic ridges and the extensive epidural exposure. Graft migration is a significant risk with uninstrumented PLIF because there is nothing to maintain the alignment and prevent relaxation of the tension that keeps the graft in place. Actions that can reduce the complications associated with PLIF include having the appropriate instruments for distraction and implantation. When performing PLIF for spondylolisthesis, the nerve roots exiting through the same foramen (e.g., the L5 root for L5-S1 PLIF) may be under significant compression and tension because of the anterolisthesis and pseudodisk. The path of the nerve root takes it directly over the desired entry point into the interspace, and the plane of the disk space causes distractors to go through the region of the axilla of this root. One way to avoid the problem is to use a drill or osteotome to remove the dorsal osteophyte lateral to the lower root and medial to the exiting root. This allows a flatter trajectory into the disk space and avoids unnecessary manipulation of an already tenuous root.

Several types of bone or cage constructs, including titanium and carbon fiber cages, femoral bone dowels, or impacted bone wedges, can be placed into the intervertebral space. Placement of cages and bone dowels from behind requires more extensive exposure than needed for PLIF with impacted bone grafts. Although the literature on this type of procedure may describe removal of only the medial facets, more surgeons find that the whole facet or most of the facet needs to be removed to provide adequate exposure and protection of the nerve root and thecal sac. Because this approach results in some posterior instability, it should be combined with some form of posterior instrumentation such as pedicle screws. The most common complications include tearing of the thecal sac or nerve root sleeve with subsequent CSF leakage, injury to the nerve root, and infection. Prevention of nerve root sleeve and dural tears requires adequate removal of the posterior elements (e.g., lamina, medial or full facets) and placement of some kind of protective retractor to prevent the threads from catching the dura. Excessive retraction of the nerve root can result in significant neurapraxia. Because of the nature of the implants and the difficulty in obtaining postoperative imaging (i.e., metallic beam-hardening artifact on CT and ferromagnetic susceptibility artifact on MRI), postoperative surveillance for infection is necessary. Another problem with use of nonbiodegradable spacer devices is the fact that the body forms a "protective" capsule around all foreign bodies that gets larger over time, thereby resulting in further impingement on the diameter of the fusion mass traveling vertically in the spacer, which reduces the strength of the fusion mass. This may explain why many studies have shown better outcomes earlier in the series and a decrease in successful outcomes more than 2 years after surgery.

Pedicle Screw Fixation

The use of pedicle screw fixation has significantly increased fusion rates over those with noninstrumented fusions.[87,308,502-504] Use of the pedicle screw fixation technique, which has undergone significant medicolegal scrutiny, has been vindicated, and it is applied to lumbar, thoracic, and cervical spinal cases. The major risks are related to misplacement of the screws, fracture of the neural elements being stabilized, injury to neural and vascular structures, and infection or poor wound healing.[290,295,308-310,495,502,503,505-518] Reduction of risk is undertaken on several fronts. Understanding the biomechanical parameters and indications can reduce the risk for surgical misadventure. Pedicle screws can be placed by relying only on anatomic parameters to determine the entry point and angulation, but for surgeons who wish to have confirmatory assistance, several imaging and image-guided techniques are available, as discussed previously.[321,507,509]

Facet Screw Fixation

Two types of facet screws can be used for segmental fixation: the Boucher technique of facet screw fixation[519,520] and the Magerl translaminar facet screw fixation.[304,521-527] The translaminar screw fixation technique is as stiff as pedicle screw fixation except in extension, in which it is less stiff than pedicle screws.[528] Fusion rates are reportedly comparable to those with pedicle screws, but the lower perioperative morbidity rates of translaminar screws make them an acceptable option for some surgeons and patients. The practice at our institution is to not place them at L5-S1 because of stress concentration or when significant spondylolisthesis is present (i.e., grade II or greater after reduction).

CONCLUSION

Spinal and cranial surgery can be made safer with a better understanding of the complications that are likely to arise. The use of various technologic advances, such as stereotactic navigation and neurophysiologic monitoring, can help improve accuracy. A thorough understanding of the types of problems encountered with a given procedure or approach makes the surgeon more wary and probably reduces the incidence of such complications. Newer techniques are being developed to improve exposure with lower morbidity, and over time it is likely that many of the procedures now commonly performed will be replaced by less invasive and more effective ones as our understanding of the underlying processes progresses.

SUGGESTED READINGS

Baumann SB, Welch WC, Bloom MJ. Intraoperative SSEP detection of ulnar nerve compression or ischemia in an obese patient: a unique complication associated with a specialized spinal retraction system. *Arch Phys Med Rehabil*. 2000;81:130-132.

Bednarik J, Kadanka Z, Vohanka S, et al. The value of somatosensory and motor-evoked potentials in predicting and monitoring the effect of therapy in spondylotic cervical myelopathy: prospective randomized study. *Spine*. 1999;24:1593-1598.

Bekar A, Tureyen K, Aksoy K. Unilateral blindness due to patient positioning during cervical syringomyelia surgery: unilateral blindness after prone position. *J Neurosurg Anesthesiol*. 1996;8:227-229.

Bergeson RK, Schwend RM, DeLucia T, et al. How accurately do novice surgeons place thoracic pedicle screws with the free hand technique? *Spine*. 2008;33:E501-E507.

Brown CA, Lenke LG, Bridwell KH, et al. Complications of pediatric thoracolumbar and lumbar pedicle screws. *Spine*. 1998;23:1566-1571.

Dickinson LD, Miller LD, Patel CP, et al. Enoxaparin increases the incidence of postoperative intracranial hemorrhage when initiated preoperatively for deep venous thrombosis prophylaxis in patients with brain tumors. *Neurosurgery*. 1998;43:1074-1081.

Geisler FH, Laich DT, Goldflies M, et al. Anterior tibial compartment syndrome as a positioning complication of the prone-sitting position for lumbar surgery. *Neurosurgery*. 1993;33:1117.

Grossman MG, Ducey SA, Nadler SS, et al. Meralgia paresthetica: diagnosis and treatment. *J Am Acad Orthop Surg*. 2001;9:336-344.

Kondziolka D, Firlik A, Lunsford L. Complications of stereotactic brain surgery. *Neurol Clin*. 1998;16:35-54.

Lall RR, Hauptman JS, Munoz C, et al. Intraoperative neurophysiological monitoring in spine surgery: indications, efficacy, and role of the preoperative checklist. *Neurosurg Focus*. 2012;33(5):E10.

McAfee PC, Regan JR, Zdeblick T, et al. The incidence of complications in endoscopic anterior thoracolumbar spinal reconstructive surgery. A prospective multicenter study comprising the first 100 consecutive cases. *Spine*. 1995;20:1624-1632.

Newman NJ. Perioperative visual loss after nonocular surgeries. *Am J Ophthalmol*. 2008;145:604-610.

Paniello RC, Martin-Bredahl KJ, Henkener LJ, et al. Preoperative laryngeal nerve screening for revision anterior cervical spine procedures. *Ann Otol Rhinol Laryngol*. 2008;117:594-597.

Raslan AM, Fields JD, Bhardwaj A. Prophylaxis for venous thromboembolism in neurocritical care: a critical appraisal. *Neurocrit Care*. 2010;12:297-309. doi:10.1007/s12028-009-9316-7.

Roth S, Tung A, Ksiazek S. Visual loss in a prone-positioned spine surgery patient with the head on a foam headrest and goggles covering the eyes: an old complication with a new mechanism. *Anesth Analg*. 2007;104:1185-1187.

Schierhout G, Roberts I. Anti-epileptic drugs for preventing seizures following acute traumatic brain injury. *Cochrane Database Syst Rev*. 2000;(2):CD000173.

Schwartz DM, Drummond DS, Hahn M, et al. Prevention of positional brachial plexopathy during surgical correction of scoliosis. *J Spinal Disord*. 2000;13:178-182.

Sonabend AM, Korenfeld Y, Crisman C, et al. Prevention of ventriculostomy-related infections with prophylactic antibiotics and antibiotic-coated external ventricular drains: a systematic review. *Neurosurgery*. 2011;68(4):996-1005. doi:10.1227/NEU.0b013e3182096d84.

Watters WC 3rd, Baisden J, Bono CM, et al. Antibiotic prophylaxis in spine surgery: an evidence-based clinical guideline for the use of prophylactic antibiotics in spine surgery. *Spine J*. 2009;9(2):142-146. doi:10.1016/j.spinee.2008.05.008; [Epub 2008 Jul 10].

Wu AS, Trinh VT, Suki D, et al. A prospective randomized trial of perioperative seizure prophylaxis in patients with intraparenchymal brain tumors. *J Neurosurg*. 2013;118:873-883.

See a full reference list on ExpertConsult.com

6

7 Coagulation for the Neurosurgeon

Shahid M. Nimjee, Andrew Crofton, Nathan Oh, Wolff Kirsch, Michael M. Haglund, and Gerald A. Grant

Pathologic hemorrhage in neurosurgery can result in devastating morbidity and mortality. This is often exacerbated in patients on anticoagulant or antiplatelet therapy. Although patients presenting with intracranial hemorrhage while on warfarin (Coumadin) is a familiar scenario to neurosurgeons and one in which there is a formula for anticoagulant reversal, patients on dual antiplatelet therapy or new anticoagulants drugs like dabigatran (Pradaxa) present new challenges.

In this chapter, we provide an overview of coagulation and platelet aggregation in the brain. We then present a list of anticoagulant and antiplatelet drugs currently used and methods to reverse their activity. Finally, we explore novel approaches to hemostasis and thrombosis that may provide neurosurgeons with new tools to improve outcomes in patients with pathologic hemorrhage.

BASIC SCIENCE OF COAGULATION

Hemostasis and Coagulation

Normal hemostasis is the product of well-regulated steps that maintain blood in a clot-free state in vessels. When vascular injury occurs, coagulation is initiated by inducing the rapid formation of a localized hemostatic plug within minutes at the site of vascular injury. Such *primary hemostasis* results from exposure of the extracellular matrix in the injured vessel. This creates a highly thrombogenic environment whereby platelets adhere to the damaged endothelium and become activated from their previously quiescent state. They subsequently release secretory granules, which induce additional platelet aggregation to form a hemostatic plug.[1] There are two mechanisms of hemostasis: the classical paradigm presents clotting as two distinct pathways that meet downstream to form a common pathway and is known as the *clotting cascade*; the second takes into account the role of platelets and proposes that clotting occurs on the surface of tissue factor–presenting cells and on platelets and is therefore known as the *cell-based model of coagulation*.

Coagulation Cascade

In the 1960s, two groups independently proposed a model consisting of sequential steps of activation resulting in thrombin generation that forms a blood clot.[2,3] This model eventually gave rise to a cascade that was divided into extrinsic and intrinsic pathways (Fig. 7-1). The extrinsic pathway starts with tissue factor and factor VIIa and only occurs extrinsically to circulating blood. The intrinsic pathway, an intravascular process, occurs through activation of factors XII, XI, and IX. At this juncture, factor VIIIa is required in both pathways to convert factor X to factors Xa and Va, which subsequently convert factor II, or prothrombin, to thrombin (factor IIa).[4]

Cell-Based Model of Coagulation

Although the coagulation cascade presents clotting neatly and correlates well with laboratory tests such as prothrombin time (PT) and activated partial thromboplastin time (aPTT), it fails to adequately explain coagulation in vivo. Alternatively, the cell-based model describes blood clotting in three overlapping phases—initiation, amplification, and propagation (Fig. 7-2).[5] The initiation phase occurs on tissue factor–bearing cells such as fibroblasts or endothelial cells. Tissue factor is an integral membrane protein localized on the cell in which it was synthesized. When vascular injury occurs, coagulation factor VII binds to tissue factor. This complex, in turn, activates factors IX and X. Factor Xa activates factor V, which then converts a small amount of prothrombin to thrombin. This amount of factor IIa is critical to amplification, when platelets come into contact with extracellular matrix proteins, principally the platelet surface protein glycoprotein Ib-IX (GpIb-IX) to von Willebrand factor (vWF), at the site of vascular injury. Factor VIII is activated and binds to vWF and is then cleaved by thrombin to release it from vWF. The activated platelet now has factors Va and VIIIa bound to its surface, which sets the stage for a prodigious amount of thrombin generation. During propagation, the tenase complex (consisting of factors VIIIa and IXa) activates factor X on the platelet surface, which binds to its cofactor, factor Va, generating large amounts of thrombin required to convert fibrinogen to fibrin.[5] Thrombin also activates factor XIII, which in turn stabilizes the fibrin meshwork by cross-linking adjacent fibrin monomers to one another.

Platelet Activation

As described previously, the interaction between coagulation factors in platelets is critical to thrombus formation, and the initial thrombin generation from the tissue factor–factor VII pathway is important for stimulating the platelet from a quiescent to an active state. Subendothelial vWF that is exposed as a result of endothelial damage binds to platelet GpIb-IX-V, resulting in platelet adhesion to the damaged endothelial surface. Thrombin produced from the tissue factor–factor VII pathway binds to the protease-activated receptor on the platelet surface by inside-out signal transduction, resulting in conversion of GpIIb-IIIa from a quiescent to an active state and further recruiting internal GpIIb-IIIa molecules to the platelet surface. This integrin binds to fibrinogen, linking activated platelet molecules to one another and resulting in platelet aggregation and formation of a platelet plug. To stabilize platelet aggregation, a number of activated molecules are released, including thromboxane A_2 (TXA_2), serotonin, and adenosine diphosphate (ADP). TXA_2 binds to its receptor on the surface of the platelet and induces inside-out signal transduction of GpIIb-IIIa, amplifying platelet aggregation. ADP is released from the granules of platelets and has two main functions: it contributes to the inside-out signal transduction to activate GpIIb-IIIa, and it binds to the G protein–coupled receptor P2Y12. This ADP-induced platelet aggregation both stabilizes and further stimulates platelet plug formation. This sets off a cascade of events within the activated platelet that generate platelet aggregation and platelet plug formation (see Fig. 7-2).

ANTIPLATELET DRUGS

Antithrombotic drugs are roughly classified into two groupings: antiplatelet drugs and anticoagulants (Table 7-1). The main classes of antiplatelet drugs include cyclooxygenase-1 (COX-1) inhibitors, phosphodiesterase (PDE) inhibitors, ADP receptor inhibitors, and GpIIb-IIIa inhibitors.

Cyclooxygenase-1 Inhibitors

Platelet activation begins with the process of adhesion between vWF exposed on the damaged endothelial surface and GpIb-IX. This, in turn, activates GpIIb-IIIa, which binds to fibrinogen and begins the process of platelet aggregation. To perpetuate aggregation, platelets secrete substances to activate receptors on the platelet surface. COX-1 binds to prostaglandin synthase, which subsequently metabolizes arachidonic acid into prostaglandin H_2 (PGH_2). PGH_2 is a precursor of TXA_2, which acts in a positive feedback loop for platelet activation and recruitment.

Acetylsalicylic acid (aspirin) is a COX-1 inhibitor that inhibits PGH_2 and thereby prevents the metabolism of arachidonic acid, which inhibits the production of TXA_2. Aspirin irreversibly binds to COX-1, inhibiting TXA_2 production for the life of the platelet. It is immediately absorbed and has a half-life of 30 minutes. Aspirin is prescribed at a dosage of 81 to 325 mg daily as standalone therapy and in combination with P2Y12 inhibitors such as clopidogrel and prasugrel.

Aspirin activity can be monitored using platelet aggregometry, a platelet function analyzer (PFA-100; Siemens Medical Solutions, Malvern, PA), or a VerifyNow (Accriva Diagnostics, San Diego, CA) aspirin assay. Platelet aggregometry can be performed using whole blood or platelet-rich plasma. The actual assay is performed using luminescence or physical impedance measured with a filament. The output measurement is a percentage of maximal inhibition. A platelet function analyzer is a whole-blood point-of-care assay, whereby the blood is placed in a cartridge and activated by epinephrine or ADP. The output measurement is in closing time. The reference closing times of epinephrine-activated cartridges are between 80 and 200 seconds, and those of ADP-activated cartridges are between 60 and 140 seconds. The maximal closing time is 300 seconds, which represents a therapeutic effect from platelet inhibition. The assay is useful in determining whether the patient is taking aspirin, but closing times between the reference range and the upper limit of the assay are not used to guide therapy.

The VerifyNow aspirin assay expresses platelet activation in the form of aspirin-reactive units (ARU). The reference range is

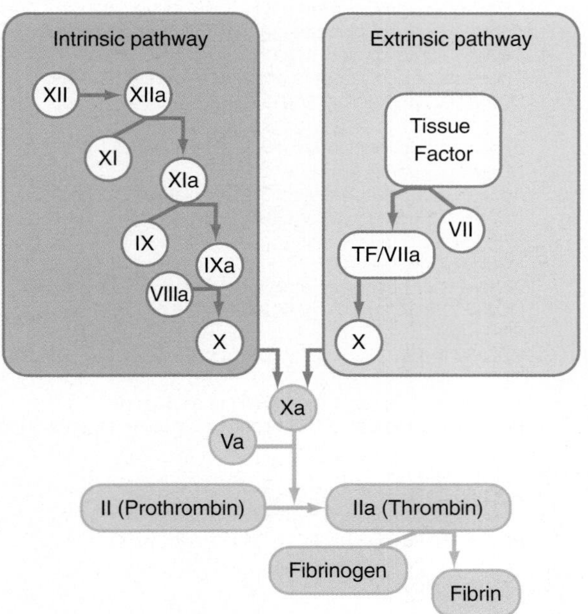

Figure 7-1. The coagulation cascade.

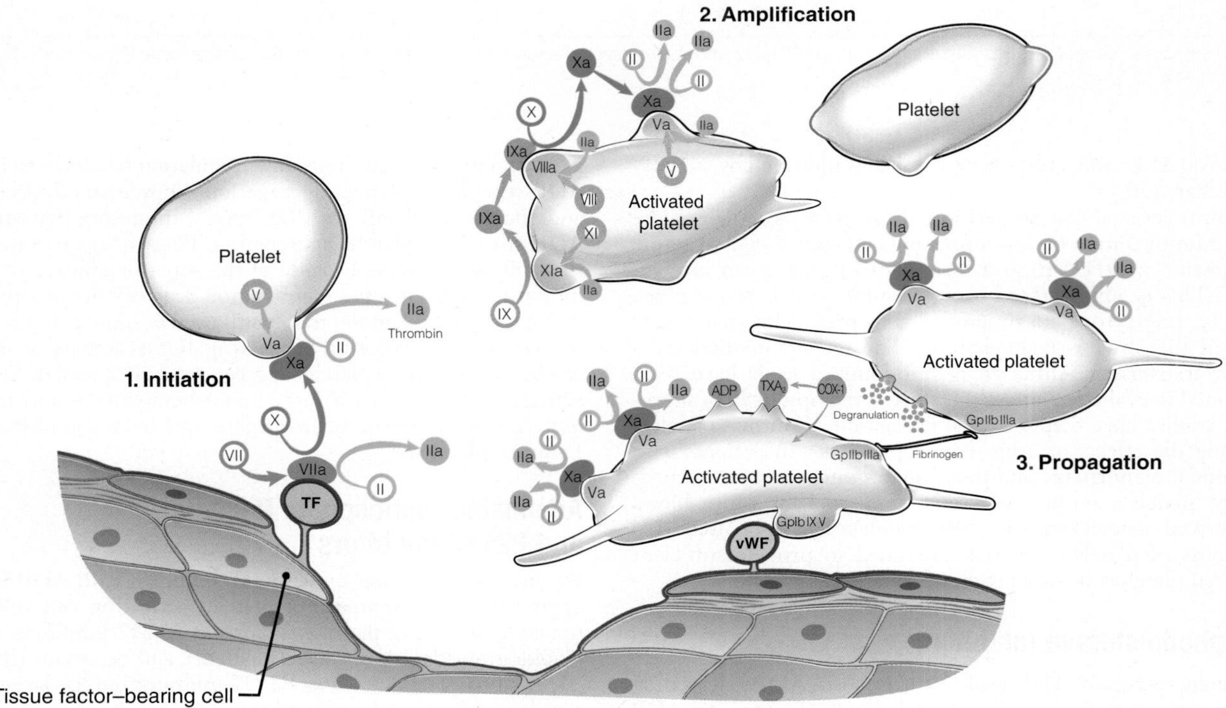

Figure 7-2. A cell-based model of coagulation that includes the role of platelets in thrombosis and coagulation factors in generating a stable thrombus. ADP, adenosine diphosphate; COX-1, cyclooxygenase-1; Gp, glycoprotein; TF, tissue factor; TXA_2, thromboxane A_2; vWF, von Willebrand factor.

TABLE 7-1 Antiplatelet and Anticoagulant Drugs and Reversing Agents

Drug	Target	Reversal Agent	Dose
Aspirin	Cyclooxygenase-1	Platelet transfusion DDAVP	Apheresis or pool platelets (>3 × 10^9 platelet/L) 1 unit DDAVP 0.3 μg/kg slow IV q12h
Dipyridamole	Phosphodiesterase type 5	Platelet transfusion DDAVP	Apheresis or pool platelets (>3 × 10^9 platelet/L) 1 unit DDAVP 0.3 μg/kg slow IV q12h
Cilostazol	Phosphodiesterase type 3	Platelet transfusion DDAVP	Apheresis or pool platelets (>3 × 10^9 platelet/L) 1 unit DDAVP 0.3 μg/kg slow IV q12h
Clopidogrel	P2Y12 receptor	Platelet transfusion DDAVP	Apheresis or pool platelets (>3 × 10^9 platelet/L) 2 units DDAVP 0.3 μg/kg slow IV q12h
Prasugrel	P2Y12 receptor	Platelet transfusion DDAVP	Apheresis or pool platelets (>3 × 10^9 platelet/L) 2 units DDAVP 0.3 μg/kg slow IV q12h
Ticagrelor	P2Y12 receptor	Platelet transfusion DDAVP	Apheresis or pool platelets (>3 × 10^9 platelet/L) 2 units DDAVP 0.3 μg/kg slow IV q12h
Abciximab	Glycoprotein IIb-IIIa	Platelet transfusion DDAVP	Apheresis or pool platelets (>3 × 10^9 platelet/L) 1 unit DDAVP 0.3 μg/kg slow IV q12h
Eptifibatide	Glycoprotein IIb-IIIa	Platelet transfusion DDAVP FFP PCC	Apheresis or pool platelets (>3 × 10^9 platelet/L) 1 unit DDAVP 0.3 μg/kg slow IV q12h FFP 1 unit PCC 50 IU/kg
Tirofiban	Glycoprotein IIb-IIIa	Platelet transfusion DDAVP FFP PCC	Apheresis or pool platelets (>3 × 10^9 platelet/L) 1 unit DDAVP 0.3 μg/kg slow IV q12h FFP 1 unit PCC 50 IU/kg
Enoxaparin	Factors Xa, IIa	Protamine	Protamine 1 mg per 1 mg LMWH (max 50 mg)
Heparin	Factors IIa, Xa	Protamine	Protamine 1 mg per 100 U heparin over last 4 hr (max 50 mg)
Fondaparinux	Direct factor Xa	rFVIIa	rFVIIa 80 μg/kg
Rivaroxaban	Direct factor Xa	PCC	PCC 50 IU/kg
Apixaban	Direct factor Xa	PCC	PCC 50 IU/kg
Bivalirudin	Direct factor IIa	None	
Lepirudin	Direct factor IIa	None	
Desirudin	Direct factor IIa	None	
Dabigatran	Direct factor IIa	None	
Warfarin	Factors II, VII, IX, X; proteins C, S	Vitamin K FFP PCC	Vitamin K IV 1-2 mg or PO 2.5-10 mg q12h Administer until corrected PCC 25-50 U/kg IV

DDAVP, desmopressin; FFP, fresh-frozen plasma; LMWH, low-molecular-weight heparin; PCC, prothrombin complex concentrate; rFVIIa, recombinant factor VIIa.

350 to 700 ARU, and a response to aspirin is indicated by an ARU of less than 550.

Aspirin reversal can be performed using two strategies. The first is administration of desmopressin (1-desamino-8-D-arginine vasopressin, or DDAVP) at a dose of 0.3 μg/kg given intravenously. This is administered over 15 minutes and can be given every 12 hours to a maximum of six doses. The major side effect of this drug is tachyphylaxis. The second method is by platelet transfusion. Although no randomized trials have been performed to evaluate platelet transfusion therapy, in vitro aggregation studies have demonstrated the action of normal platelets reversing the effects of drug-treated platelets.[7] In patients with intracranial hemorrhage and those undergoing emergent neurosurgery, platelets (either apheresis or a pool of white blood cell–derived platelets with >3 × 10^9 platelets/L) can be used.[7] Up to 5 units of platelets are recommended to provide sufficient unaltered platelets to support clot formation.[8]

Phosphodiesterase Inhibitors

Two main sources of ADP lead to thrombosis: ADP released by erythrocytes in the event of endothelial cell damage, and ADP released by secretory granules from activated platelets. ADP then binds to the platelet receptor P2Y12, resulting in platelet aggregation. PDE is an enzyme that downregulates platelet cyclic adenomonophosphate. This downregulation results in facilitating ADP-stimulated platelet aggregation. Dipyridamole (Persantin) and cilostazol (Pletal) are PDE type 3 inhibitors that attenuate ADP-stimulated platelet aggregation. These drugs are rarely used as stand-alone agents because of the superior efficacy of P2Y12 inhibitors. Aggrenox is a combination drug (25 mg of aspirin and 200 mg of dipyridamole) that is still used in some patients. There is no effective monitoring of the drug, but its activity on platelets can be assessed using platelet aggregometry. Reversal of Aggrenox activity in patients with intracranial hemorrhage and in those undergoing emergent neurosurgery can be accomplished with 1 unit of platelets.[7]

Adenosine Diphosphate Receptor and P2Y12 Inhibitors

By disrupting binding between ADP and P2Y12, ADP-induced aggregation is inhibited, but platelet activation can still occur through alternative pathways. Current P2Y12 inhibitors include clopidogrel (Plavix), prasugrel (Effient), and ticagrelor (Brilinta). Ticlopidine (Ticlid) is also a P2Y12 inhibitor but has largely been supplanted by clopidogrel and prasugrel.

The most commonly used P2Y12 inhibitor is clopidogrel, which has a half-life of approximately 7 hours and is prescribed at a dosage of 75 mg daily. Loading doses between 300 and

600 mg demonstrate an effect within 2 to 4 hours.[7] The maximal effect is realized within 4 to 7 days. Almost one third of patients who receive clopidogrel are considered nonresponders, owing in part to a mutation in cytochrome P-450, specifically CYP-2C9 and CYP-2C19, that prevents conversion of the drug into its active metabolite.[9]

Like clopidogrel, prasugrel also has a half-life of approximately 7 hours and is prescribed at a dosage of 10 mg daily for patients who weigh more than 60 kg and 5 mg for patients who weigh less than 60 kg. A loading dose of prasugrel is 60 mg. It is also metabolized by the cytochrome P-450 pathway, specifically CYP-3A4 and CYP-2B6, and it has not yet exhibited the same level of nonresponsiveness as clopidogrel.

Ticagrelor also has a half-life of approximately 7 hours, but its action is reversible on the P2Y12 receptor, requiring a maintenance twice-daily dosage of 90 mg. The loading dose is 180 mg. In contrast to clopidogrel and prasugrel, ticagrelor does not bind the ADP site on the P2Y12 receptor. It is an allosteric inhibitor. Moreover, it is not metabolized by cytochrome P-450 and therefore may have an advantage in patients with hepatic disease and in nonresponders to clopidogrel.

The activity of these drugs can be assessed by platelet aggregometry performed in both a whole-blood assay or using platelet-rich plasma. Although it is a sensitive method for monitoring platelet activity and activation, it is time-consuming and has largely been supplanted by the VerifyNow assay, which measures the effect of P2Y12 inhibitors in platelet-reactive units (PRU). Advertised as a point-of-care assay, VerifyNow is useful in evaluating patient response to clopidogrel: an estimated one third of patients have a subtherapeutic response to a standard dosage of 75 mg of clopidogrel daily. This finding allows physicians to use prasugrel or ticagrelor in this population. More recently, Delgado and colleagues demonstrated that maintaining the PRU between 60 and 140 was optimum for minimizing ischemic complications in patients undergoing flow-diversion stent placement in the treatment of intracranial aneurysm.[10]

Reversing the antiplatelet effects of P2Y12 inhibitors can occur by two strategies. The first is administration of DDAVP, which induces activation of vWF and, in turn, binds to GpIb-IX, resulting in platelet adhesion. Emergency administration is 0.3 μg/kg given intravenously over the course of 15 minutes. This can be repeated every 12 hours to a maximum of six doses. The major side effect of this drug is tachyphylaxis. The second method is platelet administration. The recommended dose is 2 units of platelets in the setting of intracranial hemorrhage or emergent need for neurosurgery.[7]

Glycoprotein IIb-IIIa Inhibitors

The binding between GpIIb-IIIa on the surface of a platelet and fibrinogen is the critical, nonredundant step that aggregates platelets to one another to form a platelet plug. Three parenteral GpIIb-IIIa inhibitors are used clinically: abciximab (ReoPro), eptifibatide (Integrilin), and tirofiban (Aggrastat).

Abciximab is a humanized mouse monoclonal antibody fragment with a plasma half-life of approximately 30 minutes but a receptor half-life that essentially lasts for days. Its primary use in neurosurgery is typically for endovascular therapy, with a bolus dose of 0.25 mg/kg given intravenously between 10 and 60 minutes before the start of a procedure. The postprocedural dose is 0.125 μg/kg per minute given intravenously for 12 hours.

Eptifibatide is a synthetic peptide with a half-life between 2 and 4 hours. It is also used in endovascular neurosurgery at a loading dose of 200 μg/kg given intravenously to a maximal dose of 22.6 mg before the start of a procedure. The drug is given by continuous infusion at 0.5 μg/kg per minute for 2 to 48 hours.

Tirofiban is a nonpeptide small molecule with a pharmacokinetic profile similar to that of eptifibatide. It has a half-life of approximately 2 to 4 hours. In endovascular neurosurgery, bolus dose ranges from 0.2 to 1.0 mg, or 0.4 μg/kg. Intravenous infusion is dosed at 0.1 μg/kg per minute for 12 hours.

No laboratory monitoring is used for these drugs, but their effect can be determined by both platelet aggregometry and platelet functional analyzer.

Reversal of GpIIb-IIIa inhibitors has as much to do with the potential side-effect profile as with actual reversal of the drug. Abciximab can cause both true thrombocytopenia and pseudothrombocytopenia. Asymptomatic mild to moderate thrombocytopenia, in which the platelet count is less than 50×10^9 platelets/L, does not require antiplatelet replacement. However, when there is clinical evidence of bleeding and the platelet count is less than 20×10^9 platelets/L, 1 unit of platelets should be administered.[7] Platelet activation can be stimulated in the case of bleeding with acute use of the drug by administering DDAVP at a dose of 0.3 μg/kg intravenously, repeated every 12 hours for up to six doses. In patients who received eptifibatide or tirofiban, an in vitro study demonstrated that administering fresh-frozen plasma (FFP) or prothrombin complex concentrate (PCC) along with platelets aided emergent reversal.[8]

ANTICOAGULANT DRUGS

The main classes of anticoagulant drugs include heparinoids, coagulation factor Xa inhibitors, thrombin inhibitors, and vitamin K–dependent coagulation factor inhibitors.

Heparin and Heparinoids

Unfractionated heparin is the most commonly used parenteral anticoagulant. It is a polyglycosaminoglycan that binds to exosite II on thrombin (factor IIa) as well as coagulation factor Xa.[11] The preference for binding to factor IIa over factor Xa is largely due to its molecular weight, which ranges from 15 to 30 kD. It has a half-life of 1 to 2 hours; therefore, after discontinuation of heparin, coagulation returns to baseline in approximately 3 to 4 hours. In endovascular neurosurgery, heparin is typically dosed at 50 to 100 units/kg administered as a bolus intravenously, with an activated clotting time (ACT) goal of greater than 250 seconds or twofold greater than baseline. Patients requiring a heparin drip are administered 600 to 1000 units initially and titrated to reach an aPTT between 65 and 85 seconds. An initial intravenous bolus dose between 4000 and 6000 units is sometimes used.

The activity of heparin is measured using an aPTT in the laboratory or an ACT as a point-of-care assay. Both measurements are in seconds, with a therapeutic value approximately twofold above baseline.

Heparin can be reversed using protamine, a positively charged molecule that binds to negatively charged heparin, preventing the binding to thrombin. The effective dose of protamine is 1 mg per 100 IU of heparin. Protamine should be dosed based on the amount of active heparin in circulation, so if 1000 IU of heparin has been administered over 2 hours, patients should receive 20 mg of protamine to fully reverse the activity of heparin.

Low-molecular-weight heparin (LMWH) is a fractionated form of heparin with a molecular weight of 8 to 15 kD.[11] The shorter length results in preference for factor Xa over factor IIa. The half-life of LMWH is approximately 4 hours, so a number of hours is usually required to return to a normal coagulation profile after drug administration. Protamine is also used to reverse the activity of LMWH, but it is only effective in reversing approximately 50% of the anti–factor Xa activity.[12] Protamine is administered at a dose of 1 mg for every 1 mg of LMWH administered over the previous 6 to 8 hours.[13]

Factor Xa Inhibitors

Two classes of factor Xa inhibitors exist: pentasaccharides and an oral direct inhibitor of factor Xa. Fondaparinux (Arixtra) is a heparin-related compound that has a half-life of 17 hours and is administered subcutaneously in a daily dosage of 2.5 mg. Rivaroxaban (Xarelto) is an orally available direct factor Xa inhibitor with a half-life of 7 to 11 hours and is prescribed at a 20-mg daily dosage.[14] Apixaban (Eliquis) is another oral direct factor Xa inhibitor with a half-life of 9 to 14 hours. It is prescribed at a 5-mg twice-daily dosage.

These drugs do not require monitoring but will increase the PT and are sensitive laboratory anti–factor X assays.

The inhibitory effect of fondaparinux can be reversed with rFVIIa at a dose of 80 µg/kg.[15,16] Rivaroxaban and apixaban reversal can be achieved using PCC at a concentration of 50 IU/kg as an intravenous bolus and following either a PT or an anti–factor Xa assay.[17]

Direct Thrombin Inhibitors

Direct thrombin inhibitors (DTIs) are compounds that bind to the active site of thrombin; they include both intravenous and oral forms and univalent and divalent classes. Argatroban is an intravenous, univalent formulation with a half-life of 50 minutes.[18] It is administered intravenously at a starting dose between 2 and 10 µg/kg per minute with a goal aPTT 1.5- to 3-fold above baseline. Bivalirudin (Angiomax) is a bivalent intravenous DTI that has a half-life of approximately 25 minutes and is administered intravenously with an initial loading dose of 0.75 mg/kg followed by 1.75 mg/kg per hour for the duration of a procedure. Maintenance postprocedural anticoagulation dosing is 0.2 mg/kg per hour for up to 20 hours after intervention.[19] Desirudin (Iprivask) is also bivalent DTI with a half-life of 120 minutes when administered subcutaneously. Its dosing regimen is 15 mg subcutaneously twice daily. Dabigatran (Pradaxa) is an orally available drug with a half-life of 12 to 17 hours and is prescribed at a dosage of 150 mg twice daily.[20]

These drugs can be monitored in surgery using an ACT and are elevated in a thrombin time assay.

Unfortunately, this is the only class of anticoagulants that cannot be reversed by currently available agents, rFVIIa,[21] or PCC.[17] In patients who require urgent neurosurgical intervention or who suffer intracranial hemorrhage, bivalent, intravenous DTIs should immediately be discontinued to return to baseline coagulation function, which can be verified with a thrombin time. Hemodialysis has been used to help with the reversal of dabigatran,[22] and both rFVIIa and four-factor PCC (FEIBA; Baxter, Bloomington, IN) are considered in life-threatening situations.[23]

Vitamin K–Dependent Clotting Factor Inhibitors

Warfarin is the most commonly prescribed oral anticoagulant. It inhibits vitamin K–dependent clotting factors in the liver, including factors II, VII, IX, and X as well as proteins C and S. Other drugs in this class include acenocoumarol, phenprocoumon, and anisindione. The half-life of these compounds ranges from 18 hours to 10 days.[24] Warfarin is prescribed at a dosage of 5 mg daily and is titrated to achieve a prothrombin international normalized ratio (INR) between 2 and 3 or 2.5 and 3.5, depending on the clinical indication.

The reversal strategy for coumarins depends on the urgency of reversal. Elective reversal entails using intravenous vitamin K, 1 to 2 mg every 12 hours. Subcutaneous injection has fallen out of favor because of its variable absorption. Anticoagulant reversal after intravenous administration begins within 2 hours of the first injection and reversal is usually achieved in 12 to 16 hours.[25] Oral administration of vitamin K at a dose of 2.5 to 10 mg can take more than 24 hours to reverse the activity of coumarin.

For urgent reversal, FFP or PCC is used. The concentration of clotting factors in PCC is 60-fold higher than that in FFP.[26] PCC includes inactivated plasma-derived concentrates of factor IX with varying amounts of factors II, VII, and X and proteins C and S and works rapidly to reverse anticoagulation by replacing the vitamin K–dependent factors. There are two types of PCC: three-factor PCC has sufficient factors II, IX, and X with low factor VII, whereas four-factor PCC has sufficient factors II, VII, IX, and X.[27] The dose administered for either variant is 20 to 50 IU/kg. Some institutions use three-factor PCC along with a small dose of rFVIIa, typically 20 µg/kg, with no difference in efficacy compared with four-factor PCC.[27]

The use of FFP is associated with increased time to administration because clinicians need to obtain a patient's ABO blood type and the FFP is given as an intravenous drip. PCC, on the other hand, is reconstituted quickly and can be given by intravenous bolus over 2 to 5 minutes. A drawback of PCC is that it can lead to a hypercoagulable state, placing the patient at risk for arterial or venous thrombosis. Although vitamin K and FFP are routinely used to reverse anticoagulation, neither provides rapid INR reversal. Therefore other options have been explored, including PCC and even rFVIIa.

In patients on warfarin who require emergent neurosurgical intervention, rFVIIa can be administered. Recombinant factor VIIa is a vitamin K–dependent glycoprotein that produces hemostasis by activating the extrinsic pathway. Recombinant factor VIIa has a rapid onset of action and a half-life of 2 to 3 hours.[28] It is administered at an initial dose of 80 µg/kg, based on research limiting the size of the blood clot in patients with acute intracranial hemorrhage.[29] Administration of FFP or PCC, as well as vitamin K, is done after the rFVIIa has been given. Although the INR normalizes quickly, it is not durable given the short duration of action, and rFVIIa does not replace other vitamin K–dependent clotting factors inhibited by warfarin. A concern associated with rFVIIa is the potential to develop acute thromboembolism.

FUTURE PERSPECTIVES

Since 2005 there have been marked advances in target-specific antithrombotic drug development. Many of these newer drugs, especially orally available direct factor Xa and thrombin inhibitors, tout their utility and efficiency as being drugs that do not need monitoring. These drugs, however, provide a significant challenge for neurosurgeons because none has a specific antidote agent to reverse the activity of the drug. This results in considerable morbidity and mortality when these patients present with intracranial hemorrhage or require emergent neurosurgical intervention.

With the premise of discovering antithrombotic drugs with matched antidotes, novel research performed since 2000 has exploited the properties of aptamers. Aptamers are nucleic acid ligands that bind to and inhibit their target protein. Their potential as drug agents was first demonstrated in 1990 by impeding HIV replication by inhibiting Tat protein–tar RNA interactions.[30] Aptamers are isolated through a process called *systematic evolution of ligands by exponential enrichment* (SELEX).[31,32] This in vitro process isolates aptamers to target proteins from a library of 10^{14} molecules.[33] Aptamers have a number of properties that make them attractive drug agents: their isolation process makes it possible to develop an aptamer to virtually any target protein, they bind to their target protein with high affinity and specificity, they can undergo postselection modification to adjust their bioavailability, and their activity can be rapidly reversed.[33] This last characteristic is achieved by designing an antidote oligonucleotide that binds to the aptamer by Watson-Crick base pairing,

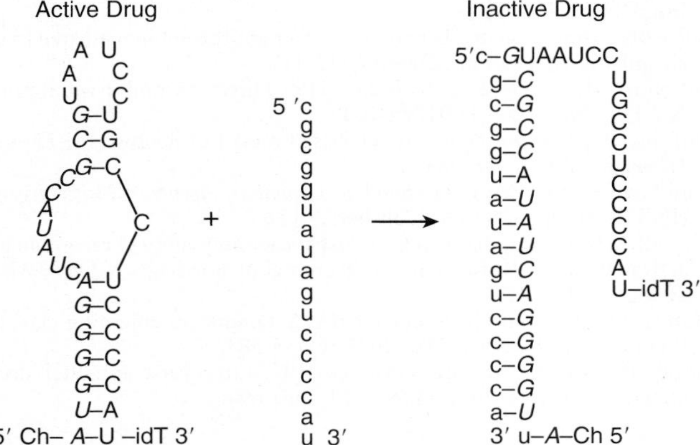

Figure 7-3. An RNA aptamer against coagulation factor IXa can be rapidly reversed by an antidote oligonucleotide (AO) that was designed based on Watson-Crick base pairing with a segment of the aptamer. The AO binds to the aptamer, preventing it from forming the necessary three-dimensional shape to bind to and inhibit factor IXa.

thereby preventing the aptamer from binding to its target protein (Fig. 7-3). There have been aptamers to coagulation factors II, IIa, IXa, and XIIa as well as to vWF.[34-40] The anti–factor IXa aptamer and matched antidote has shown promise in clinical trials as an effective, reversible anticoagulant.[41-46] Further work in this field may yield a new class of promising agents that change the way clinicians develop drugs to emphasize safety through rapid reversal as much as the antithrombotic effect of the drug.

Another major concern for neurosurgeons is intraoperative hemostasis as it pertains to coagulation. A plethora of hemostatic agents are used in neurosurgery today, including Avitene (microfibrillar collagen, C.R. Bard, Murray Hill, NJ), bone wax, Evicel (human thrombin and fibrinogen, Johnson & Johnson, New Brunswick, NJ), Floseal (bovine gelatin granules with human thrombin, Baxter), Gelfoam (porcine skin gelatin granules often combined with thrombin, Pfizer, New York, NY), Surgicel (oxidized regenerated cellulose, Johnson & Johnson), and Tisseel (human thrombin and fibrinogen, Baxter). Excellent reviews discussing neurosurgical considerations of these and other hemostatic agents are available.[47-49]

The problems with existing hemostatic materials are being recognized with their increasing application. For example, it is not often appreciated that Surgicel and other cellulose and gelatin-containing hemostats (e.g., Floseal, Gelfoam) must be removed after hemostasis is achieved when used around the spinal cord and laminectomies or around the optic nerve or chiasm because tremendous swelling can occur, exerting unwanted pressure. Similarly, the complications associated with microfibrillar collagen (Avitene), a foreign protein with a tendency to exacerbate infection, and with thrombin or thrombin-containing hemostats, which frequently lead to formation of antibodies, are underrecognized. Thrombin should be contraindicated, for example, in individuals sensitive to any of its components because febrile and antigenic reactions have been documented. Almost 20% of patients undergoing neurosurgical operations develop factor V antibodies secondary to thrombin use.[50] To overcome the negative side effects of current hemostats and improve intraoperative and postoperative hemostatic control, new hemostatic agents are being developed. The most notable novel hemostatic agents in development include chitosan, nanoparticulate agents, and combinations or derivatives of first-generation hemostatic agents like gelatin and cellulose.

Chitosan

Chitosan is the deacetylated derivative of chitin, an abundant natural biopolymer found in crustacean shells and fungi consisting of β-1,4-linked glucosamine moieties. Chitosan is a well-documented hemostatic agent whose hemostatic effect occurs *independent of the coagulation cascade* by electrostatically binding red blood cells and platelets, leading to the formation of a coagulum.[51-54] Despite a long history of being recognized as a highly hemostatic material, chitosan has yet to be widely applied in the surgical setting because of concerns regarding pyrogen contamination. Novel methods to sterilize and depyrogenate chitosan, such as nonthermal nitrogen gas plasma, are in development because conventional sterilization techniques such as dry-wet heat, gamma radiation, and ethylene oxide are contraindicated for this material. An additional advantage of nitrogen gas plasma sterilization-depyrogenation is its ability to chemically alter the surface of materials. Nitrogen gas plasma adds nitrogen groups to the surface of chitosan, which may increase its cationic nature and enhance its mucoadhesivity.[55] Chitosan has been tested in the neurosurgical setting on animal models and has been shown to be safe and nontoxic in central nervous system tissue and effectively control central nervous system hemorrhage.[56,57] Moreover, chitosan has been shown to enhance neural stem and progenitor cell growth and survival.[58] Chitosan also possesses other valuable biomedical properties, including being mucoadhesive because of its cationic nature, anti-inflammatory, antimicrobial, and resorbable. Chitosan also has analgesic and wound-healing enhancement properties. Chitosan is resorbed by a number of enzymes, including lysozyme and chitosanases.[59] Fabricating chitosan into different physical forms such as microfibrillar fleece, sponge-like pads, paper-like sheets, films, powders, flakes, and nanoparticles is easily achieved, enabling exceptional customization for different surgical applications and goals. This has significant implications for drug delivery applications in addition to hemostasis applications.

Further studies are required to characterize the surgical usefulness of chitosan as well as to identify potential side effects. However, the future is bright for chitosan because there are more than 15 different topical chitosan hemostats and antimicrobial barriers on the market for use in trauma wounds, epistaxis, and vascular access procedures and no significant complications have been reported from use of these devices.

Nanoparticulate Agents

The biomedical literature is now expanding with studies of novel nanoscale particles for numerous applications, including hemostasis. Although many regulatory and manufacturing hurdles remain before nanomedicine will be widely adopted, excellent preclinical results have been achieved with nanoparticulate hemostats. For example, Giday and colleagues demonstrated that a proprietary nanopowder composed of a granular mineral blend achieves fast, effective hemostasis after severe gastric bleeding is induced in pigs.[60] Two studies have shown that intravenous injection of poly(lactic-co-glycolic acid) (PLGA) nanoparticles dramatically improves hemostatic control after hepatectomy in rats and blast injuries in mice.[61,62] A similar study synthesized platelet-like nanoparticles and showed they reduced time to hemostasis after tail amputation in mice.[63] A nanoparticle hemostat, AC5, for neurosurgical applications based on self-assembling peptides that form nanofibers after contact with physiologic fluids and tissues is in development by Arch Therapeutics (Framingham, MA). Strong preclinical data have demonstrated that AC5 achieves rapid hemostasis in both brain and spinal cord hemorrhages in hamsters.[64,65]

First-generation hemostatic agents include collagen, fibrinogen, gelatin, thrombin, and oxidized regenerated cellulose. Second- and third-generation hemostats that are combinations of these first-generation hemostats, such as Floseal (gelatin with thrombin) and Tisseel (thrombin with fibrinogen), have emerged in recent years. Additional combination hemostats have been approved by the U.S. Food and Drug Administration, including EVARREST (oxidized regenerated cellulose coated with human fibrinogen and thrombin, Johnson & Johnson) and TachoSil (equine collagen pad coated with human fibrinogen and thrombin, Baxter), although not for neurosurgical applications.[66]

Second- and third-generation hemostats that are derivatives of first-generation hemostats are currently in preclinical development. A recent report described a cellulose derivative, carboxymethyl cellulose, which demonstrated hemostatic effectiveness similar to HemCon (Portland, OR), a topical chitosan-based hemostatic bandage used widely by the U.S. military for trauma wounds.[67,68] This study suggests that cellulose derivatives with improved hemostatic efficacy compared with commercially available cellulose-based hemostats are possible.

SUGGESTED READINGS

Adler BK. Unfractionated heparin and other antithrombin mediated anticoagulants. *Clin Lab Sci*. 2004;17:113-117.

Di Nisio M, Middeldorp S, Büller HR. Direct thrombin inhibitors. *N Engl J Med*. 2005;353:1028-1040.

Hoffman M, Monroe D 3rd. A cell-based model of hemostasis. *Thromb Haemost*. 2001;85:958-965.

Lapierre F, Wager M, D'Houtaud S. *Hemostatic Agents in Neurosurgery*. (INTECH Open Access Publisher, 2012).

Mayer SA, Brun NC, Begtrup K, et al. Efficacy and safety of recombinant activated factor VII for acute intracerebral hemorrhage. *N Engl J Med*. 2008;358:2127-2137.

Nimjee SM, Rusconi CP, Sullenger BA. Aptamers: an emerging class of therapeutics. *Annu Rev Med*. 2005;56:555-583.

Sarode R. How do I transfuse platelets (PLTs) to reverse anti-PLT drug effect? *Transfusion*. 2012;52:695-701, quiz 694.

See a full reference list on ExpertConsult.com 

8 Neuro-ophthalmology

Janet C. Rucker

Neuro-ophthalmologic symptoms and signs are common manifestations of many neurosurgical conditions and, not infrequently, are the presenting feature, the feature allowing accurate preimaging localization, or the most sensitive measure of progression. This chapter includes two sections: (1) From the Eye to the Visual Cortex: The Afferent Visual System, and (2) Ocular Motility and The Pupil: The Efferent Visual System. Each section outlines an approach to obtaining a complete history of the visual dysfunction from the patient, techniques for examination to localize the anatomic cause of the visual dysfunction, a description of the pertinent neuro-ophthalmologic anatomy, and an overview of common etiologic conditions affecting each anatomic structure. Content coverage focuses on those conditions most common in neurosurgical conditions; however, an overview of non-neurosurgical pathologies is also included to assist the neurosurgical consultant in differentiating these from the neurosurgical issues.

Broad coverage of the common causes of visual loss includes discussions of corneal pathology (as might be seen in neurosurgical patients with fifth or seventh cranial nerve involvement), retinal disorders, and a host of optic nerve disorders. Papilledema is extensively discussed, including the mechanism of vision loss in the peripheral visual field and the importance of serial formal visual field assessment. Optic nerve mimics of papilledema are discussed in a section on pseudopapilledema because the distinction between true papilledema and anomalous optic discs not related to a neurosurgical lesion may make the difference between emergent neurosurgical decompression and conservative follow-up in some patients. Additional optic neuropathies covered include ischemic, inflammatory, compressive and infiltrative, metabolic, and traumatic optic neuropathies. Visual manifestations of chiasmal and intracranial visual pathway disease follow.

The efferent visual disorder section focuses on ocular motor cranial nerve (third, fourth, and sixth cranial nerves) involvement in neurosurgical disorders with video examples but also provides a basic approach to evaluating diplopia from one end of the ocular motor pathways (extraocular muscle and neuromuscular junction) to the other (supranuclear brainstem ocular motor structures). New in this edition is coverage of the eye movement examination in coma. The eye movement section concludes with a discussion of treatment of symptomatic double vision, which is often a predominant source of degradation of visual function and quality of life in neurosurgical patients. The chapter concludes with pupillary disorders, taking the approach of the importance of initial recognition of which pupil is the abnormal pupil in anisocoria. When the larger pupil is abnormal, parasympathetic involvement for third nerve dysfunction, a tonic pupil, or pharmacologic dilation of the pupil are the most common entities. When the smaller pupil is the abnormal pupil, Horner's syndrome may be present.

In summary, this chapter provides an overview of common neuro-ophthalmic manifestations of neurosurgical conditions. References for more comprehensive topic coverage are included, as are boxes outlining neuro-ophthalmologic examination techniques as well as extensive differential localization and differential diagnostic considerations for disc edema and ocular motor cranial nerve disorders. Correct identification and localization of common visual disturbances and attention to prevention of visual morbidity in the neurosurgical patient are critical, and it is the hope that this chapter will facilitate those important goals.

Full text of this chapter is available online at ExpertConsult.com 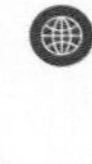

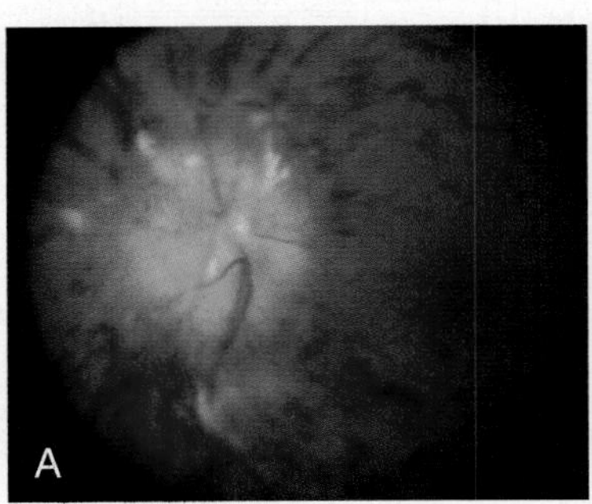

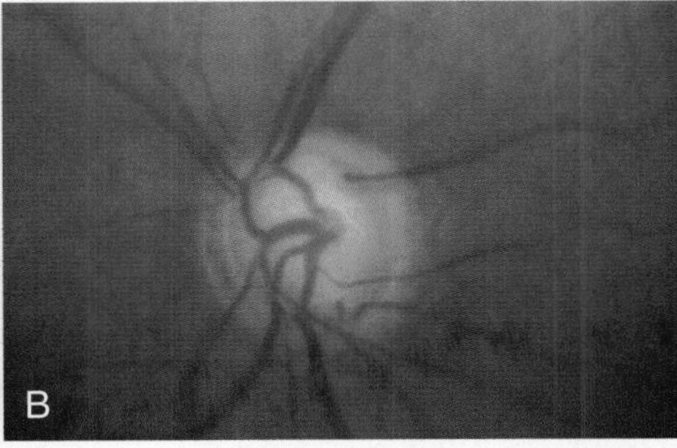

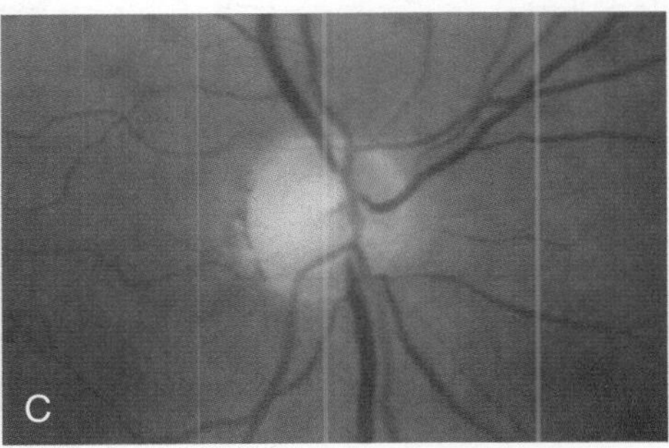

Optic disc pathology. A, Severe disc edema of the left optic disc from papilledema (raised intracranial pressure). Note the substantial blurring of the disc margins, nearly complete obscuration of the vasculature at the disc, peripapillary disc hemorrhages, and white gliosis and cotton-wool spots. **B,** Optic disc cupping from glaucoma. Note the normal color of the neuroretinal rim beyond the central yellow extensive cupping. **C,** Optic atrophy of the right optic disc.

9 Neurotology

P. Ashley Wackym

The purpose of this chapter is to review the anatomy, physiology, assessment, and differential diagnoses of hearing and balance disorders that are relevant to the practicing neurosurgeon. In the otorhinolaryngologic subspecialty of otology, neurotology, and cranial base surgery, the focus is on the anatomy, physiology, and abnormalities of the three cranial nerves that traverse the temporal bone—the cochlear, vestibular, and facial nerves—as well as specific tests of their functions.

Knowledge of cochlear anatomy and physiology serves as the foundation to assess the tools available to measure cochlear function. The following diagnostic tests and their subtest components are reviewed: audiometry, tympanometry, acoustic reflexes, auditory brainstem evoked responses, and otoacoustic emissions. The specific components of hearing and the auditory pathway that each test measures are discussed, as are auditory brainstem evoked responses in auditory neuropathy and electrically auditory evoked potentials in cochlear implant recipients. In addition, the importance of preoperative and postoperative follow-up audiologic evaluation is emphasized.

This Web-based chapter also outlines vestibular anatomy and physiology. This knowledge provides the background for understanding the following diagnostic tests and their subtest components: physical examination with nystagmus observation, positional and rotational testing, and electronystagmography/videonystagmography. Also, the correlation of individual tests with the specific components of vestibular and the vestibular pathways is reviewed.

With this background in vestibular and brainstem anatomy and physiology, the chapter then focuses on the differential diagnosis of vertigo, and both peripheral and central vestibular disorders are reviewed. Peripheral vestibular disorders include benign positional vertigo, Meniere's disease, secondary endolymphatic hydrops, vestibular neuronitis, superior semicircular canal dehiscence syndrome, posttraumatic vertigo, and drug-induced ototoxicity. Central vestibular disorders include vestibular migraine and brainstem lesions such as multiple sclerosis, vascular accidents, vertebrobasilar insufficiency, and posterior fossa tumors.

At the end of the chapter, the surgical indications for vestibular neurectomy, as well as those for cochlear and auditory brainstem implantation, are discussed.

Full text of this chapter is available online at ExpertConsult.com 

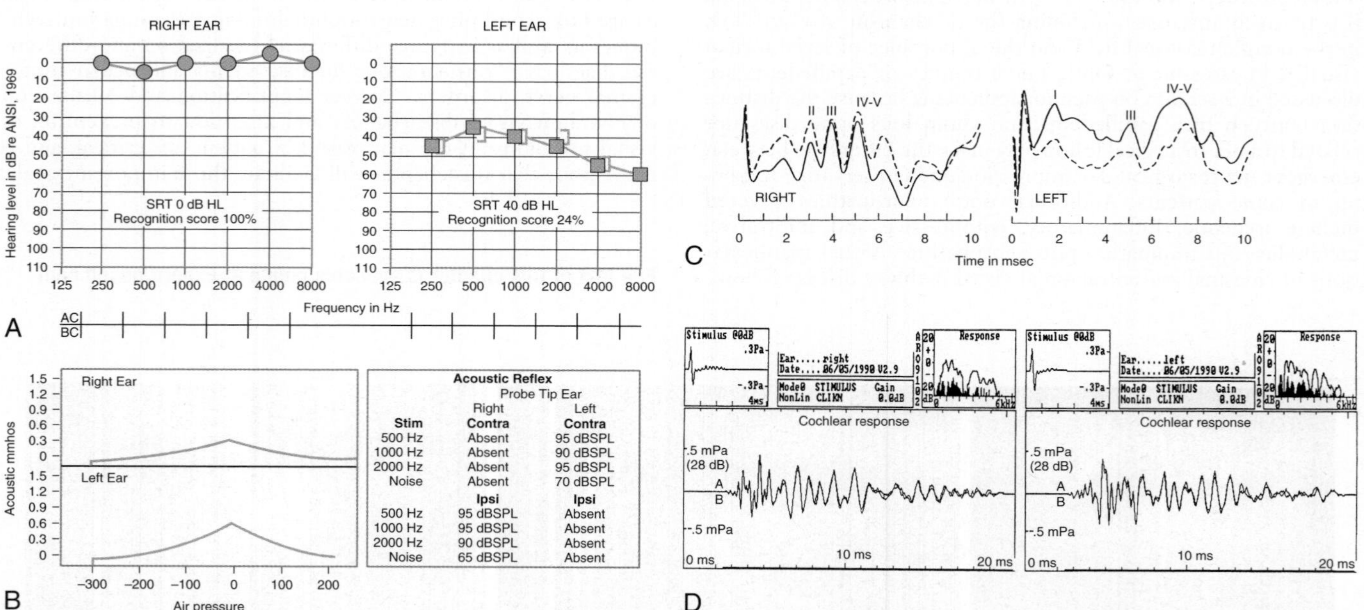

Bilateral auditory test results from a patient with unilateral (left ear) acoustic neuroma extending into the cerebellopontine angle. A, Air conduction (AC; *red circles [right ear]* and *blue squares [left ear]*) and bone conduction (BC; *open brackets opening to the left [left ear only]*) pure-tone threshold sensitivities are plotted as a function of frequency. Measures of pure tone and speech recognition show left sensorineural hearing loss and poor speech discrimination on the left. The speech reception threshold (SRT) is expressed in hearing level (HL), and the speech recognition score is the percentage of correct responses. **B,** Tympanograms and acoustic reflex threshold measures show normal middle ear impedance and absence of acoustic reflexes on the left. dBSPL, decibels of sound pressure level; mmhos, millisiemens. **C,** Auditory brainstem evoked responses at a 75-dB normalized hearing level show poor wave structure and delay of wave V on the left. **D,** Measures of otoacoustic emissions show normal cochlear function despite the sensorineural hearing loss and poor speech discrimination in the left ear. *(Published with permission; copyright © 2009, P. A. Wackym, MD.)*

10 Neurourology

Lara S. MacLachlan, Brett D. Lebed, and Eric S. Rovner

Central nervous system disorders are a frequent cause of urologic symptoms and voiding dysfunction. Appropriate recognition and timely management of urologic issues relevant to neurological conditions are important to avoid potentially irreversible adverse outcomes.

The lower urinary tract has two basic physiologic functions: low-pressure storage of adequate volumes of urine with appropriate sensation and periodic, voluntary expulsion of urine from the bladder in a coordinated and complete fashion. To provide these functions, the bladder, bladder neck, external urethral sphincter, and urethra must have coordinated activity mediated by the autonomic and somatic nervous systems.

When evaluating a patient with urologic problems secondary to a neurological condition, a thorough neurourologic evaluation should be performed. A detailed history and physical examination, including a neurological examination, are essential for assessment, accurate diagnosis, and treatment of urologic conditions resulting from neurological disease. Additional diagnostics, such as laboratory testing and various radiologic studies to evaluate the upper and lower urinary tract, often require review. Ultimately, ongoing reassessment at regular intervals is also necessary to prevent progression of urologic disease in these patients.

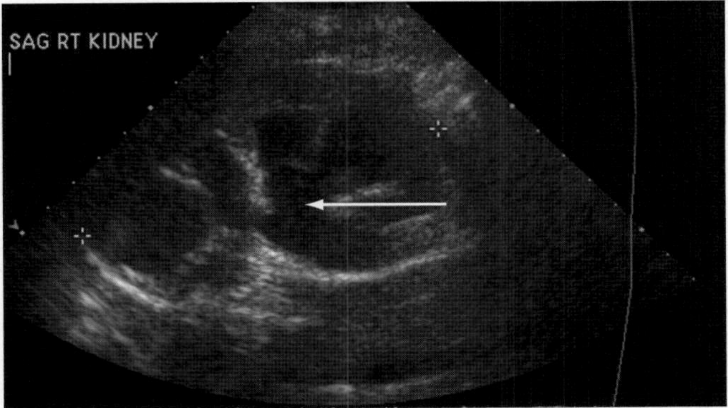

Renal ultrasound demonstrating hydronephrosis in a patient with a neurogenic bladder and poor bladder compliance. The *arrow* identifies areas of distention of the renal pelvis, calyces, and proximal ureter. Note the preserved renal parenchyma surrounding the calyces, a finding suggesting preserved renal function.

Urinary complications of neurological disease or injury can affect the filling/storage or emptying phases of micturition, or can impact both phases. The deficits are usually dependent on the area of the nervous system involved in the disease and can be grouped into supraspinal lesions, spinal lesions, suprasacral cord injury, and disease at or distal to the sacral spinal cord. Although significant variability exists within a given disease entity, characteristic symptom patterns and urodynamic findings are common, depending on the level or location of the lesion.

Once a diagnosis of the neurological or neurosurgical disease has been established and the neurourologic disturbance identified, attention should be given to the short- and long-term treatment of symptoms and prevention of long-term complications. There are four general goals in bladder management: (1) protecting renal function and upper urinary tracts, (2) minimizing lower urinary tract complications, (3) treating the bothersome symptoms of neurourologic disease, and (4) choosing a management program compatible with individual patient goals and abilities. To achieve these goals, treatment should focus on maintenance of low storage pressure, prevention of incontinence, promotion of efficient bladder emptying, and avoidance of infection. Because of the complicated and variable symptomatology of neurourologic disorders, management can be more easily divided into categories of lower urinary tract dysfunction rather than treatment of specific disease entities.

Full text of this chapter is available online at ExpertConsult.com 

11 Computed Tomography and Magnetic Resonance Imaging of the Brain

Thomas Aquinas Kim, Aleksandrs Uldis Kalnins, and Robert W. Prost

COMPUTED TOMOGRAPHY OF THE BRAIN

History and Fundamentals

Computed tomography (CT), formerly called computed axial tomography (CAT), was developed in the early 1970s by Sir Geoffrey Hounsfield and his colleagues in England.[1] It was possibly the most important advance in medical imaging after the discovery of x-rays by Professor Wilhelm Röntgen. It represented the first commercially available imaging equipment with which the emerging technologic advances in computing were used to generate digital images, displayed in gray scale. Its development revolutionized the evaluation of patients with neurological diseases and enabled noninvasive visualization of the inside of the body, which allowed detection of diseases and abnormalities and played a key role in the diagnosis, management, and treatment of patients on a daily basis in the practice of medicine all over the world.[2] Although its place in imaging of the brain and spine has been somewhat supplanted by another revolutionary technology, magnetic resonance imaging (MRI), CT remains widely used and an important first study of choice in many aspects of neurosurgery. Furthermore, because of important advances in CT technology during the last 20 years—such as multidetector configurations in newer CT scanners and the ever-increasing speed of computer technology, which enable very fast CT scanning of a patient in seconds rather than minutes—its use has strongly surged. Such advances have led to the development of CT angiography (CTA) and perfusion CT, which have become important in noninvasive evaluation of cerebrovascular diseases. In addition, portable CT scanners can provide high-quality images for point-of-care imaging in an intensive care unit setting and thereby avoid potential risks associated with transport of critically patients.

CT can be performed in various planes that depend on patient position and the CT gantry angle within its limited arc. For example, direct CT imaging of the paranasal sinuses or brain in the coronal plane can be performed with the patient in a supine position with the patient's head hanging over the edge of the CT scanner table or with the patient in the prone position and the neck hyperextended. Most commonly, however, CT imaging of the brain and spine is performed in the axial plane, with the patient in a supine position on the scanner table and the head and neck in a neutral position. The need for a direct coronal patient position has lessened since the advent of high-resolution multiplanar reconstruction capabilities on newer generation CT scanners. These reconstruction capabilities can generate axial images in 0.5- to 0.6-mm increments, which can then be reformatted into the sagittal, coronal, and oblique planes, with image quality nearly identical to that obtained from direct scanning.[3,4]

A typical routine brain CT scan consists of 5-mm contiguous axial images through the entire brain from the skull base to the vertex, without the intravenous injection of contrast material. This can be followed by another set of 5-mm axial images through the brain after the intravenous administration of a contrast agent: typically 100 mL of iodinated contrast material, injected through an 18- or a 20-gauge intravenous catheter. Scanning intervals are adjusted for clinical need and for indications such as patient age and size; need for higher resolution images of specific anatomy such as the orbits, temporal bone, and skull base; or CTA. With the newer multidetector CT scanners, these images can be reconstructed into submillimeter axial images that can be used to generate two-dimensional (2D) and three-dimensional (3D) reformatted sagittal and coronal images and thus better delineate parenchymal, vascular, and osseous anatomy.

The radiation dose delivered to patients during CT examination has become an object of significant concern because of the possibility of radiation-induced cancers, especially for pediatric patients undergoing repeated examinations. Radiation doses have been reduced 25% to 98% through the use of interactive reconstruction methods.[5] Since the introduction of these methods in 2008, all major CT manufacturers now offer dose reduction as an option. However, dose reduction can have a significant effect on image quality and must be based on the patient and the likelihood of requirements for repeated surveillance examinations.[6]

CT is most often the first study of choice in evaluation of a patient with suspected acute intracranial disease because of its ready availability, ease of use, short acquisition time, and high sensitivity for detection of acute hemorrhage and fractures. It can provide a wealth of information about the brain, including ventricular size, presence of brain edema, mass effect, presence and location of hemorrhage or masses, midline shift, evolving ischemic injuries, fractures, benign and malignant osseous disease, and evaluation of the paranasal sinuses. Its availability and short acquisition time also allow frequent repeat scanning of the brain, which can contribute to the management and follow-up of patients in the acute, subacute, and chronic phases in both inpatient and outpatient settings.[7-9]

In neurosurgery, CT of the head is used for preoperative and postoperative evaluation for hemorrhage, infarction, hydrocephalus, mass effect, and fracture and for postsurgical assessment.[10-14] CT is the study of choice in evaluating for acute hemorrhage because it has higher sensitivity and specificity for this indication than MRI does. Intracranial hemorrhage is typically described in terms of its location within the head, such as epidural, subdural, subarachnoid, intraventricular, and parenchymal; each of these different types of hemorrhages have sufficiently distinct appearances and locations. The borders of an epidural hemorrhage have a biconvex contour (Fig. 11-1A) in relation to the cranial vault and adjacent brain parenchyma, and this condition is usually the result of acute trauma associated with an acute fracture across branches of meningeal arteries that hemorrhage into the epidural space. Less commonly, rapid venous hemorrhage into the epidural space may cause an epidural hematoma. The extent of an epidural hematoma is usually limited by periosteal dural insertions at the major sutures. However, an epidural hematoma can extend across the midline in the frontal region anterior to the coronal suture because it is not limited by the dural reflections within the anterior interhemispheric fissure (Fig. 11-1C).

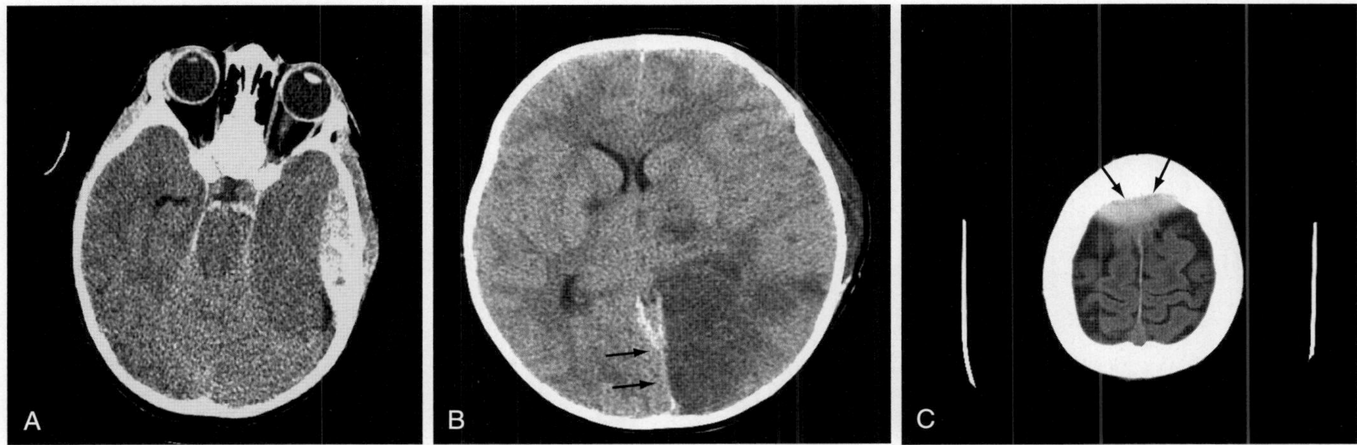

Figure 11-1. A, Non–contrast-enhanced computed tomographic (CT) image of the head, demonstrating an acute epidural hematoma over the left cerebral hemisphere. Note the biconvex contours of the hematoma. **B,** Postoperative CT shows multiple infarctions, including a large left posterior distribution infarction *(arrows)* of the cerebral artery from compression of this vessel by the epidural hematoma. **C,** In a different patient, epidural hematoma at the vertex *(arrows),* extending across the interhemispheric fissure.

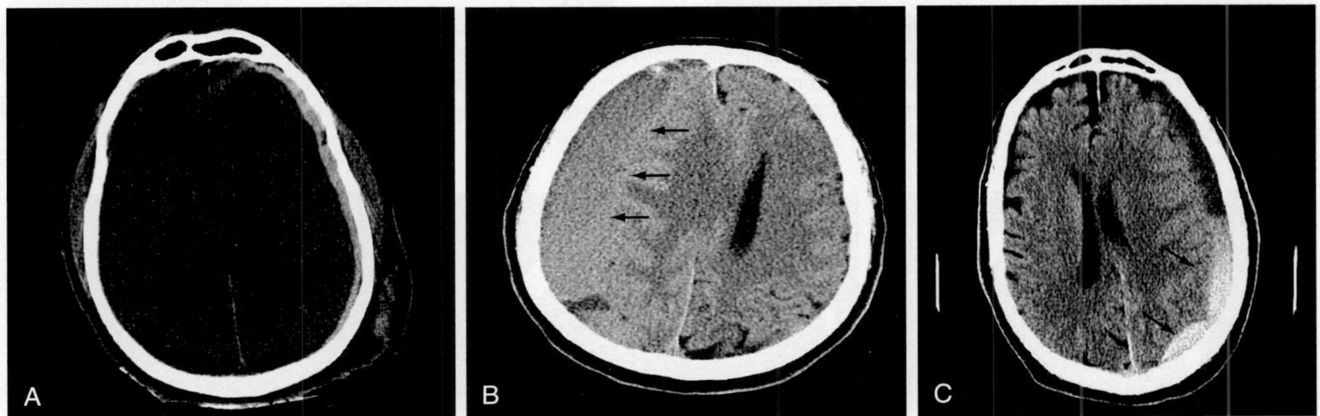

Figure 11-2. A, Non–contrast-enhanced computed tomographic (CT) image of the head, showing a thin left acute subdural hematoma (SDH). **B,** Right subacute, nearly isodense SDH *(arrows).* **C,** Acute-on-chronic SDH over the left frontal and parietal lobes.

A subdural hematoma (SDH) is more common than an epidural hematoma, particularly in older patients, and is generally associated with acute head trauma, with or without an associated fracture. Its shape is different from that of an epidural hematoma because its deeper border against the brain parenchyma is concave and approximates the contour of the adjacent cerebral hemisphere convexity. An acute SDH is typically a result of venous hemorrhage and is not limited by the periosteal dural insertions at the major sutures. However, it is limited by the midline dural reflections within the interhemispheric fissure. The density of the blood in any type of SDH—whether acute, subacute, or chronic—changes over time from hyperdense to isodense to hypodense (Fig. 11-2). However, a hyperacute SDH or an acute subarachnoid hemorrhage (SAH) in the presence of coagulopathy may sometimes appear isodense or hypodense.

Trauma is the most common cause of SAH, whereas rupture of an intracranial aneurysm is the most common nontraumatic cause of SAH. SAH extends freely within the subarachnoid spaces around the cerebral hemispheres, brainstem, and cerebellum and frequently, by reflux of cerebrospinal fluid (CSF), extends into the intraventricular spaces. It often leads to acute, subacute, or chronic hydrocephalus because the blood products disrupt and obstruct the normal CSF drainage pathways (Fig. 11-3).

Parenchymal hemorrhages have many causes, including trauma, hypertension, vascular anomalies such as arteriovenous malformation or cavernoma, infarction, neoplasm, infection, or vasculitis. They can be small or large, and they can be single or multiple; patient prognosis depends on the cause, number, size, and associated mass effect of the hemorrhage, among other variables (Fig. 11-4).

Computed Tomographic Angiography

Advances in CT scanner technology have improved the capacity for higher resolution images in the submillimeter range with shorter acquisition times. Such technologic improvements have led to imaging techniques such as CTA, which enables relatively noninvasive imaging of the major arteries and veins of the neck and brain after an intravenous injection of iodinated contrast material, rather than the traditional catheter-based intra-arterial angiogram technique. This venous injection helps avoid the small risk for complications such as vascular dissection, renal injury,

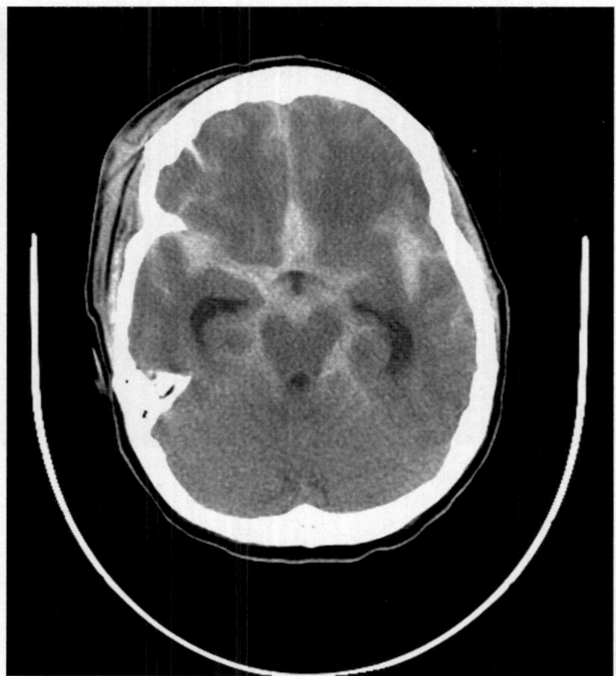

Figure 11-3. Acute diffuse subarachnoid hemorrhages within the suprasellar cistern, ambient cistern, and frontal and temporal sulci. There is dilation of both temporal horns of the lateral ventricles in association with communicating hydrocephalus.

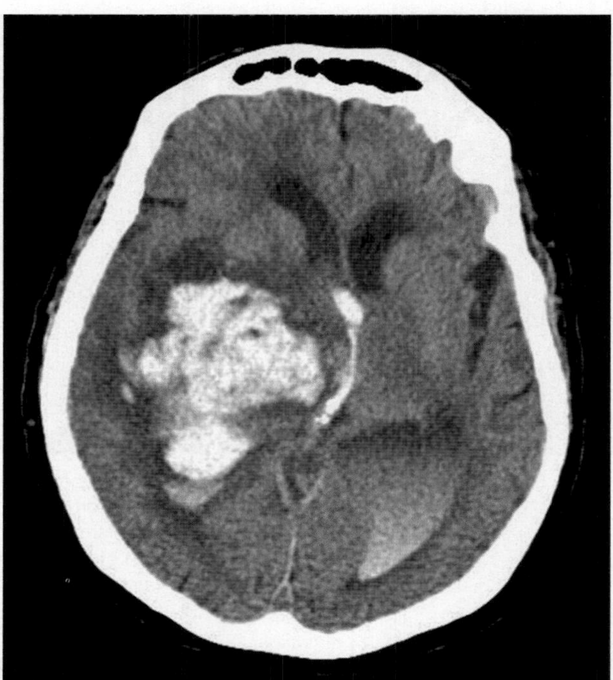

Figure 11-4. Non–contrast-enhanced computed tomographic image of the head, demonstrating an acute right thalamic hypertensive hemorrhage, midline shift to the left, intraventricular hemorrhage, and hydrocephalus.

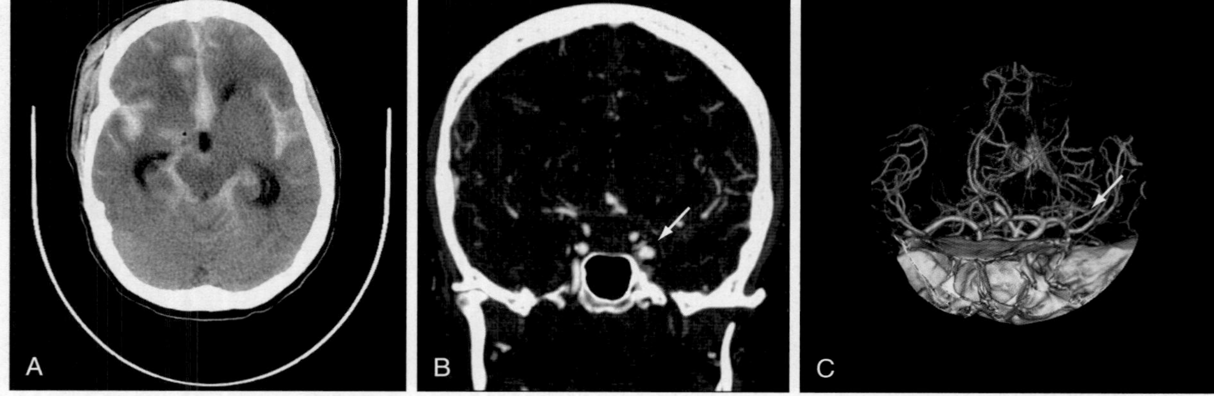

Figure 11-5. Non–contrast-enhanced computed tomographic (CT) images of the head. A, These images illustrate subarachnoid hemorrhage from a ruptured aneurysm of the anterior communicating (ACOM) artery. **B,** Coronal two-dimensional reformatted image from a CT angiogram (CTA) of the brain, demonstrating an irregular aneurysm in the ACOM artery *(arrow)*. **C,** Three-dimensional CTA reconstruction image of the aneurysm in the ACOM artery *(arrow)*.

allergic reaction, and iatrogenic embolic strokes associated with traditional catheter angiography.

CTA of the neck or brain is performed with a multidetector CT scanner, which enables rapid dynamic imaging of the anatomy of interest. Iodinated contrast material is delivered as a bolus injection through a large-bore (18-gauge) intravenous catheter. Typically, submillimeter axial images are obtained and then reformatted into 2D sagittal and coronal image data sets at 1- to 2-mm intervals. The reconstruction images are usually 3D, but interpretation of the study is based primarily on the original axial data set and the 2D sagittal and coronal reformatted images. The diagnostic sensitivity and specificity of CTA are comparable with those of catheter angiography for both the extracranial and intracranial vasculature.[15,16] Although CTA cannot entirely replace traditional catheter angiography, it is a very useful noninvasive screening study for the evaluation, management, and follow-up of patients with definite or possible aneurysms, as well as the evaluation of vasospasm, arteriovenous malformations, traumatic dissection, stroke, and atherosclerotic stenosis of the carotid or vertebral artery (Figs. 11-5 and 11-6).[17]

Perfusion Computed Tomography

Perfusion computed tomography (pCT) provides physiologic information in addition to anatomic information. pCT is performed with the latest-generation multidetector CT scanners,

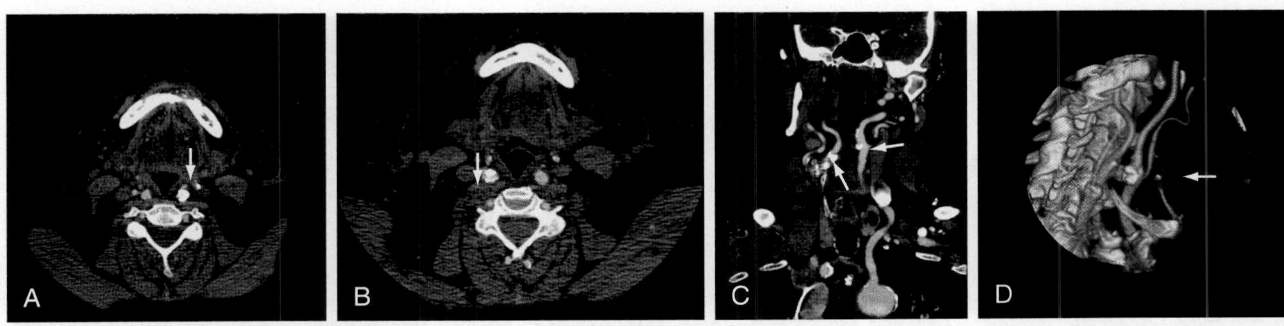

Figure 11-6. Computed tomographic angiograms (CTAs) of the neck. Source images illustrate calcified atherosclerotic stenoses *(arrows)* of the origins of the left **(A)** and right **(B)** internal carotid arteries. **C,** Coronal two-dimensional reformatted image shows calcified atherosclerotic disease of both common carotid artery bifurcations *(arrows).* **D,** Oblique three-dimensional reconstruction image shows calcified plaque in the bifurcation of the left common carotid artery *(arrow).*

which allow very rapid CT imaging of a particular anatomic area, such as the cerebral hemispheres. Iodinated contrast material is delivered in a bolus intravenous injection at a rate of 4 to 5 mL/sec, and rapid serial CT images of a chosen volume are obtained in multiple phases over an approximately 1-minute period. At the end of this acquisition, multiphase time-density curves corresponding to each voxel are generated within a 2D image of a multilevel image data set. The data from these images are further postprocessed with a mathematical algorithm that allows displays of the data in color maps that represent such physiologic cerebral perfusion parameters as cerebral blood flow (CBF), cerebral blood volume (CBV), and mean transit time (MTT). The CBF, CBV, and MTT maps generated from this CT technique are, in part, quantitative; that is, the numerical values obtained from these images may be expressed in milliliters per 100 g/min for CBF, mL/100 g for CBV, and seconds for MTT.[18] The pCT technology has been validated against other proven in vivo techniques such as xenon-enhanced CT and positron emission tomography.[19-23]

pCT has been used to evaluate acute stroke, central nervous system (CNS) neoplasms, and ischemic sequelae of SAH-related vasospasm. The most common use of pCT is for the evaluation of acute stroke. The various color maps of cerebral perfusion help determine the presence of salvageable ischemic penumbra during the first few hours after stroke, which may lead to more aggressive therapy, such as an intra-arterial thrombolysis or thrombus extraction to enable rapid recanalization of occluded large intracranial arteries (e.g., the supraclinoid segment of the internal carotid artery or the M1 segment of the middle cerebral artery) (Fig. 11-7).

The availability of physiologic data also helps in the diagnosis, management, and treatment of ruptured aneurysm and subsequent vasospasm, which may contribute to acute or subacute ischemic injury. Evaluation of affected patients has typically relied on serial clinical assessment, non–contrast-enhanced head CT, and transcranial Doppler ultrasonography. This evaluation protocol has recognized limitations; in particular, non–contrast-enhanced CT and transcranial Doppler (TCD) ultrasonography may not accurately reflect the state of cerebral perfusion at an early enough stage to allow successful intervention for reversal of oligemia and ischemia. Baseline and follow-up pCT can demonstrate the size and extent of brain areas at risk for stroke in patients in a neurological intensive care unit, often before symptoms develop and permanent infarction occurs (Fig. 11-8). For some patients, this early detection of at-risk areas may enable earlier medical and catheter-based intervention for vasospasm and thus prevent delayed ischemic injury.[19-21]

MAGNETIC RESONANCE IMAGING OF THE BRAIN

Physics and Techniques of Magnetic Resonance Imaging

History

The interaction of the intrinsic magnetic moment of the nucleus with an externally imposed magnetic field results in the phenomenon known as *nuclear magnetic resonance* (NMR). In 1946, two independent research groups—Bloch and colleagues, working with liquid water,[24] and Purcell and Hansen, working with solid paraffin[25]—detected the hydrogen nucleus resonance in bulk matter. Purcell further described the processes and time constants (T1 and T2) by which the resonance would dissipate.[26] This set the stage for the eventual development of MRI 30 years later. Between 1946 and 1976, NMR became a useful laboratory tool for probing molecular structure. Laboratory NMR instruments had small spaces for the sample, usually a small test tube. Use of NMR for larger objects, such as humans, required the development of larger magnets with larger sample spaces. The term *magnetic resonance imaging*, rather than *nuclear magnetic resonance*, is used to allay patient anxiety about a test whose name includes "nuclear."

Basic Physics of Magnetic Resonance Imaging

Why Hydrogen? Many nuclei bear a magnetic moment. Those relevant to biology include phosphorus 31, carbon 13, and sodium 23. However, all MRI systems use the resonance of the hydrogen nucleus for three reasons. First, it is easy to detect the magnetic resonance signal. The hydrogen nucleus has the largest magnetic moment of any nucleus and is therefore the most detectable. Second, the natural abundance of hydrogen is high: 99.99% for hydrogen 1. In contrast, the natural abundance of carbon 13 is 1.1% (98% of carbon is carbon 12, which has no magnetic moment). Third, hydrogen is contained in water, which is in high concentration in the body; in the brain, the concentration of water is approximately 67% by weight.

Creating the Signal. To begin, the sample is immersed in a strong, constant magnetic field. A magnet that creates the field may be one of three designs. First is the electromagnet, similar in principle to a washing machine solenoid. Bloch and colleagues[24] and Purcell and Hansen[25] used these magnets in their original experiments. However, the maximal field strength that can be achieved is limited in practical applications to

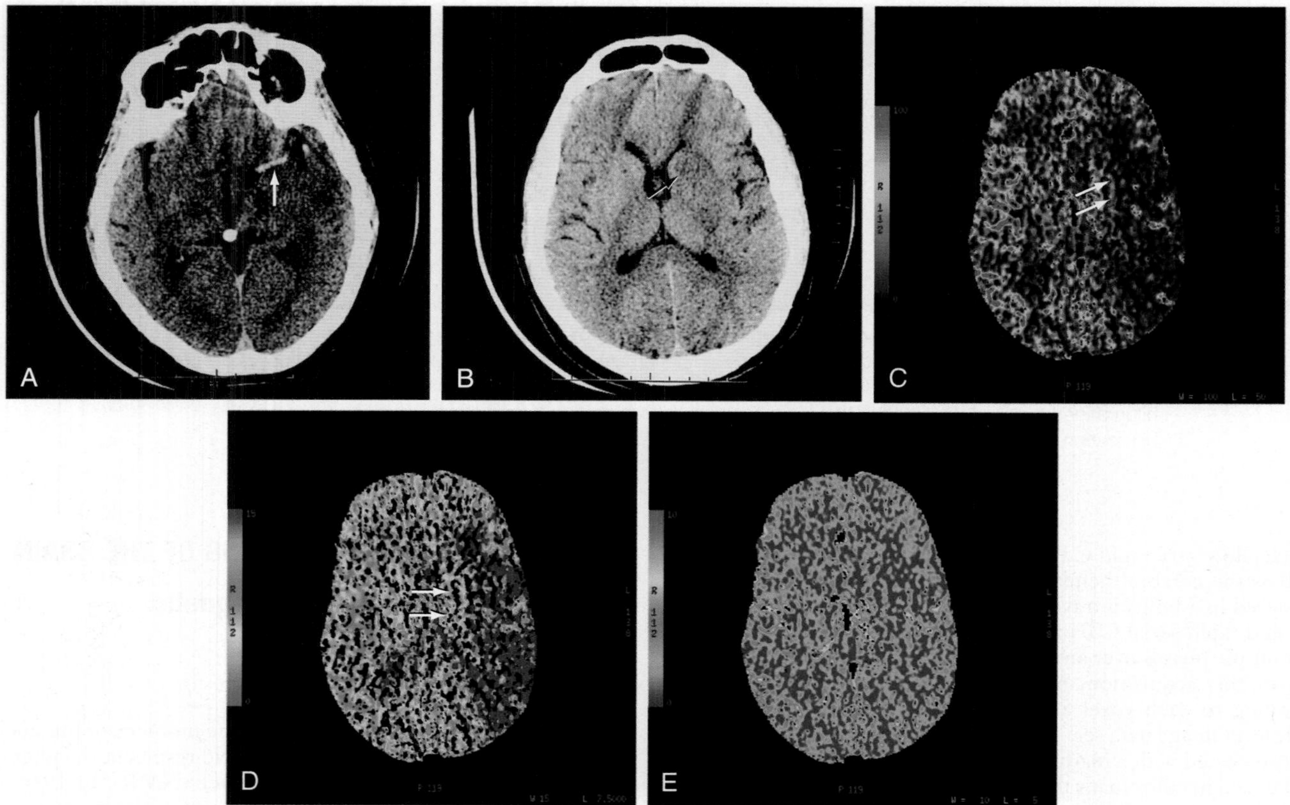

Figure 11-7. Computed tomographic (CT) images of the left middle cerebral artery (MCA). A, Non–contrast-enhanced image illustrates increased density *(arrow)* of the M1 segment of the left MCA—the "dense MCA sign"—in a patient with an acute left hemispheric stroke. **B,** Early ischemic changes exhibit hypodensity within left lenticular nuclei *(arrow).* **C,** Perfusion CT shows a perfusion defect in the left MCA distribution on a map of cerebral blood flow (CBF; *arrows).* **D,** Perfusion CT map of mean transit time (MTT) at the same level illustrates delayed MTT in the left MCA distribution *(arrows).* **E,** Perfusion CT map of cerebral blood volume (CBV) at the same level illustrates a normal perfusion pattern that is symmetrical with the contralateral MCA territory. This pattern of perfusion defects in the CBF and MTT maps and the mismatched normal perfusion on the CBV map represent salvageable ischemic penumbra within the left MCA territory.

approximately 0.4 T (1 T = 10,000 Gy). An electromagnet consumes large amounts of electricity, and its use in MRI has therefore declined.

The second magnet type is a permanent magnet assembled from ferromagnetic material. The field strength of this type of magnet is limited to 0.3 T. Permanent magnets are generally used for small, low-cost open designs. This technology tends to be used in MRI systems that accommodate large (usually >300 lb [136 kg]) or claustrophobic patients.

The third and most widely used magnet type is the superconducting magnet. This design is also similar to that of a washing machine solenoid. However, unlike the solenoid, the superconducting magnet is an alloy that conducts electricity without resistance when kept at temperatures within 15 degrees of absolute zero. An electrical current is slowly driven into the magnet. Once the current reaches the desired level, the ends of the magnet wire are connected, which forces the current to circulate continuously without loss. Magnets of this type can remain at field strength for many years without the addition of electrical current. Field strengths of up to 8 T can be achieved in these magnets, which can accommodate human subjects. Most MRI systems now use superconducting magnets, usually 1.0 to 1.5 T, although an increasing number of hospitals and imaging centers are now using 3-T clinical MRI systems.

When the sample is immersed in the strong, constant magnetic field, the spins in the sample undergo a slight polarization. This polarization, known as M0, increases with increasing magnetic field. At 1.5 T, this polarization is very slight, approximately 1×10^{-5}. This means that just 10 in 1 million nuclei are polarized.[27] The polarization competes with the randomizing effect of the thermal vibration (Fig. 11-9). Only the polarized nuclei contribute to the magnetic resonance signal; hence, MRI systems with higher field strength produce better images.

The classic model created by Bloch helps describe the motion of the spins. Spins that align with the main field precess around the direction of the main field in a manner similar to the spinning of a toy top (Fig. 11-10). The rate of this precession is a product of the intrinsic magnetic moment (the gyromagnetic ratio) of the spin and the strength of the main magnetic field. The rate of precession is known as the *Larmor* (or *resonant*) *frequency.*[28] The spins aligned along B0 are rotated into a plane transverse to the direction of the main magnetic field by the action of a time-varying magnetic field called *B1* (Fig. 11-11). The B1 field is created by the radiofrequency (RF) transmitter and the antenna, known as the *RF coil.* The frequency of the B1 field matches the Larmor frequency of the spins. The B1 field is of brief duration, typically 1 to 10 milliseconds, and is thus referred to as an *RF pulse.* The angle through which the spin is rotated is called the

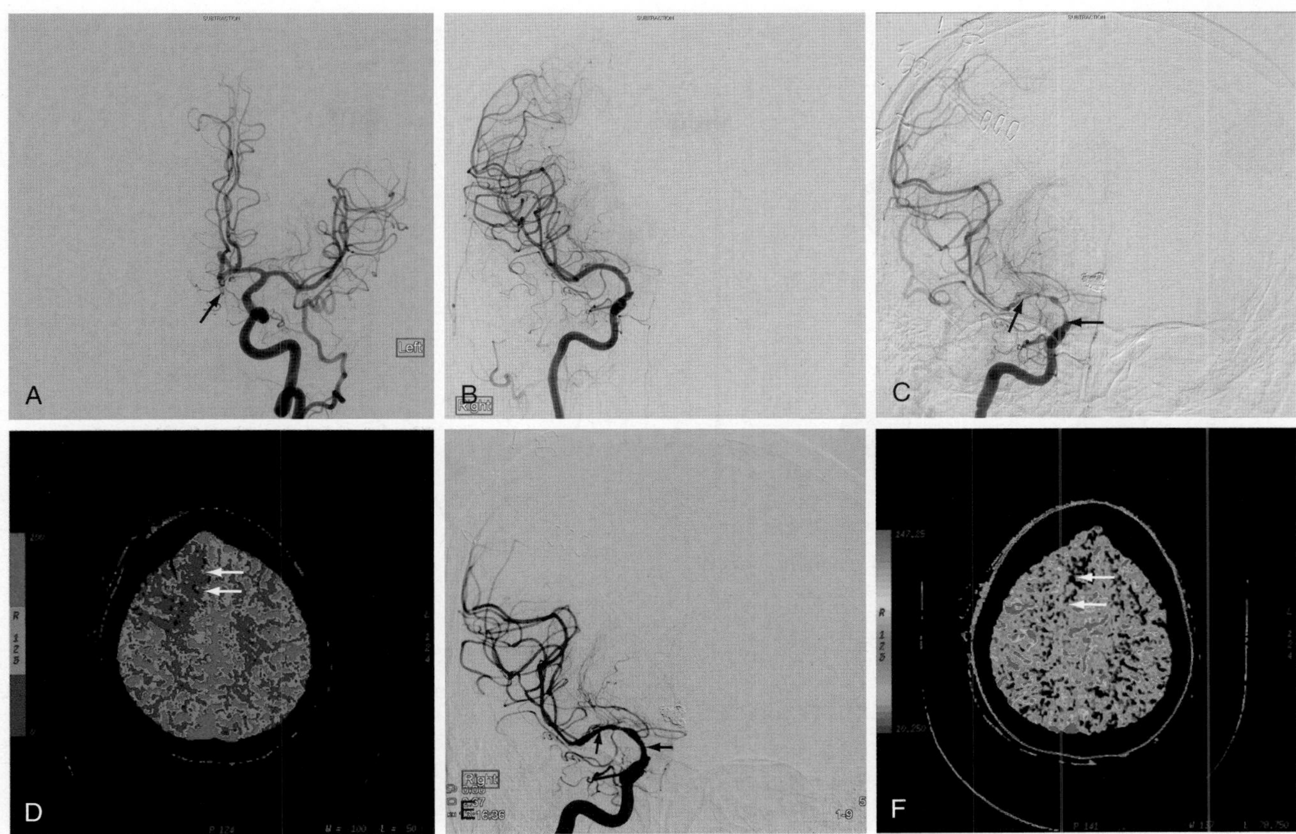

Figure 11-8. A, Anteroposterior angiogram of the left internal carotid (ICA), demonstrating a ruptured aneurysm in the anterior communicating artery *(arrow)*. **B,** Anteroposterior angiogram of the right ICA, illustrating absence of the A1 segment of the right anterior cerebral artery and no vasospasm. **C,** Anteroposterior angiogram of the right ICA 7 days after admission, showing severe vasospasm of the M1 segment of the right middle cerebral artery (MCA; *upward-pointing arrow*) and supraclinoid right ICA *(left-pointing arrow)*. **D,** Perfusion computed tomographic map of cerebral blood flow (CBF), demonstrating vasospasm-induced decreased CBF (*blue* areas) within the right frontal lobe *(arrows)*. **E,** Anteroposterior angiogram of the right ICA after intra-arterial administration of verapamil, showing improved vessel caliber of the MCA *(upward-pointing arrow)* and ICA *(left-pointing arrow)*. **F,** Follow-up perfusion computed tomographic image at the same level as in **D,** illustrating restored CBF in the right anterior frontal lobe on a CBF color map *(arrows)*.

flip angle. The flip angle depends on the duration and amplitude of the RF pulse.

Detecting the Signal. To detect the magnetic resonance signal, an RF coil is placed as shown in Figure 11-12. This may be the same coil used to transmit the B1 pulse. A time-varying magnetic field is created at the coil by the magnetic field of the precessing spins (rotated in the transverse plane) as they pass by the RF coil. Magnetic induction (Faraday's law) causes the RF coil to produce an electrical current, which can then be amplified and detected (Fig. 11-13). An interesting and important disparity should be noted. The amount of power used to produce the RF pulse is in the range of 100 to 20,000 W. The signal that is received from the object is approximately 10^{-12} W. This received signal is no greater than the signals from radio or television stations, among other sources. To prevent interference from these external sources, MRI systems are enclosed in electrically shielded rooms, which are six-sided copper boxes.

Physics: Localizing the Signal. Up to this point, the sample has been polarized and excited and a signal detected, but the location of the spins that created the signal remains unknown. Suppose that two objects are in the magnetic field, both of which create a signal. To force each object to give off a unique signal, the magnetic field can be modified to vary as a function of position along the x-axis (Fig. 11-14). The resonant frequency of the spins is a function only of the magnetic field at that point in space. Thus the spatial origin of the signal can be determined by the frequency of the received signal. In practice, to determine this, a linear gradient is created that adds to or subtracts from the main field as a linear function of offset from the origin. An MRI system has three gradients: x, y, and z. The gradient system serves two purposes in the MRI system. The first is to limit the excitation to one plane or slab (Fig. 11-15). If an RF pulse is transmitted during the time that a gradient is applied, excitation will affect only one slice or slab, the thickness of which depends on the amplitude of the gradient and the bandwidth of the RF pulse. The second purpose is to encode the spatial location of spins to form the magnetic resonance image. In a slice, the two directions of encoding required are frequency and phase. To establish location along the frequency-encoding axis, a gradient is applied during the signal readout time. To encode the orthogonal axis, a gradient is applied somewhere between the time of excitation and reception and is called *phase encoding*. One unique value of phase encoding is applied every time that the readout gradient is applied. Thus the excitation and readout must be repeated to

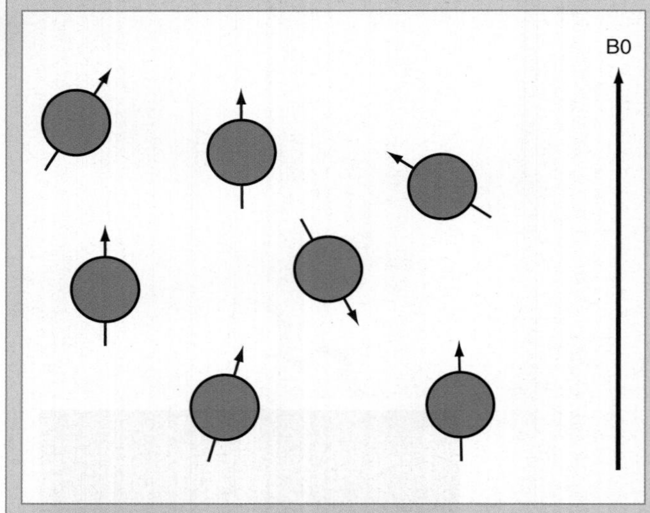

Figure 11-9. Illustration of nuclear spins in the magnetic field B0. The net alignment of spins is along B0. This is the source of M0, or longitudinal magnetization. In reality, the net aligned versus unaligned fraction is about 1/100,000 in a 1.5-T field at body temperature.

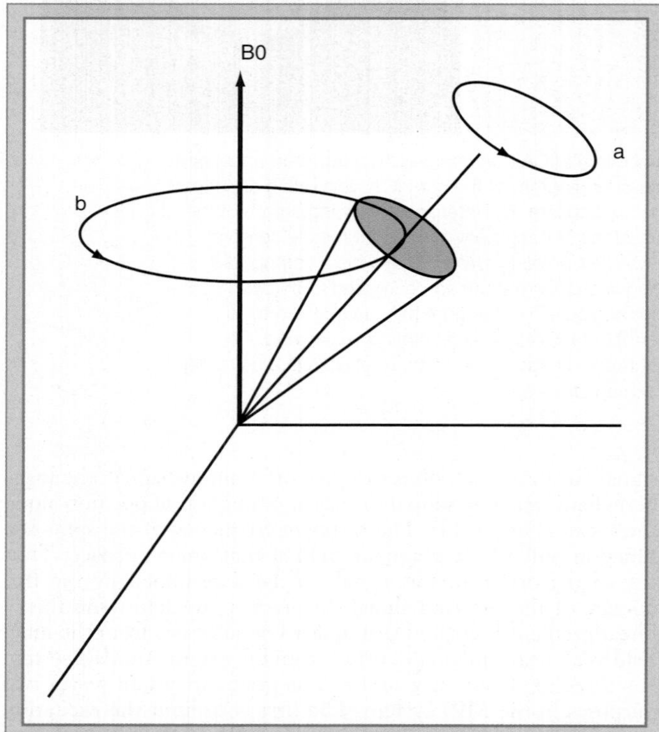

Figure 11-10. "Spinning top" model of nuclear spin. The spin of nucleus a creates the magnetic moment of the nucleus, which causes the spin to precess along circle b around magnetic field B0. The rate of this precession around B0 is called the *Larmor frequency.*

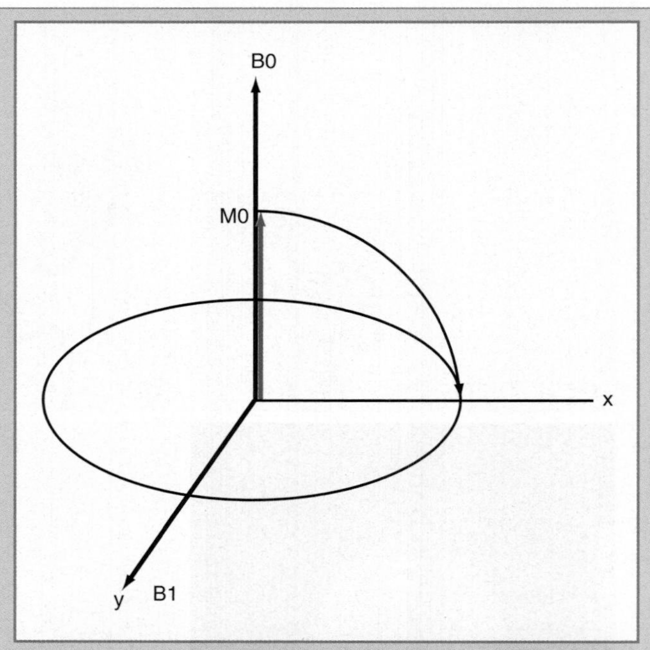

Figure 11-11. The applied (transmitted) radiofrequency magnetic field B1 causes the spin to experience a torque, which twists the M0 magnetization (causes it to nutate) into the transverse plane *xy,* where it is referred to as *Mxy.*

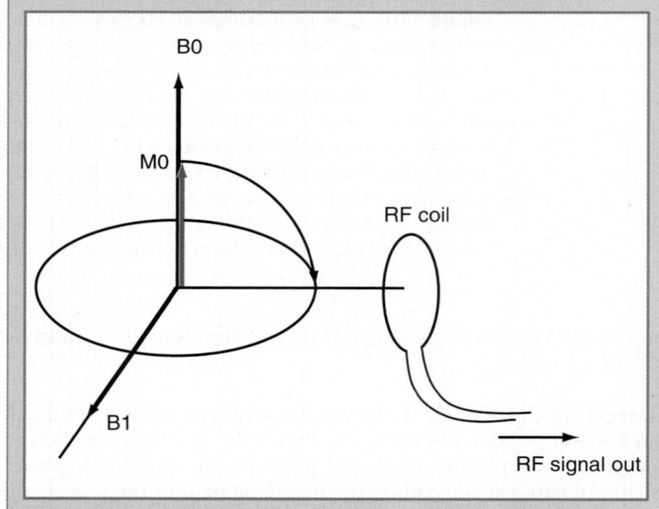

Figure 11-12. The radiofrequency (RF) coil both transmits and receives the signal from the spins in the transverse plane, where B0 and B1 are magnetic fields and M0 is the magnetization.

make an image. The rate at which the excitation is repeated is the repetition time (TR).

The Origin of Image Contrast. The intensity of a voxel in an image arises from three principal factors. The first is the number of protons in the voxel, known as *proton density*. If this were the only image mechanism, MRI would be little more than CT. However, intensity in the voxel also depends on the relaxation rates of the spins. One such rate is the longitudinal relaxation rate: T1 (Fig. 11-16A). After excitation, the magnetization in the slice returns along the axis of the main magnetic field by interaction with other nonmoving hydrogen spins, typically those attached to large molecules. The magnetization returns along B0 as an exponential function of the ratio of T1 and the rate at which the excitation is repeated: TR. The transverse relaxation rate, T2 (Fig. 11-16B), is the rate at which spins that have been excited

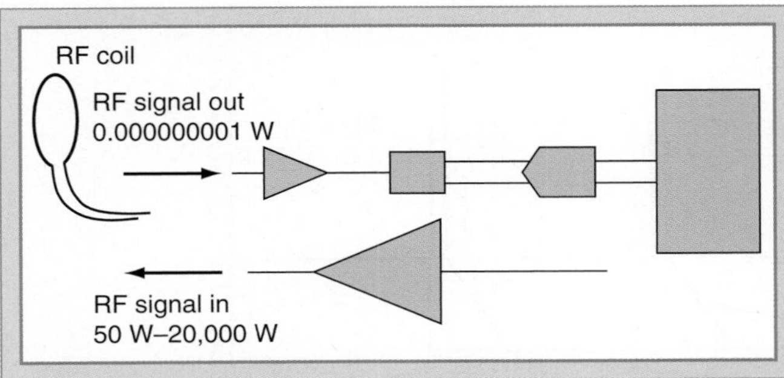

Figure 11-13. Bloch diagram of the transmit-and-receive scheme used in magnetic resonance imaging that illustrates the large disparity between the high radiofrequency (RF) power transmitted into the patient and the tiny RF signal received from the patient.

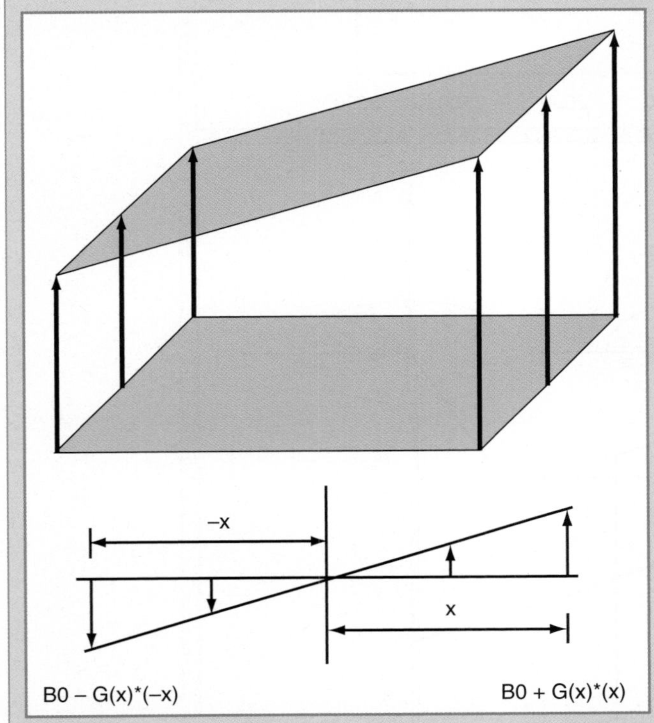

Figure 11-14. Magnetic field gradients alter the strength of the main magnetic field (B0). A single gradient (G) is designed to change the magnetic field along only one direction (along the x, y, or z axis). Three such gradients are required to localize signals in three dimensions.

into the transverse plane lose coherence. Each spin precesses at a rate that is determined by the magnetic field at the location of that spin. Macroscopic and microscopic field gradients, created by differences in the magnetic susceptibility of tissue, cause some of the excited spins to precess faster and some slower. Eventually, the spins are spread out uniformly, which produces no signal in the RF coil used to detect the spins.

Three principal image intensity factors—proton density, T1, and T2—influence the appearance of every voxel on MRI. For example, cortical bone appears hypointense on MRI because the proton density (of mobile spins) is quite low. Lung parenchyma usually appears hypointense because the T2 of lung tissue is so low that the signal is gone before it can be sampled. The long T1

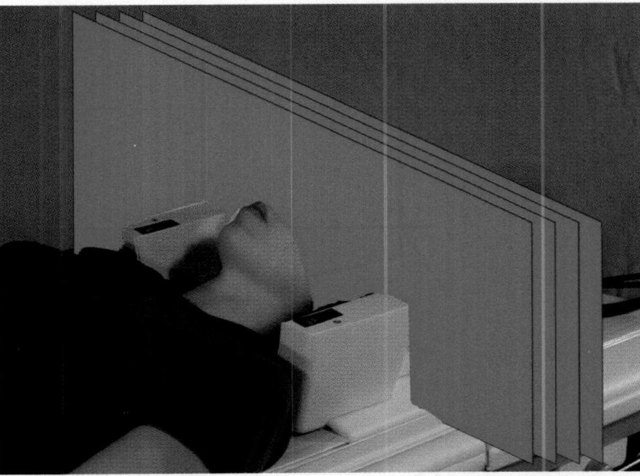

Figure 11-15. Slice selection illustrating a group of four excited axial slices relative to a patient. (Radiofrequency head coil courtesy of Midwest R.F. LLC.)

of liquid water causes CSF to appear hypointense on sequences that use short TR times.

An MRI scan user has a choice of pulse sequence parameters such as echo time (TE) and TR. Maximal contrast between structures of interest may be achieved by the appropriate choice of sequence parameters. Conversely, inappropriate choices may result in failure to detect a lesion. Other endogenous sources of contrast include blood flow (on magnetic resonance angiography [MRA]) and water-macromolecular T1-based interactions (magnetization transfer).

Spin Echo

After the spins have been rotated into the transverse plane by the initial 90-degree RF pulse (Fig. 11-17A), they begin to lose coherence because of the effects of local inhomogeneities (contributed by changes in tissue), inhomogeneities secondary to imperfections in the B0 field, and diffusion of water molecules (Fig. 11-17B). If a second RF pulse is transmitted at twice the amplitude of the first pulse, the relative direction of the spins can be reversed (Fig. 11-17C). Then, at the echo time, the spins will have nearly regained coherence (Fig. 11-17D). The effects of magnetic field inhomogeneities are thus canceled out. One loss, that caused by diffusion, cannot be reversed but is usually negligible in routine imaging. The resulting coherence produces the spin echo as described by Hahn in 1950.[29] If the 180-degree pulse is not used, the signal decreases with increasing echo time; the rate of decrease is referred to as T2*. With the 180-degree pulse included, the decrease is T2, with T2 always being greater than T2*.

The spin echo sequence is the mainstay of routine clinical imaging. By adjusting TE and TR times, the technician can select proton density–weighted images, T1-weighted images, or T2-weighted images (Table 11-1).

Gadolinium Contrast

Enhancement with exogenous contrast material is now a routine part of MRI. The material most widely used is a gadolinium chelate. The gadolinium atom is strongly paramagnetic and acts to shorten the T1 relaxation time of nearby water protons in blood.[30] The agent does not pass the blood-brain barrier; thus it is useful in detecting disruption of the blood-brain barrier by neoplasm, infection, trauma, and infarction. The T1-shortening effect is also used for rapid MRA, which is performed in a fast

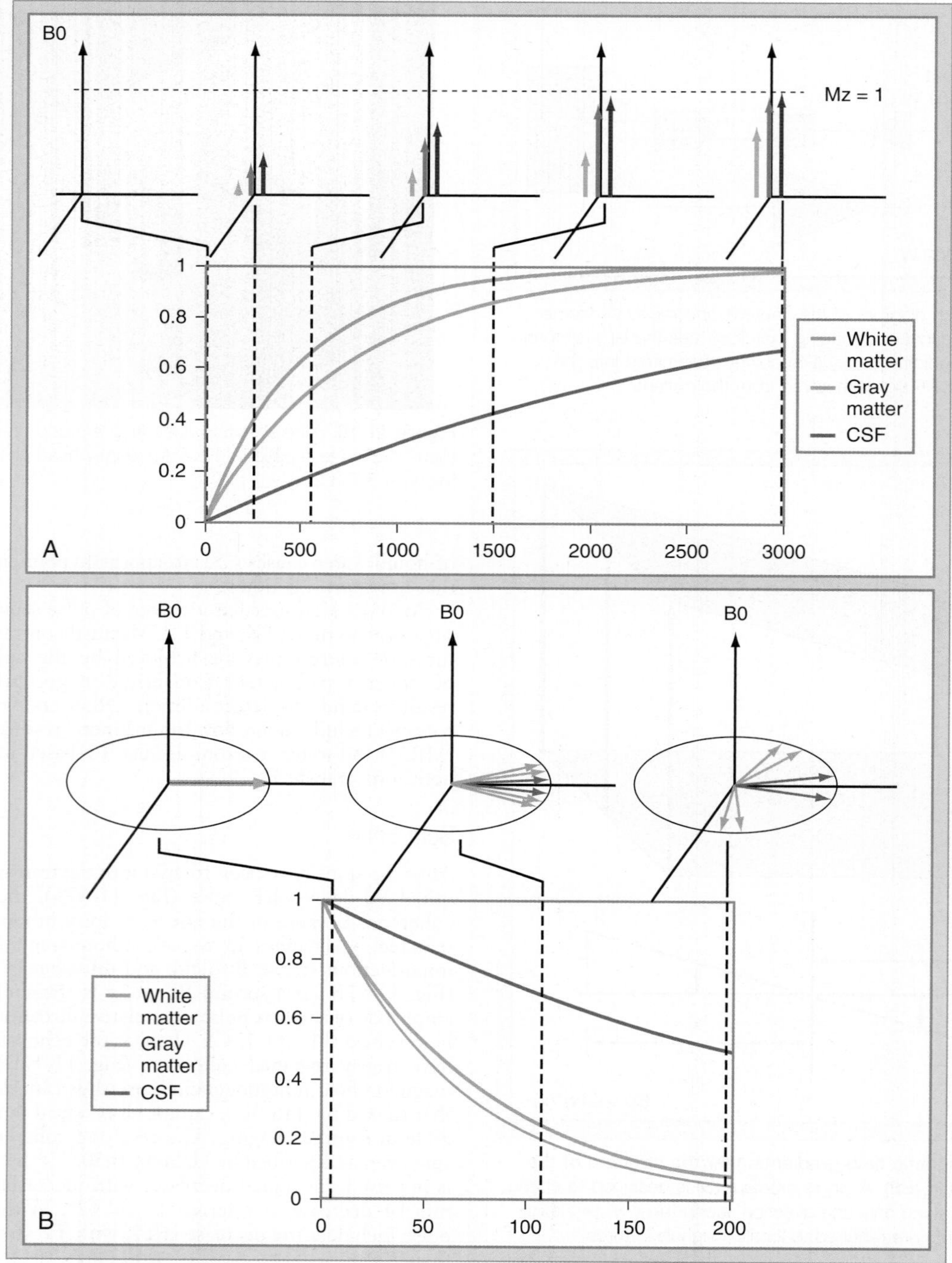

Figure 11-16. **A,** Recovery of longitudinal magnetization (Mz) versus time for three substances with different T1 values. **B,** Decay of Mx versus time for three substances with different T2 values. CSF, cerebrospinal fluid.

scanning protocol after the bolus injection of a contrast agent. In the brain, bolus injection of gadolinium with repeated echo planar imaging (EPI) has been used to image perfusion[31] and the blood volume of tumors.[32]

Fast Spin Echo Imaging

Fast spin echo (FSE) sequences decrease scan time by increasing the efficiency of data collection.[33] The increased efficiency can be used to either decrease scan time or increase the signal-to-noise ratio of the resulting images. Because of improved scan efficiency, FSE sequences are used frequently in radiology, particularly in imaging of the CNS.

To understand this improved efficiency, it is necessary to understand how the data are collected. In a conventional spin echo sequence (Fig. 11-18A), a single line of *k*-space samples (called a *view*) is collected. For images that are not fractional excitation, the number of views is equal to the matrix size in the

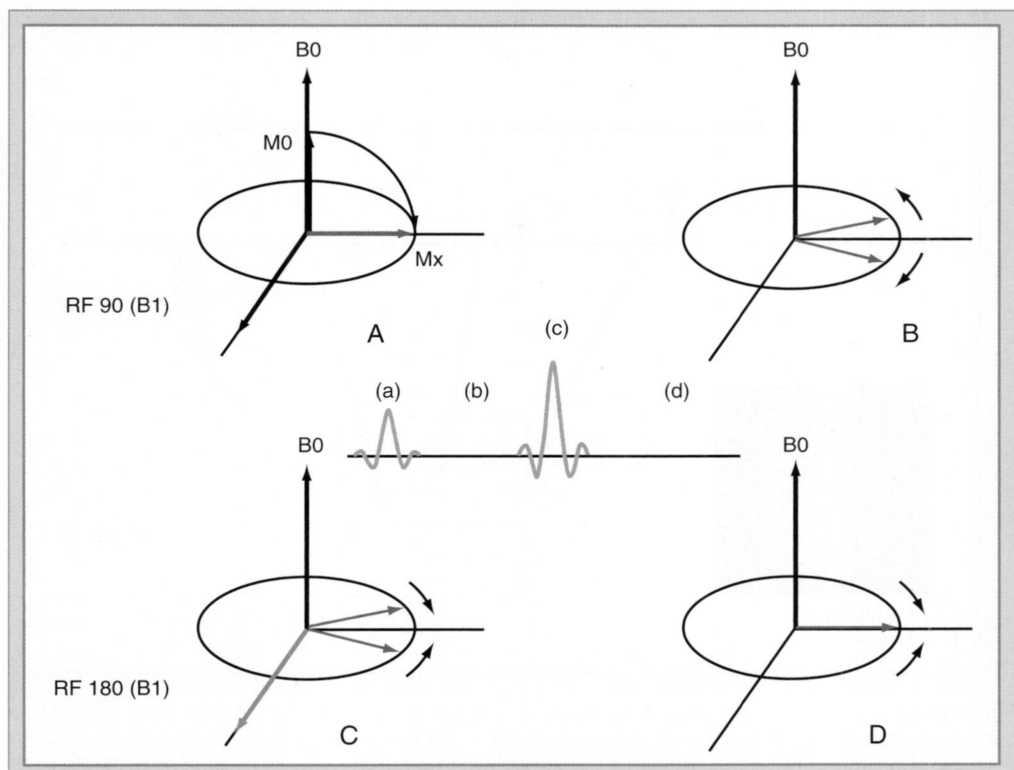

Figure 11-17. The spin echo starts with nutation of longitudinal magnetization (Mz) into the transverse plane **(A).** The magnetization decays over time **(B)** until the radiofrequency (RF) 180-degree pulse **(C)** reverses the direction of the spins, which then reform magnetization M0 at the echo time (**D**).

TABLE 11-1 Weighting of Magnetic Resonance Images

Repetition Time (TR)	Echo Time (TE)	
	Short TE	**Long TE**
Short TR	T1-weighted image	Mixed contrast—do not use
Long TR	Proton density–weighted image	T2-weighted image

phase that encodes image direction. The next view is collected at TR later, when the sequence is repeated. The entire *k*-space matrix must be collected before the images can be reconstructed. The TR is set in accordance with the desired degree of contrast (see Table 11-1). The FSE sequence collects multiple views in each TR (Fig. 11-18B). The number of views collected per TR is known as the *echo train length*. An FSE sequence with an echo train length of 4 has a total scan time that is 25% that of a conventional spin echo sequence with equivalent TR. The echo train length can be equal to the number of views in the sequence. This allows the entire image to be collected in a single TR.

The efficiency of FSE sequences is improved at the expense of image contrast purity because each view is collected at a different echo time (see Fig. 11-18B). The effect is to create image blurring that worsens with increasing echo train length or decreasing tissue T2. The relatively long T2 times of tissues in the neuraxis allow echo train length values of 16 to be used routinely. To image uncooperative patients, single-shot FSE sequences can be used, but with some increase in image blurring.

Inversion Recovery

Image contrast can be further manipulated by transmission of a 180-degree RF pulse before the pulse sequence. The effect of this pulse is to rotate the spins from their orientation along the *z*-axis from positive to negative (Fig. 11-19A). The longitudinal magnetization (Mz) signal regrows from $-z$ to $+z$ at a rate determined by the T1 of the spins. The regrowth is plotted in Figure 11-19B for several tissues. If the 90-degree RF pulse is transmitted at the time at which Mz is 0, the tissue produces no signal. Inversion recovery can be used to increase contrast between structures, such as gray and white matter, or to nullify signals that arise from protons of a known T1. A coronal image scan performed at multiple T1s is shown in Figure 11-20. The round object above the volunteer's head is a jar of mayonnaise. In fluid-attenuated inversion recovery (FLAIR) imaging,[34] this method is used to nullify the CSF signal while preserving signal from edematous tissue. The inversion pulse may be applied to a spin echo or gradient echo sequence.

Gradient Echo

The pulse that rotates Mz into the transverse plane, nominally a 90-degree pulse, does not have to be followed by an 180-degree pulse to produce an echo. In this case, the sequence is referred to as a *gradient echo* because a readout gradient is used to form the echo. When the 180-degree pulse is eliminated, sequence time is saved and TR may be made very short: as little as 6 milliseconds. In this way, the *k*-space can be filled very quickly, and the scan can be completed in a matter of seconds rather than minutes, as is the case with conventional spin echo. At the TRs

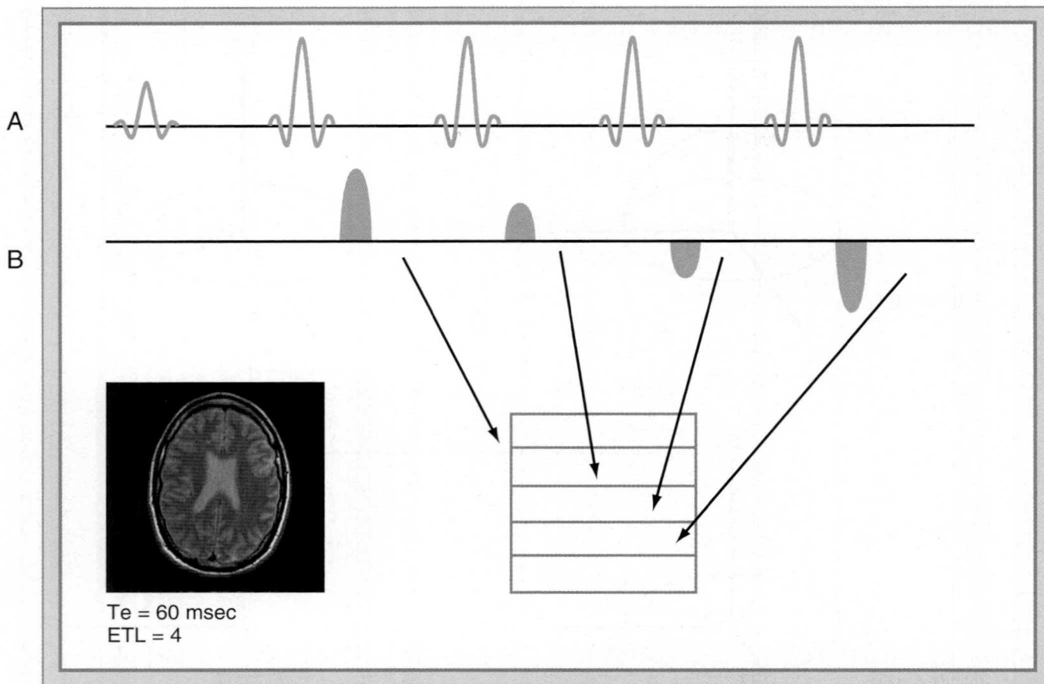

Figure 11-18. In a multiple-echo spin echo sequence (not shown here), a single phase encoding is applied for all four echoes and each echo fills in the same sample line in four separate *k*-space matrices. The sequence must be repeated a number of times equal to the resolution in the phase-encoding direction of the image. In the fast spin echo sequence, a different phase encoding is applied for each echo of the same sequence. In this way, a single *k*-space matrix is filled four times faster. This yields one image in 25% of the time required to complete the sequence. **A,** RF pulses. **B,** Phase encoding gradient waveform. ETL, echo train length; Te, echo time.

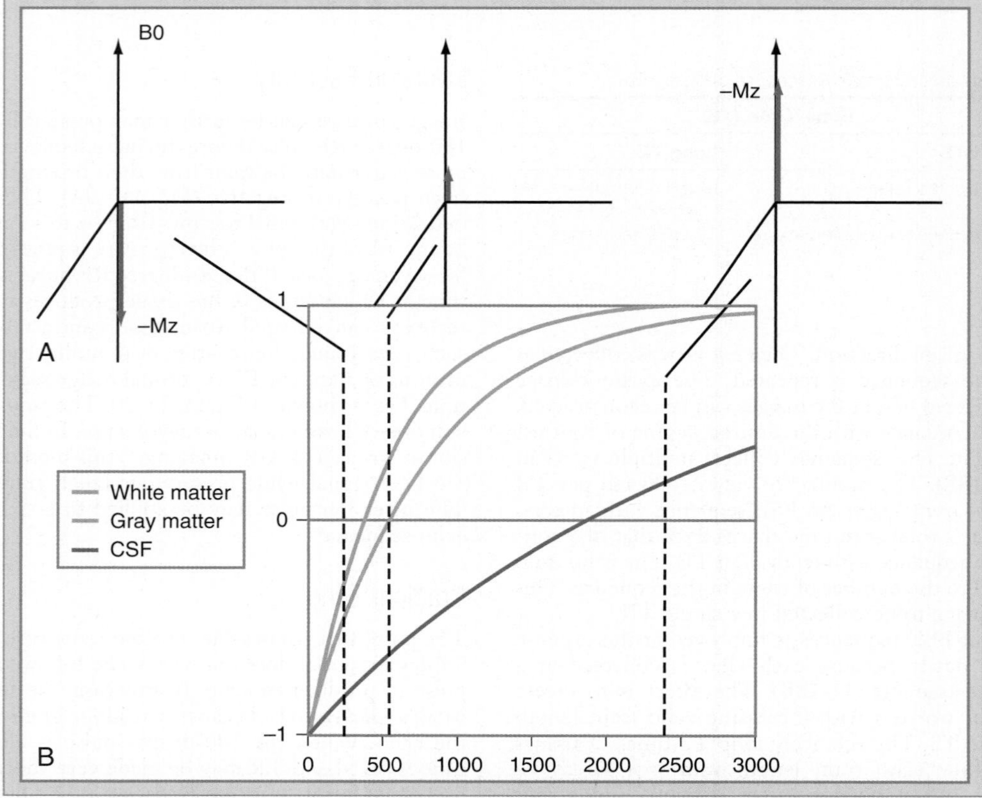

Figure 11-19. Inversion recovery sequence showing both the motion of the spins **(A)** and a plot of longitudinal magnetization (Mz) versus time **(B).** B0 is the magnetic field. CSF, cerebrospinal fluid.

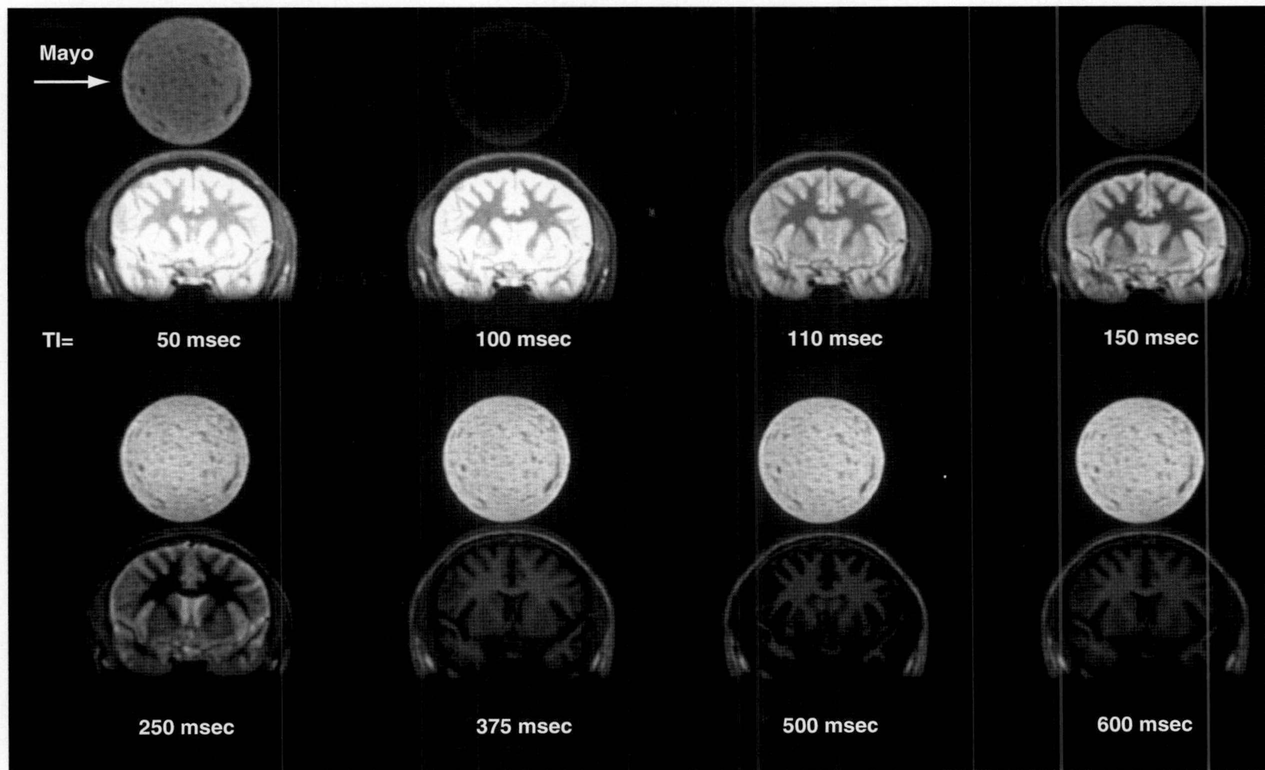

Figure 11-20. Coronal inversion recovery magnetic resonance images of a volunteer and a jar of mayonnaise. The nullifying effect of certain T1 times on various substances is illustrated: T1 of 110 milliseconds nullifies mayonnaise (Mayo), T1 of 150 milliseconds nullifies white matter, and T1 of 375 milliseconds nullifies gray matter.

used in conventional spin echo sequences, 500 to 2000 milliseconds, the magnetic resonance signal is strongest when the first RF pulse is 90 degrees. When the TR time is very short, the peak signal is obtained at a flip angle of less than 90 degrees. The flip angle becomes an important determinant of image contrast in gradient echo sequences. Low flip angles (typically 5 to 20 degrees) result in images that are more T2* weighted, whereas higher flip angles (40 to 90 degrees) result in images that are more T1 weighted.

Of importance is that gradient echo sequences do not yield the purity of contrast of a conventional spin echo sequence and that the T2 weighting in a conventional spin echo is replaced by T2* weighting in gradient echo sequences. The advantages of gradient echo are short scan times, their usefulness in MRA, and the ability to visualize hemosiderin and ferritin. MRA does not entail spin echo because flow is dephased and becomes invisible.

Echo Planar Imaging

The readout gradient used to form the echo in a gradient echo sequence can be repeated to collect additional *k*-space views in a manner similar to that of FSE.[35] Between repetitions of the readout gradient, a small phase-encoding gradient is applied that allows a different view to be collected during the subsequent readout gradient (Fig. 11-21). Only a single excitation is used to collect all the views in *k*-space. The entire image can be collected in approximately 40 milliseconds. This sequence is used in applications that are highly sensitive to even minor patient movements. As with FSE, blurring can be caused by acquisition of views at different echo times but without rephasing of the RF 180-degree pulses. This effect limits the resolution obtainable. Although a matrix of 256 × 256 may be used for an FSE image, EPI is limited to 128 × 128 or, more typically, 64 × 64 over the same field of view. Despite these limitations, EPI is essential for diffusion, perfusion, and functional MRI.

Diffusion-Weighted Imaging

Diffusion of water in the brain depends on the integrity of the cellular membrane and the osmotic balance of the neurons and astrocytes.[36] In ischemic processes, the diffusion of water first decreases because of cellular swelling, and thus the extracellular space decreases. During recovery and into the chronic stage, the loss of cell wall integrity causes the diffusion to increase.

In the discussion of the spin echo, it was noted that the 180-degree pulse could not recover signal lost because of diffusion. If the water molecule moves between the time of the gradient that is applied before the 180-degree pulse and the gradient after the 180-degree pulse, the B0 field is different. The difference in B0 field is caused by the applied gradient and the total motion of the spin in that direction. The spin precesses at a different rate before and after the 180-degree pulse, thereby resulting in an accumulated phase error at the time of readout and a loss of signal. The farther that the spin wanders (in brownian terms) between gradient lobes, the greater the signal loss. Hence, a chronic infarct is hypointense. Conversely, when the cells swell and the spin motion is reduced to less than that of normal tissue, the diffusion loss is reduced to less than that of normal tissue, and the region becomes hyperintense.

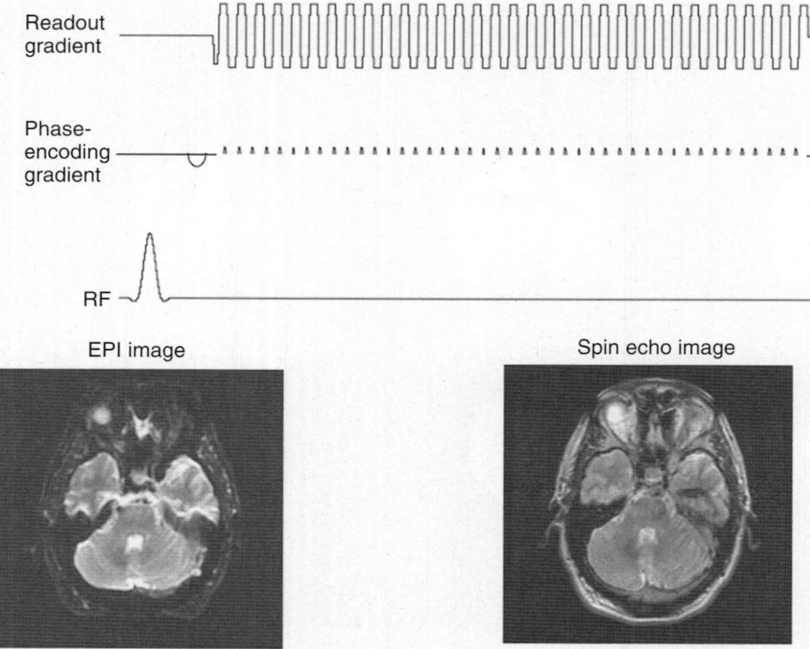

Figure 11-21. Sequence diagram and image from echo planar imaging (EPI). The readout gradient repeatedly reverses, which fills the *k*-space matrix in a single excitation. EPI is similar in concept to fast spin echo imaging, except for the repeated 180-degree radiofrequency pulses. In the absence of these pulses in EPI, susceptibility artifacts are present in areas adjacent to bone and air.

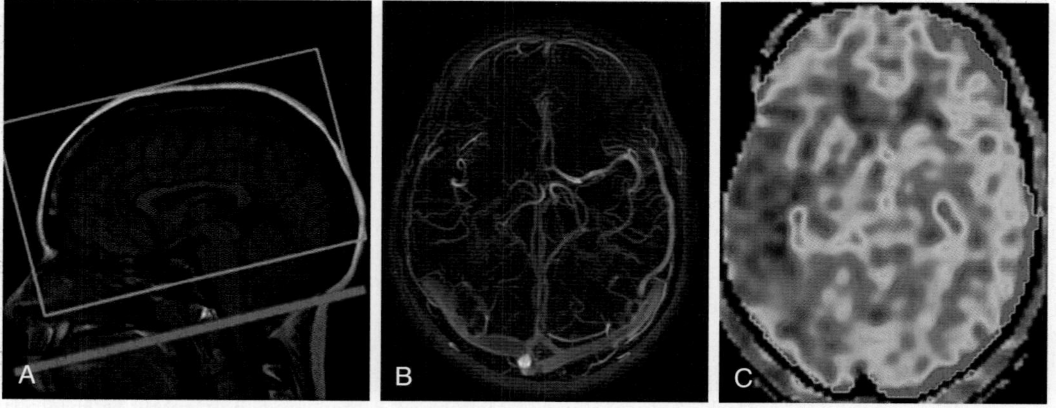

Figure 11-22. Arterial spin labeling: occluded artery. A, The *red bar* illustrates the tagging slice used to presaturate inflowing spins. **B,** Magnetic resonance angiogram of a patient with an occluded right middle cerebral artery. **C,** Perfusion image from the same patient as in **B,** showing the expected hypoperfusion (in *blue*) in the right hemisphere.

Perfusion-Weighted Imaging

There are two magnetic resonance–based approaches to measuring tissue perfusion.[37] The first method for imaging tissue perfusion is arterial spin labeling.

In the arterial spin labeling method, perfusion is derived from the change of image intensity in the parenchyma that is caused by a spatial presaturation of the blood in the carotid arteries. To generate perfusion images, an axially oriented slice in the neck is excited, followed by rapid imaging of axial slices (usually in a 3D volume) in the brain, as shown in Figure 11-22A. The slice excitation in the neck inverts (tags) the magnetization of the spins in the carotid vessels. When these spins reach the brain, they exchange magnetization with unexcited spins by perfusion and lower the image intensity in voxels in proportion to the extent of perfusion-based exchange. In this way, the perfusion effect can be directly imaged. The effect is small, and to eliminate the signal from the nonmoving spins, the scan in the brain is repeated without the tagging excitation.

Quantitative perfusion is complicated by two important problems.[38] The first is that the apparent diffusion changes if the transit time of the inverted spins is significantly different from normal. These transit times can be greater than normal in elderly patients and less than the adult normal in children. The second complicating feature is an implicit assumption that the partition coefficient of the perfusing spins between the blood and

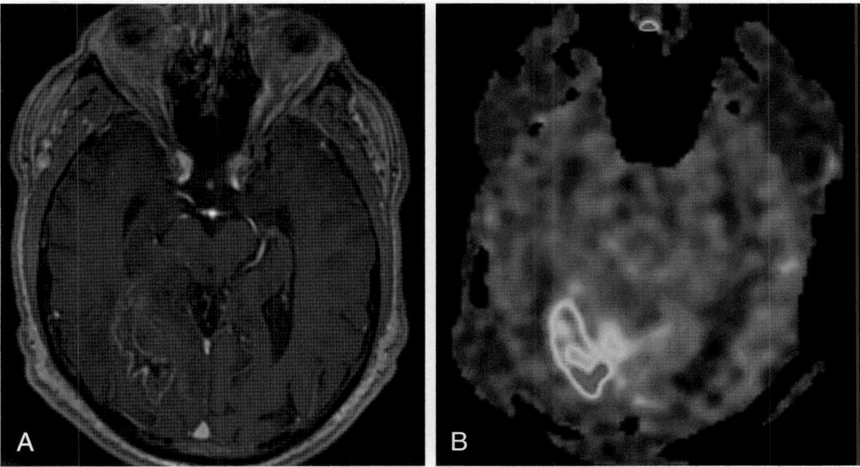

Figure 11-23. Arterial spin labeling: brain tumor. A. T1 image demonstrating contrast enhancement of the tumor. **B**. Perfusion imaging demonstrating hyperperfusion in the lesion, shown in *orange* and *red*.

parenchyma is constant. The partition coefficient is slightly different between gray and white matter. It also can change with hematocrit levels.

Typically, arterial spin labeling is used to detect regions of hypoperfusion or hyperperfusion in the brain.[39,40] The most frequent hypoperfusion effect occurs in cases of ischemic stroke or arterial occlusion. An MRA of an occlusion of the right middle cerebral artery is shown in Figure 11-22B. The arterial spin labeling image in Figure 11-22C demonstrates the resultant hypoperfusion in the right hemisphere. Hyperperfusion is most commonly observed in tumors that demonstrate angiogenic activity, as shown in Figure 11-23.[41]

The second method of perfusion-weighted imaging is by bolus injection of contrast material while EPI is repeatedly performed. Time course images from EPI are then fitted to a model of the response of the tissue to the presence of the contrast agent, and an image of perfusion is made.[41] This method, also known as a *dynamic susceptibility contrast method,* requires a rapid intravenous bolus injection of gadolinium contrast material at a rate of 4 to 5 mL/sec, usually through an 18-gauge intravenous catheter, followed by injection of normal saline.

The dynamic susceptibility contrast method is used most commonly to evaluate intracranial neoplasms. It can also be used to distinguish recurrent neoplasm from radiation necrosis in patients who underwent radiation therapy for primary brain tumors.[42]

Spectroscopy

The resonant frequency of a spin is determined not only by the B0 magnetic field and its associated imperfections but also by the molecule of which the nucleus is a part. The effect is slight but not negligible. This phenomenon is known as *chemical shift;* that is, the chemical microenvironment of a given nucleus results in a slight change in the resonance frequency of the nucleus from that expected in its pure state. The difference between the resonant frequencies of the protons in water and the hydrogen atoms in the methylene groups in lipid is about 3.5 ppm. This translates to a difference of about 220 Hz for operation at 1.5 T. Between the water proton and fat proton resonances are resonances of other moieties of interest in the brain. These include myoinositol, a sugar phosphate; choline, a key indicator of membrane turnover; creatine and phosphocreatine, part of the energy pool; glutamate and glutamine, the primary excitatory neurotransmitter and its astrocyte-recycled counterpart; *N*-acetyl aspartate, a key indicator of neuronal health; and lactate, an indicator of a shift to anaerobic metabolism. A spectrum of the resonances of the protons in these compounds is shown in Figure 11-24A. These resonances are included in every MRI of the brain. However, the concentration of each is lower than that of water by a factor of 5000 to 10,000. Detecting the resonances of the metabolites thus requires much larger voxels for spectroscopy (2 cm^3) than for MRI (1 mm^3).

Two principal methods are used to collect spectroscopic data. In the first, single-voxel spectroscopy, a voxel is selected from three successive RF pulses, and then the signal from the entire voxel is read out. In the second, chemical shift imaging, a larger volume or slice with one or more RF pulses is selected. Phase-encoding gradients are then applied in one to three directions to yield 2D or 3D spectroscopy data sets. Reconstruction allows the selected region to be subdivided into separate voxels. An individual spectrum can then be extracted from a voxel, or a resonance may be selected and an image made of that resonance. Such 2D and 3D data sets can be postprocessed to generate color maps of metabolite distributions within the volume of brain evaluated with spectroscopy (Fig. 11-24B).

Spectroscopic data can be collected for several different substances present in the body, including phosphorus, carbon, and sodium. Exogenous substances that can be detected in the body include fluorine and lithium, both of which are found in psychoactive drugs. However, proton (hydrogen) spectroscopy is the most readily commercially available because of the high abundance of hydrogen, in the form of water and other hydrogen-containing molecules, in comparison with other substances. Spectroscopy with substances other than hydrogen also requires additional hardware and software to allow what is known as *multinuclear spectroscopy*. In the MRI literature that describes human imaging, the literature volume is greatest for proton spectroscopy.

Clinical proton magnetic resonance spectroscopy (MRS) has been commercially available for more than a decade. Nevertheless, MRS remains somewhat limited in use, available only in select academic medical centers and some large community hospitals, because of the level of complexity in acquisition and postprocessing of data. However, in centers with active spectroscopy programs, clinical MRS can add value in the diagnosis, follow-up, and thus management of various neurological diseases, including epilepsy, neoplasms, demyelinating disorders, metabolic diseases, and ischemic diseases.[43,44] The clinical applications of proton

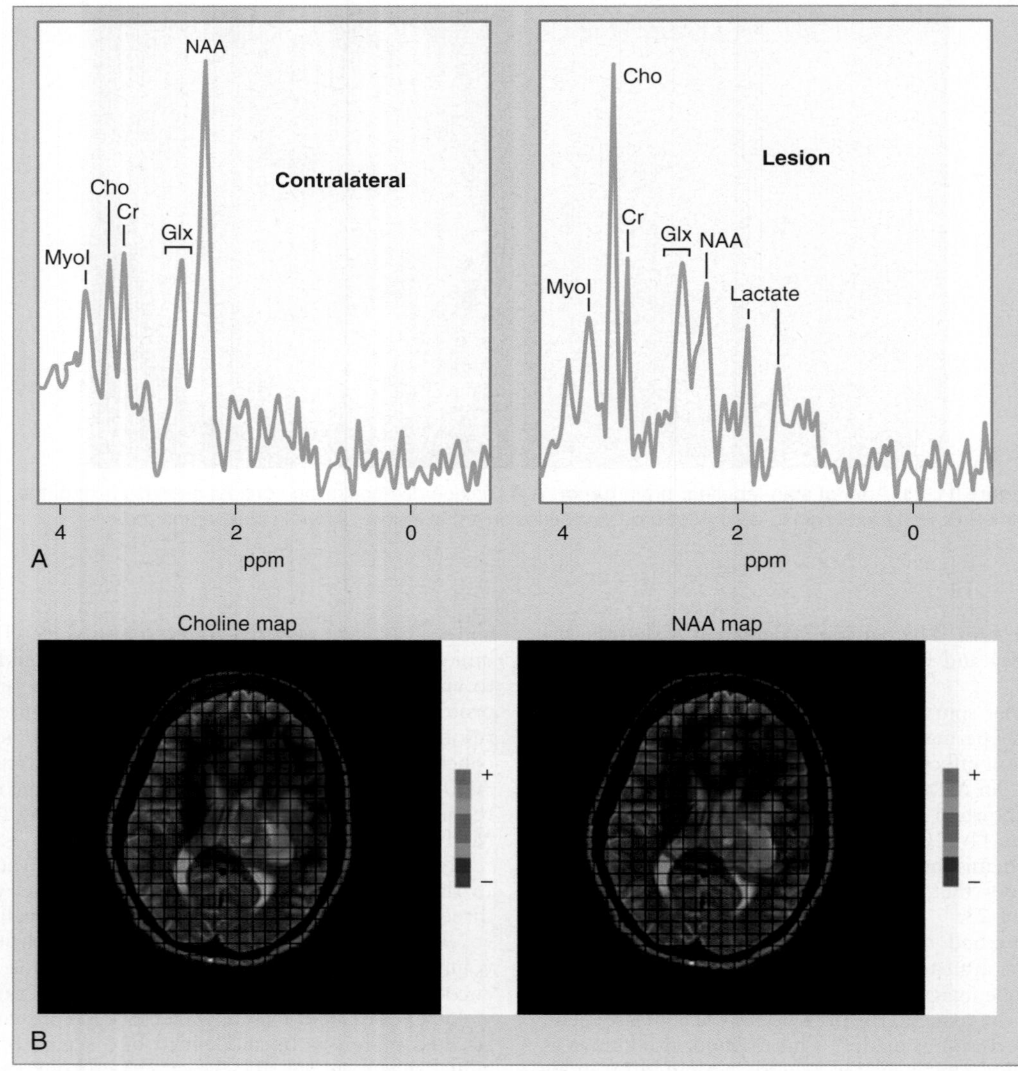

Figure 11-24. Magnetic resonance spectroscopy. A, Spectra extracted from a data set in hydrogen 1 chemical shift imaging. In the spectrum labeled *lesion,* choline (Cho) resonance is increased and *N*-acetyl aspartate (NAA) resonance is decreased. The spectra from the contralateral hemisphere show a normal pattern. Cr, creatine; Glx, glutamate and glutamine; Myo, myoinositol. **B,** Metabolite images made from the same data set used in **A.** The increased concentration of choline is seen in the lesion as the *red area.*

spectroscopy to neoplasms, stroke, and epilepsy are discussed later in this chapter.

Functional Magnetic Resonance Imaging

Functional MRI is used to image the change in the ratio of oxyhemoglobin to deoxyhemoglobin in cerebral blood in response to a stimulus.[45] Changes in the ratio within activated cortical structures are indicative of changes in the oxygen extraction fraction.[46] These changes are thought to occur in response to cortical function and the resulting upregulation of local metabolism. The change in the ratio of oxyhemoglobin to deoxyhemoglobin alters the magnetic susceptibility of the blood because deoxyhemoglobin is less paramagnetic than oxyhemoglobin. This difference is manifested as a change in T2* in activated tissue.

The effect is slight; at 1.5-T the change in image intensity is less than 6%. To prevent interference from patient motion, the data are collected with EPI techniques. Images are repeatedly acquired at the same location over the course of the application of a stimulus pattern. With the a priori knowledge of the stimulus pattern and its cross-correlation with the time course intensity data, a functional image may be made (Fig. 11-25).

Diffusion Tensor Imaging

Diffusion tensor imaging (DTI) has become a valuable presurgical planning tool because it allows the direct visualization of white matter bundles in the brain.[47] DTI exploits the spatially nonuniform microscopic motion of water in the axons to create images of the white matter tracts in brain and spinal cord.[48,49] Water molecules in volume, as in a ventricle, undergo unrestricted brownian motion, which over time is equal in all directions (isotropic). In axons, this diffusion occurs preferentially along the long dimension of the axon. Diffusion perpendicular to that long dimension is restricted and therefore reduced because the water cannot freely diffuse across the cell wall. To measure the magnitude and direction of this anisotropic diffusion, a diffusion imaging sequence is repeated with multiple combinations

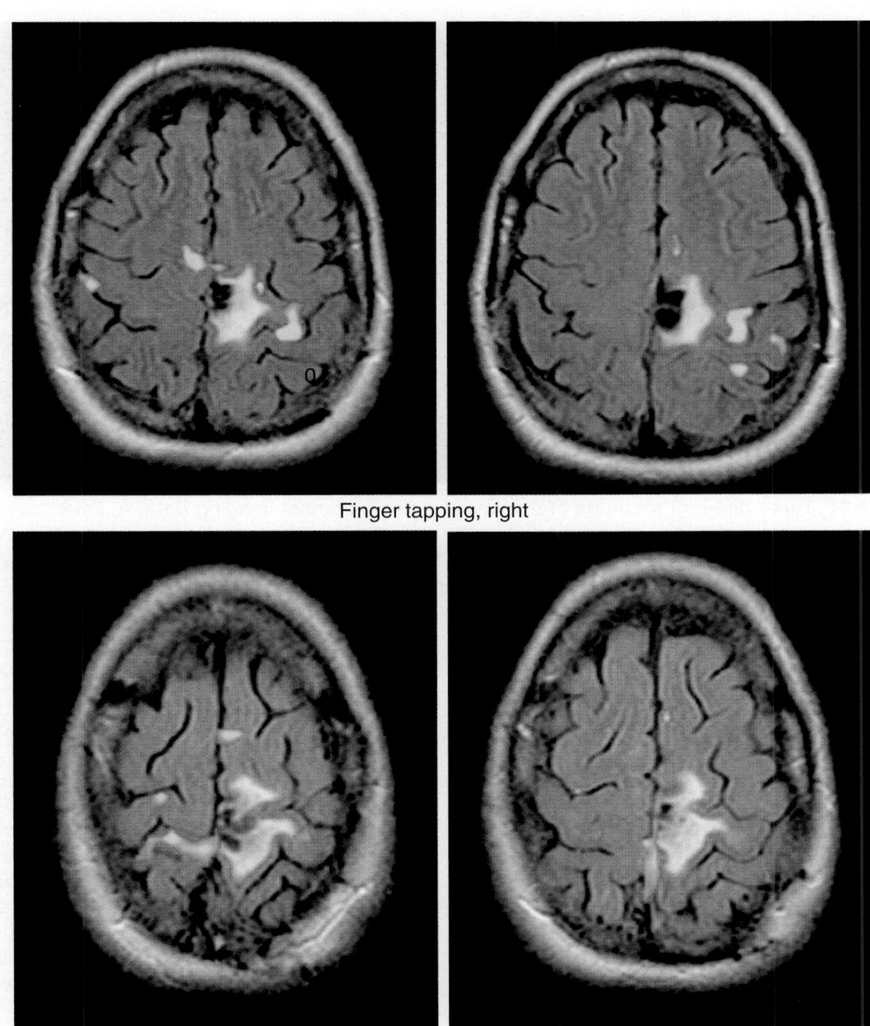

Figure 11-25. Functional magnetic resonance images of a lesion near the left motor cortex. The functional data overlie each fluid-attenuated inversion recovery image.

of diffusion gradients along the three gradient directions. The values of the combinations each form a vector in three dimensions and are chosen to create a geodesic spheroid in space. In this way, the magnitude and direction of diffusion can be determined for every voxel in the acquired diffusion image. This effect is illustrated in Figure 11-26, in which the color of the image is a function of the anisotropic magnitude and direction of the diffusion in the brain. The diffusion in the lateral ventricle is isotropic and demonstrates no color in the image. Diffusion with anisotropy directed in the left-to-right direction is color-coded red and shown in the corpus callosum. Diffusion anisotropy in the anterior-posterior direction is color-coded green.

Diffusion Tensor Imaging Display. There are three principal methods of displaying DTI data. The first and simplest is a fractional anisotropy image, in which the image intensity (in gray scale or false color) corresponds to the magnitude of the anisotropy in that voxel (Fig. 11-27A). A value of zero corresponds to isotropic diffusion, as is observed in the ventricles. A value of 1 indicates that all diffusion is oriented in one direction. This is not seen in vivo because there is always some transverse diffusion, even in the most densely packed white matter bundles.

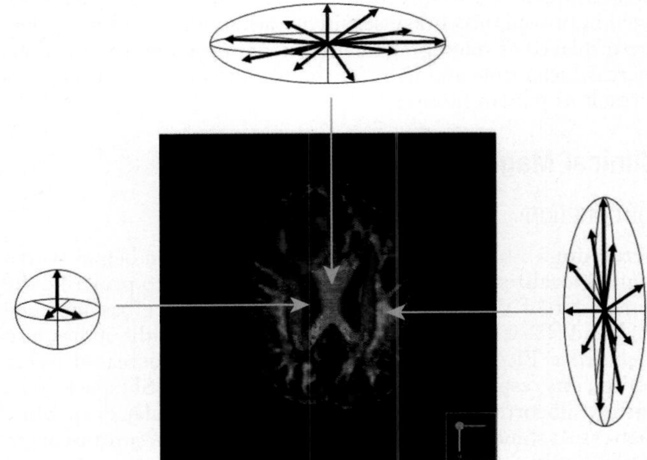

Figure 11-26. Diffusion tensor imaging with colors corresponding to the direction of diffusion anisotropy. Drawings around the image illustrate the preferential directions of diffusion, which are the basis of the anisotropy.

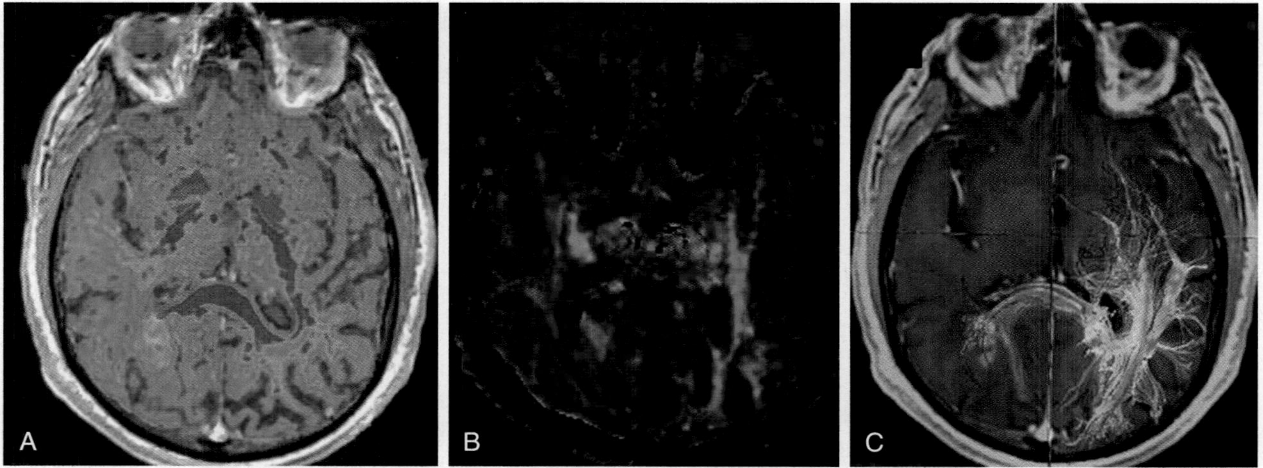

Figure 11-27. Three different methods of displaying diffusion tensor imaging data. A, False color image of anisotropy merged with the corresponding T1 image slice. *Red* represents greater anisotropy but does not indicate direction. **B,** Color eigenvector image in which the color indicates the direction of anisotropy and thus the direction of the white matter bundle. **C,** A tractographic image overlying the postcontrast image, illustrating the destruction of the white matter bundles near the right trigone.

The second method of display is to color-code the anisotropy for the coordinate axes *x*, *y*, and *z*. This creates a visually appealing and intuitive image, as shown in Figure 11-27B. This type of display does not show individual fiber bundles; it shows only the direction of the anisotropy in a given voxel.

The third method of display is tractography, wherein a 3D image of fiber bundles is created (Figure 11-27C). The volume image can be reformatted to allow the viewer to trace the bundle through the brain. Images in Figure 11-27 were obtained from a patient with a dense homonymous hemianopsia and show the destruction of white matter tracts by a neoplastic lesion.

Limitations of Diffusion Tensor Imaging. DTI is based on an EPI sequence. The EPI sequence is acutely susceptible to magnetic field inhomogeneity, which causes spatial distortions and image intensity dropouts. This effect is most severe near the inferior surfaces of the cortex and the spinal cord.[50]

The diffusion tensor weighting consists of at least 6 and sometimes as many as 256 directions of sensitization. More directions yield improved directional sensitivity, which is helpful if the data are displayed as tractographic images. However, more directions increase scan time and increase the likelihood of compromise as a result of patient motion.

Clinical Magnetic Resonance Imaging

Introduction

Screening. The usual screening MRI of the brain begins with a sagittal localizer of the brain, which is then used to prescribe the remainder of the study. Typically, the remainder has included T1- and T2-weighted axial images; more recently, it has also included a FLAIR sequence, which results in increased lesion conspicuity, especially in the areas adjacent to CSF spaces (i.e., cortex, subcortical white matter, and periventricular deep white matter). At some centers, a gadolinium intravenous contrast agent is given routinely as a part of a screening examination. At other centers, gadolinium is administered at the neuroradiologist's discretion. The contrast-enhanced sequence usually includes an axial or coronal T1-weighted image, or both. Sagittal contrast-enhanced images can also be added as needed.

In general, screening MRI of the brain includes the entire brain, orbits, and maxillofacial and skull base regions, including the craniocervical junction. Variable slice thickness, planes, and slice intervals are used. Usually, axial and coronal images are obtained as 5-mm-thick slices, with or without an interslice gap of 1 to 2 mm. Sagittal images are generally 4 to 5 mm in thickness, with a 1- to 2-mm interslice gap. Contrast-enhanced images are almost always T1 weighted because the gadolinium contrast material's enhancement characteristics (T1-shortening effect) are best observed on T1-weighted images, although its effects may also be observed and quantified on T2-weighted images.

Tailored Magnetic Resonance Imaging. There are many different ways to perform a brain MRI examination. For patients in whom clinical suspicion of disease is high, a more tailored examination instead of a screening study should be performed to increase the likelihood of detecting relevant and clinically significant abnormalities. For example, in a patient with a suspected meningioma that involves the cavernous sinus, a more tailored study that includes thin 3-mm contiguous T1-weighted coronal images before and after administration of contrast material may better define extension of the tumor in relation to the optic chiasm, pituitary infundibulum, Meckel's cave, and orbital apex. Before a tailored study, close communication between the neuroradiologist and the neurosurgeon is necessary.

Neoplasms

Gliomas. Gliomas are the most common primary brain neoplasms in both adults and children and represent approximately half to two thirds, respectively, of all brain tumors encountered in these populations. Gliomas are usually categorized into four distinct histologic subgroups: astrocytomas, oligodendrogliomas, ependymomas, and choroid plexus tumors, which include the more common papillomas and rare carcinomas and xanthogranulomas.[51,52]

The MRI appearances of gliomas are quite varied, but in some cases, these neoplasms can have very distinct appearances and locations that enable a correct preoperative radiologic diagnosis. In other cases, the MRI appearance is not specific, and a differential diagnosis is necessary preoperatively. MRI appearances can

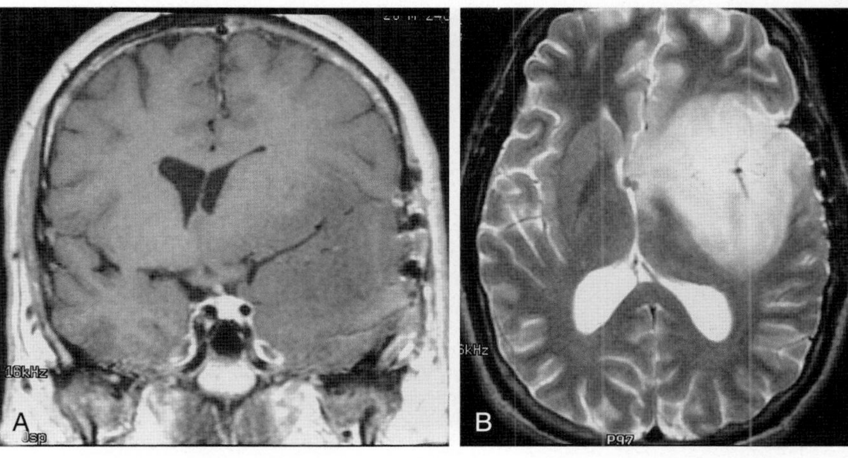

Figure 11-28. Astrocytoma. A, Spin echo, T1-weighted, contrast-enhanced coronal image demonstrating a low-grade astrocytoma as a hypointense mass in the left temporal and inferior frontal lobes that is causing superior displacement of the M1 segment of the left middle cerebral artery. **B,** Fast spin echo, T2-weighted axial image, demonstrating that the lesion involves the left basal ganglia and insula, with a mild midline shift to the right. It is homogeneously hyperintense.

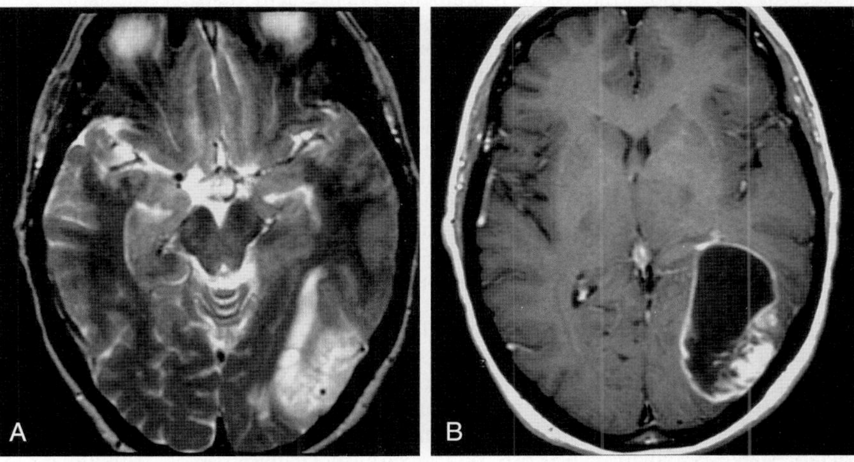

Figure 11-29. Glioblastoma multiforme. A, Fast spin echo, T2-weighted axial image demonstrating a heterogeneously hyperintense mass in the left temporal and occipital lobes. **B,** Spin echo, T1-weighted, contrast-enhanced image demonstrating a large cystic anterior component with thin peripheral enhancement and a heterogeneously enhancing solid component along the posterolateral aspect of the mass.

also vary according to the neoplasm's histologic grade: lower grade tumors usually exhibit little or no peritumoral vasogenic edema, whereas higher grade tumors demonstrate prominent vasogenic edema in association with a local/regional mass effect or herniation, or both.[53,54] However, the sensitivity and specificity of MRI in assessing the degree of histologic anaplasia of a given neoplasm are limited.

Astrocytomas represent the largest subgroup of gliomas (about 20% to 30% of all gliomas). The histologic subtypes of astrocytomas (e.g., fibrillary, protoplasmic, or gemistocytic) cannot be distinguished on MRI. However, certain subtypes—such as the cystic pilocytic astrocytomas typically found in the cerebellum in children and the subependymal giant cell astrocytomas in patients with tuberous sclerosis—may be diagnosed preoperatively on MRI because of their typical appearance, location, and clinical features. Astrocytomas are usually hypointense in relation to normal brain tissue (cortex and white matter) on T1-weighted images and mildly to significantly hyperintense in relation to normal brain on T2-weighted and FLAIR images. In general, low-grade astrocytomas are usually well circumscribed and exhibit no or minimal peritumoral edema, whereas the higher grade anaplastic or glioblastoma multiforme varieties are usually more infiltrative in appearance, have less well defined borders, and are associated with significant surrounding edema. Low-grade tumors are generally homogeneous in signal characteristics on both T1- and T2-weighted images, whereas higher grade tumors are more likely to be heterogeneous; this reflects the histologic heterogeneity associated with the cystic and necrotic changes typically found in these tumors (Figs. 11-28 and 11-29). In rare cases, certain astrocytomas demonstrate signal intensity characteristics that are similar or identical to those of CSF on T1- and T2-weighted images.[42,43] Some of these tumors are in fact predominantly cystic in composition, which explains their signal characteristics, but some are solid neoplasms whose parenchymal composition and organization (e.g., microcysts) produce signals that mimic CSF signals on MRI. Therefore, with MRI, unlike CT, lesions that appear to have the same signal as that of CSF may not be cystic.

Brainstem gliomas, which are usually of a fibrillary histologic type and more common in children, appear as poorly defined masses within the brainstem with diffuse enlargement. They frequently demonstrate exophytic growth with partial or complete circumferential encasement of the basilar artery (Fig. 11-30).[55,56] Gliomatosis cerebri, in which the neoplasm is diffusely infiltrating without a discrete mass, is another astrocytoma subtype. Many affected patients have nonfocal neurological findings, such as headache, decline in mental status, or changes in personality; on MRI, one or both cerebral hemispheres are extensively involved, with diffusely abnormal T2 hyperintensity involving the subcortical and deep white matter.

Enhancement of astrocytomas on gadolinium-enhanced T1-weighted images can be quite variable. In general, higher

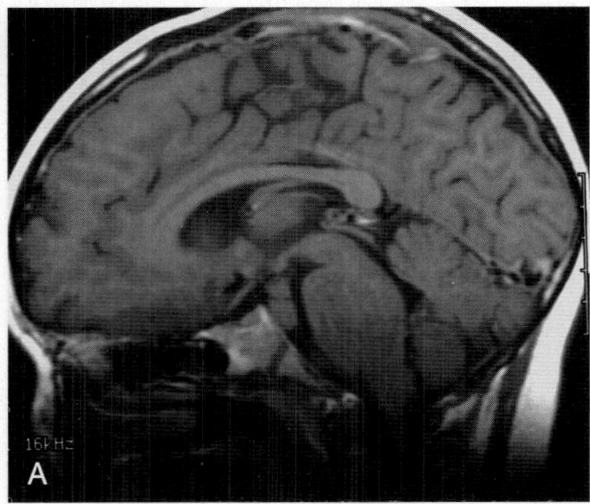
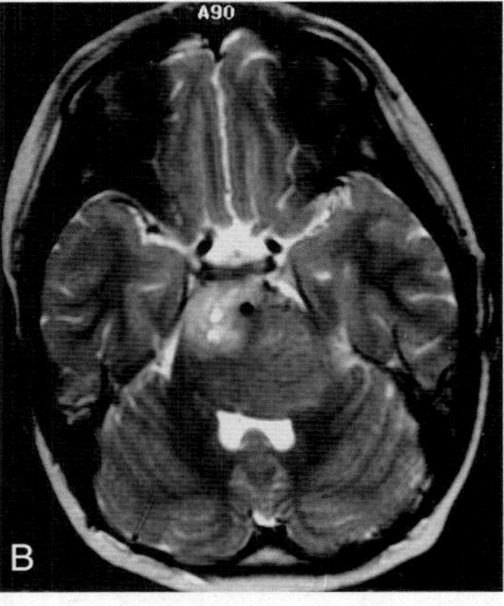

Figure 11-30. Brainstem glioma. A, Spin echo, T1-weighted, contrast-enhanced sagittal image showing a diffusely enlarged pons and upper medulla. **B,** Fast spin echo, T2-weighted axial image demonstrating heterogeneous signal characteristics in this lesion, which exhibits a mixture of hyperintense and isointense areas.

grade tumors demonstrate more prominent enhancement than do lower grade tumors.[57] However, the presence or absence of significant enhancement in a neoplasm, by itself, should not be used to suggest the degree of anaplasia. Interlobar, interhemispheric, or transtentorial macroscopic extension of astrocytomas (or any combination of such extension) and associated vasogenic edema are readily visible on MRI, especially on T2-weighted and FLAIR images. However, MRI is more limited in the assessment of microscopic tumor infiltration at the tumor margins and in defining the border between the neoplasm and its nonneoplastic vasogenic edema. T1-weighted, contrast-enhanced images can improve the sensitivity of MRI both preoperatively and postoperatively when used to look for recurrence. This might be further improved by MRS, either in single-voxel or in 2D multivoxel (chemical shift imaging) forms. On MRS, significant elevation of the amplitude of the choline peak, in relation to that of creatine or *N*-acetyl aspartate, suggests a recurrent neoplasm, whereas absence of such elevation on the background of mobile lipids and lactate suggests radiation necrosis or postsurgical changes, or both (Fig. 11-31).[58-60] Additional new MRI techniques such as perfusion MRI and activation functional MRI are now being used for preoperative evaluation of tumor and for surgical planning (Fig. 11-32).[61-64]

Oligodendrogliomas, which arise from oligodendrocytes, occur in adults, and their incidence peaks in the fourth to sixth decades. When made up predominantly or purely of oligodendrocytes, they behave in a benign manner. However, when the tumors are of mixed cell origin and contain both astrocytic and oligodendrocytic components, the astrocytic component often degenerates into a more anaplastic astrocytoma at recurrence. This occurs for about half of oligodendrogliomas. Calcifications are common in oligodendrogliomas, and histologically about 70% contain calcification.[51] On CT, calcification is visible in approximately 30% to 40% of these tumors. On MRI, calcifications are usually hypointense on T1- and T2-weighted images, but microcalcifications can demonstrate hyperintensity on T1-weighted images (Fig. 11-33). However, oligodendrogliomas, mixed oligoastrocytomas, and astrocytomas cannot be reliably differentiated by their MRI appearances.[65]

Ependymomas have protean MRI appearances with variable signal intensities on T1- and T2-weighted images, which are consistent with the variable cellularity and histologic composition found in these tumors. They are typically hypointense on T1-weighted images and hyperintense on T2-weighted images, but calcification or cystic or hemorrhagic components often result in variable heterogeneous magnetic resonance signals and enhancement (Fig. 11-34).[66] Ependymomas can be supratentorial, typically within the lateral ventricles, and infratentorial, within the fourth ventricle. They can demonstrate intraventricular or predominantly extraventricular appearances. A subtype, subependymoma, is typically manifested as a periventricular parenchymal mass.

Choroid plexus papillomas and carcinomas can develop within the ventricular system. In children, they typically occur in the atrium of the lateral ventricles, whereas in adults, they are more common within the fourth ventricle. They are generally hypointense on T1-weighted images and isointense to hyperintense with prominent enhancement on T2-weighted images (Fig. 11-35). Papillomas are well circumscribed and lobulated in contour, which corresponds to the classic cauliflower-like appearance in gross pathologic study.[67] Choroid plexus papillomas are frequently associated with communicating hydrocephalus. The cause of the hydrocephalus in these patients is debated, but it probably represents some combination of overproduction of CSF by the tumor and obstruction to normal CSF absorption by arachnoid granulations as a result of cellular debris shed from the papilloma.

Meningiomas. Meningiomas are the second most common primary brain neoplasm. They occur at any age and in both sexes but are usually found in middle-aged and older women. Meningiomas arise from arachnoid cap cells and are commonly found over the parasagittal cerebral convexity, sphenoid wing, parasellar region, tuberculum sella, olfactory groove, and cerebellopontine angle region. Meningiomas usually appear isointense in relation to gray matter on both T1- and T2-weighted MRI and can therefore be overlooked on a screening MRI study obtained without contrast enhancement.[68] Certain histologic subtypes such as syncytial and angioblastic meningiomas demonstrate hyperintensity on T2-weighted images.[69]

When gadolinium contrast material is administered, meningiomas are remarkably easy to detect because they exhibit reliably prominent and generally homogeneous enhancement (Fig. 11-36).[70] They are often associated with an enhanced thickened dura along the lateral margins of the tumor that is known as a *dural tail.*[71] In some cases, dural tails represent the margins of tumor extension, but in most cases they represent reactive dural enhancement without tumor infiltration.[72] A dural tail is not unique to meningiomas and can be observed in other neoplastic and nonneoplastic processes, including exophytic gliomas, dural metastases, lymphoma, and granulomatous infections. Meningiomas sometimes have areas of necrosis, macroscopic calcification, hemorrhage, or cystic changes. Such characteristics lead to some heterogeneity of signal and enhancement (Fig. 11-37). Most meningiomas have relatively small amounts of vasogenic edema and are frequently found with no significant edema despite their

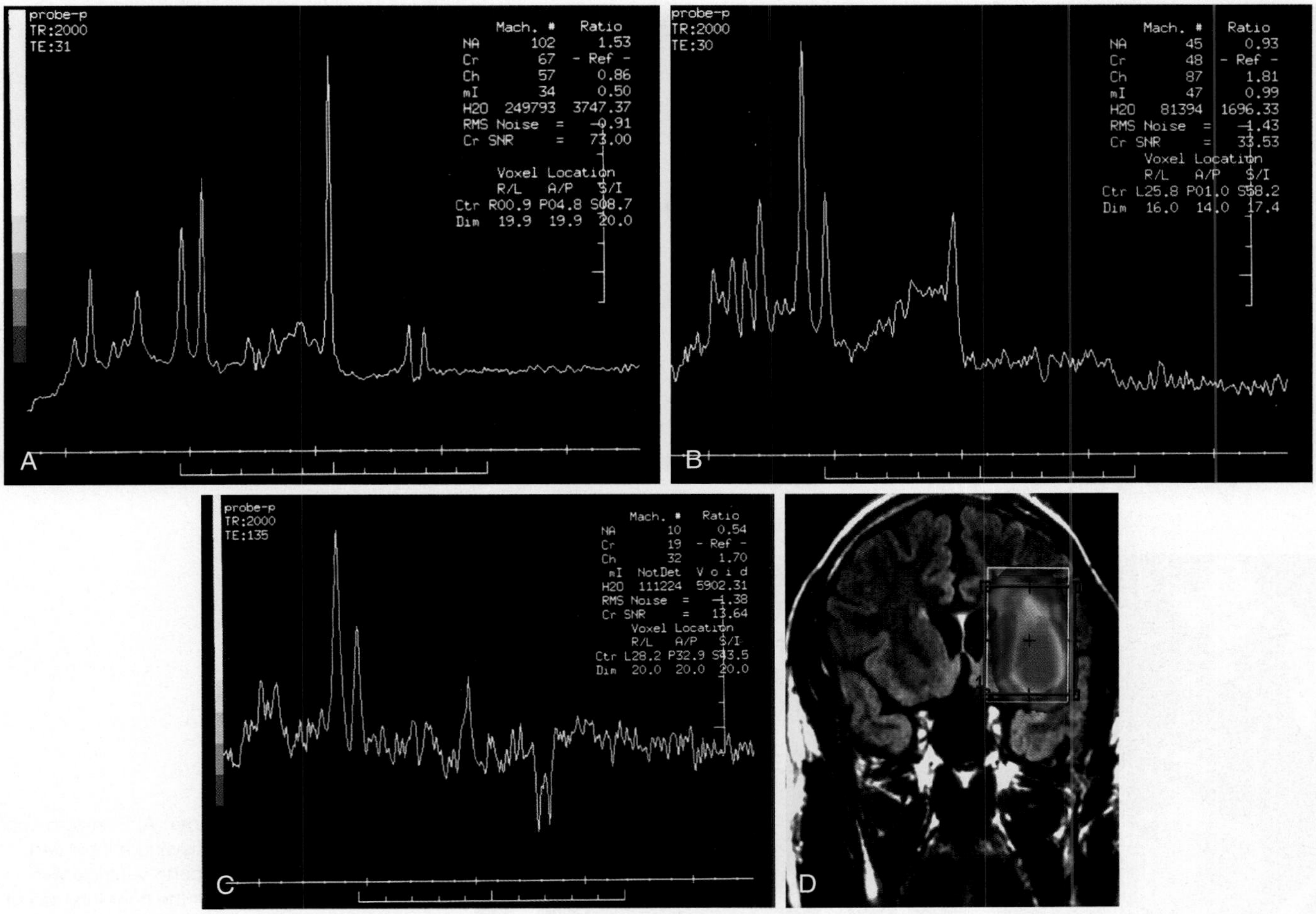

Figure 11-31. A, Single-voxel magnetic resonance (MR) spectra (recovery time [TR] = 2000 milliseconds, echo time [TE] = 35 milliseconds) from an experimental phantom showing the expected normal appearance of proton hydrogen 1 MR spectroscopy, except for the double lactate peaks. The dominant peak is for *N*-acetyl aspartate (NAA). Peaks for creatine, choline, and myoinositol are also seen (compare with the labeled normal spectra from the contralateral hemisphere in Figure 11-22A). **B,** Abnormal single-voxel MR spectra (TR = 2000 milliseconds, TE = 35 milliseconds) from a frontal lobe mass, showing reduced NAA amplitude and an increased amplitude of choline, which is consistent with a neoplasm. **C,** Single-voxel MR spectra (TR = 2000 milliseconds, TE = 135 milliseconds) from a neoplasm in a different patient, showing a similar abnormal pattern and double lactate peaks, indicative of the presence of anaerobic metabolism and production of lactate by the neoplasm. **D,** Color metabolite map for choline from multivoxel MR spectroscopy (TR = 2000 milliseconds, TE = 144 milliseconds) of a progressive high-grade astrocytoma, demonstrating an abnormally increased concentration of choline (displayed in *red*) in the left inferior frontal lobe.

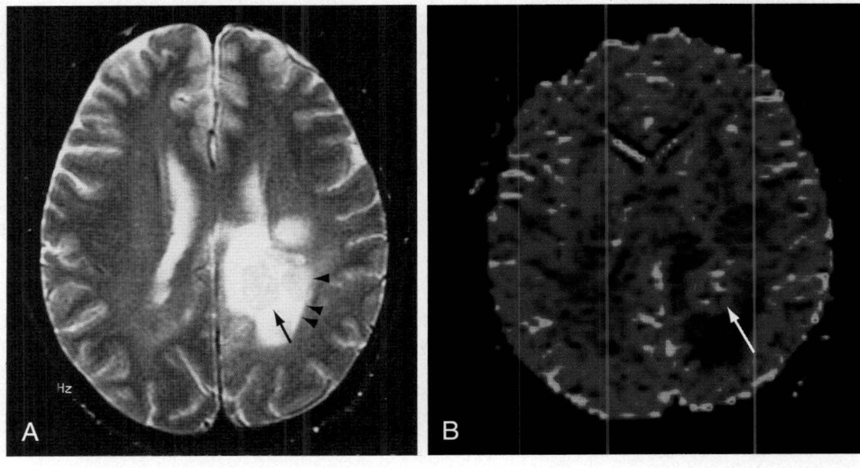

Figure 11-32. Central nervous system lymphoma. A, Fast spin echo, T2-weighted axial image at the level of the roof of the lateral ventricle shows a slightly hyperintense mass *(arrow)* surrounded by prominently hyperintense vasogenic edema *(arrowheads)*. **B,** Axial cerebral blood volume image from a perfusion magnetic resonance imaging study, demonstrating increased blood volume *(arrow)* within the mass lesion and a halo of decreased perfusion in the surrounding area of edema.

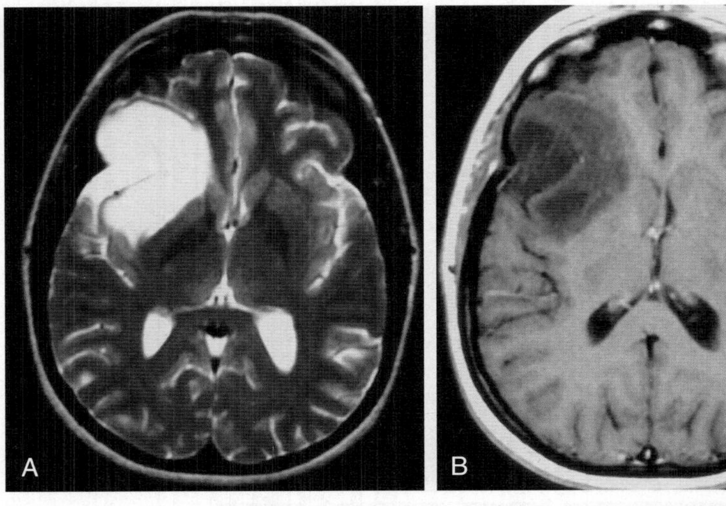

Figure 11-33. Oligodendroglioma. A, Fast spin echo, T2-weighted axial image showing a well-circumscribed, homogeneously hyperintense mass involving the right frontal lobe, insula, and basal ganglia, without significant surrounding vasogenic edema. **B,** Spin echo, T1-weighted, contrast-enhanced axial image showing a heterogeneously hypointense mass with no significant enhancement.

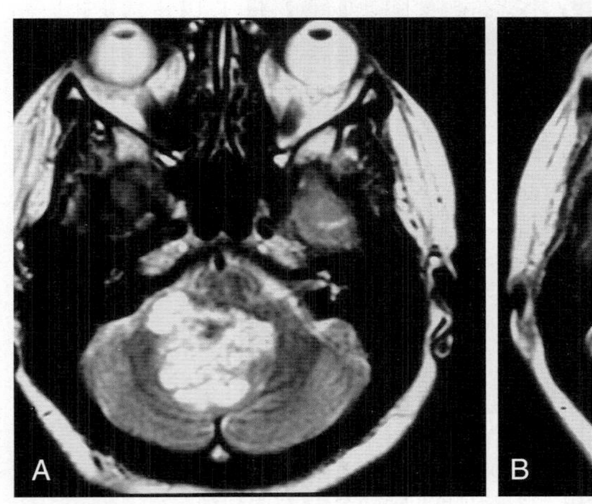

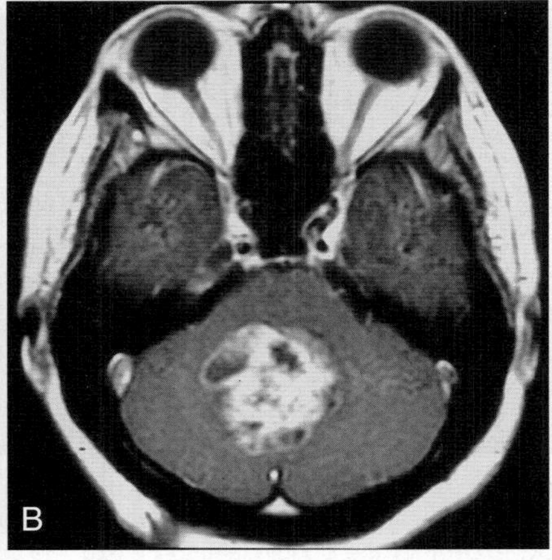

Figure 11-34. Ependymoma. A, Fast spin echo, T2-weighted axial image showing a lobulated hyperintense mass in the fourth ventricle with extension into the region of the right foramen of Luschka. **B,** Spin echo, T1-weighted, contrast-enhanced axial image demonstrating heterogeneous enhancement of this lesion.

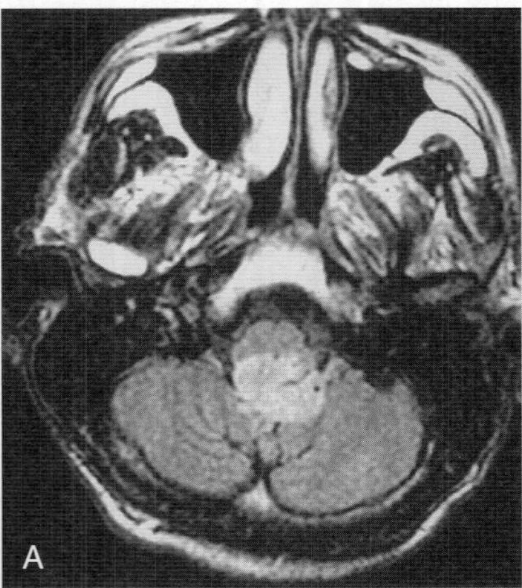

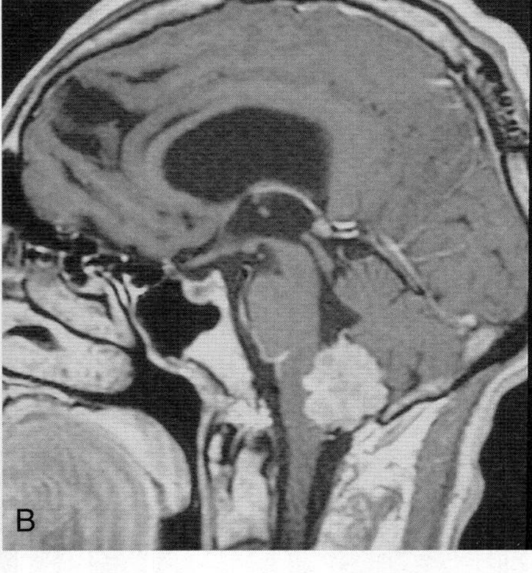

Figure 11-35. Choroid plexus papilloma. A, Fluid-attenuated inversion recovery axial image showing a homogeneously hyperintense mass in the inferior aspect of the fourth ventricle with mild distortion of the medulla and vermis. **B,** Spin echo, T1-weighted, contrast-enhanced sagittal image demonstrating prominent enhancement of this lesion.

large size. In some cases, however, they are associated with a large amount of vasogenic edema that resembles the edema observed with high-grade gliomas.[58]

Pituitary Adenomas. Pituitary adenoma is one of the more common primary neoplasms encountered in adults. The tumors may be secretory ("functioning") or nonsecretory ("nonfunctioning") adenomas. Secretory adenomas may arise from any of the secretory cell populations within the adenohypophysis, including cells that secrete prolactin, adrenocorticotropic hormone, growth hormone, or follicle-stimulating hormone/luteinizing hormone. Although histochemical evaluation reliably distinguishes these

Figure 11-36. Olfactory groove–planum sphenoidale meningioma. A, Fast spin echo, T2-weighted axial image showing a well-circumscribed, homogeneously isointense mass in the anterior cranial fossa, along the cribriform plate. **B,** Spin echo, T1-weighted, contrast-enhanced coronal image showing prominent enhancement of this lesion.

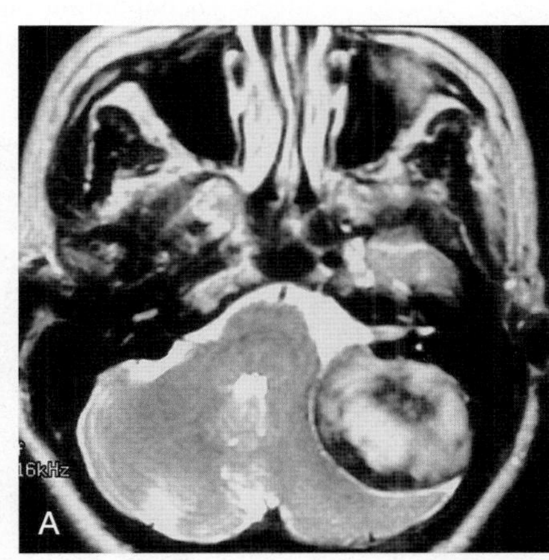

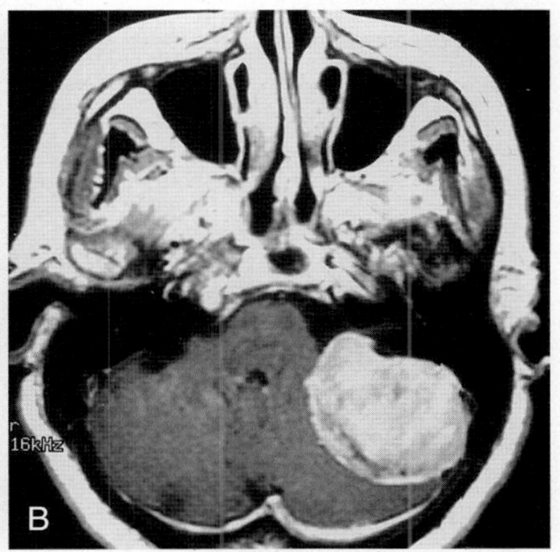

Figure 11-37. Meningioma. A, Fast spin echo, T2-weighted axial image showing a heterogeneous signal from an extra-axial mass over the left cerebellar hemisphere and extending to the left cerebellopontine angle. The mass is centered posterior to the left internal auditory canal. **B,** Spin echo, T1-weighted, contrast-enhanced image showing prominent enhancement, which is consistent with a meningioma.

subtypes, MRI cannot. However, MRI can help identify and lateralize a secretory microadenoma (<1 cm) and thus direct a transsphenoidal surgical approach. In macroadenomas (>1 cm), MRI accurately identifies the sellar, suprasellar, and parasellar extension of the tumor and its relationship to surrounding structures such as the optic chiasm, optic nerves, hypothalamus, cavernous sinuses, and the cavernous and supraclinoid segments of the internal carotid artery.

MRI evaluation of a pituitary adenoma should be a tailored examination rather than a routine screening brain examination. Furthermore, the study should be tailored differently for a microadenoma and a macroadenoma. When a microadenoma is imaged, the most important goal of the study is to identify the presence of a microadenoma to correlate with the clinical and laboratory findings. On MRI for a macroadenoma, the primary goal is to define the tumor and its relationship to the surrounding parenchymal and vascular structures.

T1 weighting with gadolinium enhancement is the most important imaging sequence for evaluating pituitary adenomas. The images should include thin (2- to 3-mm) coronal images through the sella turcica with a small field of view. With microadenomas, the gland should be scanned dynamically with a series of three to four thin coronal images, rapidly obtained over a period of 2 to 3 minutes during bolus intravenous injection of gadolinium.[73] This technique is used to identify a relatively slowly enhancing microadenoma within a rapidly and homogeneously enhancing normal pituitary parenchyma. This pattern of enhancement enables the clinician to delineate the microadenoma from normal parenchyma as a hypoenhancing/hypointense lesion on T1-weighted, contrast-enhanced images. Other imaging findings associated with a microadenoma include deviation of the infundibulum away from the side of the gland containing the adenoma, asymmetrical convexity of the superior border of the gland, or abnormal contour of the sella turcica floor.[74]

Additional imaging sequences, including T1-weighted, contrast-enhanced sagittal images and T2-weighted coronal images, are valuable in defining tumor extension and associated parenchymal changes, if present, of macroadenomas. Three-dimensional time-of-flight (TOF) MRA of the cavernous sinus and the circle of Willis can also better define the relationship between the macroadenoma and the ICAs and between the M1 and A1 segments of the middle and anterior cerebral arteries, respectively (Fig. 11-38).

Metastatic Neoplasms. MRI with gadolinium enhancement is the most sensitive imaging technique for evaluating CNS metastasis. MRI is superior to CT in tissue contrast, ease of multiplanar evaluation, and absence of artifacts, especially in the posterior fossa.[75] Neoplasms that metastasize to the brain have a wide variety of MRI appearances that depend on their cells of origin, cellular density, and associated pigments (e.g., melanin or hemorrhage). Metastatic lesions are typically localized at the gray matter–white matter junction in the cerebral hemispheres and are more frequent in the distribution of the anterior circulation than in the posterior circulation; this probably reflects differences in blood flow (Fig. 11-39). Typically, the parenchymal lesions are isointense to hypointense on T1-weighted images and isointense to hyperintense on T2-weighted images, with prominent surrounding vasogenic edema in relation to lesion size.[76] These lesions enhance moderately to prominently and are usually multiple. Some metastatic lesions—such as those from thyroid carcinoma, renal cell carcinoma, choriocarcinoma, and melanoma—are often hemorrhagic and demonstrate T1 and T2 signal changes corresponding to subacute and chronic blood breakdown products. Adenocarcinoma metastases from lung, breast, or colon cancer are occasionally associated with neoplastic cysts (Fig. 11-40). In meningeal carcinomatosis, the metastases involve the meninges and appear as a diffusely thickened enhancement of the pia or pachymeninges (Fig. 11-41) or as multiple, dura-based nodular-enhancing lesions.[77]

Schwannomas. Intracranial schwannomas arise from the Schwann cells that envelop the cranial nerves as they exit the intracranial compartment through various canals and foramina. They are more often found within the posterior fossa. The most common intracranial schwannomas arise from the vestibular divisions of the eighth cranial nerve. They are typically located within the internal auditory canal with extension through the porus acusticus into the cerebellopontine angle.[78] Depending on the size of the neoplasm, a variable degree of brainstem distortion or compression is observed, with minimal, if any, intra-axial brain edema. Tumor growth may cause bone erosion and widen the internal auditory canal and the porus acusticus. Vestibular schwannomas are usually isointense to hypointense in relation to brain tissue on T1-weighted images and hyperintense in relation to brain tissue on T2-weighted images, with prominent enhancement after intravenous gadolinium injection. When they are small (e.g., intracanalicular tumors), vestibular schwannomas typically enhance homogeneously (Fig. 11-42). However, with an increase in tumor size, cystic and necrotic foci can develop, which then contribute to more heterogeneous MRI signal characteristics and enhancement patterns (Fig. 11-43).

Vestibular schwannomas are the most common mass lesions in the cerebellopontine angle and represent about 75% of all masses in this location. The next most common mass in the cerebellopontine angle is meningioma. Meningiomas tend to exhibit more intermediate T2 signal characteristics than do vestibular

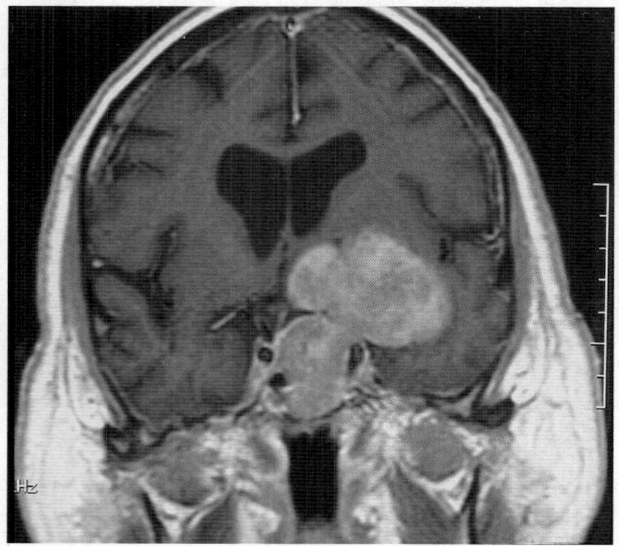

Figure 11-38. Pituitary macroadenoma. Spin-echo, T1-weighted, contrast-enhanced coronal image showing a moderately enhancing mass arising from the sella turcica with suprasellar extension, invasion of the left cavernous sinus, and a mass effect on the left anterior temporal lobe and inferior basal ganglia.

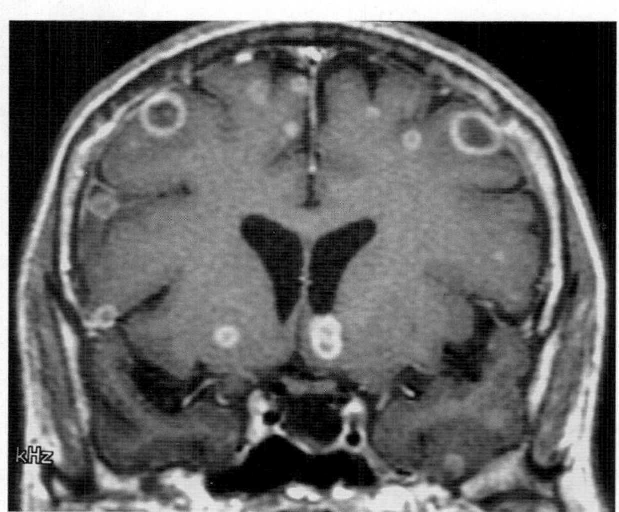

Figure 11-39. Metastases from lung carcinoma. Spin-echo, T1-weighted, contrast-enhanced coronal image demonstrating multiple ring-enhancing lesions, most of which are located at the gray matter–white matter junction.

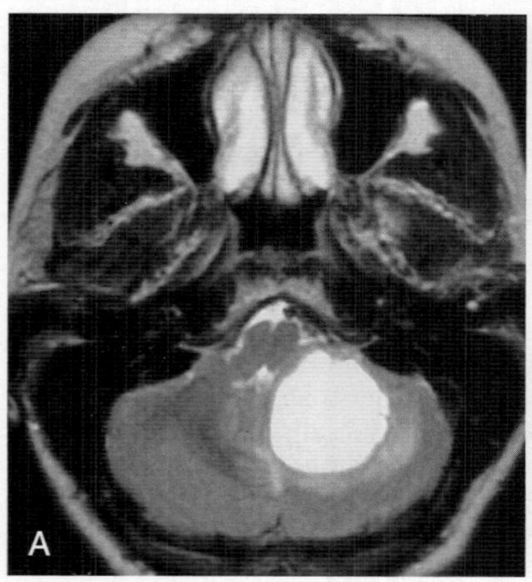

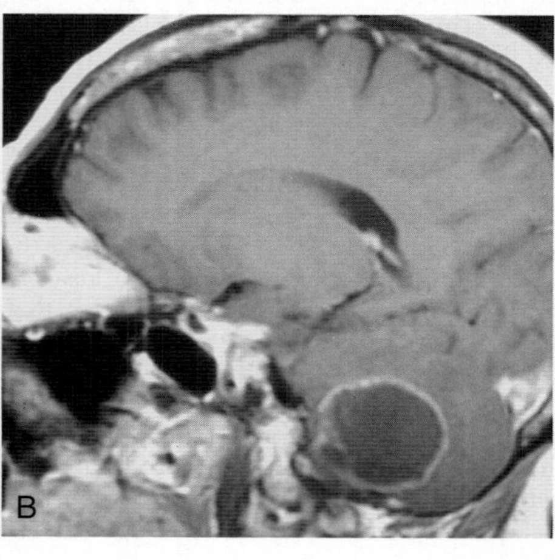

Figure 11-40. Cystic metastasis from breast carcinoma. A, Fast spin echo, T2-weighted axial image showing a cystic mass in the left cerebellar hemisphere with distortion of the adjacent medulla. **B,** Spin-echo, T1-weighted, contrast-enhanced sagittal image showing peripheral enhancement of this lesion.

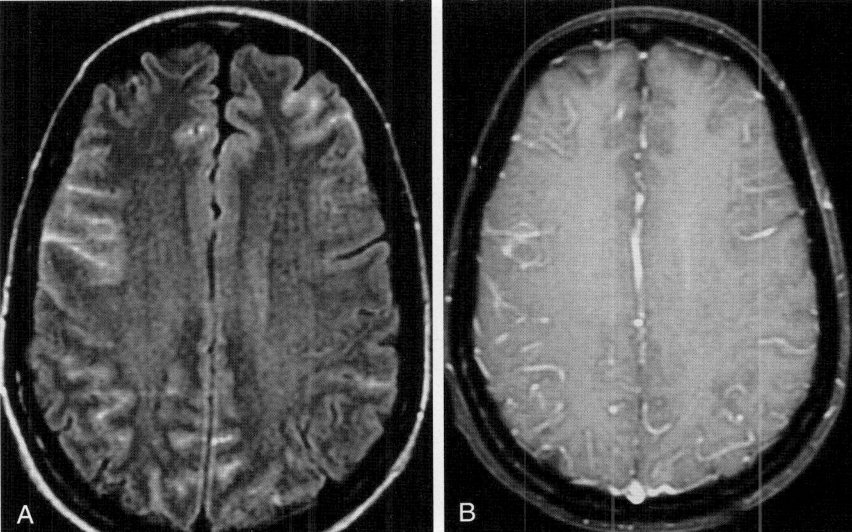

Figure 11-41. Meningeal carcinomatosis from breast carcinoma. A, Fluid-attenuated inversion recovery axial image at the level of the centrum semiovale, revealing multiple areas of abnormal hyperintensity within the sulci of both cerebral hemispheres. **B,** Spin echo, T1-weighted, contrast-enhanced, fat saturation image showing abnormal enhancement within these sulci.

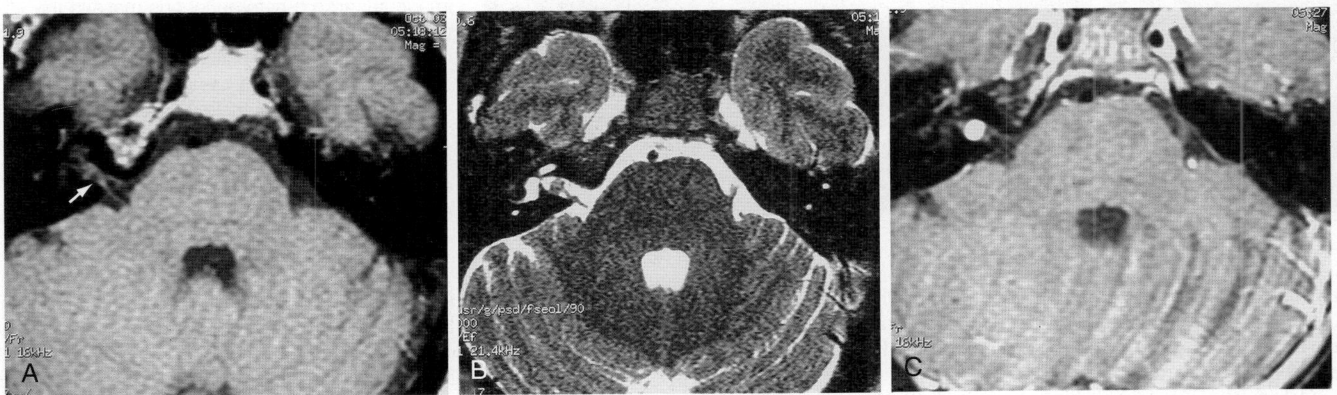

Figure 11-42. Intracanalicular vestibular schwannoma. A, Spin echo, T1-weighted, non–contrast-enhanced axial image showing a small, isointense mass with ill-defined borders in the right internal auditory canal *(arrow)*. **B,** High-resolution, fast spin echo, T2-weighted image better delineates a small, isointense intracanalicular mass. **C,** Spin echo, T1-weighted, contrast-enhanced axial image demonstrating prominent homogeneous enhancement of this mass.

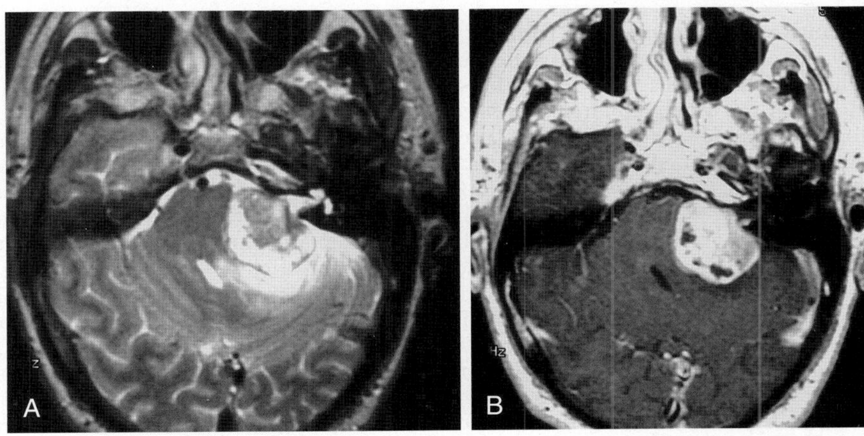

Figure 11-43. Vestibular schwannoma. A, Fast spin echo, T2-weighted axial image showing heterogeneous signal from a mass in the left cerebellopontine angle at the level of the left internal auditory canal. There is a significant mass effect on the brainstem, left cerebellar hemisphere, and fourth ventricle. **B,** Spin echo, T1-weighted, contrast-enhanced axial image showing the heterogeneous enhancement pattern of this large lesion, with minimal enhancement in the left internal auditory canal.

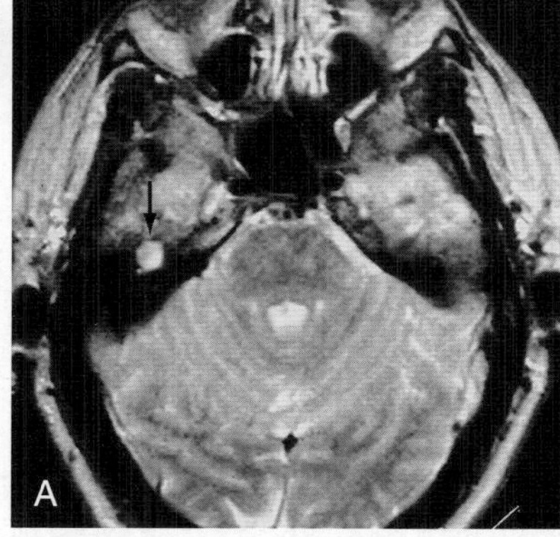

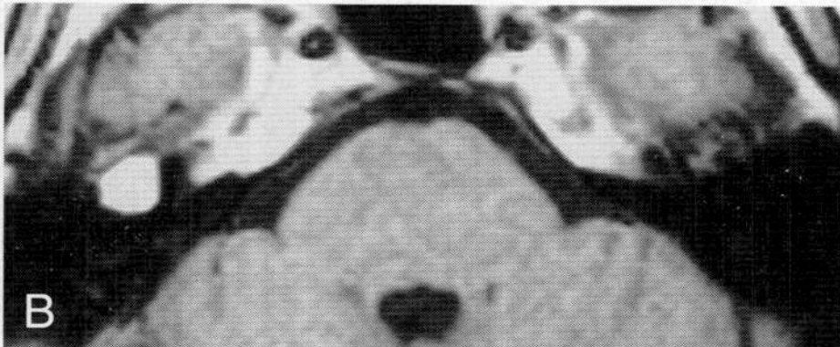

Figure 11-44. Schwannoma in the right facial nerve. A, Fast spin echo, T2-weighted axial image showing a hyperintense mass in the right petrous apex. **B,** Spin echo, T1-weighted, contrast-enhanced axial image demonstrating a homogeneously enhancing mass at the level of the geniculate ganglion.

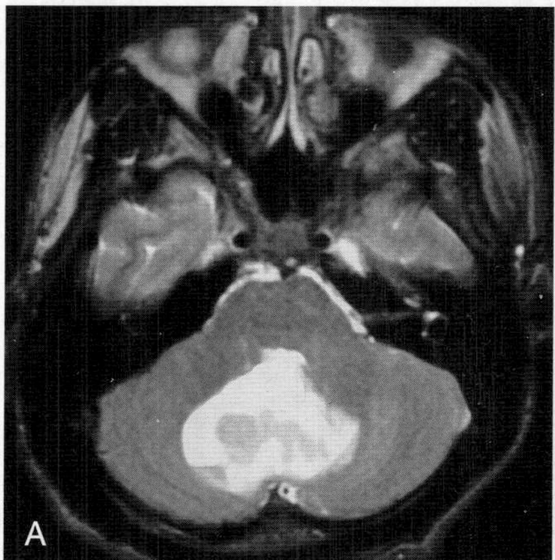

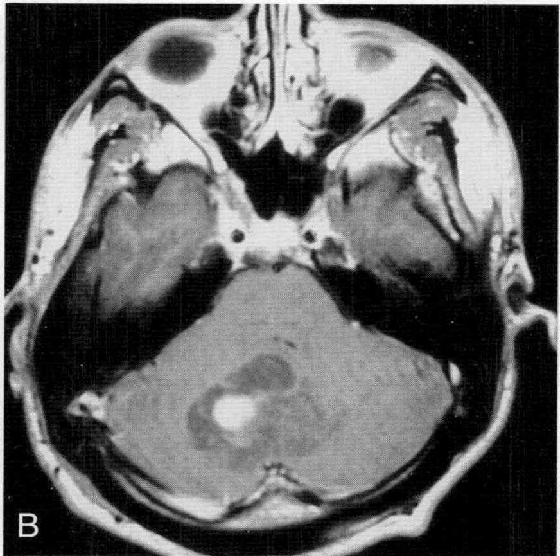

Figure 11-45. Primitive neuroectodermal tumor. A, Fast spin echo, T2-weighted axial image showing a heterogeneous mass in the posterior fossa with a cystic hyperintense anterior component and a solid isointense posterior component. This mass has nearly completely effaced the fourth ventricle. **B,** Spin echo, T1-weighted, contrast-enhanced axial image showing a central focus of prominent enhancement; in the remainder of this lesion, enhancement is variable.

schwannomas and infrequently extend into the porus acusticus. Although the epicenter of a vestibular schwannoma is at the porus acusticus, a meningioma in this area is typically located eccentric to the porus acusticus.[79]

Other intracranial schwannomas include those from the trigeminal nerve (cranial nerve V), facial nerve (VII), glossopharyngeal nerve (IX), vagus nerve (X), spinal accessory nerve (XI), and hypoglossal nerve (XII). Of these, trigeminal nerve schwannomas are the most common. Facial nerve schwannomas often appear as a lytic, enhancing mass in the petrous temporal bone in the region of the geniculate ganglion (Fig. 11-44).[80] The origin of a schwannoma that arises from cranial nerve IX, X, XI, or XII in the caudal aspect of the posterior fossa is difficult to ascertain on preoperative MRI and may be obvious only at the time of surgery.

Primitive Neuroectodermal Tumors. Primitive neuroectodermal tumors (PNETs) were first defined as large, solid hemispheric neoplasms made up of undifferentiated cells, often found in infants and young children, that, because of their locations, could not be designated as retinoblastomas, medulloblastomas, pineoblastomas, or ependymoblastomas. However, most pathologists are of the opinion that these various neoplasms have similar histopathologic features. Therefore, the designation *primitive neuroectodermal tumors* is used to describe all these undifferentiated, primitive neoplasms found in children and young adults.[40] In the posterior fossa, PNETs arise from the germinal matrices surrounding the fourth ventricle in children and along the anterolateral cerebellar hemisphere in young adults. They can also occur in the supratentorial compartment as intraventricular or intra-axial masses. PNETs are made up of small round cells and are hypercellular with a high nuclear-to-cytoplasm ratio. These characteristics contribute to their MRI signal characteristics, which are slightly hypointense to isointense in relation to brain tissue on T1-weighted images and isointense on T2-weighted images. They demonstrate moderate to prominent enhancement on T1-weighted, contrast-enhanced images. PNETs are typically homogeneous solid masses but can have cystic or necrotic components that have more heterogeneous signal and enhancement characteristics (Fig. 11-45).[81]

Infections

MRI evaluation for meningitis is limited by its marginal sensitivity. With the advent of the FLAIR pulse sequence and especially with gadolinium-enhanced FLAIR studies, sensitivity for meningeal diseases is reportedly increased, but further large-scale prospective studies are required. Normal brain MRI results do not rule out meningitis; therefore, chemical and bacteriologic examination of CSF is still needed to diagnose meningitis. However, in a patient with a highly suspected or proven meningeal infection, MRI is valuable and can help ascertain the degree of involvement and the presence of any parenchymal involvement (i.e., encephalitis, infarction, or abscess formation). MRI also can help monitor a patient's response to therapy if an objective parameter, in addition to the clinical findings, is required.[82]

Viral meningitis, when visible on MRI, is typically manifested as diffuse meningeal enhancement on gadolinium-enhanced T1-weighted images (Fig. 11-46). When encephalitis is present (e.g., herpes encephalitis), the involved parenchyma reflects the presence of cytotoxic and vasogenic edema with hypointense T1 and hyperintense T2 signal characteristics involving both gray and white matter (Fig. 11-47). Effacement of local cortical sulci, prominent leptomeningeal enhancement, and hemorrhage may also be present.[83]

Bacterial meningitis is often associated with prominent diffuse meningeal enhancement. It is typically hematogenous, but it also results from direct extension of infections in the adjacent paranasal sinuses or mastoid air cells. Complications of bacterial meningitis include subdural empyema, infarction, and parenchymal abscess. On T1-weighted images, an abscess appears as a mass with a central nonenhancing or slightly enhancing cavity with an enhancing wall of variable and irregular thickness that is surrounded by hypointense edema (which appears hyperintense on T2-weighted images). The central cavity is typically hyperintense on T2-weighted images, but it can be isointense or hypointense, depending on its contents.[84] However, these MRI appearances are similar to those observed with a necrotic neoplasm.

MRI findings can be crucial in distinguishing an abscess from a necrotic neoplasm when other clinical or laboratory data are lacking. The enhancing wall of an abscess cavity is typically thinner along its medial/deeper aspect and thicker along its lateral/superficial aspect. The extent of associated edema may be smaller with an abscess, whereas a necrotic brain neoplasm such as glioblastoma multiforme usually has a large area of surrounding vasogenic edema.[85] Newer MRI techniques such as MRS and diffusion-weighted imaging (DWI) can help differentiate abscesses from necrotic neoplasm. In MRS, spectroscopic evaluation of an abscess reveals several amino acid signatures and abundant lactate and mobile lipids. These, however, are also observed in necrotic neoplasms. On DWI, an abscess cavity typically has a restricted diffusion pattern with a low apparent diffusion coefficient and hyperintense signal on diffusion-weighted images (Fig. 11-48)[86,87]; in contrast, a cystic/necrotic neoplasm has a relatively increased apparent diffusion coefficient with hypointense signal.

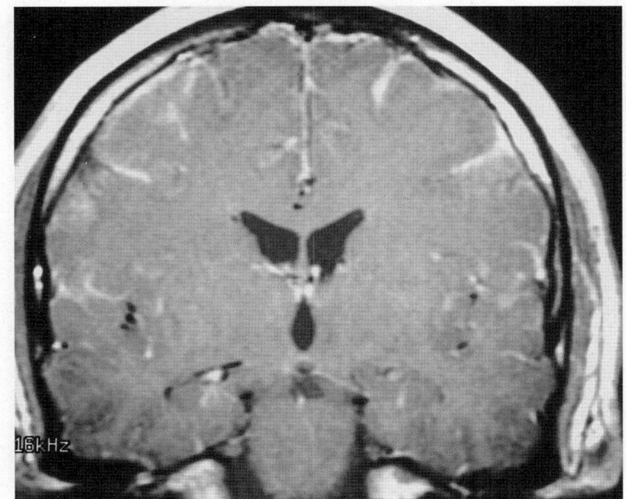

Figure 11-46. Spin echo, T1-weighted, contrast-enhanced coronal image demonstrating abnormal, thick meningeal enhancement in a patient with viral meningitis.

MRI can be used to image other infections such as tuberculosis, fungal infections, and cysticercosis. Tubercular meningitis usually involves the basal meninges and typically extends into the Virchow-Robin perivascular spaces of the basal ganglia, which may cause lacunar infarctions (Fig. 11-49).[88-90] Fungal infections involve the brain either by direct extension from contiguous structures such as the paranasal sinuses, orbits, and mastoid or by a hematogenous route. These infections are usually found in diabetic or immunocompromised patients. Meningitis and encephalitis can occur with parenchymal abscesses. In *Aspergillus* infection, the fungus has a propensity for vascular invasion, which results in hemorrhagic transformation of encephalitic foci.[91,92] Cysticercosis is an infection that results from infestation with a pork tapeworm. When these parasites die within the brain, parenchymal reaction to the dying parasites contributes to the edema, enhancement, and calcification seen on imaging. Cysticercosis appears as small, parenchymal lesions with punctate calcifications, intraventricular masses, or multiple lobulated masses that are hypointense on T1-weighted images and expand the subarachnoid spaces (racemose form; Fig. 11-50).[93,94]

Stroke and Vascular Diseases

Visualization of an acute infarction on MRI depends on several factors, including time after the ictus, stroke size, and location. Of these, time is the most important factor. The high tissue contrast of MRI has decreased the time between the occurrence of the ictus and when an acute infarction can first be identified on imaging. On T2-weighted images, acute infarction appears as a hyperintense lesion involving the cortical, white matter, or deep gray matter structures (or any combination of these). Larger cortical infarctions are associated with effacement of adjacent

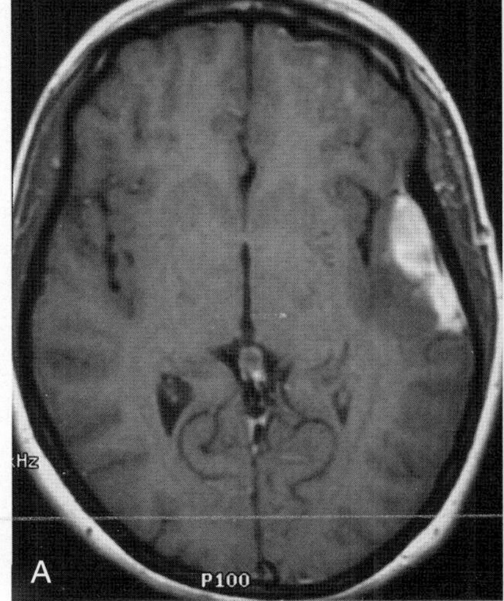

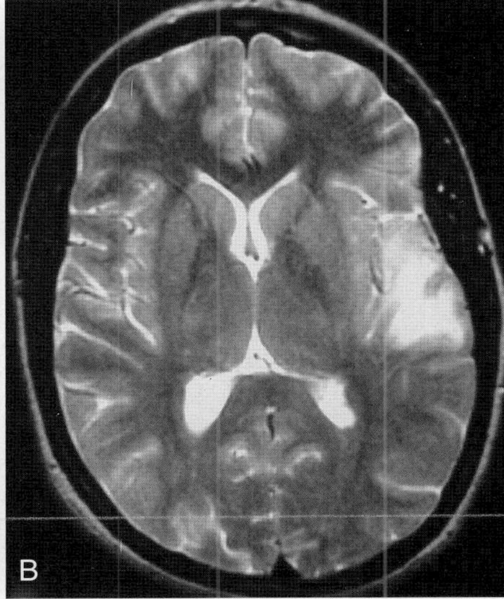

Figure 11-47. Herpes encephalitis. A, Spin echo, T1-weighted, non–contrast-enhanced axial image illustrating a lesion in the left anterior temporal lobe with a hypointense medial component and a hyperintense lateral component, which represents subacute parenchymal hemorrhage. **B,** Fast spin echo, T2-weighted axial image showing the abnormal hyperintensity of this lesion, which represents a focus of encephalitis from herpes infection.

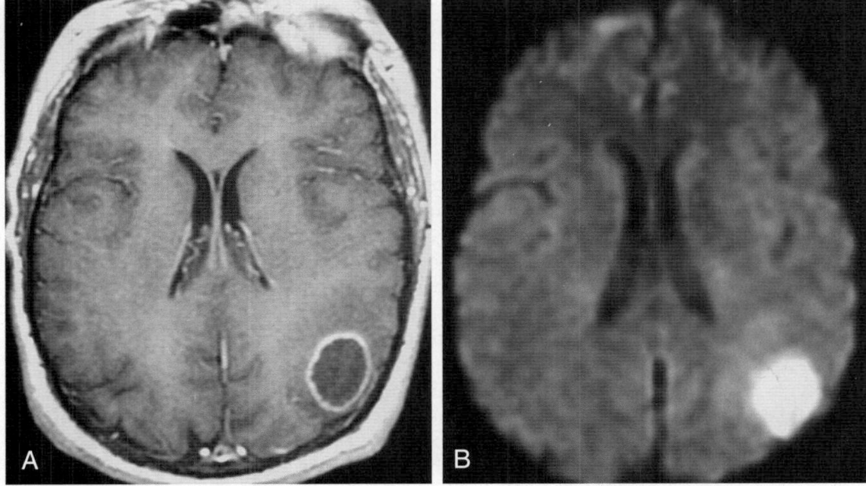

Figure 11-48. Abscess. A, Spin echo, T1-weighted, contrast-enhanced axial image showing a ring-enhancing left parietal mass with surrounding hypointense edema. **B,** Diffusion-weighted axial image revealing abnormal hyperintensity within the nonenhancing central cavity, which indicates a marked restriction of water diffusion in this lesion.

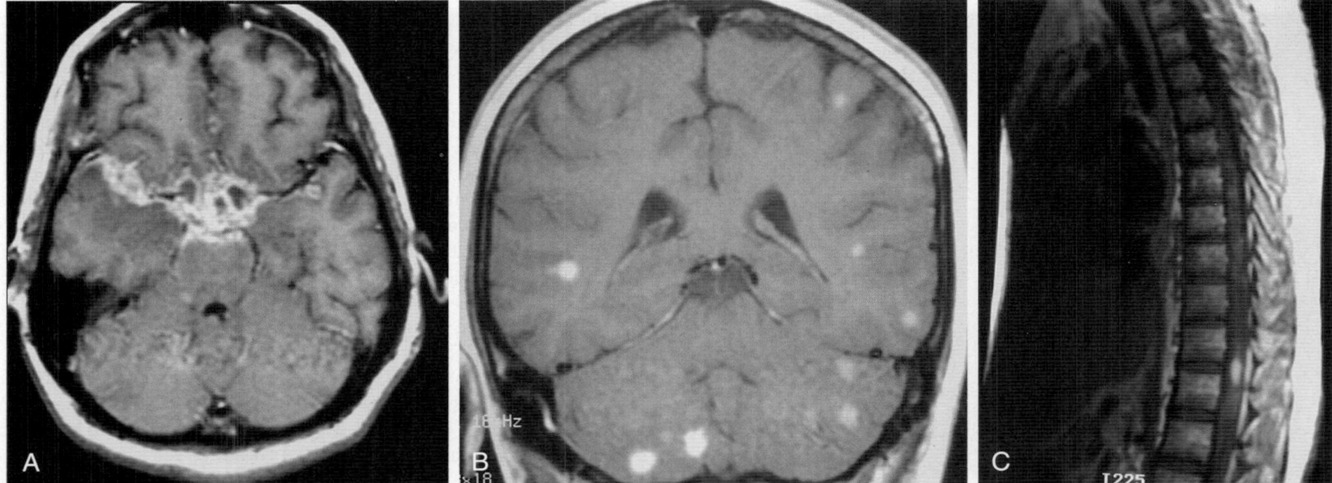

Figure 11-49. Varying appearances of tuberculosis in the central nervous system. A, Spin echo, T1-weighted, contrast-enhanced axial image demonstrating diffuse basal meningeal enhancement with edema in the right temporal lobe in a patient with tubercular meningitis. Spin echo, T1-weighted, contrast-enhanced images show multiple enhancing parenchymal nodules within the brain **(B)** and thoracic spinal cord **(C).** They represent multiple tuberculomas associated with miliary tuberculosis infection.

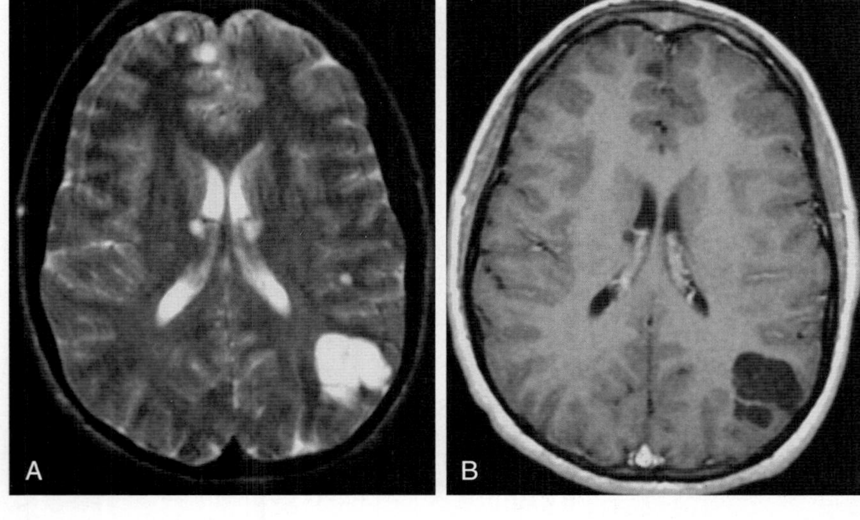

Figure 11-50. Lesions associated with central nervous system cysticercosis. Fast spin echo, T2-weighted axial image **(A)** and spin echo, T1-weighted, contrast-enhanced axial image **(B)** revealing multiple cystic parenchymal lesions at the gray matter–white matter junction and in the periventricular region. These lesions are hyperintense on the T2-weighted image and hypointense on the T1-weighted image.

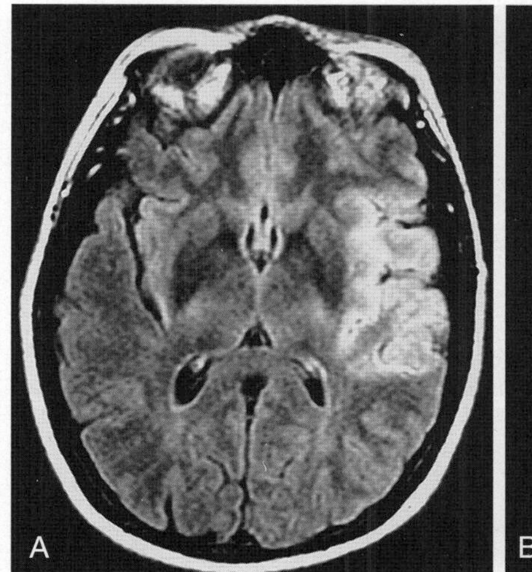

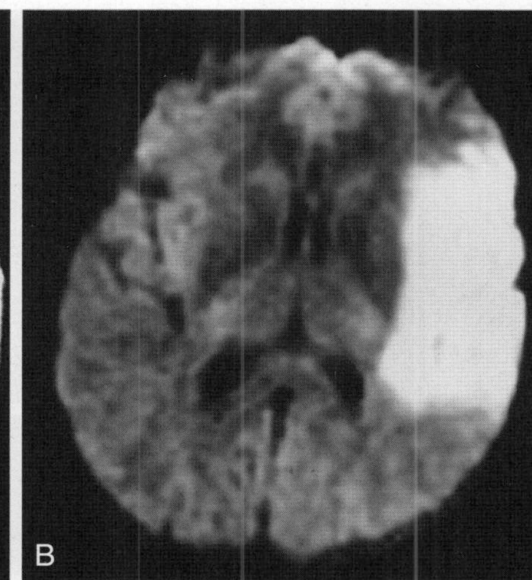

Figure 11-51. Acute infarction in the middle cerebral artery. Fluid-attenuated inversion recovery axial image **(A)** showing abnormal hyperintensity in the left frontal lobe, temporal lobe, and insula, with corresponding abnormal hyperintensity on the diffusion-weighted image **(B).**

sulci from cytotoxic edema. Abnormal hyperintensity in cortical vessels within these sulci may be the first signs of an acute infarction, even before any significant changes are apparent on T2-weighted images. Slow vascular transit time within an infarction results in loss of the normal flow void and increased signal within these vessels. Absence of a normal flow void is occasionally observed in the setting of a large infarction involving the internal carotid or anterior, middle, or posterior cerebral artery territory. With acute infarction, changes on MRI are usually evident within 24 hours of the ictus, often between 6 and 12 hours after the ictus. Cytotoxic edema increases during the first 1 to 2 weeks and resolves within 1 month. In the chronic stage, the infarcted area exhibits local volume loss with compensatory enlargement of adjacent sulci, cisterns, and ventricles along with a hyperintense signal on T2-weighted images. If hemorrhage was present during the acute or subacute stages, T1 and T2 hypointensity, representing hemosiderin and ferritin, are present in the chronic stages.

Echo planar DWI has even further decreased the time required for MRI visualization of an acute stroke.[95] In animal models, DWI can demonstrate large vascular territory infarctions (e.g., ICA or middle cerebral artery) within minutes after vessel occlusion.[96] In humans, acute infarctions can be demonstrated on DWI within 30 minutes to 1 hour. This implies that most acute infarctions should be visible on DWI by the time a patient arrives at the hospital after the onset of stroke (Fig. 11-51).[97] Once present on MRI, the hyperintense infarction on DWI persists for approximately 2 weeks, depending on size and location and the diffusion sensitivity factor (i.e., *b* value) that is used to obtain the diffusion-weighted images. After this period, subtle hyperintensity may remain and corresponds to the areas of abnormal hyperintensity on T2-weighted and FLAIR images. The degree of such hyperintensity on DWI is much less than that observed with an acute infarction. This phenomenon is known as the *T2 shine-through* effect and should not be confused with an acute infarction.[98]

Perfusion MRI, in the form of dynamic susceptibility imaging, shows promise in evaluation of cerebral perfusion, expressed as relative CBV or MTT. Again, with an echo planar technique, several hundred images of the brain can be obtained in less than 2 minutes. These raw images are then postprocessed to obtain a map of relative CBV or MTT, which is then used to qualitatively and quantitatively assess cerebral perfusion (Figs. 11-52 and 11-53). Along with diffusion-weighted images, these perfusion images can be used to determine the extent of ischemic brain tissue that is at risk for infarction. The difference between the area of abnormally low perfusion coefficient and that of abnormally low diffusion coefficient represents the ischemic penumbra that is at risk for infarction but still may be salvageable if treated.[99,100]

MRS can also play a role in acute stroke evaluation. Evidence of anaerobic metabolism (lactate production and decreased *N*-acetyl aspartate) can be detected with hydrogen 1–labeled MRS when ischemia and infarction are present. Single-voxel or 2D chemical shift imaging (multivoxel) spectroscopy can therefore define the extent of ischemic tissue that is producing significant amounts of lactate. When 2D spectroscopy is performed, a map of areas with lactate production or areas with decreased *N*-acetyl aspartate can be displayed and compared with maps of abnormal diffusion or perfusion to further delineate the cerebral tissue at risk for infarction.[101] MRS may also help predict clinical outcomes in young children with hypoxic ischemic CNS injury.[102]

Nonemergency MRI evaluation of patients with symptoms of intracranial or extracranial ischemic vascular disease usually begins with a routine brain MRI study that includes T2-weighted and FLAIR images for maximal sensitivity to detect subacute and chronic evidence of cerebral ischemic disease. MRA of the brain to evaluate the major intracranial arteries and their proximal branches is now a well-established technique. In MRA, a 3D TOF technique with added magnetization transfer pulse is typically used to improve the visualization of distal branches (Fig. 11-54). To rule out major venous thrombosis, magnetic resonance venography can be performed with either 3D TOF or phase-contrast techniques, which can easily identify the major superficial and deep venous sinuses and veins (Fig. 11-55). MRA has acceptable accuracy in evaluation of the intracranial internal carotid, vertebral, and basilar arteries, as well as the proximal branches of the anterior, middle, and posterior cerebral arteries, in the setting of significant atherosclerotic stenoses, vasospasm, or vasculitis (Fig. 11-56).[103] However, MRA is limited in its evaluation of medium-sized and small arteries. When such a disease process is clinically suspected and suggested by the results of a routine MRI study (i.e., abnormal lesions on T2-weighted or FLAIR images), conventional angiography is often warranted. Evaluation of the carotid and vertebral arteries in the neck can be performed with 2D or 3D TOF or phase-contrast magnetic resonance techniques without the use of intravenous gadolinium contrast material. The accuracy of these techniques in comparison with conventional contrast-enhanced angiography is well described.[104,105]

A newer technique involving a 3D spoiled gradient recalled (SPGR) pulse sequence obtained after rapid bolus intravenous injection of gadolinium can improve the accuracy of noninvasive magnetic resonance vascular evaluation (Fig. 11-57).[106] Like brain CTA, MRA is increasingly being used as an initial noninvasive

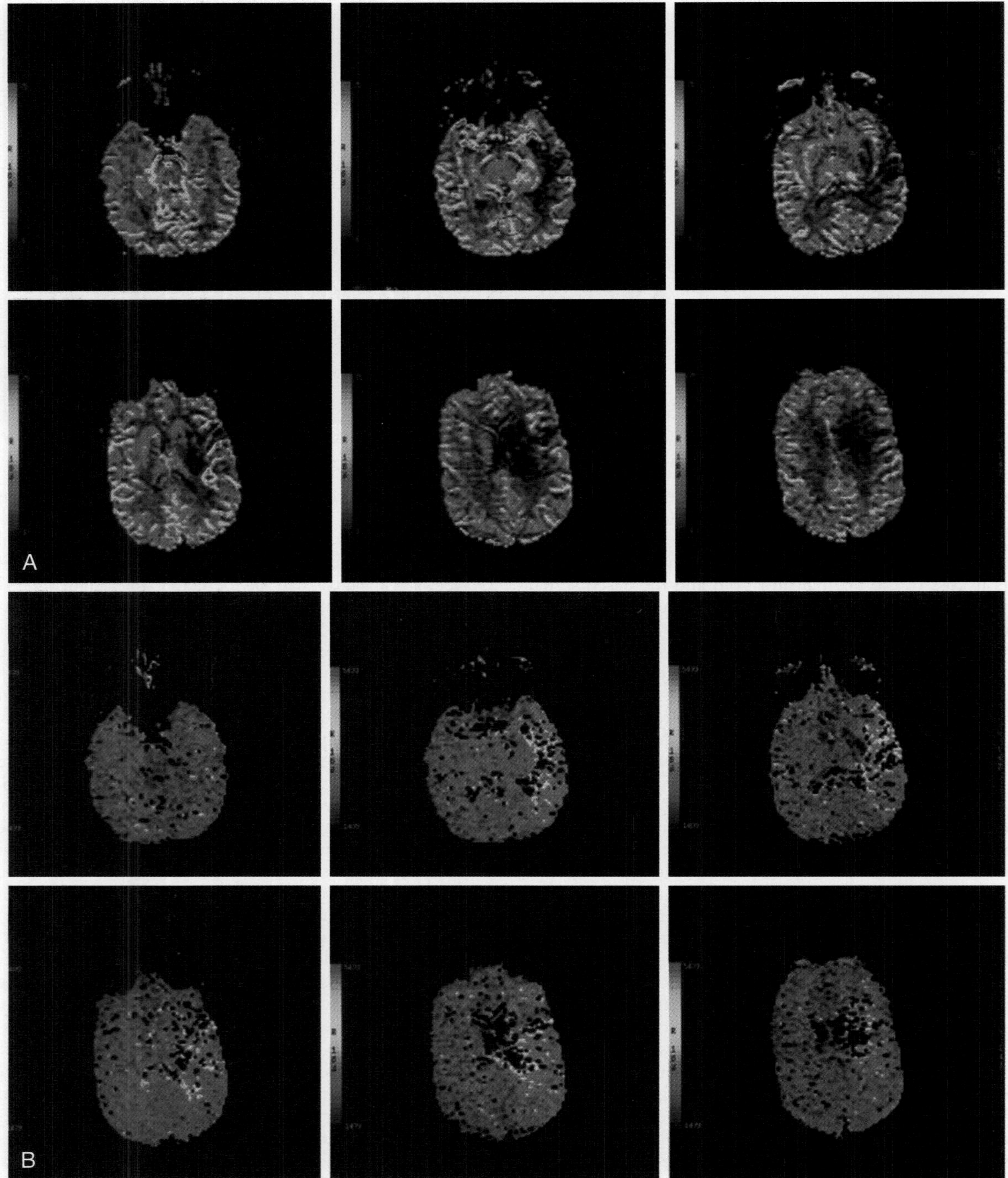

Figure 11-52. Symptoms of ischemia in the left middle cerebral artery. A, Images from a multiple-level map of relative cerebral blood volume, demonstrating decreased perfusion both in the left basal ganglia and superior temporal lobe *(dark blue)* and within the deep white matter of the left frontal and parietal lobes *(black).* **B,** Mean transit time (MTT) maps at the same levels demonstrate increased MTT (*yellow* and *green*) in the same areas.

imaging study for intracranial aneurysms or as a follow-up imaging study for untreated or treated intracranial aneurysms.[106,107] MRA or CTA of a previously coiled or clipped aneurysm can be challenging because of inherent magnetic resonance or CT artifacts generated by coils or clips. It is difficult to rule out a small recanalization or residual aneurysm on CTA because of a large amount of artifact from an aneurysm clip or coils. However, recanalization of an intracranial aneurysm previously treated by endovascular coil embolization may be demonstrated better by MRA of the brain with gadolinium bolus than by conventional TOF MRA without contrast enhancement (Fig. 11-58).[108,109]

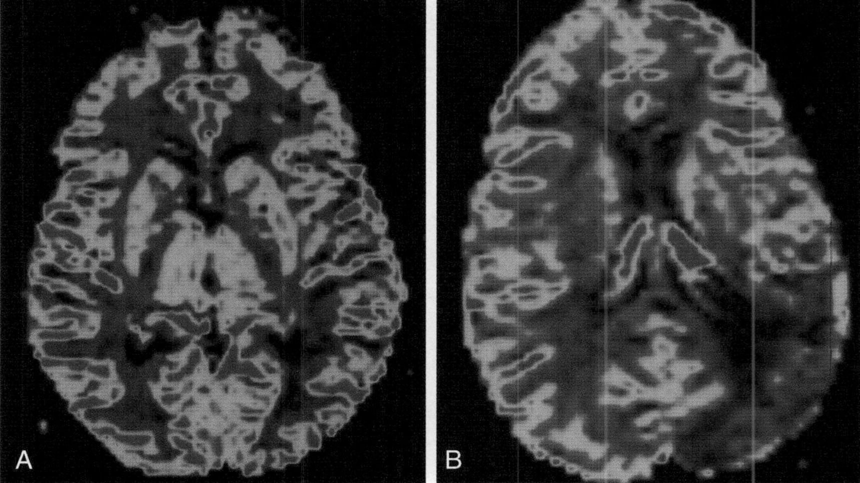

Figure 11-53. Maps of relative cerebral blood volume. A, Normal map from a perfusion magnetic resonance imaging study at the level of the basal ganglia. **B,** Map from a patient with an infarction in the left parietal and occipital lobes, demonstrating reduced perfusion *(dark blue)* within the left parietal and occipital lobes.

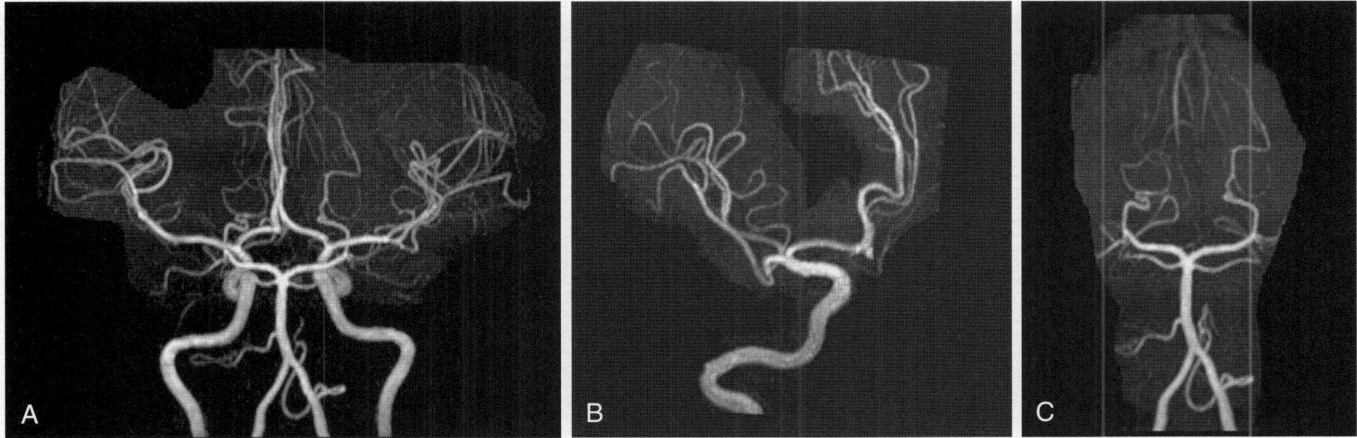

Figure 11-54. Magnetic resonance angiograms demonstrating major intracranial arteries. A, Postprocessed image from three-dimensional time-of-flight angiograms, including the A2, M2, and P2 branches of the anterior, middle, and posterior cerebral arteries. **B,** Isolated "cutout" view of the right internal carotid artery and its intracranial branches. **C,** Isolated view of the posterior circulation.

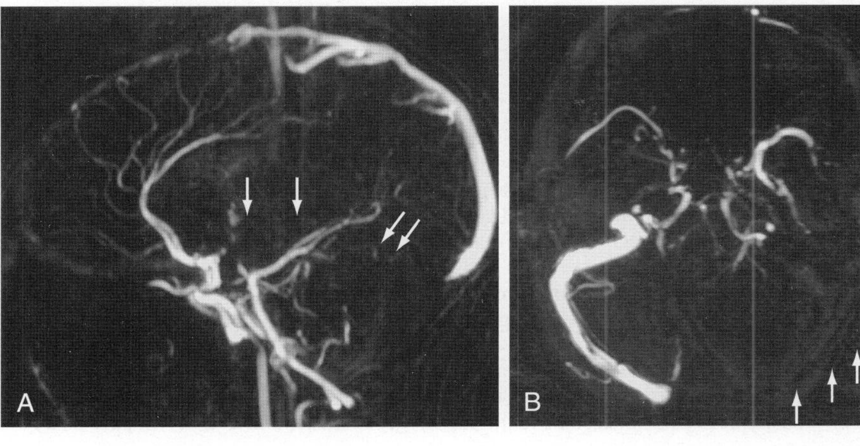

Figure 11-55. Two-dimensional time-of-flight magnetic resonance venography. A, Postprocessed sagittal image showing a normal appearance of the sagittal sinus but absence of signal from the deep internal cerebral veins, vein of Galen, and straight sinus *(arrows)*, which is indicative of thrombosis of these venous structures. **B,** Postprocessed axial image showing thrombosis *(arrows)* of the left transverse and sigmoid sinuses.

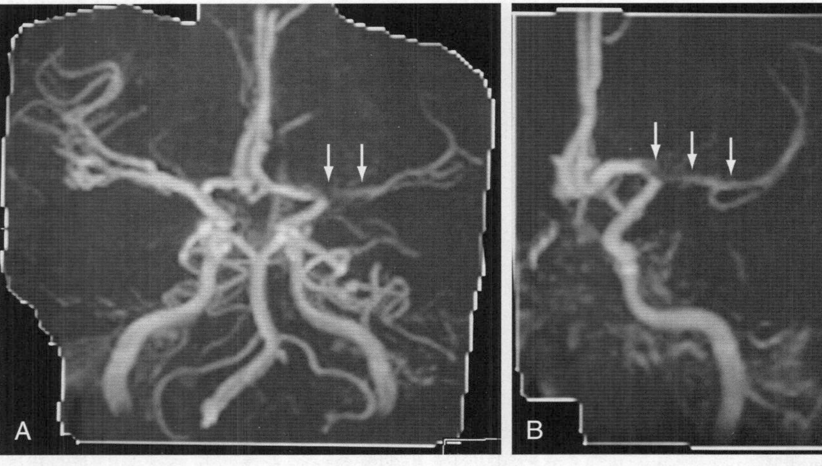

Figure 11-56. Magnetic resonance angiograms (MRAs). A, Three-dimensional time-of-flight brain MRA demonstrating reduced flow signal within the distal intracranial segment of the left internal carotid artery (ICA) and proximal left middle cerebral artery (MCA), indicated by the *arrows* (compare with the right side). **B,** Magnified MRA view of the left ICA and MCA, demonstrating thrombus within the terminal left supraclinoid ICA, the proximal A1 segment of the anterior cerebral artery, and the M1 segment of the MCA *(arrows),* with significantly diminished flow in the left MCA distribution distal to the thrombus.

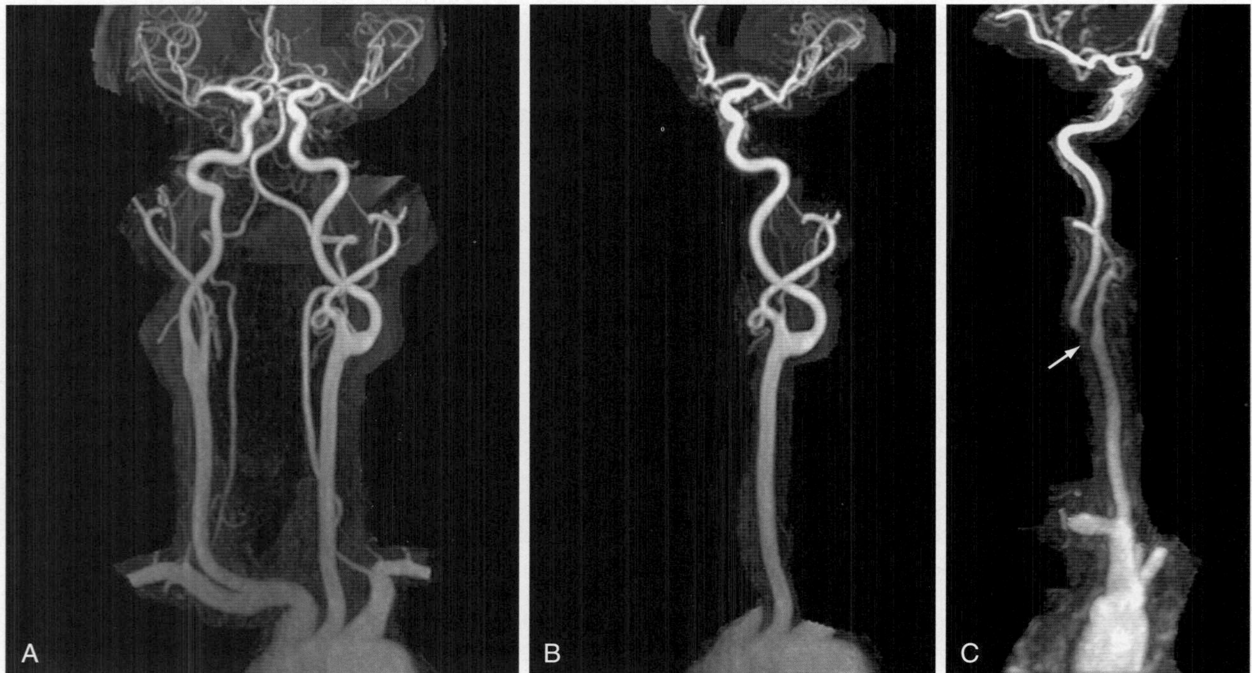

Figure 11-57. Magnetic resonance angiograms (MRAs) of the neck with gadolinium bolus. A, Three-dimensional image,demonstrating the major craniocervical arteries from the aortic arch to the proximal intracranial circulation. **B,** Isolated view of the left extracranial and intracranial carotid artery system. **C,** In a different patient, a focal stenosis *(arrow)* is visible at the origin of the right internal carotid artery.

Trauma

In cases of acute CNS trauma, evaluation for a fracture or hemorrhage is still best done with a non–contrast-enhanced CT scan. However, because of its superior tissue contrast, MRI may better define small parenchymal abnormalities on T2-weighed, FLAIR, and gradient-recalled echo (GRE) images that may not be visible on CT. GRE imaging is the most sensitive pulse sequence for acute/subacute blood breakdown products.[110] MRI also appears to be superior to CT in evaluating pathologic processes in the posterior fossa because the usual posterior fossa beam-hardening artifacts typically observed on CT are absent. MRI is also useful in the evaluation of small cortical contusions and subdural and epidural hematomas because of its higher tissue contrast and the ease of multiplanar acquisition with MRI. Small subacute SDHs, which are often isodense and therefore subtle on CT, are typically hyperintense on T1- and T2-weighted MRI and thus more conspicuous.

The MRI appearances of subdural and epidural hematomas and hygromas are variable and depend on the age and history (i.e., repeat hemorrhages). In the acute and subacute stages, T1 and T2 signal characteristics are similar to those observed with parenchymal hematomas. In the acute stage, they are isointense to hypointense on T1-weighted images and hypointense on T2-weighted images because of intracellular deoxyhemoglobin and methemoglobin; in the subacute stage, they become hyperintense on T1-weighted images and hyperintense on T2-weighted images as a result of extracellular methemoglobin. In the chronic

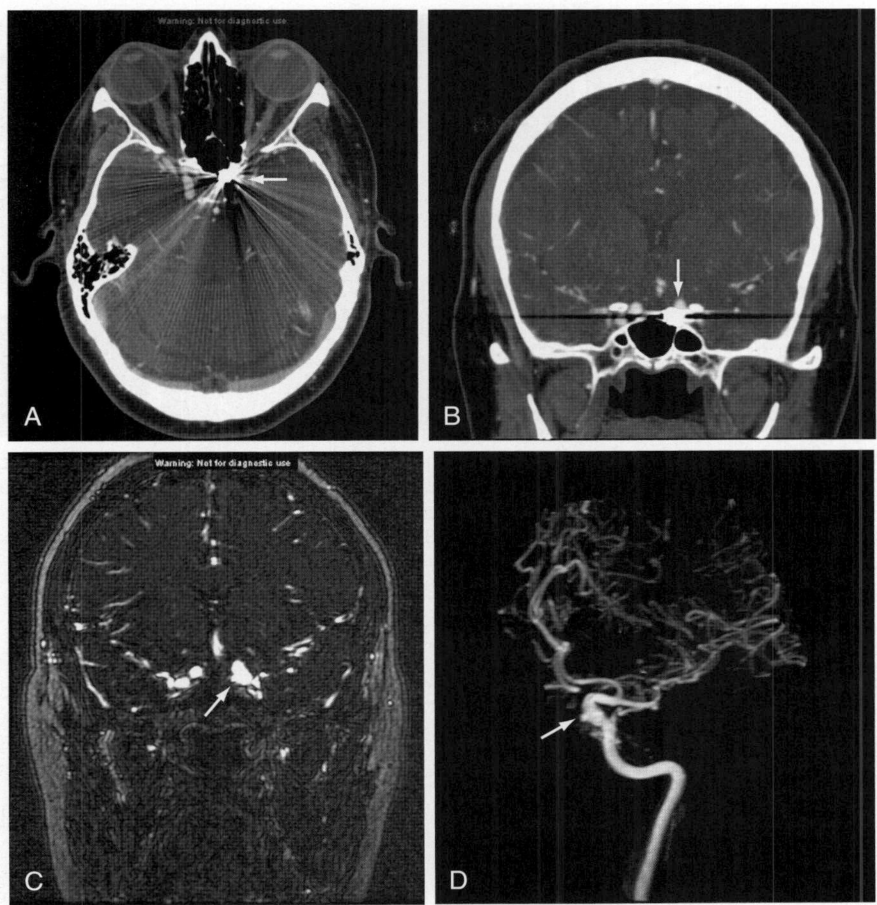

Figure 11-58. Aneurysm in the left parophthalmic internal carotid artery (ICA). A, Axial image from a computed tomographic angiogram (CTA) of the brain at the level of the anterior clinoid process, demonstrating prominent streak artifacts from previous endovascular coil embolization of the aneurysm *(arrow).* **B,** A two-dimensional coronal reformatted image from the CTA data set is compromised by artifacts, with poor visualization of the region of the aneurysm in the neck *(arrow).* **C,** Coronal image from a magnetic resonance angiogram (MRA) of the brain with gadolinium bolus, demonstrating small recurrent filling of the aneurysm *(arrow)* in the left ICA. **D,** Three-dimensional reconstruction image from the MRA data set with a cutout view of the left ICA, revealing definite small recanalization of the previously coiled aneurysm *(arrow).*

stage, parenchymal hemorrhages are hypointense on T1-weighted images and markedly hypointense on T2-weighted images as a result of susceptibility effects from intracellular ferritin and hemosiderin, which are present mostly in the interstitium and within macrophages. However, chronic SDHs (hygromas) are hypointense on T1-weighted images and hyperintense on T2-weighted images, similar to CSF. This reflects the low-density fluid collection that is typically observed on CT. Some authors suggest that MRI with a FLAIR pulse sequence has high sensitivity for acute SAH, but significant debate remains about its accuracy in the presence of frequently observed CSF flow–related artifacts associated with this pulse sequence, especially in the basal cisterns.[111-113]

MRI is especially helpful in the evaluation of diffuse axonal injury, which usually results from a high-speed acceleration and deceleration injury that causes mechanical stress on the brain and thus results in "shear" injuries.[114] The multiple, small, and subtle shear injuries at the gray matter–white matter border, along the corpus callosum, and within the brainstem that are typical of diffuse axonal injury are much better evaluated with MRI than with CT. The GRE pulse sequence, which is highly sensitive to areas of changes in susceptibility, is valuable when diffuse small parenchymal hemorrhages in the setting of trauma are evaluated. On T2-weighted and FLAIR images, these small superficial lesions at the gray matter–white matter border and the lesions in the deep pericallosal area, deep gray matter, and upper brainstem are hyperintense. If hemorrhagic, these lesions are also hypointense on GRE images because of changes in susceptibility associated with acute blood breakdown products such as deoxyhemoglobin and intracellular methemoglobin.[115] In the chronic stage, hemosiderin and ferritin result in hypointensity on T2-weighted and GRE images.[116]

Brain MRI can be useful when a patient with an acute head injury has minimal CT abnormalities but has profound neurological deficits. In addition, MRI may be helpful when an objective measure of extensive brain injury, particularly brainstem injury, is required before a patient's prognosis is discussed with the family. Newer MRI techniques such as DWI, perfusion MRI, and MRS may play additional roles in detecting areas of ischemia and infarction in cases of trauma.[117]

Acute traumatic vascular injury at the skull base that involves the ICA or vertebral artery can be quickly and noninvasively evaluated with MRI. MRI, which is highly sensitive to high-grade vessel stenosis or occlusion from traumatic dissection,

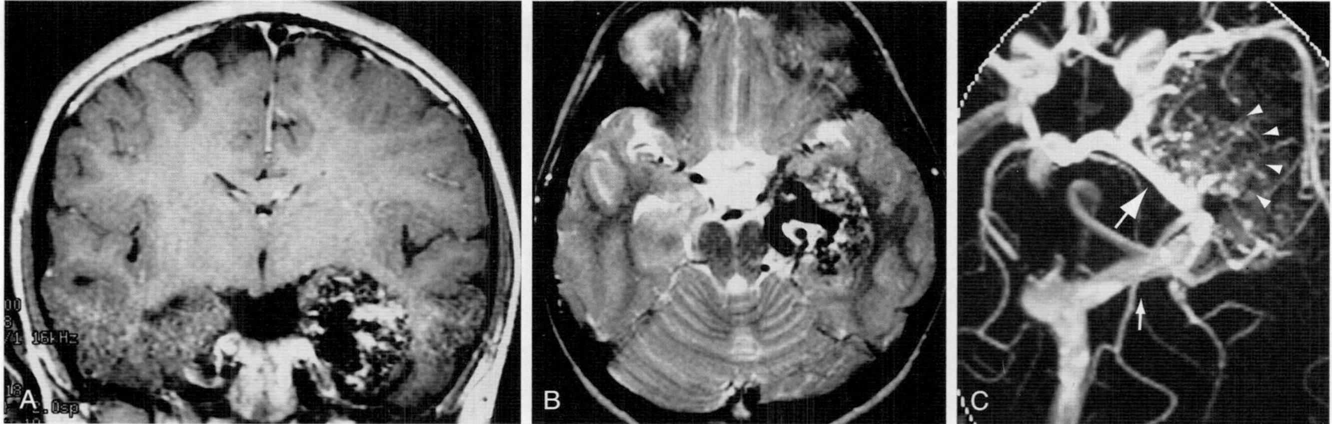

Figure 11-59. Large arteriovenous malformation in the left temporal lobe. Spin echo, T1-weighted, contrast-enhanced coronal image **(A)**; fast spin echo, T2-weighted axial image **(B)**; and postprocessed axial image from three-dimensional time-of-flight magnetic resonance angiography **(C)** illustrate the malformation with multiple flow voids within a large nidus *(arrowheads)* and prominently dilated feeding arteries *(large arrow)* and draining veins *(small arrow)*.

demonstrates the absence of normal flow void in these vessels. Additional T1-weighted images with fat saturation in the neck and at the skull base readily identify the thrombus in the false lumen with subacute methemoglobin. In the neck and the skull base, 2D/3D MRA can add additional information and display the relevant arterial tree from the aortic arch to the brain. Although conventional catheter angiography still remains the "gold standard," MRA in a possibly unstable patient who has sustained trauma can help guide clinical management and direct further conventional angiographic evaluation once the patient is stable.

Vascular Malformations

Intracerebral vascular malformations are categorized as four distinct types: arteriovenous malformation (AVM), cavernous malformation (cavernous angioma or hemangioma), developmental venous anomaly (DVA; previously known as *venous malformation* or *venous angioma*), and capillary telangiectasia. All except capillary telangiectasia are typically visible on MRI. An AVM is a vascular malformation that consists of a nidus that lacks the normal capillary network, thereby enabling direct communication between abnormally enlarged thick-walled feeding arterial channels and thin-walled draining venous channels. The vessels often lack normal smooth muscle and elastic lamina layers. AVMs are often associated with aneurysms of feeding arteries or the draining veins (venous varix). No normal parenchyma is intermixed with an AVM, although some gliosis may be observed. On MRI, an AVM appears as a complex tangle of abnormally enlarged vessels that demonstrate flow voids because of a high-flow state. Secondary findings, such as subacute and chronic blood breakdown products (methemoglobin, ferritin, and hemosiderin), can be found with corresponding areas of hypointensity on T2-weighted and GRE images.[118] Similar small hypointensity is also observed on T2-weighted images in the setting of calcifications associated with an AVM. Surrounding areas of edema, ischemia, or encephalomalacia may also be present.[119] These areas are visible on T2-weighted and FLAIR images as hyperintensity, with or without loss of volume in the case of chronic atrophy. Thin, linear cortical hyperintensity may also be observed on T1-weighted images if cortical laminar necrosis from chronic ischemia, as a result of a physiologic steal phenomenon, occurs in the parenchyma adjacent to the AVM. AVMs can also be further visualized on 2D or 3D MRA with either phase-contrast or TOF techniques (Fig. 11-59).[120] These MRI techniques can be used to diagnose AVMs and help in preoperative localization with 3D intraoperative guidance software. MRI is also useful in monitoring smaller AVMs treated by stereotactic radiosurgery (linear accelerator or Gamma Knife techniques).[121,122]

Cavernous malformations are slow-flow vascular malformations made up of abnormally large venous channels without associated abnormally enlarged feeding arteries or draining veins. They become symptomatic and also visible on MRI because they frequently bleed.[123] Typically, cavernous malformations are discrete parenchymal masses with heterogeneous hypointensity and hyperintensity on T1- as well as T2-weighted images as a result of blood breakdown products of various ages. When hemorrhage is recent, reactive hyperintense surrounding edema may be seen on T2-weighted images with associated local mass effect.[124] Multiple cavernous malformations are found in patients with vascular malformation syndromes. Because MRI, among all the imaging techniques, including conventional angiography, best visualizes these cavernous malformations, it is the study of choice in the initial evaluation and follow-up of patients with cavernomas (Fig. 11-60).

A DVA is not a pathologic vascular malformation. Instead, a DVA is a normal variant in which several prominent deep parenchymal veins drain from a normal part of the brain and then into an unusually large superficial or deep draining vein. The angiographic and MRI appearance of these malformations has been described in the literature as resembling the head of Medusa, a Greek mythologic woman whose "hair" consisted of multiple live serpents. Because this is a benign entity and requires no intervention, its recognition on imaging studies is essential. DVAs have a typical imaging appearance on T2-weighted MRI that consists of several slightly prominent vessels with flow voids that drain into a larger draining vein.[125] They are best visualized on T1-weighted, contrast-enhanced images (Fig. 11-61). DVAs may sometimes coexist with cavernous malformations. If a hemorrhage is present in the vicinity of a DVA, the cause of hemorrhage is probably an occult cavernous malformation near the DVA.

Capillary telangiectasia is a histopathologic diagnosis rather than a radiologic one. It is rarely diagnosed preoperatively. If capillary telangiectasia is visible on MRI, it appears as a nonspecific focus of hyperintensity on T2-weighted images, which may be associated with subtle enhancement on contrast-enhanced,

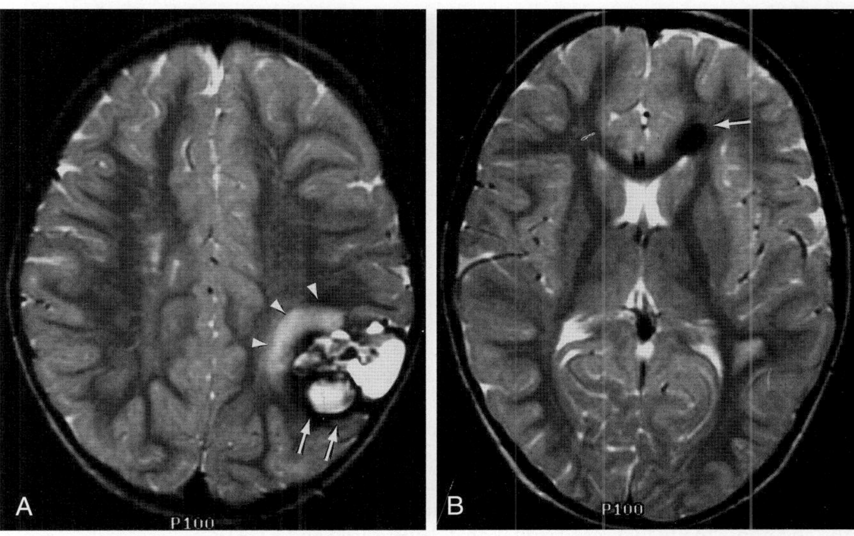

Figure 11-60. Hemorrhage from cavernous malformations. A, Fast spin echo, T2-weighted axial image showing a mass with heterogeneous signal in the left frontoparietal lobes, central hyperintensity, and a peripheral rim of hypointensity with associated surrounding hyperintensity. This is a large cavernous malformation *(arrows)* with evidence of recurrent hemorrhages; blood breakdown products of different ages are surrounded by mild edema *(arrowheads),* suggestive of a recent episode of hemorrhage. **B,** Fast spin echo, T2-weighted axial image at the level of the basal ganglia in the same patient, illustrating a focus of abnormal hypointensity, representing hemosiderin, adjacent to the left frontal horn *(arrow).* This represents a focus of old hemorrhage from a smaller cavernous malformation.

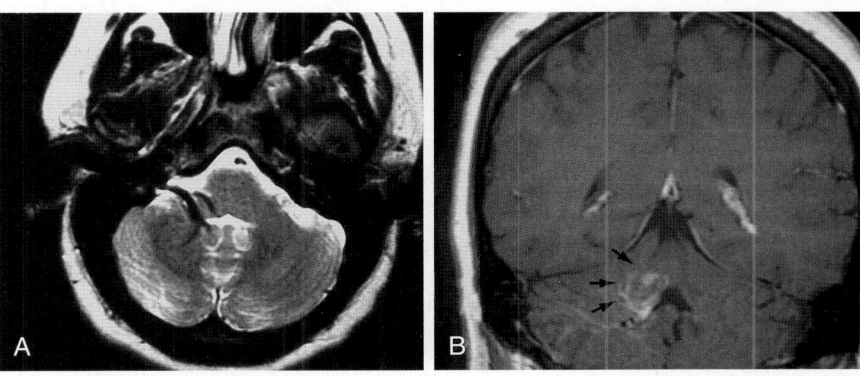

Figure 11-61. Developmental venous anomaly. A, Fast spin echo, T2-weighted axial image illustrating branching flow voids in the right brachium pontis region with extension into the adjacent cisternal space. **B,** Spin echo, T1-weighted, contrast-enhanced coronal image demonstrating a typical branching pattern of dilated veins in a developmental venous anomaly next to the fourth ventricle *(arrows).*

T1-weighted images. Multiple capillary telangiectasias are found in patients with ataxia-telangiectasia syndrome, which affects both the CNS and other viscera.[126]

Seizure and Epilepsy

Imaging of a patient with a first-time seizure usually begins with a head CT without contrast material, followed by a contrast-enhanced study if necessary. Causes of seizures such as stroke, hemorrhage, neoplasm, abscess, or benign cysts are often evaluated adequately with CT. Routine brain MRI has higher sensitivity than CT for subtle parenchymal lesions and meningeal diseases. However, in epilepsy, in which seizures are recurrent, a more tailored MRI study is required to rule out a structural substrate for epilepsy, including mesial temporal sclerosis, subtle cortical and subcortical neoplasms, or migration anomalies (heterotopias). These lesions may not be apparent on routine brain MRI examination because they are often quite small and their signal characteristics are similar to those of adjacent normal brain tissue on both T1- and T2-weighted images.

Several different MRI protocols have been developed to evaluate patients with epilepsy. These protocols usually include a type of high-resolution, 3D, and heavily T1-weighted acquisition of the whole brain. An SPGR sequence is one such pulse sequence that can be obtained at 1-mm intervals in the axial, coronal, and sagittal planes. Small slice thickness along with its heavily T1-weighted parameters accentuates the signal difference between gray and white matter and thus improves the detection of small focal heterotopias and migration anomalies.[127,128] MRI acquisition with the use of phased-array surface coils over a part of the head, instead of the usual head coil used for brain MRI, may also improve resolution and sensitivity. These surface coils have an improved signal-to-noise ratio that is usually several times greater than that obtained with a routine head coil, and they have the flexibility to be placed directly over the part of the brain that is suspected of containing the epileptic focus. They are useful in the evaluation of small cortical or subcortical lesions, which may not otherwise be visible on routine brain MRI. The advantages of surface coils are diminished for deeper structures because the signal decreases as the distance between the coil and the structure increases. Nonetheless, phased-array surface coils have been used successfully to evaluate the mesial temporal lobes in patients with complex partial seizures referable to the temporal lobes. In many such patients, MRI correlates of mesial temporal sclerosis—such as hippocampal atrophy, abnormal hippocampal hyperintensity on T2-weighted images, and disruption of the hippocampal internal architecture—are observed.[129-131] Such imaging of the mesial temporal lobes is most efficacious in a coronal or modified coronal plane perpendicular to the anteroposterior axis of the hippocampus at 1- to 20-mm intervals with T1-weighted, T2-weighted, and FLAIR images (Fig. 11-62).

Tailored MRI techniques are valuable in the preoperative imaging evaluation of patients with epilepsy. These techniques are useful particularly in the preoperative evaluation and lateralization of the seizure focus in patients with temporal lobe epilepsy. Various MRI parameters can be used to diagnose the

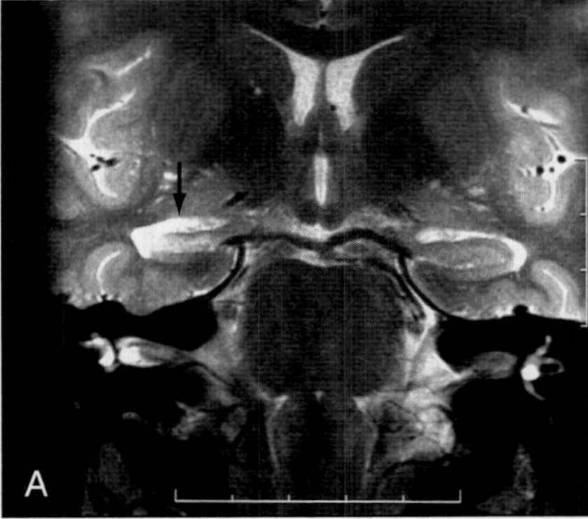

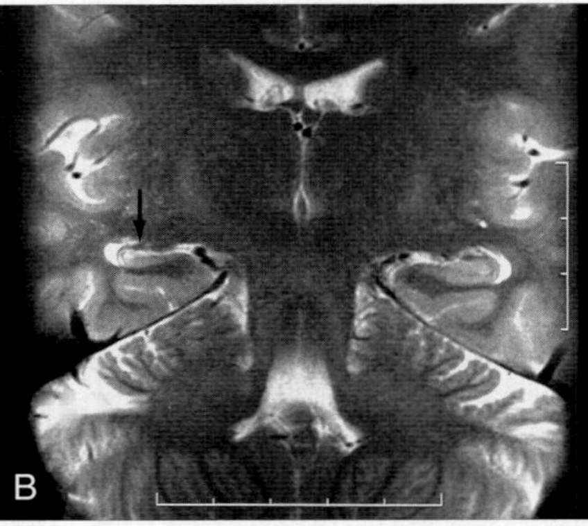

Figure 11-62. Temporal lobe epilepsy. **A,** High-resolution, fast spin echo, T2-weighted coronal image obtained with phased-array surface coils, demonstrating subtle abnormal hyperintensity in the right hippocampus *(arrow)*. **B,** A coronal image through the body of the right hippocampus, demonstrating prominent asymmetrical atrophy of the right hippocampus *(arrow)* in comparison with the contralateral left hippocampus.

presence of mesial temporal sclerosis in such patients, including qualitative techniques such as visual evaluation for asymmetrically and abnormally increased signal on T2-weighted and FLAIR coronal images, decreased hippocampal volume, and larger-than-normal size of the temporal horn of the lateral ventricle within the ipsilateral temporal lobe.

Quantitative measurements of these changes can be studied with 3D hippocampal volumetry to quantify the hippocampal atrophy and T2-weighted relaxometry to quantify the change in T2 signal. Such MRI lateralization, when possible, has significant prognostic value for patients who undergo surgery to treat medically intractable temporal lobe epilepsy. Patients with a lateralizing MRI abnormality have a significantly greater seizure-free rate after hippocampal resection and partial temporal lobectomy than do those who do not demonstrate such a lateralizing abnormality on preoperative MRI.[132,133] MRS can also be used to study the mesial temporal lobes, including the hippocampus, in temporal lobe epilepsy. Single-voxel and 2D chemical shift imaging techniques are used to obtain proton magnetic resonance spectra from the hippocampi and surrounding mesial temporal lobe structures. In MRS, to ascertain neuronal concentration and integrity, the concentration of the neuronal marker metabolite *N*-acetyl aspartate is measured with an absolute quantitative technique or, more commonly, by a ratio in which *N*-acetyl aspartate is compared with a reference metabolite such as creatine. A high accuracy rate in lateralization of the diseased hippocampus in patients with temporal lobe epilepsy is reported with the use of single-voxel or chemical shift imaging proton MRS.[58,134-136]

More recently, activation functional MRI and DTI with 2D and 3D white matter tractography are also being used as a part of preoperative evaluation and surgical planning for patients with epilepsy, especially temporal lobe epilepsy. Molecular imaging by means of receptor ligands that are visible on single-photon emission CT and positron emission tomography can also help localize areas of cortical malformations and epileptogenic foci.[137-140]

SUGGESTED READINGS

Aine CJ. A conceptual overview and critique of functional neuroimaging techniques in humans: I. MRI/fMRI and PET. *Crit Rev Neurobiol*. 1995;9:229-309.

Bradley WG, Shey RB. MR imaging evaluation of seizures. *Radiology*. 2000;214:651-656.

Burdette JH, Elster AD, Ricci PE. Acute cerebral infarction: quantification of spin-density and T2 shine-through phenomena on diffusion-weighted MR images. *Radiology*. 1999;212:333-339.

Falcone S, Post MJ. Encephalitis, cerebritis, and brain abscess: pathophysiology and imaging findings. *Neuroimaging Clin N Am*. 2000;10:333-353.

Gentry LR. Imaging of closed head injury. *Radiology*. 1994;191:1-17.

Hounsfield GN. Computerized transverse axial scanning (tomography). 1. Description of system. *Br J Radiol*. 1973;46:1016-1022.

Huda W. *Review of Radiologic Physics*. 3rd ed. Baltimore: Lippincott Williams & Wilkins; 2009.

Jack CR Jr. Magnetic resonance imaging. Neuroimaging and anatomy. *Neuroimaging Clin N Am*. 1995;5:597-622.

Lev MH, Rosen BR. Clinical applications of intracranial perfusion MR imaging. *Neuroimaging Clin N Am*. 1999;9:309-331.

Luat AF, Chugani HT. Molecular and diffusion tensor imaging of epileptic networks. *Epilepsia*. 2008;49(suppl 3):15-22.

McLean MA, Cross JJ. Magnetic resonance spectroscopy: principles and applications in neurosurgery. *Br J Neurosurg*. 2009;23:5-13.

Okahara M, Kiyosue H, Yamashita M, et al. Diagnostic accuracy of magnetic resonance angiography for cerebral aneurysms in correlation with 3D-digital subtraction angiographic images: a study of 133 aneurysms. *Stroke*. 2002;33:1803-1808.

Okazaki H. *Fundamentals of Neuropathology: Morphologic Basis of Neurologic Disorders*. 2nd ed. New York: Igaku-Shoin; 1989.

Osborne A. *Diagnostic Neuroradiology*. St. Louis: Mosby; 1994.

Ricci PE. Imaging of adult brain tumors. *Neuroimaging Clin N Am*. 1999;9:651-669.

Ross B, Michaelis T. Clinical applications of magnetic resonance spectroscopy. *Magn Reson Q*. 1994;10:191-247.

Rowley HA, Grant PE, Roberts TP. Diffusion MR imaging. Theory and applications. *Neuroimaging Clin N Am*. 1999;9:343-361.

Sorensen AG, Copen WA, Ostergaard L, et al. Hyperacute stroke: simultaneous measurement of relative cerebral blood volume, relative cerebral blood flow, and mean tissue transit time. *Radiology*. 1999;2102:519-527.

Wikström J, Ronne-Engström E, Gal G, et al. Three-dimensional time-of-flight (3D TOF) magnetic resonance angiography (MRA) and contrast-enhanced MRA of intracranial aneurysms treated with platinum coils. *Acta Radiol*. 2008;49:190-196.

Wintermark M, Dillon WP, Smith WS, et al. Visual grading system for vasospasm based on perfusion CT imaging: comparisons with conventional angiography and quantitative perfusion CT. *Cerebrovasc Dis*. 2008;26:163-170.

Wintermark M, Sincic R, Sridhar D, et al. Cerebral perfusion CT: technique and clinical applications. *J Neuroradiol*. 2008;35:253-260.

Woermann FG, Vollmar C. Clinical MRI in children and adults with focal epilepsy: a critical review. *Epilepsy Behav*. 2009;15:40-49.

Yetkin FZ, Mueller WM, Morris GL, et al. Functional MR activation correlated with intraoperative cortical mapping. *AJNR Am J Neuroradiol*. 1997;18:1311-1315.

See a full reference list on ExpertConsult.com

12 Radiology of the Spine

Todd M. Emch, Ajit A. Krishnaney, and Michael T. Modic

The first role of imaging is to provide reliable anatomic or functional information. The second—and perhaps more important—is to provide information that will guide therapeutic decision making. As a rule, patients are referred for imaging for the evaluation of pain syndromes, functional or mechanical alterations, neurological symptoms suggestive of spinal cord or nerve root involvement, trauma, and congenital abnormalities. The space (extradural, intradural, extramedullary, and intramedullary) in which the abnormality exists, although not known a priori, is an important consideration in the differential diagnosis and selection of diagnostic tests.

The different modalities are discussed in terms of their advantages and disadvantages and for which indications imaging is appropriate. Although imaging can be purely diagnostic, it can also play a role in imaging-guided procedures both for diagnostic and therapeutic aims.

Although formally interpreted by radiologists, imaging of the spine can also be considered a tool used by neurosurgeons, and they should have a high level of skill in interpreting imaging examinations. After a discussion of imaging modalities and common imaging indications, a systematic method of interpreting imaging examinations is presented, with a focus on pathology.

MODALITIES AND TECHNICAL CONSIDERATIONS

The core modalities for spine imaging include conventional radiography, computed tomographic (CT) imaging (including CT myelography), and magnetic resonance imaging (MRI). Additional imaging modalities includes bone scintigraphy, positron emission tomography, and ultrasonography (US), which may be used alone or in conjunction with radiographs, CT imaging, or MRI.

Radiography

Conventional radiography is performed primarily in the extradural space, which includes the osseous structures and, to a lesser extent, the immediately surrounding soft tissues. Conventional radiography is less expensive and easier to perform than CT imaging or MRI. It provides a convenient means of assessing alignment and gross bone integrity and can also be used for purposes of localization in procedural planning and evaluation of movement when flexion-extension views are obtained. It is capable of demonstrating the general changes involving various types of arthritis and disk space narrowing. According to appropriateness criteria, radiography is considered sufficient for the initial evaluation of recent significant trauma, osteoporosis, or back pain in individuals older than 70 years.[1]

Digital radiography, as opposed to conventional techniques, has enabled more flexible handling of images (e.g., duplication, transmission, postprocessing), as well as expedited cycle time. The latter advantage is extremely useful in the intraoperative environment because the results are available immediately after exposure, without the need for traditional processing.[2]

The disadvantages of conventional radiographic techniques are that they visualize mainly osseous structures and are relatively insensitive to soft tissue changes within the disk, ligaments, nerves, and paraspinal tissues. Bone marrow involvement must be significant and far advanced before it is demonstrable on conventional radiographs; a 30% to 75% change must occur for the abnormality to become apparent.[3,4]

Conventional radiographs of the spine can be obtained with lateral and frontal projections and with additional views, including oblique, flexion-extension, and weight-bearing.[5] In radiography, as well as fluoroscopy, ionizing radiation is used, and so this should be considered when pregnant patients and the pediatric population undergo radiography.[6]

Computed Tomographic Imaging

Since its introduction in the 1970s, CT imaging technology has evolved; currently, multidetector devices can cover larger areas in shorter examination times.[7,8] In addition, thinner sections can be used to allow the acquisition of isotropic voxels that can be processed into three-dimensional (3D) data sets, which can be reformatted into any plane without loss of resolution. Subsequent 3D multiplanar reformatted images are particularly useful for the evaluation of trauma, for assessment of fusion postoperatively and pseudoarthrosis, and for instrumentation. Window level and width manipulation can accentuate osseous or soft tissue structures.[6] CT imaging is an important tool and is the first alternative when MRI is contraindicated or unavailable.

CT imaging without contrast material is most useful for evaluation of the extradural space, including osseous structures and surrounding soft tissues. CT imaging can discriminate among various tissues by differences in attenuation and can provide high-resolution bone detail and enough soft tissue information to accurately assess degenerative disk disease and associated changes or sequelae such as herniation, stenosis, and facet arthritis. CT imaging is equivalent to MRI in the diagnosis of a lumbar herniated disk and stenosis but is less accurate in depicting marrow changes and soft tissue structures such as paravertebral lesions, intraspinal structures, or intraspinal isease.[9] The primary disadvantages of CT imaging are the overlap in attenuation with normal and abnormal soft tissue disease and, as with conventional radiography, ionizing radiation.

CT angiography (CTA) can also be obtained with the rapid injection of intravenous contrast material for the evaluation of the vasculature of the neck in cases of trauma, for evaluation of vessel dissection, or in cases in which vessels are encased or displaced by neoplasm.[10]

Myelography

Myelography, in comparison with radiography or cross-sectional imaging, is invasive because exogenous contrast material is administered into the subarachnoid space. Enhancement with contrast material produces both extradural and intradural information. Currently, non-ionic contrast material has a lower rate of complication than do previously used contrast media.[11,12] Complications include postprocedural headaches (10% to 15% of patients) and rare but possible adverse events such as nerve damage, formation of an iatrogenic epidermoid, infection, seizure, allergic reaction, and arachnoiditis. The incidence of headaches severe enough to necessitate treatment (e.g., epidural blood patch) is approximately 1%.[13,14]

To perform myelography, the patient is placed prone, and access to the thecal sac is achieved in a manner similar to that of

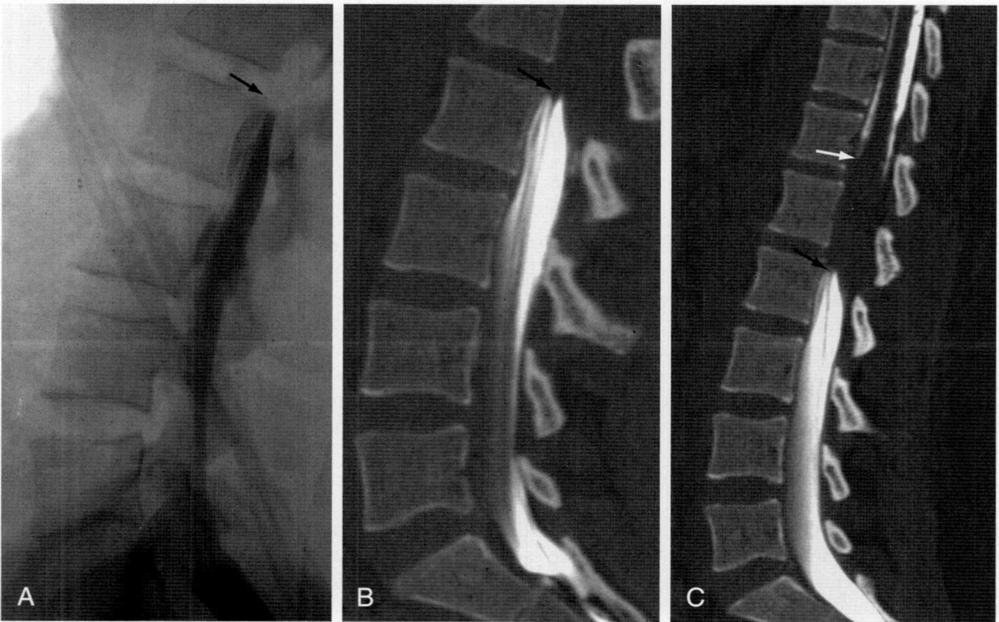

Figure 12-1. Myelographic image **(A)** and computed tomographic (CT) myelogram **(B)** demonstrate lack of cranial extension of contrast material (myelographic block) secondary to epidural extension of metastatic disease *(black arrows)*. CT myelogram **(C)** defines the superior extent of disease *(white arrow)* after intrathecal contrast injection at the C1-C2 level (not shown).

a lumbar puncture: typically at the L2-L3 or L3-L4 level from either a midline or an oblique approach. Once access is achieved, the flow of contrast material is monitored under fluoroscopic guidance during the injection. If contrast material fails to extend cranially as a result of mass effect (a myelographic block), it is necessary to obtain access to the subarachnoid space at the C1-C2 level and inject additional contrast material to define the superior aspect of the lesion (Fig. 12-1).[15]

Myelography can outline the nerve roots, spinal cord, and its coverings. Intradural and extradural disease can be identified and characterized on the basis of the character and structure of its effect on the contrast column (Fig. 12-2). Radiographic contrast-enhanced myelography is rarely performed on its own and is almost always used in conjunction with CT imaging. Conventional radiographic myelography may be useful for general anatomic appraisal in patients with complex deformities or when implanted hardware or electronic devices preclude the use of MRI or CT imaging. CT myelography provides excellent delineation of intradural structures such as the spinal cord and nerve roots and their relationship to the soft tissue and bony surroundings. It is useful in distinguishing bone changes from soft tissue changes (e.g., osteophytes and disk herniations), which may be indistinguishable on radiographic myelograms (Fig. 12-3). Multidetector CT imaging of the entire spinal axis can be performed in 20 to 30 seconds. With intrathecal contrast media, subsequent multiplanar reformatted images can provide complex 3D assessment of anatomic and pathologic abnormalities with myelogram-like images. New forms of dual-energy multidetector CT imaging can subtract out bone in both single slices and 3D multiplanar reformatted images (Fig. 12-4).

The disadvantages of plain and CT myelography concern primarily the intrathecal introduction of contrast media (toxicity and risk of allergic reaction) into the subarachnoid space, use of ionizing radiation, and limited soft tissue discrimination. Premyelography administration of anticoagulants also poses an issue; aside from aspirin, most must be discontinued.[16]

Magnetic Resonance Imaging

MRI is currently the preferred modality for most patients with significant signs and symptoms of spinal disorders.[17] It depicts excellent contrast among different types of soft tissues. MRI without contrast material is capable of evaluating the extradural, intradural extramedullary, and intramedullary spaces. MRI is noninvasive and without the risks associated with ionizing radiation. Anatomic imaging can be performed in different planes, as well as used for volume acquisitions. It is the most sensitive modality and most specific technique for identifying abnormalities of the spinal cord, nerve roots, cerebrospinal fluid (CSF) space, and soft tissues, and it also provides direct visualization of bone marrow. When used with gadolinium complexed with diethylenetriaminepentaacetic acid (DTPA), MRI has even greater sensitivity for detecting intramedullary disease, inflammatory changes, and reparative processes such as may occur with postoperative changes and trauma.[18-22] MRI is particularly efficacious for the evaluation of so-called red flag diagnoses such as osteomyelitis, neoplasia, and trauma.[17]

For evaluation of degenerative disk disease, T1- and T2-weighted images performed in the axial and sagittal planes are used, although fast spin echo, T2-weighted images have replaced conventional T2-weighted images because acquisition times are shorter. Short tau inversion recovery (STIR) or fat-suppressed T2-weighted images are also used to delineate bone marrow or soft tissue edema (Fig. 12-5).[23] Aside from conventional MRI pulse sequences that focus on morphologic features, techniques that provide physiologic or functional information include dynamic imaging, diffusion imaging, spectroscopy, and magnetic resonance neurography.[24,25]

Dynamic Imaging

Methods for dynamic imaging of the spine vary, which adds to the difficulty of determining its usefulness. Available methods

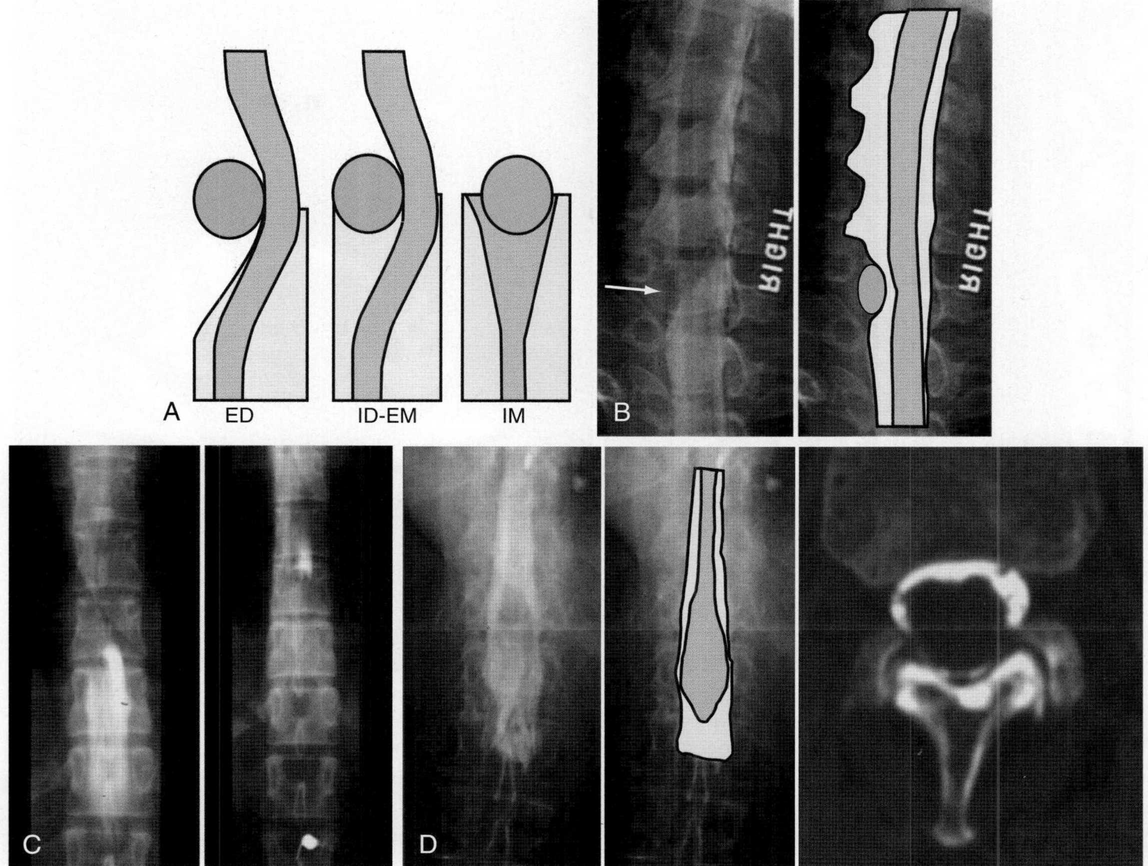

Figure 12-2. A, Diagrammatic representation of extradural (ED), intradural extramedullary (ID-EM), and intramedullary (IM) lesions of the spine. *Purple,* spinal cord; *orange,* mass; *tan,* subarachnoid space. **B,** Oblique view from a cervical myelogram demonstrating an extradural defect *(arrow)* from a herniated disk at the C6-C7 level with cutoff of the nerve root. The superimposed diagram demonstrates the typical concave inward appearance of an extradural defect. **C,** Anteroposterior (AP) radiographs from a thoracic myelogram demonstrating an intradural extramedullary lesion. Contrast agent was introduced into the subarachnoid material below the lesion on the left radiograph and at the C1-C2 level to outline the superior extent of the lesion on the right radiograph. Leftward displacement of the spinal cord silhouette is visible. **D,** *Left and middle,* AP views from a thoracic myelogram demonstrating an intramedullary mass at the conus. The contrast column in the subarachnoid space is splayed around the intramedullary mass. Computed tomographic myelogram *(right)* demonstrates the enlarged conus.

include axial loading with the patient in the supine position and the use of an upright open MRI system that allows flexion-extension imaging (Fig. 12-6).[26,27] The rationale for dynamic imaging is to identify disk protrusions or changes in spinal canal diameter that are not apparent when the conventional supine position is used for imaging.[25,26,28-30] Hiwatashi and colleagues[28] evaluated 200 patients with clinical symptoms of spinal stenosis and, in 20, found that routine and axial-loaded studies yielded detectable differences in caliber of the dural sac. Management was changed in 5 of these patients; the surgeons opted for surgery. Although dynamic imaging has benefits, its routine use appears to be outweighed by patient discomfort and added imaging time.

Neurography

Magnetic resonance neurography is used to evaluate the peripheral nerves, including the brachial and lumbar plexuses, with high-resolution T1-weighted imaging and fat-suppressed T2-weighted or STIR imaging.[24,31,32] Nerve compression, trauma, hypertrophy, neuroma, and tumor infiltration can be evaluated with magnetic resonance neurography.[33,34]

Cerebrospinal Fluid

CSF flow studies with cine MRI provide cardiac-gated gradient phase-contrast images that are displayed qualitatively as CSF flow images in a closed-loop kinematic format (Video 12-1). This same data set can be displayed quantitatively on a graph or in numerical format as analysis of values of flow velocity and volume flow rate.[35] These images demonstrate the pulsatile motion of CSF, not the bulk flow. Pulsatile flow is a result of expansion of the brain during systole and relaxation during diastole and is therefore bidirectional: CSF flows caudally (downward) during systole and cranially (upward) during diastole. Typically, the signal intensity of normal CSF flow in these studies is demonstrated as hyperintense during systole, when flow is caudal, and hypointense during diastole, where flow is cranial. These images are usually

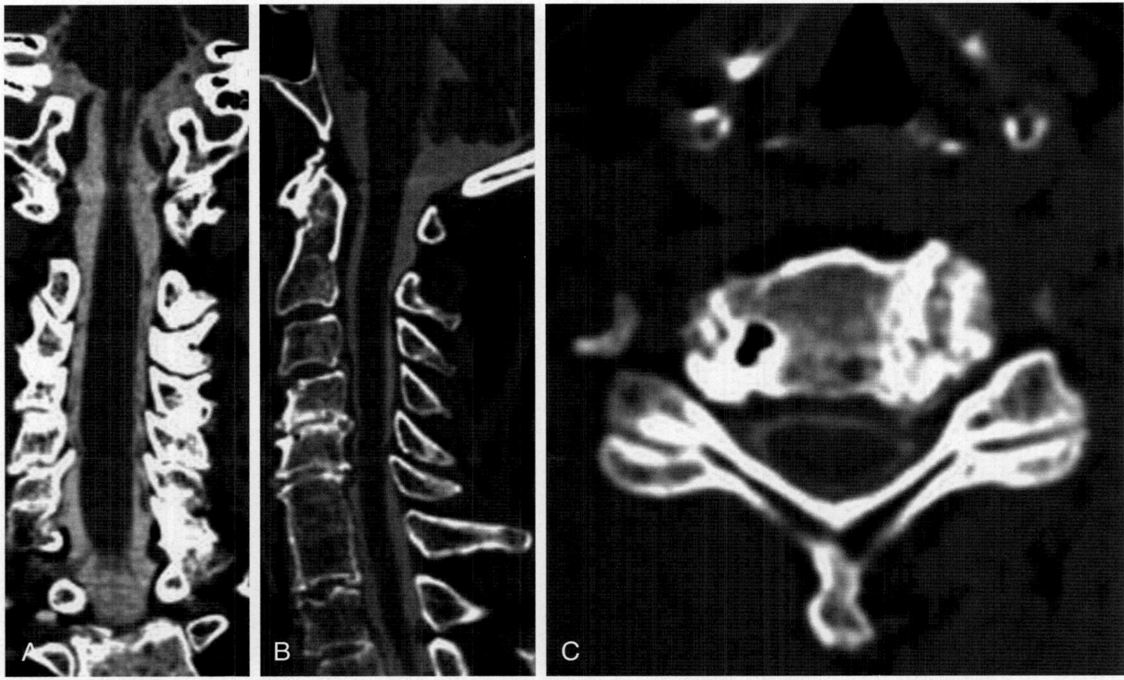

Figure 12-3. Coronal **(A)** and sagittal **(B)** multiplanar reformatted computed tomographic myelograms obtained from the axial data set **(C).** Hypertrophic degenerative changes of the vertebral body margins and uncinate processes are producing extradural indentations on the subarachnoid space.

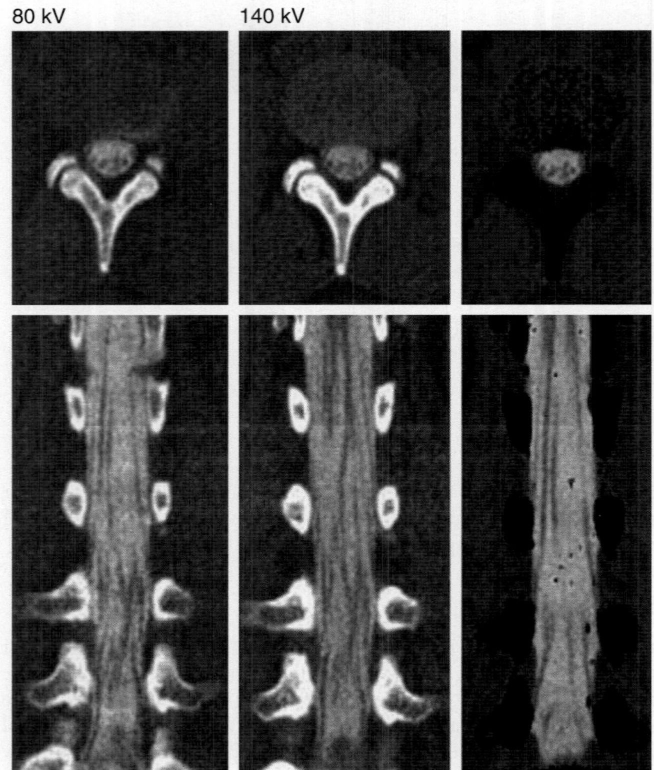

Figure 12-4. Dual-energy subtraction computed tomographic (CT) myelography. Primarily acquired axial and multiplanar reformatted coronal images through the lumbar region from a CT myelographic study were obtained with a CT scanner in which two x-ray tubes were used. Different exposure factors with 80 and 140 kV produced data sets on which subtraction *(right)* could be performed on the basis of attenuation differences related to the exposure factors.

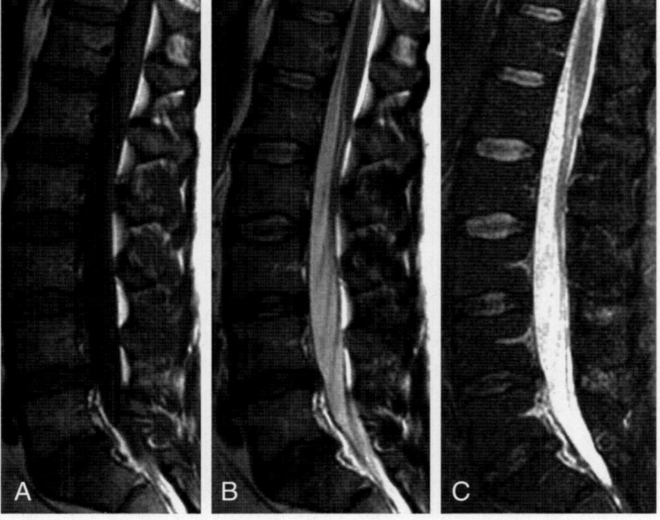

Figure 12-5. Magnetic resonance imaging (MRI) sequences. Images through the lumbar spine demonstrate the different appearances obtained with different techniques. On sagittal T1-weighted spin echo image **(A),** the vertebral body marrow has higher signal intensity than does the intervertebral disk, primarily because of the fat content of the marrow space. On T2-weighted spin echo image **(B),** the intervertebral disk has higher signal intensity than does the vertebral body because of prolonged relaxation time related to both bound and unbound water species. This change in signal is probably a reflection of the health of the proteoglycans more than the total water content. The short tau inversion recovery (STIR) sequence **(C)** demonstrates decreased signal intensity of the marrow space and is the sequence that is most sensitive to marrow involvement. Note the degenerative changes at the L4-L5 and L5-S1 levels. The decreased signal intensity of a degenerative disk is better noted on the T2-weighted and STIR sequences. Note the loss of the internuclear cleft as the degree of degeneration increases, as at the L5-S1 level.

displayed in the sagittal and axial planes. In general, the degree of pulsatile flow diminishes as it proceeds caudally.[36] Clinically, these studies are most often used for the evaluation of CSF flow in patients with Chiari I and II malformations and for the assessment of syrinx cavities (Fig. 12-7).[37,38]

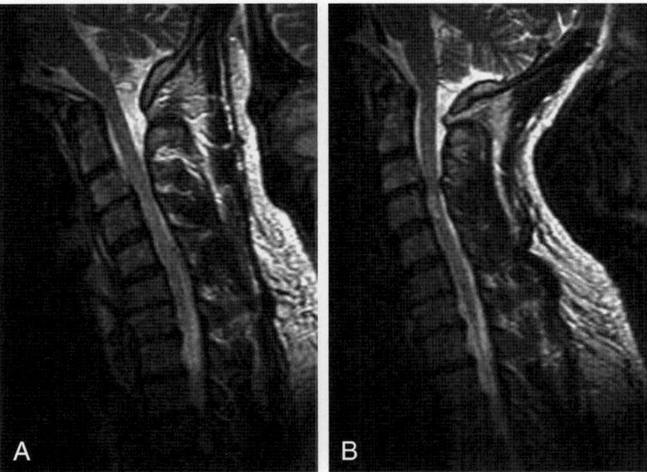

Figure 12-6. Sagittal T2-weighted spin echo images through the cervical spine in flexion **(A)** and extension **(B).** Note the decreased anterior-posterior canal diameter on the extension image (7 versus 4 mm) at the C3-C4 level.

Artifacts and Contraindications

Instrumentation, metal implanted as part of surgical procedures, and implanted electronic devices represent challenges for both CT imaging and MRI. In the case of CT imaging, metal can create beam-hardening artifacts that obscure adjacent soft tissue and osseous structures (Fig. 12-8). Multidetector studies with isotropic voxels and software used to decrease beam-hardening artifact can often decrease the image degradation caused by implanted metal.[39] Different types of metal produce different types of artifacts on MRI that may render the examination uninterpretable. The term *magnetic susceptibility* refers to the manner and amount by which a material becomes magnetized in a magnetic field. Nonferrous magnetic metals may produce local electrical currents induced by the changing field, which causes distortion of the field and artifacts. These artifacts take two main forms: geometric distortion and signal loss secondary to dephasing (Fig. 12-9). Certain techniques are more susceptible to these artifacts, and gradient echo images in particular are especially sensitive to differences in magnetic susceptibility and field homogeneity.

Although metals can cause artifacts that render the examination uninterpretable, certain indwelling devices may be a contraindication to the entire examination. Some types of aneurysm clips, cardiac valves, and vascular devices can result in harm to patients during an MRI examination. Some implantable devices may cease to function properly after an MRI study, and others may be a source of heating with deleterious biologic effects and burns. Publications and websites that track information related to contraindications are available.[39]

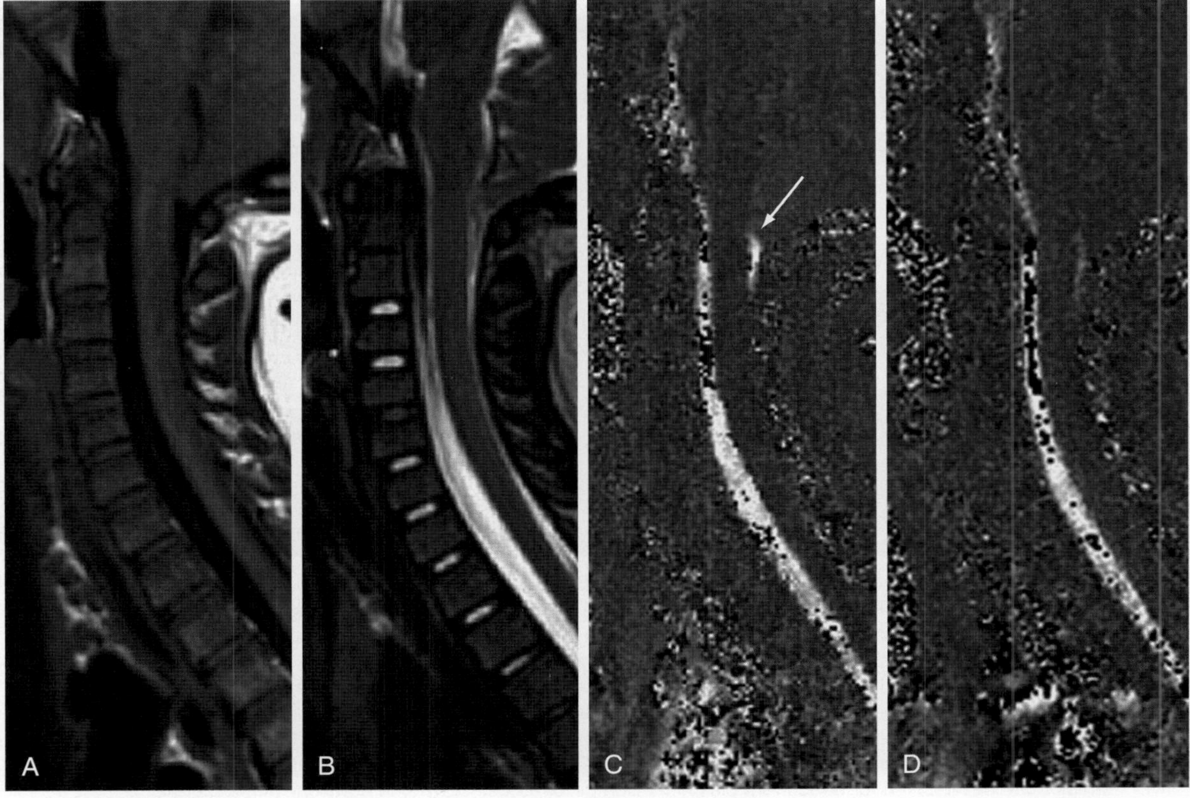

Figure 12-7. Sagittal T1-weighted **(A),** T2-weighted **(B),** and cerebrospinal fluid (CSF) flow studies (**C** and **D**) of the craniovertebral junction in a patient with a Chiari I malformation. Note that the majority of CSF flow is within the basal cisterns and ventral to the cervical cord. Only a small amount of CSF flow is identified dorsally (**C,** *arrow*).

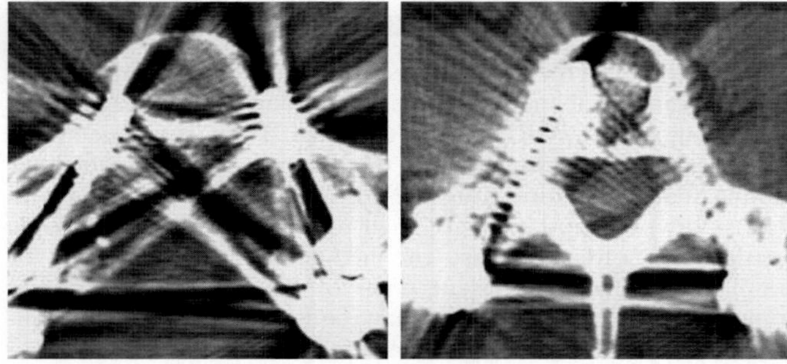

Figure 12-8. Beam-hardening artifact on axial computed tomographic images, caused by pedicle screws.

The primary disadvantages of MRI are related to its cost and safety concerns with regard to electronic devices or implants. The safety issues include heating, dislodgment, and malfunction, as well as image distortion in the presence of metal. Claustrophobia remains a significant problem that sometimes necessitates the use of machines with a larger bore and sedation or general anesthesia. The acquisition of MRI data sets takes considerable longer than that of CT imaging; patient motion also decreases the diagnostic quality of the examination.[40]

Intravenous contrast agents are commonly used with both CT and MRI examinations. Both iodinated (CT imaging) and paramagnetic substances (MRI) are cleared by the kidneys and should be used with caution or not at all in patients with impaired renal function. Although this has been common knowledge with the

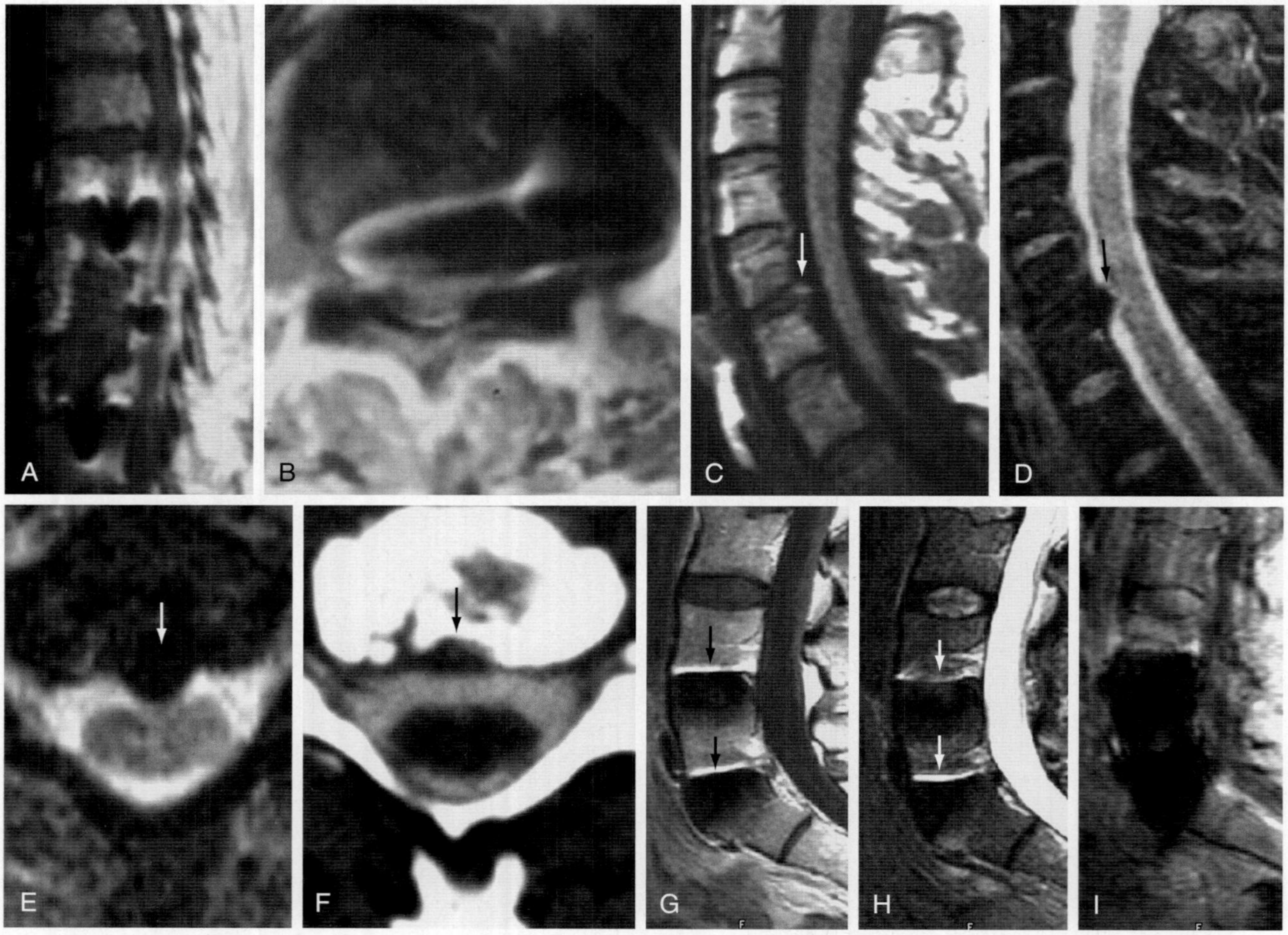

Figure 12-9. Metallic artifacts on sagittal **(A)** and axial **(B)** T1-weighted images through the thoracic spine in a patient with steel rods. There is a geometric artifact with complete distortion of the image as a result of the stainless steel. On the sagittal T1-weighted image **(C),** a small extradural defect is noted at the C5-C6 level *(white arrow).* This defect appears more prominent on the sagittal gradient echo image (**D,** *black arrow*). On the axial gradient echo image **(E),** this defect *(white arrow)* appears to be midline. Axial computed tomographic (CT) myelogram **(F)** shows postsurgical changes *(black arrow)* but no evidence of an extradural defect. These changes are secondary to a susceptibility effect produced by small shards of metal that are often noted on MRI after surgery but are too small to be visible on CT or plain radiographs. The susceptibility artifact can be mistaken for a recurrent disk herniation or for an osteophyte. In a patient with a metallic intradiscal fixation device at the L4-L5 and L5-S1 levels, note that the susceptibility artifact is less prominent on the sagittal T1-weighted sequence (**G,** *black arrows*) than on the sagittal T2-weighted image (**H,** *white arrows*). It is most prominent on the gradient echo image **(I)** because of its heightened sensitivity to field inhomogeneity and susceptibility changes.

iodinated contrast media used for CT imaging, various complications related to the use of paramagnetic contrast agents have been documented in patients with impaired renal function. Despite being uncommon, nephrogenic systemic fibrosis, a late serious adverse reaction to gadolinium, has been well documented.[39,41] In addition, allergic reactions can occur after administration of iodine or gadolinium contrast agents.[42,43]

Last, it may not be possible to perform an examination or procedure within the constraints of table weight limits and maximum open diameters of gantries in CT or MRI machinery.[44]

Spinal Angiography

Spinal angiography can be performed with MRI (magnetic resonance angiography [MRA]), with CTA, and with catheter-based digital subtraction angiography with selective arterial catheterization.[10,45,46] The last technique is still regarded as the most accurate for the detection and pretreatment characterization of vascular malformations of the spinal cord and meninges. Although it is probably associated with the highest risk among procedures for spinal imaging, the complication rate has been greatly reduced with the use of microcatheters and more experienced users. Definitive treatment of vascular lesions by endovascular means is now more common, and the examination can be better directed by information from diagnostic MRA and CTA studies, which can help focus the catheter examination.[47,48] MRA—the addition of angiography to standard MRI—does not have significantly different sensitivity, specificity, and accuracy of detection of spinal malformations, but it often provides detection of the level of a fistula or vascular malformation. CTA of the spinal axis is relatively easy to perform and is also useful in identifying the level of involvement.

Ultrasonography

The use of ultrasonography in the spine is limited because of the sound waves' difficulty penetrating bone. Its main value is intraoperative, for additional characterization and localization of disease such as spinal cord tumors, and in pediatric applications.[49] High-frequency probes that improve spatial resolution are commonly used intraoperatively because of the ability to directly approach the region of disease.[50]

Thermography, Diskography, and Computed Tomographic Diskography

Most experts believe that thermography findings are too nonspecific to be of significant value for the evaluation of spinal disorders.[17] Diskography is a technique that, by nature of direct stimulation, is thought by some experts to be able to identify painful and concordant disks.[1,51] Diskography and CT diskography are still used, especially when other imaging modalities have failed to localize the cause of pain. The morphologic information is not as critical as reproduction of a patient's characteristic pain. Although some data support its use, prospective well-controlled trials in support of its prognostic value remain absent from the literature.

Nuclear Medicine Examinations

Technetium 99m methylene diphosphonate bone scans are most useful for evaluation of the extradural space. Bone scans are a moderately sensitive test for detecting the presence of tumor, infection, or occult fractures of the vertebrae but are rarely specific for diagnosis. The yield is very low in patients in whom radiographic and laboratory results are normal and highest in those with known malignancy.[52] These scans are contraindicated during pregnancy. They are an important tool for surveying the entire skeleton for metastatic disease and can visualize as low as a 5% change in bone marrow. In lytic or aggressive lesions, however, there may be an absence of radiotracer uptake, which is indicative of a "cold" lesion; increased radiotracer uptake, in contrast, is indicative of more osteoblast activity.[53,54]

To further evaluate sites that appear positive on bone scans, single-photon emission computed tomography (SPECT) and positron emission tomography (PET) with fluorodeoxyglucose are often used in conjunction with CT imaging and are capable of improved specificity and anatomic localization, particularly in patients with malignancies.[55] While PET-CT is commonly used in disease staging, PET-MRI is an emerging technology showing diagnostic promise.[56] Indium 111 octreotide, a somatostatin analogue, demonstrates uptake in neuroendocrine tumors and meningiomas.[57]

INDICATIONS FOR IMAGING AND IMAGING FINDINGS

Although determining the proper examination to be obtained in a particular clinical context is important, clinicians must also recognize that imaging is not necessary in certain situations, such as cases of uncomplicated acute back pain and low risk trauma.[58,59]

Degenerative Disk Disease, Including Back Pain

Degenerative disk disease includes desiccation, fibrosis, narrowing of the disk space, diffuse bulging of the annulus beyond the disk space, extensive fissuring and mucinous degeneration of the annulus, end plate changes, and osteophytes at the vertebral apophyses. Conventional radiographs can identify disk space narrowing, bone changes, and malalignment. CT studies can further identify disk herniation and provide better morphologic characterization of various types of stenosis. MRI provides the greatest spectrum of morphologic findings: degenerative changes are manifested as disk space narrowing, loss of T2-weighted signal intensity from the intervertebral disk, fissures, vacuum disk changes, disk calcifications, ligamentous hypertrophy or edema, end plate marrow signal changes, osteophytosis, disk herniation, malalignment, and stenosis.[60]

Degenerative Disk Changes

The major cartilaginous joint (amphiarthrosis) of the vertebral column is the intervertebral disk. Each disk consists of the nucleus pulposus and the annulus fibrosus. In degenerative disk disease, there are alterations to disk hydration, collagen, and proteoglycans, with eventual loss of the delineation between the annulus fibrosus and nucleus pulposus.[61-63] MRI demonstrates this change as low-signal intensity on T2-weighted images (Fig. 12-10).[21] Although this low T2 signal intensity of a degenerated disk is commonly referred to as *desiccation*, absolute measurements of cadaver disks on T2-weighted images are correlated more closely with the glycosaminoglycan concentration than with the absolute water content; this finding suggests that the signal changes are a reflection of the state of water rather than of total water volume.

Annular tears or fissures occur when there is disruption of all or some of the layers of the annular lamellae. Whether these fissures are a manifestation or a cause of degenerative disk disease is not known; however, one theory suggests that once the annulus fibrosus is disrupted, there is subsequent alteration of nucleus pulposus and then the disk is replaced by fibrous tissue and cystic spaces (Fig. 12-11).[64-68]

Vacuum disk phenomena representing gas, principally nitrogen, occur at sites of negative pressure in the intervertebral disk,[69] manifested as lucency on radiographs, low attenuation on CT imaging, or low-signal intensity on MRI (Fig. 12-12).[70]

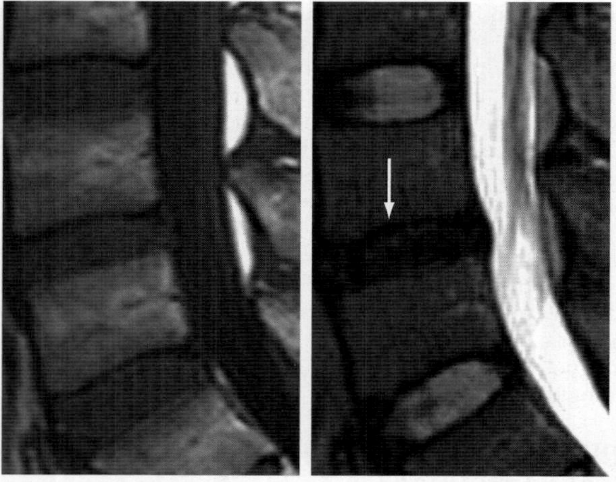

Figure 12-10. Degenerative disk disease. There is mild disk space narrowing *(arrow)* and loss of signal intensity on T2-weighted images of the L4-L5 intervertebral disk.

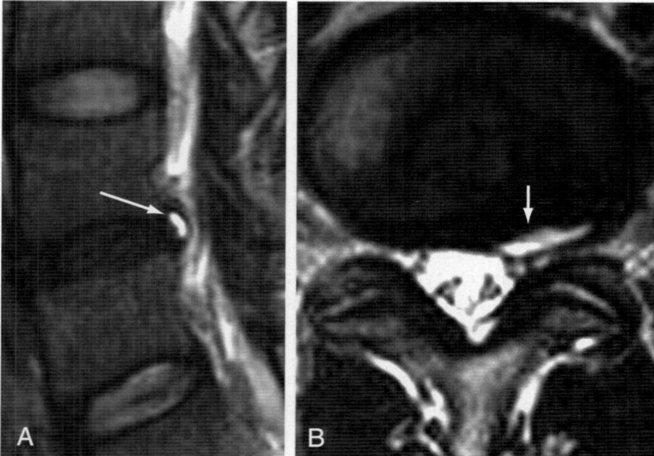

Figure 12-11. Annular tear on parasagittal **(A)** and axial **(B)** T2-weighted images through the L4-L5 intervertebral disk. Note the high-signal intensity in the outer annulus/longitudinal ligament complex, which represents the area of annular disruption *(arrows).*

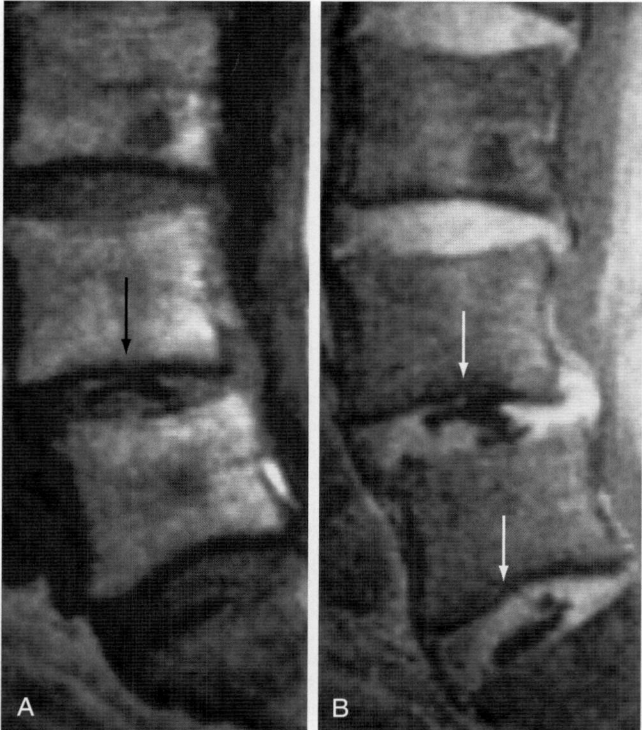

Figure 12-12. Vacuum disk phenomenon. Note the decreased signal intensity within the L4-L5 intervertebral disk, which is better depicted on the gradient echo image (**B,** *white arrow*) than on the spin echo image (**A,** *black arrows*).

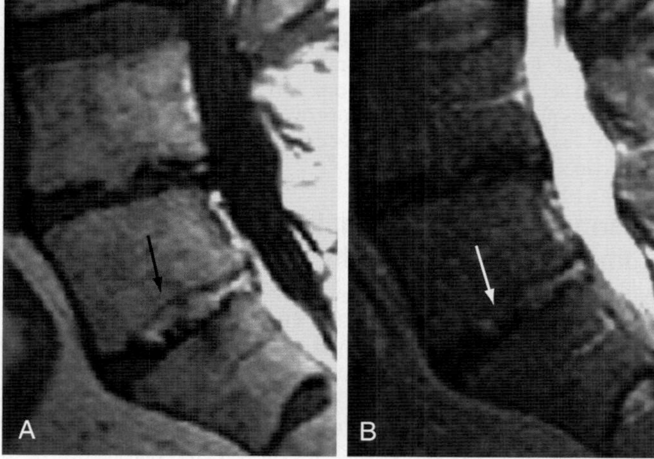

Figure 12-13. Intervertebral disk calcification ***(arrows).*** Note the high-signal intensity on T1-weighted **(A)** and T2-weighted **(B)** images at the L5-S1 level.

Intradiskal or intraosseous air is most commonly degenerative in nature; it can occur with infection, although this is uncommon.[71]

In addition, disks can calcify with degenerative disk disease. Increased density on radiographs or increased attenuation on CT imaging is the most common findings. The appearance of calcification on MRI can be variable, ranging from low in signal intensity (most common) to demonstrating T1 hyperintensity depending on the concentration of calcification (Fig. 12-13).[72] T1 hyperintensity that changes to low-signal intensity with fat saturation is thought to represent ossification with fatty marrow in severe disk degeneration or degenerative disk fusion.

Disk degeneration has been classified in a scheme that has reasonable intraobserver and interobserver agreement.[73] Although MRI demonstrates morphologic alterations in the intervertebral disk with degenerative changes, no clear correlation with symptoms has been identified as of yet.

Degenerative Marrow Changes

Changes in signal intensity of the vertebral body marrow adjacent to the end plates of degenerated disks are a long recognized and common observation on MRI of the lumbar spine.[74,75] However, despite a growing body of literature on this subject, their clinical importance and relationship to symptoms remain unclear.[76]

These marrow changes appear to take three main forms and can be simplistically thought of as edema (type I), fat (type II), and sclerosis (type III). Type I changes consist of decreased signal intensity on T1-weighted images and increased signal intensity on T2-weighted images (Fig. 12-14). They have been identified in approximately 4% of patients scanned for lumbar disease,[75] in approximately 8% of patients after discectomy,[77] and in 40% to

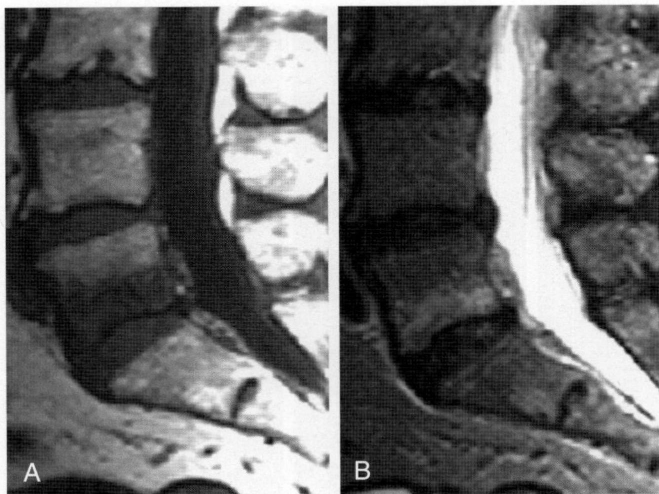

Figure 12-14. Type I degenerative marrow changes. Signal intensity of the L5 vertebral body adjacent to the degenerated disk space is decreased on the sagittal T1-weighted image **(A)** and increased on the sagittal T2-weighted image **(B).**

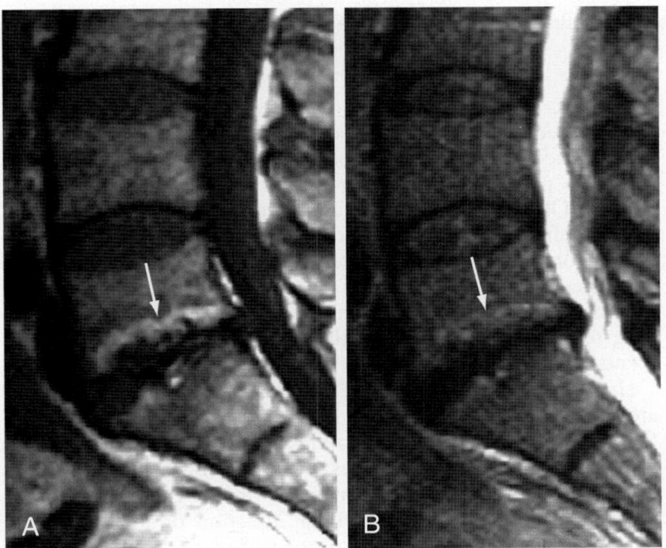

Figure 12-15. Type II degenerative marrow change *(arrows).* Signal intensity along the opposing margins of L5 and S1 is increased on both T1-weighted **(A)** and T2-weighted **(B)** images.

50% of chymopapain-treated disks, which may be viewed as a model of acute disk degeneration.[78] Histopathologic analysis of type I changes demonstrates abnormal fibrovascular tissue in the vertebral end plates, which accounts for the MRI findings, and also indicates the potential for enhancement. Type II changes are represented by increased signal intensity on T1-weighted images and isointense or slightly hyperintense signal on T2-weighted images (Fig. 12-15). These changes are present in approximately 16% of patients undergoing MRI. Type II changes comprise end plate disruption and fatty marrow replacement, which account for their MRI appearance. Type III changes are characterized by low-signal intensity on all pulse sequences and as sclerosis on radiographs. Low-signal intensity of type III end plate change represents the sparseness of marrow in areas of advanced sclerosis, which reflects the development of dense woven bone (Fig. 12-16).[79]

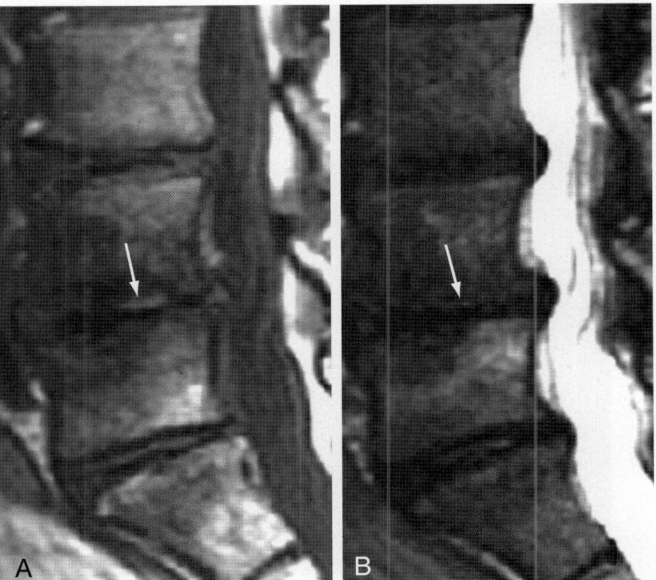

Figure 12-16. Type III degenerative marrow change *(arrows).* Signal intensity of the opposing vertebral body margins at the L4-L5 level is decreased on both T1-weighted **(A)** and T2-weighted **(B)** images.

Similar marrow changes in end plates have also been noted in the pedicles (Fig. 12-17). Although originally described as being associated with spondylolysis, they have also been noted in patients with degenerative facet disease and pedicle fractures.[80,81] The exact mechanism by which these marrow changes occur is not known. The association of these marrow changes with degenerative disk disease, facet changes, and pars and pedicle fractures suggest that they are a response to biomechanical stress.

Of these three types of changes, type I changes appear to be most dynamic, affected by ongoing underlying pathologic processes such as continuing degeneration with associated changing biomechanical stresses. Type I changes are most often associated with ongoing low back symptoms.[82-86] In a longitudinal study, the incidence of new degenerative marrow changes was 6% over a 3-year period, most being type I.[83] In a study of patients with nonoperated low back pain, Mitra and associates[84] found that 92% of type I changes converted either wholly or partially to type II changes (52%), became more extensive (40%), or remained unchanged (8%). There was an improvement in symptoms in patients in whom type I changes converted to type II.

Some diskography studies in patients with degenerative marrow changes have suggested that type I marrow changes are invariably associated with painful disks.[87,88] Other studies have failed to reproduce this association, and thus the relationship between degenerative marrow changes and diskogenic pain remains unproven.[89,90]

Multiple authors have observed a variety of inflammatory mediators in association with degenerative marrow changes. Burke and colleagues[89] observed an increase in proinflammatory mediators in the disks of patients with type I marrow changes who were undergoing fusion for low back pain. Ohtori and coworkers[91] found that the cartilaginous end plates of patients with type I marrow changes had more protein gene product (PGP) 9.5–immunoreactive nerve fibers and more tumor necrosis factor (TNF)–immunoreactive cells than did normal end plates.[91] PGP 9.5 immunoreactivity occurred exclusively in patients with diskogenic low back pain. TNF immunoreactivity in end plates with type I marrow changes was higher than in those with type

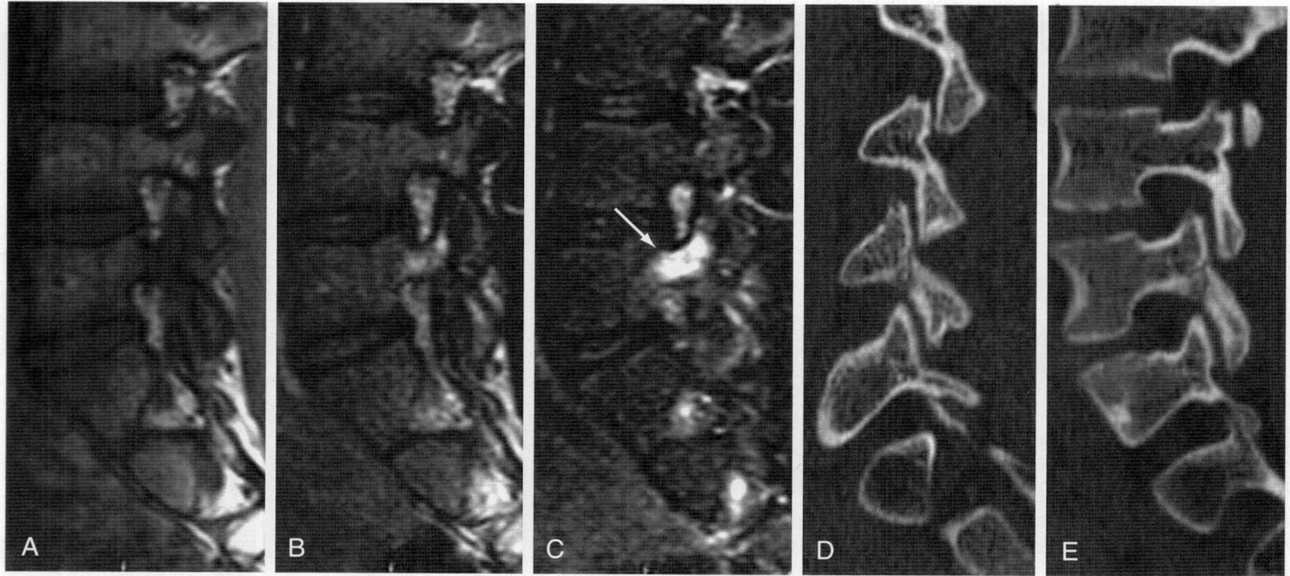

Figure 12-17. Pedicle hyperintensity/pars interarticularis fracture. Parasagittal T1-weighted **(A)**, T2-weighted **(B)**, and short tau inversion recovery (STIR) **(C)** images demonstrate high-signal intensity within the pedicle of L4, which is best appreciated on the STIR sequence (**C,** *arrow*). Parasagittal **(E)** and sagittal **(E)** computed tomographic multiplanar reformatted images demonstrate a subacute fracture through the pars at the L4-L5 level.

II marrow changes. Rahme and Moussa[76] concluded that type I marrow changes represent a more active inflammation mediated by proinflammatory cytokines, whereas type II and type III changes are more quiescent. In a study of infliximab, a monoclonal antibody against TNF-α, Korhonen and associates[92] found that it was most effective when degenerative type I marrow changes were symptomatic. Nevertheless, the relationship of degenerative marrow changes to immunobiologic and cellular response mechanisms, although probably important, remains unclear.

In a study by Toyone and colleagues,[86] segmental hypermobility was present in 70% of patients with type I marrow changes but in only 16% with type II changes.[86] The greatest evidence that these marrow changes, particularly type I, are related to biomechanical instability is probably based on observations after fusion. Chataigner and collaborators[93] suggested that patients with type I marrow changes have much better outcomes with surgery than do those with isolated degenerative disk disease and normal or type II marrow changes. In addition, conversion of type I marrow changes to either normal or type II was associated with higher fusion rates and better outcomes. Other studies support the contention that persistence of type I changes after fusion suggests pseudoarthrosis and is associated with persistent symptoms. Conversely, conversion of type I marrow changes to either normal or type II changes is associated with higher fusion rates and better outcomes (Fig. 12-18).[94-96] The conclusion is that fusion produces greater stability, reduces biomechanical stress, and accelerates the course of type I marrow changes toward improvement.

As further support that these fluid marrow changes reflect biomechanical stress, there is similar marrow conversion in the pedicles of vertebral bodies associated with symptomatic pars and pedicle fractures, as well as in severe degenerative facet joint disease. Pedicle marrow change to a normal or type II appearance is associated with improvement in symptoms.[97]

Additional research has yielded findings that type I end plate changes can be secondary to infection.[98] Stirling and colleagues[99] found positive cultures in 19 of 36 disks obtained after microdiscectomy. In 16 of those 19 disks, *Propionibacterium acnes* was isolated.[99] Albert and associates[100] found similar results by studying patients undergoing surgery for degenerative disk disease. Of the patients who underwent discectomy, 43% had positive anaerobic cultures, and 80% of those patients went on to develop new type I end plate changes. Because these findings suggested that disk herniations can provide conditions favorable for low-grade anaerobic infections, a study was performed with long-term antibiotic therapy; the treatment produced improvements over the placebo.[98]

In summary, type I end plate changes are more strongly associated with pain and underlying instability and also are predictive for a favorable outcome after stabilization surgery. Type I changes can progress to type II changes, which are more static and less associated with symptoms. Conversion of type II changes to type I changes would raise concern for infection or progression in degenerative changes. The origin of end plate changes on MRI is thought to be secondary to mechanical stresses/instability, possibly in combination with biochemical or infectious factors, although additional research is needed.

Degenerative Facet and Ligamentous Changes

The zygoapophyseal joint is composed of the superior and inferior articulating facets and, like diarthrodial synovium-lined joints, it is susceptible to arthropathy (Fig. 12-19). Loss of disk space height and altered biomechanics result in facet joint arthrosis and osteophytosis with consequent canal, foraminal, and lateral recess stenosis. Alternatively, it has been proposed that facet arthropathy can occur independently and be inherently symptomatic.[101,102] Aside from facet arthrosis, joint effusions can occur, with pain caused by irritation of nerve fibers of the synovium and joint capsule.[102] Probably as a result of osteoarthritis and instability of the facet joints, 2.3% of synovial cysts are in anterior or intraspinal locations and 7.3% are in posterior or extraspinal locations (Fig. 12-20).[103]

Ligaments of the spine are the anterior longitudinal ligament, the posterior longitudinal ligament, the paired sets of ligamenta

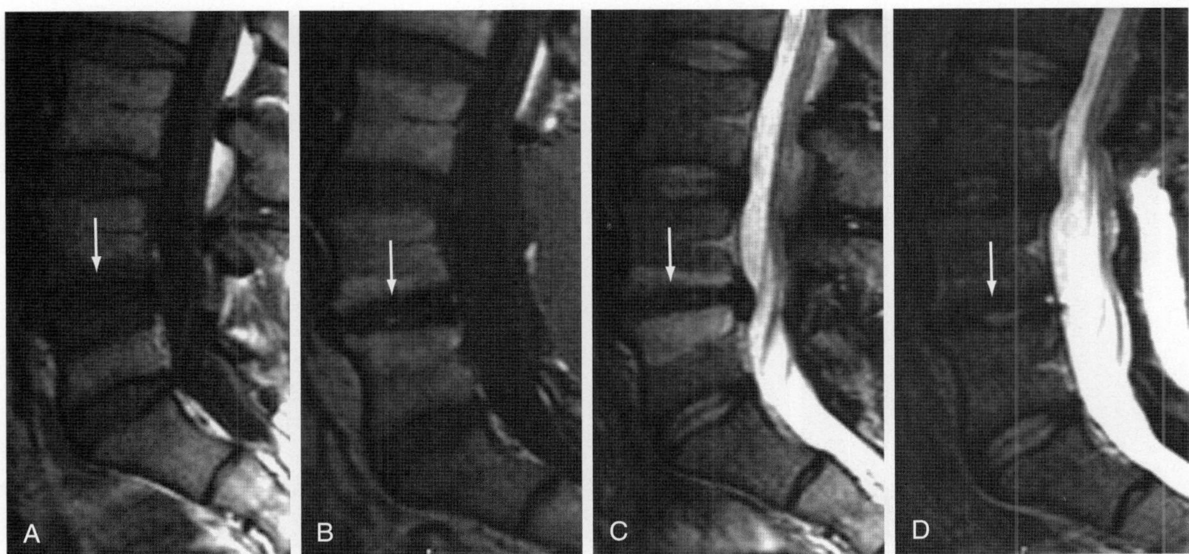

Figure 12-18. Conversion of type I marrow changes. Preoperative (**A** and **C**) and postoperative (**B** and **D**) images of the lumbar spine in a patient after lumbar fusion demonstrate typical type I marrow changes at the L4-L5 level preoperatively *(arrows).* Postoperatively, the type I changes converted to type II changes. The decreased signal on the preoperative T1-weighted image converted to an increased signal that represents lipid marrow conversion. The increased signal intensity on the preoperative T2-weighted image has resolved.

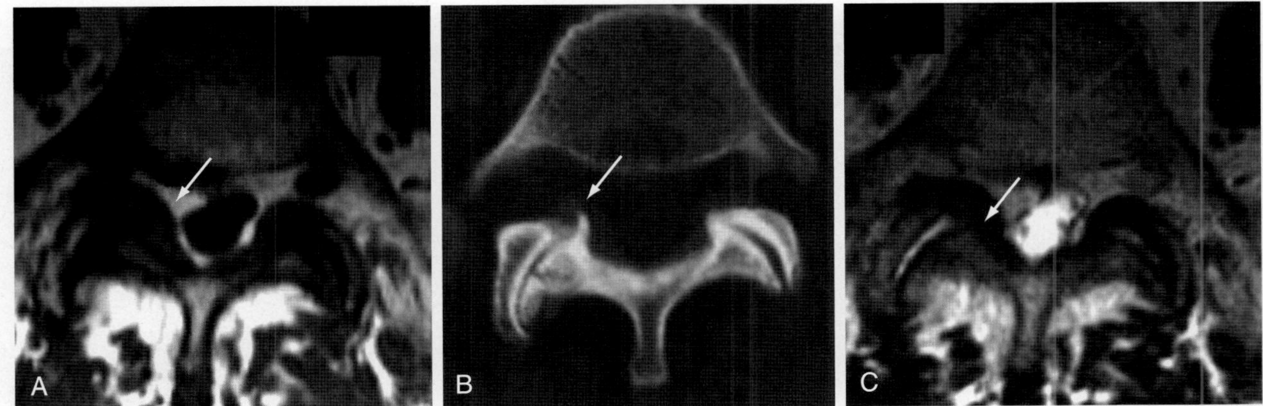

Figure 12-19. Degenerative facet changes. These changes *(arrows)* are visible on a T1-weighted image **(A),** a high-resolution computed tomographic image **(B),** and a T2-weighted spin echo axial image **(C)** through the L4-L5 facets. Note the bony osteophyte along the anterior margin of the inferior facet at L4 on the right and the degenerative facet narrowing bilaterally. The bony changes are not as obvious on the T1- and T2-weighted images, but narrowing and asymmetrical soft tissue are clearly identifiable on magnetic resonance imaging.

flava, the intertransverse ligaments, and the unpaired supraspinous ligament. Alterations in alignment can lead to ligamentous laxity, followed by subsequent deterioration with loss of elasticity, calcification, and ossification. Exaggerated lordosis or severe disk space loss in the lumbar spine leads to close approximation and contact of the spinous processes and to degeneration of intervening ligaments.[104,105]

Alignment Abnormalities

Spondylolisthesis can be classified as degenerative, isthmic, iatrogenic, and traumatic. Alterations in alignment can result from degenerative changes centered at the intervertebral disk, vertebral bodies, and facet joints, which can alter normal spinal movement. Degenerative spondylolisthesis is related primarily to degenerative changes of the apophyseal joints and is most common at the L4-L5 vertebral level (Fig. 12-21), where the orientation of the facet joints tend to be more sagittal. The pars interarticularis is typically intact. Rostrocaudal facet joint subluxation can occur when disk space is narrowed.[60]

Disk Herniation

Disk herniation is the displacement of nucleus pulposus, cartilage, fragmented apophyseal bone, or fragmented annular tissue beyond the intervertebral disk space. The opposing vertebral end plates define the superior and inferior margins of the disk space. Peripherally, the disk space is defined by the outer edges of the vertebral ring apophyses.

The term *herniated disk* and nomenclature standardization are purely morphologic; there is no implication of cause, relation to patient's symptoms, or need for treatment. Herniations can be

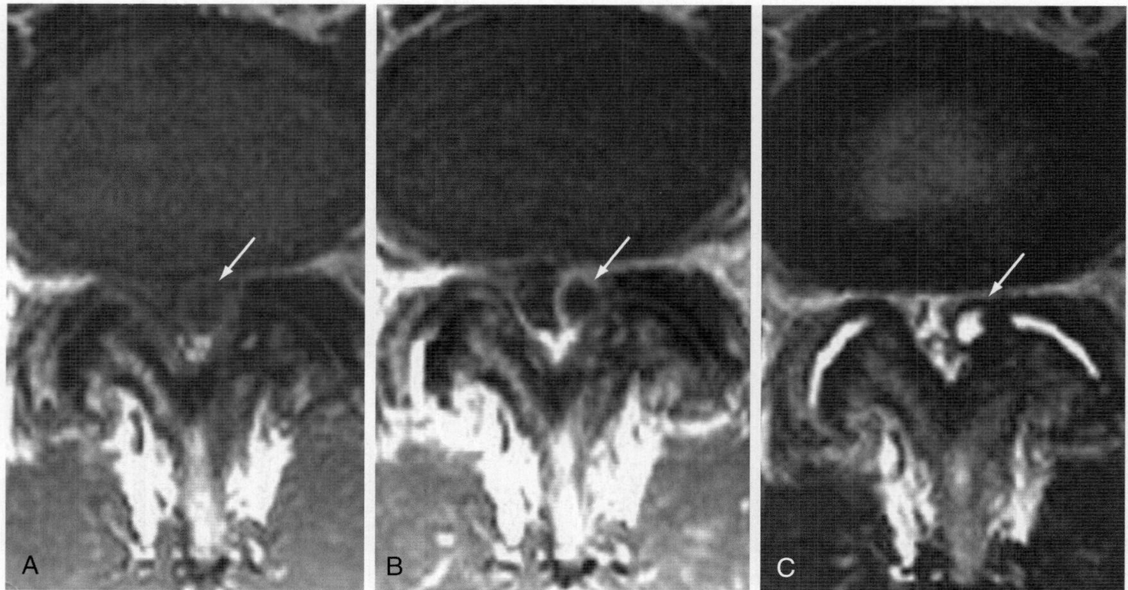

Figure 12-20. Synovial cyst. Synovial cyst demonstrated on images through the facets at the L4-L5 level. There are severe bilateral degenerative facet changes with distraction and fluid. On the axial T1-weighted image **(A)**, an ill-defined soft tissue mass is projecting medially off the left facet *(arrow)*. On the contrast-enhanced T1-weighted image **(B)**, this soft tissue mass *(arrow)* is clearly outlined by peripheral enhancement. The T2-weighted image **(C)** demonstrates that this mass *(arrow)* has high-signal intensity, suggestive of fluid.

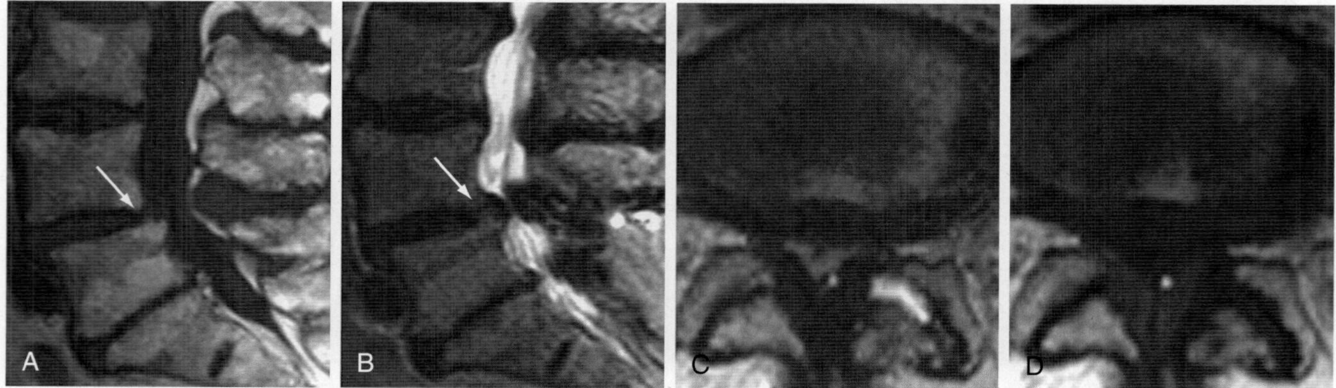

Figure 12-21. Degenerative spondylolisthesis. Sagittal T1-weighted **(A)** and T2-weighted **(B)** spin echo images of the lumbar spine demonstrate grade I spondylolisthesis of L4 on L5 *(arrows)*, as well as severe central canal stenosis and thickening of the posterior ligaments. Axial T1-weighted **(C)** and T2-weighted **(D)** images through the L4-L5 level demonstrate the severe central canal stenosis, thickened posterior ligaments, and severe bilateral degenerative facet changes.

localized or generalized, in which width of the herniation is greater than 50% (180 degrees) of the periphery of the disk.[106] Herniations occur either with disruption of the annulus fibrosus or with disruption of the vertebral end plate (Schmorl's node). Disruption of the annulus is inferred when disk material extends beyond the edges of the ring apophyses by less than 50% (180 degrees) of the circumference of the disk (Fig. 12-22). Localized displacement in the axial plane can be focal (less than 25% of the disk circumference) or broad based (between 25% and 50% of the disk circumference). Extension of disk material circumferentially (50% to 100%) beyond the edges of the ring apophyses is referred to as *bulging* and is not considered a form of herniation.

Other categories of herniations include protrusions and extrusions. If the greatest distance, in any plane, between the edges of the disk material beyond the disk space is less than the distance between the edges of the base in the same plane, the herniation is considered a protrusion (Fig. 12-23). If, in at least one plane, any one distance between the edges of the disk material beyond the disk space is greater than the distance between the edges of the base in the same plane, or when no continuity exists between the disk material beyond the disk space and that within the disk space, the herniation is considered an extrusion (Fig. 12-24). The condition in which disk material has lost continuity with the parent disk is sequestration. Displacement of disk material away from the site of extrusion, regardless of whether it is sequestrated (Fig. 12-25), is migration. There can multiple herniations at a single disk space.[107]

Schmorl's nodes, or intravertebral herniations, are herniations in the cranial or caudal plane, extending through a defect in the

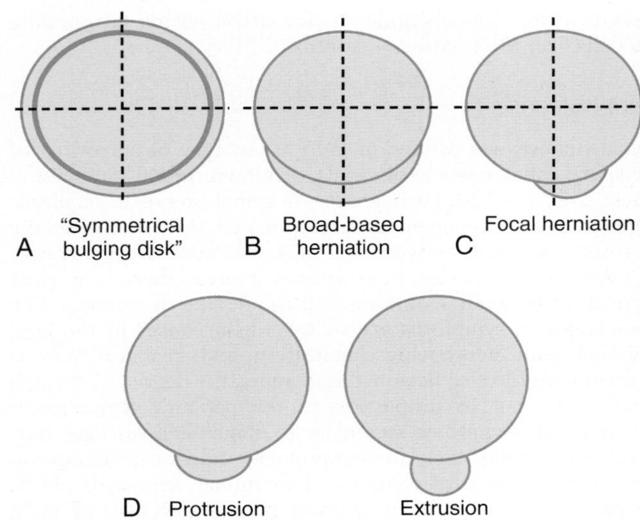

Figure 12-22. A, Symmetrical bulging disk. **B,** Broad-based herniation. **C,** Focal herniation. **D,** Protrusion and extrusion.

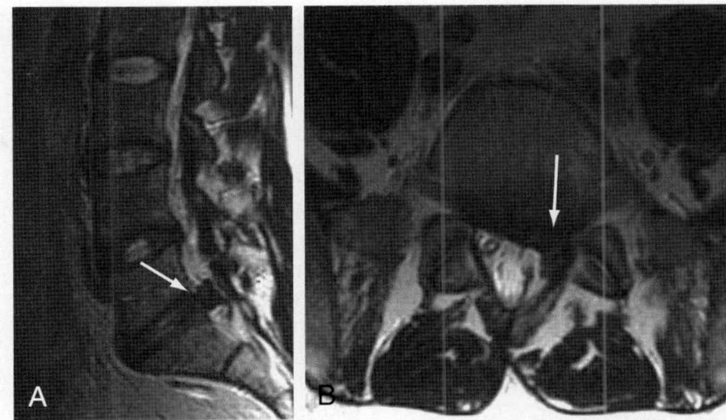

Figure 12-24. Disk extrusion. Sagittal **(A)** and axial **(B)** T2-weighted images of the lumbar spine demonstrate disk extrusion *(arrows)* on the sagittal image with a narrow base. The axial image demonstrates posterior displacement of the S1 nerve root on the left as a result of this disk extrusion.

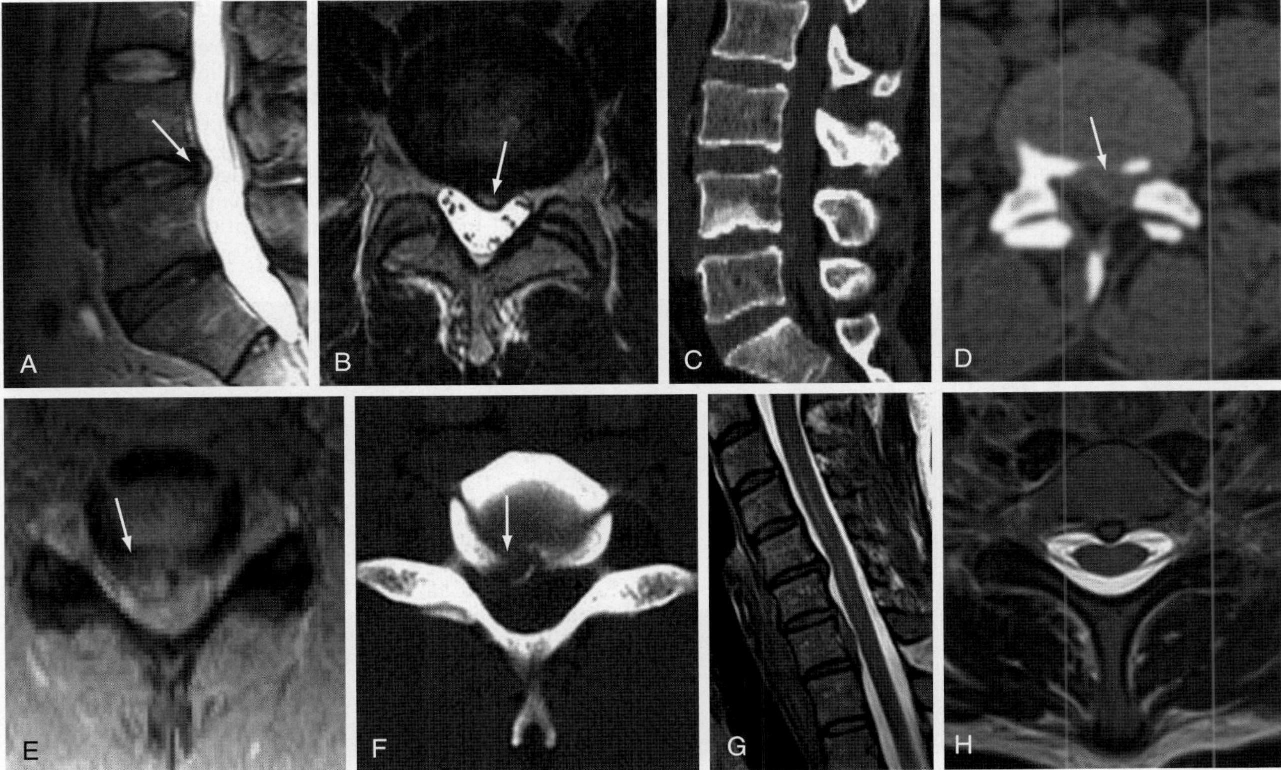

Figure 12-23. Disk protrusion. Sagittal T2-weighted image **(A)** of the lumbar spine shows that the disk extends beyond the vertebral body margins *(arrow);* the axial T2-weighted image **(B)** shows the base to be broader than the posterior extent *(arrow).* Sagittal multiplanar reformatted (MPR) computed tomographic (CT) image **(C)** through the lumbar spine demonstrates an ill-defined soft tissue mass projecting posteriorly at the L4-L5 disk level. The broad-based disk protrusion is better depicted on the axial MPR CT image **(D)** *(white arrow).* Axial gradient echo magnetic resonance image **(E)** and CT image **(F)** at the C5-C6 level demonstrate the broad-based right-sided disk protrusion *(arrows).* Sagittal **(G)** and axial **(H)** T2-weighted images of the cervical spine demonstrate disk protrusion at the C5-C6 level and disk extrusion with an inferior fragment at the C6-C7 level. The axial image through the body of C7 demonstrates the rounded soft tissue mass centrally in the anterior epidural space.

vertebral body end plate. Nonacute Schmorl's nodes, which demonstrate lack of edema on MRI, can be considered incidental findings and have been reported in 38% to 75% of the general population.[108,109] Most Schmorl's nodes are believed to occur after increased axial loading in the setting of a normal annulus fibrosus, although they can also occur when an alteration to the normal vertebral body end plate occurs secondary to neoplasm, infection, or any process that weakens the end plate or the underlying bone. Although Schmorl's nodes are considered an incidental finding when chronic in nature, some patients report a remote history of acute back pain without radiculopathy, which supports the theory that Schmorl's nodes are caused by traumatic axial loading. In cases of acute Schmorl's nodes, bone marrow edema surrounding the defect on MRI has been described.[110]

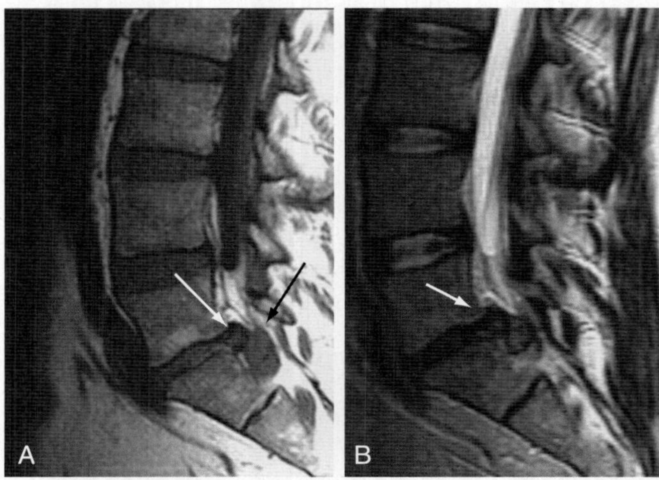

Figure 12-25. Disk extrusion and a free fragment. Sagittal T1-weighted **(A)** and T2-weighted **(B)** images of the lumbar spine reveal the disk extrusion *(white arrows)* and an inferior fragment (**A,** *black arrow*).

Spinal Stenosis

Spinal stenosis was defined in 1975 as any type of narrowing of the spinal canal, nerve root canals, or intervertebral foramina.[111] There are two broad categories of spinal stenosis: acquired/degenerative and congenital/developmental. A developmentally narrowed canal can be worsened by superimposed degenerative disk disease (Fig. 12-26). For acquired stenosis, there is no clear correlation between symptoms and the degree of stenosis. The most common symptoms are sensory disturbances in the legs, low back pain, neurogenic claudication, and weakness; pain is relieved with forward flexion. On imaging, the degree of stenosis tends to be out of proportion to the patient's symptoms.[112] Patients with symptoms secondary to spinal stenosis have narrower spinal canals than do asymptomatic individuals. Extension worsens the degree of central and foraminal stenosis by 11%, whereas flexion appears to improve it by an average of 11%. Segmental instability, which can cause static and dynamic stenosis, is considered a cause of low back pain.[113] Despite the strengths of MRI and CT imaging in defining morphologic findings in spinal stenosis and degenerative disk disease, prognostic information is lacking, and clinicians cannot predict which patients will benefit from or do well with surgery.[114]

Significance of Imaging Findings and When to Image

The goals of advanced imaging is to provide accurate morphologic information that will then guide clinical decision making.[115] Bridging these two factors is the natural history of degenerative disk disease and the high prevalence of morphologic alterations in asymptomatic individuals.[116-118] Of asymptomatic patients, 20% to 28% demonstrate morphologic abnormalities, including disk herniations and other findings of degenerative disk disease.[116-118] In a study of symptomatic patients with low back

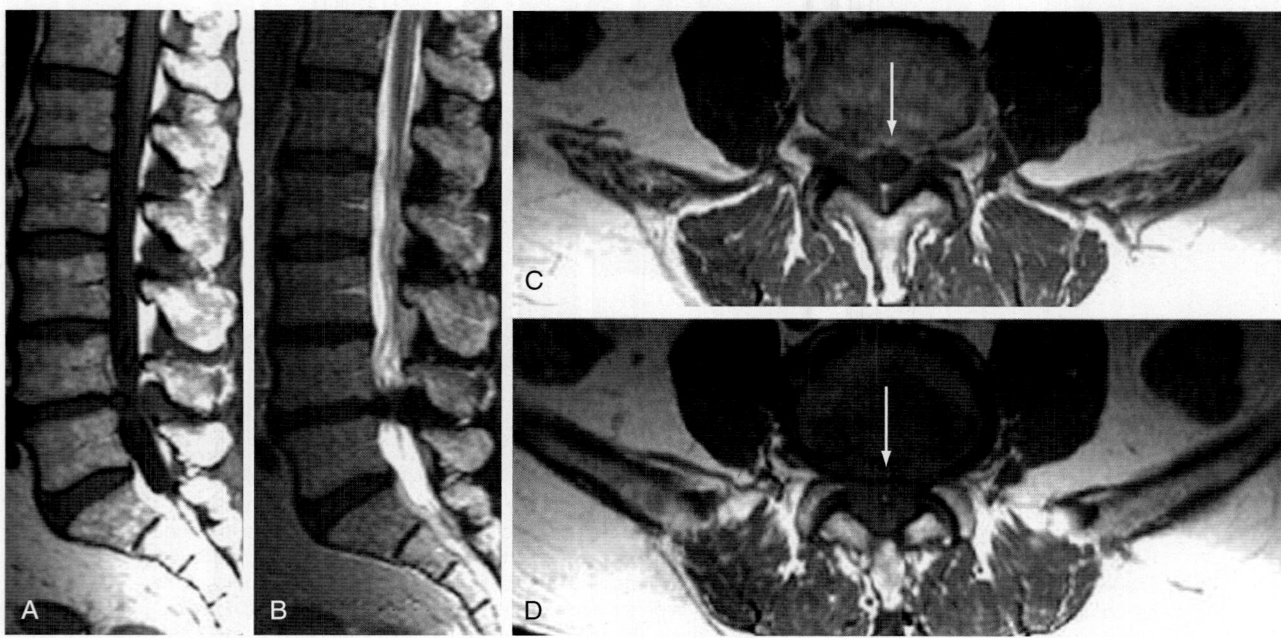

Figure 12-26. Lumbar canal stenosis. Midline T1-weighted **(A)** and T2-weighted **(B)** images of the lumbar spine. Diffuse central canal narrowing, evidence of a broad-based disk protrusion, and severe canal stenosis at the L4-L5 level are evident. Contiguous axial T1-weighted images (**C** and **D**) of the L4-L5 level demonstrate severe central canal stenosis *(arrows).*

pain or sciatica, the prevalence of disk herniation was similar in those with low back pain and those with radiculopathy at initial evaluation.[119] The prevalence of herniation, was higher among patients with low back pain (57%) and patients with radiculopathy (65%) than among asymptomatic patients (20% to 28%).[116,117] Disk herniations tend to improve over time; of patients with disk herniation at initial examination, one third exhibited significant resolution or disappearance by 6 weeks and two thirds by 6 months.[119,120]

The type, size, and location of herniation at diagnosis and changes in herniation size and type over time were not correlated with outcome. In fact, the presence of herniation on MRI was a positive prognostic finding.[119] Although the natural course is for herniations to resolve, new herniations can occur in the interim. In Modic and colleagues' study,[119] new or larger disk herniations developed in 13% of symptomatic patients over a 6-week period. The lack of prognostic value of imaging studies also applies to the conservative management of spinal stenosis; prognostic imaging findings have not been correlated reliably with surgical success or even with whether patients will benefit from surgery.[114,121] Demographic and clinical factors such as gender and work status are stronger factors for predicting the outcome of conservative treatment, whereas the structure and spinal stenosis, combined with the clinical presentation, are better predictors for outcomes after surgery.[122]

Further confounding the utility of spine imaging for degenerative disk disease involves the issue of reproducibility of reporting results. In a comparison of assessments by radiologists and clinicians, there was excellent agreement with the level of the abnormality; however, agreement was only fair ($\kappa = 0.24$) in terms of the morphologic description of the abnormality.[123] Studying radiologists for interobserver and intraobserver reliability with regard to degenerative disk disease, Arana and associates found excellent intraobserver reliability but only moderate interobserver reliability.[124]

Back pain, a common indication for obtaining imaging examinations, and its relationship to degenerative disk disease are poorly understood, but a combination of degenerative disk disease itself, including mass effect, and biochemical factors is thought to be causative.[60] In addition, degenerative disk disease has been found in asymptomatic individuals, and multiple studies have shown that imaging for uncomplicated back pain does not positively affect treatment outcomes.[118,125-128]

In a meta-analysis, Chou and colleagues[126] recommended that imaging not be obtained for uncomplicated acute or subacute back pain in the absence of "red flags" that would raise concern for underlying infection or neoplasm.[126] The rationale for not obtaining imaging is multifactorial, including the natural course of improvement of back pain,[129] the rarity of serious underlying condition in the absence of "red flags" or myelopathy,[130] the overall poor correlation of imaging findings with symptoms,[117,131] and the minimal effect on clinical decision making.[132] In addition, imaging can result in harm to the patient either from radiation exposure[58] or through the psychological effects of learning that he or she has degenerative disk disease.[133]

Metastatic Disease

In the extradural space, the most common spinal neoplasms are metastatic lesions. Conventional radiographs usually remain negative until 50% to 70% of the bone has been destroyed. Bone scans have high sensitivity with larger lesions, especially if there is cortical involvement. MRI provides coverage of the spinal axis and is more sensitive than other modalities to the presence of marrow replacement. The characteristic MRI finding in lytic metastases is decreased signal intensity of the marrow space on T1-weighted images (Fig. 12-27). This finding may be solitary, multiple, or diffuse (Fig. 12-28). In adults, the vertebral body marrow signal on T1-weighted images is normally brighter than that of adjacent disks. Reversal of this signal intensity ratio after the age of 40 is a cause for concern. Lesions on T2-weighted imaging are more variable and can range from hypointense to hyperintense. STIR sequences usually demonstrate high-signal intensity, and the appearance on diffusion-weighted images is variable. The presence of epidural disease is easily evaluated in STIR studies.

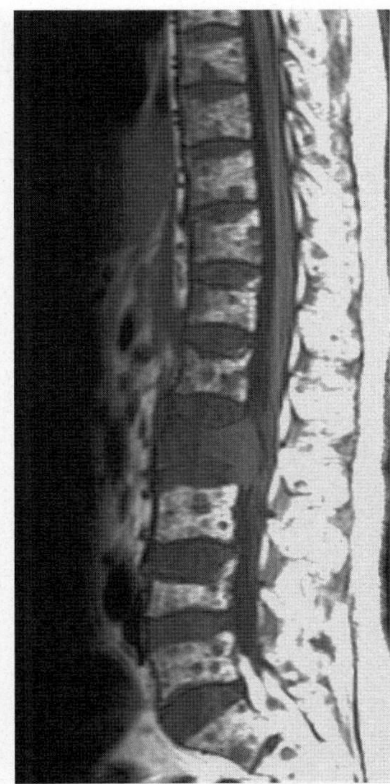

Figure 12-27. Metastases demonstrated on a sagittal T1-weighted spin echo image of the lumbar spine. Patchy and focal replacement of the marrow space is visible at all visualized levels. The marrow of the L2 vertebral body has been completely replaced, with loss of height and a convex posterior extension of the vertebral body into the spinal canal.

MRI is the imaging examination of choice and the most sensitive imaging study for the detection of marrow involvement and paravertebral tumor extension. It has, in most cases, replaced myelography for the evaluation of spinal cord compression because it depicts areas between the myelographic block. It is 95% accurate in detecting metastatic compression of the cord and cauda equina.[134-136]

Infection

In general, the early findings of disk space infection on plain radiographs consist of minimal disk space narrowing and erosion or indistinctness of the end plates. There may be adjacent paraspinal soft tissue swelling, which may be detectable in the lumbar region as enlargement of a paravertebral soft tissue shadow, in the thoracic region as a paraspinal mass, and in the cervical region as prevertebral soft tissue swelling. As the disease progresses, the disk space narrowing worsens, and destruction of the end plates becomes more obvious (Fig. 12-29). In healing, the disk space remains markedly narrowed or fuses.

Intense uptake in two adjacent vertebral bodies with loss of the disk space is visible on bone scans in patients with vertebral osteomyelitis. In the spine, it can be problematic to differentiate increased radionuclide uptake as a result of vertebral

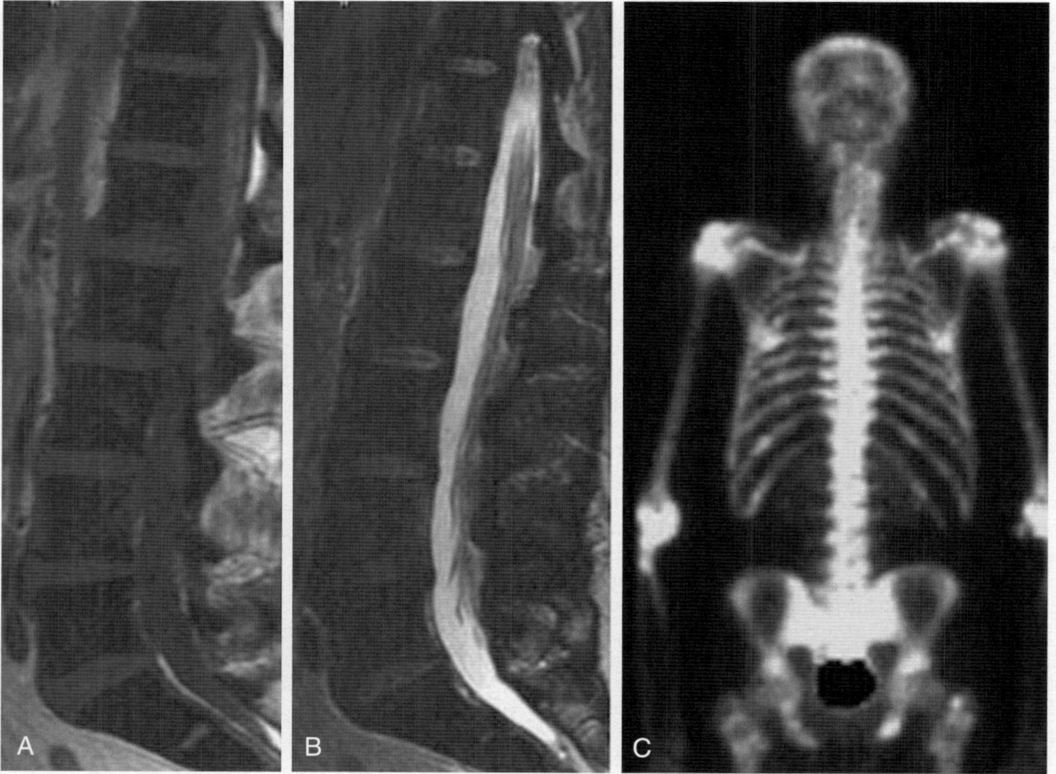

Figure 12-28. Diffuse marrow replacement from metastatic disease. Sagittal T1-weighted spin echo image **(A)** shows diffuse decreased signal intensity of the visualized osseous structures. The signal intensity of the intervertebral disk is higher than that of the vertebral body. T2-weighted image **(B)** shows diffuse decreased signal intensity of the marrow space. Whole-body technetium 99 bone scan **(C)** demonstrates diffuse increased activity throughout the spinal column.

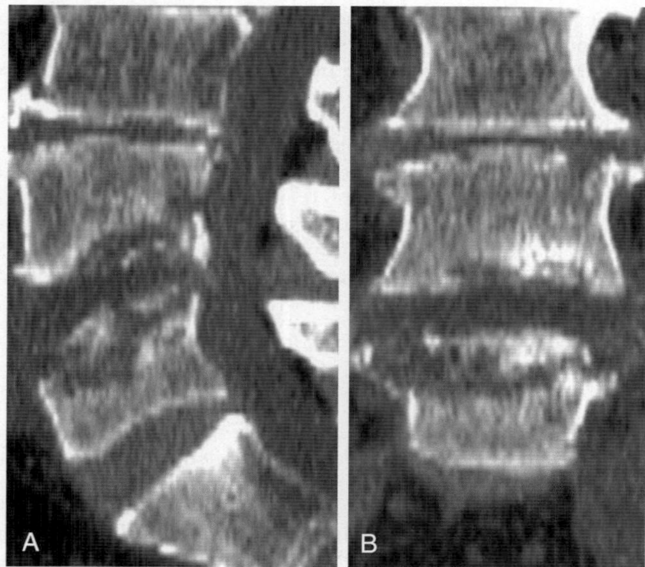

Figure 12-29. Vertebral osteomyelitis. Sagittal **(A)** and coronal **(B)** multiplanar reformatted images from a computed tomographic data set of the lumbar spine. Destructive changes of the adjacent vertebral body margins of L4 and L5 are evident, each with an irregular contour and an ill-defined soft tissue mass.

osteomyelitis from degenerative disk disease, benign compression fracture, or metastatic disease. The combination of gallium scanning or indium 111–labeled white blood cells and three-phase bone scanning may increase the specificity of imaging results. Although highly specific, indium 111–labeled white blood cells demonstrate poor sensitivity for the diagnosis of vertebral osteomyelitis. Fluorodeoxyglucose (FDG)–PET imaging demonstrates the increased glucose metabolism in the inflammatory cells that is associated with osteomyelitis. The FDG-PET scan is not affected by metallic implants and may be useful in evaluating infections in patients with hardware. FDG-PET has better resolution than does the more traditional nuclear medicine imaging and may be useful for differentiating bone infection from soft tissue infection. Low FDG uptake on PET scanning has been shown in fractures and in pseudoarthrosis; this fact may be useful in differentiating these entities from vertebral osteomyelitis. Malignancies, however, often appear similar to osteomyelitis on nuclear medicine studies because both exhibit increased uptake.

CT imaging is most useful for the detection of bone destruction and paraspinal soft tissue changes. The addition of intrathecal contrast material improves the delineation of epidural masses. CT imaging demonstrates a decrease in attenuation of the affected vertebral body and disk. CT criteria for the diagnosis of pyogenic vertebral osteomyelitis include diffuse permeative bone destruction (moth-eaten appearance), gas within the bone or adjacent soft tissues, involvement of the intervertebral disk primarily, and prevertebral soft tissue involvement.[106,111,137]

MRI has a sensitivity of 96%, a specificity of 92%, and an accuracy of 94% in the diagnosis of vertebral osteomyelitis.[138]

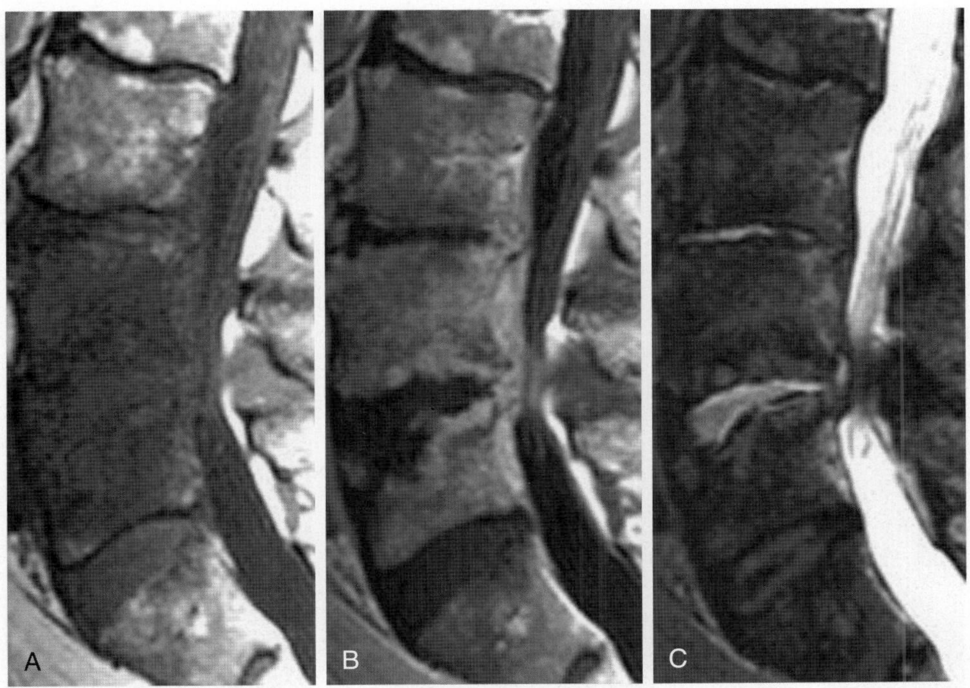

Figure 12-30. Vertebral osteomyelitis. Sagittal T1-weighted image **(A)** demonstrates decreased signal intensity of the L4 and L5 vertebral bodies with loss of end plate definition and confluent abnormal soft tissue extending across the disk space. Contrast-enhanced T1-weighted image **(B)** shows increase in marrow signal intensity and peripheral enhancement of the irregular disk space margins. Enhancement of soft tissue in the anterior epidural space is also noted. The T2-weighted image **(C)** demonstrates nonanatomic high-signal intensity within the disk space.

The classic MRI appearance of vertebral osteomyelitis includes the following characteristics: a confluent decrease in signal intensity of the intervertebral disk and adjacent vertebral bodies, with an inability to discern a margin between the two on T1-weighted images; increased signal intensity of the vertebral bodies adjacent to the involved disk on T2-weighted images; an abnormal configuration and increased signal intensity of the intervertebral disk; and the presence of paravertebral soft tissue swelling.[137] The addition of gadolinium has been found to increase the accuracy of the diagnosis of vertebral osteomyelitis in equivocal cases.[137] The involved portions of the adjacent vertebral body and disk are typically enhanced after the administration of gadolinium (Fig. 12-30).

The presence of abnormal soft tissue in a paraspinal epidural location raises the differential consideration of inflammatory phlegmon versus abscess. These soft tissue masses encroach on the central canal and foramina in varying degrees. The typical phlegmon enhances homogeneously on T1-weighted images and usually appears hyperintense on T2-weighted and STIR images. An epidural abscess characteristically demonstrates a peripherally enhancing fluid or soft tissue collection (Fig. 12-31). Epidural metastases may look like phlegmon; a large extruded disk that has migrated may demonstrate peripheral enhancement and must be differentiated from an abscess. Other differential considerations include epidural lipomatosis, which has a more characteristic fat signal on T1-weighted images, and epidural hematomas, whose appearances are more variable on T1- and T2-weighted images and usually demonstrate loss of signal on gradient echo images as a result of the presence of blood by-products. More recently, it has been suggested that restricted diffusion is characteristic of an abscess.[138,139]

Trauma

Plain radiography, MRI, and CT are all used in evaluation of the posttraumatic spinal column and are often complementary. Appropriate indications for imaging the spine in trauma include pain, neurological deficit, altered consciousness, and the presence of a high-risk mechanism of injury. The Canadian C-Spine Rule Study confirmed that "low-risk" patients (ambulatory, no midline tenderness, no immediate onset of pain, able to sit, or victims of simple rear-end motor vehicle collisions) who could actively rotate their heads 45 degrees in both directions do not require imaging.[59]

Computed Tomography

CT scanning has been shown to be significantly more sensitive and more time efficient than plain radiography for detection of cervical fractures in the setting of acute spinal trauma. Because of the widespread availability of high-quality CT scanners, the ability to acquire images rapidly, and the ability to construct multiplanar and 3D images, CT scanning is the ideal screening test for cervical fracture. The sensitivity of CT scanning for acute cervical fractures ranges from 90% to 99% with specificities of 72% to 89%. The sensitivity of plain radiography in the acute setting ranges from 39% to 94%.[140-142] Moreover, a number of studies have demonstrated limitations in the ability of plain radiography to reveal injuries to the upper cervical spine and occipital condyles.[143,144] Because of its greater sensitivity and wide availability, CT scanning is quickly becoming the initial screening modality for bone injury in the cervical spine.

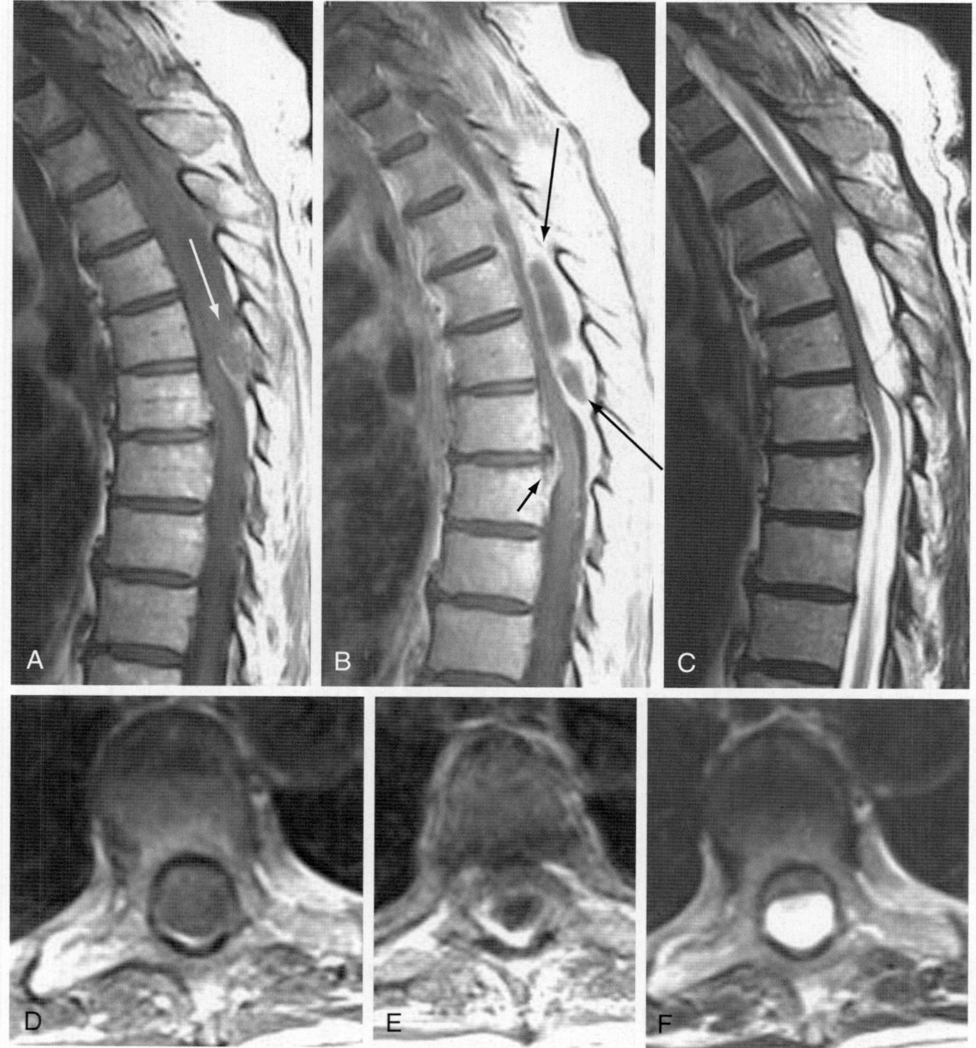

Figure 12-31. Epidural abscess. Epidural abscess on images of the thoracic spine. On T1-weighted sagittal image **(A)**, a posterior epidural mass *(arrow)* is apparent. After administration of contrast agent **(B)**, the full extent of the posterior epidural mass can be appreciated, as can the degree of spinal cord compression. Peripheral enhancement surrounds a nonenhancing loculated core, which is characteristic of an epidural abscess *(long black arrows)*. The T2-weighted image **(C)** shows more confluent high-signal intensity throughout the entire region. The epidural abscess is difficult to identify on axial T1-weighted image **(D)** through the posterior epidural mass, although the spinal cord is markedly compressed anteriorly. Its character and nature are better appreciated on axial T1-weighted contrast-enhanced **(E)** and T2-weighted **(F)** images.

CT scanning has been shown to be superior to plain radiography in assessing fractures of the thoracic and lumbar spine as well. Campbell and coauthors[145] reported that 20% of burst fractures diagnosed on CT scans were misdiagnosed as stable wedge compression fractures on plain radiographs. CT imaging is better at revealing fractures of the dorsal elements, malalignment, and intracanalicular fragments.

Radiography

CT scanning has largely supplanted plain radiography as the modality of choice for the evaluation of osseous injury to the spine. However, plain radiographs can be very useful in the evaluation of trauma injuries, particularly when CT scanning is unavailable.

Plain radiographs are also critical in the evaluation of instability in the absence of bony injury. Stability of the cervical spine is best assessed with dynamic imaging that includes flexion and extension views. An increase in the atlantodental interval or greater than 3.5-mm horizontal displacement of the vertebral body between flexion and extension can be indicative of spinal instability. This examination should be performed only on alert, cooperative patients without either neurological injury or radiographic evidence of unstable spinal injuries. Frequently, cervical mobility is limited by pain and muscle spasm at the time of the initial injury. Flexion and extension views may be more helpful when performed 7 to 10 days after the injury.[146]

Magnetic Resonance Imaging

MRI provides the best evaluation of soft tissue pathologic processes and is the only means of directly evaluating the spinal cord. The information obtained is often complementary to that of CT evaluation of the bone structures. Information about disk herniations, hematoma formation, and ligamentous and muscular injury can be instrumental in determining the appropriate treatment for the patient. MRI is indicated in cases of trauma when patients have a neurological deficit or when a soft tissue or vascular injury is suspected. STIR sequences can reveal bone edema and aid in differentiating the acuity of fractures. Heavily T2-weighted sequences can be used to evaluate for nerve root avulsions and pseudomeningocele development. MRA and fat-saturated T2-weighted sequences can be used to screen for vascular injuries. Ligamentous and soft tissue injuries are best visualized on fat-saturated T2-weighted images. The normal anterior and posterior longitudinal ligaments appear as continuous hypointense lines along the ventral and dorsal aspects of the vertebral bodies. In the presence of soft tissue injury, areas of increased T2 signal or discontinuity of the ligament may be visible. MRI is the modality of choice for the evaluation of a variety of posttraumatic conditions, including myelomalacia, spinal cord tethering, syrinx formation, and the presence of dural arteriovenous fistulas.[146]

Although MRI can be very useful in the setting of acute trauma, it has not been in widespread use of a variety of reasons. The requirement for special ventilators and monitors can often make it difficult or even impossible to image critically ill patients who have sustained trauma. MRI in patients with bullet fragments within the spine remains controversial. Most bullets are nonferrous; however, the composition of the embedded projectile is rarely known in the acute setting. In theory, a ferrous fragment may become mobile in the magnetic field, which could result in greater damage to surrounding structures, although this has never been reported. Finally, access to MRI scanners is limited and qualified technicians are scarce in the acute setting at many centers.

Postoperative Imaging

Imaging of the spine in patients who have undergone spinal surgery poses a unique set of circumstances, whether the reason for surgery was for degenerative disk disease, decompression for neoplasm or infection, or vertebral augmentation for compression fracture. If instrumentation has been used, metallic artifact may inhibit the ability to visualize the adjacent structures on MRI. Moreover, scar tissue may obscure small disk herniations or tumors. In the immediate postoperative period, loss of normal tissue planes, certain blood products, and the presence of air in the surgical area obscure neural structures on MRI.

Magnetic Resonance Imaging

The use of gadolinium frequently aids in the distinction between "normal" postoperative changes and pathologic processes. Scar tissue consistently enhances and is often associated with retraction of the thecal sac and the absence of a mass effect (Figs. 12-32 and 12-33). It may, however, produce a mass effect in some situations, and it may be contiguous with the disk space. Disks, in contrast, do not usually enhance centrally within the first 20 minutes after the injection of paramagnetic contrast medium.

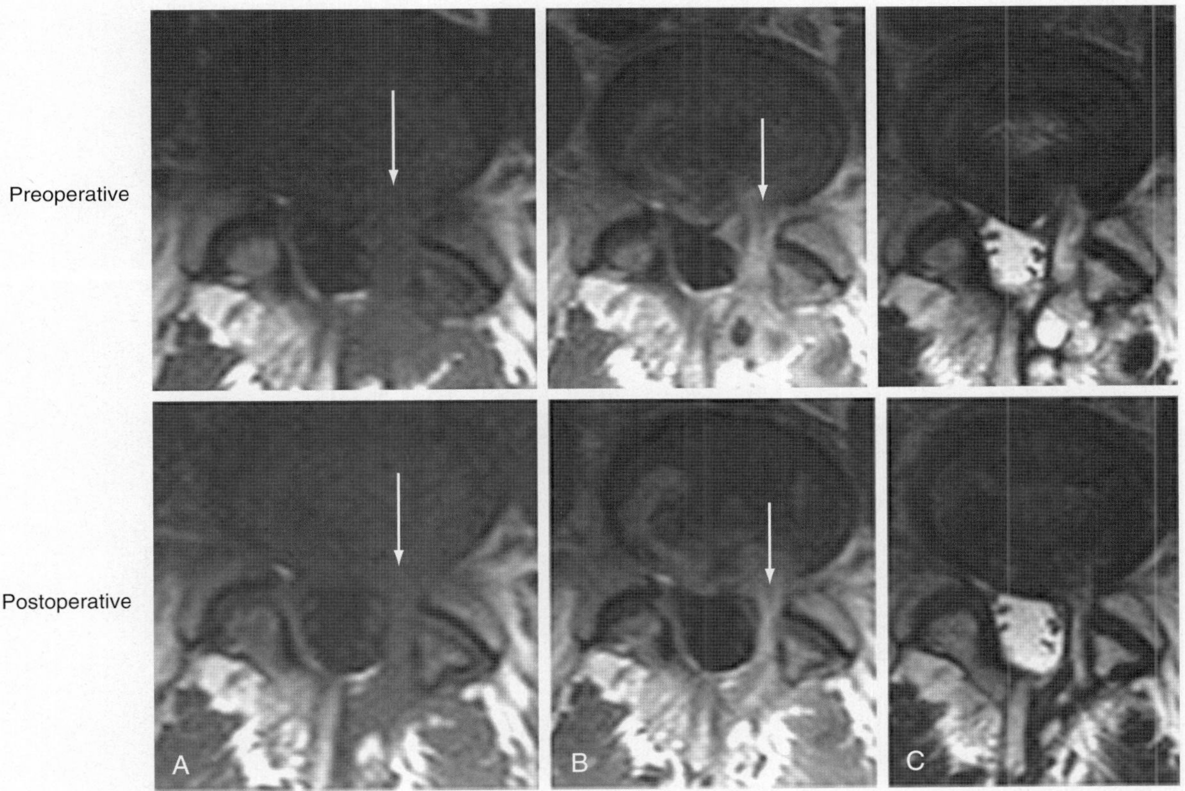

Figure 12-32. Axial T1-weighted **(A),** contrast-enhanced T1-weighted **(B),** and T2-weighted **(C)** images through the L4-L5 disk in a patient with epidural fibrosis. The immediate preoperative study demonstrated aberrant soft tissue *(arrows)* in the anterior and left lateral epidural space. This was enhanced in a relatively homogeneous manner after administration of contrast material. There was mild deformity of the thecal sac. Eight weeks postoperatively, the thecal sac had reexpanded, and the aberrant soft tissue, which continued to demonstrate homogeneous enhancement, had retracted somewhat.

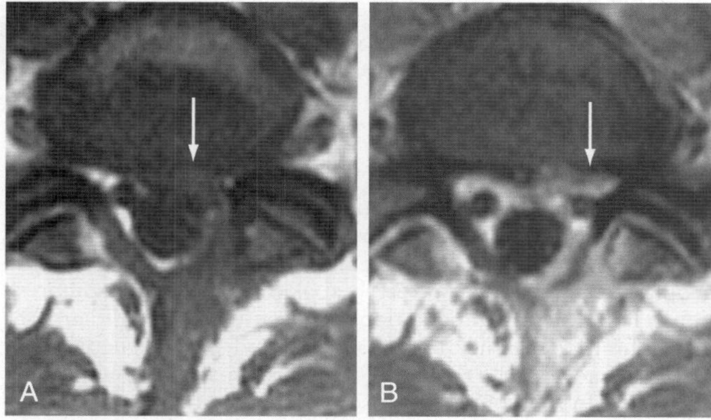

Figure 12-33. Postlaminectomy scar tissue. Scar tissue depicted on axial T1-weighted images before **(A)** and after **(B)** contrast enhancement after a left-sided laminectomy. The precontrast T1-weighted axial image shows aberrant soft tissue *(arrow)* in the left anterior epidural space. Contrast material caused relative homogeneous enhancement of this aberrant soft tissue *(arrow)* without evidence of a mass effect. This is scar tissue.

Peripheral enhancement is common both preoperatively and postoperatively (Fig. 12-34). Disks enhance centrally if imaging is delayed. This distinction can aid in the diagnosis of recurrent/residual disk herniation. Enhancing epidural scar is a common finding in the immediate postoperative period; the enhancement decreases over time.[77,147] In some reports, researchers have associated the presence of epidural scar with symptoms[148,149] and have also suggested that the presence of epidural scar is not correlated with symptoms.[150,151]

Primary differential considerations, besides scar and disk, are epidural hematoma and abscess (Fig. 12-35). In the acute period, an epidural hematoma may not have peripheral enhancement, and the signal intensity characteristics of the soft tissue mass may reflect blood by-products. Unfortunately, the signal intensity of blood by-products that are characteristic on brain imaging is not always characteristic of the spine. In particular, the high-signal intensity noted on T1-weighted images is not as frequently encountered. Epidural abscesses usually have peripheral enhancement and, in the absence of osseous changes, may be difficult to distinguish from recurrent disk herniation or hematoma.

The imaging findings of arachnoiditis are a reflection of the adhesion and clumping of nerve roots after inflammation. Group

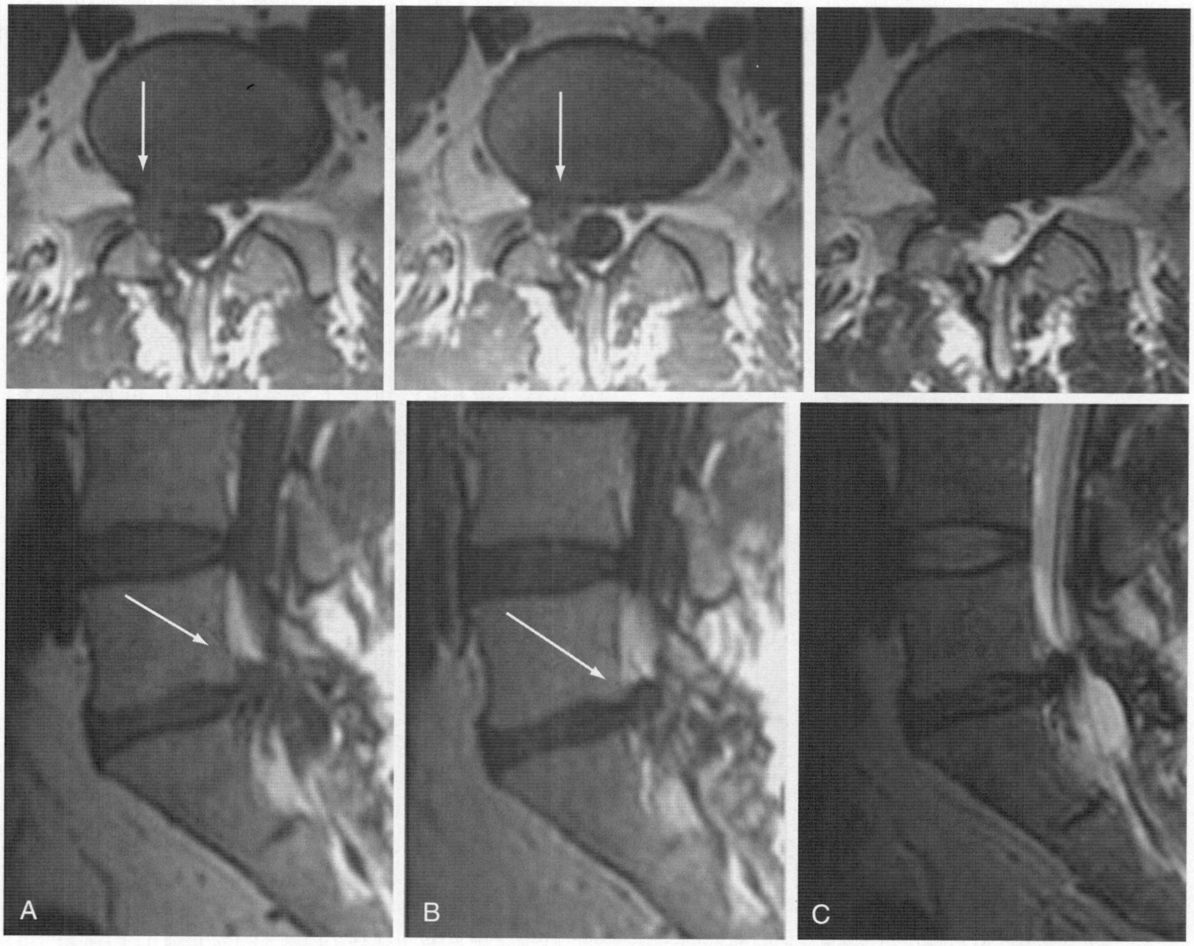

Figure 12-34. Recurrent disk herniation. Recurrent disk herniation demonstrated on images through the lumbar spine after a right-sided laminectomy at the L5-S1 level. T1-weighted axial and sagittal images before contrast enhancement **(A)** reveal aberrant soft tissue *(arrows)* in the right anterior and lateral epidural space. The contrast-enhanced T1-weighted **(B)** and T2-weighted **(C)** images demonstrate mild peripheral enhancement of aberrant soft tissue (**B,** *arrows*) surrounding a nonenhancing core.

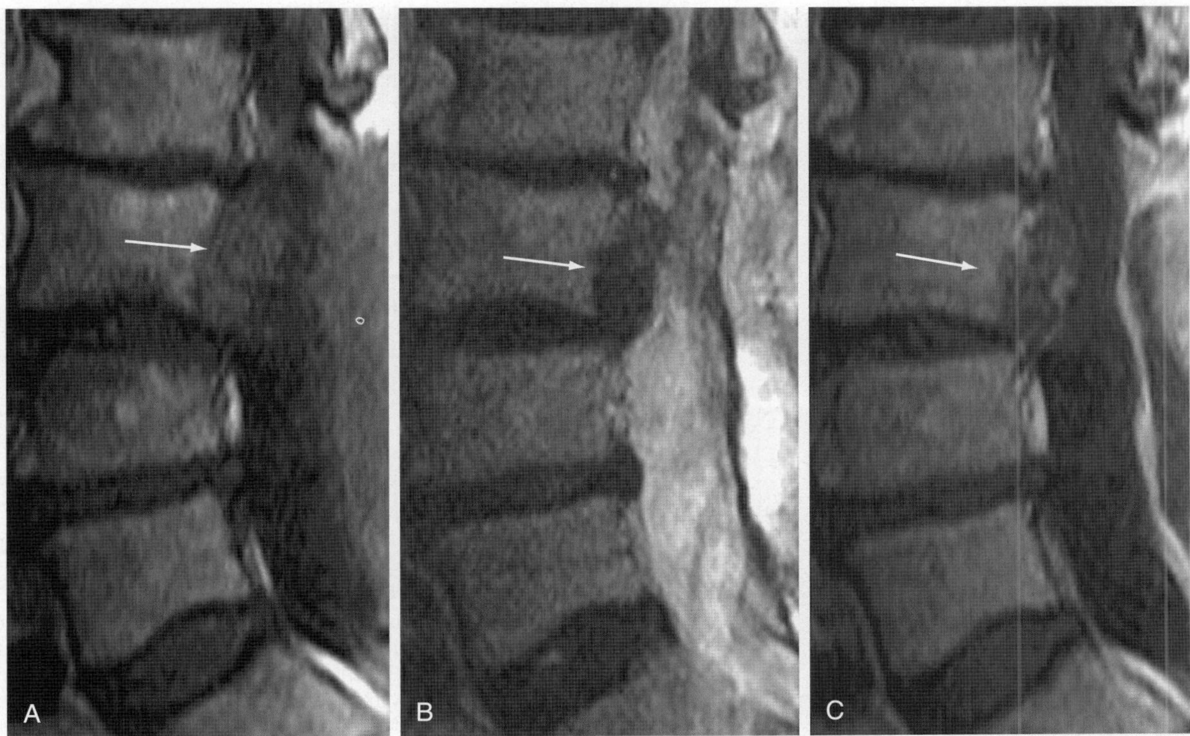

Figure 12-35. Postoperative epidural hematoma *(arrows).* Images of the lumbar spine after laminectomy. A large soft tissue mass *(arrows)* is situated in the anterior epidural space behind the body of L3. It has soft tissue signal intensity on the sagittal T1-weighted image **(A)** but markedly decreased signal intensity on the T2-weighted image **(B).** After administration of contrast agent, the T1-weighted image **(C)** shows minimal peripheral enhancement. Note the posterior laminectomy defect. This was found to be an epidural hematoma at surgery.

I arachnoiditis is manifested by clumping of individual traversing nerve roots within the thecal sac (Fig. 12-36). Group II is characterized by a featureless sac in which individual nerve roots are not identified (Fig. 12-37). There is often absence or blunting of nerve root sleeve filling. Group III is characterized by soft tissue masses that cause filling defects within the subarachnoid space and may block the flow of myelographic contrast media (Fig. 12-38). These findings of arachnoiditis are evident on plain myelography, CT myelography, and MRI. The different appearances of arachnoiditis probably represent points on a spectrum rather than different entities or stages. There may be minimal nerve root and dural enhancement, or no enhancement at all, after administration of contrast media. The differential diagnosis includes crowding of nerve roots with stenosis, leptomeningeal seeding of neoplasms, or meningitis.[152,153]

In patients with metallic implants, screw artifact can hamper visualization of the foramina and nerve roots, although the central canal is still adequately visible in most cases. Metal artifact can be minimized through a variety of techniques, including fast spin echo sequences, smaller voxel size, enlargement of the field of view, or the use of higher readout bandwidth. Moreover, geometric distortion occurs along the frequency in the coded direction. Frequency in coding directed parallel to the axis of an implant improves image quality, except at the tip.

Computed Tomography

CT imaging and CT myelography are essential tools for postoperative imaging. Screw artifact can be minimized to allow greater visualization of the foramina and lateral recesses. The presence of pseudarthrosis in patients who have undergone spinal fusion is best assessed with fine-cut CT imaging. Postprocessing of the images with sagittal and coronal reconstructions can aid in the evaluation of fusion. Hardware placement and integrity can also be assessed in this manner. Myelography can enhance the appearance of compressive and intrinsic lesions of the neural elements.

Radiography

Although largely supplanted by CT for the assessment of spinal fusion, plain radiography can be very useful in postoperative evaluation. It is cheap, fast, and effective for assessing the position and competence of spinal hardware. Moreover, 3-ft anteroposterior and lateral radiographs are essential in the evaluation of deformity and correction of deformity. Dynamic imaging with flexion and extension views is also helpful in the assessment of spinal stability and the presence of pseudarthrosis.

Congenital Abnormalities

Advances in neuroimaging of the pediatric spine have dramatically improved the ability to evaluate children noninvasively. Plain radiographs, ultrasonography, CT imaging, and MRI are the mainstays of imaging. Spinal cord tumors and infection are diagnosed earlier and more easily in children than in adults, and complex congenital anomalies of the brain and spinal cord can be completely evaluated both before and after surgery. Plain radiographs of the spine are most helpful in evaluating trauma, spinal instability, scoliosis, and spina bifida. Certain primary bone tumors of the spine are better detected initially on routine radiographs.

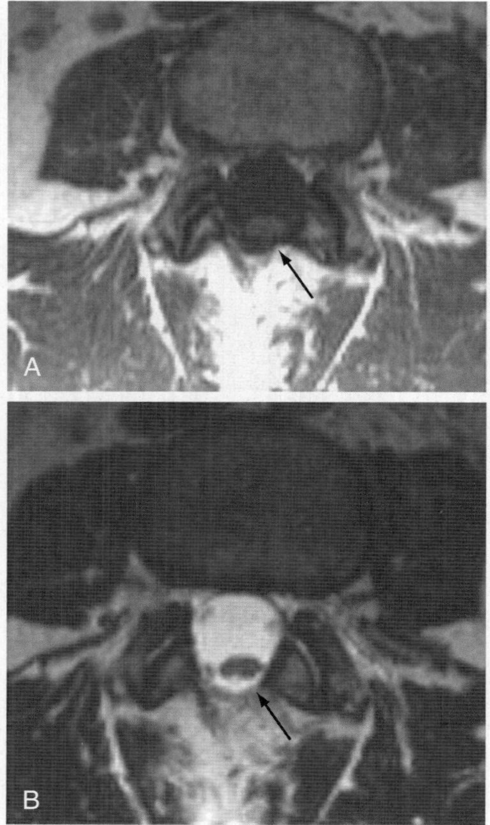

Figure 12-36. Group I arachnoiditis. Axial T1-weighted **(A)** and T2-weighted **(B)** images of the lumbar spine show evidence of a laminectomy defect. Portions of the traversing nerve roots are clumped posteriorly *(arrows).*

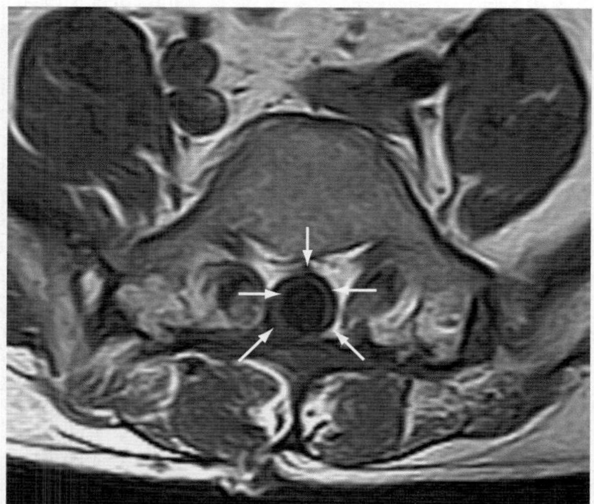

Figure 12-37. Group II arachnoiditis. Axial T1-weighted spin echo image through the lumbar spine demonstrates a laminectomy defect and a thin rim of soft tissue signal intensity *(arrows)* on the thecal sac that appears adherent peripherally. No individual traversing nerves are identified centrally.

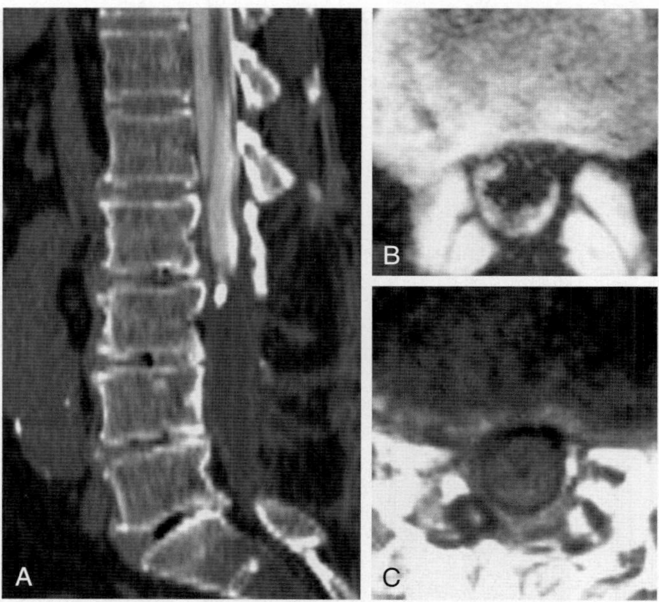

Figure 12-38. Group III arachnoiditis. Sagittal multiplanar reformatted computed tomographic (CT) myelogram **(A)** shows complete blockage of the flow of contrast material at the L2-L3 level. A laminectomy defect is visible, together with evidence of calcification along the posterior margin of the thecal sac. The axial CT myelogram **(B)** demonstrates a soft tissue mass within the thecal sac, which is evidenced by soft tissue signal intensity on the axial T1-weighted spin echo image **(C).**

In infants with a skin dimple or nevus in the presence of no or minimal neurological deficits, ultrasonography of the spinal contents is useful as the first imaging modality after plain radiographs. It is also useful intraoperatively for precise localization of intramedullary tumors, cysts, and syringomyelia. It may be performed through surgical bone defects or areas where posterior elements are congenitally absent.

CT imaging is excellent in assessing pathologic processes of bone and, with intrathecal contrast enhancement, in delineating spinal cord anatomy. As with other disease states, MRI provides the most accurate soft tissue, bone, and fluid depiction of anatomy and pathologic processes. In a child, however, greater preparation and teamwork are required because motionless examination is critical. General anesthesia or sedation is often needed in younger patients.

Spinal dysraphism is a spectrum of disorders in which midline closure of neural, bone, or other mesenchymal tissues is defective. The "open" dysraphic states include myelocele, myelomeningocele, hydromyelia, Chiari II malformations, hemimyelocele, and myeloschisis. The "closed" dysraphic states include dermal sinus, lipomeningocele, tight filum terminale, meningocele, myelocystocele, diastematomyelia, neurenteric cyst, slit notochord, and developmental tumors such as spinal lipomas.[154]

Patients with spinal dysraphism usually have cutaneous stigmata. Radiographic findings may show formation or segmentation anomalies, congenital scoliosis or kyphosis, canal widening, or osseous defects. Multislice CT imaging with multiplanar reformatting is helpful in definitive preoperative bone assessment. As noted earlier, in infants with a skin dimple or nevus and no or minimal neurological deficits, ultrasonography is of value as the first imaging modality after plain radiographs and is also used for intraoperative surgical guidance. MRI is the definitive modality for diagnosis, surgical planning, and follow-up.

In addition to ultrasonography, MRI has also proved useful in fetal imaging of congenital abnormalities. For disorders of the

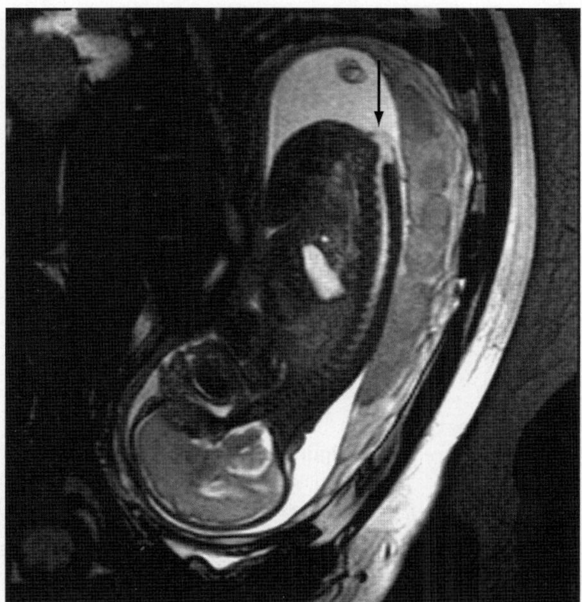

Figure 12-39. Fetal spinal dysraphism. Sagittal T2-weighted image through a fetus demonstrates spinal dysraphism with herniation of the thecal sac *(arrow)*. Resolution is not adequate for determining whether neural elements are present.

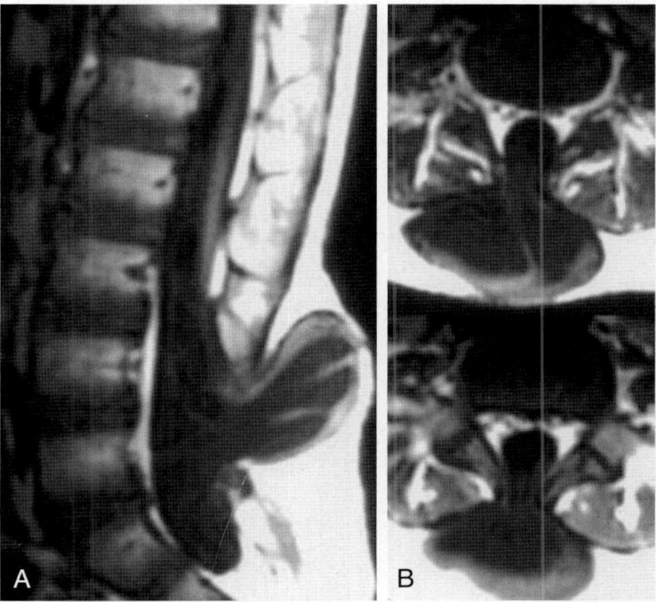

Figure 12-40. Myelomeningocele. Myelomeningocele demonstrated on sagittal **(A)** and axial **(B)** T1-weighted images through a dysraphic defect in the distal region through which both neural elements and cerebrospinal fluid have herniated. The placode is adherent dorsally, and the nerve roots are splayed more ventrally.

neural tube that have been diagnosed with ultrasonography, MRI can provide additional information in determining the level and contents of a suspected myelomeningocele and demonstrating the presence and severity of associated Chiari II malformations and ventriculomegaly in the presence of open spinal neural tube defects. MRI can be used to assess the structure of the brainstem and cortex and can provide useful prognostic information (Fig. 12-39).[155]

Open dysraphic defects are usually closed surgically within 24 to 48 hours of affected patients' birth. Subsequently, patients are referred for imaging to evaluate any change in neurological status that may be related to Chiari II malformations or other associated abnormalities. Such imaging is also performed after myelomeningocele closure or shunt implantation for hydrocephalus (Fig. 12-40).

Distinction between hydromyelia and syringomyelia is difficult if not impossible to make on imaging studies; hence the term *hydrosyringomyelia* is more commonly used. MRI demonstrates intramedullary CSF signal intensities within the spinal cord, which may be diffusely enlarged with sacculations or septations.

MRI signal intensity characteristics are useful in the assessment and differentiation of a series of disorders. In lipomeningocele and lipoma, MRI demonstrates the relationship of a T1-hyperintense lipoma and the neural elements and is useful for surgical planning (Fig. 12-41).

Dermal sinuses, or epithelial tracks extending from the skin surface into deeper tissues, often end in a dermoid/epidermoid or lipoma. Affected patients may have infection secondary to an abscess. On MRI, a dermal sinus generally appears with relative hypointensity (Fig. 12-42). Uninfected dermoid/epidermoid tumors usually do not enhance and may exhibit restrictive diffusion. They may appear hypointense in relation to CSF on MRI sequences, but their characteristics are variable. If they are infected, paramagnetic contrast material usually helps enhance the lesions.

On plain radiographs, neurenteric cysts typically appear as posterior mediastinal masses associated with vertebral body abnormalities. They are usually found in the lower cervical or thoracic region. On MRI, the signal intensity is variable, depending on the contents of the cyst. If serous, they may appear similar to CSF, but if they contain mucoid secretions, they may be hyperintense on T1-weighted MRI.

Diastematomyelia, the most common neurenteric or split notochord entity, may necessitate several imaging modalities for full anatomic delineation (Fig. 12-43). Plain radiographs may show spina bifida, intersegmental laminar fusion, anomalies of the vertebral bodies, and kyphoscoliosis. For septal definition, axial spin echo T2-weighted MRI, axial gradient echo T2-weighted MRI, CT imaging, or CT myelography may be necessary. Other commonly associated abnormalities, including a thickened filum, developmental tumors (lipomas, dermoid/epidermoid), and hydromyelia, can be depicted.

There may be a bone spur or cartilaginous spur within the cleft in the spinal cord. For accurate definition, a combination of sagittal, coronal, and axial MRI, CT imaging, or CT myelography may be necessary. The conus is located below the L2 level in more than 75% of affected patients, and a thickened filum is often associated. Hydromyelia is present in approximately 50% of affected patients, and the spinal column is almost always abnormal.[154,156,157]

Vascular Disorders

Vascular disorders of the spine can be classified as (1) vascular malformations of the spine and spinal cord and (2) parenchymal injury as a result of hemorrhage or stroke. Evaluation of patients with potential vascular disease of the spine is frequently challenging. MRI is the screening procedure of choice for detection of vascular abnormalities of the spine. It is capable of identifying spinal cord enlargement and enhancement and changes in signal intensity related to flowing blood within arterial or venous structures. The presence of blood products that may be more remote can also be identified, especially on gradient echo imaging. In addition to static imaging, both contrast-enhanced and

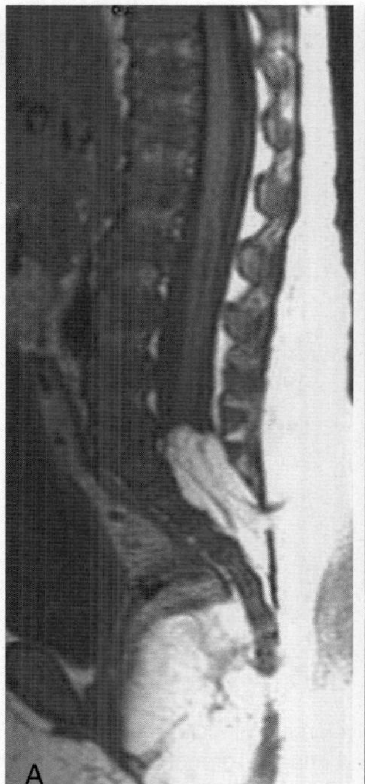

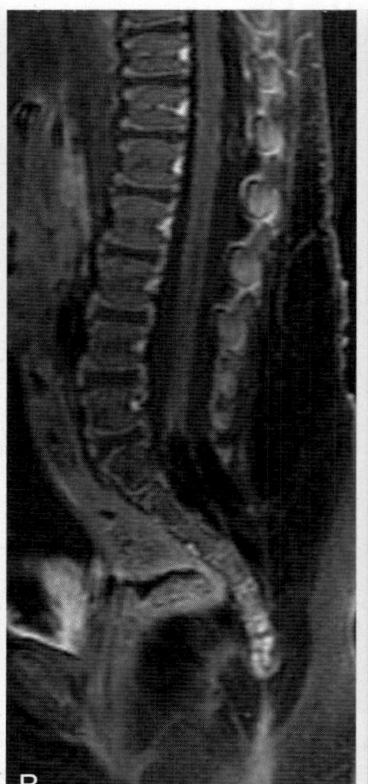

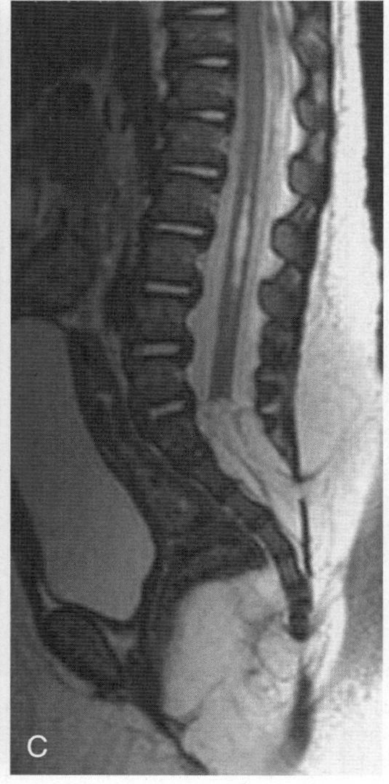

Figure 12-41. Lipomeningocele. Sagittal T1-weighted **(A),** fat-suppressed T1-weighted **(B),** and T2-weighted **(C)** images of the lumbosacral region reveal a tethered spinal cord that terminates in a lipomeningocele in the lumbosacral region that is communicating with a presacral lipoma. A syrinx cavity is present in the tethered spinal cord in the upper lumbar region.

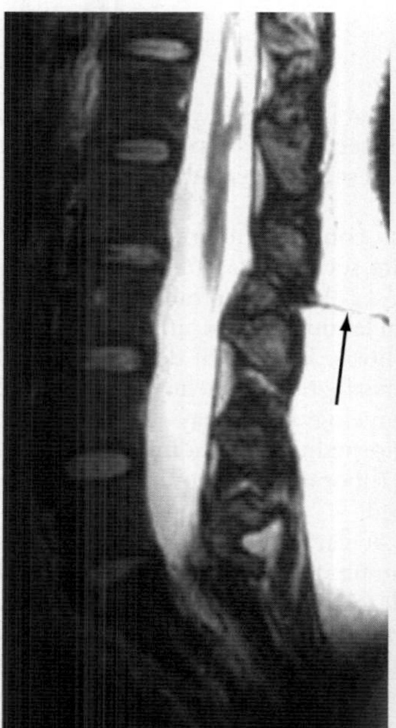

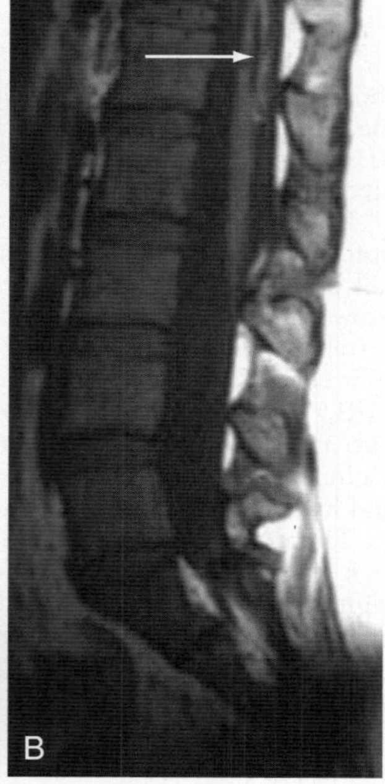

Figure 12-42. Dermal sinus. Dermal sinus visualized on sagittal T2-weighted **(A)** and T1-weighted **(B)** images of the lumbar region. A sinus tract (**A,** *black arrow*) passing intraspinally is associated with tethering of the spinal cord at the L3 level. There is a syrinx cavity within the spinal cord at the L1 level (**B,** *white arrow*).

time-of-flight techniques are available for MRA examination. MRI can reliably reveal or rule out spinal vascular abnormalities and provide important localization information, but it does not enable clinicians to accurately classify the subtypes. Even when there is good depiction of the arterial and venous anatomy with MRA techniques, catheter-based angiography is required for further therapeutic management. Once a diagnosis is made or suspected, further evaluation is warranted, with either conventional spinal angiography or CTA.

Vascular Malformations of the Spine and Spinal Cord

Spinal vascular malformations are a heterogeneous group of non-neoplastic vascular abnormalities that account for 3% to 16% of spinal mass lesions. The current classification system is based on the angioarchitecture and hemodynamics of the lesion as defined by spinal angiography. The major groups of spinal vascular malformations are spinal-dural arteriovenous fistulas (SDAVFs; Fig. 12-44), spinal cord arteriovenous malformations (SCAVMs; Fig. 12-45), perimedullary spinal cord arteriovenous fistulas (SCAVFs; Fig. 12-46), and cavernous angioma (Fig. 12-47).[158]

SDAVFs are the most common spinal vascular malformation and represent up to 80% of all spinal vascular malformations. In 80% to 90% of cases, the affected patient is male, and the malformations usually become symptomatic initially in the fourth or fifth decade of life. Anatomically, SDAVFs are arteriovenous shunts in the dura, most commonly adjacent to the intervertebral foramen or in the nerve root sleeve. The arterial supply usually arises from a dural branch of the radicular artery and drains directly into the pial veins of the spinal cord via an intradural vein. This abnormal drainage pattern results in venous hypertension and spinal cord edema. Hemorrhage with SDAVFs is rare.

There are four basic types of vascular malformations of the spinal cord: type I malformations are arteriovenous fistulas between dural branches of the spinal ramus of the radicular artery and an intradural medullary vein; type II are intramedullary glomus malformations; type III are extensive juvenile malformation; and type IV are intradural perimedullary AV fistulas. These types are described in more detail as follows:

Type I: dural arteriovenous fistula. Patients with this type are predominantly male, and it usually manifests in the fifth to eighth decades. Affected patients usually exhibit progressive radiculomyelopathy secondary to venous hypertensive myelopathy.[159] Subarachnoid hemorrhage and venous

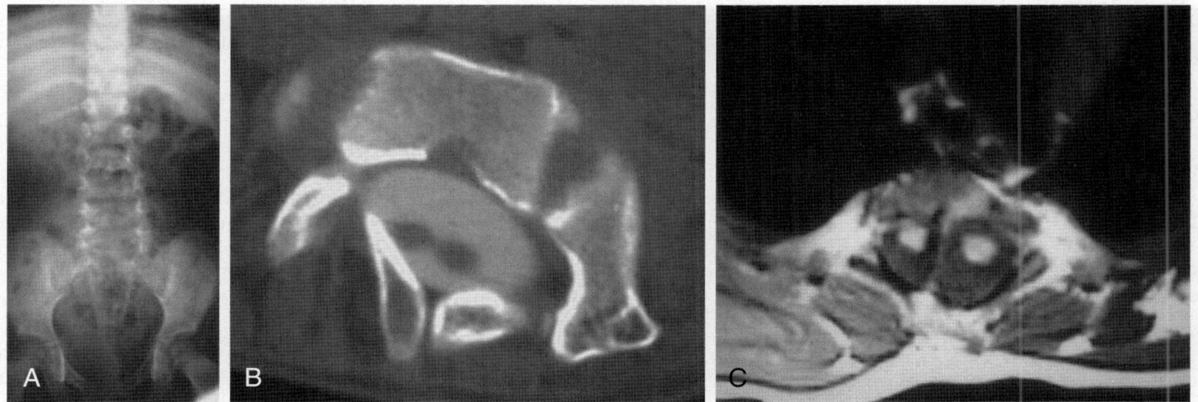

Figure 12-43. Diastematomyelia. Anteroposterior radiograph of the thoracolumbar region **(A)** and an axial computed tomographic myelogram **(B)** demonstrate spinal dysraphism with widening of the interpedicular distance in the lumbar region and anomalies of the vertebral bodies and posterior elements. Axial T1-weighted magnetic resonance image at a slightly higher level **(C)** demonstrates a septum separating two spinal cords. There appear to be two separate dural coverings.

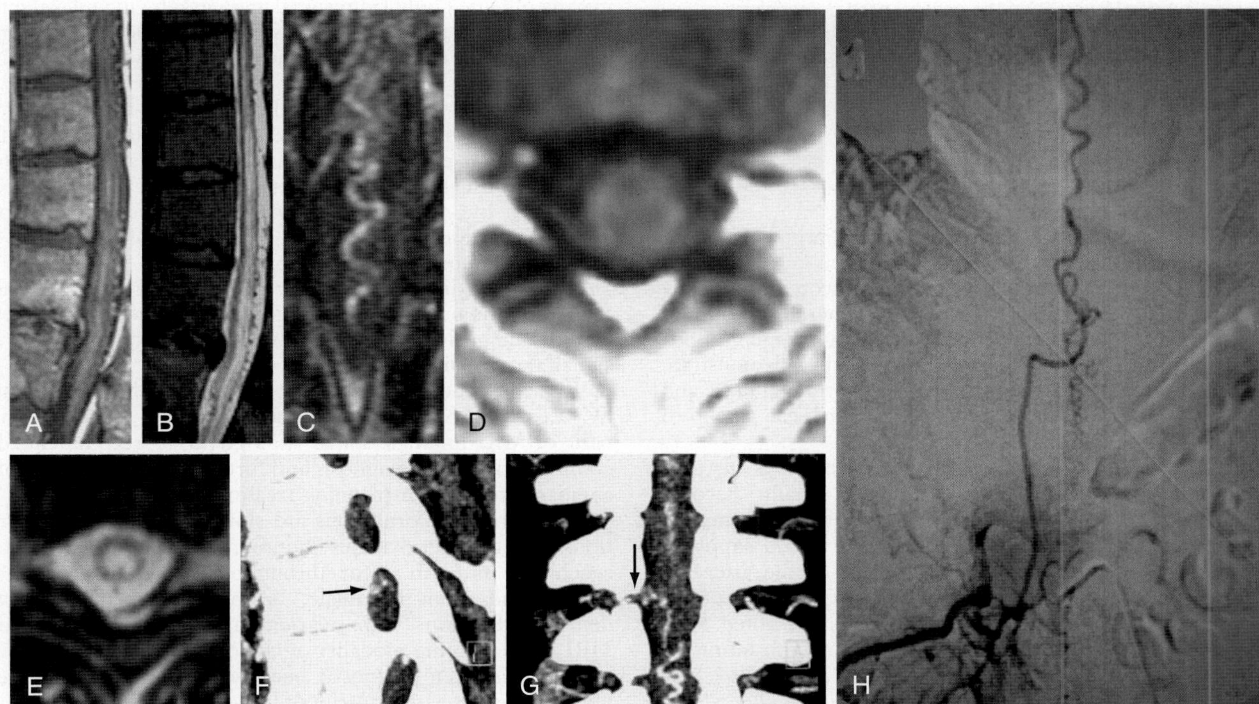

Figure 12-44. Type I dural arteriovenous fistula. Images of the distal thoracic region. Multiple enhancing vessels are noted along the surface of the thoracic cord on the T1-weighted, contrast-enhanced image **(A).** Diffuse increased hyperintensity is apparent within the spinal cord on the T2-weighted image **(B),** as are multiple small focal flow voids along the surface. Magnetic resonance angiographic image **(C)** demonstrates an enlarged draining venous plexus. Within the thoracic spinal cord, the signal intensity is decreased on the axial T1-weighted image **(D)** and increased on the T2-weighted image **(E)** centrally, secondary to the spinal cord edema. Sagittal **(F)** and coronal **(G)** multiplanar reformatted images from a computed tomographic angiogram of the thoracic cord demonstrate the prominent radicular vessel leading to the dural fistula, which then shunts into the venous plexus on the surface of the thoracic cord *(arrows).* A spinal arteriogram **(H)** demonstrates a dural fistula fed from an intercostal artery that shunts into the venous plexus along the surface of the spinal cord.

infarction are uncommon. MRI is the screening procedure of choice. Spinal cord enlargement and enhancement and central increased high signal are usually observed on T2-weighted imaging, with sparing of the cord peripherally. Low T2 signal on the cord periphery is highly suggestive of venous hypertensive myelopathy. Flow voids are encountered on the surface in 45% of affected patients.[45,160]

Type II: intramedullary glomus arteriovenous malformations (AVMs). Nineteen percent to 45% of type II AVMs are initially evaluated because of subarachnoid intraspinal

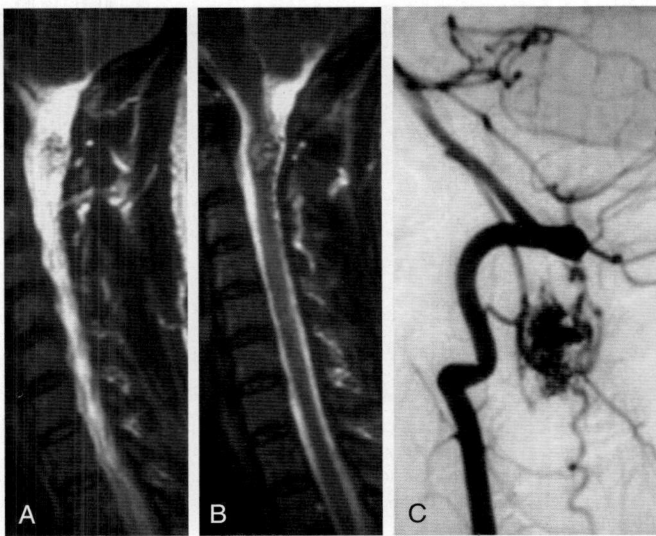

Figure 12-45. Type II arteriovenous malformation (AVM). Sagittal T2-weighted images (**A** and **B**) of the cervical cord demonstrate an intramedullary mass with heterogeneous signal at the C2 level and flow voids along the surface of the cervical cord. A lateral view from a spinal arteriogram **(C)** demonstrates opacification of the AVM nidus, which is fed from the anterior spinal artery.

hemorrhage. Arterial aneurysms are identified in more than 40% of affected patients.[161]

Type III: juvenile AVMs. These AVMs are uncommon, usually occur in the cervical region, and are generally associated with spinal cord or subarachnoid hemorrhage. Angiographically, these malformations usually demonstrate filling of the segment of the spine with intramedullary and extramedullary abnormal vasculature, which can extend to the paraspinal structures.[161]

Type IV: intradural perimedullary arteriovenous fistulas. These extramedullary malformations usually become apparent in the third to fifth decade of life and generally affect the conus and cauda equina. The blood supply is derived from the anterior spinal artery or the artery of Adamkiewicz, and arteriovenous shunting and symptoms of steal, ischemia, and venous hypertension are noted. Subarachnoid hemorrhage is a less common manifestation.[161]

MRI findings of SDAVFs include spinal cord edema and engorgement of the pial veins. Signal intensity is often abnormal in the spinal cord on T1-weighted, proton density, and T2-weighted images, although these findings are nonspecific and may occur with inflammatory and demyelinating conditions as well. A more specific finding is the presence of dilated pial vessels, best depicted on T2-weighted images as flow voids within the high-signal CSF surrounding the spinal cord.

Although MRI may be very suggestive of SDAVF, the "gold standard" for diagnosis remains spinal angiography. Selective angiography can confirm the diagnosis and provides additional information such as the level and side of the fistula, information that is essential for treatment. Occasionally, the location of the fistula may be remote from the site of greatest edema; therefore, multiple levels should be examined to ensure that the fistula is not missed. More recently, CTA has emerged as a useful, noninvasive adjunct for the diagnosis of SDAVF. In many cases the level of the fistula can be determined from CTA and be used to guide the angiographer to the appropriate levels to study selectively.

Intradural SCAVMs are thought to be congenital lesions. They occur most often in the thoracolumbar region of the spinal cord but may arise from any level. The nidus of the AVM is on or within the parenchyma of the spinal cord itself. The arterial supply arises from either the anterior or posterior spinal arteries. In many cases, dilated draining veins extend both rostrally and caudally from the nidus. Two subtypes are classically described. The more common glomus-type SCAVM consists of a relatively compact nidus confined to the spinal cord itself. In juvenile-type SCAVM, the nidus involves the spinal cord with extramedullary and extraspinal extension. Hemorrhage, either subarachnoid or intramedullary, occurs in approximately half the patients with SCAVMs.

MRI is the study of choice for noninvasive imaging of SCAVMs. Enlarged arterial vessels and an intramedullary nidus appear as flow voids on MRI. Evidence of previous hemorrhage is visible in many cases. T2-weighted sequences may show perinidal increased signal representing edema, gliosis, or areas of infarction. CTA may be helpful in delineating the location of the feeding vessels. However, conventional spinal angiography continues to be the primary study of SCAVMs and is considered mandatory before any intervention. Additional information that may be obtained only from spinal angiography includes the location of feeders and draining vessels, the presence of perinidal aneurysms, and the location of normal blood vessels rostral and caudal to the lesion.

Perimedullary SCAVFs are direct arterial-to-venous shunts located on or within the spinal cord. Arterial feeders arise from the anterior or posterior spinal arteries. They are thought to be congenital, usually become symptomatic in the second to fourth decades of life, and are manifested as progressive radiculomyelopathy, predominantly in the lower extremities. Spinal subarachnoid hemorrhage is common.

MRI is the imaging modality of choice for the diagnosis of SCAVFs. The presence of enlarged feeding and draining vessels demarcated by flow voids is the characteristic finding. Spinal cord signal abnormalities and evidence of previous hemorrhage may be present. The lack of a true nidus may help differentiate SCAVFs from SCAVMs. Once a diagnosis is suspected on the basis of MRI findings, spinal angiography is recommended for confirmation of the diagnosis and further characterization of the angioarchitecture for planning treatment.[161]

Cavernous malformations are slow-flow vascular malformations with no arteriovenous shunting. They are usually intraparenchymal and can occur throughout the spinal cord, cauda equina, and filum terminale. In most cases, they are well-demarcated lesions with surrounding hemosiderin deposition. MRI is the imaging modality of choice for cavernous malformations and is often diagnostic because of their relatively unique imaging characteristics. A rim of low-signal intensity usually surrounds the lesion and represents iron storage products. On both T1- and T2-weighted images, the lesion appears as heterogeneous signal abnormalities within the spinal cord, secondary to blood products of various ages within the lesion. Angiography is not helpful in the diagnosis of cavernous malformations (see Fig. 12-47).[162-164]

Spinal cord infarction or ischemia is a devastating entity best identified on MRI. Affected patients generally have a relatively rapid onset of paraparesis or quadriparesis. The most common causes of spinal cord infarction are related to embolic disease resulting from therapeutic intervention, aortic dissection, and hematologic diseases. T2-weighted MRI usually demonstrates nonspecific increased signal intensity involving variable lengths of the cervical or thoracic cord and may demonstrate restricted diffusion. T1-weighted images often appear normal or demonstrate slight expansion of the spinal cord (Fig. 12-48).

Please see ExpertConsult.com for an analysis of the systematic approach to interpreting imaging examination. The aim of this

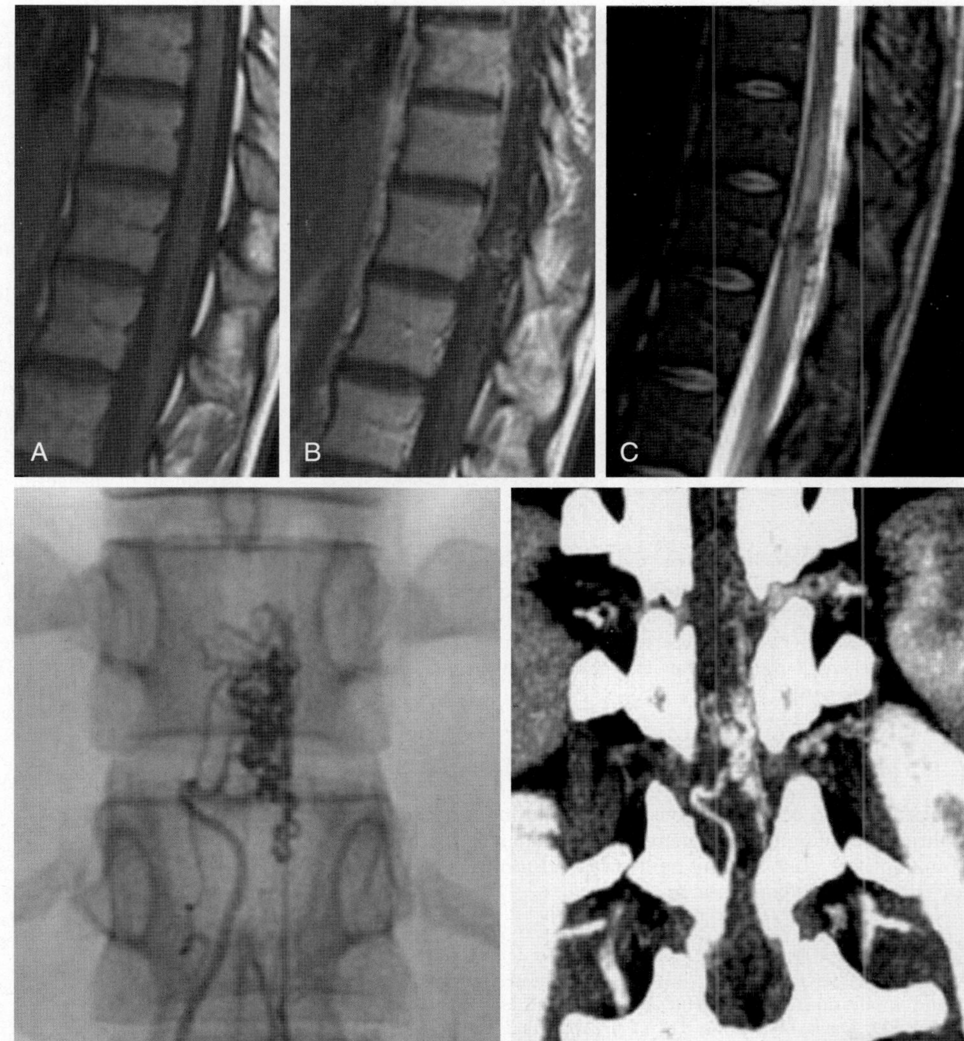

Figure 12-46. Type IV arteriovenous malformation (perimedullary fistula). Images at the level of the distal thoracic cord. T1-weighted image **(A)** shows subtle decreased signal intensity within the thoracic cord, suggestive of edema. On the contrast-enhanced T1-weighted image **(B),** multiple enhancing vessels are visible along the surface of the thoracic cord. On the T2-weighted image **(C),** signal within the cord is increased, secondary to edema; a focal low-signal presumably reflects compressed perimedullary vessels. An anteroposterior spinal arteriogram **(D)** and a computed tomographic angiogram **(E)** demonstrate filling of the vascular malformation on the surface of the cord by a radicular artery. In contradistinction to type I, shunting in this pathologic condition is at the cord level and not at the dura.

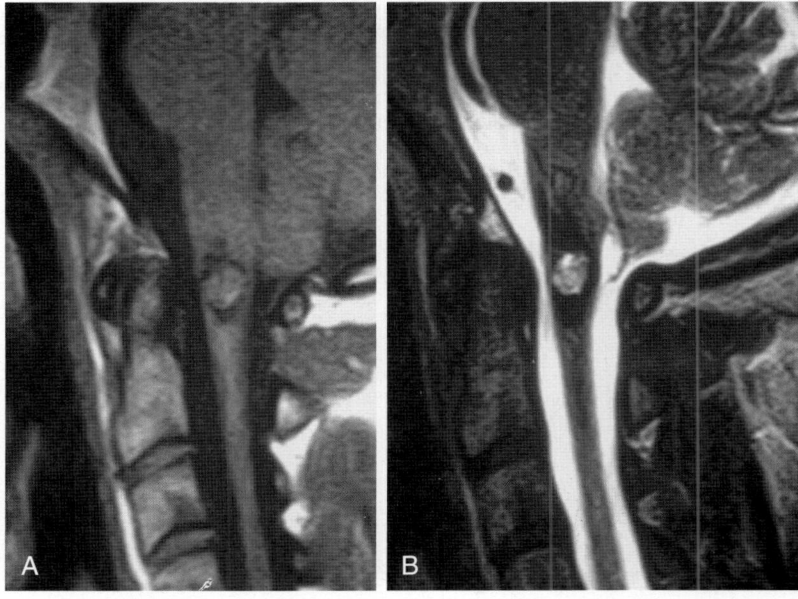

Figure 12-47. Cavernous angioma. Images at the level of the cervical medullary junction. There is a heterogeneous intramedullary mass on the sagittal T1-weighted image **(A)** with a rim with decreased signal intensity. The sagittal T2-weighted image **(B)** demonstrates a heterogeneous increased central core surrounded by a larger area of decreased signal intensity reflecting signal loss related to a susceptibility effect from remote blood by-products.

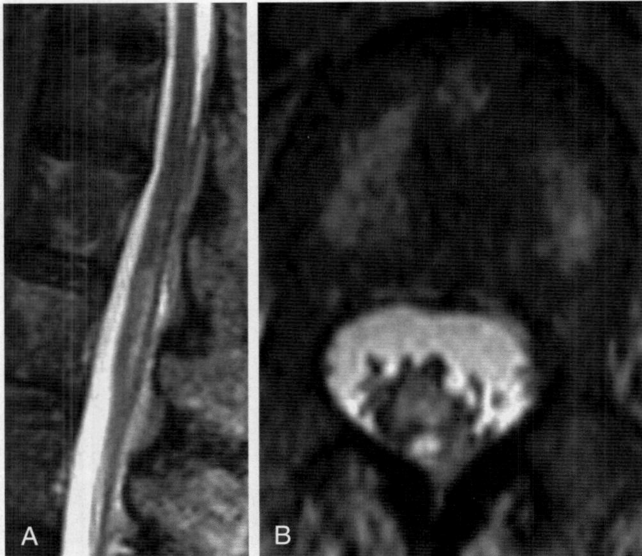

Figure 12-48. Spinal cord infarction. Spinal cord infarction noted on sagittal **(A)** and axial **(B)** T2-weighted images through the lower thoracic cord. The T1-weighted images were normal. The T2-weighted images demonstrate increased signal intensity within the distal thoracic cord.

discussion is to assist surgeons in determining whether abnormalities are benign, inflammatory, demyelinating, neoplastic, or nonneoplastic, thus helping guide the decision for surgery either for treatment or diagnostic goals.

SUGGESTED READINGS

Anson J, Spetzler R. Classification of spinal arterovenous malformations and implications for treatment. *BNI Q*. 1992;8:2-8.

Boden SD, Davis DO, Dina TS, et al. Abnormal magnetic-resonance scans of the lumbar spine in asymptomatic subjects: a prospective investigation. *J Bone Joint Surg Am*. 1990;72:403-408.

Bradley WG Jr. Low back pain. *AJNR Am J Neuroradiol*. 2007;28:990-992.

Carragee EJ, Kim DH. A prospective analysis of magnetic resonance imaging findings in patients with sciatica and lumbar disc herniation: correlation of outcomes with disc fragment and canal morphology. *Spine*. 1997;22:1650-1660.

Cook AM, Lau TN, Tomlinson MJ, et al. Magnetic resonance imaging of the whole spine in suspected malignant spinal cord compression: impact on management. *Clin Oncol*. 1998;10:39-43.

Dagirmanjian A, Schils J, McHenry M, et al. MR imaging of vertebral osteomyelitis revisited. *AJR Am J Roentgenol*. 1996;167:1539-1543.

Egelhoff JC, Bates DJ, Ross JS, et al. Spinal MR findings in neurofibromatosis types 1 and 2. *AJNR Am J Neuroradiol*. 1992;13:1071-1077.

Gilbertson J, Miller G, Goldman M, et al. Spinal dural arteriovenous fistulas: MR and myelographic findings. *AJNR Am J Neuroradiol*. 1995;16:2049-2057.

Jensen MC, Brant-Zawadzki MN, Obuchowski N, et al. Magnetic resonance imaging of the lumbar spine in people without back pain. *N Engl J Med*. 1994;331:69-73.

Korhonen T, Karppinen J, Paimela L, et al. The treatment of disc-herniation induced sciatica with infliximab: one year follow-up results of FIRST II, a randomized controlled trial. *Spine*. 2006;31:2759-2766.

Maravilla KR, Bowen BC. Imaging of the peripheral nervous system: evaluation of peripheral neuropathy and plexopathy. *AJNR Am J Neuroradiol*. 1998;19:1011-1023.

Milette PC. Reporting lumbar disk abnormalities: at last, consensus! *AJNR Am J Neuroradiol*. 2001;22:428-429.

Modic MT, Obuchowski NA, Ross JS, et al. Acute low back pain and radiculopathy. *Radiology*. 2005;237:597-604.

Modic MT, Steinberg PM, Ross JS, et al. Degenerative disc disease: assessment of changes in vertebral body marrow with MR imaging. *Radiology*. 1988;166:193-199.

Morrison JL, Kaplan PA, Dussault RG, et al. Pedicle marrow signal intensity changes in the lumbar spine: a manifestation of facet degenerative joint disease. *Skeletal Radiol*. 2000;29:703-707.

Ohtori S, Inoue G, Ito T, et al. Tumor necrosis factor–immunoreactive cells and PGP 9.5–immunoreactive nerve fibers in vertebral endplates of patients with discogenic low back pain and Modic type 1 or type 2 changes on MRI. *Spine*. 2006;31:1026-1031.

Rahme R, Moussa R. The Modic vertebral endplate and marrow changes: pathologic significance and relation to low back pain and segmental instability of the lumbar spine. *AJNR Am J Neuroradiol*. 2008;29:838-842.

Ross JS, Masaryk TJ, Modic MT, et al. MR imaging of lumbar arachnoditis. *AJR Am J Roentgenol*. 1987;149:1025-1032.

Ross JS, Obuchowski N, Zepp R. The postoperative lumbar spine: evaluation of epidural scar over a 1-year period. *AJNR Am J Neuroradiol*. 1998;19:183-186.

Schenarts PJ, Diaz J, Kaiser C, et al. Prospective comparison of admission computed tomographic scan and plain films of the upper cervical spine in trauma patients with altered mental status. *J Trauma*. 2001;51:663-668.

Shellock F. *Magnetic Resonance Procedures: Health Effects and Safety*. Philadelphia: CRC Press; 2001.

Stiel IG, Wells GA, Vandemheen KL, et al. The Canadian C-spine rule for radiography in alert and stable trauma patients. *JAMA*. 2001;286:1841-1848.

Thomsen H. Nephrogenic systemic fibrosis: a serious late adverse reaction. *Eur Radiol*. 2006;12:2619-2621.

Ulmer JL, Elster AD, Mathews VP, et al. Lumbar spondylolysis: reactive marrow changes seen in adjacent pedicles on MR images. *AJR Am J Roentgenol*. 1995;164:429-433.

Widder S, Doig C, Burrowes P, et al. Prospective evaluation of computed tomographic scanning for spinal clearance of obtunded trauma patients: preliminary results. *J Trauma*. 2004;56:1179-1184.

See a full reference list on ExpertConsult.com

13 Physiologic Evaluation of the Brain with Magnetic Resonance Imaging

Amish H. Doshi, Luke Gerke, Joseph Marchione, Pascal Bou-Haidar, and Bradley N. Delman

Although the first magnetic resonance imaging (MRI) sequences provided largely anatomic information, over the past 20 years there have been considerable advances in the development of techniques that better reflect physiology in health and in disease. With the rapid evolution of MRI, radiologists are increasingly able to suggest specific disease processes with greater confidence and accuracy. This chapter discusses some of the long established as well as newer emerging MRI techniques used today in neuroimaging.

Perfusion-weighted and diffusion-weighted imaging (DWI) allow rapid diagnosis of ischemia and infarction and can identify the so-called ischemic penumbra that might be rescued with aggressive therapy. DWI also plays a complementary role in the characterization of intracranial neoplasms, cystic or necrotic cavities such as abscesses, seizure activity, and other common pathologic entities such as demyelinating disease. Perfusion-weighted imaging refers to a number of techniques, each of which is used to estimate regional kinetics of blood flow to volumes of brain, and includes cerebral blood flow, cerebral blood volume, and mean transit time, as well as a newer non–contrast-based technique called arterial spin labeling. These techniques are discussed in detail in the full chapter.

Integrity of white matter tracts can be established with diffusion tensor imaging (DTI), and tractography allows graphic visualization of the orientation of these tracts. This technique is perhaps most clinically useful in cases in which the locations of important fiber tracts are not well defined by conventional anatomic sequences, and determining the relationship of white matter tracts relative to pathologic structural lesions (such as tumors or vascular malformations) may influence the decision to surgically intervene.

Blood oxygen level–dependent imaging exploits changes in flow and oxygenation within specific areas of the brain during specific tasks to demonstrate the site(s) and degree of brain activation and is the basis for functional MRI. Mapping of cognitive functions has clear implications for surgical planning, and preoperative identification may limit intraoperative awake testing if certain functions are localized away from the surgical bed. Functional data can be further exploited by processing in conjunction with DTI data; a site of activation can serve as a seed for DTI tractography to identify the trajectory of fibers (such as pyramidal tracts) that emanate from certain cortical areas so that they may be avoided during surgery.

Magnetic resonance spectroscopy (MRS) offers a more refined understanding of brain metabolites than anatomic sequences, and can therefore suggest areas of necrosis, areas of anaerobic metabolism, and regions of accelerated cell membrane turnover, or can identify specific metabolites characteristic of specific disease processes. MRS is now perhaps most widely used in the characterization of brain neoplasms. Recent work, however, has demonstrated the utility of MRS in other entities such as seizure disorders, Alzheimer's dementia, and demyelinating disease.

Magnetic resonance angiography (MRA) offers an important and highly accurate noninvasive evaluation of the intracranial vascular system in the diagnosis and planning of treatment of many vascular-related disease processes such as aneurysms, arteriovenous malformations, infarctions, and venous sinus thromboses. This includes phase-contrast MRA, which has become a reliable tool in evaluating a variety of conditions related to defined or suspected hydrocephalus via characterization of cerebrospinal fluid flow dynamics.

Magnetic resonance elastography (MRE) is emerging as a supplementary technique in brain MRI that has proven useful in quantitative assessment of the mechanical properties of soft tissues in vivo. Determination of tumor stiffness preoperatively can provide a significant strategic advantage in anticipating the feasibility and technical difficulty of resection and the length of the procedure. MRE is not limited to tumor assessment, and shows promise in evaluating the mechanical properties and changes in brain parenchyma in normal-pressure hydrocephalus and Alzheimer's dementia.

Positron emission tomography (PET)/MRI combines the unique features of MRI, including excellent soft tissue contrast, DWI, dynamic contrast-enhanced imaging, functional MRI, and MRS, with the quantitative physiologic information provided by PET. The practicality of PET/MRI in various clinical applications is currently being established, although the advantageous features of combined modalities can aid greatly in diagnosis, biopsy planning, assessment of tumor extent (i.e., PET may allow for detection of lesions that extend beyond territories of discrete MRI coverage), and differentiation between tumor recurrence and nonspecific findings.

Full text of this chapter is available online at ExpertConsult.com

14 Molecular Imaging of the Brain with Positron Emission Tomography

Antonio A. F. De Salles, Karlo J. Lizarraga, Alessandra Gorgulho, and William P. Melega

This chapter reviews the major principles and applications of positron emission tomography (PET) in neuropsychiatric disorders, with emphasis on neurosurgical implications.

PET allows the noninvasive evaluation of in vivo neurobiologic processes at the molecular level. PET imaging comprises (1) the production of the positron-emitting species in a cyclotron, (2) the radiopharmaceutical procedure to attach the positron-emitting species to a molecule of interest (a.k.a., tracer or probe), the most common being radioactive fluorine (^{18}F)–labeled fluorodeoxyglucose (2-[^{18}F]fluoro-2-deoxy-D-glucose, or FDG), (3) the measurement of the positron-emitting activity in a positron tomograph camera and the instrumentation for the construction of images, and (4) the tracer-kinetic model for the interpretation of temporal changes in the regional distribution, accumulation, and clearance of that positron-emitting activity.

In movement disorders, PET can identify relative decreases in the accumulation of [^{18}F]6-fluoro-L-dihydroxyphenylalanine (FDOPA) in order to differentiate among the parkinsonian syndromes, which are Parkinson's disease (PD) (asymmetric, putamen), corticobasal degeneration (asymmetric, striatum), and multiple-system atrophy and progressive supranuclear palsy (symmetric, bilateral striatum). Abnormal PET findings in the dopaminergic system could support the distinction between tremor-predominant parkinsonism and essential tremor.

PET can also provide useful information for the diagnosis of dementia. Characteristic patterns of FDG cortical hypometabolism can help identify Alzheimer's disease (AD) (bilateral temporoparietal), dementia with Lewi bodies (bilateral temporoparietal and occipital), and frontotemporal dementia and normal aging (bilateral superior temporal, superior medial frontal, cingulate, and parietal). Nonetheless, clinical correlation remains imperative because significant overlap can be observed. Finally, tracers that correlate with β-amyloid deposition are being investigated to detect AD before clinical onset.

In patients with psychiatric disease, PET studies have provided information regarding psychopharmacologic mechanisms and about neurotransmitter dysregulation, which has been used for drug development. For instance, effective antipsychotic agents demonstrate significant dopamine receptor occupancy, and antidepressants achieve high serotonin transporter occupancies at therapeutic doses. Interestingly, PET studies have been used to identify potential targets for deep brain stimulation for use in medically refractory major depression, obsessive-compulsive disorder, and posttraumatic stress disorders.

In epilepsy, PET imaging can increase the accuracy of epileptogenic foci recognition. Abnormal PET areas appear larger than the structural seizure focus. Thus, correlation of PET findings with the clinical picture, EEG results, and findings of magnetic resonance imaging (MRI) and other imaging modalities is vital.

PET studies of gliomas and brain metastases have ranged from diagnosis and grading to their postoperative assessment and differentiation from radiation necrosis, for which amino acid tracers such as FDOPA seem to be more sensitive than FDG. PET could also identify the most biologically active regions within a tumor, with potential implications for tumor targeting.

The multimodal brain imaging approach that combines high anatomic resolution data provided by MRI with low-resolution metabolic data obtained with PET has shed light on several pathophysiologic processes, expanding therapeutic options. Continuing improvements in the design of PET systems will contribute to a wider range of applications for diagnosis, therapy, and research. The combined use of gene therapy and molecular imaging will provide novel opportunities for the design and evaluation of molecular therapeutics, with the ultimate goal of improving patient outcomes.

Full text of this chapter is available online at ExpertConsult.com 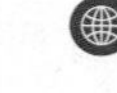

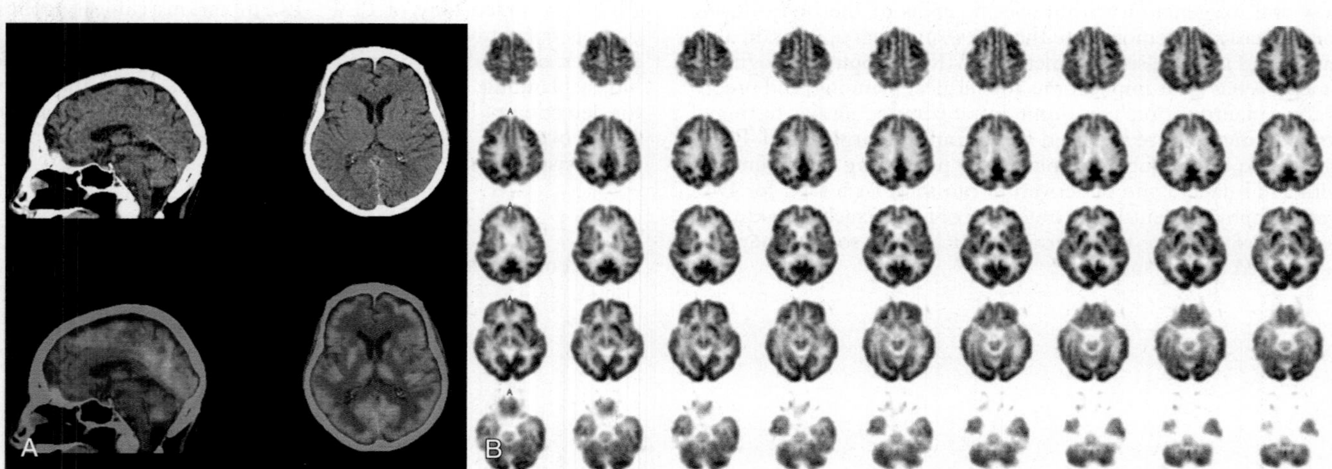

2-[^{18}F]Fluoro-2-deoxy-D-glucose (FDG) and positron emission tomography (PET)–computed tomography (CT) imaging. A, The two columns show the tomographic planes of sagittal (*left column*) and transaxial *(right column),* with CT data *(top row)* and PET data overlaid on the CT images *(bottom row).* **B,** Transaxial planes of FDG-PET images covering the superior-to-inferior extent of the brain. The *darker areas* represent regions of higher glucose metabolic rates and clearly delineate cortical and subcortical structures. *(Courtesy of D. H. Silverman, MD, PhD, Department of Molecular and Medical Pharmacology, David Geffen School of Medicine, University of California, Los Angeles. Reprinted with permission.)*

15 Intracranial Pressure Monitoring

Michael C. Huang, Vincent Y. Wang, and Geoffrey T. Manley

HISTORICAL PERSPECTIVE

The importance of intracranial pressure (ICP) was first recognized by Alexander Monro more than 200 years ago and is now referred to as the Monro-Kellie doctrine or the Monro-Kellie hypothesis.[1] The Monro-Kellie doctrine states that (1) the brain is housed in the nonexpandable skull, (2) brain parenchyma is fairly noncompressible, and (3) the volume of blood is relatively constant and outflow of venous blood is necessary for the inflow of arterial blood.[1] Later, cerebrospinal fluid (CSF) was recognized as a component of brain volume in addition to brain parenchyma and blood and was incorporated into the doctrine. If there is a new intracranial mass lesion such as a tumor or hematoma or an abnormal increase in the volume of any of the components, such as CSF (during hydrocephalus) or parenchyma (during brain edema), the volume of venous blood or CSF or both will decrease to accommodate. However, this compensatory reserve is limited, and any further increase in the volume of the pathologic lesion will lead to an increase in ICP because of the rigid, nonexpandable skull. An increase in ICP will then result in a decrease in perfusion pressure and cerebral blood flow and eventually cerebral herniation and death.[1]

For more than a century there has been clinical interest in measuring ICP. Early efforts to measure ICP were based on the observation that because the cranial and spinal CSF compartments communicate with each other, their pressure should be equal. Measurement of spinal CSF pressure through lumbar puncture should therefore reflect cranial CSF pressure, or ICP.[1,2] However, it was soon recognized that measurement of opening pressure via lumbar puncture is associated with a risk for cerebral herniation in the presence of an intracranial mass lesion and that it may not reflect ICP if there is any obstruction to CSF flow between the cranial and spinal CSF compartments.

During the first half of the 20th century, several investigators measured ventricular fluid pressure in a small number of patients.[2] Its clinical use, however, was limited until the 1960s, at which time the pioneering neurosurgeon Nils Lundberg started to measure ICP with a ventricular catheter connected to an external strain gauge pressure transducer and a standard ink-writing potentiometer recorder.[2] Drainage of CSF was also used to reduce ICP.[2] This method of ICP monitoring and CSF drainage was used in more than 400 patients, many of whom had traumatic brain injury (TBI), and marked the beginning of the modern era in ICP monitoring.[3]

Today, ICP monitoring is an integral part of neurocritical care. ICP monitoring has been used in the management of patients with TBI, subarachnoid hemorrhage (SAH), intracranial tumor, intracranial hemorrhage, stroke, hydrocephalus, central nervous system infection, and fulminant hepatic failure.[4] The Brain Trauma Foundation guidelines recommend ICP monitoring for all TBI patients with Glasgow Coma Scale (GCS) score of 8 or lower and abnormal findings on radiographic studies.[5] Consensus statements published by the Neurocritical Care Society and European Society of Intensive Care Medicine also strongly recommend the use of ICP monitoring for other acute brain injuries such as SAH and encephalitis as part of structured management protocols.[6]

Despite the adoption of ICP monitoring in the modern critical care unit and the establishment of association of intracranial hypertension with increased mortalities, the benefits of ICP-directed management strategies have been equivocal.[7-9] Recently, results from the first randomized clinical trial to evaluate ICP-directed therapy in severe TBI patients, the Benchmark Evidence from South American Trials: Treatment of Intracranial Pressure (BEST TRIP), have generated further controversy. This multicenter trial conducted in Bolivia and Ecuador compared ICP-directed management versus a novel computed tomography (CT) imaging and clinical examination–guided management protocol and found no differences in morbidity or mortality measured at 6 months after injury.[10] Analyses of the trial have scrutinized its design and challenged its generalizability given the study's locale.[11-13] Ultimately, the BEST TRIP study was not a trial of whether or not one should monitor ICP, but rather a comparison of two different management strategies for severe TBI. It highlights the need for deeper understanding of the pathophysiology of TBI and the interpretation of ICP in context of other clinical, radiographic, and monitoring information to individualize care.[6,14,15]

GENERAL PRINCIPLES AND STANDARD OF INTRACRANIAL PRESSURE MONITORING TECHNOLOGY

Since the 1960s, there has been a continuous effort to develop new technology for ICP monitoring. Nils Lundberg outlined the basic requirements for an ICP monitor, which still apply today: minimal trauma during placement, negligible risk for infection, no CSF leakage, easy to handle, reliable, and able to continue to function during various diagnostic and therapeutic procedures.[3] The Association for the Advancement of Medical Instrumentation developed the American National Standard for Intracranial Pressure Monitoring Devices, which specifies that an ICP monitoring device should have a pressure range of 0 to 100 mm Hg, accuracy of 2 mm Hg in the range of 0 to 20 mm Hg, and a maximal error of 10% in the range of 20 to 100 mm Hg.[16] Throughout the years, many different ICP monitors have been developed, but only very few are in active clinical use today.

CURRENT INTRACRANIAL PRESSURE MONITORING TECHNOLOGY

External Ventricular Drain

An external ventricular drain (EVD), or ventriculostomy drain, connected to an external strain gauge is currently the "gold standard" for measuring ICP.[16] It remains the preferred method for monitoring ICP among U.S. neurosurgeons.[17] An EVD can be placed at the bedside in the emergency department, intensive care unit (ICU), or operating room, depending on local practice tradition. Most practitioners use anatomic landmarks (freehand technique) to insert the ventricular drain into the lateral ventricle with the tip in the foramen of Monro (Fig. 15-1).[17,18] The catheter can then be tunneled subcutaneously to minimize CSF leakage and infection.[19] Ventricular fluid pressure, which represents ICP,

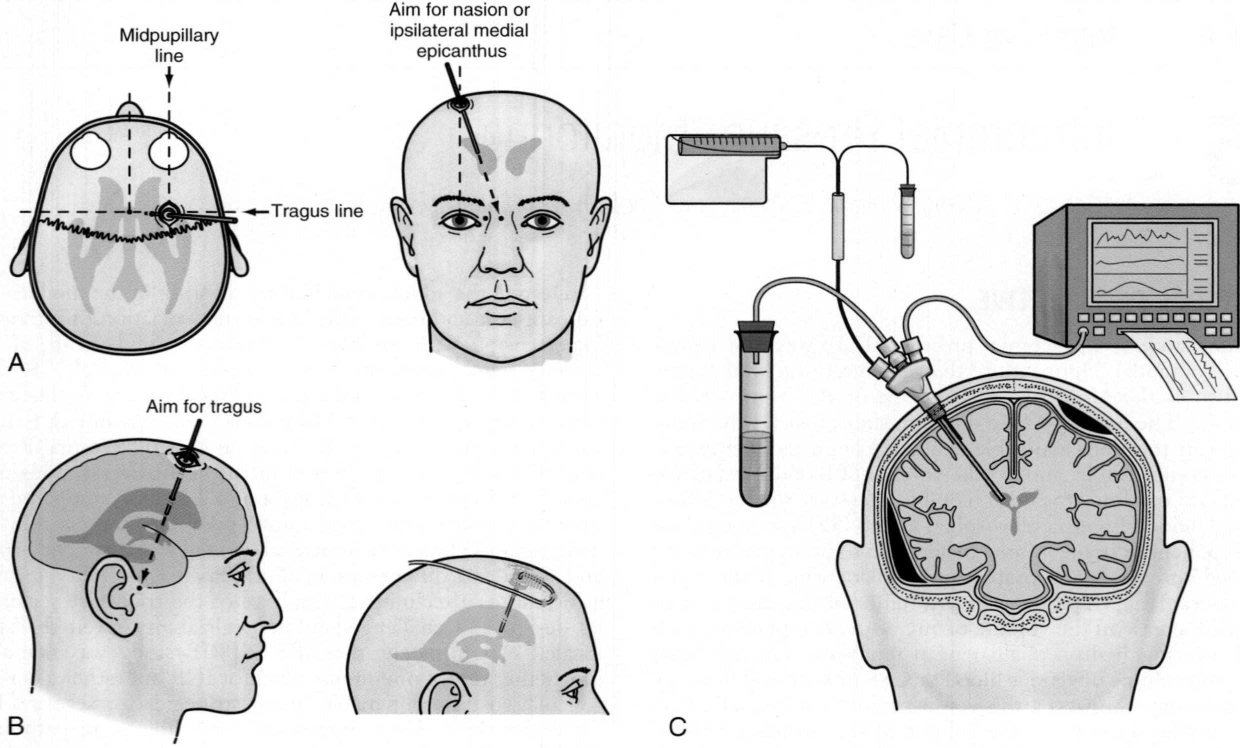

Figure 15-1. Schematic representation of landmarks used for ventriculostomy catheter placement. **A,** In the mediolateral plane, one should aim for the ipsilateral medial canthus. **B,** In the anteroposterior plane, one should aim for the ipsilateral tragus. **C,** Triple-lumen bolt with the ventriculostomy catheter, microdialysis probe, and multiparametric probe (to record tissue pH, Po_2, and Pco_2).

is transmitted to an external strain gauge transducer via the fluid-filled EVD. The strain gauge transducer can be recalibrated without manipulation of the EVD. It can be connected to many standard ICU monitoring systems and allows ICP measurements to be displayed along with other physiologic data such as pulse, blood pressure, or central venous pressure.

Advantages of the EVD as an ICP monitoring device include its extensive history, low cost, and reliability.[16,17] Most important, an EVD can also serve as a therapeutic device to remove CSF and lower ICP.[2,16] In patients with SAH or intraventricular hemorrhage, in which the elevated ICP is frequently a result of hydrocephalus, an EVD is the most appropriate ICP monitoring device, given its monitoring and therapeutic capabilities. However, an EVD has several weaknesses. Accurate placement of an EVD may be difficult with the freehand technique. In a recent survey of practicing neurosurgeons and residents, the success rate of cannulation of the ventricle was just 82%, even in the hands of practicing neurosurgeons.[17] Currently, there is an EVD placement guide available that may increase the accuracy of placement of EVDs, although it is not widely used in the neurosurgical community.[18] In some patients, it is simply not possible to place an EVD because of the small size of some ventricles or ventricular shift as a result of a mass lesion or severe edema.

Complications from EVD placement for ICP monitoring and CSF diversion include malposition, occlusion, hemorrhage, and infection. The malposition rate of EVDs ranges from 4% to 20%.[20-23] Most of the misplaced EVDs did not have any significant clinical sequelae, but about 4% of these EVDs did require replacement.[20,21,23] Occlusion by brain matter or blood clot occurs frequently, especially in patients with intraventricular hemorrhage or SAH.[20] Most of the occlusions can be resolved by flushing the EVD catheter.[20] Hemorrhage secondary to placement of an EVD occurs infrequently. Hemorrhage rates ranging from 0% to 15% have been reported in the literature, with an average rate of 1.1%.[16,21,23-25] Fortunately, most patients are asymptomatic from EVD-associated hemorrhage.[21,25] Clinically significant hemorrhage requiring surgical evacuation occurs about 0.5% of the time and results in intracerebral, subdural, and epidural hematoma.[21,23,25] Coagulopathy is thought to be associated with an increase in the hemorrhage rate, and therapeutic anticoagulants and antiplatelet agents are also known to be associated with an increased risk for hemorrhage.[26,27] In addition, laceration of a cortical artery can lead to traumatic pseudoaneurysm formation, and this complication has been reported with placement of ICP monitors.[28]

The most significant risk associated with an EVD is infection. Lozier and coworkers performed an extensive review of all the literature on infection associated with EVDs.[29] The range of infection in all the series was 0% to 22%, with a cumulative incidence of 8.8%.[19] More recent studies have found a similar rate of infection as well.[30-32] Clinical characteristics that have been identified to be associated with increased EVD-associated infection include intraventricular hemorrhage, SAH, craniotomy, CSF leakage, systemic infection, and depressed skull fracture.[29,30] Technical factors that may contribute to CSF infection include the duration of catheterization and irrigation of the catheter.[29] In 17 studies reviewed by Lozier and colleagues, 10 found an association between the duration of catheterization and infection, whereas 7 did not find such an association.[29] Careful inspection of the raw data of the latter group showed that there was an increased risk for infection after day 10 in one study.[29] More recent studies also showed an increased risk for infection with a longer duration of catheterization.[30,32,33] Most studies have reported that there are few infections during the first 5 days of drainage and monitoring with an EVD but that the infection rate increases significantly after 5 to 10 days of catheterization.[23,34,35]

Because of the relatively high rate of CSF infection in patients with EVDs, multiple interventions have been used in an attempt to minimize the infection rate. However, most studies are retrospective in nature and often do not have enough statistical power to detect small absolute differences in the incidence of infection.[29] Such interventions are discussed in the following sections.

Venue of External Ventricular Drain Placement

Lozier and coworkers analyzed five studies that looked at whether there is a difference in infection rates in EVDs placed in the operating room, ICU, or emergency department.[29] All but one of the studies revealed no significant difference in infection rate whether the EVD was placed in the operating room, ICU, or emergency department.[29] Two more recent studies also did not find statistically significant differences in infection rate related to the venue of ventriculostomy drain insertion.[32,33]

Extended Tunneling

Subcutaneous tunneling of the EVD catheter was reported by Friedman and Vries in 1980 as a way to reduce the infection rate.[19] Other investigators then extended the distance of tunneling to the upper part of the chest or abdomen and had an infection rate of 4%.[36] Two studies reported conflicting results. Sandalcioglu and Stolke reported that there was a significant difference in infection rate (83% versus 17%) for catheters that were tunneled less than 5 cm subcutaneously versus catheters that were tunneled more than 5 cm, respectively.[37] However, patient details were not available, and the infection rate of 83% in this study is significantly higher than most reported infection rates. Leung and coauthors, in contrast, did not find a significant difference in infection rate with long-tunneled EVDs.[38] Most EVD insertion kits today contain a trocar for subcutaneous tunneling in excess of 5 cm.

Prophylactic Catheter Exchange

The observation that the infection rate rises with increased duration of drainage from an EVD prompted several investigators to advocate prophylactic catheter exchange.[23,35] Several retrospective studies, however, showed that there was no benefit of prophylactic catheter exchange and that in fact there was a higher incidence of infection in the group in which catheters were routinely exchanged.[29] This was also observed in one prospective, randomized trial comparing the infection rate in a group that underwent prophylactic catheter exchange versus a control group that did not undergo prophylactic catheter exchange.[39]

Prophylactic Antibiotic Use

Many studies have analyzed the use of prophylactic antibiotics for reduction of the infection rate of EVDs. Prophylactic antibiotics can be given periprocedurally only or administered during the entire duration that the catheter is in place. Studies in the 1970s suggested that prophylactic antibiotics did reduce the infection rate when compared with no antibiotics, but two studies conducted in the 1980s and one study in 2000 did not find any reduction in the EVD infection rate in patients who received periprocedural antibiotics versus patients who did not.[29,40,41] Several other studies also compared prophylactic antibiotics given just periprocedurally versus during the entire duration when the EVD is in place. In a large retrospective study, Alleyne and colleagues did not find any significant difference in infection rates between the two groups.[42] In a prospective, randomized controlled study, however, Poon and associates did find a reduction in CSF and systemic infection in the group that received prolonged antibiotic prophylaxis.[43] It should be noted that infections that develop in patients who receive prolonged or broad-spectrum antibiotic prophylaxis, or both, for EVD placement are often caused by more virulent microorganisms such as *Candida* and gram-negative organisms.[42-53] Currently, the Guidelines for the Management of Severe Traumatic Brain Injury do not recommend antibiotic prophylaxis for EVD placement or catheterization.[45]

Antibiotic-Impregnated Catheter

A recent development in EVD catheter technology is the antibiotic-impregnated catheter. An EVD catheter impregnated with rifampin is capable of releasing rifampin in a controlled-release manner. These EVD catheters have been shown to significantly reduce bacterial adhesion versus controls in vitro and in animal models.[46] In one randomized controlled trial, Zabramski and coworkers showed that a catheter impregnated with minocycline and rifampin reduced the infection rate significantly from 9.4% to 1.3% when compared with the nonimpregnated catheter control group.[47] Although antibiotic-impregnated catheters cost significantly more than nonimpregnated catheters, one also has to consider the overall expense and length of hospital stay for patients with EVD catheter–related infections.

Fiberoptic Intracranial Pressure Monitor

Fiberoptic devices for ICP monitoring in which the catheter tip measures the amount of light reflected off a pressure-sensitive diaphragm were developed in 1980s.[48] The most widely studied fiberoptic device is the Camino fiberoptic ICP monitoring device (Integra Neuroscience, Plainsboro, NJ). The Camino fiberoptic ICP monitoring device can be placed in the subdural, intraparenchymal, and intraventricular space.

The intraparenchymal Camino ICP monitor has the most extensive clinical experience. The main strength of the intraparenchymal ICP monitor is ease of insertion. The most commonly used technique involves insertion of the monitor into the right frontal region, although it is possible to insert the probe into a region with pathology as well. However, it should be noted that compartmental pressure differentials have been observed in different regions of the brain, so the choice of where to insert the monitor is important.[49,50] Because there is no need to cannulate the ventricular system, it is possible to insert the ICP monitor even in patients with severely compressed ventricles or those with a significant midline shift. Although this device has led to more widespread use of ICP monitoring in critically injured and ill patients, there are reports of some technical issues that should be kept in mind when using these devices.

A number of early studies demonstrated that there is a high correlation between ICP measured by the intraparenchymal Camino ICP device and ICP measured by an EVD, with a correlation coefficient (r) of greater than 0.9 in both studies.[51] However, Schickner and Young found that the Camino overestimated ICP by an average of 9 mm Hg when compared with an EVD in 10 patients.[52] Nevertheless, because of its ease of insertion and low complication rate, it has gained popularity since its introduction into the market. Many large clinical series involving the intraparenchymal Camino device have been published. In most clinical series it is the sole ICP monitoring device inserted, and overall clinical experience with the Camino as an ICP monitoring device has been positive.[49-51,53,54] However, there have not been any large prospective or retrospective series that have compared the intraparenchymal fiberoptic device with an EVD as an ICP monitoring device in neurocritical care patients.

Complication rates associated with the Camino intraparenchymal device are comparatively low. In one large series of more than 1000 patients, the hemorrhage rate was just 2.5%, and the hemorrhages were all clinically silent.[53] In the same series there was no clinical infection.[53] In other series the hemorrhage rate has ranged from 0% to 5.1%.[49-51,54,55] Surgical evacuation was required in one patient in all the series.[55] The infection rate is also lower than that with an EVD. Although colonization of the catheter is frequent, meningitis occurred in just 3 patients in all the series.[50,54,55]

The most significant problem of the Camino fiberoptic device is zero drift. The device is first zeroed to atmospheric pressure (usually at room temperature) and then inserted into the brain parenchyma. Recalibration cannot be performed unless the transducer is removed from the patient, zeroed, and then reinserted. Zero drift then occurs over time, which will lead to an erroneous ICP reading. According to the manufacturer, the drift for the first 24 hours should be only 2 mm Hg and then should be 1 mm Hg for the first 5 days. However, clinical studies have shown that the daily drift is significantly larger than the manufacturer's specification. Daily drift rates of 0.5 to 3.2 mm Hg have been reported, and the maximal drift reported in most studies is usually greater than 20 mm Hg (positive or negative).[51,53-55] In most clinical series, recalibration was often needed, and this was often discovered when the clinical picture did not match the ICP reading or a negative ICP reading appeared on the monitor.[53,55] However, there has been no report of erroneous ICP reading resulting in clinical mismanagement, such as missing an enlarging mass lesion.

The Camino intraparenchymal device may be associated with mechanical problems. This was especially the case during the early study period because health care personnel were not familiar with the device and proper precaution in handling and securing the device was not taken. The fiberoptic cables are delicate and can be broken easily during transport or with patient movement. As many as 10% to 23% of the fiberoptic devices had a mechanical malfunction because of breakage of cable, dislocation of the probe, or other unknown factors.[51] More recently, the rate of mechanical complication has been lower at about 5%.[53]

Currently, the Camino fiberoptic probe can also be inserted intraventricularly or in the subdural space. The intraventricular Camino bolt allows concurrent CSF drainage and ICP monitoring through the fiberoptic Camino bolt. ICP measurement through the fiberoptic device placed intraventricularly correlates well with ICP measured through an external strain gauge, with 97% of the readings being within 5 mm Hg.[56]

The Camino fiberoptic device can also be inserted into the subdural space. The subdurally placed monitor is marketed as a postcraniotomy monitor, although there are no large-scale clinical studies to evaluate its accuracy. In addition, the Camino fiberoptic device can also be inserted with a temperature probe or brain tissue oxygen probe.

Miniature Strain Gauge

A miniature strain gauge transducer has also been developed to monitor ICP, with the Codman MicroSensor ICP Transducer (Codman, Raynham, MA) being the prototype. The Codman MicroSensor has a microchip pressure sensor at the tip of a flexible nylon cable that produces different electrical resistance based on pressure.[57] This MicroSensor can be placed in various compartments, including the ventricle, parenchyma, and subdural space. Gopinath and associates compared ICP measured by an intraventricularly placed MicroSensor with ICP measured by an EVD connected to an external strain gauge.[57] There was excellent correlation between the two measurements, with a correlation coefficient of 0.97, and 90% of the readings were within 4 mm Hg of each other.[57] Drift was minimal, with only 0.2 mm Hg of drift observed.[57] For intraparenchymal ICP measurement, the miniature strain gauge appears to be less accurate. When ICP readings measured by an intraparenchymally placed sensor were compared with ICP from a ventriculostomy drain, Signorini and colleagues found that there was a constant offset between the two ICP readings that led to erroneous ICP readings from the MicroSensor.[58] Similarly, Banister and coworkers found significant differences in ICP measurement from a parenchymal MicroSensor and a Camino ICP monitoring device.[59] Moreover, several episodes of raised ICP with clinical significance were captured by the Camino ICP monitoring device but not by the MicroSensor in this particular study.[59]

A more recent study analyzed clinical use of the miniature strain gauge in 128 patients.[60] The authors reported good clinical usefulness of the MicroSensor for ICP monitoring in neurocritical care patients, with no infection and no clinically significant hematomas noted ("several minor hematomas" were observed, however).[60] Drift was just 0.9 mm Hg in this study.[49] In 22 patients, a ventriculostomy was also performed, and ICP data from the two methods were compared.[61] The authors reported good correlation of ICP measured by the two methods ($r = 0.79$), and a Bland and Altman plot revealed good concordance.[60] Careful inspection of the raw data, however, revealed a mean difference of −1.2 mm Hg on the Bland and Altman plot, with a standard deviation of about 3 mm Hg. Inspection of the scatterplot data also revealed that a difference of more than 5 mm Hg was found frequently as well.

Two studies analyzed the MicroSensor placed in the subdural space. It was found that ICP measured by the MicroSensor placed in the subdural space had good correlation with pressure measured by a fluid-coupled transducer placed in the subdural space, as well as with pressure measured by a MicroSensor placed in the parenchyma.[62] However, this was not compared with ICP measured by either ventriculostomy or other devices. In one series from Taiwan, the MicroSensor was used to monitor ICP in 120 patients with TBI.[63] There were no complications from monitor placement.[63] Comparison of ICP measured by the subdurally placed MicroSensor with that measured by a ventriculostomy drain was done in 22 patients.[63] The observed difference in pressure was −1 to −4 mm Hg, although no statistical analysis was performed in this case.[63]

Spiegelberg Parenchymal Transducer

The Spiegelberg brain pressure monitor (Spiegelberg, Hamburg, Germany) uses an air pouch situated at the tip that is maintained at a constant volume. The pressure transducer is located in the ICP monitor, and recalibration to ambient pressure can be performed easily. Two studies evaluated the accuracy of ICP measurement of the Spiegelberg pressure sensor (intraparenchymal or subdural placement) versus ICP measured by ventriculostomy. Both studies revealed good correlation of ICP measured by the Spiegelberg pressure sensor with that measured by ventriculostomy.[61,64] The initial clinical experience in 87 patients was positive, with no infection, one small hemorrhage, and a 3.4% mechanical complication rate.[61]

Hummingbird Synergy

The Hummingbird Synergy (InnerSpace NeuroSolutions, Tustin, CA) is an access device with an integrated parenchymal ICP monitor, a ventricular drainage system, and probe ports for multimodality monitoring. The unit has a single port with a titanium bolt. Once it is secured into the cranium, the trajectory of the ventricular catheter is limited to 4 degrees of angular variation during advancement. Two additional side ports can be used to place two additional probes, such as a brain tissue oxygenation monitor, 30 mm below the dura and angled 30 degrees away from the axis of the bolt. In one series, placement of the ventricular catheter was successful 93% of the time within the first two attempts. This was associated with 10% rate of hemorrhage as identified on immediate postprocedural CT scan.[65]

In addition to the ports for the ventricular catheter and multimodality monitoring probes, the Hummingbird also has an integrated parenchymal ICP monitor. An air bladder positioned along the ventricular catheter transmits pressure waves along an air column charged with a precise amount of air. Once zeroed during the insertion process, this system provides an ICP recording with minimal artifact and is immune from positional changes. A direct comparison of the Hummingbird parenchymal and EVD measurements showed congruence within ±3 mm Hg in 93% of over 2000 recordings.[66] The Hummingbird parenchymal monitor is a viable alternative for ICP monitoring when the placement of an EVD catheter is unsuccessful because of distorted anatomy.

Telemetric Intracranial Pressure Monitoring

Bedside ICP monitoring with EVD or intraparenchymal devices offers continuous ICP recordings but has several limitations. Patients are hospitalized, usually in the ICU, and are tethered to the monitoring apparatus with limited mobility. These percutaneous devices are at risk for dislodgement during patient care and transport, and in uncooperative patients. They provide only a short-term monitoring solution and may offer limited insight in certain clinical scenarios.

Telemetric ICP monitoring systems offer the possibility of long-term ICP monitoring, especially during everyday conditions outside the hospital. Early systems were used to monitor ICPs in patients after posterior fossa tumor resection and in hydrocephalus patients after shunt insertion.[67,68] Recently an implantable telemetric ICP monitoring system produced by RAUMEDIC became commercially available. The system consists of an implantable probe, a reading device, and a portable recording device. The telemetry ICP probe consists of an intraparenchymal pressure sensor at the tip and is connected to a subgaleal transducer at the other end. The probe is implanted through a bur hole into the frontal parenchyma. Once the probe has been implanted, the ICP is measured by placing the external reader unit over the unit. ICP data are transmitted through the scalp and are finally registered by the recording device with a frequency of 1 or 5 Hz. Long-term animal testing showed reliable recording for at least 12 months.[69]

Early clinical experiences with the RAUMEDIC telemetric intraparenchymal ICP monitoring system have shown that outpatient long-term ICP monitoring is safe and can direct management decisions.[70-73] In a series of 185 patients with suspected or known hydrocephalus, the RAUMEDIC telemetric system was implanted for diagnostic purposes.[72] The patients were monitored for 3 to 409 days (mean 60.7 days). In 81% of patients with suspected ICP disorders, telemetric ICP monitoring led to definitive CSF diversion procedures. In patients with suspected shunt obstruction or overdrainage, telemetric ICP monitoring confirmed the diagnosis in 77% and 96%, respectively. There was a 5.9% overall complication rate associated with implantation of the telemetric probe. One case of intracranial abscess and two cases of superficial infection occurred. Postimplantation imaging was obtained in 160 patients. Of these, there was a 15.6% incidence of hemorrhage of any size. Only one case of postprocedural hemorrhage was associated with neurological deficits. There was a 46.9% incidence of postimplantation-associated cerebral edema as demonstrated by postprocedural imaging. Of these, eight cases were associated with implantation-related complications, including infection, abscess, and new-onset seizures.

EMERGING TECHNOLOGY

Compliance Monitor

A physiologic variable related to ICP is intracranial compliance. Compliance is defined as the change in volume per unit change in pressure. A low-compliance state means that a small change in volume will lead to a large change in pressure. A low-compliance state may therefore identify patients at risk for increasing ICP. The Spiegelberg Compliance Monitor uses the Spiegelberg brain-pressure monitor as the sensor. To measure compliance, the monitor injects a small amount of air into the air balloon pouch and measures the pressure response to this change in volume. Calculation of compliance is then based on the changes in pressure during 200 cycles. The usefulness of compliance monitoring in the clinical setting is still unknown. Limited data suggest a significant inverse relationship between compliance and ICP in patients with TBI and tumor.[74] A less clear relationship exists for patients with hydrocephalus or SAH.[74] Abnormal compliance in traumatic brain-injured patients or those with thalamic hemorrhage has been shown to return to normal with surgical intervention based on a small number of patients.[75,76] Currently, compliance monitoring is still at an experimental stage; preliminary data, however, suggest potential usefulness in the clinical setting.

Noninvasive Intracranial Pressure Monitoring

Since the 1960s there has been continuous effort to develop less invasive or noninvasive ICP monitors. CT characteristics, clinical examination findings, and monitored pressure in the epidural space have all been shown to be unreliable surrogates for ICP measurement.[77,78] There have been numerous reports of promising technologies for measuring or deriving ICP noninvasively, although none is being used clinically on a large scale. Several techniques that have been studied more extensively are discussed in the following paragraphs.

Noninvasive ICP monitoring technology can be divided into several categories. In one category, the eye or the ear is used as a window into the cranium.[79] A number of structures in the eye and the ear communicate with the CSF space and should therefore be influenced by ICP as well. The optic nerve is surrounded by subarachnoid space and a dural sheath, and the subarachnoid space will expand in the presence of increased ICP.[80] Therefore, optic nerve sheath diameter (ONSD), which can be measured by ultrasound, should correlate with ICP.[80] Although multiple studies have demonstrated a strong linear relationship between ONSD and ICP, the critical value of ONSD for detecting elevated ICP (ICP >20 mm Hg) is different in the various studies, thus limiting its potential use at this time.[80,81]

A similar principle is used by venous ophthalmodynamometry, which measures venous opening pressure (VOP), to calculate ICP.[82] In one study of 21 patients, VOP correlated well with ICP.[82] In 10 of 18 patients with ICP lower than 40 mm Hg, the calculated ICP from VOP was within 4 mm Hg of the measured ICP.[82] The biggest drawback of venous ophthalmodynamometry is that it requires dilation of the pupil to perform the measurement and thus takes away one of the most critical neurological examination parameters in a comatose patient. In addition, both ONSD and VOP measurement can be performed only intermittently and therefore can be used just as a screening tool for ICP elevation rather than as a continuous monitor.

Cochlear fluid pressure is thought to be related to ICP and can be indirectly measured by tympanic membrane displacement.[79] A number of studies have been performed to evaluate its use as a surrogate for ICP, and the results have been mixed.[79] Although there is a correlation between the two parameters, tympanic membrane displacement does not reliably predict ICP because of a wide predictive limit on linear regression.[83]

In another category, ICP measurement is based on the principle that increased ICP leads to changes in patterns of blood flow velocity in the intracranial arteries, which can be assessed by transcranial Doppler (TCD).[84] The middle cerebral artery (MCA) is considered a biologic pressure transducer whose vessel wall deflects in response to transmural pressure, modulating according to the pulsatile waveform of the cerebral blood flow velocity.[85] ICP can then be derived with various mathematical models by using the blood flow velocity data and variations in TCD waveform morphologies.[84,86] Several models have demonstrated the potential of these methods and shown that the derived ICP is within 6 mm Hg most of the time.[84,86] A recent comparison of four TCD-based algorithms for noninvasive ICP measurements against intraparenchymal monitoring in TBI patients showed moderate but significant correlations in reporting average ICP values during a single recording session. However, none of the noninvasive methods provided satisfactory accuracy for detecting ICP changes across time.[85] Limitations of the TCD-based noninvasive ICP methods include dependence on operator experience, quality of recordings, and noncontinuous recordings. Furthermore, certain fundamental characteristics of the MCA as a biologic transducer, such as its linearity, stability, and calibration coefficients, are unknown, thus limiting accuracy of TCD-based ICP estimations. Despite these shortcomings, TCD may have potential clinical usefulness for detection of cerebrovascular derangements in the setting of intracranial hypertension. As ICP increases and cerebral perfusion pressure (CPP) decreases, characteristic changes in flow velocity patterns can be detected by TCD.[87]

Delay in visual evoked potentials has also been observed in patients with increased ICP.[88] In the 1980s, the delay in visual evoked potentials was studied in pediatric patients with hydrocephalus and cerebral edema and found to have a significant correlation with ICP.[89] Currently, one commercial ICP monitor (NIP-200 noninvasive ICP monitoring system; Chongqing Hai-WeiKang Medical Instrument Company, Chongqing City, China) is available in China that derives ICP measurement from this principle. In one study, Zhao and colleagues found that ICP measurements with this monitor correlated well with ICP obtained by lumbar puncture opening pressure or ICP measured in the epidural space.[88] In another study, this monitor was used to monitor ICP and guide mannitol therapy in patients with intracerebral hemorrhage.[90] Per report, this monitor had been used in more than 2000 patients by 2005.[88]

PEDIATRIC INTRACRANIAL PRESSURE MONITORING

Only a few studies have been dedicated to the study of ICP monitoring in pediatric patients. In the Guidelines for the Acute Medical Management of Severe Traumatic Brain Injury in Infants, Children, and Adolescents, ICP monitoring is recommended only as an option for treating patients with severe TBI (GCS score <8) because there is insufficient evidence to support it as a guideline.[91] One study from the United Kingdom has shown that ICP monitoring was used 60% of the time in pediatric patients with severe TBI, which is a very high rate compared with adults.[92] However, it has been noted by others that monitoring in infants younger than 1 year is very infrequent.[93]

Techniques of ICP monitoring vary from center to center and include EVDs, intraparenchymal ICP monitors, and subdural monitors.[92,94,95] The complication rate of ICP monitoring in pediatric patients is probably comparable to that in adults. In one study, malposition of the EVD was noted 8.8% of the time.[94] Hemorrhage was observed in 17.6% of patients, although clinically significantly hemorrhage requiring intervention was observed in just one patient (1.6%).[94] Infection was observed in only 1 patient (1.6%).[94] Although the hemorrhage rate and malposition rate were higher in this study than the cumulative adult rate, only 62 patients were studied in this report.[94] For intraparenchymal monitors, the hemorrhage rate was 6.4% in one study and 10% in another study, and all of these hemorrhages were silent.[94,96] There is no report on the correlation of ICP measured by ventriculostomy versus other devices in these studies.

CONCLUSION

ICP monitoring and ICP-directed treatment remain the cornerstone of contemporary neurocritical care. Although it was developed more than 70 years ago, an EVD connected to an external strain gauge remains the most reliable, cost-effective, and accurate method for monitoring ICP. It is also the only ICP monitoring technique that allows CSF drainage as well. However, EVD placement is associated with a significant rate of infection and a small but significant rate of hemorrhage.

Intraparenchymal monitors have gained increased popularity in the past decade. These monitoring devices are easy to insert and have a low complication rate. Although these monitors have significant problems related to zero drift and mechanical failure, clinical experience with these monitors is positive regarding their use in ICP monitoring and management. Moreover, some of these intraparenchymal monitors can be inserted along with other monitoring devices such as brain temperature or brain tissue oxygenation monitoring devices for advanced neurophysiologic monitoring.

The field of ICU monitoring technology is changing at a rapid pace. Newer technologies such as wireless data transfer and noninvasive monitoring are coming to the ICU in the near future. Although it is easy to generate an enormous amount of data in the ICU, how to interpret, integrate, and use these data for managing a critically ill patient remains an art that must be mastered by every ICU physician.

SUGGESTED READINGS

Adelson PD, Bratton SL, Carney NA, et al. Guidelines for the acute medical management of severe traumatic brain injury in infants, children, and adolescents. Chapter 5. Indications for intracranial pressure monitoring in pediatric patients with severe traumatic brain injury. *Pediatr Crit Care Med*. 2003;4:S19.

Alleyne CH Jr, Hassan M, Zabramski JM. The efficacy and cost of prophylactic and periprocedural antibiotics in patients with external ventricular drains. *Neurosurgery*. 2000;47:1124.

Andrews PJ, Citerio G. Intracranial pressure. Part one: historical overview and basic concepts. *Intensive Care Med*. 2004;30:1730.

Bratton SL, Chestnut RM, Ghajar J, et al. Guidelines for the management of severe traumatic brain injury. IV. Infection prophylaxis. *J Neurotrauma*. 2007;24(suppl 1):S26.

Bratton SL, Chestnut RM, Ghajar J, et al. Guidelines for the management of severe traumatic brain injury. VI. Indications for intracranial pressure monitoring. *J Neurotrauma*. 2007;24(suppl 1):S37.

Bratton SL, Chestnut RM, Ghajar J, et al. Guidelines for the management of severe traumatic brain injury. VII. Intracranial pressure monitoring technology. *J Neurotrauma*. 2007;24(suppl 1):S45.

Chestnut RM, Temkin N, Carney N, et al. A trial of intracranial-pressure monitoring in traumatic brain injury. *N Engl J Med*. 2012;367:2471.

Davis JW, Davis IC, Bennink LD, et al. Placement of intracranial pressure monitors: are "normal" coagulation parameters necessary? *J Trauma*. 2004;57:1173.

Gelabert-Gonzalez M, Ginesta-Galan V, Sernamito-Garcia R, et al. The Camino intracranial pressure device in clinical practice. Assessment in 1000 cases. *Acta Neurochir (Wien)*. 2006;148:435.

Gopinath SP, Robertson CS, Contant CF, et al. Clinical evaluation of a miniature strain-gauge transducer for monitoring intracranial pressure. *Neurosurgery*. 1995;36:1137.

Holloway KL, Barnes T, Choi S, et al. Ventriculostomy infections: the effect of monitoring duration and catheter exchange in 584 patients. *J Neurosurg*. 1996;85:419.

Hong WC, Tu YK, Chen YS, et al. Subdural intracranial pressure monitoring in severe head injury: clinical experience with the Codman MicroSensor. *Surg Neurol*. 2006;66(suppl 2):S8.

Lozier AP, Sciacca RR, Romagnoli MF, et al. Ventriculostomy-related infections: a critical review of the literature. *Neurosurgery*. 2002;51:170.

Lundberg N. Continuous recording and control of ventricular fluid pressure in neurosurgical practice. *Acta Psychiatr Scand Suppl*. 1960;36:1.

Lundberg N, Troupp H, Lorin H. Continuous recording of the ventricular-fluid pressure in patients with severe acute traumatic brain injury. A preliminary report. *J Neurosurg*. 1965;22:581.

Poon WS, Ng S, Wai S. CSF antibiotic prophylaxis for neurosurgical patients with ventriculostomy: a randomised study. *Acta Neurochir Suppl*. 1998;71:146.

Shapiro S, Bowman R, Callahan J, et al. The fiberoptic intraparenchymal cerebral pressure monitor in 244 patients. *Surg Neurol*. 1996;45:278.

Signorini DF, Shad A, Piper IR, et al. A clinical evaluation of the Codman MicroSensor for intracranial pressure monitoring. *Br J Neurosurg*. 1998;12:223.

Wiesmann M, Mayer TE. Intracranial bleeding rates associated with two methods of external ventricular drainage. *J Clin Neurosci*. 2001;8:126.

Wong GK, Poon WS, Wai S, et al. Failure of regular external ventricular drain exchange to reduce cerebrospinal fluid infection: result of a randomised controlled trial. *J Neurol Neurosurg Psychiatry*. 2002;73:759.

Yau Y, Piper I, Contant C, et al. Multi-centre assessment of the Spiegelberg compliance monitor: interim results. *Acta Neurochir Suppl*. 2002; 81:167.

Zabramski JM, Whiting D, Darouiche RO, et al. Efficacy of antimicrobial-impregnated external ventricular drain catheters: a prospective, randomized, controlled trial. *J Neurosurg*. 2003;98:725.

See a full reference list on ExpertConsult.com

16 Principles of Neurocritical Care

Kimon Bekelis, Brandon K. Root, Imad Saeed Khan, Robert J. Singer, and Perry A. Ball

Critical care management is an integral component of neurosurgical practice. This chapter is a review of the principles of neurocritical care in the management of patients with ischemic stroke, hemorrhagic stroke, subarachnoid hemorrhage, and spinal cord injury. Critical care management of patients after head injury is covered in a separate chapter (see Chapter 349).

NEUROCRITICAL CONSIDERATIONS IN ISCHEMIC STROKE

Acute ischemic stroke leads to neuronal cell death in a matter of minutes. Therefore, therapeutic measures must commence swiftly and are best achieved at centers with expertise in the management of acute ischemic stroke and its associated complications.[1,2]

Blood Pressure

Hypertension after acute ischemic stroke is common at presentation, especially in patients with a history of hypertension. Studies have shown that the initial rise in blood pressure is temporary, and the pressure starts to decrease spontaneously 90 minutes after the onset of symptoms.[3,4] Extreme hypertension is deleterious because it may lead to encephalopathy, cardiac complications, and renal insufficiency. Accordingly, elevated blood pressure during hospitalization is linearly associated with worsened neurological outcomes.[5,6] Despite this, a moderate amount of hypertension may be beneficial in that it increases cerebral perfusion. Blood pressure management in acute stroke is thus a balance of these distinct principles, and both neurological and hemodynamic status must be monitored closely in the acute setting.

Numerous researchers have studied the effect of lowering blood pressure in the acute period after ischemic stroke, with equivocal results. Steep reduction of blood pressure is associated with worsened outcome and increased mortality rate. It is recommended that blood pressure in severely hypertensive patients (systolic blood pressure [SBP] of >220 mm Hg or diastolic blood pressure of >120 mm Hg) be decreased by about 15% over a period of 24 hours.[7]

For patients not treated with tissue plasminogen activator (tPA), there are no clear guidelines about blood pressure control. There are specific recommendations regarding blood pressure management if intravenous fibrinolytic therapy is considered: in cases of severe hypertension, the blood pressure should be gently decreased to below 180/110. After administration of intravenous tPA, blood pressure must be kept below 180/105 for at least 24 hours to decrease the risk of intracerebral hemorrhage (ICH).[7]

Glucose Control

Hyperglycemia is present in more than 40% of patients with ischemic stroke and is more common in those with a history of diabetes.[8,9] Multiple studies have shown that higher blood glucose levels, either at admission or during inpatient stay, are associated with an inferior clinical outcome, in comparison with normal glucose levels.[10-12] However, the Glucose Insulin in Stroke Trial–UK (GIST-UK), a study of the efficacy of controlling hyperglycemia after acute ischemic stroke, failed to show any clinical benefit.[13] There is no clinical evidence that targeting the blood glucose to a particular level will improve outcome; however, it is reasonable to follow the current American Diabetes Association recommendation to maintain blood glucose levels between 140 and 180 mg/dL in all hospitalized patients.[14]

Temperature

One third of all patients admitted with acute stroke are hyperthermic (temperature, >37.6°C) within the first few hours of stroke onset.[15] Hyperthermia in the setting of stroke may be linked to increased metabolic demands, increased amounts of free radicals, or enhanced release of neurotransmitters.[16] It is associated with a poor neurological outcome, and its source should be investigated.[17] In some instances, the cause of the stroke may be the cause of the hyperthermia (i.e., infective endocarditis), or it may be a complication secondary to the cerebral infarction (i.e., sepsis or pneumonia).

In one large, randomized, placebo-controlled trial,[18] investigators evaluated whether early treatment with acetaminophen improved functional outcome; they found no statistical difference between groups. The trial was stopped prematurely, but on post hoc analysis, a beneficial effect was found in patients with a baseline body temperature of 37°C to 39°C.

Induced hypothermia has shown promise as a neuroprotective therapy, although it may be associated with significant side effects that include hypotension, cardiac arrhythmias, and pneumonia. A systematic review in 2009 revealed no indication of clinical benefit or harm from the use of hypothermia in management of stroke.[19]

Nutrition and Hydration

Dehydration after ischemic stroke is common and may predispose affected patients to worsened cerebral perfusion, renal impairment, and increased likelihood of developing thrombosis. Hypervolemia, on the other hand, can also be detrimental by exacerbating cerebral edema and increasing myocardial stress. Euvolemia is therefore most desirable overall.

Intravenous fluid maintenance should be initiated for patients presenting in a euvolemic state. For dehydrated patients, rapid replacement of depleted intravascular volume, followed by fluid maintenance, is a reasonable course of action.[7] Isotonic solutions (i.e., 0.9% saline) are more suitable for this patient population than are hypotonic solutions, which may exacerbate cerebral edema. Patients with certain conditions, such as syndrome of inappropriate antidiuretic hormone or fever, require modifications to the standard hydration protocol.

Before oral administration of fluids or food is instituted, swallowing function must be assessed, to prevent aspiration pneumonia.[20] Physicians also need to be cautious when replacing fluids in patients who are vulnerable to fluid overload, particularly in patients with impaired renal clearance or heart failure. In some cases, a nasogastric or nasoduodenal tube may be inserted to provide feedings and to facilitate administration of medications. For patients who might require prolonged tube feedings, placement of a percutaneous endoscopic gastrostomy may be necessary.[21]

Cardiac Monitoring

Cardiac monitoring, which typically begins in the prehospital setting, must continue throughout the initial management period for at least the initial 24 hours after the patient's presentation.[22] The patient should be monitored for cardiac ischemia or changes on electrocardiogram (ECG), especially in cases of right middle cerebral artery (MCA) strokes affecting the insular cortex. Holter monitoring may be more effective in identifying atrial fibrillation or other serious arrhythmias.[23] Echocardiography is indicated in patients with suspected cardioembolic stroke. The efficacy of prophylactic administration of medications to prevent cardiac arrhythmias is unknown.

Antiplatelet Therapy

Administration of aspirin within 48 hours after stroke appears to significantly decrease the rate of mortality and other unfavorable outcomes.[24,25] This conclusion is based primarily on the findings that aspirin reduced the incidence of early recurrent stroke. Therefore, oral aspirin should be administered within 24 to 48 hours after the onset of symptoms. Data regarding the efficacy of other antiplatelet agents, including clopidogrel alone or in combination with aspirin therapy, are limited.

Anticoagulants

Anticoagulation with intravenous heparin is a common practice after ischemic stroke, but no studies have shown any clinical benefit.[26] In current guidelines, the American Heart Association/American Stroke Association (AHA/ASA; eTable 16-1) does not recommend the use of heparin within the first 24 hours, especially in cases of moderate to severe strokes because of the risk of hemorrhagic conversion. The usefulness of direct thrombin inhibitors such as argatroban is also not well established. In patients who receive tPA, heparin administration is contraindicated for the first 24 hours after tPA treatment.

Treatment of Acute Neurological Complications

Deterioration after initial stroke assessment occurs in up to 25% of patients. Cerebral edema, hemorrhagic transformation, and recurrent ischemia are among the possible causes.[27] The risk of sudden deterioration underscores the importance of close monitoring in a dedicated stroke center.[1,2]

Cerebral Edema

The manifestation of cerebral edema following acute stroke is variable. Many affected patients remain clinically stable, whereas others have precipitous neurological deterioration. Cytotoxic edema typically appears 3 to 4 days after stroke onset, but early reperfusion of a large infarct may lead to severe edema within the first 24 hours.[28] Medical management to minimize the development of edema includes restriction of free water, avoidance of excess glucose administration, and minimizing hypoxemia or hypercarbia. Severe cerebral edema increases the risk of elevated intracranial pressure (ICP; eTable 16-2). If this occurs, standard techniques used to manage elevated ICP, including osmotic diuresis, ventriculostomy, and hyperventilation, are recommended.[29]

Neurosurgical decompression for some patients with supratentorial infarcts should be considered. A pooled analysis of the results of three trials of the efficacy of early decompression in malignant MCA stroke (undertaken within 48 hours after presentation) showed reduction in mortality rate from 78% to 29% and significantly increased favorable outcomes for patients who underwent surgery.[30] In one trial (DEcompressive Surgery for the Treatment of malignant INfarction of the middle cerebral arterY [DESTINY] II), 112 patients 61 years of age or older with malignant MCA infarction were randomly assigned to undergo either conservative treatment or hemicraniectomy within the first 48 hours after the onset of symptoms. The results indicated significantly increased survival rates without severe disability among patients who underwent surgical decompression.[31] Emergency decompression may be advised for patients with severe supratentorial stroke and acutely worsening edema, but the likelihood of survival with severe disability needs to be discussed with the patient's family beforehand.

In cases of large cerebellar infarction, edema can cause brainstem compression or hydrocephalus. Emergency posterior fossa decompression with partial removal of the infarcted tissue is often lifesaving, and the clinical outcome is a reasonable quality of life.[32,33]

Hemorrhagic Transformation

Hemorrhagic transformation occurs in approximately 5% to 6% of patients after the use of intravenous recombinant tPA.[34-36] Hemorrhage caused by tPA usually occurs in the first 24 hours, and fatal hemorrhages most often occur in the first 12 hours.[37] If a patient shows signs of ICH, any tPA remaining in the prescription should be withheld; an emergency computed tomographic (CT) scan without contrast material should be performed, as should a type and screen; and a complete blood cell count, coagulation parameters (prothrombin time, partial thromboplastin time, international normalized ratio [INR]), and fibrinogen levels should be measured. Although there are no standardized recommendations for the management of fibrinolytic-associated hemorrhage, most protocols recommend the use of cryoprecipitate to restore the depleted fibrinogen levels.[7] Surgical evacuation may be considered, depending on the site and size of the hematoma and the patient's overall condition. Evacuation of a large hemorrhage may be lifesaving in some instances.[38]

Seizures

Seizures occur in approximately 10% of patients with ischemic stroke.[39,40] The incidence of seizures is higher among older patients, patients with preexisting dementia, and patients with hemorrhagic transformation. The reported rates for delayed or recurrent seizures vary greatly.[41,42] The data on the efficacy of anticonvulsants in the treatment of seizures in stroke patients are scarce, and current recommendations are based on the established management guidelines for seizures that may complicate any neurological illness. No studies to date have been able to show benefit of prophylactic anticonvulsant use after stroke.

NEUROCRITICAL CONSIDERATIONS IN INTRACEREBRAL HEMORRHAGE

Multiple conditions can be implicated in the development of spontaneous ICH, including chronic hypertension, amyloid angiopathy, coagulopathy, arteriovenous malformations, cavernous malformations, drug abuse (cocaine, methamphetamines, or sympathomimetic drugs), dural sinus thrombosis, underlying neoplasms, inflammatory vasculopathy, and ischemic stroke with hemorrhagic conversion.[43] Despite these varied causes, blood pressure control and reversal of coagulopathy are the common denominators in the management of acute ICH; surgical intervention can be employed in rare cases. In addition, patients should be monitored for increases in ICP and treated accordingly. The AHA/ASA made several class I recommendations for the initial management of ICH (eTable 16-3).[44]

Reversal of Coagulopathy

All anticoagulation and antiplatelet medications should be discontinued immediately after onset of ICH, and these agents should be promptly reversed if possible. Patients who take warfarin or have an elevated INR in the setting of systemic disease (e.g., liver failure) should receive fresh-frozen plasma transfusions and vitamin K to attain a goal INR of less than 1.5.[45,46] For those receiving antiplatelet therapy such as aspirin or clopidogrel (Plavix) and those with certain systemic diseases that compromise platelet function (such as uremia), data are unclear about whether platelet transfusions improve outcome.[47] Nevertheless, it is common to administer platelet transfusions to these patients, as well as to thrombocytopenic patients with platelet counts of less than 50,000, although the clinical threshold for this is widely debated. Unfortunately, there is no reversal agent for many newer classes of direct thrombin inhibitors.

Blood Pressure Control

Controlling blood pressure is essential in patients with ICH because elevated SBP increases the risk of hematoma expansion.[48,49] Despite this, decreasing pressures too much may compromise cerebral perfusion, although the clinical data regarding clear therapeutic end points are scarce. The AHA/ASA recommended the following goals for treating elevated SBP in the acute setting after spontaneous ICH[44]:

> If SBP exceeds 200 mm Hg or mean arterial pressure (MAP) exceeds 150 mm Hg, consider aggressive reduction of blood pressure with continuous intravenous infusion, with frequent blood pressure monitoring every 5 minutes.
>
> If SBP exceeds 180 mm Hg or MAP exceeds 130 mm Hg and there is the possibility of elevated ICP, then consider monitoring ICP and reducing blood pressure by using intermittent or continuous intravenous medications while maintaining a cerebral perfusion pressure of more than 60 mm Hg.
>
> If SBP exceeds 180 mm Hg or MAP exceeds 130 mm Hg and there is no evidence of elevated ICP, then consider a modest reduction of blood pressure (e.g., MAP of 110 mm Hg or target blood pressure of 160/90 mm Hg) by using intermittent or continuous intravenous medications to control blood pressure, and clinically reexamine the patient every 15 minutes.

Although several clinical trials have shown that more aggressive lowering of blood pressure (SBP <140) is safe, it remains uncertain whether this improves outcome.[50-52]

Surgical Evacuation

The usefulness of surgery is uncertain in many patients. In cases of cerebellar hemorrhage, mass effect and edema secondary to the hemorrhage can cause brainstem compression or hydrocephalus. Therefore, if neurological deterioration or hemodynamic instability occurs, surgical evacuation of the hemorrhage is often lifesaving and should be performed as soon as possible, especially when the diameter of the hematoma exceeds 3 cm.[44,53,54] Placement of an external ventricular drain (EVD) may be necessary with hydrocephalus; however, usage of this procedure without concurrent clot evacuation is not recommended because of a theoretical risk of upward herniation, and AHA/ASA guidelines oppose EVD placement alone as an initial temporizing measure in affected patients.[44]

Surgery for evacuation of supratentorial ICH is more controversial. Some evidence suggests a benefit in certain patients, although this has not been well elucidated. In the largest trial to date, the International Surgical Trial in Intracerebral Haemorrhage (STITCH),[55] patients were randomly assigned to undergo craniotomy or medical management within 96 hours of ICH; although outcomes were slightly better in the surgery recipients, this finding did not reach statistical significance, and patients with deep clots and a Glasgow Outcome Score (GCS) of less than 8 did worse with surgery. One Cochrane review of 10 studies revealed that surgery reduced the odds of death and dependency at follow-up but concluded that those findings were not robust and were limited by heterogeneity.[56] Current guidelines suggest consideration of craniotomy for patients presenting with lobar clots exceeding 30 mL and within 1 cm of the surface,[44] although decisions regarding surgery remain highly individualized. Other techniques, such as evacuation of the hemorrhage via endoscopic techniques or CT-guided aspiration, remain investigational.

NEUROCRITICAL CONSIDERATIONS IN ANEURYSMAL SUBARACHNOID HEMORRHAGE

Subarachnoid hemorrhage (SAH) secondary to cerebral aneurysm rupture can be a devastating event. The mortality rate in the first month is 45%, and 10% to 15% of affected patients die before reaching a hospital.[57] Patients who do survive the initial insult often require a prolonged course in the intensive care unit and are at risk for several major complications, which include rehemorrhage, vasospasm, hydrocephalus, increased ICP, hyponatremia, seizures, and cardiac aberrations. Despite the high rates of morbidity and mortality, outcomes have substantially improved since 2000,[58] and much of this improvement can be attributed to advances in the acute phase.

General Considerations

All patients with aneurysmal SAH should be admitted to the intensive care unit or a neurological special care unit at a high-volume center where neurosurgeons, endovascular specialists, and neurointensivists are readily available.[59,60] Because of the high risk of hemodynamic and neurological instability, the patient's vital signs and neurological examination should be serially monitored every 2 hours at minimum. Indications for endotracheal intubation include a Glasgow Coma Score of less than 8, hemodynamic instability, respiratory compromise, and inadequate control of ICP.

AHA/ASA guidelines recommend discontinuation and prompt reversal of all anticoagulant and antiplatelet treatment after initial SAH until the aneurysm is definitively secured (eTable 16-4).[61] All patients should receive thromboembolism prophylaxis with pneumatic compression boots; prophylactic subcutaneous heparin should be initiated only after treatment of the aneurysm.

Physiologic and endocrinologic abnormalities are common after aneurysmal SAH, and many are associated with a worsened outcome.[62-64] As a general rule, these derangements should be corrected as efficiently as possible. Hyperglycemia is frequent and increases the risk of vasospasm.[65] Blood glucose levels must be carefully monitored, and affected patients should be kept euglycemic with insulin if needed.[66] Hyperthermia is associated with a poor outcome, and fever should be promptly addressed with antipyretics, cooling blankets, or both.[67] Anemia should be corrected,[68] and although the criteria for transfusion varies between institutions, following daily blood cell counts and maintaining the hemoglobin above 7 g/dL is recommended. Respiratory parameters must be monitored and appropriately adjusted in the event of hypoxemia or metabolic acidosis, both of which are also common after SAH.[64]

Rehemorrhage

Aneurysmal rehemorrhage is a significant risk in the acute phase after aneurysmal SAH and is associated with a considerable increase in mortality rate.[69] Excluding the aneurysm from the circulation by either surgery or endovascular therapy is the only conclusive measure to prevent rehemorrhage. If the aneurysm remains untreated, the risk of rebleeding within the first 24 hours is 3% to 4%. On the second day, this risk is 2%, and it decreases by 0.3% on every subsequent day, for a total of 15% to 20% within the first 2 weeks.[70] The risk is higher in patients with elevated blood pressures at presentation, larger aneurysmal size, and a higher Hunt and Hess SAH grading score.[70-72]

Patients should be observed for changes in the neurological examination, new-onset seizures, or sudden hemodynamic instability, all of which can signify a new hemorrhage. Blood pressure should be closely monitored until the aneurysm is secured, and although there is no well-defined target, the AHA/ASA recommends maintaining SBP at less than 160.[61] Intravenous labetalol or hydralazine is usually effective when administered as needed, and a nicardipine drip may be used in patients resistant to one-time interventions. Additional measures commonly employed to prevent rehemorrhage include bed rest, stool softeners, maintaining low levels of external stimulation, and heavy sedation, although there is no evidence to support their efficacy.

Hydrocephalus and Intracranial Pressure

Acute hydrocephalus develops in 20% of patients with SAH. It is common at presentation, but it can develop at any point during the hospital course.[73,74] Patients with no symptoms of hydrocephalus may be closely monitored without cerebrospinal fluid (CSF) drainage. If a patient has symptoms, usually manifested as a compromised mental status, or when elevation in ICP is suspected, an EVD should be placed as soon as possible, which often results in immediate improvement. It remains common practice to initially program the EVD at a high setting (i.e., 15 to 20 cm H_2O when placed above the tragus) to avoid the possible risk of rehemorrhage until the aneurysm is treated, after which the setting is lowered (i.e., 10 cm H_2O when placed above the tragus) to allow for greater CSF drainage, although the risk of rehemorrhage from overdrainage is theoretical and may not be supported by evidence.[75]

Increased ICP is commonplace, often secondary to hydrocephalus, hyperemia, or vasodilation, and ICP should be measured hourly by transduction through the EVD. Sustained increases should be treated with elevation of the patient's head, maintenance of normocarbia, prevention of hyponatremia, and osmotic therapy with mannitol (1 g/kg) or hypertonic saline boluses. Hyperventilation has limited effectiveness beyond the short term and is usually not employed as a first resort. Decompressive craniectomy may be considered in cases refractory to the other measures just described.

Once the patient's overall condition stabilizes, the patient can be weaned from the EVD by slow raising of the drain's opening pressure while the neurological examination is monitored; if the patient's condition remains stable, the drain is ultimately clamped and removed. Nevertheless, up to 30% of patients remain dependent on CSF diversion and require permanent shunt placement.[76,77]

Hyponatremia

Hyponatremia after aneurysmal SAH is usually attributed to one of two distinct syndromes: syndrome of inappropriate antidiuretic hormone (SIADH) or cerebral salt wasting (CSW). Volume status can help the clinician differentiate between the two conditions, which is important because management often differs. SIADH is associated with normovolemia or hypervolemia and is generally treated with sodium supplementation. In contrast, CSW results in volume depletion and is effectively managed with large infusions of isotonic saline, along with sodium supplementation if necessary.

Sodium levels should be monitored every 6 to 12 hours in all patients. If needed, sodium levels can be supplemented by oral salt tablets (3 to 9 g/day), 3% saline infusions, or fludrocortisone acetate (2 mg orally or intravenously, twice daily).[78] Hyponatremia should be corrected gradually (sodium supplementation must not exceed 8 mEq over 24 hours), to prevent central pontine myelinolysis, which often manifests as acute cranial nerve palsies and quadriplegia. Fluid restriction as a means of correcting hyponatremia should be avoided in this patient population, who might require hypervolemia as part of vasospasm management.

Vasospasm

Cerebral vasospasm is the leading cause of morbidity and mortality after aneurysmal SAH. Vasospasm has two discrete definitions that are not necessarily coexistent. Radiographic vasospasm, occurring in 30% to 70% of patients, is defined as arterial narrowing of major vessels visible on angiography, irrespective of clinical symptoms. Symptomatic vasospasm, also known as delayed ischemic neurological deficit (DIND), consists of vasospasm with neurological deterioration and occurs in 20% to 30% of patients after aneurysmal SAH.[79] Clinical manifestations, which range in type and severity, include mental status changes, focal deficits, and death. The risk of symptomatic spasm is correlated with the amount of blood visible on CT scans, a history of cigarette smoking, age, and hyperglycemia.[67,80-82] A poor clinical condition may also increase risk, although data in the literature conflict.[82-84] Although its genesis is presumably related to breakdown of blood products in the subarachnoid space and pathologic changes in the vessel walls, the exact mechanism is unclear. Vasospasm typically occurs between 3 and 14 days after aneurysmal rupture; less commonly, it occurs outside this time period.[85,86] It significantly worsens overall prognosis; therefore, prevention and prompt treatment are of high importance.[87]

Nimodipine, a dihydropyridine calcium channel blocker, has been well studied and consistently shown to significantly improve clinical outcome in the setting of vasospasm.[88,89] It should be administered to all patients with aneurysmal SAH, beginning at admission and continuing through day 21. Somewhat paradoxically, it does not appear to reduce the incidence of radiographic vasospasm,[88] which suggests that its benefit may be a result of increased collateral perfusion or neuroprotective effects rather than a direct vasodilatory response. The standard dosage is 60 mg orally every 4 hours; however, transient hypotension after administration is common and should be avoided. To mitigate this effect, the dosage can be modified to 30 mg every 2 hours. Statins may reduce vasospasm by altering vasomotor reactivity or upregulating cerebral blood flow, although data in the literature are conflicting, and no randomized clinical trials have yielded data that support their usage.[90,91] Nevertheless, given the good safety profile of statins, they are commonly administered during the patient's course.

Transcranial Doppler (TCD) imaging can measure the flow velocity of intracranial vessels. As vasospasm narrows the arterial lumen and increases relative velocity, TCD imaging serves as a useful screening tool. It should be performed two to three times per week during the timeframe of significant risk, usually discontinuing 14 days after hemorrhage. Although the velocity criteria for defining spasm varies by institution, MCA mean flow velocity (MFV) that exceeds 200 cm/sec has a positive predictive value of 87%, and MCA MFV of less than 120 cm/sec has a negative predictive value of 94%.[92] This association is less clear in other vascular territories.[93] The Lindegaard ratio, expressed as MCA velocity/internal carotid artery velocity, corrects the MFV for hyperemia, which can also increase MFV as a result of increased cardiac output, anemia, or the use of vasopressors. A ratio of less than 3 is interpreted as no spasm; 3 to 4.5, as mild spasm; 4.5 to 6, moderate spasm; and higher than 6, severe spasm.[94]

Although TCD is an effective tool for both screening and monitoring, there is significant operator variability and a frequent inability to insonate intracranial vessels in some patients. Therefore, treatment for vasospasm should not be initiated on the basis of TCD values alone. The findings of the neurological examination should be closely monitored, and other potential causes of a new deficit should always be ruled out. If alternative causes are excluded, and the examination findings are correlated with TCD results, more reliable confirmatory tests should be conducted. Although digital subtraction angiography remains the "gold standard" of testing, CT angiography can also demonstrate vasospasm.[95] CT perfusion, magnetic resonance angiography, and magnetic resonance perfusion may also be effective, but their practical utility is currently limited.[96-98] When clinical findings with TCD imaging are suspect for vasospasm, many centers promptly perform CT angiography and then proceed to digital subtraction angiography with intervention if warranted.

In the setting of confirmed DIND, the standard of medical intervention is hyperdynamic therapy, also known as hypervolemic-hypertensive hemodilution (HHH). Expanding the intravascular volume, increasing blood pressure, and lowering blood viscosity, all of which increase cardiac output, are hypothesized to augment cerebral blood flow in poorly perfused areas. Despite its widespread usage, no randomized trials have proved the efficacy of HHH. Consequently, there is substantial variation in clinical routine, with no clearly defined therapeutic end points. Volume expansion can be achieved with large infusions of either isotonic crystalloid (normal saline) or colloid (albumin 5%). Goals for SBP generally range from 100 to 240 mm Hg, or a MAP of 70 to 210 mm Hg.[99] If hypertension is not achieved with volume expansion alone, vasopressors (e.g., norepinephrine, dopamine, or phenylephrine) or inotropes (e.g., dobutamine or milrinone) can be used.[100,101] Ideal parameters for blood viscosity are not clear, although a diminished oxygen-carrying capability may outweigh the beneficial effects of hemodilution if the hematocrit falls below 30%.

Regardless of each institution's specific parameters, HHH therapy is inadvisable until after the ruptured aneurysm is secured, in view of the possible risk for rerupture (see "Rehemorrhage" section). If a patient has additional, unruptured aneurysms that have not been previously secured, the risk of rupture appears low enough to proceed with HHH therapy.[102]

One important consideration is that hyperdynamic therapy, despite its function in treating symptomatic vasospasm, does not appear to prevent it.[103,104] Furthermore, it can exacerbate cerebral edema, hyponatremia, increased ICP, and pulmonary edema, for which these patients are already at considerable risk.[105,106] Therefore, hyperdynamic therapy is recommended only if DIND is confirmed; usage in isolated radiographic vasospasm or as a prophylactic measure should be avoided. On the other hand, overt hypovolemia can worsen ischemic complications.[107] In the absence of active DIND, the goal of fluid management should thus be euvolemia or mild volume expansion.

In patients who fail to improve with hyperdynamic therapy, endovascular interventions can be employed, which can reverse symptoms of delayed cerebral ischemia in 30% to 70%.[108] Direct mechanical dilation with balloon angioplasty, intra-arterial injection of vasodilators, or combination therapy is often employed.[109,110] The specifics of each endovascular strategy often depend on patient circumstances, as well as hospital capabilities and protocol.

Seizures

The incidence of seizures after aneurysmal SAH ranges from 4% to 26%.[111] Risk factors include worsened clinical grade, a greater amount of subarachnoid blood, the presence of ICH, infarction, and MCA location of an aneurysm.[112-115] Their relationship to outcome remains unclear; some studies have demonstrated that seizures are an independent predictor of poor outcome,[114,116] whereas some suggest that they are merely correlated with greater disease severity.[112]

The usage of prophylactic antiepileptic drugs remains controversial. One Cochrane review did not reveal sufficient evidence to either recommend or refute the usage of prophylactic anticonvulsants.[117] AHA/ASA guidelines maintained that the use of prophylactic anticonvulsants may be considered in the immediate posthemorrhagic period.[61]

Cardiac Abnormalities

Numerous cardiac complications after aneurysmal SAH have been well described. These include ECG changes, elevated cardiac enzymes, arrhythmias, and left ventricular dysfunction.[118,119] Although coronary vessel thrombosis and spasm may contribute, the key mechanism is probably related to hypothalamic insult, whereby a subsequent adrenergic surge and catecholamine release lead to subendocardial band necrosis.[120] The right insular cortex has also been implicated in mediating sympathetic cardiac function[121]; in one study, a greater hemorrhage burden in the right hemisphere was associated with an increased risk of cardiac aberrations.[122]

Nonspecific ECG changes are exceedingly frequent; reported prevalences range from 27% to 100%.[123] Changes in T-wave structure, increased QT interval, development of U waves, and ST-segment elevation or depression are the most common findings. These changes are not usually clinically significant in patients with SAH, and their relationship to outcome is unclear. Levels of cardiac troponins, a more specific predictor of overall cardiac function, are elevated in about 34% of patients with SAH and are associated with worsened outcome.[124,125]

Arrhythmias occur in up to half of patients with SAH but are typically benign, often manifesting as sinus bradycardia, sinus tachycardia, and premature atrial or ventricular beats. Four percent of patients develop more serious arrhythmias, such as atrial fibrillation, atrial flutter, ventricular tachycardia, ventricular fibrillation, and torsades de pointes. Clinically significant arrhythmias are associated with a high mortality rate and should be addressed promptly.[126] Patients should undergo a baseline 12-lead ECG at admission, followed by continuous telemetry monitoring through the first 2 weeks. Electrolyte levels should be monitored daily, with particular attention to potassium and magnesium. Depletion of either may provoke an arrhythmia, and correction is relatively straightforward.

The incidence of left ventricular dysfunction, as evidenced by wall motion abnormalities, ranges from 13% to 31%.[124] Neurogenic stunned myocardium, the syndrome of left ventricular dysfunction, ECG changes, and an elevation in cardiac enzymes,[127] is often reversible, in contrast to myocardial infarction which it often mimics. Treatment with inotropic agents (e.g., dobutamine or milrinone) is often effective.[128]

NEUROCRITICAL CONSIDERATIONS IN SPINAL CORD INJURY

Acute spinal cord injury (SCI) is often associated with systemic hemodynamic and pulmonary derangements, and inadequate perfusion or oxygenation of the spinal cord has the potential to worsen neurological injury.

Hemodynamics

Hypotension after acute SCI is common. SCI often occurs in the setting of other significant injuries, and the first consideration is to confirm or rule out systemic injuries that result in blood loss, such as lacerations, vascular injuries, injuries to the abdominal contents, and long bone or pelvic fractures, as the cause of the hypotension. Isolated SCI can also result in hypotension, inasmuch as the sympathetic signals from the spinal cord that increase the heart rate and the resistance in the systemic arterioles exit in the thoracic segments T1 to T4. With lesions above this level, bradycardia and hypotension can result. The administration of intravenous fluid is the first step to correct this, but because of lack of resistance in the vascular system, blood may pool within the vascular system, and pharmacologic methods become necessary to maintain hemodynamic support. Phenylephrine, whose almost exclusively α-adrenergic activity increases the tone in the vascular system, is an option, but its administration may result in reflex bradycardia because of the lack of β-adrenergic input. Norepinephrine, which has both α- and β-adrenergic activity, is often a preferable agent in this setting.

The target for blood pressure needs to be individualized. The first consideration is to ensure that perfusion is sufficient to normalize systemic markers of tissue perfusion, such as urine output, serum lactate level, and arterial pH. Placement of a central venous catheter to help assess intravascular volume and provide access for vasoactive medications can aid in the process of resuscitation. There are, however, no measurable indices of the adequacy of spinal cord perfusion and no practical way to determine perfusion pressure of the spinal cord. Arbitrary systemic MAP goals have therefore been postulated as surrogate markers of adequate spinal cord blood flow. In uncontrolled small case series of patients with acute SCI who have been managed with MAP targets between 85 and 90 mm Hg, improved neurological outcome has been claimed.[129,130] The American Association of Neurological Surgeons/Congress of Neurological Surgeons (AANS/CNS) guidelines for the management acute SCI considers this level III evidence and recommends that MAP be kept between 85 and 90 mm Hg for the first 7 days after the injury.[131] The dose of vasoactive medication needed to produce this level of pressure in some patients may produce arrhythmias or excessive vasoconstriction, especially in patients with preexisting medical comorbid conditions, and the risks and benefits of this strategy must be weighed on an individual basis. If this regimen is selected, the patient must be monitored carefully in an intensive care unit.

Pulmonary Considerations

The pulmonary consequences of SCI are reflected by the level of the spinal injury. The diaphragm is innervated by the roots of C3 to C5 roots, and so complete lesions above C3 usually result in the need for urgent intubation and mechanical ventilation. In lesions below C5, diaphragmatic function is preserved, but in the acute phase there is flaccid paralysis of the intercostal and abdominal muscles. In this setting, the chest wall collapses with diaphragmatic contraction, markedly reducing the efficiency of respiration. This results in shallow respirations that are compensated by an increase in respiratory rate, and the loss of the abdominal muscles decreases the ability to cough and clear secretions. This promotes a cycle of increasingly rapid shallow breaths, progressive atelectasis, and subsequent fatigue. During the acute phase of SCI, respiratory function must be carefully monitored, and vigorous suctioning and promotion of pulmonary toilet are crucial. Signs of progressive fatigue, such as a persistently rising respiratory rate or an increase in partial pressure of carbon dioxide, should prompt intubation. Respiratory failure occurs in about one third of patients with cervical SCI[132] at an average of 5 days after injury.[133]

The mean length of time for mechanical ventilation for patients with acute cervical SCI is about 5 weeks.[133] This is largely because the ability to wean from mechanical ventilation is dependent on the transition from flaccid to spastic paralysis of the intercostal muscles. As this occurs, the chest wall regains much of its rigidity, and inspiratory function approaches preinjury levels. This means that most patients with injury below C3 are eventually able to be weaned from mechanical ventilation,[134] but tracheostomy may need to be considered for many of these patients. Expiratory function and ability to cough, however, remain markedly diminished, and affected patients will continue to need aggressive pulmonary toilet.

16

Pharmacologic Therapy

Pharmacologic agents aimed at limiting secondary injury after SCI, such as methylprednisolone and G_{M1} ganglioside, have been studied in human trials. Unfortunately, the results of these trials have been disappointing. In the case of G_{M1} ganglioside, an initial pilot study had promising results,[135] but a subsequent larger multicenter, randomized, controlled study showed no benefit at 1 year in comparison with placebo.[136] Methylprednisolone, evaluated in the Second National Acute Spinal Cord Injury Study (NASCIS II), purportly did show a benefit.[137] However, there have been concerns about the design and conclusions of this study, and the AANS/CNS graded the results as level III evidence.[138] The use of methylprednisolone does appear to be associated with increased risk of serious complications with level I evidence. The guidelines thus recommend that neither methylprednisolone nor G_{M1} ganglioside be used in the treatment of acute SCI.[138]

Hypothermia

The use of hypothermia to limit secondary neurological injury has significant potential and has been shown to be beneficial in improved cerebral function after cardiac arrest. The value of hypothermia in acute SCI is unclear. The use of modest hypothermia (32°C to 34°C) in acute SCI has been reported to yield acceptable complication rates and improved neurological outcomes.[139-141] The AANS/CNS Joint Section on Disorders of the Spine and Peripheral Nerves classified these findings as level IV evidence and stated that the evidence is insufficient to recommend or discourage this treatment.[142]

SUGGESTED READINGS

Allen GS, Ahn HS, Preziosi TJ, et al. Cerebral arterial spasm—a controlled trial of nimodipine in patients with subarachnoid hemorrhage. *N Engl J Med*. 1983;308(11):619-624.

CAST: randomised placebo-controlled trial of early aspirin use in 20,000 patients with acute ischaemic stroke. CAST (Chinese Acute Stroke Trial) Collaborative Group. *Lancet*. 1997;349(9066):1641-1649.

Connolly ES, Rabinstein AA, Carhuapoma JR, et al. Guidelines for the management of aneurysmal subarachnoid hemorrhage: a guideline for healthcare professionals from the American Heart Association/American Stroke Association. *Stroke*. 2012;43(6):1711-1737.

The International Stroke Trial (IST): a randomised trial of aspirin, subcutaneous heparin, both, or neither among 19435 patients with acute ischaemic stroke. International Stroke Trial Collaborative Group. *Lancet*. 1997;349(9065):1569-1581.

Jüttler E, Unterberg A, Woitzik J, et al. Hemicraniectomy in older patients with extensive middle-cerebral-artery stroke. *N Engl J Med*. 2014;370(12):1091-1100.

Lindegaard KF, Nornes H, Bakke SJ, et al. Cerebral vasospasm after subarachnoid haemorrhage investigated by means of transcranial Doppler ultrasound. *Acta Neurochir Suppl (Wien)*. 1988;42:81-84.

Mendelow AD, Gregson BA, Fernandes HM, et al. Early surgery versus initial conservative treatment in patients with spontaneous supratentorial intracerebral haematomas in the International Surgical Trial in Intracerebral Haemorrhage (STICH): a randomised trial. *Lancet*. 2005;365(9457):387-397.

Vahedi K, Hofmeijer J, Juettler E, et al. Early decompressive surgery in malignant infarction of the middle cerebral artery: a pooled analysis of three randomised controlled trials. *Lancet Neurol*. 2007;6(3):215-222.

See a full reference list on ExpertConsult.com

17 The Neurosurgical Intensive Care Unit and the Unique Role of the Neurosurgeon

Richard Tyler Dalyai, Jack I. Jallo, and Robert H. Rosenwasser

Neurological surgeons have been performing neurological and neurosurgical critical care prior to those terms being in the vernacular. By the nature of the neurocritical care specialty, many of the patients who are cared for by neurological surgeons reside in the intensive care unit (ICU) because of the extent of their injury and neurological disease, whether it be cranial or spinal. There is no doubt that neurological surgeons have been instrumental in the development of this new recognized subspecialty within the field of neuroscience clinical care. The American Board of Neurological Surgery actually board certifies graduates in neurological critical care, although we all realize that this field has grown and requires additional curricular studies above and beyond the care of the central and peripheral nervous system. Many neurosurgical intensive care units (neuro-ICUs) in this country and beyond have been staffed in part by neurological surgeons with an interest in critical care, and certainly all neurosurgeons have routinely played leadership roles in the development and ongoing management of the neuro-ICU.

Neurosurgical training in America is a 7-year process and many individuals, in addition to that, take fellowships. The neurosurgical resident spends a significant part of that 7 years taking care of patients in the ICU, working with neurosurgeons as well as intensivists who are trained in the care of these patients. There are no other residency training programs where these physicians would be exposed to such high levels of critical care during the course of their residency. The Accreditation Council for Graduate Medical Education (ACGME) has developed milestones (knowledge, skills, attitudes, and other attributes) for critical care, organized in a developmental format from less to more advanced (Tables 17-1 and 17-2). These milestones provide a framework for assessing the development of competency by resident physicians in key aspects of critical care during their participation in ACGME-accredited residency or fellowship programs.[1] The main areas of focus for the neurosurgeon in the neuro-ICU have included management of subarachnoid hemorrhage (SAH), traumatic brain injury (TBI) and spinal cord injury, status epilepticus, intracerebral hemorrhage, and most recently surgical and endovascular management of vascular disease and ischemic cerebrovascular disease and surgical management of malignant middle cerebral artery infarction.

HISTORY OF THE NEURO-ICU AND HARVEY CUSHING'S CONTRIBUTIONS

Guiding principles for the practice of modern neurocritical care arguably began in one of Harvey Cushing's seminal works, "Concerning a definite regulatory mechanism of the vaso-motor center which controls blood pressure during cerebral compression." Written in 1901 in an issue of the *Bulletin of The Johns Hopkins Hospital*,[2] this study investigated in dogs the relationship of saline-induced increases in intracranial pressure (ICP) with corresponding increases in arterial blood pressure as well as partial cessation of respiration. This landmark paper shed light on the vagal and spinal reflexes of elevated ICPs, leading to discovery of the "Cushing response." The prevention of the Cushing response and elevated ICPs to prevent secondary injury remains a paramount function of neurocritical care to this day. Another of Cushing's many landmark contributions to the field was his medical observations from World War I leading to his finding that 60% of deaths resulting from penetrating head wounds were due to cerebral infections.[3] With his experience in rapid débridement, Cushing found he could lower head trauma mortality from 54% to 29% by the war's end. With this development, one of Harvey Cushing's residents, Hugh Cairns, brought about mobile head injury units that were staffed by a neurosurgeon, neurologist, and anesthesiologist. These mobile units may have been the first dedicated neuro-ICUs in history.[3]

EVALUATION OF THE NEURO-ICU PATIENT

From prehistoric patients requiring trephination to modern-day neuro-ICU patients with multiple invasive monitors, one of the most challenging tasks for physicians taking care of patients in the neuro-ICU is proper assessment. Clinical evaluation is particularly challenging when patients are unable to report medical histories or medical symptoms because of decreased mental status. Neurosurgical expertise with clinical neurological examination is particularly important in neurocritical care, especially when units are led by physicians with backgrounds in medical or surgical critical care. Neurosurgeons are needed to recognize patients' neurological signs and complications that would benefit from prompt neurosurgical interventions.

Neurosurgical evaluation must begin early, at the time of admission of a patient to the neuro-ICU. Even though most neuro-ICU patients have been initially assessed by emergency department, medical-surgical, or referring hospital staff prior to arriving in the neuro-ICU, the evaluation in the neuro-ICU should begin with the reassessment and reevaluation of each patient admitted. This starts with a careful systems-based practice for all patient transfers, with proper communication and interpersonal skills between all teams regarding the patient's neurological and systemic disorders as well as all initial interventions that have been performed outside the neuro-ICU. The tight coordination among care teams should start prior to transfer and continue throughout the patient's neuro-ICU stay in patients with multiple medical issues requiring various medical consulting and ancillary services, including respiratory, nutrition, physical therapy, and nursing teams.

Similar to the primary survey, all assessments of injury should begin with the airway, breathing, and circulation (ABCs) in assessing the airway and complications of potential intubation, vital signs of adequate ventilation, and perfusion. Particularly in patients with TBI, hypoxia or hypotension must be quickly managed and prevented. In all critically ill patients, and especially neuro-ICU patients, a careful history-taking is challenging in those with an extensive medical history or in those with diminished mental status who are unable to relay any reliable history or medical information. Information must carefully be gathered from family members, bystanders, and first responders. After a careful review of the patient's history and physical examination, neurosurgeons should review all imaging and pertinent laboratory results. In organizing this information, neurosurgeons must be able to quickly localize pathology within the neuraxis where a patient's neurological deficit may arise. For all patients in the

TABLE 17-1 ACGME Neurological Surgery Milestones for Neurosurgery Residents

Critical Care—Patient Care				
Level 1	**Level 2**	**Level 3**	**Level 4**	**Level 5**
• Performs a history and physical examination in critically-ill patients • Orders positioning, analgesics, sedation, neuromuscular blockade, intravenous (IV) fluids, and nutrition in critically-ill patients • Diagnoses and formulates treatment plans for common pulmonary diseases • Uses electrocardiogram (ECG) to diagnose cardiac arrhythmia; initiates hemodynamic monitoring • Performs a brain death examination	• Explains risks and benefits of ventilatory support • Interprets diagnostic studies (e.g., chest x-ray, brain computed tomography [CT], ECG) • Manages intracranial hypertension (e.g., hyperosmolar agents, cerebrospinal fluid [CSF] drainage) • Manages airway and performs endotracheal intubation • Inserts arterial and central venous catheters • Diagnoses and manages spinal or hypovolemic shock	• Formulates work-up and treatment plan for a comatose patient • Manages refractory intracranial hypertension (e.g., blood pressure, cerebral perfusion pressure [CPP]) • Obtains confirmatory tests and makes an accurate diagnosis of brain death • Initiates management of pneumonia or systemic infection	• Independently formulates a treatment plan for complex patients (e.g., failure of cerebral autoregulation, multiorgan failure, nonrecoverable central nervous system injury) • Diagnoses and initiates management of adult respiratory distress syndrome • Manages difficult and emergency airways • Diagnoses and manages CSF leak • Initiates management of cardiac rhythm disturbances	• Systematically reviews outcomes for neurocritical care patients • Participates in quality improvement for a neurocritical care unit • Develops a standard neurocritical care unit management protocol • Leads multidisciplinary neurocritical care team • Manages respiratory failure (e.g., mechanical ventilation, bronchoscopy) • Manages cardiac rhythm disturbances

From *Accreditation Council for Graduate Medical Education (ACGME)*. Milestones for neurological surgery. https://www.acgme.org/acgmeweb/tabid/135/ProgramandInstitutionalAccreditation/SurgicalSpecialties/NeurologicalSurgery.aspx; 2015. Accessed 14.04.15.
ACGME, Accreditation Council for Graduate Medical Education.

TABLE 17-2 ACGME Neurological Surgery Milestones for Neurosurgery Residents

Critical Care—Medical Knowledge				
Level 1	**Level 2**	**Level 3**	**Level 4**	**Level 5**
• Describes intracranial pressure (ICP), cerebral perfusion pressure, and cerebral blood flow physiology • Describes respiratory and ventilator physiology and effects on the central nervous system • Describes the pathophysiology of myocardial infarction and congestive heart failure • Describes physiology of coagulation and hemostasis • Describes principles of nutritional support • Lists indications for ICP monitoring and hematoma evacuation • Describes cerebral autoregulation	• Describes the pathophysiology and medical management of intracranial hypertension and cerebral edema • Describes modes of mechanical ventilation and management of pulmonary shunting and dead space • Describes prophylaxis for deep vein thrombosis • Describes the pathophysiology and treatment of diabetic ketoacidosis • Describes the etiology and imaging of traumatic intracranial hemorrhage and parenchymal injuries	• Describes indications for electroencephalography monitoring • Discusses indications for and risks of endotracheal intubation/ventilation • Describes the pathophysiology and treatment of systemic critical illness (e.g., hypertension, coagulopathy, electrolyte imbalance, alcohol withdrawal) • Lists indications and complications for decompressive craniectomy, cerebrospinal fluid (CSF) drainage, and barbiturate coma in traumatic brain injury (TBI)	• Describes expected outcomes after TBI and the impact of intra-cranial hypertension and of surgical intervention • Understands trans-cranial Doppler (TCD) sonography and its role in monitoring • Discusses the risks of CSF drainage, hyperosmolar therapy, and hyperventilation • Describes methods to assess intravascular volume and tissue perfusion	• Contributes to peer-reviewed literature in TBI • Describes advanced intracranial monitoring (e.g., brain tissue oxygenation, jugular venous oxygen saturation, microdialysis) • Describes advanced imaging for TBI (e.g., cerebral metabolism, perfusion) • Describes indications and risks for various methods of hemodialysis and extracorporeal membrane oxygenation

From *Accreditation Council for Graduate Medical Education (ACGME)*. Milestones for neurological surgery. https://www.acgme.org/acgmeweb/tabid/135/ProgramandInstitutionalAccreditation/SurgicalSpecialties/NeurologicalSurgery.aspx; 2015. Accessed 14.04.15.
ACGME, Accreditation Council for Graduate Medical Education.

neuro-ICU, a full review of imaging is needed to determine the extent of neurological injury as well as any systemic injuries on plain films; computed tomography (CT) of the brain, spine, chest, abdomen, or pelvis; or magnetic resonance imaging. Evaluation of patients in the neuro-ICU must also include a comprehensive assessment of pulmonary, cardiac, infectious, and hematologic illnesses or injuries and their complications. This information is necessary to develop an understanding of how these systemic illnesses and complications may impact the neuro-ICU patient's neurological disorder. This clinical evaluation is paramount in the treatment of neuro-ICU patients in all systems models of neuro-ICU care and especially when such care is coordinated and co-managed by intensivists with backgrounds other than neurosurgery.

THE ROLE OF THE ICU IN THE CARE OF NEUROSURGERY PATIENTS

Originally, the primary systems model for neuro-ICU care was a "low-intensity" model that involved direct management of neurosurgical patients almost exclusively by neurosurgeons, with limited consultation by other medical and surgical services.[4] These ICUs first developed with the need for artificial ventilator support and high-intensity nursing for neurosurgical postoperative patients. The escalation in care from that on surgical floors or intermediate-care floors generally involved a higher level of monitoring, including the use of arterial lines, mechanical ventilation, central venous access, invasive cardiac monitoring (Swan-Ganz hemodynamic monitoring), and potentially ICP monitors and ventricular drainage. These higher levels of monitoring and more frequent nursing evaluations were otherwise solely managed by the neurosurgeon with either no intensivist available or elective intensivist consultation. With the development of critical care medicine, neurosurgeons were assisted with consultation when requested by physicians specializing in critical care medicine or surgery.

Practice-of-care models were then developed in "closed" or "semiclosed" multisystem medical or surgical ICUs where patients were directly managed by a dedicated full-time intensive care team that led the management of ICU patients for the length of their ICU stay.[5] The most responsible physician would be a general medical or surgical intensivist. These specialists would directly manage all organ systems with consultation from the neurosurgical team, which would transition to primary responsibility once patients no longer had active critical care issues. Pronovost and colleagues[6] showed that staffing an ICU with critical care practitioners positively affected the outcome of ICU patients. Critical care intensivists help organize patient care, decrease resource utilization, prevent complications, and decrease length of ICU stay. Studies have suggested that ICUs with mandatory intensivist consultation have been associated with decreased hospital mortality as well as decreased hospital length of stay.[7,8] In these particular studies, critical care clinicians were experts in multiorgan system failure and critical care cardiopulmonary needs but generally were less experienced in specific neurological complications. This model, which exists in many hospitals today, mandates close involvement with a neurosurgeon to evaluate patients with complicated neurological examinations and conditions while managing specific neurological complications with which neurosurgeons have experience, such as external ventricular drains and ICP monitors, or following patients who may need a decompressive craniectomy.

Trends in medical and surgical critical care units have carried over further to the neuro-ICU with a need for specialized intensivists with knowledge of and expertise in neurological disorders as well as the systemic manifestations of disease. Starting in the 1980s, specialized neuro-ICUs were developed not only for neurosurgical postoperative patients, but also to manage TBI, intracerebral hemorrhage and SAH, status epilepticus, and ischemic stroke.[4] Neurological complications specifically monitored in the neuro-ICU setting include intracranial hypertension, cerebral edema, intracerebral hematoma expansion, cerebral vasospasm, and nonconvulsive seizures. Prompt management and avoidance of these potential complications necessitated intensivists focused on subtle changes in the neurological examination as well as expertise in managing ICP, cerebral blood flow, neuropharmacology, and electroencephalography.[4] Neurointensivists, as neurosurgeons or neurologists specializing in critical care, would be primarily responsible for the patient care. These neurointensivists require expertise not only in general ICU technologies such as mechanical ventilation but also in those technologies specific to neurological disorders, such as parenchymal brain tissue oxygen sensors and microdialysis. These new neurological monitoring devices allow for closer management of physiologic parameters. Neurosurgical intensive care has developed as a subspecialty of neurology and neurosurgery in managing multidisciplinary dedicated neuro-ICUs.

Similar to the prior studies of critical care teams, Varelas and colleagues[5] and Suarez and coworkers[9] found that neurocritical care teams in semiclosed units reduced resource utilization and reduced mortality at the same time. In a subsequent study, Varelas and associates[10] looked at the effect of appointment of a fellowship-trained neurointensivist specifically with respect to the outcomes of acute head injury and found improvements in the mortality rate, hospital length of stay, and proportion of patients discharged to home as opposed to discharged to rehabilitation or skilled nursing facilities. Although neurosurgeons have competing responsibilities in operating rooms, clinics, and other areas of the hospital, the organization of neuro-ICU care provides consistent care.[11] Varelas and associates[10] also highlighted improvements from having an experienced neurointensivist available full time at the bedside, close attention to detail, and better systems-based approaches to monitoring. These improved outcomes have been consistent with improved resource allocation and economic value of care.[12] The field of neurointensivists has continued to expand with practitioners in various subdisciplines, including neurosurgeons, neurologists, and critical care internal medicine specialists, becoming fellowship trained in neurocritical care. There is increasing evidence that specialized neurocritical care centers improve outcomes in patients with specific neurological disorders such as severe TBI,[10,13] ischemic stroke,[14] intraparenchymal hemorrhage,[15] and SAH.[16] A large systematic meta-analysis in 2011 by Kramer and Zygun[17] reported on greater than 24,000 patients and concluded that patients cared for in a neuro-ICU were more likely to have a favorable neurological outcome and lower mortality rates.

Patients in the neuro-ICU appear more likely to have received invasive intracranial or hemodynamic monitoring, tracheostomy, and nutritional support while less likely to require mechanical ventilation overall. In comparison to general ICU patients, Kurtz and coworkers[18] also found that neuro-ICU patients were less likely to receive intravenous sedation or blood transfusions. Practice modifications developed in neuro-ICUs that may improve care outcomes include hiring of specialized neurointensivists, use of temperature modification protocols, mutual rounding between neurocritical care and neurosurgical teams, implementation of SAH and TBI protocols, and the coordination of neurocritical care in a defined space.[11] Neurosurgeons maintain a cornerstone in the field and are active members in the Neurocritical Care Society because of their specialized evaluations of neurological disorders, complications, and surgical interventions. Even with the assistance of management by non-neurosurgeon neurointensivists, neurosurgeons still hold a special responsibility in the neuro-ICU in coordinating pre-, peri-, and postoperative care. Neurosurgeons are necessary to truly coordinate care and make significant decisions as to when and how to take patients to the operating room for the surgical procedures that many of these significantly acute neurological disorders mandate. Furthermore, after leaving the neuro-ICU these acutely ill patients must have a close continuity of care when transferred into lower level intermediate-care floors and when discharged into outpatient clinics. In order to provide proper continuity of care for these challenging patients, neurosurgeons closely follow, manage, and coordinate care of these patients while they are in the neuro-ICU.

ELEMENTS OF NEURO-ICU CARE

In all systems models of neuro-ICU care, general neurological evaluation, treatment, and complications avoidance are consistent needs for all neuro-ICU patients. One of the most important aspects of neurocritical care is identifying and managing intracranial hypertension and preventing secondary cerebral adverse events. Elevated ICP can lead to decreased cerebral perfusion pressure (CPP), ischemia, brain herniation, and death. Elevated ICPs should be managed with external ventricular drainage or ICP monitoring, with pharmacologic management dependent on the case scenario. While emergently addressing needs for lowering ICP, initial evaluation of intracranial hypertension should focus on determining the source of elevated pressure. The neurosurgeon has the specific responsibility of appropriately identifying mass lesions that may benefit from surgical resection or decompression. Similarly, in cases with uncontrolled intracranial hypertension or malignant edema, neurosurgeons must identify and treat patients in whom a decompressive craniectomy would be beneficial or life saving. At any time imaging data such as head CT may be repeated to evaluate for new mass lesions, edema, or cerebrospinal fluid obstruction.

A particular task for which the neuro-ICU was developed is monitoring for neurological decline, which is especially important in patients with TBI. The monitoring by the neurosurgeon, along with proper systems and nursing staff monitoring, should enable quick identification and prevention of neurological decline. Cerebral integrity can be monitored for ICP, brain tissue oxygenation, and microdialysis. Examples of causes for neurological deterioration that must be monitored for by the neurosurgeon are malignant cerebral edema, growth of intraparenchymal hemorrhages, new contusions, and extension of subdural or epidural hematomas.

The neurosurgeon must also be intimately involved with the plan of care of patients with acute SAH. This begins with initial assessment of the patient with an unrepaired aneurysm. From the clinical history, the date of bleeding and the Hunt and Hess Stroke Scale score or World Federation of Neurosurgical Societies SAH grade must be established. Evaluation of SAH patients with confusion, stupor, or coma is challenging and may necessitate neurosurgical evaluation and potentially intervention with external ventricular drainage to maintain ICP less than 20 cm of water to prevent aneurysm rerupture.[19-21] Blood pressure must be strictly controlled and maintained below a target mean arterial pressure.[22] Patients should have appropriate intravenous access, and if necessary, central access for proper volume status monitoring and use of cardiogenic inotropes and vasopressors. Intravenous fluids should be given to maintain euvolemia and a Foley catheter should be placed for volume status monitoring.[22] Electrocardiograms and cardiac troponin levels should be assessed for indications of myocardial injury. If patients are on anticoagulation (e.g., warfarin) or taking antiplatelet agents such as aspirin or clopidogrel, consideration should be given to reversal. Nimodipine should be given for vasospasm prophylaxis.[23,24] Patients should be prepared for surgery using CT angiography or digital subtraction angiography (DSA) for evaluation and planning for securing the aneurysm. This preoperative care prior to securing the aneurysm necessitates close neurosurgical evaluation and management. Neurosurgeons must ultimately coordinate the best treatment to secure the ruptured aneurysm by clip ligation or endovascular obliteration.

One of the most significant and common complications of SAH is cerebral vasospasm and resultant delayed cerebral ischemia. A neurosurgeon or neurointensivist must be closely evaluating neurological examinations to determine if there is any change or deterioration from a SAH patient's baseline examination. If a new focal neurological deficit is present, medical treatment should be initiated immediately, prior to confirmation with DSA. Permissive hypertension should be instituted and CPP goals (60 to 90 mm Hg) should be considered.[25] If indicated, patients with suspected cerebral vasospasm should undergo DSA for evaluation and potential treatment with mechanical or chemical vasodilators. In addition to neurological examinations, neurosurgeons should be closely monitoring external ventricular drainage for any significant change in output or change in bloody appearance, for a spike in blood pressure, for elevated transcranial Doppler velocity, or for any other significant changes in cardiopulmonary status. Potential complications causing changes in neurological examination must be considered, such as rebleeding, vasospasm, hydrocephalus, cerebral edema, nonconvulsive seizures, meningitis, fever, drugs, hypoxia, and delirium. The intensity and high acuity of all neuro-ICU care, especially in patients with TBI or SAH as mentioned previously, has led to research on the most consequential systems of critical care that leave room for improvement and high-quality care.

NEUROCRITICAL CARE TRAINING

The Society of Neurological Surgeons Committee on Advanced Subspecialty Training (CAST) has defined program requirements to promote a standardized, high level of neurocritical care training programs. These guidelines specify a curriculum of knowledge and clinical skills as well as training environment and administrative resources for neurosurgical residents and fellows to develop advanced proficiency in the management of critically ill neurological and neurosurgical patients.[26] Neurocritical care training programs may be established as enfolded programs during residency or after formal completion of residency. The duration of dedicated neuro-ICU care must be 12 months. Training must occur in a surgical critical care unit or neurological critical care unit with exposure to both pediatric and adult patients with traumatic injuries, cerebrovascular insults, neuro-oncologic disorders, status epilepticus, and spine and spinal cord disorders, including traumatic injuries. While physician faculty must have neurocritical care training, at least one neurosurgeon on the teaching staff must be qualified in neurocritical care.

According to the CAST document titled *Program Requirements for Advanced Training in Neurocritical Care: Neurological Surgery*,[26] the didactic curriculum must "provide the opportunity for residents to acquire advanced knowledge of the following aspects of neurosurgical critical care, particularly as they relate to the management of patients with hemodynamic instability, multiple system organ failure, and complex coexisting medical problems:

- Cardiorespiratory resuscitation
- Physiology, pathophysiology, diagnosis, and therapy of disorders of the cardiovascular, respiratory, gastrointestinal, neurological, endocrine, [and] musculoskeletal [systems], as well as of infectious diseases
- Metabolic, nutritional, and endocrine effects of critical illness
- Hematologic and coagulation disorders
- Trauma as it relates to neurological disease
- Monitoring and medical instrumentation
- Critical pediatric neurosurgical conditions
- Pharmacokinetics and dynamics of drug metabolism and excretion in critical illness
- Ethical and legal aspects of neurosurgical critical care"

The clinical curriculum should consist of neurosurgical critical care skills as defined in Table 17-3.

MODELS OF NEURO-ICU CARE

Four primary models of neuro-ICU care exist in which neurosurgeons may manage or co-manage patients (Table 17-4). In a popular traditional model, the primary responsibility for patients lies with a rotating surgical or medical intensivist (pulmonary or anesthesia critical care), with comanagement or consultation by a neurosurgeon. In academic settings, this model typically exists as a closed model with primary management of critical care issues by an intensivist. In the community setting, this model may also be seen as an open model with primary responsibility lying with the neurosurgeon, with consultation by medical/surgical intensivists.

TABLE 17-3 Clinical Components of Society of Neurological Surgeons CAST Neurocritical Care Training Programs

Respiratory	Airway management
Circulatory	Invasive and noninvasive monitoring techniques, including computations of cardiac output and of systemic and pulmonary vascular resistance; monitoring, electrocardiograms, electroencephalograms
Neurological	The performance of complete neurological examinations; the use of intracranial pressure monitoring techniques and of the electroencephalogram to evaluate cerebral function; application of hypothermia in the management of cerebral trauma
Renal	The evaluation of renal function as it relates to the neurosurgical patient and treatment paradigm
Gastrointestinal	Utilization of gastrointestinal intubation in the management of the critically ill patient; application of enteral feedings; management of percutaneous catheter devices
Hematologic	Coagulation status; appropriate use of component therapy
Infectious disease	Classification of infections and application of isolation techniques, pharmacokinetics, drug interactions, and management of antibiotic therapy during treatment of the neurological patient
Nutritional	Application of parenteral and enteral nutrition; monitoring and assessing metabolism and nutrition
Miscellaneous	Use of special beds for specific injuries; employment of pneumatic antishock garments, traction, and fixation devices

From *Society of Neurological Surgeons.* Program requirements for advanced training in neurocritical care: neurological surgery, <http://www.societyns.org/fellowships/requirements-neurocritical_care.html>. Copyright © 2008 The Society of Neurological Surgeons.

TABLE 17-4 Practice-of-Care Models for the Neuro-ICU

Traditional closed model	Primary responsibility lies with surgical/medical intensivist Academic setting
Traditional open model	Primary responsibility lies with neurosurgical attending; consult general surgical/medical intensivist Typically community setting
Open neurointensivist (telemedicine) model	Primary responsibility lies with neurosurgical attending; consult neurointensivist Typically community setting Use of telemedicine
Comanagement neurointensivist model	Dual neurosurgeon/neurointensivist responsibility Sometimes all practitioners under neurosurgical department
Closed neurosurgical managed model	Rotating CAST-trained neurosurgeons with primary responsibility for all neuro-ICU patients

CAST, Committee on Advanced Subspecialty Training; neuro-ICU, neurosurgical intensive care unit.

In the community hospital setting, a second, more recent, model evolved with the development of neurointensivists. In an open setting, neurointensivists provide consultation on matters of general and neurological critical care while neurosurgeons primary manage the neuro-ICU patients. With the advancement of telemedicine, this model incorporated satellite institutions to host neurointensivists who would be on call for all matters while a neurosurgeon would be available on site.

A third model, more common in the academic setting, was developed with dedicated neurointensivists available for primary management of neuro-ICU patients. These neurointensivists are available with specified criteria such as those mentioned previously, but neurosurgeons are also available on site for comanagement. Another contemporary development has been the primary coordination and leadership of neuro-ICU care by the department of neurosurgery, and the active involvement of neurointensivists of all primary training backgrounds within the department of neurosurgery. With this development, structure exists for involvement in all academic settings that enables better clinical communication.

A fourth model that mimics the practice of many surgical ICUs exists in some academic centers, with management by dedicated neurosurgeons who rotate for a set period with primary responsibility for all neuro-ICU patients. These neurosurgeons, who are CAST certified, enable coordination of care similar to that with general intensivists and encourage the direct involvement of neurosurgeons throughout the neurocritical care management process.

CONCLUSION

Even with the changes to neurocritical care over the past two decades, the neurosurgeon has a unique responsibility and necessary role in managing and coordinating care for patients in the neuro-ICU. Critical care medicine has developed as a specialty to diagnose, treat, and prevent life-threatening illnesses requiring invasive monitoring as well as intensive pharmacologic and mechanical organ support.[27] Specifically, neurocritical care exists to coordinate and manage this challenging patient population with medical professionals with diverse areas of expertise. The purpose of the neuro-ICU is to provide a high level of acute care for patients with neurological disorders most commonly in the pre-, peri-, and postoperative periods. This high level of care is necessary to manage or prevent injury to the central nervous system while maintaining systemic homeostasis. The fact that many of these severely ill patients with neurological disorders undergo neurosurgical operative procedures necessitates an intense involvement of neurosurgeons in their care. Neurosurgeons have been intimately involved from Harvey Cushing and the earliest neuro-ICU models to the latest "high-intensity" neuro-ICUs. Neurosurgeons must maintain a close relationship in comanaging these units to evaluate the need for and perform the procedures for which only they have training. Only with close neurosurgical involvement will neuro-ICU patients receive the highest level of care required by the extensive acuteness of their condition.

SUGGESTED READINGS

Diringer MN, Edwards DF. Admission to a neurologic/neurosurgical intensive care unit is associated with reduced mortality rate after intracerebral hemorrhage. *Crit Care Med*. 2001;29(3):635-640.

Josephson SA, Douglas VC, Lawton MT, et al. Improvement in intensive care unit outcomes in patients with subarachnoid hemorrhage after initiation of neurointensivist co-management. *J Neurosurg*. 2010; 112(3):626-630.

Knopf L, Staff I, Gomes J, et al. Impact of a neurointensivist on outcomes in critically ill stroke patients. *Neurocrit Care*. 2012;16(1):63-71.

Kramer AH, Zygun DA. Do neurocritical care units save lives? Measuring the impact of specialized ICUs. *Neurocrit Care*. 2011;14(3):329-333.

Kurtz P, Fitts V, Sumer Z, et al. How does care differ for neurological patients admitted to a neurocritical care unit versus a general ICU? *Neurocrit Care*. 2011;15(3):477-480.

Milstein A, Galvin RS, Delbanco SF, et al. Improving the safety of health care: the leapfrog initiative. *Eff Clin Pract*. 2000;3(6):313-316.

Rincon F, Mayer SA. Neurocritical care: a distinct discipline? *Curr Opin Crit Care*. 2007;13(2):115-121.

See a full reference list on ExpertConsult.com

18 Surgical Planning: An Overview

Gabriel Zada, Frank J. Attenello III, Martin Pham, and Martin H. Weiss

Comprehensive planning represents the first priority and foundation of any neurosurgical procedure. Because the nervous system has little tolerance for injury, the axiom "failing to prepare is preparing to fail" holds particularly true.

This preparation begins with clear and careful definition of technical goals and potential pitfalls of each procedure. Effective planning then allows the necessary flexibility to manage deviations from a standard operative course. By taking the necessary steps to ensure adequate preparation for a case, the neurosurgeon may prevent or avoid many significant neurosurgical complications. The experience and ability to detect and handle the most adverse intraoperative events should therefore be a self-imposed limitation for any surgeon.

Setting a practical preoperative goal also involves a clear working diagnosis. Specifically, for an intervention in a disease process to be effective, the surgical team must understand the underlying pathophysiologic process or have a targeted plan to acquire further information. The role of patient selection is critical in achieving surgical success. Unfortunately, even good patient selection and comprehensive planning cannot account for all anatomic and pathologic variables encountered during surgery. The surgeon must be amenable to potential alternative surgical goals upon encountering certain intraoperative findings or surgical pathology results. Nonsurgical diagnoses (i.e. prolactinoma, lymphoma) and alternative modalities (i.e. medical therapy, radiation based treatment) also must be considered. Surgical planning thereby seamlessly blends with a larger multimodal treatment plan to minimize morbidity and optimize timely diagnosis and treatment of disease.

This chapter aims to provide a general framework to approaching a neurosurgical procedure, specifically focusing on essential considerations and supplemental measures necessary to provide a patient with an optimal outcome.

PREOPERATIVE EVALUATION

The first task of a surgeon before any procedure is a thorough and comprehensive evaluation of the patient. Preoperative patient assessment regularly consists of a detailed and focused history, physical examination, and review of pertinent laboratory results and imaging studies. Disciplined, repetitive practice in these tasks allow for a comprehensive, detailed, and repeatable preoperative course that minimizes error. Checklists often prove useful for this comprehensive coverage.

A patient's history must begin with a clear definition of the presenting complaint. Subsequent delineation of time course and of onset of symptoms clarifies the degree of a suspected condition. In addition to establishment of pertinent positives, pertinent negatives should always be documented. This is essential in providing a record of preoperative deficits to compare with those encountered postoperatively. The side of hand dominance is an important feature to assess and document. Adherence to basic medical history taking is complete with review of medical and surgical history, medications, allergies, and familial and social history, including use of tobacco, ethanol, or illicit drugs. A general review of systems should also be included.

The physical examination includes a thorough neurological evaluation, as well as a general physical assessment. The complete neurological examination should include evaluation of mental status, speech function and understanding, cranial nerve function (including that of the first cranial nerve), motor and sensory function, and reflexes, as well as cerebellar/gait testing. Of note, the sensory examination should include evaluation of proprioception and pinprick responses. Formal visual field and acuity examination may be required if there is concern for disease anywhere along the visual tracts, from the eye itself to the occipital lobe. Rectal examination for tone, volition, sensation, and the bulbocavernosus reflex is often required in evaluating spinal disease. Specific evaluation for surgical scars in the chest or abdomen may be valuable in the planning of a procedure that extends beyond the brain or spine, such as placement of a ventriculoperitoneal shunt.

Computer documentation provides the surgeon with a useful tool for systemic and comprehensive evaluation of the history and physical examination findings. However, the surgeon must be deliberate, being cognizant of the potential for error when glossing over standard templates. Finally, many neurosurgical patients have significant comorbid conditions that necessitate evaluation preoperatively. The goals of surgery should always be considered as they relate to the patient's overall medical status and personal preferences.

Routine laboratory values, including a metabolic panel and blood cell count, are indicated before any nonemergency surgical procedure and should be obtained to screen for a number of underlying acute or chronic pathologic conditions that may pose a risk to a patient undergoing general anesthesia and surgery. The metabolic panel may suggest variations in sodium and potassium levels often noted in the neurosurgical patient population, as well as baseline renal function. Underlying anemia noted in the blood cell count must be investigated and corrected accordingly. Any suggestions of infection, such as an elevated white blood cell count, positive cultures, erythrocyte sedimentation rate (ESR), or C-reactive protein level, should be investigated and treated, especially in elective cases or if hardware implantation is planned. Before definitive surgery, particular attention should be focused on platelet count, prothrombin time (international normalized ratio), partial thromboplastin time, and bleeding time (if necessary). Any suggestions of bleeding diathesis or coagulopathy should be further investigated and corrected. Many patients currently take anticoagulant or antiplatelet agents for a number of underlying medical comorbid conditions. Discontinuation or reversal of these agents (or perhaps initiation of these agents in selected endovascular cases) should be addressed at least 1 week before surgery. Blood typing and screening, or crossmatching for packed red blood cells and blood products, should be requested from the blood bank and verified in advance. A qualitative β-human chorionic gonadotropin level should be measured for every woman of childbearing age before surgery.

Sellar disease often necessitates special preoperative consideration. Patients should undergo serum testing of a full or selective endocrine panel to evaluate any pituitary axis deficiencies. The thyroid and cortisol axes are uniquely critical, and abnormalities must be identified and corrected before any surgical procedure is performed. Ruling out nonsurgical lesions, such as prolactinomas, also necessitates judicious review of preoperative laboratory work.

Preexisting cardiac disease is common in the neurosurgical patient population. Preoperatively, a detailed cardiovascular history should be documented to assess exercise tolerance and to screen for angina or congestive heart failure. Common symptoms of heart disease are shortness of breath, chest pain, palpitations, and fatigue. Clearance by a cardiologist may be required if a patient has certain risk factors or symptoms. A 12-lead electrocardiogram (ECG) and plain chest radiographs are obtained in the majority of adult patients before elective surgery. An ECG helps detect preoperative arrhythmias, conduction defects, chamber enlargement, and myocardial ischemia. It is also helpful as a baseline for comparison with subsequent changes. The plain chest radiograph is also helpful for evaluating pulmonary infiltrates, pulmonary vessel distention, or cardiac enlargement to suggest some form of cardiac disease. If further cardiac work-up is indicated, an exercise treadmill test, echocardiography, nuclear medicine study, or coronary angiography may be performed in order to further assess the degree of cardiac risk and the need to optimize such risk before surgery. Hypertensive patients require adequate blood pressure control before elective surgery because there is a linear correlation between preoperative blood pressure and postoperative myocardial ischemia. In general, any existing cardiac risk factor must be addressed before a patient undergoes an elective neurosurgical procedure. The degree of cardiac risk, if present, should be accounted for and weighed against the urgency of the neurosurgical procedure. Any perioperative measures that may improve cardiac monitoring or function should be planned in conjunction with the anesthesia team, including normalization of electrolyte imbalances, optimization of fluid status, perioperative cardiac medications, and invasive cardiac monitoring. In the setting of baseline anemia or anticipated blood loss, especially in the setting of invasive high-risk spine surgery, large-bore intravenous access or central venous access is critical to the timely delivery of blood products and prevention of a hypovolemic intraoperative insult.

Baseline pulmonary disease is also common in the general neurosurgical population. Symptoms of pulmonary conditions include dyspnea, cough, sputum production, wheezing, or hemoptysis. Prior conditions such as recent respiratory infections, chronic obstructive pulmonary disease (COPD), and asthma must be elicited during history taking. Comorbid conditions such as asthma and COPD may hinder anesthesia during a neurosurgical procedure and must be addressed and optimized. Historical details, including a smoking history, merit special attention by the physician. Baseline oxygen saturations on routine vital signs may be a quick way to delineate pulmonary disease, inasmuch as room-air saturations below 93% are suggestive of at least mild respiratory failure. A preoperative plain chest radiograph helps show any preexisting infiltrates, atelectasis, masses, abnormal pulmonary vessels, or pneumothoraces. Further testing can be done with pulmonary function tests or a dedicated chest computed tomographic (CT) scan to rule out underlying pulmonary conditions. Perioperative medications, including steroids and beta agonists, may be indicated for patients with pulmonary disease and should be discussed with the anesthesia staff. For patients with significantly limiting pulmonary conditions, elective surgery should be postponed until pulmonary function has been maximized to reduce postoperative pulmonary morbidity. Severe ventilatory compromises may limit prone positioning for posterior fossa or spine surgery, and coincident structural lesions such as lung masses may dictate the laterality of certain neurosurgical approaches.

Some neurosurgical patients present with malnutrition or failure to thrive as a result of their disease process. Many conditions prevalent in the neurosurgical patient population render patients unable to consume a normal amount of calories to sustain normal metabolism. Because of mental status changes, weakness, paralysis, or any number of airway or cranial nerve issues, some patients rely on alternative methods of nutritional intake. These may include nasogastric tubes, percutaneous gastric tubes, or parenteral forms of intake for nutritional supplementation or full delivery. Before any neurosurgical case, a patient's nutritional status should be considered and optimized. Serum prealbumin and albumin levels can be monitored in order to assess and follow a patient's nutritional status. A clinical nutritionist can be invaluable in optimizing a patient's nutritional status before a major surgery through calculations of standard and postoperative nutritional requirements. Patients who have undergone previous surgery or radiation therapy and those taking long-term steroids may require additional caloric requirements in order to achieve adequate wound healing. Diabetes mellitus, especially in the setting of poor glycemic control, may further compromise wound healing and should be addressed during the nutritional evaluation. Screening hemoglobin A_{1c} levels may help detect this clinical scenario.

Once the evaluation of a patient's neurological and systemic disease has been thoroughly completed and a surgical plan outlined, a frank discussion with the patient and any other family members involved in the patient's care should take place. The goals of surgery and any possible barriers to these goals should be clearly and honestly delineated. For nonemergency cases, the risks and benefits of, and alternatives to, the recommended procedure should be reviewed and any additional questions answered by the surgeon. This discussion should also include a description of any permanent hardware implants that may be used, as well as the possibility of blood transfusions in high-risk cases. Time and patience are of the utmost importance during this process to ensure that the patient fully understands all aspects of the surgery. An informed consent document should then be signed by the surgeon, patient, and any witnesses present for the conversation. Additional consent for any research protocols or tissue specimen banking should also be thoroughly discussed and performed.

NEUROIMAGING STUDIES

Before the initiation or formulation of any surgical procedure, the correct battery of neuroimaging studies should be obtained and carefully reviewed by the surgeon and radiologist. Consultation with a neuroradiologist may be beneficial in selected cases when a particular diagnosis is in question, to postprocess and interpret advanced neuroimaging studies, and to confirm whether nearby anatomical structures are at risk. Preoperative images frequently include plain radiographs, CT imaging, magnetic resonance imaging (MRI), catheter angiography, or a variety of additional modalities. The surgeon should ensure that the correct sequences have been performed, have been reviewed, and are available during the procedure. The neuroimaging studies must be available in the operating room during the actual procedure because intraoperative anatomy must often be correlated with preoperative films. In addition to static images, dynamic studies of the spine such as flexion/extension views may provide insight into corresponding conditions. Although CT scanning and magnetic resonance angiography allow for a static anatomic evaluation of vasculature, catheter angiography may be helpful in defining diseases that have a time component of early or late filling. Certain pathologic entities such as arteriovenous malformations have abnormalities in flow; thus the time component must be considered in the preoperative evaluation.

Intraoperative imaging and image-guided neuronavigation are increasingly being utilized as surgical adjuncts. This intraoperative utilization of technology, however, requires additional methodical preoperative planning. Image guidance navigation systems may be used for a variety of cranial or spinal procedures, and each case may necessitate specific preoperative or intraoperative imaging sequences. The timing of acquisition of these images in relation to the operation should be considered, as some patients may require earlier admission to obtain these sequences. Intraoperative CT scanning for image-guided spine surgery or functional neurosurgery requires confirmation of machine availability and appropriate radiography technician support. Intraoperative fluoroscopy is commonly used during spine or skull base procedures. Intraoperative MRI has been used in a variety of tumor cases and similarly requires preoperative setup and appropriate use of MRI-compatible equipment in the operating room. Intraoperative catheter angiography and fluorescein angiography are commonly used during cerberovascular procedures, and operative rooms with fluoroscopy capabilities may have to be specially booked. Cannulation of the femoral artery and initial imaging for intraoperative angiography require setting up before the operation.

ANESTHESIA

Before initiating the surgical procedure, the surgeon should review the operative plan with the anesthesia team so that any appropriate preoperative or intraoperative preparations can be made. The anesthesiologist's preoperative assessment of the patient includes the patient's functional status, medical comorbid conditions, medications, allergies, and a thorough review of any cardiopulmonary symptoms or risk factors. Optimal intraoperative physiologic parameters such as blood pressure, fluid status, and temperature should be reviewed with the anesthesia team so that appropriate methods of monitoring can be placed before the start of the surgery. The proper use of ventriculostomy and lumbar drain catheters, when present, should also be reviewed with the anesthesiologist before surgery. In pediatric cases or other high-risk cases in which potential exsanguination is a concern, a plan for monitoring and transfusing blood or any additional products should be in place. Planning for autologous blood recovery systems or normovolemic hemodilution may be undertaken in cases where a significant degree of bleeding is anticipated.

Particular requirements for the administration of anesthetic medications for the procedure should be reviewed with the anesthesiologists, including the selection of paralytic agents and induction agents. This is of key importance when neurophysiological monitoring will be performed, inasmuch as many anesthetic medications can suppress electrophysiologic signals. Plans for electroencephalographic burst suppression must also be discussed with the anesthesia team before the surgery. In certain functional and tumor cases, neuroleptic anesthesia is desired so that the team can perform neurologic assessments of the patient during the operative procedure. For craniotomy or deep brain stimulator placement in which patients are awake, pain prevention requires additional preoperative preparation on the part of the anesthesia team. The perioperative administration of medications such as antibiotics, steroids, hemostatic or anticoagulation agents, antiepileptic drugs, and diuretics is frequently indicated and discussed with the anesthesia team.

A record of the patient's allergies should be readily available and alternative medications selected for existing conflicts. Any concerns regarding spinal stability should be communicated to the anesthesiologist before intubation and positioning. Fiberoptic intubation may be required in instances of cervical instability or severe spondylosis, in which the hyperextension required for standard endotracheal intubation may place the patient at risk for injury to the cervical spinal cord. Certain operative positions require additional means of monitoring that are planned before surgery. A typical example of this is the requirement for central venous Doppler monitoring for air emboli in the case of sitting craniotomies. Baseline somatosensory evoked potentials (SSEPs) and motor evoked potentials (MEPs) should be documented before and after final positioning for high-risk unstable spine surgery to further confirm safe preparation and manipulation of the patient before definitive surgical intervention.

GENERAL DETERMINATION OF SURGICAL APPROACH

In selecting a surgical approach in the majority of procedures, the surgeon should aim to provide the safest, most direct corridor with maximal access to the disease process. This approach must further minimize morbidity to structures traversed en route to and surrounding the pathologic process of interest. Surgical navigation or intraoperative motor and sensory mapping may assist in identifying critical structures to avoid. Furthermore, surgical manipulation generally minimizes retraction, traction, and compression of nervous structures. For instance, resection of extra-axial tumors is accomplished by deflection out and away from adjacent neural structures. Necessary surgical instrumentation should be anticipated, requested, and tested, preferably at least one day before the procedure. Considerations for different approaches may vary and are delineated in the following discussion.

Considerations for Cranial Procedures

Cranial procedures require careful assessment of patient positioning in conjunction with the planned surgical approach. Nursing and operating room staff should be notified of equipment for positioning that must be set up ahead of time. This may include devices for cranial fixation and for positioning of the body or extremity support. The need for extra personnel for complex positioning, such as park bench or lateral positioning, should also be announced to staff ahead of time. Neurophysiologic monitoring, including SSEPs, MEPs, and brainstem auditory evoked potential (BAER) responses, must be anticipated and discussed with the anesthesia and neuromonitoring teams before surgery. Intraoperative motor or sensory mapping, if necessary, should be anticipated and also discussed with neuromonitoring staff. Adjunct measures for brain relaxation, such as placement of a ventriculostomy catheter or lumbar drain, should be considered and placed ahead of time, when needed. Drill equipment, including electric or pneumatic set-up, as well as specific drill bits or attachments, should be selected and tested. Adjuncts for visualization, such as the operating microscope, surgical loupes, or an endoscopic system, should be selected and tested before surgery to ensure all components are in order and functional. Instruments or products required for hemostasis, such as monopolar and bipolar cautery, collagen sponge, oxidized cellulose, and thrombin, should be discussed with the operating room staff before surgery so that they are ready for use at the beginning of the procedure. If surgical navigation is to be used, it should be set up and registered, and its accuracy verified, before the procedure begins. Careful attention to physical placement of the navigation screen and camera, as well as other large equipment, should provide unhindered access and walkways for operating room personnel. Finally, when the assistance of personnel from other departments—such as plastic surgery, otolaryngology, pathology, or neurology—is needed, confirmation of their availability is courteous.

Cranial Tumor Cases

Before craniotomy for brain tumors, it is essential to prepare a clear working diagnosis and plan. Surgical goals may include a biopsy, partial resection, full resection, or a combination of these, on the basis of findings. Of note, for tumors that appear especially vascular on imaging studies, preoperative endovascular embolization may be beneficial.

When a biopsy is planned, options include stereotactic, frame-based procedures, neuronavigation-guided procedures, or open biopsy. Before biopsy, neuropathology colleagues should be notified and present for collection of the specimen. Surgical plans should include a decision algorithm for microscopic review of the frozen biopsy specimen. Pathologic features may indicate a medically treatable condition, which allows for the decision to complete the surgery without further resection. Other cases may necessitate resection, ranging from total to partial resection, with a spectrum of goals ranging from cure to cytoreduction and relief of mass effect and to palliation.

Surgical instruments necessary for tumor resection should be anticipated and may include specialized transsphenoidal or skull base sets, endoscopic equipment, and the Cavitron ultrasonic aspirator (CUSA). If a cerebrospinal fluid leak can occur near the skull base, the abdomen or thigh may be prepared for an autologous fat/fascial graft harvest (the surgeon should remember to include this in the patient consent form). Injection of fluorescein dye into the subarachnoid space may be warranted in order to improve detection of a cerebrospinal fluid leak, and this material should be ready and sometimes injected before the patient is positioned.

Operative Planning for Cerebrovascular Cases

Surgical treatment of both simple and complex cerebrovascular disease can often be facilitated greatly by thorough preoperative planning. Before open surgical intervention, the surgeon must determine the need for endovascular adjuncts. Preoperative diagnostic angiography may delineate complex vascular disease, and preoperative embolization is often required for vascular malformations.

Operating room staff should be informed of the need for equipment. A wide variety of aneurysm clips should be selected, prepared, and available to the surgeon in order to treat complex aneurysms, including various sizes and configurations of straight and fenestrated clips. The approach should proceed with a goal of sufficient exposure for both the surgical lesion and the proximal vasculature.

For vascular lesions, the surgeon must evaluate options and establish a plan in the event of intraoperative aneurysm or vascular malformation rupture. Temporary and permanent aneurysm clips should be readily available in the event of an intraoperative rupture. Methods of proximal control may include temporary aneurysm clipping, intraoperative balloon occlusion, or exposure of proximal vessels in the neck. If there is a distinct possibility for parent vessel sacrifice, a balloon test occlusion can be performed ahead of time to evaluate whether the patient can tolerate vessel occlusion. In the planning for vascular reconstruction or bypass, flow dynamics must be considered. Preoperative studies must be performed to assess whether feeder and recipient vessels are sufficient, and mapping of the vessel course with a Doppler instrument may be required. If no feeding vessel is accessible, an appropriate venous or arterial graft harvest site may be selected and prepared on the basis of the flow demand of the target distribution.

Intraoperative angiography may also be used for a variety of reasons, including proximal control, suction-decompression, and assessment of persistent filling of vascular lesions and parent vessels. Fluorescein angiography provides an alternative intraoperative measure for cerebral blood flow. Verification of distal artery patency after aneurysm ligation can be performed with a micro-Doppler flow probe, fluorescein or intraoperative angiography, or an endoscope.

Planning of Spine Procedures

For spine cases, the appropriate decision for an anterior, lateral, posterior, or combined approach must be determined. This first decision for the procedure often delineates many of the subsequent preparations for the operating room. Standard radiolucent surgical tables should be prepared and available for any of the aforementioned patient positions. Special bed adjuncts or attachments may be needed for certain procedures, such as a Wilson frame for lumbar decompression, a breaking Jackson table for lateral lumbar fusions, halo attachments for unstable cervical spinal conditions, and bed adaptors for minimally invasive tubular access.

Radiology technicians should be readily available for C-arm fluoroscopy, plain radiography, or intraoperative CT imaging for preoperative localization and image-guided navigation setup. SSEP and MEP monitoring, if desired, is set up before the procedure. Baseline and postposition neurophysiologic signals may be desired in unstable spine cases to ensure that no spinal movement has occurred to injure neurological elements. Appropriate hardware and instrumentation should be prepared, sterilized, and available before the start of the procedure. This hardware is usually specific to the case at hand and includes specialized instruments for minimally invasive approaches, spinal deformity correction, or tumor resection with subsequent spinal stabilization. If instrumentation is placed, it is the surgeon's responsibility to ensure that the appropriately sized screws, rods, cages, crosslinks, and any other equipment are promptly available and ready for use.

If the surgical plan includes bony fusion, preparations for obtaining autograft tissue (including iliac crest harvesting) should be planned. Allograft tissue should be available in inventory for placement if desired as well. Because the spinal column traverses the neck, thorax, and abdomen, special consideration should always be placed on appreciating and understanding the extraspinal anatomy that may be encountered and traversed during the spinal approach. Neurosurgeons are typically very comfortable with neural tissue and its associated bony anatomy and vasculature. However, surgical approaches to the spine may navigate around the esophagus, trachea, pleura, lungs, peritoneum, bowel, ureters, and great vessels. The neurosurgeon should be familiar and comfortable with this anatomy to prevent complications associated with those nonneurologic organ systems or should have a collaborating approach surgeon available to assist with this aspect of the operation.

CONCLUSION

Because of the complexity of neurological surgery, the surgeon must use every means available to optimize patient outcomes. Surgical success thus begins long before the surgeon sets foot in the operating theater. The foundation for this success lies in a disciplined preoperative routine, including patient's history, laboratory work-up, imaging findings, and a somber accounting of the risks with tempering of expectations. The intervention is most likely to be successful if the surgeon has regular relationships with an operating room team familiar with the nuances of required equipment and relies on other disciplines to provide context to an overall plan of care. Neurosurgery will always remain among the most audacious of human endeavors; preoperative planning provides the footing to help patients and diminish the burden of neurological disease.

SUGGESTED READINGS

Benzel EC, ed. *Spine Surgery: Techniques, Complication Avoidance and Management*. 3rd ed. Philadelphia: Saunders; 2012.

Fessler RG, Sekhar LN, eds. *Atlas of Neurosurgical Techniques: Spine and Peripheral Nerves*. New York: Thieme; 2006.

Sekhar LN, Fessler RG, eds. *Atlas of Neurosurgical Techniques: Brain*. New York: Thieme; 2006.

19 Surgical Simulation and Robotic Surgery

Christopher A. Sarkiss, Jonathan Rasouli, Warren R. Selman, and Joshua B. Bederson

In this chapter, we review several of the most commonly utilized computerized neurosurgical simulation devices and highlight key research studies to support their evidence-based use in clinical neurosurgical practice. In addition, we also focus on the utilization of robotics in neurosurgery in both cranial and spinal applications. "Simulation" is defined as a computer device that provides a surgery-like environment, including a three-dimensional visualization of various surgical scenarios. "Robotic surgery" is a surgical procedure involving a computer-enhanced device in the interface between the surgeon and the patient and introduces a varying degree of control formerly reserved for the surgeon.

Neurosurgery is an intrinsically high-risk endeavor in which even seemingly straightforward cases can be associated with complications that lead to profound disability in patients. Preoperative rehearsal in a computerized, virtual environment could potentially serve as a surrogate for some of the experience gained in practice. Historically, surgical simulation has been limited to cadaveric and animal courses, training models, or devices that test basic skills. Within the past decade, computerized surgical simulation has progressively increased in sophistication, playing a growing role in the education and training of surgeons. Computerized surgical simulation with haptic feedback in certain systems, coupled with the increased utilization of robotic-assisted microsurgery, has led to the development of a new era in the training and skill set of the 21st-century neurosurgeon.

We review the application and research of three neurosurgery-specific simulation devices currently available: NeuroTouch, Surgical Theater's 3D SuRgical Planner/Surgical Navigation Advanced Platform, and ImmersiveTouch. As the technology improves and the rehearsal scenarios become increasingly realistic, several authors foresee these devices becoming quickly adopted within day-to-day neurosurgical practice. With time, they may evolve to become a fully integrated part of a patient's neurosurgical treatment plan, improve a surgeon's confidence and familiarity in the operating room, and eventually lead to improved outcomes.

Over the past decade, surgeons have increased the utilization of robotics in various fields of surgery. While innovative and fascinating, evidence-based medicine must demonstrate true benefits to justify the use of robotics in surgery. In this chapter, we detail peer-reviewed cranial and spinal use of robotics. In addition, we survey current and future research and opportunities for growth. For robotics to become widely implemented in the neurosurgical armamentarium, it must provide the neurosurgeon and the patient with certain advantages such as smaller incisions, increased precision, decreased complications, decreased operating time, less blood loss, less postoperative pain, and decreased hospital stays.

Full text of this chapter is available online at ExpertConsult.com

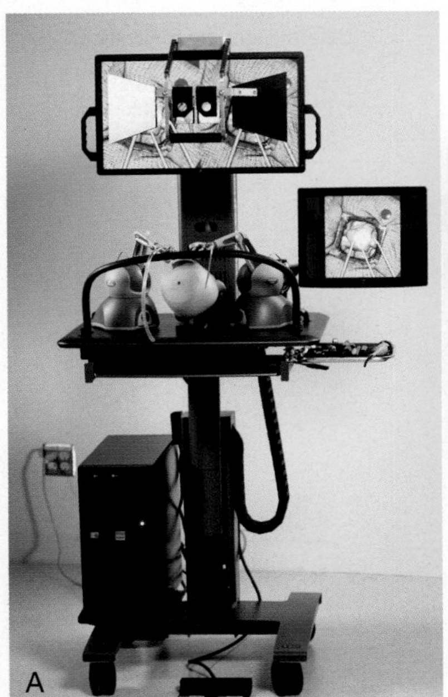
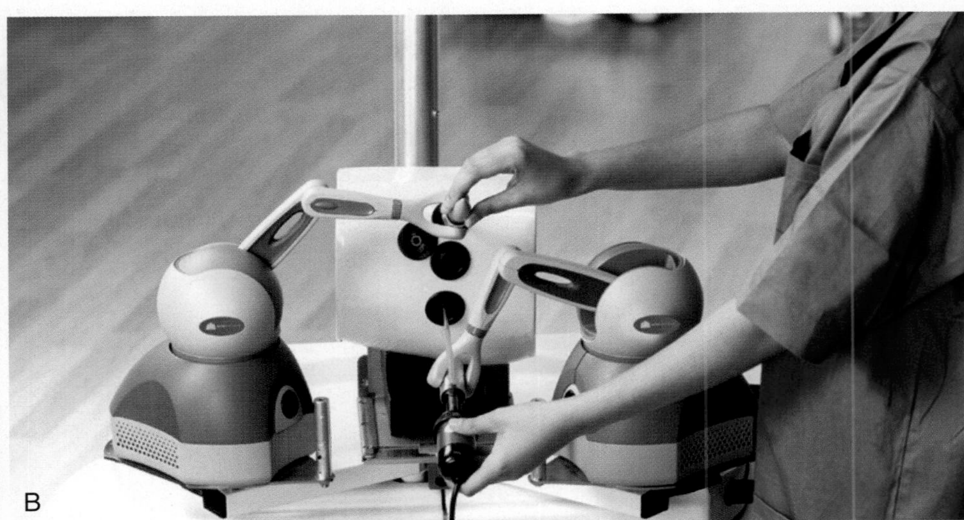

NeuroTouch simulation system. A, The NeuroTouch System developed by the National Research Council of Canada. **B,** This system includes medical simulation by the Simbionix ARTHRO Mentor (3D Systems) using the Touch haptic devices (3D Systems). *(**A,** Courtesy of the National Research Council Canada, Ottawa, Ontario. **B,** Courtesy of 3D Systems, Rock Hill, SC.)*

20 Positioning for Cranial Surgery

Irene Kim, Russell G. Strom, and John G. Golfinos

οὐκοῦν οἶσθ' ὅτι ἀρχὴ παντὸς ἔργου μέγιστον.
The beginning in every task is the chief thing.

—Plato, The Republic

The positioning of the patient is one of the most crucial steps in any cranial operation. Proper positioning allows the most direct access to the surgical target and reduces the working distance for the surgeon. It avoids brain retraction except by gravity and minimizes bleeding into the operative field. Intracranial pressure is reduced by elevating the head above the level of the heart and avoiding neck positions that obstruct venous outflow. Attentive positioning prevents pressure or traction injuries, including skin breakdown, ocular injuries, and peripheral nerve injuries.[1] The master surgeon understands the critical importance of patient positioning because errors in positioning can turn a straightforward operation into a challenging undertaking and increase the risk of a poor outcome. Young surgeons are constantly looking for "pearls" of technique to use at the climax of the dissection, yet they often fail to realize that the master surgeon has increased the likelihood of a successful operation right at the outset by paying attention to the details of the patient's position (Video 20-1).

The term *positioning* refers to the position of the surgeon as well as that of the patient. Some surgeons prefer to sit and some prefer to stand; some cases require the surgeon to both sit and stand. This chapter describes the major patient positions used in cranial surgery and how to achieve success from the very first step of the operation.

Full text of this chapter is available online at ExpertConsult.com

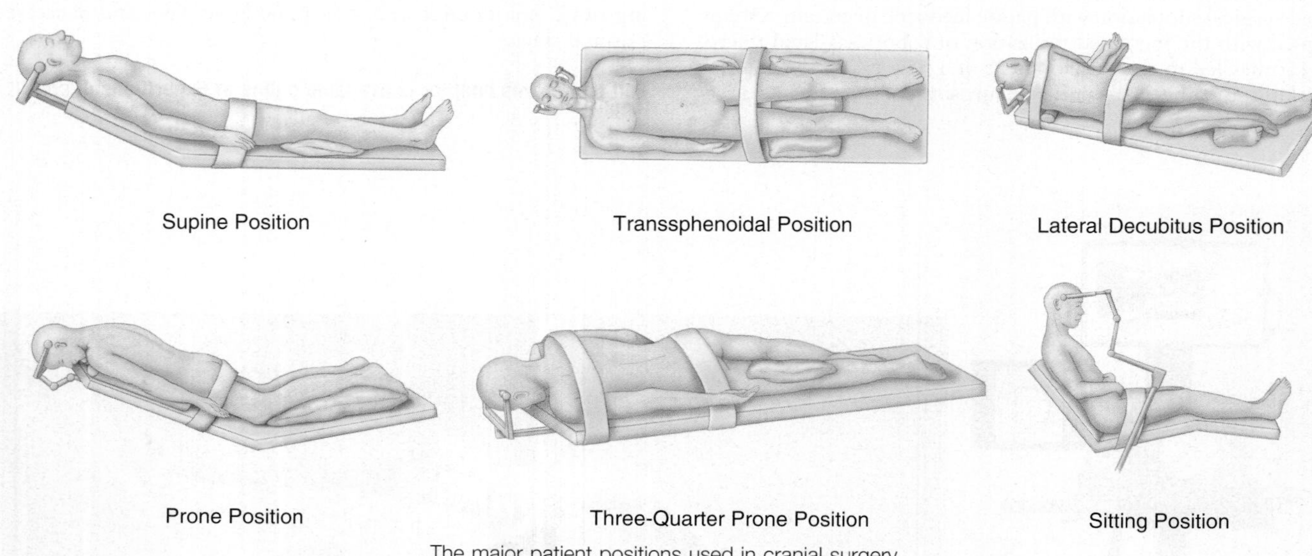

The major patient positions used in cranial surgery.

21 Positioning for Spinal Surgery

Jason A. Ellis and Peter D. Angevine

In this chapter we review the principles of patient positioning for spinal surgery. The specific equipment used, details of setup for each operative approach, and techniques for minimizing complications are addressed. The advantages and disadvantages of various operating tables, including spinal and standard operating room tables, are discussed. The utility of positioning frames such as the Wilson frame in specific situations is also presented. Head holder devices, including skull tongs and clamps, the Caspar system, and various cushions, are discussed in detail. The three standard patient positions for spinal surgery—prone, supine, and lateral—are then presented. Practical details of the equipment, setup, and general considerations needed to safely place patients in these three positions are given. Finally, an examination of position-related complications in patients undergoing spinal surgery, including spinal cord injury, vision loss, peripheral neuropathy, and soft tissue injuries, is presented. Suggestions for ways to eliminate or minimize such complications are included.

Full text of this chapter is available online at ExpertConsult.com 

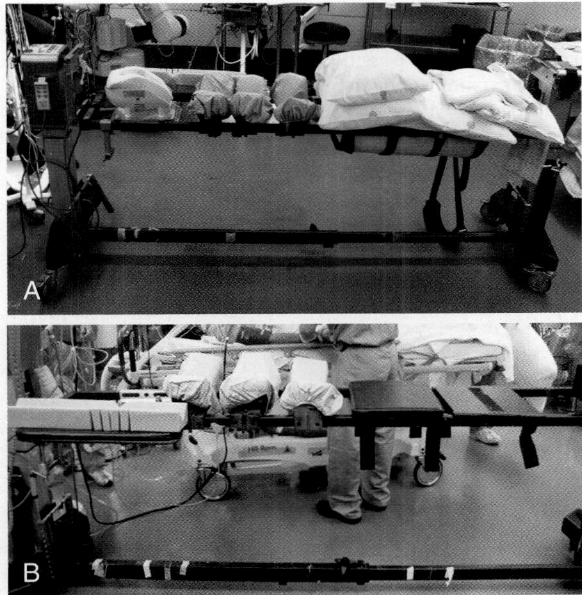

Spinal table. Modular, open-frame, radiolucent tables—shown here, a Jackson Spinal table (Mizuho OSI, Union City, CA)—are specifically designed to facilitate positioning for spinal surgery. Adjustable chest, hip, and thigh pads and movable arm boards are shown. The carbon fiber open-frame design allows for unobstructed use of fluoroscopy along the entire spinal axis. This table rotates, enabling circumferential access to the patient without need for transfer. A leg sling may be used to increase thoracolumbar kyphosis **(A)**, and a flat top may be used to accentuate lordosis **(B)**.

22 Positioning for Peripheral Nerve Surgery

Allen H. Maniker

In performing peripheral nerve surgery, as with any area of surgery, knowledge of the anatomy is of the utmost importance. The surgeon must not only understand the nerve anatomy but also be able to correlate neural structures with their target muscles and sensory distribution. Knowledge of the vascular and skeletal anatomy is also essential for planning the surgery. In much of nerve surgery, the normal anatomy is distorted from trauma, tumor, or another pathologic process, and the surgeon must understand the normal anatomy before proceeding. A properly planned incision and exposure allow for the correct identification of the vital structures, as well as room in which to perform the needed tasks. Neurosurgery of the brain and spine entails working in small, confined spaces, whereas peripheral nerve surgery often allows for the luxury of working in a more open, more exposed area. The surgeon should take advantage of this situation and make the exposure generous. Whenever possible, exposure of a nerve should include normal proximal and distal portions of the nerve to allow the surgeon to work from the normal to the abnormal areas and back to the normal area.

The specific nerve or nerves to be operated upon and the necessity of harvesting grafts will dictate much of the positioning for an operation. Should intraoperative electromyographic monitoring of muscles be utilized, the limb may be draped out of the field. If, however, the muscle contraction must be observed and no monitoring is used, the entire limb must be either exposed or covered with clear plastic drapes. In each case, the positioning and exposure must be worked out to suit the individual needs of the particular operation. In this chapter, selected nerves of the upper extremity (brachial plexus, median and anterior interosseous, radial and posterior interosseous, ulnar) and lower extremity (sciatic, peroneal, tibial, sural) are considered in turn with a brief review of anatomy, optimal positioning, and a stepwise operative exposure. More in-depth viewing of positioning for peripheral nerve surgery is available on the videos that accompany this chapter and other texts for nerves not covered in this overview.

Full text of this chapter is available online at ExpertConsult.com

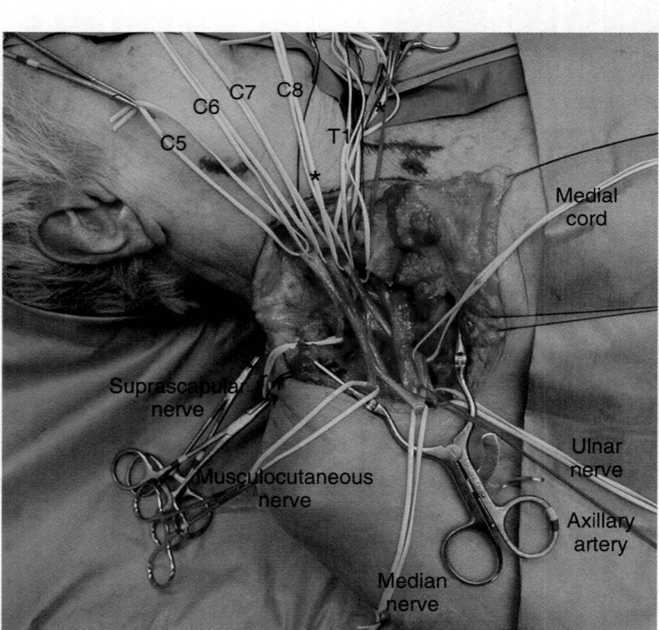

The full plexus exposed. In this cadaveric exposure, the clavicle was removed for visualization, although it is not usually done in living patients. The *asterisks* indicate the cut ends of the clavicle.

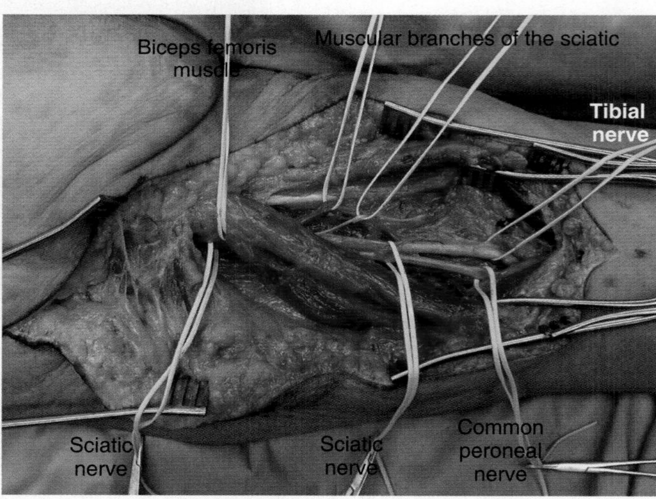

The sciatic nerve fully exposed.

23 Incisions and Closures

Elizabeth G. Zellner and John A. Persing

Uncomplicated wound healing with minimal scarring and deformity are desired outcomes in any surgical procedure. Chronic wounds, infections, or notable scarring can significantly undermine patient and family satisfaction even in the setting of a highly successful neurosurgical procedure. An understanding of basic wound healing, scalp anatomy, and principles of reconstructive surgery is helpful to achieve consistent, well-healed wounds.

The full text of this chapter, available at ExpertConsult.com, contains a basic biologic overview of wound healing, the major immunologic mediators and cell types, and the various stages of a healing wound. Although surgical scars reach up to 70% of their initial strength by 6 weeks, scar remodeling and restructuring can continue for 6 months to a year on average. Certain conditions, such as a history of radiation, aging skin in patients older than 65 years, diabetes, and chronic immunosuppression, can predispose patients to nonhealing or chronic wounds. Antibiotic use with surgical or traumatic injury should be given in an expeditious fashion to decrease the risk of infection. However, local wound irrigation and débridement can be equally important to avoid infection.

The anatomy and blood supply of the scalp are reviewed in this chapter. Understanding the vascular supply of the scalp is critical to planning surgical approaches with maximum healing potential. Over the past decade, the concept of angiosomes has developed—the idea that composite blocks of tissue are supplied by identifiable source arteries. Understanding the major and minor blood supply to the scalp allows surgeons to create both random and axial flaps (based on a certain blood supply) safely and creatively to cover a host of reconstructive problems. Any surgical incision should take into account esthetics as well as healing potential. For example, a coronal incision can be adapted as far posterior as possible, offering excellent exposure, and is also able to be well hidden, even with a receding hairline.

Closing a surgical incision involves considering the reconstructive ladder, often used by plastic surgeons to reconstruct various tissue defects. The simplest method of closing a wound is by secondary intention—or allowing the defect to close and contract on its own. This may be preferred over primary closure in contaminated, traumatic wounds of the scalp, for wounds with delayed presentation, or in high-risk medically complex patients. Management of a simple, noncontaminated incision is best achieved with primary closure, the goal being to obliterate potential dead space, distribute tension evenly along deep suture lines, and maintain suture tensile strength until tissue tensile strength is adequate. Various stylistic points of a simple closure are reviewed within the chapter. Skin grafting and flap design, from simpler random flaps that can be used throughout the scalp to more complex regional flaps for certain anatomic areas, are also reviewed within the text. A brief overview of tissue expansion and microsurgical free flaps, commonly used within the plastic surgery field, is also given.

Full text of this chapter is available online at ExpertConsult.com 

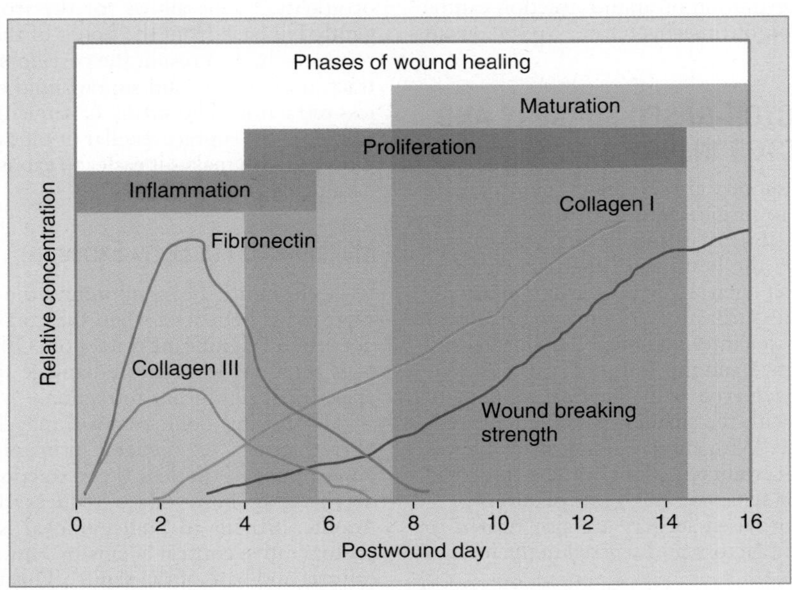

Schematic showing the production of connective tissue and resultant wound maturation over time. Fibronectin and collagen type III are initially deposited, followed later by type I collagen. *(Modified from Witte M, Barbul A. General principles of wound healing.* Surg Clin North Am. *1997;77:509.)*

24 Brain Retraction

Christina Sarris, Ryan Holland, Rachid Assina, and Charles J. Prestigiacomo

"Good illumination, unobstructed vision and a view of the whole operative field are of essential value to the surgeon. The better these conditions are, the greater precision with which he can identify the structures of pathophysiological significance."

—M. G. Yaşargil, 1958[1]

Retraction is as much art as it is science. Throughout the ages, surgeons have struggled with the concept of retraction. Used by every surgeon at some point in his or her career but truly understood by only some, retraction has just recently become a subject for scientific inquiry.

The goal of brain retraction is to allow the surgeon to safely visualize an area of interest. Early retraction was dependent on the surgeon's finger, forceps, and/or suction device. Advances in methods of brain retraction reflect the evolution of technology and have been driven by increasingly complex surgical exposures. Irrespective of the sophistication of the retraction method, avoidance of retractor-related brain injury remains a paramount goal and has recently led to an aggressive effort to minimize or eliminate the need for some forms of retraction.

This chapter initially reviews the history of brain retractor methods (online); then outlines the principles of retractor-based surgery and the avoidance of retractor injury; and closes with future developments in retractor technology.

HISTORICAL PERSPECTIVES

An illustrated history of the evolution of brain retraction can be found in the expanded version of this chapter at ExpertConsult.com.

PRINCIPLES OF RETRACTOR-BASED SURGERY AND AVOIDANCE OF RETRACTOR INJURY

The goals of retractor-based surgery are several: (1) gently create and maintain a safe corridor to surgical targets by which surgical instruments can be introduced; (2) visualize structures that are deep and usually unseen with the brain and other structures in their native state; (3) protect vital structures from injury by keeping them away from the surgical corridors of instrument transit; and (4) separate the tissue interfaces such that normal and abnormal tissue can be identified and the "surgical planes" developed. These goals must be achieved with the least amount of disruption to the structures, with the smallest possible footprint, and with no adverse sequelae. With these guiding principles as the guiding force for success, certain techniques can be employed to maximize the likelihood of achieving our goals of surgery.

The principles of retractor-based surgery are also related to patient, technical, and adjuvant factors, as discussed in the following sections.

Patient Factors

Surgical Anatomy

A clear understanding of the surgical anatomy and the natural corridors that exist in reaching the target lesion are important for minimizing retraction and optimizing visualizing. Reviewing the relevant imaging and identifying these corridors before surgery prove helpful in the positioning of the patient.

Positioning the Patient

See also Chapter 20 for further details.

Head positioning will influence venous pressure, which in turn will affect the backpressure of parenchyma on retractors. Therefore the surgeon must be cognizant of the patient's position on the operating table and especially the position of the head. Positioning should avoid hyperflexion of the neck, which might compromise venous return in the jugular veins. Placing two fingers between the chin and neck during positioning of the head will ensure proper venous return.

Ideal head positioning provides the optimal surgical approach.[28] The distance between the highest point at the skull surface and the area of interest should be minimized.[28] Whenever possible, the exposed surface of the skull should be parallel to the floor.[28] In aneurysm surgery, for example, placing the malar eminence at the higher point of the surgical field takes advantage of the force of gravity.[29] This allows for the frontal and temporal lobes to gently fall back from the bones of the anterior and middle fossa, respectively. As a result, the corridors to identifying the olfactory tract, optic nerve, and supraclinoid carotid require substantially less retraction. The sitting or semisitting position makes it easier to expose the supracerebellar or pineal region.[29] The lateral decubitus position makes it easier to expose the ipsilateral midline and paramedian lesions.[29]

Maximization of Bony Exposure

In performing the craniotomy, the concept of minimal bony exposure is beneficial when the corridors to reach the lesion do not require significant retraction. Otherwise, larger craniotomies may allow for less remote damage to brain parenchyma during episodes of significant retraction.

Maximizing bone removal may help minimize the amount of retraction.[30] A general principle is that the greater the bone removal, the less the retraction. For instance, drilling of overhanging bony edges reduces the degrees of retraction.[11] Another benefit to bone removal is the possible reduction of postoperative cortical edema by removal of large segments of the calvaria and base of the skull.[31] This technique has proven useful during certain resections. During these procedures, it is best to use the retractor on the tissue that is being removed.[32]

Dissection Corridors

If applicable, wide dissection of the subarachnoid spaces and cisterns allows for reduced retraction pressures and larger corridors. As an example, the wide opening of the sylvian fissure, in conjunction with proper head positioning, can result in excellent exposure of the supraclinoid carotid artery with minimal retraction.

Adjuvant Techniques

Fluid Diversion

Retraction on edematous brain or retraction in the setting of elevated intracranial pressure (ICP) requires more direct force and leads to potential parenchymal injury. Thus techniques that help reduce edema or increased ICP and processes that can maintain adequate cerebral blood flow (CBF) are important parts of minimizing retraction injury and achieving surgical success.

Manipulation of cerebrospinal fluid (CSF), may be another method to lessen the amount of retraction that is required. CSF drainage lessens retraction pressure.[33] CSF diversion or reduction can be accomplished by the use of dehydrating agents and/or of CSF drainage.[34] Mannitol has been shown to preserve function in a porcine model of brain retraction.[34] For some procedures, placement of a lumbar drain or external ventricular drain may be required.

Neuronavigation

The use of neuronavigation and preoperative surgical planning is complementary but not necessary for many surgeries. An additional benefit of neuronavigation is the ability to anticipate head positioning and the trajectory required to achieve a minimum amount of retraction.

Technical Aspects of Brain Retraction

Retractor Positioning

During initial placement, visualization of the entire retractor is ideal. With use of the microscope, the surgeon's attention may be drawn to the tip of the retractor, deep in the brain, while he or she inadvertently ignores the more superficial aspect of the retractor near the cortical surface where venous structures can be compromised or torn. The latter can result in a cortical injury and a slow steady (and maddening) seepage of blood into the operative field without the recognition of the source of the hemorrhage. Some surgeons therefore advocate the initial placement of the retractors under loop magnification to allow easier visualization of the entire depth of the operative field. Once initial placement is satisfactory, the microscope is used to visualize and refine final deep placement of the retractor.

Intermittent, isometric retraction results in a slow reduction in measured pressure along the surface of the retractor body and tip. This correlates to a significant reduction in cortical pressure beneath the retractor and thus minimizes cortical injury. In addition, the frequent repositioning of the retractor system during the early phases of surgery is helpful in reducing injury. The use of multiple retractors, when placed correctly, helps to reduce the risk of cortical injury while maximizing exposure and creating a larger surgical corridor.

Finding and maintaining the optimal positioning of retractors can be problematic. Rather than having a surgeon hold the retractors for the length of the operation, self-retaining retractors allow the retractor blades to stay in place without human involvement.[35] However, tightening the flexible arms to ensure stability and precision can be problematic.[36] Ideally, the brain retractor tip should be stable to within 1 mm.[37]

Attentiveness is imperative when manipulating the retractors. Surgeons must retract with the least force possible and for the briefest time necessary to accomplish the surgery.[38] Brain retractors should be manipulated when the surgeon is able to continuously visualize the retractor within the operative field through the microscope.[39] Surgeons should "walk" the retractor(s) to the proper depth on the brain parenchyma. One blade should be set first, and then the other brought parallel to it but slightly deeper.[38] The first retractor can then be advanced even closer to the target area, and so on. To a certain extent, it is better to slightly angle a retractor than to bend the blade to fit the anatomic contours of the brain.[38] However, this should not exclude the option of introducing a slight, gentle curve to the blade such that it mimics the overall contour of the surface. In so doing, great care must be given to identifying the blade's tip and ensuring that it remains in the surgeon's field of view.

Small changes in retraction pressure can be created by slightly tightening or loosening the locking nuts.[38] A micromanipulator can be added to self-retaining retractors to allow smooth adjustment of the brain spatula.[37] This micromanipulator also allows the surgeon to sense tissue resistance against the retractor as it is being adjusted.[37] Although these self-retractors have their benefits, both the adjustment knob and arm can interfere with the surgeon's hands.[36] Lastly, it is often difficult to reestablish the anatomic exposure after temporarily releasing the brain retractor.[40] This repositioning may momentarily halt the procedure.

Certain areas of the brain deserve particular attention during retraction. Small infarcts of the cortex may not lead to any clinical problems, but damage to the eloquent cortex is more likely to be associated with neurological impairment.[32] This damage to the eloquent cortex can be produced mechanically through the use of retractors.[32] Eloquent cortical areas can be identified using intraoperative electrocortical stimulation mapping or less invasive functional magnetic resonance imaging (fMRI) preoperatively.[41] When retracting on or near the optic or infraorbital nerve, gentle and short retraction should be used to avoid injury.[31] The surgeon must also be careful to avoid stretching and tearing a cortical bridging vein.[38]

Retraction Systems

Many retraction systems are highly ergonomic. All follow the basic premise of securing a frame around the patient's head, which serves as a basis from which a retractor system is built. In most cases, retractors are held in position with arms that extend from the frame system. A basic principle of retractor placement is to minimize the profile of the retractors at their interface with the retractor holders such that no devices are above the plane of the skull. This will ensure that the surgeon's hands and/or instruments do not inadvertently strike the retractor system, which is out of the visual field of the microscope.

Earlier retraction systems involved mounting the retractors directly to the skull or securing them to muscle and soft tissue.[11] These designs did not provide secure attachments, and they often interfered with the surgeon's hands.[11] Modern retraction systems attach the retractors to external frames such as head holders. The patient's head is fixed in position by three or four skull pins connected to the head holder.[42] For self-retaining systems, a semicircular basal frame is usually fixed perpendicular to the head holder.[42] Flexible retractors can then be screwed onto this frame and positioned appropriately.[42]

Flexible arms are made from several metal pieces joined together by ball-and-socket joints.[11] The length and proximity of the flexible arm to the operative field may obstruct the surgeon's hands.[11] The flexible arms should be placed close to the patient's head near the operative sight to make adjustments easier.[11] Resting a portion of the flexible arm to the frame helps ensure that the arm is not inadvertently moved.[11]

Altering Pressure

One technique to limit the decrease in cerebral perfusion that occurs during the operation is to reduce the retraction pressure. Often, the same amount of pressure does not need to be constantly applied during retraction. In fact, the pressure applied to a retractor to expose a specific area of the brain decreases with time.[33] Throughout the surgery, it may be more effective to reduce the pressure on the retractors without compromising visualization of the relevant field. In one study, the average time for a 50% reduction in required pressure was 6.6 minutes in trials of repeated retraction.[33]

Light and Magnification

The creation of the surgical corridor should result in a relatively unrestricted view of the target lesion. Proper placement of the microscope "down the pipe"—that is, the surgical corridor—will eliminate shadows and maximize light and magnification. Of note, retractor tips should always be in the visual field. This is especially important in the setting of a narrow field of view, under high magnification, where retractors can inadvertently move or be moved during the movement of instruments into and out of the surgical field.

RETRACTION INJURIES

Incidence of Retraction Injury

The incidence of retraction injury to the brain has not been well defined.[39] Perhaps a rough estimate of retraction injury can be obtained from the literature for aneurysm surgery, in which, unlike the edema of tumors, there is little to confound edema that is identified on most postoperative imaging.[39]

In his series of 1074 consecutive intracranial surgeries, Fukamachi and colleagues[43] reported detecting intracerebral hematomas in 29% of patients who underwent craniotomy for brain tumor and 8% of patients who underwent craniotomy for aneurysm surgery. Of note, 50% of hematomas were larger than 3 cm. A subsequent series of 3355 patients corroborated this finding, with the authors suggesting that 60% of the clinically prevalent hematomas detected in their series were attributable to retraction injury.[44]

Aneurysm surgery, in particular surgery of the anterior communicating artery, may shed further light on the risks of brain retraction. Recent studies have demonstrated that hematomas were detected in 2.1% of patients undergoing craniotomy for surgery of the anterior communicating artery. Additional series have described a 10% incidence of retraction injury in skull base surgery as well as visual loss during pineal surgery.[45] Infarction can be another manifestation of retraction injury. Most telling, Rosenorn[46] reported a 22% incidence of infarction at the identified vicinity of the retractor as evidenced on postoperative computed tomography (CT) scan. Thus one can summarize that retraction injury, symptomatic and asymptomatic, may occur in approximately 10% of skull base tumor operations and 5% of aneurysm operations.

Pathophysiologic Mechanisms of Retraction Injury

Injury to the brain and surrounding structures after retraction is related to mechanical deformation and perfusion of blood flow. A significant portion of mechanical disruption is secondary to disruption of perfusion. The amount of force applied per unit area (pressure) and the time over which this is applied are critical elements in determining parenchymal injury during surgical retraction. Damage results in part from decreased blood flow in the operative region. Animal studies have demonstrated this decrease in CBF near areas of brain retraction.[47] These reductions are associated with neuropathologic evidence of infarction. The infarction, however, differs from that caused by vasospasm. For instance, in one study, arterial vasospasm produced diffuse changes in large vascular areas whereas retraction caused focal changes in the region of the retractor blades.[47]

Cerebral Blood Flow

Arrest of cerebral circulation leads to cessation of neuronal electrical activity and ion hemostasis. High-energy phosphate reserves become depleted, causing membrane ion pump failure.[48] This leads to an efflux of cellular potassium and influx of sodium and water, leading to membrane depolarization. If this state of events lasts for longer than 5 to 10 minutes, irreversible cell damage will occur.[48]

The failure of basic functions such as synaptic transmission, ion pumping, and energy metabolism is dependent on residual blood flow. In accordance, tissue infarction occurs if the residual blood flow is below a critical threshold.[48] This flow threshold has been empirically estimated to be 0.15 g/min for the cerebral cortex.[48]

Rosenorn in 1979 described experiments on rats that strongly suggested that time and pressure consistently affected CBF.[49] When self-retaining brain retractors are used, regional cerebral blood flood (rCBF) decreases with increasing brain retractor pressure.[49] In animals, this decrease has led to infarcted cortical tissue and/or hemorrhaging. These infarcts are mainly caused by the direct compression of blood vessels by the retractors because even a significant increase in ICP does not produce reduction of CBF.[49] Indeed, histologic analysis of specimens with 40 mm Hg pressure of retraction for half the time of other subjects (15 minutes instead of 30) demonstrated infarction and hemorrhage. Further studies to elucidate whether the shape of the retractor affected the degree of parenchymal injury did not demonstrate any significance. Risk of infarct was significant when brain retraction pressure reached 30 mm Hg, and all animals with a brain retraction pressure of 40 mm Hg developed infarcts.[49] Venous drainage is also compromised at a brain retraction pressure exceeding 30 mm Hg.[49] These data correlated with prior studies that noted normal-amplitude somatosensory evoked potentials (SSEPs) in normotensive experimental animals when retraction pressure measured 30 mm Hg or less.

Intravascular pressure in small arterioles of the brain is approximately 30 to 40 mm Hg, whereas higher pressures are noted in larger arterioles and arteries.[50] By inference, retraction injury must result from compromise of these small arterioles and not larger arteries, which can also account for the restricted extent of retraction injury.

The decreased perfusion caused by retraction can lead to tissue hypoxia. Brain hypoxia activates both innate and adaptive immune responses via posttranscriptional activation of inflammatory signaling pathways.[51] These inflammatory responses can lead to tissue edema and destruction in the ischemic area. A cascade of events occurs after hypoxia, leading to the release of acute inflammatory mediators such as tumor necrosis factor (TNF), interleukin-1β (IL-1β), arachidonic acid metabolites, reactive oxygen species, and matrix metalloproteinases.[51] These events then lead to leukocyte extravasation, activation of complement systems, and recruitment and activation of lymphocytes such as natural killer cells.[51]

The inflammatory mediators TNF-α and IL-1β have been shown to cause neuronal damage.[51] Similarly, oxidative stress can aggravate cerebral injury.[51] The production of reactive oxygen species destroys cell membranes by inducing lipid peroxidation.[51] Conversely, antioxidants have been show to alleviate damage from brain ischemia. Natural killer cells increase neuronal excitability and synaptic transmission, leading to increased oxygen demand in dying neurons, which hastens their death. These natural killer cells also directly kill hypoxic neurons.[51]

Mechanical Disruption and Damage

Retractors can also cause damage through the direct effects of increasing pressure on the affected tissue. The forces of concern for pressure injury formation are pressure, shear, and friction.[52] High pressure gradients generate large shear forces, which contribute to the breakdown of tissue.[52] Cellular injury is therefore more pronounced at the margins of a compressed area where the pressure gradients are largest.[52] Shear forces act parallel to tissue and contribute to the mechanical breakdown of this tissue.[52] As the interface pressure against a particular region of tissue increases, the area surrounding the site is subject to an increasing pressure gradient and to higher shear forces.

A pressure gradient is also created deep to the interface pressure. As distance from the retractor increases, this gradient decreases.[52] For example, the pressure gradient at 1 cm deep is smaller than the gradient from 1 cm to 2 cm deep. Therefore, shear forces are created both in the plane of the interface pressure and in areas that lie deeper in the tissue.[52]

Based on the aforementioned observations, several studies assessed the use of intermittent retraction or multiple retractors. For example, a comparison of intermittent retraction at 40 mm Hg demonstrated less disruption to the blood-brain barrier than continuous retraction at 30 mm Hg.[39] This presumption was validated in additional studies in rats that demonstrated cortical injury with pressures of 30 to 40 mm Hg over 15 minutes as opposed to brief episodes of retraction with less than 7 minutes' duration.[39] Intermittent retraction confirmed better preservation of local CBF and histopathologic analysis. Kaido and colleagues evaluated continuous retraction, intermittent isometric retraction (subsequent retractor placement for identical exposure), and isotonic retraction (subsequent retractor placed at the same degree of pressure—30 mm Hg).[53] In their study, the authors concluded that intermittent isometric retraction reduces tissue injury in the setting of cortical vein occlusion.

Detecting Retraction Injury

Parenchymal injury secondary to retraction in noneloquent cortex may not be evident clinically or on immediate postoperative CT scans.[34,29] Delayed intracerebral hematomas may be detected several days later.[29] Therefore, retraction-induced strokes may be missed if patients are clinically stable and/or do not undergo serial postoperative scans.[29]

There are several ways to monitor CBF during the operation. Fluorescein dye (1%) can be injected into the carotid artery intraoperatively.[39] When photographs are then taken rapidly, flow patterns are produced that enable estimation of rCBF.[39] Laser Doppler and thermal diffusion measurements of CBF can also be used during the surgery.[29] In the future, retractor blades may incorporate technology that will allow online measurement of brain retractor pressure and/or CBF.

Measuring of brainstem auditory evoked potentials (BAEPs) and SSEPs can be used to monitor depression of cerebral metabolism and ischemia.[29] A linear relationship exists between SSEP amplitude and rCBF in primates.[39] The drop in SSEP amplitude and CBF is greater with increasing pressure.[29] A reduction in evoked potentials of more than 50% is likely to produce permanent injury.[29] In certain procedures, electroencephalography, BAEPs, and SSEPs can been used concurrently.[39] Another benefit is that intraoperative BAEP or SSEP monitoring can be done with little operative delay.[29] Stimulating earphones or electrodes are applied while anesthesia is being induced.[29] However, evoked potential (EP) monitoring does require the cessation of electrocautery or other sources of interference during the measurement.[29]

FUTURE DIRECTIONS

Simulation

Several simulations (for further discussion, see Chapter 19) have been developed to study the dynamic effects of brain retraction and allow neurosurgeons to practice retraction in a safe environment. These simulations incorporate both accurate neuroanatomy and realistic tactile and visual representations of retraction systems. The simulations start with a patient-specific model of the brain with increased spatial resolution in the region of surgical focus.[54] The computational model can be generated using high-resolution magnetic resonance imaging (MRI) series.[54] Regions of interest can be segmented using computer software.[54] These segments are then used to create a three-dimensional simulation of the region.

Several calculations can be made throughout the simulated surgery to increase realism. The effects of gravity on brain tissue and CSF can be calculated to simulate the slight changes in shape of the brain that are dependent on positioning of the head.[54] Because the exact shape of the brain changes according to positioning, head position must be taken into account when simulating deformation of brain tissue.

Because retractors are rigid, the deformation of the retractors is insignificant compared with the deformation of the surrounding brain tissue.[55] In accordance, these simulations must account for the deformation of tissue localized around the retractors. Algorithms have been developed to identify the physical intersection between virtual retractors and the simulated brain.[55] Once this identification has been made, the simulator can estimate the level of deformity of the tissue making contact with the virtual retractor.[55] The contacting elements identified by the algorithms also allow for haptic rendering to realistically reproduce the feel of touching a retractor to the brain.[55]

An additional calculation is needed to estimate the position of the retractor in the simulation.[54] This can be done via photographic imaging obtained through the optics of the simulator's operating microscope.[54] This enables simulators to recreate actual retractors in the virtual environment. Any movement of the actual retractors will realistically affect the simulated procedure.

Twenty-First Century Brain Retraction

The neurosurgical frontier changed dramatically from the 1980s until the present day, and neurosurgeons continue to find ways to improve visualization of the brain parenchyma during surgery while trying to minimize damage to vital structures. With novel technologies such as neuronavigation and intraoperative MRI, we have been able to advance our neurosurgical approaches, becoming more precise than ever before. Thus the demand for superior brain retraction continues to grow.

Spoon Retractors

Delicate spoon retractors were introduced in 2000 by Kyoshima and colleagues[56] for the retraction and removal of soft tissue masses. Varying in size from 5 mm to 4 cm, their concave, eggshell shape allows for upward retraction that creates significant space for visualization deep in the operative field. The advantage of these spoon retractors compared with other useful retractors such as tumor-holding clips and four-pronged hooks is that the spoons are suitable for soft tumor retraction. Also, compared with retraction with a flat brain spatula, wherein part of the mass will protrude from the flat edge of the retractor and block the operative field, spoon shapes prevent such obstruction[56] (Fig. 24-1).

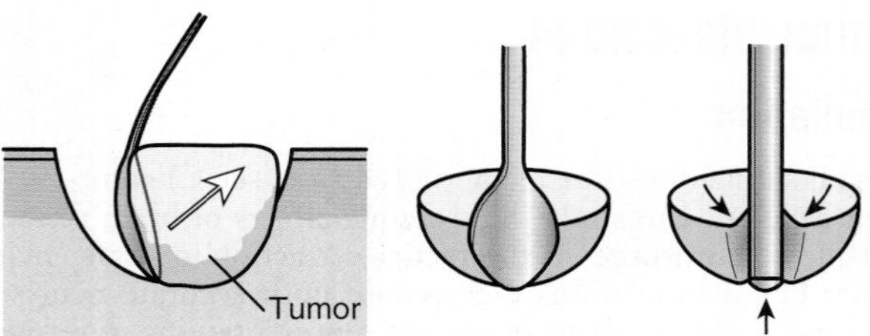

Figure 24-1. The retractor of eggshell-like concave shape enables retraction to hold a soft tumor upward *(white arrow)* creating ample space for dissecting it from surrounding structures in the depths. When an ordinary brain spatula with a flat surface is used for retracting a soft tumor, part of the tumor bulges out from the edges of the spatula, blocking the operating field *(black arrows). (From Kyoshima K, Hongo K, Kobayashi S. Spoon retractors for soft mass.* J Clin Neurosci. *2000;7:328-329.)*

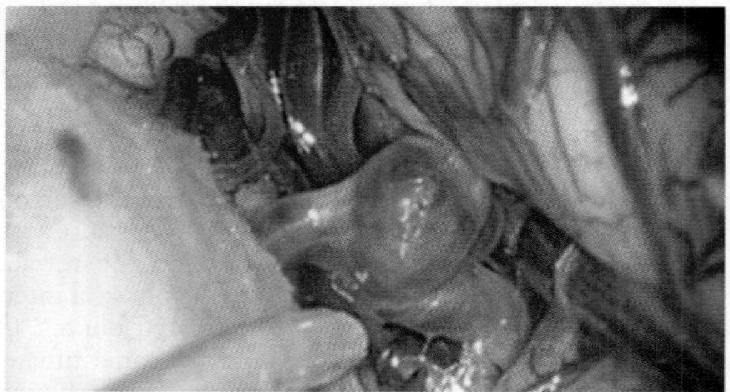

Figure 24-2. Intraoperative image obtained during dissection of a right M1 bifurcation aneurysm. The entire first portion of the operation, including sylvian fissure opening and aneurysm dissection, is performed using only the bubble retractor. *(Courtesy of Dr. Giannantonio Spena.)*

Balloon Retraction

The idea of gentle balloon inflation in the brain parenchyma has been used in various settings during the current neurosurgical era. Cokluk and colleagues[57] hypothesized that transparent microballoon dissection could gently separate healthy brain parenchyma from tumors while causing minimal damage, and they had success with tumor removal in a series of seven patients. In 2006, Serarslan and colleagues designed a device of air-filled microballoons and cotton to place between the brain surface and metal retractors to minimize parenchymal damage.[58] Giannantonio Spena and Pietro Versari have been using the small balloon tips of Fogarty catheters for gentle brain retraction for anterior circulation aneurysms, and even for midline and skull base brain tumors[35] (Fig. 24-2).

Revisiting Sponge Retraction

In the early 20th century, Ballance suggested using marine sponges for brain retraction.[10] More recently, Dagcinar and colleagues[59] took advantage of the inherent sponge characteristics of deformability and resistance to compression and used them as retractors for the modern neurosurgical era. Using simple sponge pieces along natural planes such as the sylvian fissure, they found that retraction pressure is less than provided by the self-retaining Leyla-Yaşargil retractors (Fig. 24-3). Their report suggests that these sponges, being inexpensive, easy to use, and gentle on the cortical surface, can certainly be used for complex cases. Similarly, Kashimura and colleagues[60] have reported successful use of a gelatin sponge for retraction of the temporal lobe in the subtemporal approach in 50 patients undergoing aneurysm clipping.

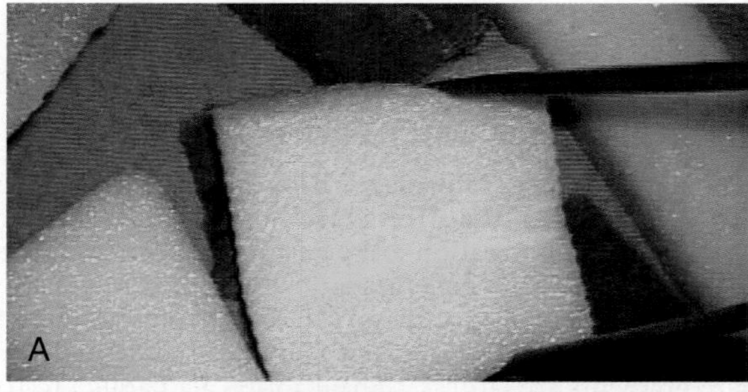

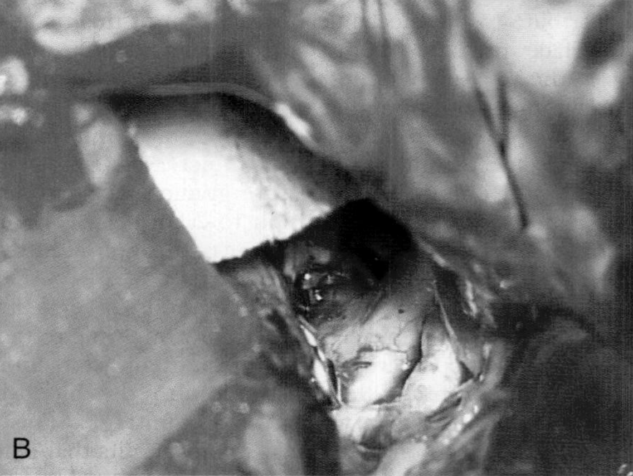

Figure 24-3. A, The sponge piece placed between the orbital roof and the frontobasal surface enables exposure of the lamina terminalis. **B,** The clip applied to the anterior communicating artery aneurysm. *(From Dagcinar A, Kaya AH, Senel A, Celik F. Sponge pieces as retractors in neurosurgical interventions.* Surg Neurol. *2007;67:493-495.)*

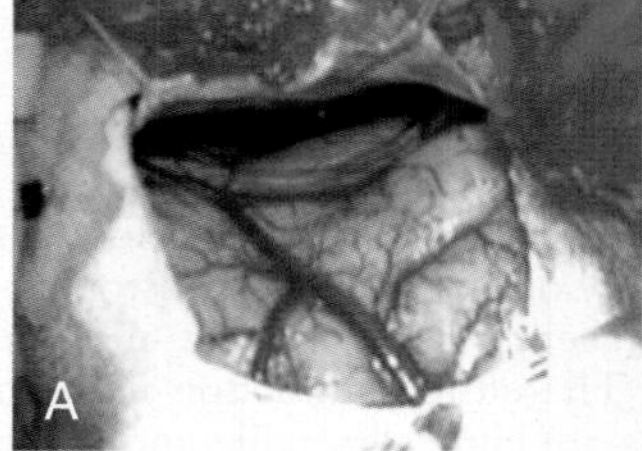

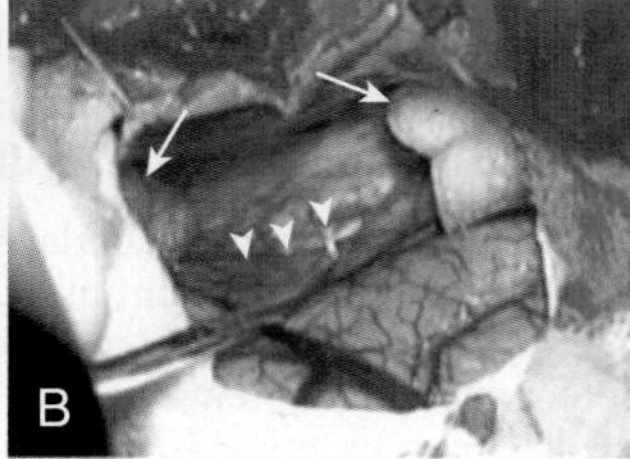

Figure 24-4. A, Intraoperative photograph of a 64-year-old man with unruptured aneurysms of the left basilar artery–superior cerebellar artery showing aspiration of the cerebrospinal fluid and slackening of the temporal lobe. **B,** Two and three pieces of gelatin sponge *(arrows)* are inserted between the dura and surfaces of the anterior and posterior temporal lobes, respectively. The free margin of the tentorium is exposed with minimal brain retraction *(arrowheads). (From Kashimura H, Ogasawara K, Kubo Y, et al. Brain retraction technique using gelatin sponge in the subtemporal approach.* Neurol Med Chir (Tokyo). *2008;48:143-146.)*

Being able to absorb a volume of water 5 to 10 times their own volume, these gelatin sponges absorb CSF during surgery and gradually swell to provide adequate brain retraction[60] (Fig. 24-4).

Tubular Retractor Systems: Minimal Invasion of the Brain Parenchyma

Tubular retractors have become popular throughout all surgical disciplines and are now being used in neurosurgery to access deep lesions of the brain. The ViewSite (Vycor Medical, Boca Raton,

FL) tubular retractor system has been successful in parenchymal retraction for both adults and children in tumor removal[17,61,62] (Fig. 24-5). Similar devices have been crafted, including a polyester cylinder for intraventricular tumor or hematoma removal, which avoids retractor injury, limits the surgical field, and protects the surrounding brain[63] (Fig. 24-6).

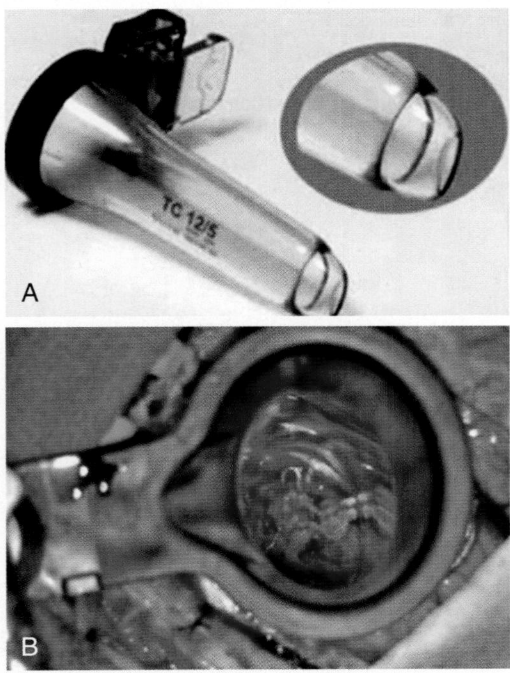

Figure 24-5. ViewSite tubular retractor system. A, Tubular retractors disperse the force of retraction over a greater surface area than do standard retractors, helping to minimize parenchymal damage. **B,** Intraoperative use of the ViewSite tubular retractor for resection of an intraventricular tumor. *(**A,** From Assina R, Rubino S, Sarris CE, et al. The history of brain retractors throughout the development of neurological surgery.* Neurosurg Focus. *2014;36:E8. Reprinted with permission from Journal of Neurosurgery Publishing Group.* ***B,*** *Courtesy of Dr. Chirag D. Gandhi.)*

Retractorless Brain Surgery: Toward a More Dynamic Neurosurgeon

Neurosurgery has trended toward more minimally invasive procedures, compared with the larger exposures advocated in the past. With endoscopic approaches and much smaller surgical fields, the use of immobile retractors is becoming less important. There is now a greater emphasis on dynamic retraction through use of the surgeon's handheld instruments.[45] Such an approach is "back to the future." Through proper use of the handheld suction device in one hand and the surgeon's operating tool in the other, enough retraction can be provided in a small window that the need to readjust fixed equipment is obviated, and the surgeon can modify his or her field of view much more rapidly[45] (Fig. 24-7). However, we must take caution with abandoning fixed retractors completely. Giuseppe Lanzino[64] has commented that countless neurosurgeons have achieved very good outcomes with use of gentle fixed retraction.

CONCLUSION

Creating safe corridors to access the deep structures of the brain defines the modern period of neurological surgery. The evolution of the retractor is a surrogate to our evolutionary understanding of how to maximize exposure and minimize the footprint in performing surgery. Although the science of retraction has become the primary focus of inquiry, it is the art of retraction

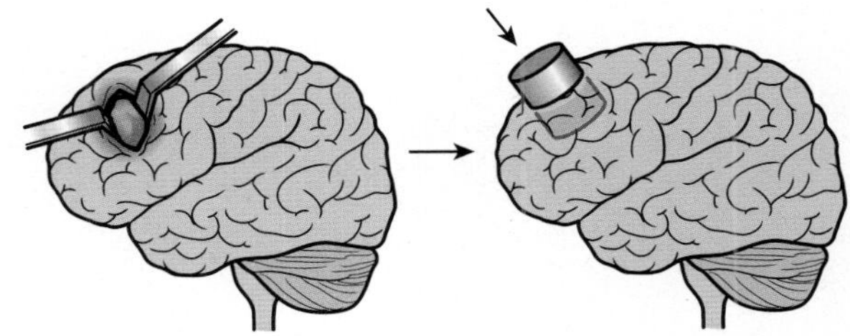

Figure 24-6. Diagram of transcylinder approach used to avoid retractor injury, limit surgical field, and protect surrounding brain during microsurgery. *(From Ogura K, Tachibana E, Aoshima C, et al. New microsurgical technique for intraparenchymal lesions of the brain: transcylinder approach.* Acta Neurochir [Wien]. *2006;148:779-785; discussion 785.)*

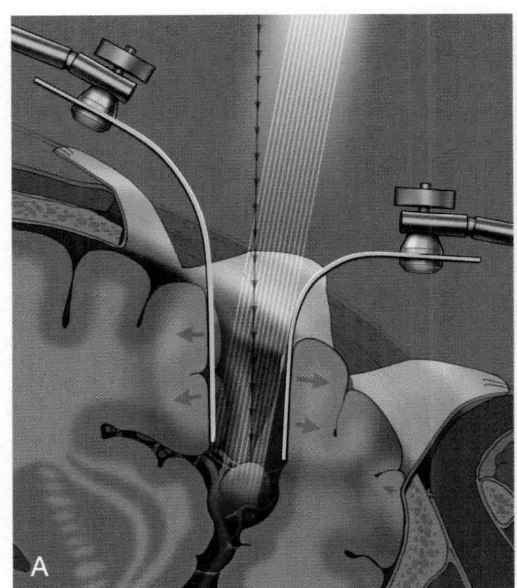

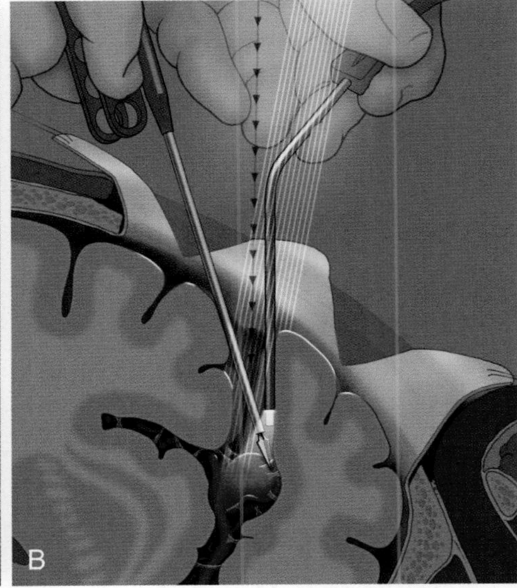

Figure 24-7. Comparison of fixed retraction and retractorless surgery in the approach to a middle cerebral artery aneurysm. **A,** Fixed retraction causes pressure-induced ischemic changes. **B,** Positioning of handheld suction can facilitate dynamic retraction. Visualization of the operative corridor is assisted by use of fiberoptic-lighted instruments. *(From Spetzler RF, Sanai N. The quiet revolution: retractorless surgery for complex vascular and skull base lesions.* J Neurosurg. *2012;116:291-300. Used with permission from Barrow Neurological Institute, Phoenix, AZ.)*

that requires true mastery. As we continue to develop newer techniques to minimize our footprint in neurosurgery, the basic tenets of our craft will not change. Safe, efficient ingress to the target and egress, visualization, protection, and separation of tissue from lesion, regardless of how we achieve them, will always be part and parcel of what we do. Without understanding these points, without respecting them, and without doing them well, we will never be able to maximize our patients' outcomes.

SUGGESTED READINGS

Goodrich JT. How to get in and out of the skull: from tumi to "hammer and chisel" to the Gigli saw and the osteoplastic flap. *Neurosurg Focus*. 2014;36:E6.

Greenblatt SH, Dagi TF, Epstein MH. *A history of neurosurgery: in its scientific and professional contexts*. Park Ridge, Ill.: American Association of Neurological Surgeons; 1997.

Spetzler RF, Sanai N. The quiet revolution: retractorless surgery for complex vascular and skull base lesions. *J Neurosurg*. 2012;116: 291-300.

Sugita K, Hirota T, Mizutani T, et al. A newly designed multipurpose microneurosurgical head frame. Technical note. *J Neurosurg*. 1978;48: 656-657.

Walker AE. *History of Neurological Surgery: Contributors*. Baltimore: Williams & Wilkins; 1951.

See a full reference list on ExpertConsult.com 

25 Visualization and Optics in Neurosurgery

Jeffrey M. Sorenson, Jon H. Robertson, Andrew W. Grande, and Matthew T. Brown

With the introduction of the operating microscope in the 1950s, a vast improvement in visualization led to a profound transformation of neurosurgery. This disruptive technology presented surgeons with an opportunity to perform more precise operations with better outcomes, but significant advances by pioneers such as Kurze, Yaşargil, and Rhoton were required before surgeons' abilities could match the improved surgical views. New instruments and surgical techniques were developed in order to delicately dissect the fine structures that became visible through the operating microscope, and the resulting need to better understand these structures gave rise to the field of microneurosurgical anatomy.

One of the earliest clinical motivations for the Rhoton laboratory was the need for better facial nerve preservation during acoustic neuroma surgery (personal communication). The view through the operating microscope, along with all of the developments it inspired, made such difficult feats possible. This link between visualization and ability has been crucial in the history of surgery and continues to drive our field forward today, not only in the operating room, but also in the laboratory and the lecture hall. Both art and technology have played an important role in such progress.

OUR UNDERSTANDING OF VISION

The quest to understand visualization has occupied many of the brightest minds since antiquity. In ancient Greece, Plato and most other prominent thinkers believed that rays emitted from the eye mediated vision. Euclid (c. 300 BC) combined this concept with his geometric principles into a theory of optics and vision whereby a cone of rays emitted from the eye traveled in straight lines to reach the subject. These rays were thought to reach out and interact with objects analogous to the sense of touch.[1] Aristotle (c. 300 BC) and others such as Avicenna (c. 1020 AD) argued against emission of rays from the eye. Democritus (c. 400 BC) and Epicurus (c. 300 BC) proposed theories in which effigies of an object were received into the eye.[2] Nonetheless, Plato's ideas prevailed for more than a millennium to follow, not the least because they were also adopted by the influential Roman physician Galen (c. 175 AD), who also incorporated the popular physiologic theory of pneuma. He believed that this vital substance originated within the cerebral ventricles and flowed through the optic nerves, then through the retina to the lens, where it produced visualization with visual rays. In this model, the lens was spherical and situated in the center of the eye. Galen's ideas became dogma that was not successfully challenged until the renaissance, when the Flemish anatomist Vesalius began to identify errors in Galen's writings through meticulous dissections. Felix Platter later gave a more detailed account of the anatomy of the eye in which the retina, rather than the lens, was considered to be the seat of vision. Johannes Kepler then explained how light rays passing through the lens could form an image on the retina, but it was still a mystery how this led to vision. Isaac Newton extended this theory by proposing that miniature vibrations within the retina were transmitted through the optic nerves to the brain, but a detailed physiologic understanding of visual processing beyond the retina did not emerge until the 20th century with the work of David Hubel and Torsten Wiesel.

Using prisms, Newton also proved that white light could be separated into component colors, which could then be mixed as desired. In the 19th century scientists such as Thomas Young, Hermann von Helmholtz, and James Maxwell deduced that the eye contains three types of receptors with distinct color sensitivities—loosely related to red, green, and blue—that combined in various proportions to produce all perceived colors. In 1861, Maxwell demonstrated that a full color image could be reproduced with separate black and white photographs taken through red, green, and blue filters and then projected together with the corresponding filters. Their trichromatic theory of color vision greatly simplified the capture and reproduction of color images because the required ingredients—filters, film emulsions, inks, and emitters—would only be needed for three colors. To this day, whether in print or on a digital display, full color images can be reproduced from three single colored images, just as Maxwell's first color photograph.

Around the time that vision scientists were learning to reproduce color perception using three colors, Charles Wheatstone realized that two images from slightly different perspectives could reproduce the effect of viewing a scene through both eyes. He invented the first stereoscope in the early 1830s, concurrent with the early development of photography. It was a simple device that employed mirrors to direct images with slightly different perspectives to each eye. Leonardo da Vinci and others before him had studied the phenomenon of binocular vision, but for reasons that are still unclear, they did not attempt to develop a stereoscopic viewer.

AUGMENTATION OF VISION

The use of lenses to magnify objects dates to antiquity. The oldest known lens, created about 750 BC, was found in the ruins of the ancient Assyrian city Nimrud, located in modern-day Iraq (Fig. 25-1). Lenses have also been found in Greek and Roman ruins; these are thought to have been used both for magnification and for burning. In the first century, after the invention of glass, the Roman philosopher Seneca wrote, "Writing, however tiny and difficult, is seen larger and clearer through a glass sphere full of water."[3] Pliny wrote about cauterizing wounds with crystal balls using solar rays.[4] If lenses were used as visual aids in the ancient world, it is a bit surprising that the invention of spectacles can only be traced as far back as 1286.[5] Another 300 years passed before Dutch spectacle makers combined lenses in a tube to create the telescope and the compound microscope in the 1590s. The scientific utility of the microscope was recognized by Robert Hooke, who in 1665 was the first to use the term *cell* when describing the magnified appearance of cork in his publication "Micrographia." Despite Hooke's achievements, early compound microscopes still had serious technical problems in their design and manufacturing because lens making was still very much a trial-and-error process. In fact, for the remainder of the 17th century, compound microscopes were outperformed by the small single spherical lens microscopes of the self-taught Dutch biologist Anton van Leeuwenhoek, who kept his manufacturing process secret, giving him a near monopoly in the field of microbiology for the remainder of his life. He was the first to describe single-cell organisms. He also examined optic nerve

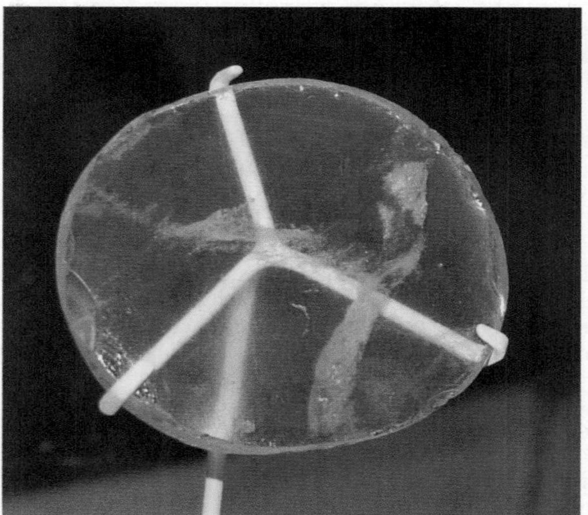

Figure 25-1. A lens found in Nimrud dating to 750 BC. *(© Trustees of the British Museum.)*

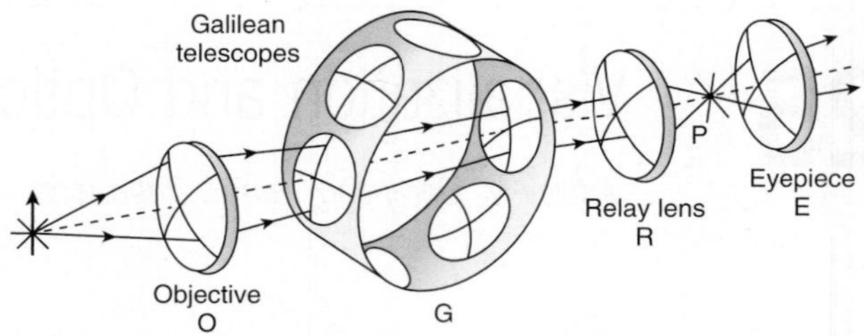

Figure 25-2. Example of a rotating Galilean system of magnification. *(From Khurana AK.* Theory and practice of optics and refraction. *2nd ed. Elsevier India, 2008.)*

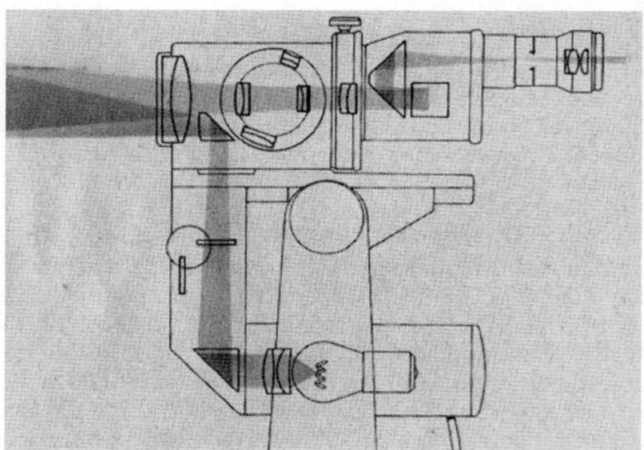

Figure 25-3. Diagram of the Zeiss OPMI 1 showing the pathway of local light source. *(From Schulze F. How the humble stereomicroscope found its way into modern surgery: the Zeiss operating microscope.* Micscape Magazine. *2012;December:1-20.)*

tissue and failed to find the hollow conduits that Galen had described.

THE OPERATING MICROSCOPE

The first described use of a microscope within the operative theater was in 1686 by Giuseppe Campani, who used a compound microscope to examine wounds and scar tissue.[6] Two more centuries would pass before the microscope was ready to assist with surgery. During that time, significant technical advancements were made in lens design in an attempt to overcome blurred images caused by several types of optical distortions. In 1730, the invention of the achromatic lens was the first step toward correcting chromatic aberration, which arises when the various colors of light in an image have different focal lengths because of a prism effect. This lens was composed of two layers of material with different refractive properties designed so that the chromatic aberration of the second material partially corrected that of the first. The problem was further reduced in 1868, when Ernst Abbe, a physicist hired by Carl Zeiss, developed an apochromatic lens using new materials. As the art and science of lens design and manufacturing progressed, so did the application of the microscope.

The use of magnification in surgery began in earnest in the second half of the 19th century with the development of loupe spectacles.[7] It was not until 1921 that the microscope made it into the operating room when Carl Nylen, an otolaryngologist in Stockholm, first used a microscope during surgery for a case of chronic otitis media.[8] His associate Gunnar Holmgren then took the initiative and developed the first binocular scope with an independent light source for use in otolaryngology.[9,10] Otolaryngologists continued to pioneer the use of the microscope in the operating room and improve on the design. As new limitations and problems became apparent, clever solutions were found. In 1938, a tripod with counterweight system was used to further stabilize the magnified view. In addition, a prism was introduced that allowed for an observer scope to be used during the procedure.[9]

Throughout the early evolution of the operating microscope, the working distance and magnification of the image remained somewhat limited. In 1948, an ophthalmologist in Chicago utilized a Bausch & Lomb microscope with a 127-mm working distance and magnifications of 3, 5, 7, and 10.5, but changing settings required replacing the eyepieces used at the head of the microscope.[9] This issue was solved through further innovation by Zeiss in 1952. Their new rotating Galilean system, developed by Hans Littman, allowed the user to change the magnification of the scope without replacing the eyepieces or changing the working distance.[6,9] The paired lenses about a rotating cylinder (Fig. 25-2) allowed for a preset change in magnification.[11] Zeiss began to market the new microscope as the OPMI 1 with rotating Galilean device, a rotating arm on a base with 100 to 405 mm of working distance, and 2.5 to 50 times magnification. The new OPMI 1 was designed for the operating room and had coaxial lighting that was superior to previous models. Further advancements were soon made to allow for greater control and utility.[9,10] In 1956, foot and hand controls were developed for axial movement and image focus. By this time, axial lighting was widely used (Fig. 25-3).[9]

Despite the continued advancements and use of the operative microscope by otolaryngologists and ophthalmologists, neurosurgeons had yet to bring a microscope into the operating theater. This changed in 1957 when Theodor Kurze, a neurosurgeon at the University of Southern California, was inspired by the work of William House, who had been pioneering microsurgical techniques for otolaryngology. After practicing microsurgical techniques in the laboratory, Kurze performed the first microneurosurgical procedure: the excision of a seventh (CN-VII) nerve neurilemmoma in a 5-year-old patient.[9,10,12] At that time, sterile drapes for the operating microscope were not well developed, leaving surgeons to improvise with materials such as sterilized plastic turkey bags, which would sometimes overheat and produce smoke during the procedure.[10] Kurze eventually performed a second procedure on his initial patient: a seventh (CN-VII) to twelfth (CN-XII) nerve anastomosis. Unfortunately, the sterile drapes for the scope were not available at the start of the case, so Kurze proceeded without the microscope. On completion of the anastomosis, the drapes had become available, and he decided to evaluate his work with the microscope. He stated that the anastomosis "looked awful," and then repaired the work with the aid of the microscope.[10] Kurze continued using the operative microscope in his practice, even transporting the scope between facilities in the back of his personal vehicle.

Although Kurze was the first neurosurgeon to use the operative microscope, R. M. P. Donaghy quickly followed by establishing the first microsurgical research laboratory in Burlington, Vermont in 1958.[10] Between Donaghy and his vascular surgery colleagues, the research laboratory was making important contributions by 1960, when they published the first use of the operative microscope for the anastomosis of small vessels. Before this work, vessels smaller than 7 to 8 mm could not be reliably repaired or joined. Also in 1960, Donaghy's interest in surgical treatments for ischemic stroke led him to perform the first open middle cerebral artery embolectomy. Later in that year, his vascular surgery colleagues, Jacobson and Suarez, published a collection of dog and rabbit carotid artery reanastamoses with a reported patency rate of 100%. Although this was an incredible development in microvascular technique, a prominent chairman of vascular surgery made the public critique that "[t]his is very nice work, but it is simply ridiculous to bring a microscope into the operating room."[10] Thus, as with most paradigm shifts, microsurgery was not universally embraced in the beginning.

Despite the lukewarm reception, work with the microscope continued to progress. Kurze and House used the scope for more than 40 middle fossa explorations and published their experience in 1962. Kurze also used the microscope for aneurysm surgery starting in 1958, although the first to publish cases of microsurgery for aneurysms were Adams and Witt in 1964, and Pool in 1965.[10] Also in 1965, Sais, a company from Buenos Aires, fitted a television camera on the observer head of the scope, allowing for recording and broadcasting. This was built on the advancements made by Zeiss with the 1961 release of the diploscope—a "true double microscope" for head-to-head work by two surgeons (Fig. 25-4).[9,13] In the same year, Zeiss released a motorized focus and zoom feature that replaced the rotating Galilean system.[9]

In 1966, a young Turkish neurosurgeon with an interest in vascular microsurgery arrived in Burlington. In Donaghy's laboratory, M. G. Yaşargil developed the superficial temporal–middle cerebral artery bypass procedure. Yaşargil eventually returned to Zurich where he was the first to perform this procedure on a human patient. Coincidentally, Donaghy repeated this feat less than 24 hours later in Vermont.[10] Yaşargil went on to help pioneer several technical advancements, such as the ability to manually tilt the microscope head (1970) and a polyaxial counterweight system with electromagnetic braking for each joint (1972), to make the operating microscope more graceful. These user-friendly features spurred wider adoption of the operating microscope and stimulated further industry-wide development.[9] Modern advancements have seen improvements in optical technology, including clearer apochromatic lenses, automatic focus, increased depth of field, and more powerful motorized zoom (Fig 25-5). The 1990s brought further neurosurgery-specific enhancements into production. Advancements in intraoperative angiography with indocyanine green fluorescence and the use of 5-aminolevulinic acid for high-grade glioma resection have been incorporated into several microscopes.[9] Stereoscopic video recording and stereotactic guidance have now become widely available.

Although often viewed as a modern tool, the endoscope has a longer history in the operating room than the microscope.

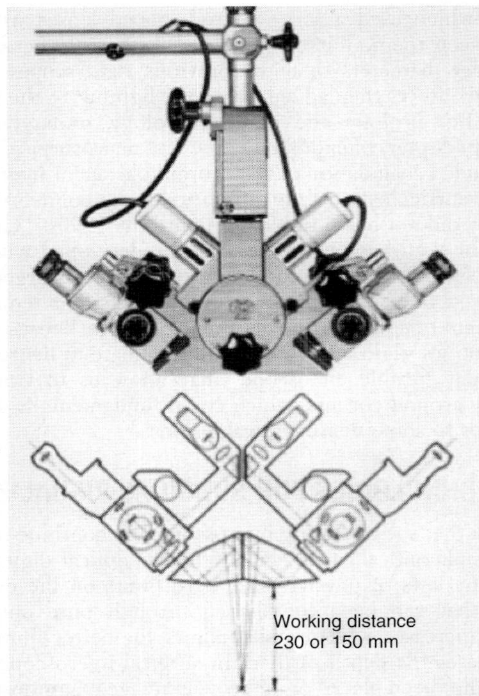

Figure 25-4. Zeiss diploscope first offered in 1961. *(From Schulze F. How the humble stereomicroscope found its way into modern surgery: the Zeiss operating microscope.* Micscape Magazine. *2012;December:1-20.)*

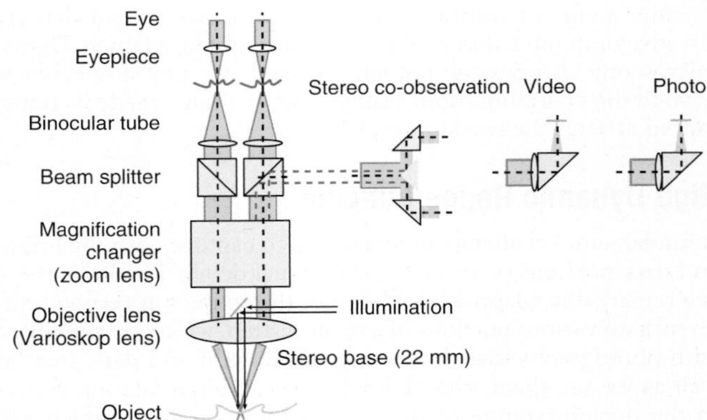

Figure 25-5. Light pathways of a modern operating microscope. *(Courtesy of Carl Zeiss Meditec AG.)*

Precursors such as the lighted speculum of Philipp Bozzini had been in use since 1806, but the field of endoscopic surgery began in 1887 with the German urologist Max Nitze, who co-invented the first operating endoscope. This device had a series of lenses within a hollow tube with a water-cooled electric lighting filament at the tip. These early endoscopes had fairly poor optics and maneuverability, so widespread adoption by gastroenterologists did not occur until the prominent British optical physicist Harold Hopkins, creator of the first viable zoom lens, developed a fiberoptic flexible endoscope in the 1950s. This allowed much more complete examinations of the gastrointestinal tract. Nonetheless, the fiberoptic scopes had resolutions that were limited by the number of fibers, which produced a pixilated image. Hopkins therefore went on to develop the rod-lens endoscope in 1959, which used a series of rod-shaped lenses with small gaps between them. This resulted in substantially better optics and smaller diameters than the previous rigid scopes used by Nitze. Karl Stores then added fiberoptic lighting to the rod-lens scopes. After urology and gastroenterology, otolaryngologists were early adopters of endoscopy. The first neurosurgical applications included coagulation of the choroid plexus for hydrocephalus, third ventriculostomy, and pituitary surgery, but neurosurgical endoscopy did not begin to blossom until the 1990s.[14] Currently, the field of skull base surgery is being redeveloped with endoscopic techniques. The endoscope provides neurosurgeons new perspectives, but like the operating microscope, it requires the development of new instruments and techniques. Because of their superior optics, rigid endoscopes still dominate in neurosurgery, but one day flexible endoscopes may allow us to work more effectively around corners, which could fundamentally alter our approaches to some neurosurgical lesions.

NEW TECHNOLOGIES FOR SURGICAL VISUALIZATION

It is likely that the operating microscope will continue to evolve from a simple optical pathway into a hybrid optical-digital device because the laws of physics place hard limits on the quality of imaging that can be accomplished through pure optics. For instance, increased aperture size allows for better illumination but decreases the depth of field. In surgical microscopes, much emphasis has been placed on improving image magnification and illumination. When this is achieved through additional lenses, wider apertures, and brighter light sources, there can be detrimental effects, such as reduced depth of field and thermal injury to tissues. With continued improvements in computing power and charged-coupled device sensors, digital microscopes may provide alternative solutions for these challenges. New technologies will undoubtedly emerge, but a few techniques for increased dynamic range of contrast and increased depth of field that are already common in digital photography might be adapted. Digital microscopy also has the potential to enhance our surgical view beyond the operating room as digital signals can already be transmitted around the world in real time.

High Dynamic Range Imaging

A fundamental challenge in imaging is to capture both the bright and dark portions of an image with equal detail. The human eye is a remarkably adaptive tool because the retina can respond differently to various portions of a scene. Often, we are disappointed with photographs that do not reproduce light and dark areas as well as we see them with the naked eye. This limitation relates to the dynamic range of the camera film or sensor, which will produce poor details in darker areas with short exposures, but loss of detail in bright areas with longer exposures. High dynamic range (HDR) imaging can overcome this limitation either with improved sensors or by combining multiple exposures with software (Fig. 25-6).

In the past few decades, microscopes have been developed with increasingly powerful lighting to adequately illuminate the darker recesses of the operative field. Light sources have included ambient light, incandescent bulbs, and then eventually halogen lamps that often melted or burned the sterile drapes.[10,15] The light source was ultimately moved to the base of the microscope with a fiberoptic connection to solve this issue. The most recent transition from the 100-W halogen lamp to the 300-W xenon bulb has enhanced illumination through the operative microscope considerably, but now the light is so intense that tissue desiccation and burns can occur.[16] A digital microscope could produce better results with less illumination by using HDR imaging to perfectly expose all parts of the image through increasingly sophisticated sensors, multiple exposure times, and manipulation of the images with software. Significant computational resources will be required to produce such enhanced video streams with acceptable latency and resolution.

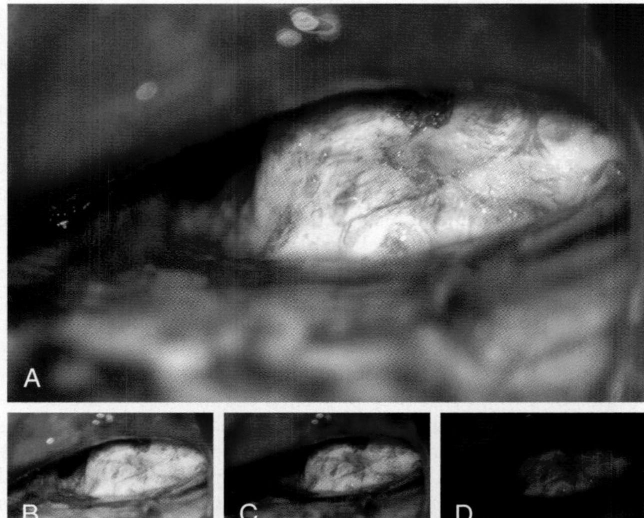

Figure 25-6. A high dynamic range photograph **(A)** has been constructed from three photographs. An overexposed image **(B)** provides good detail from the darker areas but loses detail in the lighter areas. Medium **(C)** and short **(D)** exposures do not show the darker areas well but do capture more detail in the brightest areas of the image.

Focus Stacking

Another aspect of optics that can produce frustration with operating microscopes is focusing. As the optics of the microscope are zoomed in to show more detail, the focal plane becomes increasingly narrow. The result is that portions of the surgical corridor that are slightly deeper or closer than the focal plane can be significantly out of focus. Thus, surgeons often find themselves adjusting the focus when working with deeper pathologies at high magnification. A digital microscope that is not limited by pure optics could overcome this problem by combining images at different focal planes with software (Fig. 25-7). An alternative solution is light field photography, as popularized by the Lytro camera. In such cameras, the sensor array records the angle at which light arrives in addition to the usual color and intensity information. Through software, this information allows an image to be computed at any focal plane, or with all focal planes simultaneously, so that all portions of the image are in focus. Thus, a digital operating microscope could ensure excellent illumination (through HDR) and focus (through focus stacking or light field photography) of every part of the image, exceeding the view obtained through pure optics.

Visual Annotation

In addition to delivering better quality images, a digital microscope would excel at visual annotation. Models of the patient's anatomy and pathology obtained from preoperative studies such as computed tomography, magnetic resonance imaging, or angiography can be seamlessly superimposed over live images in real time. This requires tracking the position of the microscope with a stereotactic system, which is already possible. As the brain shifts during surgery and the lesion is removed, the system would need to modify its model based on current images as well as previous data collected during the course of the surgery. Such

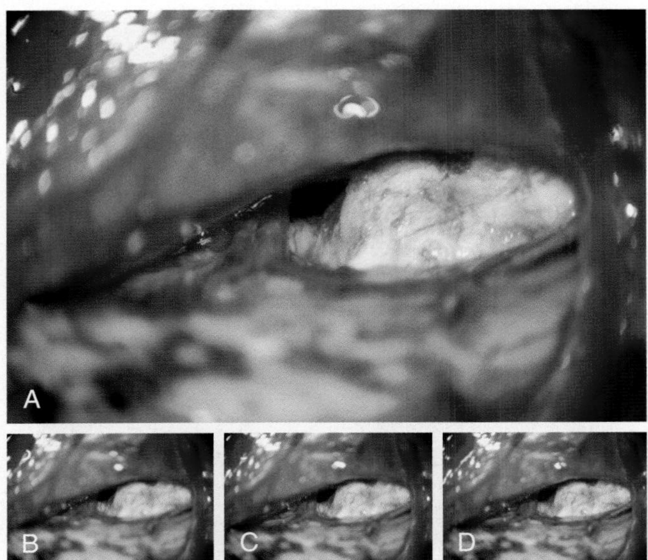

Figure 25-7. A composite photograph **(A)** with higher depth of field is created from three photographs taken at different focal planes: an image **(B)** focused on the small artery, which is deeper than the other structures; an image **(C)** focused on the deep portion of the venous complex; and an image **(D)** focused on the nerve.

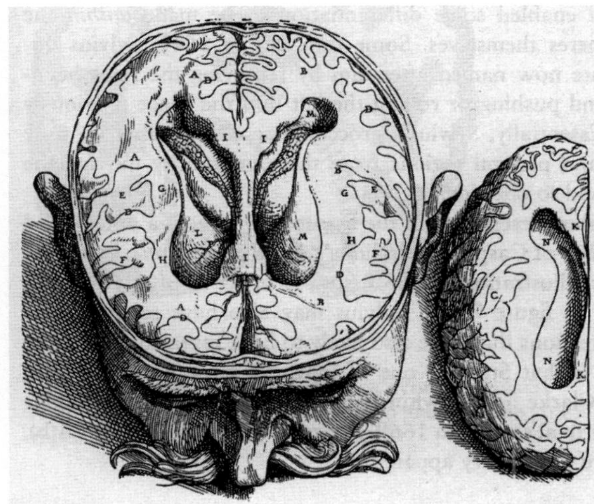

Figure 25-8. An illustration from Vesalius' Fabrica using the woodcut printing technique. *(From Vesalius A.* De Humani Corporis Fabrica Libri Septem. Book 7: The Brain. *Basel:* Ex officina *Joannis Oporini, 1543.)*

image annotation would further enhance "image-guided surgery" beyond traditional frameless stereotactic systems because the surgeon would be able to "see through" brain or tumor tissue to locate vessels or other important structures. A surgeon could peer through the brain tissue to visualize the location of an aneurysm and all related vessels prior to beginning the arachnoid dissection.

THE VISUAL RECORD

Dispel from your mind the thought that an understanding of the human body in every aspect of its structure can be given in words; the more thoroughly you describe the more you will confuse.... I advise you not to trouble with words unless you are speaking to blind men.

Leonardo da Vinci

As our ability to visually document the details of surgery and anatomic dissections improves, so does surgical education. The great Greek anatomists of Alexandria, Herophilus (335-255 BC) and Erasistratus (304-250 BC), performed extensive human dissections and vivisections during a relatively brief period before the procedures were banned. Together, they described many brain structures, including the cerebrum, cerebellum, ventricles, choroid plexus, cranial nerves, calamus scriptorius, and torcula herophili.[17] They confirmed Hippocrates' claim that the brain was the seat of thought, movement, and sensation, overturning the Aristotelian belief that it served a cooling function for the heart. Their writings have been lost to history but were extensively cited by Galen (129-199 AD), who also studied in Alexandria before becoming the personal physician of Roman emperors. Galen's works on anatomy, which were partly based on animal dissections, became the authoritative reference until the Renaissance, yet they contain no illustrations. Neither do other ancient medical texts, such as the Edwin Smith Papyrus or the writings of Hippocrates. This paucity of illustrations in the canonical texts, owing to primitive publishing technology, together with widespread prohibitions on human dissection made the study of anatomy particularly abstract and difficult for more than a millennium.

Andreas Vesalius placed the study of human anatomy onto a better footing in 1543 with the publication of his text *De Humani Corporis Fabrica Libri Septum* ("On the Fabric of the Human Body in Seven Books"). This book contained many annotated woodcut illustrations that were mass-produced by the printing press, which had been introduced to Europe only a century before (Fig. 25-8). For the first time, a high-quality illustrated anatomy textbook became accessible to a wide audience. He implored physicians to perform their own dissections, gently reminding them that the human cadaver should be the ultimate source of anatomic knowledge. Through direct observation, he was able to correct many of the errors in Galen's work. Outside of dissections, Vesalius realized that anatomic knowledge is most effectively transmitted through a visual medium, so he went to great lengths to make sure his scientific achievement was also a great work of art. The illustrations were created using refined techniques of High Renaissance artists, such as Jan Steven van Calcar, a protégé of the Venetian master Titian. Vesalius' work therefore sat squarely at the crossroads of art and science, setting the standard for all anatomy texts to follow.

The Italian polymath Leonardo da Vinci first embodied the combined artistic and scientific approach to the study of anatomy, decades before Vesalius. He performed dissections at the Santo Maria Nuova Hospital in Florence. His first anatomic illustrations were of the skull in 1489, and he later went on to draw the first accurate depiction of the human spine (Fig. 25-9). His anatomy collection eventually exceeded 200 annotated illustrations, enough to create a groundbreaking anatomy treatise, but it was never published. Instead, his anatomic works were lost until the 19th century. Michelangelo was also very interested in depicting the human body accurately in his art, leading him to perform his own dissections. In the later years of his life, he collaborated with a surgical colleague of Vesalius at the University of Padua, Dr. Realdo Colombo, who planned to create an illustrated anatomy text that would surpass Vesalius'. Unfortunately, Michelangelo never found the time, so the textbook was printed without the illustrations. Nonetheless, several other important anatomy texts were published from the University of Padua after Vesalius. In renaissance Rome, the anatomist Barolommeo Eustachi made several important contributions, such as his work that provided further clarity about the anatomy of the cranial nerves.

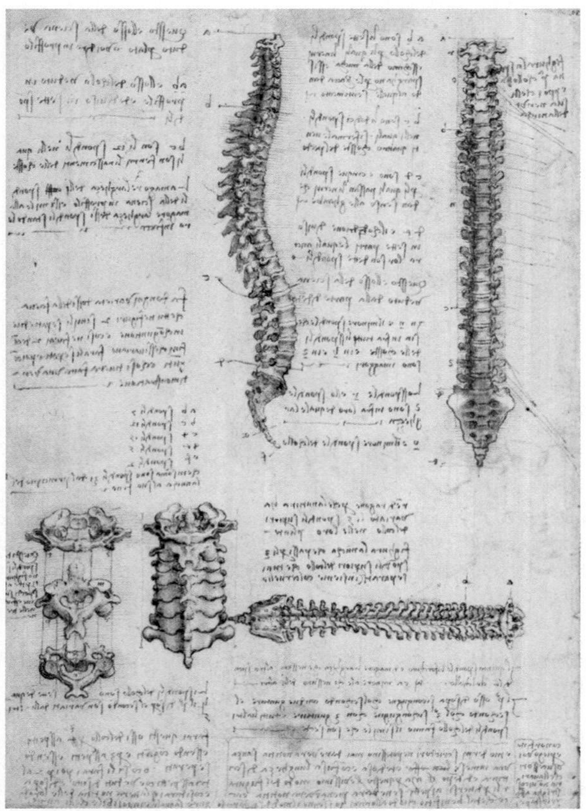

Figure 25-9. Leonardo da Vinci's drawings of the spine, which show an advanced understanding of the articulations between the cervical vertebrae. His anatomy atlas was never completed or published. *(Royal Collection Trust/© Her Majesty Queen Elizabeth II, 2014. RCIN 919007.)*

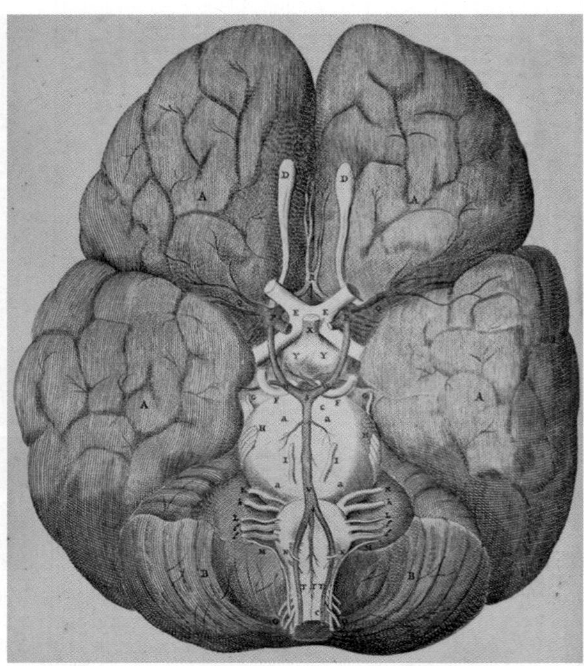

Figure 25-10. Illustration of the base of the brain showing the circle of Willis and cranial nerves as well as the finer details possible with copper plate intaglio. *(From Willis T.* Anatomy of the Brain and Nerves. *1664. Illustrated by Christopher Wren.)*

Since *Fabrica*, anatomy textbooks became artistic endeavors pushing the boundaries of technique and technology. Copper plates largely replaced woodcuttings later in the 16th century, allowing finer tones and details. With such intaglio printing, the lines of the drawing are engraved or acid-etched directly into the metal instead of being created by removing surrounding material, as with the woodcuttings that Vesalius had used. Shallow or more sparsely etched ink lines created the illusion of lighter shades even though only one color of ink was used (Fig. 25-10).

The 18th century saw the first color atlas, created by Gautier d'Agoty. This process used four different engraved metal plates to print three colors and black.[18] The process of lithography ("stone writing"), invented in 1798, would ultimately provide a quantum leap forward in the printing of images. A wax crayon drawing on limestone would preferentially accept hydrophobic ink versus the water-soaked stone. Although still tedious, this was easier and more versatile than working with metal plates or carving wood. By applying a light-sensitive chemical coating to a stone, photographic film negatives could be projected onto the surface of the stone, leaving a hydrophobic residue that would adhere to ink (photolithography). To achieve the optical illusion of shades of gray using only black ink, fine grids between the negative and the stone decomposed images by diffraction into tiny dots that would vary in size according to light intensity (half toning). Ultimately, in the 20th century, metal plates with chemical coatings replaced limestone, allowing the lithography plates to be wrapped around the cylinders of the modern printing press.

In the 19th century, Paris hosted a thriving community of artists and anatomists as well as hospitals that made cadavers readily available. It was also at the forefront of lithography. The results were beautifully illustrated anatomy atlases by anatomist-artist teams, such as Jules Cloquet and Jean-Baptiste Sarlandiere, and Jean Marc Bourgery and Nicolas-Henri Jacob; Jacob was also a pioneer in color lithography. Because chromolithography had not yet been perfected at the time of their first editions, many of their illustrations were hand painted after printing, making the atlases more expensive to produce. The beautiful dissections and illustrations in Bourgery's *Atlas of Human Anatomy and Surgery* took more than 20 years to complete (Fig. 25-11). Also in Paris, Jean Cruveilhier contributed significantly to neuroanatomy and produced seminal illustrations of neurological conditions such as meningiomas and acoustic neuromas. In Leipzig, Christian Braune developed cross-sectional anatomy by slicing frozen cadavers and making vivid color lithographic illustrations of sagittal and axial cuts (Fig. 25-12). In his later years, he mentored Max Brödel, who would go on to help launch the discipline of medical illustration.

In London, where cadavers from hospitals and workhouses had been made more plentiful by the Anatomy Act, Henry Gray collaborated with Henry Carter to produce the most famous anatomy text of the 19th century. The text was meant to be a practical and affordable guide. The illustrations made by Carter were produced by woodcutting and had a schematic quality, with labels added directly to the structures (Fig. 25-13). Gray and Carter worked very quickly, going from an idea to publishing within 3 years (1858). Despite this book's weaker artistic merit compared with the elaborate color lithographs of that century, its affordability made it very successful among students, and it is still being revised. Shortly after publication, Gray was criticized for not giving sufficient credit to Carter and previous anatomists. He died a mere 3 years later of smallpox at the age of 34 years.

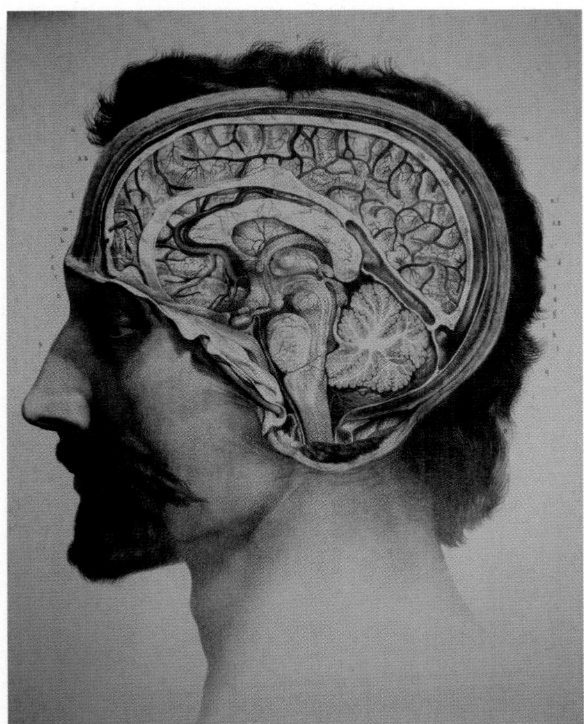

Figure 25-11. A color lithograph showing the brain. *(From Bourgery and Jacob's* Atlas of Human Anatomy and *Surgery, 1831-1854.)*

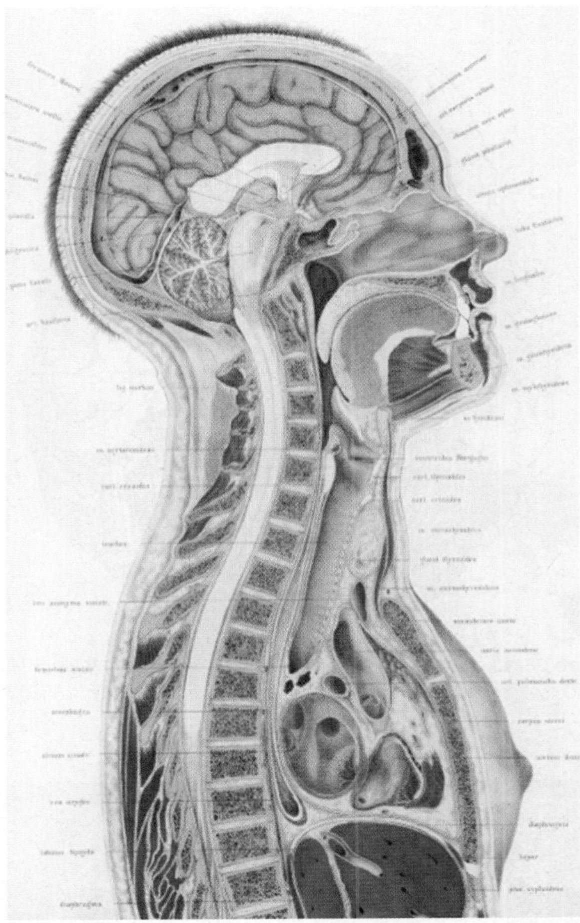

Figure 25-12. A sagittal section of the brain and spine by Christian Braune. His cross-sectional images anticipated computed tomography and magnetic resonance imaging by a century. *(From Braune C.* Topographisch-anatomischer Atlas: nach Durchschnitten an gefrornen Cadavern. *Leipzig: Verlag von Veit & Comp; 1867-1872.)*

Fine artistic technique and interpretation were carried into the 20th century by the German artist Max Brödel and the American artist-physician Frank Netter. As a child, Netter had always been intensely interested in art, but his mother saw no future in it and instead encouraged him to become a doctor. Medicine, however, became yet another inspiration for his art. During his medical studies at New York University, an anatomy instructor encouraged him to leave the cadaver laboratory, where he was making drawings, and go home to study so that he could pass the examination.[19] Nevertheless, his classmates and professors began to notice the high quality of his anatomic illustrations, which were soon in demand. He completed his surgical training but quickly left practice during the Great Depression because he found it easier to support himself making medical illustrations for pharmaceutical companies, particularly Ciba, which became his lifelong patron. The educational pamphlets he produced *(Ciba Clinical Symposia)* became very popular with physicians, so Ciba agreed to produce a series of volumes that would address a wide variety of anatomic topics *(Ciba Collection of Medical Illustrations)*. The first volume, "The Nervous System," was published in 1953, and the last volume 2 years posthumously in 1993. By thoroughly studying a topic and consulting with experts to develop a detailed understanding before starting an illustration, Netter succeeded in depicting the essential relationships between anatomy, physiology, and pathology in a manner that cannot be captured with a photograph. This unique ability has made his anatomy texts a preferred reference for medical students to this day. Netter worked with opaque watercolors (gouache), progressing from dark to light. Eduard Pernkopf also produced a beautiful, even more detailed, atlas using watercolors, but his work was subsequently stigmatized by his probable use of cadavers obtained from Nazi concentration camps.

After a demonstration in the Great Exhibition at the Crystal Palace in 1851, stereoscopy became very popular as a form of entertainment, but it did not gain much traction in medicine at that time. One of the earliest stereoscopic medical publications was Albert Neisser's *Atlas of Stereoscopic Medicine*, published in 1894. Dr. Neisser, who was known for discovering the gonorrhea bacteria, compiled a collection of stereoscopic photographs of ophthalmology patients and specimens (Fig. 25-14). The use of stereoscopy to enhance the study of anatomy began at the turn of the century when atlases such as *The Edinburgh Stereoscopic Atlas of Anatomy* (1905) and Arthur Thompson's *The Anatomy of the Eye, as Illustrated by Enlarged Stereoscopic Photographs* (1912) were published. Both of these consisted of a collection of stereoscopic photographs of anatomic specimens accompanied by labeled diagrams. With the invention of Kodachrome film in 1935, color photography became much more practical. In 1948, David Bassett, an anatomist working at Stanford University, began to collaborate with William Gruber, who had invented a popular stereoscope called the View-Master. Gruber photographed Bassett's dissections in color, and they finally completed a stereoscopic atlas in 1962 that contained more than 1000 images formatted for the View-Master stereoscope (Fig. 25-15). The atlas can still be found in many medical school libraries. Nonetheless, perhaps because of logistic concerns, stereoscopic anatomy atlases have not been widely used as core teaching materials.

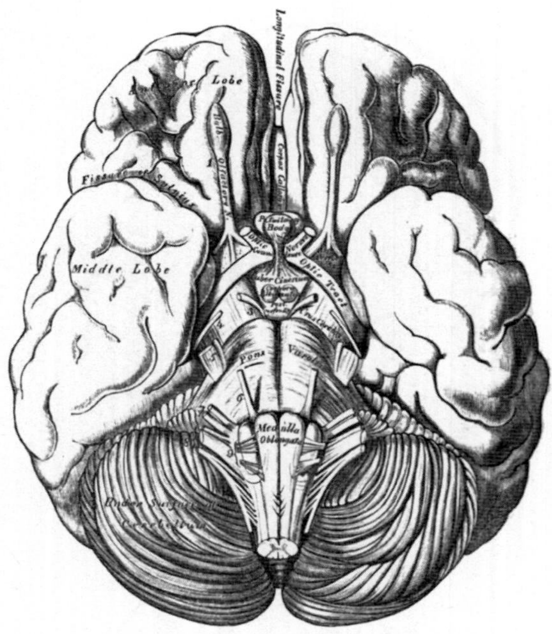

Figure 25-13. An illustration of the brain. *(From Gray H, Carter HV.* Anatomy, Descriptive and Surgical. *London: J. W. Parker, 1858.)*

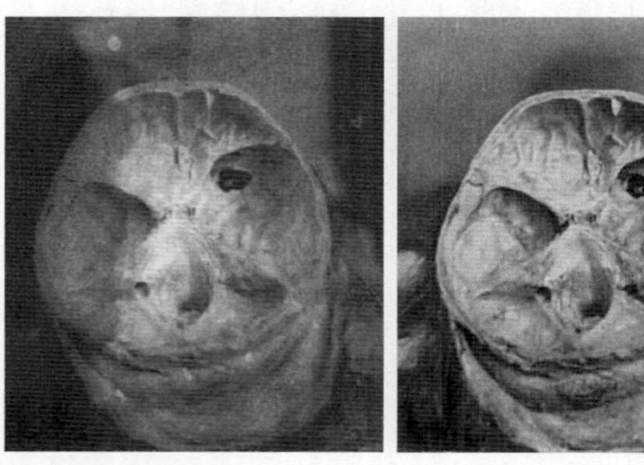

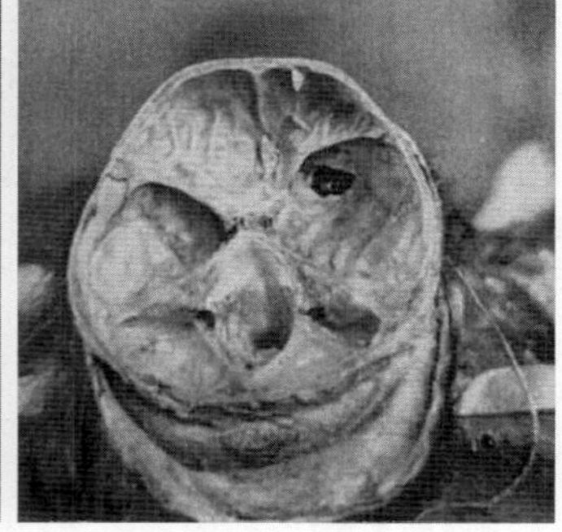

Figure 25-14. A stereoscopic photograph from Albert Neisser's book published in 1894. *(From Neisser AL.* Stereoskopischer Atlas. Sammlung photographischer Bilder aus dem Gesammtgebiet der klinischen Medizin, der Anatomie und der pathologischen Anatomie etc. *Fischer, Barth, Kassel and Leipzig, 1894.)*

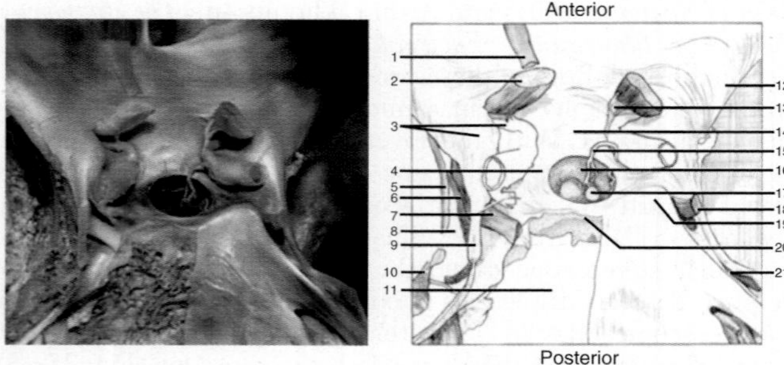

Figure 25-15. The sellar region as seen in Dr. Bassett's atlas. As with previous stereoscopic atlases, a labeled diagram was made for each image. *(Courtesy of the Lane Medical Library, Stanford University; http://lane.stanford.edu/med-history/index.html.)*

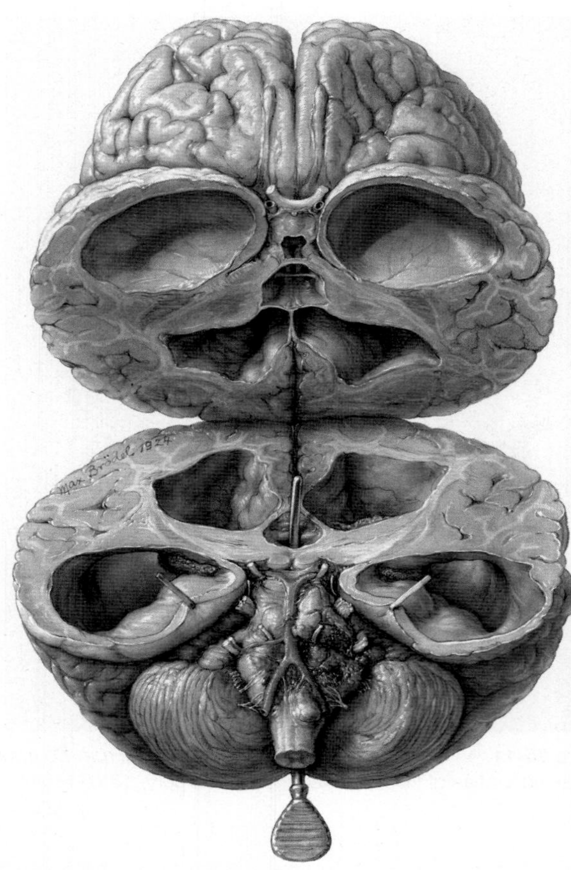

Figure 25-16. An example of the fine artistry of Max Brödel depicting hydrocephalus. Brödel worked with carbon pencil and dust, which produce an excellent chiaroscuro effect, Johns Hopkins 1924. *(Original art is No. 696 in the Walters Collection of the Max Brödel Archives in the Department of Art as Applied to Medicine, Johns Hopkins University School of Medicine, Baltimore, MD.)*

The Visual Record in Neurosurgery

> *In looking over our medical literature, one cannot help being disgusted by the inadequate character of the illustrations. I do not refer merely to artistic inefficiency, which is evident, but also to the scientific inefficiency. The remedy is simple enough, but its application is more difficult: 1. Teach the artist more medicine; 2. Teach the scientist more art."*
>
> **Max Brödel, 1907**

As medicine became increasingly subspecialized, general-purpose anatomy atlases were no longer sufficient. In the neurosurgical realm, Harvey Cushing fully embraced the role of art in communicating new knowledge and experience in his rapidly evolving field. He was also an avid collector of Vesalius' books and ultimately penned a biography of the renaissance anatomist that was published posthumously. Although Cushing often used photography, he recognized that illustrations could sometimes present the important points of anatomy and surgery more effectively.[20] He developed a fruitful collaboration with the medical artist Max Brödel, who had emigrated from Leipzig, where he had received a formal education in art and worked with the physiologist Carl Ludwig. After less than a decade at Johns Hopkins, Brödel started the first department of medical illustration and made significant contributions to several surgical fields (Fig. 25-16). Like Netter, he believed that it was necessary to carefully study his subjects before attempting to draw them, and that the artist's job was to help the viewer see what is important. Brödel carefully observed Cushing in the operating room, but like many medical artists before him, he also performed his own dissections. As a result, he was instrumental in helping to communicate Cushing's seminal work to the rest of the world. Brödel mentored Dorcas Hagar Padget, who went on to document the innovations of Walter Dandy, and Mildred Codding, who worked with Cushing after he moved to Boston. Cushing also learned much from Brödel, which helped him create his own illustrations after surgery. He would typically perform a rough sketch in the operating room with a pencil, and then later fill in the illustration with India ink in his office.[21]

In the early days of photography, there was no process to publish the images on paper. Therefore, early medical photographs had to be converted to woodcuts for publishing. The technology had matured considerably when Cushing practiced. He used photography extensively to document his operative cases, which were subsequently published in his books and archived in his brain tumor registry. Photographs of the patient taken before, during, and after their hospitalization, the tumor specimen, microscopic pathology, and drawings of the surgery were often grouped together into a montage and photographed once more as a summary of the case (Fig. 25-17). More than 10,000 5-inch × 7-inch glass plate negatives were found in Cushing's archives, which have recently been cataloged in his library at Yale. These visual records summarized a case better than a simple written report.

Microneurosurgical Anatomy

As the age of microneurosurgery unfolded in the 1960s, the operating microscope increased our capabilities in the anatomy laboratory as well in the operating room. Dr. Al Rhoton Jr. recognized a need to better understand the detailed anatomy seen through the operating microscope, so he embarked on a systematic study of microneurosurgical anatomy that would become the largest body of work of its kind. The guiding principle was that the dissections should increase understanding of anatomy enough to make neurosurgical operations more accurate and safe. He began performing dissections through the operating microscope that mimicked the view of a neurosurgical approach while revealing the relevant anatomy in much better detail than in an intraoperative view or typical cadaver prosection. As a neurosurgeon who also became an anatomist, he translated microsurgical techniques to the anatomy laboratory and also developed new techniques, resulting in dissections that were works of art tailored to the needs of neurosurgeons. His medium was primarily color photography, although he used illustrations when necessary. More than 100 neurosurgeons have traveled to Gainesville for a year or more of fellowship with Dr. Rhoton, during which they have made many original contributions to microneurosurgical anatomy. Several approaches, such as the telovelar and transchoroidal, were developed or refined in his laboratory. By 2003, Dr. Rhoton's laboratory had produced enough material to create a comprehensive microneurosurgical textbook. Published by the Congress of Neurological Surgeons, *Rhoton's Cranial Anatomy and Surgical Approaches* rapidly gained popularity (see Chapter 2).

In an effort to better reproduce the binocular view through the operating microscope, Dr. Rhoton and his fellow, Katsuta Toshiro, began making stereoscopic photographs in 1993 (Fig. 25-18). Soon after this, Dr. Rhoton began to give stereoscopic

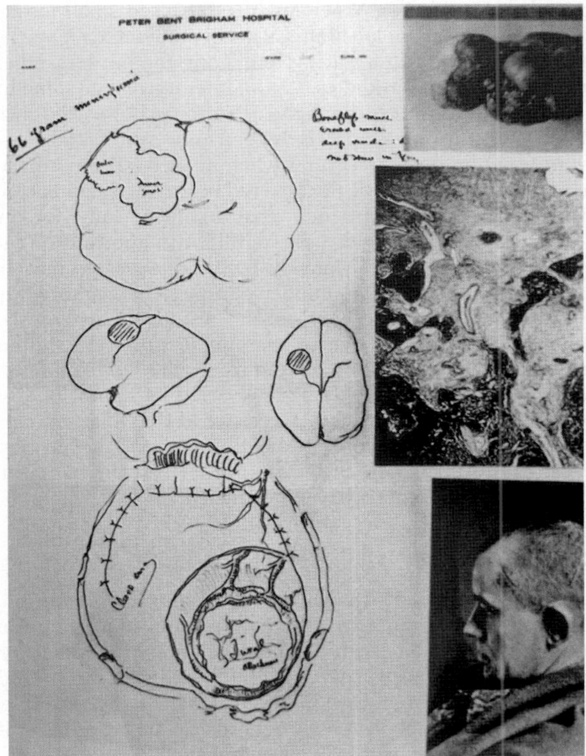

Figure 25-17. An operating room record of Harvey Cushing demonstrating a summary of a case with multiple images. *(Courtesy of the Cushing Center, Harvey Cushing/John Hay Whitney Medical Library, Yale University.)*

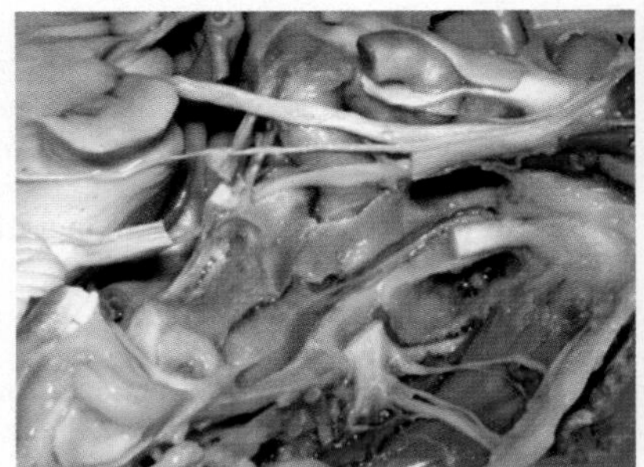
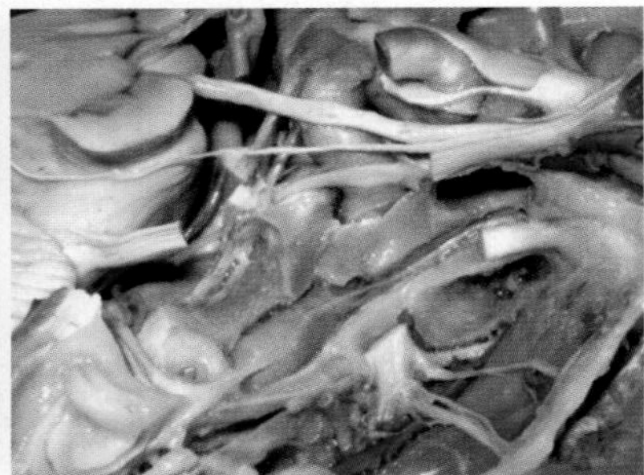

Figure 25-18. A stereoscopic photograph of the cavernous sinus region with the abducens nerve labeled with a color drawing, thereby avoiding the use of conventional labels that detract from the image. *(Courtesy of the Rhoton Collection, American Association of Neurological Surgeons [AANS]/Neurosurgical Research and Education Foundation [NREF].)*

anatomy lectures at courses and conferences using a dual-projector system with polarizing filters. The three-dimensional (3D) effect was very impressive and helped residents to better understand the complex anatomy of skull base approaches. His stereoscopic lectures were soon in high demand around the world, becoming a staple of cadaver skull base courses. As stereoscopic televisions became widely available in 2011, the Rhoton Collection was launched by the American Association of Neurological Surgeons to produce stereoscopic movies of Dr. Rhoton's lectures and to curate an online atlas containing his stereoscopic photographs that could be viewed on a wide range of devices. As with all previous anatomy atlases, labeling the anatomic structures presented a significant challenge, particularly for stereoscopic images. Since the Renaissance, anatomists such as Estienne have used lines, which made it easy to locate structures but also cluttered the image. Da Vinci and Vesalius used small letters to minimize the impact of labeling. Eustachi eliminated all markings on the images by using a grid system along the borders, labeling structures by their coordinates.[22] As an interactive digital medium, the Rhoton Collection adopted the use of superimposed drawings to define structures more precisely than conventional labels. The drawings highlight the structures when needed but are otherwise hidden, thus preserving the uncluttered beauty of the image. Such drawings have the added benefit that a student can click on an anatomic structure and cause the highlight to appear along with the name of the structure. Many thousands of drawings have been added to the Rhoton Collection to annotate the photographs. These drawings have also been used to produce the stereoscopic highlights in Dr. Rhoton's video anatomy lectures. Work is being done to allow the teaching materials in this collection to be dynamically formatted to suit a wide variety of educational situations ranging from a pocket reference on cellular phones to lectures using a stereoscopic projection system. By having the images readily available on all types of devices, their impact on neurosurgical education will be maximized.

Moving Pictures

The commoditization of video production and distribution on the Internet has significantly affected our ability to disseminate knowledge quickly. Neurosurgical journals and others such as the *New England Journal of Medicine* have adopted video as an important medium of communication because many concepts are conveyed better with video than with words or illustrations. This is particularly true for surgical procedures because the motions underlying technique cannot be fully understood with still images or a written account.

Louis Le Prince made the first film in 1887 using a movie camera of his own invention that involved 16 lenses performing exposures in rapid succession. The following year he developed a single-lens movie camera. After Le Prince's mysterious and untimely death, the Lumière brothers and Thomas Edison were influential in the early development of the film industry. Early movies were typically short and silent. Editing entailed the tedious process of cutting out unwanted segments of film with razors and rejoining it with adhesive tape. After 1927, films with audio tracks became widely available, and in 1931, a short documentary movie showing Harvey Cushing's 2000th brain tumor operation was produced with audio narration. Until recently, movie production of any kind had been expensive and labor intensive. It required a cumbersome film camera and dedicated professionals with special equipment for editing. In 1978, the senior author (JHR) began creating surgical movies through the operating microscope using 16-mm film. To document a single operation, an intraoperative cinematographer and multiple film reels were required. The film then had to be processed, cut, and spliced at a professional facility with an expensive hourly rate. The surgeon had to travel to the facility to supervise the editing sessions. Duplicates were expensive and accompanied by a loss of quality. Nonetheless, these movies had considerable impact at neurosurgical meetings because operative movies were still fairly rare.

During the 1980s, the prevalence of cameras and players using magnetic tape in cassettes, such as VCR, made filming and distribution more feasible, but editing was still a complex and expensive undertaking. Limited selections of neurosurgical videos were distributed on VCR cassettes.

In the 1990s, editing increasingly left the physical realm of razors and tape because computers could manipulate a lower quality digital copy of the original footage. These nonlinear editing (NLE) systems allowed users to jump directly to an arbitrary frame of a movie without having to mechanically roll film or tape. Because the editor was now working with digital proxy footage instead of the master tape, alternate versions could be easily cut and resequenced without worrying about damaging the master. When the editor was satisfied with the editing sequence, the software exported an "edit decision list" that was then used by a production facility to construct a master tape or film from the original footage. Introduced in 1989, the Avid NLE system ultimately revolutionized movie editing because it could be done with an Apple Macintosh desktop computer rather than the convoluted systems and mainframe computers that were previously used for NLE. Nonetheless, because it required expensive accessory hardware and remained tied to the production of a physical master tape as the final product, it was still not practical for nonprofessional users.

By the early 2000s, as digital video cameras and computers became more powerful, high-quality video production could be done entirely in the digital domain. Laptop computers ultimately became more capable than the multimillion-dollar editing suites of the 1980s. Digital cameras began to capture video at resolutions that rivaled 35-mm film. Moreover, the arrival of YouTube and other online video distribution services meant that a physical artifact was no longer required to publish a video. Thus, the traditional barriers to video production and distribution were finally eliminated. The only limitation that remains is the surgeon's time for editing.

Over the history of cinematography, 3D (stereoscopic) movies have typically been more of a novelty than a legitimate storytelling device, so widespread adoption has been slow. But for capturing the nuances of anatomy and surgery, 3D has clear benefits. In 2010, intraoperative 3D video acquisition became practical. At first, a dual-projection polarized system was used for monitoring and viewing before 3D televisions became widely available. Now, 3D surgical and anatomy videos have become popular for teaching conferences and national meetings, and most microscope manufacturers have begun to outfit microscopes with 3D video cameras. Even as public enthusiasm for 3D televisions and movies has waxed and waned, they have continued to thrive in the niche of surgical education.

Of course, education is not the only area that is enabled by high-definition and 3D video cameras. They will also enable surgeons to participate in operations without being physically present. As network bandwidth and robotic technology improve, the remote surgeon will move beyond an advisory role and become an active participant in operations anywhere in the world.

FUTURE DIRECTIONS

As in the past, improved visualization should accelerate understanding of the craft of neurosurgery at all levels. Our ability to visualize human anatomy and pathology will continue to grow in sophistication. As computing power increases, we will see the digital pathway supersede the optical pathway in the operating room. Further developments in noninvasive imaging modalities will enhance our ability to visualize derangements of the nervous system. 3D models of our patients' anatomy and proposed surgical approaches will be constructed and modified in real time. Virtual dissection and virtual surgery will become a valuable teaching tool as simulation software becomes more realistic. These simulations, together with vast online video libraries at our fingertips that contain every known variation of surgical technique, pathology, and complication, will allow neurosurgeons all over the world to climb their learning curves more quickly.

SUGGESTED READINGS

Black P, Moore MR, Rossitch E. *Harvey Cushing at the Brigham*. Stuttgart: Thieme/AANS; 1993.

Choulant L. *History and Bibliography of Anatomic Illustration*. Chicago: The University of Chicago Press; 1920.

Schulze F. How the humble stereomicroscope found its way into modern surgery: the Zeiss operating microscope. *Micscape Magazine*. 2012;1-20. <www.microscopy-uk.org.uk/mag/artdec12/fs-Zeiss-Operating-Microscopes-1.pdf>.

Schutt CA, Redding B, Cao H, et al. The illumination characteristics of operative microscopes. *Am J Otolaryngol*. 2015;36:356-360.

Udelsman R. Presidential Address: Harvey Cushing: The artist. *Surgery*. 2006;140(6):841-846.

Uluc K, Kujoth GC, Baskaya MK. Operating microscopes: past, present, and future. *Neurosurg Focus*. 2009;27(3):E4.

See a full reference list on ExpertConsult.com 

26 Advantages and Limitations of Cranial Endoscopy

Jeroen R. Coppens, James K. Liu, and William T. Couldwell

Endoscopy was first used intracranially in the treatment of hydrocephalus at the beginning of the 20th century. Since then, each new technological development has broadened interest in cranial endoscopy. The endoscope's latest renaissance has expanded its use for accessing skull base lesions via the extended endonasal approaches that involve novel reconstruction techniques using vascularized pedicled nasoseptal flaps for closure. The endoscope has proved its utility in cranial surgery and has given neurosurgeons more adaptability because it can be used alone or in combination with other open or microscopic techniques. Current indications for the use of intracranial endoscopy are reviewed, along with the limitations still encountered with the use of an endoscopic technique versus a microsurgical technique.

HISTORY OF ENDOSCOPY

The earliest use of the endoscope intracranially was reported by Victor D. Lespinasse in 1910 for the treatment of hydrocephalus.[1] Dandy[2] used the technique more extensively and became known as the father of neuroendoscopy. Interest in cranial endoscopy was driven by the lack of alternative treatments for hydrocephalus in the first half of the 20th century. Endoscopic techniques evolved from fulguration or obliteration of the choroid plexus to fenestration techniques involving the ventricles and subarachnoid planes. The first endoscopic third ventriculostomy was reported by Mixter in 1923.[3] Limited development in the technology for endoscopes, in combination with the placement of the first shunt with a valve by Nulsen and Spitz[4] in 1949, decreased the interest in cranial endoscopy until the advent of rod-lens endoscopes in 1960.[5] Better illumination and resolution of the image enabled the application of the endoscope in the context of cranial neurosurgery.

Gerard Guiot, a pioneer in intracranial and skull base endoscopy, performed the first endoscopic approach to a pituitary tumor in 1962,[6] although he later abandoned the technique because it provided inadequate visualization.[7-9] In 1973, Fukushima and colleagues[10] introduced the modern endoscope, which could be used for the biopsy of intraventricular lesions, cyst fenestration, and treatment of hydrocephalus. The use of the endoscope in transsphenoidal approaches was introduced by Guiot.[8,9] Bushe and Halves[11] were the first to report the use of a modern endoscope in pituitary surgery, in 1978. A few other reports emerged in the 1970s describing the use of an endoscope as an adjunct to the microscope in transsphenoidal approaches.[11-13] Application of the endoscope to the sella turcica did not become popular until the mid-1990s, when endoscopic sinus surgery had virtually replaced open techniques in use by otolaryngologists.[9,14] Modern endoscopic cranial surgery developed from the growth in popularity of minimally invasive surgery through keyhole approaches[15,16] in combination with the development of purely endoscopic endonasal approaches to the skull base, which led to functional endoscopic pituitary surgery.[17]

ENDOSCOPIC INSTRUMENTATION AND GENERAL PRINCIPLES

Endoscopes are generally classified as either rod-lens endoscopes or fiberoptic endoscopes (fiberscopes), according to the technology used. Rod-lens endoscopes transmit images through a series of lenses and are always rigid. They provide a clearer image and better illumination than do fiberscopes. Fiberscopes transmit images through fiberoptic threads and can be maneuvered without image distortion. The resolution of fiberscopes is proportional to the number of fibers in the endoscope. Because of the nature of optic fibers, which may be flexed without breaking, fiberscopes can be fixed or flexible. However, rigid fiberscopes allow the presence of more pixel fibers than do flexible or steerable fiberscopes.

Flexible fiberscopes have the smallest diameter, and one can be used as a stylet within a ventricular catheter. They do not have a working channel but are appropriate for visualizing catheter placement and ensuring an intraventricular position. They have not been shown to improve the surgical outcome in hydrocephalus, inasmuch as no specific location of catheter placement has been demonstrated to be superior.[18,19]

With a steerable fiberscope, the tip of the endoscope can be bent in varying degrees. A working channel is present, and its orientation is adjustable, which enables the instruments to reach all of the structures visualized. The diameter of the fiberscope varies with the number of optic fibers; the larger fiberscopes provide better image quality.

Rigid fiberscopes are available in a variety of lengths and diameters. A working channel is present, but targets can be used only on a straight line from the burr hole. The quality of vision remains inferior to that of rod-lens endoscopes.

Rod-lens endoscopes are used overwhelmingly in cranial endoscopy because of the superior quality of the image obtained. They are heavier because of the mandatory attachment of the camera and fiberoptic cable for the light source. Assorted viewing angles are available (e.g., 0-, 30-, 70-, and 120-degree angled endoscopes; Fig. 26-1). Certain types of rod-lens endoscopes have up to two working channels, through which instrumentation can be used. These working channels can also be used in addition to a trocar sheath, which enables the surgeon to use endoscopes with different viewing angles without the need to reinsert them through brain tissue. Different sheaths are available with one to multiple channels for inserting instruments, providing irrigation, or supplying suction.[20] Instrumentation in the forms of varying forceps, scissors, suction, or coagulation has been developed. The 0- and 30-degree endoscopes are the most widely used. The 0-degree endoscope minimizes the risk of disorientation, but the view through instruments inserted through the working channel remain in the periphery of the field of vision.[19] The 30-degree endoscope allows for a better control of the instruments and, with simple rotation, provides an angle of view with a surface area twice as large as that provided by a 0-degree endoscope.

The optimal use of the endoscope requires the use of a light source combined with a camera and monitor. Halogen, mercury vapor, and xenon light sources are available. The light source is connected to the endoscope via a fiberoptic cable, and its intensity can be modulated. Xenon light sources provide the best illumination for neuroendoscopy.[19] The camera is connected to the endoscope via an adapter and transmits the image to a video monitor for viewing by the rest of the surgical team. Cameras are available as a single-chip charged coupled device (CCD) or a three-chip CCD. Most systems use a single-chip CCD because of its lower cost and lighter weight, despite a lower quality image.[19] A monitor with the highest possible quality should be selected, but its resolution should not exceed that of the camera. The size of the screen should not be excessive, as a larger screen

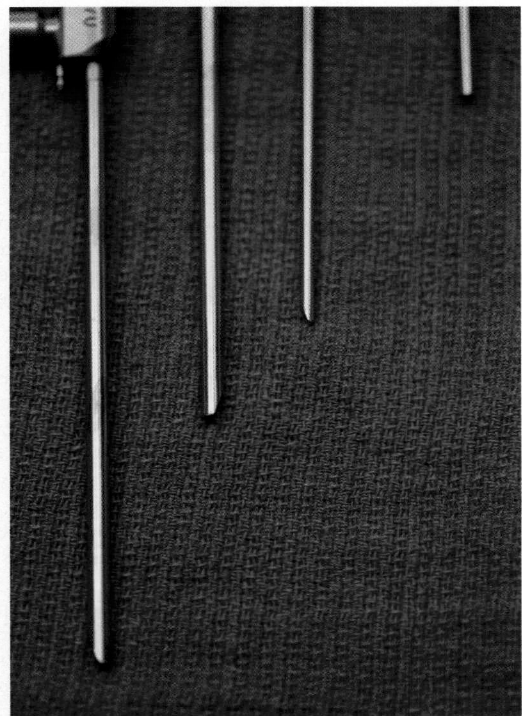

Figure 26-1. Rod-lens endoscopes are available with 0-degree or other viewing angles.

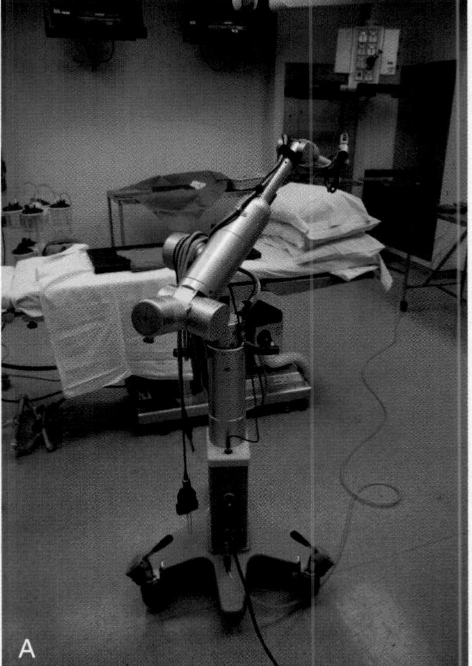

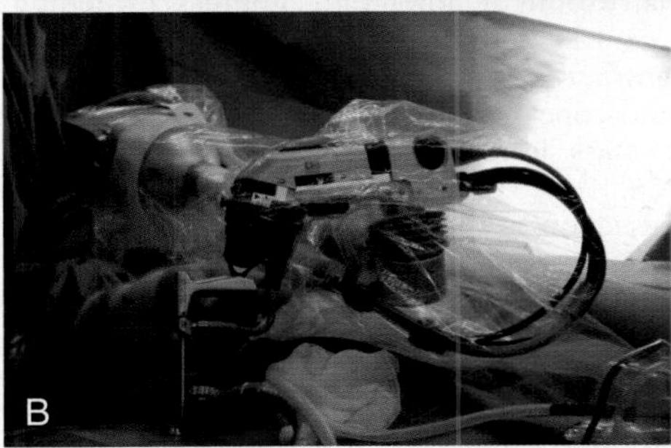

Figure 26-2. A, Olympus EndoArm (Olympus, Melville, NY), a pneumatic endoscope holder. **B,** Olympus EndoArm holding a rod-lens endoscope during surgery.

limits the quality of the image obtained. The loss of quality of the image is most pronounced in screens exceeding 13 inches (33 cm) and when a fiberscope is used.[19] Irrigation is useful in optimizing visualization and should be used in avoiding entrapment of fluid. Lactate Ringer's solution is the substance of choice for irrigation.[21]

Rigid endoscope holders may increase the surgeon's comfort during lengthy procedures, but they restrict the surgeon's freedom of movement. Holders have been developed with a combination of pneumatic and electromagnetic brakes, combining the advantages of freehand movements with the possibility of very secure and firm positioning.[22,23] Most endoscope holders need continuous manual adjustment at each of their joints, which limits their usefulness. They are usually mounted directly to the side of the operating room table, which limits the endoscope's range of movement. We have used the Olympus EndoArm (Olympus, Southend-on-Sea, U.K.), a pneumatic endoscope holder mounted on its own base, extensively (Fig. 26-2). The EndoArm consists of an arm with several ball-and-socket joints that enable movement in all planes. Movement of the joints in either direction is controlled by a single button, which gives the surgeon more fluidity in moving the endoscope.[24]

Endoscopy and Hydrocephalus

Cranial endoscopy was first used in the setting of hydrocephalus before the advent of shunt systems, when the condition was commonly fatal. Interest in the use of endoscopy has resumed because of the high rate of long-term morbidity associated with the use of shunts, most commonly shunt malfunctions and infections. In some cases, to avoid placement of a shunt system, the endoscope can be used to perform a third ventriculostomy or an obliteration of the choroid plexus. Third ventriculostomy has become an important part of the treatment of hydrocephalus, and its long-term success has varied greatly, depending on the cause of hydrocephalus. Most long-term studies cite success rates of 65% to 75% for third ventriculostomies in the treatment of hydrocephalus.[25-42]

The endoscope can also be used as an adjunct to a diversion shunt technique when a fiberscope is placed into the ventricular catheter. Adequate placement of the ventricular catheter into the ventricular system is confirmed intraoperatively. Its cost-effectiveness remains questionable, but the technique can be useful in some situations. The endoscope has also been used extensively in cases of multiloculated hydrocephalus to lower the high rates of shunt infections and revisions needed in the setting of multiple shunts.[43-45] The goal of endoscopic surgery in multiloculated hydrocephalus should be to convert the condition to uniloculated hydrocephalus that necessitates one or no shunts.[43,46] Fenestration of the septum pellucidum with the use of an endoscope may be performed to treat an isolated lateral ventricle[47,48]; in some cases, fenestration of multiple intraventricular membranes may be required,[43,46] as may aqueductoplasty or stent placement in cases of fourth ventricular outlet obstruction.[49,50]

Image guidance is helpful in keeping the surgeon oriented, and a third ventriculostomy can be performed in the same setting if the hydrocephalus is thought to be obstructive. Endoscopic control enables placement of the catheter in an optimal location, and control rates of 62% to 100% can be accomplished in loculated hydrocephalus with one or no shunt.[43,44,46,51]

Endoscopy and Tumor Resection

Gross tumor resection has been accomplished endoscopically for intraventricular tumors. Factors favorable for complete tumor resection include a soft tumor consistency, tumor diameter of less than 2 cm, moderate to low vascularity, associated hydrocephalus, histologically low-grade tumor, and tumor location in the third or lateral ventricle.[52] Tumor resection can be time consuming as it is performed in a piecemeal manner through the endoscope's working channel,[21] which in most endoscopes is limited to 2.4 mm. Complete tumor resections have been described most commonly in cases of colloid cysts.[53-57] Colloid cysts are successfully treated in 60% to 90% of cases,[52,53,57-70] and such treatment seems to carry lower morbidity rates than does open craniotomy[58-60]; however, in few endoscopic series have researchers reported any long-term follow-up past 5 years.[66] One meta-analysis showed that endoscopic resection of colloid cysts had a higher rate of incomplete resection, cyst recurrence, and reoperation than did microsurgical resection.[71] This may be because bimanual microdissection of the cyst wall from the choroid plexus attachment and internal cerebral vein cannot be achieved with the endoscopic technique. Other tumors that have been described as suitable for successful endoscopic resection have included subependymal giant cell astrocytoma, exophytic low-grade gliomas extending into the ventricles, central neurocytoma, small choroid plexus tumors, and intraventricular craniopharyngiomas.[33,52,54,72-75]

The endoscope can be used effectively in treating intraventricular mass lesions, especially when they cause hydrocephalus.[33-35,42,54,76-79] A prime example of the role of an endoscope in tumor resection is the treatment of pineal tumors. In these tumors, the endoscope can be used to obtain samples of cerebrospinal fluid (CSF) for tumor markers and cytologic study, to inspect the intraventricular cavities to detect gross intraventricular nodules not visible on magnetic resonance imaging, to obtain a biopsy specimen of the tumor, and to perform a third ventriculostomy to address the hydrocephalus. Good results in controlling hydrocephalus have been obtained.[34,80,81] Advantages of the endoscopic approach over a stereotactic needle biopsy include direct visualization of the tumor, a larger biopsy specimen, and the ability to stop the bleeding.[52]

Endoscopy can also be used as a palliative measure to treat the cystic components of certain inoperable tumors and to implant an Ommaya reservoir in locations more remote from the ventricular system.[75]

Endoscopy and Arachnoid Cysts

Endoscopy can be used to successfully treat symptomatic arachnoid cysts. Endoscopic fenestration of the cyst into the subarachnoid or intraventricular system enables the procedure to be performed through a smaller opening than is necessary with a craniotomy and obviates the need for shunt placement, which in turn prevents shunt-associated morbidity. Optimal candidates for endoscopic fenestration should have an area of continuity between the cyst wall and the ependyma or subarachnoid spaces. A large opening into the cyst wall should be created to prevent reclosure of the stoma. Symptoms can be relieved in patients with stable cyst sizes without the need for other procedures in 71% to 81% of cases.[54,75,82-84] Fenestration of the cyst in conjunction with hydrocephalus increases the ease of the procedure and enables the surgeon to perform a concomitant third ventriculostomy.[31,75,82,83,85] For arachnoid cysts of the middle fossa, fenestration into the basal cisterns is possible, but it carries some risk to the vessels of the sylvian fissure; these cysts may be best approached through a microsurgical technique.

Endoscopy and the Skull Base

The endoscope has increasingly been used in skull base surgery since the 1970s.[9,11-14] First introduced in 1978 by Bushe and Halves,[11] the endoscope was used to better visualize and reach the suprasellar extension of sellar lesions.[86-93] The speculum used in the microscopic transsphenoidal approaches limits the working space of the endoscope and other instruments, especially when the surgeon must reach far superiorly, laterally, or posteriorly into the suprasellar space.[86-91,93-96] In addition, the distal aperture of the speculum opening often limits the view through the bony sphenoid and sellar opening, and the blades of the speculum can limit the surgical freedom.

Several variations involving the use of the endoscope in transsphenoidal surgery have been reported. The endoscope has been used to make the initial approach in the sphenoid sinus, and the nasal morbidity with this approach is decreased.[97] For example, the sphenoidal approach is performed with an endoscopic rhinologic technique, and the tumor removal is performed with a standard microsurgical speculum-based transsphenoidal technique. Alternatively, the endoscope can be used for intraoperative inspection of the resection cavity after the tumor has been removed through a microsurgical approach.

The purely endoscopic endonasal transsphenoidal approach has become increasingly popular as an alternative to the microscopic techniques because it obviates the use of a nasal speculum.[17,89,98-104] This approach involves a two-surgeon (usually a neurosurgeon and an otolaryngologist), three- to four-hand technique through both nostrils (binostril approach). For treatment of pituitary tumors via the transsellar corridor, the key is to perform a maximal sphenoidotomy and posterior ethmoidectomy, as well as to create wide sellar bone opening from cavernous sinus to cavernous sinus in the lateral direction and from circular sinus to circular sinus in the vertical direction (Figs. 26-3 and 26-4). The expanded endoscopic endonasal approach can also be applied to other ventral corridors of the skull base in the sagittal plane, including the transcribriform corridor for sinonasal malignancies and olfactory groove meningiomas, the transplanum transtuberculum corridor for suprasellar craniopharyngiomas and tuberculum meningiomas, the transclival corridor for clivus chordomas and chondrosarcomas, and the transodontoid corridor for rheumatoid pannus and basilar invagination (Figs. 26-5 and 26-6).[105-109] More advanced endoscopic techniques involve treating ventral skull base lesions in the coronal plane that occupy the cavernous sinus, Meckel's cave, pterygopalatine fossa, petrous apex, infratemporal fossa, and middle fossa (Figs. 26-7 and 26-8).[110-114]

Among the advantages of the endoscopic over the microscopic technique when used in transsphenoidal approaches are a panoramic view with better illumination.[115,116] The addition of the endoscope consistently increases the area of visualization of the sellar and parasellar areas in a transethmoidal, transcolumellar, or sublabial approach, in comparison with the corresponding microscopic approach (Box 26-1; Fig. 26-9).[115] In the microscopic approaches, the advantage of the sublabial approach over the transcolumellar approach—which, in turn, improves on the transethmoidal approach—is a better anterior and superior view to address the suprasellar area.[117] The endoscope offers wider visualization in all axes, with a maximum benefit in the superior and anterior aspects (Fig. 26-10). Of note, a larger volume of visualization has been reported with an endoscopic transcolumellar approach than with a microscopic sublabial microscopic approach (see Box 26-1). Better detail in the image can be obtained with an endoscope than with a microscope because the camera source is closer to the structures of interest. Visualization in the microscopic technique is restricted by the "fixed tunnel" views offered through the openings of the nasal speculum. The microinstruments have to be used in a coaxial manner, and their

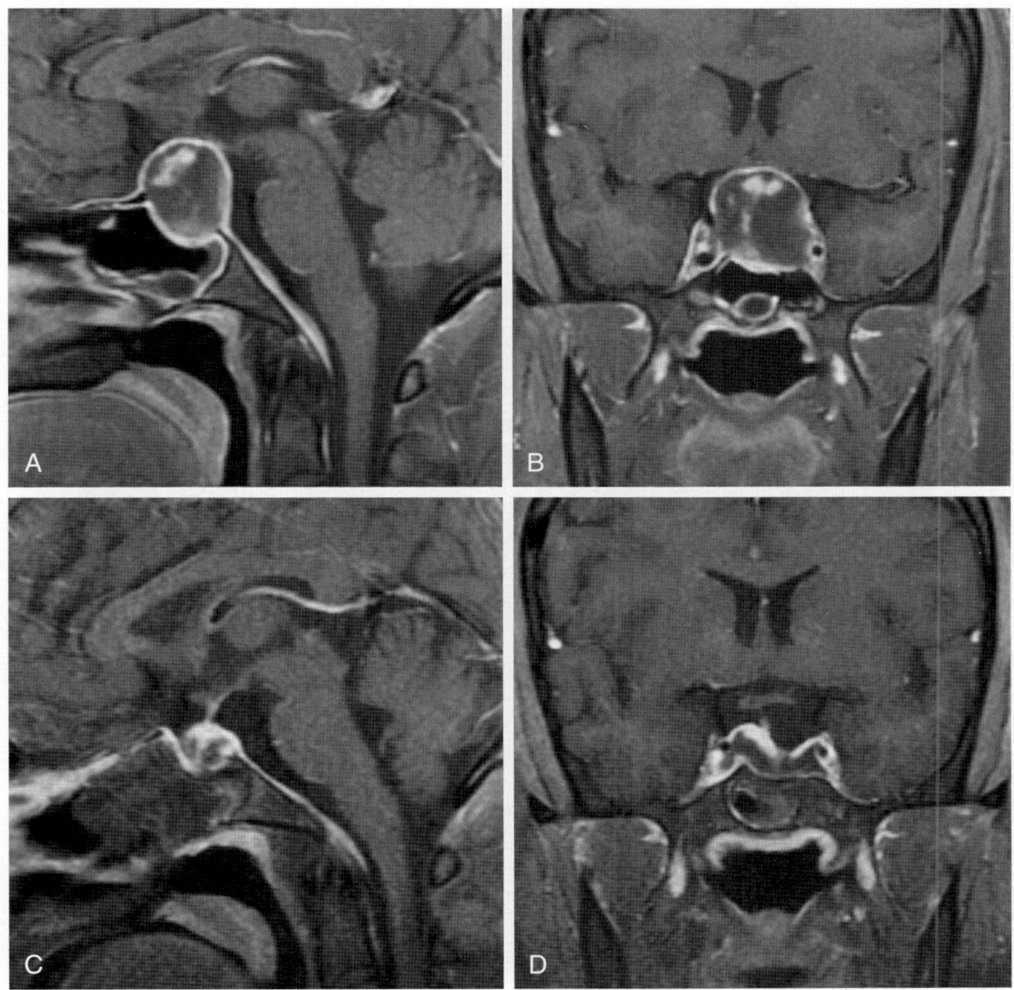

Figure 26-3. Magnetic resonance images in a patient who presented with visual loss caused by a hemorrhagic pituitary tumor. A, Preoperative sagittal view. **B,** Preoperative coronal view. **C,** Postoperative sagittal view. **D,** Postoperative coronal view. The postoperative views show complete tumor resection with decompression of the optic chiasm and preservation of the pituitary stalk after surgery with an endoscopic endonasal transsphenoidal approach.

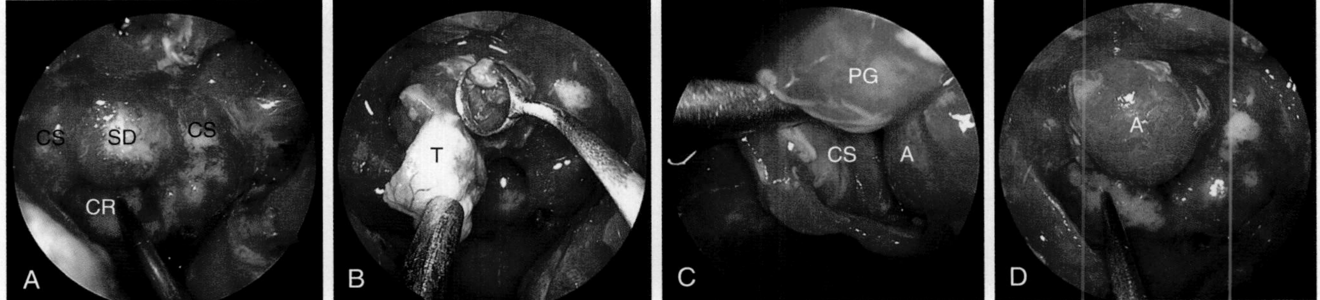

Figure 26-4. Intraoperative photographs of patient in Figure 26-3 during endoscopic endonasal transsphenoidal resection of pituitary adenoma. A, Panoramic view of the sellar dura (SD), both cavernous sinuses (CS) covered by bone, and the clival recess (CR). **B,** After the sellar dura is opened, the tumor (T) is removed with ring curettes. **C,** A 30-degree angled endoscope aimed toward the right side is used to visualize the right medial wall of the cavernous sinus (CS). The normal pituitary gland (PG) and arachnoid (A) membrane are visualized. **D,** The suprasellar arachnoid (A) membrane has descended into the sellar cavity, which signifies a meaningful decompression of the optic chiasm.

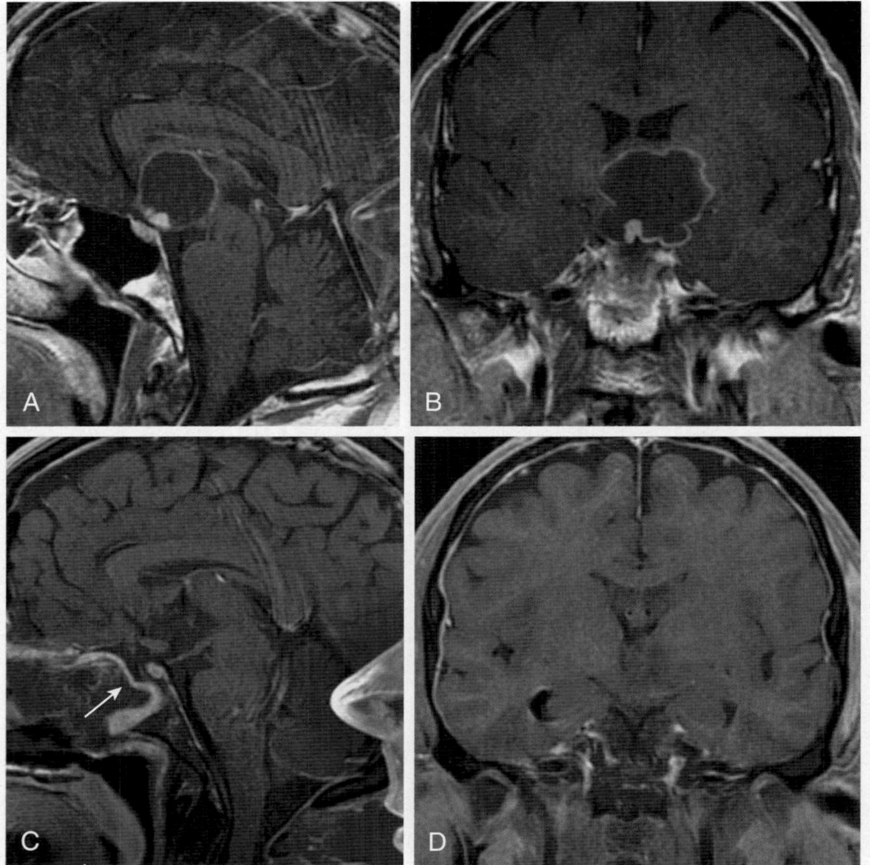

Figure 26-5. Magnetic resonance images in a patient who presented with visual loss caused by a retrochiasmatic suprasellar craniopharyngioma. A, Preoperative sagittal view. **B,** Preoperative coronal view. **C,** Postoperative sagittal view. **D,** Postoperative coronal view. The postoperative views show complete tumor resection after surgery with an extended endoscopic endonasal transsphenoidal approach via the transplanum transtuberculum corridor. The skull base defect was reconstructed with a vascularized pedicled nasoseptal flap (**C,** *white arrow*).

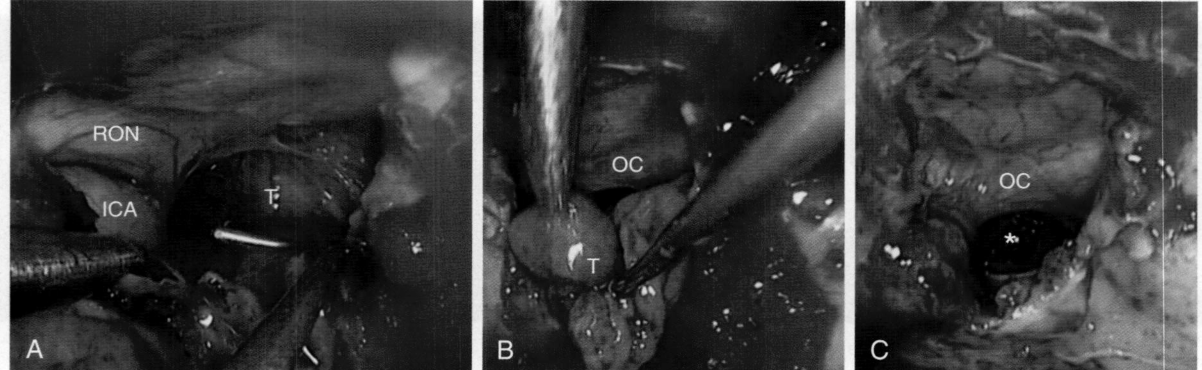

Figure 26-6. Intraoperative photographs of patient in Figure 26-5 during endoscopic endonasal resection of a craniopharyngioma. A, Exposure of the suprasellar contents, including the tumor (T), right optic nerve (RON), and right internal carotid artery (ICA), in the transplanum transtuberculum corridor. **B,** Two-handed microdissection is performed to remove the tumor (T) away from the optic chiasm (OC). **C,** Complete tumor removal and decompression of the optic chiasm (OC). The resection bed *(asterisk)* is devoid of any residual tumor.

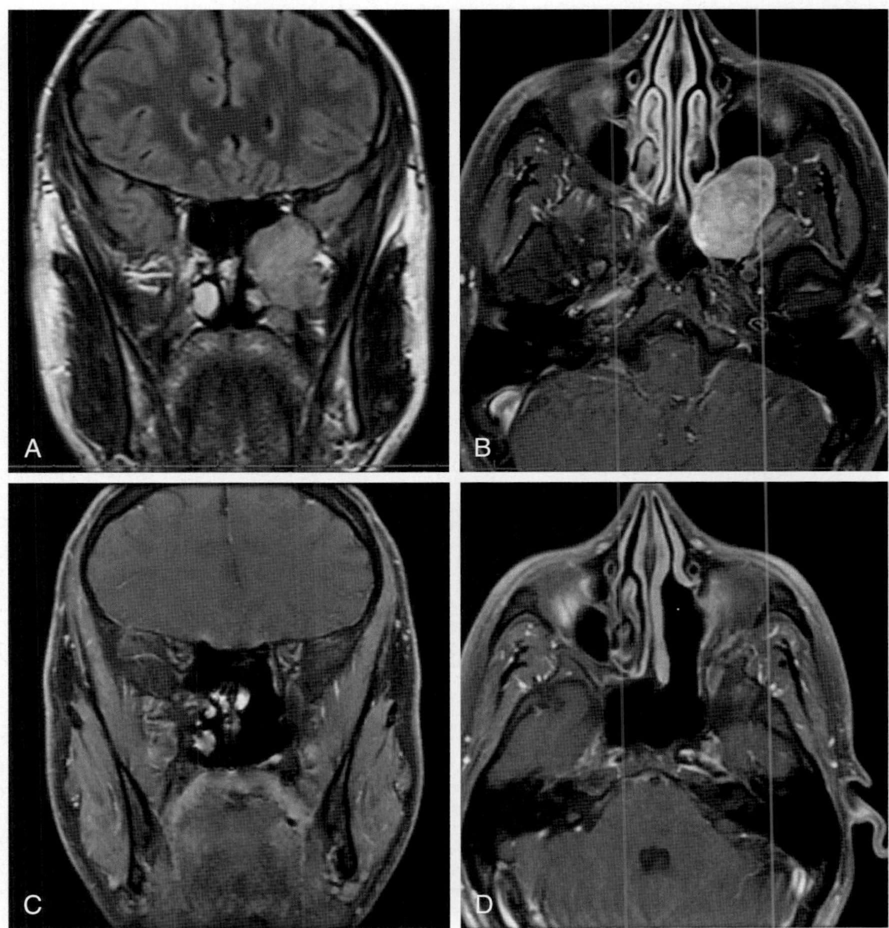

Figure 26-7. Magnetic resonance images in a patient who presented with epistaxis caused by a schwannoma of the left infratemporal fossa. A, Preoperative coronal view. **B,** Preoperative axial view. **C,** Postoperative coronal view. **D,** Postoperative axial view. The postoperative views show complete tumor resection after surgery with an endoscopic endonasal transpterygoid approach.

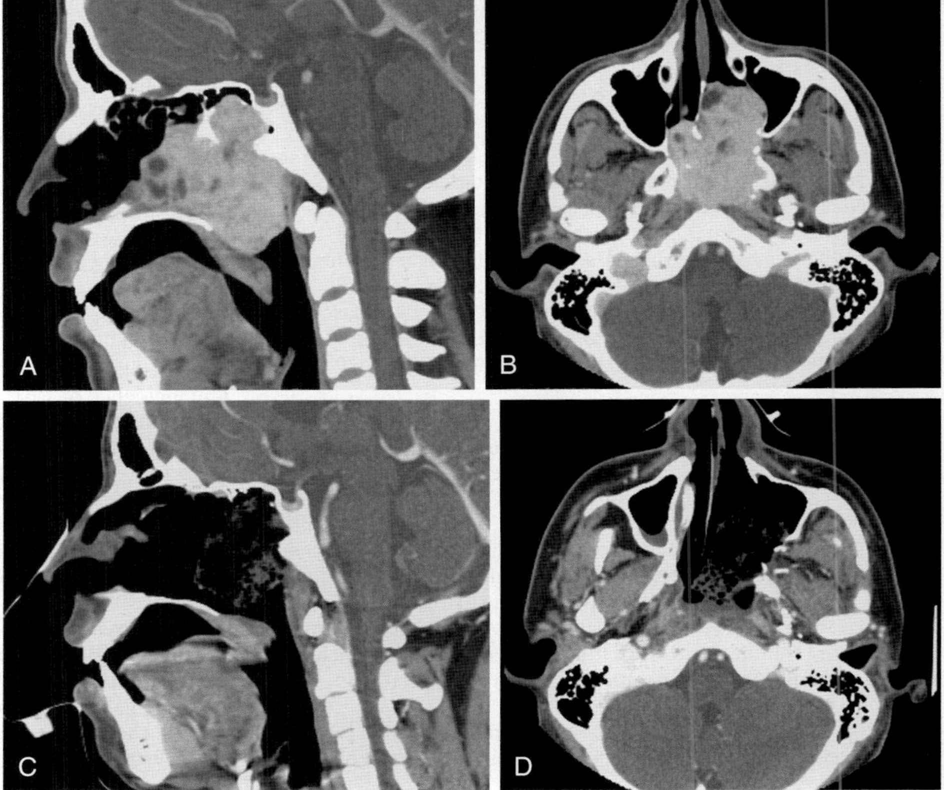

Figure 26-8. Computed tomographic angiograms in a patient who presented with epistaxis caused by a juvenile nasopharyngeal angiofibroma involving the nasal cavity, sphenoid sinus, and left pterygopalatine fossa. A, Preoperative sagittal view. **B,** Preoperative axial view. **C,** Postoperative sagittal view. **D,** Postoperative axial view. The postoperative views show complete tumor resection after surgery with an endoscopic endonasal transpterygoid approach.

BOX 26-1 Advantages and Disadvantages of the Endoscope

ADVANTAGES

Wide-angle view
Visualization at the site of surgery
Ability to look around corners with angled endoscopes
Increased area of visualization at the site of surgery

DISADVANTAGES

Lack of binocular vision with current technology
Occupying space in surgical corridor
Necessity of assistant or holder for endoscope to perform bimanual surgery
Lack of instrumentation to work through operative channel

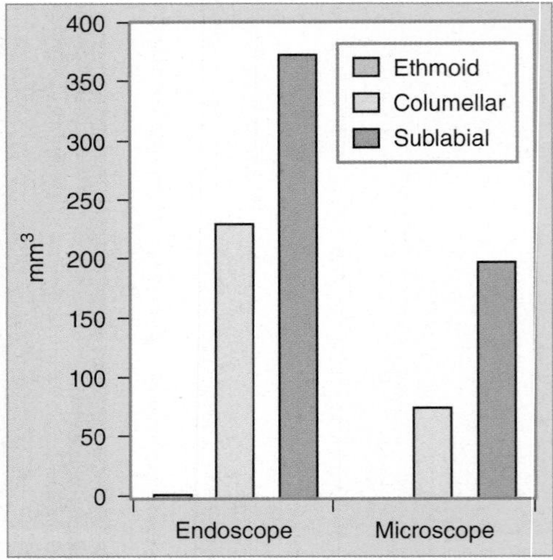

Figure 26-10. Histogram demonstrating the volume of exposure available through endoscopic and microscopic ethmoidal, columellar, and sublabial approaches. *(From Spencer WR, Das K, Nwagu C, et al. Approaches to the sellar and parasellar region: anatomic comparison of the microscope versus endoscope.* Laryngoscope. *1999;109:791-794.)*

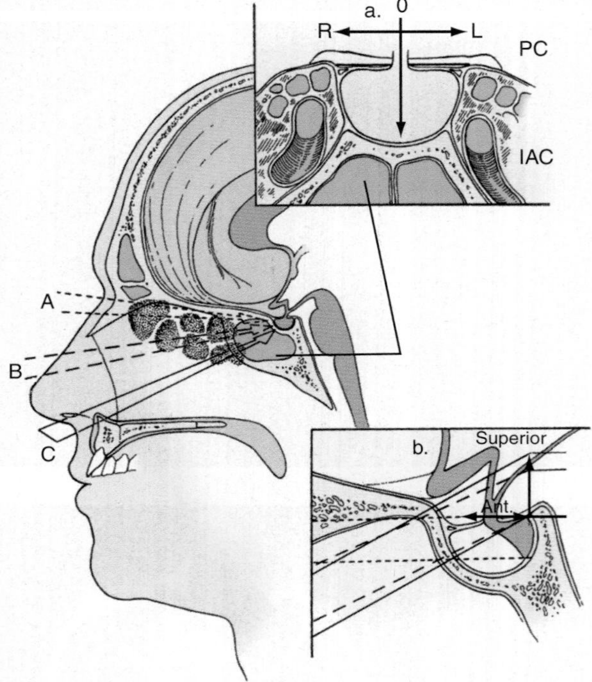

Figure 26-9. Schematic representation of the different approaches to the sellar and parasellar region. Illustrated are the transethmoidal approach (A), the transcolumellar transsphenoidal approach (B), and the sublabial transsphenoidal approach (C). Ant, anterior; IAC, internal auditory canal; L, left; PC, posterior clinoid; R, right. *(From Spencer WR, Das K, Nwagu C, et al. Approaches to the sellar and parasellar region: anatomic comparison of the microscope versus endoscope.* Laryngoscope. *1999;109:791-794.)*

reach is limited by the nasal speculum. In an anatomic study, the endoscopic binostril technique provided greater angular surgical freedom in the axial and sagittal directions than did the microscopic endonasal technique.[118] Of interest, when the sublabial incision was used for the microscopic technique, the surgical freedom was greater than with the endoscopic binostril technique in only the axial plane, not the sagittal plane. Although the sublabial exposure provides a wider surgical corridor, the risks may include more trauma to the nasal mucosa,[119] and vigorous opening of the speculum may cause optic nerve damage, facial pain, and swelling.[120]

A disadvantage of the endoscopic technique is the lack of depth perception in comparison with the binocular stereoscopic vision of the microscope. The endoscope's image is also distorted, with maximal magnification at its center and contraction at the periphery (a barrel effect of a wide-angle lens). This results in less accuracy of movements when the surgeon is learning to use the endoscope. Although this limitation is overcome with experience, the execution of the surgery by an inexperienced surgeon is slower than that when an experienced surgeon uses the microscope.[121] Continuous dynamic (in-and-out) movement of the endoscope can accommodate for the barrel effect and lack of depth perception.[115] Another operative tip to help the surgeon perceive depth is to palpate the anatomic landmarks that provide tactile feedback, such as placing the suction on the bone at the clival recess. In addition, the development of three-dimensional endoscopes has helped surgeons achieve better depth perception in endoscopic endonasal procedures; however, the images with three-dimensional endoscopes do not appear to have the same clarity and color representation as those with standard two-dimensional high-definition systems.

The initial use of the endoscope in transsphenoidal approaches to the sella was quickly expanded to address other midline lesions of the skull base because of their endonasal accessibility.[114,122-137] The initial experience with these procedures was criticized because of high rates of postoperative CSF leaks, which remain the biggest limitation of the use of an endonasal technique in comparison with other transcranial neurosurgical approaches.[96,135] The incidence of CSF leaks varies greatly with the nature of the condition treated and the degree of disruption of the arachnoid or ventricular system involved[135]; however, the incidence of postoperative CSF leakage has decreased dramatically to less than 5% with the advent of the vascularized pedicled nasoseptal flap.[138-141] It is important to use the nasoseptal flap as part of a multilayered reconstruction and to ensure that the flap makes direct contact with the bony defect, devoid of mucosal tissue, to promote graft adherence.

The increasing familiarity of neurosurgeons with endoscopes, combined with the use of angled endoscopes and more refined endonasal approaches, has extended access to the skull base from the crista galli to the upper cervical vertebrae.[142,143] Lateral extension of the approaches has also been accomplished to access the cavernous sinus,[144,145] Meckel's cave, the petrous apex, and the middle, posterior, and infratemporal fossae. The different pathologic conditions approached through an endoscopic technique to the skull base have expanded from tumor resections to the treatment of vascular lesions in selected cases.[146] Use of a three- or four-hand technique in the working space through both nostrils of the patient has been essential in accessing and treating lesions in some of these locations. Two surgeons can work simultaneously, and the working space between the endoscope and instruments is optimized.[147] All endoscopic approaches performed through both nostrils offer the surgeon better maneuverability of the instruments.[142] The surgeon is then always able to access the lesion through the contralateral nostril, which provides a more lateral reach to the lesion.[116] The use of a binostril approach may require an additional mucosal incision for endonasal approaches to access lesions anterior to the upper clivus. Lesions in the inferior part of the clivus or at the craniocervical junction can be accessed through an endonasal transchoanal approach.[142] If a continuous view is desired from the sellar area to the craniocervical junction, a binostril approach with bilateral mucosal incisions is preferable.[148]

Endonasal endoscopic approaches are not just an alternative to the microscopic transsphenoidal or extended transsphenoidal approaches. An endonasal endoscopic approach can replace transoral approaches to the odontoid and craniovertebral junction and can spare the splitting of the soft palate.[148] It can also replace the need for some craniotomy skull base approaches, such as those for some retrochiasmatic craniopharyngiomas, smaller meningiomas in the tuberculum and olfactory groove, esthesioneuroblastomas, and juvenile nasopharyngeal angiofibromas.

Increased familiarity with endonasal endoscopic approaches to the skull base has helped expand the role of the endoscope in treating craniofacial disease, which has minimized the need for disfiguring facial incisions or extensive facial osteotomies. Transsphenoidal endoscopic and transmaxillary endoscopic approaches can be combined with a bifrontal transbasal or frontotemporal craniotomy. A frontotemporal approach can be used to explore the middle fossa, pterygopalatine fossa, sella turcica, and cavernous sinus. A bifrontal transbasal approach can be used to access lesions involving the frontal, ethmoid, and sphenoid sinuses all the way to the cervical-clival junction inferiorly. Blind spots in this approach consist of the superolateral corner of the maxillary sinus, which is impeded by the orbits, and the most anterior portion of the nasal cavity, for which a transmaxillary approach and endonasal approach may be required.[149] An extended endonasal endoscopic transsphenoidal approach may also be necessary to access lesions medial to the lateral nasal walls and intracavernous carotid arteries. The combined transmaxillary and endoscopic endonasal approach can be performed via a Caldwell-Luc maxillotomy through a sublabial incision.[149] Such surgical strategies have been successfully used in the treatment of allergic fungal sinusitis,[150] esthesioneuroblastomas,[151-153] and recurrent craniofacial meningiomas.[154] Similar principles could be extended to the treatment of squamous cell carcinoma, adenocarcinoma, adenoid cystic carcinoma, chondrosarcoma, angiofibroma, and inverted papilloma.

The decision to use an endoscopic approach rather than a microscopic transcranial approach to the skull base is dependent on the lesion and local anatomic factors. The tumor size, vascularity, relationship to major vascular structures, and degree of lateral extension affect the surgeon's decision to perform the operation through an endonasal endoscopic approach. The thickness of bone at the skull base, degree of sphenoid sinus pneumatization, and size of the sella also influence the surgeon's decision.[155] Presellar and conchal-type sinuses limit the effectiveness of an extended endoscopic transsphenoidal approach.[132] Endoscopic approaches can avoid the need for brain retraction to access certain deep subchiasmatic, retrosellar, and intraventricular lesions, in comparison with a transcranial approach.

The endoscope is also used endonasally as a first-line therapy in treating CSF leaks in the anterior skull base, regardless of their cause (spontaneous or iatrogenic).[156] The use of fluorescein in imaging has increased the surgeon's ability to correctly localize the source of the leak, even at the submucosal level, and has improved the effectiveness of the repair. According to published series,[157-162] CSF rhinorrhea from anterior skull base localization was effectively treated in 85% to 100% of cases at the time of first surgery. A repeat endoscopic endonasal approach may still be appropriate for treating the leak in a significant number of cases. The graft material and technique used do not seem to independently affect the results.[163-167] When the defect is larger or if a high-flow CSF leak is identified, the surgeon should consider a multilayered repair with a vascularized nasoseptal flap. Spontaneous CSF leaks are often associated with encephaloceles arising from the ethmoid or sphenoid regions of the skull base. These encephaloceles can be successfully resected endoscopically and should be followed by multilayered reconstruction of the dural defect.[157]

Endoscopy and Craniosynostosis

The endoscope has been used successfully in the surgical treatment of sagittal, lambdoid, coronal, and metopic craniosynostosis.[168] The endoscope enables subgaleal and epidural dissection to be performed safely with less blood loss than in an open technique. This surgical treatment may be performed in children at a younger age.

Endoscope-Assisted Microneurosurgery

Endoscope-assisted microsurgery offers the surgeon the advantages of both the endoscope and the microscope. The addition of the endoscope to the microscope provides better illumination and detail in the image[15,16,84,169] while providing wider angles of visualization.[16] The craniotomy performed can be smaller, and the endoscope still provides for a wide enough view to perform the surgery according to the keyhole concept.[16]

Applications of endoscope-assisted microsurgery have been described in aneurysm surgery.[15,170-175] The endoscope provides for illumination in deep, dark corners and for clearer detail of structures. Angled endoscopes can provide the surgeon with better knowledge of the location of perforating arteries or cranial nerves around corners and behind the aneurysm sac. The endoscope can also better verify the relationship of those structures to the clip to determine whether optimal clip placement was achieved.[174]

The endoscope has similar advantages in tumor surgery.[15,176,177] The endoscope can offer a view of the relationship of the tumor to adjacent structures behind the tumor and can ensure the safe manipulation or further removal of the tumor. Visualization of the internal acoustic meatus before resection of intracanalicular schwannomas has been accomplished with the endoscope.[176] An endoscope has also been used to complete tumor resection in cases of intracranial dermoid cysts (Video 26-1).[178]

Different methods have been described to integrate the images coming from the endoscope and microscope.[16] The images can be kept separate on different monitors or can be integrated side by side through the microscope eyepieces or through high-definition liquid crystal display visors on the forehead. Most surgeons choose to place the endoscope in a holder to keep it stable in the surgical field and to prevent it from causing injury to adjacent neural structures.[16,169-172,177,179] Both of the surgeon's hands are thus free to operate instruments, but the endoscopic vision is static. Some surgeons have argued, however, that it is better to use the endoscope freehand to maintain a dynamic view, especially in aneurysm surgery.[170] Endoscope holders with pneumatic arms are the most versatile and enable the surgeon to lock or unlock all joints of the arm with one button.[24]

LIMITATIONS OF USE OF THE ENDOSCOPE IN INTRACRANIAL SURGERY

There are several limitations to the use of endoscope-assisted microneurosurgery or endoscopic surgery that are independent of the limitations previously discussed. The endoscope is more prone to accumulating debris or blood on the lens and may need to be retrieved from the surgical field more often to be cleaned when used in this setting. If the surgeon chooses to work with instruments through the endoscope's working channel, the accessible area is limited by the trajectory of the sheath. In addition, the surgical armamentarium is limited. Instrumentation can be used parallel to the endoscope to circumvent the problem, but a two- to four-hand technique is required. The endoscope can be bulky when used in conjunction with the microscope and may limit the surgeon's ability to move instruments in the field. Finally, the surgery may be slower, even when performed by experienced surgeons, largely because of the lack of three-dimensional vision with most endoscopes (the two-dimensional high-definition scopes). Accuracy with movement will match that achieved with microscopic surgery with experience.[121]

CONCLUSION

The endoscope was introduced in neurosurgery in the first half of the 20th century in the treatment of hydrocephalus. Limitations in the instrumentation, combined with poor visualization, restricted its use until the 1990s. Interest in cranial endoscopy beyond the treatment of hydrocephalus developed because it offered less aggressive approaches. Improvements in instrumentation and the increasing familiarity with endoscopes by otolaryngologists working in conjunction with neurosurgeons led to a renaissance of the use of the endoscope in skull base surgery. In certain situations, the endoscope offers some clear optic advantages over the microscope in transsphenoidal approaches, and the endoscope is increasingly used by neurosurgeons as an alternative to a craniotomy in specific cases. The choice to use the endoscope instead of microsurgical approaches must be based on the natural history of the patient's lesion and morbidity associated with either technique.

SUGGESTED READINGS

Cappabianca P, Alfieri A, de Divitiis E. Endoscopic endonasal transsphenoidal approach to the sella: towards functional endoscopic pituitary surgery (FEPS). *Minim Invasive Neurosurg*. 1998;41:66-73.

Couldwell WT, Weiss MH, Rabb C, et al. Variations on the standard transsphenoidal approach to the sellar region, with emphasis on the extended approaches and parasellar approaches: surgical experience in 105 cases. *Neurosurgery*. 2004;55:539-547.

Dandy W. An operative approach for hydrocephalus. *Bull John Hopkins Hosp*. 1922;33:189-190.

Das K, Spencer W, Nwagwu CI, et al. Approaches to the sellar and parasellar region: anatomic comparison of endonasal-transsphenoidal, sublabial-transsphenoidal, and transethmoidal approaches. *Neurol Res*. 2001;23:51-54.

de Divitiis E, Cappabianca P. Microscopic and endoscopic transsphenoidal surgery. *Neurosurgery*. 2002;51:1527-1529.

Fries G, Perneczky A. Endoscope-assisted brain surgery: part 2—analysis of 380 procedures. *Neurosurgery*. 1998;42:226-231.

Guiot J, Rougerie J, Fourestier M, et al. [Intracranial endoscopic explorations]. *Presse Med*. 1963;71:1225-1228.

Iantosca MR, Hader WJ, Drake JM. Results of endoscopic third ventriculostomy. *Neurosurg Clin N Am*. 2004;15:67-75.

Kassam A, Snyderman CH, Mintz A, et al. Expanded endonasal approach: the rostrocaudal axis. Part I. Crista galli to the sella turcica. *Neurosurg Focus*. 2005;19(1):E3.

Kassam A, Snyderman CH, Mintz A, et al. Expanded endonasal approach: the rostrocaudal axis. Part II. Posterior clinoids to the foramen magnum. *Neurosurg Focus*. 2005;19(1):E4.

Kehler U, Brunori A, Gliemroth J, et al. Twenty colloid cysts—comparison of endoscopic and microsurgical management. *Minim Invasive Neurosurg*. 2001;44:121-127.

Liu JK, Christiano LD, Patel SK, et al. Surgical nuances for removal of olfactory groove meningiomas using the endoscopic endonasal transcribriform approach. *Neurosurg Focus*. 2011;30:E3.

Liu JK, Christiano LD, Patel SK, et al. Surgical nuances for removal of tuberculum sellae meningiomas with optic canal involvement using the endoscopic endonasal extended transsphenoidal transplanum transtuberculum approach. *Neurosurg Focus*. 2011;30:E2.

Liu JK, Christiano LD, Patel SK, et al. Surgical nuances for removal of retrochiasmatic craniopharyngioma via the endoscopic endonasal extended transsphenoidal transplanum transtuberculum approach. *Neurosurg Focus*. 2011;30:E14.

Liu JK, Das K, Weiss MH, et al. The history and evolution of transsphenoidal surgery. *J Neurosurg*. 2001;95:1083-1096.

Liu JK, Decker D, Schaefer SD, et al. Zones of approach for craniofacial resection: minimizing facial incisions for resection of anterior cranial base and paranasal sinus tumors. *Neurosurgery*. 2003;53:1126-1135.

Liu JK, Patel J, Goldstein IM, et al. Endoscopic endonasal transclival transodontoid approach for ventral decompression of the craniovertebral junction: operative technique and nuances. *Neurosurg Focus*. 2015;38:E17.

Mixter W. Ventriculoscopy and puncture of the floor of the third ventricle: preliminary report of a case. *Boston Med Surg J*. 1923;188: 277-278.

Nulsen FE, Spitz EB. Treatment of hydrocephalus by direct shunt from ventricle to jugular vein. *Surg Forum*. 1952;2:399-402.

Oi S, Abbott R. Loculated ventricles and isolated compartments in hydrocephalus: their pathophysiology and the efficacy of neuroendoscopic surgery. *Neurosurg Clin N Am*. 2004;15:77-87.

Perneczky A, Fries G. Endoscope-assisted brain surgery: part 1—evolution, basic concept, and current technique. *Neurosurgery*. 1998; 42:219-224.

Rao G, Klimo P Jr, Jensen RL, et al. Surgical strategies for recurrent craniofacial meningiomas. *Neurosurgery*. 2006;58:874-880.

Spencer WR, Das K, Nwagu C, et al. Approaches to the sellar and parasellar region: anatomic comparison of the microscope versus endoscope. *Laryngoscope*. 1999;109:791-794.

Zweig JL, Carrau RL, Celin SE, et al. Endoscopic repair of cerebrospinal fluid leaks to the sinonasal tract: predictors of success. *Otolaryngol Head Neck Surg*. 2000;123:195-201.

See a full reference list on ExpertConsult.com

27 Thorascopic Spine Surgery

Ricky Raj Singh Kalra, Meic H. Schmidt, and Rudolf W. Beisse

The applications of endoscopic spine surgery have significantly expanded since the first publications in the 1990s.[1-6] Operating techniques have been standardized and unified, and today these approaches to the spine are safe and time efficient, with low complication rates and operative times that are comparable with those of open procedures with the adequate training and manual skills of the surgeon.[7] Thus endoscopic operations on the spinal column no longer represent exceptional interventions but have become standard procedures in spine surgery. Thoracoscopic techniques can be used to approach the anterior column of the spine in the area between the third thoracic vertebra and the third lumbar vertebra because endoscopic splitting of the diaphragm also allows the exposure of the upper sections of the lumbar spine. The application potential includes anterior release procedures, with incision and resection of ligaments and intervertebral disks; removal of fragmented disks or sections of vertebrae, including anterior decompression of the spinal canal; resection of metastatic spinal tumors with replacement of vertebral bodies with biologic or alloplastic materials; and ventral stabilization procedures with implants designed for use in endoscopic spine surgery. In addition, percutaneous endoscopic techniques are used for minimally invasive treatment of degenerative disk disease of the thoracic and lumbar spine.

PRINCIPLES

The principle of thoracoscopic spine surgery includes the use of a rigid endoscope and long instruments that are inserted through small incisions between intercostal spaces. The thoracic cavity is used as a preformed operative corridor after the lung has been collapsed on one side by a double-lumen, single-lung ventilation technique. The image of the operation site is transmitted onto high-definition video screens. Because a two-dimensional image is provided by the system, new skills are necessary to assess the depth and angle of the instruments used.

INDICATIONS

Overall, the indications for the technique described here are as follows:

- Anterior reconstruction of unstable fractures of the thoracic spine and thoracolumbar junction[8]
- Decompression of posttraumatic and degenerative narrowing of the spinal canal[9]
- Correction of disk-ligament instability
- Correction of posttraumatic deformity of healed fractures with or without instability[10]
- Revision surgery (i.e., for implant removal, for infection, and for implant failure and loosening)[11]
- Preparation and release of the anterior column in the presence of tumor and metastasis
- Sympathectomy for hyperhidrosis[12]
- Protruded disk removal in degenerative disk disease of the thoracic spine[6]
- Resection of metastatic spinal tumors[13]

TECHNICAL REQUIREMENTS

Trocars

Reusable, flexible, and black threaded trocars with a diameter of 11 mm are used to reduce light reflections and the pressure on the intercostal nerves and vascular bundle. Air insufflation is not required, and thus valves within the trocars are not necessary.

Image Transmission

The key to any endoscopic technique is image recording and transmission. True high-definition video technique has also revolutionized the endoscopic technique and now provides an endoscopic view comparable with microscopic images. A high-intensity xenon light source is necessary to illuminate the thoracic cavity. A rigid, long, 30-degree endoscope enables positioning of the camera far away from the working portal, thus facilitating undisturbed working and variable adjustment of the angle of vision. The intraoperative view is transmitted onto two or three flat screens (Fig. 27-1).

Instruments

Complete sets of instruments for soft tissue and bone preparation are available from contemporary instrument manufacturers (Fig. 27-2). Instruments should have a nonreflective surface and a depth scale on both sides and be ergonomically designed with big handles for safe control and handling. They are used in the *three-point anchoring technique*, which means that every sharp and potentially dangerous instrument is guided by both hands; one hand is based on the chest wall, always controlling and sometimes neutralizing unexpected forces and movements of the instrument (see Video 27-9).

Implants

Several implants for anterior instrumentation that can be used for endoscopic, mini-open, or open spine surgery are available. Most of them are based on the principle of a cannulated screw and plate system, first allowing the implantation of K wires under fluoroscopic control to be used as landmarks, followed by the insertion of screws. Biomechanically tested four-point fixation implants provide adequate angular stability, which is necessary for stand-alone anterior instrumentation (Fig. 27-3).[14]

For vertebral body replacement, bone graft (autograft or allograft) or mechanical devices can be used and filled or surrounded with the autologous bone harvested from the corpectomy site. A wide variety of expandable titanium cages are currently available.[15]

PREOPERATIVE REQUIREMENTS

Education of the Patient

The patient should be informed about the following approach-specific risks and hazards:

- Injury to the spinal cord, spinal nerves, and sympathetic trunk (deafferentation syndrome), with neurological deficits

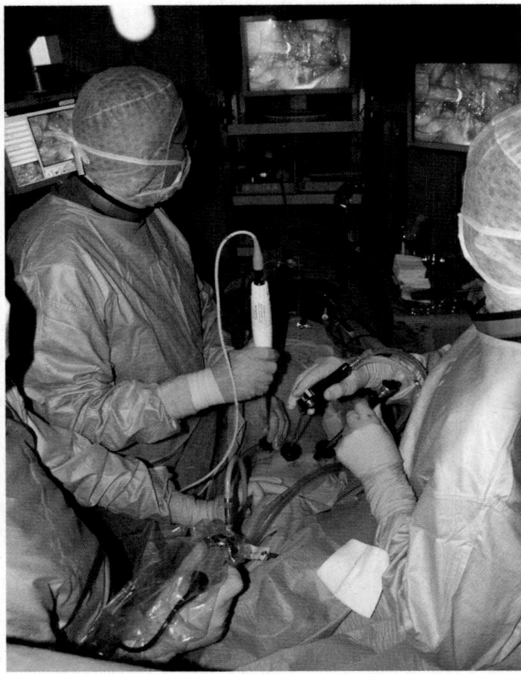

Figure 27-1. Thoracoscopic surgery at the spine. All portals, the 30-degree scope, and the instruments are inserted. The surgical team is looking at three high-definition flat screen monitors.

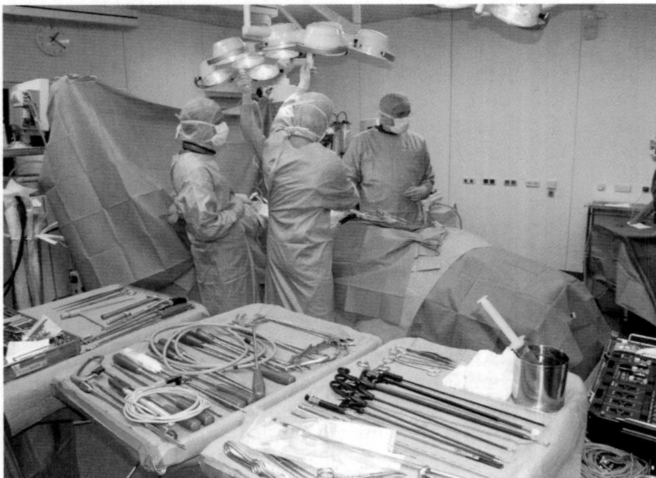

Figure 27-2. A whole set of long instruments for endoscopic soft tissue preparation and bone resection and devices for thoracoscopic implantation of a stabilizing implant. All these materials are prepared to be used for the thoracoscopic procedure.

- Injury to the greater vessels, thoracic duct, and segmental vessels
- Possibility of surgical conversion to a conventional thoracotomy
- Injury to spleen, diaphragm, and kidneys
- Port and diaphragmatic hernia

Anesthesia

A pulmonary function test and breathing therapy are commonly performed preoperatively to assess the patient's vital parameters.

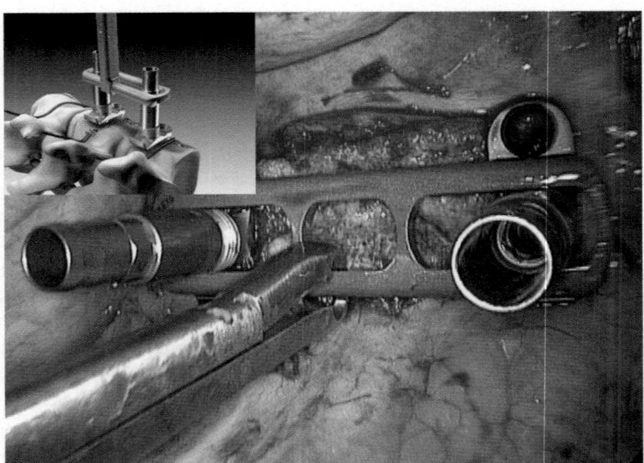

Figure 27-3. Screw and constraint plate implant for endoscopic and open instrumentation. This material is placed at the anterior column of the thoracic and lumbar spine *(inset)* (MACS TL, Aesculap, Tuttlingen, Germany).

Routine bowel preparation is commonly used to decrease intra-abdominal pressure and tension on the diaphragm. The thoracoscopic operation is performed while the patient is under general anesthesia. Double-lumen tube intubation and single-lung ventilation are applied as routine. Proper placement of the endotracheal tube is confirmed by bronchoscopy. A Foley catheter, a central venous line, and an arterial line for continuous blood pressure assessment are placed. For postoperative pain relief, a peridural analgesic is inserted in the thoracic region.

Positioning of the Patient

All endoscopic operations at the anterior column of the thoracic spine and the thoracolumbar junction are performed with the patient lying on his or her side (Video 27-1). The approach side is determined by the preoperative computed tomographic (CT) scans and depends on the position of the major vessels shown in the scans and the surgery that is planned. Because of the great variability in the vascular anatomy, firm rules are no longer set for selection of the approach side by the height of the lesion.

The patient is stabilized in the side-lying position with four supports and a special U-shaped cushion for the legs. It is possible to use a vacuum mattress, but its construction height can hamper the manipulation of instruments under C-arm control and conversion to the open procedure.

Designing the Entry Portals

As a routine, four portals are used: endoscope portal, working portal, suction-irrigation portal, and retractor portal (Video 27-2). Their location and, in particular, the position of the working portal are crucial for the endoscopic operation to proceed optimally. For this reason, the lesion is first displayed in the lateral projection (with reference to the patient's body) under precise adjustment of the image intensifier, and a marker is used to draw the injured spinal section onto the lateral thoracic wall (Fig. 27-4). The working portal is drawn in directly above the lesion. The trocar for the endoscope is marked either caudal or cranial to the working portal, depending on the height of the lesion, and follows the axis of the spine. The distance from the working portal is approximately two intercostal spaces. The entry points for suction-irrigation and the retractor are then located ventral from these portals.

After skin disinfection and sterile draping, single-lung ventilation is begun in consultation with the anesthetist. The portal in

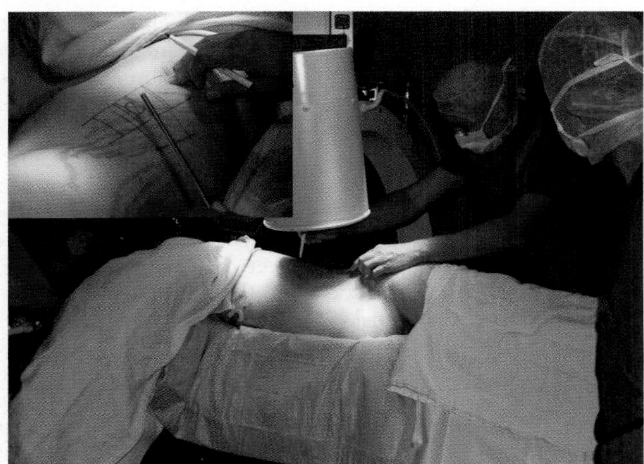

Figure 27-4. With the patient placed in a true lateral position, the affected section of the spine is accurately projected to the lateral thoracic and abdominal wall and marked with use of a C-arm amplifier *(inset).*

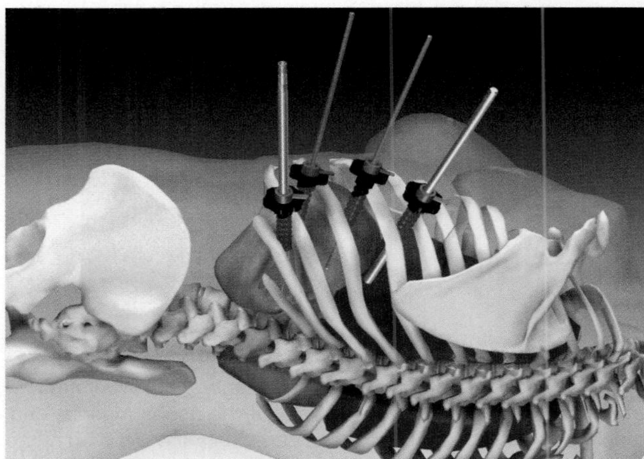

Figure 27-5. Placement of the trocars and instruments for an endoscopic intervention at the thoracolumbar spine.

the farthest cranial position is always selected as the first approach because the risk of injury to the liver, spleen, and diaphragm is comparatively minor in this position. The approach is made by the mini-thoracotomy technique, which enables examination of the immediate surroundings of the insertion site with the fingers before the trocar is introduced (Video 27-3). The rigid 30-degree endoscope is then carefully inserted, and the thoracic cavity is inspected to rule out the existence of adhesions or parenchymal lesions. The other three trocars and then the instruments are subsequently introduced under endoscopic visualization.

OPERATIVE TECHNIQUES

Approach to the Thoracolumbar Junction

This operation is also performed with the use of single-lung ventilation (Video 27-4).[8,11,16,17] The approach side is, again, decided according to the location of the major vessels, which can be identified from the preoperative CT scan. In most cases, the best approach to the thoracolumbar junction is from the left. Placement of the trocars and instruments is illustrated in Figure 27-5.

As a first step, the affected section of the spine is drawn onto the skin of the lateral abdominal and thoracic wall under image intensifier control. Careful attention is paid to correct projection of the vertebrae, whose end plates and anterior and posterior margins should be displayed in the central beam, in sharp focus with no double contour. This marking is the sole reference for subsequent placement of the portals.

The working portal is situated directly above the lesion; the portal for the endoscope is located over the spine two or three intercostal spaces away from the working portal in a cranial direction. The portals for the retractor and the suction-irrigation instruments are situated ventrally from this point.

The domelike diaphragm is firmly connected at its margins with the sternum, ribs, and spine and arches up into the thoracic cavity. Topographically, the attachment sites of the diaphragm to the spine are at the level of the first lumbar vertebra, whereas the lowest point of the thoracic cavity projects with the phrenicocostal sinus at the level of the baseplate of the second lumbar vertebra (Fig. 27-6). This makes it possible to place a trocar intrathoracically in the phrenicocostal sinus, which, after incision of the diaphragm attachment to the spine, provides access to the retroperitoneal section of the thoracolumbar junction down to

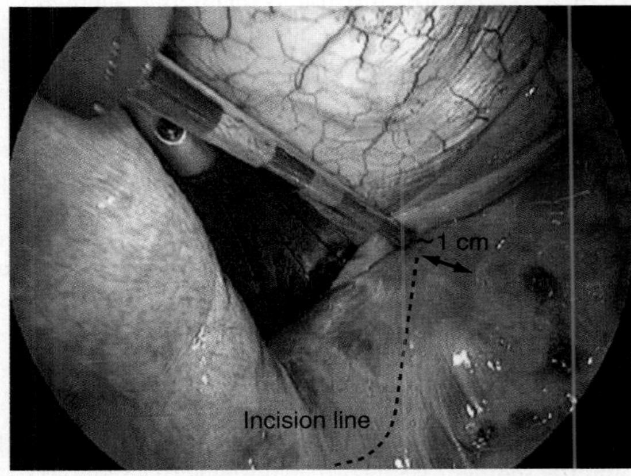

Figure 27-6. Typical operation site at the thoracolumbar section of the spine. The *interrupted line* runs parallel to the attachment of the diaphragm and indicates the location of incision for access to the subdiaphragmatic section of the thoracolumbar junction, L1, and L2.

the baseplate of the second lumbar vertebra. This requires a 4- to 5-cm-long incision along the attachment of the diaphragm; access to the L1-L2 intervertebral disk can be obtained with a shorter incision of 2 to 3 cm (Fig. 27-7).[16-18]

To prevent a postoperative diaphragmatic hernia, an incision that runs parallel to the diaphragmatic attachment is preferred. Because of the domelike architecture of the diaphragm, an increase in intra-abdominal pressure from a semicircular incision parallel to the attachment causes the resected margins to come together and to adhere spontaneously, whereas a radial incision close to the orifices of the aorta and the esophagus weakens the diaphragm fixation and causes the resected margins to gape. In addition, it is recommended that every incision in the attachment that is longer than 2 cm be sutured endoscopically to prevent hernia formation.

Endoscopic Treatment of Spinal Trauma (Anterior Reconstruction)

Landmarks

Initially, landmarks are determined under image intensifier control to serve as orientation points for the surgeon and camera

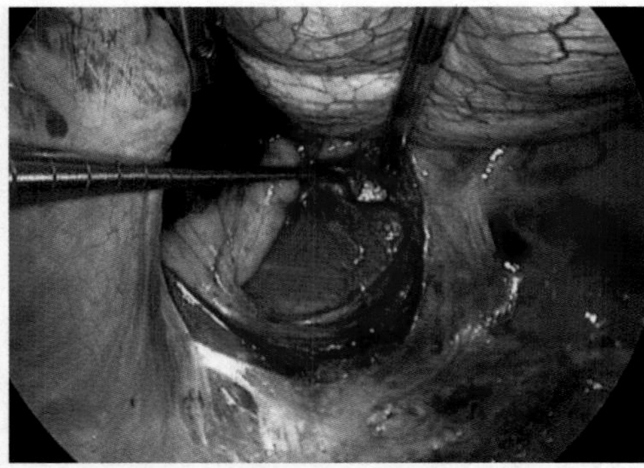

Figure 27-7. Partial detachment of the diaphragm reveals the retroperitoneal fat, the anterior border of the psoas muscle, and the spine. A fan-shaped retractor is inserted into the diaphragm gap.

operator during the subsequent course of the operation (Video 27-5). For this, the K wires associated with the implant are used; cannulated screws with integrated clamping elements then replace the K wires. If no implant is used, marker points can be set onto the parietal pleura under fluoroscopic control by use of the cautery or ultrasonic knife. Thus the K wires also define the later position of the screws, and they are placed near the end plates between the posterior and central thirds of the vertebra. To achieve this in the thoracolumbar junction region, the psoas muscle must be mobilized in a ventral-to-dorsal direction, thus avoiding irritation of the fibers of the lumbar plexus. Through positioning of the K wires near the end plates, injury to the segment vessels is avoided, and the screws are anchored in a region of higher bone density.

Preparation of the Segment Vessels

The pleura is opened along the connecting line between the K wires, and the segment vessels are exposed with a Cobb raspatory. These vessels are mobilized subperiosteally from both sides, ligated twice with titanium clips ventrally and dorsally, and raised slightly with a nerve hook. The vessels are dissected with the endoscopic hook scissors. The lateral aspects of the vertebral body and the disks are exposed with the raspatory (Video 27-6).

Cannulated Screw Insertion

The K wires are now overdrilled with a cannulated broach, and the lateral cortex of the vertebral body is opened (Video 27-7). The working trocar is exchanged for a speculum through a switching stick, and the clamping element is tightened with a screw. The length of the screw has been previously measured against the preoperative CT scan and subsequently defines whether a monocortical or bicortical screw fixation is to be attempted. The direction of the screw can be altered after removal of the K wire and checked in both planes under C-arm monitoring. The connecting line between the screws and the anterior boundary of the clamping elements now defines an area of safety within which the partial removal of the vertebral body and the disks is performed. The ventral and dorsal extents of the partial corpectomy thus defined also then correspond to the dimensions of the planned vertebral body replacement, which has a transverse diameter between 16 mm (thoracic) and 20 mm (lumbar).

The intervertebral disks are incised laterally with a long-handled knife, and the disk space is opened with a slightly offset osteotome (Video 27-8). The posterior osteotomy is then performed with a straight osteotome from disk space to disk space on the connecting line between the screws. The scale on the osteotome shows the corresponding depth, which in the anterior direction should be about two thirds of the diameter of the vertebra. The line of the anterior osteotomy runs along the anterior boundary of the clamping elements; to avoid unintentional perforation of the anterior vertebral wall (and adjacent vessels), an osteotome that is slightly angled to the rear is used. The central section of the vertebral body is now removed with a rongeur, and the removed cancellous bone is preserved for later implantation adjacent to the vertebral body replacement (Video 27-9). In cases of metastatic disease, the bone is collected and sent to for pathologic analysis as part of the specimen. With a curette and rongeurs, the intervertebral disks are then resected, and the end plates are freshened up with box cutters. When titanium cages are implanted, any weakening of the load-bearing end plates must be avoided. In monosegmental fusion with a tricortical pelvic crest graft, the subchondral bone lamella on the cranial end plate is removed to assist healing of the bone graft.

Insertion of the Bone Graft

In monosegmental reconstructions and fusion, a tricortical bone graft taken from the iliac crest is used. After the corpectomy defect has been measured, the iliac crest is prepared and exposed. With the use of an oscillating saw and chisel, the bone graft is harvested and firmly connected to a graft holder. The graft is inserted in a centered position into the defect, which has to be fluoroscopically checked in both planes (Video 27-10).

For vertebral body replacement in a bisegmental reconstruction, we mostly use the hydraulically working Hydrolift (Aesculap, Center Valley, Pennsylvania) with continuously variable distraction and adaptation of the end plates. Before the vertebra replacement is implanted, the extent and clean preparation of the implant site in the anterior sagittal direction and in its depth should be verified by palpation with a probe hook under image intensifier control.

Two Langenbeck hooks are inserted into the incision for the working portals, and the incision is widened slightly. The vertebral body replacement is then gradually introduced through the chest wall into the thoracic cavity and positioned over the defect in the vertebral body with a holder. Once again, it is determined that no soft tissue, particularly the ligated segment vessels, has slipped between the corpectomy defect and the vertebral body replacement. The vertebral body replacement device is then implanted into the planned central position in the vertebral body and distracted. The implant is surrounded with the cancellous bone harvested from the partial corpectomy or frozen allograft bone. An antibiotic medium (e.g., gentamicin-collagen) can be added to the spongiosa. After the corpectomy defect zone has been filled with spongiosa, it is covered with fibrin fleece.

Ventral Instrumentation with a Constraint Plate Implant

Because the screws and so-called clamping elements belonging to the implant were placed into position as a first step before the beginning of the partial corpectomy, the plate must be fastened and the ventral screws of the four-point fixation inserted (Video 27-11). The distance between the screws is defined with a special measuring instrument to select a plate of the correct length. This is introduced lengthwise into the thoracic cavity through the incision for the working portal, laid onto the clamping elements with a holding forceps, and there definitively fixed with nuts with a starting torque of 15 Nm. To bring the plate into direct bone contact with the lateral vertebral body wall, the bone screws are tightened. The ventral screws are inserted after temporary fixation of a targeting device and opening of the cortex. Because of the heart shape of the vertebral body, the ventral screws are usually 5 mm shorter than the dorsal screws. The fixation of the angle-stable implant ends with the insertion of a locking

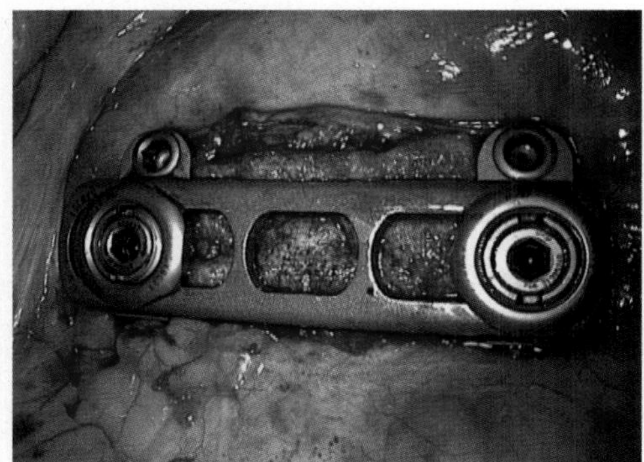

Figure 27-8. Thoracoscopic anterior instrumentation with a four-point stabilization constraint plate and screw system.

screw that locks the polyaxial mechanism of the dorsal screws (Fig. 27-8).

Final Stages of the Endoscopic Operation

In every case, radiographs are taken in both planes with the C-arm to check the decompression and position of the implants before the operation is concluded (Video 27-12). For operations on the thoracolumbar junction that include incision of the diaphragmatic attachment, an incision longer than 2 cm should be closed with endoscopic suturing. Two or three adapting sutures are sufficient, depending on the extent of the incision. The suture does not need to be watertight.

The entire thoracic cavity is again inspected endoscopically, and the site is irrigated and cleaned of blood residue.

A No. 20 Charrière thoracic drainage tube is inserted through the suction-irrigation portal. The instruments are removed under endoscopic monitoring. After consultation with the anesthesiologist, the lung is reinflated and ventilated. The complete reinflation of the lung is checked endoscopically before the endoscope is removed.

In the four incisions for the portals, adapting sutures are applied to the musculature, and suturing closes the skin. The thoracic drainage is connected to a water seal chamber, and suction of 15 cm H_2O is applied. The patient is usually extubated while still on the operating table. The chest tube usually stays in place for 24 hours. A postoperative chest radiograph is obtained immediately and again the morning after the procedure. The chest tube is placed on water seal the next morning and removed on postoperative day 2.

SPECIAL INDICATIONS

Removal of Posterior Wall Fragments: Endoscopic Anterior Decompression[9]

Depending on the level of stenosis, compression of the spinal canal can lead to a neurological deficit. The spectrum of injuries to the spinal canal, medullary cone, and cauda equina ranges from simple contusion to complete tearing of the neural structures. As long as the structures have not been severed, recovery of function and amelioration of sensory deficits may be possible in principle. Thus the indications for anterior decompression are present when significant narrowing and a neurological deficit remain after primary dorsal reduction and stabilization.

Operative Technique

Completion of the partial corpectomy and adjacent diskectomies is recommended before the canal decompression. The next step is to identify the pedicle of the fractured vertebral body. In traumatic burst fracture, the pedicles are nearly always preserved, and the retropulsed fragment usually is medial to the pedicle. Thus the retropulsed fragment is trapped between the two pedicles and is difficult to remove or reduce.

Resection of the ipsilateral pedicle with a punch is recommended before removal of the retropulsed fragment is attempted. For this reason, resection of the ipsilateral pedicle has a dual importance: it exposes the spinal canal, and it frees the retropulsed fragment from the pincer grip of the pedicles. A Cobb elevator is used to expose the ipsilateral pedicle subperiosteally and to push the nerve root away dorsally without separating the root from the surrounding soft tissue. The inferior margin of the pedicle is identified with a nerve hook, and the pedicle is transected with a punch, which can be facilitated by thinning the pedicle with a high-speed bur beforehand. Removal of the dorsocranial section of the vertebral body with the base of the pedicle exposes the posterior margin fragment and brings the dura into view. The compressing fragment can now be lifted off the dura under direct view, mobilized in the direction of the partial corpectomy, and resected. A nerve hook is used under image intensifier control to document the completeness of the posterior margin fragment resection in both planes. In cases with posterior wall resection, an expandable titanium cage is used as a vertebral body replacement because of its greater primary stability and the lower risk of dislocation. The operation concludes with the ventral instrumentation and suturing of the diaphragm attachment.

CASE STUDY 27-1

A 43-year-old man demonstrating severe back pain at the thoracolumbar junction, weakness of the lower extremities below T12, and moderate bowel and bladder dysfunction was referred to our hospital. After radiologic diagnostic studies and neurological examination, the patient was brought to the operating room for dorsal reduction and stabilization by internal fixator, followed by thoracoscopic anterior decompression and reconstruction (Figs. 27-9 to 27-11).

Removal of Protruded Herniated Disk: Endoscopic Treatment of Degenerative Disk Disease

Only 0.15% to 1% of all operative procedures for degenerative disk disease are performed to treat thoracic disk protrusion.[19-21] A specialty of the thoracic region includes a procedure to remove a "calcified disk" and one to remove an "intradural disk herniation" (Fig. 27-12). These removal procedures are technically demanding. Because the thoracic spinal canal has a smaller diameter, whereas the thoracic spinal cord has a bigger volume, there is little space to accommodate disk herniation. As a consequence, small disk protrusions might cause significant symptoms. Depending on the localization and expansion of herniation—medial, mediolateral, intraforaminal, or extraforaminal—typical symptoms of thoracic disk herniation can be described.

Operative Treatment Options

The following surgical approaches[22] are used to fit the needed level and herniation site:

- Transthoracic approach, open or endoscopic (T4-T11 level, central disk herniation, with or without calcification)
- Lateral extracavitary approach (T6-T12 level, centrolateral disk herniation)[23]

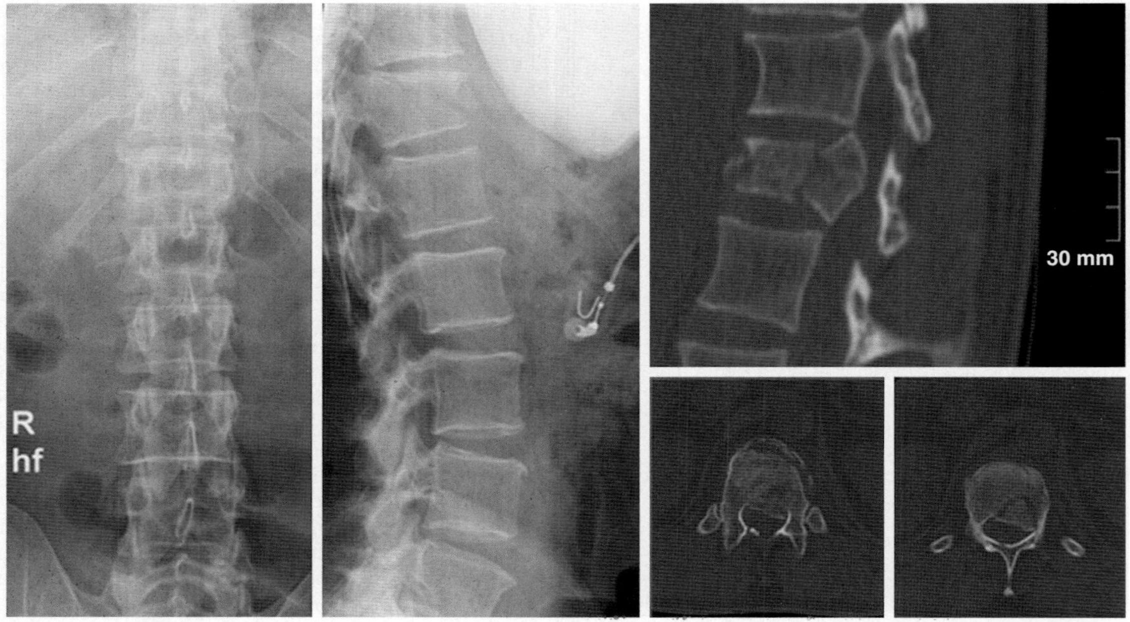

Figure 27-9. Radiographs showing L1 complete burst fracture type A 3.3 with severe compromise of the spinal canal, causing a Frankel C neurological deficit.

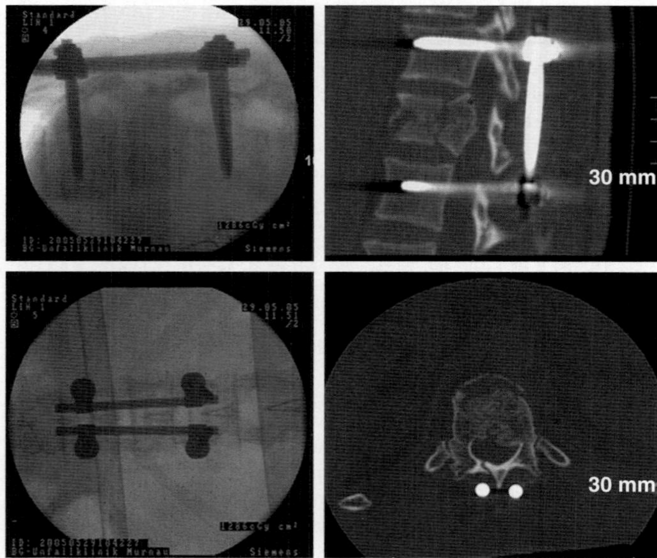

Figure 27-10. Radiographs showing dorsal reduction and stabilization by internal fixator to achieve indirect decompression by ligamentotaxis.

- Transfacet approach, pedicle preserving (all levels, centrolateral disk herniation)[22]
- Transpedicular approach (all levels, centrolateral disk herniation)[24]

Because of the high rate of morbidity with the open transthoracic approach, indications were few. The tissue-preserving thoracoscopic approach[6,12,25] is useful for greater numbers of indications, leaving centrolateral and lateral disk herniations to be approached posterolaterally. The thoracoscopic approach and operative technique are described here (Video 27-13).

Special Anatomic Considerations

The difference between the thoracic spine and the cervical and lumbar spine is the presence of rib-attached vertebrae. Except for the first thoracic vertebra, every rib articulates with the costovertebral joint through a cranial and a caudal part onto the neighboring vertebral bodies. Because of that anatomic situation, the rib head covers the dorsal disk space and the ipsilateral pedicle. Therefore, rib head removal is a key procedure for access to the disk space. The nerve root and the outgoing segmental vessels form a bundle next to the rib head caudally, riding in a bone groove along the caudal rib ventrally. The dorsal borders of most vertebrae are concavely shaped; this is confirmed preoperatively on axial CT views. Therefore, the fluoroscopic visible back wall is created by summation effect; the anatomic concave back wall is ventral to that line.

Operating Room Setup

Positioning the Patient. The side for the approach has to be dictated primarily by the localization of the disk herniation, symptoms, and the adjacent great vessels. In cases of centromedial and right lateral herniation, the approach from the right side is preferred (Fig. 27-13).

Confirmation of the Operative Site. Verification of the level of disease can be difficult before the main procedure is started. Several methods are recommended to ensure that the right intervertebral disk space is addressed. Dickman and colleagues[12] recommended a preoperative radiograph of the chest to localize the level. Large osteophytes visible on CT scans or plain radiographs can serve as surgical or radiographic landmarks. After the endoscopic procedure has started, it is recommended that the ribs be counted with use of the C-arm, beginning caudally at the 12th rib. Rib identification should be repeated several times to ensure accuracy. The pleura over the identified rib head is then cauterized. In patients with an abnormal number of ribs, close attention will prevent misidentification of the spinal level.

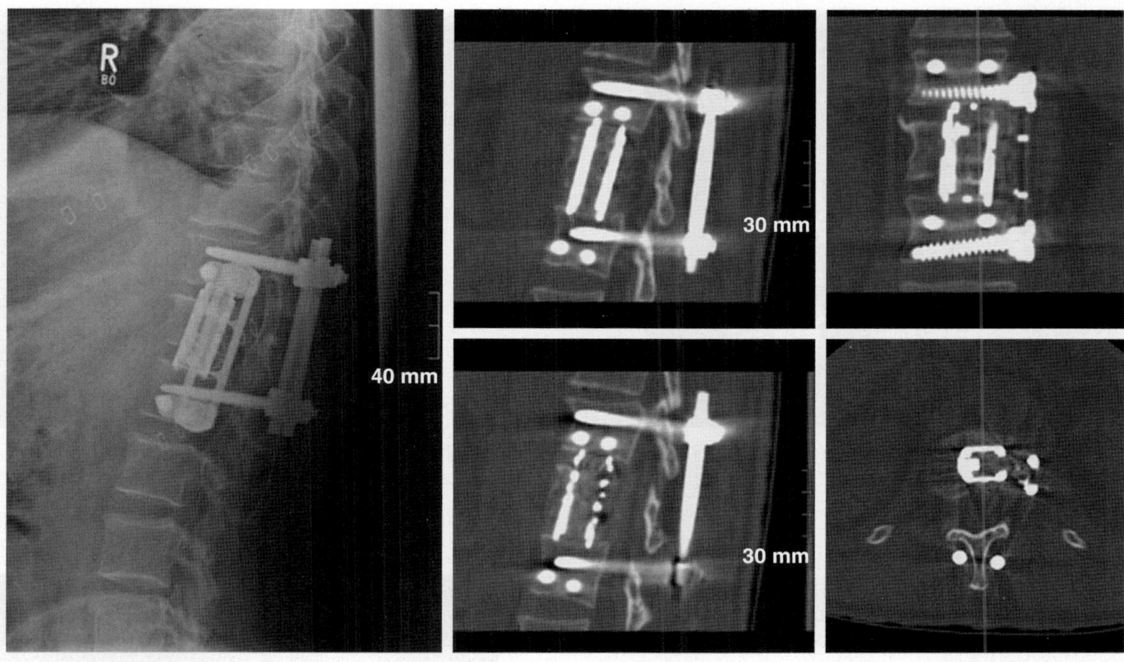

Figure 27-11. Radiographs showing thoracoscopic reconstruction of the anterior column with anterior decompression (i.e., posterior wall resection, vertebral body replacement, and anterior instrumentation).

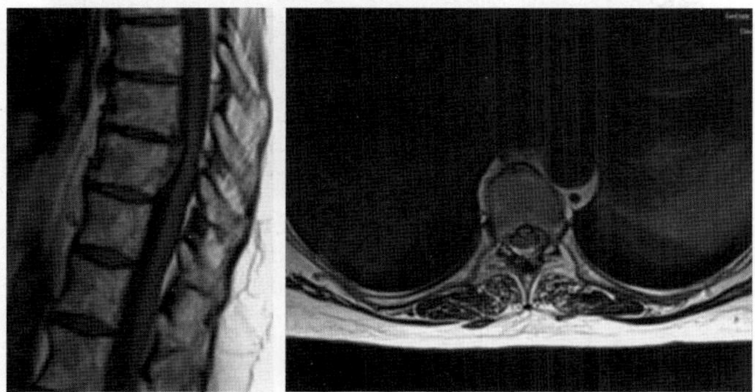

Figure 27-12. Calcified herniated disk at the T9-T10 level with severe narrowing of the spinal canal and cord in a 54-year-old woman, causing myelopathy and beltlike back pain.

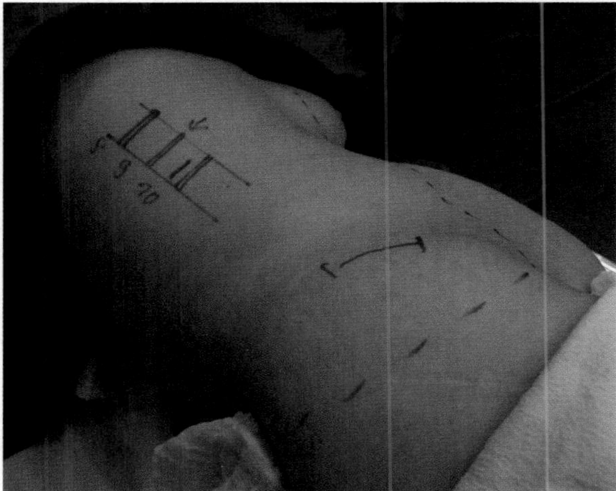

Figure 27-13. The affected segment is marked on the right chest wall before the endoscopic procedure is started. The working portal will be placed directly above the pathologic process; the 30-degree endoscope will be inserted from below.

Marking the level of interest by percutaneous placement of a tiny metallic marker that is CT guided simultaneously with the preoperative CT scan might be the most accurate way to identify easily and reproducibly the correct level during the operative procedure.[26]

Operative Technique

The general principle of the procedure is to resect the rib head of the adjacent rib and expose the pedicle and the affected intervertebral disk (Fig. 27-14). A block-shaped defect is then created in the adjacent vertebral bodies for removal of soft and calcified disk material away from the dura and into the defect. Afterward, the rib head, which usually fits into the defect, is used for a monosegmental fusion procedure to be accomplished by ventral instrumentation.

Technical and Operative Details

A lateral fluoroscopic picture is obtained to determine the level of disease and the position of the four portals. The working portal is outlined directly over the affected intervertebral space. After the approach has been made and all portals are correctly positioned, the spine is exposed by retraction of the lung with the fan-shaped retractor. The pleura over the identified and confirmed rib head is cauterized.

At this point, K wires are inserted into the vertebral bodies above and below the level selected for diskectomy (C-arm guided)

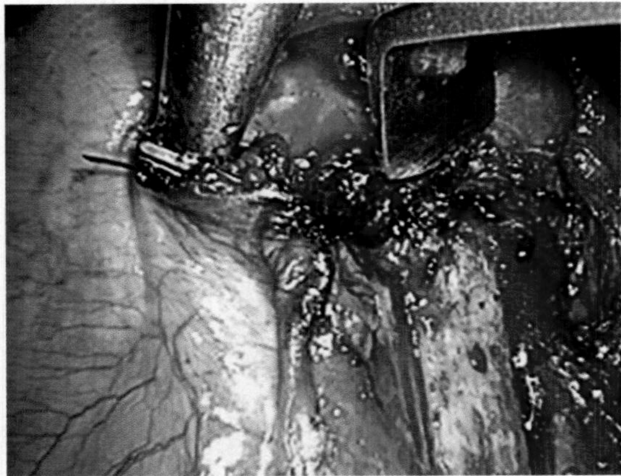

Figure 27-14. Mobilization of the rib head for access to the T9-T10 intervertebral disk and the pedicle of T10.

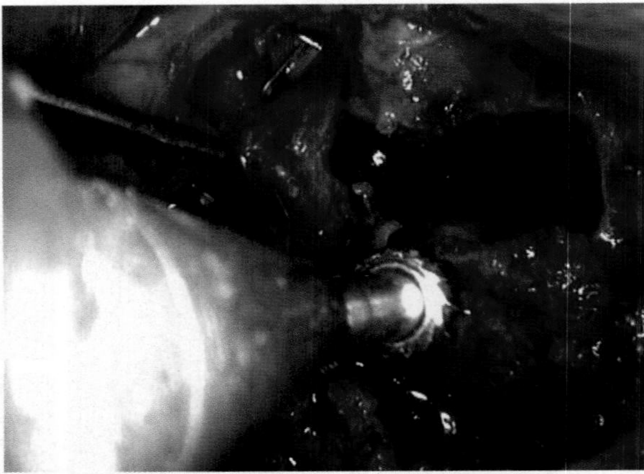

Figure 27-15. Partial corpectomy of T9 and T10 with a high-speed bur to create a defect in the vertebral bodies in front.

as landmarks according to the implant system that is used for stabilization and fusion. The procedure includes partial removal of the disk, combined with a more or less extended bone defect at the adjacent vertebral bodies; distinct instability thus can be expected. Therefore, a monosegmental fusion with anterior instrumentation is advised.

After trap-door incision of the pleura over the identified disk space and the adjacent one, the segmental vessels of at least the lower adjacent vertebra are prepared, ligated with clips, and transected. If mobilization of the aorta is needed, the segmental vessels are ligated and dissected at multiple levels. The capsular and ligamentous structures of the rib head are cut with a Cobb elevator, and the rib head is mobilized. The pleura is opened along the course of the proximal rib, and the proximal 2 cm of the rib is resected. The rib head is preserved and used as bone graft for later fusion. The pedicle can now be exposed to identify the neuroforamina above and below.

Partial corpectomy is performed with a high-speed diamond bur or an osteotome. A well-defined, block-shaped central defect involving the upper and lower thirds of the adjacent vertebral bodies is created. Initially, the posterior vertebral body wall is preserved (Fig. 27-15).

Once the base of the pedicle caudal to the intervertebral disk space is identified, the thickness can be reduced with a diamond bur to weaken the pedicle and to facilitate the transection with Kerrison rongeurs. Dickman and colleagues[12] recommended starting at the upper rim of the pedicle because there is less bleeding from the epidural venous plexus. Under direct endoscopic view of the dura, the posterior wall is then dissected off the dura and carefully pushed into the corpectomy site or thinned out with a high-speed diamond bur. The sequestered part of the disk is then removed with dissectors and rongeurs. If an intradural disk is calcified and herniated, the intradural part of the sequestrated disk has to be carefully separated from the arachnoid mater with microdissection (Fig. 27-16). Even if this is not possible without tearing the dura, the base of the calcified disk can be thinned with the diamond bur, leaving only a shell of calcification attached to the dura but free to move without bone or soft tissue impingement. Complete decompression of the dural sac across the vertebral body to the level of the contralateral pedicle is confirmed by direct endoscopic view and radiologically by fluoroscopy with use of a nerve hook in an anteroposterior projection. After decompression, the dura is covered with Gelfoam. The corpectomy defect is reconstructed, with the rib head harvested at the first step. The size of the graft is determined with an endoscopic measurement of the defect.

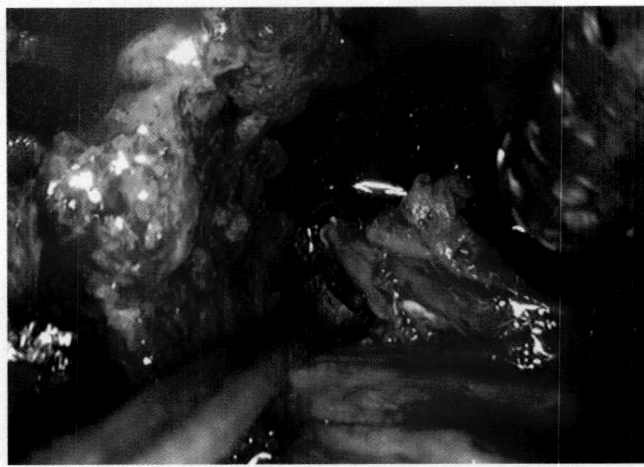

Figure 27-16. After the pedicle of T10 has been dissected, the posterior vertebral wall, including the calcified herniated disk, is carefully dissected from the dura and pushed into the vertebral defect in front.

We routinely perform a monosegmental endoscopic anterior fixation with a constrained screw-plate system to achieve a solid bony fusion of the segment.

Resection of Metastatic Spinal Tumors in Thorax and Thoracolumbar Junction: Special Considerations

Minimally invasive thoracoscopic surgery in patients with metastatic disease plays a significant role in minimizing surgical morbidity and recovery time. In many patients, the goal of surgery shifts from gross total resection to neuroelemental decompression and stabilization, followed by fast recovery and adjuvant chemotherapy and radiation.

Surgical considerations in patients with metastatic spinal disease include preoperative consultations with the surgical oncologists to minimize or, in cases of multiple lesions, combine surgical interventions. Intraoperatively, autologous bone must not be used for fusion mass. All bone removed should be sent for pathologic analysis and replaced with allograft material.

Primary lung cancer is a contraindication to thoracoscopic surgery for metastatic disease. Scarring of the lung, previous chest surgery, and thoracic lesions limit the extent of surgical corridor available in the thorax. In affected patients, management must be through an open or posterior approach.

CONCLUSION

In recent years, endoscopic procedures on the spine have become an alternative to standard spine surgery. Through the transdiaphragmatic approach, it has been possible to open up the thoracolumbar junction, including the retroperitoneal segments of the spine, by way of an endoscopic technique. With the extension of the technique to the retroperitoneal sections of the thoracolumbar junction, the indications for the endoscopic technique have increased substantially; the techniques now include complete fracture treatment with vertebral body replacement and ventral instrumentation, as well as anterior decompression of the spinal canal in posttraumatic, metastatic, and degenerative pathologic processes. The complication rate of the endoscopic procedure is of the same scale as that for open procedures; one clear advantage is the reduced morbidity associated with the minimally invasive technique.

SUGGESTED READINGS

Alberico AM, Sahni KS, Hall JA Jr, et al. High thoracic disc herniation. *Neurosurgery*. 1986;19:449-451.

Albrand OW, Corkill G. Thoracic disc herniation. Treatment and prognosis. *Spine*. 1979;4:41-46.

Awwad EE, Martin DS, Smith KR Jr, et al. Asymptomatic versus symptomatic herniated thoracic discs: their frequency and characteristics as detected by computed tomography after myelography. *Neurosurgery*. 1991;28:180-186.

Beisse R. Video-assisted techniques in the management of thoracolumbar fractures. *Orthop Clin North Am*. 2007;38:419-429.

Beisse R. Endoscopic surgery on the thoracolumbar junction of the spine. *Eur Spine J*. 2006;15:687-704.

Beisse R, Muckley T, Schmidt MH, et al. Surgical technique and results of endoscopic anterior spinal canal decompression. *J Neurosurg Spine*. 2005;2:128-136.

Beisse R, Potulski M, Beger J, et al. Development and clinical application of a thoracoscopic implantable frame plate for the treatment of thoracolumbar fractures and instabilities. *Orthopäde*. 2002;31:413-422.

Beisse R, Potulski M, Bühren V. Endoscopic techniques for the management of spinal trauma. *Eur J Trauma*. 2001;27:275-291.

Beisse R, Potulski M, Temme C, et al. [Endoscopically controlled division of the diaphragm. A minimally invasive approach to ventral management of thoracolumbar fractures of the spine.]. *Unfallchirurg*. 1998; 101:619-627.

Beisse R, Trapp O. Thoracoscopic management of spinal trauma. *Oper Tech Neurosurg*. 2006;8:205-213.

Dickman CA, Rosenthal DJ, Perin NI. *Thoracoscopic Spine Surgery*. New York: Thieme; 1999.

Horowitz MB, Moossy JJ, Julian T, et al. Thoracic discectomy using video assisted thoracoscopy. *Spine*. 1994;19:1082-1086.

Kim DH, Jahng TA, Balabhadra RS, et al. Thoracoscopic transdiaphragmatic approach to thoracolumbar junction fractures. *Spine J*. 2004;4: 317-328.

Knop C, Bastian L, Lange U, et al. Complications in surgical treatment of thoracolumbar injuries. *Eur Spine J*. 2002;11:214-226.

Knop C, Lange U, Bastian L, et al. Biomechanical compression tests with a new implant for thoracolumbar vertebral body replacement. *Eur Spine J*. 2001;10:30-37.

Le Roux PD, Haglund MM, Harris AB. Thoracic disc disease: experience with the transpedicular approach in twenty consecutive patients. *Neurosurgery*. 1993;33:58-66.

Mack MJ, Aronoff RJ, Acuff TE, et al. Present role of thoracoscopy in the diagnosis and treatment of diseases of the chest. *Ann Thorac Surg*. 1992;54:403-408.

Mack MJ, Regan J, Bobechko WP, et al. Applications of thoracoscopy for diseases of spine. *Ann Thorac Surg*. 1993;56:736-738.

Maiman DJ, Larson SJ, Luck E, et al. Lateral extracavitary approach to the spine for thoracic disc herniation: report of 23 cases. *Neurosurgery*. 1984;14:178-182.

McAfee PC, Regan JR, Zdeblick T, et al. The incidence of complications in endoscopic anterior thoracolumbar spinal reconstructive surgery. A prospective multicenter study comprising the first 100 consecutive cases. *Spine*. 1995;20:1624-1632.

Regan JJ, McAfee P, Mack M. *Atlas of Endoscopic Spine Surgery*. St. Louis: Quality Medical; 1995.

Rosenthal D, Marquardt G, Lorenz R, et al. Anterior decompression and stabilization using a microsurgical endoscopic technique for metastatic tumors of the thoracic spine. *J Neurosurg*. 1996;8:565-572.

Rosenthal D, Rosenthal R, Simone A. Removal of a protruded disc using microsurgery endoscopy. *Spine*. 1994;19:1087-1091.

Stillerman CB, Chen TC, Day JD, et al. The transfacet pedicle-sparing approach for thoracic disc removal: cadaveric morphometric analysis and preliminary clinical experience. *J Neurosurg*. 1995;83:971-976.

See a full reference list on ExpertConsult.com

28 Cranioplasty

Matthew A. Piazza and M. Sean Grady

In this chapter, we review the clinical indications, preoperative assessment and timing of cranioplasty, and the methods of autologous bone flap storage. We also analyze the properties of commonly used implants, as well as newer materials and composites. In addition, we illustrate the technical aspects of both autologous and methyl methacrylate cranioplasty with accompanying videos, and we discuss cranioplasty complications and their management.

Cranioplasty for reconstruction of skull defects is a common neurosurgical procedure and should be a skill of every neurosurgeon. An understanding of the clinical indications for and timing of cranioplasty, the availability of various materials for reconstruction, appropriate surgical technique and perioperative management, and knowledge of potential complications are critical for proper surgical decision making and a successful outcome.

Beyond the reestablishment of normal cranial architecture and the protective barrier of the skull, cranioplasty may also restore normal cerebrospinal fluid dynamics in patients who have undergone large decompressive craniectomies for elevated intracranial pressure. Moreover, the timing of cranioplasty depends largely on the clinical indication for the original craniectomy procedure. Patients undergoing decompressive surgery for elevated intracranial pressure may require delayed cranioplasty, whereas patients with lesions involving the skull can generally tolerate immediate cranial reconstruction. Patients under consideration for cranioplasty should undergo preoperative laboratory evaluation, be free from infection and hemodynamically stable, and undergo cranial imaging, preferably non–contrast-enhanced computed tomographic imaging of the head with bone windows. In the case of autologous cranioplasty, proper aseptic storage of the bone flap is essential. Before reimplantation of the stored bone flap, preliminary procedures are the norm.

The ideal nonautologous material is malleable, sterilizable, nonmagnetic, radiolucent, lightweight, and easily secured to existing skull. Various materials are available for cranial reconstruction, including autologous materials, ceramics, polymers, metallic implants, and composite materials, each with its own advantages and disadvantages.

A successful surgical outcome relies on meticulous dissection and separation of the scalp flap and temporalis muscle from the underlying dura or dural substitute, adequate removal of fibrous tissue from the bony edge of the skull defect, and, if applicable, proper preparation of the bone substitute. Cerebrospinal fluid aspiration may occasionally be necessary to allow brain relaxation intraoperatively. Some patients may ultimately require shunting.

While cranioplasty is a common and usually well tolerated neurosurgical procedure, the neurosurgeon should be cognizant of the potential complications after cranioplasty, which include but are not limited to autologous bone resorption, surgical site infection, postoperative seizures, and the development of subdural collections or hydrocephalus.

Full text of this chapter is available online at ExpertConsult.com

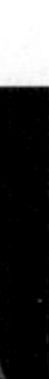

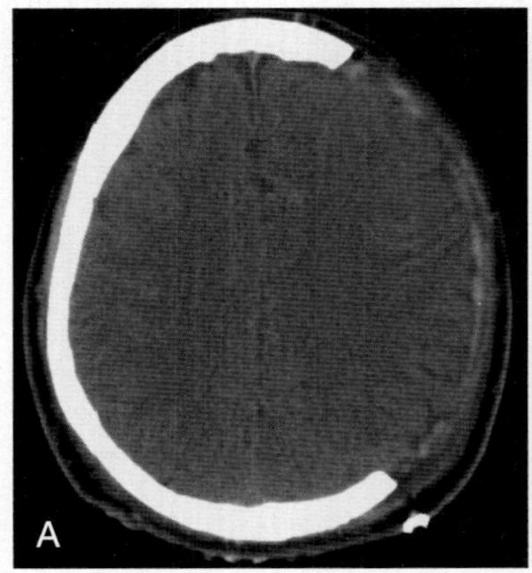

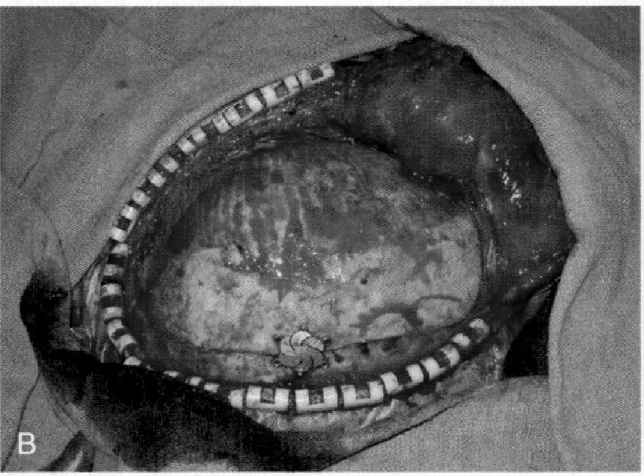

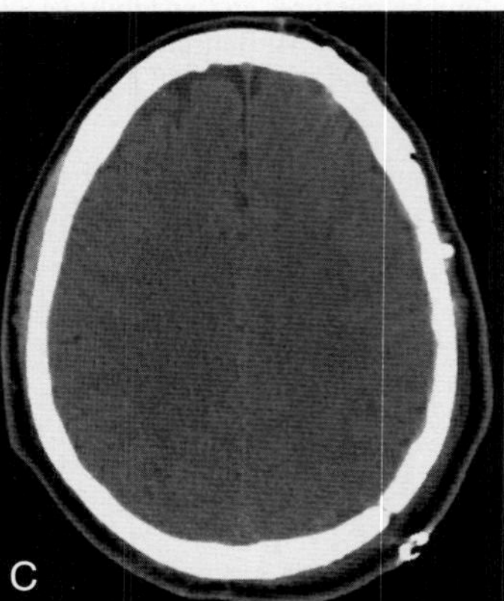

Cranioplasty after left decompressive hemicraniectomy for intractable intracranial hypertension. **A,** Preoperative computed tomographic scan demonstrating left skull defect. **B,** Intraoperative photograph of autologous bone flap secured to native skull with plating system. **C,** Postoperative computed tomographic scan demonstrating cranioplasty.

PART 6 Geriatric Neurosurgery: Normal Pressure Hydrocephalus and Chronic Subdural Hematoma

Evaluation and Management of Hydrocephalus

29 Production and Flow of Cerebrospinal Fluid

Conrad E. Johanson

This chapter reviews the physiology and pharmacology involved in cerebrospinal fluid (CSF) production and flow. Such information is essential for the rational treatment of hydrocephalus and increased intracranial pressure. Judicious management of CSF dynamics in neural disorders entails significant advances in molecular medicine and imaging. Successful control of intracranial pressure (ICP) is linked to intimate knowledge of CSF production, flow, and motion within the ventricular-subarachnoid spaces. Choroid plexus, the main source of fluid formation, is a strategic pharmacologic target. Molecular physiology expression and functional analyses have delineated the choroid epithelial sodium, chloride, and bicarbonate transporters that generate CSF; thus, the newly discovered Na^+-HCO_3^- cotransporter helps to maintain cerebroventricular volume and CSF ion homeostasis. Recent advances in medicinal control of CSF formation center on the role of neurohumoral factors (e.g., endogenous atrial natriuretic peptide [ANP]) in modulating water fluxes across the epithelium of the blood-CSF barrier. As ICP rises, the titer of ANP in CSF increases proportionally. By a putative servo-like feedback mechanism on choroid plexus ANP receptors, the elevated level of ANP in CSF reduces sodium transport, fluid formation, and ICP. This inhibitory mechanism involves enhanced cyclic guanosine monophosphate generation in the choroidal epithelium and consequent inhibitory effects on aquaporin 1. For the next generation of diuretic agents to curtail CSF excesses, agents will include those structurally related to acetazolamide, furosemide, and bumetanide to interfere with water movement across aquaporin 1 water channels in choroid plexus. On the other hand, the observed CSF production *increase* at night, to flush the brain of harmful catabolite waste products, raises the question of how cyclical changes in CSF neurotransmitters and hormones results in greater CSF flow nocturnally. Knowledge of neuroendocrine-driven diurnal and nocturnal rhythms will expedite drug development for better control of extracellular fluid movements and thus ICP. In aging, normal-pressure hydrocephalus (NPH), and Alzheimer's disease (AD), the CSF formation and turnover rates *decrease*. The curtailed CSF dynamics in neurodegeneration prompts the question of whether pharmacologic countering by augmenting the sluggish CSF flow in geriatric patients could benefit the failing brain metabolism and functions. Accordingly, an essential area of CSF pharmacology is to identify new agents to finely control fluid movements through brain in both high-pressure hydrocephalus and the lower incremented ICP in NPH and AD. New physiologic insights inform on controlling CSF clearance across the resistive arachnoidal interfaces with venous blood and lymph. A challenge to quantitative magnetic resonance imaging assessments is distinguishing the profiles of CSF dynamics (choroidal fluid production, transependymal flow, and arachnoidal drainage) in NPH compared with AD to manage better the brain fluid imbalances in late-life stages. Increasing attention focuses on how the age sensitivity of CSF flow into Virchow-Robin spaces interacts with interstitial fluid movement into the proposed glymphatic drainage sites around cortical-subarachnoid space veins. Novel therapies are on the horizon for manipulating central regional fluid movements in hydrocephalus, pseudotumor cerebri, cerebral edema, and aging-associated neurodegeneration.

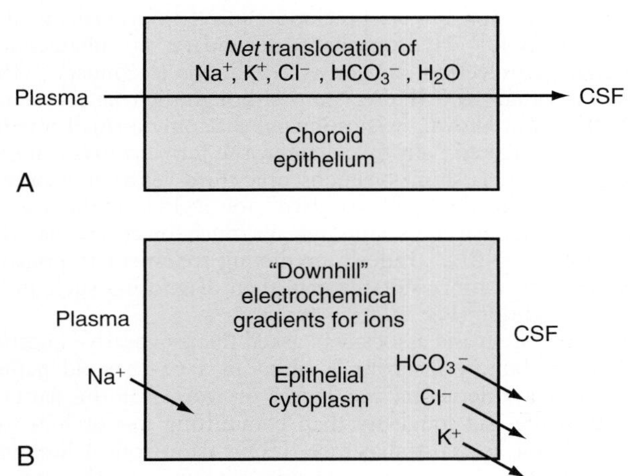

Ionic gradients across choroid plexus membranes that drive secretion of cerebrospinal fluid (CSF). A, The continual streaming across choroid plexus of the CSF, a fluid rich in Na^+, K^+, Cl^-, and HCO_3^-, occurs as the result of regulated transport and permeability to various ions and water. **B,** Active extrusion of Na^+ by choroid plexus into CSF sets up a downhill gradient for Na^+ across the opposite basolateral membrane. This inward Na^+ gradient promotes transfer of plasma-derived Na^+ into the choroidal epithelium through ion cotransport or exchange. Cl^-, HCO_3^-, and K^+ ions that are loaded into choroid plexus are subsequently released through channels or cotransporters down their respective electrochemical gradients into ventricular CSF. *(From Johanson CE, Duncan JA 3rd, Klinge PM, et al. Multiplicity of cerebrospinal fluid functions: new challenges in health and disease.* Cerebrospinal Fluid Res. *2008;5:10.)*

Full text of this chapter is available online at ExpertConsult.com 

30 Clinical Evaluation of Adult Hydrocephalus

Luke Macyszyn and Sherman C. Stein

Any discussion of hydrocephalus evaluation must begin with classification. This is necessary both to help organize the clinician's thinking and to direct the evaluation itself. Among the many classification systems are those divided by the various causes of hydrocephalus, by whether intracranial pressure (ICP) is elevated or normal, and by whether the hydrocephalus is communicating or noncommunicating.

The cause of hydrocephalus in a particular case is often revealed by the associated signs and symptoms; suspecting the cause guides the choice and timing of diagnostic studies. In most cases in adults, hydrocephalus is acquired; common causes include infection, hemorrhage (subarachnoid or intraventricular), trauma, obstruction by mass lesions, and postoperative causes, particularly after procedures at the skull base, the posterior fossa, and within the cerebral ventricles.

Whether ICP is high or normal often dictates how the hydrocephalus manifests. High ICP causes headache, nausea, and vomiting, as well as papilledema and abducens nerve palsy. Common symptoms when ICP is normal are cognitive impairment, gait disturbance, and urinary incontinence. It must be remembered that ICP may gradually fall over time; many cases of untreated high-ICP hydrocephalus can resolve if left untreated. These cases can be considered secondary normal-pressure hydrocephalus (NPH). Whether a patient's hydrocephalus is communicating or noncommunicating may influence symptoms and treatment.

Two related groups have been described. Cowan and associates[1] reviewed symptoms in young and middle-aged adults with hydrocephalus and elevated ICP. They found that symptoms included elements usually attributed to both high-ICP hydrocephalus and NPH: headaches and impairments in gait, cognition, and bladder control. Larsson and colleagues[2] studied adults whose hydrocephalus was chronic and became apparent only gradually or after sudden clinical deterioration.[2] Some of these patients had received cerebrospinal fluid (CSF) shunts in childhood, but the hydrocephalus was believed to be "compensated" or "arrested." In others, the only sign suggesting the long duration of the hydrocephalus was an abnormally large head[3] or neuroimaging evidence of congenital aqueductal stenosis.[4]

Evaluation of high-pressure hydrocephalus is usually straightforward. History and associated findings guide neuroimaging studies in determining cause and treatment. NPH secondary to one of the causes listed previously is often identified by history or is apparent during CSF or neuroimaging studies. It is idiopathic NPH (iNPH) that presents diagnostic challenges and is the subject of the balance of this chapter.

In the 1960s, when iNPH was first described,[5,6] it appeared to be a unique entity. The clinical triad of gait disturbance, dementia, and urinary incontinence was considered pathognomonic.[7] A reasonable pathophysiologic process was described; it appeared to fully explain the disease and its manifestations.[8] Diagnostic studies that were based on the proposed pathophysiologic process were considered valuable confirmatory adjuncts in distinguishing NPH from cerebral atrophy (hydrocephalus ex vacuo). However, it was not long until this diagnostic paradigm was questioned. When ventricular shunts were inserted, the predictive power of some or all of physical and laboratory findings was found to be unimpressive or absent.[9,10] Test after test was proposed as the definitive diagnostic tool. To date, none has found universal support.

For most diseases, the evaluation of diagnostic tests is straightforward. The clinician needs only to calculate the disease's prevalence and compare the accuracy of the operating characteristics (sensitivity and specificity) of competing tests to make a given diagnosis. These values, in addition to the availability, invasiveness, and costs of various tests, allows the clinician to rate them and to choose treatment most suitable for a particular patient.

However, this approach falls far short in the case of NPH. Almost all evaluations of predictive tests involved shunt insertion only in cases with certain diagnostic criteria, thus creating self-fulfilling prophecies. When some patients are denied treatment, clinicians know nothing about how they might have responded. Furthermore, operating characteristics of a diagnostic test can be evaluated only in the presence of a diagnostic "gold standard," a surefire means of determining whether the disease is present.[11] Unfortunately, no findings are pathognomonic for NPH. There are not even any characteristic postmortem findings for NPH in the brain parenchyma, the meninges, or the CSF spaces.[12,13] Evidence of Alzheimer's disease or cerebrovascular changes, or both, are often discovered in cortical biopsy specimens from patients thought to have NPH.[14,15] The presence of these other diagnoses, however, does not always preclude clinical improvement after shunt insertion.[15] Hydrocephalus secondary to subarachnoid hemorrhage, infection, and other conditions (secondary NPH) usually responds to CSF diversion. Although the true prevalence of NPH is not known, it is estimated that only a small fraction of cases are treated.[16] In this chapter, the term *treatment* means CSF diversion via shunt or endoscopic third ventriculostomy. A practical diagnostic "gold standard" for iNPH might also be treatment responsiveness, although at a much lower rate than that for secondary NPH.[17] Indeed, predicting treatment responsiveness might be a more suitable goal than diagnosing such an ill-defined condition (Fig. 30-1).

In 2006, Stein and associates[18] asked the provocative question of whether blindly inserting a shunt in a 65-year-old patient with moderate dementia was better or worse for the patient's quality of life and longevity than committing her or him to a nursing home for custodial care. Using data from a literature review, they projected the probable outcomes to the patient, considering expected results of custodial care versus various likelihoods of shunt response and complications. Average rates of reported shunt response and complications suggested that empirical shunt insertion resulted in a robustly higher quality of life for the hypothetical patient than did custodial care.[18] In a companion article, Burnett and colleagues[19] compared empirical shunt insertion to various diagnostic tests for NPH in use at the time. They were able to show that employing any of the tests to screen for shunt response would not improve quality of life; in fact, most tests worsened it by condemning potential shunt responders to custodial care. Furthermore, even a theoretical test that perfectly predicted shunt response could be cost effective (to the patient and to society) only if it could be performed at very low cost.[19]

Nevertheless, in most reviews of the topic since 2005, authors have discussed a menu of diagnostic approaches with little reflection on their predictive values[20-28]; only a few have recognized how little value these tests have.[29-33] The popularity of hydrodynamic testing is reflected both in reviews[34-36] and in guidelines[37,38] that emphasize its usefulness. With that in mind, we review the

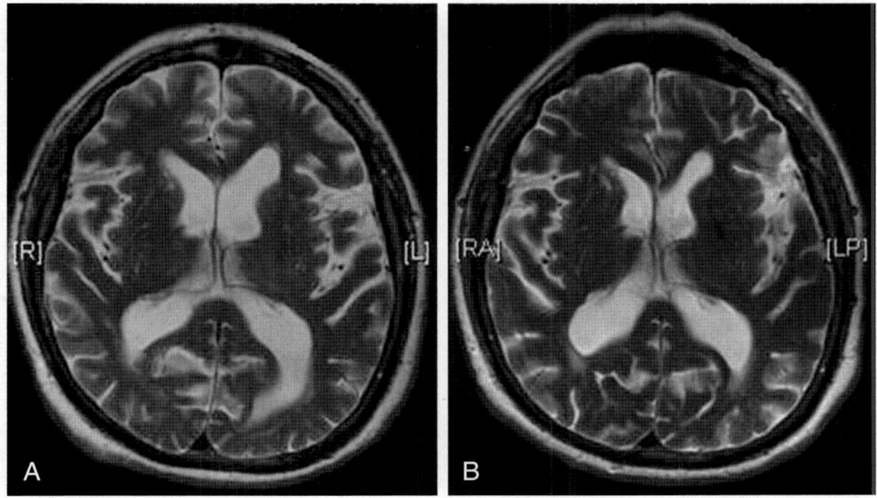

Figure 30-1. A, Preoperative T2-weighted magnetic resonance image of normal-pressure hydrocephalus (NPH). **B,** Postoperative scan in a patient with NPH and a good outcome (ventricular catheter not well demonstrated at this level).

TABLE 30-1 Reported Sensitivity and Specificity of Tests for Idiopathic Normal-Pressure Hydrocephalus

Series	Test	No. of Cases	Sensitivity	Specificity
Tullberg et al, 2000[72]	CSF sulfatide concentration	43	0.74	0.94
Shiino et al, 2004[65]	MRI spectroscopy	21	1.0	0.88
Farace and Shaffrey, 2005[73]	Neuropsychology tests and high-volume spinal tap	32	0.83	0.77
Marmarou et al, 2005[74]	External ventricular drainage	102	0.95	0.78
Marmarou et al, 2005[74]	R_{out}	102	0.75	0.63
Burnett et al, 2006[19]	R_{out}: pooled literature average	NA	0.86	0.69
Kawaguchi et al, 2011[58]	CT cisternography	82	0.52-0.95	0-0.40
Yamada et al, 2013[67]	CBF change after acetazolamide	25	0.85	0.4
Wikkelsø et al, 2013[48]	R_{out}: different cutoffs	115	0.31-0.92	0.06-0.88
Wikkelsø et al, 2013[48]	High-volume spinal tap	115	0.52	0.59
Virhammar et al, 2014[75]	Callosal angle	109	0.67	0.67

CBF, cerebral blood flow; CSF, cerebrospinal fluid; CT, computed tomographic; MRI, magnetic resonance imaging; NA, not available; R_{out}, resistance to CSF outflow.

current state of tests being proposed to assist in the diagnosis of NPH or in predicting treatment responsiveness, or both.

DIAGNOSTIC TESTS

Burnett and colleagues[19] reviewed the state of various tests proposed for the diagnosis of NPH. The following discussion is intended primarily to update and supplement that earlier review, in which no evidence of a dispositive test was found. Table 30-1 summarizes reported accuracy of various tests in predicting treatment response of suspected iNPH. With few exceptions, references cited in this table are case series in which subjects with negative results rarely received treatment. Therefore, positive and negative predictive power of the tests cannot be calculated.

PHYSICAL AND NEUROBEHAVIORAL FINDINGS

Of the classic triad of impaired gait, dementia, and urinary incontinence, only gait disturbance is currently considered useful in predicting treatment response,[39] and computerized analysis of gait shows improvement after successful shunt insertion.[40] In NPH, gait gradually becomes wide based, with reduced step height and stride. The perceived difficulty of raising the feet has been termed *magnetic gait.*[41] Similar gait defects in patients with Parkinson's disease can be distinguished by their tendency to exhibit festination (progressive involuntary acceleration with continued walking) and by the associated tremor, rigidity, and akinesia.

Neurobehavioral changes in NPH feature apathy or anxiety, in contrast to the delusions, agitation, depression, and irritability common with Alzheimer's disease.[42] Cognitive testing has shown a predominance of executive disorders, attention deficits, and visuoperceptual and visuospatial dysfunction in NPH, along with memory impairment.[43] Saito and colleagues[43] also emphasized that frontal lobe deficits predominate in NPH, whereas impaired memory is the signature finding in Alzheimer's disease. Hellstrom and associates[44] suggested that certain neuropsychological tests—namely, the Grooved Pegboard, the Rey Auditory Verbal Learning test, and the Stroop test—predict treatment outcome in NPH. Furthermore, they reported that test performance improved after successful shunt insertion. Certain occupational and physical therapy assessments have also been reported to predict shunt response.[45]

Pressure Dynamics of Cerebrospinal Fluid

Since the original hypothesis that NPH resulted from partial or temporary CSF obstruction,[8] resistance to CSF outflow (R_{out}) has been considered a useful measurement. Several studies of the correlation between R_{out} and treatment response have been reported.[46-48] Unfortunately, the reported sensitivity of this parameter ranges widely in the literature, ranging between 40% and 100%, there being considerable overlap in test results between shunt responders and nonresponders. It is unresolved whether this failure is the result of a lack of test standardization or a faulty hypothesis.

Another popular procedure is to monitor the clinical and neuroimaging response to a spinal tap with large-volume CSF drainage. Measurements have shown improvement in decreased cerebral perfusion values[49] after high-volume CSF removal, particularly in the dorsolateral frontal and left mesiotemporal regions.[50] The recent European iNPH Multicentre Study[48] revealed high positive predictive values of both lumbar CSF drainage and R_{out} determinations (a positive test result is correlated with good treatment outcome). A disappointing finding was that the negative predictive values of both tests were low; in other words, many subjects proved shunt-responsive despite negative test results. The authors suggested that a positive test result might support the decision for surgery, whereas a negative test result did not reliably exclude a positive shunt response. Gupta and Lang[51] noted that clinical improvement after large-volume tap was no better than after a sham puncture, which raised further questions about the predictive value of the procedure.

Neuroimaging

Lebret and associates[52] reported on MRI image segmentation to calculate the relative volumes of cerebral ventricles and subarachnoid spaces. The subarachnoid-to-ventricular volume ratio is diminished in patients with NPH, in comparison with healthy subjects (Figs. 30-2 and 30-3). It is unknown whether there is any correlation with treatment response. Structural changes thought to be predictive of NPH include an empty sella, "mismatch sign" (much narrower subarachnoid space than the amount of ventriculomegaly would indicate),[53] and a callosal angle of less than 63 degrees.[54]

Cardiac gated, phase-contrast MRI can depict the flow of CSF and can be used to calculate CSF flow rates in suspected NPH.[55] Increased flow velocities through the cerebral aqueduct have been correlated with decreased cerebral compliance but not with shunt response.[56,57] Computed tomographic cisternography has sensitivity and specificity approximately similar to those of a large-volume spinal tap.[58] It has been suggested that functional MRI might improve prediction of treatment response.[59,60]

Diffusion tensor imaging shows that fractional anisotropy values of the corticospinal tract are significantly increased in patients with NPH in comparison with both healthy controls and patients with Alzheimer's and Parkinson's diseases.[61] Hattori and associates[61] hypothesized that this may account for the gait disturbance in NPH. On the other hand, fractional anisotropy appears to be reduced in the thinned corpus callosum of patients with NPH,[62,63] and similar changes have been reported in the hippocampus, albeit without change in hippocampal volume.[64] It is hypothesized that future techniques may create a functional MRI biomarker that can aid the clinician in diagnosis and prediction of treatment response.[59,60] Shiino and colleagues[65] reported that the MRI spectroscopy of white matter can help predict treatment response. A literature review suggested that evidence supporting the use of MRI spectroscopy was stronger than that for other neuroimaging techniques,[60] but further study is needed.

Measures of Cerebral Blood Flow or Metabolism

Single photon emission computed tomography (SPECT) has been used to classify patterns of diminished cerebral blood flow (CBF) in suspected NPH. In one large multicenter trial, there was no correlation between preoperative CBF pattern and shunt response.[66] SPECT has also been used to measure the response of CBF to an acetazolamide; a CBF increase of less than 40% has been suggested to predict shunt response.[67] A positron emission tomographic (PET) study of a small cohort showed that regional cerebral oxygen metabolism is significantly lower in the basal ganglia of patients with NPH than in that of age-matched controls.[68]

Levels of neurofilament protein are elevated in the ventricular CSF of patients with NPH and decrease after shunt insertion.[69] In an extensive review of metabolic derangements in NPH, Kondziella and colleagues[70] suggested there may be a "point of no return," beyond which the metabolic changes can no longer be

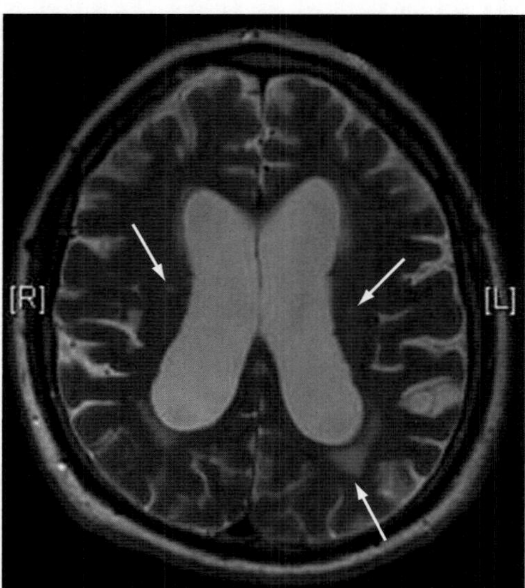

Figure 30-2. T2-weighted magnetic resonance image of normal-pressure hydrocephalus: ventriculomegaly, periventricular lucency *(inferior arrow)*, and white matter hyperintensities (*superior arrows;* see text for debate regarding white matter hyperintensities).

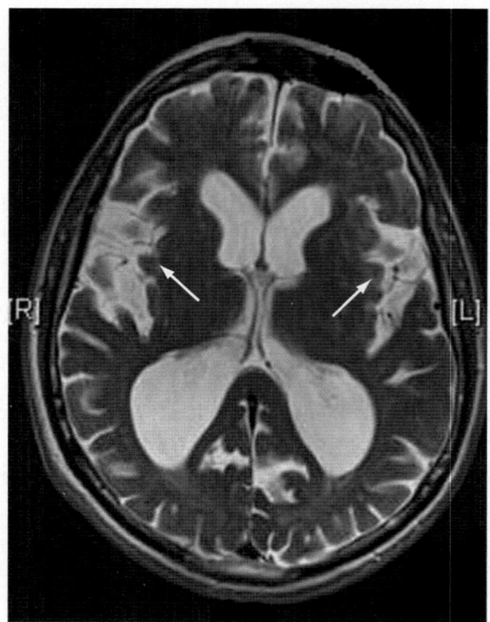

Figure 30-3. T2-weighted magnetic resonance image of normal-pressure hydrocephalus and enlarged perisylvian fissures *(arrows)* without generalized atrophy.

reversed by the restoration of CSF flow. If this hypothesis is correct, no single test can be expected to predict treatment response in all cases, and a combination of biochemical and other studies may be needed.

CONCLUSION

Evaluation of hydrocephalus for adult patients in whom a cause is known or suspected is determined by the underlying cause and the degree of intracranial hypertension. It is difficult to draw firm conclusions for iNPH, however. Because NPH is such an uncertain diagnosis, we recommend that any test for it be judged by the test's accuracy at predicting clinical improvement after treatment. Of the diagnostic procedures currently in use for NPH, none can be considered the diagnostic "gold standard." Many such procedures tested have shown disappointing sensitivity and specificity in predicting treatment response. Some tests have strong advocates, but some of the same tests have generated equally strong opposition. A number of tests discussed previously seem promising but cannot be considered dispositive. We recommend judging a test by its ability to predict response to CSF diversion, rather than by its correspondence with an unverified pathophysiologic pattern.

It is understandable that clinicians caring for patients with suspected NPH would prefer some confirmation of likely effectiveness before recommending surgery. However, evaluating the predictive power of any of these diagnostic tests is limited by their lack of validation. In almost every study published in which shunt outcome was assessed after testing, the findings were weakened by the almost-universal practice of limiting surgery to patients with positive test results. This introduces selection bias[71] and creates a self-fulfilling prophecy. If patients with negative test results are not offered treatment, they cannot demonstrate how they would have responded.

This is not a trivial concern. Withholding a potentially valuable therapy from patients on the basis of unproven screening criteria carries an associated cost. These losses involve both economic and quality-of-life issues. Some of the patients denied treatment deteriorate in custodial care, and the cost to themselves, their families, and society is higher than if they had received hydrocephalus treatment. Although we currently recommend shunt placement for all patients with potential NPH, the search continues for predictive tests and combinations of findings that improve shunt success rates. We recognize that there is no consensus on the matter, and we understand that performing confirmatory tests for NPH provides a degree of comfort to physicians and patients' families alike.

SUGGESTED READINGS

Begg CB, Greene RA. Assessment of diagnostic tests when disease verification is subject to selection bias. *Biometrics*. 1983;39(1):207-215.

Burnett MG, Sonnad SS, Stein SC. Screening tests for normal-pressure hydrocephalus: sensitivity, specificity, and cost. *J Neurosurg*. 2006;105(6):823-829.

Gupta A, Lang AE. Potential placebo effect in assessing idiopathic normal pressure hydrocephalus. *J Neurosurg*. 2011;114(5):1428-1431.

Jaraj D, Rabiei K, Marlow T, et al. Prevalence of idiopathic normal-pressure hydrocephalus. *Neurology*. 2014;82(16):1449-1454.

Kiefer M, Unterberg A. The differential diagnosis and treatment of normal-pressure hydrocephalus. *Dtsch Arztebl Int*. 2012;109(1-2):15-25.

Marmarou A, Young HF, Aygok GA, et al. Diagnosis and management of idiopathic normal-pressure hydrocephalus: a prospective study in 151 patients. *J Neurosurg*. 2005;102(6):987-997.

Relkin N, Marmarou A, Klinge P, et al. Diagnosing idiopathic normal-pressure hydrocephalus. *Neurosurgery*. 2005;57(3 suppl):S4-S16.

Stein SC, Burnett MG, Sonnad SS. Shunts in normal-pressure hydrocephalus: do we place too many or too few? *J Neurosurg*. 2006;105(6):815-822.

Virhammar J, Laurell K, Cesarini KG, et al. The callosal angle measured on MRI as a predictor of outcome in idiopathic normal-pressure hydrocephalus. *J Neurosurg*. 2014;120(1):178-184.

Wikkelsø C, Hellstrom P, Klinge PM, et al. The European iNPH Multicentre Study on the predictive values of resistance to CSF outflow and the CSF Tap Test in patients with idiopathic normal pressure hydrocephalus. *J Neurol Neurosurg Psychiatry*. 2013;84(5):562-568.

See a full reference list on ExpertConsult.com

31 Shunting

Marvin Bergsneider

Hydrocephalus is a commonly encountered disorder that occurs either as a primary condition or as the sequela to an intracranial hemorrhage, a space-occupying lesion, or meningitis. For more than a half century, a cerebrospinal fluid (CSF) shunt has been the mainstay of treatment for hydrocephalus. Although many consider shunting a relatively simple procedure, problems with CSF shunts are common, costly, and sometimes debilitating. Within the first year, shunts fail at extraordinary rate of up to 40% and show nearly a 10% infection rate.[1-4] The shunt operation has one of the highest associated complication rates in neurosurgery. Furthermore, cases of hydrocephalus can be some of the most complex and challenging clinical scenarios facing a neurosurgeon.[5,6]

The aim of this chapter is to help neurosurgeons choose the type of shunt, valve setting, and shunt location that will offer the highest probability of a good outcome, while avoiding complications and revisions, in adult patients with hydrocephalus (see Chapters 197, 198, and 201 for discussions of pediatric hydrocephalus and pediatric shunts). Unfortunately, there are scant level I and II evidentiary data on which to base guidelines pertaining to shunting methods and materials for adult hydrocephalus patients. Our recommendations are therefore derived from personal experience (more than 6000 outpatient encounters and 800 surgical procedures on adult hydrocephalus patients over a 20-year period), insight drawn from our own clinical studies,[7-9] and information gleaned from the literature.

Although this chapter is entitled "Shunting," neurosurgeons should always consider endoscopic third ventriculostomy (ETV) as an alternative when appropriate[7,10] (see Chapter 32 for more information on the role of third ventriculostomy in adults and children). Proceeding automatically with a shunt operation, particularly in patients presenting with shunt failure, potentially robs the patient an opportunity to live shunt-free. Clinicians should investigate the etiology and ventricular anatomy in every case of hydrocephalus. In some cases, even patients with presumed "communicating" hydrocephalus instead have a ventricular obstruction that clinicians can readily visualize using modern high-resolution magnetic resonance imaging (MRI) technology (such as the CISS or FIESTA sagittal sequences)[7,11,12] (see Chapter 30). Adult patients shunted in early childhood have a particularly high incidence of noncommunicating (intraventricular) hydrocephalus in our experience.

KEY POINT

In the initial evaluation of a newly diagnosed hydrocephalus patient or a previously shunted one, an essential component of the evaluation is to determine whether an ETV (or related procedure) should be considered.

Historically, probably the most challenging unwanted consequence of shunted hydrocephalus has been, and continues to be, CSF overdrainage. In infants, shunting effectively eliminates the forces that normally expand the skull. Later in childhood, this results in an abnormally small cranium adding to the risk of craniocerebral disproportion. In older children and young adults, chronic overdrainage can result in slit-like ventricles, which, in turn, negatively influence intracranial compliance and predispose to ventricular shunt obstruction owing to apposition of the ependymal wall or choroid plexus. In older adults, overdrainage can manifest as subdural fluid collections or "spinal headaches." Each of these conditions increases the likelihood of a shunt revision, which then introduces the specter of shunt infection. The shunt valve currently has the greatest influence on CSF overdrainage.

VALVE DESIGN AND TERMINOLOGY

Probably the most important component of a shunt system is the valve. Neurosurgeons can choose from more than 125 commercially available valves.[13] Since the 1960s, the predominant theme in the evolution of valve design has been the goal of preventing CSF overdrainage. This includes the introduction of antisiphon devices (ASDs), flow-restricting elements, multistage valves, and adjustable valves. It is important to understand that manufacturers have little or no direct in vivo intracranial pressure (ICP) or CSF flow data to back up advertised claims such as "preventing excessive flow while allowing constant physiological drainage,"[13a] or "regulates flow through the valve at a rate close to that of CSF secretion, therefore minimizing the risks of under or overdrainage."[13b] Our studies[8] demonstrate that the in vivo behavior of even the simplest shunt, the ventriculoperitoneal (VP) shunt with a standard differential-pressure valve (DPV), is poorly predicted by the first-order, steady-flow equations that are the basis of the many valve designs.

In our opinion, there is no single valve mechanism, design, or arrangement that is clearly the "best," nor one that will be adequate for every hydrocephalus patient. There are some valves and valve settings, however, that are poorly suited for adult hydrocephalus and will likely result in a higher complication rate.

Hydrocephalus is a heterogeneous disorder with a wide range of ICPs, ventricular compliance, CSF profiles, and other features across patients. For most pediatric patients, most valve designs work satisfactorily at least in the short term. For unclear reasons, adult hydrocephalus is less forgiving, presumably owing to the less elastic brain in addition to the augmented effect of gravity-dependent drainage. Knowledge of valve design and function can greatly help in preventing and managing complications. The following is a primer on shunt valve design and characteristics with which every neurosurgeon placing shunts should be familiar.

The Differential-Pressure Valve

The basic building block of most shunt valves is a differential-pressure "check valve" mechanism. The basic design of John Holter[14] continues in some form more than a half century after its development. In most modern valve designs, it consists of a tiny sphere situated on a ring, with a spring pushing the sphere downward on the ring. CSF passes through the ring orifice, elevating the ball if the pressure exceeds the pressure exerted by the spring. This creates a one-way flow mechanism because reverse flow will not occur as the ball seats down onto the ring.

Fluid flow depends on the *differential pressure* across the ring: not necessarily the absolute CSF pressure. For example, if the spring is exerting 100 mm H_2O of pressure downward, CSF will flow if the difference between the inlet and outlet pressure is greater than 100 mm H_2O, regardless whether the inlet pressure is positive or negative.

A common misconception is that the valve opening pressure must be lower than the measured CSF pressure for CSF to flow across the valve. Our in vivo studies have demonstrated that the interaction between CSF pressure and valve function is not straightforward and that, in general, more CSF drainage occurs than one might naively predict. We studied a group of patients with idiopathic normal-pressure hydrocephalus (NPH) in whom the mean preoperative recumbent ICP was 164 ± 64 mm H_2O. Each patient underwent a VP shunt with a standard DPV (as the only valve mechanism) initially set at an opening pressure of 200 mm H_2O. Whereas one might predict that no CSF flow would occur at this valve setting, the postoperative ICP was statistically lower at 125 ± 69 mm H_2O ($P = .04$).[8]

The concepts of CSF opening pressure (which, by default, is a mean pressure), and bulk CSF flow have been the standards of hydrocephalus pathophysiology teaching for decades. The reality, however, is that the ICP waveform is pulsatile, with superimposed significant elevations of ICP occurring because of coughing and Valsalva maneuvers as well as intrinsic vasomotor changes. The phenomenon of how CSF flow can occur with valve pressure settings exceeding the "measured" CSF pressure (ICP, ventricular or lumbar pressure) can be explained by the combination of pulsatile-dynamic ICP physiology interacting with a one-way DPV.

The interaction between pulsatile ICP and the one-way valve mechanism (inherent to DPVs) is paramount to the understanding of shunt overdrainage. Our continuous ICP recordings demonstrate that peak ICPs often exceed 200 mm H_2O among patients with a mean ICP of 164 mm H_2O.[7] Even taking into account distal intra-abdominal pressure, one-way CSF egress occurs during these peaks across the DPV. The minute boluses of CSF exiting the cranial vault with every pulsation exceeding the valve pressure results in a reduction of the *mean* ICP. This "check valve" one-way flow mechanism acts like a tiny pump of sorts, theoretically resulting in more drainage through a DPV set at zero compared with a valveless shunt. This phenomenon is amplified with the use of valve pressure settings lower than the *mean* preoperative ICP and likely accounts in large part for excessive CSF drainage in clinical practice.

KEY POINT
There is a basic misconception that the valve opening pressure must be lower than the mean ventricular pressure for the shunt to flow.

Most commercially available CSF shunt valves contain a DPV mechanism in one form or another. For some, it is the sole valve mechanism, whereas in others, it is the first in-series component of the valve assembly. Examples of ball-spring valves are the Strata Valve (Medtronic, Minneapolis, MN), Codman Hakim Programmable and Precision Valves (DePuy Synthes, West Chester, PA), and the proGAV (Aesculap, Center Valley, PA). A simpler, less accurate mechanism consists of a valve mechanism derived from two apposing semirigid membranes. These valves, which include the Medtronic, Pudenz (Integra, Plainsboro, NJ), and Codman distal slit valves, are manufactured and then individually tested to determine the approximate opening pressure. They are then segregated into different bins covering a range of pressures. For example, the "medium-pressure valve" bin would contain valves ranging from 50 to 90 mm H_2O opening pressure.

Adjustable ("Programmable") Valves

A "programmable," or adjustable, valve is created by adding a mechanism that enables precise changes of the spring tension of a DPV. There are several competing designs enabling this, all incorporating a magnetic actuation of a rotor. Strictly speaking, these valves are not truly programmable and are better considered as merely *adjustable* valves. Adjustable valves arose from the realization that fixed-pressure DPVs result in either overdrainage

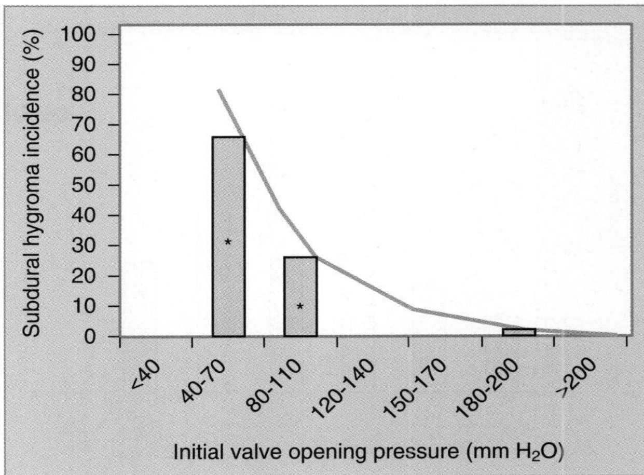

Figure 31-1. Estimated risk for subdural hygroma formation with idiopathic normal-pressure hydrocephalus. The Dutch Normal-Pressure Hydrocephalus Study[15] documented subdural hygroma (effusion) incidences of about 70% and about 30% with low- and medium-pressure differential-pressure valves, respectively (data signified with *asterisk*). We encountered a 4% incidence among patients with an initial valve setting of 200 mm H_2O. Combining these data sets results in a nearly linear relationship between valve opening pressure and subdural hygroma incidence. The hygroma incidence for other valve designs and arrangements has not been well documented. *(From Bergsneider M, Miller C, Vespa PM, et al. Surgical management of adult hydrocephalus.* Neurosurgery. *2008;62:SHC643-660.)*

or underdrainage in a significant number of adult patients. The Dutch Normal-Pressure Hydrocephalus Study,[15] a prospective, randomized study, demonstrated that subdural hygromas occurred in 71% of patients with fixed low-pressure valve shunts compared with 34% in patients randomized to medium-pressure shunts. Given the likelihood that expanding or large subdural hygromas pose a risk for subdural hematoma, this is one example showing that there is clearly a risk for selecting too low of an opening pressure. The analysis of our series of 114 consecutive idiopathic NPH patients, each treated with an initial valve opening pressure of 200 mm H_2O, revealed a subdural hygroma incidence of 4%.[7] As shown in Figure 31-1, combining the results of the Dutch Normal-Pressure Hydrocephalus Study with our experience suggests a seemingly exponential relationship between subdural hygromas and valve opening pressure.

Another justification for the routine use of adjustable valves is based on the range of "final" valve opening pressures when these valves are used. In our retrospective evaluation of 114 consecutive NPH patients surgically treated with a CSF shunt, the histogram distribution of the final valve opening pressure revealed a roughly gaussian distribution, with most patients in the 120 to 140 mm H_2O range (Fig. 31-2).[7] This finding closely agrees with other large NPH studies.[16] With the wide distribution of final valve pressures shown in Figure 31-2 (from <40 to >200 mm H_2O), it is difficult to fathom how a fixed-pressure valve could adequately serve this population unless there were a way of selecting the appropriate valve pressure preoperatively. Although some have suggested algorithms to do so,[16,17] none has been independently evaluated or validated.

KEY POINT
Most adult hydrocephalus patients with adjustable valves will require at least one valve adjustment, highlighting the risk for and downside of using a fixed-pressure valve design.

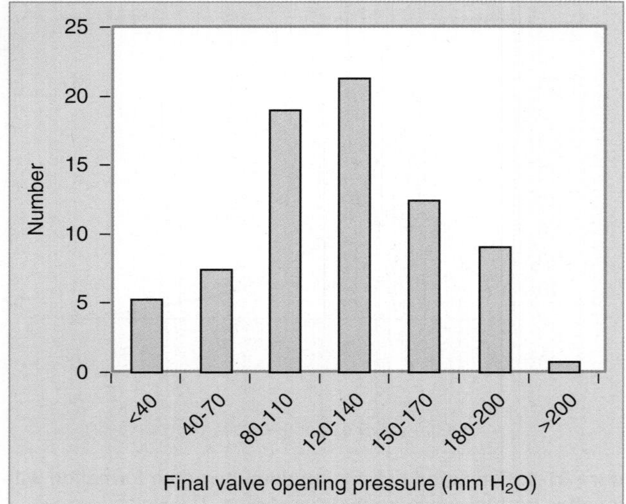

Figure 31-2. Range of valve opening pressures in the treatment of idiopathic normal-pressure hydrocephalus (iNPH). Histogram of final differential valve opening-pressure values showing a gaussian distribution centered at approximately 140 mm H_2O. The wide range of valve opening pressures required indicates that no single valve opening pressure is appropriate for the treatment of iNPH. *(From Bergsneider M, Miller C, Vespa PM, et al. Surgical management of adult hydrocephalus.* Neurosurgery. *2008;62:SHC643-660.)*

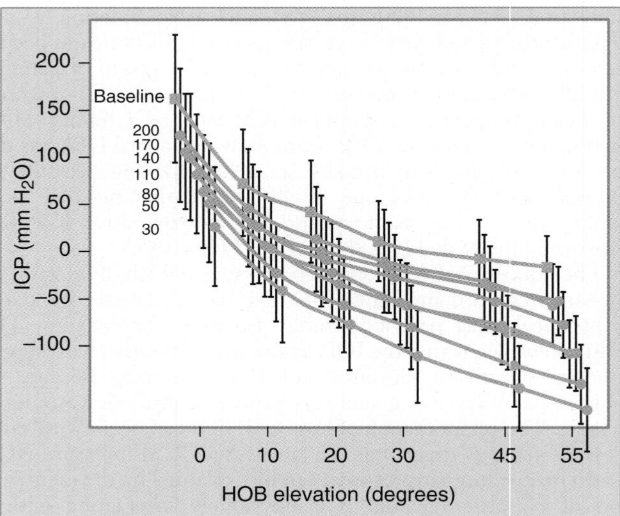

Figure 31-3. Intracranial pressure (ICP) (mean ± standard deviation) versus head-of-bed (HOB) elevation curves through the full range of differential-pressure valve opening pressures (200, 170, 140, etc.) measured from idiopathic normal-pressure hydrocephalus (iNPH) patients treated with a ventriculoperitoneal shunt. The preshunt baseline curve *(thicker line, filled square)* was obtained from the same group of patients. Note that the preoperative and postoperative curves roughly parallel one-another, demonstrating the limited role of "siphoning" as the cause of overdrainage in iNPH patients. *(Courtesy of Bergsneider M, Yang I, Hu X, et al. Relationship between valve opening pressure, body position, and intracranial pressure in normal pressure hydrocephalus: paradigm for selection of programmable valve pressure setting.* Neurosurgery. *2004;55:851-858; discussion 858-859.)*

Some neurosurgeons remain reluctant to use adjustable valves on a routine basis (or at all). Indeed, a prospective, randomized trial of predominantly pediatric patients comparing the Codman Hakim adjustable valve and a standard DPV failed to demonstrate a difference in shunt failure rates.[4] The results of this study, however, do not necessarily apply to adult hydrocephalus. Arguments that these valves are unreliable, or malfunction more frequently than fixed valves, are not supported by any clinical study (nor our clinical experience with the implantation of more than 600 of these devices). Perhaps the biggest drawback is cost. Currently, adjustable valves are 2 to 3 times more expensive than fixed-pressure valves, and there is no clinical study comparing cost-effectiveness. A direct comparison of cost utilization would have to factor in the morbidity associated with repeat operations and associated operative risks when using fixed-pressure valves.

Another drawback of adjustable valves has been MRI compatibility. Because the rotors harbor permanent magnets, some valve designs (first generation) have a higher susceptibility to large magnetic fields, especially MRI scanners. In our practice, we specifically use valves with locking mechanisms in patients in whom it is anticipated that future MRI studies are required (e.g., any patient with a brain tumor). Table 31-1 summarizes characteristics of the most commonly used adjustable valves.

Antisiphon, Flow-Restricting, and Gravitational Devices

Soon after the first DPVs were implanted in the 1950s, CSF overdrainage complications were recognized.[13,18-20] Early studies[18] documented significantly negative ICPs in shunted patients in the upright position. At the time, it was assumed that overdrainage complications (such as subdural hematomas) were due to this gravity-dependent drainage (which was originally terms "siphoning"). Over the ensuing years, multiple device types have been manufactured to counteract excessive drainage, most of which are add-on devices placed immediately distal, in series, with the primary DPV mechanism.

In our opinion, the etiology of shunt-related CSF overdrainage is multifactorial and heterogeneous, with an excessive emphasis being placed on the role of siphoning. Our ICP studies in idiopathic NPH patients,[8] as well as others,[15] suggest that historically the primary problem as been the use of DPV settings that were too low, with gravity-dependent drainage being a compounding phenomenon. It is important to note that, as any person assumes an upright position, ICP decreases whether they have a shunt or not. As a matter of fact, in the standing position, healthy adults have a slightly subatmospheric ICP (measured level with the foramen of Monro). When you place a shunt with solely a DPV, the curve of ICP compared with head-of-bed elevation in shunted patients nearly parallels that of the preshunt state (Fig. 31-3).[8] In other words, a shunt with a DPV essentially lowers the ICP nearly equally across the head-of-bed angulation range. The degree of ICP reduction is largely a function of the valve opening pressure, again supporting the notion that shunt overdrainage occurs primarily as a result of valve pressure selection.

KEY POINT

In vivo ICP data suggest that the etiology of shunt overdrainage with DPVs is in many, if not most, cases a result of a valve opening-pressure selection that is too low, rather than so-called siphoning.

Even with the use of properly selected DPV opening-pressure settings, gravity-dependent drainage can still be problematic, albeit in a minority of patients. Currently, it is not possible to

TABLE 31-1 Characteristics of Commonly Used Adjustable Valves

Valve Manufacturer	Valve Model	Variations	Primary Valve Mechanism Type	Ease of Adjustment	MRI Susceptibility	Valve Opening Pressure (range, mm H_2O)	No. of Gradations	Integral Antisiphon, Flow-Restricting, or Gravitational Device	Antisiphon or Gravitational Valve Name	Clinical Considerations
Codman	Hakim Programmable	Various form factors	Ball-spring DPV	Typically easy. Not possible to read valve setting. Large cumbersome suitcase.	High	30-200	17	No		
Codman	Hakim Programmable with SiphonGuard	Various form factors	Ball-spring DPV	Same as above	High	30-200	17	Yes	SiphonGuard	No studies demonstrating efficacy of SiphonGuard
Medtronic	Strata	Various form factors	Ball-spring DPV	StrataVarius adjustment tool very easy to use	High		5	Yes	Siphon Control Device	Siphon control device mechanism may fail if thick scar forms over it. Use in low-pressure hydrocephalus states may be contraindicated
Medtronic	Strata NSC	Various form factors	Ball-spring DPV	Same as above. Must insert separate SIMM card.	High			No (NSC means no siphon control)		
Sophysa	Polaris	Range of adjustable opening pressures	Ball-spring DPV	Can be very challenging with thick scalp	Very low	10-140, 30-200, 40-300, 50-400	5	No		
Aesculap	proGAV		Ball-spring DPV	Can be very challenging with thick scalp. Moderately painful for most patients.	Very low			No		
Aesculap	proGAV with ShuntAssistant (also called proSA)		Ball-spring DPV	Same as above	Very low			Yes	ShuntAssistant	
Integra	Orbis Sigma II		Self-adjusting pin in orifice design: flow restricting	Not externally adjustable	None	N/A		Basic design is flow restricting		No clinical evidence demonstrating clinical efficacy.

DPV, differential-pressure valve; MRI, magnetic resonance imaging.

31

predict which patients will require a second valve mechanism in addition to the DPV.

The ASD design is the oldest, consisting of a membrane that is mechanically coupled to the subcutaneous tissue overlying it.[21] The pressure differential between the internal valve lumen and the atmosphere, transmitted across the skin and ASD membrane, determines the flow-pressure characteristics of the ASD device. When the intraluminal pressure becomes significantly negative relative to atmospheric pressure, the membrane is drawn inward, interacting with other fixed components of the ASD and thereby creating an increased ASD-valve pressure gradient. A newer generation ASD design (termed a *siphon control device*) is found in the Delta Chamber Valve (Medtronic),[22] which is incorporated in the Delta Valve (fixed pressure) and the Strata Valve (adjustable DPV). For patients suffering from overdrainage headaches, the addition of an ASD can be very effective.[23]

For some hydrocephalus patients, the presence of an ASD is detrimental.[24-29] This so-called low-pressure hydrocephalus syndrome, of which the incidence has not been quantified but presumed less than 5%, occurs in both children and adults. Given the low incidence of low-pressure hydrocephalus, we do not feel that this “risk” constitutes a contraindication for the general use of products with ASDs. For clinicians who routinely use ASD devices, however, it is important that they become familiar with the signs and symptoms of low-pressure hydrocephalus.[7,24]

KEY POINT

A patient who fails to improve clinically (or deteriorates), continues to have significant ventriculomegaly that does not change, has low measured ICP, or has a patent shunt with an ASD should not be diagnosed as a nonresponder until the diagnosis of low-pressure hydrocephalus has been ruled out.[24]

Another approach taken to counteract shunt overdrainage is the incorporation of a CSF flow-restriction mechanism. The premise is that shunt overdrainage can be averted if the rate of CSF drainage is limited. There are several different design approaches to achieve flow restriction. The Orbis-Sigma II Valve (Integra) was designed to directly address flow restriction by using a multistage needle-valve design. Depending on the differential pressure, a needle is raised or lowered through a small orifice. The diameter of the needle at any given point will determine the cross-sectional area through which the CSF can flow. The manufacturer claims that in stage I, it functions as a low-pressure DPV to minimize underdrainage complications. When conditions favor postural or vasogenic overdrainage, the needle moves to stage II, and the valve functions as a flow regulator to maintain flow within physiologic limits. Lastly, the manufacture claims that if ICP elevates abruptly, the valve opens widely to function as a safety valve, allowing rapid CSF flow.

There is scarce in vivo clinical evidence, however, to support the efficacy of an ASD or the Orbis-Sigma Valve design. A large, prospective, randomized study comparing a standard DPV, the Delta Valve, and the Orbis-Sigma Valve (the original design, predating the Orbis-Sigma II) found no statistical difference in the rate of ventricular reduction, the final ventricle size, or the incidence of clinical shunt failure.[1,30] In a retrospective study comparing the Orbis-Sigma Valve with a standard DPV in NPH, Weiner and colleagues[31] found no significant difference in the time to initial malfunction (shunt survival) between the Orbis-Sigma Valve and the DPV shunts. There were three subdural hematomas and one infection in the Orbis-Sigma Valve group compared with no complications in the DPV group (P = .11). Nearly 90% of all patients experienced improvement in gait after shunting, regardless of the valve system that was used. The Orbis-Sigma II valve was studied in a single-armed, prospective, multicenter clinical study that included 270 adult hydrocephalic patients.[32] Shunt obstruction occurred in 14% of patients. The probability of having experienced a shunt failure-free interval at 1 year was 71%, and at 2 years, it was 67%, with no difference in shunt survival in pediatric versus adult groups. According to the authors, overdrainage occurred in only 2% of patients, although their definition of overdrainage was very narrow. Clinical underdrainage was not assessed.

Another approach to flow restriction is the incorporation of an add-on high flow resistance element. The Codman SiphonGuard (DePuy Synthes) is a coiled helical device that is placed immediately distal to a DPV (adjustable or fixed pressure). The SiphonGuard device is unaffected by scar tissue encapsulation or external pressure. According to the manufacturer, “When excessive flow is detected, the primary pathway closes and flow is diverted to the high resistance secondary pathway. The secondary pathway decreases the flow rate by 90% while maintaining a drainage rate within physiological ranges, which prevents the damaging complications due to overdrainage.”[13a] To our knowledge, to date there are no published clinical studies evaluating the SiphonGuard device in vivo. In vitro bench-top testing from an independent laboratory[33] demonstrates that switching between the primary and secondary pathways was initiated at a fluid flow rate between 700 and 1800 μL/min.

Miyake and associates[17] created an externalized loop connected to an indwelling VP shunt and measured CSF flow rates in patients with NPH. They assessed the Codman adjustable (DPV) and Orbis-Sigma valves. They demonstrated that shunt flow differed across patients, but in general, flow increased as the adjustable valve setting was lowered regardless of whether the patient was recumbent or sitting. At higher opening pressures of the adjustable valve (140 to 200 mm H_2O) in the recumbent position, the flow was intermittent, whereas at the lowest setting of 30 mm H_2O, the flow rate was 100 to 200 μL/min. In the sitting position, the shunt flow rates were higher, ranging from 200 to 600 μL/min. Based on these data in which measured CSF flow rates did not exceed 600 μL/min, it is unclear whether the flow-restricting circuit in the SiphonGuard would be activated at all in NPH. Similar flow data do not exist for younger hydrocephalus patients to our knowledge, although presumably the flow rates may be higher than in NPH patients. For the Orbis-Sigma Valve, the flow rates were very similar to the adjustable valve set at 200 mm H_2O in both the recumbent and sitting positions. This actual in vivo flow data would appear to contradict the Orbis-Sigma manufacturer’s concept that in stage I, it functions as a low-pressure DPV. There are no in vivo data available to either confirm or refute the manufacturer’s claims regarding stage II and III activity.

Medtronic manufactures a peritoneal catheter with a smaller internal diameter, which also achieves a fixed added flow resistance. This catheter is intended to be used in conjunction with a DPV. To date, there have been no published clinical studies addressing the clinical efficacy or pitfalls of this approach. Interestingly, Sotelo and colleagues[34] reported the use of a valveless shunt that incorporated solely a peritoneal catheter with a highly precise cross-sectional internal diameter of 0.51 mm to limit CSF flow (a much higher resistance compared with the Medtronic catheter). At the end of the observation period of 44 ± 17 months, the failure rate of the shunting device was 14% for the high-resistance valveless shunt compared with 46% for controls (P < .0002). Shunt endurance was 88% for patients with the valveless shunt and 60% for patients with conventional valve shunts. Signs of overdrainage developed in 40% of patients treated with valved shunts, but apparently were not observed in patients with the high-resistance valveless shunt.

Another approach to combat overdrainage has been with the so-called gravitational devices. This is accomplished through a mechanical mechanism using dense spheres that divert the CSF into one of two parallel DPVs. When the patient is in the recumbent position, the opening pressure is zero, whereas CSF is diverted to a DPV with a higher opening pressure in the upright position. This approach is not new (the Integra Horizontal-Vertical Valve has been marketed for more than two decades), but recent improved designs have offered a graded transition.

Aesculap manufactures both fixed (ShuntAssistant) and adjustable (proSA) gravitational valves. When used alone without a series adjustable DPV, the fixed gravitational devices have shown mixed results with regard to preventing overdrainage or underdrainage clinical conditions.[35,36] It was subsequently recommended that these gravitational devices be used in series distal to an adjustable DPV, although this, too, has been beset with technical problems.[37] Our anecdotal experience with the add-on Aesculap ShuntAssistant (fixed) valve is that although it could be effective in alleviating overdrainage headaches, underdrainage symptoms led to a large proportion of these devices being explanted.

The combination of an adjustable DPV together with the proSA allows the maximal degree of shunt management. Analogous to the concept that a fixed-pressure DPV does not allow tailoring to individual patient needs, it is likely that addressing the heterogeneous overdrainage problems (in patients in whom an adjustable DPV failed) is best done with an adjustable gravitational device. We have encountered NPH patients who cannot tolerate further lowering of an adjustable DPV because of overdrainage symptoms (headache, hearing loss) and yet who fail to improve clinically (gait, bladder control). The use of the adjustable DPV and the proSA has been highly effective in correcting both the simultaneous overdrainage and underdrainage states in many of these cases in our anecdotal experience. In other patients with chronic headaches without postural dependence, this approach has not been effective. A major drawback to the combined adjustable valve approach is high cost. See Table 31-2 for a summary of antisiphon, flow-restricting, and gravitational device characteristics.

MANAGING SHUNT OVERDRAINAGE AND UNDERDRAINAGE

Overdrainage

The term *overdrainage* means different things to different people. In our view, it is a condition that is caused by excessive CSF drainage or intracranial hypotension *and* is of clinical significance. Overdrainage typically manifests as either postural headaches (with or without nausea or other ill feelings) or imaging evidence of pathologic subdural fluid collections.

Overdrainage headache symptoms are equivalent to a post–lumbar puncture or "spinal" headache. We know from the lumbar puncture literature that, depending on needle size and design, the incidence of post–dural puncture headaches is 1% to 30%.[38] Presumably, most subjects after lumbar puncture experience some period of intracranial hypotension, but only a minority are sensitive to the state. This means that the mere presence of negative ICP is not pathognomonic of overdrainage. In fact, our studies and others [8,18] document that some degree of intracranial hypotension is the norm in shunted patients (data exist primarily for DPV shunts), but only a small percentage complain of postural headaches.

KEY POINT

In shunted patients undergoing continuous ICP monitoring, the finding of negative ICPs in the upright position is not diagnostic of shunt overdrainage; there must be accompanying symptoms to establish this diagnosis.

The determination of postural headaches is straightforward in most cases. The patient will have clearly recognized that the headache (or other) symptoms occur within minutes of assuming an upright position and are alleviated immediately with recumbency. ICP monitoring is not needed in such cases. Furthermore, postural headaches can occur in the setting of unchanged ventricle size, a reduction in ventricle size, or the presence of subdural fluid collections. Increasing the DPV opening pressure (by at least 30 mm H_2O) usually alleviates postural headache symptoms within 1 hour of the intervention. The use of adjustable valves obviates the need for a shunt revision in most of these cases. In the situation in which the patient is already at the maximal valve opening pressure of an adjustable valve (or has a fixed-pressure or other valve), a shunt revision is typically required to either add an ASD or gravitational device or, with the latter scenario, change the valve to an adjustable valve with a higher range of pressures. As mentioned previously, adjustable gravitational valves offer the greatest leeway in management and have been shown to be highly effective in alleviating overdrainage symptoms.[39] When postural headaches are mild, conservative measures such as hydration often can bide patients over until their body re-equilibrates and the symptoms abate spontaneously.

Less commonly, headache may not be the main symptom of shunt overdrainage. Some patients complain of only nausea, whereas others have difficulty concentrating. For patients who have new-onset headaches not present before the shunt operation, there should be a clinical suspicion of overdrainage even if there is no clear postural relationship.

In general, overdrainage headaches do not occur in a delayed manner. In other words, a patient who has been doing fine for months will not spontaneously present with overdrainage symptoms. Exceptions to this rule might include new subdural fluid collection or inadvertent shunt adjustment (such as with an MRI).

The development of subdural fluid collections is a second possible manifestation of shunt overdrainage. Subdural hygroma (also known as effusions) formation is relatively common in the shunted NPH population. Small subdural hygromas (<5 mm) are usually asymptomatic[15] and are often associated with improvement in NPH symptoms because their presence only occurs in conjunction with reduction of the ventricular system. As a result, the presence of a subdural hygroma is not by itself diagnostic of shunt overdrainage. Expanding or large subdural hygromas are more worrisome, and many would agree they are a risk factor for the development of acute hemorrhage (subdural hematoma). A non–trauma-related subdural hematoma in a shunted patient is obviously an overdrainage presentation.

It is our observation that shunted patients undergoing a contrast-enhanced MRI sometimes show diffuse pachymeningeal enhancement—the same finding that is used to diagnose spontaneous intracranial hypotension. Given that most shunts generate some degree of intracranial hypotension, this enhancement pattern is not necessarily indicative of clinical overdrainage. If postural symptoms are present, however, then the finding may support an overdrainage diagnosis.

"Slit" or collapsed ventricles are typically a manifestation of *chronic* overdrainage. Not all patients with slit (or unilateral slit) ventricles have symptoms, but it is generally agreed that this state increases the risk for ventricular shunt obstruction. The apposition of the ventricular catheter to the ventricular wall increases the chance of ingrowth of ependymal cells or choroid plexus. The adult slit ventricle syndrome is an ill-defined disorder, but the key components are a symptomatic, shunted patient with slit or collapsed ventricles seen on computed tomography or MRI. Its incidence is unknown, but it represents about 5% of the non-NPH evaluations in our clinic.[7] Although relatively few in number, these patients represent a disproportionate amount of clinical

TABLE 31-2 Antisiphon Device, Flow Restriction, and Gravitational Valve Characteristics

Valve Manufacturer	Valve Model	Form Factors	Mechanism	Adjustable?	Ease of Adjustment	MRI Susceptibility	Valve Opening Pressure (range, mm H_2O)	No. of Adjustment Gradations	Integration with DPV	Available as Stand Alone?	Clinical Considerations
Codman	SiphonGuard	Low profile, cylindrical	At flow rates exceeding 0.7-1.5 μL/min, primary pathway closes and flow is diverted to the high resistance secondary pathway	No	N/A	None	N/A	N/A	Available integrated with various Codman valves	Yes	Lack of clinical study documenting efficacy or corroborating manufacturer claims
Medtronic	Delta Chamber	Low profile, button sized	Siphon control device is a membrane housed within chamber that changes flow resistance relative to atmospheric pressure	No	N/A	None	N/A	N/A	Integrated into Strata II and Delta valves	Yes	Siphon control device mechanism may be ineffectual due to scar formation or in low pressure hydrocephalus states
Aesculap	ShuntAssistant	Low profile cylindrical	Tantalum spheres direct CSF to differential pressure valve in upright position. Supine valve pressure always zero.	No	N/A	None	Various upright pressure level settings available: 100, 150, 200, 250, 300, and 350	N/A	No	Yes	Unclear how to determine which model to use for any given patient
Aesculap	proSA	Moderate low profile	Same as ShuntAssistant	Yes	Programming device causes moderate discomfort and can be very challenging with thick scalp	None at 3 Tesla	Upright pressure level setting adjustable between 0 and 400	24	No	Yes	Combined with adjustable DPV provides highest degree of management options but at greatly added cost

CSF, cerebrospinal fluid; DPV, differential pressure valve; MRI, magnetic resonance imaging.

effort expended, with frequent emergency department visits and requests for office visits. The syndrome occurs more commonly in patients who have been shunted for many years, either as an adult or in childhood. Additionally, it is our observation that a significant proportion of patients with adult slit ventricle syndrome have previously unrecognized noncommunicating hydrocephalus.

Common symptoms of adult slit ventricle syndrome include intermittent headaches that become more frequent and intense over time. The etiology of these intermittent headaches has been unclear but may be related to periods of insufficient CSF drainage. In addition, collapse of the ventricular system lowers intracranial compliance, further amplifying elevations in ICP during shunt underdrainage. At shunt revision, the typical intraoperative finding is near-total, but not complete, obstruction of the ventricular catheter (typically only one or two holes are patent). Left untreated, the symptoms may progress to more continuous headaches, presumably owing to completed mechanical obstruction of the shunt system. Therefore the slit ventricle syndrome is actually an underdrainage syndrome created by a preceding period of overdrainage.

Significant hearing loss is an uncommon complication of CSF shunting. One small prospective study showed a significant increase in the mean threshold in most frequencies and the pure tone average after VP shunt placement.[40] In our experience, the hearing loss is reversible with valve pressure adjustments.

Underdrainage

In many cases, shunt underdrainage is easy to recognize. This includes patients who were obviously symptomatic from hydrocephalus and then fail to improve after shunt surgery, or see a return of their symptoms with clinical deterioration. Similarly, interval enlargement of the ventricles is diagnostic of underdrainage.

The patient in whom the association between clinical findings and ventriculomegaly is uncertain and who fails to improve after shunt surgery (or only minimally improves) represents a clinical challenge. This is especially problematic in NPH patients because there always exists some doubt in the diagnosis. As a result, the failure to improve might be attributed to an incorrect diagnosis (an underrecognized weakness of many NPH clinical studies).

For example, what if there is no clinical improvement in a suspected NPH patient despite the valve being brought down to its lowest setting? After confirming shunt patency, many might consider such a patient a nonresponder and therefore by inference misdiagnosed. For patients in this scenario who remain with significant ventriculomegaly, the low-pressure hydrocephalus state should be considered.[25,29] In these patients, clinical improvement strongly coincides with reduction in the ventricular size, and only with significant negative ICP does reduction in the ventricular size occur. Not surprisingly, this state occurs with higher incidence in patients with ASDs.[24-29]

In NPH, if imaging reveals a reduction in ventricular size, then a patient should be considered a nonresponder if no clinical improvement has occurred. Downward adjustments in valve opening pressure are unlikely to benefit the patient and instead increase the risk for subdural hematoma.

If underdrainage is suspected, shunt obstruction is always a consideration. Based largely on the experience with pediatric hydrocephalus, many neurosurgeons use nuclear medicine isotope studies to determine shunt patency.[41-44] At our center, however, we have found fewer indications for this study, and it is now rarely obtained. The primary reason is that the results of the study seldom alter the clinical decision tree, and second, it cannot differentiate mechanical from *functional* shunt overdrainage.

> **KEY POINT**
> In NPH, documenting shunt patency with a nuclear medicine isotope study is not diagnostic of a shunt nonresponder. Functional underdrainage must be considered.

VALVE SELECTION

There are no evidenced-based guidelines to support any recommendations. If the prospective pediatric hydrocephalus valve studies[1,3,4,30,45] were extrapolated to the adult population, no one valve design would appear to hold an advantage. Most would agree that NPH is clearly a distinct entity from pediatric hydrocephalus forms, and therefore the relevance of the previously mentioned studies can be challenged. Based on peer-reviewed published clinical studies and our own large experience, we see no reasonable justification for not using an adjustable valve for NPH. Although adjustable valves are not the panacea, the use of a nonadjustable valves for the treatment of NPH exposes the patient to an unacceptable underdrainage or overdrainage risk.

In our view, the more difficult question pertains to the younger adult age group (18 to 65 years). Our routine practice includes the use of an adjustable valve for all adult patients, although admittedly, there are fewer published data to support this practice. What is not known is whether the added cost can be justified relative to the selective benefit in this cohort. Because we have no way of differentiating which patients might or might not benefit from the use of an adjustable valve, we do not feel that the cost of the device should dictate the decision. An adjustable valve will be equivalent or better than a standard fixed DPV for any given adult patient.

The next question is whether an adjustable valve should be used alone or in conjunction with another device. There is no evidence demonstrating that valve designs incorporating an ASD, a flow-restricting device, or a gravitational device lower the incidence of overdrainage complications. In our opinion, what is important is that the clinician understand the potential pitfalls and risks of each valve type (including the stand-alone DPV) and be able to recognize possible shunt overdrainage and underdrainage states.

The second decision in valve selection is choosing the initial opening pressure. Our experience since the 1990s is largely limited to the use of an adjustable, stand-alone DPV. For NPH, it is our experience that about 2% will have clinical overdrainage despite a valve pressure setting of 200 mm H_2O, and the other 2% will underdrain at a setting as low as 30 mm H_2O. As mentioned previously, an additional small percentage experience simultaneous overdrainage and underdrainage problems at various valve settings. An adjustable valve with a range from 10 to 240 mm H_2O therefore meets the needs of most NPH patients based on our experience.

In our practice, for NPH patients the valve is initially set at 200 mm H_2O unless they are of short stature, in which cases settings as low as 140 mm H_2O are used. The opening pressure is sequentially lowered, typically by 30 mm over 2 to 3 weeks to effect. In a prospective double-blind, randomized, controlled, dual-center study using a VP shunt with an adjustable valve, patients were randomized to an initial setting of 200 mm H_2O with gradual reduction versus maintaining a fixed setting of 120 mm H_2O.[46] An equal percentage (~22%) experienced a shunt complication; 9 had subdural hematomas, 3 mechanical obstructions, and 1 infection. The frequency of overdrainage symptoms was significantly higher for a valve setting of 120 mm H_2O or less compared with a setting of greater than 120 mm H_2O. The adjustment group had a higher improvement rate (88%) than the fixed group (62%) ($P = .032$).[46]

We recommend that younger, non-NPH patients receive even higher opening-pressure settings (upper opening pressures of 300 or 400 mm H_2O) or, alternatively, incorporate an adjustable gravitational device in series with the standard adjustable valve (30 to 200 mm H_2O).

SHUNT CONFIGURATION

Cerebrospinal Fluid Access

For routine shunt placement, we prefer a frontal (precoronal) ventricular puncture shunt rather than a posterior or occipital shunt. A retrospective analysis of shunt operations from the United Kingdom Registry Study that frontal catheters were adequately placed in 67% of cases, whereas occipital catheters were adequate in 52%.[47] The use of frameless stereotaxis has been shown to improve optimal catheter placement,[48] and we routinely use it for patients with a bifrontal distance (maximal distance of lateral frontal horns) of less than 40 mm. The tip of the catheter should reside just anterior to the ipsilateral foramen of Monro[49] to keep it away from the choroid plexus. Time to failure has been shown to be significantly affected by the accuracy of catheter placement, with a 66% higher risk with poor placement relative to optimal placement.[50] If the ventricles are large, the catheter is first positioned orthogonal to the skull, then slightly angled about 5 degrees anteriorly before the freehand insertion. The ideal depth is typically 5 cm of catheter at the dura.

Occipital ventricular catheter placement offers the marginal advantage of avoiding the retroauricular "turn the corner" incision necessary with frontal shunts. A disadvantage is that the adjustable valve can end up in the suboccipital region, making it difficult or impossible to readjust. For occipital shunt placement, a third incision should be considered anterior and superior to the ventricular catheter incision, thereby situating the adjustable valve over the occipital retroauricular region. With this configuration, the subgaleal catheter ascends cranially before making the turn at the third incision caudally to connect with the valve.

As a general rule, every shunt incision should be carefully planned so that it does not directly overlie a shunt component. Failure to do so increases the risk for skin breakdown. We routinely place a modified titanium bur hole cover (one sector removed) over the frontal bur hole site after the catheter is situated. This prevents dimpling of the skin into the bur hole, which can result in poor cosmesis and sometimes discomfort.

Some neurosurgeons routinely use ventricular endoscopy to assist ventricular shunt placement. A recent multicenter trial demonstrated no benefit from this strategy.[51] In our opinion, endoscopy is not a substitute for stereotaxis. A poor initial trajectory may not be remediable by attempted endoscopic catheter placement.

Distal Site

Since 1995, our center has performed a similar number of VP and ventriculoatrial (VA) shunts. We and others have found a nearly identical complication rate between the two techniques.[7,52] We use a pragmatic decision-making process. If the patient is not obese and has no history (or low probability) of peritoneal adhesions, then a VP shunt is offered. Otherwise, a VA shunt is recommended. There is a growing literature regarding laparoscopy-assisted peritoneal catheter placement for obese patients and patients with peritoneal adhesions.[53-57] Laparoscopy can virtually eliminate the complication of retraction of the peritoneal catheter into the subcutaneous pocket underlying the wound. The perception that the infection rate is higher with VA shunts compared with VP shunts is not supported by the literature.[7,58] Shunt nephritis, an immune-complex–mediated glomerulonephritis, is an extremely rare complication that results from long-term, subacute bacteremia (typically an indolent species such as *Staphylococcus epidermidis*).[59]

Our techniques for VP and VA shunt placement are shown in Videos 31-1 and 31-2, respectively. For VA shunts, we routinely use a modified percutaneous technique[60-62] and place the catheter tip in the superior vena cava just above the atrium to minimize the risk for sinus arrhythmias. We routinely use intraoperative fluoroscopy to confirm optimal placement of the catheter tip. For patient in which radiographic confirmation cannot be used, we use an electrocardiographic (ECG) localization technique.[63] This may occur because of positioning constraints or interference with a pacemaker. In brief, the atrial catheter, once placed, is attached sterilely to intravenous tubing primed by the scrub nurse with bicarbonate saline. A Jahar electrode is interposed in the tubing and carefully secured to the anesthesia drapes so that the anesthesiologist can secure an ECG monitoring lead. This arrangement ensures sterility by maintaining all intraluminal components on the surgical field. The ECG tracing is then monitored as the atrial catheter is advanced. Typically, the P wave enlarges as the atrium is approached, then becomes biphasic as the sinoatrial node is reached. Withdrawing the catheter 1 cm then places the catheter tip at the distal superior vena cava.

INFECTION AVOIDANCE

Nearly every prospective pediatric population shunt study has reported an infection rate of about 8%.[1,3,4,51] Less information is available about infection rates for adults. There are clearly multiple contributing factors for shunt infections, but given the highest incidence within the first month of surgery, a "contamination" most likely occurs at the time of the shunt surgery. A study by Kulkarni and associates[64] suggested that many are iatrogenic and identified surgical glove breaks as one of the likely and common culprits.[65]

KEY POINT
Double gloving by all surgical staff and surgeons should be considered standard of care for all shunt operations.

Meta-analyses support the routine use of perioperative intravenous antibiotics.[66,67] We routinely used cephalozin (Ancef), although an argument could be made for an antibiotic with better CNS penetration. There are few or no data based on randomized trials demonstrating that any preoperative or intraoperative interventions (other than preoperative antibiotics) influence the rate of shunt infections.

We routinely remove the hair (with clippers) over the surgical areas after the patient is anesthetized. Our rationale is that there is greater assurance that the surgical preparation solution will cleanse and make contact with all surfaces exposed after draping if the hair has been removed. Although thorough cleansing of the hair may be achievable in young children with fine hair, we do not believe this is achievable in most adults with thicker hair.

For "healthy" patients undergoing a primary, uncomplicated shunt operation, basically we employ only the previously mentioned measures. For other patients, we use a tailored approach. Before every shunt operation, we investigate the risk factors for shunt infection. These include any of the following: malnourishment, diabetes mellitus, open sores or wounds, hospitalization for more than 24 hours, shunt revision within 3 months, and immunosuppression (including steroids). If possible, a shunt operation should be postponed for patients with active infections, such as a urinary tract infection, until the infection is resolved. In many cases, it is prudent to enlist the aid of an infectious diseases consultant. High-risk patients undergo a more extensive preoperative skin preparation. These include intensive care unit (ICU) patients with an external ventriculostomy, patients with history of a shunt operation within 30 days, patients with a tracheostomy, and patients with a history of problematic skin infections. After clipping the hair as described earlier, all adhesive residues along the tract are removed using an adhesive remover solvent. This is particularly important in neurosurgical ICU patients who have had ventriculostomies, electroencephalogram leads, or recent craniotomies. These adhesive residues are not removed by the standard sterile preparation, and in our opinion, the space underlying them may be contaminated by virulent nosocomial organisms. After the adhesive residue is removed, we gently cleanse the skin with a mild detergent before a final surgical "sterile" preparation with povidone-iodine or chlorhexidine.

Clinical studies strongly support the routine use of antibiotic-impregnated catheters. A retrospective review of hospital discharge and billing records from 12,589 consecutive cases from 287 U.S. hospital systems of adult and pediatric patients undergoing de novo ventricular shunt placement revealed a significant reduction in infection in adult patients who received antibiotic-impregnated catheters (2.2% versus 3.6%; $P = .02$).[68] Analysis of the same data set revealed tremendous cost savings with the use of these catheters as well.[69] An analysis by Eymann and colleagues[70] suggests that, despite the incremental implant costs associated with the use of antibiotic impregnated catheters, the overall reduction in infection-related costs made their use cost beneficial. We routinely use antibiotic impregnated catheters for all shunt operations.

A third tier of antimicrobials is the instillation of intrathecal (intraventricular) antibiotics at the time of the shunt operation.[71] This better addresses the possibility of CSF "contamination" at the time of surgery. Many of the common skin bacteria associated with shunt infections, such as coagulase-negative staphylococci and *Propionibacterium acnes*, are highly sensitive to antibiotics, and therefore giving a high concentration of intraventricular antibiotics is likely beneficial. Since 2013, we have routinely used intrathecal antibiotics for all higher risk shunt operations (as defined previously). The antibiotic solution (tobramycin 8 mg and vancomycin 10 mg in 6 mL of saline) is prepared by the hospital pharmacy in a sterile hood.

A wound breakdown or CSF leak increases the risk for (or is a sign of) shunt infection.[64] The importance of planning the incision sites and configurations, so as to not overlie any shunt hardware, cannot be overemphasized. We do not use monopolar electrocautery (and avoid any coagulation) on skin incisions. Meticulous closure of the wounds is also important. For scalp wounds, after an interrupted layer of absorbable galeal sutures, we routinely close the skin using a 3-0 (or 4-0) running vertical mattress suture to best appose and align the skin edges.

Although usually straightforward, shunt placement carries one of the highest complication rates among neurosurgery operations. Attention to detail and careful planning and surgical technique can mitigate many risk factors.

KEY POINT
Patient morbidity related to a shunt infection (or a poorly placed shunt) is high, and therefore the operation deserves the same attention to detail and degree of resident supervision as any major neurosurgery operation.

Shunt Allergies

True shunt allergies are rare. CSF often demonstrates persistent eosinophilia (3% to 36%) with negative cultures. Recurrent shunt failure is a common presentation. Pathologic examination of the ventricular catheter often demonstrates mechanical obstruction by inflammatory debris consisting of eosinophils and multinucleated giant cells. There are documented cases of immune responses to unpolymerized silicone in the literature.[72-74] There are several management strategies. One is to consider an ETV and remove the offending shunt. A second is to use a shunt system with hyperextruded silicone components (Medtronic). According to the manufacturer, many shunt allergies arise from a reaction to the oils used during the silicone manufacturing.

MISCELLANEOUS CONDITIONS AND CLINICAL CHALLENGES

High Protein Concentration or Cell Count in the Cerebrospinal Fluid

High CSF protein concentration alone does not appear to increase the incidence of shunt obstruction.[75] It is the cell count (which is often associated with a high protein concentration) that is more problematic. Ideally, the fewer the total cells the better, specifically white blood cells. Issues such as pleocytosis chronicity must be considered, and therefore it is not possible to assign (an arbitrary) cutoff point for cell number. For example, in a patient with coccidioidomycosis meningitis, you may have to accept CSF cell counts in the hundreds.

The Patient Undergoing Anticoagulation or Antiplatelet Therapy

We make every effort to normalize the clotting profile before shunt implantation. Antiplatelet therapy is stopped at least 8 days before surgery. Patients on anticoagulants must be fully reversed and, if necessary, temporarily placed on enoxaparin (Lovenox), which is then discontinued 24 hours before surgery. A normal partial thromboplastin time and international normalized ratio (INR) are documented before skin incision. After surgery, anticoagulants can be restarted as early as 3 to 5 days postoperatively.[76] It is critical to maintain a tightly controlled INR. Aspirin or clopidogrel (Plavix) is begun 7 to 10 after surgery. In our opinion, combined aspirin and clopidogrel are contraindicated after shunt surgery because of the high risk for subdural hematoma.

The Hemicraniectomy Patient

Managing hydrocephalus in a patient with a hemicraniectomy is challenging. This hypercompliant state is prone to both shunt underdrainage and overdrainage situations in the same patient, depending on body position. If possible, it is advisable to perform the cranioplasty before the shunt placement or as soon as possible if a shunt is already present. During this cranioplasty, we place multiple central dural tack-up sutures every 2 cm. Failure to do so greatly increases the risk for an epidural hematoma after the shunt is placed (or if already present).

Shunt Operations Associated with Other Procedures

For patients undergoing a lengthy craniotomy (such as for tumor resection), we avoid placing a shunt at the same operation. There is typically a higher CSF cell count associated at the time, and the longer operative time increases the risk for shunt infection.

Continuity Care of the Pediatric Hydrocephalus into Adulthood

The transition from the pediatric to the adult neurosurgeon can be very stressful for the patient and family because a lifelong bond is seemingly broken. Based on our experience, the following observations and recommendations are offered: (1) Shunt failure in early adulthood in a patient who has not had a shunt revision since early childhood is frequently a highly challenging scenario. Shunt underdrainage and overdrainage are frequent, and therefore the combination of adjustable DPV and gravitational valves should be considered. (2) Always assess for the potential use of ETV. Long-term shunting does not necessarily equate to shunt dependence. (3) Seek guidance from pediatric neurosurgery colleagues, preferably the referring one if possible.

In a small retrospective study, 10% of pediatric patients had become shunt independent before adulthood. Twenty-two percent of shunts remained intact without revision for up to 35 years (mean functional intactness of 23 years). Seventy-five percent of patients worked on a daily basis, and 45% lived independently.[77]

ROLE OF ENDOSCOPIC THIRD VENTRICULOSCOPY

There exists a controversy regarding the efficacy of ETV in adult patients with extraventricular ("communicating") hydrocephalus, particularly in NPH.[78-81] In a 2008 multicenter clinical trial, Gangemi and colleagues[82] reported a nearly 70% rate of (marginal) clinical improvement, with a low complication rate, in patients with communicating NPH treated with ETV. This study was criticized because their patients had not systematically undergone a lumbar drainage trial preoperatively, and therefore the extent of expected improvement was not known. In a recent randomized clinical trial comparing ETV to VP shunt for NPH, Pinto and associates reported that VP shunt is a superior method because it had better functional neurological outcomes 12 months after surgery.[83] (For further information and a discussion of ETV, see Chapter 32.)

As mentioned previously, evidence of physical ventricular obstruction should be sought in all patients to assess whether ETV is an option.[84,85] Even if the ETV results in shunt independence, theoretically the conversion of ventricular to extraventricular hydrocephalus should lower the risk for subdural hematoma formation by more evenly equalizing the intraventricular and subarachnoid pressures following the ETV.

With regard to ETV technique in adults, principally it is the same.[10] Video 31-3 demonstrates the technique we use.

Disclosure

The author has received travel stipends from Codman and Shurtleff, Medtronics, Aesculap, and Sophysa. The author has served on Advisory Boards for Codman and Shurtleff and Medtronics. Clinically, the University of California, Los Angeles, Adult Hydrocephalus Center uses Codman, Medtronic, Sophysa, Aesculap, and Integra products.

Acknowledgment

Eric Stiner, MD, contributed a significant effort in the writing of the previous edition of this chapter while he was a neurosurgery resident at the University of California, Los Angeles.

SUGGESTED READINGS

Drake JM. Does double gloving prevent cerebrospinal fluid shunt infection? *J Neurosurg*. 2006;104:3-4.

Drake JM, Kestle JR, Milner R, et al. Randomized trial of cerebrospinal fluid shunt valve design in pediatric hydrocephalus. *Neurosurgery*. 1998;43:294-303.

Dusick JR, McArthur DL, Bergsneider M. Success and complication rates of endoscopic third ventriculostomy for adult hydrocephalus: a series of 108 patients. *Surg Neurol*. 2008;69:5-15.

Ellegaard L, Mogensen S, Juhler M. Ultrasound-guided percutaneous placement of ventriculoatrial shunts. *Childs Nerv Syst*. 2007;23:857-862.

Eymann R, Chehab S, Strowitzki M, et al. Clinical and economic consequences of antibiotic-impregnated cerebrospinal fluid shunt catheters. *J Neurosurg Pediatr*. 2008;1:444-450.

Goodwin CR, Kharkar S, Wang P, et al. Evaluation and treatment of patients with suspected normal pressure hydrocephalus on long-term warfarin anticoagulation therapy. *Neurosurgery*. 2007;60:497-501.

See a full reference list on ExpertConsult.com

32 The Role of Third Ventriculostomy in Adults and Children: A Critical Review

Walavan Sivakumar, James M. Drake, and Jay Riva-Cambrin

The daily incorporation of the endoscope into neurosurgical practice represents a paradigm shift toward a minimally invasive surgical approach to neurological disease. The ability to view deep-seated cerebral target structures with a close-up and wide-angle view has revolutionized the surgical management of ventricular, sellar, and parasellar disease. In this chapter, we will review the use of endoscopic third ventriculostomy (ETV) in both adult and pediatric hydrocephalus.

COMPARISON OF ADULT AND PEDIATRIC HYDROCEPHALUS

Epidemiology

Despite the large societal effect of adult and pediatric hydrocephalus, the current literature has a dearth of scientific data on adult hydrocephalus. Much more is known about the incidence, prevalence, epidemiologic factors, inpatient hospitalization, health care costs, and mortality associated with hydrocephalus in children. Simon and colleagues[1] estimated that there are nearly 40,000 admissions for hydrocephalus each year in the United States, with approximately 400,000 hospital days and $2 billion per year in hospital charges for the care of pediatric hydrocephalus alone. Although hydrocephalus accounts for more inpatient utilization than do comparable chronic conditions like cystic fibrosis, Gross and colleagues found that it receives only 4% of the National Institutes of Health (NIH) funding.[2] Studies such as this have identified pediatric hydrocephalus as an area that needs greater research efforts. After confirming these results in the NIH Research Portfolio Online Reporting Tools (RePORT) database, Gross and associates[2] recommended that researchers consider partnerships, when appropriate, with small businesses, as well as other non-NIH sources of funding.

Tisell and colleagues[3] conducted a cross-sectional study to evaluate the incidence of adult hydrocephalus in Sweden. They identified 891 adult patients with new diagnoses of and receiving treatment for hydrocephalus during a 3-year period; that number represented an incidence of 3.6 per 100,000. Tisell and colleagues also found that the incidence increased over the 3 years of study. In a North American setting, Patwardhan and Nanda[4] used the Nationwide Inpatient Sample database to ascertain that 8305 new cases of pediatric and adult hydrocephalus were treated in the United States in 2000. The rate of inpatient mortality secondary to hydrocephalus was 2.7%, and the overall cost to the health care system was estimated to be $1.1 billion in 2000. Bondurant and Jimenez[5] used a similar database to estimate the overall prevalence of hydrocephalus in the United States at 125,000 cases in 1988, with 36,000 cerebrospinal fluid (CSF) shunt operations being performed each year. Neither of these studies specifically addressed the adult population, inasmuch as pediatric cases were amalgamated into the patient set.

The causes and incidences of hydrocephalus differ vastly between children and adults. Tisell and colleagues[3] found that the most common subtypes of adult hydrocephalus diagnosed were normal-pressure hydrocephalus (NPH; 47%); acquired communicating high-pressure hydrocephalus from bleeding, such as post-subarachnoid hemorrhage (15%); adult-onset aqueductal stenosis (10%); other noncommunicating hydrocephalus (e.g., tectal glioma; 9%); and communicating hydrocephalus acquired from trauma (5%). The Hydrocephalus Clinical Research Network, which is a 10-center network dedicated to studying pediatric hydrocephalus, gathered unpublished data that indicate that the five most common causes of pediatric hydrocephalus are intraventricular hemorrhage resulting from premature birth (22%), myelomeningocele (16%), posterior fossa tumor (11%), aqueductal stenosis (8%), and congenital communicating hydrocephalus (8%).[6]

PATIENT SELECTION AND OUTCOMES

Pediatric Hydrocephalus

The overall success rate of ETV is between 50% and 90% at 1 year,[7-10] primarily because hydrocephalus has such a heterogeneous set of causes, which vary with the age of the population being studied. For example, the success rate of ETV for children with hydrocephalus secondary to tectal gliomas is 88%,[9] whereas ETVs done in the context of intraventricular hemorrhage associated with prematurity succeed in only 0% to 33% of cases.[11,12] Therefore, careful patient selection is absolutely essential in maximizing the chances of success and minimizing the complications inherent in ETV.

Young age (less than 6 months) is associated with a lower success rate, independent of cause; however, this age effect either plateaus or diminishes after the age of 2 years, perhaps because of cranial maturation.[8,13] The literature indicates that the success rate for ETV is high in patients older than 2 years with noncommunicating hydrocephalus caused by aqueductal stenosis, tectal glioma, and posterior fossa tumors.[8,9] On the other hand, the success rate in patients with hydrocephalus caused by intraventricular hemorrhage in association with prematurity or postinfectious hydrocephalus appears to be lower; thus its use in these populations is somewhat controversial.[11,12,14]

In 2009, Kulkarni and associates[14] evaluated 618 pediatric patients who underwent ETV procedures in 12 pediatric institutions and used the data to develop the ETV Success Score. According to a regression model developed from a training set and later confirmed in a validation set, age, cause of hydrocephalus, and the existence of a previous CSF shunt are important and independent factors in predicting ETV success (Figure 32-1). Older patients with primary pathologic process near the region of the aqueduct of Sylvius without a history of previous ventricular shunting tended to have the most favorable prognosis. The ETV Success Score is now used preoperatively at our institution for patient evaluation and counseling.

The most important factor in selecting adult patients for ETV is the subtype of hydrocephalus itself. Treatment with ETV appears to offer the most benefit for late-onset idiopathic aqueductal stenosis (LIAS), secondary noncommunicating hydrocephalus, NPH, and conversion of a shunt in a patient who was treated for hydrocephalus as a child.[15] To date, the ETV Success Score has not been validated in the population of adults with hydrocephalus.

ETV SUCCESS SCORE

= Age Score + Etiology Score + Previous Shunt Score
≈ percentage probability of ETV success

SCORE	AGE ↓ +	ETIOLOGY ↓ +	PREVIOUS SHUNT ↓
0	<1 month	Postinfectious	Previous shunt
10	1 month to <6 months		No previous shunt
20		• Myelomeningocele • Intraventricular hemorrhage • Nontectal brain tumor	
30	6 months to <1 year	• Aqueductal stenosis • Tectal tumor • Other etiology	
40	1 year to <10 years		
50	≥10 years		

Figure 32-1. The ETV Success Score can be calculated to closely approximate the percentage possibility of successful endoscopic third ventriculostomy (ETV). *(From Kulkarni AV, Drake JM, Mallucci CL, et al. Endoscopic third ventriculostomy in the treatment of childhood hydrocephalus.* J Pediatr. *2009;155:254-259.e1.)*

Adult Hydrocephalus

Late-Onset Idiopathic Aqueductal Stenosis

LIAS, also known as "delayed" or "compensated" aqueductal stenosis, is a type of triventricular hydrocephalus with little or no flow through the aqueduct of Sylvius and a normal to small fourth ventricle. This form of hydrocephalus occurs in adult patients in the absence of space-occupying lesions or previous insults to the central nervous system (e.g., previous meningitis). LIAS represents approximately 3% to 10% of all cases of hydrocephalus in adults.[16] In a meta-analysis of 190 patients, Tisell[17] found that clinical symptoms included headaches (70%), cognitive impairment (55%), urinary incontinence (40%), gait disturbance (28%), diplopia (15%), and endocrine dysfunction (12%). Fukuhara and Luciano[16] evaluated 31 patients and added papilledema, swallowing difficulty, Parinaud's syndrome, and seizures to this list. Of interest is that the patient population tended to consist of two groups: a younger cohort (mean age of 33 years), presenting primarily with headache and signs and symptoms of raised intracranial pressure, and an older cohort (mean age of 63 years), with larger ventricles and NPH-like symptoms (cognitive impairment, urinary incontinence, and gait disturbance).[16]

Patients with LIAS respond to ETV, if properly selected on the basis of clinical presentation, radiologic findings of triventricular hydrocephalus, and minimal subarachnoid spaces. Success typically results in a complete or near-complete resolution of preexisting signs and symptoms and no need for further CSF diversion procedures. The preponderance of the literature suggests that the success rate of ETV in these patients is 50% to 86.5%; several authors have reported a success rate of approximately 80% with 6 to 22 months of follow-up.[10,17,18]

Secondary Noncommunicating Hydrocephalus

Secondary noncommunicating adult-onset hydrocephalus is defined as obstructive hydrocephalus resulting from a lesion impeding the CSF pathway.[17] The first choice for treatment of such lesions is removal or partial resection of the lesion to reestablish CSF flow; however, in many cases, this is not possible or warranted. In these cases, ETV may be a feasible alternative. Pineal region tumors, tectal gliomas, and posterior fossa tumors are the most common types of mass lesions that cause secondary noncommunicating hydrocephalus in both adults and children. Rare entities such as thalamic masses, cerebellar infarctions, and neurocysticercosis have also been described.[18,19] Dusick and associates[15] reviewed a series of 108 adult patients who underwent ETV for treatment of hydrocephalus and found that a mass lesion was an indication for the procedure in 47 (43.5%). Their overall success rate for this indication was 76.6%, although the median follow-up period was short (8 months). In their study, pineal region masses were the most prevalent indication for ETV, and the success rate in these cases was 71%. Both these incidence and success rates are compatible with those reported in other similar studies.[20-22] Success rates for ETV to treat patients with tectal gliomas are even higher (81% to 88%), although 18% of these patients may require a second ETV for ostomy blockage.[9,23] Tectal gliomas are uncommon and, in general, represent only about 4% of all cases treated with ETV, both pediatric and adult.[23] Arachnoid cysts, especially those found in the suprasellar region, prepontine region, third ventricle, or posterior fossa, can often cause obstructive hydrocephalus. Dusick and associates[15] found that ETV was successful in treating this cause of hydrocephalus in 86% of cases.

Frequently, ETVs for tectal and pineal region masses are paired with an endoscopic biopsy of the lesion through the third ventricle. Despite a high rate of success with the ETV itself, diagnostic rates for the masses are generally lower (69% to 90%). Complications associated with biopsy are generally documented at approximately 18%.[7,20] Common complications of these types of biopsy include intracerebellar and intraventricular hemorrhages, upgaze palsies, ventriculitis, and sodium balance disturbances.[7,20]

Normal-Pressure Hydrocephalus

The diagnosis and treatment of idiopathic normal-pressure hydrocephalus (iNPH) remain controversial in the neurosurgical literature. This condition is characterized by a gradual blockage of CSF drainage, which causes the slow buildup of fluid and a less dramatic increase in fluid pressure. Patients with iNPH are, in general, elderly patients with a triad of clinical signs and symptoms: (1) gait abnormalities such as a "magnetic" or "festinating" gait, (2) bladder incontinence, and (3) cognitive impairments or dementia. In 2005, the iNPH guidelines study group attempted to create guidelines for the diagnosis and treatment of NPH but were unable to establish clear evidence-based guidelines based on class I studies.[24] Findings on magnetic resonance imaging (MRI) include ventriculomegaly, focal subarachnoid space enlargements, and an open aqueduct, without evidence of a macroscopic blockage of CSF flow.[25,26] Most authors have used an open aqueduct as a criterion for NPH diagnosis. The fourth ventricle is of normal size in 35% of patients with an open aqueduct, slightly enlarged in 37%, and grossly enlarged in 27%.[27]

Diagnosis of NPH can be supported by results of formal neuropsychological testing, results of gait testing, clinical improvement after a lumbar CSF tap test[28] or an external CSF lumbar drainage test,[25] or a high-pressure steady-state plateau found on lumbar infusion test.[28] There is as yet no consensus as to which of these tests either defines the diagnosis or predicts good outcomes after CSF diversion.

The use of ETV is controversial for the management of NPH. Detractors of its use in this context note that CSF shunts have a high success rate in patients with NPH[25,29,30] and ETVs do not lower intracranial pressure enough to maximally improve clinical outcome. Proponents emphasize that use of ETV enables these patients to be free of hardware and point out that CSF shunts cause frequent complications in these patients, including infection, overdrainage symptoms, a need for revision, and subdural hematomas.[27,30]

Reported success rates of ETV in patients with NPH have varied considerably: from 21% in a study of 14 patients[29] to 87% in a study of 15 patients with 27 months of follow-up[30]; Gangemi and colleagues[27] had a success rate of 69% in their series of 110 patients with NPH treated with ETVs at four centers and monitored for a minimum of 2 years. A successful procedure was defined as resulting in a significant improvement in clinical symptoms. Of these 110 patients, another 22% had no change clinically and 9% deteriorated. Potential predictors of success included a shorter duration of symptoms and milder symptoms, but neither patient age nor the size of the fourth ventricle was predictive of response.

Secondary Endoscopic Third Ventriculostomy for Revision of Pediatric-Onset Hydrocephalus

Many adult patients with aqueductal stenosis, previous posterior fossa tumors, or intraventricular hemorrhage secondary to prematurity underwent placement of a shunt as children because their diagnosis preceded the recent ETV resurgence or because they required treatment before the age of 1 year, at which point ETVs have been demonstrated to have a poor success rate.[8] If these patients present with a shunt malfunction as adults, ETV with shunt removal is a viable option in lieu of shunt revision. Most studies show a success rate of about 70% in these patients at a median follow-up of 36 months,[22,31] although success rates vary with each study's selection criteria (underlying cause for each ETV). This may explain why other studies show similar initial success rates that diminish rapidly to 25% at 2 years.[32] Another consideration in assessing whether ETV is appropriate in an adult patient who has a shunt is that the complication rate is much higher (31%) for ETVs performed after shunt malfunction than for ETVs performed as a primary procedure (8%).[33]

A special consideration should be made for patients with myelomeningocele who have an implanted shunt. Use of ETV as a primary procedure for treating hydrocephalus in affected children was rare because it can be technically challenging and has poor rates of success (11% to 37%).[11,34] Nevertheless, when ETV is undertaken in the setting of shunt malfunction in older children or adults with myelomeningocele, the success rate increases to 63% to 93%.[11,34]

PREOPERATIVE IMAGING

We recommend performing MRI preoperatively. The MRI sequence of most value is the high-resolution sagittal T2-weighted image, which allows visualization of the floor of the third ventricle to identify thickness, bowing, and the proximity to both the clivus and the basilar arteries. T2-weighted imaging can help to identify when membranes beneath the ventricular floor, such as the membrane of Liliequist, are thickened and require fenestration. The sagittal view also demonstrates whether flow through the aqueduct is obstructed. Other factors that should be examined include the relative size of the fourth ventricle, the presence of ventricular or compressive lesions, and the presence of blood products or other debris in the ventricular system.

Some authors also rely on the sagittal cine phase-contrast sequence to identify the absence of flow through the cerebral aqueduct for ETV patient selection.[35] We do not place much emphasis on the cine imaging because we have found it to overestimate the level of CSF flow through the aqueduct. In these cases, ETV candidates who might have otherwise benefited from this procedure might not be offered the treatment.

Additional considerations in the pediatric population include anatomic variations noted in patients with spina bifida, Chiari malformation, and Dandy-Walker malformation and its variants. Variations affecting surgical feasibility and success may include agenesis of the corpus callosum, fused fornices, thickened massa intermedias, thickened third ventricular floors, and Chiari type 2 malformations.[36]

RADIOLOGIC OUTCOMES

In general, the success of an ETV is measured by resolution of clinical signs and symptoms and absence of the need of a repeat procedure (either repeat ETV or CSF shunting). The diminution of ventricle size after an ETV is usually considered a much smaller factor in judging success, if it is used at all; however, there are growing concerns that persistently enlarged ventricles even without signs of raised intracranial pressure may have chronic cognitive consequences.[37,38] In a study that included both children and adults who underwent ETV, Fukuhara and associates[35] demonstrated that only 25% of patients' ventricles diminished in size the day after surgery, those of 52% were diminished 6 months later, and those of 58% were diminished 1 year later. Other authors have found a significant correlation between diminution of ventricular size and clinical improvement.[39] Wellons and colleagues[40] described a decreased ratio of frontal horn to occipital horn in 89% of pediatric patients who underwent ETV and an increase in all patients who experienced ETV failure. Despite these improvements in ventriculomegaly, however, in most cases ventricles remain larger than normalized correlates for age and sex, which is contrary to findings from patients with shunts.[41]

OPERATIVE TECHNIQUE FOR ENDOSCOPIC THIRD VENTRICULOSTOMY

Operating Suite

Ideally, the patient on the operating table should be in the center of the operating suite. The patient's head should be turned away from the door, in an attempt to reduce the possibility of infection. The endoscopy tower should be placed at the patient's feet facing the patient's head and the surgeon. This is critical to ensure the surgeon's comfort and to monitor visibility at all times while the surgeon is facing the operative field. Setting the light source to 40% intensity seems to optimize anatomic visualization and minimize glare off the ventricular walls. Proper focus aperture and white balancing should also occur at this time. Any equipment problems should be detected and corrected before skin opening.

Irrigation is necessary in neuroendoscopy and serves to clear the operative field, maintain ventricular volumes/working space, and stop low-pressure venous bleeding. Irrigation can be used in either a continuous or an intermittent manner, whereby the operative assistant controls the flow or delivers boluses through a 50-mL syringe. We recommend continuous irrigation with 1-L bags of Ringer's lactate heated to 37.5°C and hung on an intravenous drip pole next to the monitor with tubing tracking along the patient's body. In this setup, the flow of irrigation can be controlled either by the scrub nurse with a stopcock or by the circulator, who can also raise or lower the intravenous drip pole or place a pressure bag around the intravenous solution to increase flow. We use intraoperative ultrasonography in every case. The ultrasound machine is positioned at the head of the bed with the probe's wire clamped to the instrument tray, directly accessible to the surgeon.

The patient is placed in the supine position with the head on a donut foam headrest or a horseshoe head frame, depending on the patient's size. The neck is slightly flexed to maintain proper cerebral venous drainage and kept in a midline position to help the endoscope operator maintain orientation at all times. For ETV with choroid plexus coagulation (CPC), the flexible endoscope is preferred and positioned preoperatively in the endoscope holder.

Operative Techniques

A curvilinear incision is usually made around a point 2 to 3 cm to the right of the midline and 1 cm in front of the palpated coronal suture. Distortional ventricular anatomy may necessitate a left-sided approach. An extended burr hole is made to a diameter of approximately 2 cm to allow the use of the ultrasound probe, as well as to provide a large enough dural area in which to make a linear incision. Options for opening include a cruciate dural opening or a small (3-4 cm) craniotomy to allow definitive dural closure.

The cortical surface is coagulated, and a brain needle is placed in the right lateral ventricle under ultrasound guidance. The use of the ultrasound imaging for entry into the ventricle ensures a precise trajectory aimed at the foramen of Monro. A proper trajectory allows access to the third ventricle with minimal torsion on the cortical mantle and on the thalamic and forniceal aspects of the foramen of Monro. The brain needle is then removed, and ultrasound guidance is used to place the endoscope sheath/trocar down the tract. After the light source and irrigation are activated, the endoscope is then placed into the sheath.

Anatomic Considerations

Knowledge of ventricular anatomy is paramount and should be reviewed with the surgical assistants before the operation. The lateral ventricle venous anatomy gives visual confirmation as to which ventricle the endoscope has entered. The thalamostriate vein runs along the lateral wall, converging with the anterior septal vein before entering the foramen of Monro as the internal cerebral vein. The choroid plexus, together with the superior choroidal vein, runs along the floor of the lateral ventricle (Figure 32-2).

When the foramen of Monro is entered, the surgeon must ensure that traction is not placed along the margins. The anterior and medial circumference of the foramen of Monro is the fornix, which should be carefully monitored for traction because injury to it can cause disturbance in short-term memory. The posterior and lateral circumference represents the thalamus and choroid plexus, which should also be monitored, although the thalamus is much more resistant to slight traction.

The floor of the third ventricle is generally thin and translucent in the hydrocephalic patient. After the third ventricle is entered, the paired mammillary bodies should be evident midway along the floor, with the basilar complex usually just anterior to them in the midline (Figure 32-3). The infundibular recess is usually evident as a pinkish-orange spot on the anterior midline floor. Slightly posterior to this recess is a white rectangular transverse band of the dorsum sella. The ideal spot for fenestration through the floor of the third ventricle is midway between the basilar complex and the dorsum sella in the midline. The oculomotor and the abducens (deeper) nerves can at times be visualized laterally along the ventricular floor. In some patients, the ventricular floor is thicker and somewhat opaque. In this scenario, the infundibular recess, clivus, and basilar pulsations are usually visible, and the fenestration can be directed over the bony aspect of the clivus in the midline for maximal safety.

Procedure

The fenestration through the floor of the ventricle is made bluntly with a blunt trocar, closed forceps, or laser wire. Sharp fenestration and cautery are not recommended because both these techniques increase the risk to the basilar artery complex. Some authors maintain that fenestrations may create tension along the walls of the third ventricles and increase the risk for postoperative hypothalamic dysfunction,[32] but we have not found this to be problematic. Others use a small Doppler probe to locate the basilar complex definitively before fenestration, especially in patients who have opaque third ventricle floors.[39]

The fenestration is then dilated to 4 to 6 mm in diameter with the use of a double-balloon catheter, Fogarty balloon, spreaders,

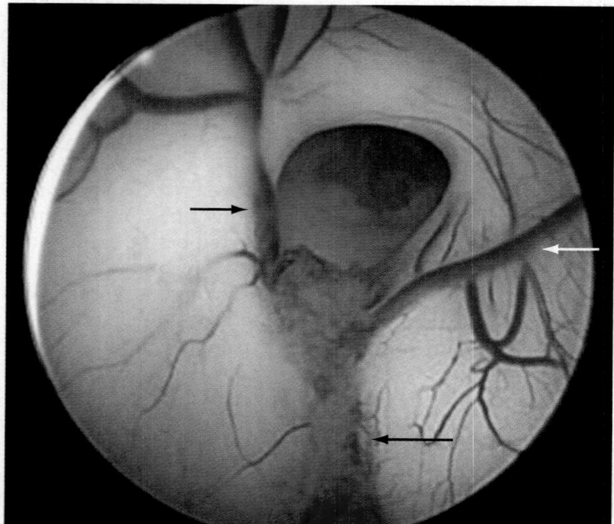

Figure 32-2. Endoscopic view into the right lateral ventricle. The thalamostriate vein *(white arrow)* runs along the lateral wall converging with the anterior septal vein *(top short black arrow)* before converging and entering the foramen of Monro as the internal cerebral vein. The superior choroidal vein *(bottom long black arrow)* is also seen coursing through the choroid plexus. *(Courtesy of T. T. Wong, MD.)*

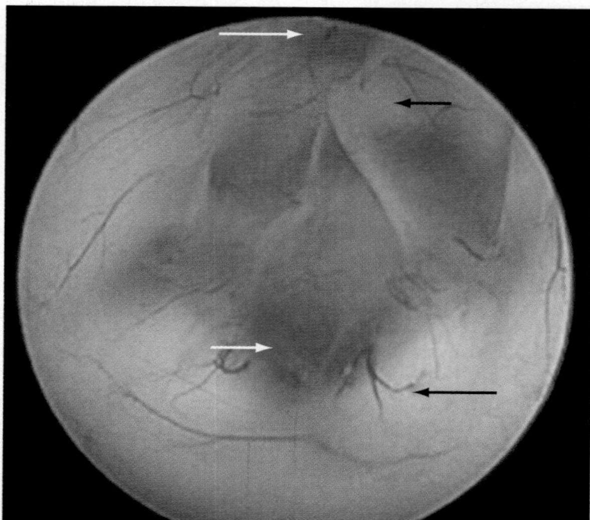

Figure 32-3. Endoscopic view of the floor of the third ventricle. The ideal spot for fenestration is in the midline, midway between the dorsum sella *(top short black arrow)* and the basilar artery *(bottom short white arrow)*. The paired mamillary bodies *(bottom long black arrow)* and the infundibular recess *(top long white arrow)* are also seen. *(Courtesy of T. T. Wong, MD.)*

or forceps. The endoscope is then perched atop the ostomy to inspect the subarachnoid spaces for membranes such as the membrane of Liliequist. These, too, must be carefully fenestrated, or the operation will be at risk of failure. A rule of thumb is that if the endoscope can fit within the fenestration, it is large enough. After the fenestration, the floor of the third ventricle should pulsate and flap with respiration and heart rates. These pulsations have been shown to be a strong predictor of ETV success.[40]

Endoscopic Third Ventriculostomy and Choroid Plexus Coagulation (for Infants Younger than 2 Years)

Warf and associates[42] found that addition of CPC to the ETV increased success rates from 47% to 82% in African infants younger than 1 year. The ETV–CPC combination was subsequently found to be successful in a North American setting; the Hydrocephalus Clinical Research Network achieved a 52% success rate 12 months after surgery[43] in children younger than 2 years. This outcome was corroborated by Warf himself at Boston Children's Hospital, where he found a 57% overall success rate in the population of infants with hydrocephalus.[44]

When CPC is planned, the trajectory of the endoscope is measured to allow for a septostomy and access to the contralateral choroid plexus. We usually begin with the ipsilateral choroid plexus. Beginning at the foramen of Monro, and taking great care to avoid cauterizing the fornix, we coagulate the choroid plexus posteriorly toward the ipsilateral temporal horn. The glomus is enlarged in a subset of these patients, and patience is necessary to ensure a circumferential cauterization of all visualized vessels. Next, a septostomy is performed, and the choroid plexus is coagulated from the foramen of Monro to the temporal horn.

The flexible endoscope is recommended for all cases of ETV-CPC. Kulkarni and associates[43] found that they were able to cauterize more than 90% of the choroid plexus in the lateral ventricle in 88% of patients with the flexible endoscope but just 14% of patients when the rigid endoscope was used. When more than 90% of choroid plexus was cauterized, the success rate increased from 51% to 82%. Especially in the temporal horn, care is taken to reverse all endoscopic manipulation when the endoscope is retracted, to ensure minimal injury to surrounding neural tissue.

Closure and Postoperative Issues

Once any ETV procedure is completed, the endoscope should be withdrawn slowly to inspect for hemorrhage and contusions before final removal. Some authors use fibrin glue or Gelfoam sponge (Pfizer) to occlude the tract through the cortex. This can prevent subdural hygromas and CSF leakage. We do not routinely occlude the tract; rather, we close the dura mater in a watertight manner. If the dura cannot be closed primarily, a piece of dura regeneration matrix is sutured in a watertight manner to the native dura.

The use of external ventricular drains postoperatively is controversial. Many surgeons use them to measure the intracranial pressure postoperatively or as an emergency safety valve in the case of patient deterioration or ETV failure. Detractors point out that an external drain can promote leakage and wound pseudomeningocele and, if open, may not allow the necessary pressure to encourage flow through the ventriculostomy, which causes false-negative failures. Our goal is to limit the use of external drains except in select cases in which the patient presents in a morbid state, at high risk for failure, or at high risk for hemorrhage during and after the procedure.

Many centers encourage the use of subcutaneous burr hole reservoirs after ETVs. These can be tapped in emergency scenarios or potential infections and can also be used postoperatively to measure intracranial pressure[39,41]; however, ventricular reservoirs may encourage the patency of the cortical tract and thus encourage CSF leak. Their use may also disallow the possibility of rendering the patient free of hardware. We do not routinely place ventricular reservoirs at our institution.

As stated previously, ventriculomegaly in patients who have undergone ETV decreased at a much slower rate and to far less an extent than in patients with implanted shunts.[38] Therefore, we obtain postoperative imaging (fast-sequence MRI) 6 to 8 weeks after surgery, rather than the day after, as is our practice in patients with shunts. More recently, we have initiated the practice of performing postoperative MRI with thin-cut sagittal T2-weighted images to directly observe CSF pulsations through the third ventricular floor. Typical in-hospital stays for patients after ETV vary between 1 and 3 days, with most patients going home on postoperative day two; this is longer than their counterparts with shunts.

COMPLICATIONS

Preoperative informed consent and postoperative patient monitoring require a detailed understanding of both the types and the frequencies of complications associated with ETV. Despite allowing the patient to be free of hardware and therefore invulnerable to shunt infection, ETVs are certainly not without risk, especially in the short term. The risk of ETV failure, described previously, ranges from 10% to 50% in most studies.[45] This variation is potentially the result of the wide range of causes of hydrocephalus. The overall rate of complications from this procedure varies from 5.8% to 16%; the rate of permanent morbidity is less than 3%.[46] The variation in these percentages is based primarily on indications for the ETV, cause of hydrocephalus, and the presence of comorbid conditions. In addition, complication rates may be associated with center and surgeon experience, and vigilance in reporting may be variable as well.[47]

Major complications that should be disclosed to the patient before surgery include CSF leakage (1% to 6% of cases), meningitis (1% to 5%), cranial neuropathies (1% to 2%), seizures (1%), and medical and endocrinologic complications (2% to 9%) (Table 32-1). Overall hemorrhage rates vary from 1% to 8.5% and include intraventricular bleeds that necessitate either the abandonment of the procedure or reoperation (when hemorrhage is blocking the ostomy), postoperative hematoma, and catastrophic basilar injury (<0.2% of cases[45,46]). Adverse effects of hypothalamic injuries, especially pathologic weight gain, are generally underreported and include diabetes insipidus, amenorrhea, and precocious puberty.[32]

ETV must be considered a treatment, not a cure, for hydrocephalus; therefore, patients who undergo ETV require follow-up just like their counterparts with shunts. This is especially important because rapid delayed deterioration has been reported in more than 1 per 200 patients who have undergone ETV.[7] Sixteen such cases have been reported, with a staggering mortality rate of 81%. All of the survivors except one have been disabled as a result of the rapid deterioration.[4]

REPEATED ENDOSCOPIC THIRD VENTRICULOSTOMY AFTER PRIMARY FAILURE

When ETV treatment fails, affected patients present with the usual constellation of signs and symptoms of raised intracranial pressure. Increased ventricular size in comparison with the initial postoperative baseline is noted on computed tomography or MRI. Persistent wound pseudomeningoceles and delayed CSF leaks are also highly suggestive of ETV failure.

Patients with ETV failure should undergo MRI with high-resolution T2-weighted sagittal sequencing. This sequence allows

TABLE 32-1 Reported Rates of Complications in Patients after Endoscopic Third Ventriculostomy

Study	Patient Population	Sample Size	CSF Leak (%)	Meningitis (%)	Severe Hemorrhage (%)	Hypothalamic Injury (%)	Cranial Neuropathy (%)	Seizure (%)	Rapid Delayed Deterioration/ Death (%)	Wound Infection (%)	Medical Complications (%)	Overall Complication Rate (%)
Drake et al.[8]	Pediatric (age 0-20 yr)	368	3.6	2.8	1.4	1.4	1.4	1.4	0.5	—	—	13.6
Jenkinson et al.[31]	Adult (age 16-79 yr)	190	1	0	2	—	1	—	0	—	—	5.8
Hader et al.[33]	Pediatric and adult	131	6.1	5.3	2.3	6.1	2.3	1	—	1.5	—	16*
Gangemi et al.[27]	Adult NPH only	110	1.8	—	3.6	—	—	—	0	1	—	6.4
Dusick et al.[15]	Adult (age 17-88 yr)	108	—	1	1.9	—	—	1	1.9	—	8.3	14.8
Amini et al.[45]	Adult	36	3	3	0	0	0	0	—	0	0	14
Kulkarni et al.[43]	Pediatric	36	—	6	0	0	0	0	3	—	—	9

CSF, cerebrospinal fluid; NPH, normal-pressure hydrocephalus. "0" indicates that the authors clearly stated that they found no such complications; "—" indicates that such complications were not discussed or reported.

*8% for primary endoscopic third ventriculostomies (ETVs) and 31% for ETVs in lieu of shunt revisions.

the clinician to evaluate the ventricle size, the presence or absence of an interruption in the floor of the third ventricle (ostomy), and whether a flow void exists through the opening. If the opening is present with or without a flow void, serial lumbar punctures to encourage flow through the ostomy can be considered.[43] If there is no resolution after two or three attempts, then CSF shunting is mandated. In a patient in whom neither an opening nor a flow void is seen on MRI, a reexploration or repeat ETV is warranted. During the reexploration, if an opening is visualized and is of adequate size, then conversion to a CSF shunt is suggested. In cases in which the ostomy is occluded either by debris or by scar tissue, a refenestration is warranted. Gangemi and colleagues[27] reported that of the 10 (of 110) patients who worsened clinically after primary ETV, 4 were found to have occluded ostomies on MRI and agreed to undergo a repeat ETV procedure. All 4 improved clinically.

CONCLUSION

The use of ETV has increased in both adult and pediatric hydrocephalus, with success rates varying from 50% to 90%. Patient selection is key to achieving clinical success. Conditions that are most favorable for ETV consideration in the adult population are LIAS, secondary (lesional) obstructive hydrocephalus, NPH, and possibly secondary ETV revisions in patients with pediatric-onset hydrocephalus who have a shunt. The success of ETV depends on detailed knowledge of the intricacies of each of these causes and their success rates, awareness of the potential risks and complications, and expertise in normal and anomalous ventricular anatomy. Early data suggest that in the infant population (<2 years old) with noninfectious hydrocephalus, adding CPC may further bolster the success rates of this procedure.

SUGGESTED READINGS

Amini A, Schmidt RH. Endoscopic third ventriculostomy in a series of 36 adult patients. *Neurosurg Focus*. 2005;19(6):E9.

Beems T, Grotenhuis JA. Long-term complications and definition of failure of neuroendoscopic procedures. *Childs Nerv Syst*. 2004;20(11-12):868-877.

Bergsneider M, Miller C, Vespa PM, et al. Surgical management of adult hydrocephalus. *Neurosurgery*. 2008;62(suppl 2):643-659.

Brockmeyer D, Abtin K, Carey L, et al. Endoscopic third ventriculostomy: an outcome analysis. *Pediatr Neurosurg*. 1998;28(5):236-240.

Drake JM. Endoscopic third ventriculostomy in pediatric patients: the Canadian experience. *Neurosurgery*. 2007;60(5):881-886.

Dusick JR, McArthur DL, Bergsneider M. Success and complication rates of endoscopic third ventriculostomy for adult hydrocephalus: a series of 108 patients. *Surg Neurol*. 2008;69(1):5-15.

Fukuhara T, Vorster SJ, Luciano MG. Risk factors for failure of endoscopic third ventriculostomy for obstructive hydrocephalus. *Neurosurgery*. 2000;46(5):1100-1109.

Furlanetti LL, Santos MV, de Oliveira RS. The success of endoscopic third ventriculostomy in children: analysis of prognostic factors. *Pediatr Neurosurg*. 2012;48(6):352-359.

Gangemi M, Mascari C, Maiuri F, et al. Long-term outcome of endoscopic third ventriculostomy in obstructive hydrocephalus. *Minim Invasive Neurosurg*. 2007;50(5):265-269.

Gross P, Reed GT, Engelmann R, et al. Hydrocephalus research funding from the National Institutes of Health: a 10-year perspective. *J Neurosurg Pediatr*. 2014;13(2):145-150.

Jallo GI, Kothbauer KF, Abbott IR. Endoscopic third ventriculostomy. *Neurosurg Focus*. 2005;19(6):E11.

Jenkinson MD, Hayhurst C, Al-Jumaily M, et al. The role of endoscopic third ventriculostomy in adult patients with hydrocephalus. *J Neurosurg*. 2009;110(5):861-866.

Kulkarni AV, Drake JM, Mallucci CL, et al. Endoscopic third ventriculostomy in the treatment of childhood hydrocephalus. *J Pediatr*. 2009;155(2):254-259.e1.

Kulkarni AV, Riva-Cambrin J, Browd SR, et al. Endoscopic third ventriculostomy and choroid plexus cauterization in infants with hydrocephalus: a retrospective Hydrocephalus Clinical Research Network study. *J Neurosurg Pediatr*. 2014;14(3):224-229.

Marmarou A, Bergsneider M, Relkin N, et al. Development of guidelines for idiopathic normal-pressure hydrocephalus: introduction. *Neurosurgery*. 2005;57(3 suppl):S1-S3.

Simon TD, Butler J, Whitlock KB, et al. Risk factors for first cerebrospinal fluid shunt infection: findings from a multi-center prospective cohort study. *J Pediatr*. 2014;164(6):1462-1468.e2.

Simon TD, Riva-Cambrin J, Srivastava R, et al. Hospital care for children with hydrocephalus in the United States: utilization, charges, comorbidities, and deaths. *J Neurosurg Pediatr*. 2008;1(2):131-137.

Stone SS, Warf BC. Combined endoscopic third ventriculostomy and choroid plexus cauterization as primary treatment for infant hydrocephalus: a prospective North American series. *J Neurosurg Pediatr*. 2014;14:439-446.

Teo C, Jones R. Management of hydrocephalus by endoscopic third ventriculostomy in patients with myelomeningocele. *Pediatr Neurosurg*. 1996;25(2):57-63.

Warf BC, Tracy S, Mugamba J. Long-term outcome for endoscopic third ventriculostomy alone or in combination with choroid plexus cauterization for congenital aqueductal stenosis in African infants. *J Neurosurg Pediatr*. 2012;10(2):108-111.

See a full reference list on ExpertConsult.com

33 Pathophysiology of Chronic Subdural Hematomas

R. Loch Macdonald

DEFINITIONS

A chronic subdural hematoma (CSDH) has been defined as liquefied hematoma in the subdural space with a characteristic outer membrane and occurring, if known, at least 3 weeks after head injury.[1] A subdural hygroma contains cerebrospinal fluid (CSF) and, in some definitions, is xanthochromic, which means that bleeding occurred at some point. Because the arachnoid may be dehiscent, some CDSHs can contain CSF, and there is a spectrum of subdural collections from CSDH to hygromas or effusions. Because some CSDHs evolve from acute subdural hematomas, these entities also represent a spectrum.

EPIDEMIOLOGY

The incidence of CSDH is not well known. On Awaji Island in Japan, the incidence of CSDH was 13 per 100,000 per year for 1986 to 1988 inclusive.[2] It increased with age, from 3.4 per 100,000 annually among those younger than 65 years to 58 per 100,000 annually among those older. Balser and associates[3] estimated the incidence from admissions to the Veterans Affairs hospital system in the state of New York between 2000 and 2012. They derived an age-standardized annual rate of 39 per 100,000. They found that 203 of 695 (29%) underwent surgery and that the recurrence rate was 11%. The annual incidence was 21 per 100,000 in the Miyagi Traumatic Head Injury Registry for 2005 to 2007 inclusive.[4] The most common cause was motor vehicle crash in younger patients and ground-level fall in elderly patients.

Factors associated with increased risk of CSDH are as follows[5-7]:

- Increasing age
- Alcohol consumption
- Male sex
- Use of anticoagulant or antiplatelet drugs
- Alzheimer's disease and other neurological diseases associated with brain atrophy
- Systemic disease associated with brain atrophy, such as liver and kidney disease
- Dialysis
- Conditions associated with craniocerebral disproportion, such as the period after ventriculoperitoneal shunting for hydrocephalus
- Conditions associated with low intracranial pressure, such as lumbar CSF drainage and spontaneous intracranial hypotension (the latter often being secondary to spontaneous spinal CSF leakage)
- Lumbar puncture
- Spinal anesthesia
- Spinal surgery complicated by dural tears

Beck and colleagues[6] noted that older patients are more likely to develop CSDH as a result of minor trauma in association with brain atrophy, whereas younger patients (younger than 60 years) often present with no history of trauma and with minimal brain atrophy. Beck and colleagues searched for spinal CSF leakage in a consecutive series of 27 patients younger than 60 years who had undergone surgery for CSDH and found a CSF leak in 7 (26%).

CAUSE

The most common theory of the cause of CSDH is that minor inertial brain injury causes movement of the brain within the skull and tears bridging veins as they traverse the cell layer of the dural border (Figs. 33-1 and 33-2).[8] Torn bridging vein stumps with clotted ends have been reported at surgery, although this is probably uncommon and is not usually observable because treatment is usually with a burr hole.[9] In these cases, early computed tomographic (CT) scans would show a hyperdense, acute subdural hematoma, and the CSDH evolves from this acute hematoma.[10] About two thirds of patients with CSDH report a history of trauma in the months before diagnosis.[11-13]

There is no subdural space (see Fig. 33-2). The dura mater is separated from the arachnoid by a thin layer of dural border cells.[14] The dural border cell layer contains flattened, elongated cells connected by desmosomes with amorphous extracellular matrix and limited extracellular fibers (i.e., collagen). This structure makes that cell layer a natural cleavage plane in which the dura mater is easily separated from the arachnoid.[15] During craniotomy and opening of the dura, the most common plane of separation of the meninges is within the dural border cell layer. Evidence that CSDH forms in the dural border cell layer includes electron microscopic studies showing dural border cells in the outer and inner CSDH membranes.[14,16,17]

In addition, the walls of veins traversing from the cortex to the dura are thinnest where they pass through the dural border cell layer.[8] Yamashima and Friede[8] examined the ultrastructure of bridging veins in four human autopsy specimens. The segment of the veins traversing the dural border cell layer was thinner than the subarachnoid portion. The vessel walls were as thin as 10 µm, in comparison with 50 to 200 µm in the subarachnoid space. The veins in this segment had a single layer of endothelial cells, only a thin layer of collagen in places, and no surrounding arachnoid trabeculae. As they traverse from the potentially mobile brain to the fixed points in the dural sinuses where they drain, they are thus predisposed to tearing in the virtual subdural space.

Development of CSDH from subdural hygroma was noted by Japanese neurosurgeons in the 1960s and 1970s and was presumed to result from CSF leakage into the dural border cell layer, which stimulates formation of the outer membrane granulation tissue (Fig. 33-3).[10,18]

Another hypothesis about the evolution of subdural hygroma to CSDH is that any shearing injury to the dural border cell layer—including hemorrhage from bridging veins, CSF accumulation, or even shearing forces associated with normal activities in patients predisposed by platelet/vessel or coagulation disorders or craniocerebral disproportion—can incite a wound healing response that leads to CSDH.[8] In support of this hypothesis are cases in which an elderly patient has a minor head injury. An initial CT scan in the first day or so appears unremarkable, but the patient returns weeks later with a CSDH (Fig. 33-4). Also, only about two thirds of affected patients recall a head injury.[11-13] This suggests that more minor daily activities, such as coughing and straining or even increased tension on the dural border cell layer in the setting of brain atrophy, could cause shearing through

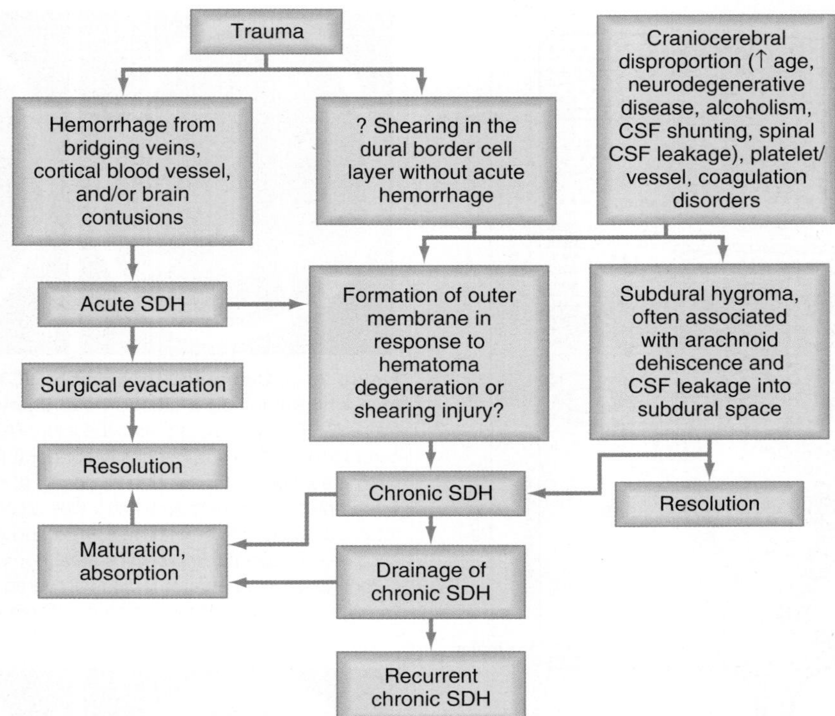

Figure 33-1. A flowchart of the clinical factors that contribute to formation of a chronic subdural hematoma. CSF, cerebrospinal fluid; SDH, subdural hematoma.

this layer, inciting a wound healing response. Incidental findings of thin subdural neomembranes in 46 (4%) of 1044 consecutive autopsy specimens support this but do not exclude the possibility that a forgotten trauma led to a CSDH that spontaneously resolved.[8,19]

Congenital and acquired platelet/vessel and coagulation disorders are associated with increased risk of CSDH, as well as with recurrence after surgery.[13,20]

PATHOLOGY

CSDHs are encapsulated, flattened structures usually located over one cerebral convexity, although they are bilateral in about 19% of cases.[21] The median volume of fluid in CSDHs was 96 mL (range, 33-270 mL) in 28 patients who underwent surgery in one series and 93 mL (range, 20-170 mL) in another series of 19 patients with 22 CSDHs.[22,23] There is an outer membrane that may be up to 10 mm thick. The membrane closely resembles granulation tissue that develops after injury to the dermis. It develops by proliferation from cells of the dura and probably of the dural border cell layer with ingrowth of dural capillaries. It contains numerous thin-walled sinusoidal blood vessels, fibroblasts, mast cells, eosinophils and myofibroblasts.[14,24-26] Some of the fibroblasts assume a contractile phenotype; these are known as myofibroblasts. There are reports of smooth muscle cells in the outer membrane.[27] Cells resembling those of the dural border cell layer are found in the outer and inner membranes. Ultrastructurally the blood vessels have endothelial fenestrations, gap junctions, an incomplete basement membrane, and an incomplete layer of pericytes.[28] They range in diameter from a few to 80 μm. This newly formed vasculature is susceptible to bleeding, probably spontaneously but also secondary to inflammation and fibrinolytic activity in the CSDH fluid. The extracellular space contains erythrocytes that also can be seen traversing endothelial cell gaps, a disorganized collagenous network, and other cells mentioned previously.[24] Erythropoiesis, as determined by presence of erythroblasts, in outer CSDH membranes is documented but not known to be of any clinical importance.[29]

The evolution of CSDH appears to parallel cutaneous wound healing, with phases of clotting of any extravasated blood, inflammation, proliferation and formation of granulation tissue, and remodeling and healing with fibrosis. The time course is different, however, and may be difficult to define because no inciting event can be determined in about a third of cases and rebleeding can occur, which will potentially begin another cycle of the wound healing response.

The inner membrane is a thin (30-300 μm thick), relatively avascular layer of cells adherent to the residual dural border cells and arachnoid cells. The cells are fibroblasts and dural border cells.[14,17,30] Yamashima and Yamamoto[30] examined 10 cases in which electron microscopy revealed 30- to 300-μm layers of flattened cells resembling dural border layer cells, containing extracellular collagen, elastin, granular material, some blood pigments, and fibrin.

CSDHs contain fluid ranging from yellow to dark brown, described as like coffee, red wine, or engine oil.[31] Takahashi and associates[32] found that CSDH fluid initially contains decreasing numbers of intact blood cells, but these numbers increase again after weeks because of recurrent hemorrhage into the CSDH. The fluid otherwise resembles serum biochemically.

PATHOGENESIS

Theories about why CSDHs enlarge over time include (1) the idea of a self-perpetuating cycle of recurrent hemorrhage, fibrinolysis, inflammation, and angiogenesis and (2) the concept of osmotic and oncotic pressure gradients between CSDH fluid and CSF or blood.

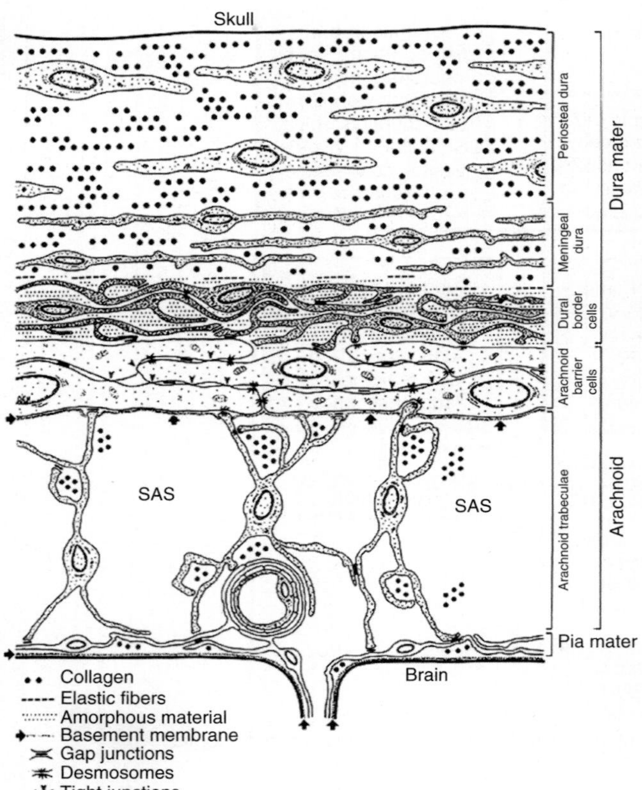

Figure 33-2. Diagram of the meninges showing the important anatomy of each layer. Collagen (*large dots* indicate locations, but not the structure, of the collagen) is relatively abundant in both layers of the dura mater and arachnoid trabeculae but notably sparse in the dural border cell layer. Cells of the cell layer of the dural border adhere to each other by desmosomes but are otherwise not supported by robust extracellular collagen. This results in a natural cleavage plane through this layer, separating the dura mater from the arachnoid and giving the impression of a subdural space. The dural border cells also adhere to the arachnoid barrier cells, which themselves are strongly united by tight junctions and desmosomes. SAS, subarachnoid space. *(From Haines DE. On the question of a subdural space.* Anat Rec. *1991;230(1):3-21.)*

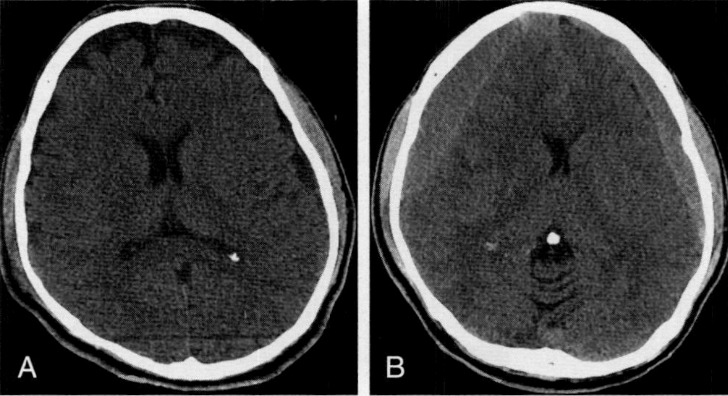

Figure 33-3. Computed tomographic (CT) scans in a 27-year-old man who sustained a closed-head injury after being struck by a train. A CT scan 3 hours after the injury **(A)** showed bilateral cerebrospinal fluid (CSF)–density subdural fluid collections (subdural hygromas) and scalp swelling bilaterally at sites of superficial injury. He was confused but recovered and was discharged after 2 days. He returned 69 days later with headache and gait unsteadiness, and another CT scan **(B)** showed bilateral homogeneous hypodense chronic subdural hematoma. He recovered fully after the creation of bilateral burr holes and insertion of closed-system drains.

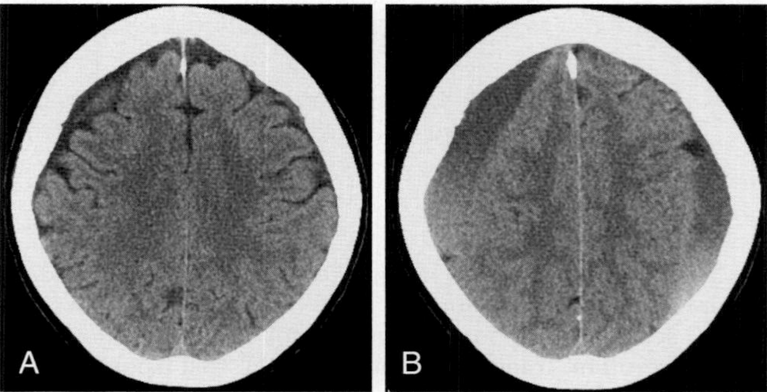

Figure 33-4. Computed tomographic (CT) scans in a 77-year-old man who fell and sustained a minor head injury. A CT scan hours after the injury **(A)** showed no acute bleeding and no subdural hygromas. He presented 20 days later with headache, confusion, and unsteady gait. A follow-up CT scan **(B)** showed a bilateral layering type of chronic subdural hematoma.

Recurrent Hemorrhage, Fibrinolysis, Inflammation, and Angiogenesis

The meninges are derived from embryonic mesoderm and, as with other mesodermal tissues such as dermis, the response to injury is the same for the initial hemorrhage or, in theory, a shearing injury in the border cell layer of the meninges. In wound healing and CSDH, extravasated blood, if any, undergoes platelet activation, which causes the release of platelet-derived growth factor, and clotting, which causes the release of thrombin, and fibrinogen.[33,34] Many of these substances have been measured in CSDH fluid with variable results that are difficult to interpret because when the CSDH started is often unknown and recurrent cycles of bleeding will start new cycles of the clotting/fibrinolysis/inflammation/angiogenesis cycle that overlap with other phases already ongoing. The blood also undergoes hemolysis. In general, platelet-derived growth factor, basic fibroblast growth factor, and transforming growth factor β, among other cytokines, assist in generating inflammation with recruitment of polymorphonuclear leukocytes, mast cells, and macrophages.[35-37] A proliferative phase follows, characterized by proliferation of fibroblasts and myofibroblasts, collagen formation, and angiogenesis. The outer membrane is probably vascular, whereas the inner membrane is thin and avascular because the CSDH forms in the dural border cell layer with the inner meningeal layer of the dura mater next to where the outer membrane forms, and this layer of the dura has a well-developed capillary network.[38] The proliferative phase produces varying amounts of granulation tissue, which histologically and ultrastructurally is very similar to that in chronic human cutaneous wounds and the outer CSDH membrane.[39] Fibrinolysis is activated, and hemorrhage from the neovascular system may be increased by tissue plasminogen activator (tPA) and matrix metalloproteinases synthesized by cells in the outer membrane, as in other granulation tissue.[40-42] The outer membrane contains tPA, which activates plasminogen to plasmin and causes fibrinolysis.[43-45] Active matrix metalloproteinases can degrade collagen and lead to bleeding from the neovascular system.[46]

The most plausible explanation for enlargement of CSDH is recurrent hemorrhage into the subdural fluid from the outer membrane. Fibrinolysis and inflammation are probably pathophysiologically important and are known to interact. Evidence for this is that fresh blood is frequently observed on CT scans of

CSDH.[37] Intact erythrocytes are found in CSDH fluid.[47] Ito and associates[48,49] found chromium 51–labeled erythrocytes in CSDH fluid 6 to 24 hours after they were injected systemically in 50 humans. They calculated that fresh daily bleeding accounted for about 7% of the CSDH volume; the values were higher in cases of laminar (mixed) or layered types of CSDH, as noted on CT scans, than in cases of homogeneous low-density CSDH. Recurrent bleeding is from the thin-walled blood vessels in the granulation tissue of the outer membrane. Light and electron microscopic studies have shown that these blood vessels may consist of a single layer of endothelial cells with a poorly developed or no basement membrane.[50,51] They are sometimes surrounded by inflammatory cells and fresh blood. The endothelial cells may be separated by gap junctions through which erythrocytes are passing.

The composition of CSDH fluid is consistent with blood that has entered the CSDH and then undergone coagulation, followed by fibrinolysis and hemolysis.[52,53] The fluid contains low concentrations of coagulation factors, including fibrinogen,[23,49,54] and increased concentrations of substances indicative of fibrinolysis, such as fibrin degradation products[23,49,55,56] and tPA.[54,57,58] The low concentrations of fibrinogen, plasminogen, and α_2-plasmin inhibitor (α_2-antiplasmin); the increased concentrations of fibrin degradation products and tPA; and the prolonged prothrombin and partial thromboplastin times are characteristic of blood that has clotted.[23,57,59,60] Evidence that fibrinolysis has been activated includes the low concentrations of α_2-antiplasmin and plasminogen and the increased concentrations of the plasmin–α_2-antiplasmin complex.[61,62] Because the half-life of plasmin is 100 msec, the concentration of plasmin–α_2-antiplasmin complex is used as a marker of fibrinolysis.

Several groups of researchers found varying profiles of proinflammatory and anti-inflammatory cytokines and chemokines in CSDH fluid.[36,37,63-67] Most investigators found that CSDH fluid had higher concentrations of interleukin (IL)–6 and IL-8 and usually increased levels of tumor necrosis factor α. Stanisic and colleagues[64] measured these and additional cytokines in 56 patients with CSDHs and reported that concentrations of IL-2R, IL-5, IL-6, and IL-7 (proinflammatory cytokines) and of IL-10 and IL-13 (anti-inflammatory cytokines) were higher in CSDH fluid than in systemic blood. In contrast to other reports, concentrations of tumor necrosis factor α, IL-1β, IL-2, and IL-4 were significantly lower in CSDH fluid than in peripheral blood. The ratio of proinflammatory to anti-inflammatory cytokines was higher in CSDH fluid than in peripheral blood. In general, inflammation increases vascular permeability and attracts leukocytes.[54] Results of immunohistochemical studies suggest that the source of the cytokines is the outer membrane. IL-6 is a proinflammatory cytokine that increases vascular permeability and whose expression is stimulated in fibroblasts and epithelial cells by thrombin. IL-8 is chemotactic for polymorphonuclear leukocytes and lymphocytes.

The kinin-kallikrein system consists of numerous proteins and peptides that interact with the coagulation and inflammatory cascades and that also have been implicated in the pathophysiologic process of CSDH.[54] Activated coagulation factor XII (Hageman factor), as well as plasmin, converts prekallikrein to kallikrein, which in turn converts high-molecular-weight kininogen to bradykinin. Bradykinin is a potent vasodilator that also increases vascular permeability. The prekallikrein probably enters CSDH fluid via the neovascular vessels of the permeable outer membrane (exudation) or through recurrent hemorrhage. The presence of bradykinin with low concentrations of prekallikrein in CSDH fluid suggests that the kallikrein-kinin system is activated.[54]

Platelet-activating factor is a chemoattractant that also stimulates release of tPA from endothelial cells, may increase vascular permeability, and attracts and degranulates eosinophils.[68] In one study, it was found at increased concentrations in CSDH fluid from 34 patients, and in immunohistochemistry studies, it was localized to the sinusoidal neovascular vessels of the outer membrane.[69]

Angiogenic and growth factors, including vascular endothelial growth factor and basic fibroblast growth factor, have been detected in CSDH fluid and the outer membrane.[36,58,66,70,71] The findings are consistent with the wound healing response and formation of granulation tissue, including matrix metalloproteinases 2 and 9, whose levels are elevated in CSDH fluid and which stimulate production of vascular endothelial growth factor and basic fibroblast growth factor.[71] A likely source of matrix metalloproteinases are the proliferating fibroblasts in the outer membrane. Vascular endothelial growth factor stimulates angiogenesis and vascular permeability; in immunohistochemistry study, it was localized by the outer membrane fibrous tissue and inflammatory cells.[72] It also increases tPA production in endothelial cells, which would contribute to recurrent hemorrhage.[58] Basic fibroblast growth factor mediates cell proliferation and migration and stimulates synthesis of enzymes that break down extracellular matrix and plasminogen.

Fibrin degradation products are potent stimulators of angiogenesis. Growth factors also stimulate formation of provisional extracellular matrix composed of fibronectin, fibrin, and hyaluronic acid. Collagen is formed during healing of wounds and of CSDH. Transforming growth factor β mediates collagen synthesis during wound healing, and its levels were increased in CSDH fluid in one study.[73] High concentrations of procollagen propeptides of types I and III collagen were found in CSDH fluid.[15,74]

Osmotic and Oncotic (Colloid Osmotic) Pressures

Gardner[75] suggested that a difference in osmolarity between CSF and the CSDH fluid caused the CSDH to enlarge by imbibing CSF. Subsequent theories invoked oncotic pressure gradients between intravascular plasma and CSDH fluid.[76] The osmotic/oncotic pressure gradient theory is not supported by studies showing there is no difference in osmolarity or oncotic pressure among CSDH fluid, plasma, and CSF.[76] Osmolality is related to the number of molecules in the fluid regardless of molecular weight, whereas oncotic pressure (colloid osmotic pressure) is pressure across a membrane that is impermeable only to molecules above a higher molecular weight, such as albumin. Weir[77] measured the osmolality of CSDH fluid from 23 patients and found that it was the same as that of serum and CSF. The fluid contained albumin but not prealbumin (transthyretin, found in CSF), and thus it resembled serum, which led him to conclude that the most likely reason for the delayed development of symptoms in cases of CSDH was recurrent bleeding, effusion of albumin, or bleeding from a damaged vein. Oncotic pressure also was the same in CSDH fluid and venous blood and was highly correlated with the protein content of the CSDH fluid.[76]

Although recurrent hemorrhage is probably the most important process that leads to CSDH enlargement, it is likely that exudation (leakage of serum, fibrin, and white blood cells across blood vessels as a result of inflammation) and transudation (fluid accumulation with low protein content as a result of oncotic pressure differences and not inflammation) contribute in part to the pathogenesis of CSDH.[15,78]

APPEARANCE ON COMPUTED TOMOGRAPHY AND MAGNETIC RESONANCE IMAGING

Relationships between the appearance of CSDHs on CT scan and the contents of the CSDH fluid have been examined.[37] It has been suggested that CSDHs are hypodense in the early stage, isodense or of high density in the mature stage, of mixed density in the progressive stage, and of low density in the resolving phase

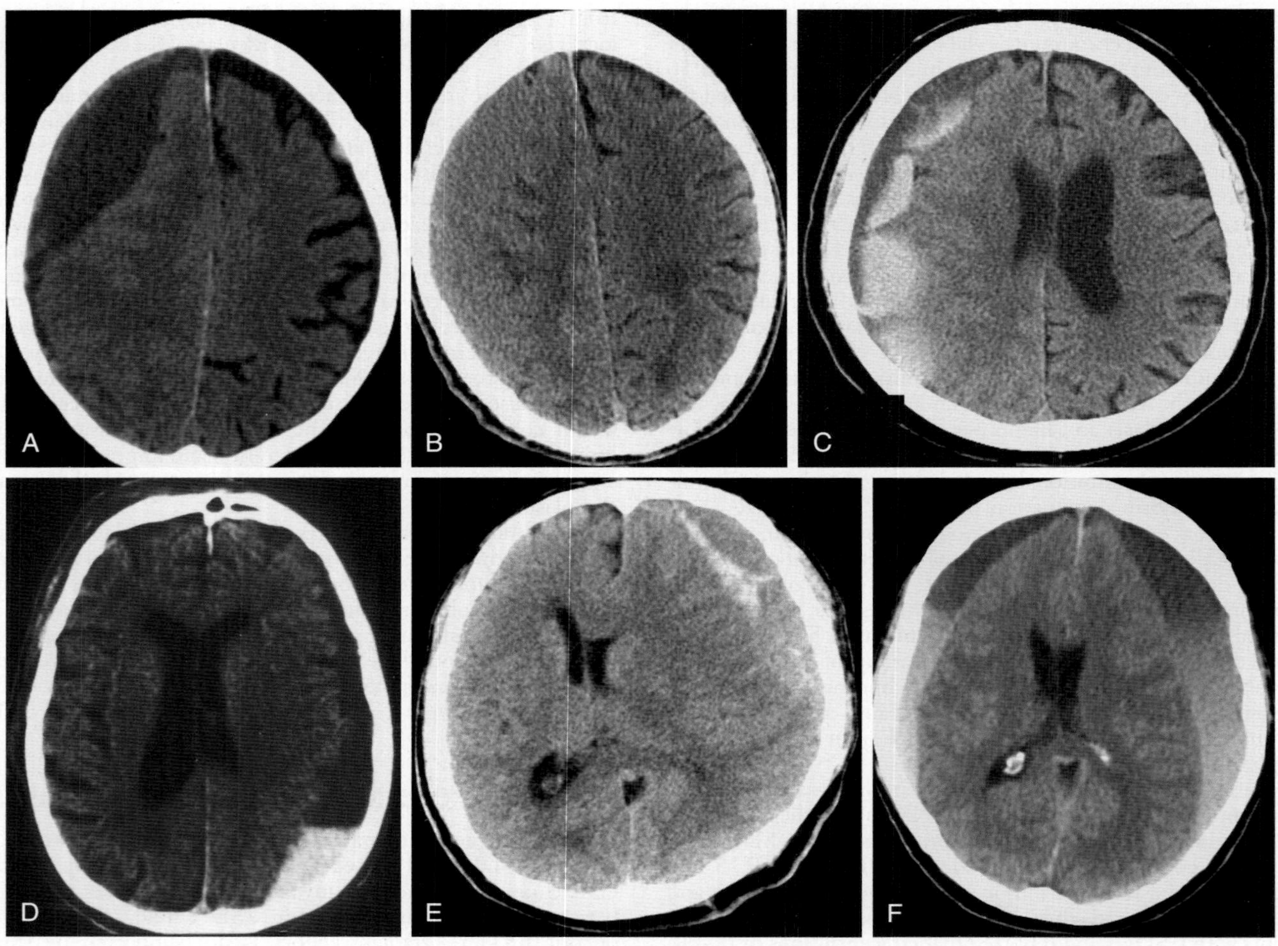

Figure 33-5. Different appearances of chronic subdural hematoma on computed tomographic scans. Homogeneous hypodense **(A)**, homogeneous isodense **(B)**, trabeculated **(C)**, layering separated **(D)**, laminar **(E)**, and layering gradated **(F)** appearances.

TABLE 33-1 Classification of Chronic Subdural Hematoma on Computed Tomography[80,91]

Type	Characteristics
Homogeneous	Homogeneous hypodense, isodense, or hyperdense hematoma Risk of enlargement and recurrence: 10%-15%
Laminar (mixed)	Thin, high-density layers usually along the inner membrane Higher risk of enlargement Risk of recurrence similar to that of the homogeneous type
Layered (separated or gradation)	Two components of different density: low density anteriorly and high density posteriorly If margin is distinct, hematoma is the separated subtype; if margin is indistinct, hematoma is the gradation type Highest risk of growth and recurrence
Trabecular (multilocular)	Mixed density with high-density septations, usually with low-intensity or isointense background Low risk of growth and recurrence

(Fig. 33-5; Table 33-1).[37,79,80] In the evolution from an acute subdural hematoma to a CSDH, the lesion would obviously start as a hyperdense acute hematoma. Evolution from a subdural hygroma would likely start as a homogeneous low-density CSDH. Most of the density is ascribable to hemoglobin in the fluid. With time, the hematoma becomes less dense. Hemorrhage into the fluid would increase the density diffusely (making the fluid isodense or hyperdense); in cases of recurrent bleeding, there may be a layer of increased density along the surface of the brain with less dense fluid more superficially (laminar, or mixed, type). As fibrinolysis proceeds and the CSDH matures, the layered appearance develops. The trabecular stage represents resolution of the CSDH.

The CT appearance may be correlated with the risk of growth or recurrence, or both, after surgery. The homogeneous stage is thought to have a low risk of rebleeding.[80] This implies that many CSDHs must spontaneously resolve. Laminar and separated CSDH were most likely to enlarge over time, and the separated subtype had the highest rate of enlargement and of recurrence. The trabecular stage was associated with low rates of growth and recurrence.[20,81] Some researchers, however, have not found that CT appearance is predictive of CSDH growth or recurrence.[82]

In contrast to current CT technology, magnetic resonance imaging (MRI) may be a more sensitive test to detect CSDH. As with CT scanning, MRI appearance has been correlated with risk of recurrence after treatment.[83] In one series of 199 patients with 230 CSDHs, 3% exhibited recurrence—defined as reaccumulation within 6 months to at least the same size as before surgery—with high intensity on T1-weighted images, and 12% exhibited recurrence with isointensity or low intensity. The researchers also noted that the increased risk of recurrence was statistically insignificant with a CT appearance of the layered type, in comparison with appearances of high density, isodensity, low density, and mixed density.

Fukuhara and colleagues[84] reported that certain MRI findings were associated with risk of recurrence. El-Kadi and colleagues[84a] suggested that the reason recurrence was higher with a high-intensity MRI appearance was that this appearance characterizes the early proliferative phase of CSDH with neovascularity in the outer membrane. In the later proliferative stage, the CSDH has a high-intensity homogeneous appearance and enlarges by another mechanism, such as transport of plasma or CSF into the CSDH; at that stage, the risk of rebleeding is lower. Fujisawa and associates[85] noted that MRI appearance was useful for differentiating CSDH from empyema and subdural hygroma. They performed CT scanning and MRI on 44 patients with 60 CSDHs. They classified CT and MRI appearances as low density/intensity, isodensity/isointensity, high density/intensity, layered density/intensity, and mixed density/intensity. The MRI appearance was determined on T1- and T2-weighted images. This resulted in 25 different patterns, of a possible 125. The CSDH fluid was found to have biochemical features of hemolysis, with higher concentrations of potassium, glutamate oxaloacetate transaminase, bilirubin, and lactate dehydrogenase than in peripheral blood. The authors did not comment on the risk of recurrence in relation to CT or MRI appearance.

NATURAL HISTORY AND RECURRENCE AFTER SURGERY

Data about the natural history of CSDH are limited. In one study of 24 patients with CSDH, 5 had headache and cognitive decline but were considered to not have increased intracranial pressure.[86] These 5 patients did not undergo surgery, and the CSDH spontaneously resolved in all 5. The authors considered such resolution more likely to occur in patients older than 70 years with thin, asymptomatic, low-density CSDH.[87]

Recurrence is defined, as mentioned earlier, as return of symptoms within some time after surgery (variably defined as up to 6 months) with or without expansion of the CSDH or with expansion of residual postoperative CSDH.[83] It is reported in 9% to 27% of patients.[88,89] Risk factors for recurrence have been reported to include congenital or acquired platelet/vessel and coagulation disorders, intracranial hypotension, older age, brain atrophy, bilateral CSDH, CT appearance (density and type), diabetes mellitus, absence of a drain, postoperative accumulation of subdural air, inflammatory cytokine concentrations in the CSDH fluid, and alcohol abuse.[63,82,89]

Several investigators used multivariate analysis to determine independent risk factors for recurrence of CSDH after surgery. Chon and coworkers[82] studied 420 patients with CSDH, of whom 92 (22%) experienced recurrences. Recurrence was more likely with more postoperative midline shift, diabetes mellitus, history of seizures, increased preoperative width of hematoma, and anticoagulant therapy. Another report concluded trabecular appearance on CT scan, history of seizures, increased width of hematoma, and no history of diabetes mellitus were associated with recurrence.[90] These results conflict with other findings in that the trabecular type has usually been associated with low risk of recurrence. Patients with diabetes have increased blood viscosity, which could lead to recurrence by increasing CSDH fluid oncotic pressure, but they also may have augmented platelet aggregation, which would decrease recurrence. On the other hand, diabetes is a well-known factor that impairs wound healing in general.[33] Recurrence is probably caused by multiple interacting factors, including failure of the brain to reexpand after drainage. Fukuhara and colleagues[84] measured brain tissue elastance in 14 patients with CSDH; in patients with larger residual CSDH a month after surgery, elastance was higher, which indicates that the brain was stiffer and less compliant. Increasing age was also correlated with increasing elastance.

CONCLUSION

CSDH most commonly develops in patients with craniocerebral disproportion as a result of multiple possible underlying conditions. Platelet/vessel and coagulation disorders increase the risk of CSDH development. Minor trauma causes shearing in the dural border cell layer that may injure cortical veins bridging to the dura, where their walls are thinnest as they pass through the dural border cell layer.[66] Injury and possible acute bleeding essentially creates a cut through the dural border cell layer. The response is similar to the cutaneous wound healing response. There is an inflammatory response to injury with proliferation of the mesenchyme-derived dural border cells. A layer of granulation tissue forms adjacent to the dura (the outer membrane), characterized by inflammation and angiogenesis with thin-walled sinusoidal blood vessels, inflammatory cells, fibroblasts, and myofibroblasts. A thin inner membrane encapsulates the hematoma but does not proliferate much because it lacks inherent vascularity. The hematoma initially clots, but then fibrinolysis and hemolysis occur, and the enclosed CSDH cavity probably prevents clearance of fibrinolytic enzymes, inflammatory cytokines, and angiogenic factors, which leads to cycles of inflammation, fibrinolysis, angiogenesis, and rebleeding. As with cutaneous wounds, healing usually occurs, but if the balance of factors promoting healing—such as intact coagulation, removal of some of the CSDH fluid by surgery, and resolution of craniocerebral disproportion—is outweighed by ongoing inflammation, bleeding, and lack of brain reexpansion, then the CSDH expands or recurs.

SUGGESTED READINGS

Chen JC, Levy ML. Causes, epidemiology, and risk factors of chronic subdural hematoma. *Neurosurg Clin N Am*. 2000;11(3):399-406.

Haines DE. On the question of a subdural space. *Anat Rec*. 1991;230(1):3-21.

Lee KS. Natural history of chronic subdural haematoma. *Brain Inj*. 2004;18(4):351-358.

Nakaguchi H, Tanishima T, Yoshimasu N. Factors in the natural history of chronic subdural hematomas that influence their postoperative recurrence. *J Neurosurg*. 2001;95(2):256-262.

Santarius T, Kirkpatrick PJ, Ganesan D, et al. Use of drains versus no drains after burr-hole evacuation of chronic subdural haematoma: a randomised controlled trial. *Lancet*. 2009;374(9695):1067-1073.

Stoodley M, Weir B. Contents of chronic subdural hematoma. *Neurosurg Clin N Am*. 2000;11(3):425-434.

Weigel R, Schmiedek P, Krauss JK. Outcome of contemporary surgery for chronic subdural haematoma: evidence based review. *J Neurol Neurosurg Psychiatry*. 2003;74(7):937-943.

See a full reference list on ExpertConsult.com

34 Medical and Surgical Management of Chronic Subdural Hematomas

Aswin Chari, Angelos G. Kolias, Nicholas Borg, Peter J. Hutchinson, and Thomas Santarius

EPIDEMIOLOGY

Chronic subdural hematoma (CSDH) can be defined as a predominantly hypodense or isodense crescentic collection along the cerebral convexity on cranial computed tomography (CT), which has to be differentiated from subdural empyema and hygroma. This chapter deals with the diagnosis and management of adult CSDH only, because pediatric CSDH is a separate disease entity with distinctive etiology and management.

CSDH is a disease of the elderly; mean age at presentation in a randomized controlled trial from our institution was 76.8 years (range 36-95 years) and there is a 3 : 1 male-to-female ratio across all age groups.[1] The incidence of CSDH is quoted at about 10/100,000 per year[2-4] and is rising as a result of the combination of an aging population and the increasing use of anticoagulant and antiplatelet medications.

PATHOGENESIS

CSDH arises at the dural border cell layer, a thin layer of cells between the dura mater and arachnoid mater with less extracellular collagen and intercellular connections prone to separation (Fig. 34-1).[5-8] Development of CSDH requires a predisposing factor of a shrinking volume within the cranial vault (e.g., the elderly atrophic brain, the alcoholic brain, or the overdraining cerebrospinal fluid shunt) and a precipitant trauma that can often be so minor that it is not identified in the history. Two possible etiologies have been hypothesized,[9,10] although there remains debate about what proportion of CSDH arises from each.[5]

The first etiology is an acute subdural hematoma (ASDH). These usually occur in the context of trauma resulting from tearing of the bridging veins that traverse the dural border cell layer or, less commonly, tearing of cortical arteries or veins. An ASDH that is not surgically evacuated in the acute setting will usually be resorbed; in certain cases, this process is incomplete and the hematoma becomes chronic as the acute clot lyses (Fig. 34-2). Chronic hematomas expand as a result of a local inflammatory reaction,[11,12] causing fibrinolysis of the clot[13] and the production of angiogenic factors that promote neovascularization and bleeding from fragile capillaries.[5,12,14] Studies have demonstrated that roughly 20% of conservatively managed ASDHs will become chronic, although the factors that predispose to this transformation have not been identified.[15,16] In clinical practice, it would seem sensible to rescan any small, asymptomatic ASDH only if there is symptomatic progression. Especially in the elderly patient with comorbidities, it is less of a physiologic strain to undergo bur-hole craniostomy to evacuate a CSDH than a large craniotomy to evacuate an ASDH.

The second etiology is from a subdural hygroma, a collection of cerebrospinal fluid in the subdural space caused by the splitting of the dural border cell layer at points of tension between the dura mater and arachnoid mater. This has been shown to occur spontaneously, especially in asymmetrical skulls where the tension may not be spread evenly.[9] In the subdural space, neomembranes form through proliferation of the dural border cells and neovascularization occurs. Hemorrhage and the resulting inflammatory response from these new vessels leads to the formation and expansion of a CSDH.[9]

A range of risk factors have been identified, including advancing age, a history of falls or minor head injury, use of anticoagulants or antiplatelet drugs, bleeding diatheses, alcohol (contributing to globalized brain atrophy, higher risk of falls, and hepatogenic coagulopathy), epilepsy, low intracranial pressure states, and hemodialysis.[14,17-20]

Perhaps the most important risk factor that has contributed to the increasing incidence of CSDH is the use of anticoagulant and antiplatelet medication. The widespread use of these agents has made quantification of risk difficult,[18] but they have been shown to increase the incidence of both "atraumatic" (whereby the trauma is so minor that it is not recollected) and recurrent CSDH.[21-23]

CLINICAL PRESENTATION

CSDH can present heterogeneously, and symptom onset and progression can vary from days to weeks. Common presenting symptoms and signs include headache, limb and gait disturbance, hemiparesis/hemiplegia, cognitive decline, and confusion (Table 34-1).[1] It is important to remember, however, that a significant proportion (20% to 30%) of CSDHs may be completely asymptomatic and discovered incidentally. Consciousness level at presentation is usually normal or only slightly altered, although a minority (20%) may present with a Glasgow Coma Scale (GCS) score less than 13.[1] In the Cambridge Chronic Subdural Hematoma Trial, 20% of patients were on anticoagulants and 32% on antiplatelet agents at presentation; approximately 20% of patients had bilateral collections.[1] In a majority of cases, a history of minor trauma may be elicited, although this may be so minor that it is not recollected. The time from trauma to presentation varies from days to weeks and, in frequent fallers, it may be difficult to identify which fall was associated with the initiation and development of the CSDH.

There is evidence to suggest that prognosis can be predicted by the GCS, GCS motor score, and modified Rankin Scale at admission.[1,24,25] An alternative to the GCS used in many CSDH studies is the Markwalder Grading System[19]; although historically popular, it is rather imprecise in its descriptions. We therefore recommend a combination of the GCS, focal neurological signs, and a functional outcome measure (e.g., modified Rankin Scale) to provide a comprehensive approach to assessing patients both at admission and at follow-up, especially in academic contexts.

DIAGNOSIS

The mainstay for diagnosis is CT. CSDH is seen as a hypodense (<30 Hounsfield units) crescentic collection along the convexity but may have isodense (subacute, 30-60 Hounsfield units) or hyperdense (acute, >60 Hounsfield units) components.[26,27] Subacute CSDH may be overlooked, especially if it is bilateral or does not cause midline shift. Features that can be helpful include medial displacement of the gray matter–white matter interface and failure of the convexity sulci to reach the inner table of the

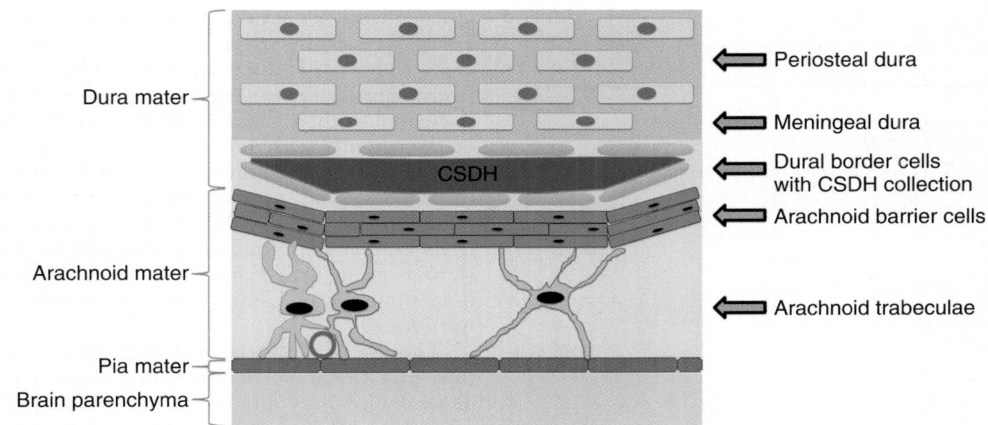

Figure 34-1. Schematic diagram of the meninges illustrating the dural border cell layer, a thin layer of cells between the dura mater and arachnoid mater with less extracellular collagen and intercellular connections prone to separation, where chronic subdural hematoma (CSDH) forms. *(Modified from Santarius T, Kirkpatrick PJ, Kolias AG, et al. Working toward rational and evidence-based treatment of chronic subdural hematoma.* Clin Neurosurg. *2010;57:112-122.)*

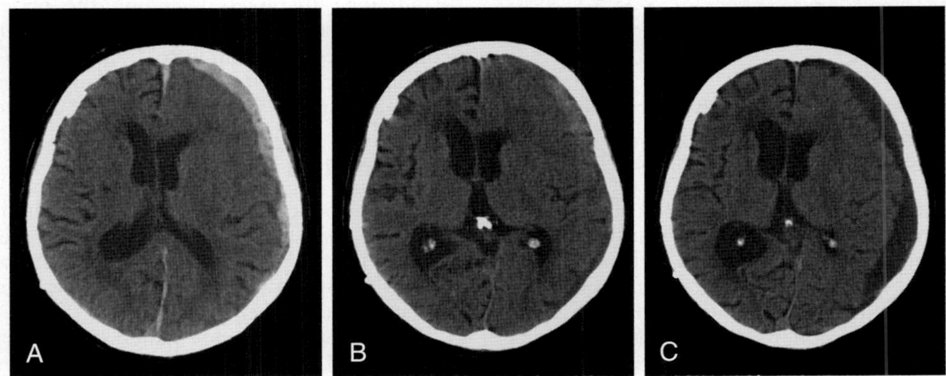

Figure 34-2. Example of evolution of acute into chronic subdural hematoma (SDH) in a 90-year-old male on warfarin presenting with reduced consciousness after a fall. **A,** Initial computed tomography (CT) scan showing a left-sided hyperdense (acute) SDH. **B,** Follow-up CT scan 9 days postinjury showing isodense (subacute) SDH as the clot organizes. **C,** Follow-up CT scan 27 days postinjury showing expanding homogeneous hypodense (chronic) SDH suitable for bur-hole evacuation.

skull.[27] Differentials for a hypodense crescentic collection include subdural hygroma (discussed earlier) and subdural empyema. The clinical picture and magnetic resonance imaging will help making the correct diagnosis.

Nakaguchi and colleagues categorized CSDH into four subtypes (homogeneous, laminar, separated, and trabecular), hypothesizing that they were four stages in the natural history of the disease process (Fig. 34-3).[28] They found higher recurrence rates in the separated subtype (36%) and lower recurrence rates in the trabecular subtype (0%) as compared to the homogeneous (15%) and laminar (19%) subtypes,[28] findings that have since been corroborated.[29] However, this has not led to a stratified approach to the treatment of CSDH in routine clinical practice.

Magnetic resonance imaging does not currently have a role in routine clinical practice and is usually performed when other diagnoses were originally suspected.

MANAGEMENT

Preoperative Optimization

The typical patient undergoing surgical intervention for CSDH is often an elderly patient with multiple comorbidities. Those who are taking anticoagulant and antiplatelet medications often have significant cardiovascular disease, and therefore they must undergo a thorough anesthetic assessment to determine suitability and risk of general anesthesia. The assessment should include a cardiorespiratory examination, routine blood tests (complete blood count, urea and electrolytes, clotting studies), and an electrocardiogram; further tests such as a chest radiograph and echocardiography may be required in selected patients. This assessment can aid decisions about whether or not surgical intervention is appropriate and, if so, the type of surgical intervention (see "Conservative Management" section later). Medical optimization, such as treatment of concomitant lower respiratory tract infections or optimization of cardiovascular medications, may be required prior to surgical intervention if the clinical situation allows.

Correction of Coagulopathy and Thrombopathy

Correction of coagulopathy or thrombopathy is crucial to reduce the risks of bleeding during operative intervention and of recurrence. It is not thought to have an effect on the CSDH itself because there is usually no acute bleeding to stop; however, reversal of coagulopathy should occur in nonoperatively managed

TABLE 34-1 Presenting Symptoms and Admission Glasgow Coma Scale (GCS) Score of Patients with Chronic Subdural Hematoma (CSDH)*

	n	%
PRESENTING SYMPTOMS (N = 205)		
Gait disturbance and falls	116	(55.5%)
Mental deterioration	71	(34.0%)
Limb weakness	71	(34.0%)
Acute confusion	67	(32.1%)
Headache	36	(17.2%)
Drowsiness or coma	20	(9.6%)
Speech impairment	12	(5.7%)
Nonspecific deterioration	7	(3.3%)
Collapse	2	(1.0%)
Seizure	2	(1.0%)
Incontinence	1	(0.5%)
Visual disturbance	1	(0.5%)
Vomiting	1	(0.5%)
GCS AT PRESENTATION (N = 202)		
13-15	163	(80.7%)
9-12	25	(12.4%)
3-8	14	(6.9%)

*Data from a prospective randomized controlled trial at our institution examining the role of subdural drains in addition to bur-hole craniostomy for treatment of CSDH.[1]

patients to prevent further expansion. (For further discussion of coagulation, see Chapter 7.)

Most often, the coagulopathy or thrombopathy is iatrogenic. Vitamin K antagonists (e.g., warfarin) can be reversed using a combination of prothrombin complex concentrate (PCC), fresh frozen plasma, and parenteral vitamin K. Most institutions have local protocols to guide clinicians based on the patient's international normalized ratio (INR), clinical state, and timing of pending surgical intervention. For the patient with CSDH in need of urgent surgical intervention, we would advise a combination of PCC and parenteral vitamin K; ideally, the INR should be rechecked prior to surgery and should be less than 1.4.

For the new oral anticoagulants (e.g., dabigatran, rivaroxaban, and fondaparinux), the new European Heart Rhythm Association guidelines suggest that time is the best antidote; if possible, surgery should be delayed until 24 hours after the last dose and this should be extended to 48 hours if the patient has renal impairment and is on a direct thrombin inhibitor (e.g., dabigatran). If urgent intervention is clinically indicated, there may be a role for PCC to reverse these new agents.[30]

With regard to antiplatelet therapy, there is evidence to support delaying treatment by 7 to 10 days to allow the production of fully functional platelets.[23] If treatment cannot be delayed, the American Society of Hematology guidelines recommend platelet transfusion,[31] although there is little evidence for this or any other form of platelet augmentation in this setting.[14,32]

Other sources of clotting and platelet dysfunction may exist in this population, and these should be treated in conjunction with hematologists.

Adjuvant Treatments

There are two main adjuvant medical therapies used for the treatment of CSDH: steroids and antiepileptic medications.

Given the current evidence base, it is unclear whether steroids have a role to play in the management of CSDH and, if so, whether their role is as pre- or postoperative adjunctive therapy or as monotherapy instead of surgery in selected patients.[24,33-37] In the Netherlands, where the use of steroids is frequent, multivariate analysis on a cohort of 496 consecutive patients showed that an increased duration of preoperative steroid use was independently associated with lower recurrence risk, supporting a role for steroids as preoperative adjuvant therapy.[24] Another study, which used a 2-week course of adjuvant steroids postoperatively, suggested a trend for lower recurrence rate in these patients compared to those treated surgically only.[34] In a Spanish cohort of 95 patients with mild symptoms (Markwalder Grade 1-2) treated with steroids only, over three quarters were successfully managed without surgery.[35] Because the current evidence is based solely on retrospective data, a number of randomized controlled trials are currently underway that will help clarify the role of steroids in the management of CSDH.[38] Currently, they are not used routinely in United Kingdom practice[39] or locally in our institution.

The use of prophylactic antiepileptic medication was examined in a Cochrane review, which found a highly variable, but generally low, pre- and postoperative seizure incidence (2.3% to 17% and 1.0% to 23%, respectively).[40] In the three retrospective studies that were analyzed, preoperative antiepileptic prophylaxis was shown to reduce postoperative seizure rate but not discharge outcome.[41] Hence, there is currently no evidence to advocate the use of prophylactic antiepileptic medication in this patient population.

Many other agents have been suggested as adjunctive or stand-alone therapies, including the platelet-activating factor receptor antagonist etizolam,[42] tranexamic acid,[43] and angiotensin-converting enzyme inhibitors.[44] Although none is used routinely, the efficacy of angiotensin-converting enzyme inhibitors in the management of CSDH is the subject of an ongoing trial.

Conservative Management

In general, nonoperative treatment is offered to patients in whom operative risks are believed to outweigh the benefits of surgery. This includes asymptomatic patients with small collections at one end of the spectrum and moribund patients with poor baseline function at the other end.

For the asymptomatic patients with small collections, there are no fixed management guidelines. During the initial admission, efforts must be made to reverse coagulopathy and/or thrombopathy and a course of steroids may be tried (see "Correction of Coagulopathy and Thrombopathy" and "Adjuvant Treatments" sections for further details). Following discharge, repeat CT scanning may be performed either at fixed intervals (e.g., every 2 weeks) until resolution of the hematoma or until it becomes symptomatic, at which point surgical intervention should be undertaken; an alternative, more pragmatic approach may be to rescan the patient only if he or she becomes symptomatic.

At the other end of the spectrum, patients managed conservatively because of either a poor baseline or high surgical risk should be managed in conjunction with other specialties, especially geriatricians and palliative care teams. Importantly, the patient (whenever possible) and the next of kin should be consulted about the appropriateness of escalation of care should the patient deteriorate.

Surgical Intervention

In general, there is consensus that patients with symptoms that can be attributed to a radiologically confirmed CSDH should be treated surgically. Surgical treatment of symptomatic CSDH results in a rapid improvement of patient symptoms and a favorable outcome in over 80% of patients.[14] Coupled with relatively low surgical risk, surgical evacuation is currently the mainstay of management for symptomatic patients.

Three primary surgical techniques are used: (1) twist-drill craniostomy (TDC), involving small openings (<10 mm) made using a twist drill; (2) bur-hole craniostomy (BHC), involving openings of 10 to 30 mm; and (3) craniotomy, involving larger

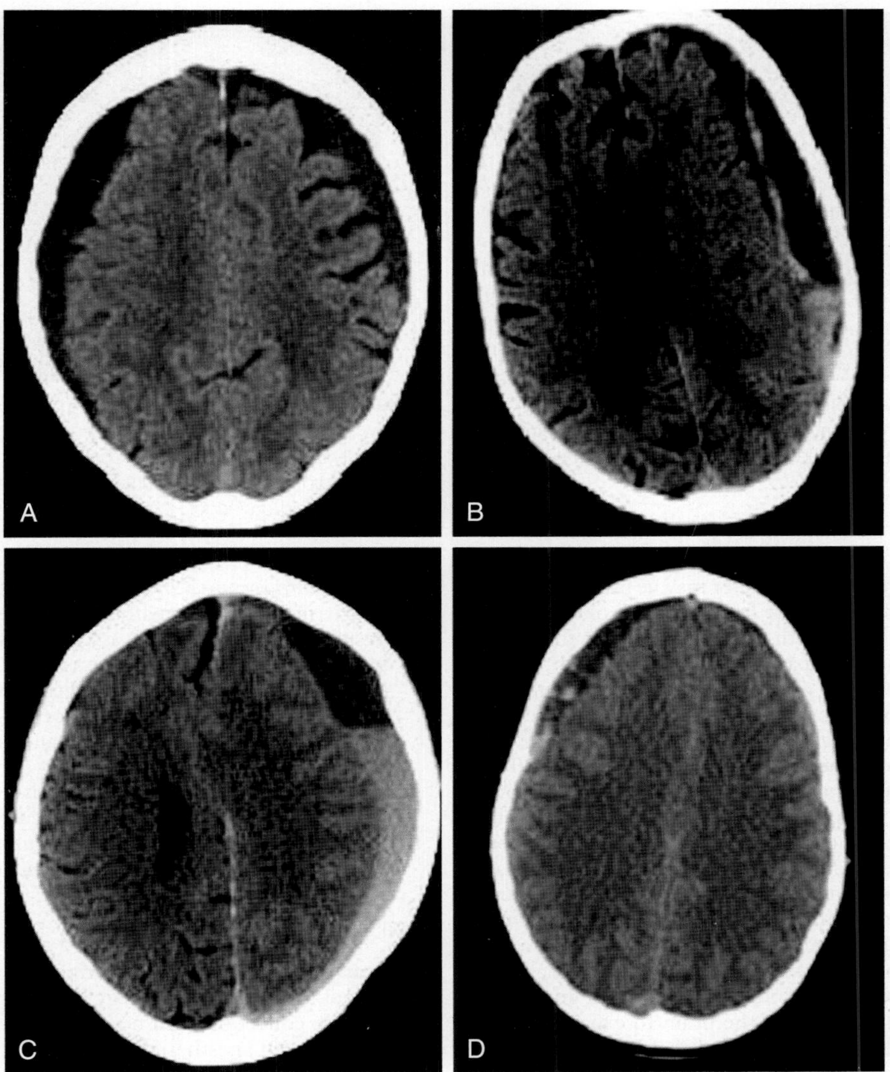

Figure 34-3. Computed tomography scans demonstrating classification of chronic subdural hematomas according to their internal architecture (as proposed by Nakaguchi and colleagues[28]). **A,** Homogeneous. **B,** Laminar. **C,** Separated. **D,** Trabecular. *(Modified from Santarius T, Kolias AG, Hutchinson PJ. Surgical management of chronic subdural haematoma in adults. In: Quiñones-Hinojosa A, ed.* Schmidek & Sweet Operative Neurosurgical Techniques: Indications, Methods, and Results. *6th ed. Philadelphia: Saunders; 2012.)*

openings.[45] Within each of these three broad categories, a number of specific techniques have been described and are used by individual surgeons.[5,39,45] Usually one or two techniques are used by a surgeon or institution to treat most cases of presenting CSDHs. Although it is likely that certain techniques are more suitable for certain subtypes of CSDHs, this has not been shown in published literature, and the choice of technique is probably determined by institutional tradition more than any other factors. The following sections describe the techniques as used and viewed based on the experience from our institution.

Bur-Hole Craniostomy

Indications. BHC is by far the most common technique performed at our institution for CSDH unless there are multiple membranes or a significant acute component to the hematoma, in which case mini-craniotomy would be used.

Anesthesia. BHC is usually performed under general anesthesia but may be performed under local anesthesia.

Technique (Video 34-1). The patient is placed supine on a horseshoe headrest and the head and shoulders are tilted to the contralateral side, ideally with the frontal bur hole being placed at the highest point of the head. This may be difficult to achieve in an elderly patient with a stiff neck, in which case operating table tilt may be useful. Two bur holes are placed over the maximum width of the hematoma, roughly 7 cm apart. Usually, there is one frontal and one parietal bur hole, both of which are just superior to the superior temporal line (Fig. 34-4); a common mistake is to place the bur holes too medially. The dura and outer membrane of the CSDH are incised, releasing hematoma fluid, which is classically described as "engine-oil" colored but may resemble blood, serum, or cerebrospinal fluid. The subdural collection cavity is then irrigated liberally with saline until the

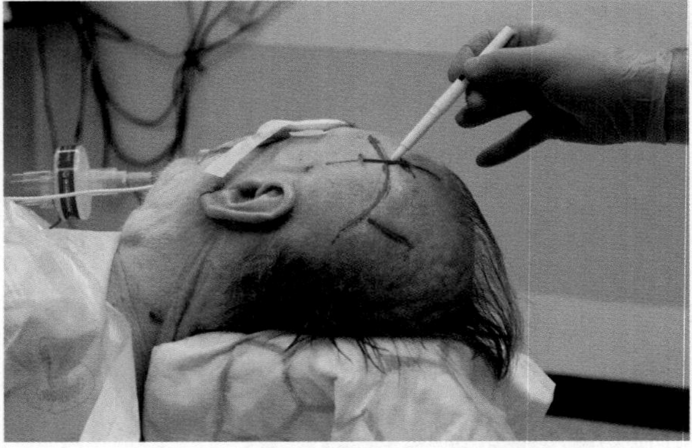

Figure 34-4. Preoperative photograph illustrating the positioning of incisions for bur-hole craniostomy. Note that there is one parietal and one frontal bur hole, both positioned slightly superior to the superior temporal line *(red line).*

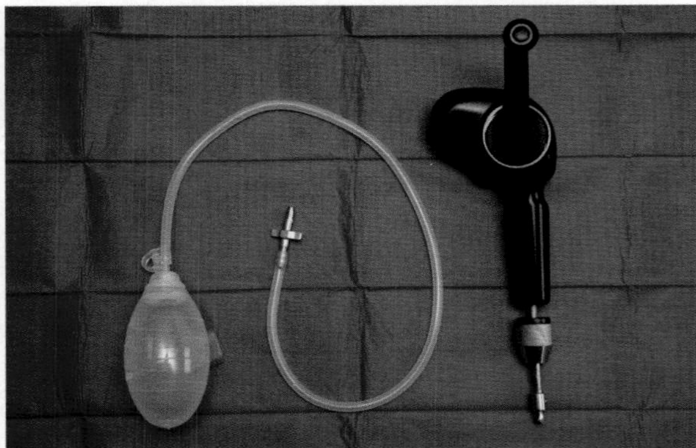

Figure 34-5. The Subdural Evacuating Port System is one of two new hollow screw systems that have been used as modifications of the original twist-drill craniostomy technique. The screw is screwed into the skull and attached to a Jackson-Pratt drain under slight negative pressure to aid drainage.

effluent runs clear; a soft, flexible catheter may be used to augment thorough irrigation in areas remote from the bur holes, although it does carry risks associated with blind insertion of the tubing into subdural space. First the parietal wound is closed: the bur hole is plugged with a thick wafer of absorbable sponge (e.g., gelatin sponge) to aid hemostasis and improve the seal. Next the scalp is closed in two layers, galeal and cutaneous. A soft silicone drain is then inserted into the subdural space via the frontal bur hole. The cavity and drainage tubing are filled with saline prior to closure to aid brain reexpansion through the combination of brain pulsation and the siphoning effect of the drain. It is therefore important that the drain tubing is at least 50 cm long and the drainage bag is positioned below the level of the patient's head. Air trapped in the subdural space and tube may dampen the efficacy of the drain, and hence brain reexpansion, and so may increase recurrence. The drain is removed after approximately 48 hours.[1,27] This is an arbitrary period, thought to be a good compromise between the time given to the brain to expand and the risk of infection related to the presence of the drain, and may be shortened if there is no drainage or lengthened if there is ongoing drainage. If a blood clot blocks the drain, it may be possible to dislodge it by wrapping the drain's soft tubing around a pen several times (see end of Video 34-1). There may be instances in which rapid brain reexpansion prevents safe insertion of the subdural drain; in these instances, a drain is not inserted.

Discussion. The series reported by Markwalder and associates in 1981 brought BHC into prominence as a first-line alternative to craniotomy for the treatment of CSDH,[19] and surveys in the United Kingdom, Canada, and the Netherlands suggest that this is the most popular technique currently in use.[39,46,47] It seems to provide the best balance between maximal efficacy and minimal invasiveness. A randomized controlled trial from our unit confirmed that the use of a subdural drain in a closed drainage system for approximately 48 hours decreased recurrence from 24.3% to 9.3% ($p = 0.003$) and 6-month mortality from 18.1% to 9.6% ($p = 0.042$).[1] However, uncertainties remain about a number of aspects of the technique:

- *Number of bur holes:* Although systematic reviews have found no difference in outcome between one and two bur holes,[48,49] we tend to create two bur holes under general anesthesia because this provides better exposure while being less invasive than a full craniotomy. One bur hole may be considered if the CSDH is more localized or the procedure is performed under local anesthesia, for example.
- *Use of intraoperative irrigation:* There is evidence suggesting that irrigating the hematoma cavity leads to better outcomes despite the potential risks associated with introducing air and infection.[50-52] Although saline is currently used, there is preliminary evidence of reduced recurrence with both thrombin and tissue plasminogen activator as irrigation fluid. These clearly have opposite purposes, and further evidence is thus required.[53,54]
- *Use of drains:* Although there is high-quality evidence that the use of subdural drains reduces recurrence,[1] preliminary evidence suggests that subgaleal and subperiosteal drains may be equally effective,[55-57] but further evaluation is required.

Twist-Drill Craniostomy

Indications. TDC is not performed at our institution but may be used as a less invasive strategy in patients with a predominantly hypodense collection with no membranes thought to be unsuitable for general anesthesia.

Anesthesia. Local anesthesia is used for TDC.

Technique. TDC may be performed at the bedside on the ward or in the neurocritical care unit. After injection of local anesthesia, one or more twist drill holes are placed over the maximal width of the hematoma. The dura and outer membrane are then pierced with a spinal needle and a drainage system is placed. A number of different systems are available, including subdural irrigating and nonirrigating drains and hollow screw systems (see "Discussion" section for further details). As with the BHC technique, drains may be removed after approximately 48 hours.

Discussion. The TDC technique was first published by Tabaddor and Shulman, who found it to be superior to BHC and craniotomy in their cohort of 21 patients.[58] Authors have advocated for its safety and efficacy in comparison to BHC,[59-63] especially in elderly patients with multiple comorbidities who were thought unsuitable for general anesthesia.[64,65] A recent modification to the original technique involves the insertion of a hollow screw to set up a closed drainage system (Fig. 34-5). This technique, unlike the traditional TDC technique, does not require the blind insertion of a catheter in the subdural space, subverting the risks of brain laceration and bleeding from cortical vessels. Preliminary evidence from a systematic review of 796 patients treated with this technique suggests efficacy and safety profiles similar to those of TDC, but level I evidence is pending.[66-68]

Craniotomy and Mini-craniotomy

Indications. At our institution, craniotomy is currently reserved for patients with a significant acute component to the collection, multiple membranes, or recurrent CSDH, but some use mini-craniotomy as a method of choice.

Anesthesia. General anesthesia is used for craniotomy and mini-craniotomy.

Technique. The patient is placed supine with the head on a horseshoe headrest. The head and shoulders are tilted roughly 45 degrees to the contralateral side, as with the bur-hole technique, aiming for the frontal half of the craniotomy to be in the highest point of the head. A free bone flap of varying sizes is created over the hematoma, providing maximal access. (Usually the term *craniotomy* is used if the flap is 6 cm or greater and *mini-craniotomy* is used if the flap is less than 6 cm.) The dura and outer membrane are opened and the cavity is irrigated liberally with saline. As with BHC, a soft silicone drain may inserted subdurally, and the bone flap is replaced and secured. The drain is removed after approximately 48 hours.

Discussion. Historically, craniotomies were associated with significant morbidity and mortality. In modern practice, large craniotomies have been replaced by smaller mini-craniotomies,[69,70] but even these continue to be associated with significant morbidity and mortality for the treatment of primary CSDH; a recent study showed in-hospital mortality of 13.5%.[70] In modern practice, mini-craniotomies are often reserved for recurrent CSDH with extensive organization and membrane formation[71,72] or primary evacuation of a CSDH that has a significant acute component. However, some surgeons use mini-craniotomy as the treatment of choice for the majority of CSDHs. Exact indications of this technique require further refinement, and the efficacy and risk profile of mini-craniotomy need to be compared to those of bur-hole drainage.

Anesthesia

Choice of anesthesia (general versus local) is largely dependent on choice of surgical technique; although most surgeons would prefer to perform craniotomy or mini-craniotomy under general anesthesia, BHC and TDC are performed under either general or local anesthesia. In our institution, we tend to perform BHC under general anesthesia unless there are contraindications or it is deemed to be too high risk.

There are arguments to support both anesthetic techniques. Although common medical risks are probably greater with general anesthesia (no formal evaluation has been published to date), it is overall more comfortable for the patient and the surgeon. Opting for comfort is not merely a frivolous indulgence; operating on an anxious, confused, or otherwise agitated patient can significantly affect the quality of technical execution of the procedure. Local anesthesia is generally associated with less physiologic stress and may reduce length of stay and the delay between admission and operation. In recent years, conscious sedation has arisen as a viable intermediate, facilitating patient comfort while reducing the risks associated with a general anesthetic.[73]

Outcomes

In general, surgical outcomes in CSDH are favorable, with the majority of patients improving postoperatively. In a trial setting, good functional outcomes are achieved in more than 80% of patients. At 6 months, about 10% of patients experience a recurrence and mortality is about 5%.[1] Comparison of techniques comes from three large meta-analyses.[14,45,74] Although they reach subtly different conclusions, general consensus is that craniotomy is associated with less recurrence than the other two techniques, but a higher rate of morbidity and mortality. Although TDC has the lowest morbidity and mortality rates, recurrence is higher. Therefore, BHC is generally recommended because it provides the balance between efficacy and risks (Table 34-2). It has to be kept in mind that the data, particularly those pertaining to craniotomy, are somewhat outdated, as discussed previously.

All three studies, and indeed any attempt at meta-analysis in CSDH, are limited by the paucity of level I evidence in the field. To date, we have identified only 13 published prospective randomized controlled trials in the field, and small numbers, variable surgical techniques, and heterogeneous outcome measures limit comparisons among these trials. In addition, outcome measures in these studies have tended to focus on either recurrence or a "good outcome" with heterogeneous definitions for both, limiting the potential for cross-study comparisons. The focus needs to shift to homogenize these outcome measures, concentrate on functional outcomes (such as the modified Rankin Scale), and ensure that future studies are high-quality prospective studies that facilitate evidence-based treatment options for CSDH.

Postoperative Care

Stipulation of early postoperative bed rest of CSDH patients remains a controversial issue, with roughly half of surgeons for or against it in surveys.[39,46] Whereas bed rest is thought to reduce recurrence rates by promoting brain expansion, early mobilization is thought to decrease medical complications associated with immobility, specifically venous thromboembolism and hospital-acquired infections. A large study with historical controls found no significant difference in recurrence rates but increased medical

TABLE 34-2 Comparison of Efficacy, Morbidity/Complications, Recurrence, and Mortality of the Different Techniques in Contemporary Meta-analyses[14,45,74]

		Successful Outcome	Morbidity/Complications	Recurrence	Mortality
Almenawer et al.[74] (2014)	BHC	86.0%	7.2%	10.5%	3.5%
	TDC	90.2%	5.5%	14.5%	3.6%
	Craniotomy	80.3%	10.2%	6.2%	6.8%
Ducruet et al.[14] (2012)	BHC	84.9%	9.3%	11.7%	3.7%
	TDC	93.5%	2.5%	28.1%	5.1%
	Craniotomy	74.4%	3.9%	19.4%	12.2%
Weigel et al.[45] (2003)	BHC	79.1%	3.8%	12.1%	2.7%
	TDC	88.1%	3.0%	33.0%	2.9%
	Craniotomy	67.8%	12.3%	10.8%	4.6%

BHC, bur-hole craniostomy; TDC, twist-drill craniostomy.

complications in the delayed mobilization (after 3 days) group as compared to the early mobilization (on the first postoperative day) group.[75] In our practice, we place no restriction and actively encourage mobilization as soon as possible, with physiotherapy assistance if necessary; even short periods of bed rest can set an elderly patient back physically and mentally.

As with all hospital inpatients, all CSDH patients with impaired mobility should receive thromboprophylaxis. Thromboembolism-deterrent stockings should be applied to all patients upon admission if not contraindicated. Prophylactic-dose low-molecular-weight heparin should also be prescribed if the patient is immobile postoperatively; if a drain is left in situ postoperatively, the low-molecular-weight heparin can be commenced once the drain is removed.

With regard to restarting anticoagulant and antiplatelet medication, there are still many unknowns, such as if and when to restart medication and, if so, whether the postoperative anticoagulant target (INR) or dose should be the same as that given preoperatively.[76] Currently these decisions are made on an individual patient basis; advice from a physician or general practitioner is often useful, and factors to be considered include the indication for anticoagulation, patient age and comorbidities, and risk of further falls and head injury. An objective method that can be used for patients taking warfarin for atrial fibrillation is to compare their CHA_2DS_2-VASc thromboembolism risk scores without anticoagulation and the HAS-BLED bleeding risk scores with anticoagulation to quantify relative risks (Fig. 34-6).[76] Limited individual studies advocate for safe resumption of warfarin as little as 3 days post-CSDH.[77] There are few data about the new oral anticoagulant medications, but the current European Heart Rhythm Association guidelines suggest they can be safely restarted 10 to 14 days after an intracranial hemorrhage.[30]

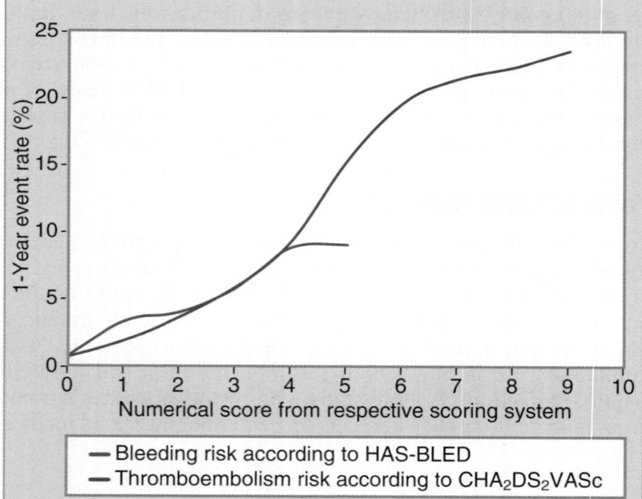

Figure 34-6. Comparison of 1-year bleeding risk according to the HAS-BLED (*h*ypertension, *a*bnormal renal and liver function, *s*troke, *b*leeding, *l*abile international normalized ratio, *e*lderly, and *d*rugs or alcohol) score and 1-year thromboembolism risk according to the CHA_2DS_2-VASc (congestive heart failure; *h*ypertension; *a*ge >75 years; *d*iabetes mellitus; prior *s*troke, transient ischemic attack, or thromboembolism; *v*ascular disease; *a*ge 65-74 years; and *s*ex *c*ategory) score in patients with atrial fibrillation. Note that the numerical values correspond to almost identical risks and, assuming that a bleed and thromboembolism are associated with similar morbidity and mortality, a decision on whether or not to restart anticoagulation may be made based on a comparison of these scores. *(Modified from Chari A, Clemente Morgado T, Rigamonti D. Recommencement of anticoagulation in chronic subdural haematoma: a systematic review and meta-analysis.* Br J Neurosurg. *2013;28:2-7.)*

Follow-up

In our unit, CSDH patients are generally discharged from the hospital when mobile or returning to their baseline function; they may be transferred back to a regional hospital to facilitate further rehabilitation if they are stable from a CSDH point of view. Routine early postoperative CT scans are not performed unless clinically indicated. Patients are seen in the clinic at 2 to 3 months, with a CT scan to screen for subtle symptomatic residual collection. At this stage the vast majority of patients are discharged from follow-up.

Complications and Prognosis

Perhaps the most important complication of CSDH is recurrence necessitating reoperation because it has been shown to affect postoperative functional outcomes[1] and quality of life.[22] Recurrence rates in the literature vary widely from 0 to 76%,[14,45] but contemporary consensus is that the reoperation rate is 10% to 20%. Factors that have been associated with recurrence include bilateral CSDH,[78,79] preoperative anticoagulant[18,21,29] and antiplatelet[18] medication, intraoperative visualization of poor brain reexpansion and thick membranes,[80] postoperative persistence of midline shift,[29] and intracranial air,[81] although data for these come from small studies with low events-per-variable ratios and thus have to be interpreted cautiously.

Procedure-specific complications include focal brain injury, postoperative acute subdural or intracranial hemorrhage, seizures, surgical site infection, subdural empyema, and tension pneumocephalus.[82] Nonsurgical complications include hospital-acquired infections (respiratory and urinary), venous thromboembolism, myocardial infarction, and stroke. In the elderly population, even trivial complications may result in serious adverse outcomes, and effort must be made to prevent these where possible and diagnose and treat them early when they occur.

Mortality ranges between 0 and 32% and morbidity between 0 and 25%, although contemporary figures would suggest that operative mortality ranges around 2% to 5%.[14,45] A number of studies have retrospectively examined morbidity and mortality from CSDH and identified age, GCS or clinical state (Markwalder Grade) at presentation, presence of medical comorbidities (including liver and renal dysfunction), and coagulopathy as important prognostic factors.[17,80,83-85]

FUTURE RESEARCH AREAS

In spite of CSDH being one of the most common neurosurgical conditions, there remain a number of unanswered questions surrounding its management in terms of preoperative, intraoperative, postoperative, and adjuvant care (Fig. 34-7). Despite being abundant, the literature on CSDH is limited by a paucity of high-quality studies. In order to reach evidence-based treatment decisions in CSDH, there must be a drive to conduct robust, high-quality studies answering clinically important questions that will facilitate improvement in outcomes.

Particularly, CSDH is currently approached as a single entity, with little potential to tailor treatment according to individual patient and hematoma characteristics. Further research in this field needs to focus on providing solid data to allow formulation of an evidence-based individualized treatment plan for each patient that maximizes functional outcomes while minimizing risks for this common neurosurgical condition.

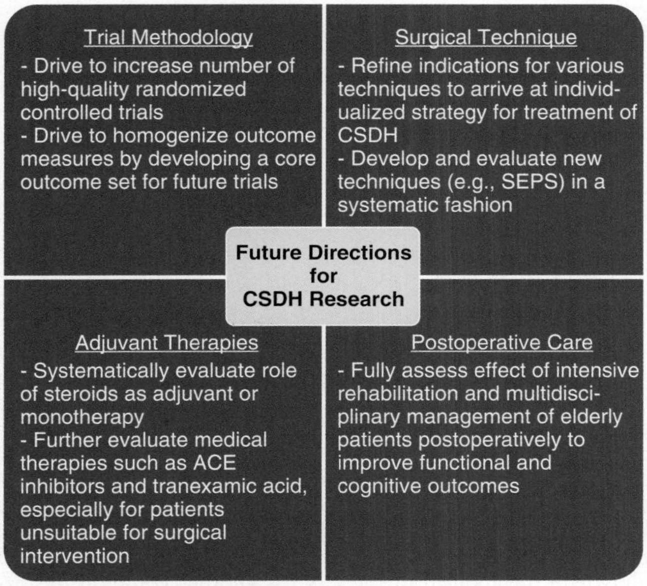

Trial Methodology	Surgical Technique
- Drive to increase number of high-quality randomized controlled trials - Drive to homogenize outcome measures by developing a core outcome set for future trials	- Refine indications for various techniques to arrive at individualized strategy for treatment of CSDH - Develop and evaluate new techniques (e.g., SEPS) in a systematic fashion
Future Directions for CSDH Research	
Adjuvant Therapies	**Postoperative Care**
- Systematically evaluate role of steroids as adjuvant or monotherapy - Further evaluate medical therapies such as ACE inhibitors and tranexamic acid, especially for patients unsuitable for surgical intervention	- Fully assess effect of intensive rehabilitation and multidisciplinary management of elderly patients postoperatively to improve functional and cognitive outcomes

Figure 34-7. Future research areas in chronic subdural hematoma (CSDH). ACE, angiotensin-converting enzyme; SEPS, Subdural Evacuating Port System.

CONCLUSION

Current consensus is that symptomatic CSDH is best treated by surgical evacuation, and although BHC is generally accepted as first line for surgical treatment worldwide, further work needs to be done to refine indications for the different surgical techniques. In addition, there is a need to better define the role of adjuvant therapies such as steroids. Given that the burden of CSDH is set to rise in the coming years, there is an expressed need to improve outcomes for this common neurosurgical condition.

SUGGESTED READINGS

Almenawer SA, Farrokhyar F, Hong C, et al. Chronic subdural hematoma management: a systematic review and meta-analysis of 34829 patients. *Ann Surg*. 2014;259:449-457.

Berghauser Pont LM, Dirven CM, Dippel DW, et al. The role of corticosteroids in the management of chronic subdural hematoma: a systematic review. *Eur J Neurol*. 2012;19:1397-1403.

Chari A, Kolias AG, Bond S, et al. Twist-drill craniostomy with hollow screws for evacuation of chronic subdural haematoma: a systematic review. *J Neurosurg*. 2014;121:176-183.

Ducruet AF, Grobelny BT, Zacharia BE, et al. The surgical management of chronic subdural hematoma. *Neurosurg Rev*. 2012;35:155-169, discussion 169.

Horn EM, Feiz-Erfan I, Bristol RE, et al. Bedside twist drill craniostomy for chronic subdural hematoma: a comparative study. *Surg Neurol*. 2006;65:150-153, discussion 153-154.

Santarius T, Kirkpatrick PJ, Ganesan D, et al. Use of drains versus no drains after burr-hole evacuation of chronic subdural haematoma: a randomised controlled trial. *Lancet*. 2009;374:1067-1073.

Santarius T, Kirkpatrick PJ, Kolias AG, et al. Working toward rational and evidence-based treatment of chronic subdural hematoma. *Clin Neurosurg*. 2010;57:112-122.

Weigel R, Schmiedek P, Krauss JK. Outcome of contemporary surgery for chronic subdural haematoma: evidence based review. *J Neurol Neurosurg Psychiatry*. 2003;74:937-943.

See a full reference list on ExpertConsult.com

35 Basic Science of Central Nervous System Infections

Jeffrey M. Tessier and W. Michael Scheld

Infections within the central nervous system (CNS) are generally divided into specific clinical categories on the basis of the anatomy of the infection (parenchymal, meningeal, parameningeal) and the presence of space-occupying lesions (e.g. abscess, empyema) or diffuse inflammation (e.g. meningitis, encephalitis). CNS infections can also be categorized according to etiology: bacterial, viral, fungal, parasitic, or prion related. Given the substantial structural and functional defenses that prevent infection of the CNS by any of these agents, specific mechanisms have evolved among neuroinvasive pathogens that facilitate their entry into and survival in the CNS. Opportunistic infection of the CNS may occur when host structural and/or functional defenses are impaired; this is a common mechanism for post-neurosurgical CNS infections such as shunt infection, brain abscess, and bacterial meningitis.

Pathogens enter the CNS directly (e.g., through trauma, neurosurgery), via passage across the blood-brain or blood–cerebrospinal fluid barrier (e.g., bacterial meningitis caused by *Escherichia coli*), or via retrograde transport along neural structures (e.g., rabies). Once entry has been achieved, the invading organism must survive the onslaught of immune effectors that are present in or recruited into the CNS in response to the invasion. Examples of immune effectors normally present in the CNS are astrocytes and microglia, both of which cellular elements are involved in the recruitment of additional cellular and humoral defenses from outside the CNS. Both of these cell types clearly play important roles in the defense against and pathogenesis of CNS infections caused by a wide array of neuropathogens; these roles are discussed in more detail in the full chapter. The interactions between the host immune response and the invading pathogens produce a complex and dynamic "battlefield," leading to varying degrees of both structural and functional damage to the CNS. Examples of immune effectors involved in both defense of and damage to the CNS are matrix metalloproteinases, enzymes that are capable of degrading important components of the blood-brain barrier (e.g., type IV collagen) and altering both host immune responses via modification of cytokine/chemokine molecules and their downstream consequences. Dysregulation of glutamate metabolism in the CNS is another common mechanism for altered CNS function and structural damage during infections caused by several different pathogens (e.g., human immunodeficiency virus [HIV], pneumococci). Many neuroinvasive pathogens damage CNS components directly via toxin production; the critical roles played by pneumolysin, a pore-forming cholesterol-dependent cytolysin, in the pathogenesis of pneumococcal meningitis are discussed in this chapter as an example of pathogen-mediated direct damage to the CNS.

In addition to addressing basic mechanisms involved in the broad pathogenesis of CNS infections like meningitis and encephalitis, this chapter also addresses the biology of pyogenic brain abscesses and similar space-occupying diseases that are encountered by the neurosurgeon. The chapter concludes with a discussion of the role of biofilms in cerebrospinal fluid (CSF) shunt infections and potential therapeutic targets that may provide additional benefits in the treatment of these difficult complications of neurosurgical CSF management.

Full text of this chapter is available online at ExpertConsult.com

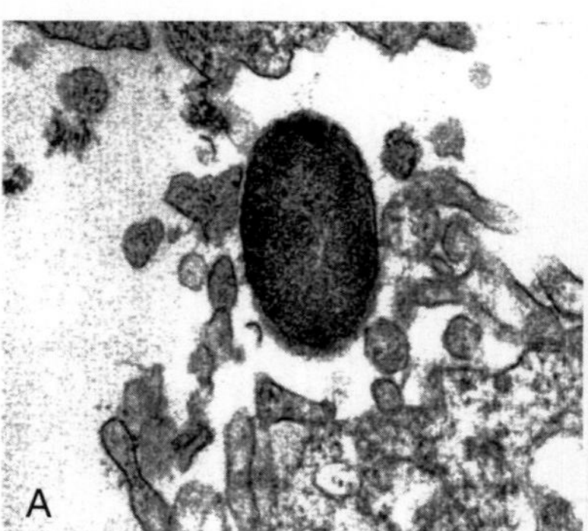

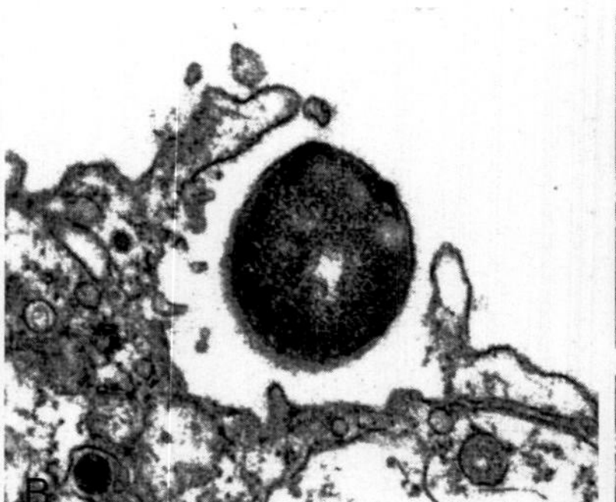

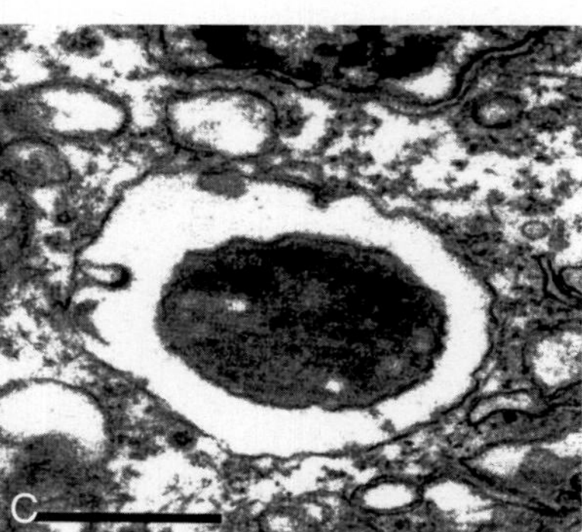

Transmission electron micrographs of *Escherichia coli.* K1 strain RS 218 undergoing attachment (**A**) and internalization (**B** and **C**) into human brain microvascular endothelial cells. Scale bar, 1 μm. *(From Kim KS. Microbial translocation of the blood-brain barrier.* Int J Parasitol. *2006;36:607-614.)*

36 Postoperative Infections of the Head and Brain

Mary L. Pisculli, Frederick G. Barker II, and Christopher J. Farrell

Before Lister's 1867 introduction of surgical antisepsis, nearly 80% of operations were followed by infections at the surgical site and almost half of the patients died after operation.[1] Despite considerable advances in our understanding of the pathogenesis of surgical infection, the introduction of rigorous aseptic practices within the operating room, and the use of prophylactic antibiotics for clean operations, infection after neurosurgical intervention remains an all too frequent occurrence. Although mortality rates have decreased markedly, postcraniotomy infections commonly require prolonged antibiotic treatment and additional surgical interventions for successful eradication and frequently result in significant morbidity, prolonged hospitalization, and increased health care expenses. The economic burden of postoperative infections is significant: the median hospital charge for patients with a surgical site infection (SSI) attributable to methicillin-resistant *Staphylococcus aureus* (MRSA) is almost $100,000, triple that for uninfected surgical patients,[2] and the overall cost of SSIs is believed to account for up to $10 billion annually in health care expenditures.[3]

The diagnosis of infection after craniotomy is often challenging. Many of the typical correlates of infection are nonspecific in the postoperative setting, and recognition of infection may frequently be delayed. An accurate understanding of the clinical, laboratory, and radiographic manifestations of postcraniotomy infection is critical to enable timely medical and surgical intervention and to limit the neurological sequelae of infection. This chapter examines these manifestations and discusses the tenets of effective therapy. The epidemiology of postcraniotomy infections is also discussed, along with a review of the factors conferring an increased risk for infection and the strategies that have proved to decrease the incidence of postoperative infection. Infections related to cerebrospinal fluid (CSF) shunting procedures are not included in this chapter.

EPIDEMIOLOGY AND ETIOLOGY

Postoperative infections are typically categorized according to anatomic site (Table 36-1). The Centers for Disease Control and Prevention (CDC) defines *superficial incisional infections* as those limited to the skin and subcutaneous tissue, whereas *deep incisional infections* may involve the subgaleal space and bone flap. *Deep organ space infections* include subdural empyema, brain abscess, and meningitis/ventriculitis. According to data from the CDC's National Nosocomial Infection Surveillance (NNIS) program, superficial infections are responsible for 60% of SSIs after craniotomy. Meningitis is the most common deep organ space infection, representing 22% of postcraniotomy infections, whereas other intracranial infections, including subdural empyema and brain abscess, account for 14%.[4] The incidence of infection after craniotomy is difficult to estimate from the neurosurgical literature because of differences in definitions and methodology. Several large prospective studies have reported postcraniotomy infection rates ranging from 1% to 10%, with the higher rates occurring in the absence of antibiotic prophylaxis.[4-11] In a study restricted to elective procedures, McClelland and Hall[8] reviewed the postoperative courses of 1587 patients who underwent cranial operations over a 15-year period performed by a single surgeon and found an impressively low rate (0.8%) of postoperative infection.

In accord with other studies,[6,12-14] McClelland and Hall[8] identified *S. aureus* as the causative agent for approximately half of the infections that develop after craniotomy. Infections after craniotomy are most commonly associated with gram-positive bacteria, *S. aureus*, and coagulase-negative staphylococci. Isolation of *Propionibacterium acnes*, an anaerobic gram-positive bacillus, from neurosurgical specimens had been dismissed as a contaminant because it is commensal scalp flora; however, the role of *P. acnes* as a causative agent of postcraniotomy infections is now established. Earlier reports likely underestimated its pathologic role owing to its often indolent clinical manifestation and the difficulties associated with microbiologic isolation of the organism, specifically the need to hold the anaerobic culture for 10 days.[15] Other bacteria isolated from postcraniotomy infections include enterococci, *Streptococcus* spp., *Pseudomonas aeruginosa*, *Acinetobacter* spp., *Citrobacter* spp., *Enterobacter* spp., *Klebsiella pneumoniae*, *Escherichia coli*, miscellaneous other gram-negative bacilli, and yeast. Gram-negative bacteria have been isolated in 5% to 8% of postcraniotomy infections as well as within polymicrobial infections.[16] Although direct spread from contiguous areas of infection is common, the causative agents tend to vary according to the site of infection and the antimicrobial spectrum of administered perioperative antibiotics.[7] Yang and colleagues[17] retrospectively identified 31 patients with brain abscesses after neurosurgical procedures and found the most prevalent pathogens to be a single gram-negative bacillus (*Enterobacter cloacae*, *K. pneumoniae*, *E. coli*, *P. aeruginosa*, *Proteus mirabilis*, and *Salmonella* species) or a polymicrobial infection (including *E. coli*, *E. cloacae*, *P. mirabilis*, *S. aureus*, *S. epidermidis*, *Acinetobacter baumannii*, *K. pneumoniae*, *Citrobacter diversus*, and viridans streptococci), followed by infection with streptococcal and staphylococcal spp. Gram-negative bacilli are also the most common causes of postoperative meningitis, accounting for 29% to 38% of nosocomial episodes of this infection.[18,19]

RISK FACTORS FOR INFECTION AND PREVENTIVE STRATEGIES

The majority of postsurgical infections are due to contamination of the wound with bacteria from the patient's skin. Although the magnitude of contamination and the virulence of the contaminating organism certainly contribute to the rate of infection, all surgical wounds become inoculated with bacteria to some extent at the time of surgery, but in only a small percentage of patients does this contamination lead to clinical infection.[20,21] Although it is unlikely that all postoperative infections can be completely prevented, many of the factors influencing the development of infection may be modifiable, including those attributable to the patient and others related to the surgical intervention itself.

Host defense mechanisms, which represent the primary barrier to establishment of infection, may be impaired in patients undergoing craniotomy. The brain is a relatively immune privileged site, and low levels of antibody and complement contribute to make the brain less efficient than other organs of the body at eradicating infection. Furthermore, many of the underlying pathologies leading to neurosurgical intervention may significantly impair immune function. For example, patients with malignant gliomas express a variety of immune defects, including increased secretion of immunosuppressive cytokines.[22] In addition, many of the

TABLE 36-1 Epidemiology, Clinical Presentation, and Treatment Recommendations for Postoperative Cranial Infections

Location of Infection	Etiology (Most Common)	Signs and Symptoms	Treatment Options
Superficial incisional	*Staphylococcus aureus*, coagulase-negative staphylococci	Incisional erythema, tenderness, suppurative drainage	Local débridement ± oral/intravenous antibiotics*
Subgaleal space and bone flap	*Staphylococcus aureus*, coagulase-negative staphylococci, *Propionibacterium acnes*	Incisional erythema, tenderness, suppurative drainage Exposed bone flap/hardware	Local débridement Intravenous antibiotics Bone flap removal *with either delayed cranioplasty or immediate titanium cranioplasty*†
Autogenous/synthetic cranioplasty	*Staphylococcal* spp, *Propionibacterium acnes*, gram-negative bacilli	Incisional erythema, tenderness, suppurative drainage Exposed bone flap/hardware	Local débridement Intravenous antibiotics Bone flap removal
Subdural empyema	*Staphylococcal* spp, gram-negative bacilli, *Streptococcus* spp	Superficial infection Encephalopathy Seizures	Local débridement Intravenous antibiotics
Brain abscess	Gram-negative bacilli, *Staphylococcal* spp, *Streptococcus* spp	Encephalopathy Seizures Nausea/vomiting Focal neurological deficit	Local débridement Intravenous antibiotics
Meningitis	Gram-negative bacilli	Headache Meningismus Fever	Intravenous antibiotics Cerebrospinal fluid leak repair ± corticosteroids

*Intravenous antibiotics with increased institutional incidence of methicillin-resistant *S. aureus*.
†Prolonged (≥3 months) oral antibiotic therapy, depending on organism susceptibility pattern.

adjunctive therapies used for treating brain tumors, such as corticosteroid administration, chemotherapy, and irradiation, may result in immune compromise. Other frequent indications for craniotomy, such as trauma, have also been shown to be profoundly immunosuppressive.[23]

General surgical and infection control studies have identified other host factors that influence the risk for SSI, including advanced age, obesity, hypoalbuminemia, diabetes mellitus, and poor functional status.[3,24-26] Gianotti and associates[27] demonstrated the importance of nutritional status in oncologic surgery by showing that malnourished patients had improved resistance to infection after as little as 5 days of enteral nutrition. Even though earlier reports suggested an increased rate of postoperative infection after general surgical procedures in patients infected with human immunodeficiency virus (HIV),[28,29] retrospective studies performed since the advent of highly active antiretroviral therapy (HAART) have not demonstrated an association between SSI rates and HIV infection.[30-32]

The increased rate of SSIs associated with the preceding factors has been attributed to nonspecific deficits in host defense. Obesity and the associated potential impairment of antibiotic tissue penetration may also limit the efficacy of preventive antimicrobial therapy.[33] Although the influence of many of these individual intrinsic preoperative factors on the rate of SSI after neurosurgical intervention has not been established in prospective studies, optimization of immune function through minimization of corticosteroid use, adequate nutritional support, and perioperative glucose control may all be potentially beneficial in the prevention of postcraniotomy infections. Additional patient endogenous risk factors that have been found to increase the risk of infection after craniotomy are a preoperative American Society of Anesthesiologists (ASA) classification 2 or higher and a concomitant (including remote) infection at the time of craniotomy.[34]

Several factors specific to craniotomy have been identified as raising the risk for postoperative infection. In a prospective multicenter trial, Korinek[5] identified postoperative CSF leakage and early subsequent reoperation as independent risk factors for SSI, suggesting that careful attention to closure techniques and meticulous hemostasis may potentially result in lower rates of postoperative infection. Multiple studies have established CSF leakage as a major risk factor for infection.[6,9,11,14,35-37] Korinek[5] also identified the following independent predictors of postoperative infection after craniotomy: surgery lasting longer than 4 hours, emergency surgery, clean-contaminated and contaminated surgery, and neurosurgical intervention in the preceding month. Valentini and colleagues[38] observed a relative risk (RR) of 12.6 for postoperative infection in elective clean craniotomies lasting 2 hours and an RR of 24.3 for procedures lasting longer than 3 hours. The association between longer duration of surgery and infection has not been defined precisely, but plausible explanations include greater complexity of the surgery and prolonged exposure of the wound to bacterial contamination.

The association of a variety of other risk factors with infection after craniotomy has been less reliably demonstrated; placement of drains or intracranial pressure monitors, poor neurological status, paranasal sinus entry, diabetes mellitus, and foreign body implantation (other than shunts) have been identified as risk factors in some retrospective studies.[5,9,14,34,38,39] Synthetic dural substitutes are foreign bodies and might represent a potentially greater risk factor for infection than an autologous graft material such as pericranium, temporalis fascia, or fascia lata. Evidence demonstrating increased rates of infection with the use of synthetic dural substitutes, however, is limited. Malliti and colleagues[40] reported a statistically nonsignificant higher incidence of deep wound infections after craniotomy with the use of a nonresorbable polyester urethane synthetic dural graft (Neuro-Patch, B. Braun, Boulogne, France). Postoperative CSF leaks were also significantly more frequent when the synthetic dural substitute was used, thus limiting the ability of this study to determine whether use of the dural substitute independently increased the risk for infection. The presence of a nonresorbable dural substitute may also impair successful treatment of an infected wound because a graft may become colonized and its removal may be required to eradicate the infection. A variety of nonautologous, resorbable collagen dural substitutes are currently available, and their relationship with surgical infection has not been well explored. McCall and coworkers[41] reported the uncomplicated use of several of these materials in a small number of patients in the setting of contaminated wounds, a finding suggesting that they may not impede clearance of infection. The use of Gliadel wafers (Arbor Pharmaceuticals, Atlanta, GA), which contain 1,3-bis-(2-chloroethyl)-1-nitrosourea (BCNU), for the treatment of malignant gliomas has also been associated with an increased incidence of postoperative infection. McGovern and associates[42] reported a 28% rate of infection in cases associated with insertion of BCNU wafers between 1996 and 1999; however, incidence of infection appeared in part to be associated with inadequate antibiotic prophylaxis. A subsequent report with a larger patient population (n = 1013) did not reveal any statistically significant differences in the rate of postoperative infection with BCNU wafer use.[43]

Cranioplasty and bone flap replacement procedures represent an aberrant category of neurosurgical interventions, with multiple reports demonstrating infectious complications rates approaching 30%.[44-47] Although some studies have suggested a relationship between cranioplasty material (autograft vs. allograft) and SSI, a systematic review by Yadla and coworkers[44] failed to demonstrate a significant difference based on type of prosthesis or timing of bone flap replacement. More extensive evaluation of the strategies used to avoid SSI associated with these procedures is discussed in Chapter 28.

Multiple prospective randomized clinical studies and a meta-analysis have validated the effectiveness of preoperative antibiotics in reducing the incidence of SSIs after craniotomy.[12,35,36,48,49] Cairns described the first trial of a modern prophylactic antibiotic in neurosurgery in 1947 when he reported sprinkling a "light frosting" of penicillin powder directly onto the brain in 670 patients and deemed the results superior to those of historical controls.[50,51] In 1979, Malis[52] demonstrated the ability of a prophylactic antibiotic regimen (vancomycin and an aminoglycoside) to reduce the incidence of SSI after craniotomy. Since these initial reports, a variety of antibiotic regimens have been used for effective surgical prophylaxis. Guidelines for a standardized approach to antimicrobial prophylaxis in surgery have been developed and updated in an effort to prevent SSI (and their associated morbidity, mortality, and additional health care costs and length of hospitalization) without adverse consequences to both the patient and the microbial milieu of the patient or the hospital.[16] The Surgical Care Improvement Project (SCIP) outlines the following three performance measures for monitoring appropriate antimicrobial prophylaxis use: selection of an appropriate antibiotic, its administration within 1 hour before incision (2 hours to allow for the administration of vancomycin and fluoroquinolones), and discontinuation of the antibiotic within 24 hours after surgery is completed.[53] The choice of an agent with an appropriately narrow spectrum of coverage against relevant pathogens should be guided by individual institutional data on frequently recovered pathogens and their resistance profiles. For clean neurosurgical procedures, a single dose of cefazolin is recommended. Vancomycin may be used as an alternative agent in the setting of MRSA colonization or for a patient with a documented β-lactam allergy.[16] Antibiotics with short half-lives such as cefazolin should be readministered every 3 to 4 hours during prolonged surgery to ensure adequate drug levels throughout the period of potential contamination, including the time of wound closure.[16] Use of antibiotics beyond 24 hours postoperatively has not shown a greater benefit and may increase the risk for other nosocomial infections as well as promote the emergence of multidrug-resistant pathogens.[53,54]

With the rise of resistant pathogens, in particular MRSA, attention is being placed on the perioperative management of neurosurgical patients with MRSA colonization. A review of 1000 neurosurgical admissions identified the following risk factors for MRSA infection: male sex, malignancy, diabetes, prior MRSA infection, immunosuppressed state, and traumatic injury.[55] Le and associates[56] observed an MRSA colonization rate of 19% in patients undergoing cranioplasty after prior decompressive craniectomy, which was more than three times higher than that for all patients admitted to their neurosurgical intensive care unit. After institution of a cranioplasty-specific protocol that included a change in perioperative antibiotic administration from cefazolin to vancomycin, the rate of SSI decreased from 24% to 3%.[56] Although the institution of MRSA-specific antibiotic prophylaxis appears to benefit neurosurgical patients identified with MRSA colonization or prior MRSA infection, its widespread use may lead to further development of resistance.[57] MRSA screening and decolonization protocols have been increasingly implemented but the optimal strategy for neurosurgical cranial procedures has not yet been determined.[16]

Other perioperative risk reduction considerations include surgical site preparation and environmental control within the operating room. Although no evidence has been found that preoperative hair removal reduces the incidence of postoperative infection, any hair removal that is performed should be done as close to the time of surgery as possible, and clippers used rather than a razor to minimize the number of bacteria that colonize the inevitable small cuts and abrasions that develop from shaving.[58-60] Several antiseptic skin preparations have been used (chlorhexidine, iodophor compounds, alcohol), but no agent has been definitively shown to be more effective than another.[61] To provide effective antisepsis, these agents must remain on the skin until they dry naturally, with avoidance of any pooling. Theoretically, adhesive barrier drapes with antiseptic embedded within the adhesive may prevent bacterial contamination of the surgical site throughout the operative procedure; however, their ability to reduce the incidence of SSI has not been proven.[62] Similarly, there is no reliable evidence to support having the patient bathe or shower preoperatively with an antiseptic skin product.[63]

Measures to decrease bacterial contamination in the operating room (OR) environment may help to reduce SSIs, although it is difficult to ascertain the independent effects of these measures from the literature.[64] Both the number of health care workers within the operating room and traffic throughout the procedure should be kept to a minimum because bacterial shedding increases with activity and can potentially result in increased airborne contamination. Ensuring adequate ventilation minimizes the particulates and bacteria in the perioperative environment, and the use of high-efficiency particulate air (HEPA) filters has been shown to reduce the rate of SSI development after orthopedic implant surgery.[65] Effective cleaning and disinfection of the operating room environment is also imperative to decrease pathogen transmission. Using ultraviolet markers and environmental cultures, Munoz-Price and associates[66] evaluated OR contamination and cleaning practices at an academic medical center and demonstrated bacterial contamination, including by multidrug-resistant organisms, on more than half of tested surfaces. After implementation of ongoing performance feedback measures and increased attention to cleaning of high-touch areas and anesthesia equipment, the percentage of cleaned surfaces increased to 82%.

PRINCIPLES OF TREATMENT

Immune defenses within the brain are rarely adequate to control infection once it has been established. Postoperative infections tend to be particularly difficult to resolve because of the complex anatomic changes resulting from craniotomy and the frequent involvement of virulent organisms. Early and decisive intervention is critical to limit morbidity, and the keystone of successful treatment is effective source control (i.e., drainage of abscesses and infected fluid collections and débridement of necrotic tissue). Once source control has been achieved, initiation of appropriate antibiotic therapy is necessary to eliminate any residual local infection.

The antibiotic regimen and duration of treatment should be selected in consultation with infectious diseases specialists and based on the capacity of the antibiotic to penetrate the infected tissue effectively and exhibit activity against the suspected pathogen. Bactericidal rather than bacteriostatic agents are generally preferred because of the inefficient opsonization and phagocytic capabilities within the brain.[67] Most antibiotic agents enter the central nervous system (CNS) predominantly by passive diffusion down a concentration gradient, with physical barriers such as the blood-brain and blood-CSF barriers functioning as the primary determinants of drug distribution. Inflammation at the site of infection may facilitate entry of drugs across these barriers and into the brain, but not all postoperative infections are accompanied by marked inflammation, and concomitant treatment with corticosteroids may further impair drug entry.[68] Other inherent physiochemical properties of the antimicrobial agent may affect its penetration into the CNS, including molecular weight, lipophilicity, plasma protein binding, and ionization state. Ultimately, adequate dosing to achieve maximal bactericidal activity depends on the susceptibility of the causative organism (its minimal bactericidal concentration [MBC]). Often, in the absence of data from prospective randomized clinical trials evaluating the success rates of specific antibacterial agents, recommendations for the treatment of postcraniotomy infections are based largely on the results of previous experience, along with consideration of the complex physiologic, bacteriologic, and pharmacologic factors involved.

As postoperative infections may have severe neurological sequelae or cause death, empirical treatment of postoperative infections should include coverage for the full spectrum of potential pathogens, including resistant gram-positive organisms (e.g., MRSA) and nosocomial gram-negative bacilli (e.g., *Pseudomonas* and *Acinetobacter* spp.). Infections that may have an anaerobic component (brain abscess, paranasal sinus approach) should also be treated empirically with metronidazole. Suitable empirical regimens for postcraniotomy infections typically include a combination of vancomycin and a drug such as a third- or fourth-generation cephalosporin that has antipseudomonal activity (e.g., ceftazidime, cefepime), with the addition of metronidazole when anaerobic infection is possible. Owing to activity against gram-negative and anaerobic bacteria, a carbapenem (e.g., meropenem) may be substituted for the combination of a third-generation cephalosporin and metronidazole.[69] Antibiotic selection should be tailored once species identification and results of susceptibility testing by a microbiologic specimen are available.

β-Lactam antibiotics (penicillins, cephalosporins, carbapenems) have poor penetration into the CSF in the absence of meningeal inflammation, but higher systemic doses can result in therapeutic CSF concentrations.[67] Third- and fourth-generation cephalosporins (specifically cefotaxime, ceftriaxone, and ceftazidime) are often used for the treatment of CNS and postcraniotomy infections because of their low toxicity and excellent in vitro activity against many of the responsible bacterial pathogens. Administration of these agents in high doses achieves therapeutic concentrations within brain abscess cavities.[70] High-dose β-lactamase inhibitors such as sulbactam and tazobactam are also effective in protecting the coadministered penicillin agent and have been shown to provide benefit in the treatment of *A. baumannii* meningitis.[67] The carbapenems, such as imipenem and meropenem, also cover a broad antimicrobial spectrum and have been used successfully for the treatment of bacterial brain abscesses.[69,71,72] Imipenem, however, is associated with an increased seizure risk relative to meropenem (and other β-lactams), so its use should be carefully considered for the treatment of CNS infections.[67,69,73] As a class, β-lactam antibiotics are proconvulsive and, for this reason, their use via intraventricular injection is not recommended.

Vancomycin has weaker activity against staphylococcal infections relative to β-lactams and decreased penetration into the CNS owing to its high molecular weight (1449 daltons).[67] Even in the presence of significant inflammation, concentrations of vancomycin may be critically low at the site of infection,[74] and substitution of a β-lactamase–resistant penicillin (e.g., nafcillin, oxacillin) for vancomycin is appropriate, except in the setting of resistance or hypersensitivity.

Newer agents that may prove useful for the treatment of resistant staphylococcal infections include linezolid and daptomycin. Linezolid has bacteriostatic activity against both MRSA and vancomycin-resistant enterococci and bactericidal activity against most streptococci. Linezolid, which has excellent bioavailability, may be administered intravenously or orally. Experience with this agent for the treatment of postcraniotomy infections is limited but it may play a role in the treatment of resistant gram-positive infections and in the setting of treatment failure.[75] Potential side effects include myelosuppression and irreversible peripheral neuropathy.[67] Daptomycin, a novel cyclic lipopeptide antibiotic, has shown better in vitro microbicidal activity against MRSA than either vancomycin or linezolid and has been primarily used and approved by the U.S. Food and Drug Administration (FDA) for the treatment of skin and soft tissue infections. Animal models of meningitis suggest that it may be an effective therapeutic agent in a setting of meningeal inflammation, but human studies of its efficacy in neurosurgical infections are lacking.[76,77]

Rifampin is a broad-spectrum antimicrobial that may have a role in the adjunctive treatment of bone flap osteomyelitis or infections associated with foreign body implantation. These types of infections are notoriously difficult to eradicate because of their resistance to host defense mechanisms and poor penetration of antimicrobials. Most foreign body infections are caused by staphylococci growing in biofilms consisting of bacteria clustered together in an extracellular matrix attached to the foreign body.[78] Depletion of metabolic substances within the biofilm causes the microbes to enter a slowly growing (sessile) state. Dormant microbes within the biofilm are up to a 1000 times more tolerant of [most] antimicrobial agents than their free-living (planktonic) counterparts.[79-81] Rifampin is one of just a few agents that can effectively penetrate biofilms and kill organisms in the sessile phase of growth. Because of the rapid emergence of resistance to it, rifampin must always be used in combination with a second active agent. In vitro data, experimental animal models, and several randomized clinical trials suggest that dual therapy that includes rifampin may be better than monotherapy for orthopedic hardware–related staphylococcal infections in terms of bone sterilization and cure rates.[82,83] This experience makes adjunctive therapy with rifampin an attractive consideration for difficult postcraniotomy staphylococcal infections associated with retained hardware or osteitis. Caution must be used with rifampin therapy because of its very large number of drug interactions. Through cytochrome P-450 enzyme induction, rifampin increases the metabolism of many substrates, including antiseizure drugs, anticoagulants, and immunosuppressive and chemotherapeutic agents.[84]

From a pharmacokinetic viewpoint, fluoroquinolones (levofloxacin, ciprofloxacin, moxifloxacin) are attractive agents for the treatment of CNS infection because of their lipophilicity and low molecular weight. For sensitive gram-negative aerobic bacilli, fluoroquinolones (in particular, ciprofloxacin) are useful; however, their therapeutic utility is limited in other infections owing to a high rate of bacterial resistance in nosocomial infections and (albeit modestly) increased seizure potential and to limited data regarding their clinical effectiveness for postoperative CNS infections.[67]

Aminoglycosides have excellent activity against aerobic gram-negative bacilli, including *P. aeruginosa*, as well as synergistic activity with β-lactams against aerobic gram-positive cocci. Systemic use of aminoglycosides is limited by their toxicity profile and a narrow therapeutic window. Their penetration into CSF and across the blood-brain barrier is poor.[85] Polymyxins (e.g., colistin) also have activity against a broad array of gram-negative bacilli but fell out of favor because of nephrotoxicity. As a result of the retained activity of polymyxins against multidrug-resistant gram-negative bacilli, including *P. aeruginosa* and *A. baumannii*, this class again plays a role in infections that are difficult to treat. As with the aminoglycosides, the distribution of systemically administered polymyxins to CSF is poor, and their toxicity does not allow for an increase in systemic doses. Intraventricular antibiotic administration bypasses the blood-brain barrier, can achieve much higher CSF concentrations than systemic administration, and has been used successfully in multiple case reports.[86-88] Intraventricular antibiotic dosing has been associated with neurotoxicity, however, in experimental animal models and a small number of case reports.[89,90] Currently, there are no well-established data to support adjunctive intraventricular administration of an antimicrobial when a systemically delivered agent can achieve adequate microbicidal concentrations in CSF.

SUPERFICIAL INCISIONAL INFECTIONS

Clinical Manifestations

Superficial infections after craniotomy comprise a collection of anatomically distinct infections that may extend from the skin to the epidural space. The potential for these infections to extend to the underlying bone flap and through the dura mandates rapid effective treatment with close monitoring to ensure a response to therapy and resolution of infection.

Superficial infection is the most common infectious complication after craniotomy. Although every surgical patient is at risk for postoperative infection, a variety of factors may contribute to create an environment that is suboptimal for wound healing and more favorable for infection, including repeat operative intervention, poor tissue quality, impaired vascular supply, radiation injury, nutritional deficiencies, and the presence of foreign bodies. The role of foreign material in facilitating infection was first reported by Elek and Conen,[91] who demonstrated that the presence of suture material increased the skin abscess–causing virulence of coagulase-positive staphylococci by 10,000-fold. Continuous activation of granulocytes by foreign bodies may lead to local impairment of phagocytic ability, thereby reducing the amount of bacterial contamination needed to establish infection.[15]

Superficial infection typically manifests as local erythema, swelling, and tenderness at the craniotomy site with possible suppurative drainage (Fig. 36-1). With progressive infection, systemic signs such as malaise, fever, and chills may develop. Exposure of the underlying bone flap or metallic hardware (Fig. 36-2) indicates deep organ space infection, whereas the presence of neurological symptoms such as meningismus, altered mental status, and new focal deficits, strongly suggests the coexistence of intracranial infection. The most common pathogenic agents of superficial wound infections are gram-positive cocci, including *S. aureus*, coagulase-negative staphylococci, and *P. acnes*.[37,92]

Diagnostic Imaging and Laboratory Data

The presence of a superficial wound infection is often clinically apparent; however, imaging studies can frequently assist in defining the anatomic extent of infection (especially extension through the dura) as well as identifying possible precipitating factors such as entry into the mastoid air cells or paranasal sinuses during craniotomy. Computed tomography (CT) or magnetic resonance imaging (MRI) may reveal fluid collections in the subgaleal or epidural space that require surgical evacuation or demonstrate extension of infection beyond the dura and into the subdural space or brain parenchyma. Imaging studies may also show evidence of bone flap destruction suggestive of osteomyelitis. Unfortunately, diffusion-weighted MRI, which is very sensitive for the detection of spontaneous intracerebral abscesses, is frequently unreliable in diagnosing the presence of superficial infection after craniotomy.[93]

Measurement of the erythrocyte sedimentation rate (ESR) or C-reactive protein (CRP) concentration may provide some assistance in detecting infection and monitoring the response to therapy. These acute-phase reactants are normally elevated after craniotomy and return toward baseline by the fifth postoperative day.[94] Although these markers are highly nonspecific, prolonged elevation or a secondary increase in their levels may indicate the development of infection.

Treatment

Treatment of superficial wound infections depends on the extent of infection. Superficial cellulitis, a spreading infection of subcutaneous tissue without deeper infection of the subgaleal space or bone flap, is generally treated with oral or intravenous antibiotic therapy. Oral agents typically used to treat gram-positive bacterial

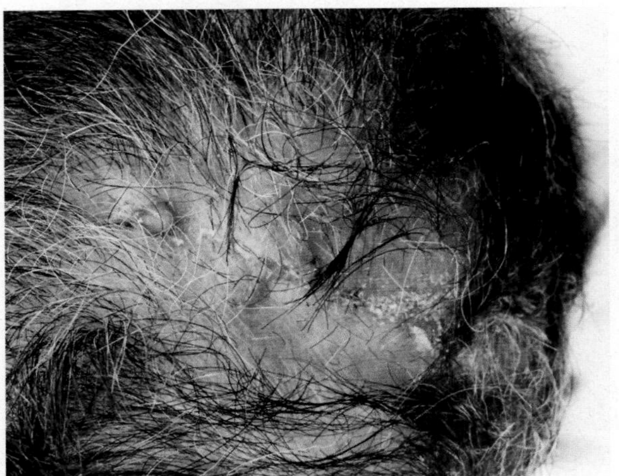

Figure 36-1. Purulent drainage from a superficially infected craniotomy incision with surrounding erythema.

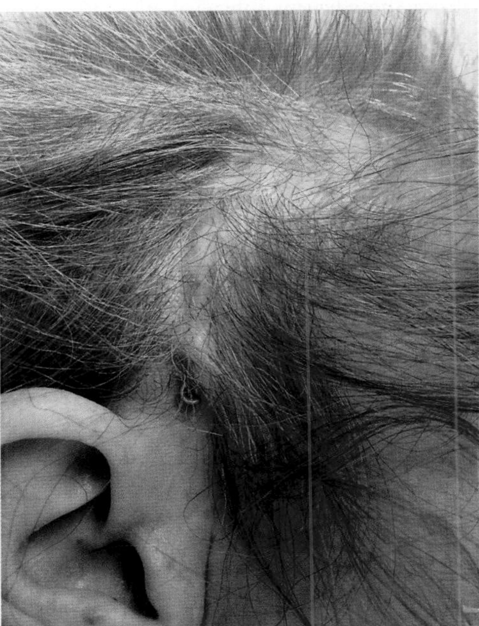

Figure 36-2. Skin breakdown at the inferior aspect of the craniotomy incision with exposed titanium hardware.

infections include first-generation cephalosporins (e.g., cefazolin) or beta-lactamase–resistant penicillins (e.g., dicloxacillin) in the absence of known MRSA colonization or infection. In patients with rapidly spreading infection, prominent systemic symptoms, or significant comorbidity, initial antibiotic therapy should be administered by the intravenous route with expanded coverage for nosocomial pathogens until the symptoms improve.[95,96]

Hyperbaric oxygen (HBO) therapy is sometimes used to treat complicated superficial infections, including those involving the bone flap. HBO therapy increases oxygen tension in infected tissues, thereby improving oxidative killing of aerobic bacteria by phagocytic cells and providing a direct bactericidal effect on anaerobic organisms such as *P. acnes*. Larsson and associates[99] used HBO to treat postcraniotomy infections successfully in 15 of 19 patients without removing the bone flap and in 3 of 6 patients with acrylic cranioplasties.[97] HBO therapy has shown some utility in the treatment of poorly healing, secondarily infected wounds such as those frequently associated with radiation injury.[98] Irradiation may impair wound healing by multiple mechanisms, including microvascular injury and ischemic damage, fibroblast dysfunction, and alterations in the synthesis of growth factors.[99] In addition to helping clear the infection, HBO therapy may also promote neoangiogenesis and reverse the vascular compromise present at the wound.[7,100] Limitations of HBO therapy include the cost of treatment and the need for multiple sessions. The possibility of increased tumor growth with the use of HBO in patients with malignancy has been raised as a potential concern, although clinical and experimental evidence of a tumor-stimulatory effect is lacking.[101-105] The use of local rotational or pedicled flaps or vascularized myocutaneous free flaps represents another potential treatment option for chronic postoperative infections that cannot be eradicated with conventional surgical débridement and bone flap removal.[106]

DEEP INCISIONAL INFECTIONS: SUBGALEAL SPACE AND BONE FLAP

Clinical Manifestations

Infection of the bone flap most often results from either direct bacterial inoculation at the time of surgery or extension of infection from the adjacent subgaleal (Fig. 36-3A) or epidural (Fig. 36-3B) compartment. Development of infection within the devascularized bone flap presents increased challenges for treatment, and any superficial infection extending to the subgaleal space must be presumed to have contaminated the bone flap. Infections occurring after cranioplasty are included in this category, and this topic is more extensively discussed in further chapters.

Diagnostic Imaging and Laboratory Data

A high index of suspicion is necessary to diagnose bone flap infection because laboratory markers and imaging findings are often nonspecific. The majority of infections of autogenous cranioplasties after decompressive craniectomy are attributable to commensal skin flora; however, a significant proportion are due to nosocomial gram-positive and gram-negative organisms.[95] Late presentations of indolent infections are also possible, with cases of *P. acnes* infection reported at 300 days postoperatively.[95] Reliance upon ESR and CRP level as evidence of infection should be avoided because a rise in CRP level can be detected in only one third of patients with postoperative infection after cranioplasty.[95]

CT and MRI studies may show the presence of subgaleal or epidural infection with bone flap destruction suggestive of osteomyelitis (Fig. 36-4). Hardware failure with surrounding bone lucency may also indicate infection.

Treatment

Devitalization and devascularization of the bone flap at the time of craniotomy present a unique challenge in the treatment of infection because of impaired delivery of host defense mechanisms and antibacterial agents. Treatment options include antibiotic therapy alone, surgical débridement with removal of the bone flap, and débridement with replacement of the bone flap or other cranioplasty material such as titanium mesh. Prolonged antibiotic therapy may control the clinical manifestations of infection but rarely leads to complete eradication, with frequent recrudescence after discontinuation of the antibiotic. Removal of the infected bone flap followed by delayed cranioplasty offers the best chance of clearing the initial infection; however, this treatment approach entails multiple surgical interventions and at least temporary cosmetic deformity while predisposing to the possibility of subsequent brain injury with a long-term risk for cranioplasty infection.[107-109] Several small case series have reported clinical resolution of infection with preservation of the bone flap.

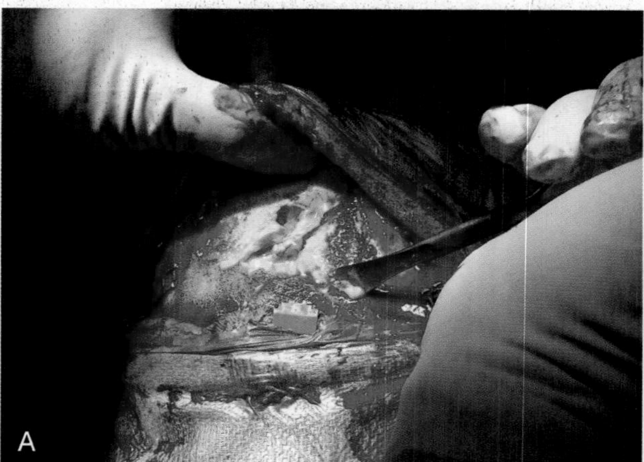

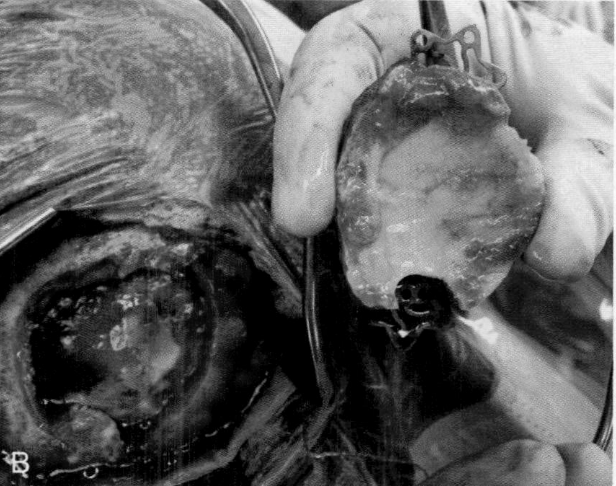

Figure 36-3. A, Surgical débridement of a superficial postcraniotomy infection in a patient who had undergone multiple craniotomies and radiation treatments for malignancy. There is spread of infection to the underlying bone flap, with erosion and adjacent purulent material in the epidural space. **B,** Epidural infection with contamination of the undersurface of the devascularized bone flap.

Bruce and Bruce[110] reported salvage of the bone flap in 11 of 13 patients through simple mechanical débridement of the bone flap to remove any necrotic or purulent debris and soaking of the bone in antibiotic-containing solution and povidine.[110] Similarly, Kshettry and associates[111] demonstrated successful resolution of infection in 10 of 12 patients treated with immediate titanium mesh cranioplasty at the time of initial surgical débridement (Fig. 36-5).[111] The majority of patients in this study, however, were treated with an antimicrobial regimen consisting of prolonged (4 to 6 weeks) intravenous antibiotic therapy followed by oral antibiotic therapy. Two patients were treated with indefinite oral antibiotic therapy for continuous suppression of infection. Closed-suction antibiotic solution irrigation systems have also been used to treat bone flap osteomyelitis, with varying degrees of success.[108,112] In the selection of the therapeutic approach for each patient, the risks associated with salvaging the bone flap and preventing a cranial defect must be weighed against the hazards of the infection itself as well as of prolonged antibiotic administration.

DEEP ORGAN SPACE INFECTIONS

Subdural Empyema

Clinical Manifestations

Although spontaneously occurring subdural empyema is typically accompanied by fever and headache, followed by the rapid development of focal neurological deficits, altered mental status, and seizures, this fulminant manifestation is rarely seen in patients in whom subdural empyema develops after craniotomy.[92,113] Hlavin and associates,[18] in reviewing their experience in 27 patients with postoperative subdural and epidural empyemas, found that only a third were febrile and that 85% were without headache. The most common findings were evidence of superficial wound infection and the presence of diffuse encephalopathy. In almost half the patients, the subdural empyema occurred more than 1 month after the craniotomy. Seizures were present in 25% of patients with postoperative subdural empyema.

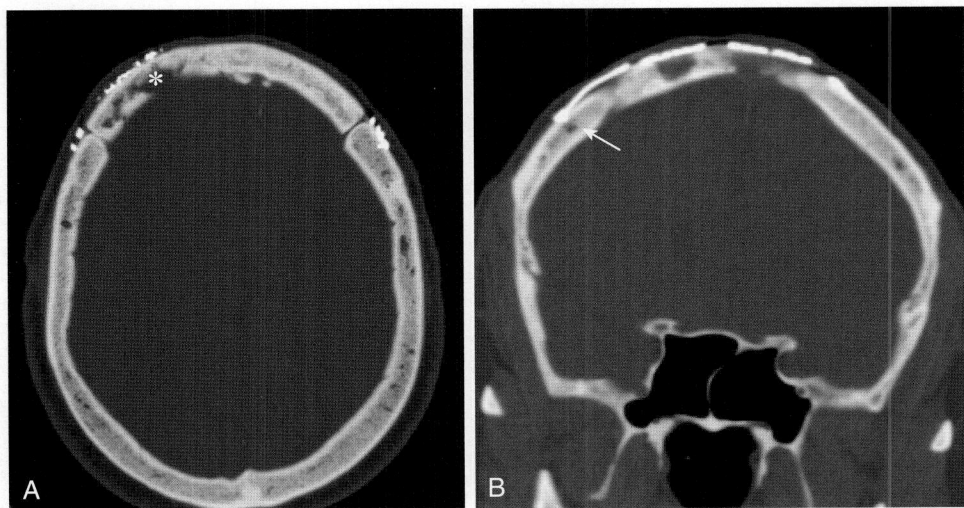

Figure 36-4. A, Axial computed tomography (CT) scan demonstrating erosion of bone flap *(asterisk)* indicative of osteomyelitis. **B,** Coronal CT scan showing failure of titanium screws with surrounding bone lucency *(arrow).*

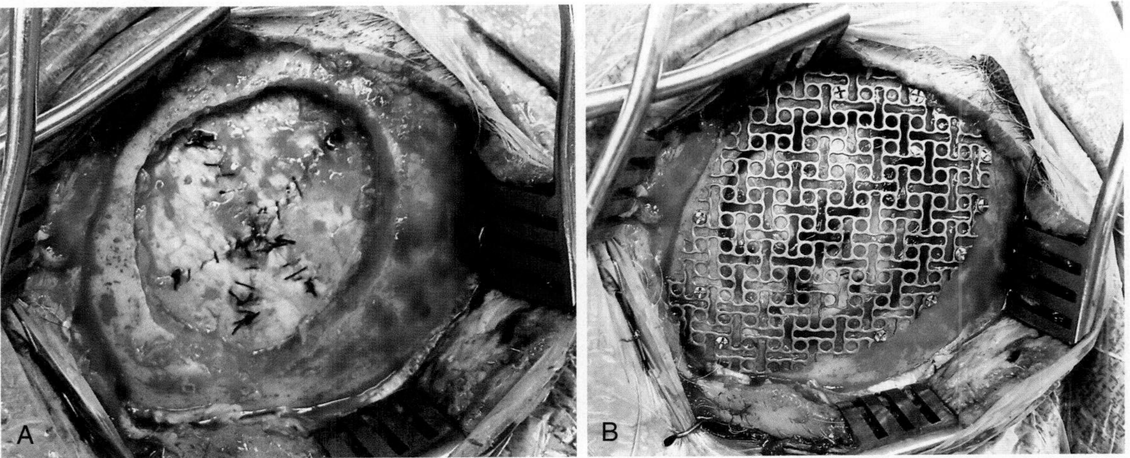

Figure 36-5. A, Débridement of the epidural infection and removal of the infected bone flap and hardware. **B,** Immediate titanium mesh cranioplasty performed at the time of infection débridement.

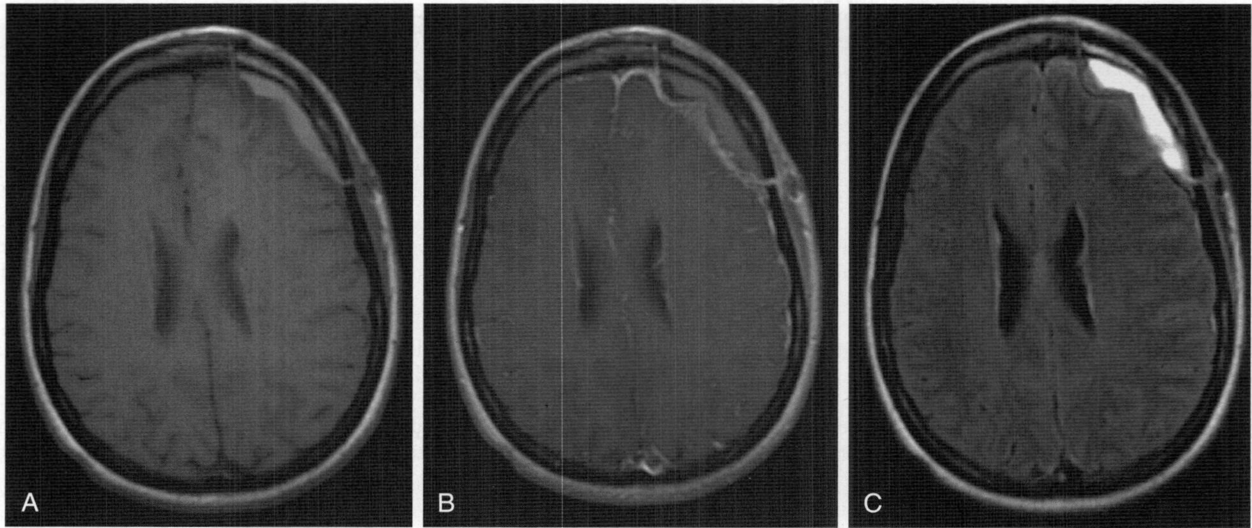

Figure 36-6. A, T1-weighted axial magnetic resonance (MR) image reveals a hyperintense subdural fluid collection that developed after craniotomy for aneurysm repair. The fluid collection enhances peripherally with gadolinium **(B)** and, because of higher protein content, exhibits increased signal intensity on fluid-attenuated inversion recovery (FLAIR) MR sequences **(C)** relative to cerebrospinal fluid. A craniotomy was performed to drain the collection, and frank purulence was encountered in the subdural space.

Diagnostic Imaging and Laboratory Data

Sterile extra-axial fluid collections are commonly noted on postoperative imaging studies, and their differentiation from infected purulent fluids (empyema) may be difficult in the absence of overt clinical signs. In subdural empyema, non–contrast-enhanced CT typically demonstrates a crescent-shaped fluid collection that is slightly more dense than CSF and located beneath the craniotomy flap or adjacent to the falx. Increased signal intensity is usually seen on T1-weighted and fluid-attenuated inversion recovery (FLAIR) MRI sequences because of the increased protein concentration of an empyema relative to CSF. Peripheral enhancement of the fluid collection is common (Fig. 36-6). Unfortunately, these imaging characteristics are nonspecific and may also be seen with postoperative hematomas or sterile effusions. The presence of restricted diffusion on MRI may be helpful, although the absence of restricted diffusion does not exclude the presence of infection; 29% of confirmed postoperative subdural infections did not demonstrate diffusion abnormalities in one study.[93] Progressive enlargement of the fluid collection or unexplained edema in adjacent cerebral cortex may be helpful in identifying the existence of infection.

Laboratory data findings in patients with subdural empyema are typically nonspecific. Hlavin and associates[18] found an elevated white blood cell count in 63% of their patients with postoperative infections, whereas ESR values were often within the normal range. CSF findings may be normal or may show evidence of a parameningeal reaction but rarely yield definitive evidence of infection. Additionally, lumbar puncture is frequently contraindicated in the setting of subdural empyema because of the possibility of cerebral herniation. In one study of 280 patients with spontaneous subdural empyemas who underwent lumbar puncture, 33 were thought to have experienced neurological deterioration as a direct result of the procedure.[114]

Treatment

Although postoperative subdural empyemas tend to have a more insidious course than spontaneous infections, early diagnosis and aggressive treatment are necessary to prevent intraparenchymal spread of infection and to avoid complications such as thrombophlebitis and venous infarction. Surgical drainage is usually necessary because antimicrobial agents do not reliably sterilize the empyema.[113] The goals of surgery are to evacuate the purulent collection completely and, when significant edema is associated with the infection, to achieve adequate decompression of the brain. Although the optimal surgical approach (craniotomy versus bur-hole drainage) is debated, craniotomy is generally advocated because it ensures maximal drainage of the collection and allows inspection of adjacent anatomic areas and removal of the bone flap if necessary.

Empirical antibiotic therapy should be started as soon as material for Gram stain and culture has been obtained, or earlier if surgical intervention must be delayed. The antibiotics chosen should be active against both skin flora and gram-negative bacilli because the latter have been shown to account for about half of subdural empyemas after craniotomy.[18] Vancomycin plus a third-generation cephalosporin with good activity against *Pseudomonas*, such as ceftazidime, is a frequently used empirical regimen, with adjustment according to individual institutional profiles of resistance. The duration of antibiotic therapy is typically 4 to 6 weeks. The role of imaging, especially diffusion imaging, in the evaluation of response to therapy or duration of therapy has been only minimally explored.[115,116]

Brain Abscess

Clinical Manifestations

Localized intraparenchymal abscesses may develop after craniotomy as a result of direct bacterial seeding or by extension of more superficial infection through an incompetent dura. Although the development of a brain abscess after craniotomy is rare, it is likely that a common postoperative sequela, such as a small fluid collection or a compromised area of contused or ischemic brain, serves as a nidus for abscess formation. Once infection has been established, abscess development begins as a localized area of cerebritis characterized by perivascular

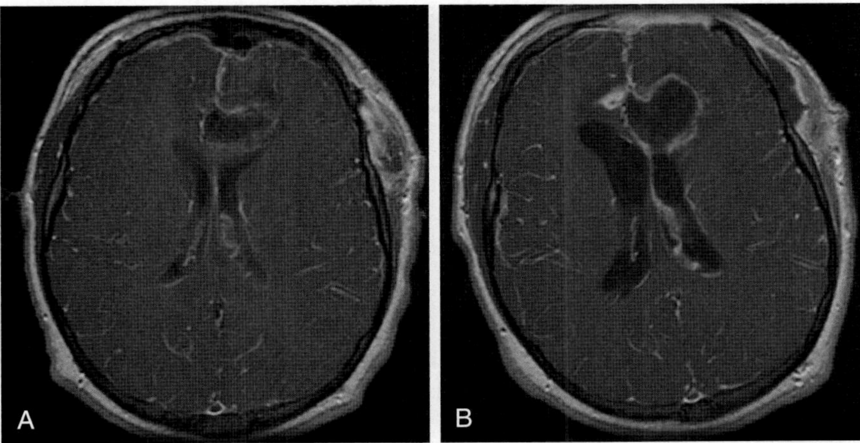

Figure 36-7. Purulent drainage developed after craniotomy for a left frontal cavernous malformation. **A,** T1-weighted axial magnetic resonance (MR) image after gadolinium administration demonstrates enhancement within the extra-axial space and the resection cavity. A craniotomy with drainage of purulent material from the epidural and subdural compartments was performed, and treatment with intravenous antibiotics was started. Five days later, severe headache and worsened mental status developed. **B,** MR image shows rupture of the intraparenchymal abscess into the adjacent lateral ventricle.

inflammation and edema formation. It then progresses to a discrete focus of necrotic, purulent material surrounded by a well-vascularized capsule composed of fibroblasts and reactive collagen.[117]

Clinically, the classic triad of headache, fever, and focal neurological deficit is rarely present, and the signs and symptoms of postoperative abscess are frequently nonspecific. Fever is present in only about half of affected patients, and its absence should not be used to exclude the diagnosis.[17,117-120] Symptoms, which are often related to the presence of an expanding, irritative mass lesion, include altered level of consciousness, nausea, vomiting, and seizures. In a series of 31 patients with nosocomial brain abscess after neurosurgical intervention, Yang and coworkers[17] reported that 17 had a disturbance in consciousness. The prognosis is much poorer in patients with significant alterations in mental status or rapid progression of symptoms, and a high degree of suspicion is necessary to recognize the existence of infection as early as possible.[121] Seizures develop in about 20% of patients with spontaneous brain abscess and appear to occur at a similar rate with postoperative abscesses.[17,119,122]

Abrupt worsening of preexisting headache accompanied by new onset of meningismus may indicate rupture of a brain abscess into the cerebral ventricle, a condition associated with a high mortality rate that may require more aggressive medical and surgical intervention. Intraventricular rupture of a brain abscess (IVROBA) may also manifest clinically as sudden neurological deterioration with obtundation or coma (Fig. 36-7). The pathophysiology of this decline is probably multifactorial, including both the development of severe widespread meningoencephalitis and alterations in CSF flow causing an increase in intracranial pressure. Zeidman and colleagues,[123] in an extensive review of the literature from 1950 to 1993, identified 129 reported cases of IVROBA with a combined mortality rate of 85%. Furthermore, although the overall mortality for brain abscesses decreased significantly over successive decades, the mortality rate for IVROBA remained consistent throughout this period. Lee and colleagues[124] reported the latest data on IVROBA outcome in a series of 62 patients treated between 1986 and 2005. The observed mortality rate was 27%; however, the overall rate of poor neurological outcome, consisting of severe disability, persistent vegetative state, or death, was nearly 50%.

Clinical and radiographic identification of patients at increased risk for intraventricular rupture should prompt more urgent surgical intervention and decrease the incidence of IVROBA and its sequelae. Neither the specific infecting organism nor abscess size is associated with risk for rupture, although multiloculated abscesses have been correlated with increased risk.[124] Not surprisingly, decreased distance from the abscess capsule to the ventricular wall has also been demonstrated to correlate with the rate of intraventricular rupture.[124,125] These data correspond to findings in pathologic studies revealing that abscess capsule formation tends to be more complete on the cortical side of a brain abscess than on the ventricular side, a difference that probably contributes to the increased rate of intraventricular rupture with deep-seated abscesses.[126] The presence of localized ventricular enhancement on CT has also been shown to herald impending intraventricular rupture and clinical deterioration.[127] Once IVROBA has occurred, radiographic imaging often reveals diffuse ependymal and meningeal enhancement and the presence of debris within the ventricles (see Fig. 36-7). Hydrocephalus accompanies IVROBA in about 50% of cases, and septation of the ventricles may occur as a delayed complication of intraventricular rupture.[124,128] Takeshita and colleagues[127] found that all 20 of their patients with IVROBA reported prodromal symptoms of severe headache and meningeal irritation before the onset of rapid clinical decline.[127] Decreased morbidity seems to be associated with IVROBA in patients taking antibiotics or with sterile abscesses at the time of rupture, supporting rapid initiation of antimicrobial therapy in patients exhibiting prodromal symptoms or with abscesses adjacent to the ventricular system.[125,127]

Diagnostic Imaging and Laboratory Data

Because of the often nonspecific clinical symptoms associated with brain abscess and the frequent absence of fever, neuroimaging typically plays a dominant role in the diagnosis of postoperative intraparenchymal infection. Imaging studies can also help define the anatomic extent of infection to guide surgical intervention and assist in evaluating the response to therapy. The radiographic features of brain abscess depend on its stage of progression. During the cerebritis stage, CT reveals a poorly defined area of low attenuation with a mass effect and significant edema. As a

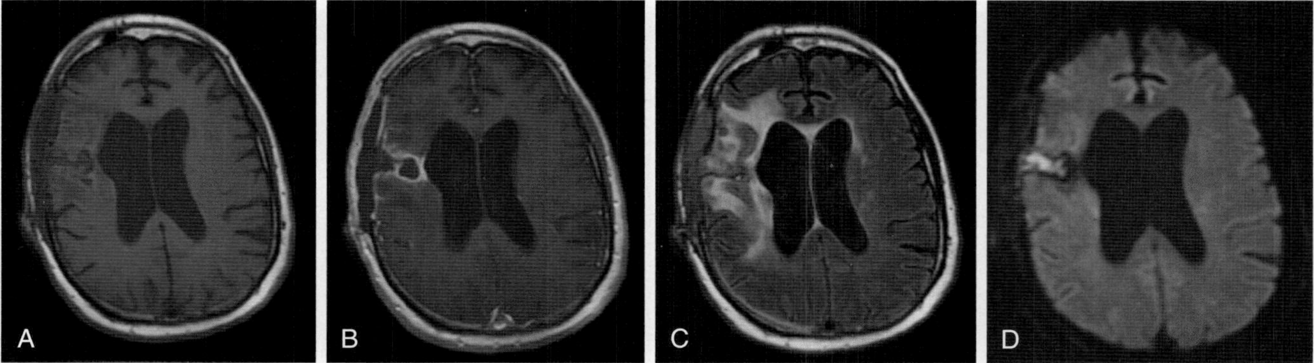

Figure 36-8. One month after resection of a right frontal glioma, this patient exhibited confusion and lethargy. T1-weighted axial magnetic resonance (MR) images obtained before **(A)** and after **(B)** gadolinium administration demonstrate enhancement of the resection cavity and surrounding meninges, and the fluid-attenuated inversion recovery (FLAIR) sequence **(C)** shows significant surrounding edema. Abnormal restricted diffusion on diffusion-weighted MR image **(D)** suggests infection. Craniotomy confirmed the presence of purulent material in the subdural and intraparenchymal locations.

capsule begins to form around the infection, peripheral enhancement increases and the center of the lesion becomes progressively hypodense. Cerebritis typically appears on MRI as an area of high signal intensity on T2-weighted images with patchy gadolinium enhancement.[129] Subsequent capsule development is characterized on T1-weighted images as a ring of gadolinium enhancement surrounding a necrotic cavity of low signal intensity (Fig. 36-8). Concurrent treatment with corticosteroids, radiation therapy, and chemotherapy may alter the radiographic progression of abscess development. Corticosteroids have been shown in experimental models to reduce the thickness of the abscess capsule and the extent of contrast enhancement on both CT and MRI.[117] Additionally, the presence of peripheral enhancement around a resection cavity is often nonspecific in the postcraniotomy setting and may reflect residual or recurrent tumor, treatment effect, infarction, or resolving hematoma.

Diffusion-weighted MRI has demonstrated a high degree of specificity and sensitivity in differentiating spontaneous abscess from other ring-enhancing lesions, and its application to the diagnosis of postoperative brain abscess may prove useful. In a retrospective analysis, we reviewed the diffusion-weighted imaging findings in 50 patients with microbiologically confirmed postoperative infections and found evidence of abnormally restricted diffusion in all patients with intraparenchymal infection; much higher false-negative rates on diffusion-weighted imaging were found with more superficial infections, such as epidural or subgaleal abscesses.[93] Importantly, the presence of restricted diffusion is not specific for infection, and correlation with apparent diffusion coefficient and T2-weighted MRI sequences or CT is necessary to evaluate for blood products that may cause a "T2 shine-through effect," in which the infection appears bright on diffusion-weighted images. The role of other advanced MRI sequences potentially useful for the diagnosis of infection, such as spectroscopy and perfusion imaging, has largely been unexplored in the postoperative setting.[130,131]

As with clinical and radiographic manifestations of postcraniotomy brain abscess, there are no laboratory findings that definitively establish the diagnosis. Peripheral leukocytosis is frequently absent, and although the ESR and CRP concentration are usually elevated, normal values may occur in patients with proven infection.[132,133] Blood cultures seldom yield a causative organism but should be performed to assess for a possible hematogenous source of infection. Lumbar puncture is frequently contraindicated because of increased intracranial pressure and the risk of cerebral herniation, and CSF analysis is rarely helpful in the setting of an unruptured brain abscess, typically revealing only a nonspecific elevation in protein level and cell count.[120]

Treatment

The approach to treatment of postoperative brain abscesses is similar to that for spontaneous abscesses, although the increased frequency of bacterial pathogens resistant to multiple antibiotics and the extension of infection into adjacent anatomic compartments in the postoperative setting may complicate treatment. The general goals of treatment are to relieve the mass effect, improve clinical symptoms, and fully resolve the infection. In most cases, a combination of surgical drainage and a prolonged course of intravenous antibiotics is required. Surgical options include open operative drainage or excision of the lesion and stereotactic aspiration. Both options have been used successfully in the treatment of postcraniotomy abscess, although stereotactic aspiration of brain abscesses is associated with a higher incidence of recurrence and the need for repeat surgical intervention.[100,134] Additionally, postcraniotomy abscesses are often multiloculated, a feature that predicts a higher chance of recurrence after initial drainage.[135] Open surgical excision also facilitates débridement of any associated parameningeal infection and removal of necrotic debris or foreign bodies.

Once specimens have been obtained for Gram stain and aerobic and anaerobic culture, empirical antibiotic therapy should be started on the basis of Gram stain results and institutional data regarding the probable causative agents and their antibiotic resistance patterns. Empirical treatment with vancomycin and a third- or fourth-generation cephalosporin with antipseudomonal activity (e.g., ceftazidime, cefepime) is appropriate, although studies comparing the relative efficacy of various treatment regimens have not been performed. Metronidazole may be added to the empirical regimen for coverage of anaerobic organisms, especially if an otic, paranasal sinus, or mastoid source of infection is suspected on the basis of the surgical intervention performed or a history of head trauma with skull base fractures. In patients with contraindications to therapy with a cephalosporin or metronidazole, meropenem may be used as an alternative empirical agent.[69] In critically ill patients in whom urgent surgical drainage is not possible, initiation of broad-spectrum antibiotic therapy before culture results are available may be necessary. Mampalam and coworkers[136] reported, however, that 30% of patients who received antibiotics preoperatively had sterile culture results, thus potentially leading to inappropriate medical treatment or the need for prolonged therapy with multiple antibiotics. In some instances, Gram stain findings may still help guide antimicrobial therapy.

High-dose intravenous antibiotics have conventionally been administered for 6 to 8 weeks in patients with brain abscesses. Frequently, this treatment is followed by a course of oral antibiotic therapy if a suitable agent is available, although the efficacy and necessity of this approach have not been established. Shorter-course therapies have also been reported to be effective,[119,134] and length of treatment should be guided by the virulence of the causative organism, clinical therapeutic response, and serial neuroimaging findings. Progressive enlargement of the abscess or failure of the abscess to become smaller despite treatment of a susceptible organism with an appropriate antibiotic should prompt repeat surgical drainage and microbiologic reassessment. Several reports have also advocated placement of drains into the abscess for postsurgical drainage and intracavitary administration of antibiotics for difficult to treat infections[117,137,138]; however, this form of therapy should be used with caution given the minimal evidence in support of its efficacy and the potential for neurotoxicity, including seizures. Brain abscesses associated with intraventricular rupture may also require more aggressive treatment to reduce morbidity and mortality. Intraventricular administration of antibiotics may be considered for the treatment of bacterial infections susceptible only to antibacterials with poor blood-CSF penetration. Multiple reports have demonstrated increased CSF antibiotic concentrations, successful clearance of ventricular infection, and minimal toxicity after intraventricular administration of antibiotics, most commonly vancomycin, aminoglycosides, and colistin.[86,139-143]

Adjunctive corticosteroid treatment may be indicated in patients with significant cerebral edema related to cerebral infections with signs of impending herniation. Additionally, given the high incidence of seizures associated with brain abscess, administration of seizure prophylaxis should be considered until the infection has resolved.

Bacterial Meningitis

Clinical Manifestations

Bacterial meningitis is relatively uncommon after neurosurgical procedures, complicating less than 1% of craniotomies.[8,13] Although the clinical course of nosocomial meningitis tends to be less fulminant than that of community-acquired meningitis, rapid diagnosis and implementation of antimicrobial therapy are critical because the mortality rate may exceed 20% if treatment is delayed.[144,145] The typical symptoms of meningitis tend to be present in patients with postoperative bacterial meningitis, including fever, headache, and neck stiffness; however, these symptoms may also occur in patients without infection after craniotomy, especially of the posterior fossa.

Complicating the diagnosis of postoperative meningitis is the clinically similar condition of a sterile postoperative meningitis presumed to be due to chemical irritation, as first described by Cushing and Bailey[146] in 1928. Subsequent investigators have shown that aseptic (chemical) meningitis is responsible for 60% to 75% of all cases of postoperative clinical meningitis and that it occurs most frequently in children and after posterior fossa surgery.[145,147] Despite its frequent occurrence, the etiology of aseptic meningitis remains incompletely understood, but it is presumed to be caused by irritation from blood breakdown products or from factors released by surgical materials such as dural substitutes. Diagnosis of aseptic meningitis requires negative results of CSF Gram staining and sterile culture results, and the patient must recover fully without the administration of antibiotics. Corticosteroids typically provide symptomatic relief in patients with aseptic chemical meningitis.

Diagnostic Imaging and Laboratory Data

Unfortunately, differentiation between chemical and bacterial meningitis is frequently problematic, and no single clinical sign or diagnostic test distinguishes between the two entities with certainty. Neuroimaging studies rarely assist in the diagnosis of postoperative meningitis because the characteristic imaging sign, meningeal enhancement, can also be seen in up to 80% of post-craniotomy patients who do not have infections.[148] CT or MRI may, however, reveal secondary complications of meningitis, including hydrocephalus, parameningeal abscess, and ischemia/infarction related to vasculitis and thrombosis of superficial vessels.

CSF culture data remain the "gold standard" for diagnosis of postoperative bacterial meningitis, although the definition of health care–associated meningitis used by the CDC allows for a diagnosis of meningitis without positive CSF culture results in the setting of other clinical findings (increased white cell count, elevated protein, and/or decreased glucose concentration in CSF; or organisms seen on Gram stain of CSF; or organisms cultured from blood) and if a "physician institutes appropriate antimicrobial therapy."[149] CSF Gram staining is highly insensitive for infection. Several studies have shown that Gram staining results are positive in only 25% to 50% of cases of culture-confirmed bacterial meningitis.[19,150] CSF hypoglycorrhachia and pleocytosis with neutrophilic predominance are common findings in both aseptic meningitis and bacterial meningitis, although one study found that CSF white blood cell counts greater than 7500 cells/μL and glucose concentrations lower than 10 mg/dL were not present in any patient with aseptic meningitis.[150] Unfortunately, laboratory findings within this range were not very common in patients who did have confirmed bacterial infections.

A variety of alternative diagnostic tests have been investigated to better distinguish between these two entities, with several retrospective studies identifying CSF lactate concentrations greater than 4 mmol/L and interleukin-1β (IL-1bβ) levels greater than 90 ng/L predicting the presence of bacterial meningitis with good sensitivity and specificity in postsurgical patients.[151,152] Elevated CSF lactate probably results from a combination of bacterial production, anaerobic glycolysis, and metabolism by CSF leukocytes,[153] whereas IL-1β is a key inflammatory mediator in the response to meningeal infection.[154] Data regarding the clinical utility of these newer assays are promising, but until they have been well validated in prospective studies, the recommendation remains that all patients with clinical and laboratory features consistent with postoperative meningitis receive empirical antibiotic treatment until CSF culture results are confirmed to be sterile (Table 36-2).[145,155]

TABLE 36-2 Cerebrospinal Fluid (CSF) Analysis of Bacterial and Chemical (Aseptic) Meningitis

CSF Marker	Finding(s) in Bacterial Meningitis	Finding(s) in Chemical (Aseptic) Meningitis
Gram stain	Positive (25%-50% of cases)	Negative
White blood cell count	Increased	Increased (<7500 cells/μL)
Neutrophil %	Increased	Normal or increased
Lymphocyte %	Normal or slightly increased	Normal or increased
Protein level	Increased	Increased
Glucose level	Decreased	Decreased (>10 mg/dL)
Other markers	Lactate > 4 mmol/L Interleukin-1β (IL-1β) positive	Lactate < 4 mmol/L IL-1β negative

Treatment

The choice of agent for empirical coverage depends on local bacterial infection and resistance patterns; however, typically the combination of vancomycin and a third-generation cephalosporin with antipseudomonal activity (e.g., ceftazidime) is appropriate. If the patient is not deteriorating clinically, CSF culture results remain sterile, and the treating clinician believes the original clinical syndrome to have been consistent with aseptic chemical meningitis, antibiotics may be discontinued after several days, provided that antibiotic therapy had not been started before CSF was obtained for culture. Using this algorithm, Zarrouck and colleagues[145] demonstrated that the duration of antibiotic treatment of aseptic meningitis could be decreased from a mean of 11 days to 3.5 days, with no cases of diagnosed aseptic meningitis later proving to have been misdiagnosed bacterial meningitis.[145] However, the possibility of misdiagnosis suggests that the patient should be kept under close clinical observation for a time after treatment with antibiotics is stopped.

Once the infecting pathogen has been isolated and its susceptibility profile determined, antibiotic therapy can be modified for optimal treatment. The duration of treatment may depend on the offending organism and its antibiotic susceptibility pattern as well as on other complicating factors, such as the presence of parameningeal foci or the patient's underlying immune status. The clinician may wish to add corticosteroids to the regimen, given the evidence that they are beneficial in many cases of sporadic bacterial meningitis; however, no trials have evaluated their use for postoperative bacterial meningitis specifically. Failure to improve after the institution of appropriate antibiotic therapy for a susceptible organism should prompt further CSF evaluation and measurement of CSF antibiotic concentrations.

CONCLUSION

The development of infection after craniotomy is a relatively rare occurrence, and prospective, randomized data evaluating the relative efficacy of various medical and surgical interventions are limited. The consequences, however, of a missed diagnosis or improper treatment can be devastating. As the management of postcraniotomy infections continues to become increasingly complex with the emergence of highly resistant bacteria and implantation of foreign devices, close cooperation among neurosurgeons, infectious disease specialists, and hospital infection control services is critical to achieving the best possible outcomes and reducing neurological morbidity.

SUGGESTED READINGS

Alexander JW. The contributions of infection control to a century of surgical progress. *Ann Surg*. 1985;201:423.

Barker FG 2nd. Efficacy of prophylactic antibiotics for craniotomy: a meta-analysis. *Neurosurgery*. 1994;35:484.

Bratzler DW, Dellinger EP, Olsen KM, et al. Clinical practice guidelines for antimicrobial prophylaxis in surgery. *Surg Infect (Larchmt)*. 2013;14:73.

Bruce JN, Bruce SS. Preservation of bone flaps in patients with postcraniotomy infections. *J Neurosurg*. 2003;98:1203.

Darouiche RO. Treatment of infections associated with surgical implants. *N Engl J Med*. 2004;350:1422.

Durand ML, Calderwood SB, Weber DJ, et al. Acute bacterial meningitis in adults. A review of 493 episodes. *N Engl J Med*. 1993;328:21.

Farrell CJ, Hoh BL, Pisculli ML, et al. Limitations of diffusion-weighted imaging in the diagnosis of postoperative infections. *Neurosurgery*. 2008;62:577.

Forgacs P, Geyer CA, Freidberg SR. Characterization of chemical meningitis after neurological surgery. *Clin Infect Dis*. 2001;32:179.

Hlavin ML, Kaminski HJ, Fenstermaker RA, et al. Intracranial suppuration: a modern decade of postoperative subdural empyema and epidural abscess. *Neurosurgery*. 1994;34:974.

Korinek AM. Risk factors for neurosurgical site infections after craniotomy: a prospective multicenter study of 2944 patients. The French Study Group of Neurosurgical Infections, the SEHP, and the C-CLIN Paris-Nord. Service Epidemiologie Hygiene et Prevention. *Neurosurgery*. 1997;41:1073.

Korinek AM, Golmard JL, Elcheick A, et al. Risk factors for neurosurgical site infections after craniotomy: a critical reappraisal of antibiotic prophylaxis on 4,578 patients. *Br J Neurosurg*. 2005;19:155.

Kshettry VR, Hardy S, Weil RJ, et al. Immediate titanium cranioplasty after debridement and craniectomy for postcraniotomy surgical site infection. *Neurosurgery*. 2012;70:8.

Kurz A, Sessler DI, Lenhardt R. Perioperative normothermia to reduce the incidence of surgical-wound infection and shorten hospitalization. Study of Wound Infection and Temperature Group. *N Engl J Med*. 1996;334:1209.

Larsson A, Engstrom M, Uusijarvi J, et al. Hyperbaric oxygen treatment of postoperative neurosurgical infections. *Neurosurgery*. 2002;50:287.

Lee TH, Chang WN, Su TM, et al. Clinical features and predictive factors of intraventricular rupture in patients who have bacterial brain abscesses. *J Neurol Neurosurg Psychiatry*. 2007;78:303.

Malis LI. Prevention of neurosurgical infection by intraoperative antibiotics. *Neurosurgery*. 1979;5:339.

Mathisen GE, Johnson JP. Brain abscess. *Clin Infect Dis*. 1997;25:763.

McClelland S 3rd, Hall WA. Postoperative central nervous system infection: incidence and associated factors in 2111 neurosurgical procedures. *Clin Infect Dis*. 2007;45:55.

Nau R, Sörgel F, Eiffert H. Penetration of drugs through the blood-cerebrospinal fluid/blood-brain barrier for treatment of central nervous system infections. *Clin Microbiol Rev*. 2010;23:858.

Seydoux C, Francioli P. Bacterial brain abscesses: factors influencing mortality and sequelae. *Clin Infect Dis*. 1992;15:394.

Takeshita M, Kagawa M, Izawa M, et al. Current treatment strategies and factors influencing outcome in patients with bacterial brain abscess. *Acta Neurochir (Wien)*. 1998;140:1263.

Tanner J, Woodings D, Moncaster K. Preoperative hair removal to reduce surgical site infection. *Cochrane Database Syst Rev*. 2006;(3):CD004122.

Zarrouk V, Vassor I, Bert F, et al. Evaluation of the management of postoperative aseptic meningitis. *Clin Infect Dis*. 2007;44:1555.

Zeidman SM, Geisler FH, Olivi A. Intraventricular rupture of a purulent brain abscess: case report. *Neurosurgery*. 1995;36:189.

See a full reference list on ExpertConsult.com

37 Postoperative Infections of the Spine

Vijay M. Ravindra, Michael A. Finn, Meic H. Schmidt, and Andrew T. Dailey

Infection after surgical intervention for spinal disorders is a feared complication and can contribute significantly to patient morbidity. Surgical site infections (SSIs) are now the most frequent hospital-acquired infections, their rate having surpassed those of urinary tract infections, ventilator-acquired pneumonias, central line infections, and *Clostridium difficile* infections.[1] It is estimated that the 500,000 SSIs that occur annually account for more than $10 billion in U.S. health care expenditure.[2] Thus, routes to prevent infection, facilitate early diagnosis, and provide adequate treatment are of interest. Although these infections are infrequently encountered after spinal intervention, reported in between 1% and 5.4% of cases,[3-9] certain subpopulations, such as patients with trauma or cancer, may have much higher infection rates.[6,10-12] The estimated cost of postoperative infection varies widely in the literature, and amounts in excess of $100,000[13] have been reported in cases that necessitate multiple washouts and extended hospitalization with prolonged administration of intravenous antibiotics, which may in turn necessitate placement in a skilled nursing facility. It is also difficult to estimate the physical and social effect on the patient, who may be subjected to repeated washout and revision procedures and prolonged courses of intravenous antibiotic treatment. Clearly, spine surgeons must make progress toward minimizing the incidence and impact of postoperative infections through increased efforts in utilizing sterile technique, reducing surgical times, reducing soft tissue trauma, and using antibiotic prophylaxis and application of local antibiotics at the completion of the procedure. In addition, familiarity with current state-of-the art diagnostic tests, imaging evaluation, and treatment methods is essential.

INCIDENCE

Infections of the disk or bone with extension into the epidural space have been reported after invasive procedures of the spine, both open surgical interventions, as for scoliosis, and closed diagnostic procedures, such as lumbar diskography. This chapter focuses on infections occurring after open surgical procedures performed with either a traditional open approach or more modern, minimal-incision surgical techniques. These infections represent a subgroup of all spinal infections, and they may be further divided into several smaller subgroups. The risks, symptoms, and treatment paradigms for spinal infection vary, depending on the region of the intervention (cervical, thoracic, or lumbar), the approach (anterior, posterior, or lateral), and whether instrumentation was used.

Noninstrumented Spinal Procedures

Noninstrumented spinal surgery includes anterior and posterior decompressive procedures and is usually confined to short stretches of the spinal column; most often, only a single level is treated. Although noninstrumented procedures may include fusions, most fusion procedures are now supplemented with instrumentation.

Lumbar diskectomy is one of the most common procedures performed on the spine and usually improves clinical symptoms.[14] Fortunately, rates of infection are low; in most series, researchers have reported rates of 1% or lower.[15,16] In newer series of endoscopic minimally invasive diskectomy, researchers have reported even lower rates of infection,[17,18] with one group reporting no infections in the treatment of 262 patients.[18] Infection may occur superficially, in the skin or muscle tissue, or in the disk space itself. The former type is easier to treat and often becomes obvious after 1 to 2 weeks; however, because of the avascular nature of the disk, discitis may take several weeks to months before it is diagnosed, particularly with less virulent organisms, such as *Propionobacter acnes*. The clinical symptoms of back pain may be accompanied by fever; elevation in erythrocyte sedimentation rate (ESR) or C-reactive protein (CRP) level; in later stages, radiographic changes with disk degeneration; and, in progressive cases, end plate degeneration.

Patients undergoing laminectomy without fusion also have a low incidence of infection; rates are commonly reported at approximately 2%.[19] Infection may be superficial to the fascia or deep to it, with involvement around the epidural space. Laminoplasty techniques are associated with higher rates of infection, although they are probably most appropriately considered instrumented procedures because of the small plates used for expansion of the canal.[20]

Noninstrumented posterior spinal fusion is associated with a higher rate of infection than that for decompressive procedures.[6,21] This outcome is attributable to longer operating times, greater blood loss, greater soft tissue destruction, and the placement of devascularized allograft.

In the cervical spine, single-level decompression with foraminotomy is associated with a low infection rate, with reported rates approaching 0%.[22] More invasive posterior laminectomy can have higher infection rates with foraminotomy alone, reported at approximately 2%, although infection rates for laminoplasty and for laminectomy with fusion are much higher. Anterior cervical surgery is usually performed with instrumentation, although occasionally anterior cervical foraminotomy or anterior cervical diskectomy and fusion are performed without cervical plating. Infection rates for the anterior cervical approach, however, are extremely low with and without the use of instrumention[23]; thus, it is difficult to discern any real difference between the two techniques. Similar findings have been shown for cervical arthroplasty, with most researchers reporting a 0% infection rate.

Finally, relatively small interventional procedures such as chemonucleolysis or diskography are associated with an infection rate of up to 4% in the absence of preoperative antibiotics. Fortunately, this incidence can be dramatically decreased with the use of a two-needle technique and prophylactic antibiotics.[24-27]

Instrumented Spinal Procedures

The use of instrumentation in posterior spinal procedures increases the incidence of postoperative infection to approximately 3% to 7% in many series.[4,28-31] Spinal instrumentation increases the risk of infection by acting as a site of secondary seeding for organisms, rather than as a source of inoculation.[32] One study revealed that of 21 patients undergoing hardware removal for noninfectious reasons, 11 exhibited positive growth on cultures.[33] Although most infections occur in the immediate postoperative period, a number of reports have shown that infections can occur years after surgery.[34-37] Colonization of the implants is probably commonplace, and biofilm formation may protect these organisms, predisposing patients to delayed infection.[38]

The type of instrumentation may affect the probability of clinical infection. Patients with older steel implants are more susceptible to colonization and delayed spinal infections.[37] Furthermore, corrosion and fretting at cross-connector sites have been associated with foreign body reactions and with the development of a local environment favorable for the growth of endogenous or low-virulence bacteria.[35,37,39,40] This association has not been reported with newer titanium implants, which are resistant to corrosion and have greater resistance to colonization.

Anterior instrumented spinal procedures are associated with lower rates of infection, and when infections occur, they tend to be superficial.[23,41-43] The low incidence of infection with the anterior approach is probably attributable to minimal soft tissue trauma and subsequent muscle necrosis. Although the anterior approach itself is associated with a low risk of infection, the anterior-posterior approach to the spine has the highest rates of infection,[44] a finding probably attributable to the greater length and complexity of the surgery.

Minimally invasive surgery is a rapidly expanding field in spine surgery. The goal of minimally invasive spinal surgery is to minimize soft tissue trauma and blood loss and thereby hasten patient recovery and decrease the risk of infection. Initial results are promising,[45,46] although most series have been small and no reduction in wound infection has been conclusively demonstrated.[47] Further experience with these techniques will clarify the extent of reduced infection risk with these methods.

Finally, the implantation of intrathecal drug delivery systems and spinal cord stimulators is associated with an approximately 5% risk of infection.[48,49] With these devices, infection occurs in the pump or stimulator pocket in many cases; infection of the intraspinal component can lead to meningitis or epidural abscess.[48-50] These infections tend to occur early, usually within the first 2 weeks to 2 months after surgery, and are treated by removal of the complete system.

INFECTIOUS RISK FACTORS

Patient-, surgery-, and disease-specific factors play a role in determining the risk profile for each particular case (Table 37-1).

TABLE 37-1 Infection Risk Factors

Condition	Increased Risk
PATIENT-SPECIFIC FACTORS	
Age	>20 yr
Diabetes mellitus	Glucose intolerance
Malnutrition	Albumin level <3.5 mg/dL Total lymphocyte count <1500/mL
Obesity	
Alcoholism	
Tobacco use	
Urinary/fecal incontinence	
Immunocompromised state	Steroid use Rheumatoid disease
DISEASE-SPECIFIC FACTORS	
Malignancy	
Trauma	Spinal cord injury
SURGICAL FACTORS	
Posterior approaches	Staged anterior-posterior procedures
Length of surgery	>5 hr
Number of levels	
Estimated blood loss	>1 L Blood transfusion
Postoperative stay in intensive care unit	
Preoperative hospital stay	

Patient-Specific Factors

Important among patient-specific factors are medical comorbid conditions, including increasing age, obesity, diabetes, poor nutritional status, and alcohol and tobacco use.[8,44,51-54] Other factors associated with an increased risk of postoperative infection include steroid use, rheumatoid disease, and an immunocompromised state.[44,55,56]

Obesity is a frequent comorbid condition in the population of patients undergoing spine surgery and can lead to poor outcomes regardless of the indication, pathologic process, or technicalities of the procedure. Several studies have demonstrated the increased risk for infection among obese patients undergoing spine surgery.[44,53,55,57,58] Obese patients are subject to longer operative times; greater amounts of retraction forces, which in turn causes increased soft tissue necrosis; greater amounts of poorly vascularized fatty tissue with decreased oxygen tension; decreased immune defense in adipose tissue; and poor tissue concentrations of prophylactic antibiotics.[32,59-61] In addition, overweight and obese patients have been found to have an increased risk of postoperative complications (e.g., superficial wound infection, pulmonary embolism) in relation to patients of normal weight.[62] Moreover, obesity and diabetes are closely related and may be present simultaneously.

Malnutrition is a well-known factor that predisposes patients to infection. It has been demonstrated to impair immune response and delay wound healing. Klein and colleagues[51] reported that 25% of patients undergoing elective lumbar surgery had laboratory evidence of malnutrition and that 11 of 13 infections occurred in these patients. Other authors have also reported a high rate of infection in malnourished patients undergoing spinal surgery,[63] as well as the development of malnutrition in some patients during their hospital stay after spinal surgery, which is of particular concern for patients undergoing staged procedures.[64] Commonly used indices of malnutrition are a serum albumin value of less than 3.5 mg/dL and a total lymphocyte count of less than 1500/mL.[65] Malnutrition may also be related to malignancy and trauma, two conditions associated with higher rates of infection. Other indices, including skinfold thickness, transferrin levels, arm muscle circumference, and weight-height ratio, can also be used to assess nutritional status.[66]

Diabetes impairs wound healing and predisposes to wound infection in spinal and other surgical procedures.[8,44,67-69] Postoperative wound infections have been reported to occur in up to 24% of diabetic patients undergoing spine surgery.[44,68] Mechanisms by which diabetes is thought to contribute to infection risk include increased glucose concentrations in wound fluids, the presence of dysfunctional polymorphonuclear neutrophils and macrophages, impaired lymphocyte chemotaxis, and delayed wound reepithelialization.[70-73] Impaired glucose tolerance without overt diabetes has been correlated with wound infection complications as well.[8,55] Although studies of deep sternal SSI in cardiothoracic procedures have demonstrated an ability to reduce this risk with strict perioperative glucose control, no such study exists in the spine literature.[74,75]

Finally, tobacco use has been demonstrated as a risk factor for wound infection in several studies.[76-78] Hypothesized mechanisms include deprivation of oxygen to tissues, impaired wound healing, and deficient neutrophil function.[79-81]

Surgery-Specific Factors

Several surgical variables other than those discussed earlier may predispose patients to infection. Many of these variables are correlated with the magnitude of the surgery itself. Therefore, it is not surprising that a high number of levels treated, long length of surgery, high procedural complexity, and high amount of blood loss have all been associated with an increased risk of infection.[4,28,53,67,82,83] Operative times longer than 5 hours and blood loss greater than 1000 mL are each associated with an increased rate of infection.[67,82]

The use of a Cell Saver system (Haemonetics, Braintree, MA) has been inconsistently correlated with infection risk. Blood that has been processed by the Cell Saver system has been shown to be contaminated in 37% of various surgical procedures[84] and has been correlated with infection in series of patients undergoing spinal surgery.[34] The use of blood transfusion, however, has been correlated with infection in numerous studies, and this risk may be independent of the amount of blood loss.[34,85,86]

Other surgical risk factors include revision surgery, the use of allograft material, and surgery extending to the sacrum or pelvis. Increased risk in surgery in the sacral or pelvic region may be attributable to urine and fecal contamination.[28,87,88] Finally, the involvement of two or more resident surgeons in the procedure has been correlated with increased infectious risk in one study.[55] Although not completely explored, this variable is probably a reflection of the length and complexity of the procedure rather than a truly independent risk factor.

Prolonged presurgical hospitalization and postoperative stays in the intensive care unit are also risk factors for wound infection. Blam and associates[11] reported that patients staying in the intensive care unit for more than 1 day had a 6- to 13-fold greater risk of postoperative infection than did patients who did not stay in the intensive care unit. Wimmer and colleagues[67] showed that extensive presurgical hospital stay was significantly associated with infection.

Disease-Specific Factors

Infection rate has repeatedly been linked to the disease state of the patient. The presence of malignancy appears to be associated with the highest incidence of infection, reported to be as high as 20% in some series.[6,10] This rate has been reported to be even higher in patients undergoing radiation therapy before open surgery.[89-92] The higher rate of postoperative infection in this population is multifactorial: poor nutritional status, the length and complexity of surgical procedures necessary for spinal reconstruction, and the use of adjunctive therapies such as corticosteroids all contribute to the dramatically elevated risk of infection.

Traumatic spinal injury is also associated with a significantly higher risk of infection, especially in the presence of a complete neurological injury.[11,12] The risk in affected patients is multifactorial, including prolonged stay in the intensive care unit, urinary or fecal incontinence, and the need for complex instrumentation to stabilize the patient.[8] However, early surgery and hypervigilance with these patients have reduced the rates of infection to less than 5%.

CLINICAL FINDINGS

The manifestation of spinal infection depends on whether the infection is superficial or deep. Superficial infections occur above the lumbodorsal fascia in the dermis and subcutaneous tissues and usually manifest in the immediate postoperative period with erythema, purulent drainage, local tenderness, and separation or dehiscence of the wound edges. Affected patients may exhibit a low-grade fever, and laboratory evaluation may reveal elevated ESR and CRP levels and elevated white blood cell count (WBC). The presence of these indices is variable, however. For example, Levi and colleagues[4] reported an average temperature of 37.5°C and a WBC count of 10.2 ($\times 10^6$ cells/mL) in 17 patients with postoperative infections. If the wound is open or purulence is expressible, Gram stain and cultures collected aseptically are often useful in revealing the pathogen and targeting treatment.

Deep infections have a much more variable manifestation. They may manifest in the immediate postoperative period—some authors have reported most manifesting 2 to 3 weeks postoperatively—or in a delayed manner, several months to several years after surgery.[35,37] Patients with an acute manifestation often have symptoms, with significant pain, fever, anorexia, and night sweats. The wound overlying a deep infection can appear completely normal or, if the infection tracks superficially, can be purulent. Patients with a delayed manifestation often present with increasing back pain, wound drainage, and erythema but may lack fever altogether.[37,93]

Spinal epidural abscess is a rare complication of spine surgery that may occur in an acute or delayed fashion with increased back pain, fever, and neurological deficit.[94,95] Patients with spinal epidural abscess may have a rapid neurological decline, and the presence of any neurological deficit should raise concern for this process.[96]

EVALUATION

Laboratory evaluation, physical examination, and radiographic studies are the key to the diagnosis of postoperative spinal infections. Laboratory evaluation should include WBC, ESR, and CRP evaluation, as well as cultures and Gram stain if there is an open wound with purulent drainage. The complete blood cell count may include an elevated WBC with a preponderance of neutrophils in an acute infection, but this is not always the case, especially in patients with a delayed manifestation.[93,97] The ESR is reliably elevated in the setting of infection, but it may be difficult to interpret in the immediate postoperative period. ESR values normally rise to a maximum of 102 mm/hr after spinal fusion surgery and 75 mm/hr after disk surgery on postoperative day 4 before declining to normal levels 2 to 4 weeks postoperatively.[97] Patients with infection have persistently elevated ESR values, usually 2 standard deviations greater than the mean.[97] Infections with low-grade pathogens, such as *Propionibacterum* species, may, however, be associated with low or normal ESR values.[98] Furthermore, serial ESR values with trends can additionally be useful data in tracking the response to treatment of infection. CRP level may also be useful in diagnosing and monitoring infection and subsequent treatment response. A normal elevation of CRP level is also seen in the immediate postoperative period; however, this elevation is more rapid, and the level returns to baseline more rapidly than that of ESR, although complete normalization may take up to 2 weeks in the postoperative period (Fig. 37-1).[99,100] In addition, CRP values are elevated more frequently in the setting of infection with low-grade pathogens than are ESR values.[98]

Accurate diagnosis of bacterial pathogens is critical in the treatment of postoperative infections. Antibiotic therapy should be withheld until after specimens are taken for Gram stain and culture. These specimens can be easily taken from draining or open wounds, but the skin should be prepared carefully before specimen collection to prevent contamination by normal skin flora. If débridement is planned, specimens should be taken from both superficial and deep parts of the wound. When obtaining a direct specimen is difficult, blood cultures may aid in the diagnosis of a pathogen. Alternatively, computed tomography (CT)–guided or open biopsy may be helpful; a diagnosis is obtained in more than 30% to 50% of biopsies.[101-103] Enoch and associates[104] found a positive culture in 36% of samples and successfully determined bacterial causes of infection; however, they did speculate that a large majority of negative cultures result from the use of prior antimicrobial therapy.

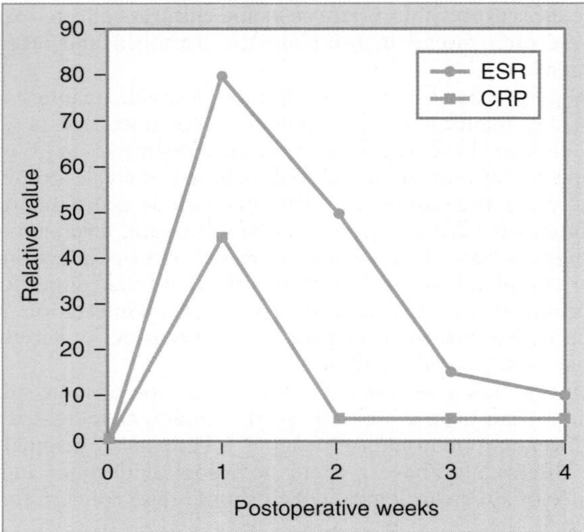

Figure 37-1. Graph showing normal postoperative spikes in erythrocyte sedimentation rate (ESR) and C-reactive protein (CRP). Note that the decline of ESR values is variable and that normalization takes between 2 and 4 weeks.

Imaging Diagnosis

Use of appropriate imaging modalities may aid in the diagnosis of infection, as well as in the assessment of spinal instrumentation and fusion, which may be compromised with infection. Immediate postoperative imaging may be difficult to interpret because normal postoperative inflammatory changes mimic those found in infection. Imaging in this setting is thus an adjunct in diagnosis, and the results can be valuable in the context of clinical examination and laboratory findings.

Plain Radiography and Computed Tomography

Plain radiographs are useful in the assessment of spinal alignment, paravertebral soft tissue swelling, and bone response to infection. They may have limited utility in the immediate postoperative period. Early bone changes in response to infection manifest approximately 2 to 3 weeks postoperatively with evidence of disk space narrowing, bone destruction, and blurring of end plates. This is followed by vertebral body collapse or sclerosis of end plates and bone ankylosis in the more chronic setting.[105] Increased soft tissue swelling, especially in the retropharyngeal space after anterior spinal surgery, may indicate the presence of an abscess. Plain radiographs are also useful in the evaluation of the integrity of spinal hardware; lucency around screws is indicative of loosening, hardware failure, or pseudoarthrosis.

CT reveals a sequence of bone changes similar to that of radiographs, but it provides improved anatomic detail (Fig. 37-2) and can better reveal paraspinal masses and epidural collections.[105] When performed with contrast enhancement, CT can accurately delineate the presence of an abscess. In addition, CT can provide information for the planning of procedures, either open débridement or CT-guided biopsy.[106] CT myelography may aid in the diagnosis of epidural or subdural empyema in cases in which magnetic resonance imaging (MRI) is unavailable, contraindicated, or difficult to evaluate because of hardware artifact.[107]

Nuclear Medicine

Bone scans with technetium 99m–labeled methylene diphosphonate can help diagnose and localize an infection, but the sensitivity and specificity of this technique are limited because other

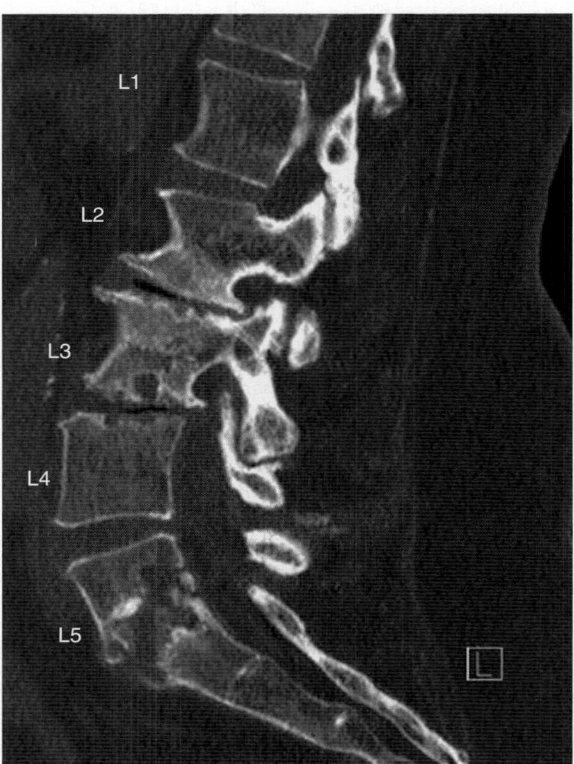

Figure 37-2. Sagittal computed tomographic scan of a patient with discitis of L5 to S1. Note end plate sclerosis, vertebral body collapse, and focal kyphosis.

conditions, such as trauma, tumor, or vascular insult, may have increased uptake and because uptake may be negative in areas of decreased blood flow or bone tissue.[105,108] A three-phase bone scan may increase the sensitivity and specificity of this test.[109] A scan with indium 111– or technetium 99m–labeled leukocytes (tagged WBC scan) may help in diagnosing infection when other factors, such as fracture, may cause false-positive results on bone scanning.[109,110]

Experience with fluorine 18 fluorodeoxyglucose–positron emission tomographic (PET) scans shows some promise, but it is difficult to differentiate tumor from infection.[111,112] PET scans may be particularly useful in the postoperative setting; a negative PET scan can rule out infection.[113]

Magnetic Resonance Imaging

MRI is the imaging modality of choice for evaluating spinal infections because it has high sensitivity and specificity of approximately 95% in the diagnosis of spinal infections, including osteomyelitis.[114-116] Early MRI findings in the setting of infection include bone marrow edema, whose signal manifests as hypointensity on T1-weighted sequences and hyperintensity on T2-weighted/short tau inversion recovery (STIR) sequences.[116,117] These findings can be nonspecific; however, the observation of end plate erosion with loss of end plate integrity, disk space narrowing, and disk space hyperintensity on T2-weighted sequences dramatically increases the sensitivity in diagnosing infections.[118] In addition, the signal of the disk space cleft, normally of low intensity, is lost on T2-weighted sequences in infection.[105] The addition of contrast enhancement is useful in confirming the presence of infection, delineating the extent of infection, and differentiating infection from solid granulation tissue, the latter most often having a homogeneous pattern of enhancement

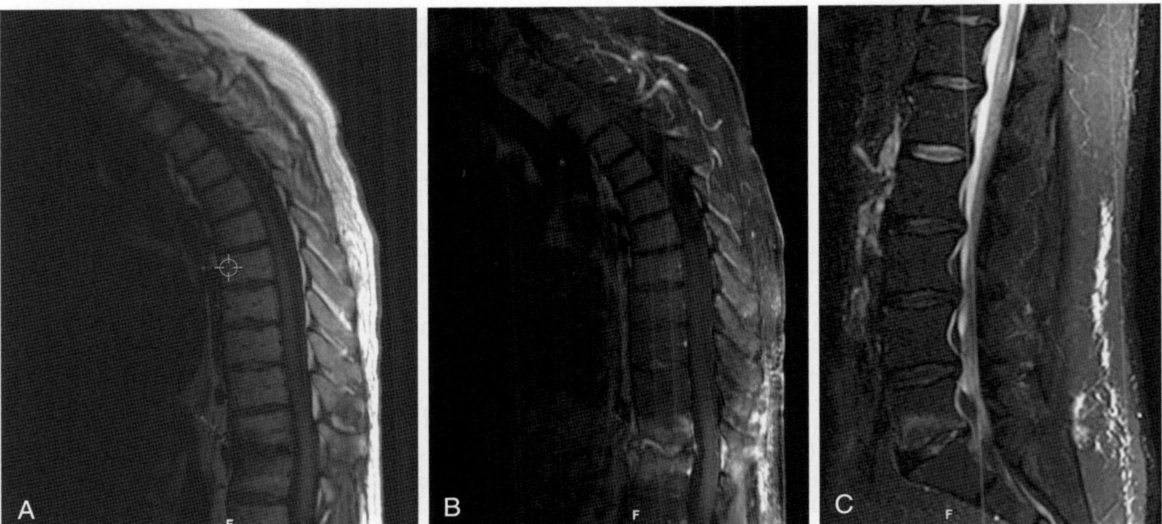

Figure 37-3. Magnetic resonance images (MRIs) of thoracic discitis. A, Sagittal T1-weighted noncontrast MRI. **B,** Sagittal T1-weighted contrast-enhanced MRI. Note hypointense signal intensity in vertebral bodies and avid enhancement with the administration of contrast material. **C,** Sagittal T2-weighted sequence MRI in a patient with postoperative L5-S1 discitis. Note hyperintense signal in adjacent end plates.

(Fig. 37-3).[117-120] MRI can also aid in detecting soft tissue masses associated with infection, such as paraspinal or epidural abscesses. The presence of an associated mass increases the likelihood of infection to 98%.[118]

Some of these MRI findings, including increased vertebral body edema and contrast enhancement, may be present in the normal postoperative setting[121,122]; however, the presence of an adjacent soft tissue mass in this setting strongly indicates the diagnosis of infection. Conversely, the absence of the MRI findings listed previously is strongly correlated with the absence of infection.[122]

BACTERIOLOGIC STUDY

Skin flora are the most common causative organisms in postoperative spinal infection with *Staphylococcus* species, particularly *Staphylococcus aureus*, which is the most frequently detected organism.[4,30,56,123] However, methicillin-resistant *S. aureus* (MRSA), gram-negative organisms, and mixed flora are detected in sufficient frequency to recommend withholding antibiotics until adequate culture specimens have been obtained and then providing treatment with broad-spectrum antibiotics until culture results are confirmed. Abdul-Jabbar and colleagues[124] reported on the common pathogens found in SSIs from a high-volume academic spine group. *S. aureus* was the organism most commonly isolated (45%), followed by *Staphylococcus epidermidis* (31%) and then all gram-negative flora (30%). Overall, methicillin-resistant organisms were found in 34% of cases and were more commonly found after revision surgery than after primary surgeries. Delayed infections occur with bacteria of low virulence, most commonly with *Propionibacterium* species and *S. epidermidis.*[37,98,125] Isolation of *Propionibacterium* species in cultures can take up to a week, and this bacterium might play a role in acute infections as well.[98]

TREATMENT

The treatment of postoperative spinal infections is not standardized, and there is much debate in the literature concerning management. Two areas of debate are (1) whether to remove instrumentation and (2) whether to utilize adjuncts to débridement and washout, including vacuum-assisted closure (VAC) (i.e., wound VAC), continuous irrigation systems, and implanted antibiotic beads. Despite these ongoing discussions, it is clear that optimal outcome requires prompt diagnosis and aggressive treatment.

Nonoperative Treatment

Some superficial wound infections can be treated with local wound care and antibiotics and may not necessitate a return to the operating room. In the absence of frank wound breakdown, purulent drainage, or fluctuance, empirical antibiotic treatment aimed at skin flora may be adequate. Follow-up monitoring is important to ensure that symptoms resolve with treatment and there is no progression to deeper tissues and structures.

Postoperative discitis may also be treated nonoperatively. Diagnosis of infecting pathogens should be obtained via blood cultures, which are positive in up to 50% of cases,[126] or from CT-guided tissue biopsy before antibiotic therapy is initiated. Once cultures have been obtained, broad-spectrum antibiotics are started until specific organisms are identified and antibiotic therapy can be narrowed accordingly. If culture results do not indicate the causative organism, broad-spectrum antistaphylococcal coverage should be provided because of the probability and overwhelming presence of this organism.[127] Use of an external brace and relative rest can also help mitigate the symptoms of mechanical back pain in postoperative discitis.[128] Although evidence-based recommendations for duration of antibiotic therapy are lacking, a course of intravenous antibiotics for 6 weeks, followed by oral antibiotics for 6 weeks, is commonly prescribed, along with an orthotic brace for comfort.

Medical treatment is usually successful, although surgical treatment is indicated in cases of poor clinical response to medical treatment, continued back pain, or instability. The surgical goal in such instances should be thorough débridement of infected tissue, including infected bone, and stabilization with bone graft and titanium instrumentation. Cervical and thoracic discitis or osteomyelitis often necessitate débridement with an anterior approach, which may be difficult in patients with significant medical comorbid conditions. To reach the bone and disk space, the soft tissues must be dissected, which is often difficult, and additional assistance from an access surgeon may be required, particularly in the setting of chronic infection. Thoracoscopic approaches have also been described in treating thoracic infections, with acceptable morbidity.[129,130]

Surgical Débridement

For wounds that have broken down, have purulent drainage, or are fluctuant or otherwise raise concern for deep extension, operative exploration is usually required; the goals are (1) diagnosis of the infective agent, (2) débridement of nonviable tissue, and (3) assurance of stabilization. Preoperative antibiotics are withheld until adequate culture specimens have been obtained, and the entire length of the wound is opened. Preoperative imaging can be used to determine the extent of débridement; evidence of deep infection mandates opening of the lumbodorsal fascia. Although some authors recommend opening the fascia in all cases,[32] it may be left closed in cases in which it is intact and infection and wound breakdown are probably only superficial, according to preoperative imaging and intraoperative findings. Alternatively, some authors have suggested aspirating the subfascial compartment with a needle and obtaining an intraoperative Gram stain, with the results guiding the need to open this layer.[28,83] The lumbodorsal fascia should be opened only after thorough débridement and irrigation of the superficial compartment. Cultures from the deep compartment should be taken separately and labeled as such.

Aggressive débridement should be undertaken in each open compartment. Loose bone fragments, gel foam or fibrin sealant remnants, and necrotic muscle and fat should be meticulously removed. All areas involved in the operation should be inspected. If the disk space was subjected to instrumentation, it should be viewed, culture specimens taken, and débridement performed. At the conclusion of débridement, healthy soft tissue—as evidenced by adequate vasculature and perfusion—should be exposed.

The issue of instrumentation removal has been a significant controversy in the setting of infection, with some authors recommending removal in all or most cases,[3,36,37,98,123,125,131] and others reporting successful treatment with maintained instrumentation.[30,31,83,132-135] Some authors even reason that stability provided by maintenance of instrumentation may aid in the clearing of infection.[135,136] Recurrent infections with retained hardware have been reported in the setting of delayed infections and in cases of scoliosis and traumatic fracture treatment with steel constructs. Newer titanium implants are not associated with this phenomenon and have been used with success in stabilizing the infected spine.[134,137] Furthermore, the removal of hardware in an unstable spine is not a viable option, and we therefore recommend the maintenance of hardware in all cases in which spinal stability and fusion maturation are in question.

On completion of débridement, the integrity of the fusion construct should be confirmed by visual inspection and manual manipulation. If instrumentation is found to be loose, either on manual inspection or preoperative radiographic assessment, it must be removed, and an alternative means of fixation must be used. In the case of pedicle screw fixation, a screw of larger diameter can be used as a "rescue screw." Structural allograft tissue used in the initial construct may also be left in place, but loose chips of bone should be removed.[134,138] If, however, the infection has manifested in a delayed manner and the fusion is solid, the surgeon should consider removing instrumentation.[9] Careful follow-up is needed because loss of correction has been observed with instrumentation removal despite solid bone fusion.[37,125,131,139] Infection is also associated with an increased rate of pseudarthrosis, and this complication, although not strictly correlated with a negative clinical outcome, should be assessed in the follow-up period.[83,140]

Before closure, the wound should be thoroughly irrigated. We often use a low-pressure pulsatile irrigator with copious amounts (9 L) of antibiotic solution.[141,142] Primary wound closure should be performed if possible. Some authors recommend closing wounds in a delayed manner or allowing healing to occur by secondary intention[133,143,144]; however, this mandates a return to the operating room and exposure of the wound to the risk of secondary infection.[31] The wound should be closed in layers around a drain to eliminate dead space. Some authors have advocated for additional washouts in 2 to 3 days until purulent collections are no longer identified.[32] We have found this to be unnecessary in most patients and use clinical examination and laboratory findings to guide this decision.

Treatment of Infections in the Intrathecal Pump and Spinal Cord Stimulator

For infections in the intrathecal pump and for spinal cord stimulator infections, treatment typically involves removal of the device and, initially, broad-spectrum antibiotics with gradual narrowing of antibiotic coverage once culture results have been obtained.[48] Removing intrathecal drug delivery devices is, however, associated with drug withdrawal symptoms. [48] There have been reports of nonoperative treatment in such cases, even in the setting of meningitis[49,145-147]; however, there is no clear evidence to recommend this course of treatment. Although novel techniques such as the injection and infusion of antibiotics into the drug delivery system are appealing in this setting, the efficacy of such measures has not been firmly established, and further experience is needed before nonsurgical treatment of neuroprosthetic devices can be recommended.

Wound Vacuum-Assisted Closure

There have been numerous reports of wound VAC use in the general, orthopedic, and plastic surgery literature,[148-150] but the application of VAC for spinal wounds is a more recent phenomenon. In VAC, negative pressure is applied to the wound, which leads to removal of third-space fluid, improvement of blood flow, stimulation of angiogenesis, stimulation of granulation tissue development, and reduction in bacterial load.[151-154] The VAC device is composed of a polyurethane sponge, a plastic sealant drape, and a negative-pressure suction device. The sponge should be placed within the confines of the wound bed, with care taken to ensure that it contacts all area of the wound, thereby leaving no dead space, while at the same time avoiding skin contact. The sealant should cover the surrounding area to prevent loss of suction, and the device is then activated with approximately 125 mm Hg of suction. VAC dressings are replaced every 2 to 4 days, as needed, by a skilled nurse or in the operating room. Once the infection has been eradicated and the wound edges appear healthy, the patient can be returned to the operating room for delayed primary wound closure.

Although a randomized controlled trial has yet to prove the efficacy of this technique in spinal surgery, potential advantages include more rapid resolution of infection, fewer trips to the operating room for wound washout, no need for frequent dressing changes in open wounds, and decreased likelihood of reliance on closure by secondary intention.[155] Potential complications include significant blood loss, hypoalbuminemia, toxic shock syndrome, retained sponges, and possible cerebrospinal fluid leak.[156]

Irrigation-Suction Technique

The application of an irrigation-suction apparatus has also been reported.[4,157] This involves closure of the wound over the irrigation catheters and placement of drains separately in both the deep and superficial compartments of the wound. An antibiotic solution, chosen on the basis of Gram stain and culture results, is used for irrigation at a rate of up to 50 mL/hr, and the suction catheter is attached to a medium-pressure Hemovac drain. The drains are left in place for 5 to 7 days, at which point the irrigation drains are removed, and the Hemovac drain is removed a day later.

Although no randomized controlled trial has proved the efficacy of this technique, it is appealing in that it provides continuous antibiotic irrigation of the wound bed, does not necessitate leaving the wound open, and does not necessitate numerous return trips to the operating room.

Other Surgical Techniques

Other surgical adjuncts to treat infection are the use of antibiotic beads and muscle flaps. The placement of antibiotic beads in the surgical bed in the treatment of spinal infections has been reported with promising results.[83] High local concentrations of antibiotics are provided with this technique, which has also been shown to be effective in the treatment of open and contaminated fractures.[158,159]

In severe cases of wound breakdown, rotational muscle flaps may be necessary to cover the wound and aid in wound healing by reducing dead space and enhancing antibiotic and oxygen delivery. These can be particularly useful in the setting of chronic infections with repeated wound breakdown and in cases of persistent cerebrospinal fluid leaks with incompetent dura and unresolved wound drainage. Potential donor sites for spinal coverage include the latissimus, trapezius, gluteus, and paraspinal muscles. The help of a plastic surgeon is required for such reconstructions.[160-162]

Antibiotic Therapy

Treatment with broad-spectrum antibiotics should be started after adequate culture specimens have been obtained. The chosen antibiotics should cover skin pathogens and take into account local resistance patterns. Results of a Gram stain can guide initial therapy, but broad coverage should be used until final culture results are obtained. Once cultures are finalized, the choice of antibiotic is narrowed for each specific organism. There are currently no standardized length-of-treatment recommendations for postoperative spinal infections, but most authors recommend 4 to 6 weeks of intravenous antibiotic therapy, typically followed by a course of oral antibiotic therapy. An infectious disease specialist should be enlisted to guide appropriate therapy. Response to treatment is monitored with clinical examination (increasing back pain and persistent fever indicate potential treatment failure) and laboratory evaluation. ESR, CRP, and WBC values are checked regularly and should show a trend to normal with effective therapy. Serial imaging can be used to evaluate for progression of neural compression, but caution should be used when evaluating infectious response to antibiotics because imaging findings can lag behind treatment response by several months.

PREVENTION

The most effective way of dealing with postoperative infections is prevention. A comprehensive preoperative, intraoperative, and postoperative approach to prevention must be undertaken to minimize the risk of this devastating and costly complication.

Preoperative optimization of controllable risk can aid in the reduction of infection, especially in elective cases. Preoperative smoking cessation is linked to a decreased risk of surgical complications, although the length of cessation needed to have an effect is not clear.[163] Because nutritional status is a major risk factor for the development of infection, nutritional intake should be assessed and optimized preoperatively.[51,52] Abnormal serum albumin or total lymphocyte count[164-170] values may prompt a delay of elective surgery while deficiencies are corrected with the aid of a nutritionist or internist. Concomitant infections should be identified and treated before surgery if possible. The presence of a urinary tract or respiratory infection may increase the risk of operative wound infection, especially in the setting of instrumentation, and elective cases are usually delayed until these infections are eradicated.

Hair shaving during skin preparation has received a great deal of attention in the cranial literature; one randomized trial in the spine literature showed an increased risk of infection in patients whose heads are shaved preoperatively.[171] Potential mechanisms by which skin shaving may increase infection risk include the loss of protective skin flora and the creation of microabrasions that may facilitate bacterial colonization.[171,172] If the presence of hair interferes with the surgical approach, it should be removed with clippers and not a razor, to mitigate skin abrasions caused by microtrauma.

The use of prophylactic antibiotic medications in spinal surgery has been the standard of care since its description by Horwitz and Curtin in 1975.[21] They reported a significant decrease in postoperative infection with the use of prophylactic antibiotics.[21] Since then, six randomized studies have been conducted to examine the efficacy of antibiotics in preventing infection. Although none of these studies demonstrated a significant benefit alone, all revealed trends toward reduced infection with prophylaxis,[173-178] and when collective data were pooled in a meta-analysis, a significant overall reduction in infection rate from 5.9% to 2.2% was obtained.[179]

Prophylactic antibiotics traditionally cover skin flora and take into account local resistance patterns, as well as history of patient reactions to antibiotics. Some authors additionally recommend screening even low-risk patients for MRSA preoperatively.[180] First-generation cephalosporins, such as cefazolin, are the most commonly used prophylactic agents because of their reactivity with gram-positive skin flora, as well as with gram-negative bacteria such as *Escherichia coli*. The use of second- and third-generation cephalosporins is reserved for the treatment of infection rather than prophylaxis.[181] Patients who are MRSA-positive or allergic to cephalosporins should be given a glycopeptide, such as vancomycin, and gentamicin. Antibiotics should be administered approximately 30 minutes to 1 hour before skin incision to ensure adequacy of blood levels at the time of skin incision and readministered at half the dose every 4 hours or with every 1500 mL of blood loss during surgery if cephalosporins are administered or every 8 hours if a glycopeptide and gentamicin are administered.[55,180,182-184] Dosage of medications should be based on patient weight; those weighing more than 80 kg, for example, should receive 2 g of preoperative cefazolin.[55,182]

Patients undergoing procedures involving the disk space, such as diskography or diskectomy, should also receive antibiotic prophylaxis, although the optimum choice of drug is unclear. Several animal and human studies indicate that β-lactam antibiotics and cephalosporins have poor penetration into the disk and nucleus, whereas clindamycin, aminoglycosides, and glycopeptides have been shown to have good penetration.[27,164-170] Good results have been reported in retrospective studies in which antibiotics were administered directly into the disk space during the procedure, mixed either with contrast material in diskography or with a sponge at diskectomy.[24,185] Randomized trials have not been conducted to validate the efficacy of either method of prophylaxis; therefore, the treating physician should give careful thought to each method. In a large retrospective study of 3063 patients, Kaliaperumal and colleagues[186] found that the incidence of spondylodiscitis was lower with standard microsurgical technique with antiseptic irrigation into the disk space than with standard microdiskectomy.

Several intraoperative measures may play a role in reducing infectious risk. The maintenance of strict aseptic technique is critical. This involves participation of all operating room staff to minimize operating room traffic. Periodic release of tissue retractors may reduce ischemic damage to paraspinal musculature,[187,188] which may in turn reduce tissue necrosis, improving wound healing and reducing infection rates. Using two sets of gloves (double gloving) is highly recommended in spinal procedures, especially those requiring instrumentation. Yinusa and associates[189] recorded glove puncture in 63.6% of spinal operations, the highest incidence for any type of orthopedic surgery. The rate of puncture of the inner glove with double gloving was significantly lower than that for puncture of single gloves.

Intraoperative irrigation of the wound is cited as a prophylactic measure. Bacitracin irrigation has been shown to be more beneficial than saline irrigation in a contaminated canine osseus tissue model.[190] Antibiotic irrigation has demonstrated promising results in general and orthopedic surgical procedures and is used widely.[191-194] The most robust evidence to date is that of Chang and colleagues,[195] who performed a prospective randomized trial with dilute (0.35%) povidone-iodine solution to irrigate tissues before bone grafting. They reported a reduction in infection, from 3.4% with saline irrigation to 0% with povidone-iodine irrigation, without any adverse effects. This trial has not been reproduced, but the use of povidone-iodine irrigation is simple, and the results of the single study are strong enough to recommend routine use. It is important to irrigate the spinal wound before decortication because bacitracin and povidone-iodine solution have a cytotoxic effect on osteoblasts at elevated concentrations.[196]

Vancomycin Powder

Local delivery of antibiotics to the wound bed and the bone graft during surgery is an attractive option because the penetration of antibiotics in surgical wounds may vary as a result of tissue ischemia, seroma, and hematoma.[197] Vancomycin powder has been previously used in cardiothoracic, orthopedic, and vascular surgery with lowered rates of SSIs. Vancomycin powder has a relatively low hospital cost, is easy to manipulate and deliver, and has broad coverage against the typical organisms in superficial and deep spinal wound infections.[198] In a meta-analysis of data concerning spinal SSIs and vancomycin powder, Khan and associates[199] found that it may be protective against SSIs (relative risk = 0.34; 95% confidence interval, 0.17-0.66; $P = .021$); to prevent one SSI, the number needed to treat was 36. Interestingly, a subgroup analysis of the same study revealed that patients who had implants had a reduced risk of SSIs with vancomycin powder ($P = .023$) whereas those who had noninstrumented spinal operations did not ($P = .226$). In a cohort of 112 patients undergoing posterior cervical fusion for spondylotic myelopathy, Caroom and colleagues[197] found a significant decrease in the rate of infection among the patients who received vancomycin powder (0%), in comparison with the control group ($P = .007$; power, 81%). Although the side effect profile for systemic vancomycin therapy is well known, the effects of vancomycin powder applied locally are not well understood. A high-peak concentration occurs with the direct intrawound application of antibiotic powder without a carrier and has been shown to have cytotoxic effects in animal models[200-202]; this finding has yet to be shown in humans.

Initially, Sweet and associates[203] reported on 1732 consecutive thoracic and lumbar posterior instrumented spinal fusions; 21 deep wound infections occurred among the 821 control patients, who received intravenous cephalexin (2.6%), whereas there were 2 deep wound infections among the 911 patients who received intravenous cephalexin with vancomycin powder. The reduction in wound infections was statistically significant ($P < .0001$), and there were no adverse complications related to vancomycin powder use. O'Neill and colleagues[204] demonstrated similar efficacy of vancomycin powder in patients who underwent posterior spinal fusion for traumatic injuries. They found a statistically significant difference in infection rate between the patients who received vancomycin powder (0%) and those who did not (13%; $P = .02$) and no untoward side effects in 110 patients. They posited that using vancomycin powder is an effective method in reducing costly and harmful postoperative wound infections. Molinari and associates[198] reported a 0.99% rate of deep spinal wound infections among 1512 patients who underwent spinal surgery and received 1 g of vancomycin powder before closure of the wound.

Not all reports on the use of vancomycin powder have demonstrated a benefit. Vancomycin powder may not provide benefit in patients undergoing surgery to correct spinal deformity. Martin and colleagues[205] demonstrated that there was no significant difference in rates of deep wound infection between the patients who did not receive vancomycin powder (5.3%) and those who did (5.1%; $P = .936$) among 306 patients undergoing posterior spinal deformity surgery. Thus, other methods are needed to reduce the incidence of SSIs in this population.

Although there is compelling evidence in support of the use of vancomycin powder, the exact dose and patient population it should be used in remain open to debate. Ghobrial and associates[206] studied the microbial trends associated with intraoperative vancomycin powder and found that its use may increase the incidence of gram-negative or polymicrobial spinal infections; in addition, it may be correlated with postoperative seroma formation caused by sterilized fluid and subsequent negative cultures.

Several postoperative measures have been proposed to decrease the risk of infection, although none have been studied in randomized controlled trials. The use of a postsurgical drain is controversial. Some researchers have reported a reduction in infection, whereas others have reported an increased incidence of infection, and still others have reported no change.[34,207] In cases in which a drain was used, the use of antibiotic prophylaxis has not been shown to be beneficial.[180] Other postoperative measures that may reduce the risk of infection are the application of a sterile dressing, strict glucose control,[8,55,74] and ensuring adequate nutrition.[10,51]

The use of postoperative antibiotics is controversial. A retrospective study demonstrated no difference in infection rate when postoperative antibiotics were continued for 24 hours in comparison with their continuation for 5 to 7 days. Infections occurring in the setting of prolonged administration were, however, more likely to be with resistant organisms.[181]

SUGGESTED READINGS

Chang FY, Chang MC, Wang ST, et al. Can povidone-iodine solution be used safely in a spinal surgery? *Eur Spine J*. 2006;15:1005-1014.

Fraser RD, Osti OL, Vernon-Roberts B. Iatrogenic discitis: the role of intravenous antibiotics in prevention and treatment. An experimental study. *Spine*. 1989;14:1025-1032.

James SL, Davies AM. Imaging of infectious spinal disorders in children and adults. *Eur J Radiol*. 2006;58:27-40.

Klein JD, Hey LA, Yu CS, et al. Perioperative nutrition and postoperative complications in patients undergoing spinal surgery. *Spine*. 1996;21:2676-2682.

Lee MC, Wang MY, Fessler RG, et al. Instrumentation in patients with spinal infection. *Neurosurg Focus*. 2004;17(6):E7.

Levi AD, Dickman CA, Sonntag VK. Management of postoperative infections after spinal instrumentation. *J Neurosurg*. 1997;86:975-980.

Mangram A, Horan T, Pearson M, et al. Guideline for prevention of surgical site infection, 1999. Centers for Disease Control and Prevention (CDC) Hospital Infection Control Practices Advisory Committee. *Am J Infect Control*. 1999;27:97-132.

Mehbod AA, Ogilvie JW, Pinto MR, et al. Postoperative deep wound infections in adults after spinal fusion: management with vacuum-assisted wound closure. *J Spinal Disord Tech*. 2005;18:14-17.

Olsen MA, Mayfield J, Lauryssen C, et al. Risk factors for surgical site infection in spinal surgery. *J Neurosurg*. 2003;98:149-155.

Olsen MA, Nepple JJ, Riew KD, et al. Risk factors for surgical site infection following orthopaedic spinal operations. *J Bone Joint Surg Am*. 2008;90:62-69.

Rubinstein E, Findler G, Amit P, et al. Perioperative prophylactic cephazolin in spinal surgery: a double-blind placebo-controlled trial. *J Bone Joint Surg Br*. 1994;76:99-102.

Weinstein MA, McCabe JP, Cammisa FP Jr. Postoperative spinal wound infection: a review of 2,391 consecutive index procedures. *J Spinal Disord*. 2000;13:422-426.

Wimmer C, Gluch H. Management of postoperative wound infection in posterior spinal fusion with instrumentation. *J Spinal Disord*. 1996;9:505-508.

Wimmer C, Gluch H, Franzreb M, et al. Predisposing factors for infection in spine surgery: a survey of 850 spinal procedures. *J Spinal Disord*. 1998;11:124-128.

See a full reference list on ExpertConsult.com

38 The Use and Misuse of Antibiotics in Neurosurgery

Ciro Vasquez, Kristen E. Jones, Matthew A. Hunt, and Stephen J. Haines

THE IMPORTANCE OF ANTIBIOTICS IN NEUROSURGERY

Few neurosurgeons would be willing to practice modern neurosurgery without the ready availability of antibiotics. These drugs have made it possible to treat infections of the brain, meninges, and surgical site effectively and to salvage excellent results from what would otherwise be devastating complications of neurosurgical operations. Although some still argue—based on the extraordinary results of Harvey Cushing, who reported one infection in 149 patients (0.7%)—that careful technique overcomes almost all sources of infection, a very special understanding of the available evidence is required to deliberately omit perioperative antibiotic prophylaxis in modern neurosurgical practice.[1] Antibiotics are an integral part of the daily life of the neurosurgeon.

Like all other neurosurgical interventions, however, antibiotics carry with them cost and risk. A superficial understanding of their use and the evidence underlying their applications can lead to excessive use, ineffective use, and other forms of misuse that should be avoided if excellence in practice is to be achieved. In this chapter, we review appropriate use and discuss common misuses of antibiotics in neurosurgical practice.

RISKS OF ANTIBIOTIC ADMINISTRATION

Antibiotic therapy in the neurosurgical patient is implemented in various situations, including prophylaxis for procedures, empirical treatment of a presumed infection, or treatment of a specific infection. The administration of antibiotics is not without consequence, however. Adverse drug reactions that may result include central nervous system (CNS) toxicities, systemic toxicities, allergic reactions, side effects, and drug-drug interactions.* Moreover, there is the potential for antibiotic resistance with careless administration. Tables 38-1 and 38-2 summarize commonly used antibiotics in neurosurgery, along with their local and systemic toxicities, side effects, drug-drug interactions, and potential for resistance.

GENERAL PRINCIPLES OF ANTIBIOTIC USE

Neurosurgeons are involved in the treatment of infections not only of the CNS itself but also of the surrounding structures. These include the cranial soft tissues, skull, and paranasal sinuses; the spine, intervertebral disks, and paraspinal soft tissues; and the tissues and body cavities utilized for the insertion of hardware. Fortunately, many of the infections with which neurosurgeons must deal are extradural. This fact simplifies treatment, in that delivery of antibiotics does not depend on the physiology of the either the blood-brain barrier (BBB) or the blood–cerebrospinal fluid barrier (BCSFB). However, these brain barriers present an obstacle to the entry of antibiotics and require special consideration when treating an infection inside them.

*For detailed information on adverse effects of common antibiotics in neurosurgery, please see the previous version of this chapter.[2]

The Blood-Brain and Blood–Cerebrospinal Fluid Barriers

The BBB is formed by the endothelial cells of the cerebral vasculature, supported by astroglia and pericytes, with tight junctions between the endothelial cells and minimal fenestrations or bulk transport across the cells. The BCSFB is located at the epithelial layer of the choroid plexus, not at the endothelium, but is similar in character with tight junctions between the epithelial cells. For both of the barriers, active influx and efflux transporters located on the endothelial/epithelial cell surface may drastically alter the distribution of an antibiotic into the desired compartment.[3,4]

Factors such as increasing molecular weight, ionization, plasma protein binding, metabolism at the barrier, and presence of efflux transporters will decrease the permeability of substances across the brain barriers.[4,5] Other factors such as increased lipophilicity, influx transporters, and inflammation can increase the permeability of the barriers to antibiotics.[6] Antibiotics may cross into the cerebrospinal fluid (CSF) or brain parenchyma more readily at the initiation of treatment, but as the inflammatory response to the infection abates, either from the antibiotic treatment or from administration of other medications such as dexamethasone, the ability of an antibiotic to cross the brain barriers will diminish.[7,8] However, this effect may not alter outcome.[9-13]

The overall goal of antibiotic treatment is to deliver an adequate concentration of the drug to the proper compartment.[14-16] This may be accomplished in several ways. First, the dose of the drug may be increased. This method is helpful in drugs with low systemic toxicities and relatively low permeability across the brain barriers, such as β-lactam antibiotics. Second, the choice of antibiotics may be altered to a drug that has greater penetration into the CNS, such as chloramphenicol or the quinolones. Third, antibiotics may be delivered directly across the brain barriers (usually by indwelling ventricular or lumbar catheters). This method is especially helpful when using antibiotics such as vancomycin or the aminoglycosides, which have higher systemic toxicities and poor permeability across the brain barriers that limit the systemic dose that may be administered.

An excellent review of the BCSFB and BBB has been published by Nau and colleagues.[17]

Pharmacokinetics of Antibiotic Delivery

Effective antibiotic dosing is achieved by understanding the pharmacokinetics of antibiotics, which depends on the systemic pharmacokinetics, as well as on the behavior of the antibiotic in its access to and elimination from the CNS. It is important to bear in mind that most data relating to antibiotic pharmacokinetics in the CNS come from studies on CSF and meningitis, with much less data for the brain parenchyma itself.[18,19] A few studies have used microdialysis assays for brain interstitial concentrations of antibiotics themselves, but these studies had small numbers of patients, were conducted in patients with other underlying brain injuries, and had limitations in methods.[20-22]

In determining the proportion of antibiotic reaching the CNS, careful interpretation of experimental data is required.

TABLE 38-1 Antibiotic Neurotoxicity

Antibiotic	Seizure	Central Nervous System	Peripheral Nervous System	Other/Systemic
Sulfonamides		Kernicterus in infants		Psychiatric syndromes*
		Ataxia		
Quinolones	✓	Headache	Polyneuropathy	Psychiatric syndromes
		Dizziness	Exacerbation of myasthenia gravis	
		Insomnia		
		Pseudotumor cerebri		
Penicillins	✓	Encephalopathy (intrathecal)	Exacerbation of myasthenia gravis (ampicillin)	Psychiatric syndromes
		Lethargy	Arachnoiditis (intrathecal)	Hoigne's syndrome†
		Multifocal myoclonus		
Cephalosporins	✓	Encephalopathy		Psychiatric syndromes
		Aseptic meningitis		Hypersensitivity reaction
Carbapenems	✓			Nausea and vomiting
Aminoglycosides		Anosmia	Neuromuscular blockade	Nephrotoxicity
		Aseptic meningitis		Ototoxicity
Polymyxins	✓	Encephalopathy	Neuromuscular blockade	Nephrotoxicity
	(Intrathecal)	Ptosis, diplopia	Paresthesias	Ototoxicity
		Dysphagia		
		Areflexia		
		Chemical meningitis		
Vancomycin		Vestibular toxicity		Ototoxicity
Tetracyclines		Pseudotumor cerebri	Neuromuscular blockade	
		Vestibular toxicity	Exacerbation of myasthenia gravis	
Chloramphenicol		Encephalopathy	Optic neuropathy	Bone marrow suppression
			Peripheral neuropathy	Aplastic anemia
				Gray baby syndrome
Macrolides			Exacerbation of myasthenia gravis	Psychiatric syndromes
				Ototoxicity
Linezolid			Peripheral neuropathy	
			Optic neuropathy	
Rifampin		Headache, confusion, ataxia	Numbness, muscular weakness	Gastrointestinal symptoms

*Psychiatric syndromes include depression, hallucinations, anxiety attacks, and psychosis.
†Hoigne's syndrome: symptoms of panic attacks, acute psychosis with seizures or hallucinations.

TABLE 38-2 Selected Drug Interactions

Antibiotic	Warfarin	Anticonvulsants	Other
Quinolones	Potentiate		Potentiate theophylline and caffeine
Carbapenems			Potentiate theophylline, quinolones, metronidazole, ganciclovir, or cyclosporine seizure threshold reduction
Chloramphenicol	Potentiates	Prolongs half-life of phenytoin, phenobarbital	Prolongs half-life of cyclosporine
Macrolides (erythromycin)	Potentiate	Prolongs half-life of carbamazepine	Prolong half-life of theophylline, alfentanil, triazolam, midazolam, digoxin
Rifampin	Antagonizes		Speeds catabolism of oral contraceptives, cyclosporine, itraconazole, digoxin, verapamil, nifedipine, simvastatin, midazolam, and human immunodeficiency virus–related protease inhibitors

Many studies looking at this proportion used simple plasma-CSF ratios at a single time point. These ratios can vary widely during a dosing cycle and can be quite misleading.[19,23] The most useful data come from using plasma-CSF AUC ratios ("AUC" is the area under the drug concentration–time curve) in intermittent dosing, or steady-state concentrations during continuous infusion. For β-lactam antibiotics, the AUC ratio generally ranges from 0.01 to 0.1. Less hydrophilic antibiotics, such as rifampicin, trimethoprim-sulfamethoxazole, and the fluoroquinolones, have ratios that range from 0.1 to 0.9. Vancomycin and the aminoglycosides also have low penetration into the CSF, with ratios less than 0.1.[19,24] However, data suggest that these ratios may be different in treatment of infections of the brain parenchyma (i.e., brain abscess). One study showed equivalent levels of the antibiotic in the abscess fluid and the plasma 6 hours after administration; however, these are also time point ratios, not AUC ratios.[25]

Concentrations of antibiotics throughout the CSF are not constant. Ventricular CSF will have a lower concentration of protein and antibiotic than lumbar CSF because the CSF produced in the ventricles has not yet mixed with exuded extracellular fluid from the brain parenchyma. Therefore, CSF concentrations of antibiotics rely on the permeability of both the BBB and the BCSFB. Penetration of antibiotics through the blood-lesion barrier (specifically the blood-abscess barrier) will vary with the stage of formation of the abscess, the relative vascularity of the lesion, and even the etiology of the lesion. However, it is impossible to differentiate the individual contributions of the blood-lesion barrier and the surrounding BBB to antibiotic concentrations using measurement of antibiotic levels within abscesses.[18,25-27] The half-life of the antibiotic in the CSF is also an important consideration. Most antibiotics are not metabolized in the CSF. Elimination comes either through diffusion back through the BBB and BCSFB, or from turnover of the CSF. Generally, the CSF half-life of antibiotics is significantly longer than the plasma half-life. The CSF half-life of antibiotics may also be increased in CNS infections because of decreased turnover of CSF. Conversely, in patients with CSF shunts or external CSF drains, the CSF half-life may be quite variable because the circulation of CSF is altered.[28,29]

Central Nervous System Toxicity of Antibiotic Therapy

Antibiotics may be toxic to the CNS when administered systemically, or when administered directly to the CNS via an intrathecal route or through antibiotic irrigation. Systemic administration of almost any class of antibiotic may cause CNS toxicity, including encephalopathy, seizures, psychiatric symptoms, cranial nerve injury, and ataxia.[30,31] Table 38-1 lists CNS toxicities of commonly used antibiotics.

Intrathecal antibiotics may also have significant neurological toxicities, although the most commonly used intrathecal antibiotics, vancomycin and gentamicin, appear to have relatively low toxicity when administered intrathecally. Additionally, discerning these effects may be difficult in the face of a coexisting serious CNS infection.[31] Intraventricular vancomycin appears to be relatively free of toxicity, even at high CSF levels.[32] Intraventricular gentamicin may have CNS toxicity, causing ototoxicity or epilepsy; however, these effects are not clearly related to CSF levels of gentamicin.[33,34] Intraventricular administration of β-lactam antibiotics may cause effects similar to those occurring when they are administered systemically, especially seizures.[35]

ANTIBIOTIC PROPHYLAXIS

Systemic Antibiotic Prophylaxis

Antibiotic prophylaxis should be considered in relation to the inherent risk of infection of the procedure under consideration. The standard approach to estimating the risk of infection in the site of surgery is the classification endorsed by the Centers for Disease Control and Prevention (CDC) (Table 38-3).[36] Expected infection rates range from less than 1% in clean wounds with antibiotic prophylaxis to 6% to 10% in dirty wounds, even with antibiotic treatment.[37]

Clean wounds in neurosurgery are generally subdivided into those with and without implantation of a substantial foreign body. The prototypical neurosurgical foreign body is the shunt. Clean shunt implantations utilizing antibiotic prophylaxis have approximately an 8% to 10% infection rate, a rate much higher than non–foreign body operations.[38]

The use of antibiotics in contaminated and dirty wounds is considered therapeutic, not prophylactic. A full therapeutic course is recommended. Limiting antibiotics to perioperative use in these wound categories would be considered misuse.

Clean and Clean-Contaminated Neurosurgical Procedures

The value of systemic antibiotic prophylaxis in clean neurosurgical operations is supported by level I evidence from multiple randomized clinical trials and a high-quality meta-analysis.[39] The same is true of systemic antibiotic prophylaxis for shunt operations.[40,41] Additional meta-analyses have supported its value in preventing meningitis after craniotomy[42] and in spine neurosurgery.[43]

The value of systemic antibiotic prophylaxis in clean-contaminated operations has not been adequately studied to allow a confident conclusion to be reached. In this regard, the current accepted practice in transnasal surgery varies from limited perioperative use[44] to use as if the procedure were contaminated (i.e., therapeutic doses for a therapeutic duration).[45]

It is not feasible to study the differential effectiveness of various antibiotics. If one antibiotic reduces the expected infection rate to 1% and another is twice as good (infection rate of 0.5%), a study of over 5000 patients would be required to have a reasonable chance (power of 0.8) of finding that result to be statistically significant ($P \leq .05$). While the duration of prophylactic antibiotic administration in neurosurgery has not been specifically studied in a randomized trial, the general principles of systemic prophylactic antibiotic administration are well established in many disciplines.[36] These principles are as follows[46]:

- Use an antibiotic directed at the most common organisms implicated in postoperative infection for the specific operation in the institution in which the operation takes place.
- Administer the antibiotic intravenously timed so that a bactericidal level is obtained at the time of incision.
- Repeat the antibiotic dose at intervals so that bactericidal serum levels are maintained during the operation.
- Do not continue the antibiotic more than a few hours after the end of the operation.
- Vancomycin should be avoided unless no other antibiotic meets the above criteria.

The value of systemic antibiotic prophylaxis in reducing the rate of infection after neurosurgical operations is well established with evidence of the highest quality. Failure to use antibiotics in this way requires justification with evidence of similar quality.

External Ventricular Drains

There is insufficient evidence to support a firm conclusion about the value of systemic antibiotic prophylaxis in reducing infections associated with external ventricular drains.[47] A prospective, randomized trial conducted by Pople and colleagues comparing the

TABLE 38-3 Classification of Surgical Site Infection

Wound Class	Description	Examples
Clean	Uninflamed, uncontaminated, no trauma or infection, primarily closed with no break in sterile technique	Craniotomy for tumor Microlumbar diskectomy
Clean-contaminated	Entry into alimentary, respiratory, or genitourinary tract under controlled circumstances; no contamination; minor break in sterile technique	Transnasal hypophysectomy
Contaminated	Nonpurulent inflammation, recent trauma, gastrointestinal tract contamination, major break in sterile technique	Depressed skull fracture with overlying laceration Dropped bone flap
Dirty	Purulent inflammation, perforated viscus, fecal contamination, trauma with devitalized tissue, foreign bodies or other gross contamination	Open depressed skull fracture with in-driven foreign bodies Epidural abscess Brain abscess

Data from Mangram AJ, Horan TC, Pearson ML, et al. Guideline for Prevention of Surgical Site Infection, 1999. Centers for Disease Control and Prevention (CDC) Hospital Infection Control Practices Advisory Committee. *Am J Infect Control.* 1999;27:97-132.

infection rate with the use of antibiotic-impregnated catheters to that with standard catheters showed that there was no significant reduction in the infection rate (2.5% in antibiotic-impregnated and 2.8% in standard catheters).[48] Similarly, Mikhaylov and coworkers[49] and Wright and associates[50] retrospectively reviewed the incidence of catheter-associated infection.

Meta-analyses by Thomas and colleagues[51] and Sonabend and associates[52] demonstrated that the use of prophylactic antibiotics and antibiotic-impregnated ventricular drains had a protective effect and decreased the number of infections, with a statistically significant reduction in catheter-associated infections. This was supported in an observational study by Harrop and colleagues wherein the incidence of infection was decreased after implementation of antibiotic-impregnated catheters.[53] This is an area in which further study could be useful.

Cerebrospinal Fluid Fistula

A Cochrane Systematic Review has examined the value of systemic antibiotic prophylaxis for preventing meningitis in patients with basilar skull fracture and confirmed the long-held view that the practice is ineffective.[54]

Prophylaxis in Spine Surgery

In 2012 the CDC guidelines for prophylactic antibiotic use in spine surgery were reviewed and new recommendations were made after reviewing published meta-analyses and systematic reviews. A grade B recommendation (fair evidence, level II or III studies) was given to the use of prophylactic antibiotics preoperatively for reduction of infection in patients undergoing spine surgery. For instrumented spine surgery, a grade C recommendation (poor-quality evidence, level IV or V studies) was given.[55] Current practice is to administer a single dose of cefazolin based on weight.[56] No antibiotic has demonstrated superiority over other agents for prophylactic use.[57] In cases of complex spine surgery or when there are associated patient comorbidities, the addition of gram-negative coverage, topical intrawound application of vancomycin or gentamicin,[43] and the redosing of antibiotics are advisable. Redosing can be done every 3 to 4 hours to maintain therapeutic levels during the procedure. There is no recommendation as to the duration of prophylactic antibiotic treatment after spine surgery, and therefore no scientific reason to deviate from the CDC guidelines. General practice is to discontinue administration after 24 hours, although no statistical significance was seen in a study comparing 48 hours of prophylaxis to 72 hours.[58]

Topical Antibiotic Prophylaxis

The topical use of antibiotics during neurosurgical procedures to prevent postoperative infection has a long history, but has not been studied with sufficient rigor to produce a definitive conclusion about its effectiveness. Two reviews have been published.[59,60]

When they first became available, antibiotics were sprinkled into the wound in powdered form. In 1947, Pennybacker and colleagues reported a reduction in infection rates to modern levels (0.9%),[61] but a large review of practice at Massachusetts General Hospital in 1966 did not confirm this benefit.[62] Similarly, Sweet and associates showed a decrease in the rate of deep wound infections with the addition of 1 g of vancomycin.[63] However, this finding was not supported by a prospective randomized trial by Molinari and coworkers, in which there was no statistically significant reduction in wound infection with concomitant use of vancomycin powder in the surgical wound.[64]

The principles of topical antibiotic prophylaxis are similar to those for systemic antibiotic prophylaxis: the antibiotic(s) should be active against the most likely infecting organisms in the institution in which they are used, and bactericidal concentrations with minimal toxicity should be used.[65]

The issue of toxicity requires special considerations for topical administration. The tendency of penicillin to produce seizures when applied to the cerebral cortex is well known, and therefore topical penicillins should be avoided.[66] Limited study of the effect of topical application on the cerebral cortex suggests that bacitracin and metronidazole have the lowest likelihood of producing epileptiform activity.[67] pH is likely to be an important parameter, and topical solutions applied directly to the nervous system should be adjusted to physiologic pH where possible.

Cerebrospinal Fluid Shunts

Topical antibiotic prophylaxis is commonly used during CSF shunt procedures in two ways: (1) irrigation of the wound and filling the shunt with antibiotic solution, and (2) the use of antibiotic-impregnated shunt catheters. The topical use of solutions has the same quality of evidence as it does in other neurosurgical procedures (see earlier). Reviews of the prevention of CSF shunt infection have examined the evidence regarding antibiotic-impregnated shunt catheters and concluded that the evidence did support their effectiveness in reducing shunt infection rates.[40,68,69] In a meta-analysis of 14 studies, of which one was a controlled cohort, one a randomized controlled trial, and all but one having level III data, Klimo and associates found that seven studies showed antibiotic-impregnated catheters to be protective and seven showed no statistical benefit.[70] Overall, shunt-related infection was 2.63 times more likely using standard catheters than antibiotic-impregnated catheters, but when the studies were analyzed according to their institutional statistics, the heterogeneity was reduced to nonsignificant levels.[70] However, there is concern of a shift of causative agents with antibiotic-impregnated catheters.

ANTIBIOTIC TREATMENT

Regarding the treatment of common neurosurgical infections, a review of the literature reveals a lack of properly designed randomized controlled studies evaluating the different treatment regimens. Therefore, the majority of the evidence regarding the effectiveness of the different antibiotic therapies is classified as only level III evidence. The recommendations come from the experiences of individuals and groups who have found success in the way they manage a certain infection.

Soft Tissue Infections

Initial treatment of soft tissue infections in most cases should be directed against staphylococci and streptococci. Oral antibiotic therapy with a semisynthetic penicillin, a first-generation cephalosporin, clindamycin, or erythromycin should be considered.[71] If methicillin-resistant *Staphylococcus aureus* (MRSA) is suspected, then vancomycin should be used until cultures prove otherwise. The duration of antimicrobial therapy is dictated by how the infection responds and typically should continue for 7 to 10 days.

Necrotizing Soft Tissue Infections

Because of the polymicrobial nature of necrotizing soft tissue infections, empirical treatment with broad-spectrum antibiotics is often initiated. A number of different regimens may be used to achieve broad-spectrum coverage. The most common patterns include the following[72]:

1. Penicillin or ampicillin plus anaerobic coverage (clindamycin or metronidazole)

2. Vancomycin plus anaerobic coverage and gram-negative coverage (an aminoglycoside or aztreonam or third-generation cephalosporin)
3. Ampicillin-sulbactam with additional gram-negative coverage
4. Imipenem with additional coverage

The most common antibiotic prescribing error is inadequate coverage of *Enterococcus*, which optimally requires ampicillin or vancomycin plus an aminoglycoside.[72]

Meningitis

Meningitis is a medical emergency and carries a high mortality rate. Delay in initiating treatment is associated with increased risk for death.[73] Three general requirements of antimicrobial therapy for bacterial meningitis include (1) use of bactericidal drug(s) effective against the offending organism, (2) use of drugs that have good CSF penetration, and (3) structuring the regimen to optimize bactericidal efficacy based on the pharmacodynamics of the antibiotics chosen.

Empirical antibiotic treatment should be initiated in patients with suspected bacterial meningitis. This should be directed at the most likely bacteria based on age of patient and host factors.[74] It must cover both gram-positive and gram-negative organisms (*Klebsiella pneumoniae* and *Pseudomonas aeruginosa*)[74] (Table 38-4). Appropriate therapy, pending CSF culture results, is vancomycin (15 to 20 mg/kg intravenously every 8 to 12 hours, not exceeding 2 g per dose or a total daily dose of 60 mg/kg; vancomycin serum trough levels should be 15 to 20 μg/mL) plus ceftazidime (2 g intravenously every 8 hours) *or* cefepime (2 g intravenously every 8 hours) *or* meropenem (2 g intravenously every 8 hours).[74]

Empirical therapy should continue in all patients with clinical and laboratory features suggestive of postoperative meningitis, with discontinuation at 48 to 72 hours if the CSF cultures are negative.[74] Aseptic meningitis is defined by a negative CSF culture on the third day. Intravenous antibiotic therapy should be aimed at a presumed pathogen if the Gram stain is diagnostic. If a gram-positive organism is seen in a patient with head trauma after a neurosurgical procedure, with a neurosurgical device, or with a CSF leak, *S. aureus* and coagulase-negative staphylococci are more common and therapy with vancomycin is warranted. If a gram-negative bacillus is isolated, ceftazidime, cefepime, or meropenem is warranted because *P. aeruginosa* and *Acinetobacter* species are more common. For *Acinetobacter*, meropenem is a better choice because there are reports of resistance to cephalosporins.[74]

Unfortunately, there have been reports of the emergence of resistant gram-negative bacilli (resistant *Enterobacter*[75-78] and *Acinetobacter*[79-81] species) that have plasmid-encoded or inducible chromosomal β-lactamases that hydrolyze extended-spectrum cephalosporins.[82] In these cases, amikacin can be added, although this does not always prevent the development of resistance, as Chow and coworkers have described in their study.[83] Therefore, for β-lactamase–producing Enterobacteriaceae or *Acinetobacter* species, an extended-spectrum carbapenem such as meropenem may be employed because these organisms tend to be resistant to multiple antibiotics. Moreover, Parodi and colleagues have reported good clinical and microbiologic responses with carbapenems for *Enterobacter* meningitis.[84] However, this antibiotic must be used judiciously because carbapenem-resistant *Enterobacter* strains have been reported.[85] For resistant *Acinetobacter* meningitis, Nguyen and colleagues demonstrated that intravenous imipenem and amikacin with or without intrathecal amikacin could be used successfully with the caveat that all patients must have their ventriculostomy catheters removed as part of the treatment.[80] Although their study had a small number of cases, Rodriguez Guardado and coworkers demonstrated that intravenous and intrathecal colistin is an option and is as safe and effective as carbapenems in the treatment of nosocomial meningitis caused by *Acinetobacter*.[86] Furthermore, a review by Falagas and associates documented that therapy with intraventricular and intrathecal polymyxins alone or in combination with systemic antimicrobial agents is effective against gram-negative meningitis.[87]

As mentioned previously, gram-negative bacilli have the potential to develop resistance to β-lactam antibiotics; therefore, CSF needs to be sampled at regular intervals to ensure that it is being sterilized. When the response to systemic antibiotic treatment is poor during treatment of gram-negative meningitis, the use of intraventricular antibiotics in combination with intravenous antibiotics should be considered early. The most commonly

TABLE 38-4 Recommendations for Empirical Antimicrobial Therapy for Purulent Meningitis Based on Patient Age and Specific Predisposing Condition (A-III)

Predisposing Factor	Common Bacterial Pathogens	Antimicrobial Therapy
Age		
<1 mo	*Streptococcus agalactiae, Escherichia coli, Listeria monocytogenes, Klebsiella* species	Ampicillin plus cefotaxime or ampicillin plus an aminoglycoside
1-23 mo	*Streptococcus pneumoniae, Neisseria meningitidis, S. agalactiae, Haemophilus influenzae, E. coli*	Vancomycin plus a third-generation cephalosporin*,†
2-50 yr	*N. meningitidis, S. pneumoniae*	Vancomycin plus a third-generation cephalosporin*,†
>50 yr	*S. pneumoniae, N. meningitidis, L. monocytogenes,* aerobic gram-negative bacilli	Vancomycin plus ampicillin plus a third-generation cephalosporin*,†
Head trauma		
Basilar skull fracture	*S. pneumoniae, H. influenzae,* group A β-hemolytic streptococci	Vancomycin plus a third-generation cephalosporin*
Penetrating trauma	*Staphylococcus aureus,* coagulase-negative staphylococci (especially *Staphylococcus epidermidis*), aerobic gram-negative bacilli (including *Pseudomonas aeruginosa*)	Vancomycin plus either cefepime, ceftazidime, or meropenem
Postneurosurgery	Aerobic gram-negative bacilli (including *P. aeruginosa*), *S. aureus,* coagulase-negative staphylococci (especially *S. epidermidis*)	Vancomycin plus either cefepime, ceftazidime, or meropenem
Cerebrospinal fluid shunt	Coagulase-negative staphylococci (especially *S. epidermidis*), *S. aureus,* aerobic gram-negative bacilli (including *P. aeruginosa*), *Propionibacterium acnes*	Vancomycin plus cefepime,‡ vancomycin plus ceftazidime,‡ or vancomycin plus meropenem‡

Modified from Tunkel AR, Hartman BJ, Kaplan SL, et al. Practice guidelines for the management of bacterial meningitis. *Clin Infect Dis.* 2004;39:1267-1284.
*Ceftriaxone or cefotaxime.
†Some experts would add rifampin if dexamethasone is also given.
‡In infants and children, vancomycin alone is reasonable unless Gram stains reveal the presence of gram-negative bacilli.

used intraventricular agents include gentamicin, amikacin, and polymyxin E (colistin) (Table 38-5).[82,88]

As results from cultures are confirmed for susceptibility, the antibiotic treatment should be adjusted accordingly. Practice guidelines for pathogen-specific antimicrobial therapy of bacterial meningitis have been published by the Infectious Diseases Society of America[89] along with recommended dosages (Tables 38-6 and 38-7). The length of treatment is most often 2 weeks after cultures have been negative when treating gram-negative bacilli.[90,91] Other authors have recommended a treatment duration between 2 and 4 weeks.[82,92,93] When treating *S. aureus*, 2 weeks of treatment is reasonable. However, the duration of therapy should always be individualized based on the patient's clinical response to treatment.

Adjuvant Therapy with Dexamethasone

Because of the increased release of inflammatory factors associated with lysis of bacterial cell walls, as well as the induction of an inflammatory reaction by live pneumococci, the use of an antiinflammatory agent is justified. Agents such as dexamethasone (0.15 mg/kg every 6 hours for 2 to 4 days) and methylprednisolone should inhibit the cyclooxygenase pathway of arachidonic acid. If the organism is not *Streptococcus pneumoniae*, the medication should be discontinued.[74]

TABLE 38-5. Recommended Dosages of Antimicrobial Agents Administered by the Intraventricular Route (A-III)

Antimicrobial Agent	Daily Intraventricular Dose (mg)
Vancomycin	5-20*
Gentamicin	1-8†
Tobramycin	5-20
Amikacin	5-50‡
Polymyxin B	5§
Colistin	10
Quinupristin/dalfopristin	2-5
Teicoplanin	5-40‖

Modified from Tunkel AR, Hartman BJ, Kaplan SL, et al. Practice guidelines for the management of bacterial meningitis. *Clin Infect Dis.* 2004;39:1267-1284.

NOTE: There are no specific data that define the exact dose of an antimicrobial agent that should be administered by the intraventricular route. Virtually all intrathecal use of antibiotics is considered "off label."

*Most studies have used a 10- or 20-mg dose.

†Usual daily dose is 1 to 2 mg for infants and children and 4 to 8 mg for adults.

‡The usual daily intraventricular dose is 30 mg.

§Dosage in children is 2 mg daily.

‖Dosage of 5 to 10 mg every 48 to 72 hours.

TABLE 38-6 Recommendations for Specific Antimicrobial Therapy in Bacterial Meningitis Based on Isolated Pathogen and Susceptibility Testing

Microorganism, Susceptibility	Standard Therapy	Alternative Therapies
Streptococcus pneumoniae		
Penicillin MIC		
<0.1 μg/mL	Penicillin G or ampicillin	Third-generation cephalosporin,* chloramphenicol
0.1-1.0 μg/mL†	Third-generation cephalosporin*	Cefepime (B-II), meropenem (B-II)
≥2.0 μg/mL	Vancomycin plus a third-generation cephalosporin*,‡	Third-generation cephalosporin* plus fluoroquinolone§ (B-II)
Cefotaxime or ceftriaxone MIC ≥1.0 μg/mL	Vancomycin plus a third-generation cephalosporin*,‡	Fluoroquinolone§ (B-II)
Neisseria meningitidis		
Penicillin MIC		
<0.1 μg/mL	Penicillin G or ampicillin	Third-generation cephalosporin,* chloramphenicol
0.1-1.0 μg/mL	Third-generation cephalosporin*	Chloramphenicol, fluoroquinolone, meropenem
Listeria monocytogenes	Ampicillin or penicillin G‖	Trimethoprim-sulfamethoxazole (B-III)
Streptococcus agalactiae	Ampicillin or penicillin G‖	Third-generation cephalosporin* (B-III)
Escherichia coli and other Enterobacteriaceae**	Third-generation cephalosporin (A-II)	Aztreonam, fluoroquinolone, meropenem, trimethoprim-sulfamethoxazole, ampicillin
*Pseudomonas aeruginosa***	Cefepime‖ or ceftazidime‖ (A-II)	Aztreonam,‖ ciprofloxacin,‖ meropenem‖
Haemophilus influenzae		
β-Lactamase negative	Ampicillin	Third-generation cephalosporin,* cefepime, chloramphenicol, fluoroquinolone, aztreonam
β-Lactamase positive	Third-generation cephalosporin (A-I)	Cefepime (A-I), chloramphenicol, fluoroquinolone, aztreonam
Staphylococcus aureus		
Methicillin susceptible	Nafcillin or oxacillin	Vancomycin, meropenem (B-III), linezolid, daptomycin
Methicillin resistant	Vancomycin¶	Trimethoprim-sulfamethoxazole, linezolid (B-III), daptomycin
Staphylococcus epidermidis	Vancomycin¶	Linezolid (B-III)
Enterococcus species		
Ampicillin susceptible	Ampicillin plus gentamicin	—
Ampicillin resistant	Vancomycin plus gentamicin	—
Ampicillin and vancomycin resistant	Linezolid (B-III)	—

Modified from Tunkel AR, Hartman BJ, Kaplan SL, et al. Practice guidelines for the management of bacterial meningitis. *Clin Infect Dis.* 2004;39:1267-1284.

MIC, minimum inhibitory concentration.

NOTE: All recommendations are grade A-III (Infectious Diseases Society of America–U.S. Public Health Service grading system), unless otherwise indicated.

*Ceftriaxone or cefotaxime.

†Ceftriaxone/cefotaxime-susceptible isolates.

‡Consider addition of rifampin if the MIC of ceftriaxone is greater than 2 μg/mL.

§Gatifloxacin or moxifloxacin.

‖Addition of an aminoglycoside should be considered.

¶Consider addition of rifampin.

**Choice of a specific antimicrobial agent must be guided by in vitro susceptibility test results.

TABLE 38-7 Recommended Dosages of Antimicrobial Therapy in Patients with Bacterial Meningitis (A-III)

Antimicrobial Agent	Total Daily Dose (Dosing Interval in Hours)			
	Neonates 0-7 Days Old*	Neonates 8-28 Days Old*	Infants and Children	Adults
Amikacin†	15-20 mg/kg (12)	30 mg/kg (8)	20-30 mg/kg (8)	15 mg/kg (8)
Ampicillin	150 mg/kg (8)	200 mg/kg (6-8)	300 mg/kg (6)	12 g (4)
Aztreonam	—	—	—	6-8 g (6-8)
Cefepime	—	—	150 mg/kg (8)	6 g (8)
Cefotaxime	100-150 mg/kg (8-12)	150-200 mg/kg (6-8)	225-300 mg/kg (6-8)	8-12 g (4-6)
Ceftazidime	100-150 mg/kg (8-12)	150 mg/kg (8)	150 mg/kg (8)	6 g (8)
Ceftriaxone	—	—	80-100 mg/kg (12-24)	4 g (12-24)
Chloramphenicol	25 mg/kg (24)	50 mg/kg (12-24)	75-100 mg/kg (6)	4-6 g (6)‡
Ciprofloxacin	—	—	—	800-1200 mg (8-12)
Gatifloxacin	—	—	—	400 mg (24)§
Gentamicin†	5 mg/kg (12)	7.5 mg/kg (8)	7.5 mg/kg (8)	5 mg/kg (8)
Meropenem	—	—	120 mg/kg (8)	6 g (8)
Moxifloxacin	—	—	—	400 mg (24)§
Nafcillin	75 mg/kg (8-12)	100-150 mg/kg (6-8)	200 mg/kg (6)	9-12 g (4)
Oxacillin	75 mg/kg (8-12)	150-200 mg/kg (6-8)	200 mg/kg (6)	9-12 g (4)
Penicillin G	0.15 mU/kg (8-12)	0.2 mU/kg (6-8)	0.3 mU/kg (4-6)	24 mU (4)
Rifampin	—	10-20 mg/kg (12)	10-20 mg/kg (12-24)‖	600 mg (24)
Tobramycin†	5 mg/kg (12)	7.5 mg/kg (8)	7.5 mg/kg (8)	5 mg/kg (8)
TMP-SMZ¶	—	—	10-20 mg/kg (6-12)	10-20 mg/kg (6-12)
Vancomycin**	20-30 mg/kg (8-12)	30-45 mg/kg (6-8)	60 mg/kg (6)	30-45 mg/kg (8-12)

Modified from Tunkel AR, Hartman BJ, Kaplan SL, et al. Practice guidelines for the management of bacterial meningitis. *Clin Infect Dis.* 2004;39:1267-1284.
TMP-SMZ, trimethoprim-sulfamethoxazole.
*Smaller doses and longer intervals of administration may be advisable for very low-birth-weight neonates (<2000 g).
†Need to monitor peak and trough serum concentrations.
‡Higher dose recommended for patients with pneumococcal meningitis.
§No data on optimal dosage needed in patients with bacterial meningitis.
‖Maximum daily dose of 600 mg.
¶Dosage based on trimethoprim component.
**Maintain serum trough concentrations of 15 to 20 μg/mL.

Empyema

Subdural empyema is a surgical emergency. Antibiotics alone do not reliably sterilize the empyema; therefore, surgical intervention is necessary in order to obtain cultures to guide the antibiotic treatment and to decompress the site if there is increased intracranial pressure or spinal cord compression. There have been reports of conservative management with antibiotic therapy alone; however, the circumstances in which conservative management is effective are when the infection is small and in a supratentorial location and there are no neurological findings.[94,95]

The antibiotic treatment plan should be geared toward the pathogen that was isolated in the culture. If there is suspicion of *S. aureus* as the causative agent, empirical therapy with vancomycin should begin, with a change to nafcillin if cultures are found to contain methicillin-sensitive *S. aureus* (MSSA). For an infection caused by a gram-negative bacillus, a third-generation cephalosporin (such as cefepime or ceftazidime) or a carbapenem (e.g., meropenem) is an appropriate choice for treatment. If an anaerobe is suspected, metronidazole is recommended; however, it is not needed if meropenem has been started. Given the difficulty in culturing anaerobes, anaerobic coverage should be maintained even if another organism is cultured.

In children with a subdural empyema, if the organism is unknown, oxacillin plus ceftriaxone plus metronidazole is an appropriate combination.[96] Other centers have used a combination of cefotaxime, amoxicillin, and metronidazole or linezolid with acceptable results.[97,98]

Although there are no current guidelines for duration of treatment, it is generally recommended that intravenous administration last for 3 to 4 weeks, with continuation of oral antibiotics depending on the specific patient.[95] Other practices recommend 6 weeks of intravenous therapy followed by 4 to 6 weeks of oral therapy.[94]

TABLE 38-8 Empirical Treatment for Bacterial Brain Abscess

Predisposing Factor	Antimicrobial Therapy
Otitis media or mastoiditis	Metronidazole plus third-generation cephalosporin*
Sinusitis	Metronidazole plus third-generation cephalosporin*,†
Dental infection	Penicillin plus metronidazole
Penetrating trauma or postneurosurgery	Vancomycin plus third-generation cephalosporin*,‡
Bacterial endocarditis	Vancomycin plus gentamicin
Congenital heart disease	Third-generation cephalosporin*
Undetermined	Vancomycin plus metronidazole plus third-generation cephalosporin*

Modified from Tunkel A. Brain abscess. In: Mandell G, Bennett J, Dolin R, eds. *Principles and Practice of Infectious Diseases.* 7th ed. Philadelphia: Churchill Livingstone; 2010:1265-1278.
*Ceftriaxone or cefotaxime.
†Add vancomycin if methicillin-resistant *Staphylococcus aureus.*
‡If *Pseudomonas aeruginosa,* use ceftazidime or cefepime.

Brain Abscess

Although there are no current practice guidelines for the treatment of brain abscesses, surgery is recommended for lesions greater than 2.5 cm in diameter.[99-101] For lesions less than 2.5 cm, the largest lesion should be aspirated and the fluid sent for culture. Other practices include recommending solely antibiotic therapy but only if the lesion is less than 2.5 cm in diameter, there are no signs of increased intracranial pressure, and the source of infection has been isolated.[99-104] Empirical antibiotic therapy should be initiated according to the patient's predisposing condition, the presumed pathogen, and the frequency of isolation of certain organisms (Table 38-8).[105]

New antibiotics have been reported as being effective in the treatment of brain abscess. Third-generation cephalosporins (cefotaxime, ceftriaxone, ceftizoxime, and ceftazidime) have shown good treatment results; cefotaxime has the highest CSF penetration. In cases of resistant pathogens, the carbapenems (imipenem and meropenem) have shown appropriate intra-abscess penetration. Imipenem is less favorable because of an increased risk for seizures. When there is uncertainty as to pathogenesis, the empirical regimen should include vancomycin, metronidazole, and a third-generation cephalosporin.[100,102,106,107] In posttraumatic and postsurgical abscesses, empirical therapy should account for the possible presence of staphylococci and gram-negative rods.[100] *Proteus*, *Escherichia coli*, and *Serratia* species, which are common causes of cerebral abscesses in neonates, should be covered with a combination of cefotaxime and gentamicin or amikacin. As cultures and sensitivities are reported, the antibiotic regimen should be tailored accordingly.

When there is isolation of *Streptococcus milleri* from the brain abscess, high-dose penicillin G is the antibiotic of choice; alternatives include a third-generation cephalosporin (cefotaxime or ceftriaxone).[95] Anaerobic organisms (except *Bacteroides fragilis*) also respond to penicillin G. In cases of isolation of *B. fragilis*, metronidazole should be added to the regimen in addition to a third-generation cephalosporin. An *S. aureus* regimen should include vancomycin, subsequently changed to nafcillin if MSSA is cultured. Some practices include vancomycin in their empirical regimen because of the high incidence of MRSA organisms. There are no studies that compare the duration of antibiotic treatment.

Ventriculitis

The initial antibiotic regimen should include broad-spectrum coverage for possible resistant gram-positive and gram-negative organisms. Appropriate antibiotic therapy may include vancomycin plus a cephalosporin with antipseudomonal coverage, such as cefepime or ceftazidime. Alternatively, vancomycin can be combined with meropenem to achieve similar coverage. The use of intraventricular vancomycin has also been reported to be successful in the treatment of ventriculitis caused by *Staphylococcus* and *Enterococcus* species.[108,109]

Intravenous polymyxin E (colistin) may be an option for gram-negative organisms, such as *Acinetobacter* and *Pseudomonas*, that are resistant to first-line antibacterial treatments.[110] Case reports have also documenting the success of intrathecal colistin in the treatment of resistant *Acinetobacter* ventriculitis.[111-113]

Shunt Infections

No randomized control trial has been conducted to determine the appropriate antibiotic regimen for shunt infection. Several factors that need consideration in the treatment of shunt infections include removal of hardware, the selection of antibiotic therapy, need for intrathecal use of antibiotics, duration of antibiotic therapy, and duration of treatment.

Current recommendations for treatment of shunt infections are based on guidelines for management of bacterial meningitis.[114] Initial antibiotic selection should be broad spectrum and include coverage for MRSA and *Staphylococcus epidermidis* along with coverage for resistant gram-negative organisms such as *Pseudomonas* species, which have a propensity to adhere to foreign material.[115] Empirical antibiotic therapy should consist of vancomycin to cover gram-positive organisms along with a cephalosporin with antipseudomonal activity, such as cefepime or ceftazidime.[116-118] Rifampin can also be added for gram-positive shunt infections that fail to clear on vancomycin monotherapy.[115] Intrathecal administration of vancomycin or aminoglycosides may need to be initiated for shunt infections that are difficult to eradicate and fail to clear by systemic therapy.[115] The British Society for Antimicrobial Chemotherapy has recommended that, after shunt externalization, intraventricular vancomycin (20 mg/day) be administered in combination with intravenous or oral rifampicin.[119] Gentamicin is another agent that has been commonly used intrathecally (1 to 2 mg/day in infants and 4 to 8 mg/day in adults), in combination with an intravenous agent such as a β-lactam, to treat infections caused by a gram-negative organism. The appropriate dosage is determined by the inhibitory quotient. This is calculated by the trough CSF concentration divided by the minimum inhibitory concentration, and it should exceed 10 to 20. It is noted that the trough value is obtained 24 hours after administration of the antibiotic dose and before the next dose.

For the treatment of *Propionibacterium acnes*, small studies have documented success with intravenous penicillin combined with shunt externalization and replacement.[120] An alternative treatment of gram-positive shunt infections is with intravenous linezolid, which has been demonstrated to be successful in case reports.[121,122] Linezolid possesses many attractive features that may increase its use, such as excellent CSF penetration and broad-spectrum activity. Additionally, Cruciani and colleagues demonstrated that intraventricular administration of teicoplanin was effective in seven patients with staphylococcal neurosurgical shunt infections.[123]

Infection with Spinal Instrumentation

Despite a moderate infection rate of 2% to 20% after spinal instrumentation,[124] there are no current guidelines for treatment of deep wound infections in the setting of spinal instrumentation. Current practice is to preserve the spinal instrumentation, although the presence of a biofilm surrounding the instrumentation and the duration of infection play critical roles in determining the need for removal of the hardware.[124-127]

Empirical antibiotic therapy should be directed against staphylococcal species along with gram-negative organisms. Initial treatment with vancomycin and a third-generation cephalosporin until culture and susceptibility results become available is appropriate. When there is débridement with implant retention, the treatment must include antibiotics with good efficacy against adherent bacteria, such as rifampicin and the fluoroquinolones.[126]

The duration of antibiotic therapy for postoperative infection following spinal instrumentation is still debated. Kowalski and associates recommended an initial 4- to 6-week course of intravenous therapy followed by up to 1 year of oral therapy in difficult-to-eradicate infections.[128] Other authors recommend shorter courses of oral therapy (6 to 12 weeks).[126,129-131]

Vertebral Osteomyelitis and Diskitis

Diagnosis and management of vertebral osteomyelitis and diskitis are very similar and therefore are discussed together in this section. Needle aspiration biopsy is generally not recommended when there is a clinical diagnosis that correlates with radiologic findings and there is a positive blood culture.[132] However, a biopsy is recommended when blood cultures are negative or when there is concern that the blood pathogen may differ from the findings of needle aspiration.[133,134] If the initial biopsy does not reveal a pathogen, empirical treatment should be started against common bacterial agents, taking into consideration that false-negative cultures are frequent when antibiotics have been started before obtaining a culture. If no improvement is noted, open surgical biopsy is recommended. Other practices recommend open biopsy before antibiotic treatment if initial cultures are negative.[133,134]

If the organism found is MSSA, recommended treatment is with nafcillin or oxacillin (1.5 to 2 g intravenously every 4 hours);

if the organism is MRSA, recommended treatment is with vancomycin (15 to 20 mg/kg every 8 to 12 hours). If the pathogen is *Streptococcus* that is sensitive to penicillin, the recommendation is treatment with either ceftriaxone (1 to 2 g intravenously every 24 hours) or penicillin G (12 to 18 million U/day by continuous infusion in outpatients or in six divided doses daily for inpatients). If there is intermediate or full resistance to penicillin, an expert in infectious diseases should be consulted. For gram-negative bacilli, either a third-generation cephalosporin (ceftriaxone 1 to 2 g intravenously daily or ceftazidime 2 g intravenously every 8 hours or cefotaxime 2 g every 6 hours), or a fourth-generation cephalosporin (cefepime 2 g intravenously every 12 hours), or a fluoroquinolone (ciprofloxacin 400 mg intravenously every 12 hours) is an appropriate option.[134]

Previous studies have recommended that antibiotics be administered for a minimum of 6 to 12 weeks.[135-137] Gasbarrini and colleagues have recommended that a minimum of 6 weeks of intravenous antibiotics be administered followed by 6 weeks of oral antibiotics.[138] For tuberculous vertebral osteomyelitis, the current standard of practice is to initiate isoniazid and rifampin for a 6- to 9-month period.[139] Nussbaum and coworkers have recommended that the course of treatment be at least 12 months in duration and consist of at least two antituberculous drugs.[140]

Osteomyelitis of the Skull

Initial antibiotic therapy should be directed against staphylococci with vancomycin plus a third-generation cephalosporin to cover gram-negative bacilli. If there is a concern for the presence of anaerobes, metronidazole should be initiated. Once the culture and susceptibility results become available, the antibiotic therapy can be modified. Intravenous antibiotic treatment should be continued for at least 4 weeks and possibly be followed by an additional oral course of antibiotics.[141]

SURGICAL CARE IMPROVEMENT PROJECT MEASURES

Surgical Care Improvement Project (SCIP) measures were introduced in 2006 with the goal of reducing surgical postoperative infection rates. There are currently three measures that pertain to antibiotic use in surgical interventions: prophylactic antibiotic received within 1 hour prior to incision, prophylactic antibiotic selection for surgical patients, and prophylactic antibiotics discontinued within 24 hours after surgery end time. Also included in the measures is appropriate hair removal for surgical patients.

There is grade A-I evidence to support the recommendation to administer antibiotic prophylaxis in all three measures.[142-146] A study by Cataife and colleagues, in which SCIP compliance rates were evaluated in 295 hospital groups, showed that those hospitals with higher compliance rates had significant lower surgical site infection rates when compared with those with lower compliance rates.[142] However, the timing of stopping the use of antibiotics did not have an impact in the reduction of infection rates. These findings were also supported by a retrospective study in which the infections rates were analyzed after the implementation of SCIP guidelines in colorectal surgery.[147] Guidelines from the CDC recommend that no hair should be removed because there is no associated statistically significant surgical site infection rate reduction,[148,149] and several studies have confirmed this finding.[150,151]

CONCLUSION

Antibiotics are essential to modern neurosurgical practice. Like all drugs, they have important risks and their misuse can lead to serious problems for individual patients. Irresponsible use by the profession can even lead to public health concerns. Judicious use and adherence to basic principles of appropriate usage optimize their value in the treatment of neurosurgical patients. Basic principles include the following:

1. Antibiotics should be used only for the prevention or treatment of susceptible infections.
2. The choice of antibiotic should be guided by the most likely infecting organisms and directed by culture results whenever possible.
3. Antibiotics should be used for their shortest effective duration.
4. The risks associated with antibiotic administration must be considered every time they are used.
5. Dose and frequency of administration should be guided by principles of pharmacokinetics and, in serious infections, measured antibiotic levels.

Failure to follow established basic principles can lead to antibiotic misuse that can range from ineffective (using an antibiotic in a way that it cannot work) to harmful (superinfection with an organism resistant to all known drugs). The following is a list of a few such misuses of antibiotics in neurosurgery:

- *Intraventricular administration of chloramphenicol*
  - It penetrates the BBB very well.
  - It requires hydrolysis in the liver to be active.
- *Routine use of vancomycin for prophylaxis*
  - Most infections are not caused by MRSA.
  - Vancomycin penetration into the CSF is variable and frequently poor in the absence of inflammation.
  - Indiscriminant prophylactic use contributes to the emergence of vancomycin resistance, which threatens to become a major public health problem because alternative antibiotics for vancomycin-resistant organisms are not widely available.
- *Assuming that good CSF penetration in the presence of meningeal inflammation is equivalent to good penetration of the CNS in the absence of inflammation*
- *It can't hurt*
  - See the toxicities and interactions listed in Tables 38-1 and 38-2.
- *More is better*
  - Excessive use leads to selecting resistant organisms, which makes treatment more difficult.
  - Superinfections (e.g., *Clostridium difficile*) hurt patients.

Adherence to basic principles and appropriate consultation with specialists in infectious diseases can optimize the use of antibiotics in neurosurgical practice.

SUGGESTED READINGS

Arlotti M, Grossi P, Pea F, et al. Consensus document on controversial issues for the treatment of infections of the central nervous system: bacterial brain abscesses. *Int J Infect Dis*. 2010;14(suppl 4):S79-S92.

Berenguer CM, Ochsner MG Jr, Lord SA, et al. Improving surgical site infections: using National Surgical Quality Improvement Program data to institute Surgical Care Improvement Project protocols in improving surgical outcomes. *J Am Coll Surg*. 2010;210(5):737-741, 741-743.

Cataife G, Weinberg DA, Wong HH, et al. The effect of Surgical Care Improvement Project (SCIP) compliance on surgical site infections (SSI). *Med Care*. 2014;52(2 suppl 1):S66-S73.

Harrop JS, Sharan AD, Ratliff J, et al. Impact of a standardized protocol and antibiotic-impregnated catheters on ventriculostomy infection rates in cerebrovascular patients. *Neurosurgery*. 2010;67(1):187-191, discussion 191.

Hawn MT, Richman JS, Vick CC, et al. Timing of surgical antibiotic prophylaxis and the risk of surgical site infection. *JAMA Surg*. 2013;148(7):649-657.

Hendaus MA. Subdural empyema in children. *Glob J Health Sci*. 2013;5(6): 54-59.

Mikhaylov Y, Wilson TJ, Rajajee V, et al. Efficacy of antibiotic-impregnated external ventricular drains in reducing ventriculostomy-associated infections. *J Clin Neurosci*. 2014;21(5):765-768.

Miksić NG. Spinal infections with and without hardware: the viewpoint of an infectious disease specialist. *Eur J Orthop Surg Traumatol*. 2013; 23(suppl 1):S21-S28.

Sarmast AH, Showkat HI, Bhat AR, et al. Analysis and management of brain abscess; a ten year hospital based study. *Turk Neurosurg*. 2012;22(6):682-689.

Zimmerli W. Clinical practice. Vertebral osteomyelitis. *N Engl J Med*. 2010;362(11):1022-1029.

See a full reference list on ExpertConsult.com

39 Brain Abscess

Allan R. Tunkel, H. Richard Winn, and W. Michael Scheld

This chapter comprehensively reviews brain abscess, cranial subdural empyema, and cranial epidural abscess. For each entity, we outline the epidemiology and pathogenesis, etiology, clinical findings and diagnosis, and management.

BRAIN ABSCESS

Epidemiology and Pathogenesis

Brain abscess is defined as a focal intracranial infection that is initiated as an area of cerebritis and evolves into a collection of pus surrounded by a vascularized capsule. In later series, the incidence has ranged from 0.4 to 0.9 cases per 100,000 population, with rates increased in immunocompromised patients. Organisms can reach the central nervous system (CNS) by spread from a contiguous source of infection (25% to 50% of cases), hematogenous dissemination (20% to 35% of cases), or trauma; brain abscess is cryptogenic in about 10% to 35% of patients.

Etiology

The probable infecting pathogen in patients with brain abscess depends on the pathogenesis of the infection and the presence of various predisposing conditions. The most common bacterial causes are streptococci (aerobic, anaerobic, and microaerophilic), which are isolated in up to 70% of cases. Multiple organisms are cultured in 14% to 28% of those patients with positive culture results. The incidence of negative culture results has ranged from 0% to 43%; previous use of antimicrobial therapy may account for such results. Brain abscess caused by *Nocardia* species may occur as part of a disseminated infection in patients with cutaneous or pulmonary disease; most have defects in cell-mediated immunity such as corticosteroid therapy, organ transplantation, human immunodeficiency virus (HIV) infection, or neoplasia. *Mycobacterium tuberculosis* has increasingly been observed to cause brain abscess, with cases reported in patients with HIV infection and solid organ transplantation, although tuberculous brain abscesses can be seen in both immunocompromised and immunocompetent patients. The incidence of fungal brain abscess has been rising as a result of the increased use of corticosteroid therapy, broad-spectrum antimicrobial therapy, and immunosuppressive agents.

CLINICAL FINDINGS AND DIAGNOSIS

The clinical manifestations of brain abscess may run the gamut from indolent to fulminant; most are related to the size and location of the space-occupying lesion within the brain and the virulence of the infecting organism. The classic clinical triad—fever, headache, and focal neurological deficits—is seen in less than 50% of patients. The specific neurological findings in brain abscess are also defined by location within the CNS.

Magnetic resonance imaging (MRI) is the diagnostic neuroimaging procedure of choice in patients with brain abscess; on diffusion-weighted images, restricted diffusion may be seen and may distinguish abscesses from necrotic neoplasms. A major advance in neuroimaging is the ability to perform stereotactic MRI- or CT-guided aspiration to facilitate microbiologic diagnosis. At the time of aspiration, specimens should be sent for Gram stain, routine aerobic and anaerobic culture, modified acid-fast smears, acid-fast smears and culture, and fungal smears and culture.

MANAGEMENT

The initial approach to management of a patient with a suspected brain abscess is a multidisciplinary one that involves a neuroradiologist, neurosurgeon, and infectious disease specialist. After aspiration of abscess material and submission of specimens for special stains, histopathologic examination, and culture, empirical antimicrobial therapy should be initiated on the basis of stains of the aspirated specimen and the probable pathogenesis of infection. The combination of metronidazole and a third-generation cephalosporin is commonly used in patients with bacterial brain abscess; in patients in whom *Staphylococcus aureus* is also considered a probable pathogen, vancomycin is added pending identification of the organism and in vitro susceptibility testing. In patients with no clear predisposing factors, administration of vancomycin, metronidazole, and a third- or fourth-generation cephalosporin is reasonable. In patients in whom infection due to *Nocardia* is suspected (e.g., after organ transplantation), trimethoprim-sulfamethoxazole or sulfadiazine should be added. If *Aspergillus* infection is suspected, voriconazole is recommended.

Once the infecting pathogen is isolated, antimicrobial therapy can be modified for optimal treatment; however, because of the pathogenesis of infection, some bacteria may be isolated as part of a mixed infection. Surgical therapy is often required (either bur-hole aspiration or complete excision after craniotomy) for the optimal approach to patients with bacterial brain abscess, although certain groups of patients may be treated with medical therapy alone; such groups include those with medical conditions that increase the risk associated with surgery, those with multiple abscesses, those with abscesses in a deep or dominant location, those who have coexisting meningitis or ependymitis, those in whom early reduction of the abscess with clinical improvement occurs after antimicrobial therapy, and those in whom abscess size is less than 2.5 cm to 3 cm. Patients with fungal brain abscess, especially those who are immunocompromised, have a high mortality rate despite combined medical and surgical therapy; especially in those with mold infections of the CNS, the approach to management must include early diagnosis, administration of antifungal therapy, neurosurgical assessment and intervention, and management of immunologic impairment.

CRANIAL SUBDURAL EMPYEMA AND EPIDURAL ABSCESS

Epidemiology and Etiology

Cranial subdural empyema refers to a collection of pus in the space between the dura and the arachnoid; the most common predisposing conditions are otorhinologic infections. The etiologic agents in patients with cranial subdural empyema include aerobic streptococci, staphylococci, aerobic gram-negative bacilli, and anaerobic streptococci and other anaerobes. *Cranial epidural abscess* refers to a localized collection of pus between the dura mater and overlying skull; the pathogenesis and bacterial etiology

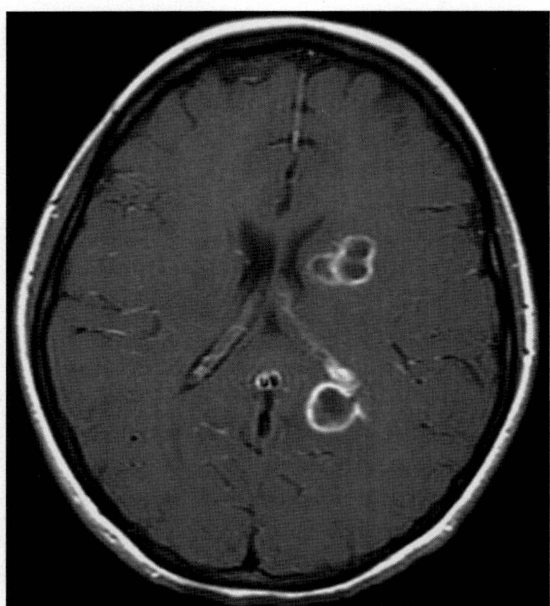

Axial contrast-enhanced T1-weighted magnetic resonance image demonstrating two rim-enhancing masses of the left periventricular white matter that represent abscesses. The intraventricular enhancement is suggestive of ventriculitis. *(Courtesy of Stanley Lu, MD, Monmouth Medical Center, Long Branch, NJ.)*

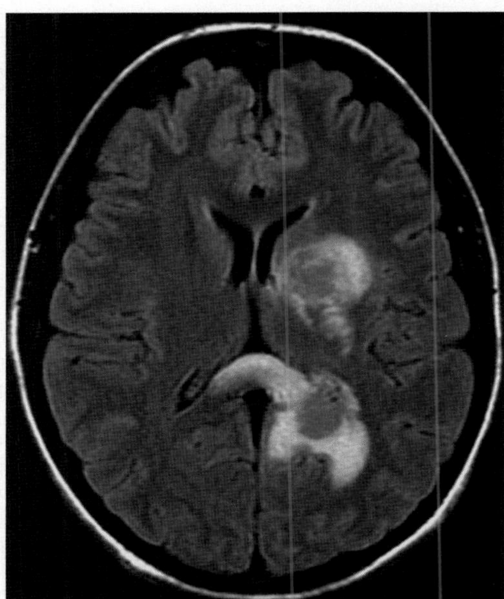

Axial fluid-attenuated inversion recovery (FLAIR) image of the patient in the previous figure demonstrating vasogenic edema surrounding each lesion. *(Courtesy of Stanley Lu, MD, Monmouth Medical Center, Long Branch, NJ.)*

are usually identical to those described for cranial subdural empyema.

Clinical Findings and Diagnosis

The clinical presentation in patients with cranial subdural empyema may be rapidly progressive, with symptoms and signs related to increased intracranial pressure, meningeal irritation, or focal cortical inflammation. The clinical manifestations of cranial epidural abscess may be insidious and are usually overshadowed by the primary focus of infection; the findings are generally insidious because the dura is closely apposed to the inner surface of the cranium such that the abscess usually enlarges too slowly to produce the sudden onset of major neurological deficits seen in patients with cranial subdural empyema.

MRI, the diagnostic imaging procedure of choice, usually demonstrates a crescentic or elliptical area of hypointensity below the cranial vault or adjacent to the falx cerebri; MRI is superior to CT because it provides better clarity of morphologic detail and may detect the presence of a subdural empyema that is not seen on CT. MRI is also the diagnostic imaging procedure of choice in patients with cranial epidural abscess; it usually demonstrates a superficial, circumscribed area of diminished intensity with pachymeningeal enhancement.

Management

Cranial subdural empyema is a surgical emergency because antimicrobial therapy alone does not reliably sterilize the empyema. The goals of surgical therapy are to achieve adequate decompression of the brain and to evacuate the empyema completely. In a large series of patients in which the efficacy of drainage after CT-guided bur holes was compared with craniectomy or craniotomy drainage, mortality rates were higher in patients treated by only drainage via bur holes (23.3%) than in those who underwent craniectomy (11.5%) or craniotomy (8.4%); patients who underwent drainage via bur holes or craniectomy required more frequent operations to drain recurrent or remaining pus and exhibited higher mortality rates and worse outcomes. Regardless of the method of drainage, once purulent material is aspirated, initial antimicrobial therapy should be based on the results of Gram staining and the pathogenesis of the infection. Management of cranial epidural abscess also requires a combined medical and surgical approach; for surgical drainage, craniotomy or craniectomy is generally preferred over bur-hole placement or aspiration of purulent material through the scalp.

Full text of this chapter is available online at ExpertConsult.com

40 Meningitis and Encephalitis

Sherise D. Ferguson and Ian E. McCutcheon

Meningitis is inflammation of the meninges. It can be caused by a variety of microbial entities, including but not limited to bacteria, viruses, and fungi. Even in the era of advanced antibiotics and available vaccinations, meningitis remains a serious disease that continues to impose significant morbidity and mortality. *Encephalitis* is inflammation of the brain parenchyma, predominantly the result of viral pathogens; bacterial encephalitis also occurs, but at a lower incidence. This chapter, which can be found in full on ExpertConsult.com, focuses on the epidemiology, pathogenesis, and treatment of meningitis and encephalitis.

Both community-acquired and nosocomial forms of bacterial meningitis are discussed. Community-acquired meningitis is a serious cause of infectious mortality and morbidity worldwide. The epidemiology, presentation, and complications of meningitis from typical pathogens are explored here in detail. Pyogenic infections of the meninges originate either by hematogenous spread of bacteria or by direct extension from bacterially colonized cranial structures adjacent to the meninges. Although the exact mechanisms governing bacteria-host interaction are not completely understood, the current literature is reviewed in this chapter with a focus on bacterial transgression of the blood-brain barrier. Rapid diagnosis of meningitis is critical for early initiation of appropriate treatment and has a direct effect on patient outcome; hence the salient features of laboratory work-up are also covered. The recommended antibiotic regimens for common pathogens are described as well.

In addition to bacterial and other infections, this chapter covers aseptic meningitis and encephalitis, that is, inflammatory conditions affecting these structures that are not caused by an easily identifiable infectious agent. The multiple infectious etiologies associated with aseptic central nervous system inflammation include viruses, fungi, parasites, protozoa, and *Rickettsia* species. The epidemiology, transmission, clinical features, and treatment of meningitis and encephalitis caused by these entities are presented in detail.

Full text of this chapter is available online at ExpertConsult.com

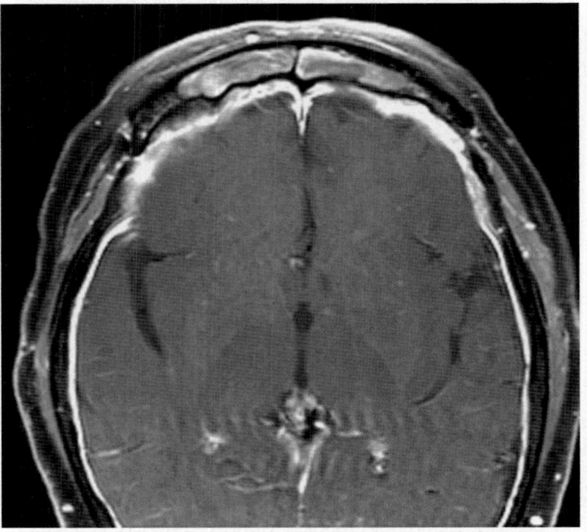

Recurrent meningitis due to persistent cerebrospinal fluid (CSF) leak through skull base. A 53-year-old woman with Cushing's disease underwent subtotal resection through a transbasal approach for tumor resection; a CSF leak developed 1 month later. The leak persisted over the next 9 months, during which time she suffered three separate bouts of meningitis, the first of which was culture-positive for *Streptococcus intermedius*. This axial T1-weighted magnetic resonance image, with contrast administration, was obtained during the third episode. It shows diffuse enhancement over the brain convexities and falx cerebri, a classic finding in active bacterial meningitis. The expanded extracerebral space is consistent with ongoing intracranial hypotension from the loss of CSF. Of note, the frontal sinus shows mucosal thickening and enhancement consistent with paranasal sinusitis. However, there is no breach in the posterior wall allowing direct contact between the sinus cavity and intracranial compartment, so the meningitis must be ascribed to the ongoing CSF leak.

41 Acquired Immunodeficiency Syndrome

M. Kelly Nicholas, John Collins, and Rimas V. Lukas

This chapter is a review of acquired immunodeficiency syndrome (AIDS) with the goal of providing the neurosurgeon with a comprehensive understanding of the human immunodeficiency virus (HIV) and how it relates to the practice of neurosurgery.

AIDS is caused by infection with HIV. HIV can affect the nervous system both directly and indirectly. Both the central nervous system (CNS) and the peripheral nervous system can be directly affected by HIV. Direct infection of the nervous system can manifest as acute retroviral syndrome with symptoms consistent with aseptic meningitis. This manifestation is transient and self-limited. Chronic HIV infection can lead to the development of HIV-associated encephalopathy, a dementing illness. In addition, it can lead to HIV-associated myelopathy. HIV infection is also associated with an increased risk of stroke. Immune reconstitution with highly active antiretroviral therapy (HAART) can lead to an overly robust immune response, the immune reconstitution inflammatory syndrome (IRIS), which can affect the CNS. In the peripheral nervous system, HIV can cause a wide range of neuropathies and myopathy. HAART can also cause neuropathy and myopathy.

HIV may also affect the nervous system indirectly via its effects on the immune system. Patients with HIV infection are at increased risk for a variety of infections and neoplasms that are infrequent in the general population. These include infections of the brain parenchyma or the cerebrospinal fluid by unicellular parasites, such as *Toxoplasma* species; fungi, such as *Cryptococcus* species; mycobacterial species; viruses, such as JC virus and cytomegalovirus; and bacteria, such as *Treponema* and *Bartonella* species. Infected patients are also at much greater risk for the development of CNS lymphoma, which is often associated with concomitant Epstein-Barr virus infection.

Full text of this chapter is available online at ExpertConsult.com

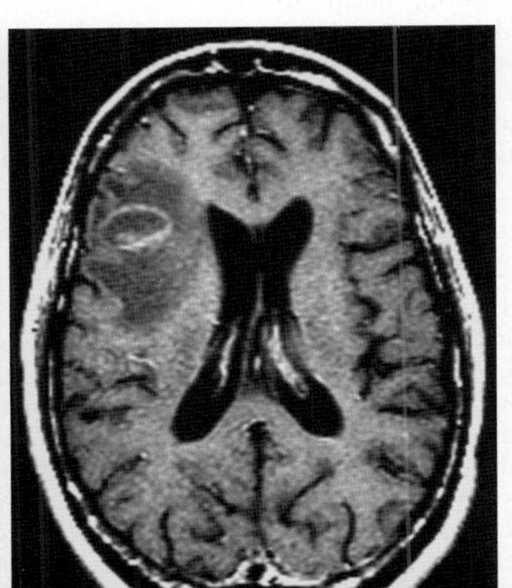
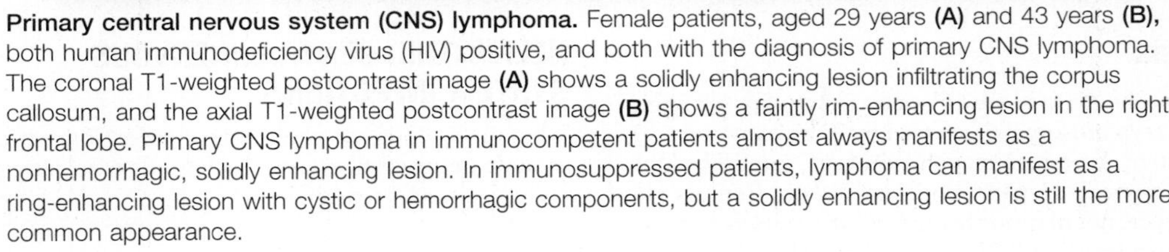

Primary central nervous system (CNS) lymphoma. Female patients, aged 29 years **(A)** and 43 years **(B),** both human immunodeficiency virus (HIV) positive, and both with the diagnosis of primary CNS lymphoma. The coronal T1-weighted postcontrast image **(A)** shows a solidly enhancing lesion infiltrating the corpus callosum, and the axial T1-weighted postcontrast image **(B)** shows a faintly rim-enhancing lesion in the right frontal lobe. Primary CNS lymphoma in immunocompetent patients almost always manifests as a nonhemorrhagic, solidly enhancing lesion. In immunosuppressed patients, lymphoma can manifest as a ring-enhancing lesion with cystic or hemorrhagic components, but a solidly enhancing lesion is still the more common appearance.

42 Parasitic Infections

Oscar H. Del Brutto, Juan J. Figueroa, and Hector H. Garcia

Parasitic diseases of the central nervous system (CNS) affect millions of people in the developing world, where most infections are linked to poverty and related conditions. In addition, increased tourism and immigration have turned some formerly geographically restricted parasitic infections into widespread conditions.

PROTOZOAL CENTRAL NERVOUS SYSTEM INFECTIONS

The most common protozoal infections affecting the CNS include malaria, toxoplasmosis, trypanosomiasis, and amebiasis by free-living ameba or by *Entamoeba histolytica*.

Malaria

Plasmodium infections have a complex biologic cycle in which humans are infected through the skin during a blood meal by a female *Anopheles* mosquito. Cerebral malaria is a major cause of mortality in the world, mostly in Africa. Fever is the initial complaint, followed by progressive somnolence associated with seizures, extensor posturing, and disconjugate gaze. Retinal hemorrhages suggest a poor prognosis. Up to 25% of patients die despite medical care. Permanent sequelae, more common in children, include mental retardation, epilepsy, blindness, and motor deficits.

Toxoplasmosis

After the acquired immunodeficiency syndrome (AIDS) epidemic, toxoplasmosis has become a highly common parasitic disease of the CNS. *Toxoplasma gondii* is a protozoan acquired by the ingestion of contaminated cat feces or by eating undercooked meat. In AIDS patients, CNS toxoplasmosis most often results from reactivation of a dormant infection with *T. gondii*. Immunocompromised hosts may present with an acute encephalitic syndrome or, more frequently, a subacute disease characterized by focal signs associated with seizures and intracranial hypertension. Neurological symptoms rarely develop in immunocompetent hosts, although an acute encephalitic syndrome progressing to coma occurs in some cases.

Trypanosomiasis

There are two different *Trypanosoma* diseases in humans: sleeping sickness or African trypanosomiasis, caused by *Trypanosoma brucei*, and Chagas' disease or American trypanosomiasis, caused by *Trypanosoma cruzi*. In African trypanosomiasis, *T. brucei* enters the human body by direct inoculation through a bite of its vector, the tsetse fly; it then invades the CNS and remains latent for a long time. Thereafter, the disease enters into a stage in which the symptoms (fever, hepatosplenomegaly, and cervical lymphadenopathy) suggest activation of the reticuloendothelial system. Somnolence, apathy, involuntary movements, and rigidity then appear. The neurological manifestations progress to dementia, stupor, coma, and death.

In the case of American trypanosomiasis, triatomine bugs ("kissing bugs"), found mostly in the genus *Triatoma*, are the vector for *T. cruzi*. These insects infect humans by biting them to feed on their blood and defecating in the area. *T. cruzi* parasites in the insect's feces are then exposed to the bite wound or facial mucosae (eyes, mouth), usually by the bitten person when scratching. More rarely, infection can be acquired through uncooked food contaminated with infected bug feces, from blood/organ donation, or congenitally from an infected mother. CNS disease is rare and occurs mostly in immunocompromised individuals. Chronic disease is not usually associated with primary neurological complications; however, cardioembolic brain infarcts develop in some patients as a result of chagasic dilated cardiomyopathy. In addition, immunocompromised patients can experience reactivation of chronic infections, which results in a rapidly fatal meningoencephalitic syndrome similar to that observed in acute infections.

Free-Living Amebae

Free-living amebae may invade the CNS. *Acanthamoeba* spp. and *Balamuthia mandrillaris* affect mainly immunocompromised patients, and they invade the CNS by the hematogenous route from a primary infection of the skin or the respiratory tract. In contrast, *Naegleria fowleri* infection occurs in normal hosts and is acquired during swimming in warm fresh water; the parasites enter through the nasal cavity and migrate through olfactory nerves to the CNS. *Acanthamoeba* spp., *Sappinia pedata*, and *B. mandrillaris* produce a subacute to chronic granulomatous amebic encephalitis characterized by low-grade fever, focal signs, seizures, intracranial hypertension, and behavioral changes, eventually progressing to loss of consciousness, coma, and death. *N. fowleri* causes primary amebic meningoencephalitis, a fulminant disease resembling acute bacterial meningitis that carries a grim prognosis.

Amebiasis by *Entamoeba histolytica*

The intestinal parasite *E. histolytica* normally causes dysenteric diarrhea or liver abscesses. It may invade the CNS from the colon or liver in patients with severe infections (usually in the setting of advanced systemic amebiasis) and produce a multifocal encephalopathy.

HELMINTHIC CENTRAL NERVOUS SYSTEM INFECTIONS

The most common helminthic infections affecting the CNS include neurocysticercosis, hydatid disease, paragonimiasis, schistosomiasis, and toxocariasis.

Cysticercosis

Cysticercosis occurs when humans become intermediate hosts of *Taenia solium* by ingesting its eggs from contaminated food or fecal-oral contamination. CNS invasion is known as neurocysticercosis (NCC). The most common presentation of parenchymal NCC is epilepsy, but many other focal neurological signs have been described. Extraparenchymal NCC presents with intracranial hypertension (frequently associated with obstructive hydrocephalus) or focal neurological deficits.

Echinococcosis (Hydatid Disease)

There are two main forms of echinococcosis: cystic hydatid disease (caused by *Echinococcus granulosus*) and alveolar hydatid disease (caused by *Echinococcus multilocularis*). In both cases humans acquire the infection by accidental ingestion of *Echinococcus* eggs. After entering the body, the eggs transform into cysts that grow in the liver, lungs, heart, and CNS.

Cystic hydatid disease results in seizures or increased intracranial pressure of subacute onset, often in association with focal neurological deficits. Orbital involvement is manifested as proptosis and ophthalmoplegia. In alveolar hydatid disease *(Echinococcus multilocularis)*, neurological manifestations (focal neurological deficits, seizures, and intracranial hypertension) progress more rapidly and are more severe than with cystic hydatid disease. Spinal cord involvement is more common in cystic hydatid disease than in alveolar hydatid disease, but it may be observed in both.

Paragonimiasis

Humans acquire the infection by ingesting metacercariae of flukes of the genus *Paragonimus* in undercooked crustaceans. Metacercariae liberate larvae, which cross the intestinal wall and migrate to the lungs, where they mature into adult worms. Erratic migration of worms along the jugular veins and carotid arteries or hematogenous dissemination of larvae results in CNS involvement. Most patients have acute meningitis that may or may not be associated with focal neurological signs as a result of cerebral infarction secondary to arteritis. Other patients with parenchymal brain granulomas have seizures, focal neurological deficits, and intracranial hypertension. Cerebral hemorrhages may occur along tracks of larval migration or as a result of the necrotizing vasculitis that occurs during granuloma formation. Spinal paragonimiasis is associated with radicular pain, weakness, and sensory disturbances.

Schistosomiasis (*Schistosoma mansoni, haematobium,* and *japonicum*)

Schistosomiasis, or infection with the flukes *S. mansoni*, *S. haematobium*, or *S. japonicum*, affects approximately 200 million individuals, mostly in sub-Saharan Africa. CNS infection is a rare complication caused by embolization of eggs or adult worms to the brain or spinal cord microcirculation. CNS symptoms reflect multifocal inflammatory granulomatous lesions and include seizures, focal neurological deficits, mass effect, or diffuse encephalitis. Nodular, ring-enhancing intraparenchymal lesions are seen on computed tomography or magnetic resonance imaging. Occasionally, *S. mansoni* eggs in the medulla may cause progressive transverse myelitis as a result of granulomatous lesions.

Toxocariasis (*Toxocara canis* and *cati*)

Toxocariasis is a cosmopolitan nematode infection caused by *T. canis* or *T. cati*. Most infected humans are asymptomatic, and human disease is mostly related to complications of larval migration. Larvae originate from the intestine and migrate through the circulatory system. Apparently, symptomatic CNS invasion is infrequent. However, it has been associated with seizures, motor and sensory problems, meningitis, encephalitis, and other neurological syndromes.

Full text of this chapter is available online at ExpertConsult.com

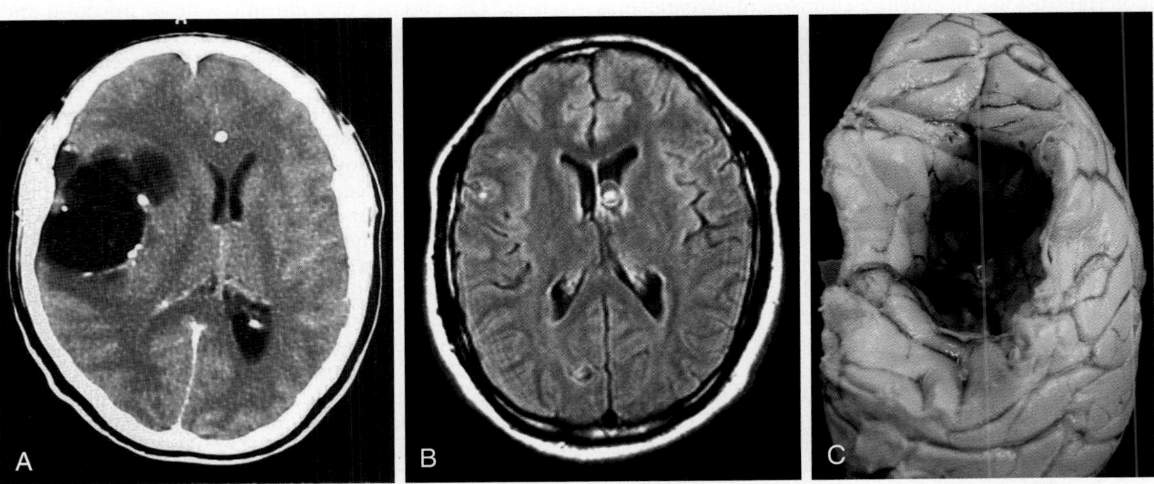

A, "Giant" cysticercal cyst in the right sylvian fissure. **B,** Intraventricular cysticercus. **C,** Brain impression after surgical excision of a hydatid cyst. *(Courtesy of the Neuropathology Museum, Instituto de Ciencias Neurologicas, Lima, Peru.)*

43 Surgical Risk of Transmittable Disease

Donald E. Fry

The first reports of transmission of blood-borne pathogens from patients to surgeons occurred more than 60 years ago.[1,2] These early reports of "serum hepatitis" were generally viewed with a detached attitude by surgeons as reflecting something that occasionally happened, and these events did not arouse concern about occupational risks. With the recognition of hepatitis A virus (HAV) and hepatitis B virus (HBV) as distinct viral pathogens and the development of specific antibody detection methods, the scope of HBV infection among patients and among surgeons was appreciated. Surgeons had a disproportionately higher prevalence of HBV positivity than did the general population, and it was rapidly appreciated that transmission of the infection from patients to surgeons (and other health care workers [HCWs]) was far more common than had been realized. Moreover, a nonserotyped hepatitis was identified, indicating yet another form of transmissible hepatitis that occurred after blood transfusion and other forms of percutaneous blood exposures.[3] This nonserotyped hepatitis was labeled non-A, non-B hepatitis (NANBH).[4] During the 1970s, evidence was mounting that surgeons and other HCWs were exposed to multiple potential hepatitis viruses, but an attitude of indifference persisted with respect to these risks.

In 1981,[5] acquired immunodeficiency syndrome (AIDS) was first reported, and subsequent investigations characterized human immunodeficiency virus (HIV) as the putative agent. HIV infection was associated with sexual contact, but it also became apparent that blood transfusion and other mechanisms of percutaneous exposure from blood contamination were sources of viral transmission. During the 1980s, it became apparent that nearly 1 million people in the United States had HIV infection and that clinical AIDS was a uniformly fatal disease.[6] Furthermore, it became apparent that HIV infection was a latent disease that otherwise healthy-appearing people carried for a number of years before clinical AIDS was evident.[7] It was also recognized that those with latent infections were reservoirs for transmission of the virus to others. Events surrounding the recognition of AIDS led to great concern and anxiety in the surgical profession about the occupational risks for both AIDS and hepatitis infection. Demands for testing of patients before operations surfaced, and denial of care of HIV-infected individuals was feared as part of the aftermath.

More than 30 years have passed since the first AIDS cases were reported, and many events have tempered the great fears that surfaced about the occupational risks for this infection in the 1990s. Occupational transmission has been proved to be very uncommon. The development of highly active antiretroviral therapy (HAART) has not eradicated HIV infection but has provided long-term quality of life for many patients.[8] HAART has dramatically reduced circulating viral loads in infected patients and has reduced further the risks for transmission among those receiving treatment. With respect to hepatitis, a highly effective HBV vaccine has been developed from recombinant technology that has dramatically reduced the risk for occupational HBV infection for surgeons. Although no vaccine has yet been developed for hepatitis C virus (HCV) infection, considerable research effort has resulted in effective treatments for many of these infections.

Unfortunately, these many positive developments have now re-created lassitude and indifference about occupational infection in the operating room. Old bad habits are resurfacing, and accepted principles for prevention are being ignored. The objective of this chapter is to emphasize to neurosurgeons that continued vigilance is necessary because both known and, in all likelihood, unknown transmissible agents remain in the surgical environment. This sense of awareness of both known and unknown risks requires a commitment to avoiding blood exposure when providing neurosurgery care.

HEPATITIS

The past 30 years have yielded a dramatic expansion in our understanding of the world of hepatitis infection. Currently six distinct hepatitis viruses have been identified (Table 43-1). There remains a probability that at least one additional virus will be characterized. At the present time, only HBV and HCV appear to be of great occupational concern to surgeons. Most of the following discussion is limited to HBV and HCV infection.

HAV is transmitted by the fecal-oral route and is usually acquired after ingestion of contaminated water or food products.[9] It is an RNA virus that causes an acute and frequently severe acute hepatitis syndrome. Infected individuals with the hepatitis syndrome (jaundice, malaise) are acutely ill, but the disease is seldom lethal except in elderly and infirmed patients. Importantly, after HAV clinical infection has resolved, there is no state of chronic infection in the aftermath of the acute infection. The absence of a chronic state of infection and the infrequently identified transmission of HAV from blood or blood products do not make this a virus of occupational concern in health care.

Hepatitis E virus had been identified primarily in Southeast Asia but is now identified globally.[10] Like HAV, it is transmitted by the fecal-oral route, and there is no chronic infection after resolution of the acute infection. A vaccine for hepatitis E has been developed but is currently only available in China.[11] Occupational blood exposure is not associated with a risk for HEV infection.

Hepatitis D virus (HDV), also known as the delta agent, is an incomplete RNA virus that cannot cause infection or replicate without the coexistence of concurrent acute or chronic HBV infection.[12] HDV infection is not commonly identified in the United States. It is principally seen among the intravenous drug abuse population. HDV infection amplifies the severity of the underlying HBV infection. HDV is a blood-borne pathogen and theoretically could be an occupational risk for HCWs if preexistent HBV infection were present. Effective vaccination against HBV infection eliminates this risk.

Hepatitis G virus is the most recently identified agent (hepatitis F was putatively identified but has not been validated).[13] It is considered the same as the GB virus, for which the "GB" initials came from the index infected surgeon who was the source of virus used in early studies. It is blood borne and is found commonly with HBV and HCV infection. It has genetic homology to HCV. It is infrequently found as the sole agent in clinical hepatitis infection, and many have challenged its actual role in human hepatitis infection. It is present in as many as 1.4% of blood donors and persists in a chronic state for many years.[14] The full scope of its clinical relevance and occupational transmission risk continues to be debated.

TABLE 43-1 Features of Known Hepatitis Viruses as Currently Identified

Type of Hepatitis	Route of Genome	Viral Family	Transmission	Occupational Risk
A	RNA	Picornaviridae	Fecal-oral	No chronic infection; no risk for occupational infection
B*	DNA	Hepadnaviridae	Blood-borne	More than 1 million chronically infected patients in the United States; documented vaccination eliminates the risk
C*	RNA	Flaviviridae	Blood-borne	About 3-5 million chronically infected patients in the United States; no vaccination; avoiding exposure is the only preventive strategy
D	RNA	Viroid	Blood-borne	Not identified as occupational risk; requires coexistent HBV infection; no risk with HBV vaccination
E	RNA	Caliciviridae	Fecal-oral	No chronic disease; not common in United States; no occupational risk
G	RNA	Flaviviridae	Blood-borne	Commonly called GBV-C; not associated with infection; not considered an occupational risk

GBV-C, GB virus C; HBV, hepatitis B virus.
*Only hepatitis B and hepatitis C are considered occupational pathogens.

Hepatitis B Infection

HBV infection is the most thoroughly studied of the blood-borne hepatitis viruses in humans. HBV is a DNA virus that is very efficiently transmitted with exposure to blood or blood products. Before the era of effective vaccination, HBV infection was the most common and most serious of occupational infections for surgeons. A single hollow percutaneous needlestick injury is associated with a 25% to 30% risk for transmission to the naïve host.[15] Intravenous drug abuse with shared needles has been a major source of transmission of the infection. HBV is a sexually transmitted disease, and a national initiative to vaccinate pediatric and adolescent populations against HBV is underway.[16] Effective screening of the blood supply has virtually eliminated contaminated units of transfused blood as a source of new cases of HBV infection.

Access of the HBV virus to the host results in binding and internalization of the virus within hepatocytes. Viral replication occurs at varying rates after infection. In only about 25% of acute infections is there a clinically discernable hepatitis syndrome.[17] Most cases are either characterized by a mild malaise without jaundice or have a completely indolent character. Among all acute infections, about 5% of cases result in chronic sustained infection that persists indefinitely.[18] The incidence of chronic infection is not related to whether acute infection was identified, meaning that many individuals with chronic disease are unaware of their disease status. This chronic state of infection is associated with sustained damage to the liver, although selected cases may have a persistent viremia without evidence of continued liver damage. Hepatocellular carcinoma, portal hypertension, and end-stage liver disease from hepatic cirrhosis are the consequences for many patients with the chronic disease.[19] The individual with chronic HBV infection is a reservoir for virus that can infect others. It is currently estimated that 1 million people in the United States have chronic HBV infection,[20] with many millions more in the international community infected.[21]

HBV infection among surgeons in the era before the availability of the vaccine was common. In a 1996 study, about one third of surgeons in practice for more than 10 years had serologic evidence of prior HBV infection.[22] About one third had been vaccinated, but one third had no antibody on serology and remained vulnerable to acute infection. In the late 1980s, the Centers for Disease Control and Prevention (CDC) estimated that 250 HCWs died annually from the consequences of occupationally acquired chronic HBV infection that had obviously been contracted many years previously.[23] A current estimate identifies about 200 deaths annually in the United States from occupationally acquired HBV infection.[24]

In the 1980s, a highly effective HBV vaccine was developed using attenuated virus from infected patients.[25] Recombinant technology rapidly emerged and resulted in development of an equally effective vaccine that was not derived from human sources. The vaccine is administered in three doses, with the second and third doses given 1 and 6 months after the initial administration. About 95% of individuals have an appropriate antibody response to the surface antigen of HBV. Documentation of the antibody response is essential, and revaccination is necessary for those who do not seroconvert from the initial immunization effort. Revaccination after a failed initial attempt has a 30% to 50% probability of being successful.[26] Vaccination of all surgeons and HCWs is necessary, and not being vaccinated is unacceptable.

Hepatitis C

HCV was identified in 1989 and has for the most part been the virus responsible for NANBH.[27] HCV is an RNA virus with multiple different serotypes. It is a source of occupational infection for surgeons and HCWs, but is less efficiently transmitted than HBV. A percutaneous needlestick from a hollow needle has about a 2% risk for transmission of the virus.[28] HCV has many of the same epidemiologic characteristics as HBV with respect to high-risk populations of patients and means of infection within society.[29] Screening of the blood supply for antibody to the virus has dramatically reduced the risk for transfusion-associated infection.

The clinical sequelae after infection of the hepatocyte follow similar patterns to HBV. Like HBV, most acute HCV infections are clinically indolent and not associated with a clinical picture of hepatitis.[30] However, unlike HBV, rates of chronic HCV infection are 60% to 80%.[31] The natural history of chronic disease is highly variable, with some patients progressing to end-stage liver disease or hepatocellular carcinoma while others have chronic antigenemia but do not have an evolving pattern of liver damage.[32] Still others may have spontaneous resolution of the infection at a later time. HCV has an unpredictable time course. Individuals who are antigen positive are infectious to others. Three to 5 million people in the United States have chronic HCV infection,[33-35] and HCV has become the leading cause of disease leading to hepatic transplantation.[36,37]

There is no vaccine for HCV, although progress has been made with antiviral treatment for this infection.[38] The HCV infection results in a circulating antibody that is not thought to neutralize the virus. There are multiple different serotypes of the virus, and reinfection can occur with the same viral type in patients who cleared the initial infection. The prospects for a vaccine are challenging when even acute infection does not confer protective immunity for the host against future infection. The antibody response may be delayed up to 6 months after acute infection, which makes HCV detection in the blood supply more difficult among donors with recent acute infection.

HUMAN IMMUNODEFICIENCY VIRUS

HIV is a retrovirus.[39] It is an RNA virus, and as a consequence of the enzyme reverse transcriptase, a complementary DNA (cDNA) is produced from the RNA template after the virus invades the target cell. The incorporation of the viral cDNA into the host cell genome becomes the basis for the synthesis of viral proteins and replication of new viral units. The CD4-positive lymphocyte becomes the major target of the virus, and the lysis and loss of these cells are a fundamental issue in the immunodeficiency state that evolves with subsequent clinical AIDS. The acute infection may be characterized by a modest and nonspecific viral syndrome or by no discernable symptoms. The progression of the natural history of the infection without treatment is 10 years or longer before AIDS emerges.

HIV infection is transmitted by sexual contact and by intravenous drug abuse. Vertical transmission from infected mothers to newborns has been dramatically reduced in frequency in the United States by the use of antepartum antiretroviral therapy.[40] Transmission secondary to blood transfusion has essentially been eliminated with effective screening procedures in the United States and Western Europe. HIV infection remains an international pandemic, especially in the African continent where preventive strategies have been ineffective and treatment of established infection has been unavailable. About 1.1 million people are living with HIV infection in the United States, and this number has continued to increase.[41] About 16% of HIV-infected individuals are unaware of their infection. More than 636,000 have died since the recognition of the disease.[42]

Considerable effort has been extended into the evaluation and prevention of occupational HIV infection among HCWs. A serologic survey of more than 3000 orthopedic surgeons at a national meeting identified only two cases of HIV infection, both of which were in individuals with nonoccupational risks for infection.[43] Prospective evaluation of mucous membrane and percutaneous exposure events among HCWs has documented 57 cases of occupational infection (Table 43-2).[44] Transmission is considered a 0.3% risk from a percutaneous exposure among HCWs.[45] Epidemiologic evaluation of HCWs who have developed HIV infection but who do not have nonoccupational risk factors for the disease has resulted in the identification of 143 cases of probable occupational transmission (Table 43-3). At this time, no documented infections have been transmitted from patient to surgeon in the United States from percutaneous exposure events in the operating room. Epidemiologic evaluation has identified six probable infections among surgeons that were identified in the 143 cases mentioned previously. Compared with HBV and HCV, the efficiency of transmission in the health care setting is much less with HIV. Long-term survivors with successful treatment of HIV infections are being seen with greater frequency, although concern about the effects of long term antiretroviral treatments makes the emergence of resistant strains a constant threat. Multiple efforts have been and are currently being attempted to prevent HIV infection with a vaccine. The changing antigenic presentation of the virus from the constant mutation process has made stable antigen targets for vaccine development quite elusive.

TABLE 43-2 Number of Patients with Documented Seroconversion to HIV Following a Specific Exposure Incident*

Occupation	No. of Documented Occupational HIV Infections
Nurses	24
Clinical laboratory workers	16
Physicians, nonsurgical	6
Nonclinical laboratory workers	3
Housekeeping and maintenance workers	2
Surgical technicians	2
Embalmer and morgue technician	1
Health aide or attendant	1
Respiratory therapist	1
Dialysis technician	1
TOTAL	57

HIV, human immunodeficiency virus.
*All patients had a negative serology at the time of the exposure event and then seroconverted to a positive HIV status following the event.

PREVENTION OF OCCUPATIONAL INFECTION

Occupational infection with one of the discussed viruses has been the result of percutaneous or mucous membrane exposure to contaminated blood. Transmission events have generally occurred in the setting of percutaneous exposure to blood when the infectious status of the patient was unknown. Because patients may not be aware of their infectious status and social risk factors for infection are commonly not discovered during the preoperative evaluation of a surgical patient, it is generally recommended that standard preventive measures be employed in the care of all patients. Application of enhanced or relaxed preventive measures based on the surgeon's presumption of patient risk is not dependable and is discouraged. Preventive strategies are grouped into three categories: personal protective barriers, technical considerations, and prompt response to exposure events. Of greatest importance is maintaining vigilance and constant awareness when using sharp instruments in the operating room. Many injuries are due to carelessness and could have been prevented by the surgeon and others in the operating room environment having a keen appreciation of the dangers of avoidable behavior that leads to a percutaneous injury to self or a colleague.

Personal Protective Barriers

Much has been made of the value of using eye shields and in the use of double gloving to prevent blood contact with the skin or mucous membranes of the surgeon. Every surgeon has had the experience of an arterial or irrigation spray in the face during an operation. Protective eye and face shields are available in every

TABLE 43-3 Number of Health Care Personnel Thought to Represent Possible Seroconversions for Occupational HIV Infection*

Occupation	No. of Possible Occupational HIV Infections
Nurses	36
Clinical laboratory workers	17
Health aides or attendants	15
Housekeepers and maintenance workers	14
Nonsurgical physicians	13
Emergency medical technicians	12
Other technicians and therapists	9
Surgical physicians	6
Dental workers and dentists	6
Dialysis technicians	3
Surgical technicians	2
Embalmers and morgue technicians	2
Respiratory therapists	2
Others	6
TOTAL	143

HIV, human immunodeficiency virus.
*These cases were identified from the epidemiologic evaluation of health care workers who reported to Centers for Disease Control and Infection with HIV infection but were determined after case evaluation not to have nonoccupational risk factors for the infection.

operating room and are mandated by the U.S. Occupational and Safety Health Administration.[46] Observations made in many operating rooms give testimony to the lassitude about occupational infection when one sees inadequate or no eye protection being used during operations in which eye exposure is a real risk.

Double gloving has been shown in many studies to prevent blood contact onto the hands of surgeons.[47-49] A recent extensive review of the literature has documented the preponderance of evidence that supports the use of double gloves, especially during operations with anticipated blood loss or with a long duration of surgical time.[50] If the surgeon washes his or her hands with isopropyl alcohol after a lengthy craniotomy or a major spine procedure, all of the stinging around the cuticles and elsewhere will be validation that nonintact skin is present. Sustained blood contact on the hands with nonintact skin means that occupational infection is a potential risk. Double gloving will prevent blood contact, and the use of indicator systems permits prompt recognition when the glove barrier has been breached.[51] It has been argued that double gloving may interfere with the dexterity of the surgeon, but recent data indicate no significant difference in two-point discrimination or dexterity between study subjects with single or double gloves.[52]

In a previous study, 90% of blood contact with the skin of the operating room team occurred on the hands and forearms[53] (Table 43-4). Reinforcement of the forearms with sleeve covers, combined with double gloving that extends above the level of the seam of the glove-cuff of the surgical gown, provides a double ply of protection to the area of the body most vulnerable to blood contact during operations. Use of sleeve covers is most appropriate during operations within the chest or abdomen but certainly is worth consideration during craniotomy for trauma and major spine procedures, in which significant blood loss can be anticipated. Wearing a plastic apron under the surgical gown and trauma boots that cover the feet up to the level of the knee should also be considered when intracranial hematomas are being surgically managed.

Technical Considerations

Safe surgery means a zero tolerance for avoidable behavior that leads to percutaneous injury. Sharp instruments must be handled with respect. Blunt needle technology has been shown to reduce injuries[54] and has been endorsed by the American College of Surgeons[55] and the National Institute for Occupational Safety and Health.[56] A recent comprehensive review of the literature identified considerable evidence to support the use of blunt needles to prevent exposure of the surgical team to blood and body fluids.[57] The use of the surgical "way station" (e.g., Mayo stand) for the passage of loaded needle holders has been a common strategy for the hands-free passage of scalpels and loaded needle holders and will prevent injury to the surgeon and to scrub personnel from direct hand-to-hand exchanges.[58] Use of the electrocautery instead of the scalpel may reduce risks from knife injury. Some have advocated that selected common procedures can be done without any sharp instruments in the surgical field.[59] Others have advocated the use of safety scalpels with retraction devices to reduce percutaneous injuries in the operating room, but these have not been demonstrated to be effective.[60] Towel barriers to cover bony edges of the cranial vault or spicules of bone in spine procedures can minimize inadvertent abrasions, glove tears, and punctures from these structures. Drills, saws, and rongeurs are all part of selected procedures and require attention to avoid injury. Avoiding injury in the operating room is more about attitude than technique.

Response to Exposure

Exposure events will occur. They should be recognized promptly and managed at the opportune moment. Blood contamination of the hand or forearm should ideally be managed by a surgical scrub of the site, but events at the time of the exposure commonly make this impractical. Glove violations or needle punctures at a minimum require removal of the glove, irrigation of the site with povidone iodine or isopropyl alcohol, and then regloving. Eye exposures should be rinsed promptly with sterile saline solution. Blood breakthrough of the surgical gown should result in removal of the gown, irrigation of the exposed skin, and regowning.

When exposure has occurred to a patient with known or suspected infection, a specific course of action is necessary. A current serology for the index viruses needs to be done for the exposed surgeon to document that preexistent disease is not present.[61] Unfortunately, most exposure events occur with patients for whom the serology is not known, and often the surgeon's perception of the risk of the event precludes definitive documentation of preexistent viral infection.

For known HBV exposures the recommendations remain the same as published in 2001 and begin with current knowledge of the antibody status of the exposed surgeon. Prior vaccination with a positive antibody response for the HBV surface antigen means that nothing further needs to be done. If the serology indicates a weak reaction or no antibody response, then a dose of the HBV immunoglobulin and a "booster" dose of the HBV vaccine should be given. If the exposed individual has not had a prior course of full vaccination, then a dose of the HBV immunoglobulin and

TABLE 43-4 Frequency of Blood Contact and Exposure in the Operating Room*

Type of Operation	Total Cases Studied	No. of Blood Contact Cases	Total Personnel with Blood Contact	No. Personnel Blood Exposure
Orthopedic	201	56 (28%)	71	19
Gynecologic	81	24 (30%)	32	8
General surgery	75	19 (25%)	25	7
Otolaryngology	58	10 (17%)	13	1
Pediatric surgery	50	11 (22%)	22	3
Trauma/burn	45	21 (47%)†	37	7
Neurosurgery	43	11 (26%)	16	6
Cardiothoracic	26	15 (58%‡	36	6
Cesarean delivery	25	12 (48%)†	25	5
Others	80	11 (14%)	16	1
TOTAL	684	190 (28%)	293	63

*In a prospective study, a 4-week period of surgical care at the University of New Mexico Hospital was evaluated for the frequency of blood contact with the skin of any member in the operating room, or blood exposure from either a percutaneous or mucous membrane event.[53]

†$P < .05$.

‡$P < .025$.

the HBV vaccine should be administered. It is recommended that the HBV immunoglobulin be administered as soon as possible after the exposure event. The HBV immunoglobulin is 70% to 90% effective if given within 7 days of the exposure event.[62] The exposed surgeon should complete the three-dose regimen of vaccination, which includes the second and third dose 1 and 6 months after the initial administration. If the surgeon is positive for the *core antibody* of HBV, then the surgeon has had prior HBV infection. If this is a new finding for the surgeon, then the presence of the core antigen for HBV needs to be evaluated because the surgeon may have unrecognized chronic infection. With the increased emphasis on HBV vaccination, there should be very few chronic HBV infections discovered after an exposure event in the operating room.

Because there is no vaccine for HCV, the exposed surgeon should have an immediate blood specimen drawn to establish whether prior HCV infection exists. Repeat studies are then done at 1, 3, and 6 months. Serologic studies for the HCV antibody have been the traditional method for identifying infection with HCV; RNA counts are then used to document the infection in those who are seropositive. Many exposed clinicians prefer have HCV RNA testing directly rather than the antibody screening method. No prophylactic HCV antiviral treatment is recommended until evidence of active infection is documented.

There is no vaccine for HIV, but some epidemiologic evidence supports the use of prophylactic antiretroviral therapy for known or suspected exposures.[63] Postexposure prophylaxis is recommended when the source patient is documented to be HIV positive. The treatment should be continued for a full course with three drugs, and serologic evaluation for seroconversion is then completed.[64]

What should be the response to a severe exposure event when preexistent infection of the patient is not suspected? A safe course of action is to request serologic testing of the index patient. Most patients will give permission, especially if they know that the surgeon is also being tested. When serologic information about the index patient is not available, the surgeon may be advised to have appropriate serologic follow-up. Relative to the risk for HIV infection, the surgeon will have to decide whether to receive antiretroviral therapy. Indeed, surgeons engaged in invasive procedures with significant exposure rates to patient blood (e.g., intracranial trauma, spine surgery) and those treating populations of patients who have high prevalence rates of infection (e.g., trauma patients) need to know their serologic status for all viral pathogens of concern and undergo repeated testing on an annual basis.

THE INFECTED SURGEON

A great source of debate during the 1990s was whether surgeons who had contracted one of the blood-borne viral infections should continue to engage in invasive procedures. Some have argued for routine testing of physicians and surgeons and recommend suspension of privileges for those who test positive. Others have pointed to an absence of evidence to demonstrate that infected surgeons are a risk to their patients. The identification of a Florida dentist who apparently transmitted HIV infection to several of his patients, presumably by intention, ignited the controversy.[65,66] Many states passed laws requiring various levels of action against physicians known to harbor HBV or HIV infection. Although the intensity of the debate has receded, many punitive laws about infected surgeons remain.

There are many clusters of HBV infection that have been transmitted from infected surgeons and dentists to patients.[67-69] Since 2007, there have been only two identified transmissions to patients from infected surgeons.[70,71] The common feature for transmission is a surgeon with a high concentration of viral units per milliliter of blood. The e-antigen of HBV has been a marker to identify such surgeons. The e-antigen of HBV is a degradation product of the viral nucleocapsid and is seen in patients with active viral replication in the liver.[72] Because an epitope of the HBV virus has been identified that is not associated with the e-antigen,[73] actual viral counts in blood are considered a better predictor of the risk for transmission to patients. The current threshold for infection risk is more than 1000 International Units (IU)/mL, which is also 5000 Genomic Equivalents (GE)/mL.

The CDC has modified its previous recommendations and now recommends that actual viral thresholds as identified previously be used in evaluation of the chronic HBV-infected surgeon.[74] Surgeons are not considered to pose a risk when their viral concentrations are less than 1000 IU/mL. The CDC recommends a review of surgical practice by institutional expert panels for surgeons who exceed this level in the development of their own policies on this question. Surgeons who test positive for e-antigen and those who exceed the viral concentration threshold should continue to adhere to the recommendations of the American College of Surgeons and have an expert local panel convened to make recommendations about future surgical practice (Table 43-5).[75]

Although many cases of HBV transmission to patients from infected surgeons have been identified, only four surgeons have been associated with transmission of HCV infection to patients.

TABLE 43-5 Key Points for Emphasis from the Statement on the Surgeon and Hepatitis by the American College of Surgeons

Point of Emphasis on Hepatitis Infection	Comment
Surgeons have an ethical obligation to care for patients with HBV or HCV infection.	Hepatitis infection is not covered by the Americans with Disabilities Act. The moral imperative remains while exercising appropriate standards of infection control in the health care setting.
Surgeons should know their HBV and HCV infection status.	Significantly improved antiviral chemotherapy for these infections is currently available. Future additional therapies are being pursed.
Surgeons who test positive for the e-antigen of HBV are a potential risk to their patients.	These surgeons should be evaluated by an expert panel to make recommendations about the prevention of infection to patients.
All surgeons should know their antibody status for HBV infection and should be immunized against HBV infection.	There can be no excuse for not being vaccinated against HBV infection. Documentation of an antibody response to vaccination is important.
HCV-infected surgeons can safely continue to practice surgery.	The surgeon with HCV infection should adhere to all standards of infection control in the care of patients. It is advisable to seek expert advice about currently available treatment for the infection.
All surgeons should seek expert consultation when a documented or suspected exposure event has occurred to a chronic HBV or HCV infected patient.	The surgeon should confer with local experts or call the National Clinicians' Postexposure Prophylaxis Hotline at 1-888-448-4911 or visit their website at http://www.nccc.ucsf.edu/Hotlines/PEPline.

HBV, hepatitis B virus; HCV, hepatitis C virus.

Data from *American College of Surgeons*. Statement on the surgeon and hepatitis. <https://www.facs.org/about-acs/statements/22-hepatitis>; April 1, 2004 Accessed 22.10.15.

The most notable case was from Spain.[76] A cardiac surgeon with high blood viral counts (10^7 viruses/mL) was identified in the transmission of infection to at least five patients. Single surgeon-to-patient transmissions of HCV infection have been reported from a cardiac surgeon from the United Kingdom,[77] and single transmissions have been reported from Germany involving a gynecologist[78] and an orthopedic surgeon.[79] No occupational infection has occurred at this time from a neurosurgeon to a patient.

Surgeons and other physicians have been vectors in the transmission of infection even though they may not be infected with HCV themselves. Several clusters of nosocomial transmission of HCV infection to patients have occurred from contaminated multiple-dose vials,[80,81] contaminated radiopharmaceuticals,[82] unsafe injection practices,[83] reused needles and syringes,[84] and poor hand hygiene.[85]

To date, no occupational transmission of HIV infection has occurred in the United States except for the dental cases noted previously. A single case report from France identifies a potential transmission from an HIV-infected orthopedic surgeon.[86] Studies of patients from the practices of surgeons with HIV infection have not identified evidence of transmission.[87] The position of the American College of Surgeons with respect to the HIV-infected surgeon continues to be a valid one (Table 43-6).[88] It is important for HIV-positive surgeons to know that they have infection so that effective treatment can be given. The attitude of the 1990s, that not knowing was the best recourse, is clearly not valid at this point.

LEGAL ISSUES

It is understandable that issues of transmissible infection passing from surgeons or other HCWs to patients would generate some legal issues. The legal and political issues were triggered by recommendations from the CDC for the prevention of HIV and HBV infection during "exposure-prone invasive procedures."[89] Among these recommendations, the CDC advised that "exposure-prone procedures should be identified by medical/surgical/dental organizations and institutions at which the procedures are performed." Moreover, "HCWs who are infected with HIV or HBV (and are e-antigen positive) should not perform exposure-prone procedures unless they have sought counsel from an expert review panel and been advised under what circumstances, if any, they may continue to perform these procedures. Such circumstances would include notifying prospective patients of the HCW's seropositivity before they undergo exposure-prone invasive procedures." This led to the passage of Public Law 102-141 by the U.S. Congress in October 1991, which required states to implement the CDC recommendations, or their equivalent, as a condition for the receipt of Public Health Service funds. All the states complied, although laws were very different from state to state. Although the furor and passion about this subject have waned, fines and imprisonment remain in the law of many states for surgeons who do not follow the requirements established by the CDC in 1991.

A more serious issue for neurosurgeons and for surgeons in general is the Americans with Disabilities Act (ADA).[90] The ADA was passed in 1990 and prohibits discrimination on the basis of a person's disability, which specifically includes patients with HIV or AIDS. The Act specifically prohibits private providers of public accommodations (dental or medical services) from discrimination based on the defined disability. The Supreme Court of the United States ruled in favor of a lawsuit filed by an HIV-positive patient in 1998 in *Bragdon v. Abbott*.[91] In this case a dentist refused to fill a cavity for the patient in his office but rather chose to do it in the hospital because of concerns about safety from HIV infection. The Court ruled that the patient posed no direct threat to the dentist and that damages were incurred in the discriminatory expense of having the dental work performed at a hospital.

In yet another case, a private neurosurgery group was required to pay $40,000 in monetary compensation and a $10,000 civil penalty to the United States.[92] A neurosurgeon in the group allegedly refused to provide care for an HIV-positive patient who had a back condition. An Assistant Attorney General stated, "The Department of Justice will not stand idly by when doctors refuse medical services, including surgery to people with HIV disease. A discriminatory refusal of medical care is especially egregious where, as here, the refusal affects a population so dependent on the availability of medical services."

The moral of the case law just discussed is that all surgeons must provide standard treatment for HIV patients regardless of

TABLE 43-6 Key Points for Emphasis in the Statement on the Surgeon and HIV Infection from the American College of Surgeons

Point of Emphasis on HIV Infection	Comment
Surgeons have an ethical obligation to give care to HIV patients.	It is not only an obligation, it is the law that you *must* provide care for HIV-infected patients based on the Americans with Disabilities Act.
Contemporary standards of infection control practice should be used in all venues of patient care.	In the era of other nosocomial pathogens that can be transmitted in the course of patient care, infection control practice is essential in all patient contacts.
HIV-infected surgeons may continue to practice with invasive procedures under the provisions that standards of infection control are employed and the surgeon is physically fit to practice.	HIV-infected surgeons, especially when given highly effective antiretroviral chemotherapy, should have privileges to practice in the same context as having diabetes or hypertension. Functional considerations of health should dictate. When there are questions, the surgeon's personal physician or a locally convened group of experts in HIV should provide recommendations about the continuation of surgical practice.
Postexposure prophylaxis with antiretroviral chemotherapy is recommended.	Although the data are not completely convincing, exposure to an HIV-infected patient, or an unusually severe exposure event to a patient of unknown serology, should initiate the triple-drug prophylaxis regimen. Questions can be addressed to the National Clinicians' Postexposure Prophylaxis Hotline at 1-888-448-4911 or at http://nccc.ucsf.edu/clinician-consultation/pep-post-exposure-prophylaxis/.
All surgeons should know their HIV status.	Because effective treatment is available, surgeons should be tested. The attitudes of the early 1990s, when treatment was less effective and restrictions of practice loomed in the background, have passed.
All surgeons and the leadership in U.S. surgery must remain sensitive to the issues of patient safety and workplace risks of HIV infection.	Individual surgeons and the national organizations that represent them should maintain an interest in all developments surrounding HIV, its treatment, and transmission. All should maintain an interest for patient safety.

HIV, human immunodeficiency virus.
Data from *American College of Surgeons*. Statement on the surgeon and HIV infection. <https://www.facs.org/about-acs/statements/13-hiv-infection>; May 1, 2004 Accessed 22.10.15.

TABLE 43-7 Sources of Iatrogenically Transmitted Creutzfeldt-Jakob Disease among 469 Patients

Source of Iatrogenic Disease	No. of Cases	Comment
Surgical procedures:		
Dura mater grafts	228	A total of 123 cases came from Japan.
Surgical instruments	4	Three cases came from the United Kingdom and 1 from France. All had standard sterilization following the index procedure.
Electroencephalogram needles	2	Both cases came from Switzerland.
Corneal transplants	2	One case came from Germany and one from the United States.
Hormone therapy:		
Growth hormone	226	A total of 119 cases came from France, 65 cases from the United Kingdom, and 29 cases from the United States.
Gonadotropin	4	All four cases came from Australia.
Blood transfusion	3	All 3 cases came from the United Kingdom.

From Brown P, Brandel J-P, Sato T, et al. Iatrogenic Creutzfeldt-Jakob disease, final assessment. *Emerg Infect Dis*. 2012;18:901-907.

their own personal attitudes. It is a violation of the ADA to refer HIV patients to another surgeon because of personal feelings about the patient's viral infection. It is important to emphasize that the surgeon's risk for occupational infection is small with appropriate infection control practice and that refusal of care to these patients may have severe consequences.

FUTURE CONSIDERATIONS

It is unlikely that all risks from blood-borne pathogens have been fully described.[93] Additional potential hepatitis viral threats remain.[94] HCV has accounted for only about 80% of the NANBH virus infections.[95] Another hepatitis virus likely exists. The TT virus has been described in Japan,[96] and although its significance as a pathogen to humans is not clear, its presence gives testimony that other undefined viruses are potentially present in the blood of our patients. The SEN virus is yet another novel virus that may be a hepatic pathogen[97] and is transmissible from patient to patient.[98]

New acute viral disease entities have stormed on the clinical scene from all over the world and must be considered a threat. West Nile virus infection has been transmitted by transfusion and must be considered a potential occupational pathogen during the viremic phase of the disease.[99] Severe acute respiratory syndrome (SARS)[100] and the Asian Avian influenza[101] epidemic are examples of acute infections that are not viewed as blood-borne pathogens but must have an asymptomatic viremic phase that may make them transmissible. The efficiency of international travel makes these scenarios plausible.

Perhaps the most intriguing of future issues in blood-borne transmissible disease is prion disease, or "infectious proteins." Transmission from a diseased host to a naïve recipient of the abnormal neuroprotein results in the development of the new variant of Creutzfeldt-Jakob disease (CJD).[102] The abnormal prion particle is only protein and has no DNA or RNA. It is thought to transmit disease by the abnormally folded pathogen protein serving as a template, which results in the normally occurring prion protein assuming the abnormal configuration. The disease has not yet been fully defined, but transmission results in some hosts having the progressive degenerative CJD, whereas others may be chronic asymptomatic carriers of the protein while being "infectious" to others.[103] The major source of iatrogenic transmission has been from dura mater grafts and the administration of growth hormone (Table 43-7).[104,105] Four cases of transmission have occurred from contaminated neurosurgical instruments. Reports of newly recognized cases of iatrogenic transmission of CJD have diminished in number and have been associated with remote exposures. Transmission of CJD from exposure events of the past decade has not been identified. This near elimination of transmissions is likely due to the identification of patients with suspected disease, the use of disposable instruments, quarantine of nondisposable instruments when disease is suspected, and rigorous sterilization procedures of instruments used when disease is confirmed.[106] Clinical[107,108] and experimental[109] evidence implicates transfusion as a means for transmission. Occupational transmission is a potential consideration either from handling infected tissues or from blood exposure from patients with clinical or asymptomatic disease.

In the final analysis, human blood contains many known and unknown transmissible hazards that pose a potential risk to neurosurgeons. It can only be concluded that blood is a potentially toxic substance and that the clinical surgeon must exercise due diligence in the avoidance of blood contact or percutaneous injury in the course of providing surgical care.

SUGGESTED READINGS

Alter HJ. Emerging, re-emerging and submerging infectious threats to the blood supply. *Vox Sang*. 2004;87(suppl 2):S56-S61.

Berguer R, Heller PJ. Preventing sharps injuries in the operating room. *J Am Coll Surg*. 2004;199:462-467.

Brown P, Brandel J-P, Sato T, et al. Iatrogenic Creutzfeldt-Jakob disease, final assessment. *Emerg Infect Dis*. 2012;18:901-907.

Centers for Disease Control and Prevention. *Surveillance of occupationally acquired HIV/AIDS in healthcare personnel, as of December 2010*. <http://www.cdc.gov/HAI/organisms/hiv/Surveillance-Occupationally-Acquired-HIV-AIDS.html>.

Department of Justice. *Neurosurgery group pays $50,000 to settle HIV discrimination claim with Justice Department*. Available at: <http://www.usdoj.gov/opa/pr/2000/December/709cr.htm>.

Esteban JI, Gomez J, Martell M, et al. Transmission of hepatitis C virus by a cardiac surgeon. *N Engl J Med*. 1996;334:555-560.

Fry DE, Harris WE, Kohnke EN, et al. The Influence of Double-Gloving on Manual Dexterity and Tactile Sensation of Surgeons. *J Am College Surg*. 2010;210:325-330.

Harpaz R, von Seidlein L, Averhoff FM, et al. Transmission of hepatitis B virus to multiple patients from a surgeon without evidence of inadequate infection control. *N Engl J Med*. 1996;334:549-554.

Makary MA, Pronovost PJ, Weiss ES, et al. Sharpless surgery: a prospective study of the feasibility of performing operations using non-sharp techniques in an urban, university-based surgical practice. *World J Surg*. 2006;30:1224-1229.

Shapiro CN, Tokars JI, Chamberland ME, American Academy of Orthopaedic Surgeons Serosurvey Study Committee. Use of hepatitis-B vaccine and infection with hepatitis B and C among orthopaedic surgeons. *J Bone Joint Surg Am*. 1996;78:1791-1800.

Thomas JG, Chenoweth CE, Sullivan SE. Iatrogenic Creutzfeldt-Jakob disease via surgical instruments. *J Clin Neurosci*. 2013;20:1207-1212.

U.S. Public Health Service. Updated U.S. Public Health Service guidelines for the management of occupational exposure to HBV, HCV, and HIV and recommendations for postexposure prophylaxis. *MMWR Recomm Rep*. 2001;50(RR–11):1-52.

See a full reference list on ExpertConsult.com

Overview and Future Opportunities

Michel Kliot, Pierre J. Magistretti, Robert M. Friedlander, and Michael M. Haglund

Science is ever evolving. As illustrated in this 7th edition of *Youmans and Winn Neurological Surgery*, the techniques are changing much faster than the questions posed. Although the anatomy of the human brain has not changed since physicians acquired the ability to study it, the ability to visualize pathways, at both gross and microscopic levels, has changed dramatically, as has the ability to probe its depths and treat its pathology. Chapter 1, dealing with the history of neurosurgery, traces the origin of physicians' understanding that action, thought, and perception originate in and are mediated by structures of the nervous system. Chapter 1 also shows how attempts to treat its maladies have been refined over time, from chiseling away at the cranium with crude chisels to using the microscope in combination with navigation systems. In Chapters 2 and 3, the authors discuss how the frontiers of gross and three-dimensional anatomy have been expanded. To paraphrase one of neurosurgery's greatest practitioners, Professor Gazi Yaşargil, the most important thing for a surgeon to learn is "anatomy, anatomy, and anatomy" (personally heard at one of his lectures in Boston in the late 1970s).

As important as neuroanatomy is to the neurosurgeon, the same can be said of the basic and clinical sciences to the neurosurgeon who aspires to be a clinician scientist. In this "Basic and Clinical Sciences" section, Chapters 44 through 57 cover a gamut of topics ranging from molecular biology to neurosurgical epidemiology. Chapter 44 ("Molecular Biology and Genomics: A Primer for Neurosurgeons") presents the basics of molecular biology that underlie current approaches to understanding the biological behavior of tumors at the level of alterations in DNA structure and RNA expression. Chapter 45 ("Optogenetics and Clarity") highlights two new and exciting techniques that are revolutionizing research in the neurosciences. Through the selective introduction of light-activated receptors into the membranes of neurons, optogenetics has made it possible to activate specific populations of neurons in a manner that allows scientists to both create and correct abnormalities that mediate important functions and behaviors. Through the selective removal of lipids from the brain, clarity is allowing scientists to peer into the three-dimensional depths of the brain and create panoramic maps with selective stains and molecular probes. The end result is not only informative but esthetically beautiful.

In Chapter 46 ("Neuroembyology"), the authors describe some of the molecular pathways that underlie the amazingly complex unfolding of the development of the nervous system. Chapter 47 ("Stem Cell Biology") is an exploration of the persistence of embryonic cells in the adult nervous system and their potential role in diseases, such as brain tumors, as well as recovery after injury. Chapter 48 ("Neurons and Neuroglia") is a description of the important roles that neurons and glia play in creating and maintaining the complex circuitry and physiologic functions in the nervous system. In Chapter 49 ("Cellular Mechanisms of Brain Energy Metabolism"), the authors describe the molecular pathways that provide necessary energy for the brain and how imbalances result in impaired function and in extreme cases cell death. In Chapter 50 ("Cellular and Molecular Responses in the Peripheral and Central Nervous Systems: Similarities and Differences"), the authors compare and contrast the responses of the adult central and peripheral nervous systems to injury and how these differences lead to different outcomes.

Chapters 51 ("The Blood-Brain Barrier"), 52 ("Physiology of the Cerebrospinal Fluid and Intracranial Pressure"), 53 ("Cerebral Edema"), and 54 ("Extracellular Fluid Movement and Clearance in the Brain: The Glymphatic System") deal with different aspects of the very important homeostatic mechanisms that maintain and regulate the flow of fluid in the brain and contribute to such important parameters as cerebral blood flow, perfusion pressure, and intracranial pressure. Chapter 55 ("Altered Consciousness") makes the transition from brain anatomy and physiology to human behavior by discussing the different levels of consciousness ranging from being comatose to being alert. Chapter 56 ("Neuropsychological Testing") is a description of the battery of tests that are available both to evaluate patients and to determine the efficacy of treatments. In Chapter 57 ("Neurosurgical Epidemiology and Outcomes Assessment"), the authors describe the tools that neurosurgeons can use to determine the prevalence and incidence of the disorders that they treat, as well as the success or failure of treatments and interventions. Other relevant basic and clinical science topics can be found in portions of some of the more clinical chapters in other sections of this book.

CONTROVERSIES AND UNRESOLVED QUESTIONS

The basic and clinical scientific discoveries and techniques described have increased neurosurgeons' understanding of how the nervous system is constructed, functions normally, functions abnormally when perturbed by disease or trauma, and can potentially be repaired with thoughtful medical and surgical interventions. Larger issues with potentially great therapeutic effects remain to be answered and addressed more fully by discovery in the laboratory and clinic; these issues include the following:

- Methods of protecting the nervous system after traumatic and ischemic injury.
- Methods of reducing the metabolic needs of the nervous system rapidly, especially when it is deprived of its oxygen supply, usually through interruption of blood flow.
- Methods of regulating cellular proliferation and cellular migration to better control or arrest the growth and spread of tumor cells.
- Methods of more selectively targeting and eradicating tumor tissue.
- Methods of enlisting the body's own defenses to combat disease, such as the immune system in eradicating tumors.
- Methods of reducing intracranial pressure to maintain adequate blood flow.
- Methods of better treating altered flow dynamics of cerebrospinal fluid, as in, for example, the setting of hydrocephalus.
- Methods of selectively altering the blood-brain barrier so as to enable the penetration of useful drugs in regions where they may be of benefit.
- More precise methods of manipulating brain tissue by means of robotic techniques.

In terms of understanding how the brain actually works to produce the mind—a primary interest of many physicians who entered this field—a lot remains to be discovered. Currently, neurosurgeons are at a stage analogous to trying to understand light emanating from a light bulb before the discovery of electromagnetic waves. Scientists could study the electricity running through the filament that gives rise to the light that passes through the glass. But it was possible to study light itself only after scientists had an understanding of electromagnetic waves and photons that allowed them to measure and quantify directly light itself. Neurosurgeons' efforts to understand the mind from the brain are currently analogous to trying to understand a recording of a Beethoven symphony by studying the components of a MP3 player. It is hoped that breakthroughs and paradigm shifts in the future will help neurosurgeons understand the mind from the brain at both conceptual and physical levels.

The role of basic and clinical research is vital not only in the education of neurosurgery residents but also in developing and fostering an expectation within them that they can and should contribute to the evolution and advancement of their chosen field and profession. Research is the impetus that drives new discoveries and therapies. The very fact that questions always far outnumber answers keeps neurosurgeons humble and expectant, as well as being a wonderful antidote to boredom and preventing their work from becoming stale and lackadaisical. In addition to providing the very best care available to patients now, research provides hope, both to patient and to physician, that one day currently intractable medical problems will become more manageable and treatable. Research should nourish the intellect and spirit of neurosurgeons, irrespective of the status of their training or their site of practice, while simultaneously motivating self-improvement. It also provides hope to counteract the devastating consequences when disease overcomes the best therapeutic efforts. Research is a precious endeavor that needs to be nurtured and promoted, especially in times when clinical efforts are measured more in terms of relative value units than in terms of patients' well-being and physicians' professional fulfillment.

44 Molecular Biology and Genomics: A Primer for Neurosurgeons

Kevin Y. Miyashiro and James H. Eberwine

The central nervous system (CNS) is arrayed as a series of precisely positioned, functional microcircuits that rely on a vast catalog of gene products to be spatially and temporally deployed to specific subcellular domains. Understanding the concerted action of combinatorial gene sets expressed by discrete sets of cells and, increasingly, by single cells continues to be one of the most enduring fundamental challenges in contemporary neuroscience. By building on the technical foundations of pioneering molecular biology work now decades past, new breakthroughs in today's "omics" techniques are transforming the landscape of CNS research. The filtering of three innovative concepts of the Human Genome Project—decreased assay cost, miniaturization of assays, and the development of highly parallel assays assessing targets on a large scale—into other techniques, namely genome-wide association studies and molecular fingerprints assessing RNA abundance, have spurred the widespread adoption of these "omics" technologies. With more recent methodologic advances in genome editing with CRISPR, transcriptomics with RNA sequencing (RNA-Seq), and proteomics with new top-down approaches, we foster, more than ever, rich and detailed depictions of our understanding of the molecular mechanisms underlying cellular function. Here, we review the historical foundations of molecular biology, its formative influence on our current knowledge of the CNS, and an abridged survey of cutting edge techniques available for the neuroscientist's toolbox.

Full text of this chapter is available online at ExpertConsult.com 

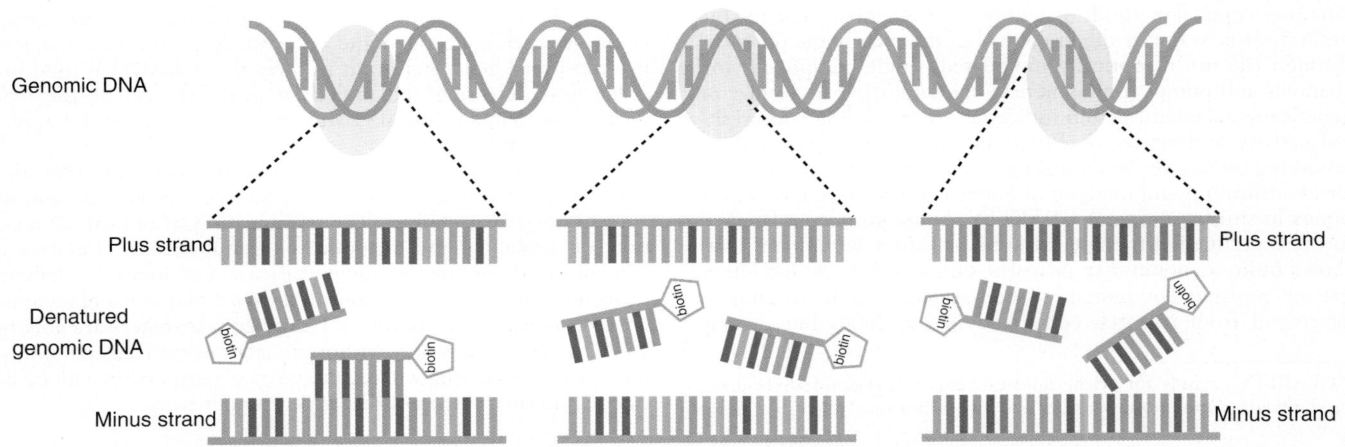

The basic tools of molecular biology are based on molecular hybridization. A cartoon schematic of molecular hybridization shows the basic principle in practice illustrated with a portion of genomic DNA. When genomic DNA is transferred to a solid-phase support such as nylon or nitrocellulose in a Southern blot, the DNA is denatured so that labeled probes may hybridize to the single-stranded genomic DNA sequence. We highlight three representative areas of the genomic DNA, each having a different sequence. The length of these sequences, as well as the probes, is not drawn to scale, and they would contain many more base pairs than depicted. A probe, labeled here with biotin, that has nucleotide complementarity to genomic sequence will bind with specificity.

45 Optogenetics and CLARITY*

Lief E. Fenno, Brian Hsueh, David Purger, and Paul S.A. Kalanithi†

In the 18th century, Luigi Galvani demonstrated that electricity was the central currency of neural activity, through a series of insightful experiments in which he used frog muscle. This finding was rapidly adapted to diagnostic evaluation in the clinic. By the early 20th century, electrode recordings defined patterns of neural activity in both health and disease (e.g., epileptiform and interictal abnormalities on the electroencephalogram). The integration of a current source made electrodes capable of altering neural function. However, after more than a century, the resolution of electrical recording and stimulation of the central nervous system remains limited, to a similar extent as in these early experiments; specifically, it is still not possible to identify or target prespecified populations at the single neuron level.

To address these shortcomings, the development of new tools and techniques has enabled unprecedented insight into the workings of the nervous system through the ability to optically control and assess neural activity in healthy and diseased specimens at the intact, whole-brain level with subcellular resolution. As a result, clinical, governmental, and business organizations are interested in applying new results and further expanding neuroscience knowledge. Some of these novel approaches may be put to therapeutic or diagnostic use. This chapter serves as a general introduction to optical methods that allow neuroscientists to study the brain in three ways: by direct control of the membrane potential through the use of optically modulated, single-component ion channels and pumps (optogenetics); by employing molecular or genetically encoded calcium indicators for recording subthreshold activity and action potentials in intact specimens; and by rendering tissue samples completely transparent to allow molecular identification and imaging of entire circuits, nuclei, or whole brains in situ by means of CLARITY. Although not yet applied in the experimental therapeutic arena, all three techniques have shown utility in nonhuman primates, human cell lines, and either live or postmortem human tissue samples. These techniques developed from research conducted in the 2000s but quickly became entrenched as new standards in laboratory practice. Collectively, they have revolutionized neural readout and control and have enabled experimental approaches that were only dreamed of until the turn of the century; the influence on neurological surgery has great potential.

The addition of these optical methods to the neuroscience "toolbox" has significantly contributed to addressing questions that might have been described by Galvani as being "very much involved in darkness." Together, they represent approaches that enable precise control of and data collection from defined neural populations and molecular profiling of intact specimens to include the entire human brain. Their rapid development has renewed interest in and focus on neuroscience (e.g., the BRAIN Initiative).

The effect of these methods on medicine and surgery is likely to be via two separate avenues. The less direct but more immediate primary application is through a continued elucidation of fundamental principles of neurological health and disease. As is noted throughout the extended online text, questions regarding the basis of disease, ranging from the molecular to behavioral levels, have been addressed, with the use of myriad model organisms and human tissue resources. The second avenue is direct therapeutic application. With the control and readout agents being genetically encoded and acknowledging practical barriers to widespread gene therapy, it is likely that CLARITY, used for intact tissue clearing and molecular profiling, will be the first technology applied clinically, with immediate potential for application in pathology.

As the implementation of these techniques improves and matures, they will give researchers an even greater degree of control over their subject. The combination of optical stimulation or silencing and readout for simultaneous closed-loop control of thousands of genetically or topologically defined neurons in intact model organisms is now a tangible and demonstrated experimental approach. However, researchers are able to apply the techniques only within the laboratory. Translation into therapeutic modalities will require years of partnership with dedicated clinicians, a process that is now under way.

*"CLARITY" stands for "*c*lear *l*ipid-exchanged *a*crylamide-hybridized *r*igid *i*maging/*i*mmunostaining/*i*n situ hybridization-compatible *t*issue h*y*drogel."
†Deceased.

Full text of this chapter is available online at ExpertConsult.com

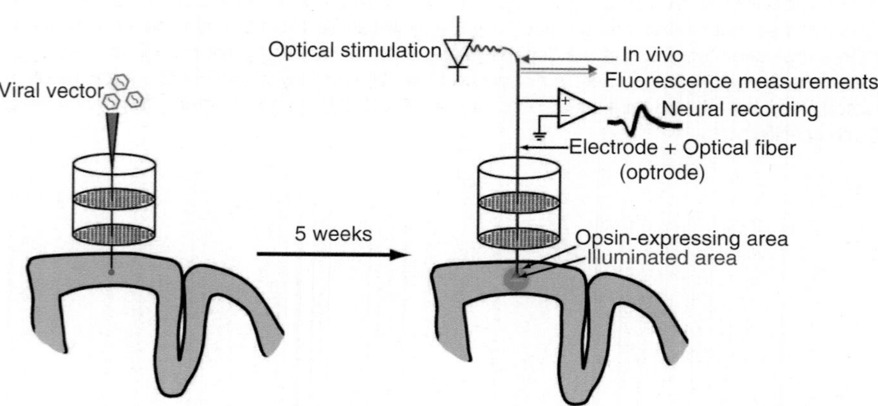

Optogenetic control of cortical activity in nonhuman primates. Primates are injected with virus-carrying optogenetic tools to sensitize defined populations of neurons to light. *(Modified from Diester I, Kaufman MT, Mogri M, et al. An optogenetic toolbox designed for primates.* Nat Neurosci *2001;14:387-397.)*

46 Neuroembryology

Harvey B. Sarnat, Laura Flores-Sarnat, and Joseph D. Pinter

Neuroembryology is the study of the development of the nervous system, from gastrulation when the neural plate is recognized for the first time and the body plan of bilateral symmetry and cephalization is established by the primitive streak, until maturity. Three axes of the body and of the future neural tube and central nervous system (CNS) are established at the time of gastrulation, with gradients of genetic expression in each. In general, two gradients of maturation occur in each axis: rostrocaudal or caudorostral in the longitudinal axis; dorsoventral or ventrodorsal in the vertical axis; and mediolateral or lateromedial in the horizontal axis. Most malformations of the CNS follow one or more gradients in these axes and can be explained on this basis, and genetic programming of the neural tube follows these gradients. For example, sonic hedgehog *(SHH)* follows a ventrodorsal gradient, but the families of paired homeobox genes *(PAX)* and of bone morphogenic protein *(BMP)* follow a dorsoventral gradient, both acting in the vertical axis. They are alternatively called *ventralizing* or *dorsalizing* genes or genes that produce dorsal or ventral programming of the neural tube. Other genes important in the early development of the neural tube are the various segmentation genes that provide compartments through which neurons of the same type can be concentrated to form cranial nerve nuclei, for example, and to limit cellular migration in the longitudinal axis. These compartments are called *neuromeres;* the eight neuromeres of the hindbrain and spinal cord are called *rhombomeres.* Examples of genes of segmentation include the families of engrailed *(EN)*, wingless *(WNT)*, homeobox *(HOX)*, and Krox *(KROX)*. The spinal cord is not intrinsically segmented, despite regional differentiation of specific structures of the preganglionic sympathetic and parasympathetic nervous systems and formation of specific motor neurons in particular parts, such as the phrenic nerve in C4 and the urethral and anal sphincters in S4. Apparent segmentation is produced by grouping of nerve roots and blood vessels entering and leaving the spinal cord, imposed by the segmentation of somites from earlier continuous longitudinal columns of somitomeres. (For further information on molecular genetics and neuroembryology, see Chapter 186.)

Neurulation is the dorsal midline closure by fusion of the neural folds to form the neural tube. It is initiated in the cervical region and extends both rostrally and caudally. The final closure is at multiple sites, not a single site as previously thought, but in the regions of the anterior and posterior neuropores. The bending and folding of the neural plate to form a tube is mediated in part by cellular sliding and intercellular adhesion molecules and also by the wide base of the floor plate ependymal in the ventral midline that creates wedge-shaped cells with a narrow ventricular apex; hence, physical forces contribute much to the bending and formation of a tube. The dorsal surfaces of the neural plate and folds become the central canal and eventually differentiate into ependyma at the ventricular or central canal surface, but initially form neuroepithelium with many mitoses at the ventricular surface. Ependymal differentiation arrests all mitotic activity, and the neuroepithelium becomes postmitotic premigratory neuroblasts and glioblasts. The central canal throughout the spinal cord initially is not a narrow canal but rather a tall and large ventricular lumen that becomes smaller and narrower with neuropil growth.

The region caudal to the posterior neuropore, which becomes the conus medullaris, does not close by folding but is a solid cone of neuroepithelium within which a central canal burrows; this conus region is called *secondary neurulation.*

Neural induction is the influence of the neural tube on development of nonneural structures. It is mediated by neural crest, initiated at the lateral margins of the neural plate and folds, and, at the time of neurulation, emanates from the dorsal midline of each of the three primitive cerebral vesicles: prosencephalic, mesencephalic, and rhombencephalic with its specializations of cardiac and gastrointestinal neural crest. Nearly all craniofacial development is induced from the neural tube by neural crest cells, which do not differentiate into their variety of tissues until reaching their final site.

Regional differentiation of structures along the length of the neural tube is accompanied by differentiation of specific types of cells, both neurons and glia. Neuronal maturation includes the formation of membrane ion channels and an energy supply by Na^+,K^+–adenosine triphosphatase (ATPase) to maintain a resting membrane potential capable of depolarization. Receptors for chemical neurotransmitters also must form in the membranes. Transmitter synthesis involves a great increase in ribosomes and mitochondria and a mechanism to transport the transmitter from its site of biosynthesis in the soma along the axoplasm to the axonal terminal. Molecules for assembly into synaptic vesicles also must be transported. Microtubules and neurofilaments are part of the cytoskeleton, but also serve other functions such as axoplasmic flow. The development of neurites, axonal pathfinding, and synaptogenesis are additional processes of neuronal maturation. Finally, neurons produce specific nuclear and cytoplasmic proteins characteristic for each type of neuron, and these proteins can be recognized by immunocytochemical antibodies to demonstrate their expression and localization in tissue sections of developing brain. In some malformations certain types of neurons are selectively affected and others spared. The loss of equilibrium between excitatory and inhibitory neurons in the cerebral cortex, for example, may contribute to epileptogenesis.

Genetically determined malformations may be germline mutations that occur at the time of fertilization and are present in every cell, although not expressed in all (e.g., *LIS1* causing lissencephaly 1), or postzygotic somatic mutations that affect some but not all clones of progenitor cells (e.g., hemimegalencephaly). Not all malformations of the nervous system are genetically determined. Some result from fetal exposure to teratogenic toxins and drugs, x-irradiation, hypoxia or ischemia, intrauterine infections, vitamin and dietary deficiencies, and other adverse prenatal events that interrupt normal developmental processes.

Our growing understanding of the molecular genetic details of normal and abnormal brain development has made it clear that classification systems for disorders based on morphology or genetic mutations alone are inadequate. Descriptive morphogenesis must be integrated with patterns of genetic expression. Timing of onset of developmental processes, gradients of expression of genetic expression along the axes of the neural tube, and conceptualization of malformations as disorders of normal developmental processes are primordial for insight into neuroembryology, both normal and aberrant. Recent advances in molecular genetics, neuroimaging including fetal brain, and neuropathology all contribute to better understanding of brain malformations and ultimately to approaches to prevent and treat disorders of the developing nervous system.

Full text of this chapter is available online at ExpertConsult.com 

47 Stem Cell Biology in the Central Nervous System

Philip J. Horner and Samuel Emerson

The central nervous system has long been thought to be a fixed substrate of neural processes and synapses with limited plasticity. Over the last few decades it has been shown that the brain has a particularly striking reserve for plasticity and perhaps repair: the adult neural stem cell. Originally described in the 1960s, neural stem cells have been more recently derived and characterized in the culture dish. Neural stem cells originate from ventricular zones in the brain and subependymal zones in the spinal cord. Two regions of the brain contain a renewable resource of stem cells that seed the brain with progenitor cells that create new nerve cells and connections in the hippocampus and olfactory bulb. The process of neurogenesis in these regions continues throughout the life span, but their capacity for creating significant autologous replacement of neurons following neural injury is quite limited. In this chapter, we review the location and molecular makeup of neural stem cells and review their response to injury. In addition, we consider the latest approaches to harness neural stem cells and their progeny to engineer new brain cells and circuitry to heal the injured nervous system.

Full text of this chapter is available online at ExpertConsult.com 

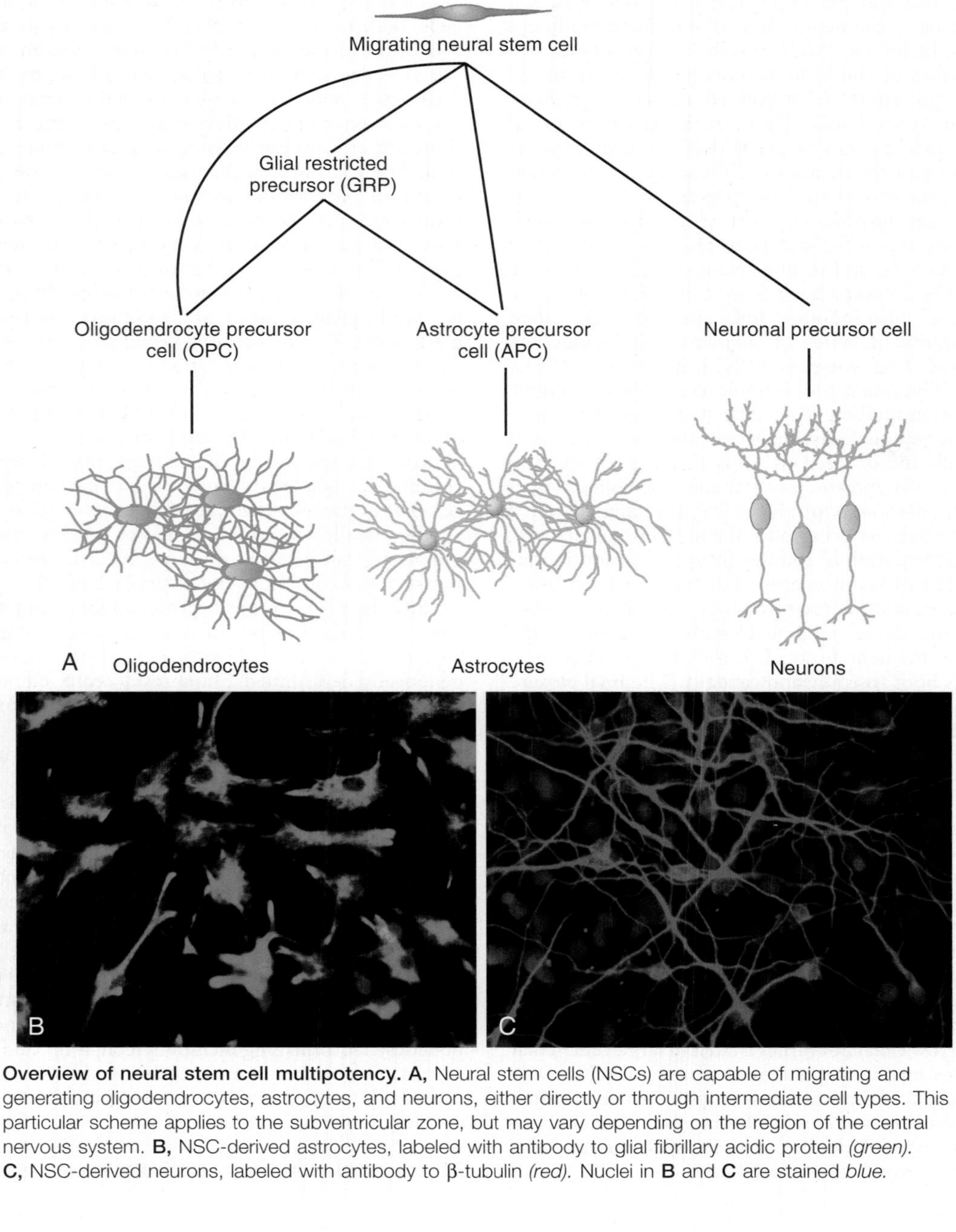

Migrating neural stem cell
Glial restricted precursor (GRP)
Oligodendrocyte precursor cell (OPC)
Astrocyte precursor cell (APC)
Neuronal precursor cell
A Oligodendrocytes
Astrocytes
Neurons
B
C

Overview of neural stem cell multipotency. A, Neural stem cells (NSCs) are capable of migrating and generating oligodendrocytes, astrocytes, and neurons, either directly or through intermediate cell types. This particular scheme applies to the subventricular zone, but may vary depending on the region of the central nervous system. **B,** NSC-derived astrocytes, labeled with antibody to glial fibrillary acidic protein *(green).* **C,** NSC-derived neurons, labeled with antibody to β-tubulin *(red).* Nuclei in **B** and **C** are stained *blue.*

48 Neurons and Neuroglia

Bruce D. Trapp and Karl Herrup

This chapter provides an overview of the diversity and some basic description of the structure of each of the major cell types. The cells of the brain are a virtual menagerie of cell types, and within each type there is substantial variation in properties such as size and shape. This applies most obviously to the neuronal cells, but it is also true for the nonneuronal, neuroglial, cells. We begin with the neuron and its major compartments—the dendrite, cell body, axon, and synapse. Each of these subdomains of the neuron has its own specialized function and unique physiology. The dendrite serves as the antenna of the cell; it is the primary site for receiving input from upstream neurons. It responds to these inputs with small changes in membrane potential that sum as they propagate along the neuronal membrane. The cell body is the site where these potential changes meet and sum to determine whether to pass the information along to the next cell by means of an action potential. The axon is the conduit along which the axon potential travels to reach the downstream targets of the neuron. Like the dendrite, it has a highly specialized composition of membrane channels whose proper functioning allows a strong membrane depolarization to propagate, often at great distances, without diminishing. The synapse is a pairing of the axon terminus and the downstream target (most often the dendrite of another neuron). At this specialized structure the action potential of the axon triggers the release of a small aliquot of neurotransmitter that interacts with target receptors, often on the dendrite of another neuron, and the process is thus repeated.

Although the neuron is the primary cell responsible for transmitting information over long distances, it is not alone in the brain. Several other nonneuronal cell types known as *neuroglia* are intermingled with the neurons and are indispensable for their proper functioning. We review the major neuroglial cell types and summarize their interactions with one another and with the nerve cells. Astrocytes form an anastomosing network that surrounds the neurons and the vasculature of the brain. They are heavily involved in maintaining the ionic and nutritional environment in which the neurons function, in particular at the synapse, where they also serve to clear neurotransmitters such as glutamate. Radial glia serve a guidance role during development and are a source of precursors during development and beyond. Oligodendrocytes are responsible for creating the myelin of the central nervous system (CNS), the fatty coating of the neuronal axon that allows for rapid, salutatory conduction of the action potential. In the peripheral nervous system (PNS), this same function is carried out by a neural crest-derived cell known as a Schwann cell. Microglial cells are the mediators of the innate immune system of the brain and function in ways very similar to macrophages in the periphery.

In the aggregate, these elements and their basic interactions are the cellular toolkit the brain uses to achieve the functions described in later chapters.

Full text of this chapter is available online at ExpertConsult.com

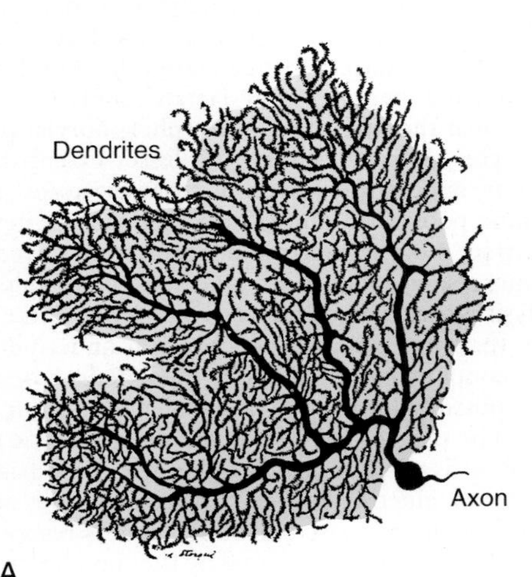

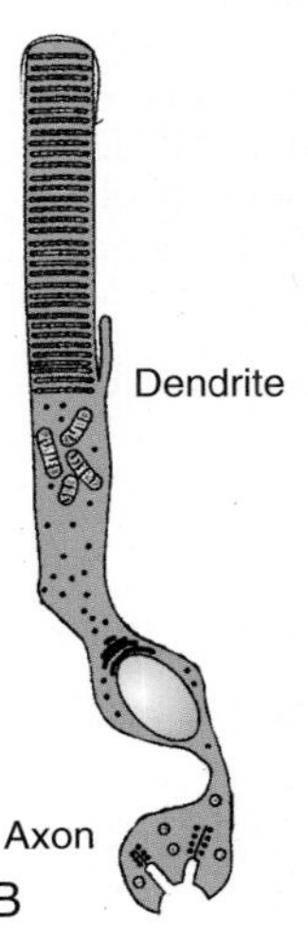

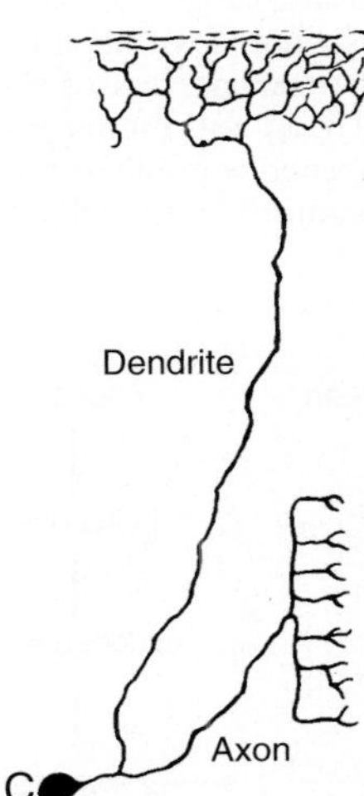

Three examples of the structural diversity among the cells known as neurons. A, Cerebellar Purkinje cell. This cell is the most traditional in its shape, with a clear dendritic domain, a large cell body, and a single axon that leaves the cell opposite the main dendritic shaft. **B,** Rod photoreceptor. The light-sensitive stacks of photopigment-containing membrane are at the *top*, and the short, stubby axon is at the *bottom*. **C,** Dorsal root ganglion neuron. The peripheral process is at the *top*; the ganglion itself, containing the cell body, is at the *lower right*; and the central process is deployed within the central nervous system at the *lower right*. *(**A,** Modified from Truex RC, Carpenter MB.* Human Neuroanatomy. *Baltimore: Williams & Wilkins; 1970. **B** and **C,** Modified from Hof P, Trapp BD, de Vellis J, et al. The cellular components of nervous tissue. In: Zigmond M, Bloom FE, Landis SC, et al, eds.* Fundamental Neuroscience. *San Diego: Academic Press; 1999:41–69.)*

49 Cellular Mechanisms of Brain Energy Metabolism

Albert H. Gjedde and Pierre J. Magistretti

The activity of the human brain depends on a sufficient supply of glucose and oxygen, as well as other substances, delivered by the blood flow to the brain, and on the steady removal of the products of metabolism such as carbon dioxide and lactate and other metabolites. The directions of delivery in turn depend on the concentrations and pressures of the substances in the vascular and tissue compartments. Except for extreme exertions, concentrations and pressures of key metabolites in brain tissue are maintained within narrow limits, the needs of changing brain function being met by changes of flux rather than concentration or pressure. Current evidence suggests that this regulation is accomplished without a rigid association between the changes of oxygen consumption, glucose combustion, and blood flow associated with variable brain function. The claim that increases of blood flow occur simply to satisfy the demands for oxygen and glucose during neuronal excitation must therefore be regarded as one-dimensional.

Energy budget estimates suggest that most of the brain's demand for energy turnover reflects the steady-state magnitude of graded membrane depolarization rather than action potential generation and propagation. The increased energy turnover is required to maintain the graded depolarization of neuronal membranes associated with changing sodium and potassium conductance. Conversely, it is not the case that increased energy turnover is required to sustain the instances of membrane hyperpolarization caused by decreased conductance of sodium or increased conductance of potassium or chloride.

Glucose, pyruvate, and lactate occupy single tissue compartments with uniform concentrations, but the pathways and enzymes responsible for glycolysis and oxidative phosphorylation are unevenly distributed within and among the main cell populations. When the transporters of the main metabolites (glucose transporter [GLUT] and monocarboxylate transporter [MCT]) establish homogeneous pools of the glycolytic metabolite pools, it is thermodynamically impossible for the effective properties of the lactate dehydrogenase (LDH) subtypes in vivo to differ spatially among the different compartments of cells. The glycolytic breakdown of glucose ("aerobic glycolysis") and the oxidative phosphorylation of adenosine diphosphate (ADP) by adenosine triphosphate (ATP) synthase in mitochondria ("oxidative phosphorylation") occur at physically distinct sites that necessarily require the transfer of products of glycolysis from sites of aerobic glycolysis in cytosol to sites of oxidative phosphorylation in mitochondria. When the transfer distance varies among the cellular compartments, varying degrees of delay and accumulation of the intermediates can be detected, particularly during acute increases of metabolic rate, as reflected in part in the astrocyte-neuron lactate shuttle (ANLS) activity.

The bulk of current knowledge of cerebral metabolic rates, volumes of cells, and distribution of glycolytic and oxidative activities in vitro and in vivo in rodents and humans implies that cell bodies and extensions in the form of terminals, synapses, and end-feet differ substantially, with at least four identifiable compartments, representing glial cell bodies, glial extensions into the neuropil ("astropil"), neuronal cell bodies with the associated proximal dendrites, and the distal dendrites extending into the neuropil, and with an oxidative gradient from the neuronal cell bodies, through neuronal and astrocytic extensions into the neuropil, to the cell bodies of astrocytes, where the glycolytic component of metabolism is held to be the greatest.

Substantial pyruvate and lactate generation and accumulation occur when the less oxidative compartments are activated more than the more oxidative neuronal sites. In the early stages of activation, there is demand for glutamate removal of a magnitude that exceeds the low oxidative capacity of the neuropil and astrocytes. Although the resulting pyruvate and lactate accumulation is influenced by lactate exchange across the blood-brain barrier, the accumulated pyruvate and lactate pools are available for common use at the sites of oxidative phosphorylation in neurons and astrocytes. Astrocytes, and to a lesser extent distal parts of the neurons, appear to contribute more pyruvate and lactate to the common pools than do the proximal parts of neurons, which in turn extract more pyruvate and lactate from the common pool.

The increase in blood flow appears to be coupled to the rate of glycolysis rather than oxygen consumption. There is increasing evidence that the putative mechanism underlying the flow-glycolysis coupling is a calcium ion–mediated astrocytic response, aided and possibly initiated by a signal arising from lactate accumulation. The physiologic reason for the glycolytic mediation of blood flow activation is not clear because flow has a moderate effect only on glucose delivery. Instead, it now appears more likely that it is the increased glycolysis that is responsible for the increase of blood flow as mediated by the signaling role of lactate, rather than the direct demand for increased blood flow. This sequence of events inverts the flow-metabolism coupling sequence from the conventional flow-oxygen-glucose series to the revised glucose-flow-oxygen steps.

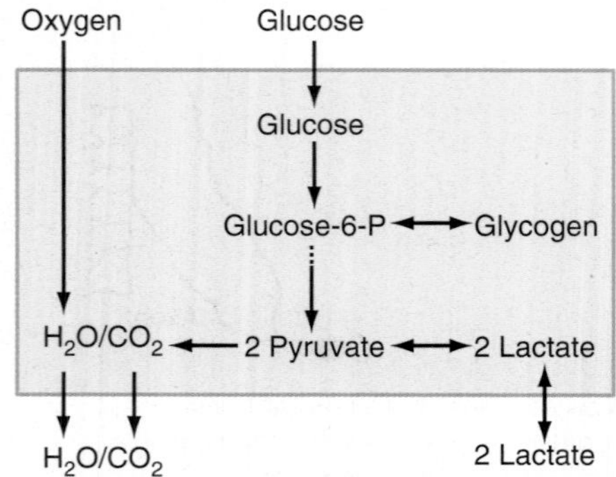

Simplified illustration of the main metabolic pathways active in mammalian brain. Glucose-6-P, glucose-6-phosphate.

Full text of this chapter is available online at ExpertConsult.com

50 Cellular and Molecular Responses in the Peripheral and Central Nervous Systems: Similarities and Differences

Rajiv Saigal, Harjus Singh Birk, and Michel Kliot

In this chapter, we review and compare the cellular and molecular responses in the peripheral nervous system (PNS) and central nervous system (CNS). In addition, we discuss opportunities for intervention that could potentially serve as new means of therapy.

PERIPHERAL NERVOUS SYSTEM RESPONSE TO INJURY

Damage to a peripheral nerve can be characterized using a three-tiered system that includes neurapraxic, axonotmetic, and neurotmetic injuries. The mildest form, neurapraxic injury, is characterized by myelin damage in which fast recovery is feasible. Axonotmesis is a medium-grade injury in which axon damage may be present but the surrounding structures remain intact. The most severe type of injury is neurotmesis, in which both axonal continuity and the surrounding structures are disrupted and, as a result, axonal regeneration is impeded. Neurapraxic- and axonotmetic-related peripheral nerve injuries may be able to undergo recovery.

Cell Body Survival and the Peripheral Nervous System Axonal Pathway

After axonal injury takes place, neurotropic factors become prevalent in the distal peripheral nerve stump and help promote survival of both sensory and sympathetic neurons. Neurotrophins stimulate the migration of and enhance the response of Schwann cells to aide in axonal regeneration. After axotomy, Schwann cells become active within 24 hours and release monocyte chemoattractant protein-1, a protein that recruits macrophages for axonal and myelin debris clearance. An important mediator in wallerian degeneration is calcium influx after injury, because it helps restore membrane integrity and promote regeneration. This makes calcium modulation a possible target for regeneration after axonal injury.

Extracellular Matrix Proteins and Cellular and Molecular Response in the Peripheral Nervous System

In addition to the role of neurotropic factors and calcium modulation in promoting regeneration after axotomy, the matrix proteins of the basal lamina and endoneurium also aid in this process. Specifically, the basal lamina contains laminin B, laminin 2, and laminin 10 that have neurite-promoting properties in the distal nerve stump. Once the process of axonal regeneration is initiated, glial growth factor mediates the maturation of immature peripheral nerve cells.

Axonal Regeneration in the Peripheral Nervous System and Factors Influencing Target Reinnervation in End Organs

External electrical stimulation has been show to promote regeneration in the PNS. Specifically, 1 hour to 2 weeks of 20-Hz stimulation of injured axons helps stimulate recovery and reduces regeneration time from 10 weeks to 3 weeks in an animal model of PNS injury. Electrical stimulation activates cyclic adenosine monophosphate channels that enable axonal regrowth. Regeneration following peripheral nervous system injury is challenging because the target specificity is needed for functional recovery, but is not always achieved.

CENTRAL NERVOUS SYSTEM RESPONSE TO INJURY

Key biologic differences make CNS regeneration and recovery more difficult than that in the PNS. In the CNS, oligodendrocytes produce inhibitory molecules, such as neurite outgrowth inhibitor (Nogo)-66, myelin-associated glycoprotein, and oligodendrocyte myelin glycoprotein. Unlike PNS Schwann cells, oligodendrocytes do not initiate clearance of injured debris or activate immune cells to assist in this process. Unlike PNS macrophages, CNS microglia have a limited and delayed response to injury. Glial scar formation is common in the CNS, a result of intermediate filament and chondroitin sulfate proteoglycan production in the CNS. Secondary injury resulting from the inflammatory response is an important factor in the CNS. Astrocytes express nuclear factor-κB and produce proinflammatory molecules, including transforming growth factor-β2, chemokine (C-C motif) ligand 2, and interferon-γ–inducible protein-10.

OPPORTUNITIES FOR INTERVENTION

Opportunities to intervene clinically in promoting recovery from either PNS or CNS injury can be grouped into (1) prevention of cell death, (2) regeneration, and (3) enhanced plasticity. Delivery of anti-inflammatory molecules and neurotrophins has proven promising in animal models for limiting cell death. Antibodies may be used to disrupt growth-inhibitory molecules such as Nogo-A. The glial scar may be disrupted with chondroitinase ABC or matrix metalloproteinases. The mammalian nervous system has marked capacity for plasticity. Electrical stimulation and rehabilitation appear to enhance this plasticity after injury. Although many of these strategies have shown promise in animal models of PNS and CNS injury, there is need for further development and research in order to demonstrate efficacy in humans.

Full text of this chapter is available online at ExpertConsult.com 

51 The Blood-Brain Barrier

Briana C. Prager, Shahid M. Nimjee, Gerald A. Grant, Chaitali Ghosh, and Damir Janigro

This chapter, available in full at ExpertConsult.com, reviews the blood-brain barrier (BBB), an important component of the neurovascular unit. The blood-brain barrier (BBB) is made of specialized endothelial cells, basement membrane, neurons, and the following neuroglial structures: astrocytes, pericytes, and microglia. The BBB connects and interacts with peripheral intravascular signals, cerebrospinal and interstitial fluids, and the parenchymal environment to mediate a complex system of exchange, transport, and clearance. Perturbation of BBB integrity plays a role in a human brain pathology, and the potential effect of BBB cells is more widespread and complex than initially believed. For example, the pathogenesis of multiple sclerosis is dependent on extravasation of leukocytes through the BBB and into the parenchyma, and therapeutics targeted at increasing BBB integrity, such as interferon-β, have been relatively effective in reducing the rate of relapse. Ischemic stroke, originally viewed as inducing some short-term mechanical disruption of the BBB, has been shown to lead to chronic inflammation and thus increased BBB permeability, potentially contributing to long-term detrimental sequelae. As such, treatments are now being identified and studied to target maintaining integrity at the BBB.

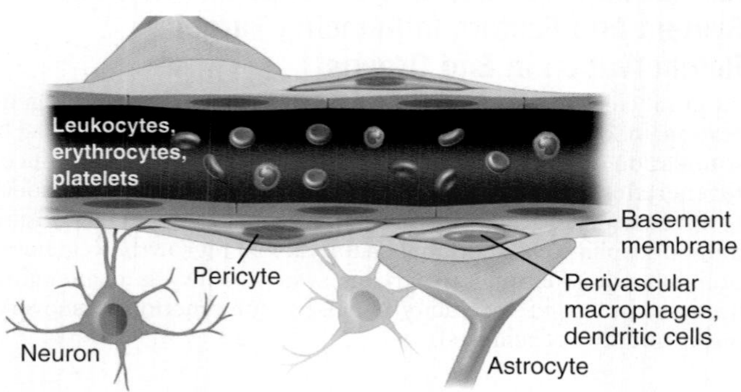

Schematic of a "neurovascular unit," which consists of endothelial cells, astrocytes, pericytes, macrophages, microglia, neurons, the basement membrane, and the extracellular matrix.

Full text of this chapter is available online at ExpertConsult.com 

52 Physiology of the Cerebrospinal Fluid and Intracranial Pressure

Andrew Beaumont

A wide variety of neurological and neurosurgical conditions are associated with disordered physiology of the cerebrospinal fluid (CSF) and intracranial pressure (ICP). The position of the brain within a rigid structure, namely the skull, creates a unique physiologic environment in which changes in intracranial volume ($V_{INTRACRANIAL\ SPACE}$) can create pathologic elevations in ICP.

The basic physiologic tenets of this concept were put forward in the Monro-Kellie doctrine, or hypothesis, which can be expressed as follows:

$$V_{CSF} + V_{BLOOD} + V_{BRAIN} + V_{OTHER} = V_{INTRACRANIAL\ SPACE} = (\text{CONSTANT})$$

where V_{CSF} is volume of CSF, V_{BLOOD} is volume of blood, V_{BRAIN} is volume of brain, and V_{OTHER} is volume of any abnormal component, such as a tumor. This equation provides a general framework for understanding pathologic causes of elevated ICP and also its treatments.

ICP is equivalent to CSF pressure. ICP is therefore reflective of the balance among CSF formation, volume storage or compliance, and fluid absorption. The ICP has a natural waveform that is influenced by cardiac and respiratory cycles. Physical principles can define a pressure-volume index (PVI), which is the calculated volume in milliliters (mL) that would need to be added to the intracranial volume to increase ICP by a factor of 10. Reduced intracranial compliance lowers the PVI, and smaller changes in volume result in greater changes in pressure. Under non–steady-state dynamics, added intracranial volume can be compensated for initially by reduction of one of the other elements, until this compensation is overwhelmed. Thereafter PVI is reduced and elevations in ICP are more pronounced.

Elevations in ICP reduce cerebral perfusion pressure (CPP), which in turn can affect autoregulation and may limit tissue blood flow or even trigger a hyperemic response. Correlation between spontaneous waves of ICP and blood pressure has been shown to relate to autoregulation. Measurement of this correlation (pressure reactivity index [PRx]) can therefore provide information about autoregulation that can help guide therapy choices.

There are not good data to support a definition of optimal cerebral blood flow under pathologic conditions. It is clear that ischemia resulting from raised ICP causes more swelling, which in turn elevates ICP further. The end point of unchecked ICP elevation is herniation and brain death.

Several technologies are available for measuring ICP, and although clinical guidelines have been published, there is no general consensus on patient selection, timing, or duration of ICP monitoring. Although the importance of ICP control is well recognized, clinical trials have failed to demonstrate survival benefits in disease state with use of ICP monitoring. Novel noninvasive monitoring techniques for measuring ICP have been developed, including evaluation of pupil reactivity, use of transcranial Doppler ultrasonography, electroencephalography (EEG) and magnetic resonance imaging (MRI). The "gold standard" remains pressure transduction through a ventriculostomy.

Treatments for raised ICP can be grouped according to their site of action within the framework of the Monro-Kellie doctrine. V_{CSF} can be treated with CSF diversion, either temporary (external ventricular drainage) or permanent (CSF shunt). Medications such as acetazolamide can reduce CSF production, and their use is a first-line treatment option in idiopathic intracranial hypertension (ICH). V_{BLOOD} can be reduced by hyperventilation, head of bed elevation, and also sedatives or barbiturates. Sedatives and barbiturates reduce tissue oxygen utilization and therefore may be beneficial for reducing blood flow but also permitting tolerance of lower oxygen delivery. The major contributor to V_{BRAIN} is cerebral edema, treatment of which can include mannitol, blood pressure control, steroids, and hypothermia.

Using this framework to understand the non–steady-state dynamics of raised ICP allows rational choice of treatments. Future developments will begin to define other physiologic parameters in conjunction with ICP that can help guide specific disease-targeted therapies. Even within a single type of disease, such as traumatic brain injury, the pathophysiology may be greatly heterogeneous, making treatment decisions more difficult.

Full text of this chapter is available online at ExpertConsult.com

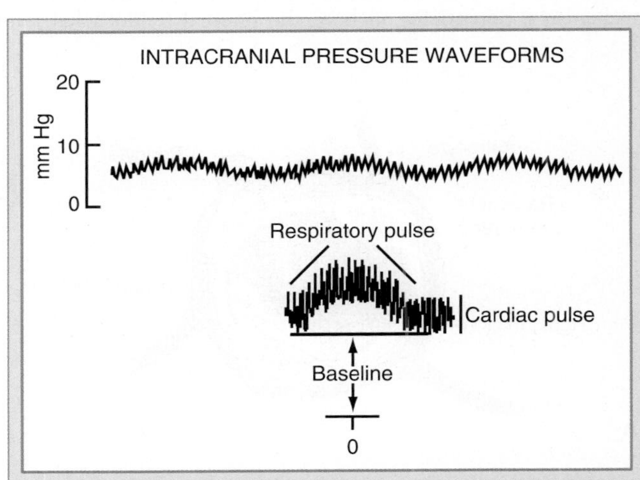

Normal intracranial pressure (ICP) waveform. The baseline pressure level is affected by rhythmic components caused by cardiorespiratory activity. Fluctuation of mean arterial pressure with heart rate causes small amplitude rapid pulsation, and respiration causes larger-amplitude fluctuations of lower frequency. ICP is completely described only by information about both the baseline level and the pulsatile components.

53 Cerebral Edema

Robert J. Weil and Edward H. Oldfield

OVERVIEW AND HISTORICAL BACKGROUND

Cerebral edema represents the accumulation of excess fluid in the intracellular or extracellular spaces of the brain. It can result from a variety of physiologic and pathologic processes and is frequently responsible for much of the morbidity and mortality associated with brain tumors and a variety of other disorders, including trauma, infarction, hemorrhage, and infection. A basic conception of the barriers that exist between and among blood, cerebrospinal fluid (CSF), and the brain is required to fully understand cerebral edema. In this chapter, we outline the physiology of the blood-brain barrier (BBB) and describe and discuss the principal types and causes of cerebral edema. Reviews that outline the history of research and recent advances in this area and that provide detailed summaries beyond the scope of this chapter are cited in the references.

THE BLOOD-BRAIN BARRIER

The principal component of the BBB is the endothelial cells that line the cerebral microvasculature. The tight junctions between adjacent endothelial cells in the brain, which are nonpermissive in comparison to those in the systemic circulation, prevent the paracellular transport of most molecules. Although small substances, such as oxygen and carbon dioxide, and small lipophilic molecules, such as ethanol, may diffuse freely through the lipid membranes that constitute the BBB, larger, bulkier, more complex or hydrophilic molecules require active, transcellular transport mechanisms, potentially on both the luminal (endothelial) and abluminal (brain) membranes, to enter the brain. The active transport mechanisms require energy in the form of adenosine triphosphate (ATP).

MOLECULAR EVENTS IN CEREBRAL EDEMA

Cerebral edema is a common end result of a variety of neurological and systemic disorders. Most classifications of cerebral edema describe four categories: *cytotoxic*, or cellular swelling secondary to cell injury; *vasogenic*, which results from vascular leakage through a disrupted BBB and consequently increased fluid and altered concentrations of ions, peptides, and macromolecules in the extracellular space; *interstitial*, which occurs with transependymal flow of CSF in patients with hydrocephalus; and *osmotic*, when the brain is hyperosmolar relative to plasma and thus induces water to flow passively across an intact BBB along its concentration gradient. It may be difficult to separate edema into these distinct classes in every patient because more than one of these types exist simultaneously as a result of the nature and timing of the underlying disorder. Because interstitial edema and osmotic edema have fewer causes or are uncommon in neurosurgical patients, our principal focus in this chapter is on vasogenic and cytotoxic edema.

Tissue swelling—edema—may be intracellular or extracellular. It has the potential to result in profound shifts in the relative volumes occupied by the cellular and interstitial elements. Continued redistribution of water, ions, peptides, and other neuroactive substances within and between the cells of the central nervous system (neurons, glia, microglia, and endothelial cells) may exacerbate the severity of the edema. These failures lead to a variety of molecular events and cascades that potentiate cerebral and BBB dysfunction.

Full text of this chapter is available online at ExpertConsult.com

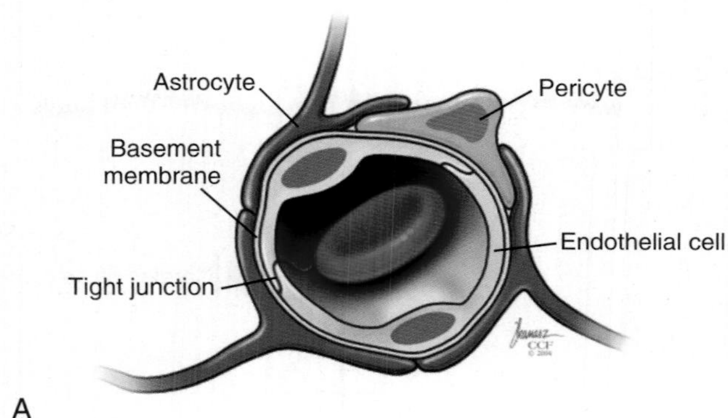

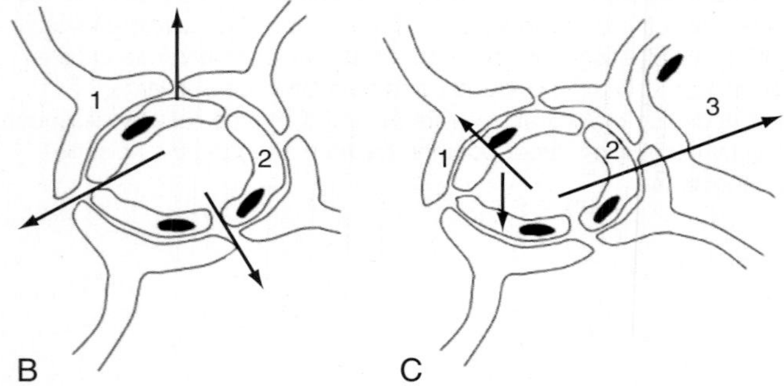

Microscopic representations of the blood-brain barrier (BBB) and the two most common forms of cerebral edema. A, The BBB is created by compact apposition of endothelial cells to create a barrier between the vascular system and the brain parenchyma. This is reinforced by numerous pericytes. A thin basement membrane surrounds the endothelial cells and provides both structural support and a dense physical barrier between the circulation and the microenvironment of the brain. Astrocytes extend cellular processes (astrocytic "foot processes") that cover the basement membrane, which enhances the BBB by limiting the ability of macromolecules or circulating cells to gain access to the central nervous system. **B,** In vasogenic edema, increased permeability of the capillaries, through dehiscent or incompetent tight junctions, leads to exudation of a plasma ultrafiltrate and water into the extracellular space. *Arrows* demonstrate flow through the tight junctions and into the extracellular space. **C,** In cytotoxic edema, depletion of energy and metabolites leads to failure of the sodium-potassium adenosine triphosphatase (Na^+,K^+-ATPase) pump and accumulation of sodium within the cells (astrocytes and endothelial cells, as well as neurons); water follows the concentration gradient into the cells, which swell in response. *Arrows* demonstrate the path of water into cells from the vascular space. 1, Astrocytes and astrocytic foot processes; 2, endothelial cells; 3, neurons. *(**A,** Reprinted with permission, Cleveland Clinic Center for Medical Art & Photography © 2005-2010. All Rights Reserved.)*

54 Extracellular Fluid Movement and Clearance in the Brain: The Glymphatic Pathway

Jeffrey J. Iliff and Richard Deren Penn

The brain and spinal cord are composed of distinct fluid compartments, including the blood column, the cerebrospinal fluid (CSF), the interstitial fluid (ISF), and the intracellular compartments. Fluid movement between these compartments is tightly controlled by barrier structures such as the blood-brain barrier (BBB) and blood-CSF barrier. Recent insights into the physiology of fluid movement within and around the brain suggest that interactions between the CSF and the ISF are more extensive and functionally significant than previously anticipated.

The movement of interstitial solutes through the brain is governed by the processes of diffusion and bulk flow. The relative contribution of these two processes, depending on solute size, charge, polarity, and binding to extracellular matrix and BBB efflux transporters, is detailed.

Fluid from the CSF and ISF compartments readily exchange, both across the ependymal and pial surfaces separating them and along specific anatomic pathways, including perivascular spaces surrounding cerebral blood vessels and white matter tracts. The anatomic bases of these bulk flow pathways and the driving forces believed to propel bulk flow are defined.

Recent studies detailing the glymphatic system suggest that CSF from the subarachnoid space rapidly recirculates into and through the brain along perivascular spaces surrounding penetrating cerebral arteries, whereas ISF in turn is cleared from the brain along perivascular spaces surrounding large-caliber draining veins. The exchange of CSF and ISF along these perivascular pathways is dependent on water transport through perivascular astrocytic end-feet and appears to be a feature primarily of the sleeping brain. Studies detailing glymphatic pathway function in the rodent brain are covered.

Glymphatic pathway function plays a key role in interstitial waste clearance, solute distribution, and peripheral immune surveillance within the intact brain. Impairment of glymphatic pathway function appears to occur in the aging brain, after ischemic or traumatic brain injury, and after subarachnoid hemorrhage and is presumed to occur in conditions featuring BBB disruption such as brain tumors. The involvement of glymphatic pathway dysfunction in the development and resolution of cerebral edema is discussed, as is its proposed role in the development of neurodegenerative conditions such as Alzheimer's disease.

Because the ISF is the fluid compartment through which central nervous system (CNS)-targeting therapeutics must move, and because perivascular glymphatic pathways provide a low-resistance pathway for the exchange of CSF and ISF, the biology of the glymphatic system and its dysfunction in the setting of disease have important implications for the delivery of CNS therapeutics, including in the setting of intrathecal delivery, convection-enhanced delivery (CED), and the use of trans-BBB delivery pathways such as "Trojan horse" approaches, including BBB receptors. Understanding the effect that these pathways have on the movement of fluid through brain tissue, and how different disease processes influence these mechanics, will be important for the development of effective drug-delivery approaches, such as CED, to target CNS disease.

Full text of this chapter is available online at ExpertConsult.com

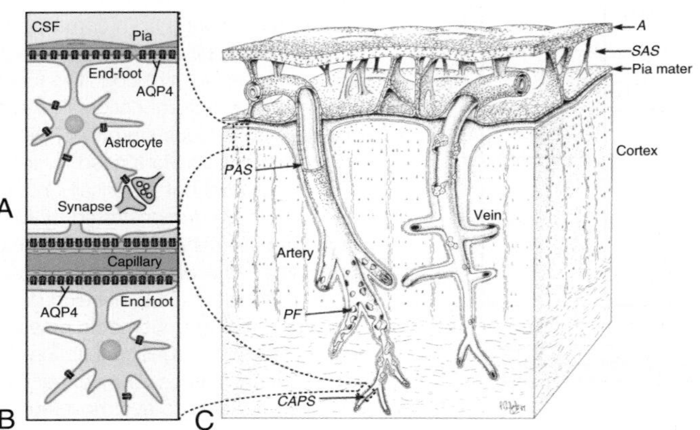

Apposition of astrocytic end-foot processes with paravascular and perivascular spaces. A, Astrocyte end-feet form the glial limitans facing the subpial spaces and express high levels of the water channel aquaporin 4 (AQP4). **B,** Perivascular astrocytic end-feet ensheath the cerebral microcirculation and express AQP4 at high levels in the vessel-facing perivascular membrane. **C,** Diagram showing relationships between pia mater and penetrating cerebral blood vessels. Leptomeningeal vessels are ensheathed by a layer of the pia mater, forming a paravascular space (PVS) between the pial sheath and the vessel wall that runs through the subarachnoid space (SAS). In penetrating arteries, this PVS follows the vessel into the brain, becoming perforated and fusing with the basement membrane of the distal arteriole, before the terminal capillary bed (CAPS). The PVS surrounding veins does not enter the brain, but rather reflects back on the pia mater, rending the PVS surrounding veins continuous with the subpial space. A, arachnoid membrane; CSF, cerebrospinal fluid; PAS, peri-arterial space; PF, pial fenestrations. *(**A** and **B,** Modified from Nagelhus EA, Ottersen OP. Physiological roles of aquaporin-4 in brain.* Physiol Rev. *2013;93:1543-1562.* ***C,*** *Modified from Zhang ET, Inman CB, Weller RO. Interrelationships of the pia mater and the perivascular (Virchow-Robin) spaces in the human cerebrum.* J Anat. *1990;170:111-123.)*

55 Altered Consciousness

Nicholas D. Schiff

Altered consciousness after brain injury is associated with several clinical syndromes, including coma, vegetative state (VS), minimally conscious state (MCS), akinetic mutism, and other related conditions. In this chapter a clinically oriented review is presented with emphasis on mechanisms that underlie altered consciousness at the neuronal "circuit" level. A brief taxonomy of altered states of consciousness is presented introducing the major categories of disorders of consciousness: coma, VS, and MCS. A general strategy to assess patients with disorders of consciousness and formulate a diagnosis and prognosis based on mechanistic principles is provided to guide the clinician. Important factors reviewed in this approach include the considerable differences in probabilities and time frames of recovery from coma, VS, or MCS and how this should influence decision making and clinical judgment. The approach is briefly framed in the context of evolving knowledge of specific cellular and circuit-level factors that underlie the pathophysiology of impaired consciousness, including the important role of the anterior forebrain mesocircuit and brain mechanisms underlying forebrain arousal. A closing section of the chapter reviews the potential contribution of new neuroimaging modalities and theoretical models to the diagnostic assessment of patients with disorders of consciousness. The widely emerging use of functional neuroimaging techniques utilizing magnetic resonance imaging and positron emission tomography in research-based assessments of disorders of consciousness has identified many surprising and challenging new findings. However, the translation of these observations into clinical practice has an uncertain path. Although limited preservation of cerebral network activity may be identified and graded, judging the cognitive level in patients with disorders of consciousness is not possible using nonbehavioral proxies such as functional magnetic resonance imaging. Nonetheless, some individual results demonstrate clear dissociation from clinical assessments and provide an urgent challenge to the practicing clinician. The syndrome of cognitive-motor dissociation (CMD) is defined and discussed with an emphasis on how clinical assessments aimed at locating patients at risk for CMD may develop.

Full text of this chapter is available online at ExpertConsult.com 

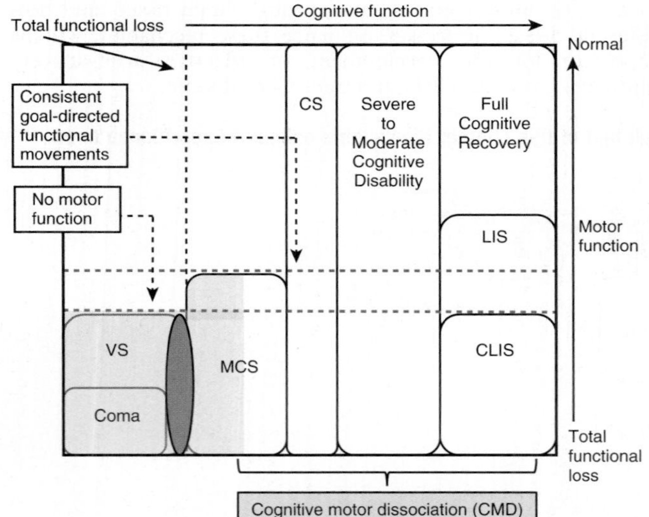

Taxonomy of disorders of consciousness after structural brain injuries. The distinctions among clinical disorders of consciousness can be best captured on a two-dimensional axis by comparing degree of impaired cognitive function against degree of motor function. At the bottom left of the figure, the functional equivalence of coma and vegetative state (VS) as unconscious brain states in which no behavioral evidence of consciousness is present and both cognitive and motor function are absent (VS differing from coma by intermittent eyes open periods) is indicated by their placement to the left of the vertical dashed line, indicating total loss of cognitive function, and below the dashed red line, indicating no motor function. The dark purple oval between coma/VS and minimally conscious state (MCS) indicates a transition zone where fragments of behavior untied to sensory stimuli may be observed prior to the unequivocal but potentially intermittent behavioral evidence of consciousness demonstrated by MCS patients; recovery of consistent goal-directed behaviors marks emergence from MCS above the dashed green line. After emergence from MCS, recovery patterns include the confusional state (CS), in which patients cannot be formally tested using standard neuropsychometric measures, are disoriented, and exhibit a limited range of cognitive function. Locked-in state (LIS) designates normal conscious awareness but severe motor impairment limiting communication channels typically to eye movements. LIS is not a disorder of consciousness, and LIS patients retain normal cognitive function by definition. The light purple zone encompassing coma, VS, and the left half of the MCS region shows cognitive motor dissociation (CMD), a clinical syndrome of patients with behavioral examinations consistent with coma, VS, or limited nonreflexive behaviors seen in MCS who demonstrate command following in examinations utilizing novel neuroimaging technologies (see chapter discussion). This syndrome indicates a wide range of uncertainty of cognitive capacity, marked by the brackets; in patients without any behavioral response, it is not possible to independently judge level of consciousness across the range of VS to the complete locked-in state (CLIS) without surrogate measures. The gap between the dashed green line and the dashed red line indicates the presence of inconsistent functional movements and a restricted range of uncertainty in establishing cognitive level from MCS to CLIS/LIS.

56 Neuropsychological Testing

Jordan H. Grafman

In this chapter, the rationale for, and methods used in, neuropsychological assessment of patients undergoing neurosurgery are described. The neuropsychological assessment of patients is justified for both clinical and research-driven reasons, and examples of each are provided.

It is vital to appreciate the scope of services and research methods that neuropsychology can offer (Table 56-1), and these methods are illustrated early in the chapter, along with a brief description of differences between the role of a clinical neuropsychologist or cognitive neuroscientist in the neurosurgical management of patients. Intervention techniques provided by neuropsychologists are described. Complex tasks, which are often necessary to quantify an ability or deficit, are referenced. The best predictors of functional outcome after brain damage are social and executive function status and not motor or sensory disorders.

Later in the chapter, the importance of quantifying performance and using neuropsychological tests to predict real-life behaviors is reviewed. A substantial proportion of the chapter is dedicated to noting how advances in cognitive neuroscience are contributing to clinicians' ability to evaluate and intervene with patients undergoing neurosurgery. The neuropsychological assessment of cancer patients serves as an example of how the application of various neuropsychological techniques can provide valuable information for the neurosurgical team, the patient's family, and, of course, the patient. The chapter concludes with mention of new cognitive neuroscience findings, with a particular focus on neuroplasticity and opportunities to integrate them into the neurosurgical management of patients.

Full text of this chapter is available online at ExpertConsult.com 

TABLE 56-1 Some Potential Uses of Neuropsychology

Type of Neuropsychological Input	Practitioner	Goal
Broad-based or targeted neuropsychological evaluation	Clinical neuropsychologist	Characterizing the patient's cognition, social skills, personality, and mood Prediction of outcome
Repeated neuropsychological evaluations	Clinical neuropsychologist	Characterizing recovery of function over time Documenting presurgical and postsurgical (or other intervention) changes in function
Neuropsychological rehabilitation	Clinical neuropsychologist (providing supervision)	Targeted or general improvement in some aspect of neuropsychological function Facilitating functional outcome
Neuropsychological monitoring during surgery	Clinical neuropsychologist or cognitive neuroscientist	Characterizing brain areas concerned with specific neuropsychological functions for clinical or research purposes
Postsurgical neuropsychological testing with implanted electrodes (e.g., on-off stimulation)	Cognitive neuroscientist or clinical neuropsychologist	Characterizing brain areas concerned with specific neuropsychological functions for research purposes
Postsurgical neuropsychological testing on groups of patients with specific excisions (e.g., anterior temporal lobe)	Cognitive neuroscientist or clinical neuropsychologist	Characterizing brain areas concerned with specific neuropsychological functions for research purposes

57 Neurosurgical Epidemiology and Outcomes Assessment

Catherine Miller, Hugh Garton, Frederick G. Barker II, and Stephen J. Haines

In this chapter, we focus on the application of statistical and epidemiologic principles to neurosurgical diagnosis, measurement, outcomes assessment and improvement, and critical review competence, which together provide the skill set necessary to develop an evidence-based approach to clinical practice. As the evidence base for neurosurgery evolves, its influence on the practice of neurosurgery will increase. The neurosurgeon who wishes to provide the best care for his or her patients must become familiar with the tools to access the rapidly growing base of high-quality evidence regarding neurosurgical practice.

The chapter begins by reviewing the potential sources of error encountered during clinical research, and how these biases affect study design as well as outcomes. We debate multiple methods employed to deal with confounding variables, such as standardization, stratification, matching, and randomization. The use of accurate statistical analysis in outcomes assessment is imperative to arrive at a correct conclusion. Definitions of several fundamental principles of statistical analysis are given and their applications discussed.

We then address how statistics and probability are involved in the diagnosis of neurosurgical illness. Diagnosis requires the development of a list of possible explanations for the patient's complaints to form a differential diagnosis. Through the work-up of a patient, the probability of particular diagnoses is weighed against history and examination findings. The properties of diagnostic tests such as sensitivity, specificity, predictive value, and likelihood ratios are reviewed, and we demonstrate how to calculate and interpret each property.

Neurosurgeons are becoming increasingly aware of the need to offer concrete scientific support for their medical practices. Tradition and reasoning from pathophysiologic principles, while important in generating hypotheses, are not a substitute for scientific method. Determining how and what outcomes should be measured is necessary to develop improved outcome assessments. We examine techniques of outcome measurement and many of the available measurement instruments used in neurosurgery.

Clinical researchers and clinicians using clinical research must be familiar with the various research designs available and commonly used in the medical literature. To better understand the features of study design, it is helpful to consider factors that limit the ability of a study to answer a question. We list specific study designs with descriptions of the usefulness and pitfalls of each study method. Because randomized clinical trials provide the best evidence for clinical practice, we offer a brief summary of the design of these trials.

We finally broach the topic of how to evaluate newly developed technologies. The chapter ends with a review of the well-defined process of evaluation and introduction of new drugs, as well as the application of this process to the introduction of new surgical techniques.

Full text of this chapter is available online at ExpertConsult.com

Symptoms, Signs, and Predictive Values

Context	Symptom/Sign	PPV (95% CI if Available)	Sensitivity	Specificity	NPV	Prevalence of the Disorder	Reference
Sciatica, evaluation for lumbar HNP	Typical description of sciatic pain	71%	46%	84%		46%	22
	Straight-leg raise	51%-90%	91% (78%-97%)	32% (17%-52%)		46%-89%	22
	Crossed straight-leg raise	97%-100%	32% (16%-54%)	98% (94%-99%)		74%-89%	22
	Weak tibialis anterior	93%	54%	89%		74%	22
	Weak extensor hallucis longus	91%	62%	50%		89%	22
	Sensory loss	66%-87%	28%-0.6%	57%-65%		58%-89%	22
						See also Deyo et al.	12
Evaluation for increased ICP	Loss of spontaneous venous pulsations	75%	100%	87%	100%	47%	23
Evaluation for ICP >15 mm Hg in patients with craniosynostosis	Papilledema	87%	32%	98%	74%	14%	24
Evaluation for shunt failure in pediatric patients	Failure of CSF shunt pumping chamber to depress and refill appropriately	21%	18%-20%	81%-83%	78%-81%	18%-22%	25
	Seizure	2.9%					26
Evaluation of children after first shunt placement for shunt failure within 5 months after shunt placement	Irritability	78% (61%-90%)	39%	96%	82%	26%	27
	Fluid tracking around shunt	75% (51%-91%)	21%	98%	77%	26%	27
	Decreased level of consciousness	100% (59%-100%)	10%	100%	75%	26%	27
	Bulging fontanelle	92% (79%-98%)	51%	98%	85%	26%	27

CI, confidence interval; CSF, cerebrospinal fluid; HNP, herniated nucleus pulposus; ICP, intracranial pressure; NPV, negative predictive value; PPV, positive predictive value.

Overview and Controversies

Robert A. McGovern, Guy M. McKhann II, Itzhak Fried, Andrew W. McEvoy, Steven V. Pacia, Dennis D. Spencer, and Nitin Tandon

This introductory chapter has two components: an initial overview of the contents of the epilepsy section and a discussion of various controversial topics related to epilepsy that neurosurgeons, irrespective of their experience, face when caring for patients with epilepsy. Our goal was to incorporate new and recent information into every chapter. The addition of new topics has also increased the comprehensive nature of the epilepsy section. Since publication of the previous edition, a number of techniques have begun to change epilepsy surgery, with more minimally invasive monitoring approaches and treatment options. These techniques are highlighted in this "Epilepsy" section, and their pros and cons are pointed out in the "Controversies in Epilepsy" section of this introductory chapter.

OVERVIEW

The "Epilepsy" section, divided into five parts, is designed to review progress and advances in the field.

Part 1, "Basic Science of Epilepsy," focuses on electrophysiologic properties of the central nervous system (Chapter 58), animal models responsible for scientific advances (Chapter 59), and malformations of cortical development frequently observed in patients with epilepsy (Chapter 60). These basic sciences are directly relevant to epilepsy and for the practicing neurosurgeon.

Part 2, "Approach to the Patient," deals with the clinical evaluation and monitoring. The diagnosis and classification of seizures are covered in Chapter 61, and antiepileptic medications are described in Chapter 62. Chapter 63 is a review of the application and value of external electroencephalography (EEG).

Part 3, "Preoperative Evaluation for Epilepsy," extensively reviews the preoperative work-up. Chapters 64 and 65 focus broadly on the preoperative assessment of epilepsy patients and the neuroradiologic evaluation. Subsequent chapters elaborate on more specific aspects of the preoperative evaluation: magnetoencephalography (MEG)/magnetic source imaging (Chapter 66), single-photon emission computed tomography (SPECT; Chapter 67), and Wada testing (Chapter 68).

Part 4, "Intraoperative Mapping and Monitoring for Cortical Resections," begins with Chapter 69, in which the authors present and analyze these intraoperative techniques, including motor, sensory, and language regions. Chapter 70 outlines the investigation of human cognition in patients undergoing epilepsy surgery.

Part 5, "Specific Operative Approaches," contains reviews of these approaches and many intraoperative videos. These chapters cover the gamut of operative approaches utilized in the treatment of epilepsy. Chapter 71 is a discussion of intracranial monitoring with subdural grid and strip recording, and Chapter 72 focuses on stereotactic implantation of EEG depth electrodes (stereoelectroencephalography [SEEG]). Then surgical techniques for the follow procedures are reviewed: corpus callosotomy, multiple subpial transections, and topectomy (Chapter 73); extratemporal epilepsy (Chapter 74); standard temporal lobectomy (Chapter 75); selective approaches to mesial temporal lobe epilepsy (Chapter 76); and hemispheric disconnection procedures (Chapter 77). Subsequently, chapters deal with radiosurgical treatment for epilepsy (Chapter 78) and electrical stimulation for epilepsy (Chapter 79). Chapter 80 deals comprehensively with surgical outcomes and complications.

CONTROVERSIES IN EPILEPSY

Of the many controversies in the field of epilepsy, we have chosen to focus on those that are most directly relevant to epilepsy surgeons, epilepsy surgery pathology, and the general care of patients with epilepsy who undergo neurosurgery.

Do Animal Models of Epilepsy Mimic the Human Disease?

An ideal animal model of epilepsy would reproduce the relevant features of the human condition.[1,2] These include behavioral seizures of similar age at onset and type, EEG abnormalities, focal pathologic features, behavioral comorbidity, and response to antiepileptic therapy. It is not surprising that no animal model meets all of these criteria successfully.

Some of the most common epilepsy surgical pathologies are mesial temporal sclerosis (MTS); malformations of cortical development (MCDs), including focal cortical dysplasia; focal neocortical (stroke, posttraumatic) epilepsies; and low-grade primary brain neoplasms such as ganglioglioma or dysembryoplastic neuroepithelial tumor (DNET). There are many models of MTS, including most prominently kindling and drug-induced (kainic acid and pilocarpine) models. The kindling model provides evidence that "seizures beget seizures," a long-held tenet of human epilepsy.[3] This propagative nature of epilepsy is not universally proven or accepted but remains a primary motivation for stopping epilepsy as soon as possible in patients. The drug-induced models of MTS remain useful, particularly for their time course and pathologic alterations in relation to the human condition.[4,5]

For MCDs, there are both induced and genetic models. Brain lesions can be induced by chemicals, freezing, or irradiation, and all of these models have relative strengths and weaknesses. For some rare monogenetic conditions, mouse models recapitulate aspects of both the pathologic mechanisms and seizures of the human condition (see Chapter 59). Over the past two decades, a variety of alterations affecting the mammalian target of rapamycin (mTOR) pathway have been implicated in various forms of MCD. Further investigation of these and related models will advance the understanding of mTOR pathway disorders in humans.[6] There are limited animal models of chronic focal neocortical epilepsy and low-grade tumor–induced epilepsy.

In order to develop better models of human epilepsy, investigators first have to better understand the human condition that they are actually modeling. For example, in human neocortical epilepsy, it is becoming clear with advances in neuroimaging that many cases previously thought to be "magnetic resonance imaging

(MRI) normal" actually arise from very subtle MCDs that can be detected only with advanced imaging paradigms or high–field strength magnets.[7] As epilepsy surgery becomes less invasive and more attention is directed toward primary lesioning procedures such as laser interstitial thermal therapy (LITT) or Gamma Knife radiosurgery, there will be less human tissue to investigate for pathophysiologic conditions. It is thus imperative to continue to develop animal models that better recapitulate the various subtypes of human epilepsy.

Is Levetiracetam Safe and Efficacious for Patients Undergoing Neurosurgery or with Status Epilepticus?

Since its release, levetiracetam (Keppra) has been increasingly used for treatment and prevention of seizures in hospitalized patients. This is not surprising in view of its availability in intravenous form, an incidence of allergic reactions lower than that of older drugs such as phenytoin,[8] its efficacy for partial and generalized seizures,[9] its favorable pharmacokinetics,[10] and its minimal effects on blood pressure.[11] In addition, several small series have demonstrated levetiracetam to be as equally effective as phenytoin for seizure treatment and prophylaxis for patients undergoing neurosurgery.[12-15] According to most of these reviews, levetiracetam has few drawbacks, except for cost, which may be comparable with that of older drugs such as valproate and phenytoin, depending on how often blood levels are measured.[16,17]

Unfortunately, well-controlled comparative efficacy data for patients taking levetiracetam versus both older agents (phenytoin and valproate) and newer agents (lacosamide) after neurosurgery are unavailable. Although data about the adjunctive use of levetiracetam in status epilepticus are more plentiful, the efficacy rates vary widely, from 44% to 94%; retrospective studies have demonstrated greater efficacy than have prospective ones.[18] To date, class I data do not exist to support the choice of levetiracetam over any other antiepileptic drug (AED) after the generally accepted use of benzodiazepines as first-line treatment of status epilepticus.[19] In addition, although levetiracetam appears to have an overall favorable intensive care unit profile, mood and cognitive side effects are well described, including the development of postictal psychosis in three of 50 patients treated with levetiracetam and lorazepam for status epilepticus.[20] This finding warrants further validation but may be underreported. Finally, levetiracetam has also produced conflicting results in animal models of status epilepticus.[21,22]

In summary, levetiracetam has been an enormously popular and useful AED for various populations of patients with seizures and epilepsy. However, efficacy and safety data for neurosurgical and status epilepticus patients remain incomplete. Fortunately, at least one large-scale, multicenter study of status epilepticus is under way,[23] as is a prospective multicenter registry for status epilepticus, to help answer these questions.[24]

Can Antiepileptic Medications Be Discontinued after Successful Epilepsy Surgery?

Tapering or discontinuing AEDs in any patient with a seizure disorder is difficult and anxiety provoking for patients and physicians. After the extensive diagnostic evaluations and prolonged hospitalizations necessary for successful epilepsy surgery, patients desire a life without medication side effects, regular blood tests, and numerous physician visits. Unfortunately, creating guidelines for AED discontinuation after epilepsy surgery is inherently difficult. Resective procedures are often tailored to the epileptogenic zone and its proximity to functional or eloquent cortex; thus some resections are "more complete" than others. Causes, such as trauma, may give rise to multiple epileptogenic foci in the same patient, some amenable to resection and others still necessitating AEDs to maintain seizure control. As a result, blanket recommendations for AED discontinuation that are based on prespecified periods of seizure control with AEDs are likely to fall short in some cases.[25]

In a survey of Canadian epileptologists, the most important factors influencing the decision to withdraw AEDs after surgery were negative EEG findings, patient preference, and unilateral MTS.[26] Conversely, the desire to drive, abnormal EEG patterns, persistent auras, seizures after discharge, and presurgical multifocal, bilateral, or diffuse findings were reasons to continue AED therapy. In this survey, most physicians required a seizure-free period of more than 1 year before AED reduction can be considered. However, studies have demonstrated differing seizure recurrence rates after AED tapering according to duration of seizure freedom. One review of 97 pediatric epilepsy surgery cases concluded that 84% of patients who were seizure free at 6 months would achieve long-term seizure freedom off medication.[27] In contrast, in an earlier study, 36% of patients had seizures by 5 years when AEDs were discontinued, in comparison with only 7% of patients taking AEDs.[25]

Although all breakthrough seizures related to AED tapering carry a small risk of injury, an even greater fear is that patients could return to a permanent medically refractory state. Again, studies conflict with regard to the magnitude of this risk. A 2005 pediatric study of 260 children identified 3 children whose seizures became medically refractory after postoperative seizure freedom for more than 1 year.[28] In contrast, a large European collaborative study of epilepsy surgery in children concluded that AED withdrawal had no influence on long-term outcome or cure.[29] A very different conclusion was reached in a more recent series of 609 patients who underwent epilepsy surgery, of whom 35% failed to achieve a 2-year remission if seizures occurred during AED tapering.[30]

The goal of resective epilepsy surgery is complete seizure freedom without functional impairment, as well as freedom from the burden of AED therapy. Clearly, many patients achieve seizure freedom and are able to diminish or discontinue AEDs. However, until more information is gathered from well-controlled long-term studies, AED discontinuation after epilepsy surgery continues to be a difficult decision that must be carefully individualized.

What Is the Optimal Neuroimaging Evaluation in a Candidate for Epilepsy Surgery?

Structural Imaging

The outcomes after epilepsy surgery are heavily influenced by whether a lesion was resected. A large meta-analysis of 42 publications about 3557 patients revealed that in cases with a lesion discernible on MRI, 69% of patients undergoing temporal lobe resection and 66% of those undergoing extratemporal resections were seizure free, whereas in patients without discernible lesions, 45% of those undergoing temporal lobe resection and 34% of those undergoing extratemporal resections were seizure free. Overall, the odds of being seizure free after surgery are 2.5 times higher in patients with lesions demonstrated on MRI or histopathologic study (odds ratio, 2.5; $P < .001$).[31] In addition, nonlesional patients undergoing surgery have a greater possibility of both new cognitive deficits as well as continued, unchanged intractable epilepsy.[32]

Identification of anatomic abnormalities and epileptogenic lesions is a crucial component of the presurgical evaluation in patients with medically refractory epilepsy, and high-quality MRI imaging in the evaluation of epilepsy is therefore essential. A dedicated MRI epilepsy protocol optimized for lesion detection is crucial, as is a retrospective assessment of cases with equivocal

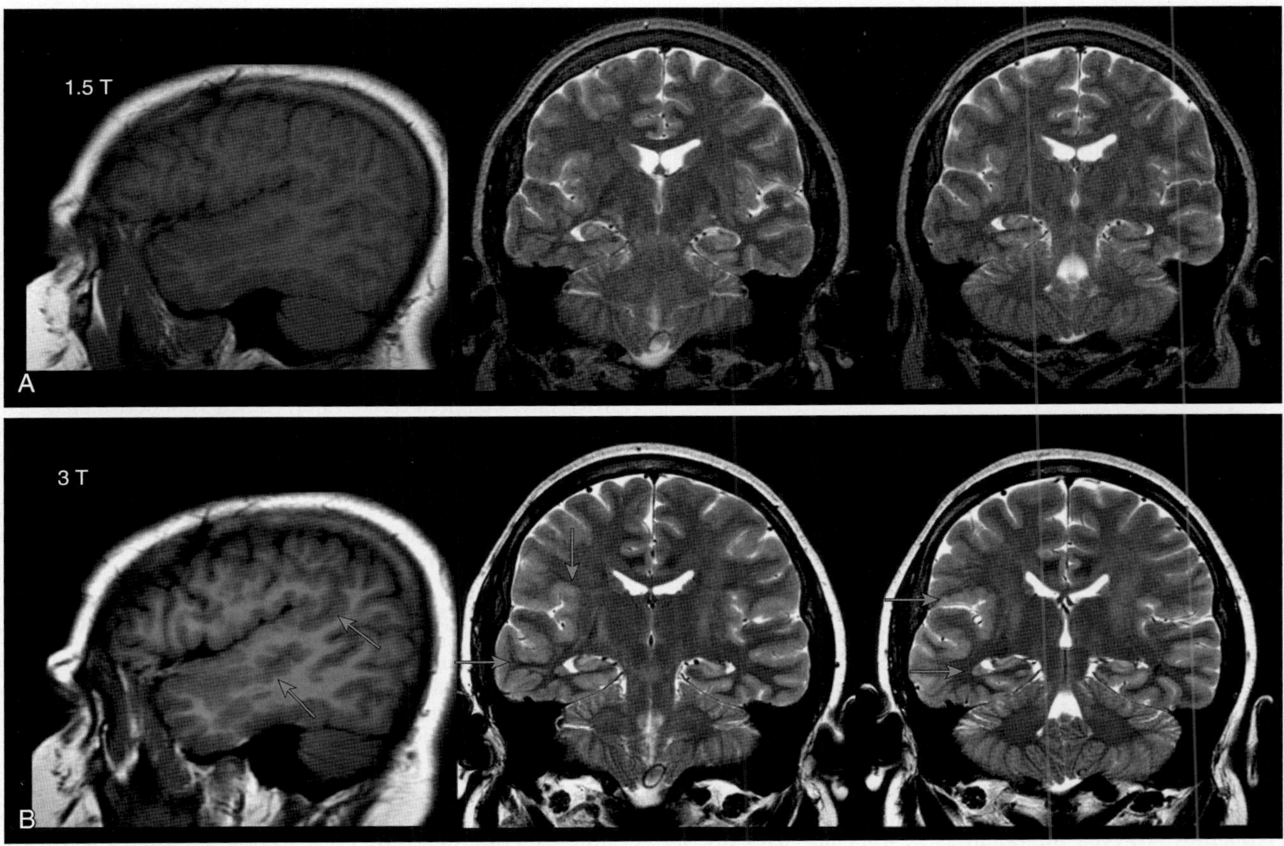

Figure III-1. Sagittal and axial T1-weighted images obtained on 1.5-T and 3-T magnetic resonance scanners. The 3-T images **(B)** clearly depict polymicrogyria along the sylvian fissure and superior temporal sulcus, as well as subependymal heterotopic nodules and aberrant right temporal lobe sulcation *(arrows).* These findings are only hinted at in the 1.5-T scans **(A).** For comparison, 3-T images through the contralateral hemisphere demonstrate a normal appearance of the cortex.

findings or thought to be nonlesional on MRI imaging driven by results of scalp EEG, MEG, semiology, and positron emission tomography/SPECT studies.[33] Such imaging should be performed on a 3-T (or higher) scanner whenever possible, and the imaging protocol should ensure that high-resolution images are obtained through the whole brain (Fig. III-1).

Is Wada Testing Still Necessary before Temporal Lobe Epilepsy Surgery?

The Wada test has proved to be an important tool in the presurgical evaluation of epilepsy surgery since the 1960s. However, epilepsy centers have been reevaluating its role because of concerns about complications related to the invasive nature of this procedure; problems with its reliability and validity; and difficulties with a worldwide shortage of sodium amytal.

Clinical practice varies widely with regard to the proportion of presurgical candidates undergoing the Wada test (from zero to 100%). The availability of noninvasive alternatives, particularly functional MRI, but more recently MEG and transcranial magnetic stimulation, have at the very least led many centers to question the use of the Wada test on a case-by-case basis to ensure that the risk-benefit ratio is appropriate for every patient.[34]

Functional MRI is being used exclusively in some centers to lateralize and localize language in candidates for epilepsy surgery. The use of tailored resections to spare language and memory function, along with the widely practiced technique of craniotomy while the patient is awake has led many centers to question the need for a Wada study.

It has become more widely accepted that no patient has become amnestic after temporal lobe resection if results of other tests (volumetric MRI, T2-weighted relaxometry, and baseline neuropsychological function) indicated that the structure and function of the contralateral mesial temporal structures were intact. The risks with the Wada test seem to outweigh the chances of postoperative amnesia syndrome in many patients with temporal lobe epilepsy. However, despite advances in functional imaging, the Wada test for lateralizing language remains important in cases with a higher probability of atypical hemispheric dominance: that is, left-handed patients and those with large left hemispheric lesions acquired early in life.[35-37]

Minimally Invasive versus Maximally Resective Epilepsy Surgery: What Will Improve Safety and Outcomes?

The extent of resection in nonlesional cases is a matter of balancing epileptogenicity against function.[38-40] The goals of resective surgery are to maximize seizure outcomes and to minimize the double-negative outcome of a new cognitive deficit in addition to unchanged and still intractable epilepsy. The approach of large en bloc resections or large disconnections should be used only in patients with truly devastating epilepsies; other patients should undergo a careful evaluation with intracranial techniques (described later). In the United States and parts of western

Europe, intracranial monitoring has traditionally consisted of subdural electrode arrays. However, as a result of improvements in neuroimaging and stereotactic robotic technology, SEEG has been used in an increased number of epilepsy centers in preference to subdural recording in many clinical situations. Because of less invasiveness and lower rates of morbidity, many patients and families unwilling to consider a large craniotomy for subdural monitoring are amenable to SEEG implantation. A strategy favoring electrode monitoring implantations over large up-front resections provides the opportunity to more readily consider less extensive resective options, as well as other approaches such as neuromodulation or nonresection. A pediatric SEEG series in which minimal resections were carried out in accordance with this general philosophy showed a 60% rate of seizure freedom at 2 years postoperatively.[41]

When Is Invasive Brain Recording Necessary? Which Technique Is Preferable: Subdural Recording or Stereo-Electroencephalography?

The decision to proceed with surgical resection requires locating the seizure focus, a prerequisite to formulating a surgical plan. Initially, noninvasive techniques are used in an attempt to localize the seizure focus. Scalp EEG often provides sufficient information about the side and hemispheric region of the seizure focus. In addition, MRI can demonstrate discrete lesions, such as hippocampal sclerosis observed in mesial temporal lobe epilepsy (MTLE), subtle gray and white matter changes in focal cortical dysplasia, tumors, or vascular malformations. In cases in which the results of seizure semiology, scalp EEG, and MRI are definitively concordant, patients may undergo surgical resection without invasive monitoring.

Frequently, however, the noninvasive work-up yields discordant results, and a seizure focus cannot be identified definitively. In these cases, invasive electrocorticography should be used to localize the focus and guide surgical treatment.[42] Subdural electrodes can be placed over the regions of putative seizure onset, and then the grids or strips can be monitored extraoperatively for seizure activity, propagation, and interictal spiking. This technique has the advantage of significantly improved spatial resolution in comparison with scalp EEG because of its placement directly on the cortical surface and increased electrode density over the presumed epileptogenic sites. In addition, subdural electrodes are used for stimulation-based mapping of adjacent eloquent cerebral regions. Unfortunately, there are a host of complications typically associated with placement of subdural electrodes, such as infections (3%-4%),[43,44]; hemorrhages, including subdural, epidural, and intraparenchymal hematomas (2%-4%); and cerebrospinal fluid leak (5%-10%).[43,44]

Whereas subdural electrode placement is limited to recording from the cortical surface, SEEG affords the advantage of recording from deep epileptic foci, more readily allows for bilateral implantation, and can better define the epileptogenic zone in three dimensions; thus it potentially improves the ability to localize an epileptic focus. In addition, its less invasive nature underlies its potential for fewer complications than does open subdural implantation surgery. A meta-analysis demonstrated a much lower prevalence of infectious (0.8%) and hemorrhagic (1%) complications after SEEG in comparison with subdural monitoring.[45] The question becomes one of which cases are better suited to SEEG than to subdural implants.

For subdural recordings, the ideal indications include superficial neocortical lesions for which further delineation of the epileptogenic zone is needed or are in eloquent areas such as language centers that need to be mapped. In addition, in children younger than 3 years, SEEG is technically more difficult to perform because of skull thickness, and subdural implants may be necessary. SEEG is ideal for lesions such as deep sulcal focal cortical dysplasia or those involving the limbic system, such as insula, cingulate cortex, or medial parietal lobe. In addition, SEEG is particularly useful in nonlesional cases in which extensive unilateral or bilateral implants are needed or in which the patient has undergone a prior craniotomy or in whom prior epilepsy surgery failed.

Placement of both subdural and SEEG electrodes is generally safe and effective for localizing an epileptic focus in patients with discordant findings on noninvasive imaging. Although complications are an accepted aspect of each procedure, they can be minimized. For subdural grid placement, meticulous surgical technique, generous duroplasty, and careful postoperative sterility can all help minimize infection and mass effect–related complications of subdural electrode implants. Careful preoperative surgical planning through the use of fused contrast-enhanced MRI and computed tomography–based volumetric images helps minimize the risk of intraoperative hemorrhage for placement of SEEG depth electrodes. Because SEEG electrode placement is less invasive, research will probably continue to demonstrate that this technique has a lower complication rate. However, studies must also demonstrate that SEEG electrode placement results in comparable seizure freedom rates.

ATL versus SAH versus LITT versus SRS for MTLE

A multidisciplinary team can use an alphabet soup of surgical options to treat MTLE. Significant evidence indicates that open surgical approaches for epilepsy—anterior temporal lobectomy (ATL) and selective amygdalohippocampectomy (SAH)—are superior to continued medical therapy in patients with pharmacoresistant MTLE. Two randomized, controlled trials have demonstrated seizure freedom rates of 60% to 70% at 2 to 5 years after temporal lobe surgical resection, in comparison with 0% to 10% of patients continuing medical therapy.[46,47] For these patients, open surgical resection is defined as either removal of the anterior two thirds of the temporal lobe (standard ATL) or a more selective resection of mesial temporal structures (SAH).

Selective Amygdalohippocampectomy versus Anterior Temporal Lobectomy

Because lateral temporal neocortex is thought to be intimately involved in verbal memory and visual naming, researchers in neuropsychological studies have attempted to examine the potential benefits of sparing this cortex in SAH, particularly in dominant temporal lobe surgery. Indeed, the result of years of cognitive outcomes research has shown that patients undergoing dominant ATL tend to have persistent deficits in verbal memory and word finding.[48,49] In addition, those with MTS generally have worse cognitive baselines and exhibit less of a decline than do those without MTS documented on MRI and pathologic study, whereas those without MTS tend to have higher baseline cognitive scores and exhibit a more severe decline postoperatively.[50]

In many retrospective studies, investigators have compared seizure outcomes, cognitive outcomes, or both after ATL with those after SAH, but in no published prospective, controlled trials have patients been randomly assigned to undergo either ATL or SAH. These studies are weakened by the fact that many neurosurgeons in the field began performing mostly SAH surgeries after 2005 and have mainly compared data from ATL procedures performed at the beginning of the study period with those from SAH procedures toward the end of the study period.[51,52] Nevertheless, some patterns have become apparent when the literature is examined in totality.

First, almost every direct comparison study has shown equivalent seizure freedom rates (60%-90% at 3-6 years of follow-up) between SAH and ATL in adult patients,[51,53-57] with exceptions.[58] In addition, studies describing only SAH[59-63] have shown seizure freedom rates similar to those in historic ATL data.[64] Second, most cognitive outcome studies in which SAH and ATL were compared have shown slightly better results for SAH, although a meta-analysis did not reveal a difference between surgical approaches.[65] The most consistent finding across multiple retrospective studies is a lesser decline in verbal memory after dominant lobe SAH than after ATL[51,57,66]; in some studies, a higher percentage of patients actually exhibited improvement in verbal memory postoperatively.[55] Other studies have demonstrated improved nonverbal memory in nondominant SAH in comparison with ATL,[52,67] as well as improved immediate recall.[57] Of interest, one reason that patients who undergo SAH still demonstrate verbal memory and language difficulties may be "collateral damage" (T2/fluid-attenuated inversion recovery [FLAIR] signal change) along the surgical approach route: one group showed that an increase in damage to this tissue was predictive of worse memory outcome.[68] Again, however, some studies have shown no difference between techniques.[69-71] In an effort to improve on both the neuropsychological outcomes and complications associated with open surgery, less invasive therapeutic options have been developed.

Laser Interstitial Thermal Therapy

LITT is a technique in which a laser fiber is stereotactically implanted into the region of choice and progressively heated in order to thermally ablate the region under MRI guidance. This process allows for the generation of nearly real-time observation of lesion creation. There are a few advantages afforded by this approach. First, this technique allows for the ablation of deep subcortical regions that may be difficult to access surgically while the lesion is observed in nearly real time. Second, the minimally invasive nature of this approach provides for shorter hospital stays and, potentially, fewer complications in comparison with traditional open surgical approaches. Third, given the ability to generate a lesion in nearly real time with image guidance, this technique has the potential benefit of limiting cognitive deficits postoperatively.

Because LITT remains a new technique, the literature on its use for MTLE is limited. In one case series, 13 patients from 16 to 64 years of age received stereotactic laser amygdalohippocampotomy for medically refractory mesial temporal seizures.[72] Of the 9 patients with MTS documented on MRI, 6 were seizure free on follow-up (5-26 months); however, only one of the four patients without MTS documented on MRI attained seizure freedom. In a more recent case series, Kang and colleagues[73] demonstrated slightly more pessimistic findings: 8 (53%) of 15 patients were seizure free at 6 months and only 4 (36%) of 11 patients at 1 year. All but 1 of their patients had MTS. Adverse events that occurred during both studies included the development of homonymous hemianopia in 2 patients and the development of an acute subdural hematoma in 1 patient and an intraparenchymal hematoma in another, both of which resolved without evacuation. One patient also developed a transient fourth cranial nerve palsy. As expected, postoperative hospital stay was short, ranging from 1 to 3 days. In terms of neuropsychological data, Drane and associates[74] compared outcomes in 19 patients who received LITT for MTLE with outcomes of standard open surgical resections. LITT recipients demonstrated improved visual naming in comparison with patients who underwent open surgery. Kang and colleagues[73] also examined cognitive outcomes in their case series and found preservation of contextual verbal memory postoperatively but declines in noncontextual memory, although these data were available for only 6 patients and could not be compared with those of patients undergoing open surgical resection. As discussed previously, the theoretical benefit of LITT is obvious, but more research is needed to further elucidate this matter.

Stereotactic Radiosurgery

Stereotactic radiosurgery (SRS) is a technique in which a source of ionizing radiation is directed at a stereotactically defined target in order to create a lesion in the tissue. This approach affords many of the same advantages of LITT. Because of its noninvasive nature, patients go home the same day, although the procedure does not enable the surgeon to visualize the lesion in real time. Of importance, however, is that unlike the effect of LITT, the effect of SRS on seizure frequency is delayed; a maximum reduction in seizures is typically observed 12 to 18 months after treatment.[75] During this time, seizures continue to occur, and the risk of associated morbidity and mortality (sudden unexplained death in epilepsy) probably remains.[76,77]

Two large, prospective SRS studies with long-term follow-up[78,79] have been conducted in groups of 15 and 30 patients, respectively. In both studies, the investigators used similar treatment protocols, with a marginal dose of 24 Gy and the total volume of the 50% isodense target area between 5.5 and 9 mL. Both studies showed similar outcomes, with 60% and 67% freedom from seizures (Engel classes IA and IB) rates at 8 and 2 years' follow-up, respectively. Few neuropsychological outcome studies of SRS for MTLE have been performed, although the large, prospective studies just discussed mainly showed no difference in cognitive outcomes after SRS. The most detailed data come from an American multicenter prospective trial,[80] which showed no overall differences in language or verbal memory for dominant lobe SRS, although patients did show mild decreases in confrontation naming and noncontextual verbal memory. Régis and colleagues[77] reported stable or improved cognitive outcomes in all patients, but detailed data were not made available. However, 55% of these patients had the lowest baseline cognitive outcome score; therefore, it was impossible for them to decline according to this measure. The issue of long-term cognitive outcome therefore, is probably still in question for SRS in MTLE.

In view of the options just presented, the treating neurosurgeon is confronted with a number of possibilities to offer patients with MTLE who are referred for surgical evaluation. Because of similar outcomes of open surgical approaches, a surgeon's comfort with one surgical approach over another has traditionally been a reasonable strategy for producing good patient outcomes. Now, however, different possibilities arise. No matter how efficient or comfortable a surgeon is with an open surgical resective technique, no patient undergoing SAH or ATL will go home the same day or the next, as would a patient undergoing LITT or SRS. On the other hand, although this is still a preliminary finding, seizure freedom rates in patients receiving LITT appear to be lower than those in patients undergoing open surgical resection. Meanwhile, patients undergoing SRS will continue to experience seizures for a period of months. Thus a comprehensive epilepsy evaluation must be undertaken by neurologists and neuropsychologists, and the benefits and risks of each approach must be thoroughly discussed with each individual patient. These steps are essential for the modern neurosurgeon to decide on treatment.

Electrical Stimulation: What Kind and Where?

The notion of using electricity to modulate aberrant cerebral electrical activity is conceptually appealing and one that will probably enable physicians to treat many more epilepsies than resective procedures can. However, despite the availability of three devices (two that have received approval by the U.S. Food and Drug Administration and one that has CE marking in the European Economic Area), the effectiveness of these devices in providing durable relief from seizures has been limited. In addition, these devices incur significant and recurring costs, and they limit the types and field strengths at which MRI scans, which might help evaluate the epilepsy further, can be obtained.

In randomized prospective studies, the rate of success with vagus nerve stimulation in mean seizure reduction was approximately 25% to 35%. Longer term open-label, uncontrolled data suggest 50% responder rates at 1 to 5 years.[81,82] In a pivotal U.S. trial of anterior thalamus deep brain stimulation,[83] the median rate of seizure reduction was 40%, with further reduction to 56% on unblinded extension at 25 months. A double-blind randomized controlled trial of responsive neurostimulation[84] showed a mean seizure reduction of 37.9% among patients who received active stimulation, in contrast to 17.3% in the sham control group, but a 50% reduction was achieved in equivalent numbers (29% and 27%, respectively) of these groups.

On average, only approximately 3% to 5% of patients undergoing any kind of neuromodulation become seizure free. A common feature with other neurostimulation studies is that the responder rate increases in the open-label phase, reaching approximately 50% to 60% at 2 years. It is possible that plasticity is induced by the longer duration of stimulation, but it is also possible that the effect on mood is durable and that the close clinical follow-up of these patients' compliance with medical therapy also has an effect. In the community setting, the use of vagus nerve stimulation/responsive neurostimulation on patients who have not undergone a systematic evaluation at a tertiary epilepsy program is inappropriate. With current technology, resective epilepsy surgery is designed with a primary goal of seizure cure, whereas stimulation techniques have a primary goal of seizure palliation.

Neural stimulation devices will probably have a more meaningful role in the future as the paradigms for seizure sensing and for neurostimulation are optimized, on the basis of an understanding of the neurobiologic features of epileptic networks, to yield treatment effects more robust than current effects. In addition, seizure detection may eventually be coupled with other therapeutic modalities such as focal cooling or focal drug delivery to improve patient outcomes.

Tumor Surgery versus Epilepsy Surgery for Patients with Glioma and Epilepsy: Is Invasive Monitoring Needed?

Epilepsy and tumors can manifest with a great degree of clinical overlap. Repeated seizures are a common presenting symptom of some brain tumors, and patients suffering from medically refractory epilepsy may be found to harbor a tumor. Interestingly, the time interval between seizure onset and surgery differs markedly between these groups (Fig. III-2). Because long progression-free survival can be achieved with early aggressive management of low-grade tumors, durable seizure control in these patients is imperative.

Epilepsy is a common neurological manifestation in patients with primary infiltrative brain tumors, occurring in 60% to 100% of patients with low-grade tumors and 25% to 60% of those with high-grade gliomas.[85,86] Seizures probably arise in neocortical regions at the infiltrating margin of gliomas, where invading tumor cells intermingle with neurons and induce alterations in neuronal physiologic properties. Currently, the therapeutic approach most effective in ameliorating seizures in patients with glioma is to maximize tumor resection to include the infiltrating tumor margins.[87] However, when therapy fails and the tumors recur, patients usually present with new or worsening seizures.[88]

The location of tumors plays an important role in the management of tumoral epilepsy. Although the traditional surgical strategy in tumor-related epilepsy is a lesionectomy, more extensive resection may be indicated for tumors in the temporal lobe.[89-91] Seizures commonly accompany tumors that are situated predominantly in the frontal, temporal, and insular regions, as well as those that are located close to the cortical surface.[92] Tumors that are in the temporal lobe or in the perirolandic region carry the greatest risk for seizure occurrence, especially with incomplete resections, but also with complete resections.[93]

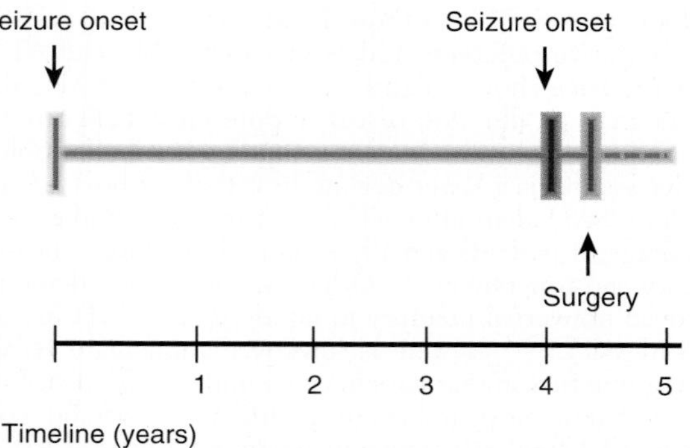

Figure III-2. Timeline demonstrating the spectrum of seizure onset and timing of surgery in patients with tumor-related epilepsy. In *orange* is the time of seizure onset in a patient with epilepsy resulting from a brain tumor. In *blue* is the first seizure in a patient who presents with a mass and has a seizure. *Red* indicates the timing of surgery.

The presence of residual neoplasm, periresection gliosis, or hippocampal sclerosis may account for persistent seizure activity in these cases.[94] Decisions regarding the extent of resection depend on the status of and localization of sensorimotor, language, and memory functions and are individualized on the basis of the neuropsychological profile and functional state of the patient. In some patients with tumors, the epileptogenic zone may be remote from the tumor itself, and invasive intracranial recordings or intraoperative electrocorticography may be helpful for tailoring the resection. It is reasonable in the majority of cases of tumoral epilepsy to begin treatment by maximizing the extent of tumor resection, using mapping techniques and intraoperative electrocorticography as indicated. Epilepsy persistence after maximal tumor resection can then be managed as an epilepsy problem, with the possibility of invasive monitoring, if further surgical resection is an option from a risk-benefit perspective.

Will Imaging Make Intracranial Monitoring Obsolete?

There is no doubt that imaging techniques at higher field strength will help elucidate the epileptogenic zone structurally, neurochemically,[95] and, someday, perhaps functionally.[96] Thus far there has been no compelling evidence that purely structural imaging at higher fields will result in better delineation of brain regions with potential for seizure genesis,[97] but such advances are probably a matter of time and innovations in magnetic resonance physics. The aberrant connectivity and hemodynamics of dysplastic cortical tissue should be particularly amenable to detection. The use of automated morphometric analyses that have already shown promise in detecting subtle dysplasia at 3 T[7,98] will probably also benefit from higher field strength. However, it is unlikely that these imaging techniques will demonstrate how the regions detected in this manner contribute to the generation of seizures. In at least the foreseeable future, such imaging techniques will probably serve principally as a means of refining intracranial electrophysiologic targeting in the nonlesional neocortical epilepsies. The epilepsy alchemist's goal is to determine a metabolic or physiologic imaging biomarker that can reliably predict the epileptogenic zone interictally and help make intracranial monitoring obsolete in the future.

See a full reference list on ExpertConsult.com

58 Electrophysiologic Properties of the Mammalian Central Nervous System

Rebecca L. Achey, Guy M. McKhann II, and Damir Janigro

The study of excitable cells is, for a number of reasons, a fascinating one. Interest in electrophysiology and neuronal function spans many medical specialties because these excitable cells are those by which we move, think, and perform complex yet automatic tasks such as cardiovascular regulation. It is for these reasons that electrophysiologic studies have attracted the foremost physiologists of the last century. Despite these outstanding contributions, several fundamental issues in neuroscience remain unresolved. Traditionally, clinical electrophysiology has used a more holistic approach than nonclinical neurophysiology. Clinical insight into brain function (or dysfunction) is commonly achieved today by increasingly sophisticated imaging techniques, allowing real-time observations. The booming advancement of molecular biology and its fundamental contribution to medicine in general, and neuroscience in particular, has unveiled an incredible level of ordered complexity in neuronal function. Basic scientists are producing a large quantity of molecular data, spanning from investigations of the role of a single protein in the electric behavior of neurons to genetic markers of neurological disease. In spite of the immense popularity of these approaches, it is important to remember that the electrical properties of individual neurons and the neuronal environment are the final effectors of brain activity and that diseases of the brain derive from abnormalities at the cellular level. It is thus foreseeable that novel discoveries in neuroscience will continue to emerge as innovations in electrophysiologic signaling recording propel the field forward.

A typical brain-computer interface (BCI) system. The patient performs motor imagery that generates a specific pattern of brain activity to serve as a signal for the BCI. Signal acquisition occurs via electroencephalography (EEG), electrocorticography (ECoG), or intracortical signaling recording. Signal input from the different recording methods is digitized and processed via feature extraction and algorithmic translation by the computer. The algorithm then outputs device commands that can be used to operate a robotic arm, environmental controls, communication devices, wheelchairs, and other assistive devices for neurorehabilitation. *(Modified from Wolpaw JR, Birbaumer N, McFarland, et al. Brain-computer interfaces for communication and control.* Clin Neurophysiol. *2002;113:767-791; and Leuthardt EC, Schalk G, Moran D, et al. The emerging world of motor neuroprosthetics: a neurosurgical perspective.* Neurosurgery. *2006;59:1-14.)*

Central nervous system (CNS) function is dependent on homeostatic mechanisms that precisely regulate the extracellular level and concentration of neurotransmitters, ions, pH, and other variables. The neuronal cell membrane is a complex biochemical entity that interfaces between the cell and its environment. Its functions include the directional transport of specific substances and the maintenance of chemical gradients, particularly electrochemical gradients, across the plasma membrane. These ion gradients can be of high specificity (e.g., sodium versus potassium ions) and of great functional significance (e.g., in the production of action potentials). In addition, CNS function is supported by numerous nonneuronal mechanisms responsible for the control of extracellular and intracellular homeostasis (glial cells, cerebral vasculature). It has become increasingly evident that pathophysiologic changes in ion channel function play a major role in the development of certain disorders of the nervous system.

This brief introductory chapter on CNS electrophysiology does not attempt to explain in detail the complex biophysical properties underlying communication between individual neurons or transduction of environmental and sensory signals into electrical activity in specific regions of the brain or spinal cord. Several excellent textbooks deal with specific aspects of CNS function and electrophysiology, and recent publications describe in a concise yet comprehensive manner the complex properties of ion currents responsible for neuronal excitation. This chapter provides the reader with succinct background information on the electrical properties of neurons, and in addition focuses on other aspects of brain function relevant to modern understanding of the pathophysiologic changes occurring in the diseased brain. These include the description of some of the mechanisms involved in brain homeostasis, the genesis of synchronous activity by electrotonic and/or ephaptic interactions, and molecular changes in ion channels underlying neurological diseases. Because complete referencing of such a broad topic would entail a bibliography of thousands of citations, relevant recent reviews, textbooks, and a nonexhaustive compilation of representative work is included.

Full text of this chapter is available online at ExpertConsult.com 

59 Animal Models of Epilepsy

Maria Elisa Calcagnotto, Wyatt Potter, and Scott C. Baraban

In this chapter, available in full on ExpertConsult.com, we review models designed to mimic three broad classes of epileptic disorders: temporal lobe epilepsy, epilepsy associated with a brain malformation, and focal epilepsies.

Epilepsy affects a sizeable portion of the population worldwide and is responsible for a heavy social and economic burden.[1] Given that most epileptic disorders are attributed to uncontrolled and often medically intractable seizures, it is evident that further experimental studies offer hope for a deeper understanding of the underlying pathophysiology and, ultimately, better treatments. To achieve these goals, human studies, albeit of great value, may not be sufficient owing to both ethical and practical limitations.[2] As such, it is not surprising that animal models were developed and have significantly contributed to the epilepsy research literature. A common concern with all animal models is how reliable they are in mimicking the human condition. Are the anatomic and electrophysiologic similarities with human epileptic disorders real or superficial? To what extent can findings in animal research be extended to humans? And, perhaps most important, what new insights can be gained from animal model studies that cannot be predicted from clinical studies? In the design and interpretation of animal models, it is important to remember that epilepsy is not a single disease, a syndrome, or a homogeneous entity. Although a common feature of epilepsy is the tendency to have spontaneous epileptic seizures,[3] the many ways in which seizures are generated (and manifest) are quite varied. Seizures are caused by excessive and abnormal neuronal discharge; they can be motor, sensory, or autonomic. Epilepsy etiologies range from genetic to acquired to idiopathic.[4] Epilepsy symptoms are varied because they depend on the brain areas involved in a certain type of seizure, as well as on the stage of brain maturation. The type of seizure and presence of other symptoms can be used to define a specific *epileptic syndrome*. Because epilepsy involves many levels of structure and activity in the brain, from molecules to networks, with causes that range from genes to environmental insults, there is no surprise that many epilepsy models are needed.

A good model of epilepsy should reproduce as many salient aspects as possible for a specific type of human epilepsy.[5,6] Ideally, the model should demonstrate spontaneous behavioral seizures of the type (e.g., partial, absence, tonic-clonic) its human counterpart exhibits, as well as electroencephalographic (ictal and interictal discharges, focal or generalized) and structural (if any) brain abnormalities similar to those seen in the human epilepsy it mirrors. The etiology (e.g., cortical malformation [CM], genetic predisposition, focal gliosis) should, if possible, be the same as well. If the human epilepsy has a specific age of onset, the model should do the same. The animal model should have behavioral comorbidities (such as memory deficits or developmental retardation) that parallel the human. Finally, the model in question should respond to antiepileptic drugs (AEDs) in a manner similar to the human condition after which it is modeled. Although these goals are scientifically sound, few (if any) animal models actually fulfill all these criteria.

Animal Models	Advantages/Strengths	Disadvantages/Weaknesses
Temporal Lobe Epilepsy (TLE)[243]: Stimulus Induced		
Kindling	Process of epileptogenesis is easily controlled and reliably measured Minimal mortality Precision of epileptogenic focus Induced structural alterations are similar to the human TLE	Long time course to develop spontaneous seizures Uncertainty of developing spontaneous seizures Labor- and time-intensive Risk of losing or damaging the chronic electrode implantation Difficult to apply in mice or neonatal, infant rats
TLE: Chemically Induced		
Pilocarpine	Several network and neurochemical similarities between human TLE	Produces lesions in neocortical areas Variability and high mortality Time constraints and costs
Kainate	Induces habitually hippocampus-restricted injuries	Time constraints and costs
Cortical Malformation (CM)[244,245]: Injury Models		
Methylazoxymethanol (MAM)	Similar deficits found in dysplastic tissue samples from patients with focal cortical dysplasia and epilepsy Inexpensive and easy to handle Reproducible results	Does not mimic the etiology of a clinical malformation Rare spontaneous recurrent seizures
Irradiation	Presence of recurrent spontaneous seizures Reproducible results	Special hardware laboratory and training personnel
Freeze	Easy to develop Produces focal cortical alterations similar to human CM Reproducible results	Lack of recurrent spontaneous seizures
CM: Genetic Models		
tish Mutant rat	Similar seizure onset zone to the subcortical band heterotopia in humans Presence of recurrent spontaneous seizures	Gene responsible for this phenotype remains unknown Phenotype involves quite different molecular and cellular mechanisms
Reeler mutant	Severe disruption of brain development similar to humans	Lack of recurrent spontaneous seizures
Lis1 mutant	Exhibit significant hippocampal malformations and slowed migration of interneuron precursors Presence of spontaneous electrographic seizures	Display no neocortical abnormality
Focal[5,241]		
Aluminum	Induces spontaneous partial seizures similar to humans	Long and unpredictable latency period before clinical and electrographic onset of spontaneous seizures Use of monkeys
Ferrous	Short period to develop spontaneous recurrent seizures Alterations in cerebral tissue similar to posttraumatic epilepsy in humans	Labor intensive

60 Malformations of Cortical Development

Gregory G. Heuer and Peter B. Crino

This chapter will provide an overview of the neuropathologic, cell biologic, and molecular features of select malformations of cortical development (MCD).

Over the past two decades, there have been major advances in understanding the causes of MCD and the potential links to epilepsy, neurobehavioral disorders, and intellectual disabilities. MCD are highly associated with medically intractable epilepsy. In many cases, patients will require resective surgery to remove the tissue lesion as a therapeutic approach. This has provided a unique opportunity for direct investigation into abnormalities in gene sequence, mRNA expression, and protein translation that can be used for therapeutic discovery. There are currently more than 25 unique genes that have been identified as causative for MCD affecting a wide variety of encoded proteins (i.e., cell signaling, transport, cytoskeletal proteins). Mouse models have been generated for many as a strategy to study the pathogenic effects of these mutations. Some of the identified mutations occur as de novo or inherited germline events in some MCD, such as tuberous sclerosis complex and lissencephaly, and are encoded on autosomal or X chromosomes. In contrast, a growing body of evidence shows that a number of MCD result from somatic mutations that occur in neuroglial progenitor cells during brain development. Somatic mutations are not inherited and result in sporadic focal brain abnormalities of varying size (i.e., focal cortical dysplasia [FCD], hemimegalencephaly), but no other manifestations in the rest of the body.

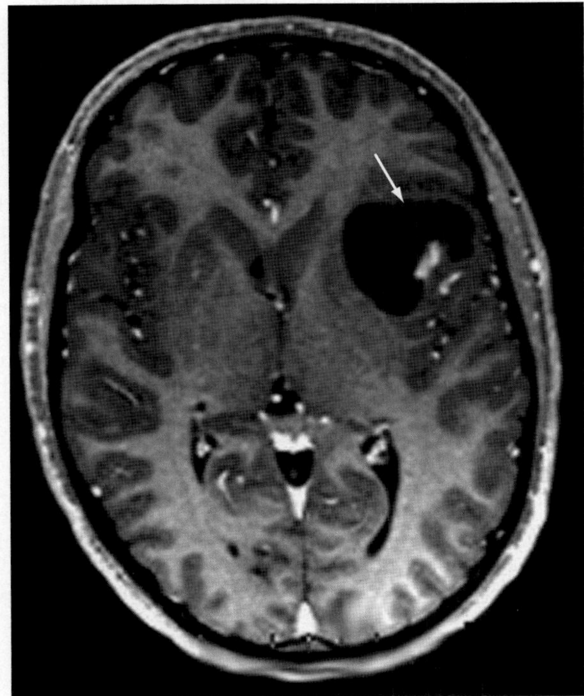

Magnetic resonance image depicting a left frontal ganglioglioma *(arrow).* T1-weighted image after intravenous gadolinium.

Perhaps most exciting has been the growing association between a number of focal MCD subtypes and mutations in regulatory genes within the mammalian target of rapamycin (mTOR) pathway. These disorders, referred to as *mTORopathies*, are best represented by the paradigm disorder, tuberous sclerosis complex (TSC), in which there are focal MCD known as tubers in 80% of patients. TSC is an autosomal dominant disorder, but can result from de novo mutations in either the *TSC1* or *TSC2* genes. The encoded proteins, TSC1 and TSC2, are negative regulators of mTOR via an intermediate protein, Rheb, and serve to modulate mTOR signaling in response to growth factors and nutrient levels in the cell. Mutations in either TSC1 or TSC2 lead to constitutively activated mTOR signaling in the brain. Aberrant mTOR activation during embryonic brain development causes disordered assembly of the cerebral cortex, improper connectivity, and hyperexcitability (seizures). Early clinical trials with mTOR inhibitor compounds, such as sirolimus and everolimus, have led to decrease seizures in TSC patients. Interestingly, over the past 5 years, somatic mutations in other mTOR associated genes such as *PTEN*, *PI3K*, *AKT3*, *DEPDC5*, and *NPRL3* have been associated with FCD type IIa and IIb, all culminating in constitutive mTOR activation. Amazingly, several of these genes are also associated with hemimegalencephaly, a hemispheric form of FCD. These findings provide a number of "actionable genotypes" to approach therapeutically with mTOR inhibitors.

Another family of MCD that has seen major advances has been lissencephaly and diffuse MCD syndromes. The first gene identified for lissencephaly, a devastating brain malformation associated with severe intractable seizures and profound cognitive disability, was *LIS1*, in association with the recessive Miller-Dieker lissencephaly syndrome. Over the next 10 years, mutations in a number of other functionally linked, but also distinct, genes have been identified including *DCX*, *filamin A*, and *ARX*. Subsequently, mutations in several tubulin (e.g., *TUBA1A*) isoforms have been linked to lissencephaly subtypes. These findings suggest that lissencephaly may represent a spectrum of phenotypes resulting from a broad range of genotypes. At this point, these molecular findings have not yielded new therapeutic targets.

Whereas antiepileptic drugs remain an important treatment approach for seizures in MCD, many individuals with epilepsy associated with MCD will be refractory to medications, despite attempts at rational polytherapy. In these individuals, the mainstay of treatment remains resective epilepsy surgery to remove the MCD and functionally disconnect the aberrant cortical network. In some cases, disconnective surgery (e.g., corpus callosotomy) can be used to help atonic or tonic seizure semiologies. Device-based approaches, such as the vagus nerve stimulator and responsive neurostimulation, have not proved to be particularly effective.

Full text of this chapter is available online at ExpertConsult.com 

61 Diagnosis and Classification of Seizures and Epilepsy

Jeremy J. Moeller and Lawrence J. Hirsch

Seizures and epilepsy are among the most commonly encountered neurological disorders. The worldwide annual incidence of epilepsy diagnoses is approximately 50 per 100,000,[1] and survey data suggest that approximately 1% of people in the United States have epilepsy.[2] Isolated seizures are even more common. In North America and Western Europe, 2% to 5% of children have a febrile convulsion before the age of 5 years, and in other parts of the world, the lifetime incidence of febrile convulsions is 10% or higher.[3] An additional 3% to 4% of people may experience an acute symptomatic seizure in their lifetime.[4] Neurosurgical disorders are among the most common causes of both acute symptomatic and unprovoked seizures. In addition, up to two thirds of patients with epilepsy may not achieve freedom from seizures with antiepileptic drugs (AEDs),[5,6] and many of these patients may have a disorder that can be treated surgically.[7]

Seizures and epilepsy are challenging to diagnose for several reasons, including the difficulties in obtaining an accurate and complete history, the numerous disorders that mimic epilepsy, and ongoing debate about defining and classifying seizures and epilepsy syndromes.

In this chapter, we review the classification and diagnosis of seizures, with a focus on practical application in the neurological or neurosurgical clinical setting.

DEFINITION OF EPILEPSY

Epilepsy and seizures are manifestations of brain dysfunction that can be the result of a broad range of underlying causes; therefore, establishing a unifying definition for either of these terms has been challenging. The International League Against Epilepsy (ILAE) has produced several publications regarding the definitions of epilepsy and seizures.[8-10] Definitions of epilepsy and seizures can be divided into *conceptual definitions*, which are useful for communication with patients and in neurology education, and *operational or practical definitions*, which can be used in clinical practice and research.[8]

The conceptual definition of an epileptic seizure is "a transient occurrence of signs and/or symptoms due to abnormal excessive or synchronous neuronal activity in the brain" (Box 61-1).[9] In many clinical situations, it is not possible to identify direct evidence of "abnormal excessive or synchronous neuronal activity," and so a clinical judgment is based mainly on history, physical examination findings, and results of investigations as outlined in the "Diagnosis of Seizures and Epilepsy" section of this chapter. Furthermore, electrographically confirmed seizures can occur without any detectable signs or symptoms. Thus this conceptual definition is impractical for clinical use.

The conceptual definition of epilepsy is also outlined in Box 61-1. This definition has been translated into an operational (practical) definition for use in the clinical or research setting. According to this definition, only one seizure may be necessary for the diagnosis of epilepsy, particularly if there is a high (>60%) risk of recurrent seizures in the next 10 years. For example, a patient with a tumor or vascular malformation who has had one unprovoked seizure would be at high risk of subsequent seizures, and epilepsy could therefore be diagnosed. In addition to defining epilepsy on the basis of one or more seizures, the ILAE considers patients to have epilepsy if they have an "epilepsy syndrome," diagnosed on the basis of the clinical situation, electroencephalographic (EEG) results, and other findings. In most cases, epilepsy syndromes are associated with obvious seizures, but in some exceptional epilepsy syndromes, patients may have epilepsy without obvious behavioral seizures, as with continuous spikes and waves during sleep and Landau-Kleffner syndrome.[9] In these clinical situations, EEG reveals evidence of seizures on EEG, and neurological examination reveals other abnormalities, but discrete clinical seizures may not be evident.

Discussions about definitions are not esoteric; a diagnosis of an unprovoked seizure, epilepsy, or both can have major implications for treatment decisions, driving and occupational status, and patient self-perception and psychosocial well-being.[8]

Fisher and associates' report[8] provided some case examples of the application of the current ILAE definition in several specific clinical scenarios.

Controversies in the Classification of Epilepsy and Seizures

The classification of seizures and epilepsy has been the subject of debate and discussion in those who treat people with epilepsy for more than a century. Jean-Étienne Dominique Esquirol first described a differentiation between "le grand mal" and "le petit mal" as early as 1815,[11] and although these terms are not part of any modern classification system, they are still frequently used by patients and occasionally by health care providers to describe seizures. The ILAE first developed a widely used classification system for seizures in the 1960s,[12] and multiple revisions of this system have been attempted since. The most widely used classification system for epileptic seizures is based on a report by an ILAE commission published in 1981.[13] For epilepsy syndromes, the most widely used classification system was published in 1989.[14] As a result of subsequent developments in the understanding of epilepsy and seizures, multiple revisions of these classification systems have been proposed[15-17]; these have included attempts to abandon outdated terminology and concepts. Each of these systems has been met with some resistance among epilepsy specialists, and none have been widely adopted in clinical practice.[18] For the purposes of this chapter, the traditional 1981 and 1989 classification systems are used, with comments on proposed updated terminology as appropriate.

Classification of Seizures

The 1981 classification system distinguished among three main types of seizures: partial (focal) seizures, generalized seizures, and unclassified epileptic seizures.[13] Although the specific terms and some details have changed with subsequent proposed revisions, the distinction between partial (focal) and generalized seizures remains clinically important. The pathophysiologic assumption of this distinction is that, at onset, partial (focal) seizures involve

BOX 61-1 Definitions of Epilepsy and Seizures*

CONCEPTUAL DEFINITION OF A SEIZURE[9]

An epileptic seizure is a transient occurrence of signs or symptoms due to abnormal excessive or synchronous neuronal activity in the brain.

CONCEPTUAL DEFINITION OF EPILEPSY[9]

Epilepsy is a disorder of the brain characterized by an enduring predisposition to generate epileptic seizures and by the neurobiologic, cognitive, psychological, and social consequences of this condition. The definition of epilepsy requires the occurrence of at least one epileptic seizure.

OPERATIONAL (PRACTICAL) CLINICAL DEFINITION OF EPILEPSY[8]

Epilepsy is a disease of the brain defined by any of the following conditions:

1. At least two unprovoked (or reflex) seizures occurring >24 hours apart
2. One unprovoked (or reflex) seizure and a probability of further seizures similar to the general recurrence risk (at least 60%) after two unprovoked seizures, occurring over the next 10 years
3. Diagnosis of an epilepsy syndrome

Epilepsy is considered to be resolved for individuals who had an age-dependent epilepsy syndrome but are now past the applicable age or those who have remained seizure free for the last 10 years, with no seizure medications for the last 5 years.

*Definitions from the International League Against Epilepsy (ILAE).

abnormal excessive synchronous brain activity in one part or hemisphere of the brain, whereas in generalized seizures, the abnormal activity is widespread virtually instantaneously after onset: in essence, involving both hemispheres immediately.[13] Focal seizures can be divided into seizures without impairment of awareness (*simple partial seizures* in the 1981 classification) and those with impairment of awareness (*complex partial seizures*). Figure 61-1 demonstrates a schematic representation of different seizure types, including terminology from both the 1981 and 2010 classification systems.

A different course of investigation and treatment might be chosen on the basis of whether the seizures appear to arise from a focal brain abnormality or from more widespread brain dysfunction. Many medications are effective primarily against focal-onset seizures, whereas others are effective against both focal and generalized seizures.[19] Some antiseizure medications can exacerbate generalized seizures, especially myoclonic and absence seizures; these drugs include commonly used medications such as carbamazepine, phenytoin, and oxcarbazepine. The presence of focal seizures warrants careful examination and neuroimaging to identify a structural abnormality as a possible cause.[14]

Classification of Epilepsy Syndromes

The 1989 classification system for the epilepsy syndromes is based on both seizure types (distinguishing between generalized and partial/focal seizures) and on the presumed cause of the seizure disorder.[14] Seizure disorders were described as symptomatic, cryptogenic, or idiopathic. The term *symptomatic* is most straightforward and is used to describe an epilepsy syndrome with a known underlying disorder of the central nervous system (CNS) that could be reasonably expected to cause the patient's seizures. The term *cryptogenic* is used when a presumed underlying symptomatic cause has not yet been identified. The term *idiopathic* was used to identify syndromes in which there was no underlying cause with the exception of a possible genetic predisposition. With advances in genetics, functional neuroimaging, and the understanding of the pathophysiologic processes of epilepsy, these terms have become problematic. As yet, unfortunately, no alternative system has been widely adopted, although a new one was proposed in 2010.[16]

From a practical clinical perspective, the distinction between localization-related epilepsy and generalized epilepsy syndromes is still useful. As mentioned previously, investigation and treatment will depend strongly on this distinction in classification.

DIAGNOSIS OF SEIZURES AND EPILEPSY

Initial Diagnostic Approach and Differential Diagnosis

Two questions of particular importance in the evaluation of a patient presenting with a seizure are the following:

1. Was the event a seizure?
2. If so, was it provoked?

The answers to these two questions will have a profound effect on subsequent diagnostic testing, management, and prognosis. In most cases, a thorough history and a careful physical examination (along with selected diagnostic tests) are sufficient to answer these two questions. In some cases, as discussed later, the answers remain elusive, and expert consultation or specialized diagnostic procedures are necessary.

Was the Event a Seizure?

In the evaluation of a patient with seizures, it is important to consider the differential diagnosis. In two population-based studies in the United Kingdom, 18% to 22% of patients with a diagnosis of epilepsy had another possible explanation for their episodes.[20,21] In a study of patients referred to a specialty clinic after the diagnosis of first unprovoked seizure, 27% (136 of 496) either did not have epilepsy or had acute symptomatic seizures.[22] By far, the most common causes of episodes misdiagnosed as seizures are syncope and psychogenic nonepileptic spells (PNES).[20-22] Some clinical features that may help distinguish seizures from syncope and nonepileptic attacks are included in Table 61-1, and a differential diagnosis of seizures is outlined in Table 61-2. Diagnosis of syncope may be made on the basis of history alone, but additional diagnostic tests,—including electrocardiography, prolonged cardiac rhythm monitoring, echocardiography, or tilt-table testing—may also be required.[23] A cardiology consultation is often helpful in guiding investigations and treatment of presumed neurocardiogenic syncope. The "gold standard" for the diagnosis of psychogenic nonepileptic spells is identification of a characteristic episode on video-EEG monitoring.[24] The interval between onset and diagnosis of PNES is 7 to 10 years; most affected patients receive multiple treatments for epileptic seizures before being referred for specialist consultation and video-EEG monitoring.[25,26]

Obtaining a reliable history of episodes associated with transient loss of consciousness can be challenging. The patients themselves are not able to provide many details about what happened during the event, and eyewitnesses can be unreliable. In one study, students were shown videos of both seizures and syncope, without prior warning, and then asked to provide details about the events afterward. Only 44% to 60% of observable items were recalled correctly, and up to 23% of students provided an observation of something that was not observable.[27] In other words, many students recalled seeing something that did not occur.

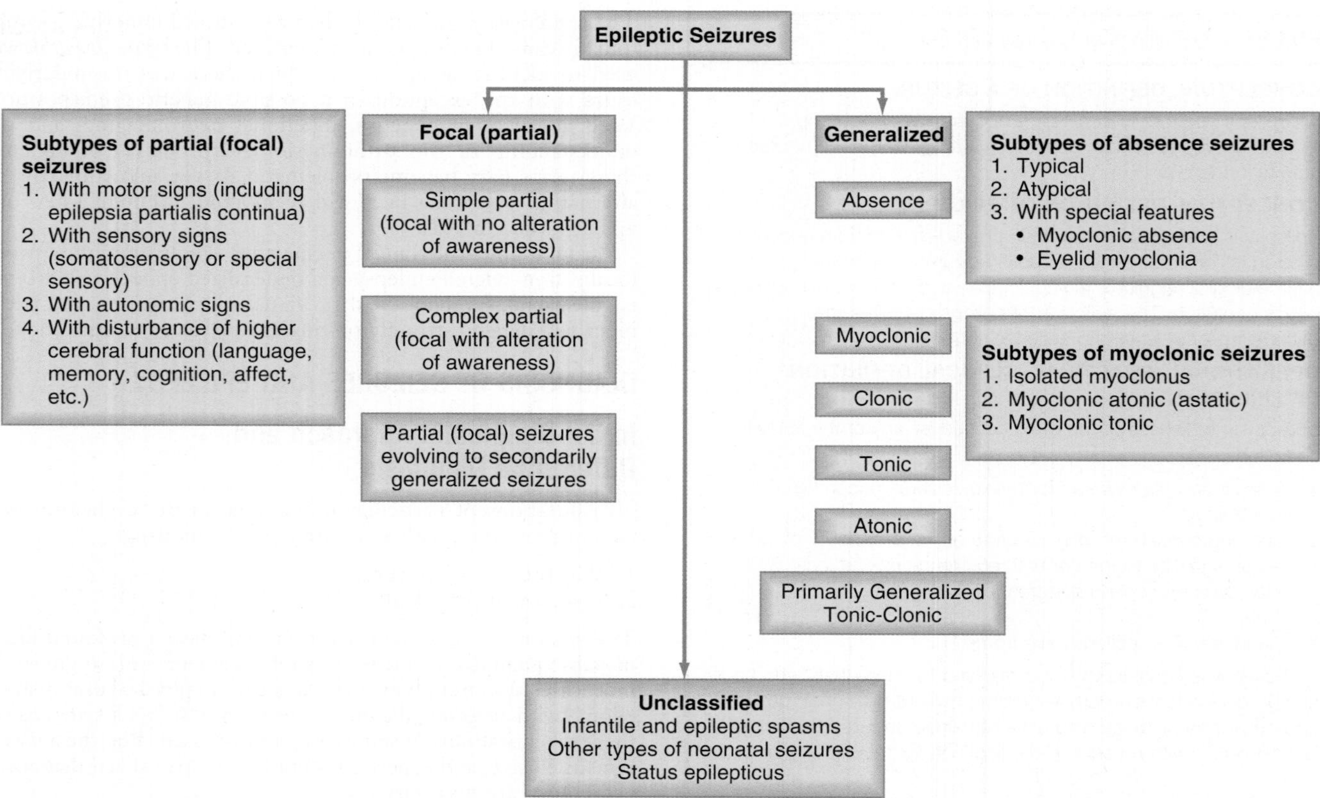

Figure 61-1. International League Against Epilepsy (ILAE) classification of epileptic seizures. *(Modified from Proposal for revised clinical and electroencephalographic classification of epileptic seizures. From the Commission on Classification and Terminology of the International League Against Epilepsy.* Epilepsia. *1981;22:489-501; and from Berg AT, Berkovic SF, Brodie MJ, et al. Revised terminology and concepts for organization of seizures and epilepsies: report of the ILAE Commission on Classification and Terminology, 2005-2009.* Epilepsia. *2010;51:676-685.)*

Although the major distinguishing features of seizures, syncope, and PNES are outlined in Table 61-1, a few items warrant additional discussion:

1. "All that shakes is not a seizure": Many health care providers with limited experience in epilepsy and related disorders believe that abnormal movements (shaking, twitching, stiffening) are a relatively rare phenomenon in syncope. In fact, these movements are very common: in a landmark German study, 59 healthy students volunteered to self-induce syncope through a combination of maneuvers (squatting, hyperventilation, Valsalva maneuver, standing up), and the subsequent movements were analyzed on video.[28] Of the students who experienced complete loss of consciousness, 90% had myoclonus, and many had other abnormal movements, including head turn, repetitive purposeless movements, gaze deviation, and vocalizations. In some cases, the myoclonic jerks were multifocal and dramatic (although uniformly short in duration, at most 15 seconds), in a way that could superficially resemble a seizure to an inexperienced or emotionally distressed observer. One of the features most useful for distinguishing a generalized tonic-clonic seizure from syncope or other nonepileptic phenomena is a *sustained tonic phase*, which is generally absent during syncope and almost always present in generalized tonic-clonic seizures. This is also one of the features most reliably and accurately recalled by eyewitnesses.[27] In addition, a loss of postural tone and a brief period of complete immobility precedes abnormal movements in syncope, but not in most seizures.
2. Urinary incontinence: Questions about urinary incontinence are a staple of most providers' standard seizure history; however, the presence or absence of urinary incontinence is unlikely to be helpful in distinguishing epileptic seizures from either syncope or PNES. In five studies, the incidence of urinary incontinence in seizures was compared with that in either syncope or PNES; a pooled analysis[29] of the results of all five showed that this component of the history is of no value in establishing a differential diagnosis. In other words, from a practical perspective, urinary incontinence is equally likely to be reported in syncope, PNES, and seizures.
3. Tongue bite: Questions about tongue biting are another staple in the typical seizure history. Tongue bite is more likely in seizures than in PNES, but this feature is not associated with high sensitivity or specificity. Lateral tongue bite is much more likely to occur in seizures, and thus an epileptic seizure is statistically more likely to be diagnosed.[30]
4. Other injuries: Injuries, including serious injuries such as lacerations, fractures, dental injury, and burns, can occur with PNES, and the presence of a serious injury does not necessarily help distinguish a nonepileptic event from an epileptic seizure.[31] The occurrence of serious injuries in PNES is evidence of the involuntary (although poorly understood) nature of these attacks in patients with this disorder.[24] Certain types of injuries may be more likely to occur in the tonic phase of a generalized tonic-clonic seizure than in either PNES or syncope; therefore, they may be helpful distinguishing features on physical examination or with investigations. Posterior dislocation or fracture of the shoulder or shoulder instability

TABLE 61-1 Clinical Features of Generalized Tonic-Clonic Seizures, PNES, and Syncope

Timing	Generalized Tonic-Clonic Seizure	PNES	Syncope
Before the event	• Possible warning • Symptoms suggestive of simple or complex partial seizure • Myoclonus or other abnormal movements	• Possible warning • Possible acute psychological stressor	• Lightheadedness • Pallor and diaphoresis • Tunnel vision • Roaring sound in ears • Sensation of warmth in the body • Provoking factors: fear, pain, sudden emotional distress, position change, palpitations
During the event	• Prominent tonic phase • "Ictal cry" • Loss of consciousness • Eyes usually open • Duration: typically 1-2 min	• Asynchronous movements • Stopping-and-starting cadence • Opisthotonic posturing, pelvic thrusting, side-to-side head movement • Eyes often closed • Often bizarre movements (frontal lobe epilepsy must be considered) • Preserved awareness despite bilateral motor manifestations • Behaviors that are modifiable by the examiner • Weeping	• Generally brief (<15 sec), although can be longer if patient is held upright or has persistent hypotension • Myoclonus: common; tonic posturing: less common • Eyes usually open, often with upward eye deviation
After the event	• Stertorous breathing (noisy, wet, slow respirations) • Decreased muscle tone • Prolonged sleepiness or confusion (at least several minutes and often longer) • Sore muscles and headache • Lateral tongue bite, petechial rash on face and upper chest • Possible shoulder dislocation or vertebral compression fracture • Elevation of serum CK level after 12-24 hr	• Shallow, rapid respirations • Lateral tongue bite: less common • Rapid recovery or "pseudosleep" (prolonged unresponsiveness with eyes closed) • Possible emotional distress or weeping	• Rapid recovery (within a few seconds) once blood pressure normalizes • Gradual return of vision and hearing (patients describe sounds initially distant and then gradually increasing to normal volume) • Nausea, pallor, diaphoresis: may be ongoing • Possible urinary incontinence • Prolonged confusion or altered mental state: can be explained by a head injury if the patient fell during syncope

Data from Azar NJ, Tayah TF, Wang L, et al. Postictal breathing pattern distinguishes epileptic from nonepileptic convulsive seizures. *Epilepsia.* 2008;49:132-137; Brown RJ, Syed TU, Benbadis S, et al. Psychogenic nonepileptic seizures. *Epilepsy Behav.* 2011;22:85-93; Lempert T, Bauer M, Schmidt D. Syncope: a videometric analysis of 56 episodes of transient cerebral hypoxia. *Ann Neurol.* 1994;36:233-237; Hirsch LJ, Pedley TA. Syncope, seizures and their mimics. In: Rowland LP, Pedley TA, eds. *Merritt's Neurology.* 12th ed. Philadelphia: Lippincott Williams & Wilkins; 2010:15-21.
CK, creatine kinase; PNES, psychogenic nonepileptic spell.

may occur after recurrent seizures,[32] and vertebral compression fractures have also been reported.[33] The presence of petechiae on the face and upper chest is also likely a useful indicator that an epileptic seizure has occurred, and this probably results from the transient intense Valsalva phenomenon that can occur during the tonic phase of a generalized tonic-clonic seizure.[34] The presence of unexplained injuries such as tongue bite, thoracic compression fracture, shoulder injury, or petechiae upon awakening may be an indicator of unrecognized nocturnal convulsions.[32,34,35]

Misdiagnosis of epilepsy can have serious consequences. In a Canadian study of patients with neurocardiogenic syncope misdiagnosed as seizures, AEDs were administered to 35% of patients, including several pregnant women.[36] Misdiagnosis of PNES has been followed by adverse reactions to nonindicated AEDs, loss of pregnancy, frequent harmful invasive procedures, and even death.[37-39] Up to 25% of patients with status epilepticus who were admitted to the neurological intensive care unit may have had nonepileptic attacks (i.e., "pseudo–status epilepticus").[40] Possibly because of the disinhibiting effects of benzodiazepines, such patients often receive much higher doses of benzodiazepines and are more likely to require long-term central venous access than patients with true status epilepticus.[37,40] For these reasons, we strongly recommend adhering to the American Academy of Neurology practice parameter guidelines and promptly referring any patient with atypical spells, or spells that have continued despite treatment with one or two appropriate AEDs, to a specialized epilepsy center for further investigation.[41]

If the Event Was a Seizure, Was It Unprovoked?

Epilepsy would not be diagnosed if the only manifestations were acute symptomatic seizures. Acute symptomatic seizures are also known as *provoked seizures, reactive seizures* or *situation-related seizures.*[42] Acute symptomatic seizures are defined as "seizures occurring in close temporal relationship with an acute CNS insult, which may be metabolic, toxic, structural, infectious or due to inflammation."[42] The definition of a "close temporal relationship" may depend on the acute insult or clinical condition. In some cases, the clinical scenario is clear: an acute symptomatic seizure can diagnosed definitively if the patient's serum blood glucose level is 30 mg/dL (1.7 mmol/L) or lower at the time of the seizure. Some situations are less clear; a task force of the ILAE proposed that seizures should be considered acute symptomatic if they occur within 7 days of the onset of an acute cerebrovascular syndrome, but what of the patient who has a seizure on day 8?[42]

The First Seizure

One of the most challenging aspects of epilepsy diagnosis is determining the risk of recurrence after a single unprovoked seizure. Overall, the long-term risk of a recurrent seizure in a patient who has a single unprovoked event is between 40% and 50%.[43-46] Of those who are going to have a recurrent seizure, more than 50% will have it within 6 months, and 80% to 90% will have it within 2 years.[43,44,46] Put another way, if a patient remains seizure free without AED treatment for at least 6 months

TABLE 61-2 Differential Diagnosis of Seizures

Etiologic Category	Diagnosis	Clinical Features
Cardiovascular	Syncope	See Table 61-1 for details
Cerebrovascular	TIA, limb shaking	Nonrhythmic, coarse, 3- to 12-Hz shaking of arm, leg, or both contralateral to severe carotid stenosis
		May occur upon standing or with other causes of hypoperfusion
	TIA with aphasia or other negative neurological symptoms	A single transient episode of aphasia or unilateral weakness or numbness is often considered a TIA; however, clinicians should consider focal seizures with recurrent, stereotyped episodes that leave no residual neurological deficit and no evidence of infarction on neuroimaging
	Transient global amnesia	Prolonged spell (hours) with normal behavior except for amnesia; personal identity always intact (if not, psychogenic amnesia should be suspected)
Psychogenic	PNES	See Table 61-1 for details
	Panic attack, hyperventilation	Often with environmental trigger
		Severe fear
		Hyperventilation with perioral cyanosis, bilateral hand paresthesias, carpopedal spasm
		No complete LOC
		Dyspnea
		Palpitations
		>5 min in duration
		Associated depression and phobias, especially agoraphobia
	Fugue attacks	Can be difficult to distinguish from nonconvulsive status epilepticus without EEG
Sleep disorder	Cataplexy	No LOC
		Other features of narcolepsy present (daytime somnolence, hypnagogic hallucinations, sleep paralysis)
		Triggered by emotion, especially laughter
	Other sleep phenomena	Somnambulism, night terrors, confusional arousals, enuresis, REM behavior disorder, hypnagogic hallucinations, periodic limb movements
		All can be difficult to distinguish from seizures without a reliable witness; video-EEG monitoring or polysomnography is necessary
Other	Migraine	Slow progression of neurological symptoms over >5 min and prolonged duration (usually 20-60 min)
		Subsequent headache may be absent
	Hypoglycemia	Long prodrome; rapid recovery only when treated
	"Drop attacks"	Can result from cataplexy, cervical spine disease, basilar ischemia, vertigo attacks, seizures (myoclonic, tonic, atonic, rarely focal), or syncope
	Staring/behavioral spells in patients with static encephalopathy or dementia	Sometimes difficult to distinguish from seizures without video-EEG monitoring

Modified from Hirsch LJ, Pedley TA. Syncope, seizures and their mimics. In: Rowland LP, Pedley TA, eds. *Merritt's Neurology*. 12th ed. Philadephia: Lippincott Williams & Wilkins; 2010:15-21.

EEG, electroencephalography; LOC, loss of consciousness; PNES, psychogenic nonepileptic spells; REM, rapid eye movement; TIA, transient ischemic attack.

after the index event, the risk of a recurrent seizure is less than 20%; if the patient remains seizure free for at least 2 years, the risk of recurrence is less than 10%.[47]

By convention, and in most studies, a single "event" is considered one or more seizures within a single 24-hour period. Therefore, a patient could have several seizures (or even status epilepticus) in a 1-day period, but they would still be considered only one seizure event. In terms of cause, the risk of recurrence is probably not any higher in patients with multiple seizures in a 24-hour period than in those with only one seizure at presentation.[48]

In almost every study of first seizures, the two most important predictors of seizure are the presence of epileptiform abnormalities on EEG and an underlying neurological disorder, as manifested by an abnormality on neurological examination or neuroimaging.[46,49] In one large study, the probability of recurrent seizures within 5 years was 30% in patients with a normal EEG finding and no neurological disorder, 56% in patients with either an abnormal EEG finding or an underlying neurological disorder, and 73% in patients with both an abnormal EEG finding and a neurological disorder.[49] Therefore, it is possible to make a diagnosis of epilepsy after a single seizure if EEG, neurological examination, neuroimaging, or other factors indicate a high risk of recurrence.[8] For this reason, we recommend that all patients with a first unprovoked seizure have a careful neurological examination, at least routine EEG, and neuroimaging, preferably magnetic resonance imaging (MRI).[50]

Other factors that may be associated with a higher risk of seizure recurrence, at least in some studies, include a first seizure during sleep, a family history of epilepsy, and a history of febrile seizures.[45,46] However, it is possible that with any of these factors, some or all of the additional risk of recurrent seizure could be attributed to either an abnormal EEG finding or an underlying neurological disorder that could be identified on physical examination or neuroimaging. In one study multivariate analysis techniques were used to control for codependent variables such as EEG or neuroimaging findings, none of the factors just listed was an independent predictor of a higher risk of recurrent seizures.[49] A history of traumatic brain injury can be a risk factor for epilepsy, but the increased risk probably is clinically significant only for moderate and severe brain injuries (loss of consciousness for 30 minutes or more, skull fracture, or evidence of traumatic changes on brain imaging).[51] The increased risk of seizures remains elevated long after the initial injury: at least up to 10 years after injury in patients with moderate brain injury and even after 10 years in patients with severe brain injury.[51]

Although this chapter does not focus on treatment, it is worthwhile to mention two large trials in which patients were randomly assigned to receive either immediate treatment with AEDs or delayed treatment, in which an AED would be started only after a recurrent seizure.[43,44] In general, immediate treatment with an AED lowered the risk of recurrence in a given time period by about half. Although early treatment with AEDs could delay the recurrence of seizures, there was no difference between the groups with regard to long-term freedom from seizure. The long-term prognosis after a first seizure is good in most patients: approximately 90% achieve long-term freedom from seizures after a first seizure, with or without medications.[43,44]

Investigations

Initial Investigations

Figure 61-2 contains our recommendations for the initial approach to diagnosing a possible seizure in the emergency setting, with an emphasis on distinguishing seizures from other seizure-like events and determining whether the seizure was provoked or unprovoked.

Most "routine" laboratory investigations (serum electrolyte, calcium, and magnesium measurements; toxicology screen) are intended to identify acute provoking factors. Serum prolactin levels have been shown to rise in the 10 to 20 minutes after seizures, particularly generalized tonic-clonic seizures, and do not rise after PNES. Abnormal elevation of the prolactin level within 10 to 20 minutes of the inciting event (defined in most studies as at least twice a baseline level, which can be determined 6 or more hours after the event or, to control for diurnal variations, 24 hours after the seizure) may be helpful in distinguishing generalized tonic-clonic seizure from PNES.[52] However, a normal prolactin level does not necessarily exclude the possibility of seizures. In addition, serum prolactin levels can increase after syncope, and so an elevated prolactin level would not be helpful in distinguishing seizures from syncope.[52] Serum prolactin levels drop quickly 10 to 20 minutes after the event, and so we would not recommend routine testing of serum prolactin more than 20 to 30 minutes after a seizure-like episode. Other laboratory values may also be abnormal after seizures; these include anion-gap metabolic acidosis (almost always seen right after a convulsive seizure and resolving rapidly), elevated white blood cell count (demargination), elevated creatine kinase (CK) level (most helpful >24 hours after the event), elevated ammonia level, and increased amount of neuron-specific enolase. However, none of these factors has sufficient discriminative value to reliably distinguish seizures from nonepileptic phenomena in routine clinical settings.[53,54]

If the patient is experiencing back pain or shoulder pain, routine radiographs may be useful for detecting evidence of seizure-related injuries, such as shoulder dislocation or vertebral compression fracture.[32,33]

Electroencephalography

EEG is of particular use in the evaluation of patients with seizures for three main reasons: (1) providing additional evidence that the spell was epileptic, if epileptiform discharges are present on EEG; (2) providing additional information about epilepsy subtype; and (3) determining the likelihood of recurrent events after a first seizure. As mentioned previously, the presence of epileptiform discharges on an EEG indicates a significantly higher risk of subsequent seizures.[43,44,46] EEG findings may also be helpful in determining whether a patient has a focal or generalized epilepsy syndrome. For example, the presence of focal epileptiform discharges on EEG might suggest a focal seizure disorder, and such a finding may prompt additional evaluation for focal abnormalities on neuroimaging. Generalized discharges on EEG would be suggestive of a generalized seizure disorder, and the presence of

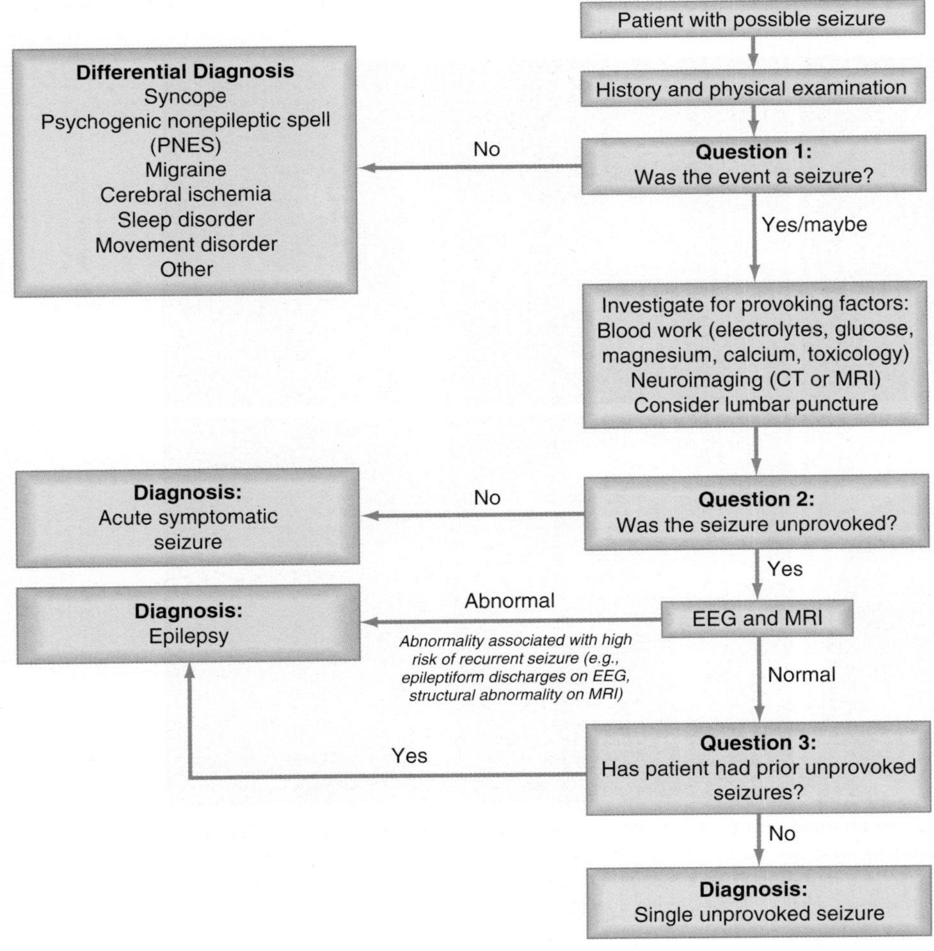

Figure 61-2. Initial diagnostic approach to suspected seizure. CT, computed tomography; EEG, electroencephalography; MRI, magnetic resonance imaging.

focal lesions might be less suspect. However, in rare cases, a focal lesion can generate discharges that appear generalized on scalp EEG, a phenomenon known as *secondary bilateral synchrony* and most common with frontal lobe foci.[55]

A normal EEG does not rule out the diagnosis of epilepsy or seizures. The likelihood of finding epileptiform discharges on a single routine EEG recording has been reported to be between 8% and 50%.[50] The rate of abnormalities is in the higher end of this range, approximately 50%, if the EEG is performed within 24 hours of the first seizure.[22] The likelihood of identifying an epileptiform abnormality can increase to 80% to 90% with serial EEG recordings.[56,57] Prolonged EEG recording—either outpatient ambulatory EEG or inpatient video-EEG monitoring—reveals similar amounts of epileptiform discharges as does serial EEG recordings, and in 95% of patients with interictal epileptiform abnormalities, the abnormalities are seen within the first 48 hours of recording.[58,59] However, approximately 10% of patient with epilepsy never demonstrate interictal abnormalities on scalp EEG, probably because the focus of the seizure is very small or because the focus is in a region of cortex inaccessible to scalp electrodes, such as the depth of a sulcus, the cingulate cortex or medial brain regions, the mesial temporal lobes, the orbitofrontal cortex, and the insular cortex. In one study of simultaneous scalp and intracranial EEG recordings, synchronous discharges involving less than 10 to 20 cm^2 were unlikely to generate a spike on scalp EEG.[60]

It is important to interpret EEG results in the context of the entire clinical scenario. Benign or nonspecific EEG patterns are commonly misinterpreted as indicative of underlying epilepsy.[61-63] If the EEG findings appear inconsistent with the clinical presentation, we recommend repeated or prolonged EEG or a review of the EEG recording by an experienced fellowship-trained or board-certified electroencephalographer.

Video-EEG monitoring is the "gold standard" in the diagnosis of seizures and nonepileptic spells. As mentioned previously, any patient who continues to have episodes despite adequate trials of one or two AEDs should be referred for video-EEG monitoring to clarify the diagnosis and possibly for consideration of epilepsy surgery. The reasons we recommend early referral are that (1) the patient may be having not seizures but rather PNES, syncope, or some other seizure "mimic," and (2) after failure of two or three trials of appropriate AEDs at appropriate doses, the likelihood of obtaining freedom from seizures with additional AEDs is low (about 5%), and epilepsy surgery may be a consideration.[5]

Neuroimaging

Either computed tomography (CT) or MRI should be considered in all patients presenting with a first seizure, particularly those presenting with partial (focal) seizures and those who demonstrate focal abnormalities on examination.[50,64] CT may be appropriate in the emergency setting, in which MRI is not easily available, and the purpose is to identify an acute provoking factor, such as hemorrhage or acute infarction. MRI is much more sensitive for subtle abnormalities and should be considered in all patients with focal or recurrent unprovoked seizures.

Many subtle MRI abnormalities are associated with focal epilepsy, and these abnormalities frequently go undetected on "routine" studies. It is important to provide as much detailed clinical information as possible to the neuroradiologist in the MRI referral. For example, if a patient has clinical features suggesting an onset in a specific hemisphere or lobe, the radiologist may pay particular attention to this region. There are generally accepted protocols for MRI evaluations of epilepsy, with specific sequences designed to best identify the types of focal abnormalities commonly associated with refractory seizures.[65] Figure 61-3

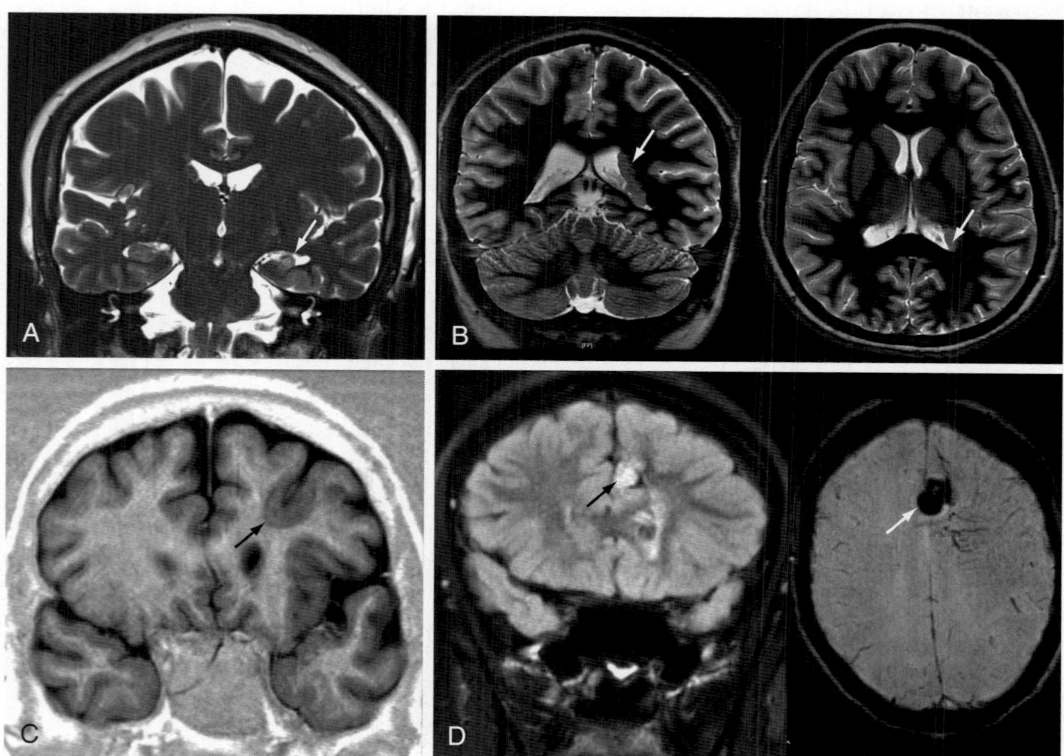

Figure 61-3. Magnetic resonance imaging: appearances of common lesions associated with epileptic seizures. Each lesion is indicated by an *arrow.* **A,** Mesial temporal sclerosis. **B,** Periventricular nodular heterotopia. **C,** Focal cortical dysplasia in the depth of a sulcus. **D,** Cavernous malformation. *(**C,** Courtesy Dr. R. Mark Sadler, Dalhousie University, Halifax, Nova Scotia, Canada.)*

shows some focal abnormalities on MRI that are commonly associated with epilepsy.

Functional neuroimaging techniques—for example, interictal and ictal single photon emission computed tomography, positron emission tomography, and specialized MRI techniques such as functional MRI, volumetric analysis of MRI, and diffusion tensor imaging—can all play an important role in the evaluation of a patient for possible epilepsy surgery, and this is discussed further in other chapters.[66]

CONCLUSIONS

Seizures and epilepsy can be difficult to diagnose and even more difficult to classify. In the initial diagnostic evaluation, is important to obtain a thorough history, conduct a careful physical examination, and arrange investigations as the history and examination findings warrant. We believe that it is important for clinicians to be flexible about the initial diagnosis in patients with apparent seizures. When seizures persist despite adequate initial treatment, referral to an epilepsy specialist for consideration of video-EEG monitoring is important for confirming the diagnosis and exploring other treatment options, including the possibility of epilepsy surgery.

SUGGESTED READINGS

Berg AT, Berkovic SF, Brodie MJ, et al. Revised terminology and concepts for organization of seizures and epilepsies: report of the ILAE Commission on Classification and Terminology, 2005-2009. *Epilepsia*. 2010;51(4):676-685.

Blume WT, Lüders HO, Mizrahi E, et al. Glossary of descriptive terminology for ictal semiology: report of the ILAE task force on classification and terminology. *Epilepsia*. 2001;42(9):1212-1218.

Brown RJ, Syed TU, Benbadis S, et al. Psychogenic nonepileptic seizures. *Epilepsy Behav*. 2011;22(1):85-93.

Duncan JS. Imaging in the surgical treatment of epilepsy. *Nat Rev Neurol*. 2010;6(10):537-550.

Fisher RS, Acevedo C, Arzimanoglou A, et al. ILAE official report: a practical clinical definition of epilepsy. *Epilepsia*. 2014;55(4):475-482.

Krumholz A, Wiebe S, Gronseth G, et al. Practice parameter: evaluating an apparent unprovoked first seizure in adults (an evidence-based review): report of the Quality Standards Subcommittee of the American Academy of Neurology and the American Epilepsy Society. *Neurology*. 2007;69(21):1996-2007.

Kwan P, Brodie MJ. Early identification of refractory epilepsy. *N Engl J Med*. 2000;342(5):314-319.

Lempert T, Bauer M, Schmidt D. Syncope: a videometric analysis of 56 episodes of transient cerebral hypoxia. *Ann Neurol*. 1994;36(2): 233-237.

Proposal for revised classification of epilepsies and epileptic syndromes. Commission on Classification and Terminology of the International League Against Epilepsy. *Epilepsia*. 1989;30(4):389-399.

Proposal for revised clinical and electroencephalographic classification of epileptic seizures. From the Commission on Classification and Terminology of the International League Against Epilepsy. *Epilepsia*. 1981; 22(4):489-501.

See a full reference list on ExpertConsult.com

62 Antiepileptic Medications: Principles of Clinical Use

Danielle A. Becker and Steven V. Pacia

Since the early 1990s, many new antiepileptic drugs (AEDs) have become available to treat seizures. However, 33% of patients with epilepsy continue to suffer seizures despite proper medical management.[1] Several newer agents have advantages over older medications with regard to efficacy, safety, pharmacokinetic profile, and drug-drug interactions. Because of the increasing awareness of long-term side effects with established older drugs such as phenytoin, newer agents are often tried first for seizure management. In addition, many newer medications have fewer drug-drug interactions and necessitate less routine laboratory monitoring.

In this chapter, we review the pharmacologic features and mechanisms of action of commonly prescribed AEDs, including their pharmacokinetic properties, drug interactions, recommended treatment doses, preoperative and postoperative uses, side effects, and safety profiles. Approaches to AED management of the neurosurgical patient are discussed, as are recommendations for initiating, monitoring, and discontinuing medication.

CLINICAL PHARMACOLOGIC FEATURES OF ANTIEPILEPTIC DRUGS

Many AEDs are available today, and choosing a drug on the basis of side effect profiles and interactions can be challenging. Medications have varying protein-binding properties and may induce or inhibit metabolic enzymes that affect elimination pathways. These pharmacokinetic interactions must be considered in the selection of an AED. The pharmacokinetic properties for the most commonly used AEDs are summarized in Table 62-1. The mechanisms of action of these drugs are summarized in Table 62-2. Intravenous formulation and infusion rates are presented in Table 62-3.

Hepatic enzyme induction or inhibition and protein-binding displacement may necessitate dose adjustments and careful clinical monitoring. Phenytoin, phenobarbital, and carbamazepine are cytochrome P-450 (CYP) enzyme inducers with the degree of enzyme induction proportional to dose. The inducers' enhancement of hepatic metabolism may result in subtherapeutic concentrations of other AEDS and medications, such as warfarin, that are also metabolized by CYP. However, induction is not strictly additive when multiple inducers are administered simultaneously. When an inducer is removed, serum concentrations of an affected drug may rise, which increases the likelihood of toxic side effects. Conversely, an AED that inhibits hepatic enzyme activity, such as valproic acid, may decrease the rate of metabolism of a CYP enzyme–metabolized drug, usually in a dose-dependent manner. The enzymatic inhibition effects typically occur within 24 hours of addition of the inhibitor. Protein-binding displacement occurs when one drug has less affinity for plasma proteins and tissue than does another. Rising unbound drug concentrations can result in acute toxicity. Clinically important protein-binding interactions occur frequently with phenytoin and valproic acid.

Antiepileptic Drugs

Phenytoin

Although the use of phenytoin has declined since 2000, it is still widely used, especially in the inpatient and emergency department settings. It is a wide-spectrum AED that is used to treat partial seizures, generalized convulsive seizures, status epilepticus, and neonatal seizures, but it has limited efficacy for absence, clonic, myoclonic, tonic, or atonic seizures.[2] Phenytoin is often first-line treatment for status epilepticus because it can be given intravenously and loaded rapidly.

Phenytoin has a nonlinear relationship between maintenance dosing and steady-state concentrations. In the higher therapeutic ranges, small dose elevations can increase serum concentrations significantly. In addition, the rate of elimination of phenytoin declines with higher serum concentrations. A typical maintenance dosage is 300 to 400 mg/day.

Phenytoin is a potent hepatic enzyme inducer and may lower the levels of other medications. It may result in more rapid elimination of AEDs, including carbamazepine, valproic acid, felbamate, lamotrigine, topiramate, and zonisamide, as well as other classes of medication, including anticlotting agents (warfarin), oral contraceptives, and some chemotherapeutic agents. Phenytoin is also highly protein bound, which, when displaced, may result in higher free phenytoin levels (i.e., when phenytoin is displaced from the protein molecule, there is more of the drug free floating in the circulating blood); this in turn renders total serum levels uninterpretable and has the potential for toxic side effects. Free levels of phenytoin are elevated in patients with hypoalbuminemia, a frequent occurrence in renal disease; therefore, dosage reductions in such patients are necessary. Phenytoin is excreted in both urine and feces as metabolites.

Although phenytoin is relatively safe, intravenous infusion has been associated with bradycardia and hypotension,[3] as well as local skin necrosis, known as *purple glove syndrome*.[4] These infrequent but serious consequences can be avoided through the use of fosphenytoin for intravenous administration, with an infusion rate up to 150 mg/min (3 mg/kg/min) instead of 50 mg/min (1 mg/kg/min) for phenytoin. Typical side effects associated with phenytoin, especially at high serum concentrations, include nystagmus, ataxia, diplopia, drowsiness, and hepatotoxicity. These side effects tend to be dose related. Adverse effects associated with chronic use include gingival hyperplasia, hirsutism, peripheral neuropathy, and bone demineralization. Patients who have been taking phenytoin for several years should undergo a bone density study. Idiosyncratic reactions, including a lupus-like syndrome and aplastic anemia, although rare, have been documented.[5]

Carbamazepine and Oxcarbazepine

Carbamazepine is used for the treatment of focal onset seizures, both partial and secondarily generalized, and has an excellent side effect profile.[6]

Carbamazepine has linear elimination kinetic properties and is cleared almost entirely via hepatic metabolism. Although it induces its own metabolism, the effect is delayed; therefore, carbamazepine must be increased slowly over the first 3 to 4 weeks of treatment. Therapy may be initiated with 100 to 200 mg/day and subsequently increased to a target dose of 600 to 800 mg/day. Most responsive patients need twice-daily dosing. If higher doses are needed, toxicity may be avoided by administration of the medication three times a day or with the use of an extended-release preparation. Elderly patients require lower dosages than do younger adults to achieve adequate serum concentrations.[7] Serum drug levels are a useful guide, although in patients with poorly controlled epilepsy, the dose may have to be increased to

TABLE 62-1 Pharmacokinetic Parameters of Antiepileptic Drugs

Drug	Vd (L/kg)	Protein Binding (%)*	T ½ (hour)	Therapeutic Range (mg/L)†	Active Metabolite	Adult Daily Dose Range‡ (mg/day)	Intravenous Form
Carbamazepine	0.8-2	75	12-17	4-12	Yes	600-800	No
Felbamate	0.75	25	20-23	30-60	No	1200-3600	No
Gabapentin	0.85	0	5-9	2-20	No	900-3600	No
Lamotrigine	1.0	55	12-60	2-20	No	200-400	No
Levetiracetam	0.5-0.7	<10	6-8	12-46	No	1000-3000	Yes
Oxcarbazepine	0.7-0.8	45	1-2.5	10-35	Yes	600-1800	No
Phenobarbital	0.55	45	36-118	10-40	No	60-180	Yes
Primidone	0.75	20-30	3-7	5-10	Yes	500-1000	No
Phenytoin	0.75	90	7-42	10-20	No	300-400	Yes
Topiramate	0.65	15	21	5-20	No	200-400	No
Valproic acid	0.16	70-93§	6-17	50-100	Yes	500-1000	Yes
Zonisamide	1.5	40	27-70	10-40	No	100-400	No
Lacosamide	0.6	<15	13	—	No	200-400	Yes
Perampanel	—	95-96	70-105	—	No	4-12	No
Rufinamide	0.7	30	6-10	—	No	2400-3200	No
Eslicarbazepine acetate	0.87	<40	13-20	—	No	800-1200	No
Clobazam	1.4	85	11-77	—	Yes	20-40	No

T ½, elimination half-time; Vd, volume of distribution.
*Fraction bound to serum proteins.
†Therapeutic range of serum concentration.
‡Dose schedule may vary according to half-life and release form.
§Concentration dependent.

TABLE 62-2 Mechanism of Action of Antiepileptic Drugs

Drugs	Na⁺ Channel Block	Enhance GABA	Ca^{2+} Channel Block	Glutamate Receptor	Other
Phenytoin	NaF, NaP				
Carbamazepine	NaF				
Ethosuximide	NaP		T-type		
Benzodiazepine		$GABA_AR$, Increased frequency of chloride channel opening			
Phenobarbital		$GABA_AR$, Prolongs chloride channel opening	HVA	AMPA	
Valproic acid	NaF, NaP	Increased turnover	T-type		
Gabapentin/ Pregabalin		Increased turnover	HVA (α2δ)		
Lamotrigine	NaF		HVA		
Levetiracetam		Reverses DMCM	HVA		SV2A modulation
Topiramate	NaF, NaP	$GABA_AR$	HVA	KA/AMPA	
Zonisamide	NaF	+	T-type		
Rufinamide	NaF				
Clobazam		$GABA_AR$ agonist			
Vigabatrin		Inhibits GABA-transaminase			
Lacosamide	NaS				
Perampanel				AMPA receptor antagonist	
Felbamate		Positive modulator of $GABA_AR$ by enhancing Cl-current		Binds and opens NMDA receptors Blocks non-NMDA receptors	Weak inhibitory effects on GABA-receptor binding, benzodiazepine receptor binding

AMPA, α-amino-3-hydroxy-5-methyl-4-isoxazole-propionic acid; DMCM, methyl-6,7-dimethoxy-4-ethyl-β-carboline-3-carboxylate (a negative allosteric modulator of $GABA_AR$); GABA, γ-aminobutyric acid; $GABA_AR$, type A GABA receptor; HVA, high voltage activated; KA, kainate; NaF, fast sodium current; NaP, persistent sodium current; NaS, slow inactivation of sodium channels; NMDA, N-methyl-D-aspartate; SV2A, synaptic vesicle protein 2A.

the maximum that is clinically tolerated, independent of plasma level. Carbamazepine is a CYP enzyme inducer and therefore increases the metabolism of other medications, including hormonal contraceptives. There is no intravenous preparation of carbamazepine.

Typical side effects associated with carbamazepine include nausea, dizziness, drowsiness, diplopia, weight gain, rash, and hyponatremia. Rare side effects include more severe allergic reactions, including Stevens-Johnson syndrome and toxic epidermal necrolysis. Risk of allergy is higher with rapid titration. Cross-reactivity for anticonvulsant hypersensitivity syndrome, characterized by fever, skin rash, and internal organ involvement, can be as high as 80% among carbamazepine, phenytoin, and phenobarbital.[8] Transient leucopenia may also be seen in the first few

TABLE 62-3 Antiepileptic Drugs with Intravenous Formulation

Medication	Infusion Rate	Cautions
Phenytoin (Dilantin)	IV injection at <50 mg/min	Cardiac monitoring (rate, rhythm, blood pressure) and close clinical observation are recommended during and after dose administration.
Fosphenytoin (Cerebyx)	IV infusion at <150 mg PE/min	
Valproic acid (Depakote)	IV infusion over 60 min; recommended infusion rate, generally 20 mg/min	Monitor CBC, LFT measurements, and serum ammonia level.
Phenobarbital (Luminal)	Maximum rate of slow IV injection for adults: 60 mg/min in less acute situations and 75-100 mg/min for status epilepticus	
Levetiracetam (Keppra)	Infusion over 15 min Can be safely administered IV in 5-min period as add-on to regular status epilepticus treatment.	
Lacosamide (Vimpat)	Infusion over 30-60 min	
Midazolam (Versed)	1-mg/mL formulation recommended to facilitate slow injection (rapid- or single-bolus IV administration not recommended)	
Propofol (Diprivan)	IV infusion 20 mg every 10 sec until induction onset (approx 1-2 g/kg). Maintenance: IV infusion, 100-200 cg/kg/min (approx 6-12 mg/kg/hr)	Significant accumulation may occur with long-term use. The longer the infusion and higher the dose are, the longer is the time to awakening from drug cessation. Longer emergence times may occur in obese patients.

CBC, complete blood cell count; IV, intravenous; LFT, liver function test; PE, phenytoin equivalents.

months of titration of carbamazepine in 10% to 20% of patients. Persistent leucopenia has been reported in 2% of patients taking carbamazepine and has been shown to be reversible with discontinuation of the medication.[9]

Oxcarbazepine is an analogue of carbamazepine and is often used as an alternative to carbamazepine because it has similar clinical characteristics. Oxcarbazepine is also a CYP enzyme inducer, but to a lesser degree than carbamazepine. Oxcarbazepine may be initiated at a dose of 300 mg twice daily in adults and 5 to 10 mg/kg/day in children. For adults, the recommended monotherapy dosage is 600 to 1200 mg/day, and adjunctive therapy dosing is 1200 mg/day or higher, if needed, which may be increased at weekly intervals.[10] There is no intravenous preparation for oxcarbazepine.[7] The side effects of oxcarbazepine are similar to, although somewhat milder than, those of carbamazepine and include somnolence, dizziness, ataxia, diplopia, and blurred vision. Of importance, clinically significant hyponatremia, defined as a serum sodium level lower than 125 mEq/L, has been observed in 2.5% of patients taking oxcarbazepine.[10] Hyponatremia is more common with oxcarbazepine than carbamazepine, and its onset is often dose dependent.[11]

Valproic Acid

Valproic acid was approved for use in the United States in 1978 and has been used for the treatment of epilepsy since then.[12] It is a first-line agent for primary generalized epilepsy. Valproic acid is effective against generalized seizure types, including absence, myoclonic, and tonic-clonic seizures. It is also effective in treating partial seizures, seizures associated with Lennox-Gastaut syndrome, infantile spasms, neonatal seizures, and febrile seizures.[13,14]

Valproic acid inhibits the activity of CYP2C9, a CYP isoform in human liver microsomes. Inhibition of CYP2C9 by valproic acid prolongs the elimination of phenytoin, phenobarbital, diazepam, amitriptyline, and many other medications.[15] However, its metabolism can also be accelerated by CYP enzyme–inducing drugs. In adults, its half-life ranges from 13 to 16 hours in the absence of enzyme-inducing medications.[16,17] The initial target dose of valproic acid is 15 mg/kg/day (500 to 1000 mg/day). Valproic acid may need to be titrated upward by 5 to 10 mg/kg/day at weekly intervals, especially in the setting of enzyme-inducing medications. Valproic acid has a high affinity for serum proteins and can therefore displace other medications from protein, resulting in the presence of higher free fractions of other drugs in the blood.[18]

Valproic acid has been associated with various side effects. Transient hair loss, weight gain, and dose-related tremor are fairly frequent side effects. Drowsiness, lethargy, and confusional states may occur, but usually with valproic acid levels higher than 100 mg/L. In rare cases, valproic acid has been associated with acute mental status changes that can progress to stupor or coma.[19,20] Case studies have demonstrated that the stupor or confusion appears a few days after efficacious drug plasma levels are attained and disappears 24 to 72 hours after valproic acid is withdrawn. Neither toxic levels of valproic acid nor significant elevations in blood levels of the other coadministered anticonvulsant drugs have occurred. The mechanism underlying this change in mental status is unknown, but it is thought to be related to the addition of valproic acid to other existing anticonvulsants. The acute mental status change is thought to be independent of the hyperammonemia often associated with the use of valproic acid. Of importance, L-carnitine supplementation has been beneficial in acute valproic acid overdoses and is now recommended for routine supplementation in a subgroup of pediatric patients treated with valproic acid.[21]

Gastrointestinal (GI) side effects including nausea, vomiting, GI distress, and anorexia also occur in the setting of valproic acid administration but can be reduced with the enteric-coated tablets available. Fatal hepatotoxicity and pancreatitis are two rare but serious complications necessitating laboratory monitoring. Thrombocytopenia may result from valproic acid and improves with dose reduction. Valproic acid has also been associated with altered platelet function and disturbances of hemostasis, which may cause excessive bleeding. Valproic acid is therefore sometimes withdrawn before elective surgery. However, several studies did not find evidence of excessive perioperative bleeding in patients who remained on valproic acid during surgery.[22] Additionally, in women of child-bearing age, valproic acid is associated with an increased risk of neural tube defects, as well as an increase in the risk for polycystic ovaries and endocrine disturbances. Most recently, valproic acid was linked to lower IQ scores in children exposed to valproic acid in utero.[23] The effect appeared to be dose dependent.

Phenobarbital and Primidone

Phenobarbital has been used to treat seizures since 1912 and primidone since 1952. Although the use of phenobarbital in industrialized nations has declined, largely because of its side effects, it remains an important AED worldwide because of its lower cost and long half-life. Phenobarbital and primidone have similar chemical structures and are used to treat partial and secondarily generalized seizures. Phenobarbital is still used frequently for status epilepticus and neonatal seizures.

Phenobarbital is eliminated through hepatic metabolism and renal excretion. It has first-order/linear kinetic properties. The elimination half-life averages 80 to 100 hours in adults and newborns, but it is shorter in infants and children (63 to 69 hours).[24] For maintenance dosing, we suggest 2 to 5 mg/kg/day (60 to 180 mg/day). Phenobarbital is not highly protein bound (45%). Treatment with primidone results in the buildup of levels of phenobarbital and therefore has effects similar to those of phenobarbital. However, it has a much shorter half-life, and daily dose requirements (500 to 1000 mg/day) are, on average, more than five times greater than those for phenobarbital. Phenobarbital and primidone are CYP enzyme inducers and therefore increase the metabolism of other medications. Phenobarbital is available in both intravenous and intramuscular preparations, which are useful in the treatment of neonatal seizures, status epilepticus, and alcohol withdrawal seizures.

In comparison with many other AEDs, phenobarbital and primidone are associated with more sedative and behavioral side effects. They are more likely to cause dose-related neurotoxic reactions than systemic toxicity, but the latter does occur. Neurotoxicity is characterized by dysarthria, ataxia, incoordination, and nystagmus. Children tend to exhibit less sedation and more hyperactivity, aggressiveness, and insomnia than do adults. These effects occur in up to 50% of all children taking phenobarbital.[25] Depression may also complicate phenobarbital and primidone therapy.[26]

Felbamate

Felbamate was approved in the United States in 1993 for use either as monotherapy or as adjunctive therapy for patients older than 14 years with partial seizures, with or without generalization. It has also been approved for use as adjunctive therapy in patients with Lennox-Gastaut syndrome of all ages.[27] The use of felbamate has been limited because of its potentially serious toxic effects, which include aplastic anemia[28] and hepatotoxicity.[29] As a result, felbamate is often reserved for patients with refractory seizures that have responded poorly to other medications.

The recommended daily dose of felbamate is 1200 mg/day (15 mg/kg/day) for the first week. It may be titrated upward weekly by doubling of the dose in the second week and then, if necessary, tripling of the initial dose in the third week. Felbamate is well absorbed orally. It is metabolized in the liver and excreted through the kidneys. Its elimination half-life is 20 hours with monotherapy but decreases to 13 to 14 hours in the presence of enzyme-inducing AEDs.[30] It also acts as a CYP enzyme inhibitor and causes elevations of serum levels of phenytoin and valproic acid. As a result, it may be necessary to reduce the dose of other AEDs when felbamate is introduced. Felbamate also has a low protein-binding capacity and thus is unlikely to displace other medications from plasma proteins. At doses higher than 1200 to 1600 mg/day, felbamate exhibits first-order pharmacokinetic properties. Peak plasma concentrations are reached within 3 hours of oral administration.[31]

Typical side effects of felbamate include nausea, vomiting, anorexia and weight loss, somnolence, and insomnia/stimulation. Before recommendations for careful laboratory monitoring were published, aplastic anemia occurred in 1 per 5000 patients, and hepatic necrosis occurred in 1 per 7000 to 1 per 22,000.[32] Serious toxicity may be avoided by careful screening of complete blood cell counts and liver function test measurements.[29] Most life-threatening reactions occur in the first 6 to 12 months of treatment. Many clinicians recommend bimonthly laboratory testing for the first 6 months of treatment, followed by monthly testing for the next 6 months, followed by testing every 6 to 12 months thereafter.[33] Since the advent of serial blood monitoring, more than 35,000 new patients have started taking felbamate, with no reports of aplastic anemia or liver failure.[33]

Gabapentin and Pregabalin

Gabapentin was initially approved in the United States in 1993 for adjunctive treatment of partial seizures, with or without secondary generalization. It has since been approved as monotherapy for seizures in approximately 40 countries outside the United States. Gabapentin is effective against refractory focal seizures, as well as benign epilepsy of childhood with centrotemporal spikes. Pregabalin is similar to gabapentin and is approved in the United States for use for treatment of focal onset and secondarily generalized seizures. However, pregabalin has better bioavailability.[34] Both AEDs are now prescribed more frequently for pain than for epilepsy.

Gabapentin and pregabalin differ from other AEDs in that they are eliminated entirely through the kidneys, mainly unchanged, and therefore have no pharmacokinetic interactions. Renal clearance is linear in relation to the creatinine clearance. The initial target doses for gabapentin are 900 to 1800 mg/day (30 mg/kg/day). Higher doses up to 3600 mg/day are well tolerated. The daily dose should be divided into three administrations per day. The typical adult dosage for pregabalin is 150 mg/day the first week, with a titration up to 300 mg/day the second week, 450 mg/day the third week, and then 600 mg/day. Gabapentin and pregabalin are not protein bound.

The most common adverse effects reported with gabapentin and pregabalin are somnolence, dizziness, dry mouth, peripheral edema, and blurred vision. Modest weight gain and adverse behavioral effects in children have also been reported.[35,36]

Lamotrigine

Lamotrigine is indicated for use as adjunctive therapy for partial seizures, primary generalized tonic-clonic seizures, and generalized seizures associated with Lennox-Gastaut syndrome.[37] It is also effective against absence seizures and juvenile myoclonic epilepsy. In addition, conversion to monotherapy is indicated for adults with partial seizures who are taking carbamazepine, phenytoin, phenobarbital, primidone, or valproic acid. However, it has not been approved for initial monotherapy in the United States.

Lamotrigine is metabolized in the liver by conjugation with glucuronic acid, and 90% of the administered dose is excreted as metabolites in the urine. Approximately 55% is protein bound. The half-life is relatively long, 12 to 14 hours, and the drug can therefore be administered twice daily. This half-life extends up to 60 hours in the setting of adjunct therapy with valproic acid, whereas serum levels are markedly reduced by enzyme-inducing drugs. Patients typically start lamotrigine therapy at 25 mg/day during the first 2 weeks of treatment. The average daily dose is 200 to 400 mg/day. It is important to have a slow titration schedule at 1- to 2-week intervals initially to reduce the occurrence of severe rash, including Stevens-Johnson syndrome.

The most common side effects associated with lamotrigine are dizziness, nausea, and headache. The side effect of most concern is serious rash, which is more frequent when lamotrigine is initiated at higher dosages or when the dosage is rapidly increased.[38] Development of a serious rash is more common in conjunction with dual lamotrigine and valproic acid therapy, as a result of elevated serum lamotrigine levels. Patients allergic to carbamazepine and phenytoin are at increased risk for rash.[39] Nevertheless, lamotrigine has been associated with a favorable psychotropic profile, improving mood and protecting against adverse mood effects of other medications.[40-42] In addition, because of the lack of effects on bone density and hormone concentrations, together with a relatively low risk of birth defects when it is taken during pregnancy, this drug is an important option for women.

Topiramate

Topiramate was initially approved in the United States for use as adjunctive therapy for partial-onset seizures. It was subsequently approved for treatment in children and adults with partial-onset seizures, primary generalized tonic-clonic seizures, and the multiple-seizure types associated with the Lennox-Gastaut syndrome. It is approved in the United States as monotherapy in adults and children 10 years of age and older.

The metabolism and clearance of topiramate is increased by CYP enzyme–inducing drugs. Topiramate can reduce the efficacy of oral contraceptives when taken at doses higher than 200 mg daily. Topiramate is eliminated via the kidneys and has low protein binding in the serum. It has a relatively long half-life, of 19 to 23 hours. It is rapidly absorbed, reaching peak plasma concentration levels within 1 to 4 hours at doses of 100 to 400 mg/day. Initial dosing should be started at 25 to 50 mg/day (0.5 to 1.0 mg/kg/day) with increased weekly dosing by the same amount until a target dose of 200 to 400 mg/day is achieved.

Slow titration of topiramate helps reduce side effects, including somnolence, impaired concentration, confusion, verbal memory and word-finding problems, and paresthesias. Topiramate may also cause anorexia, weight loss, nephrolithiasis, metabolic acidosis, and reduced sweating in children.

Levetiracetam

Levetiracetam was approved in the United States in 2000 as adjunctive therapy for partial epilepsy. It is currently approved for treatment of partial and secondarily generalized seizures, primary generalized tonic-clonic seizures, and myoclonic seizures in juvenile myoclonic epilepsy.

Levetiracetam has a favorable pharmacokinetic and safety profile. The pharmacokinetic properties are linear, and levetiracetam is not protein bound (<10%). Its metabolites are not pharmacologically active and are excreted renally. Levetiracetam is absorbed rapidly and can reach peak plasma concentrations within 1 hour after an oral dose. Because its half-life is 6 to 8 hours, this medication is usually administered twice daily. A typical starting dose is 250 to 500 mg twice daily in adults and 20 mg/kg/day in children. Maintenance dosing is typically 1000 to 3000 mg/day in adults and 30 to 40 mg/kg/day in children. Levetiracetam may also be administered intravenously.

Levetiracetam has not been associated with life-threatening adverse effects. The most common complaints are somnolence, dizziness, and behavioral problems, including emotional lability, depression, agitation, hostility, anxiety, and aggression.[43] Levetiracetam is rarely associated with allergic reactions.

Zonisamide

Zonisamide was approved in the United States in 2000 and is effective against partial and secondarily generalized seizures, primary generalized tonic-clonic seizures, Lennox-Gastaut syndrome, juvenile myoclonic epilepsy, absence seizures, infantile spasms, myoclonic astatic epilepsy (Doose's syndrome), and progressive myoclonic epilepsy.

Zonisamide has a half-life of 50 to 69 hours and is typically administered daily. It is metabolized by the liver. Peak plasma concentrations are achieved within 2 to 5 hours of oral administration.[44] It has linear pharmacokinetic properties and is more than 50% protein bound. Although it has no effects on other AEDs, its metabolism is accelerated by phenytoin, carbamazepine, phenobarbital, primidone, and valproic acid. The initial suggested starting dosage is 100 mg/day in adults and 1.0 to 2.0 mg/kg/day in children with a target dosage of 100 to 400 mg/day in adults.

Zonisamide may cause drowsiness, fatigue, ataxia, psychomotor slowing, behavioral or psychiatric disturbance (or both), anorexia, and weight loss. Zonisamide is a sulfa drug and may cause allergic rash; thus it should be avoided by patients with hypersensitivity to sulfonamides. As with topiramate, metabolic acidosis, hypohidrosis, nephrolithiasis, and paresthesias may occur with zonisamide.

Lacosamide

Lacosamide was approved in the United States in 2008 for use as adjunctive therapy in adults with complex partial seizures.

Lacosamide has a fast rate of absorption, minimal metabolism by CYP enzymes, low protein binding, and a low potential for drug-drug interactions. Forty percent of lacosamide is excreted unchanged renally. Lacosamide can reach peak plasma concentration as soon as 30 minutes and as late as 4 hours after oral administration. Initial titration dosing starts at 100 mg/day during the first week, followed by weekly titration in 100-mg increments to the targeted dose of 200 to 400 mg/day. However, doses as high as 400 to 600 mg/day may be necessary for seizure control in some patients with refractory disease.[45,46] The half-life of lacosamide is approximately 13 hours, and twice-daily dosing is recommended. Lacosamide is available in an intravenous formulation and may prove beneficial for status epilepticus, but definitive studies are ongoing.

Side effects of lacosamide include dizziness, nausea, vomiting, headache, ataxia, fatigue and diplopia.

Newly Approved Antiepileptic Drugs

Perampanel. Perampanel (Fycompa) is used as an adjunctive therapy to treat partial-onset seizures, with or without secondarily generalized seizures, in people 12 years of age and older. The most common side effects of perampanel include dizziness, sleepiness, tiredness, irritability, falls, nausea, problems with muscle coordination, problems walking normally, vertigo, and weight gain. This drug has also been associated with new or worsened aggressive behavior (including homicidal behavior). The usual adult daily dosage is 4 to 12 mg/day.

Rufinamide. Rufinamide (Banzel) is used to treat patients with Lennox-Gastaut syndrome, including complex partial seizures, generalized tonic-clonic seizures, absence seizures, tonic seizures, and atonic seizures. The most common side effects are fatigue/somnolence, nausea, vomiting, headache, dizziness, decreased appetite, and rash. Rare but serious side effects include hypersensitivity syndrome, associated with rash; swelling and liver abnormalities; and abnormalities in blood cell counts and liver function. The usual adult daily dosage is based on weight. For adults who weigh 50.1 to 70 kg, the recommended daily dose is up to 2400 mg/day; for adults who weigh more than 70 kg, the recommended daily dose is up to 3200 mg/day.

Eslicarbazepine Acetate. Eslicarbazepine acetate (Aptiom) is approved in the United States as an adjunctive therapy to treat partial-onset seizures, with or without secondary generalization. Common side effects include dizziness, ataxia, impaired coordination, tiredness, trouble concentrating, vision problems, and abnormal liver function. Like oxcarbazepine, eslicarbazepine acetate may be associated with hyponatremia. The usual adult daily dosage is 800 to 1200 mg/day.

Clobazam. Clobazam (Onfi) is approved in the United States for adjunctive treatment for seizures associated with Lennox-Gastaut syndrome in patients 2 years of age or older. The most common side effects include sleepiness, drooling, constipation, cough, pain with urination, fever, aggressiveness, difficulty sleeping, slurred speech, and respiratory difficulty. Clobazam has also been associated with dizziness and cognitive slowing, which may improve over time. Like other benzodiazepines, clobazam can cause withdrawal symptoms if it is stopped abruptly. The usual adult daily dosage is 20 to 40 mg/day.

Use of Anesthetics

Midazolam and Propofol

Anesthetic agents may be useful in treating status epilepticus or in patients in the intensive care unit (ICU) who are agitated or prone to hyperventilation. If status epilepticus persists longer than 1 hour despite the use of conventional AEDs, intravenous anesthetic agents may be necessary to terminate seizures in an intubated patient monitored in the ICU. Consensus guidelines support the use of midazolam or propofol as first-line agents in patients with either refractory generalized convulsive or focal status epilepticus.[47,48] Midazolam is often used in this setting (0.2 mg/kg IV bolus then 0.05 to 0.5 mg/kg/hr infusion). However, propofol (1 to 2 mg/kg/hr infusion with overall at a rate <5 mg/kg/hr) is also an excellent choice in this setting because of its shorter half-life and association with less sedation.[49-51] Propofol has a rapid onset and a short duration of action as well.[52] Propofol should be used cautiously and ideally for a limited time period, with an infusion rate not exceeding 67 μg/kg/min.[53] Propofol infused at rates of less than 5 mg/kg/hr is relatively safe, although metabolic acidosis may occur in children after prolonged use, and deaths have been attributed to propofol infusion syndrome.[54,55] The mortality rate with midazolam may be lower than that with propofol. One small study of 20 patients showed comparable seizure control with midazolam and propofol, but the mortality rates were 57% with propofol and only 17% with midazolam.[50] Larger studies are needed to validate this finding.

INITIATION AND DISCONTINUATION OF ANTIEPILEPTIC DRUGS

Decision to Initiate Antiepileptic Drug Treatment

AEDs reduce the risk of recurrent seizures but they do not alter underlying disease or affect long-term outcome.[56] Therefore, the decision to initiate AED treatment is based on an estimated risk of recurrent seizures in comparison with the risks of chronic AED use. Studies have shown that although the risk of a recurrence after a single unprovoked seizure was 14% at 1 year and 34% at 5 years,[57] the risk of recurrence after two unprovoked seizures was 73% at 4 years.[58] Thus treatment after a second unprovoked seizure is common practice, especially for children with nonfebrile seizures.[59,60] Nevertheless, AED treatment after a single unprovoked seizure should be considered in the setting of the following risk factors: epileptiform abnormalities on electroencephalography (EEG); a remote symptomatic cause, identified through clinical history or neuroimaging; and abnormal neurological examination results, including focal findings.[57,61]

An AED is chosen on the basis of its known efficacy for a given seizure type or epilepsy syndrome. In most cases, history, imaging, and EEG help determine whether a seizure was the result of localization-related or generalized epilepsy. Most seizures that occur in neurosurgical patients are due to lesions such as tumors, infarctions, hemorrhages, or gliosis. Therefore, a drug with established efficacy for partial or localization-related seizures would be chosen as initial therapy. Fortunately, the number of appropriate agents available is increasing.

Before an AED is selected, the side effect profile, the patient's age and gender, and the presence of any comorbid conditions should be considered. Dose titration is guided by seizure control and side effect tolerance. Certain drugs (e.g., lamotrigine) must be titrated slowly because of the risk of allergy and therefore are usually not initiated as first-line therapy in patients with high risk of seizure recurrence and immediate need for therapy who are undergoing neurosurgery. AEDs appropriate for intravenous loading are listed in Tables 62-1 and 62-3. Once an AED is selected, the dosage should be increased to the safest tolerated level before it can be considered a treatment failure. Of course, target dosage varies with patient population. For instance, elderly patients may require lower doses because of lower clearance rates and enhanced sensitivity to side effects. If treatment with an AED has failed, either for lack of efficacy or because of intolerable side effects, a second drug must be titrated to a therapeutic dose before the initial drug is tapered. The persistence of seizures does not always indicate complete AED failure. AEDs are often partially effective, limiting the spread, frequency, and duration of seizures. As a result, partial seizures may become dangerous secondarily generalized seizures when AED doses are subtherapeutic or when AEDs are stopped suddenly.

Drug levels can help guide treatment but should never replace clinical observation and judgment. Drug levels also allow monitoring of compliance. Additional laboratory tests should be performed before the start of any AED treatment, including a complete blood cell count and a comprehensive metabolic panel, which includes liver function tests (LFTs). A comprehensive metabolic panel should be routinely checked with the use of carbamazepine and oxcarbazepine to monitor for hyponatremia. The complete blood cell count and liver function should be checked routinely in patients taking valproic acid or felbamate.

Special Neurosurgical Considerations

Craniotomy and Perioperative Antiepileptic Drugs

Between 20% and 50% of all patients who undergo neurosurgery have a seizure in the first week after surgery.[62,63] The American Academy of Neurology (AAN) has not made recommendations regarding perioperative prophylaxis, but it does recommend that all AEDs be tapered and discontinued in the first week postoperatively in patients who have not had a seizure.[64] Phenytoin has been shown to reduce the risk of seizures in the first postoperative week on average by 44%.[65] However, phenytoin can cause hematologic suppression and increase plasma clearance, as well as decrease bioavailability of dexamethasone.[66]

Levetiracetam has replaced phenytoin in many neurological ICUs. In addition, for patients undergoing craniotomy, levetiracetam has advantages over phenytoin, including lesser drug-drug interactions, good tolerability with fewer side effects, rapid titration, and lower risk of allergy than with phenytoin. In a study by Milligan and associates,[67] 1 of 105 patients taking levetiracetam and 9 of 210 patients taking phenytoin had seizures within 7 days of surgery. Levetiracetam was also associated with fewer adverse effects (1% of those taking levetiracetam, 18% of those taking phenytoin).

Trauma and Antiepileptic Drugs

The risk of developing posttraumatic epilepsy (PTE) is correlated with the severity of brain injury and duration of loss of consciousness (LOC). In one large review of patients with head trauma who lost consciousness after impact, the relative risk of developing PTE was 1.9 for those with LOC for less than 30 minutes, 2.9 for those with LOC for 30 minutes to 24 hours, and 17.2 for those with LOC that lasted more than 1 day.[68] Other factors that increased the risk of late PTE included depressed skull fracture, penetrating trauma, intracranial hemorrhage, advanced age, and early posttraumatic seizures. Because of the high incidence of early posttraumatic seizures with severe traumatic brain injury, affected patients should receive prophylactic AEDs in the first week after injury.[69] Although phenytoin is effective against early posttraumatic seizures, levetiracetam may be preferable because of its better side effect profile and better adverse event profile.[70]

Brain Tumors and Antiepileptic Drug Therapy

Patients with brain tumors who present with seizures should begin AED therapy immediately. The risk of seizure recurrence after a single seizure is higher in patients with evidence of a structural brain lesion.[71] Although evidence supports the initiation of AEDs in the setting of seizures, AED prophylaxis has not been proven to reduce the incidence of epilepsy.[72] The need for perioperative (up to 1 week postoperative) prophylactic AED treatment is not as well established. The decision to initiate AEDs for perioperative prophylaxis should be influenced by tumor size and location. Seizures occur more frequently when tumors are located in the frontoparietal, frontotemporal, parasagittal, and temporal regions.[73] In patients who may require chemotherapy, a non–CYP enzyme–inducing AED, which will not diminish serum chemotherapy agent levels, is preferred.

As with intraparechymal brain tumors, large randomized studies of perioperative AED management have not been conducted for patients with meningiomas. One review of 626 such patients revealed 90% of patients to be seizure free at 48 months.[74] Persistent seizures were associated with parasagittal and sphenoidal locations, as were uncontrolled preoperative seizures.

The AAN found that long-term prophylaxis with AED treatment does not reduce the frequency of seizures in patients with newly diagnosed brain tumors and, in fact, increases adverse side effects and interactions with chemotherapy. However, the AAN did not take a definite stand regarding perioperative prophylaxis.

Decision to Discontinue Drug Treatment

Discontinuation of treatment is also based on a risk-benefit analysis. The decision to discontinue AEDs is usually discussed after a 2-year period of seizure freedom for children with epilepsy. For adults, the decision is often based on numerous factors, including whether the patient is driving and the patient's occupation. Seizures are more likely to recur after cessation of treatment if the patient has a history of known remote symptomatic epilepsy associated with a prior neurological insult, seizure onset after the age of 12 years, a family history of epilepsy, focal or generalized slowing on EEG, or a history of complex febrile seizures. The risk of recurrent seizures after 2 years of seizure freedom varies according to the risk factors just described and whether the interictal EEG is persistently abnormal.[75]

Studies have shown that the rate of drug tapering does not alter the seizure recurrence risk at 2 years. However, slow tapering is advisable, if possible, in order to reduce the risk of withdrawal effects. In addition, because seizure tends to recur early, during or shortly after the withdrawal of AEDs,[76] smaller partial seizures (as opposed to stronger generalized seizures) may occur if the AED levels decline slowly. The majority of the patients who have recurrent seizures become seizure-free and achieve remission after the AEDs are restarted.[77]

In patients who have achieved seizure freedom after epilepsy surgery, the decision to alter medication regimens is not usually considered until 1 year after surgery, unless the medications produce intolerable side effects. The decision to discontinue a medication completely after surgery is not typically addressed until 2 years after surgery. Studies have shown that 60% of adult patients with medically refractory epilepsy who became seizure free after resective surgery remained seizure free when their AEDs were tapered off.[78] Of those who had recurrent seizures after the tapering of AEDs, the majority regained freedom from seizures after resuming therapy.[79] Risk factors associated with lower rates of seizure freedom after AED tapering include longer duration of epilepsy, normal appearance on preoperative magnetic resonance imaging, and occurrence of postoperative seizures before initiation of AED withdrawal.[80]

SUGGESTED READINGS

Annegers JF, Coan SP. The risks of epilepsy after traumatic brain injury. *Seizure*. 2000;9(7):453-457.

Berg A, Shinnar S. The risk of seizure recurrence following a first unprovoked seizure: a quantitative review. *Neurology*. 1991;41:965-972.

Brodie MJ, Ditcher MA. Antiepileptic drugs. *N Engl J Med*. 1996;334:168-175.

Claassen J, Hirsch LJ, Emerson RG, et al. Treatment of refractory status epilepticus with pentobarbital, propofol, or midazolam: a systematic review. *Epilepsia*. 2002;43:146-153.

Hauser WA, Rich SS, Lee JR, et al. Risk of recurrent seizures after two unprovoked seizures. *N Engl J Med*. 1998;338(7):429.

Hwang H, Kim KJ. New antiepileptic drugs in pediatric epilepsy. *Brain Dev*. 2008;30:549-555.

Karceski S, Morrell MJ, Carpenter D. Treatment of epilepsy in adults: expert opinion, 2005. *Epilepsy Behav*. 2005;7(suppl 1):S1-S64.

Schiller Y, Cascino GD, So EL, et al. Discontinuation of antiepileptic drugs after successful epilepsy surgery. *Neurology*. 2000;54:346-349.

Shaw MD, Foy PM. Epilepsy after craniotomy and the place of prophylactic anticonvulsant drugs discussion paper. *J R Soc Med*. 1991;84:221-223.

Temkin NR. Prophylactic anticonvulsants after neurosurgery. *Epilepsy Curr*. 2002;2(4):105-107.

See a full reference list on ExpertConsult.com

63 Continuous Electroencephalography in Neurological-Neurosurgical Intensive Care

Applications and Value

Jens Witsch, Emma Meyers, and Jan Claassen

The goal of critical care medicine is to ensure the patient's survival with little or no disability. Because the patient's status is in a continuous flux, it is crucial to detect changes that are associated with worsening of the patient's condition and ideally may be reversed. All vital organ functions should be monitored, and any change should be diagnosed in real time. Currently, monitoring and fast analysis of cardiac and pulmonary function are established practices in any intensive care unit. On admission, every patient is connected to a continuous electrocardiogram monitor, pulse oximeter, and blood pressure monitors. However, there is no standardized and ubiquitously applied way of monitoring brain function. Even in many specialized neurological-neurosurgical intensive care units (neuro-ICU), the most commonly used measure to evaluate brain function is repeated neurological examination, which is often unreliable, especially in deeply sedated patients. Imaging modalities may be more specific, such as computed tomography (CT) to diagnose hemorrhages or magnetic resonance imaging (MRI) to diagnose acute strokes. However, because imaging is not performed continuously, temporal resolution is lacking. Conversely, invasive monitoring of intracranial pressure or brain oxygen may allow assessment of brain physiology in real time, but spatial resolution is poor.

Continuous electroencephalography (cEEG) monitors brain function and reflects changes in large regions of the brain in real time. It may be used to detect seizures, monitor the effects of therapeutic interventions, detect newly developing ischemia, and aid in prognostication. Indications for cEEG include convulsive or nonconvulsive status epilepticus (NCSE), acute stroke, traumatic brain injury (TBI), and post–cardiac arrest syndrome (PCAS) (Table 63-1), among others.[1,2]

The complexity of the electroencephalography (EEG) signal and, therefore, the necessity of interpretation by specialized electrophysiology staff entail relatively high manpower and cost, which have impeded the widespread application of cEEG. Furthermore, technical challenges such as appropriate data collection and data storage limit the routine use of cEEG to relatively specialized neuro-ICUs. However, with advances in computer technology, these obstacles are being overcome, making cEEG a promising diagnostic tool for routine clinical neurological intensive care use.

ELECTROENCEPHALOGRAPHY-RELATED INFRASTRUCTURE IN INTENSIVE CARE UNITS

EEG-related infrastructure in the ICU may be subdivided into *basic*, *advanced*, and *highly advanced* standards. Requirements for *basic* emergent EEG include the capability to connect a spot EEG at all times and to provide standard EEG reading at least once a day or within 2 hours of performing the study on demand.

An *advanced* EEG laboratory must include, in addition to the basic requirements, the capability of Web-based expert interpretation of EEG studies at all times and the capacity to provide EEG reads on demand within 1 hour of performing the study. Furthermore, it requires daily maintenance of the EEG recording equipment and the option to upgrade spot EEG to continuous EEG recording.

In addition to advanced EEG laboratory requirements, *highly advanced* EEG laboratories should provide, or at least aim for, the capability to perform EEG reads in real time, to carry out invasive EEG monitoring, to combine EEG recordings with multimodal monitoring (MMM), and to have an informatics structure in place that allows interpretation of the EEG-MMM data in a synchronized fashion. Different types of electrodes (needle or disk electrodes, MRI-compatible electrodes) should be available, if needed.[3]

In this chapter, we review current indications for cEEG and its potential uses in critically ill patients. First, we describe nonconvulsive seizures (NCSzs), NCSE, and convulsive status epilepticus (CSE) in neuro-ICU patients in general, followed by the incidence of NCSzs in common specific neuro-ICU conditions, including TBI, subarachnoid hemorrhage (SAH), intracerebral hemorrhage (ICH), acute ischemic stroke (AIS), PCAS, and infectious and noninfectious encephalopathies.

The final paragraphs are dedicated to the role of EEG in the detection of ischemia and periodic discharges (PDs) and to the use of cEEG as part of MMM. The use of cEEG as an aid in predicting neurological outcomes is discussed. Important indications for continuous EEG monitoring are summarized in Table 63-1.

DETECTION OF NONCONVULSIVE SEIZURES AND STATUS EPILEPTICUS

Nonconvulsive Seizures and Nonconvulsive Status Epilepticus

Definitions

Seizures in ICUs are very common. Often, they are nonconvulsive and associated with poor outcome.[4,5] Figure 63-1 shows an EEG trace of an NCSz.

Status epilepticus (SE) is a prolonged seizure. Recent guidelines have defined SE as at least 5 minutes of ongoing clinical or electrographic seizure activity or recurrent seizures without recovery to baseline between seizures.[4] This definition is based on the observation that most seizures that last longer than 5 minutes do not cease spontaneously.[6-12] In NCSE there are usually no obvious clinical findings (e.g., rhythmic jerking of the extremities) apart from a decreased level of consciousness, which is a nonspecific finding in the neuro-ICU setting, associated with the seizure activity seen on EEG, although subtle clinical signs may be present (see "Diagnosis" section).

Etiology

The causes of NCSzs and NCSE in neuro-ICU patients may vary by age and patient group and are generally similar to the causes of convulsive seizures (see later), including structural lesions,

TABLE 63-1 Indications for Continuous Electroencephalography Monitoring

Indication	Rationale	References
Recent clinical seizure or SE without return to baseline >10 min	Ongoing nonconvulsive status despite cessation of motor activity,18%-50%	36, 45, 43, 194
Coma, including post–cardiac arrest	Frequent nonconvulsive seizures, 20%-60%	38, 195
Epileptiform activity or periodic discharges on initial 30-min EEG	Risk for nonconvulsive seizures, 40%-60%	194, 196
Intracranial hemorrhage including TBI, SAH, ICH	Frequent nonconvulsive seizures, 20%-35%	197
Suspected nonconvulsive seizures in patients with altered mental status	Frequent nonconvulsive seizures, 10%-30%	1, 38, 198

EEG, electroencephalography; ICH, intracerebral hemorrhage; SAH, subarachnoid hemorrhage; SE, status epilepticus; TBI, traumatic brain injury.
Modified from Brophy GM, Bell R, Claassen J, et al. Guidelines for the evaluation and management of status epilepticus. *Neurocrit Care*. 2012;17:3-23.

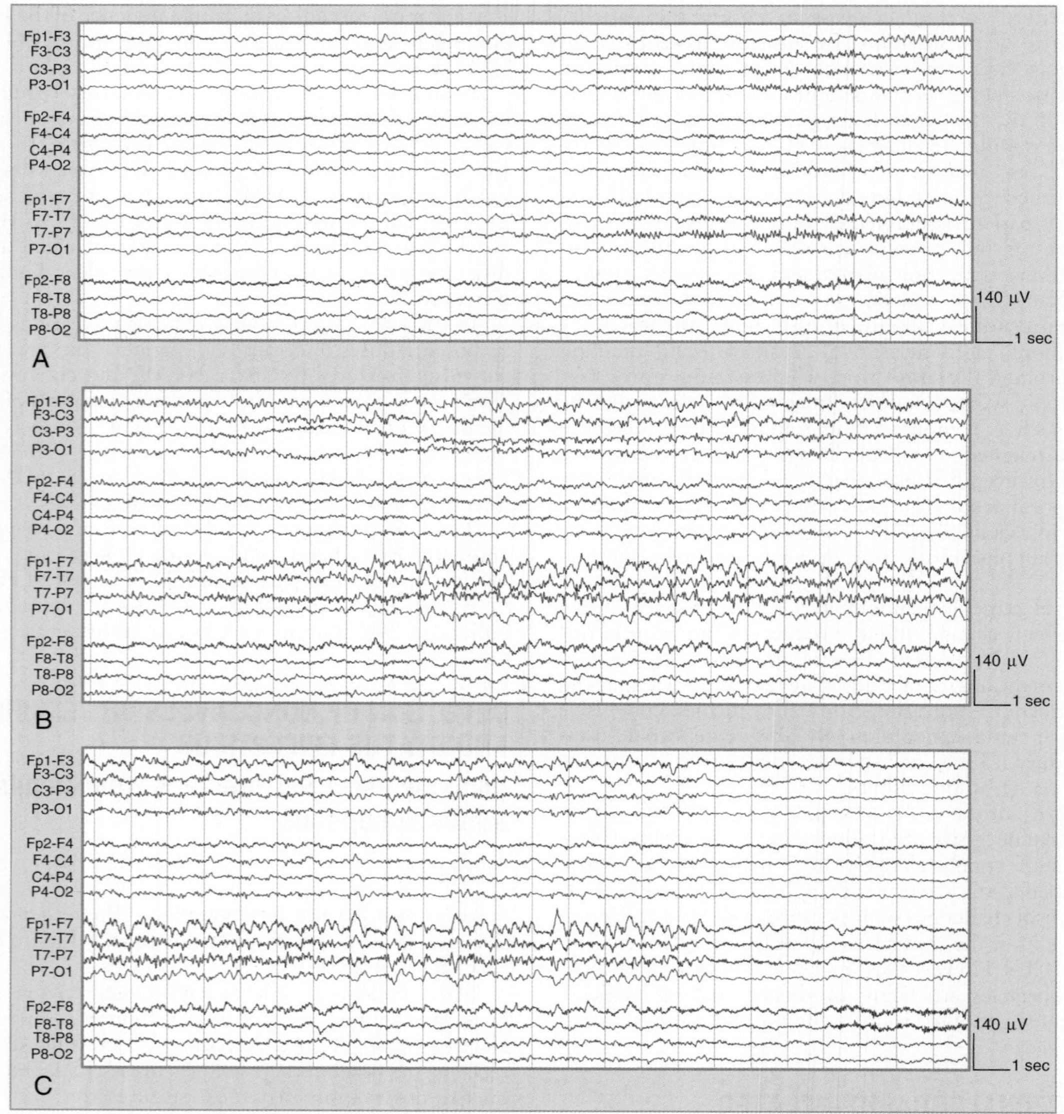

Figure 63-1. Gradual appearance of a left-sided nonconvulsive seizure in a 64-year-old man with a right-sided parietotemporal central nervous system B-cell non-Hodgkin's lymphoma, treated conservatively. The patient was admitted for recurrent episodes of confusion. **A,** Baseline electroencephalogram with bifrontal fast activity slowly evolving into a left-sided frontotemporal seizure (**B**), which spontaneously ceases (**C**).

infections, metabolic derangements, toxins, drug withdrawal, and epilepsy, all of which are common diagnoses in critically ill patients.[13] Inflammation, frequently seen after acute brain injury, may be a unifying underlying cause of NCSzs by lowering the seizure threshold and starting a vicious cycle of seizure induced inflammation.[14] As a physiologic consequence, NCSzs are associated with elevation of intracranial pressure, brain tissue hypoxia, and increasing mass effect. Further studies have shown correlations between NCSzs and elevation of neuron-specific enolase, interstitial glutamate, and pyruvate.[15-22]

Incidence

Depending on the underlying condition, NCSzs may occur in up to one third of neurological critical care patient populations after acute brain injury.[1,5,21,23-37] Major studies investigating NCSzs in various patient populations using cEEG are summarized in Table 63-2.

Diagnosis

Coma is the most common clinical presentation of NCSE in an ICU setting,[4] and clinical diagnosis of NCSzs and NCSE is often hindered by the fact that many neuro-ICU patients are comatose as a consequence of the acute brain injury or sedation. In one study including 236 ICU patients with coma of any kind, NCSE was found on EEG recording in 8% of patients.[38] Thus NCSE should be part of the differential diagnosis in all comatose patients. Subtle clinical signs that have been associated with NCSzs and NCSE include face and limb myoclonus, nystagmus, eye deviation, pupillary abnormalities, and autonomic instability, but these signs are sparse or absent in many cases.[39-42] Therefore clinical examination as a sole diagnostic modality is not reliable, and complementary EEG recordings are indispensable to the diagnosis of NCSzs and NCSE. The EEG criteria for definite NCSzs are outlined in Box 63-1.

Convulsive Status Epilepticus

CSE is defined as prolonged seizure activity on EEG (see "Definitions" section under "Nonconvulsive Seizures and Nonconvulsive Status Epilepticus") accompanied by the tonic-clonic movements of the extremities, mental status impairment, and

TABLE 63-2 Studies Using Continuous Electroencephalography Monitoring for Detection of Nonconvulsive Seizures in Critical Care Patient Populations

Study	Design	Population	No. of Participants	NCSzs (Frequency)	Other Findings
Dennis et al., 2002[28]	R CS	SAH	233		3% NCSE (31% or 8 of 26 with EEG)
Claassen et al., 2006[66]	R CS	SAH	116	15%	11% NCSE
O'Connor et al., 2014[199]	R CS	SAH	69	10% (in unselected patients)	18% in patients with clinical suspicion for seizures; 9% in patients without suspicion for seizures
Lindgren et al., 2012[200]	R CS	SAH	28	7%	
Vespa et al., 2003[21]	P CS	AIS	46	6%	
Vespa et al., 2003[21]	P CS	ICH	63	28%	
Claassen et al., 2007[24]	R CS	ICH	102	18%	7% NCSE
Carrera et al., 2006[32]	P CS	AIS	100	2%	3% PEDs
Vespa et al., 1999[48]	P CS	TBI	94	22% (convulsive and nonconvulsive; in 12% purely nonconvulsive)	
Ronne-Engstrom and Winkler, 2006[26]	R CS	TBI	70	33%	
Olivecrona et al., 2009[27]	P CS	TBI	47	0%	8.5% clinical seizures before EEG
Crepeau[201]	R CS	PCAS	62	8%	
Knight[202]	R CS	PCAS	33	33%	82% patients with seizures died during hospitalization (50% without seizures died)
Mani et al., 2012[90]	R CS	PCAS	38	24%	7 of 9 NCSzs patients had NCSE
Rossetti et al., 2001[85]	P CS	PCAS	34	15%	6% GPEDs
Sadaka et al., 2015[203]	R CS	PCAS	58	5%	All NCSz patients (n = 3) had NCSE
Carrera et al., 2008[31]	R CS	CNS infection (64% viral)	42	33%	40% PEDs
Jordan, 1993[33]	R CS	Mixed neuro-ICU		34%	
Claassen et al., 2004[34]	R CS	ICU/ward	570	18% (exclusively nonconvulsive)	
Pandian et al., 2004[1]	R CS	Mixed neuro-ICU	105	No denominator	
Kramer et al., 2012[74]	R CS	Mixed neuro-ICU (GCS ≤12)	34	44%	
Shafi et al., 2012[204]	R CS	All patients receiving continuous EEG, mostly mixed neuro-ICU population	242	29%	Findings on early (first 30 min) screening EEG in 190 patients without early seizures: PEDs 11%; triphasic waves 13%
Ponten et al., 2010[205]	P CS	Mixed neuro-ICU (56% PCAS)	50	4%	
Das et al., 2009[206]	R CS	Mixed neuro-ICU	54	19%	NCSE in 3 of 10 NCSz patients; spikes/sharp waves in 6%; PLEDs in 9%; GPEDs in 4%
Amantini et al., 2009[35]	P CS	TBI, ICH, SAH	68	3%	
Drislane, 2000[36]	R CS	All NCSE	91	No denominator	
Oddo et al., 2009[207]	R CS	Medical ICU	201	10%	17% PEDs
Kurtz et al., 2014[168]	R CS	Surgical ICU	154	16%	5% NCSE, 29% PEDs
Tanner et al., 2014[208]	R CS	Mixed ICU (GCS 8)	170	8%	
Kamel et al., 2013[209]	R CS	Medical and surgical ICU	105	11%	

AIS, acute ischemic stroke; CNS, central nervous system; CS, case series; EEG, electroencephalography; GCS, Glasgow Coma Scale; GPEDs, generalized periodic discharges; ICH, intracerebral hemorrhage; ICU, intensive care unit; NCSE, nonconvulsive status epilepticus; NCSz, nonconvulsive seizures; neuro-ICU, neurological intensive care unit; PEDs, periodic epileptiform discharges; PLEDs, periodic lateralized epileptiform discharges; P, prospective; PCAS, post–cardiac arrest syndrome; R, retrospective; SAH, subarachnoid hemorrhage; TBI, traumatic brain injury.

BOX 63-1 Criteria for Definite Nonconvulsive Seizures*

Any pattern lasting at least 10 seconds and satisfying any one of the following three primary criteria:

PRIMARY CRITERIA

Repetitive generalized or focal spikes, sharp waves, spike and wave complexes at ≥3/sec

Repetitive generalized or focal spikes, sharp waves, spike and wave or sharp and slow-wave complexes at <3/sec and the secondary criterion

Sequential rhythmic, periodic, or quasi-periodic waves at ≥1/sec and unequivocal evolution in frequency (gradually increasing or decreasing by at least 1/sec, e.g., 2-3/sec), morphology, or location (gradual spread into or out of a region involving at least two electrodes). Evolution in amplitude alone is not sufficient. Change in sharpness without other change in morphology is not enough to satisfy evolution in morphology.

SECONDARY CRITERION

Significant improvement in the clinical state or appearance of previously absent normal electroencephalographic patterns (such as posterior-dominant "alpha" rhythm) temporally coupled to acute administration of a rapidly acting antiepileptic drug. Resolution of the "epileptiform" discharges leaving diffuse slowing without clinical improvement and without the appearance of previously absent normal electroencephalographic patterns would not satisfy the secondary criterion.

*Satisfying these criteria is adequate for confirming nonconvulsive seizure activity. However, failing to meet these criteria does not rule out nonconvulsive seizure activity; clinical judgment and correlation are required in this situation.

Modified from Chong DJ, Hirsch LJ. Which EEG patterns warrant treatment in the critically ill? Reviewing the evidence for treatment of periodic epileptiform discharges and related patterns. *J Clin Neurophysiol*. 2005;22:79, Tab 2, as modified from Young GB, Jordan KG, Doig GS. An assessment of nonconvulsive seizures in the intensive care unit using continuous EEG monitoring: an investigation of variables associated with mortality. *Neurology*. 1996;47:83.

potential transient neurologic deficits in the postictal phase.[4] The etiology of CSE does not essentially differ from that of NCSE (see "Etiology" section under "Nonconvulsive Seizures and Nonconvulsive Status Epilepticus").

CSE is, in principle, a clinical diagnosis that does not always require EEG confirmation. However, EEG may be necessary to differentiate between CSE and psychogenic seizures or cerebral herniation, which may both be accompanied by rhythmic movements of the extremities as well. Even if the diagnosis of CSE is established, such as by the use of spot EEG, and CSE has been successfully terminated by benzodiazepine administration, NCSz or NCSE persists in 48% and 14% of cases.[43,44] Again, coma is the most common clinical presentation in patients with ongoing nonconvulsive epileptic brain activity following the termination of CSE, which in this situation is particularly nonspecific because many patients may be comatose postictally or as a consequence of benzodiazepine administration. In one prospective randomized controlled trial, patients with ongoing SE experienced a twofold higher mortality than those without ongoing epileptic activity.[45] cEEG should therefore be routinely recorded, after termination of CSE, to rule out persistent epileptic brain activity.

Treatment of Status Epilepticus and Nonconvulsive Seizures

Although it is still a matter of debate whether NCSzs should be treated, and in the past there were also controversies about treatment of SE,[46,47] today there is no question that treatment of SE is a medical emergency, which is reflected in current guidelines.[4] It has been shown multiple times that SE is associated with a worse outcome, and duration of SE and delay to reaching the diagnosis are each independent predictors of worse outcome.[48,49] Emergent treatment of SE includes intravenous administration of benzodiazepines, which have been shown to have the highest efficacy. Nasal, rectal, and buccal modes of administration are possible when intravenous access is not available. Class I, level A evidence is available for lorazepam and midazolam.[4,45,50-53] For details of emergent and urgent treatment of SE as well as treatment of refractory SE, please refer to current guidelines.[4]

Traumatic Brain Injury

Authors who did not use cEEG but determined seizures solely on clinical grounds have shown seizure incidences within the first week after TBI of between 4% and 14% and a 15% incidence in patients with severe TBI.[54-56] In two cEEG studies that included 94 and 70 TBI patients, respectively, purely nonconvulsive seizures were found in one eighth[48] to one third of patients.[26]

In a large retrospective study including 570 critically ill patients, of 51 patients in the TBI subgroup, 9 (18%) had NCSzs and 4 (8%) had NCSE.[34] In another study including 47 patients with severe TBI undergoing intubation, sedation cEEG monitoring, and ICP monitoring, seizures were seen in 8% of patients before the start of sedation. When patients were sedated, no seizures were detected.[27] A recent study of pediatric ICU patients showed electrographic seizures in 43% after TBI.[57]

Although post-TBI seizures have been associated with increases of ICP,[23] it is unclear whether treatment of seizures may improve clinical outcome after TBI. It is unlikely that conclusive data will be available in the future because the occurrence of post-TBI seizures correlates highly with the severity of TBI[58] and poor outcome is overshadowed by TBI severity as the most important cofactor.

Subarachnoid Hemorrhage

Convulsive and nonconvulsive seizures are frequent in aneurysmal SAH.[59] The occurrence of convulsive seizures at SAH onset has been associated with total SAH blood volume on CT scan.[60] Their frequency varies in different studies between 3% and 21%.[29,59-65]

In a large study on electrographic seizure detection in critically ill patients including a subgroup of 108 SAH patients, seizures were detected in 19% of SAH patients, and 92% of seizures were nonconvulsive.[34] In another study of 479 SAH patients, electrographic seizures were detected in 11%.[14] Other authors report seizure detection rates as low as 3% in a population of 233 patients, possibly because only 26 patients had EEG monitoring. Out of these 26 patients, 8 (31%) had NCSzs.[28]

Intracortical depth electrodes are more likely to detect seizures than surface EEG recordings. In a study including 90 poor-grade SAH patients, NCSzs were found on depth electrode measurements in 38% of patients and on surface EEG measurements in 8% of patients.[18]

Other common EEG findings in SAH include PDs, which have been found in 28% in a cohort of 109 SAH patients.[66] PDs are discussed in more detail at the end of this chapter.

Factors associated with NCSzs were poor admission Hunt and Hess Scale grade, parenchymal bleeds, large amounts of cisternal blood, delayed cerebral ischemia (DCI), aneurysm clipping, and anterior circulation aneurysm,[29,67] whereas advanced age, coma, brain edema, and hydrocephalus were associated with a higher risk for NCSE.[5,28] In a recent study, inflammation following SAH, as reflected in clinical symptoms and in serum biomarkers of inflammation, was causally linked to the occurrence of NCSz.[14]

Antiepileptic drug prophylaxis and treatment of NCSzs in SAH remain a matter of debate because clinical data on the subject are still sparse. Whether convulsive seizures in the context of SAH worsen outcome is controversial. One study of 381 SAH patients showed an association of clinical seizures at SAH onset and poor outcome at 6 weeks,[60] although a recent study in a larger sample of 1479 patients showed an association of SAH-onset seizures with in-hospital complications (including subsequent seizures), but could not confirm an association of SAH-onset seizures with poor outcome or epilepsy 3 months after SAH.[68]

In a series of 116 aneurysmal subarachnoid hemorrhage patients undergoing cEEG monitoring, absence of sleep architecture and presence of periodic lateralized epileptiform discharges (PLEDs) were associated with poor outcome.[66] In another study of 48 SAH patients, epileptiform discharges on EEG, occurrence of NCSE, and nonreactive EEG background predicted poor outcome.[18] Additionally, NCSz may be partially responsible for the poor outcomes in SAH complicated by pronounced inflammatory responses.[14] More studies correlating electrographic seizure burden and outcome are necessary to discern optimal treatment regimens.

Intracerebral Hemorrhage

The risk for in-hospital convulsive seizures following ICH ranges from 3% to 19%.[24,28,69-72] NCSzs occurred in 18% to 21% of patients with ICH in two studies using cEEG.[21,24] The occurrence of hematoma expansion increases seizure risk by at least 30% in the first 24 hours after admission.[24] Lobar location of hemorrhage and midline shift also predict higher seizure rates.[21] PDs were found in 17% of patients[24] and were more frequently associated with cortical ICH (29%) than with deeper hematomas (8%).

In a study of a mixed patient cohort (N = 5027) including AIS and ICH patients, the occurrence of convulsive seizures was associated with increased morbidity and mortality at follow-up. Only 65% of stroke patients with seizures were discharged alive, and 30-day and 1-year stroke fatalities were significantly higher in patients with seizures than in those without seizures. Factors associated with seizures were stroke severity and hemorrhagic stroke.[73]

NCSzs may predict worse outcome in ICH patients, but available data are not sufficient to determine whether seizures independently influence outcome.[21,24,74,75] The occurrence of PDs, on the other hand, was independently associated with worse outcome.[24]

Acute Ischemic Stroke

A recent epidemiologic study of more than 10,000 patients found clinically apparent convulsive seizures at stroke onset in 2.0% and poststroke seizures (during hospitalization) in 1.5% of patients.[76] Other studies found rates of acute seizures between 2% and 9% after AIS.[69,71,77-80] Studies using cEEG have found higher incidences.[21,34] In one series, 11% of 56 patients with ischemic stroke undergoing cEEG had seizures; these seizures were purely nonconvulsive in 5 of 6 patients.[34] Other authors using cEEG in ischemic stroke patients reported NCSz frequencies of 6% (in a cohort of 46 patients)[21] and 17% (in a cohort of 100 patients).[32] In that study, only stroke severity was independently associated with the occurrence of seizures.

In a mixed stroke patient cohort (76% ischemic stroke patients), 6.5% of patients were found to have early electrographic seizures within 24 hours after stroke onset, and 6.0% had PLEDs.[37] Although there is consensus that electrographic seizures in ICH patients should be treated, prophylactic antiepileptic drug treatment is not generally recommended in patients after ICH or ischemic stroke.[81] Acute, clinically apparent seizures are associated with increased mortality in patients with ischemic stroke.[69,80,82] Other studies have used quantitative EEG to predict functional outcome after AIS,[83] but the relationship between NCSz and outcome after AIS is currently still unknown. Further research is needed to establish the role of cEEG in prognostication after AIS.

Hypoxic-Ischemic Injury and Post–Cardiac Arrest Syndrome

The neurological intensive care section of the European Society of Intensive Care Management recommends routine EEG monitoring in patients with PCAS during therapeutic hypothermia (TH) and for 24 hours after rewarming.[84] Continuous EEG after cardiac arrest not only enables seizure detection but also is an important instrument for prognostication in patients after cardiac arrest[85-87] (see "Electroencephalography and Prognostication in Post–Cardiac Arrest Syndrome" section).

TH after cardiac arrest has been widely implemented as a potential means of neuroprotection and requires sedation and muscular relaxation, so convulsive seizures and CSE may be masked by neuromuscular blockade in these patients. Thus cEEG has a crucial role in detecting nonconvulsive and (otherwise) convulsive seizures because clinical judgment may be even less reliable in these patients than in other comatose ICU patients.[88]

Convulsive and nonconvulsive seizures are common after cardiac arrest, occurring in 10% to 30% of patients[34,89] with[85,87,90-97] or without[98-104] TH. Postanoxic status epilepticus occurs in 10% to 12% of patients, as shown in two separate studies including 51 and 101 patients.[95,97] One study showed that patients with postanoxic status epilepticus who have preserved brainstem reflexes, intact somatosensory evoked potentials, and reactive EEG background activity may benefit from aggressive treatment of status epilepticus.[86]

Electroencephalography and Prognostication in Post–Cardiac Arrest Syndrome

Prognostication is, in general, a promising application of continuous EEG. This is especially true in patients with PCAS, for which prognostication is expected to solve pressing ethical and financial issues.

However, as with all other diagnostic modalities used to prognosticate a condition, cEEG should be integrated into the decision process as one of many sources of data to help reduce prognostic uncertainty. Among many potential applications, the following briefly describes the role of EEG in approaching a prognosis after cardiac arrest.

The routine use of TH[105] has led to changes regarding the accuracy of widely accepted prognostication tools in cardiac arrest survivors. Examples include the motor response as part of the neurological examination, which may take longer to recover in hypothermia-treated patients, and the serum marker for neuronal injury, neuron-specific enolase, which has a higher cutoff for prediction of poor outcome in patients receiving TH.

EEG-specific features indicating a higher probability of poor outcome after cardiac arrest include burst suppression, generalized suppression, status epilepticus, and nonreactivity. Most studies on the prognostic value of these features predate the use of TH.[85-87,93,94,96,98-104,106-123] More recently, however, studies not only have established the value of EEG under TH conditions[87,91-94,96,106,113,114,124] but also have supported the hypothesis that EEG might have greater prognostic accuracy under TH conditions.[87,109,125-129] In contrast, a recent study has shown that somatosensory evoked potentials do not add prognostic significance when included with the neurological examination, serum neuron-specific enolase levels, and EEG parameters.[130] However, more studies are needed to confirm the superiority of cEEG over somatosensory evoked potentials.

With regard to the effect of seizures on clinical outcome, postanoxic status epilepticus was shown to be an independent predictor of mortality.[92] In one study, two types of status epilepticus were identified in patients after cardiac arrest: one developing from burst suppression, and one from a continuous EEG background pattern, with the latter type being associated with a more favorable prognosis.[93,113]

Infectious and Noninfectious Encephalopathies

Seizures are a common complication of infectious processes involving the brain and occur more frequently in viral[131,132] than bacterial infections.[133,134] Furthermore, seizures may be found in noninfectious encephalopathies, including metabolic derangements (hypoglycemia, hyperglycemia, hyponatremia, hypocalcemia), drug intoxication or withdrawal, uremia, liver dysfunction, posterior reversible encephalopathy syndrome, and sepsis.

Two studies including 62 patients with bacterial meningitis and 42 patients with varying infectious etiology (27 viral, 8 bacterial, 7 fungal and parasitic) reported clinically apparent seizure rates of 13% and 12%,[31,135] respectively. In addition, the authors reported a remarkably high rate of seizures without clinical correlate: NCSzs occurred in 9 of 42 patients (21%).[31] In another series of critically ill patients, infectious and toxic-metabolic encephalopathy accounted for 6% and 7% of cases, respectively. Twenty-nine percent of infectious and 18% of toxic metabolic patients had electrographic seizures.[34]

In one large cohort (N = 393) of critically ill patients with an admission Glasgow Coma Scale score of 12 or lower, electrographic seizures were present in 10% of the patients with central nervous system infections. In this study, only 34 patients underwent cEEG monitoring. The remaining patients had at least one routine EEG, but no cEEG, which suggests that seizure frequency was underestimated rather than overestimated. Epileptiform discharges and PDs were detected in 28% and 18% of patients, respectively.[74]

In the increasingly diagnosed entity of anti–*N*-methyl-D-aspartate (NMDA) receptor encephalitis, the EEG pattern of "extreme delta brush" has been described. In a study of 23 patients with anti-NMDA receptor encephalitis who underwent cEEG monitoring, the occurrence of this pattern was associated with prolonged illness.[136] However, it is unclear whether this relatively new EEG pattern should be considered harmful in and of itself.

Few data on treatment, outcome, and prognosis in the context of encephalopathy-related seizures exist. However, in one large study that included 671 patients with bacterial meningitis, the occurrence of seizures was independently associated with mortality.[137]

DETECTION OF ISCHEMIA

Patients with severe strokes are frequently admitted to intensive care. However, ischemia may develop secondarily in many primarily nonischemic conditions in the neuro-ICU (e.g., SAH, TBI, and meningitis). In particular, DCI after SAH accounts for a considerable portion of disability and mortality. Conversely, hyperperfusion may occur, which can lead to reperfusion injury—for example, in hypoxic brain injury, after reopening of an occluded vessel in acute ischemic stroke, or in the aftermath of TBI, when vasoreactivity may be altered. In many patients, both ischemia and hyperperfusion are physiologic variables modifiable by interventions such as raising or lowering systemic blood pressure.[138,139] What is needed is a measure of blood flow in the brain, in other words, the *end-organ response*.

Reductions in blood flow are associated with slowing of EEG background activity.[140-142] A study in 1973 showed that continuous EEG was shown to correlate well with cerebral blood flow in patients undergoing carotid endarterectomy. The ICU environment is very different from the controlled circumstances of the operating room. In ICU patients, baseline EEG measurements are not available; depending on the underlying condition, sedation regimens are more variable than during scheduled surgery, and sedation is regularly discontinued per protocol, which causes fluctuations in EEG measurements.

The following section summarizes the role of EEG in detecting ischemia after SAH and AIS.

Ischemia Detection in Subarachnoid Hemorrhage

In patients with high-grade SAH, DCI may not be detected by changes in the clinical examination[143,144] but has been shown to affect outcome.[145] Thus detecting developing ischemia early is a crucial step toward improving outcome in poor-grade SAH patients. However, to date there is no reliable monitoring tool to detect DCI in real time. Brain imaging is a discontinuous diagnostic measure and thus is not adequate for that purpose. Duplex and Doppler ultrasonography can, in principle, be repeated several times a day as a quasi-continuous diagnostic tool. However, it has the inherent limitation of only detecting blood flow velocities in the larger cerebral vessels, which do not necessarily correlate with cerebral blood flow in the brain parenchyma. Moreover, even in larger vessels, increases in flow velocities are not necessarily related to vessel stenosis. They can often not be attributed to a specific cause, or they may be the correlate of compensatory hyperperfusion (e.g., in collateral vessels) or the response to systemically administered adrenergic substances in patients with impaired cerebral autoregulation.[146,147] A retrospective study including 580 SAH patients with vasospasm according to transcranial Doppler criteria had poor specificity, clearly exceeding the incidence of angiographic and symptomatic vasospasm and DCI. In addition, vasospasm detected by angiography or transcranial duplex sonography was not associated with clinical outcome.[148]

Early studies, partly in small patient cohorts, have shown that cEEG and quantitative electroencephalography (qEEG) may substantially contribute to the detection of DCI in SAH patients.[149-152] EEG recordings change when cerebral blood flow decreases: initially there is a loss of fast frequencies, followed by an increase of slow frequencies, and, ultimately, diffuse background attenuation.[139,150] For the purpose of ischemia detection, qEEG is considered a useful technique because it makes slow changes easier to track over time (Fig. 63-2). However, the question of which algorithm is most suitable for ischemia detection using EEG is controversial. Most algorithms are based on fast Fourier transformation analysis and compare different proportions of the spectral power of the EEG (e.g., alpha-to-delta ratio [ADR]), changes in total power, composite alpha index, and relative alpha variability.[22,153,154] In one study of 78 poor-grade SAH patients, it was shown that the change of ADR was the most suitable parameter to distinguish between patients who develop DCI (median ADR: 24% decrease) and those who do not (median ADR: 3% increase).[153] A recent study using the composite alpha index has reported sensitivities of 67% to predict clinical deterioration and 50% to predict clinical improvement.[154] Further studies are needed to test already existent ischemia detection algorithms as well as to explore new detection methods; subsequently, the assumption that early ischemia detection translates to better clinical outcome will need to be tested.

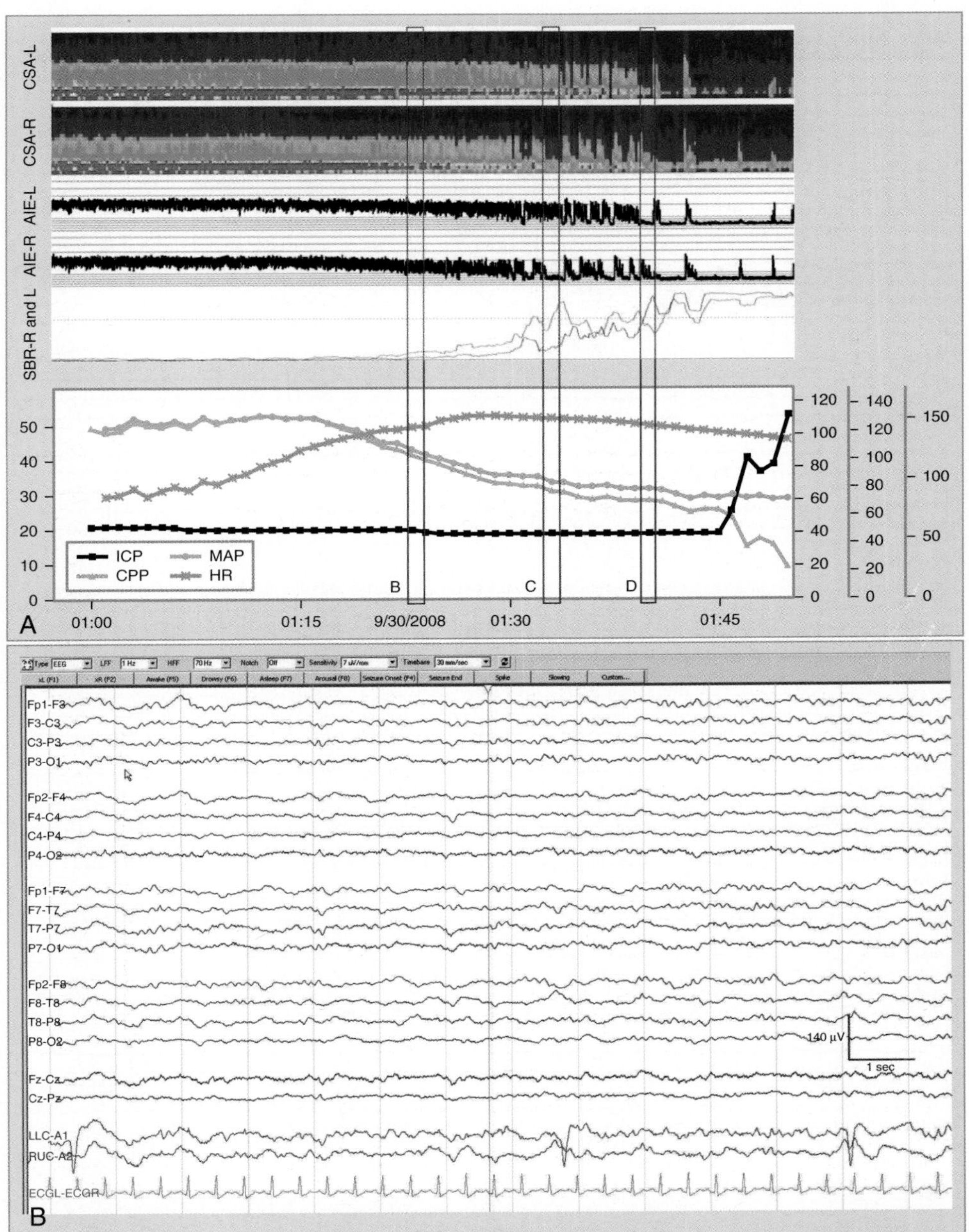

Figure 63-2. Quantitative electroencephalography (qEEG) analysis during a drop in cerebral perfusion pressure (CPP). A 55-year-old-man was admitted with intraventricular hemorrhage and pneumonia. Refractory hypotension developed and resulted first in a drop in mean arterial pressure (MAP) and a delayed increase in intracranial pressure (ICP). qEEG analysis, with 1 hour shown here, demonstrates gradual attenuation of all frequencies in the compressed spectral array (CSA; *top two rows* of qEEG, with time on the *x*-axis and frequency on the *y*-axis), a bit more prominent and earlier on the right **(A)**. Amplitude-integrated electroencephalography (AIE) reveals a gradual decline in both the minimal and maximal amplitudes per epoch, and the suppression-burst ratio (SBR) depicts the increasingly suppressed electroencephalogram (EEG) background. The raw EEG changes from diffuse background slowing and mild right hemisphere attenuation **(B)**, to marked attenuation on the right **(C)**, and then to a severely suppressed background (now more severe on the left; **D**) within approximately 1 hour. The EEGs in **B, C,** and **D** correspond to the times marked on the qEEG **(A)** with the same letters. HR, heart rate. *(Modified from Kurtz P, Hanafy KA, Claassen J. Continuous EEG monitoring: is it ready for prime time?* Curr Opin Crit Care. *2009;15:99.)*

Continued

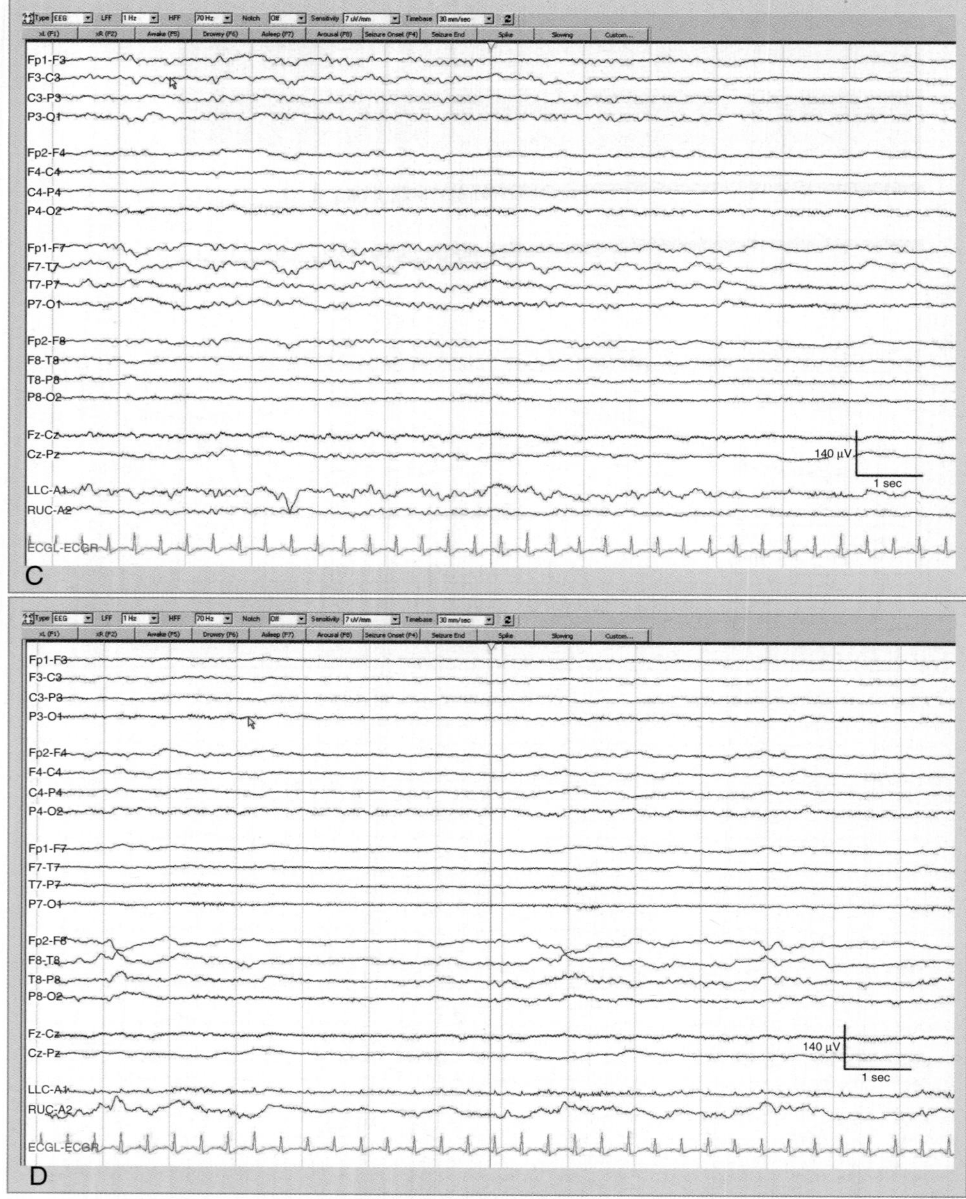

Figure 63-2, cont'd.

Ischemia Detection in Acute Ischemic Stroke

Secondary ischemia after acute ischemic stroke may occur in a considerable portion of patients, depending on the stroke subtype.[155,156] In transient ischemic attack and minor stroke patients, the risk for recurrent cerebral ischemia in the 7 days after the attack or stroke has been reported to be as high as 8% to 10%.[157-159] In these patients, as in patients with symptomatic high-grade carotid stenosis who await surgery, continuous monitoring to detect recurrent ischemia with the goal of preventing new infarctions is desirable. In theory, ischemia detection using cEEG after AIS is possible. Drops in cerebral perfusion pressure in patients with severe ischemic and hemorrhagic strokes have been associated with a reduction in high frequency power on cEEG recordings.[160]

Moreover, spatial extent of infarcted brain tissue and long-term outcome after stroke have been correlated with qEEG measures.[60,95-97] Still, brain imaging, particularly MRI, remains the diagnostic "gold standard" because it is superior in detection of repeat ischemia with higher spatial resolution. Further studies are needed to evaluate the role of cEEG in this context and define its potential role as part of multimodality ischemia detection.

PERIODIC DISCHARGES

It is important to note that widely used terminology regarding PDs changed in 2012 (Table 63-3). We will employ the new terminology except when referring to studies published before 2013.[161]

The increasing use of cEEG in intensive care units over the past decades has brought more attention to periodic EEG patterns that occur frequently but that often may not be clearly categorized as "ictal" or "interictal." This etiologic uncertainty has led to the term *ictal-interictal continuum*.[162]

Many abnormal EEG patterns on the ictal-interictal continuum have been described following acute brain injury, of which periodic discharges (PDs) are the most relevant for their high incidence in neuro-ICU patients.[163,164] PDs, as other rhythmic

TABLE 63-3 Periodic Discharges: Old and New Terminology

Old Term	New Term
Triphasic waves, most of record	Continuous (2/sec) GPDs (with triphasic morphology)
PLEDs	LPDs
BIPLEDs	BIPDs
GPEDs/PEDs	GPDs

BIPDs, bilateral independent periodic discharges; BIPLEDs, bilateral independent periodic lateralized epileptiform discharges; GPDs, generalized periodic discharges; GPEDs, generalized periodic epileptiform discharges; LPDs, lateralized periodic discharges; PEDs, periodic epileptiform discharges; PLEDs, periodic lateralized epileptiform discharges.

Modified (abbreviated) from Hirsch LJ, LaRoche SM, Gaspard N, et al. American Clinical Neurophysiology Society's standardized critical care EEG terminology: 2012 version. *J Clin Neurophysiol*. 2013;30:1-27.

or periodic EEG patterns, are distinguished according to their localization and the presence or absence of bihemispheric synchronicity and may be classified as generalized periodic discharges (GPDs), lateralized periodic discharges (LPDs), bilateral independent periodic discharges (BIPDs), or multifocal (Mf) discharges.[161]

Some evidence exists that PDs, like seizures, are accompanied by an increase in cerebral perfusion and glucose metabolism,[165-167] but whether PDs cause additional harm or merely represent an epiphenomenon of an already severely injured brain remains unclear. Systematic large studies correlating the occurrence of PDs with changes in brain metabolism have not been completed.

In a prospective series of 232 ischemic and hemorrhagic stroke patients undergoing single or serial spot EEG recordings, PDs were found in 10%.[37] In another retrospective series using cEEG in 154 surgical intensive care patients, PDs were identified in 29% of cases.[168] In a series of 102 ICH patients, PDs were reportedly found in 17% of cases (LPDs 13%, GPDs 6%, bilateral independent periodic discharges [BIPDs] 1%),[24] and, in a series of 103 SAH patients, in 23% of cases (LPDs 19%, GPDs 7%, BIPDs 4%).[169]

Because of the uncertainty about their pathophysiologic significance, it is unclear whether patients with PDs should be treated with antiepileptic drugs. Prospective trials investigating this question currently do not exist. There are conflicting data about PDs and clinical outcome, with some studies indicating an unfavorable influence of PDs on outcome,[170-173] and others not finding this.[174,175] In one study of GPDs in a mixed cohort of 200 neuro-ICU patients and 200 controls matched for age, etiology, and level of consciousness, the occurrence of GPDs was strongly associated with the occurrence of NCSzs and NCSE. NCSE, in turn, was independently associated with poor functional outcome, whereas GPDs were not.[175]

ELECTROENCEPHALOGRAPHY AND INVASIVE BRAIN MONITORING

Scalp Electroencephalography for Multimodal Monitoring Devices

There are several arguments for adding continuous scalp EEG recordings to other multimodality monitoring (MMM) devices. Seizures are very common in neuro-ICU patients, occurring frequently with SAH, TBI, ICH, and PCAS. Furthermore, seizures may significantly affect clinical outcome.[17,18,23] In particular, seizure detection in comatose patients relies heavily on EEG recordings because clinical examination may reveal little or no evidence of ongoing seizure activity.

In contrast to EEG, other MMM devices provide localized measurements of, for example, brain tissue glucose or oxygen concentration. Adding scalp EEG to MMM provides a global picture of brain physiology in the ICU patient. Without EEG, inexplicable alterations of brain interstitial glutamate and lactate pyruvate ratios, intracranial pressure, regional cerebral blood flow, and brain tissue hypoxia due to seizures may be incorrectly interpreted.[17-19,23]

Intracranial Electroencephalography Monitoring

When interpreting EEG data from ICU patients, it must be taken into account that the ICU environment is rife with sources of noise and artifacts to EEG recordings, including various electronic devices in the vicinity of the EEG electrodes, poor long-term electrode contact, and unstable recordings, all of which may result in a low signal-to-noise ratio. These limitations have decreased the sensitivity and specificity of bedside alarm systems and thus have impeded their implementation in the daily clinical routine. They can, however, be at least partially overcome by the use of intracranial brain surface EEG recordings in the form of subdural strip electrodes or intracortical depth electrodes. Intracranial EEG electrodes have a similar safety profile as other invasive monitoring techniques.[176]

Depth EEG may detect cortical spreading depression[177-180] and seizures that are only partially detected by scalp EEG[84,181] (Figs. 63-3 and 63-4). Furthermore, depth EEG may provide explanations for otherwise unexplained changes seen on MMM that may be related to seizures.[18,19,181,182]

A study of 14 patients with both scalp and intracortical depth EEG recordings underlined the importance of depth EEG by pointing out striking discrepancies between the two EEG modalities. In 6 patients with seizures on depth EEG, no seizures were found on scalp EEG.[181] In another series of 48 SAH patients, 43% of seizure events on depth EEG (n = 29) had no detectable correlate on scalp EEG. In the same series, seizures or background attenuation on depth EEG were independent predictors of death or severe disability 3 months after discharge in a multivariate model controlling for age, admission Hunt and Hess Stroke Scale score, Acute Physiology and Chronic Health Evaluation (APACHE) II score, and SAH sum score.[18]

Cortical Spreading Depolarization

Cortical spreading depolarization and depression are slow electrophysiologic phenomena occurring after acute brain injury.[183] Spreading depolarizations are believed to lead to transient ischemia and infarctions and thus contribute significantly to the disease and disability burden in patients.[184-187] Associations have been found between cortical spreading depolarization and DCI after SAH[184,186,188,189]; ischemia, fever, and hypotension after TBI[180,185,190]; brain injury in penumbral tissue[180]; seizures after acute brain injury[191]; and herniation after AIS.[179] Cortical depolarizations are best recorded by subdural strip electrode measurements, but correlates of spreading depolarizations may be detectable on surface scalp electrode EEG[192] and on intraparenchymal depth electrode EEG recordings.[193]

CONCLUSION AND FUTURE DIRECTIONS

Continuous EEG provides a global measure of brain function, increases the seizure detection rate in ICU patients, and is of particular use in comatose patients who are otherwise difficult to evaluate. It has a role in monitoring treatment success, such as in patients after termination of CSE, and contributes important prognostic information in conditions such as posthypoxic encephalopathy after cardiac arrest. Therefore cEEG recordings are increasingly implemented in the daily clinical routine in neuro-ICUs. Future research is needed to improve the efficiency of EEG review and to enhance the identification of clinically relevant data, making this information accessible to the treating physicians and nurses in a timely manner. To this end, it is

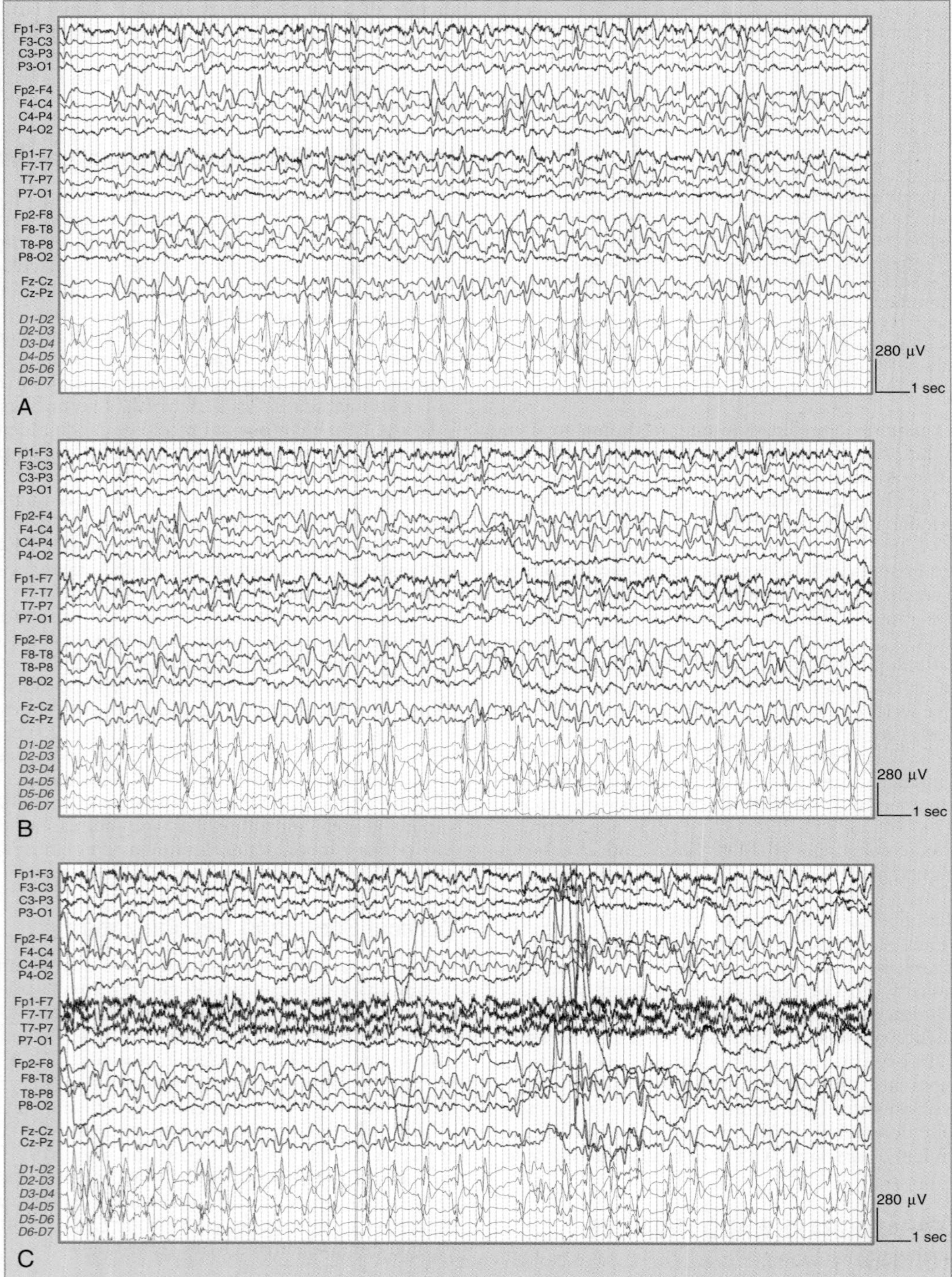

Figure 63-3. Seizure on depth electrode recordings, not clearly detected by scalp electrode recordings. Electroencephalogram (EEG) in a 70-year-old woman who was found fallen down and confused on her bathroom floor with subsequent deterioration of her level of consciousness (Glasgow Coma Scale score of 5 on admission). Computer tomography showed diffuse subarachnoid hemorrhage with intraventricular extension, diffuse cerebral edema, and mild midline shift to the right (2 mm) (Hunt and Hess score of 5, Modified Fisher score of 4). Subsequent cerebral angiography showed a right-sided posterior cerebral communicating artery aneurysm. The patient underwent successful clipping of the aneurysm. The EEG traces presented here were recorded 6 days after symptom onset. The patient showed epileptiform discharges on continuous EEG early in the course, which were treated with levetiracetam, valproic acid, and midazolam. The patient's condition finally improved, and she was discharged to rehabilitation. **A-C,** Depth electrode traces (*blue traces at bottom)* show a focal seizure. Meanwhile, scalp electrode recordings show bilateral, sharply contoured delta waves with a right frontoparietal focus **(A-C)** and superimposed left-sided frontotemporal fast activity 20 seconds later **(C),** but no clear seizures.

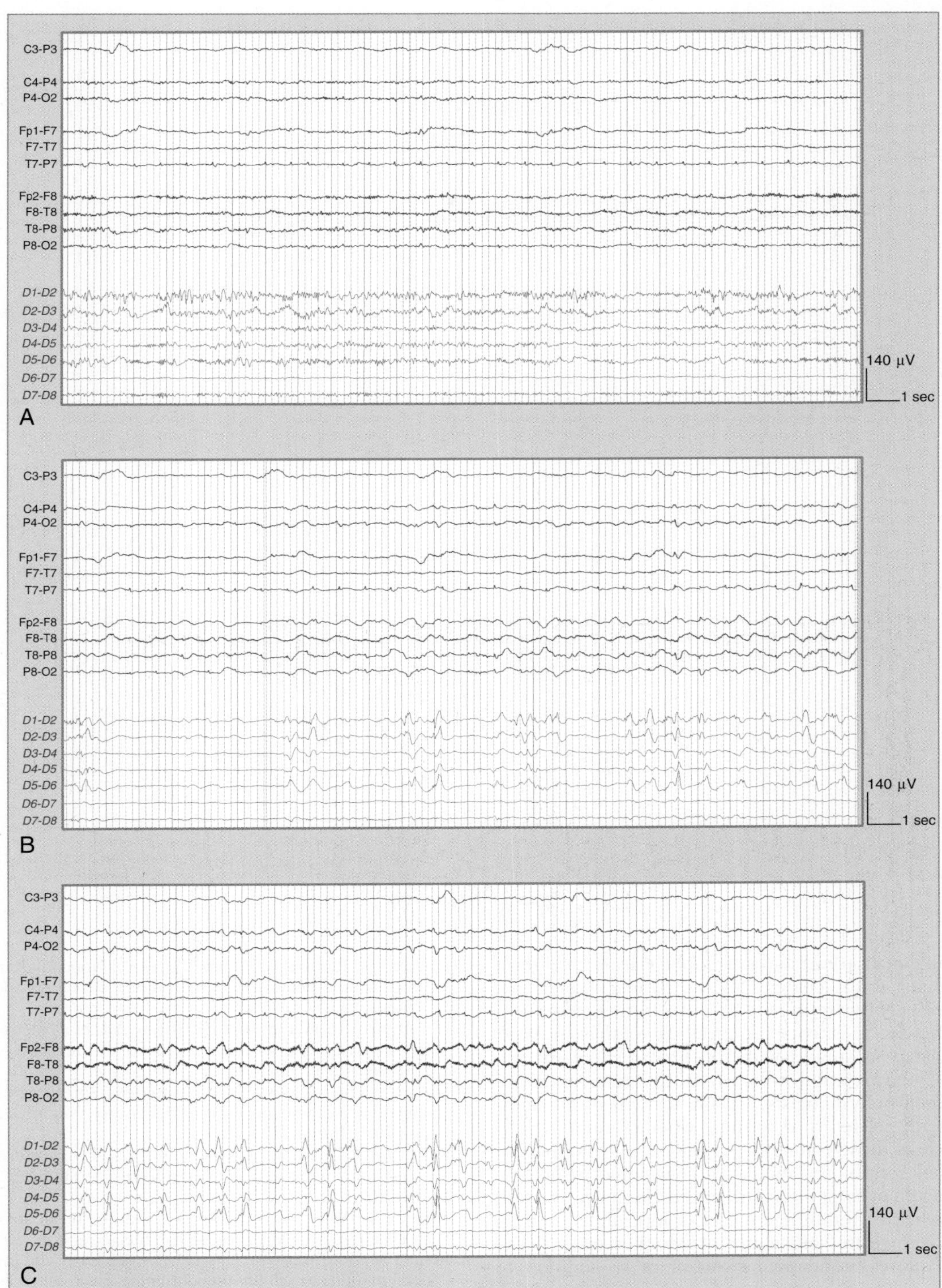

Figure 63-4. Superiority of depth electroencephalogram (EEG) recordings for seizure detection compared with scalp EEG recordings. A 69-year-old man with subarachnoid hemorrhage (Hunt and Hess score of 5) due to a ruptured anterior communicating artery aneurysm. EEG depth recordings *(blue traces at bottom)* show baseline EEG **(A)** and gradual appearance of synchronized epileptiform discharges **(B-C)** evolving into seizure activity **(D-E).** Meanwhile, scalp EEG recordings show pronounced slow delta waves **(B)** and faster synchronous right-sided activity **(C-E),** which, however, do not qualify as periodic epileptiform discharges or seizures.

Continued

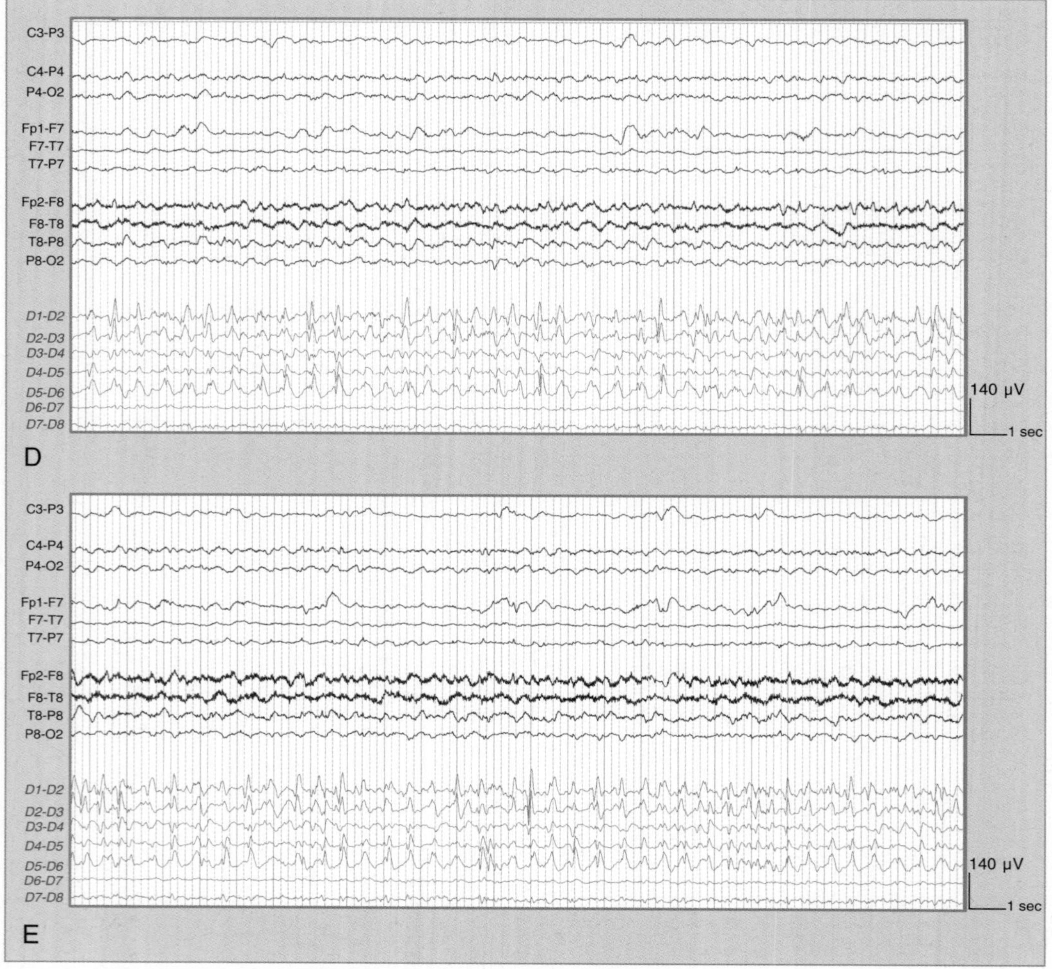

Figure 63-4, cont'd.

desirable to implement trend and threshold alarms to inform hospital staff about status changes in the patient's condition. Some modern EEG software already provides features like automated spike detection. Sensitivity and specificity of these features should be evaluated in studies with the final goal of making pragmatic EEG interpretation, which is still largely conducted only by trained neurophysiologists, feasible at the bedside. Additionally, studies are needed to determine whether certain EEG phenomena, such as those commonly classified as being part of the ictal-interictal continuum, should be considered pathologic and therefore should prompt intervention. Furthermore, it is still to be clarified whether the different cEEG modalities of scalp and depth EEG correlate sufficiently or whether depth EEG should be used more frequently instead of or in addition to scalp EEG.

Acknowledgement

We would like to acknowledge the contributions of this chapter's coauthors from the last edition, Drs. Lawrence J. Hirsch and Hiba Arif.

Funding Source

JW's work is supported by the German Research Council (DFG, research scholarship Wi 4300/1-1).

SUGGESTED READINGS

Claassen J, Mayer SA, Kowalski RG, et al. Detection of electrographic seizures with continuous EEG monitoring in critically ill patients. *Neurology*. 2004;62:1743-1748.

Claassen J, Perotte A, Albers D, et al. Nonconvulsive seizures after subarachnoid hemorrhage: multimodal detection and outcomes. *Ann Neurol*. 2013;74:53-64.

DeLorenzo RJ, Waterhouse EJ, Towne AR, et al. Persistent nonconvulsive status epilepticus after the control of convulsive status epilepticus. *Epilepsia*. 1998;39:833-840.

Dreier JP. The role of spreading depression, spreading depolarization and spreading ischemia in neurological disease. *Nat Med*. 2011;17:439-447. doi: 10.1038/nm.2333.

Rossetti AO, Oddo M, Logroscino G, et al. Prognostication after cardiac arrest and hypothermia: a prospective study. *Ann Neurol*. 2010;67:301-307.

Towne AR, Waterhouse EJ, Boggs JG, et al. Prevalence of nonconvulsive status epilepticus in comatose patients. *Neurology*. 2000;54:340-345.

Vespa PM, Boscardin WJ, Hovda DA, et al. Early and persistent impaired percent alpha variability on continuous electroencephalography monitoring as predictive of poor outcome after traumatic brain injury. *J Neurosurg*. 2002;97:84-92.

Vespa PM, Miller C, McArthur D, et al. Nonconvulsive electrographic seizures after traumatic brain injury result in a delayed, prolonged increase in intracranial pressure and metabolic crisis. *Crit Care Med*. 2007;35:2830-2836.

Waziri A, Claassen J, Stuart RM, et al. Intracortical electroencephalography in acute brain injury. *Ann Neurol*. 2009;66:366-377.

Westover MB, Shafi MM, Bianchi MT, et al. The probability of seizures during EEG monitoring in critically ill adults. *Clin Neurophysiol*. 2014. pii: S1388-2457(14)00362-9.

See a full reference list on ExpertConsult.com

64 Evaluation of Patients for Epilepsy Surgery

Imad M. Najm

In this chapter, we discuss the techniques and process used to provide surgical resection recommendations for patients with medically refractory epilepsy.

GOALS OF PRESURGICAL EVALUATION OF PATIENTS WITH EPILEPSY

The main aim of epilepsy surgery is complete resection (or disconnection) of the cortical areas or networks responsible for the generation of seizures (epileptogenic zone [EZ]), leading to complete seizure control in patients in whom multiple antiepileptic medications have failed. Therefore an accurate and comprehensive mapping of the anatomo-electro-clinical (AEC) network defining the epileptic condition is the main goal of the presurgical evaluation.[1,2] Because the EZ may overlap with functional (eloquent) cortex, an additional (and equally important) aim of the presurgical evaluation is mapping the extent of the EZ and its possible overlap with clinically testable functional regions.[3,4] To presurgically define the anatomic location of the EZ and its proximity to possible cortical and subcortical eloquent areas, various noninvasive tools are available. They include recorded seizure semiology, scalp electroencephalography (EEG) (recording of ictal and interictal epileptic patterns), high-resolution magnetic resonance imaging (MRI), positron emission tomography (PET), ictal single-photon emission computed tomography (SPECT), neuropsychological testing, and magnetoencephalography (MEG).[5]

CLINICAL APPROACH AND TECHNIQUES USED IN THE PRESURGICAL EVALUATION

Clinical Approach

Epilepsy surgery evaluation should be considered after the diagnosis of pharmacoresistant epilepsy (recently defined as a failure to respond to two or more adequately chosen and used antiepileptic medications).[6]

A detailed history taken from the patient first (in particular the details of the aura, if present) is the most important (and most cost-effective) part in the process of epilepsy surgery evaluation. Historical details of the seizure semiology and the sequence of events during a seizure should be sought (from family members or witnesses) and later compared with the seizures recorded during prolonged electroencephalographic and video monitoring. Questions regarding birth history, febrile convulsions, head injuries, central nervous system (CNS) infections, and other possible causes of seizures should be asked. Medication trials, doses used, and their side effects should be reviewed. In addition, a family history should be taken with particular reference to seizures and other neurological illnesses.

A neurological examination should uncover focal neurological abnormalities (which may constitute the anatomopathologic substrate of the epilepsy).

Necessary Techniques for the Localization of the Epileptogenic Zone

Multiple techniques may be used to achieve the aforementioned goals. In our opinion, the two most important and necessary studies to be performed in all patients considered for epilepsy surgery are high-resolution MRI and scalp-video electroencephalographic monitioring.

High-Resolution Magnetic Resonance Imaging

Further validation of the anatomic hypothesis is achieved through imaging (the identification of lesion on MRI). A high-resolution MRI scan that includes at least volume acquisition T1-weighted and fluid-attenuated inversion recovery (FLAIR) sequences to document the presence of hippocampal sclerosis, cortical dysplasia, or other potentially epileptogenic brain lesion(s) should be performed. The interpretation of the MRI studies should be done by a subspecialty-trained board-certified neuroradiologist who is active in epilepsy surgery programs because recent studies have shown a higher detection rate by subspecialized neuroradiologists than by those working in non–epilepsy surgery centers.[7] In most instances, gadolinium is not necessary unless a tumor or mass lesion is found.

Scalp-Video Electroencephalographic Monitoring

Prolonged video-EEG recordings in a dedicated epilepsy monitoring unit are needed to confirm the diagnosis of epilepsy (through interictal and ictal EEG epileptic patterns) and generate hypotheses on the network structures that may be involved in seizure generation and progression (through analysis of the captured seizure semiology) leading to the formulation of a clear AEC hypothesis. It is helpful to the physicians working in the EEG/video monitoring unit to have the MRI scan before the monitoring is done. The information from the history, neurological examination, and MRI scan is needed in the planning of the monitoring. For example, a patient with an olfactory aura, automotor (complex partial) seizures, and right hippocampal atrophy and increased FLAIR signal on MRI probably should have closely spaced bitemporal electrodes (International 10/10 System) applied with the standard International 10/20 scalp electrodes and sphenoidal electrodes inserted at the beginning of EEG/video monitoring. In this patient, the recording of only a small number of seizures (one or two) would suffice if they were of right temporal origin. A second patient with a sensory aura in the left hand and right hippocampal atrophy on MRI scan should have 10/10 electrodes placed over the right posterior frontal or anterior parietal region in addition to the temporal and sphenoidal electrodes (because of the distinct possibility of a posterior perisylvian EZ). A third patient with bilateral hippocampal atrophy on MRI, bitemporal spikes, and multiple seizures would have to be recorded (because of the higher risk of bitemporal independent seizures). Although a lesion seen on MRI is very helpful in the epilepsy surgery evaluation and may correlate with a good surgical outcome, a normal MRI does not by itself exclude a patient from epilepsy surgery; it does, however, make the presurgical evaluation significantly more complicated and expensive.

Patient Management Conference

The epilepsy patient management conference is an integral element of any comprehensive pediatric or adult epilepsy surgery program. At Cleveland Clinic, as at many other epilepsy centers, all of the epilepsy team's specialists collaborate to provide a multidisciplinary discussion, to generate hypotheses on the localization of the EZ and its presumed pathologic cause, and to formulate a set of recommendations to be discussed with the patient and family.

Historically at Cleveland Clinic, 40 to 60 professionals gather for a 2-hour early morning conference every week to review six to eight cases in detail, with the main goals being to determine whether and how to proceed with resective epilepsy surgery or further evaluation with implanted electrodes. Participants include pediatric and adult epileptologists, epilepsy neurosurgeons, neuroradiologists, functional imaging specialists, MEG specialists, neuropsychologists, psychiatrists, bioethicists, researchers, social workers, nurse practitioners, and physicians in training. The patient's primary epileptologist leads the discussion, which is often quite vigorous in the more controversial and challenging cases. As thoughts and opinions are respectfully aired, a group consensus on a set of recommendations and options is forged for informed consent.

Clearly, this demanding case conference schedule represents a significant commitment of unbillable physician work time. In the current climate of health care reform and limited resources, the benefits of case conferences must outweigh the cost. At Cleveland Clinic, we firmly believe that they do—for the following reasons:

1. *Case discussion and consensus building are the cornerstones for standardization of care.* Everyone brings a certain set of biases and opinions to the table. By hearing different perspectives and points of view, we modify our own approach to include the insights and experience of others. This brings all members of the team closer together in a synergistic collaboration and prevents major deviations from accepted norms and standards of practice.
2. *Case conferences provide a venue for reviewing all the critical studies with all the appropriate experts at the same time, to ensure that nothing is missed.* For example, an MRI may at first yield no clues to localization of the EZ, until the epilepsy-focused neuroradiologist's eyes are directed by other consultants to a specific area of interest. Everyone working in epilepsy surgery has had the experience of discovering a subtle depth-of-sulcus malformation or other anomaly only after reviewing the results from other tests. The live collaboration among different specialists in EEG, seizure semiology, MRI, PET, MEG, ictal SPECT, postprocessing studies (such as voxel-based morphometry), and outcome data leads to greater insight and optimized surgical outcomes.
3. *Case-based discussions advance the medical knowledge of every participant and cultivate a more erudite medical team.* With today's rapid advances in genomics, neurophysiology, surgery, imaging, and other disciplines, no one physician or specialist is an expert in everything. Even within the relatively narrow field of epilepsy medicine, experiences and acumen differ in some areas based on whether one cares for children or adults. What better way could there be to learn from our colleagues than to frame the discussion around the care of an actual patient?
4. *Forging a consensus opinion transforms an individual's opinion into a group decision, so the burden of responsibility is shared in difficult cases.* Vetting difficult decisions with respected peers provides the strength and confidence that are needed to expand the candidate pool and practice medicine on the cutting edge, where evidence-based data are not always available.
5. *Synchronizing everyone's opinion at case conferences leads to consistent presentation of the consensus recommendations to the patient and family.* At Cleveland Clinic, as at most epilepsy centers, the options concerning surgery are often discussed with the patient and family by various members of the team at different times. When the primary epileptologist, in-patient hospital epileptologist, and epilepsy neurosurgeon are all on the same page, the patient feels the strength of a team approach.
6. The comprehensive summary from a formal presentation at the epilepsy patient management conference becomes an indispensable document in the medical record. A standardized work sheet summarizing the relevant clinical and laboratory data facilitates astute discussion by all team members during the conference. The report is modified during the conference as additional findings and ideas come to light, and then completed with the addition of the consensus opinion and plans after the conference. The resultant summary document is a key overview of all the elements leading to the surgical decision, which serves as the touchstone for future care at the home institution or other centers.
7. The epilepsy patient management conference may ameliorate the medicolegal risk inherent in providing advanced care in challenging cases. By ensuring that nothing is missed on public review of the clinical and laboratory test results, by synchronizing everyone's opinion so that a consistent message is delivered during discussion with the patient and family, by optimizing communication among all members of the team, and by providing meticulous documentation in the medical record, the epilepsy patient management conference may reduce the likelihood of litigation in the case of an unavoidable suboptimal outcome.

Please see ExpertConsult.com for more information on the Cleveland Clinic's core prescreening committee approach.

Evolution of the Patient Management Conference during an Era of a Changing Health Care Landscape

Pending the findings of the video-EEG evaluation, the MRI, and patient management discussion, additional studies may be needed. These studies may include one or more of the following:

1. *FDG-PET:* PET imaging has been used since the 1980s in the presurgical evaluation of patients with pharmacoresistant focal epilepsies (PFEs). Various reports have shown the benefits and limitations of the technique and the postprocessing and co-registration of the data.[8-19] PET scanning is considered routine in many epilepsy centers but is no longer done on every patient at Cleveland Clinic Epilepsy Center. For example, in a right-handed patient with MRI features consistent with right hippocampal sclerosis and concordance of semiology and EEG, the patient would most likely proceed to surgery without a PET scan or a language lateralizing procedure. When indicated (in particular in the setting of a normal MRI), PET may identify one or more focal areas of hypometabolism that may point to focal cortical dysfunction or a dysfunction in a larger network. These focal areas of dysfunction, if consistent with the anatomic hypothesis, may bring further credence to an AEC hypothesis of the epileptogenic network and subsequently guide the planning of further tests (e.g., invasive evaluation).

2. *Subtraction ictal SPECT scan* co-registered with MRI (SISCOM or related technique) three-dimensional reconstruction: Ictal SPECT has been used in the presurgical workup of patients with pharmacoresistant epilepsy since the 1990s.[20-30] Ictal SPECT may be most helpful in patients with focal epilepsy who have normal MRI findings and in those with extensive focal cortical dysplasia (FCD).[31,32] Because more often than not the ictal SPECT uncovers multiple areas of activation, its interpretation should take into account the fact that the areas of hyperperfusion could be part of the larger cortical-subcortical networks in the brain and should be interpreted as such. In the setting of an MRI that did not uncover focal lesions, these findings may be extremely helpful in the design of a three-dimensional stereo-electroencephalography (SEEG) depth electrode invasive implantation.
3. *MEG:* When available, MEG can be helpful in source localization of EEG dipoles of interictal discharges in patients with MRI-negative focal epilepsies. MEG is used principally for the localization of interictal epileptiform activity because the chance of recording a seizure during MEG is very small unless the patient is having frequent daily seizures or a seizure is coincidentally recorded.[33] Multiple studies have reported on the usefulness of MEG in the presurgical evaluation of patients with pharmacoresistant epilepsy.[34-57] We recently showed MEG to be a useful tool to localize the EZ and guide invasive evaluation and surgical resection in a group of patients with medically intractable and nonlesional neocortical epilepsy.[35,47,58-64] MEG also provides functional data, including sensorimotor and language cortex localization, that may be correlated with interictal epileptiform activity with high spatial resolution.
4. *Postprocessing of MRI and MEG data:* Voxel-based morphometric (morphometric analysis program [MAP]) analysis of the MRI has been used as a postprocessing tool for the localization of MRI lesions.[65-71] Patients with MRI-negative PFE are most challenging for surgical management. We recently used a voxel-based MRI postprocessing technique, implemented using a MAP, aiming to facilitate detection of subtle FCD in MRI-negative patients.[56] In addition, we examined the concordance between MAP-identifiable regions and results of MEG-based magnetic source imaging (MSI). The detection rate of subtle changes by MAP was 48% (12 of 25 patients). Once MAP-positive areas were resected, patients were more likely to be seizure-free (P = .02). Seven patients had a concordant MSI correlate. Patients in whom a concordant area was identified by both MAP and MSI had a significantly higher chance of achieving a seizure-free outcome after complete resection of this area (P = .008). In the nine resected MAP-positive areas, pathology revealed FCD type Ia in seven and FCD type IIb in two. These studies show the promise of MAP in identifying subtle FCD abnormalities and increasing diagnostic yield of conventional MRI visual analysis in presurgical evaluation of PFE. Concordant MRI postprocessing and MSI analysis leads to the noninvasive identification of a structurally and electrically abnormal subtle lesion and thus helps uncover an epileptogenic focus that can be surgically targeted.
5. *fMRI* may help localize some functional areas of the brain and their relationships to a suspected EZ. fMRI is replacing the Wada test at many epilepsy centers to aid in determining the side (and sublobar localization) of language dominance and may possibly be useful for memory assessment.[72-86] A potential advantage of speech fMRI over Wada is its ability not only to lateralize speech, but also to anatomically localize cortical speech regions (both anterior and posterior speech areas). fMRI is also a promising technique for cortical localization of interictal epileptiform activity (EEG-fMRI), but EEG recordings with time-locked fMRI are technically challenging and the significance of interictal spiking in ictal zone localization is not entirely clear.[87-92]

The noninvasive studies achieve the goal of identification of the epileptogenic area and its possible anatomic cause in a sizable number of surgical patients (around 70% of the patients who were operated on at Cleveland Clinic in 2012) (unpublished data). But a formulation of a clear AEC hypothesis may not be possible in some patients, or an AEC hypothesis is generated but the exact location of the epileptogenic area within the network, its extent, or its overlap with functional (eloquent) cortex remains unclear. These patients may be candidates for an invasive evaluation using either subdural grids (SDGs) or SEEG depth electrodes.

Invasive Evaluation Techniques in Presurgical Evaluation

Rationale

Noninvasive techniques are helpful in identifying the general area of the EZ in a large number of patients but do not fully define its sublobar localization and/or its extent. For patients with lesions on MRI that are likely to cause seizures, the inherent weakness of these techniques is less critical when the EZ is anatomically distant from eloquent areas of the brain (e.g., nondominant anterior temporal pole). On the other hand, when MRI-identified lesions occur within potentially eloquent areas of the brain (e.g., central lobe, dominant temporoparietal area), clear localization and mapping of the extent of EZ and its potential overlap with sensorimotor or speech areas are needed for safe surgical resection. In patients with MRI-negative epilepsy, noninvasive techniques may point to the general area of epileptogenicity or identify the epileptic network but may not accurately localize or map the EZ and its function. As a result, direct cortical recording and electrical stimulation mapping is indicated for these patients.

Indications for Invasive Evaluation

Based on these limitations of noninvasive localization techniques, invasive evaluation should be considered in any of the following cases:

1. The MRI does not show a cortical lesion in a location that is concordant with the electroclinical or functional hypothesis generated by the video-EEG recordings (so-called MRI-negative cases).
2. The anatomic location of the MRI-identified lesion (and at times the location of a clearly hypometabolic focal area on PET) is not concordant with the electroclinical hypothesis. Such cases include deeply seated brain lesions such as periventricular nodular heterotopia or deep sulcal lesions. In addition, scalp EEG recordings in 85% to 100% of patients with FCD show interictal spikes that range in their distribution from lobar to lateralized and from difficult to localize to diffuse (including generalized spike-wave patterns in some cases of subependymal heterotopia).[93,94] The spatial distribution of interictal spikes is usually more extensive than the structural abnormality as assessed by intraoperative inspection or MRI visual analysis.[93]
3. There are two or more anatomic lesions with the location of at least one of them being discordant with the electroclinical hypothesis, or both lesions are located within the same functional network and it is unclear if one or both of them are epileptic.
4. The generated AEC hypothesis (MRI-negative or MRI-identifiable lesion) involves potentially eloquent cortex. The identification of the EZ, mapping of its extent, and

determination of its relationship with potentially eloquent cortex are not typically resolved in these cases. Such cases include suspected FCD as the possible pathologic substrate for the epilepsy.[95]

In these instances, an invasive evaluation would lead to the formulation of a clear resective surgical strategy. The recommendation for invasive monitoring and its type should always be made after a detailed discussion of all the findings of the noninvasive tests during the patient management conference. Areas and networks of coverage and sampling are determined based on a well-formulated AEC hypothesis based on the results of the noninvasive studies.

Choice of Invasive Method

Two extraoperative invasive methods have been used to accomplish these goals: SDG electrodes and stereotactically placed EEG depth electrodes (SEEG). The indication for and choice of the invasive method depend on MRI findings and a clear AEC hypothesis (Fig. 64-1).

Subdural Grid Implantation Method. Prolonged intracranial recordings were initially reported in 1939 when Penfield and colleagues used epidural single-contact electrodes in a patient with an old left temporoparietal fracture in whom pneumoencephalography disclosed diffuse cerebral atrophy.[96] Decades later (1980s-1990s), the use of SDG arrays became more popular in North America after multiple publications demonstrated their safety and efficacy.[97-100] Before that, most invasive techniques used in North America involved extraoperative recordings from epidural electrodes or intraoperatively placed neocortical surface electrode recordings.

Principles of and Indications for Placement of Subdural Electrodes. Extraoperative mapping with the SDG method (which includes SDGs and strips) has the main advantage of allowing an optimal coverage of the subdural space adjacent cortex with adequate and continuous cortical surface functional mapping capabilities.[4,100-102] A major strength of subdural electrodes is the comprehensive anatomic coverage of cortical surfaces, which allows accurate anatomic electrical and functional mapping of the areas of coverage. Limitations of SGDs include inadequate, partial, or incomplete intrasulcal, deep brain (e.g., insular, posterior orbitofrontal), and interhemispheric (e.g., cingulate gyrus) coverage and the relative difficulty of multilobar, three dimensional, and large–functional network sampling.[103] These characteristics are highlighted in the published results on the successes and failures of SDG implantation.[104] The best resective surgical outcomes after SDG implantation are achieved in patients with clear cortical lesions (in particular tumors), those who underwent lobar resections, and those in whom the SDG implantations were for the main purpose of functional mapping.[104,105] On the other hand, the worst outcomes were seen in patients with no clear lesions on the MRI, those with nonspecific histopathology, and those who underwent either sublobar or multilobar resections.

These characteristics suggest that the best candidates for extraoperative invasive evaluation with SDG are patients with clear cortical surface lesion(s) (excluding the interhemispheric, cingulate gyrus, deep sulcal, and mesial frontal or temporal regions), in particular those patients in whom the main indication for the invasive evaluation is electrofunctional or eloquent cortex mapping in the setting of a cortical lesion.

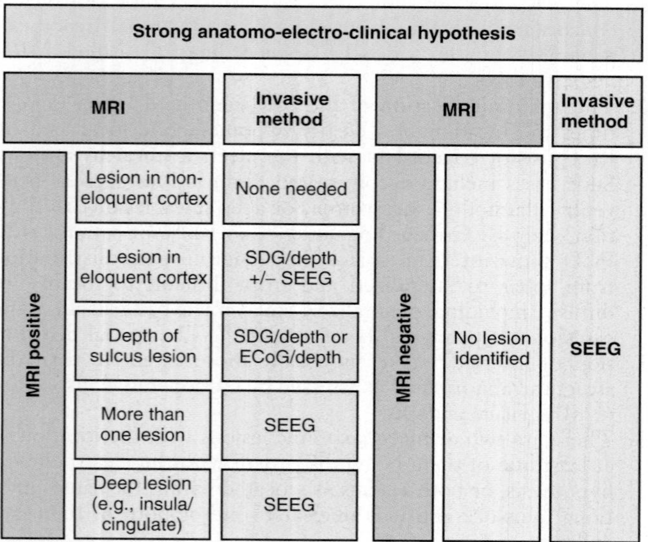

Strong anatomo-electro-clinical hypothesis
MRI
Invasive method
MRI
Invasive method
MRI positive
Lesion in non-eloquent cortex
None needed
Lesion in eloquent cortex
SDG/depth +/– SEEG
Depth of sulcus lesion
SDG/depth or ECoG/depth
More than one lesion
SEEG
Deep lesion (e.g., insula/ cingulate)
SEEG
MRI negative
No lesion identified
SEEG

Figure 64-1. Indications for invasive evaluation and choice of the method. EcoG, electrocorticography; MRI, magnetic resonance imaging; SDG, subdural grid; SEEG, stereo-electroencephalography.

Stereo-Electroencephalography Method. The SEEG method was developed in France by Jean Talairach and Jean Bancaud during the 1950s and has been mostly used in France and Italy, as the method of choice for invasive mapping in refractory focal epilepsy.[106,107] The principle of SEEG is based on AEC correlations, with the main aim being to reconstruct the three-dimensional spatial-temporal organization of the epileptic discharge within the brain based mainly on seizure semiology. The implantation strategy is individualized, with electrode placement based on a preimplantation hypothesis that takes into consideration the primary organization of the epileptiform activity and the hypothetical functional epileptic network that may be involved in the propagation of seizures. For these reasons, the preimplantation AEC hypothesis is the most important element in the process of planning for SEEG electrode placement. If the preimplantation hypothesis is incorrect, the placement of the depth electrodes will be inadequate and the interpretation of the SEEG recordings misleading. The most important characteristic of SEEG methodology is that it enables precise recordings from deep cortical and subcortical structures and multiple noncontiguous lobes, as well as bilateral explorations, while avoiding the need for large craniotomies.[95,108-112]

The SEEG technique was originally described as a multiphase and complex method using the Talairach stereotactic frame and the double-grid system in association with teleangiography.[113,114] Despite its long-reported successful record, with almost 60 years of clinical use, the technical complexity regarding the placement of SEEG depth electrodes may have contributed to its limited widespread use in centers outside Europe. Taking advantage of new imaging and computational innovations, commonly available in many surgical centers, more modern and less cumbersome methods of stereotactic implantation of depth electrodes can be applied on a routine basis.

Principles and Technique of Implantation. The development of an SEEG implantation plan requires the clear formulation of a specific and testable anatomo-electro-functional hypothesis. This hypothesis is typically generated during the patient management conference based on the results of the various noninvasive evaluation tests. At Cleveland Clinic, a final tailored implantation strategy is generated during a separate presurgical implantation meeting. Depth electrodes would sample the anatomic lesion (if identified), the more likely structure(s) of ictal onset, the clinically active regions, and the possible pathway(s) of onset and propagation of the electrical seizure activity (functional networks). The area of ictal onset (EZ) could be the one corresponding to the first clinical sign or could be a spread area from a clinically silent ictal onset zone within a functional network. For these reasons, a three-dimensional reconstruction of the network nodes upstream and downstream from the hypothesized clinical onset region is an essential component of the presurgical implantation strategy.

Indications for Electrode Placement. In addition to the general indications for invasive monitoring, specific indications can be considered to choose SEEG instead of other methods of invasive monitoring. These criteria include the following:

1. The possibility of a deep-seated or difficult-to-cover location of the EZ in areas such as the mesial structures of the temporal lobe, opercular areas, cingulate gyrus, interhemispheric regions, posterior orbitofrontal areas, insula, and depths of sulci.
2. A failure of a previous subdural invasive study to clearly outline the exact location of the seizure onset zone. The failure to identify the EZ in these patients may occur for multiple reasons that include the lack of adequate sampling from a deep focus or a clinically silent focus upstream from the EZ.
3. The need for extensive bihemispheric explorations (in particular in focal epilepsies suspected to be arising from the interhemispheric or deep insular regions).
4. Presurgical evaluation suggestive of a multilobar functional network involvement (e.g., limbic system) in the setting of normal MRI.

In these scenarios, SEEG may be considered as a more appropriate option. As mentioned earlier, SEEG has the advantages of allowing extensive and precise deep brain recordings and stimulations. In reoperations, mainly in patients who have undergone a previous subdural evaluation, it is likely that the majority of the earlier epilepsy surgeries failed because of difficulties in accurately localizing the EZ. These patients pose a significant dilemma for further management, having relatively few options available. Further open SDG evaluations may carry the risks associated with encountering scar formations, while still having the limitations related to deep cortical structure recordings. A subsequent evaluation using the SEEG method may overcome these limitations, offering an additional opportunity for seizure localization and sustained seizure freedom.[103] The main disadvantage of the SEEG method is the more restricted capability for performing functional mapping. Because of the limited number of contacts located in the superficial cortex, a contiguous mapping of eloquent brain areas cannot be obtained as in the subdural method mapping. To overcome this relative disadvantage, the functional mapping information extracted with the SEEG method is frequently complemented with other methods of mapping, such as diffusion tensor imaging or awake craniotomies.[95]

CONCLUSION

The presurgical evaluation of patients with pharmacoresistant epilepsy can often be accomplished through noninvasive methods (in particular video-EEG recordings and high-resolution MRI). An increasing number of other noninvasive techniques (e.g., PET, ictal SPECT, MEG, fMRI, EEG-fMRI) and postprocessing methods (voxel-based morphometry, SISCOM) enable the identification of the EZ, as well as mapping of functional areas of the brain. Invasive techniques may be necessary for more precise localization of seizure onsets, better delineation of the EZ, and accurate cortical functional mapping. A comprehensive presurgical evaluation of epilepsy requires the expertise of subspecialists from various disciplines. As a result, multidisciplinary patient management conferences are critical for proper management of patients with pharmacoresistant epilepsy and optimization of postresection functional and seizure outcomes.

SUGGESTED READINGS

Avanzini G. Discussion of stereoelectroencephalography. *Acta Neurol Scand Suppl*. 1994;152:70-73.

Ito T, Otsubo H, Shiraishi H, et al. Advantageous information provided by magnetoencephalography for patients with neocortical epilepsy. *Brain Dev*. 2015;37:237-242.

Najm IM, Bingaman WE, Luders HO. The use of subdural grids in the management of focal malformations due to abnormal cortical development. *Neurosurg Clin N Am*. 2002;13:87-92, viii-ix.

Rosenow F, Luders H. Presurgical evaluation of epilepsy. *Brain*. 2001;124:1683-1700.

Salamon N, Kung J, Shaw SJ, et al. FDG-PET/MRI coregistration improves detection of cortical dysplasia in patients with epilepsy. *Neurology*. 2008;71:1594-1601.

Talairach J, Tournoux P, Musolino A, et al. Stereotaxic exploration in frontal epilepsy. *Adv Neurol*. 1992;57:651-688.

Wang ZI, Alexopoulos AV, Jones SE, et al. Linking MRI postprocessing with magnetic source imaging in MRI-negative epilepsy. *Ann Neurol*. 2014;75:759-770.

See a full reference list on ExpertConsult.com 

65 Neuroradiologic Evaluation for Epilepsy Surgery: Magnetic Resonance Imaging

Anna Miserocchi, Mark Nowell, and Andrew W. McEvoy

"Preliminary observations on magnetic resonance imaging in refractory epilepsy," published in 1984,[1] marked the advent of the use of magnetic resonance imaging (MRI) in the diagnosis of epilepsy. Since then, the continuous technical development of structural and functional MRI has revolutionized the investigation and treatment of patients with epilepsy. In this chapter, we give an overview on the structural cerebral abnormalities seen on MRI that most commonly underlie epilepsy, and we explore the advances of functional MRI, diffusion tensor imaging, electroencephalography in combination with functional MRI, and magnetic resonance spectroscopy. This chapter also describes the generation and utility of three-dimensional (3D) multimodality imaging in epilepsy treatment, and outlines the increasing use of interventional MRI as an adjunct to surgical treatment.

MAGNETIC RESONANCE IMAGING IN EPILEPSY

Indications

Drug-resistant epilepsy is a chronic, debilitating disorder that is potentially curable with surgery.[2,3] The success of surgery relies on the correct identification of the epileptogenic zone, defined as the cortical area that needs to be resected or disconnected in order to achieve freedom from seizures.[4] Structural imaging of the brain makes up part of the comprehensive presurgical evaluation, which also includes history and examination, scalp video telemetry (video-electroencephalography), and neuropsychological and psychiatric assessment.[5]

The Neuroimaging Commission of the International League Against Epilepsy published the first consensus statement on this topic in 1997: the rationale to image the brain in patients developing epilepsy is to identify underlying pathologic processes early and to assist the formulation of syndrome-based and etiologic diagnoses.[6]

Structural MRI is the workhorse of imaging in epilepsy and should be conducted in all patients with epilepsy, except those with a definite diagnosis of idiopathic generalized epilepsy or benign rolandic epilepsy of childhood with centrotemporal spikes.[7] Indications for MRI include the following:

1. The onset of partial seizures, at any age.
2. The onset of generalized or unclassified seizures in the first year of life or in adulthood.
3. Evidence of a fixed deficit on neurological or neuropsychological examination.
4. Difficulty obtaining seizure control with first-line antiepileptic drugs.
5. Loss of seizure control or a change in the pattern of seizures.

Epilepsy Protocol

Three-tesla MRI scanners provide high-resolution images and whenever possible should be preferred over 1.5-T scanners. Images should be acquired in an oblique coronal orientation perpendicular to the long axis of the hippocampus. The entire brain should be included in the field of view to avoid missing subtle peripheral findings. Routine MRI sequences[3,7] include the following:

- Volumetric T1-weighted dataset with slices of 1- to 2-mm thickness
- Axial and sagittal high-resolution T2-weighted dataset with slices of 2- to 3-mm thickness
- Coronal fluid-attenuated inversion recovery (FLAIR) sequence in the same plane
- Three-dimensional FLAIR sequences
- Coronal T2*-weighted gradient echo sequence (sensitive to paramagnetic substances such as hemosiderin, useful for ruling out hemorrhagic lesions such as cavernomas)

The routine MRI acquisition protocol in the diagnosis of epilepsy should be standardized to provide a widespread standard of care and also to encourage multicenter collaboration in clinical practice and research.

Optional Sequences

Many advanced MRI techniques are available and in use in different institutions:

- Magnetization transfer imaging: images are obtained with and without magnetization transfer to derive a magnetization transfer ratio. This ratio is a measure of the magnitude of exchange of magnetization between free protons in bulk water and tightly bound protons on macromolecules such as myelin or membrane. A low magnetization transfer ratio, caused by gliosis, is a sensitive marker of mesial temporal sclerosis.
- T2-weighted relaxometry imaging: dual-echo T2-weighted imaging is performed, and the voxelwise T2 relaxation time is calculated according to the formula

  $$\text{T2 relaxation time} = (\text{TE2} - \text{TE1})/(\ln[\text{SI1}/\text{SI2}]),$$

  in which SI1 and SI2 are the signal intensities in the early and late echo images, with echo times TE1 and TE2, respectively.[3] The T2 relaxation time is a useful identifier of hippocampal abnormality. The T2 relaxation time is higher in patients with mesial temporal sclerosis than in patients with a normal hippocampus, and an intermediate value can be observed in patients without qualitative MRI evidence of hippocampal sclerosis.[8] In comparison with the normal hippocampus, in mesial temporal sclerosis the normal anterior-to-posterior T2 relaxation time gradient is accentuated (from higher to lower value).[9]
- Diffusion-weighted imaging (DWI): areas of restricted diffusion, such as infarcts, abscesses, or necrosis, are highlighted. In cases of persistent seizures, restricted diffusion is also seen in the seizure onset zone and along the areas of propagation of discharges that cause the seizures. The restricted diffusion represents seizure-induced cytotoxic edema.[10]
- Magnetic resonance spectroscopy (described later).

The use of gadolinium is not recommended on a routine basis unless images are suggestive of a tumoral lesion.

STRUCTURAL CEREBRAL ABNORMALITIES IDENTIFIED WITH MAGNETIC RESONANCE IMAGING

Hippocampal Sclerosis

Mesial temporal lobe epilepsy is the most common form of epilepsy in adults,[11] and hippocampal sclerosis or mesial temporal sclerosis is the main pathologic process associated with it. When hippocampal sclerosis is correctly identified and surgically treated, the rate of success in achieving seizure freedom is high (60% at 5 years[12]).

An essential requirement in a dedicated MRI protocol in a patient with mesial temporal lobe epilepsy is thin-slice (1- to 3-mm) images (T1- and T2-weighted) perpendicular to the long axis of the hippocampus. Additional sequences such as 3D double-inversion recovery can be helpful in identifying abnormal white matter changes in the anterior temporal lobe.[13]

Hippocampal sclerosis is demonstrated as hippocampal atrophy on coronal T1-weighted images and as increased signal intensity on T2-weighted images (Fig. 65-1).

Features associated with hippocampal sclerosis are as follows:

- Temporal horn dilatation, caused by volume loss of the hippocampus
- Atrophy of the structures that form the outflow tracts from the hippocampus (inferiorly, the parahippocampal gyrus; posteriorly, the ipsilateral fornix connected to the ipsilateral mammillary body)
- Atrophy of the structures indirectly connected with the hippocampus (the remainder of the temporal lobe, the thalamus, and the caudate nucleus)[3]

Qualitative visual inspection of MRI by neuroradiologists expert in the field is sufficient to detect hippocampal sclerosis in 80% to 90% of the cases.[14] A careful assessment of the whole brain is mandatory because in 8% to 22% of the patients, a second disease process can be found, represented mainly by focal cortical dysplasia (FCD).[14]

The limitation with sole visual inspection is that hippocampal sclerosis can be missed if it is mild or bilateral. The assessment of hippocampal sclerosis can be greatly improved by quantitative measures of hippocampal volumes and hippocampal T2 signal.[15]

Jack and colleagues[16] showed that manually measuring the hippocampal volume can improve sensitivity, enabling detection of atrophy in 75% to 90% of the hippocampi on the side that is congruent with the electrical onset of the seizures.

A significant difference in hippocampal volume (expressed as difference or ratio) between the two sides is a reasonable indicator of unilateral hippocampal sclerosis. However, there are disadvantages to comparing the volumes of the two hippocampi, including the inability to detect bilateral hippocampal sclerosis and the possibility of false lateralization in patients with an epileptogenic lesion that expands the hippocampus. These issues can be partially addressed by the establishment of hippocampal volume reference values in a normal control population.[17]

In clinical practice, the manual segmentation to assess the volume of the hippocampi is a tedious, time-consuming process, which is dependent on the expertise of the examiner, with some interrater variability.[18] There is much interest in the use of automated analyses that can reproduce similar results, making the process less time consuming and more reliable.[18-21] Coan and associates[22] compared visual analysis, volumetry, and T2 signal of the hippocampus with 3-T MRI in a population of 203 patients affected by mesial temporal lobe epilepsy. They concluded that quantitative techniques were advantageous, with new detection of hippocampal sclerosis in 28% of the patients with mesial temporal lobe epilepsy.

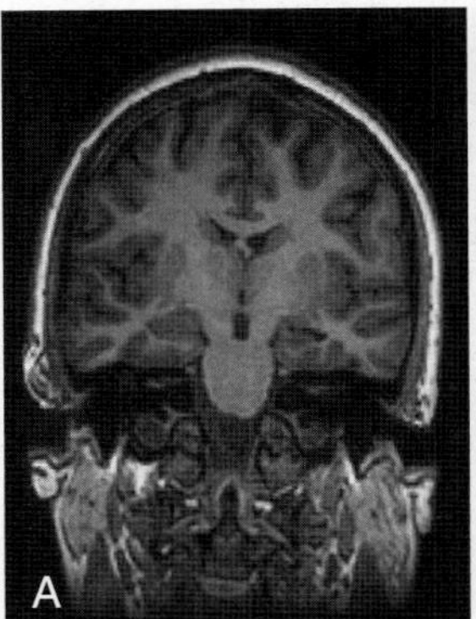

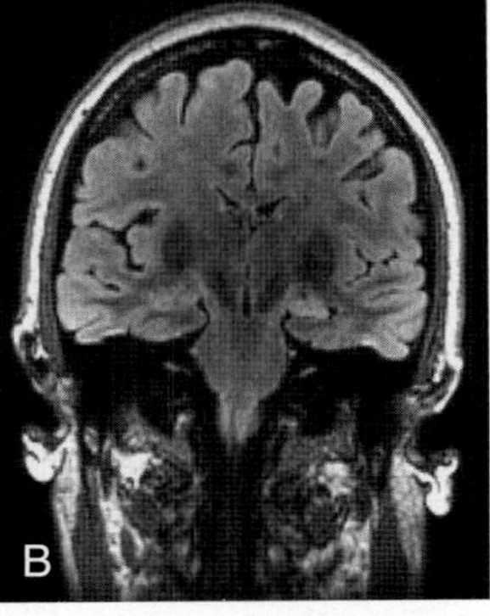

Figure 65-1. Hippocampal sclerosis. A, Coronal T1-weighted image showing left hippocampal volume loss with secondary dilatation of the temporal horn. **B,** Coronal T2-weighted fluid-attenuated inversion recovery (FLAIR) image showing increased signal in the left hippocampus.

Malformations of Cortical Development

Malformations of cortical development (MCDs) can be divided into three groups:

- Group I: malformations resulting from abnormal proliferation of neuronal and glial cells. This group includes microcephaly and macrocephaly, FCDs without and with balloon cells (Taylor dysplasia types IIa and IIb, respectively), hemimegalencephaly, tuberous sclerosis, dysembryoplastic neuroepithelial tumors, gangliogliomas, and gangliocytomas.
- Group II: malformations resulting from abnormal neuronal migration. This group includes lissencephaly and heterotopias.
- Group III: malformations resulting from abnormal cortical organization. This group includes polymicrogyrias, schizencephaly, FCDs type I, and mild MCDs.[23]

In this chapter, we first describe the MRI characteristics of the less frequent MCDs, in accordance with the classification by Barkovich and colleagues,[23] and then we dedicate a specific section to FCDs.

Group I

Tuberous sclerosis can manifest with multiple tubers or hamartomas containing balloon cells, visible on MRI as a cortical thickening with hyperintense T2 signal (Fig. 65-2). Most affected patients have subependymal nodular tubers that can show calcifications and occasionally enhancement. Subependymal giant cell astrocytomas can also be present, and they have to be differentiated from subependymal tubers because of their less benign natural history.[3,24] For this purpose, a contrast-enhanced scan is recommended because subependymal giant cell astrocytomas typically show uniform enhancement. Other distinctive features are that they are generally located near the foramen of Monro, and they tend to grow over time, which leads to obstructive hydrocephalus in 15% of cases.

In *hemimegalencephaly*, hemispheric enlargement is associated with ipsilateral ventriculomegaly and may be associated with changes in signal intensity of white matter, heterotopia, and cortical thickening[3] (see Fig. 65-2).

Group II

Lissencephaly literally means "smooth brain," and the condition is characterized by a lack of development of gyri and sulci. On MRI, the lissencaphalic brain appears agyric, and the sulci and sylvian fissures are shallow. The cortex is usually thickened (pachygyric).

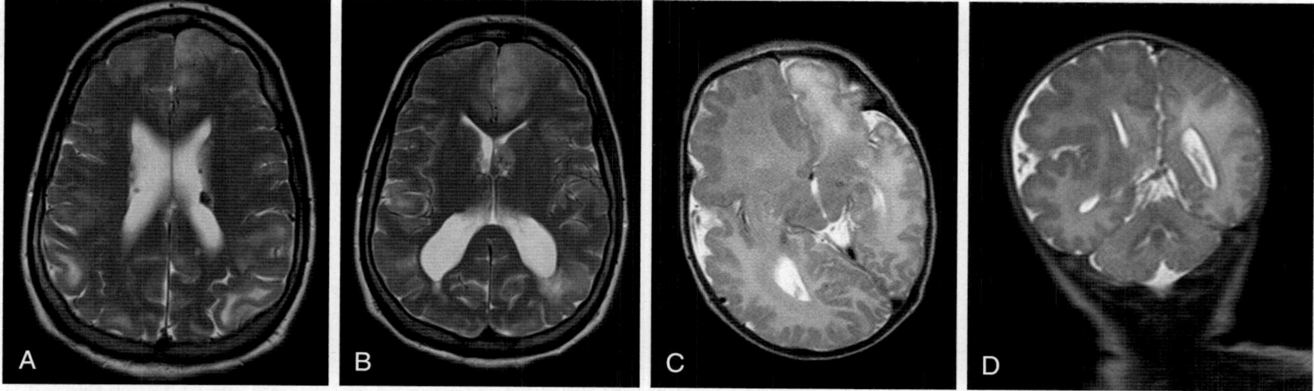

Figure 65-2. Malformations of cortical development, group I. A, Axial T2-weighted image showing multiple calcified periventricular nodules in the lateral ventricles, which give rise to the candle guttering sign, typical of tuberous sclerosis. Multiple hyperintense cortical tubers are also visible. **B,** Axial T2-weighted image showing a subependymal giant cell astrocytoma in the left frontal horn of the lateral ventricle, which caused obstruction to the foramen of Monroe; multiple cortical tubers are also visible. Axial **(C)** and coronal **(D)** T2-weighted images showing hemispheric asymmetry associated with loss of gray-white matter differentiation and thickened cortex on the right, in keeping with widespread right hemispheric malformation (hemimegalencephaly). The hyperintense signal in the left hemisphere represents normal myelination pattern in a 12-month-old child.

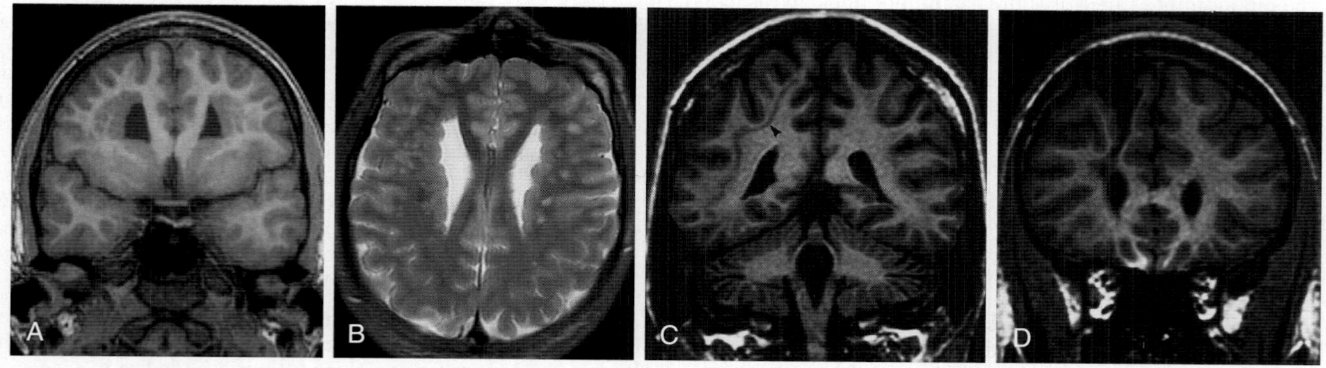

Figure 65-3. Malformations of cortical development, group II. Coronal T1-weighted image **(A)** and axial T2-weighted image **(B)** showing extensive bilateral subependymal nodular gray matter heterotopia. **C,** Coronal T1-weighted image showing extensive band heterotopia in the right cerebral hemisphere. **D,** Coronal T1-weighted image showing schizencephaly that extends to the right ventricle.

Heterotopia is the presence of gray matter in abnormal sites and may be localized (nodular) or generalized (band; Fig. 65-3). Nodular heterotopias produce a signal that is isointense in relation to gray matter and should be distinguished from tubers that can be isointense or hypointense in relation to gray matter on T1-weighted images and hyperintense on T2-weighted images. Subependymal nodular heterotopias, which are commonly bilateral and most frequently located in the occipital horn of the lateral ventricle, are found predominantly in female patients. The associated seizures are usually partial in nature.[25]

Generalized or band heterotopias are often described as a double cortex. They consist of a ribbon of gray matter within white matter, which runs parallel to the overlying cortex, which may be normal or macrogyric.

Group III

Polymicrogyria (literally, "many small folds") is a term used to describe multiple small convolutions on the hemisphere surface that can be unilateral or bilateral.

Schizencephaly (from *schizein,* meaning "to split") is a cleft in the brain that connects the ependyma of the lateral ventricle with the pial surface on the convexity of the brain. Abnormal gray matter lines the cleft and its walls and can either be separated (open lip) or apposed (closed lip). This should be distinguished from porencephaly, which is usually the result of a destructive brain injury and is lined with gliotic matter.

Mild Malformations of Cortical Development. Krsek and colleagues[34] described the imaging characteristics in a group of patients in whom histopathologic analysis showed mild MCD. Mild MCD was always located in the temporal lobe, and the most frequent MRI features, seen in 29% of the cases, were lobar hypoplasia and atrophy. Other signs, such as blurring of the junction between gray and white matter or white matter signal changes, were infrequent, and changes in cortical thickness and "funnel" track sign described for FCD type II were usually not seen.[34] For these reasons, it is very difficult to distinguish mild MCD from FCD type I.

Focal Cortical Dysplasia

FCDs are the most common group of MCDs in patients presenting with intractable epilepsy and the most common cause of epilepsy in children.[26,27]

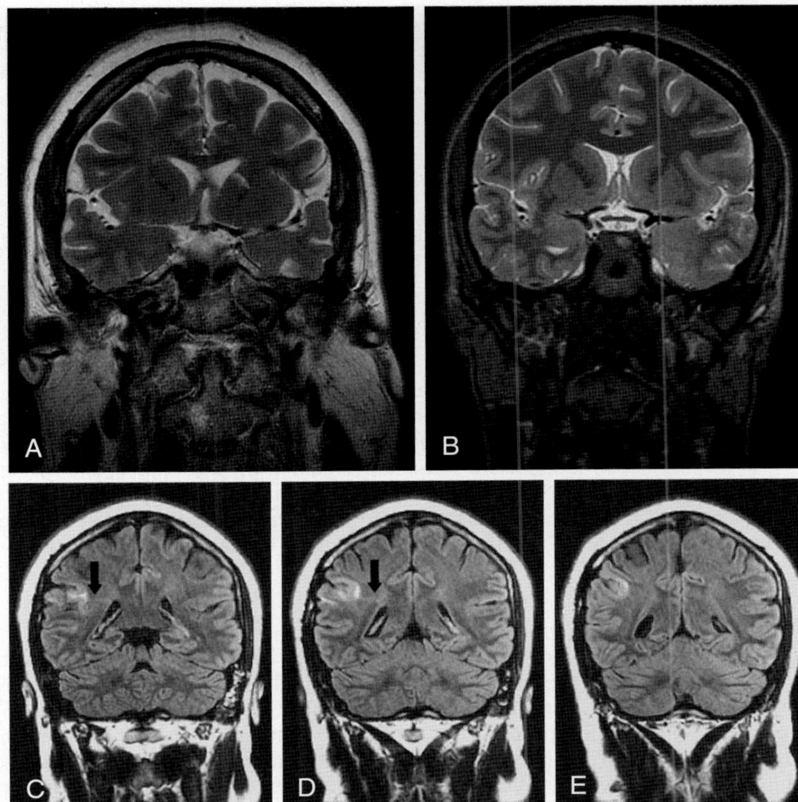

Figure 65-4. Focal cortical dysplasia (FCD). A and **B,** Coronal T2-weighted images showing hypoplasia of the left temporal pole and loss of gray-white matter differentiation, in keeping with presence of FCD. **C** to **E,** Type II FCD: coronal T2-weighted fluid-attenuated inversion recovery (FLAIR) images showing funnel track hyperintensity (**C** and **D,** *arrows*) extending from the cortex of the right supramarginal gyrus to the ventricle.

Imaging findings of FCDs can be subtle. Therefore images have to be reviewed taking into consideration a full knowledge of the patient's epilepsy, semiologic findings, and neurophysiologic characteristics. In cases of a negative MRI, other advanced imaging modalities—such as fluorodeoxyglucose positron emission tomography (FDG-PET), interictal single photon emission computed tomography (SPECT), and magnetoencephalography—should be considered to try to locate any subtle regional abnormality. Coregistration of structural MRI with advanced imaging tools allows the user to assess the spatial concordance of positive findings and also to reevaluate a "negative" MRI with the benefit of this new information.[28]

A number of researchers have attempted to identify the different imaging characteristics of the various subtypes of FCDs (Fig. 65-4). Colombo and associates[29] reported the following findings:

FCD type I, which can be completely cryptogenic. In this subtype, common findings are hypoplasia or atrophy at a lobar or sublobar level. They are frequently associated with subcortical white matter volume loss, which has an increased signal on T2-weighted images and T2-weighted FLAIR images and a decreased signal on T1-weighted images. Cortical thickness is usually preserved, although there can be mild blurring at the junction between gray and white matter. FCD type I is most frequently located in the temporal lobe, is associated with hippocampal sclerosis in more than 70% of the cases,[25,30] and is the FCD most commonly associated with developmental tumors. If structural MRI shows mass effect, cystic components, or calcifications, a tumor should be suspected, and the MRI should be repeated with gadolinium contrast material.

FCD type II, which is characterized by increased cortical thickness and blurring of the junction between gray and white matter on T1- and T2-weighted images. The subcortical area can show an increased signal on T2-weighted and FLAIR images and a decreased signal on T1-weighted images. This abnormality creates a "funnel" track between the cortex and the ventricle, which is typical of type II FCDs and explains why the condition is also termed *transmantle dysplasia*.[31] Other associated findings are abnormal cortical gyration and sulcation with increased T2 signal of the affected cortex (which remains hypointense in comparison with the underlying white matter). It is not possible to distinguish type IIa (FCD with dysmorphic neurons)[32] from IIb (FCD with dysmporphic neurons and balloon cells) on MRI,[32] although type IIb is often better delineated. In contrast to type I, type II FCD often occurs in extratemporal areas, with a predilection for the frontal lobe.[33]

Age and Imaging of Focal Cortical Dysplasia

Colombo and associates[29] reported the importance of the age of the patient in the selection of the most appropriate sequences to evaluate blurring and cortical thickness. In adults, in whom myelination is complete, T2-weighted, T1-weighted, and T1-weighted inversion recovery sequences are suitable for this purpose. In infants younger than 6 months, myelination is incomplete, which means that immature white matter can appear isointense in relation to the cortex on T1- and T2-weighted images. However in areas of FCD, the white matter almost always looks hyperintense in relation to the dysplastic area on T2-weighted images. Because the contrast between cortex and white matter is maximal before myelination begins, if seizures

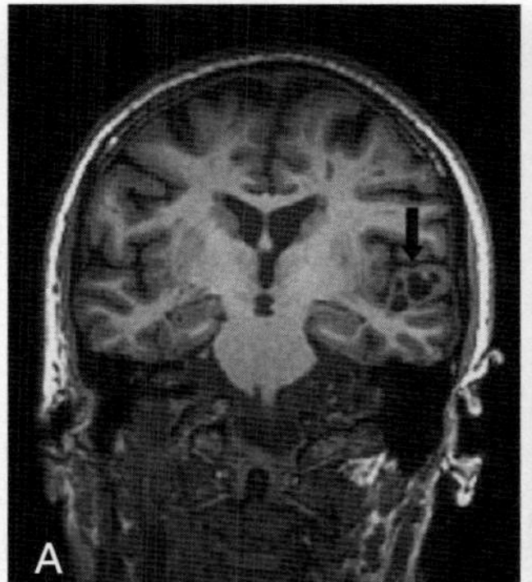

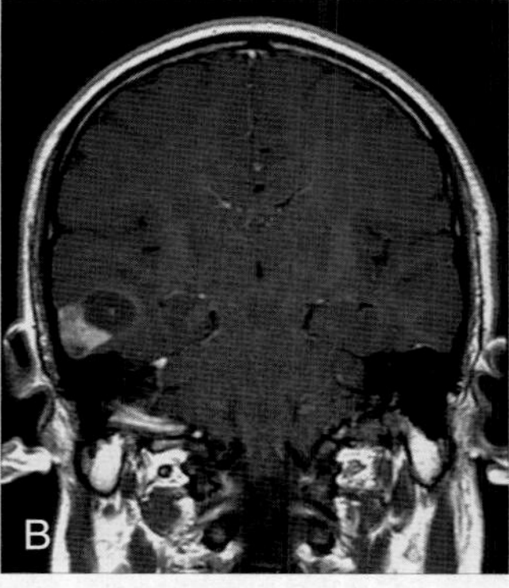

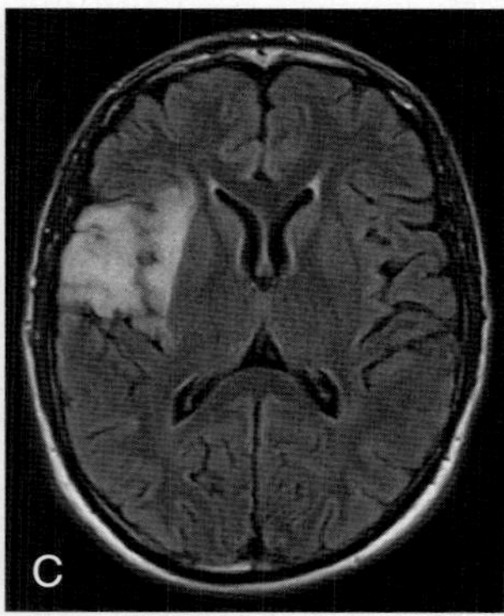

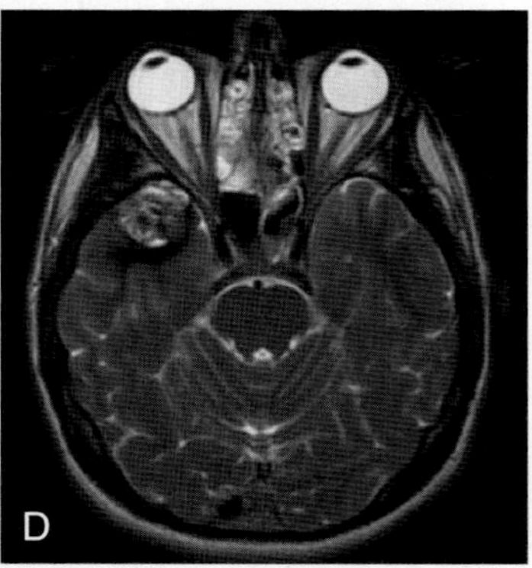

Figure 65-5. Tumors and vascular lesions. A Coronal T1-weighted image showing a hypointense multicystic cortical lesion *(arrow)* in the left superior temporal gyrus, consistent with a dysembryoplastic neuroepithelial tumor (DNET). **B,** Coronal T2-weighted image showing a right temporal cyst with a mural nodule, consistent with a ganglioglioma. **C,** Axial T2-weighted fluid-attenuated inversion recovery (FLAIR) image showing extensive increased signal abnormality, centered in the right insular region and extending into the temporal area, representing a low-grade glioma. **D,** Axial T2-weighted image showing the characteristic "popcorn" appearance of a cavernoma in the right temporal pole.

start before the age of 6 months, a scan should be obtained immediately so that the hypointense FCD on T2-weighted images clearly stands out from the hyperintense white matter. During the myelination process that occurs between ages 6 and 18 months, the contrast between gray and white matter diminishes, and FCDs are less visible. In case of a "negative" MRI, a scan should be repeated at 30 months, when the myelination is largely completed.

Tumors

Any tumor can be a possible cause of seizures. In the setting of chronic epilepsy, tumors represent 25% to 35% of the cases. In young adults and children, the most common tumors associated with epilepsy are dysembryoplastic neuroepithelial tumors (DNETs) and gangliogliomas (Fig. 65-5). In 70% of cases, they are located in the temporal lobe.[35]

DNETs manifest as focal, well-circumscribed cortical masses that may scallop the adjacent inner calvarial area and extend in the subcortical area. DNETs have a characteristic wedge-shaped, multicystic appearance that is hypointense on T1-weighted images and hyperintense on T2-weighted images. In a third of the cases, calcification and faint focal punctate or ring enhancement is present. Hyperintense FLAIR signal surrounding the lesion is characteristic.

Gangliogliomas have low signal on T1-weighted images and high signal on T2-weighted images. The most common appearance is a circumscribed cyst with mural nodule; the next most common is a solid tumor expanding the cortex. In half of the cases, calcification and enhancement are present.[3]

Low-grade gliomas present as isointense to hypointense on T1-weighted images in comparison with white matter. They seem to arise from the white matter and cause gradual expansion of the adjacent cortex with localized mass effect. They are hyperintense on T2-weighted images and FLAIR sequences. They usually do not enhance with contrast material, although the absence of enhancement does not exclude tumor progression.[36]

Vascular Malformations

The most common vascular malformations associated with epilepsy are cavernomas, which manifest with seizures in 50% of cases.[37,38] Because cavernomas contain no neural tissue, seizures are thought to arise from the surrounding hemosiderin secondary to hemorrhage. On MRI, cavernomas have a characteristic "popcorn" appearance, resulting from the different stages of hemorrhage on T1- and T2-weighted images (see Fig. 65-5). The imaging sequences of choice for cavernomas are gradient echo and susceptibility-weighted images, in which the blood products show a typical blooming hypointensity.[39]

Arteriovenous malformations also manifest with seizures in 25% of cases. The fast flow within such malformations is easily visible as flow voids on T2-weighted images, although the "gold standard" investigation is formal cerebral angiography.

Transient Changes on Magnetic Resonance Imaging in Relation to Seizures

Complex partial and generalized status epilepticus can cause transient changes on MRI, with focal areas of hyperintensity on T2-weighted images. To distinguish these conditions from underlying structural disease, it is necessary to repeat imaging at a later date when the patient has been seizure-free for a reasonable period of time.[40]

Structural Magnetic Resonance Imaging and Cognition in Epilepsy

Language and memory have been studied extensively in relation to structural imaging in temporal lobe epilepsy.[41] There appears to be a relationship between hippocampal volume and memory dysfunction: reduced left-sided volumes are associated with impairments in verbal learning and memory, and normal left-sided volumes are associated with greatest postoperative memory decline.[42] Similarly, on the right side, reduction in amygdala volume is associated with visual memory loss.[43]

Patients with temporal lobe epilepsy also exhibit a more global reduction in the volume of cerebral tissue, most evident when the volume of white matter tissue is measured across frontal, temporal, and parietal lobe regions, but not occipital lobe regions. This reduction in volume of white matter is strongly associated with cognitive impairment.[44]

In patients with temporal lobe epilepsy, increased amygdala volume may be associated with depression, dysthymia,[45,46] and psychosis,[47] and decreased amygdala volume may be associated with interictal aggression.[48]

FUNCTIONAL IMAGING

Functional Magnetic Resonance Imaging

Functional MRI (fMRI) is a technique for mapping areas of function to the cortical surface. It can be used to map language,[49] motor function,[50] memory,[51] and epileptic activity.[52] The technique indirectly detects focal areas of increased neuronal activity by identifying increased cerebral blood flow when the patient performs specific tasks known as functional paradigms (i.e., finger tapping in hand motor fMRI, verbal fluency in language fMRI).

Through echo-planar imaging sequences, a series of scans of the entire brain are generated that are sensitive to changes in blood oxygen level–dependent (BOLD) signal. The BOLD signal represents the ratio of oxyhemoglobin concentration to deoxyhemoglobin concentration. These have different signal characteristics on T2-weighted imaging. A greater concentration of oxyhemoglobin in comparison with deoxyhemoglobin produces a high BOLD signal and identifies an area with increased neuronal activity as a result of localized hyperperfusion.[53] A BOLD signal is created for each region of interest during a specific activity and is then compared with the signal in the same region in the resting state. Signal averaging over multiple acquisitions provides a map of the likelihood that function is present in this area. This signal map is coregistered with conventional MR to provide spatial and anatomic resolution (Fig. 65-6).

There are a number of limitations to this technique. First, the area of BOLD activation is greatly influenced by thresholding and can be widespread or focal. Second, there is no direct relationship between BOLD intensity and cortical eloquence. Third, areas that do not surpass the chosen threshold are not necessarily functionally inert. Finally, the area of BOLD activation might not be crucial to the execution of the task, and the task itself may not accurately reflect functional ability. For these reasons, the surgeon must exercise caution in the interpretation of the fMRI in individual patients.

Motor Function

Motor fMRI can be validated by comparison with direct cortical stimulation. In one study, preoperative motor fMRI was compared with direct cortical stimulation in 25 patients with perirolandic tumors, with an 84% correlation.[54]

Anatomically, because of the arcade of pial membranes and cortical vessels, identification of the central sulcus by inspection can be difficult intraoperatively. Motor fMRI is therefore useful in verifying gyral functional anatomy, especially in the context of perirolandic disease that may cause some migration of function. Motor fMRI can also be used to identify regions of interest necessary for generating corticospinal tractography.

Language

The intracarotid amytal (Wada) test is the traditional "gold standard" investigation to determine the laterality of language and memory function.[55] However, this technique has two limitations: (1) it is an invasive study and carries a 0.6% risk of stroke, and (2) the study is dependent on the internal carotid artery's being the sole blood supply to the functional area tested, with no hemispheric crossover. Language fMRI is being increasingly used to determine the laterality of language dominance.[56]

Expressive language is assessed with verbal fluency and verb generation tests, and receptive language function is assessed with a reading comprehension task. Verbal fluency tests commonly generate stronger and wider activations than do verb generation tasks.[49] Receptive language paradigms commonly show bilateral activation. A degree of functional reorganization has been observed: functions originating from regions close to the diseased area are more likely to relocate contralaterally, and functions originating from regions distant from the diseased area are more likely to remain in the ipsilateral hemisphere.[57] Various methods to quantify the lateralization of BOLD signals have been suggested, including counting the voxels above a set threshold and determination of the BOLD signal in anatomically defined areas.[58] The most effective measures are those that do not rely on thresholding.[56] Most often, the lateralization of function is clear from visual inspection.

Language fMRI shows high levels of concordance with the Wada test in lateralizing language function.[59] Because it is cheap, noninvasive, and repeatable, many centers have abandoned the Wada test in favor of language fMRI for lateralization of function. However, the usefulness of fMRI in localizing language function is less clear. If a resection close to the language cortex is being considered, the critical area should still be mapped through direct stimulation, either with implanted electrodes postoperatively or in the awake patient at surgery.

Electroencephalography–Functional Magnetic Resonance Imaging

Electroencephalography (EEG)–fMRI is a multimodal imaging technique that can be used to localize the region of the brain responsible for generating epileptiform discharges. This is done

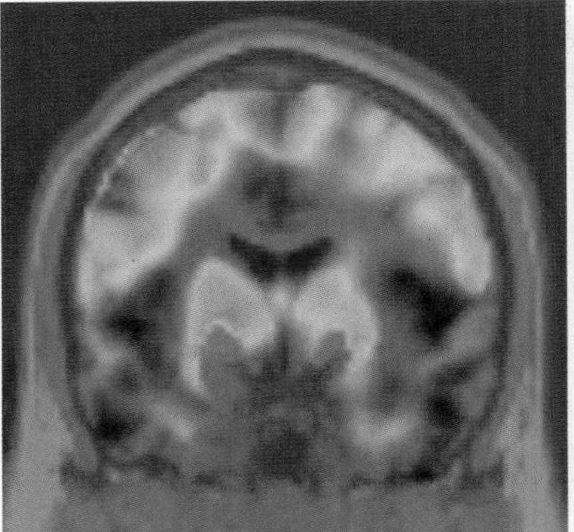
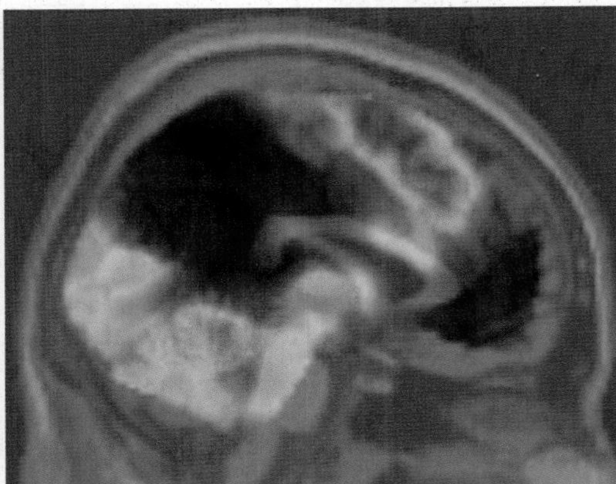
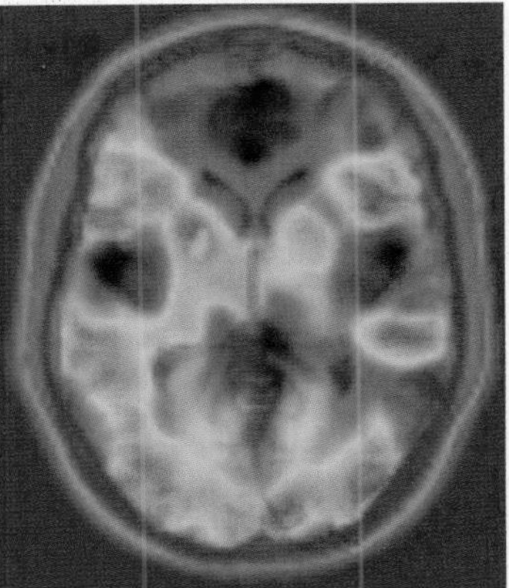

Figure 65-6. Functional magnetic resonance images. Unthresholded ictal statistical parametric maps for verbal fluency task, overlaid on T1-weighted magnetic resonance images. *Red* indicates positive activation, and *blue* indicates negative activation.

by mapping changes in hemodynamic BOLD levels associated with interictal and ictal epileptiform discharges. The "task" or "functional paradigm" in this case is the presence of epileptic activity.

EEG-fMRI is a noninvasive technique that has the significant advantage of combining the high spatial resolution of fMRI with the excellent temporal resolution of EEG. The main limitation with the technique is the requirement for epileptiform activity during the scanning, which leads to a low yield in selected patients. A new technique (Grouiller's method) addresses this limitation by incorporating voltage maps of epileptic spikes obtained previously during long-term EEG recordings into the EEG obtained in the scanner.[60] In an ideal situation, EEG-fMRI would be obtained during the ictal phase. This possibility remains confined to exceptional cases for practical constraints: technical factors, such as the patient's moving in the scanner; safety reasons; and the probability that the patient would have a seizure while undergoing the MRI.

Typically studies last between 10 and 40 minutes, with a corresponding limit on the positive yield. Of adults with refractory focal epilepsy and frequent interictal epileptiform discharges (IEDs), 50% have an IED during EEG-fMRI recording, and 50% of those individuals show a significant IED-related BOLD signal change.[61]

EEG-fMRI has been incorporated in a few centers in the presurgical evaluation of patients under trial conditions. Concordance between BOLD signal and electroclinical localization of the epileptogenic zone is reasonable in 40% to 60% of patients.[62] There is great interest in using EEG-fMRI in patients with structurally normal MRIs to identify potential regions for further investigations, such as focused anatomic MRI or electrode implantation.

However, there is currently not enough evidence for wider uptake of EEG-fMRI into clinical application. In one study, 76 patients undergoing presurgical evaluation underwent EEG-fMRI, and the locations of the IED-BOLD signal were correlated with resection margins and surgical outcome.[52] In only 21 were IEDs recorded, which demonstrates the low yield with this technique, and only 10 proceeded to resective surgery. Of those 10, 7 were seizure free after surgery, and there was concordance between the BOLD signal and resection in 6 of the 7. In the remaining 3 patients, who continued to suffer with seizures postoperatively, the BOLD signal lay outside the resection zone. This suggests a possible negative predictive value for EEG-fMRI, whereby lack of concordance is predictive of poor surgical outcome.

In summary, more prospective studies are required in which EEG-fMRI is used for localization in the presurgical evaluation of patients who proceed to surgery and achieve postoperative freedom from seizures.

Diffusion-Weighted Imaging

DWI is a magnetic resonance method that maps the diffusion of water in biologic tissues, so that each voxel has an intensity that reflects the best measurement of the rate of water diffusion. DWI is used to delineate the white matter pathways of the brain through a technique called *tractography*[63] (Fig. 65-7).

Water diffusion anisotropy (direction) in the white matter is defined by axonal alignment. Water diffuses preferentially in a direction parallel to the longitudinal axis of the axon, and diffusion is restricted perpendicular to the axis. Each voxel can therefore be expressed mathematically as a diffusion ellipsoid or tensor. The long axis of adjacent tensors can be "tracked" to progressively reconstruct the 3D orientation of nerve fibers that represent white matter connectivity. The translation of the tensors into neural trajectories can be achieved through various algorithms, which can be broadly classified as deterministic and probabilistic.

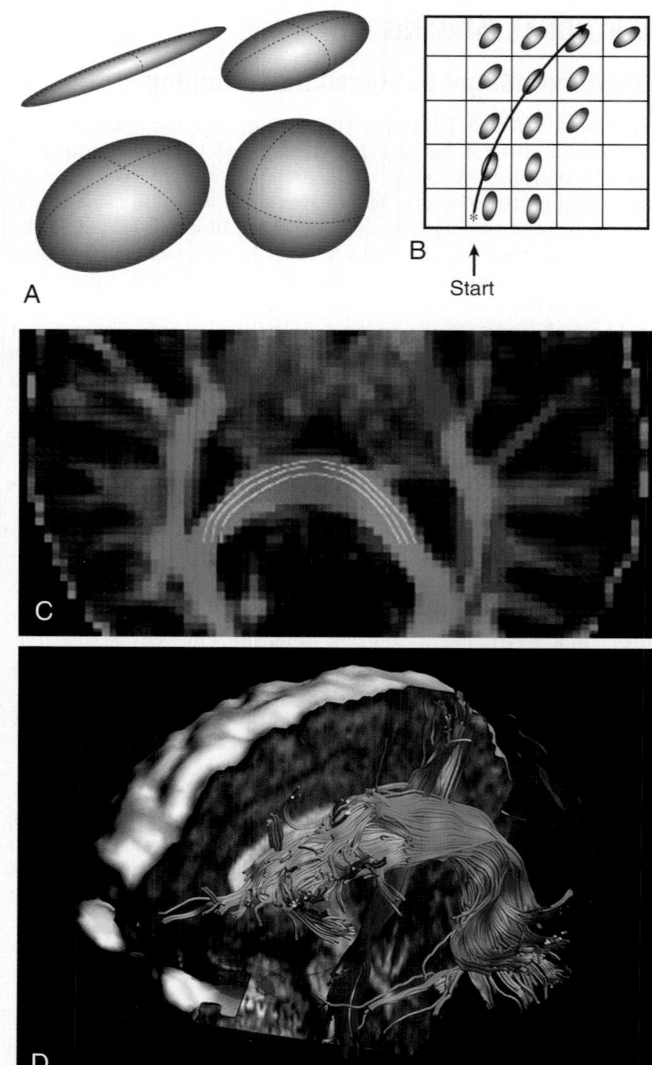

Figure 65-7. Principles of tractography. A, Diffusion ellipsoids (tensors). When there is no directionality, the fractional anisotropy is zero (spherical). A typical tensor of a white matter tract is cigar-shaped. When there are crossing fibers, the ellipsoid becomes flattened, resulting in pancake-shaped tensors. **B,** Tracking starts at a pixel, and continues along the ellipsoids as long as the adjacent vectors are strongly aligned. **C,** Axial image of color fractional anisotropic map, showing posterior corpus callosum. **D,** Tractography of the left arcuate fasciculus and corticospinal tract. *(Image created in ExploreDTI; courtesy of Sjoerd Vos, Epilepsy Society, London.)*

The most common approach used clinically is deterministic line propagation or streamline techniques, whereby neural connections are mapped in at least two arbitrary regions of interest in 3D space. Tracking of the fibers is terminated when one of these *stop criteria* is met:

1. A pixel with low fractional anisotropy is reached.
2. A predetermined trajectory curvature between two contiguous vectors is reached.

The advantage of this technique is that the processing is fairly simple and rapid.

The deterministic method has two main disadvantages. First, it is inadequate in processing voxels containing multiple fiber orientations, providing unreliable orientation estimates that delineate pathways that do not exist and failing to identify tracts that do. Because crossing fibers occur in approximately 90% of white matter voxels, this issue is very important.[64]

Second, DWI is a low signal-to-noise ratio technique, which can also affect the reliability of the estimated orientations. The provision of a single best-fit orientation, at the expense of other possible orientations, can lead to misleading results.

Probabilistic techniques were developed to deal with the issues of crossing fibers and low signal-to-noise ratios. Many of these techniques are adaptations of simple streamline approaches but include estimates of fiber orientation uncertainty. These enable more robust tractography and are increasingly used in modern clinical practice.[65,66]

The probabilistic approach has two main disadvantages. First, it is slower, and so it cannot be used interactively. Second, it may be harder to interpret visually, inasmuch as the generated tracts represent a 3D volume of potential connectivities. Anatomic knowledge is necessary to determine which fibers are anatomically incorrect and to filter them out.

Both methods of tractography are hampered by difficulties of validation. Validation can be achieved either by comparison with known neuroanatomy or by comparison with results of intraoperative electrophysiologic testing. Although both methods underestimate the fiber tracts, the probabilistic method seems slightly better in this regard.[63] Both methods are also hampered by poor interuser reproducibility; small differences in the regions of interest selected lead to considerable variation in the white matter tracts generated.

Tractography has been clinically applied most frequently to the surgical treatment of brain tumors. The corticospinal pathway is the most commonly generated tract for the treatment of tumors that lie close to the motor cortex. There is now good experience in the use of tractography exported into neuronavigation systems to aid the decision-making process during tumor resection.[65,67]

In the context of epilepsy surgery, diffusion tensor imaging (DTI) is obviously applicable to lesional cases close to eloquent cortex tissue. However, in nonlesional cases, DTI can help in evaluating the relationship between the epileptogenic area and the subcortical fibers. This is beneficial not only for surgical planning but also for neurophysiologic purposes to better understand the possible connectivity underlying the electrical spread of the seizure.

There are also reported cases of the utility of DTI in the postoperative evaluation of disconnection surgery. Choudhri and associates[68] reported that postoperative DTI in patients undergoing corpus callosotomy can confirm whether the intended fibers have been disconnected, which helps in the planning for possible further surgical intervention versus other therapies.

Toda and colleagues[69] reported the utility of DTI in a case of hemispherotomy, in which, 3 months after surgery, clonic convulsions returned. MRI showed that the genu of the corpus callosum was unsectioned, and DTI tractography confirmed the presence of callosal fibers in the genu of the corpus callosum. After additional section of the corpus callosum, the patient remained seizure free.

Acquiring DTI images in intraoperative MRI will clearly have a huge potential in evaluating disconnection procedure at the time of surgery.

MAGNETIC RESONANCE SPECTROSCOPY

Magnetic resonance spectroscopy (MRS) is an analytic method that enables the identification and quantification of metabolites within a radiologic area of interest. The spectra produced by MRS provide chemical and physiologic information, rather than anatomic data. In MRS, the resonance frequency of a nucleus supplies chemical information, which may be displayed as a spectrum of signal intensity against frequency. Therefore, the area under the tracing indicates the amplitude of the signal at that frequency. In the human brain, protons of hydrogen 1 (^{1}H) nuclei are the most used because of their high sensitivity and abundance.

Other nuclei may be used to obtain magnetic resonance spectra, including phosphorus 31 (^{31}P), fluorine 19 (^{19}F), carbon 13 (^{13}C), and sodium 23 (^{23}Na).

The ^{1}H-MRS acquisition usually starts with anatomic images in order to select a volume of interest in which the spectrum will be acquired. The volume of brain from which magnetic resonance spectra are obtained may be defined with two different techniques:

- Single-voxel, in which data are acquired from a single volume of interest
- Multivoxel (also known as *spectroscopic imaging* or *chemical-shift imaging*), in which the main difference is to simultaneously acquire many voxels and a spatial distribution of the metabolites within a single sequence

A more comprehensive description of this technique and its application in epilepsy is given elsewhere.[70,71]

We have described so far the use and the potential of MRI in detecting lesions that can be a possible cause of seizures. However, seizures can derive from a wide spectrum of causes, such as metabolic diseases and genetic diseases, most of which do not necessitate surgical treatment.

In patients with seizures and a suspected metabolic disease, such as mitochondrial disorders and creatine deficiencies, MRS may be indicated to screen for metabolic derangements. The metabolic work of brain cells during seizures is increased, which causes the demand for oxygen and nutrients to exceed supply. MRS detects this imbalance, identifying abnormal accumulation of lactate and *N*-acetyl aspartate (NAA).[72]

From a surgical perspective, MRS has two main areas of application. First, it may be useful in the diagnosis of an epileptogenic lesion. In difficult cases, ^{1}H MRS has a potential role in the preoperative differential diagnosis and can improve the accuracy and the level of confidence in differentiating a tumor from a FCD.[73] A tumor would show the following characteristics:

- Reduced levels of NAA. This metabolite is a neuronal marker, and its reduction denotes destruction of normal brain tissue. Its reduction leads to decreased NAA/creatine ratios.
- Increased levels of choline. This is usually evidenced by an increase in the choline/NAA and choline/creatine ratios.
- Minor changes in creatine levels.[70]

Decreased NAA/creatine ratios can also be a common finding in FCD; however, the relatively normal choline/creatine ratio may help to distinguish FCD from a neoplasm.[71]

The other application of MRS is in patients with unremarkable structural MRI findings. Cendes and colleagues[74] performed ^{1}H MRS and magnetic resonance volumetric analyses of the temporal lobes of 100 patients with medically refractory temporal lobe epilepsy. Proton magnetic resonance spectroscopic imaging can detect and quantify focal neuronal damage or dysfunction based on reduced signals from the neuronal marker NAA, which would reveal a reduced NAA/creatine ratio. In 100 patients with temporal lobe epilepsy and normal MRI findings, Cendes and colleagues performed MRS, quantitatively measured amygdala and hippocampal volumes, and assessed concordance with EEG lateralization. MRS findings alone were correlated with the lateralization determined by EEG in 86% of patients, better than MRI volumetry alone (83%). Moreover, MRS findings were abnormal in 12 patients in whom MRI volumetric analysis depicted normal findings.

MULTIMODALITY IMAGING IN EPILEPSY SURGERY

Principles of Multimodality

Three-dimensional multimodality imaging (3DMMI) is the use of different tools that provide distinct, complementary information to solve a common complex problem. The fundamental concept is that the integration of different data sets into a single 3D platform confers an added value over the consecutive presentation of the same data sets in series or in parallel. Most of the information implemented in 3DMMI derives from the postprocessing of MRI images; however, other imaging modalities can be integrated and displayed, which adds essential patient-specific information.

Application to Epilepsy Surgery

Because 3DMMI requires the simultaneous analysis of multiple data sets and the consideration of how each data set relates to another (Fig. 65-8), it is ideally suited to the planning of epilepsy surgery. It allows for the optimal evaluation of the spatial concordance of a site of seizure localization established through different modalities, as well as the relationship of the structural, functional and electrophysiologic changes to the anatomic features in the area. It also allows the determination of the proximity of the epileptogenic zone to eloquent cortex tissue or the functional deficit zone (i.e., the area of the brain that shows abnormal functioning in the interictal period as a result of a structural lesion, the functional consequences of the persisting epileptic condition, or both).[75]

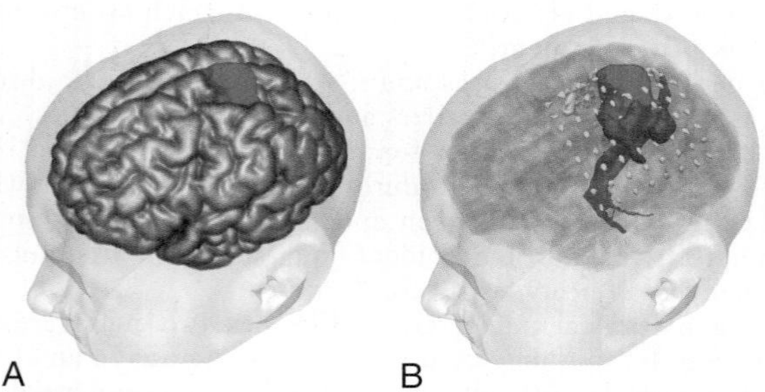

Figure 65-8. Three-dimensional visualization of patient data in EpiNav software. A, Models of scalp *(white),* volume rendering of brain *(brown),* and segmentation of tumor *(red).* **B,** Addition of hand motor area *(dark green)* and foot motor area *(light green)* on functional magnetic resonance imaging, corticospinal tractography *(blue),* and implanted electrodes *(yellow).*

In a prospective study, the usefulness of 3DMMI in the presurgical evaluation of patients undergoing intracranial EEG was assessed.[76] Disclosure of the use of 3DMMI changed some aspect of management in 43 (80%) of 54 cases, which supports the notion that the use of 3DMMI substantially influences clinical decision making.

The following common steps are followed to generate 3DMMI data:

1. Image acquisition
2. Image coregistration
3. Segmentation of regions of interest
4. 3D visualization as surface or volume renderings

Because identification of a structural lesion is a strong predictor for achieving freedom from seizures after surgery,[77,78] any imaging technique or postprocessing tool that can unmask a previously cryptogenic structural abnormality is highly valued.

In the field of pediatric epilepsy, the use of FDG-PET, diffusion tensor images, and magnetic source images has significantly improved lesion detection and localization, helping identify focal cortical dysplasia, tuberous sclerosis, hemimegalencephaly, mesial temporal sclerosis, neoplasms, Rasmussen's (chronic focal) encephalitis, perinatal infarction, and Sturge-Weber syndrome.[79]

Similarly, voxel-based morphometric analysis of cortex, in which individual brain anatomy is compared to a normal database, can identify areas of interest for further investigation[80] (Fig. 65-9). Data from these regions can then be manually segmented, registered with structural MRI, and exported into neuronavigation systems for targeted recordings with depth electrodes.

Several groups have reported on their use of 3DMMI in epilepsy surgery.[81-84] Murphy and associates[82] reported on a carefully selected cohort of 22 patients, deemed to have difficult cases, who underwent 3DMMI-guided surgery between April 1999 and October 2001. Criteria for patient selection were no lesion visualized on the conventional MRI, multiple lesions, or one very large lesion that could not be resected safely without risk of significant postoperative morbidity. Murphy and associates used PET, FLAIR MRI sequences, SPECT, and subtraction ictal

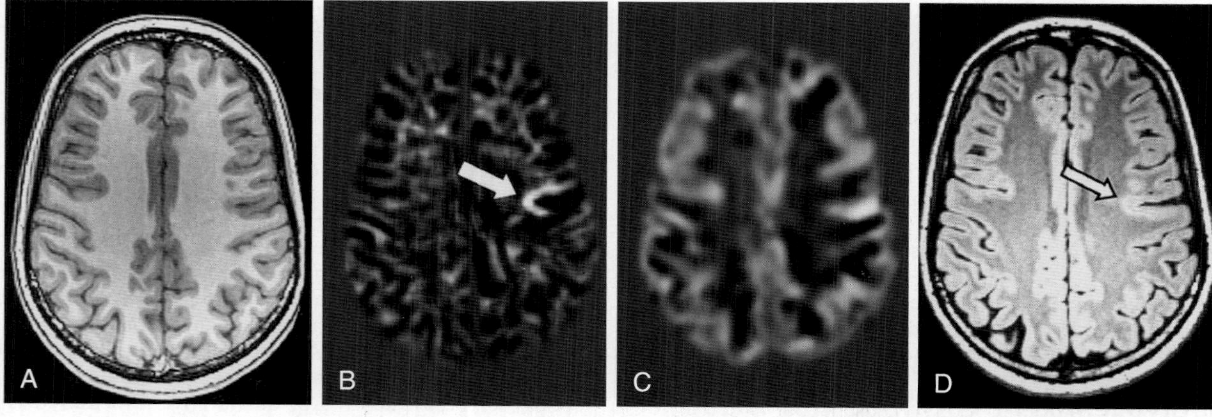

Figure 65-9. Axial view of magnetic resonance postprocessing, demonstrating left frontal area of focal cortical dysplasia. A, T1-weighted image. **B,** Junction image (*arrow* indicates lesion). **C,** Extension image. **D,** High-resolution fluid-attenuated inversion recovery (FLAIR) image (*arrow* indicates lesion). *(From Wellmer J, Parpaley Y, Von Lehe M, et al. Integrating magnetic resonance imaging postprocessing results into neuronavigation for electrode implantation and resection of subtle focal cortical dysplasia in previously cryptogenic epilepsy.* Neurosurgery. *2010;66[1]:187-194.)*

SPECT coregistered with MRI (SISCOM); imaging was coregistered with the use of a Unix-based workstation and commercially available software package (Analyze) and then downloaded onto a neuronavigation system for use in the operating room. Postoperative computed tomography was used to incorporate data from the implanted electrodes into 3DMMI. They suggested that the value of functional imaging was the unmasking of previously cryptic regions of interest, and the value of integration was to place this new information in an anatomic and surgically accessible framework. With these added gains, 3DMMI improved outcomes in more difficult cases, such as nonlesional extratemporal epilepsy. The seizure outcomes were recorded as class I ("free of disabling seizures) of the Engel Epilepsy Surgery Outcome Scale in 17 of 22 patients, although mean length of follow-up was only 27 months.

The use of 3DMMI encompasses not only new functional modalities to unmask new regions of interest but also modalities to demonstrate vascular anatomy. The incorporation of robust vascular imaging into the anatomic imaging is a prerequisite to the technique of stereo-electroencephalography (SEEG), first described by Talairach and colleagues[85] and performed today in many centers in Europe and the United States.[84,86-89] There is currently great interest in developing new noninvasive techniques of blood vessel segmentation to further reduce the risk of the SEEG procedure.[90] 3D segmentation of blood vessels also has value in open craniotomies, in which it can be used as a road map to gyral anatomy.[91]

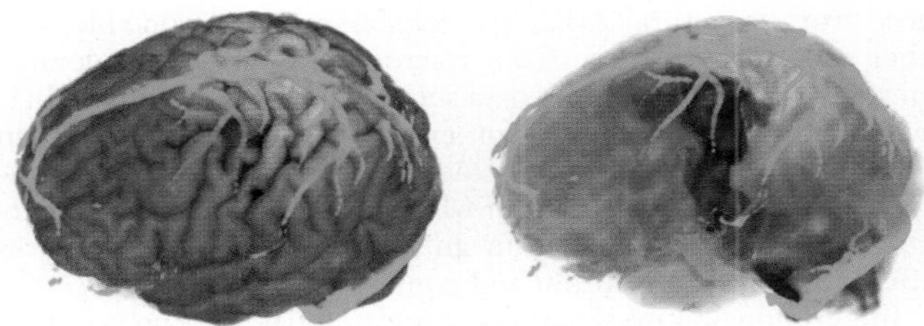

Figure 65-10. Three-dimensional multimodality imaging. Volume rendering of cortex *(gray)*, displayed in AMIRA software with the following associated modalities: focal cortical dysplasia (FCD) *(red)*, hypometabolism on fluorodeoxyglucose positron emission tomography *(pink)*, hand motor area on functional magnetic resonance imaging (fMRI) *(green)*, corticospinal tractography *(purple)*, veins *(cyan)*, and language fMRI *(orange)*. *(From Nowell M, Miserocchi A, McEvoy AW, et al. Advances in epilepsy surgery.* J Neurol Neurosurg Psychiatry *2014;85[11]:1273-1279.)*

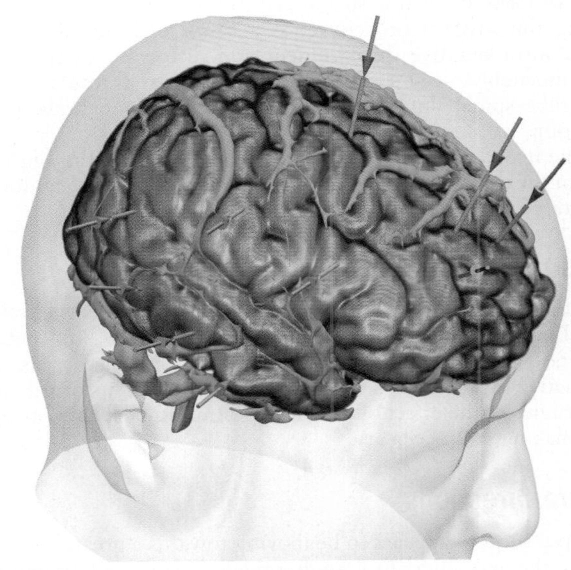

Figure 65-11. Planning tools in epilepsy. Stereo-electroencephalographic planning in EpiNav software with volume rendering of cortex *(brown)*, veins segmented from magnetic resonance venogram *(cyan)*, and implanted depth electrodes *(yellow)*.

Current Practice

The generation of 3DMMI currently takes place in three different ways:

1. Basic planning on commercially available neuronavigation systems (StealthStation S7 Navigation System, Medtronic, Minneapolis; Brainlab products, Brainlab, Feldkirchen, Germany)
2. Specialized planning software as an adjunct to neuronavigation software (StealthViz planning station, Medtronic, Minneapolis; iPlan, Brainlab)
3. Stand-alone specialized planning software packages (e.g., Amira, Visualization Sciences Group, Bordeaux, France)

Neuronavigation systems offer the most user-friendly and the simplest experience, although they are limited in their functionality with regard to data processing and analysis, visualization, and presentation. Software such as StealthViz and iPlan augment these systems, offering tools for coregistering functional and structural imaging, running deterministic tractography, and performing advanced brain and blood vessel segmentation. The most versatile systems are the stand-alone specialized planning software packages that are developed outside of industry. Examples include BioImageSuite, developed at Yale University; 3D Slicer, developed at Harvard University; Analyze, developed at the Mayo Clinic; and Amira. These are used in a range of disciplines in basic and clinical science. The major advantage of these packages is that they are not dedicated to solving specific, well-defined problems. This "nonspecialization" means that they include added flexibility in the processing, manipulation, and display of data sets, and they have an added range of tools to choose from (Figs. 65-10 and 65-11). However, with this flexibility comes the disadvantages that the software is not particularly intuitive and is difficult to integrate into a clinical environment.

Barriers to Widespread Adoption

There are three barriers to the widespread adoption of 3DMMI in clinical practice: (1) organizational infrastructure, (2) accuracy, and (3) validity.

Organizational Infrastructure

3DMMI is a complex addition to any clinical pathway; organizations must make considerable changes to accommodate this technology. The first requirement is the availability of the range of imaging modalities, along with the time and expertise to perform relevant preprocessing of data. The second requirement is a dedicated service of data integration and validation, which requires specialist training and can be costly in terms of employee hours. The third requirement is a common consensus by the entire multidisciplinary team to engage with the program, accepting that adoption is accompanied by a learning curve in how best to present and use the data. There are significant start-up and running costs with 3DMMI, and to date there is no evidence that this is a cost-effective tool in clinical practice.

Accuracy

The old adage by Aristotle "You get out what you put in" is especially pertinent to 3DMMI because some data sets, such as those from structural MRI, are reliable and reproducible, and other sets, such as those from tractography, have considerable interuser variability.[92] Some data sets are further limited by their own biophysical principles; for example, the BOLD signal in fMRI is an indirect measure of neuronal activity, and tractography is based on presumption of white matter connectivity. Interpretation of these data within an integrated data set requires differential levels of caution and confidence.

Integration and presentation of multimodal imaging is a stepwise process of spatial coregistration, and each step carries a margin of error. For this reason, it is essential that coregistration is checked manually and that errors in anatomic localization, such as laterality, are checked at each stage.

For 3DMMI to be available to the neurosurgeon in the operating room, the data sets are exported to a neuronavigation system, and a further registration takes place between the 3D model and the patient's head. This adds a further margin of error, which is dictated by the neuronavigation software and quality of registration.

The accuracy of this spatial registration further deteriorates during the surgical procedure, as a result of brain shift. This is the intraoperative displacement and distortion of the brain that inevitably occurs during operations, as a result of loss of cerebrospinal fluid, gravity, brain swelling, and brain tissue resection.

The neurologist or neurosurgeon must consider the aggregation of these margins of error as the use of this additional tool is integrated into clinical practice.

Validity

A further barrier to the widespread use of 3DMMI is the lack of class I evidence that it provides real clinical utility. This method does not lend itself easily to randomized controlled trials, and alternative evaluations, such as comparison with historical cases and studies of the effect of disclosure of multimodal data on decision making, are necessary.[76]

Future Directions

Epilepsy surgery appears to be moving towards a greater emphasis on the use of SEEG, multimodality data, and potentially minimally invasive treatments.[93] 3DMMI is likely to become increasingly important in supporting these image-guided pathways and in the generation of new computer-assisted tools.[94,95] Many groups have reported their own custom-designed methods, with the use of a range of different software platforms to achieve a 3DMMI solution. The challenge for the future is to create a dedicated umbrella platform that houses a comprehensive set of tools, is powerful and versatile, and is simple to use. This should support all stages of the care pathway: from presurgical evaluation, through planning of intracranial EEG and neurophysiologic assessment, to definitive surgical treatment.

INTERVENTIONAL MAGNETIC RESONANCE IMAGING

Interventional MRI (iMRI) is an operating modality that is used in an MRI facility. It allows the surgeon to acquire scans intraoperatively before head closure. Benefits include determination of the performed resection, detection of residual lesion, and reregistration of neuronavigation software to correct for brain shift.

Increasingly, iMRI has been employed in specialized neurosurgical centers to aid surgical treatment, with obvious benefit in cases involving lesions. The key prognostic factors for seizure outcome in this subset of patients are histologic features and the complete excision of the lesion.[96-98] Therefore, the identification of a residual lesion intraoperatively can avoid the need for second-look surgery, improve patient outcomes, and be cost effective (Fig. 65-12).

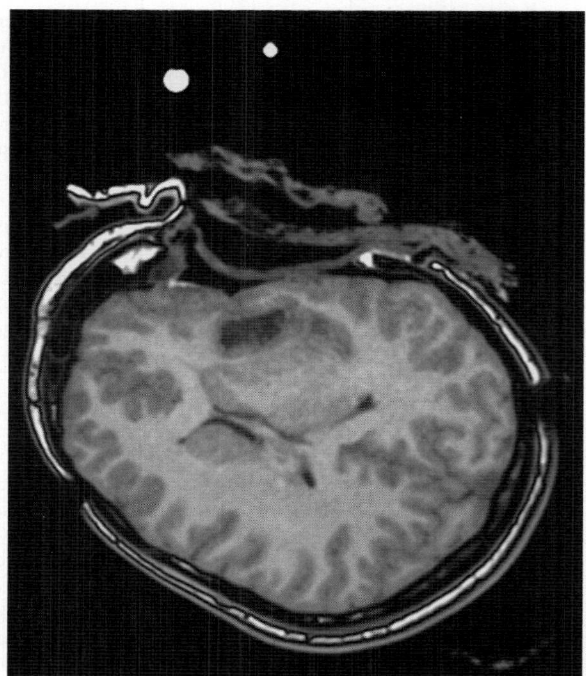

Figure 65-12. Intraoperative magnetic resonance image. Axial T1-weighted image acquired intraoperatively, showing a residual of lesion (epidermoid) in the right sylvian fissure.

Roessler and associates[99] reported on a series of 88 patients with lesional temporal lobe epilepsy who underwent surgery with iMRI. Pathologic features included low-grade tumors (gangliogliomas and DNETs), cavernomas, and FCDs, but patients with hippocampal sclerosis were excluded. The first iMRI took place when the surgeon thought that the lesion had been completely excised; intraoperative scans showed residual lesions in 25% of the patients (22 incomplete resections). A second intraoperative image showed complete resection in an additional 19 of these 22 patients. The authors concluded that as a direct effect of iMRI, overall resection rate was increased by 21.6%, and complete resection was achieved in 96.6% of the patients.

Sommer and colleagues[100] reported on a series of 25 cases of lesions in extratemporal locations affected by drug-resistant epilepsy. The lesions were located close to eloquent brain areas, and surgery was performed with iMRI and with the incorporation of fMRI and DTI. The iMRI helped identify an incomplete resection in 20% of the patients and facilitated a total resection in the entire cohort. The authors highlighted the fact that in previously reported similar series, complete resection rates ranged from 71% to 85% and that the functional outcome in their series was significantly improved in comparison with those of previously published studies.[101-103] This emphasizes the potential importance of incorporating functional imaging and iMRI to reduce the risk of postoperative neurological deficits.

Winston and associates[104] analyzed data from a cohort of 21 patients who underwent anterior temporal lobectomy for refractory epilepsy, with the use of iMRI with display of preoperative tractography of the optic radiation in the operative microscope. Tractography has previously demonstrated considerable variability in the anterior extent of the Meyers loop, ranging from 24 to 43 mm from the temporal pole in one study.[105] In this study, iMRI was used to generate transformation parameters, which were then applied to the preoperative tractographic findings to correct for brain shift.[104,106] The primary question was the severity of postoperative visual field defect and whether this was severe enough to prevent patients from driving in the future (according to the U.K. Driver and Vehicle Licensing Agency[107]). A comparison was made with an historical cohort of patients who underwent surgery by the same neurosurgeon in a conventional operating room and without the display of tractography. The percentage of patients who developed a contralateral superior quadrantanopia was significantly lower among the patients in the iMRI cohort, none of whom were prevented from driving, than among the historical cohort (13%; Fig. 65-13).

Despite the clear advantages highlighted previously in cases of lesions, the real challenge now is that epilepsy surgery is becoming more "nonlesional." In MRI-negative cases, surgeons often operate at depth and with few clear anatomic landmarks. iMRI allows surgeons to confirm the anatomic boundaries of the resection and can help in determining whether the epileptogenic area has been satisfactorily resected.

For both lesional and nonlesional cases, the possibility of integrating functional studies such as fMRI, DTI, and additional data (such as a segmented lesion or previously implanted electrodes that have identified the epileptogenic focus) and displaying the findings in the operative field through the microscope has a number of potential advantages (Fig. 65-14).

Epilepsy surgery is performed on a heterogeneous patient group, and class I evidence is therefore difficult to achieve for any surgical intervention. However, it is our opinion that iMRI is an excellent addition to the surgeon's armory and makes for safer and more effective resective epilepsy surgery.

CONCLUSION

The role of MRI in neuroradiologic evaluation of epilepsy surgery has evolved over time and elegantly represents the technologic advances made in the field.

First, structural MRI is absolutely crucial in the diagnosis of epileptogenic lesions because it guides further surgical management. The development of quantitative methods, including voxel-based morphometry, has increased the sensitivity of MRI as a diagnostic tool.

Second, the development of functional MRI and diffusion MRI has enabled the localization of eloquent cortical areas and white matter tracts. In epilepsy surgery, this is valuable information with regard to language lateralization, and it helps guide

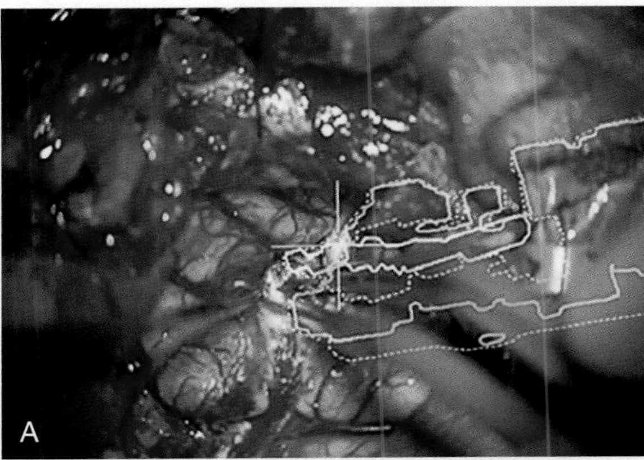

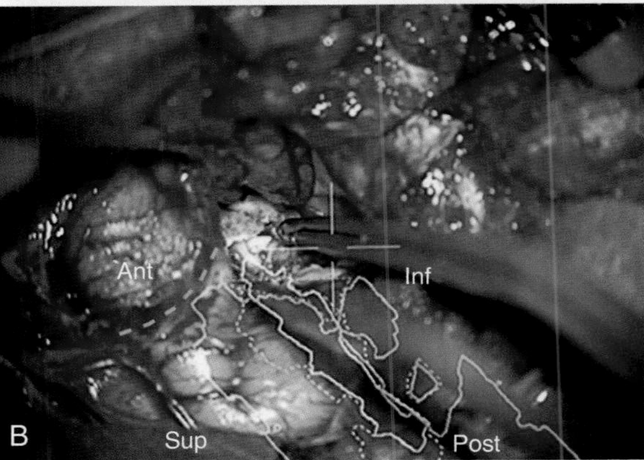

Figure 65-13. Combined use of tractography and interventional magnetic resonance imaging during anterior temporal lobe resection. View down the microscope during the approach of the temporal horn of the ventricle for access to the mesial temporal structures, with optic radiation tractography *(yellow outline)* and model of the ventricle *(white outline)* shown. The *solid lines* refer to the structure in the focal plane, and *dotted lines* refer to the maximum extent below this. The *blue dotted line* shows the line of resection anterior to the display of the optic radiation. **A,** Ventricle not opened. **B,** Ventricle opened and hippocampus visualized. *(From Winston GP, Daga P, White MJ, et al. Preventing visual field deficits from neurosurgery.* Neurology. *2014;83[7]:604-611.)*

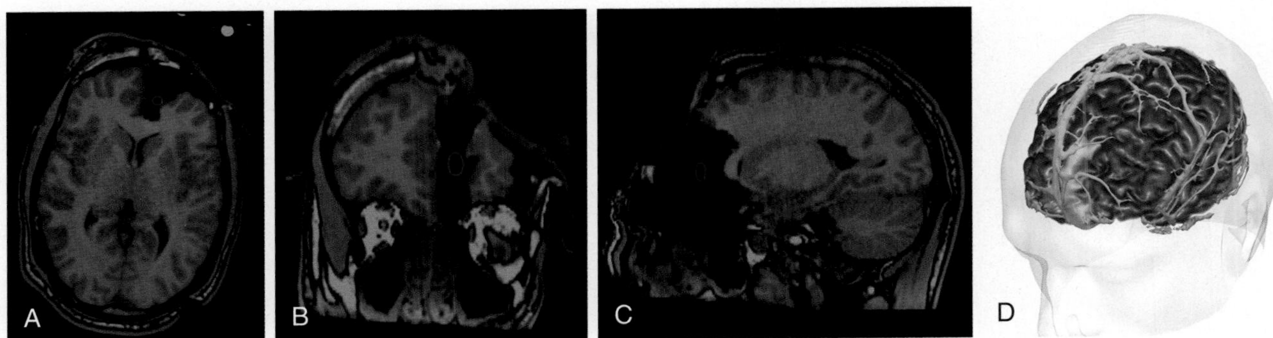

Figure 65-14. Intraoperative magnetic resonance imaging in nonlesional cases. Axial **(A),** coronal **(B),** and sagittal **(C)** T1-weighted images showing resection and model of electrode contact from previous stereo-electroencephalographic implantation that should be included in the resection (**B** and **C,** *red circles*). **D,** Three-dimensional EpiNav model of the brain *(gray)* with veins *(cyan),* scalp *(white),* and planned resection model *(yellow).*

surgeons in transiting white matter pathways in the operative field. The twinning of functional MRI to EEG is an interesting development that may further enhance the presurgical evaluation of affected patients. To best achieve the full benefit of using these different imaging modalities, they are coregistered into a single space and visualized in 3D (3DMMI).

Finally, the advent of iMRI means that MRI no longer is only concerned with diagnostics but also plays a therapeutic role in the operating room. The use of iMRI gives the surgeon confidence in resection as the operation progresses, accounting for brain shift and improving gross total resection rate. Although this tool is expensive and not yet widely available, it marks a further advance in the use of MRI in the treatment of epilepsy.

High-field MRI scanners (higher than 3 T) are being commercially developed. Currently research studies have been performed with 7-T MRI on postoperative specimens. Radiologic findings acquired at 7 T have revealed anatomic details similar to those obtained by histopathologic examination of the same specimen.[108,109]

In the future, the clinical use of high-field MRI scanners might improve the preoperative evaluation of patients with epilepsy, with the potential to identify structural abnormalities in cases previously considered nonlesional.

SUGGESTED READINGS

Barkovich AJ, Kuzniecky RI, Jackson GD, et al. A developmental and genetic classification for malformations of cortical development. *Neurology*. 2005;65(12):1873-1887.

Cardinale F, Cossu M, Castana L, et al. Stereoelectroencephalography: surgical methodology, safety, and stereotactic application accuracy in 500 procedures. *Neurosurgery*. 2013;72(3):353-366.

Colombo N, Salamon N, Raybaud C, et al. Imaging of malformations of cortical development. *Epileptic Disord*. 2009;11(3):194-205.

Cossu M, Cardinale F, Castana L, et al. Stereo-EEG in children. *Childs Nerv Syst*. 2006;22(8):766-778.

de Tisi J, Bell GS, Peacock JL, et al. The long-term outcome of adult epilepsy surgery, patterns of seizure remission, and relapse: a cohort study. *Lancet*. 2011;378(9800):1388-1395.

Duncan JS. Imaging and epilepsy. *Brain*. 1997;120(Pt 2):339-377.

Engel J Jr, McDermott MP, Wiebe S, et al. Early surgical therapy for drug-resistant temporal lobe epilepsy: a randomized trial. *JAMA*. 2012;307(9):922-930.

Englot DJ, Han SJ, Berger MS, et al. Extent of surgical resection predicts seizure freedom in low-grade temporal lobe brain tumors. *Neurosurgery*. 2012;70(4):921-928.

Farquharson S, Tournier JD, Calamante F, et al. White matter fiber tractography: why we need to move beyond DTI. *J Neurosurg*. 2013;118(6):1367-1377.

Gotman J, Benar CG, Dubeau F. Combining EEG and FMRI in epilepsy: methodological challenges and clinical results. *J Clin Neurophysiol*. 2004;21(4):229-240.

Hammers A, Heckemann R, Koepp MJ, et al. Automatic detection and quantification of hippocampal atrophy on MRI in temporal lobe epilepsy: a proof-of-principle study. *Neuroimage*. 2007;36(1):38-47.

Likeman M. Imaging in epilepsy. *Pract Neurol*. 2013;13(4):210-218.

McDonald CR. The use of neuroimaging to study behavior in patients with epilepsy. *Epilepsy Behav*. 2008;12(4):600-611.

Nowell M, Miserocchi A, McEvoy AW, et al. Advances in epilepsy surgery. *J Neurol Neurosurg Psychiatry*. 2014;85(11):1273-1279.

Nowell M, Rodionov R, Zombori G, et al. Utility of 3D multimodality imaging in the implantation of intracranial electrodes in epilepsy. *Epilepsia*. 2015;56(3):403-413.

Recommendations for neuroimaging of patients with epilepsy. Commission on Neuroimaging of the International League Against Epilepsy. *Epilepsia*. 1997;38(11):1255-1256.

Roessler K, Sommer B, Grummich P, et al. Improved resection in lesional temporal lobe epilepsy surgery using neuronavigation and intraoperative MR imaging: favourable long term surgical and seizure outcome in 88 consecutive cases. *Seizure*. 2014;23(3):201-207.

Rosenow F, Luders H. Presurgical evaluation of epilepsy. *Brain*. 2001;124(Pt 9):1683-1700.

Tassi L, Colombo N, Garbelli R, et al. Focal cortical dysplasia: neuropathological subtypes, EEG, neuroimaging and surgical outcome. *Brain*. 2002;125(Pt 8):1719-1732.

Thornton R, Laufs H, Rodionov R, et al. EEG correlated functional MRI and postoperative outcome in focal epilepsy. *J Neurol Neurosurg Psychiatry*. 2010;81(8):922-927.

Vattoth S, Manzil FF, Singhal A, et al. State of the art epilepsy imaging: an update. *Clin Nucl Med*. 2014;39(6):511-523.

Winston GP, Daga P, White MJ, et al. Preventing visual field deficits from neurosurgery. *Neurology*. 2014;83(7):604-611.

Woermann FG, Barker GJ, Birnie KD, et al. Regional changes in hippocampal T2 relaxation and volume: a quantitative magnetic resonance imaging study of hippocampal sclerosis. *J Neurol Neurosurg Psychiatry*. 1998;65(5):656-664.

Woermann FG, Jokeit H, Luerding R, et al. Language lateralization by Wada test and fMRI in 100 patients with epilepsy. *Neurology*. 2003;61(5):699-701.

Yogarajah M, Focke NK, Bonelli S, et al. Defining Meyer's loop–temporal lobe resections, visual field deficits and diffusion tensor tractography. *Brain*. 2009;132(Pt 6):1656-1668.

See a full reference list on ExpertConsult.com

66 Magnetoencephalography (MEG)/Magnetic Source Imaging (MSI)

Anto Bagić and Susan M. Bowyer

MAGNETOENCEPHALOGRAPHY PRINCIPLES

Magnetoencephalography (MEG) is a noninvasive and painless procedure that involves no external magnetic field, electricity, x-rays, or radioactivity.[1-5] It is also known as magnetic source imaging (MSI) based on its most established form of clinical application, in which source estimates (dipoles) are coregistered with the patient's magnetic resonance image[6] (see Fig. 66-1). Although, strictly speaking, MSI is a specific type of MEG application and not necessarily its synonym,[7] interchangeable use of these two terms currently prevails.[8,9] MEG is a direct, noninvasive neurophysiologic technique for studying the brain based on measuring magnetic fields primarily associated with the summated postsynaptic intradendritic electric currents subtending normal and pathologic cerebral processes that are reflected outside of the skull.[1-4] Directed flow of the electrically charged particles involved in normal or pathologic interactions of neurons in the form of electric currents is inseparably associated with magnetic fields that are recorded using supersensitive magnetic sensors.[3] Parallel orientation of the dendrites (cortical pyramidal cells) is the critical prerequisite for a spatial summation of these otherwise undetectable electric potentials (and corresponding fields), and synchronous firing is critical for temporal summation of the infinitesimal electric field generated by each individual cell to produce the still miniscule but summated magnetic fields that are detectable by the supersensitive sensors used in MEG systems[10-14] (Fig. 66-1). Because the strength of the magnetic fields produced by the brain is extremely low, very specialized instrumentation is required to detect these signals as well as to be shielded from the overpowering magnetically hostile (e.g., hospital) environment.[3,4,15] These sensing devices contain small coils (or chips) that function as flux transformers and are coupled to superconducting quantum interference devices (SQUIDs) that operate on two phenomena of quantum physics: superconductivity and tunneling.[3,4,15,16] Most modern systems include more than 300 of these specialized sensors arranged in a helmet-shaped configuration.[4,15] By analyzing the complex patterns of the signals recorded by the sensors, the location, strength, and orientation of the sources can be estimated[17,18] (see Fig. 66-1). However, the true neuronal source extent cannot be assessed even with currently available advanced source imaging techniques.[19,20] In today's clinical practice related to epilepsy, it is preferable to use a combination of the localization results from both the magnetoencephalogram and the simultaneously recorded electroencephalogram,[9,21,22] because they are complementary and most informative when combined appropriately.

MEG uses extensive spatial sampling, enabled by hundreds of sampling locations surrounding the brain, in contrast to the 20 to 30 electrodes used in traditional routine electroencephalography (EEG). This sampling volume along with the fact that magnetic fields by their nature are not filtered (smeared), weakened (reduced), or distorted by the intervening tissues (cerebrospinal fluid, meninges, skull, and scalp)—that is, the tissues surrounding the brain are "transparent" for magnetic fields—make MEG a superior technique for localizing the brain's activity very accurately using simple models.[4,5] This is particularly helpful when dealing with a complex clinical reality involving altered anatomy, as in postoperative and posttraumatic scenarios in which EEG signals are distorted and may provide misleading localization.[23-25]

Unlike EEG, which measures an amplified potential difference between two electrodes placed on the scalp, MEG measures summated, very weak magnetic fields. SQUIDS, used to measure these fields, require cooling to attain the state of superconductivity. This is currently achieved by their immersion in liquid helium, which attains a temperature near absolute zero (−269°C, −452°F, or 4.2°K). An important practical consideration is the necessity for a weekly consumption of 80 to 100 L of helium to keep the system functional, and this is a considerable cost. Different helium recycling systems are available but as of yet are not widely used in the MEG field.

Dealing with extremely weak signals is just one problem that MEG technology has to solve; the other is the overpowering and fluctuating magnetic "noise" of the external environment, which is 10^7 to 10^9 times greater than the magnetic field of the brain. (Of note, the magnetic field of the Earth is about 50 million times stronger than that of the brain, but because it is a steady field, it is not recorded by the MEG sensors.) This cardinal problem of environmental noise is solved by placing the MEG system in a magnetically shielded room that deflects the magnetically hostile influence sufficiently to enable an adequate recording. In some locations MEG systems are installed near extremely unfriendly magnetic environments such as underground railways; such placement may require additional means of "active shielding" in which current is used to cancel the detected magnetic noise from the environment.

As the fundamental laws of physics (i.e., Maxwell's equations) teach us, the relationship between the electric current and its inseparable corresponding (induced) magnetic field is governed by the *right-hand rule:* If one curls the fingers around the current-conducting wire and extends the thumb pointing in the direction of the current flow, the curled fingers point in the direction of the magnetic field. This depicts the orthogonal mutual perspective from which EEG (concerned with electric current) and MEG (concerned with magnetic field) are "viewing" the same cerebral sources. Thus the role of geometry is very important in MEG, and the sources are divided into *tangential* or *radial* with respect to the overlying skull (see Fig. 66-1). According to the right-hand rule, a tangential source (one that has the mean geometric orientation parallel to the overlying skull) will be associated with a magnetic field that spreads orthogonally through the skull and will most likely be detected by the MEG sensors. A radial ("outward") source (one that has the mean geometric orientation orthogonal to the overlying skull) will induce a magnetic field that will spread parallel to the overlying skull and will most likely remain inside the skull and thus not reach the MEG sensors. Consequently, MEG is sensitive to the sources in cerebral sulci (e.g., sylvian fissure, superior temporal sulcus) and large cortical planes (e.g., inferior temporal or frontal) because they have tangential orientation, as opposed to EEG, which prefers the gyral and fissural sources that have exclusively or predominantly radial ordination (see Fig. 66-1).

Even more than 40 years after the first SQUID MEG recording by Cohen,[2] the most common clinical use of MEG is in MSI.[5,26-28] MSI provides a best estimate of the location of cortical activity that is occurring at any instant in time.[3] This application

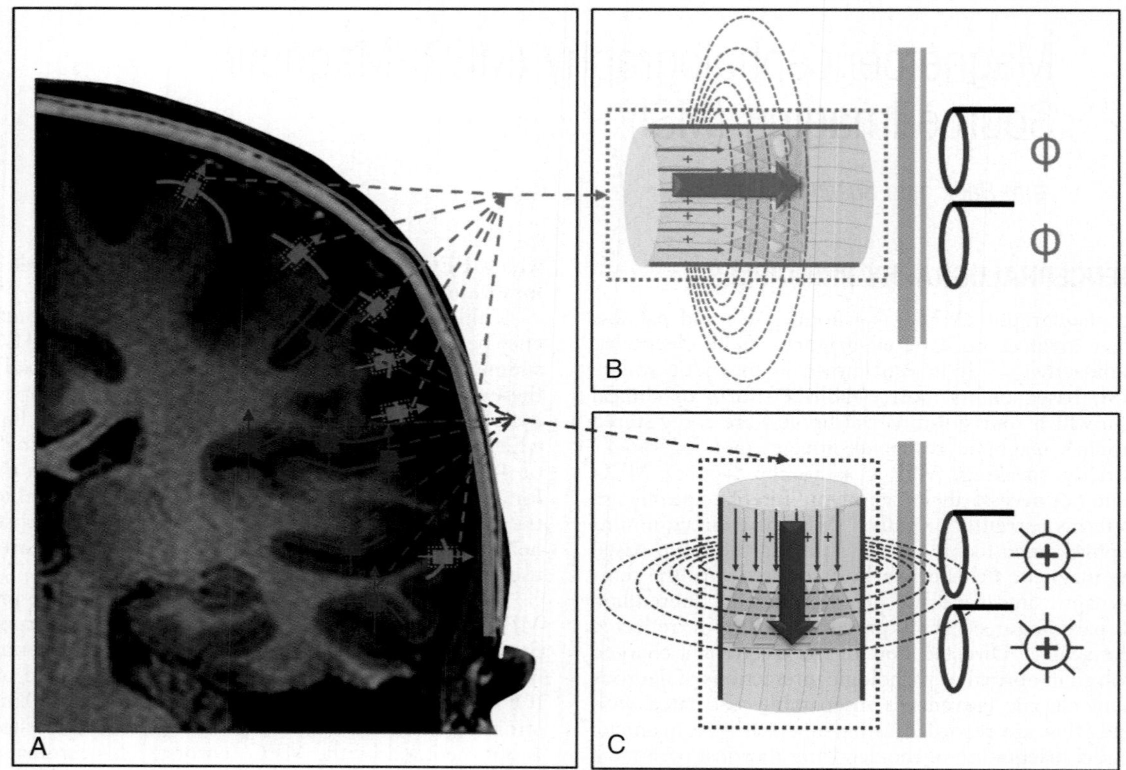

Figure 66-1. Principles of magnetic source imaging. With respect to their prevailing geometric orientation toward overlying skull (*thick light brown line* on panels **A, B,** and **C**), cerebral sources can be divided into tangential (*blue;* mostly banks of the fissures or basal planes of the lobes) and radial (*red;* mostly crests of the gyri). For this purpose, a source is represented by a box (with an *arrow* representing a current flow direction) containing tens of thousands of parallel and simultaneously firing pyramidal cells (panels **B** and **C**). Because pertinent currents follow a longitudinal dimension of the sources, the orientation matters because it reflects the orientation of the currents (vector) that produce orthogonal magnetic fields according to the right-hand rule (i.e., if an extended thumb points in the direction of prevailing current flow, the curved fingers point in the direction of corresponding magnetic fields). Therefore, in the case of the radial source *(red box, red lines),* resulting magnetic fields *(broken red ellipsoids)* do not get reflected outside of the skull, and in the case of the tangential source (*blue box* and *blue lines*), resulting magnetic fields *(broken blue ellipsoids*) do get reflected outside of the skull. Sufficient temporal and spatial summation *(thick arrows)* of miniscule currents *(thin arrows)* is required for generating fields detectable outside of the skull.

uses a sphere as the head model, and a point-like dot called an equivalent current dipole (ECD) as a source model in the iterative statistical computation process that generates possible source locations based on the measured magnetic field data[3] (see Fig. 66-1). It has been demonstrated that MEG can attain localization accuracy of 2 to 3 mm.[29-36] Of course, cerebral sources are not dots, and many sources can coexist; "dots" on magnetic resonance imaging (MRI), sometimes called "a probability cloud," may be misleading because they indicate not the extent but rather the complexity of the source (Fig. 66-2).

In addition to single ECDs,[37] many other methods of MEG analysis are utilized in research and some are advancing into clinical practice. Synthetic aperture magnetometry[38-40] is a beamforming technique that applies a spatial filter to the recorded magnetoencephalogram to determine the cortical location, minimum norm estimates is a current distribution technique that determines where the current is flowing in the cortex,[41-43] and MUltiple SIgnal Classification (MUSIC) is an algorithm used for frequency estimation.[44,45] Emerging evidence[43,45-47] suggests that other methods besides single ECD may yield similar results. More recent advances in signal processing are providing software packages and approaches that can use the MEG data to detect the underlying functional and effective connectivity in the brain.[48-52]

Compared to EEG, the advantages of MEG include that it is free of biologic references, requires no electrodes, and is able to detect a smaller activated area (about 6 cm^2 versus >10 cm^2). Also, its signals are not distorted by the skull or other intervening tissues, it is amenable to simpler clinically useful source modeling, and it provides superior spatial sampling because it covers the whole head with a few hundred sensors.[5,22,53] On the negative side, it is an immobile, expensive instrument that has to be housed inside a magnetically shielded room and kept "cold" even when not in use. In addition, it is susceptible to metallic and movement artifacts, it is sensitive to tangential sources only, it has a lower sensitivity to deep sources, and it involves labor-intensive data analysis procedures to provide imaged results.[5,53]

Because MEG is considered and used clinically primarily as a localizing tool, a frequently asked question is "What is the localization accuracy of MEG?" Overall, the source extent, complexity, and depth have a considerable effect on its localization accuracy. Probably some of the best answers came in the early days of the clinical use of MEG, in the 1980s. The position of a virtual current dipole placed at a known location in a model

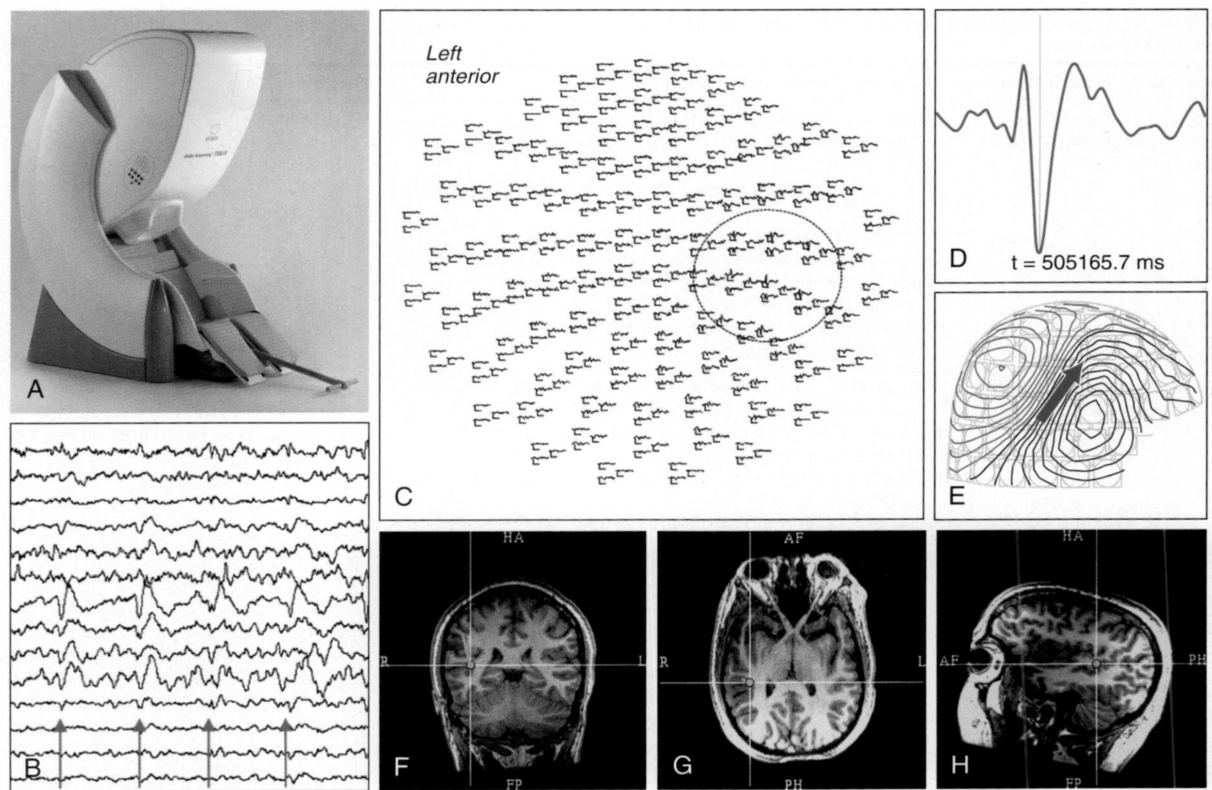

Figure 66-2. Overview of magnetoencephalography (MEG). A, A currently available MEG system positioned for recording in the seated position (Elekta Neuromag Oy, Helsinki, Finland). **B** and **C,** A MEG tracing from the right temporal region **(B)** contains multiple spikes (marked by *red arrows*), one of which can be better appreciated spatially on the head panel **(C)** in the area marked by the *circle.* **D** and **E,** Morphology of the spike can fully be explored **(D),** and its corresponding field projected on the right side of the head **(E).** The accepted position of the model of the spike's most prominent peak source (i.e., dipole) in three radiologic projections is shown in panels **F, G,** and **H.** *(A, Photograph courtesy of Elekta.)*

was determined with an accuracy of approximately 2 mm,[36] and an accuracy of approximately 3 mm in locating a current dipole source was demonstrated in different scenarios by several groups.[34-36,54,55] Romani and colleagues[31] were able to "separate sources" a few millimeters apart while studying a tonotopic map of the human auditory cortex, and Hari and associates[32] demonstrated "millimeter accuracy" while studying the organization of the somatosensory cortex. However, it its worth repeating that—at this time—irrespective of its claimed and/or true sensitivity and localizing accuracy, MEG does not provide even a rough estimate of the source size.

BRIEF OVERVIEW OF CLINICAL MAGNETOENCEPHALOGRAPHY

Generally speaking, for patients with epilepsy, this tool enables identification of epileptogenic tissue noninvasively[5,56] (see Table 66-1). Alone or combined with presurgical mapping of eloquent cortices of interest[57] (see Box 66-1), MEG creates neuronavigational maps that can be used by surgeons in real time during a surgical procedure, and that assist in delineation of parts of the brain to preserve or remove.[58-61]

Although MEG has been in clinical use for a few decades, the road to greater advances from a research to a clinical tool is still evolving. So far, over 175 MEG systems have been installed worldwide; the current cost of the system, with a magnetically shielded room, is close to $3 million. In the United States, an annual service contract ranges from $80,000 for the basic preventive maintenance and minimal support to $125,000 for complete maintenance (planned and unplanned), including replacement parts, full support, and guaranteed uptime. Helium prices fluctuate periodically and remain vastly disparate across the MEG sites and suppliers. The need for 80 L/wk plus extra for the annual maintenance procedure amounts to more than $80,000 annually in some regions.

In the United States, only two indications are approved for reimbursement within the Current Procedural Terminology (CPT) codes (American Medical Association, Chicago, IL). One is the use of MEG for recording of spontaneous epilepsy localization, billable as CPT 95965: Magnetoencephalography (MEG), recording and analysis; for spontaneous brain magnetic activity (epileptic cerebral cortex localization). The other is use of MEG for presurgical mapping of eloquent cortices (language, sensory, motor, auditory, and visual), billable as CPT 95967: Magnetoencephalography (MEG), recording and analysis; for evoked magnetic fields, single modality (e.g., sensory, motor, language, or visual cortex localization). Epilepsy surgery, particularly nonlesional neocortical, has been the key driver of the dissemination and wider acceptance of MEG in clinical practice in the preceding two decades.[8] Recently, MEG has been increasingly used in presurgical mapping[62] (Table 66-1 and Fig. 66-3).

Subject preparation is a critical step before a MEG scan, and involves a comprehensive survey for any ferromagnetic sources, ranging from any implants in patients (a vagus nerve stimulator,

TABLE 66-1 Ten Common Evidence-Based Magnetoencephalography (MEG) Indications in Presurgical Evaluation of Patients with Drug-Resistant Epilepsy

Evidence-Based MEG Indication	Evidence-Based Justification	Remarks
1. Lacking or imprecise hypothesis regarding a seizure onset	Additional nonredundant localizing information is provided by MEG in about one third of cases undergoing presurgical evaluation.[100,249] MEG-exclusive spikes are seen in 47% of patients without EEG spikes.[250-252] Retrospective MSI-guided review of MRI may disclose previously concealed lesions in up to 50% of patients.[8,88,250] Areas of interictal MEG spiking are associated with PET abnormalities in MRI-negative TLE.[253] ECD properties correlate with cortical thinning in left mesiotemporal epilepsy.[254]	Without MEG, these patients are frequently excluded from a complete presurgical evaluation or may be exposed to extensive invasive investigations that may not be entirely appropriate.
2. Negative MRI with a mesial temporal onset suspected	MSI-guided re-review of MRI may lead to a positive finding in up to 50% of seemingly negative MRIs.[8] MEG can detect mesial temporal spikes in about 85% of patients with mesial TLE.[255] MEG spike orientation may help in distinguishing mesial TLE from lateral TLE.[5,256-260] Spike orientation may predict epileptogenic side across cerebral sulci.[261] Vertical or horizontal MEG spikes in the anterior temporal pole indicate a higher chance of mesial TLE.[255]	MEG findings may help in identifying more surgical candidates, obviate a need for ICM in some cases, or at times lead to a direct resection.
3. Multiple lesions on MRI	An example of this is a patient with TS, where MEG was shown to be more accurate than an ictal scalp EEG[85] in identifying the epileptogenic zone, as well as recognizing the most active lesion (rarely identifiable with a scalp EEG),[85,86,112] and overall very useful in identifying suitable candidates for surgery[5,85,86,262] with a good long-term outcome.[263]	In the not too distant past, these patients would not have been considered for resective surgery. MEG contributed considerably to the change in clinical practice leading to identifying more surgical candidates in TS and similar populations, at times completely avoiding or better planning ICM, and performing more complete resections leading to more favorable surgical outcomes.
4. Large lesion on MRI	Large lesions introduce diagnostic complexity by changing the anatomy and making a scalp EEG unreliable.[5] MEG can identify an (the most) active part of a lesion or perilesional tissue.[5] MEG is more accurate than an ictal scalp EEG in patients with large lesions and altered anatomy.[5] MSI can guide a choice of an optimal access trajectory[264] and helps delineate the extent of resection of the epileptogenic zone.[109]	Because large lesions may not be amenable to complete resections, it is critical to know what part of perilesional areas are (most) active and thus tailor the degree of resection according to the highest likelihood of seizure improvement or full control in spite of incomplete resection.
5. Diagnostic or therapeutic reoperation	Operative or traumatic skull defects distort electric fields,[265] making spike identification difficult[266] and EEG susceptible to erroneous localization.[267] MEG is more accurate than an ictal scalp EEG in patients with altered anatomy because magnetic fields are relatively unaffected by the structure of the skull and MEG sensitivity and localization accuracy remain unaltered.[5]	MEG is not only overall superior to EEG in this setting, but may identify and localize incompletely resected parts of the original target area or a separate previously unsuspected epileptogenic focus (see Figs. 66-3E and 66-5).[100]
6. Ambiguous EEG findings suggestive of "bilateral" or "generalized" pattern	Propagation of interictal epileptiform EEG activity can lead to erroneous source localizations.[268] MEG helps distinguish between the primary focus and propagated activity,[25,269,270] and MEG spikes propagation may have prognostic implications for epilepsy surgery.[270]	These may be among the most complex patients considered for epilepsy surgery. In these settings, a working hypothesis may not be supported sufficiently to accept the risks of ICM, and having a clarification of localizing ambiguity may be a decisive factor in making an optimal decision.
7. Intrasylvian onset suspected	In spite of their overall complex anatomy, the major horizontal intrasylvian cortices (e.g., Heschl's gyrus and planum temporale) facilitate MEG sensitivity to the respective sources.[5] MEG can identify intrasylvian spikes in EEG-negative cases[228,271-273] or a single intrasylvian epileptogenic focus in patients with ambiguous EEG, such as in LKS, where MEG sensitivity is high (68%-100%)[228,274] and MSI-aided surgery may lead to a significant clinical improvement.[228,273]	Without MEG, these patients are frequently excluded from a complete presurgical evaluation or may be exposed to extensive invasive investigations that may not be entirely necessary.
8. Interhemispheric onset suspected	MEG can detect spikes from the interhemispheric area,[223,275,276] is more sensitive to frontal[277] and occipital[278] sources than EEG, and can lateralize medial frontal[276] and occipital[278] spikes even when the EEG is nonlateralizing. Almost 90% of ECoG spikes were associated with MEG spikes.[223]	Because frontal lobe epilepsy has the worst surgical outcome, and various EEG ambiguities may occur, the acquisition of additional noninvasive localizing information is essential.

TABLE 66-1 Ten Common Evidence-Based Magnetoencephalography (MEG) Indications in Presurgical Evaluation of Patients with Drug-Resistant Epilepsy—cont'd

Evidence-Based MEG Indication	Evidence-Based Justification	Remarks
9. Insular onset suspected	Because it is suspected that insular epilepsy may be accountable for failures of a significant number of TLE surgeries,[5,279] and MEG spikes can be captured in over 64% of patients with insular epilepsy,[271,280-282] MEG findings can improve diagnostic accuracy, substantiate ICM, and justify its risks.[5,271]	As a result of the low sensitivity of scalp EEGs to insular spikes, and the suspected frequent misdiagnosis of insular epilepsy as temporal, leading to a failure of anterior temporal lobectomy, the value of MEG is very high and may be decisive in justifying the risks of ICM and avoiding a surgical failure.
10. Negative (i.e., spikeless) EEG	MEG identifies interictal spikes in 47% of patients without EEG spikes.[250-252]	It is very important to avoid a misconception that patients with no spikes on EEG are unlikely to benefit from MEG and that MEG should be ordered only for "frequent spikers."

ECD, equivalent current dipole; ECoG, electrocorticography; EEG, electroencephalography; ICM, intracranial monitoring; LKS, Landau-Kleffner syndrome; MRI, magnetic resonance imaging; MSI, magnetic source imaging; PET, positron emission tomography; TLE, temporal lobe epilepsy; TS, tuberous sclerosis.

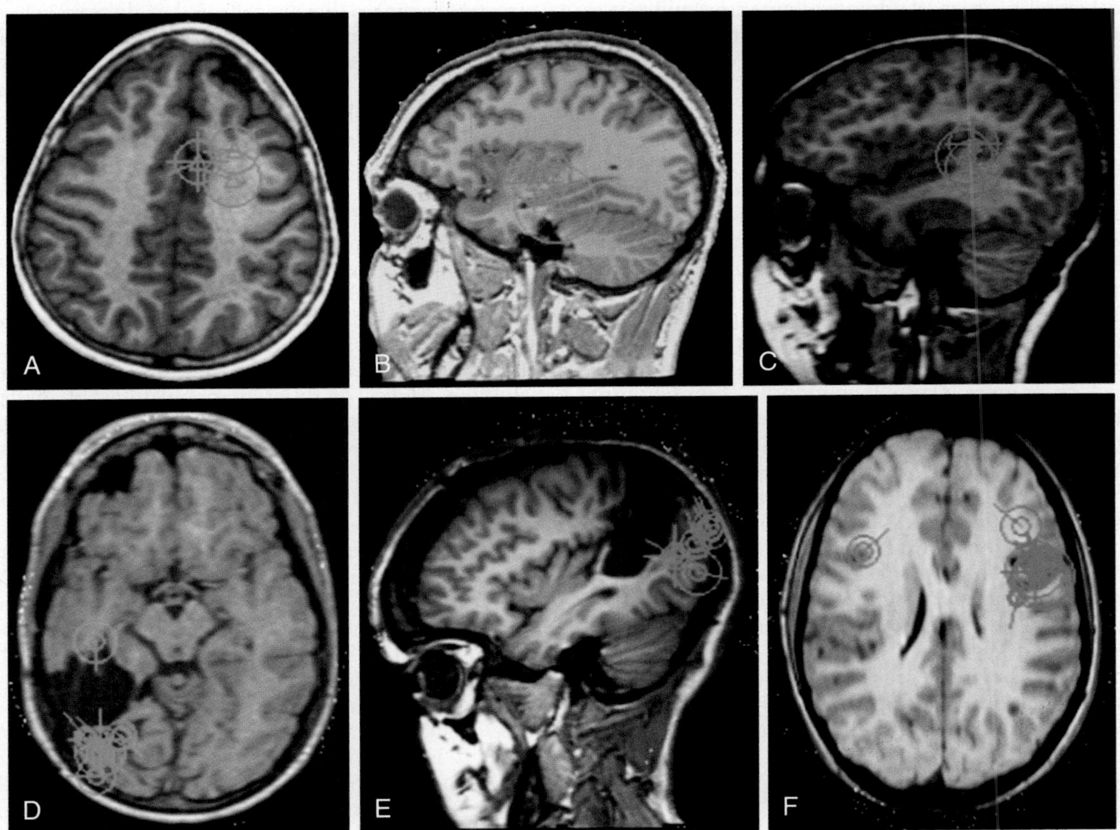

Figure 66-3. Magnetoencephalography (MEG) utilization scenarios. Each of these images is from a different patient. **A,** Clustered MEG indicating a well-lateralized (left) interhemispheric focus. **B,** Insular epilepsy. **C,** Posterior intrasylvian focus. **D,** Large area of encephalomalacia. **E,** Previous resection. **F,** Tuberous sclerosis; note the MEG spike clustering around the epileptogenic tuber. *(From Kharkar S, Knowlton R. Magnetoencephalography in the presurgical evaluation of epilepsy.* Epilepsy Behav. *2015;46:19-26.)*

rods, screws, plates, shunts, pumps, tooth fillings, dentures, nonremovable jewelry, etc.) to clothes, shoes, hair accessories or jewelry, and hair sprays, mousses, and gels. Most magnetic artifacts can be prevented by the removal of the potential source(s) and/or by a demagnetization procedure (also known as degaussing). If unavoidable artifacts are recorded, particularly those from extracranial sources (e.g., heartbeats, vagus nerve stimulator–related sources), these can be removed after the recording using specialized software such as independent component analysis, principal component analysis, or Maxfilter.[63-66] Most scans require the patient to keep very still; to this end, sleep is a powerful ally for the personnel working on the data acquisition, and appropriately instructed parents may help to calm and control children while sitting or resting next to them in a magnetically shielded room without causing considerable artifacts. Usually patients are sleep deprived prior to coming in for the MEG scan.[67] Cognitively impaired subjects unable to cooperate sufficiently and very young children may have to be sedated to ensure a technically adequate recording. If the best approach—a still patient—fails, continuous head position tracking tools are now a standard part of advanced whole-head MEG systems,[68,69] and their practical usefulness has been demonstrated.[69,70]

Clinicians should be aware of some potential drawbacks of exploiting MEG results.[5] If *multifocal epilepsy* is thought to be present, MEG may fail to detect epileptogenic zone(s) in the areas of its suboptimal sensitivity (e.g., deep sources such as those in the cingulate gyrus) or may disclose epileptogenic tissue that is not responsible for the patient's habitual seizures (e.g., propagated activity or secondary foci), and thus should not be used to exclude the epileptogenic potential of those areas. This requires placing competently interpreted MEG results in the specific clinical context expertly. Conversely, if a *single epileptogenic focus* is presumed based on consistently stereotypical semiology, MEG may identify propagated or secondary activity without disclosing the primary source and thus result in a different type of false localization. Because benign variants are not yet systematically studied and understood in MEG, this may be an explanation for at least some "bilateral" or "contralateral" MEGs. Ultimately, a spikeless (i.e., negative) MEG study should be considered with the full appreciation of its methodologic limitations and not as definite proof of the absence of epileptogenic potential.

ROLE OF MAGNETOENCEPHALOGRAPHY IN EPILEPSY SURGERY

Considering its nature, MEG provides interictal recordings and identifies an *irritative zone*. However, seizures are captured in approximately 10% of MEG recordings,[71-73] and this may assist in localizing an *ictal onset zone*, although this is not the primary purpose of MEG.[5,56] If no interictal activity is captured, pharmacologic activation of interictal epileptiform discharges may be considered to increase the yield of MEG-EEG recordings, but this is not accepted practice.[56,67,74] Repeating a study after sleep deprivation with or without antiepileptic drug manipulation may be considered as a more plausible option.[67,74,75] Importantly, patients with a negative scalp EEG should be referred for a MEG study and not deprived of it, because 47% of those without EEG spikes may have MEG spikes.[5,56] A very brief general overview of the role of MEG in epilepsy surgery is provided here, with detailed specific clinical examples illustrated by the figures and described in their captions. For clarity, 10 common evidence-based MEG indications in presurgical evaluation of patients with drug-resistant epilepsy are detailed in Table 66-1.

Irrespective of still-evident variability in presurgical evaluation of patients with drug-resistant epilepsy,[56,76-79] and of discouraging dilemmas in the interpretation of diagnostic accuracy studies during a presurgical work-up for epilepsy surgery,[80,81] four general roles for MSI in (pre)surgical decision making have been proposed[56]:

1. Supplementing sufficient new and/or supporting clinical information to propel the patient further along presurgical evaluation ("Eligibility to go forward in surgery evaluation")
2. Guiding selection of appropriate patients for proceeding directly to intracranial monitoring (ICM) or surgery ("Patient selection beyond eligibility")
3. Improving the accuracy and overall yield of ICM and surgical outcome ("Affect probability of cure")
4. Complementing other noninvasive tests with sufficient nonredundant information to obviate the need for ICM ("Skip intracranial EEG")

Multiple supporting examples for each of these four roles are detailed in Table 66-1 and Figures 66-2, 66-3, 66-4, 66-5, and 66-9.

In evaluation of pharmacoresistant epilepsy, MEG is typically utilized during phase 1 of the presurgical evaluation, which includes long-term scalp video-EEG monitoring, MRI, neuropsychological testing, and eventually positron emission tomography (PET) and/or single-photon emission computed tomography (SPECT).[5,56,77,82] In this phase, MEG is used in order to determine early if surgery is a feasible option.[5,56,82] Currently, MEG/MSI is primarily used in patients who are not obvious safe surgical candidates: those with normal or nonlesional MRI findings, conflicting electroclinical and radiologic data, or dual or multifocal pathologies, or those with lesion(s) adjacent to eloquent cortices.[5,56] MEG can be used to screen patients with MRI-detected focal or hemispheric lesions and concordant electroclinical data with an acceptable risk-benefit ratio for surgical candidacy as well as to formulate a working hypothesis about the physiology of the underlying seizures[5,56,82] (see Table 66-1 and Figs. 66-3, 66-4, 66-5, and 66-9). Even in patients with clear lesions on MRI, the MRI finding itself may not be sufficient to proceed to surgery, because association of the lesions with the epilepsy needs to be proven.[5,56,83-85] MEG provides evidence for and also distinguishes between epileptogenic and nonepileptogenic lesions in cases of several or diffuse lesions.[83,86,87] In patients with seemingly normal MRI scans, MEG can disclose subtle structural changes that are reflected in abnormal electromagnetic activity[5,8,20,88,89] and suggest further diagnostic work-up, including an expert visual reevaluation of existing or differently protocolled MRI[8] (Fig. 66-4) or the use of postprocessing methods such as voxel-based morphometry.[90]

Patients with ambiguity regarding a hypothesized epileptogenic zone may require ICM (also known as phase 2 presurgical evaluation).[5,56,91,92] The very high sensitivity of ICM is limited by its "tunnel vision": an electrode has a very limited field of view (i.e., several millimeters) and a seizure onset zone may be easily missed if placement of electrodes is not optimal,[56,91-94] which seems to be a relatively frequent occurrence.[93] The results of preoperative MEG analysis can be used not only to direct the placement of intracranial EEG electrodes but also to optimize the extent of resection and improve surgical outcomes.[95-101] Multiple studies of different populations of epilepsy patients confirmed in various clinical contexts that the completeness of removal of MEG spike-generating regions correlates with better surgical outcome[58,99,102-109] (Fig. 66-5), and that single and tighter clusters of MEG dipoles herald better surgical outcome.[99,105,110-112] Possible practical implications of these findings are that tightly clustered spikes designate epileptogenic tissue involved in seizure inception (i.e., seizure onset zone), and scattered MEG spikes reflect irritated cortex.[5,99,107] Consequently, in spite of some passionate proponents of the poorly understood and somewhat dispraised term "a (complete) clusterectomy,"[106,109] this may suggest that removal of the irritated cortex may not always be required for seizure freedom.[5]

Overall, referral of patients for epilepsy surgery is suboptimal[113,114] in spite of class I evidence,[115] but this may explain only one aspect of what may be multifactorial underutilization of MEG.[5,56,74] Physicians' insufficient familiarity with the evidence for the value of MEG in various clinical scenarios, the lack of understanding of its pertinent end user practicalities, reluctance to depart from "what we have always done," and occasional logistic limitations may also be involved. Considerable progress would be made if at least all epilepsy patients undergoing ICM and those who have failed surgery and may benefit from reoperation would be referred for MEG[5,56]; in these patients, MEG may also contribute to prognostication and counseling (see Table 66-1). Importantly, experts suggest that no patient should be denied surgery solely based on the results of a MEG study within the context of current clinical MEG practice.[56]

Although MEG is not currently used routinely for diagnosing epilepsy,[116] but rather is used as a localizing tool that advances neurophysiologic and topologic understanding of a particular clinical reality, a study that assessed the routine use of MEG as a component of the primary diagnostic process for epilepsy[117] gleaned relevant findings supporting the earlier use of MEG in

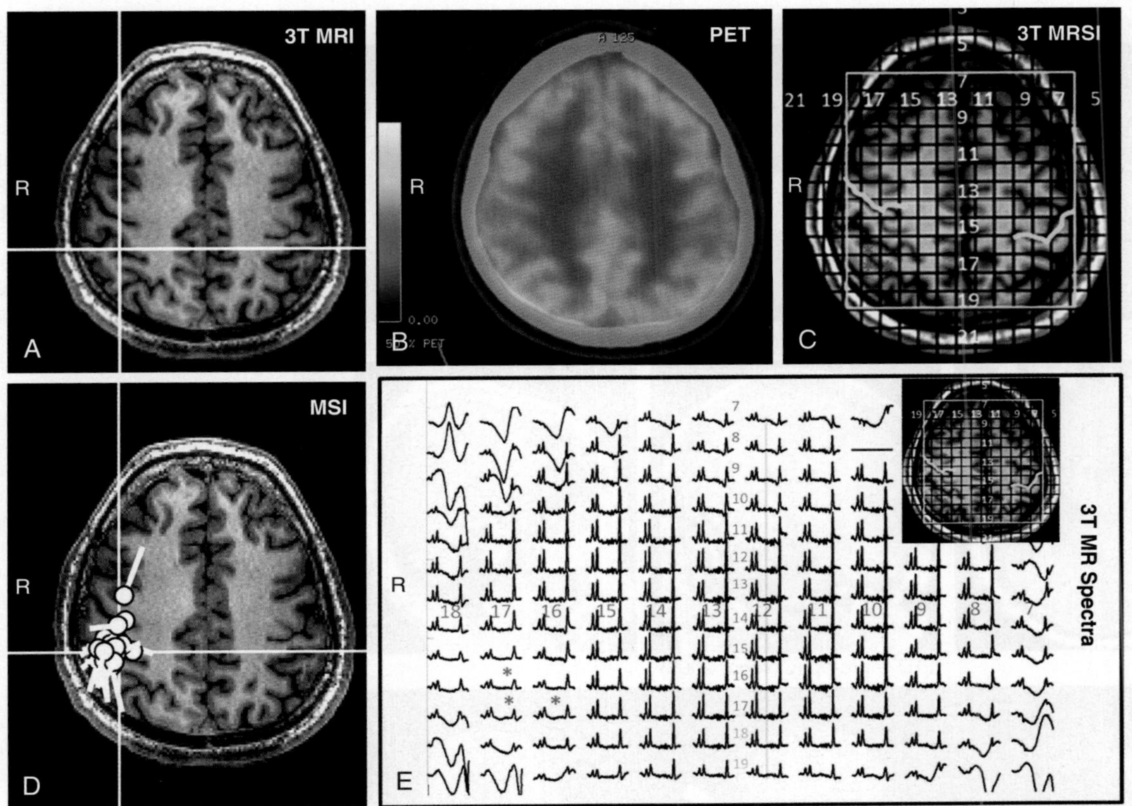

Figure 66-4. Nonlesional extratemporal epilepsy. A 29-year-old male presented with a history of a fall in childhood (his only known seizure risk factor), headaches, hypertension, depression, burns on his chest (a result of gang violence), lumbar spine surgery (in 2012), prolonged P-R interval, and epileptic seizures since the age of 5 years. He had failed two antiepileptic medications (lamotrigine, carbamazepine) and continued to experience seizures on his current three (divalproex, levetiracetam, topiramate). In consideration of epilepsy surgery, he underwent a standard presurgical evaluation that included 1.5-T and 3.0-T brain magnetic resonance imaging (MRI) with epilepsy protocols, routine electroencephalography (EEG), video-EEG, neuropsychological testing (NPT), fluorodeoxyglucose–positron emission tomography (FDG-PET), and magnetoencephalography (MEG)-EEG. This patient had truly nonlesional extratemporal epilepsy. There were no structural abnormalities on 1.5- and 3.0-T brain MRI with epilepsy protocols (**A**) (including magnetic source imaging [MSI]–guided re-review of the MRIs) and a normal FDG-PET (**B**). However, there were positive findings from an MSI study (**D**), indicative of significant cerebral dysfunction and epileptic potential expressed through the right inferior parietal lobule, and from a congruent 3-T magnetic resonance spectroscopy (MRS) (**C** and **E**) indicative of significant metabolic abnormality in the right inferior parietal lobule. *Yellow lines* seen on the scout image in panels **C** and **E** outline the estimated position of the central sulcus. *(MRS images in panels **C** and **E** were kindly provided by Julie W. Pan, MD, PhD; University of Pittsburgh Comprehensive Epilepsy Center, Pittsburgh, PA; methods used were previously published.*[201]*) (From Bagić A. Look back to leap forward: the emerging new role of magnetoencephalography (MEG) in nonlesional epilepsy.* Clin Neurophysiol. *2016;127:60-66.)*

presurgical evaluation.[56] Specifically, in a tertiary referral center outpatient cohort of 51 patients with presumed neocortical epilepsy and inconclusive EEG, MEG yielded a higher diagnostic gain (63% versus 57%) toward the clinical diagnosis as "gold standard" and a lower false-negative rate (27% versus 38%) compared with the diagnostic standard of care—a sleep-deprived EEG.[117] However, even in its most established form as a localizing tool, MEG remains underutilized in the presurgical evaluation for epilepsy surgery.

APPLICATIONS OF MAGNETOENCEPHALOGRAPHY IN FUNCTIONAL MAPPING IN NEUROSURGERY

In principle, MEG can localize any eloquent cortices that can be activated in a time-locked manner with sufficient reproducibility to enable averaging of individual responses time-locked to the stimulus in order to increase the signal-to-noise ratio, allowing for identification of the specific waveform above the background brain activity (Box 66-1).[10,11,29,30,37,57,118-125] Clinically established functional mapping modalities are language, somatosensory, motor, auditory, and visual.[57] In order to improve and standardize the clinical MEG practice, the world's first MEG clinical practice guidelines were published by the American Clinical Magnetoencephalography Society in 2011,[67,126,127] and Clinical Practice Guideline 2 is focused on functional brain mapping.[57]

It is critical to keep in mind that the size of activated brain areas visualized using various source localization techniques does not reflect the size of the source that eventually produced the modeled activity or the extent of cerebral regions subtending a tested function.[3,41,125,128,129] One illustrative example is shown in

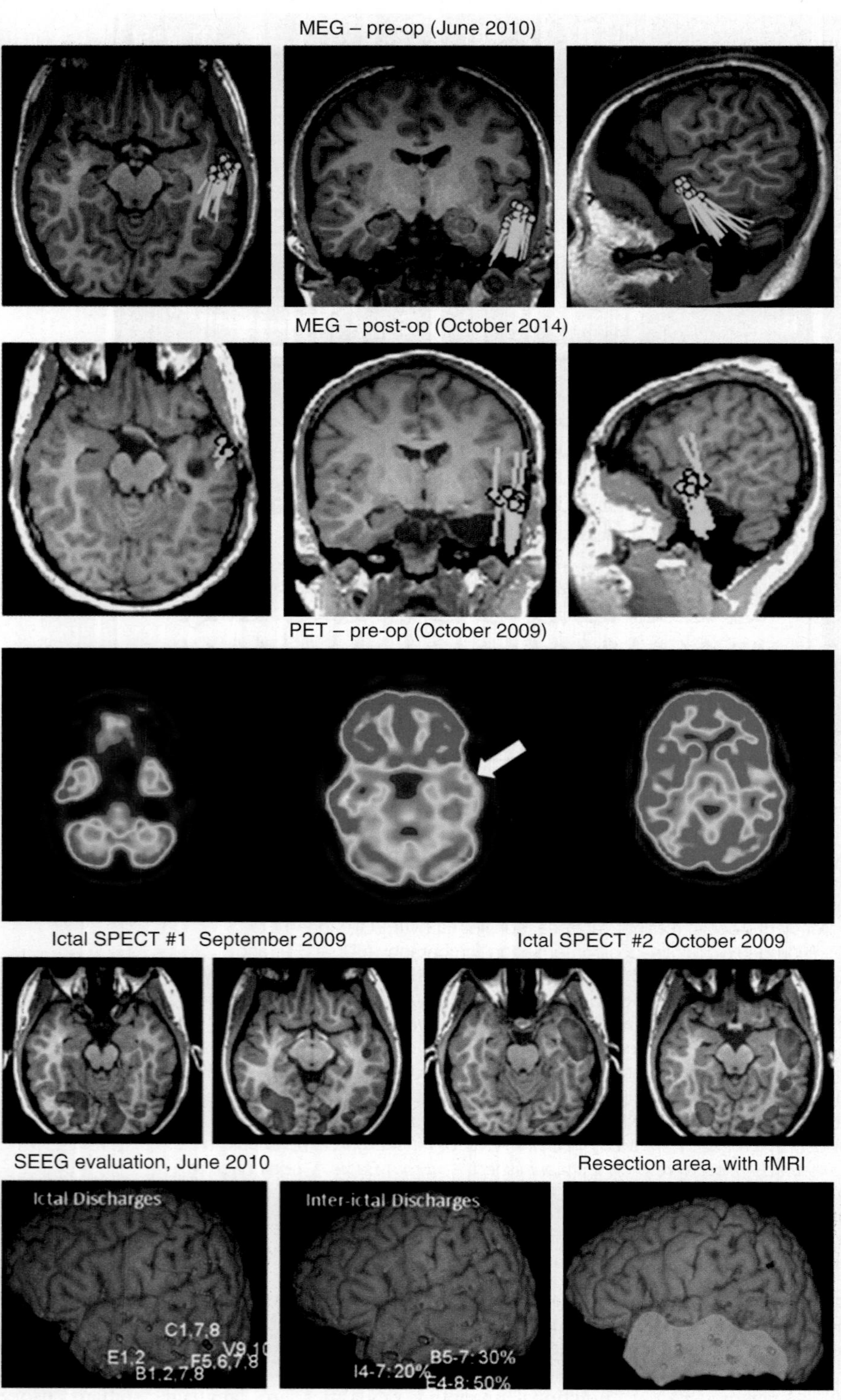

Figure 66-5. Example of comprehensive use of magnetoencephalography (MEG)/ magnetic source imaging in multimodal evaluation of a complex case of drug-resistant epilepsy. Seizures, which began in this young man at age 4½ years, were characterized as type A (right hand jerking, maintained awareness but inability to respond), and type B (increased heart rate followed by a dialeptic seizure). He had no epilepsy risk factors and a normal magnetic resonance imaging study. His first video-electroencephalography (VEEG) evaluation at an outside hospital at the age of 9 captured unclear events that appeared to implicate the right frontal region, and a second noninvasive VEEG evaluation recorded 10 seizures from the right central region. At age 10, scalp VEEG monitoring was carried out at the Cleveland Clinic, where left temporal sharp waves were found, but seizures were recorded from both the left temporal and right central-parietal regions, prompting a magnetoencephalography (MEG) study. The MEG study identified interictal discharges (mostly MEG-unique) in the left anterior temporal lobe (left superior temporal sulcus), positron emission tomography (PET) showed left anterior temporal hypometabolism *(arrow),* and conflicting results were found in two ictal single-photon emission computed tomography (SPECT) scans (the first bi-occipital, right greater than left, and the second left lateral temporal). Because of the nonconcordant data, and concern about left temporal language, the patient had an invasive evaluation with stereo-electroencephalography (SEEG) in June 2010 at age 15, which showed seizures arising from the left hippocampus and lateral temporal region. He underwent a left anterior temporal lobectomy, and after an initial postoperative seizure, was seizure free for 2 years. Unfortunately, seizures then recurred, and were similar to those before the first surgery but far more frequent. A second postoperative MEG in 2014 demonstrated abundant consistent interictal discharges (now entirely without EEG correlates) in exactly the same region as the first, in the left superior temporal gyrus, above the resection cavity. *(The case is generously provided by Richard C. Burgess, MD, PhD, Cleveland Clinic, Cleveland, OH.)*

Figure 66-6, where MEG provides critical functional landmarks by mapping motor, somatosensory, and auditory cortices, while they are integrated with various kinds of structural images for a safe preoperative plan. In the past, the most common application of functional mapping was the localization of the central sulcus.[123] This is particularly important in situations in which normal anatomic landmarks may be displaced or blurred.

ECDs provide seeming simplicity and deceptive clarity for the neuronavigational maps[59-61,130,131]—and dangerously simplistic clinical reasoning.[5,22,132] One has to keep in mind that other methods based on distributed source models provide images that resemble functional MRI (fMRI); an example of language lateralization using the Multi-Resolution FOCal Underdetermined System Solution (MR-FOCUSS) is shown in Figure 66-7.[133,134]

However, because ECD does not represent "the center" for respective function,[5,22,132] none of the methods provides source size information.[19,20,135]

Somatosensory Mapping

The somatosensory system is well understood,[30,32,33,136,137] and somatosensory evoked fields (SEFs) are the most frequently performed mapping modality in clinical practice.[74] Electrical skin stimulations have been most widely used in MEG mapping of the somatosensory cortex,[32] whereas tactile stimulations—mainly delivered using a pneumatic device[138,139] or the most recently introduced "brush stimulator"[140]—are also well established and used for stimulation of specific nerves[33,141] or dermatomes.[37,122,142-144] Among these, median nerve stimulation is very robust and the most frequently used procedure for identification of the somatosensory cortex and for hand representation,[57] whereas tibial nerve stimulations are usually used for mapping cortical representation of the lower extremities.[57] The entire sensory homunculus was mapped with MEG over two decades ago,[37,122,143,144] and the invention of the handheld brush (tapping) stimulator[140] provides a practical solution for stimulating virtually any skin point on the body in a time-locked manner for the purpose of flexible and customized somatosensory MEG mapping commensurate with a specific clinical scenario.

For clinical purposes, the primary (SI) and secondary (SII) somatosensory cortices can be reliably and reproducibly mapped with MEG[32,33,119,120] because the first identifiable component of the SEF, occurring with a latency of about 20 msec (hence the N20m), is robust and easily evoked[123,142,145,146] even in patients under anesthesia or those in a coma.[142,146] However, the SEF may be reduced in brain tumor patients with recognized sensory or motor deficits.[147] It has been well established that the N20m generator is located in the anterior wall of the somatosensory gyrus (Brodmann's area 3b),[120,121,125,142,146,148,149] and MEG identification of the central sulcus has been validated using other functional imaging methods[150-152] as well as with the gold standards of invasive procedures.[60,97,98,137] For example, one study of 30 patients with space-occupying lesions in the proximity of the central sulcus reported "complete" (100%) agreement of MEG findings with a conventional phase reversal, and demonstrated the practicability of MEG-guided neuronavigation[60] (see Fig. 66-6).

BOX 66-1 Possible Benefits of Magnetoencephalography in Presurgical Evaluation of Patients with Operable Lesions

- Localize eloquent cortices of interest noninvasively in patients without structural abnormalities.[62,123,133,178,283]
- Establish spatial relations of the lesion(s) with eloquent cortices noninvasively.[62,123,133,139,178,283]
- Detect the functional tissue within the tumor (e.g., diffusely growing gliomas).[284-286]
- Identify displaced anatomic landmarks (central sulcus, sylvian fissure, etc.).[137,160,287,288]
- Assist in choosing an optimal surgical trajectory.[61,123,264]
- Overall, define the key elements of a comprehensive neuronavigational map as a prerequisite for planning an optimal surgical trajectory and safe intraoperative navigation and operation.[61,62,123,130,131,264]

Motor Mapping

Active,[145,153] passive,[154] or imagined[155,156] movements are associated with movement-related magnetic fields, also known as motor evoked fields.[57] Evaluation of motor functions requires appropriate motor and cognitive cooperation of the subject in order to execute a sufficient number (usually 100 to 500) of repetitive self-paced or cued (visually or auditorily) movements,

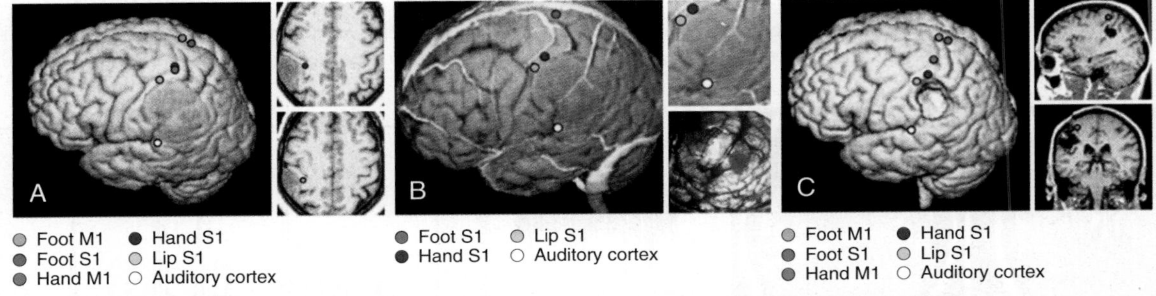

Figure 66-6. Three-dimensional (3D) integration of brain anatomy and function to facilitate intraoperative navigation around the sensorimotor strip. A, *Left.* A 3D surface rendering of the brain of a patient with a tumor in the sensorimotor region. The left parietal grade 2 oligoastrocytoma is readily identifiable. The equivalent current sources of responses to median nerve (MN-SEFs), tibial nerve (TN-SEFs), and lip (Lip-SEFs) somatosensory evoked fields and to auditory evoked fields (AEFs), and the magnetoencephalographic-electromyographic (MEG-EMG) coherences for right wrist and ankle extensions are displayed on the surface. *Right.* Sources of SEFs to median nerve and lip stimulation, displayed on two horizontal magnetic resonance imaging (MRI) sections. Note the distortion of functional cortical anatomy by the slowly growing tumor. **B,** *Left.* A 3D surface rendering of the patient's brain, including cortical veins and sources of SEFs and AEFs. *Right, top.* Enlarged section of 3D MRI surface rendering. *Right, bottom.* Corresponding brain surface during surgery. The veins are readily identifiable and allow the localization of both the somatosensory cortex *(left)* and the tumor area (*right, bottom*) (vein bifurcation over the tumor is marked with an *arrow*). **C,** *Left.* Postoperative surface rendering of the patient's brain. Sources of MEG-EMG coherences for right wrist and ankle extensions, and MN-SEFs, TN-SEFs, Lip-SEFs, and AEFs, are displayed on the surface. *Right.* Sagittal and coronal sections of the postoperative MRIs, with sources of median nerve SEFs and hand MEG-EMG coherence. *(From Mäkelä JP, Kirveskari E, Seppä M, et al. Three-dimensional integration of brain anatomy and function to facilitate intraoperative navigation around the sensorimotor strip.* Hum Brain Mapp. *2001;12:180-192.)*

or accomplish a sufficient degree of isometric contraction.[57,153] Furthermore, because movement-related magnetic field responses are harder to consistently evoke than somatosensory responses, two different motor paradigms may be required to increase the yield, and the familiarity of the MEG team with motor mapping subtleties is critical.[57] A required time locking of the onset of motor activity being mapped, for the purpose of necessary averaging, may be accomplished by a self-paced button press, a trigger photo-optic switch, simultaneously recorded EMG, visual or auditory cueing, or a three-axis accelerometer attached to the index finger.[57,139,153] MEG activity peaking between 20 or 30 and 40 or 50 msec before the onset of physical movement reflects the activity in the primary motor cortex that is modeled,[57] and coherence peaks at 20 Hz when isometric contractions are used.[153,157-160] The main advantage of MEG over fMRI and PET in terms of motor mapping is the ability of MEG to isolate pure motor activity of interest (i.e., in the precentral gyrus) as a result of its superior temporal resolution[157-160] (see Fig. 66-6).

Language Mapping

Although capable of accurate localization of the specific local or regional activation involved in various phases and aspects of language processing,[134,161-168] MEG is primarily used clinically for determining the language-dominant hemisphere in patients preparing for surgical interventions (craniotomy; stereotactic or radiosurgical procedures).[62,133,169-173] For this purpose, various types of linguistic stimuli can be presented acoustically or visually in order to activate language-specific areas and evoke language-related responses (late responses, i.e., with latency >150 msec) following the primary auditory and visual responses (early responses, i.e., with latency <150 msec).[174-176] The number of artifact-free language evoked magnetic fields from speech comprehension and/or production necessary to attain an adequate signal-to-noise-ratio usually ranges between 50 and 100.[57] Irrespective of the modality of stimulation, including some variability related to the stimulation paradigms,[57] language stimuli evoke a large, usually lateralized, response that may start about 150 msec after the stimulus and last to about 750 msec, but usually peaks between 400 and 500 msec.[57,152,175,176] More specifically, activity between 150 and 250 msec is presumably reflective of elemental feature processing and integration, activity peaking at a latency between 210 and 420 msec after the stimulus usually reflects Wernicke's area activity, and activity peaking at a latency between 400 and 700 msec typically corresponds to Broca's area, with occasional exceptions[152,175,176] (see Fig. 66-7).

The determination of hemispheric dominance for language is based on establishing a relative difference in MEG activity of interest evoked by the linguistic stimuli in each hemisphere. The degree of difference is finally expressed as a *laterality index* irrespective of whether (single or multiple) ECD,[170,171] distributed source models such as MR-FOCUSS,[133] or synthetic aperture magnetometry[177] is used. Language laterality determined by MEG was validated against gold standards such as Wada testing[133,134,170,171,177,178] and cortical stimulation mapping[166,179] and correlated with their results between 80% and 95%.[57,62] In fact, language lateralization is one of the fastest rising applications of MEG in presurgical mapping, and it is replacing logistically demanding and invasive procedures such as Wada testing (also known as the intracarotid amobarbital procedure) in many centers with direct access to MEG.[62] Available evidence suggests at least the noninferiority of MEG to the intracarotid amobarbital procedure,[180] along with the previously outlined logistical advantages.[62] Although MEG is a direct neurophysiologic method, unlike fMRI, reported regional activations should be taken with the same caution as they are with fMRI.[164,181] Noninvasive presurgical functional brain mapping is most useful if the *essential language areas* (i.e., areas whose removal may lead to a language deficit), as opposed to *participating language areas* (i.e., areas that are activated during language paradigms, but whose removal would not lead to a language deficit), are clearly identified and distinguished.[176] Inventing noninvasive methods capable of this worthy task remains an aspired goal in the functional neuroimaging field.[62,176] An example of language lateralization using MR-FOCUSS is shown in Figure 66-7. Figure 66-8 provides an example of MEG-based algorithm for presurgical lateralization of language functions.

Visual Cortex Mapping

Visual evoked fields are primarily indicated for localization of the primary visual cortex before brain operations.[29,57] Unlike SEFs,

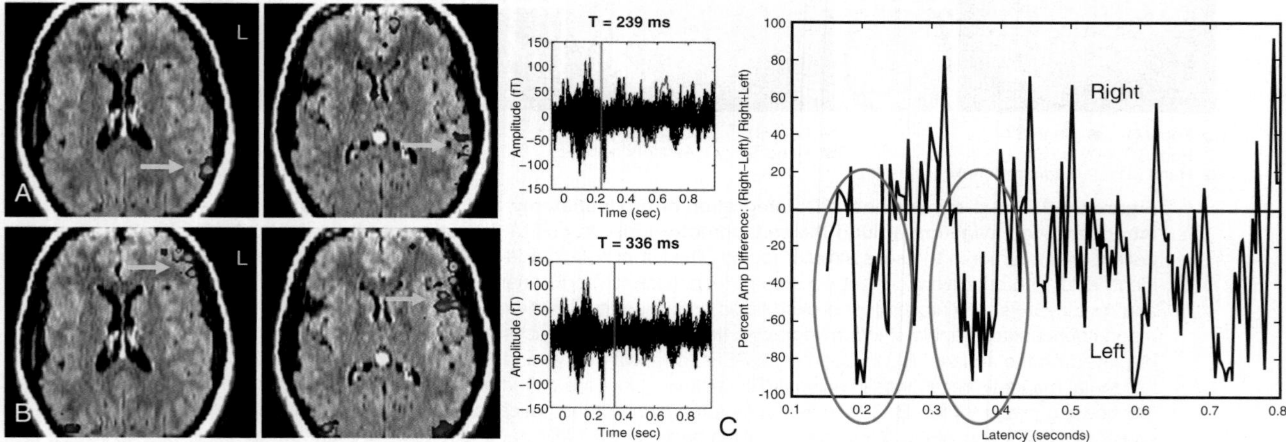

Figure 66-7. Example of language localization and lateralization by magnetoencephalography mapping with the Multi-Resolution FOCal Underdetermined System Solution (MR-FOCUSS). A, Activity in Wernicke's area was detected in the left superior temporal gyrus at 239 msec after picture onset in this picture naming task. **B,** Activity in Broca's area as detected in the left inferior frontal gyrus at 336 msec. **C,** Laterality was negative indicating left hemisphere activity. *Yellow arrows* point to the activated areas of interest. *Red circles* enclose Wernicke's and Broca's latencies. [Laterality index ranges from 0.15 to 0.8 sec. Amplitude was 20% greater on the left hemisphere (graph shown). Activity was seen 39% more of the time in the left hemisphere.]

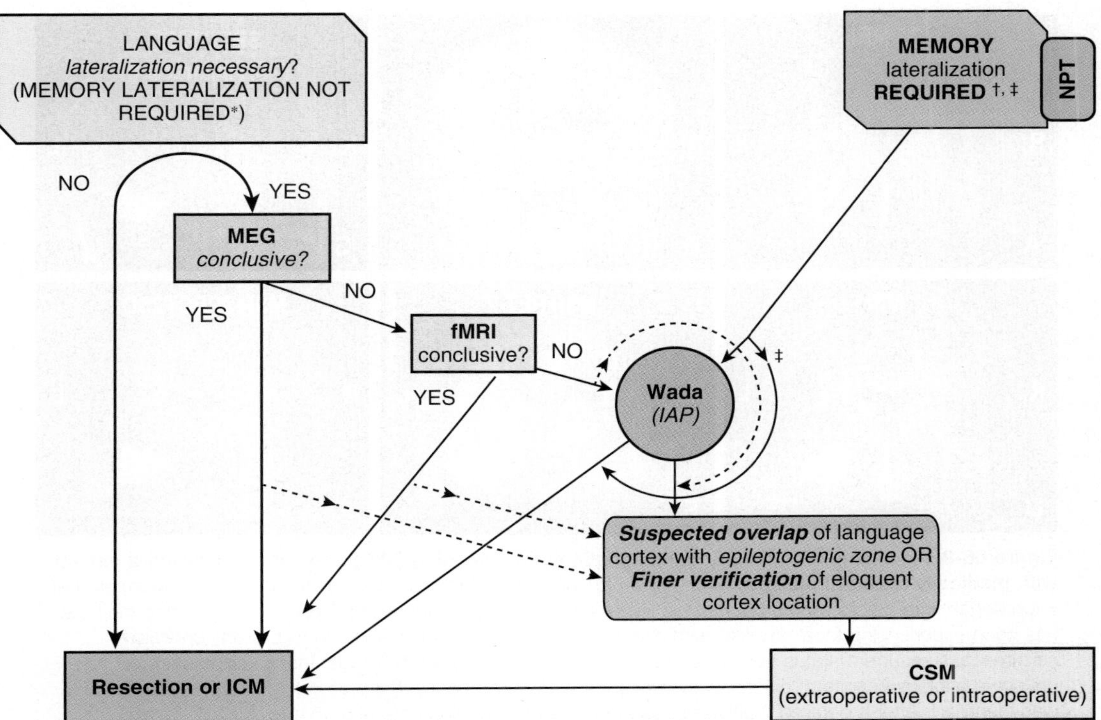

Figure 66-8. Magnetoencephalography (MEG)-based algorithm for presurgical lateralization of language functions. *For example, extratemporal epilepsy, well-lateralized right temporal lobe epilepsy (TLE) with hippocampal sclerosis (HS), TLE with planned lesionectomy. †For example, left TLE, TLE without HS, TLE with bilateral discharges, TLE with poor baseline memory. ‡No agreement exists regarding a true need for memory lateralization and the respective value of Wada testing. CSM, cortical stimulation mapping; fMRI, functional MRI; IAP, intracarotid amobarbital procedure; ICM, intracranial monitoring; NTP, neuropsychological testing.

for the purpose of visual cortex mapping, adequate cooperation of the patient, including satisfactory sleep before testing, is crucial. A specialized presentation computer with appropriate dedicated software and projector meeting the strict requirements for fast response (i.e., refresh rate) along with a reliable recording of the trigger signal with 1-msec accuracy for time locking is used to deliver stimulation images of predefined characteristics (field extent, pattern, frequency of reversal, contrast, luminance, check size, and field size to produce the appropriate subtended visual angle) on a properly positioned back-projection screen.[57] The stimulation parameters have been well established in the extensive conventional scalp visual evoked potential and outlined in the respective guidelines.[182-185] Sufficient cooperation of the patient is required to acquire 200 to 500 individual responses to yield 100 to 200 artifact-free averaged responses and to reliably identify, model, and localize the P100m.[57] Currently, visual evoked fields are used relatively infrequently in clinical practice.

Auditory Cortex Mapping

Tonotopic organization of the auditory cortex was revealed by MEG over 30 years ago,[31] and the auditory system has been well studied with MEG ever since.[187-189] In current clinical practice, auditory evoked fields (AEFs) are primarily indicated for localization of the primary auditory cortex on the superior temporal gyrus.[57] Commonly, 1000-Hz tones lasting 50 to 200 msec are presented monaurally with interstimulus intervals of 1 to 2 seconds and jitter under 100 msec at 60 dB above the subject's hearing threshold. Contralateral masking white noise presented at a 40- to 50-dB hearing level is used to prevent inadvertent cross-stimulation of the contralateral ear.[57] Ordinarily, 200 to 500 trials may be required to yield about 100 acceptable artifact-free trials for averaging to reliably identify, model, and localize the N100m component of the AEF. Older patients with increased hearing threshold level as a result of presbycusis represent a particular challenge for delivering adequate auditory stimulation. Otherwise, mapping the auditory cortex requires no active cooperation from a patient. Currently, AEFs are used only relatively infrequently in clinical practice; an example is provided in the caption of Figure 66-6.

MULTIMODAL INTEGRATION OF MAGNETOENCEPHALOGRAPHY WITH OTHER DIAGNOSTIC TESTS

Epilepsies are a prototype neurological entity in which structural and functional imaging not only plays a cardinal role in diagnosis and particularly surgical treatment but also is the foundation of many recent advances. The goal of imaging methods such as MRI, PET, and SPECT (see Figs. 66-4, 66-5, and 66-9) in clinical epileptology has been to obviate the need for invasive investigations, and the same objective continues to be pursued equally enthusiastically with MEG/MSI decades later. Multimodal neuroimaging has become a commonplace in modern epilepsy centers worldwide,[101,190-194] yet current multimodal neuroimaging has not attained a level of integrated imaging.

In spite of progress in three-dimensional functional and morphologic imaging and the fusion of data from MRI, SPECT, PET, and MEG-EEG,[195] including a single-session quadrimodal imaging procedure accomplished recently,[194] there is no study

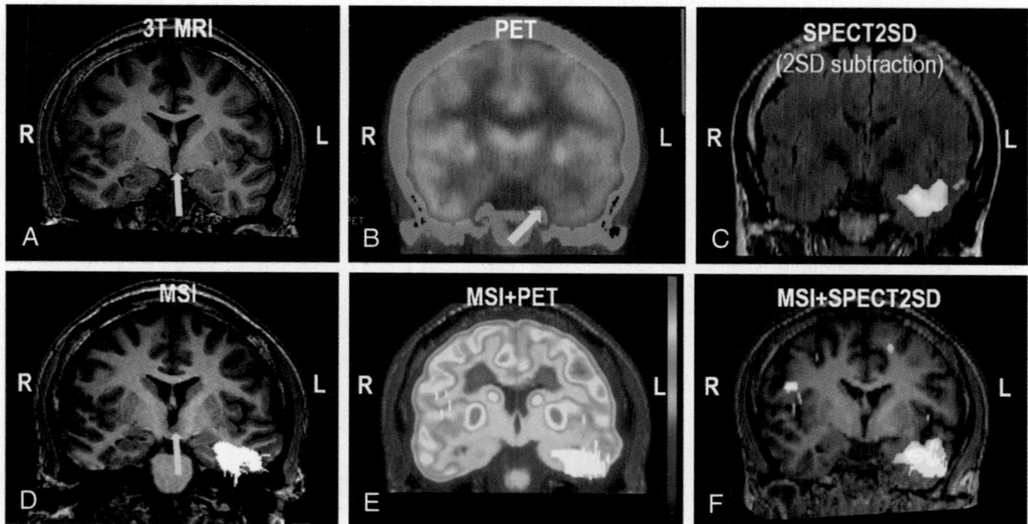

Figure 66-9. An example of multimodal magnetic source imaging (MSI) integration involving a patient with medically resistant epilepsy. A 21-year-old right-handed male had started to experience seizures that often began with a tickle in the back of his throat and laughing or giggling at 9 years of age. Since then, he has been experiencing focal seizures with alteration of awareness, focal evolving to bilateral convulsive seizures, and recurrent status epilepticus in spite of multiple antiepileptic drugs; these seizures are of unknown etiology in spite of extensive evaluation. It was only recently that his left hypothalamic hamartoma was identified. After a detailed multidisciplinary consideration of his comprehensive evaluation, it was recommended that he undergo radiosurgery, which led to no improvement of his frequent seizures. Currently, the family is pondering a laser ablation. Magnetoencephalography (MEG), 3-T magnetic resonance imaging (MRI), and indirect functional methods (positron emission tomography [PET], single-photon emission computed tomography subtraction with 2 standard deviations threshold [SPECT2SD]) were completely congruent in revealing a very active left anterior temporal irritative (and ictal) zone. Because evidence suggests that removal of brain regions containing MEG clusters leads to a favorable surgical outcome,[58,104,106,108-110] and the patient has already failed radiosurgery, it remains to be seen if this patient will need an operation in order to attain seizure freedom.

that addresses the issue systematically. A recent health technology assessment revealed that "clinical research into imaging for the localization of epileptic foci is abundant but not adequately informative."[80] Paradoxically, in spite of the fast proliferation of imaging studies, it seems that the evidence for a true effect of a specific imaging test on decision making is at best weak.[81]

MEG in the form of MSI is very amenable to multimodal integration[101,191,192] and can supplement not only structural studies,[8,89,196,197] but also metabolic[77,89,190,196-198] and vascular[77,190,198-200] studies (Fig. 66-9; see also Figs. 66-4 and 66-5). Traditionally, the timing is the most valuable contribution of MEG to non-EEG studies that are generally vastly inferior to MEG in this respect.[56,129,192] Yet, in nonlesional cases, localization supplied by MSI combined with magnetic resonance spectroscopy[8,201] (see Fig. 66-4) may lead to new insights into untangling relationships between the microstructure of the brain unrevealed by routine structural imaging and the brain's normal and abnormal function.[201] Furthermore, as we advance through an era of network science,[52,202,203] assessing functional and effective connectivity with MEG may yield invaluable new insights into understanding the mechanisms of epilepsies,[204,205] localizing epileptogenic foci,[199,206,207] selecting surgical candidates,[208] and ultimately bringing about the practical usefulness of individualized connectomes.[203]

FUTURE DIRECTIONS IN CLINICAL MAGNETOENCEPHALOGRAPHY

In epileptology, further practical MEG improvements are primarily necessary in refining source characterization and making it more intuitive and understandable to the end users,[5,22,126,209] specific definition and characterization of benign MEG variants,[22,209,210] improved understanding and clinical use of infraslow[211-215] and ultrafast[214-222] activity, more systematic exploration of distributed source models and their validation against accepted standards,[45,47,223] MEG characterization of specific epilepsies,[205,221,224-233] and systematic correlation of MEG findings with clinical outcomes.[80,81,99,103-106,206,208,234-236] Importantly, MEG may provide major advancements in understanding network properties and overall dynamics of various epilepsies.[48,52,233,237-241]

Broader application of MEG in presurgical functional brain mapping requires more education and improved understanding of the technology, and streamlined "results delivery logistics" in terms of the digital data display versatility and cross-platform compatibility for which technical prerequisites already exist but may not be implemented by the vendors, or embraced by the local information technology entities. These long-overdue improvements are practically at hand and may require only an organizational tune-up rather than a major structural overhaul. On the procedural end, standardized and validated integrated stimulation protocols enabling faster and eventually simultaneous mapping of multiple functional modalities, along with software improvements making the modeling procedures and reporting routines simpler and more robust, would be greatly beneficial. On the receiving end, seamless and versatile data communication, display, and integration are of particular importance for neurosurgeons.

With present-day neuromagnetometers, it is possible to expand the frequency range of interest from infra-slow fluctuations[212] up to very-high-frequency (about 600 Hz) oscillations.[216,242-244] Continuous head position monitoring and novel artifact suppression methods[64-66] facilitate recordings from poorly cooperative subjects, such as infants, hyperactive children, and restless adults; even artifacts caused by deep brain stimulation can be efficiently suppressed.[245]

Future MEG studies, building on the vast and methodical work of the first four decades of MEG research, aim for an increasingly comprehensive view of brain function, especially in regard to its network and processing dynamics. These studies will explore the added value of combined recordings such as MEG-fMRI, will proceed to increasingly real-life experimental designs such as the neuroscience of social interaction[129] and multisensory stimulation, and will exploit new, efficient computational methods, such as decoding of task- and stimulus-specific neural patterns.[246-248] The genetics of MEG signals also represents a promising line of ongoing and future research.

CONCLUSION

MEG is an established, reliable, noninvasive, and direct neurophysiologic method capable of providing nonredundant, otherwise noninvasively unobtainable and clinically meaningful localizing information in about one in three patients undergoing an evaluation for epilepsy surgery, and of mapping eloquent cortices with clinically meaningful accuracy in patients with operable lesions preparing for surgical treatments. In its most frequently used form as MSI, MEG not only improves presurgical evaluations of patients with drug-resistant epilepsy, but is increasingly replacing more invasive methods in brain mapping where effective new algorithms and protocols are well established. Considering the richness of MEG data and the recent progress in advanced methods, including network research, the new applications may enter the clinical arena in the near future. Timing is the critical element of brain function across the human life span and the entire spectrum of brain conditions, and MEG is uniquely suited "to address these time-sensitive issues of human brain function."[129]

Acknowledgments

We are thankful to Mr. Michael R. Czachowski for his help with coregistration of various imaging modalities.

SUGGESTED READINGS

Ebersole JS, Ebersole SM. Combining MEG and EEG source modeling in epilepsy evaluations. *J Clin Neurophysiol.* 2010;27:360-371.

Hari R, Salmelin R. Magnetoencephalography: from SQUIDs to neuroscience. Neuroimage 20th anniversary special edition. *Neuroimage.* 2012;61:386-396.

Kharkar S, Knowlton R. Magnetoencephalography in the presurgical evaluation of epilepsy. *Epilepsy Behav.* 2015;46:19-26.

Knowlton RC, Razdan SN, Limdi N, et al. Effect of epilepsy magnetic source imaging on intracranial electrode placement. *Ann Neurol.* 2009; 65:716-723.

Mäkelä JP, Forss N, Jääskeläinen J, et al. Magnetoencephalography in neurosurgery. *Neurosurgery.* 2007;61(1 suppl):147-164, discussion 164-5.

Papanicolaou AC, Rezaie R, Narayana S, et al. Is it time to replace the Wada test and put awake craniotomy to sleep? *Epilepsia.* 2014;55: 629-632.

Sutherling WW, Mamelak AN, Thyerlei D, et al. Influence of magnetic source imaging for planning intracranial EEG in epilepsy. *Neurology.* 2008;71:990-996.

Tenney JR, Fujiwara H, Horn PS, et al. Comparison of magnetic source estimation to intracranial EEG, resection area, and seizure outcome. *Epilepsia.* 2014;55:1854-1863.

See a full reference list on ExpertConsult.com

67 Single-Photon Emission Computed Tomography in Epilepsy Surgery Evaluation

Jamie J. Van Gompel, Benjamin H. Brinkmann, and Gregory D. Cascino

Focal epilepsy, the most common of seizure disorders, may be amenable to surgery if the seizure onset zone can be identified and if its ablation is expected to result in low morbidity.[1] Localization, therefore, is the key to surgically remediable epilepsy syndromes.[2] In lesional epilepsy cases, this can be relatively straightforward with standard magnetic resonance imaging (MRI).[3] In nonlesional cases, however, and those with discordant features, alternative techniques such as single-photon emission computed tomography (SPECT) are sometimes used to localize seizure onset.[4] The most frequent use of SPECT would be in nonlesional epilepsy patients in whom the semiology appears focal as a way of localizing a potential target for implantation of intracranial electrodes. No epilepsy center would resect a SPECT focus simply based on its presence and correlation with semiology, but rather epilepsy centers would use it as an implantation target for intracranial electrodes to prove seizure onset before resective surgery.

SPECT is an imaging technique that assesses cerebral blood flow by deposition of a metabolized radiopharmaceutical in the brain. Technetium 99-m ethyl cysteinate diethylester (ECD; Neurolite) or hexamethyl propylene amine oxime (HMPAO; Ceretec) is distributed to brain tissue in proportion to cerebral perfusion, is deposited, and remains stable for up to 4 hours after injection.[5] This deposition is used to indicate areas that are either hyperperfused during a seizure (called *ictal SPECT*) or hypoperfused after or between seizures (called *postictal* or *interictal SPECT*) (Fig. 67-1). The technique is time and resource intensive but can be extremely valuable in hemispheric lateralization and seizure onset localization and can help achieve the ultimate goal of epilepsy surgery: rendering patients seizure free, with as little comorbidity as possible.

Other techniques such as positron emission tomography (PET) and magnetoencephalography (MEG) are available to aid in seizure localization. Each technique has its own limitations: PET relies on the detection of metabolic abnormality in the seizure focus, and MEG on the detection of interictal discharges. Both of these studies are essentially interictal. The perceived advantage of subtraction ictal SPECT coregistered to MRI (SISCOM) and SPECT is that these investigations are an attempt to image the seizure, not a patient with epilepsy between seizures. These investigations should be seen as complementary in the evaluation of epilepsy.

ICTAL SINGLE-PHOTON EMISSION COMPUTED TOMOGRAPHY

Two tracers are commonly used in this technique: technetium 99m-hexamethylpropyleneamine oxime (^{99m}Tc-HMPAO, Ceretec) and ^{99m}Tc-bicisate (Neurolite).[6] Notably, there appears to be no difference in imaging outcomes, sensitivity, or specificity between these tracers.[7] These agents have high first-pass brain extraction, with nearly complete deposition in target tissues within 30 to 60 seconds of intravenous injection.[6] Thus, this technique allows an assessment of cerebral blood flow at a single point in time as the tracer first passes through the brain.

As a practical example, we use the following hypothetical situation: a patient undergoing video electroencephalogram (EEG) monitoring alerts unit staff after experiencing the first signs of the aura that most commonly accompanies a "typical" seizure. Fifteen seconds into that seizure, a technician is able to inject the tracer agent, while the seizure continues for an additional 40 seconds (a seizure lasting 55 seconds, in total).[6] The patient is then taken to the nuclear medicine department, typically within 4 hours, and is scanned using a tomographic gamma camera capable of detecting the gamma ray emissions of the deposited radiopharmaceutical. It is assumed that areas of high isotope deposition (indicating increased cerebral blood flow) correlate with the general localization of the seizure.

With this technique, both the timing of the injection and whether the semiology was representative of the patient's seizures are critical to understand whether the ictal SPECT image gives a true picture of the patient's epilepsy. Initially, tracer injection within 100 seconds of ictal onset was thought to be critical to identify the seizure onset zone.[8] However, further studies with larger patient numbers suggest that an injection less than 45 seconds from ictal onset is critical. Longer seizures do not allow for a later injection time.[4] In cases in which the tracer has been injected too late, the imaging may be falsely localizing, or the seizure focus may actually be hypoperfusing rather than the expected hyperperfusion due to seizure onset zone metabolic burnout.[9] Ictal SPECT has been shown to be most valuable in lobar localization and hemispheric lateralization (see Fig. 67-1A).[10]

ICTAL AND INTERICTAL SINGLE-PHOTON EMISSION COMPUTED TOMOGRAPHY

If one had access to only one SPECT study, the first choice would certainly be a well-injected ictal SPECT. In this circumstance, the seizure onset zone can be expected to be identified by hyperperfusion or increased signal. However, a separate interictal SPECT is typically performed to provide a baseline context for the ictal perfusion. Sometimes, the seizure onset zone may exhibit decreased perfusion interictally, although this is not as reliable as hyperperfusion in the ictal scan. In general, interictal SPECT has proved to have low sensitivity and a high false-positive rate in patients with temporal and extratemporal seizures.[11]

SISCOM

Subtraction of a patient's interictal SPECT from the ictal SPECT image, with subsequent fusion to an MRI, has been termed *SISCOM*. This methodology is thought to enhance the anatomic accuracy of the SPECT image as well as demonstrating more accurately the focus of hyperperfusion associated with the seizure.[6] Further, it enhances surgical planning because of the computer-generated estimation of the SPECT abnormality projected over the high-resolution anatomy of the MRI.[2] This method has been shown to aid the consensus decision-making process in epilepsy surgery (Fig. 67-2).[12]

STATISTICAL PARAMETER MAPPING STATISCOM

More recent advances in SPECT seizure imaging involve statistical comparisons between the patient's SPECT scans and a set of paired SPECT scans from normal subjects (Fig. 67-3).[13,14] statistical parametric mapping (SPM) provides a general framework for

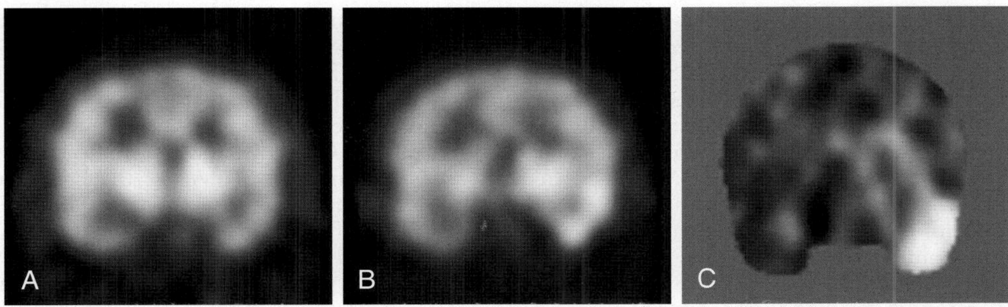

Figure 67-1. A, Interictal, or baseline single-photon emission computed tomography (SPECT). **B,** Ictal SPECT. **C,** The ictal-interictal subtraction image (masked to exclude extracerebral activity) from a 39-year-old woman with recurring left temporal seizures after a selective neocortical resection at age 19 years. The tracer was injected 21 seconds following onset in a seizure lasting 5 minutes. The subtraction image shows increased tracer deposition, and hence blood flow, in the left temporal lobe along the margin of the prior resection. The assumption is that seizures continue to arise in the left temporal lobe.

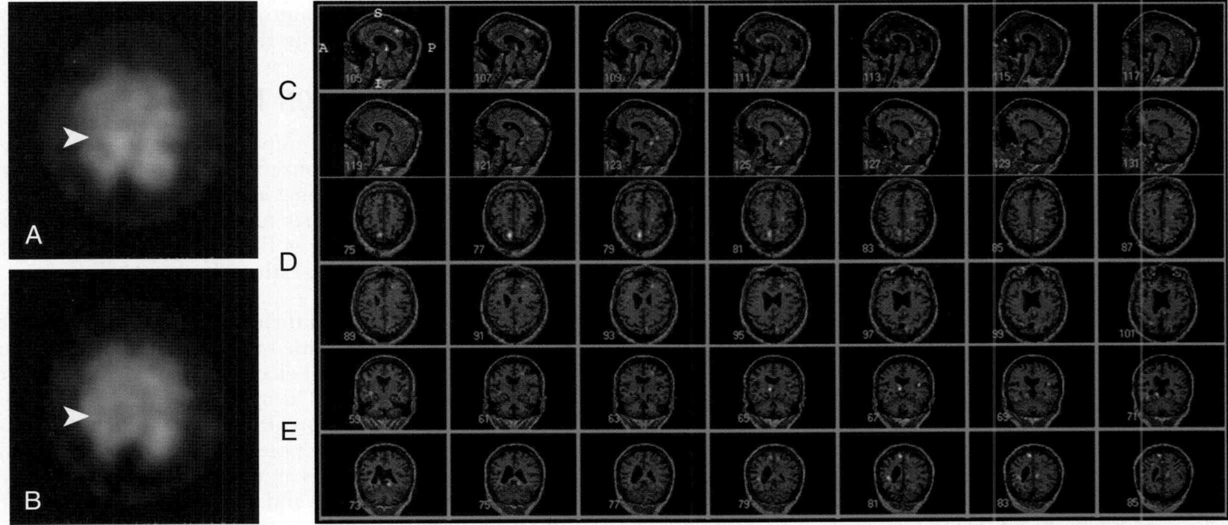

Figure 67-2. Axial single-photon emission computed tomography (SPECT) source images showing a region of hyperfusion *(arrowheads)* in ictal SPECT **(A)** and hypoperfusion **(B)** on interictal SPECT. This patient had a prior parietal resection that failed, and continued to have reflex seizures (a seizure induced by standing), involving the motor cortex. Subtraction ictal SPECT coregistered to MRI (SISCOM) sagittal **(C),** axial **(D),** and coronal **(E)** images show the markedly hyperperfused area in the leg area of motor cortex. Other areas of image tracer deposition, which are not concordant with clinical epilepsy, although they may be involved in the seizure network, are typically not targeted.

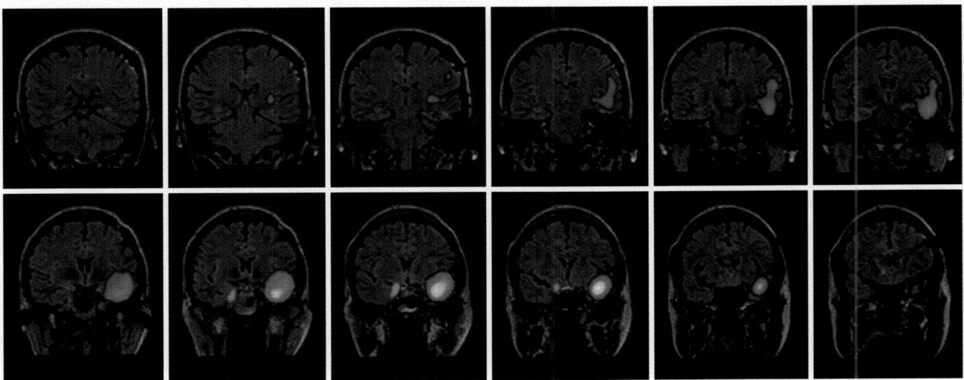

Figure 67-3. Statistical parameter mapping (SPM)-based ictal single-photon emission computed tomography (SPECT) analysis (statistical ictal SPECT coregistered MRI (STATISCOM) from a patient with left temporal lobe epilepsy. These SPM-based methods identify statistically significant differences between the ictal and interictal SPECT scans in a patient compared with a group of paired SPECT scans from normal volunteers.

comparing groups of images. Recently developed techniques to perform this statistical testing with ictal and interictal SPECT images include ictal SPECT analysis by SPM (ISAS) and statistical ictal SPECT coregistered to MRI (STATISCOM).[15] These techniques seek to determine any significant perfusion differences between a patient's scan and normal variations seen within a neurologically normal population. STATISCOM can potentially further improve the accuracy in identifying the seizure onset zone compared with SISCOM, but more data are needed to further delineate the value of this technique.[15]

LIMITATIONS OF SINGLE-PHOTON EMISSION COMPUTED TOMOGRAPHY

SPECT is a very time- and resource-intensive study. Patients are typically brought into the hospital for video EEG, and their medications are tapered down, as needed, to allow typical seizures to occur. To capture the perfusion increase associated with the seizure, the radioisotope agent must be injected as soon as possible after seizure onset. Several mechanisms are employed to enhance the injection timing for SPECT. The patients are given a signal button that allows them to alert monitoring staff to an imminent seizure. In addition, continuous video EEG recordings are viewed and interpreted by a technician trained to identify the early signs of seizure. In either circumstance, after a seizure is identified, personnel in the monitoring unit must immediately inject the predrawn radiotracer intravenously. The video is then used, along with the EEG, to estimate the injection time relative to the seizure's onset. Obviously, this imaging method is best suited for patients with long auras or seizure prodromes. If there is a long delay in the injection of the tracer agent, there is concern that the perfusion changes may represent propagated activity and seizure spread, rather than defined seizure onset.[16]

Moreover, SPECT data often demonstrate more than one hyperperfused brain region, making interpretation difficult. The coregistration for this technique requires careful review to avoid inaccuracy in the SPECT or MRI overlays. Consequently, SPECT data tend to be used for guidance of electrode implantation to a lobar location rather than an exact localization for surgical resection. More advanced techniques, such as STATISCOM, may mitigate these issues. Further, increased perfusion in the cerebellum, thalamus, or basal ganglia, which is often seen, may be real, but its significance is not well understood. There are reports of thalamic activation associated with lateralization; however, this is not widely accepted.[17] Deep activation does not affect surgical implantation strategies and potential resective procedures at our institution (Mayo Clinic). Further, deep activation is not currently used for targeting other therapies, such as deep brain stimulation.

OUTCOME PROCEDURES ASSOCIATED WITH SINGLE-PHOTON EMISSION COMPUTED TOMOGRAPHY

SPECT localization as part of the surgical assessment process has been reported to be an independent predictor of postresective Engel class I outcomes in both temporal and extratemporal nonlesional cases.[10,18] In patients with temporal lobe seizures, the sensitivity of SPECT relative to diagnostic evaluation was 0.44 for interictal (injection intentionally given without recent seizure), 0.75 for postictal (injection within 5 minutes of seizure), and 0.97 for ictal SPECT (injection less than 45 seconds from seizure onset) in a large metanalysis of the literature.[19] Similar results have been obtained relative to surgical outcome. In a large series (N = 155) of patients from our institution, where 68% were extratemporal and 50% were nonlesional, SISCOM was concordant with the ultimate resected surgery site in 70% of cases and indeterminate or discordant in all others.[2] Desai and colleagues compared concordant preoperative hypometabolic areas of PET imaging and ictal SPECT imaging with the confirmed intracranial EEG foci and found PET to be 56% sensitive and SPECT to be 87% sensitive.[20] In a series of patients (N = 51) evaluated by both ictal SPECT and SISCOM, there was a higher rate of localization of the seizure focus with SISCOM (39% versus 88%, respectively; $P < .05$). With SISCOM, there was less interobserver variability as well as improved seizure outcomes compared with SPECT interpretation in the same individuals.[4]

TAKE-HOME POINTS FOR THE SURGEON

- SPECT is a reliable and important imaging technique facilitating hemispheric lateralization and lobar or sublobar localization in many nonlesional epilepsy cases.
- Ictal SPECT, unlike other functional imaging modalities of epilepsy evaluation such as PET and MEG, is an attempt to image the seizure itself, rather than an epileptogenic brain between seizures.
- SPECT alone is not a sufficient imaging modality, but when there is concordance with semiology it provides adjunctive data to guide intracranial electrode implantation. It is critical that the surgeon have a firm understanding of factors that would make a SPECT or SISCOM study unreliable or misleading, such as a late or potentially postictal injection.
- SPECT imaging remains an important tool in developing an implantation hypothesis and, if used correctly, can improve surgical success.

SUGGESTED READINGS

Brinkmann BH, O'Brien TJ, Mullan BP, et al. Subtraction ictal SPECT coregistered to MRI for seizure focus localization in partial epilepsy. *Mayo Clin Proc.* 2000;75(6):615-624.

Devous MD, Thisted RA, Morgan GF, et al. SPECT brain imaging in epilepsy: a meta-analysis. *J Nucl Med* 1998;39(2):285-293.

O'Brien TJ, So EL, Mullan BP, et al. Subtraction peri-ictal SPECT is predictive of extratemporal epilepsy surgery outcome. *Neurology.* 2000;55(11):1668-1677.

Sulc V, Stykel S, Hanson DP, et al. Statistical SPECT processing in MRI-negative epilepsy surgery. *Neurology.* 2014;82(11):932-939.

See a full reference list on ExpertConsult.com

68 Wada Testing

Marla J. Hamberger

Depending on the location of the epileptogenic zone, resective epilepsy surgery frequently carries a risk for cognitive decline, and Wada testing is used to predict the nature and degree of this risk. The procedure remains unstandardized, and thus the term *Wada test* refers not to a specific paradigm but rather to a class of procedures involving brief anesthetization of one cerebral hemisphere to enable assessment of cognitive function of the contralateral, nonanesthetized hemisphere. Accordingly, the procedure serves as a crude, reversible analog of the proposed resection.[1]

Originally developed in the 1940s by Juhn Wada and Theodore Rasmussen to determine hemispheric language dominance,[2] the procedure remains the "gold standard" in this regard. However, both the role and use of Wada testing in the evaluation for epilepsy surgery have changed over time. Following several cases of amnesia and severe memory impairment after bilateral and unilateral temporal lobe resection,[3-5] Wada testing was modified to include assessment of hemispheric memory function to identify patients at risk for postoperative amnesia.[6] For the next few decades, virtually all surgical candidates underwent Wada testing as part of the presurgical evaluation. This intense use of the procedure generated an explosion of Wada-related research in the 1990s, providing a wealth of data regarding procedural issues, reliability, validity, safety, and utility. Nevertheless, issues in each of these domains remain controversial.

PROCEDURES

Pre-Wada Procedures

Patients referred for Wada testing typically have pharmacologically refractory epilepsy, with seizures that arise from the temporal lobe, and thus these patients are at risk for language (if seizures arise from the dominant hemisphere) and memory decline.[7-9] Therefore Wada testing involves, primarily, assessment of language and memory during the period of hemianesthesia. A comprehensive neuropsychological evaluation performed, ideally, within several weeks before the procedure provides the examiner with information regarding baseline language and memory, which aids interpretation of language and memory performance during the period of hemianesthesia. It is also helpful for patients to be familiarized with Wada procedures at the time of the neuropsychological evaluation. This increases the likelihood of good cooperation and reduces anxiety, which, if significant, could interfere with the patient's ability to comply with the procedure. On the day of the Wada procedure, an abbreviated practice session ensures that the patient understands the instructions, is not in a postictal state, and is functioning at his or her baseline level.

Scalp electroencephalogram (EEG) leads may be applied to assist in monitoring the effect of hemianesthesia and, when needed, to ascertain the presence of seizure activity or whether the patient is in an awake or sleep state.[1] Before the anesthetizing agent is administered, carotid angiography is performed to determine the presence or degree of cross flow to the contralateral hemisphere, the extent of perfusion of the posterior cerebral artery (PCA), and potentially dangerous neurovascular patterns that would result in perfusion to the brainstem. The catheter that was used for angiography remains at the proximal segment of the internal carotid artery (ICA) in preparation for injection of the anesthetic agent.

Wada Procedure: Cognitive Testing

Despite variations, there are some basic commonalities in Wada procedures across most epilepsy surgery centers (see eFig. 68-1 for sample protocol). Wada procedures take place in a neuroradiology suite, with the patient lying supine on a procedural table. Before the injection of the anesthetic (see later for agents and dosages), the patient is instructed to raise both arms, typically gripping the physicians fingers for a baseline measure of grip strength. In some centers the lateralized epileptogenic hemisphere is injected first because ipsilateral anesthetization is considered to yield the most critical information with respect to memory, that is, whether the contralateral hemisphere can support learning and memory.[10] When it is determined that the hemianesthetic effect has taken hold several seconds after the initial injection (i.e., contralateral hemiplegia, unilateral EEG slowing), testing begins, and it proceeds at a relatively quick pace to ensure sufficient testing during the brief hemianesthetic interval. This consists of a combination of speech-language and memory testing conducted within 3 to 5 minutes. When the language-dominant hemisphere is injected, the patient typically exhibits an initial speech arrest, yet might be able to vocalize. Orally presented commands (e.g., point to your nose) serve to test speech comprehension and can also serve as auditory verbal memory stimuli (e.g., what did the examiner ask you to do?). However, most Wada memory items are dually encodable by verbal or visual means, typically consisting of either real (e.g., comb, watch) or pictured items.[11,12] Patients are asked to name and remember these items, thereby serving the dual purpose of testing both language (i.e., naming) and memory encoding (for later recall or recognition testing). Some centers also include unnamable visual stimuli for a "purer" test of visual memory. Although the memory component of the Wada was intended to predict amnesia and not gradations in memory decline, "pure" verbal or visual stimuli have been used in attempts to predict "material-specific" memory decline (i.e., nonamnestic postoperative memory reduction limited to verbal or visual memory). The number of memory items presented varies among centers, generally ranging from 4 to 12.[13,14]

Intermittently during the procedure, typically following presentation of two to three test items, the hemianesthetic effect is monitored by EEG and grip strength. After presentation of memory items, language is typically assessed further by repetition of phrases and sentences, comprehension questions, and possibly reading. With dominant hemisphere injection, recovery of speech and language is typically characterized by paraphasic speech errors before full return to baseline. The point at which the hemianesthetic effect is considered no longer adequate varies among centers (e.g., full return versus partial return). After full neurological recovery (i.e., baseline EEG, speech and motor function), memory is tested, either by free recall or, more often, by recognition memory testing using either multiple-choice arrays or forced-choice, yes/no recognition. The memory score is typically expressed as a fraction or percentage correct (e.g., 7/10 or 70%), with some centers reducing the score by a penalty for false-positive recognition responses and some centers adding a point as a handicap for performance after the language-dominant hemisphere injection.[15] Another variation involves the inclusion of confidence ratings for each memory response. This provides information regarding the strength of the memory response and has been incorporated into the memory asymmetry score[15] (see "Memory Asymmetry" section).

INTERPRETATION OF WADA TESTING RESULTS

Language

It is necessary for the surgical team to know whether the epileptogenic hemisphere supports language. This information may determine whether the patient requires cortical language mapping, the extent of the resection, and how the patient will be counseled regarding postoperative cognitive outcome. Further, in the event of a surgical complication, it is useful to know whether the surgery involved the dominant or nondominant hemisphere.

Although most right-handed individuals are left hemisphere dominant for language, the ability to predict hemispheric language dominance is reduced in epilepsy because structural or functional lesions can cause intrahemispheric or interhemispheric reorganization.[16-22] Although Wada testing is considered the gold standard for determining language dominance, the actual testing techniques are not standardized. Some centers determine hemispheric language representation based on qualitative observations, such as occurrence of speech arrest or presence of paraphasic errors, whereas others use more empirically based scoring methods with calculated laterality indexes.[1,10] There is some agreement that the absence of language disruption after both left and right hemisphere injections is not sufficient to conclude bilateral language representation because this could merely reflect inadequate perfusion of the anesthetic. Rather, it is generally accepted that the presence of paraphasic speech errors following both left and right injections is the best indicator of bilateral language representation.[6,23,24] Certainly, in the context of epilepsy, the rate of atypical language organization is higher than in the normal population.[22] Interestingly, it appears that when language does shift, in whole or in part, to the right hemisphere, expressive and receptive functions are more likely to shift together, whether the shift-inducing pathology is in the left frontal or left temporal region.[25]

Memory

Pass versus Fail

One commonly hears the question, "Did the patient pass the Wada?" Within the culture of an epilepsy surgery center, this is shorthand for asking whether Wada memory performance was sufficient for the patient to undergo anteromedial (or medial) resection of the temporal lobe that is generating seizures—that is, whether there is virtually no risk for postoperative amnesia. In general, if the patient "passes" recognition memory testing for items that were presented during ipsilateral hemianesthesia, this is taken as evidence that the contralateral temporal lobe has adequate learning and memory capacity, and thus the patient has "passed the Wada." Of course, the next logical question is: What is a passing score?

As noted earlier, the Wada test remains unstandardized, and pass/fail criteria vary across centers, as do other aspects of the procedure. Whereas some centers consider 50% correct responses sufficient for passing, others require 67% or 75%.[10,15,26] Yet even among centers with the same accuracy criterion, the actual performance required varies, depending on the number of memory items presented, use of handicap or penalty scoring, and testing format (e.g., free recall, forced choice, multiple choice). Furthermore, some centers might accept a poor memory score as a passing Wada test, as long as the contralateral memory score is not significantly higher[27,28] (see "Memory Asymmetry" section).

In evaluating memory performance, it is important to consider the quality of the procedure and factors that could potentially confound performance and thus complicate interpretation. To varying degrees, some patients become obtunded, confused, emotionally labile, or inattentive following unilateral injection of the less affected hemisphere.[29] These reactions may render a patient unable to attend to and, consequently, unable to encode memory items, which would invalidate a memory assessment.

Memory Asymmetry

Most epilepsy surgery programs that use Wada testing conduct both ipsilateral and contralateral injections.[10,30,31] However, some centers perform only the ipsilateral injection, reasoning that the only critical information needed for the patient to proceed to surgery is the memory performance during the simulated surgical effect.[32] When both hemispheres are tested, the ideal hemispheric Wada memory pattern consists of strong memory following injection of the ipsilateral or affected hemisphere and weak memory following injection of the contralateral hemisphere. Wada memory performance is considered asymmetrical if left and right memory performances differ by a minimum of 20%.[31] This asymmetry indicates that the contralateral hemisphere has adequate learning and memory capacity, whereas the ipsilateral temporal region cannot support new learning, and therefore the patient has little to lose after ipsilateral resection. Wada memory asymmetries in this direction have been shown to predict postoperative memory performance,[15,27,31] lateralization of seizure onset,[33,34] and medial versus lateral neocortical seizure onset.[35] On the other hand, a reversed memory performance asymmetry (i.e., poor memory following the ipsilateral injection and strong memory following the contralateral injection) suggests that the contralateral hemisphere is unable to support new learning and that resection of functional ipsilateral medial structures would result in significant memory decline, most likely postoperative amnesia.[27,28,36] In fact, it has been asserted that a significant reversed asymmetry is the only cause for concern with respect to postoperative amnesia and that memory "failure" following ipsilateral injection without significant (reversed) asymmetry is not predictive of postoperative amnesia[27,28] (see "Validity" section).

ANESTHETIC AGENTS AND DOSAGES

The Wada procedure was developed using sodium amobarbital, and this remained the primary anesthetic used in Wada testing until a global shortage of amobarbital occurred in 2003. In response to this shortage, followed by ongoing difficulty obtaining amobarbital, many major epilepsy surgery centers began using alternate anesthetic agents such as etomidate,[37,38] propofol,[39] secobarbital sodium,[40] and methohexital.[41,42]

Amobarbital dosages in the early decades of Wada testing tended to be in the 150- to 200-mg range, delivered as a single bolus. During the past 10 to 15 years, dosages have been reduced to the 100- to 125-mg range, although certain antiepileptic drugs, mainly carbonic anhydrase inhibitors, have been shown to raise the threshold of the amobarbital anesthetic effect.[43,44] Amobarbital is considered a short-acting drug, with peak effect lasting 4 to 8 minutes. However, most clinicians would agree that patients frequently demonstrate a residual sedative effect with amobarbital that can sometimes compromise the patient's ability to comply with the second ICA injection.

Both methohexital and etomidate are shorter acting relative to amobarbital. The absence of prolonged sedation has been accepted as a welcome change; however, a shorter acting agent provides less time for testing. Dosages of these agents generally range from 2 to 6 mg, with some centers using continuous drug administration or multiple consecutive injections to lengthen the testing interval. Nevertheless, continued experience with these agents indicates that improvements in techniques are still evolving.[38] Most relevant, the behavioral, EEG, and neurological effects of these anesthetics are similar, and results of language and memory testing appear to be equivalent to those obtained with amobarbital.[41] Despite concern of methohexital increasing the risk for seizures, this appears to be relevant only at high doses (25 to 50 mg); in fact, intravenous injections of methohexital have been shown to be useful for pharmacologic activation of epileptiform EEG abnormalities during electrocorticography.[45,46] Fortunately, low doses of intra-arterial methohexital used for Wada testing have not been associated with activation of interictal spikes or seizures.[41]

SAFETY

Risks of Wada testing have been estimated using cerebral angiography risk data and therefore include stroke, femoral neuropathy, internal artery spasm, and arterial dissection. Complication rates in large, prospective series have been reported as low as 0.34% for neurological complications and 0.3% for dissections in the cervical arteries.[47] Another study reported 2.63% for neurological complications, including 0.14% with permanent disability.[48] However, analysis of a series of 677 consecutive patients who underwent Wada testing revealed a considerably higher complication rate, although these investigators may have used a broader operational definition for complications.[49] Specifically, adverse events occurred in 74 patients (10.9%) and included encephalopathy (7.2%), seizure (1.2%), stroke (0.6%), transient ischemic attack (0.6%), localized hemorrhage at the catheter insertion site (0.6%), carotid artery dissection (0.4%), allergic reaction to contrast (0.3%), bleeding from the catheter insertion site (0.1%), and infection (0.1%). Persistent deficits (i.e., greater than 3 months) occurred in four patients (0.6%)—three patients with stroke and one patient with dissection. Risk factors for complications included older age for stroke and dissection and younger age for seizures. In addition to the more inclusive list of adverse events, the complication rate may have been higher than previous reports from cerebral angiography because of prolonged time of an indwelling catheter and additional manipulation with injection of anesthetic. These authors cautioned that the surgical team must weigh the gain of reliable and valid information against the risk for complications when considering a patient for Wada testing.

WADA TESTING IN CHILDREN

Wada testing in children presents a set of additional and unique challenges[50]; however, pediatric cerebral angiography is a commonly performed procedure, and successful Wada testing has been reported in children as young as 5 years of age.[51,52] Although all patients should be made fully familiar with Wada procedures beforehand, this is particularly important for children. Baseline Wada testing performed in the angiography suite allows the child to become familiar with the physical environment, Wada personnel, and nature of the tests. The practice session also enables the examiner to determine each child's appropriate level of difficulty for Wada test items.

Whereas adults typically undergo pre-Wada angiography with only local anesthetic for the femoral artery puncture, children often do not tolerate the introduction of the catheter under local anesthesia. There is some concern that administration of a sedating agent during catheterization would interfere with subsequent cognitive testing. However, retrospective review of 24 pediatric Wada procedures in children as young as 6 years using propofol during angiography revealed smooth and rapid recovery from anesthesia.[39] In this series, Wada testing was initiated within 15 to 25 minutes of cessation of propofol, with successful testing completed in all 24 patients. The dosage of amobarbital in pediatric patients has been reported to range from 60 to 130 mg,[53] although the overall, mean dosages reported tend to be similar to those used in adults (100 to 125 mg). Pediatric experience is limited for the newer agents, yet a literature review revealed a tendency toward mildly lower dosages for children than those used for adults.[41]

Although most attempts at Wada testing in children are successful, there is a sizable minority of children for whom the procedure fails. Rates of successful Wada testing in children range from 50%[54] to 83%,[53] depending on a variety of factors. Risk factors identified for unsuccessful Wada testing in children include full-scale intelligence quotient of less than 80, young age (<4 years), and seizure onset from the left dominant hemisphere (presumed by right-handedness). Information regarding language processing in the nonepileptogenic hemisphere is the most readily obtainable information among younger children because this involves testing the "healthy" hemisphere, without the need to ensure memory encoding.

PERFUSION PATTERNS

The memory component of the Wada test is intended to mimic the effect of removal of memory-related, medial temporal structures, mainly the hippocampus. However, standard Wada testing involves an ICA injection, which typically perfuses only the anterior one third of the hippocampus. The posterior portion of the hippocampus is supplied primarily by the vertebrobasilar system through the PCA. In only about 9% of patients, the PCA arises from the ICA.[55] Thus the importance of arterial perfusion patterns with respect to hemispheric memory assessment is controversial. It has been asserted that ICA injection renders the hippocampus dysfunctional, despite the absence of complete perfusion. This position is based on hippocampal depth electrode recording of slow EEG activity throughout the hippocampus following ICA injection, possibly reflecting functional deafferentation of the hippocampus from surrounding anesthetized cortex.[56] However, EEG slowing can also be found in contralateral regions after ICA injection, which are unlikely dysfunctional, owing to deafferentation. Single-photon emission computed tomography studies have shown reduced cerebral blood flow only in regions perfused by anterior and middle cerebral arteries.[57] There are several reports of direct PCA injections; however, this carries a higher risk for stroke and therefore is not commonly performed.[58,59] Finally, some studies suggest that perfusion of the PCA does not appear to influence Wada memory findings.[60,61] Hence, this issue remains unresolved.

RELIABILITY

Questions regarding reliability of Wada testing refer mainly to the reproducibility of Wada memory results. Given that memory "failure" following the ipsilateral (epileptogenic) hemisphere injection could render a patient inoperable, repeating the procedure is relatively common.[62] That many patients pass the repeat procedure after having failed the first has raised questions regarding the reliability of Wada testing. However, in evaluating the reliability of Wada testing, it is critical that the reasons underlying the improved performance be considered. For example, positive changes in the patient's state can result in improved memory performance (e.g., reduced anxiety, improved attention related to lower dosage of anesthetic agent or duration since prior seizure). In these cases, improved memory performance does not reflect the reliability of the procedure. Results from studies investigating reliability have been consistent, including the largest series reported of 630 Wada procedures over 10 years.[62] In this series, improved memory performance following the second injection was frequently related to correction of external factors that rendered the first procedure technically unsatisfactory. When the same procedural complication recurred, or when the procedure was, again, technically satisfactory, outcomes were unchanged. Overall, 79% of the ipsilateral and 73% of the contralateral pass/fail outcomes were consistent. Thus the Wada procedure, when technically accurate, appears to be highly reliable for both ipsilateral and contralateral testing.

VALIDITY

Difficulty in assessing the validity of Wada memory testing has been an ongoing topic of discussion since its inception.[63-65] To accurately determine whether the procedure identifies individuals at risk for postoperative amnesia or significant memory decline requires knowledge of the natural occurrence, or base rate, of the phenomenon. This information has, essentially, been unobtainable because the decision to recommend surgery is typically based, in part, on the results of Wada memory testing. Thus the outcome variable (postoperative memory) is confounded with the predictor variable (Wada memory performance).[10] Determination of the base rate of amnesia and the ability of Wada testing to identify patients at risk for amnesia would require a large series of patients to undergo medial temporal resection without consideration of Wada results. Historically, this has been considered unethical (but see changes in use discussed in the next section). Furthermore, another difficulty in the assessment of validity is that the base rate of postoperative amnesia is likely to be quite low, with estimates of approximately 1%.[10] To date, thousands of temporal lobe resections have been performed, yet literature review reveals only seven reported cases of amnesia following unilateral temporal lobe resection (although to some extent, this may be due to reporting bias).

Reports of false-positive Wada memory results have also fueled questions regarding the validity of Wada memory testing.[66] Wyllie and colleagues reported 4 patients who failed Wada memory testing without developing postoperative amnesia (yet they did exhibit postoperative memory decline).[51] Similarly, Kubo and colleagues reported 10 patients who failed Wada memory testing following both ipsilateral and contralateral injections, without postoperative amnesia.[26] However, as noted earlier (see "Memory Asymmetry" section), reversed Wada memory asymmetry has been associated with poorer memory outcome[27] and poorer seizure outcome[67] and is reported to have occurred in one case of postoperative amnesia.[28]

CHANGES IN THE USE OF WADA TESTING AND POSSIBLE ALTERNATIVES

Given questions regarding the validity of Wada testing, together with safety concerns associated with an invasive procedure, it is not surprising that the inclusion of Wada testing in the evaluation for epilepsy surgery has decreased considerably over the years.[63] Results from a 1992 international Wada survey indicated that 85% of the 71 epilepsy surgery center participants conducted Wada testing with all temporal lobe epilepsy surgery candidates.[68] This is in stark contrast to results of a 2008 survey of 92 centers from 31 countries, which found that only 12% of centers conduct Wada testing with all temporal lobe epilepsy surgical candidates.[63] Moreover, this more recent survey found that more than 30% of centers never or rarely use Wada testing.

Several factors likely contributed to this marked change. First, despite the variability in Wada testing practices, some consistent findings emerged from the surge of Wada testing research in the 1990s. Perhaps most relevant, under certain circumstances, Wada testing results failed to provide additional information beyond that which was already known from the basic, noninvasive, presurgical evaluation.[69-72] Specifically, when data from EEG, structural magnetic resonance imaging, seizure semiology, and neuropsychological testing are consistent with each other, implicating the same epileptogenic region, with no reason to suspect atypical language organization (based on handedness and, possibly, postictal language testing), it is unlikely that Wada memory or language results would yield new information that is not already evident from these other sources. Straightforward patients such as these are now less frequently referred for Wada testing. Table 68-1 presents theoretical case examples indicating how the Wada test may or may not contribute to the presurgical work-up.

The reduction in Wada testing might also be related to the increase in surgical centers outside of North America, where the decision to conduct a Wada procedure is less influenced by legal considerations and liability concerns (i.e., in the context of postoperative complications).[63] Moreover, despite the significant decline in in Wada testing, there does not appear to have been a significant change in postoperative memory or language outcome. Finally, advances in neuroimaging have led to increased efforts to develop noninvasive alternatives. Although, like Wada testing, functional neuroimaging is fraught with limitations and controversies, numerous studies have aimed to develop functional magnetic resonance imaging (fMRI) protocols to lateralize language and predict postoperative memory, with the ultimate goal of replacing the Wada procedure.[66]

Functional Neuroimaging

In contemplating fMRI as an alternative to Wada testing, it is important to consider critical differences between disruptive and activation techniques. Wada testing, a disruptive method, enables the examiner to determine whether the temporarily "lesioned"

TABLE 68-1 Theoretical Case Examples: Contribution of Wada Results to Surgical Decision Making

EEG	MRI	NP	Postictal Language	Hand	Wada
Left temporal	MTS	Verbal memory impairment, naming impairment	Dysphasic >1 min	R	All data suggest left/dominant medial temporal onset. Wada is unlikely to provide additional information.
Left temporal	WNL	WNL	Intact	L	Work-up raises question of atypical language organization; Wada will clarify.
Left or right temporal	WNL	Both verbal and visual memory are below expectation	Not tested	N/A	Poor global memory raises concern that one (nonsurgical) temporal lobe will be unable to support learning and memory. Wada will clarify.
Right temporal	WNL	Verbal memory impairment	Unclear	N/A	EEG is inconsistent with NP results; pattern raises question of right language dominance or, if left hemisphere is dominant, potential inability of left temporal region to support learning and memory. Wada can clarify language lateralization and hemispheric memory support.

EEG, electroencephalography; L, left; MRI, magnetic resonance imaging; MTS, mesial temporal sclerosis; N/A, not applicable; NP, neuropsychology; R, right; WNL, within normal limits.

area is essential for the function under investigation. On the other hand, fMRI reveals regions that are activated during, or that participate in, a given function, indirectly, by the blood oxygen level–dependent (BOLD) signal; thus it is unknown whether the regions that are activated are critical for the particular function.

It is also important to note that just as Wada techniques vary among centers, fMRI paradigms vary as well. For language lateralization, some centers use word-generation paradigms, whereas others employ tasks, such as semantic decision, reading, comprehension, or naming, or advocate the use of multiple language tasks.[73-75] The fMRI memory tasks are even more variable with respect to the nature of test stimuli (e.g., verbal versus visual) and task demands (implicit versus explicit memory tasks).[76] Selection and definition of relevant regions of interest and approaches to thresholding vary among centers as well.[66] Additionally, just as some patients are unable to undergo Wada testing because of issues such as vascular anomalies or allergy to contrast material, patients with claustrophobia, obesity, slow processing speed, severe inattention, cranial anomalies resulting in macrocephaly, or cognitive impairment are not well suited for fMRI.[75] Patients with vagal nerve stimulators can undergo fMRI on a 1.5-Tesla but not a 3-Tesla scanner. Thus, similar to Wada testing, fMRI has its own set of limitations and sources of variability.

Language

Because Wada testing is used for lateralization and not localization of language, fMRI is a reasonable alternative to consider. Laterality indexes can be calculated for both Wada testing (i.e., performance) and fMRI (activated voxels) data. Despite differences in the nature of the data used to calculate these indexes, concordance rates between Wada and fMRI language results are considered high: 75% to more than 90%.[77] In the largest sample of epilepsy patients reported to date (N = 229), discordant results were observed in 14% of patients, with discordance highest among patients who were classified as having bilateral language with either method.[78] Thus, when language lateralization is the only question at hand (i.e., not hemispheric memory), the use of fMRI in place of Wada testing is largely accepted, at least as a first step. It is generally recommended that bilateral activation on fMRI during language localization tasks be followed up with Wada testing for more definitive results.[64,66]

Memory

The application of fMRI, an activation method, could be considered more problematic, or at least more controversial, with regard to hemispheric memory. Whereas Wada testing allows direct testing of memory capability of the contralateral temporal region, fMRI provides only correlative, activation data. Nevertheless, considerable efforts have been aimed toward developing fMRI paradigms to replace Wada memory testing, primarily in the prediction of verbal memory decline following dominant temporal lobe resection. Although some paradigms have shown promise in this regard,[79,80] hemispheric memory capacity has proved more challenging than language lateralization.[81] Interestingly, a different approach using degree of language lateralization to predict postoperative verbal memory has demonstrated predictive value.[82] This contribution was shown to be similar to that obtained with Wada language lateralization, yet carries the advantage of a noninvasive method. Perhaps most relevant, much of the predictive variance (54%) was accounted for by preoperative memory performance and age at epilepsy onset, both noninvasive, readily available measures (see Binder[81] for a comprehensive review of fMRI and Wada memory testing).

CLOSING COMMENTS

Wada testing has received considerable attention, and findings from this large body of research can be used to guide whether and how to conduct the procedure. In clinical practice, the decision to conduct Wada testing should be made on a case-by-case basis. Factors to consider include the patient's age, level of education, state of general and arterial health, mental health and ability to comply with an awake and invasive procedure, cognitive function, and concordance versus discordance among other components of the presurgical work-up. If results from other procedures are concordant, it is unlikely that Wada testing will provide further information that would modify the clinical course, and perhaps it might not be worth the risk of an invasive procedure. On the other hand, if findings are discordant, results of Wada testing could potentially clarify the inconsistency or provide an additional piece of the puzzle that would contribute to the surgical decision.

SUGGESTED READINGS

Hamberger MJ, Cole J. Language organization and reorganization in epilepsy. *Neuropsychol Rev*. 2011;21:240-251.

Hermann BP, Wyler AR, Somes G, et al. Pathological status of the mesial temporal lobe predicts memory outcome after left anterior temporal lobectomy. *Neurosurgery*. 1992;31:653-657.

Janecek JK, Swanson SJ, Sabsevitz DS, et al. Language lateralization by fMRI and Wada testing in 229 patients with epilepsy: rates and predictors of discordance. *Epilepsia*. 2013;54:314-322.

Kapur N, Prevett M. Unexpected amnesia: are there lessons to be learned from cases of amnesia following unilateral temporal lobe surgery? *Brain*. 2003;126:2573-2585.

Loring DW, Meader KJ, Lee GP, et al. Wada memory asymmetries predict verbal memory decline after anterior temporal lobectomy. *Neurology*. 1995;45:1329-1333.

Rausch R, Babb TL, Engel J Jr, et al. Memory following intracarotid amobarbital injection contralateral to hippocampal damage. *Arch Neurol*. 1989;46:783-788.

Scoville WB, Milner B. Loss of recent memory after bilateral hippocampal lesions. *J Neurol Neurosurg Psychiatry*. 1957;20:11-21.

See a full reference list on ExpertConsult.com

69 Motor, Sensory, and Language Mapping and Monitoring for Cortical Resections

Sandra Serafini, Ben Waldau, and Michael M. Haglund

Whether in the presence or absence of a lesion, a patient with epilepsy who is deemed a good candidate for resective surgery will often undergo pre-resection cortical stimulation mapping to remove maximum pathologic tissue while simultaneously minimizing postoperative functional deficits in motor, sensory, or language abilities. This chapter reviews the basics of functional mapping, including motor, sensory, and language mapping and monitoring for cortical resections. The major motor, sensory, and language areas that should be taken into account during surgery are listed in Table 69-1.

The organization of motor and sensory function was first described by Penfield and Rasmussen, and a schematic representation of summary results was published in 1950.[1] This description has been extensively relied upon to provide an expectation of the area of cortex devoted to specific motor or sensory functions (Fig. 69-1), typically with good correspondence between anatomic and functional correlation in the normal population. It is not unusual, however, for motor and sensory areas to be displaced by a variety of pathologies, including epileptic foci and mass lesions,[2,3] that introduce variability in the exact functional location from patient to patient. Magnetic resonance imaging (MRI) scans are extremely helpful in predicting the relationship of motor cortex to a tumor by identifying a few constant MRI landmarks. On T2-weighted axial images near the convexity, a pair of mirror-image lines nearly perpendicular to the falx may be readily identified and represent the central sulcus.[4,5] The hand "knob" typically appears as an "omega"—a structure referred to by Paul Broca as the "pli de passage Moyen" and easily visualized on MRI scans. Large lesions may compress the central region and distort this sulcal anatomy, but the landmark is usually identified by comparing it with the unaffected contralateral hemisphere on T1- and T2-weighted images.[6-11] Although less precise, a midline sagittal image and a lateral parasagittal image may be viewed with respect to the marginal ramus of the cingulate sulcus and a perpendicular line drawn from the posterior roof of the insular triangle to identify the rolandic cortex.

The anterior suprasylvian region can have varying sulcus topography, and a classification based on anatomic landmarks has been published by Ebeling and coworkers.[12] Correlation has been shown between the structure of the frontal operculum as seen on MRI and the location of the speech-motor area (commonly referred to as Broca's area); however, approximately 50% of cortical stimulation patients have speech arrest not in the frontal operculum, but rather in the ventral portion of the precentral gyrus. The visibility of both structures allows preoperative prediction of this location.[13]

Patients with dense hemiparesis are not good candidates for mapping the motor pathways intraoperatively, regardless of the type of stimulation used. Volitional movements of the face and extremities may be stimulated by cortical and subcortical mapping intraoperatively, but children younger than 5 to 7 years often have an electrically inexcitable cortex when a direct stimulating current is applied with a bipolar electrode.[14,15] Complex stimulating paradigms may still, however, bring out the excitability of pediatric motor cortex.[16] With the use of somatosensory evoked potentials (SSEPs), phase reversal over the central sulcus is available if direct stimulation mapping cannot be accomplished easily.[17-21] Insertion of a subdural electrode array under general anesthesia followed by extraoperative mapping may allow the mapping of motor, sensory, language, and ictal seizure onsets in young children and in uncooperative adults. These techniques may be contraindicated in patients with significant cerebral edema from malignant gliomas or metastatic tumors and may expose patients to the risks of a second craniotomy with the added morbidity and the possibilities of the collection of blood or cerebrospinal fluid underneath the electrodes, or of delayed infection.[22]

Removing an epileptic focus or lesion in the language-dominant hemisphere poses particular challenges because there is a lack of specific correspondence between anatomic landmarks and language beyond broad perisylvian areas such as inferior frontal, superior and middle temporal, or inferior parietal gyri. Additional variability is likely to be introduced from an epileptic disorder, particularly with an early age of onset.[23,24] Although cortical areas necessary for motor, sensory, or language function are usually discreet,[25] where a distance of only a few millimeters may be the difference between function or lack of function, our experience is also consistent with reports of infrequent "transition zones" where cortical stimulation induces only occasional word-finding disruption.[26] Because of this combination of individual variability, variability resulting from pathology, and small, discrete functional areas, it becomes necessary to map out motor, sensory, and language areas for each patient to create a tailored map from which resection margins can be decided.

FOUNDATIONS OF LANGUAGE MAPPING IN EPILEPSY SURGERY

Stimulation mapping during language measurement in awake adults has shown several features of the cortical organization of language that appear to be independent from brain lesions or other disorders such as epilepsy.[22] Several of these features must be taken into account during resection planning within the dominant hemisphere. Although there is a high degree of localization of sites with consistent evoked errors in one language measure (and thus essential for function), there exists a broad variance across the patient population in terms of the exact locations of these sites. In a series of 117 patients undergoing intraoperative stimulation mapping in the left dominant perisylvian cortex during visual naming, Ojemann and colleagues found that most patients had essential sites with surface areas of 2 cm or less, with only 16% having an area of essential language sites as large as 6 cm.[27] Bilingual or multilingual patients may show a more diffuse pattern of language sites, across a variety of ages of acquisition and levels of proficiency.[28-31] It has also been shown that localization of American Sign Language differs slightly from that of naming in hearing patients proficient in sign language.[32] The discrete localization is evident in both the frontal and temporoparietal sites and has been demonstrated with visual naming and word and sentence reading as language measures. Some sites have

TABLE 69-1 Areas Identified by Functional Mapping

Motor pathways	Primary motor cortex, subcortical corona radiata, internal capsule, cerebral peduncle
Supplementary motor area	Motor cortex and descending motor pathways
Insula	Dominant: language localization and subcortical motor pathways Nondominant: subcortical motor pathways
Language localization	Dominant hemisphere: inferior and posterior frontal, superior and middle temporal gyri; supramarginal, angular, temporal insula; subcortical arcuate fasciculus; inferior occipitofrontal fasciculus
Sensory pathways	Primary sensory cortex
Intractable seizures	Electrocorticography, grid mapping of ictal onsets

very discrete boundaries, whereas others have a surrounding area in which occasional errors are evoked, suggesting a more graded transition from cortex unrelated to language to cortex potentially related to a different language function.[33,34]

In most patients, several essential perisylvian areas are involved in language function. In Ojemann and colleagues' series, two thirds of the patients had two sites; in a quarter, three sites were present.[27] Usually, there was one frontal site and one or more temporoparietal sites; however, in approximately 10% of patients there was no frontal language site, and around another 10% had no temporoparietal language site. Although a majority of patients have temporoparietal language sites, the critical issue here is the large variance between patients, even with a single language task such as visual confrontation naming.

This considerable variance in language localization is illustrated in Figure 69-2. The percentage of essential language sites in the entire series is shown in the circles and demonstrates a range in the temporoparietal region of 2% to 36% of patients with essential language sites in a single area.[27] Of note is the 14% of essential language sites in the anterior superior temporal gyrus and the 5% of such sites in the anterior middle temporal gyrus, in front of the central sulcus. In the posterior language area, no local area was crucial for language in more than about a third of the patients. This variation in language localization is substantially greater than the morphologic variability in the perisylvian cortex, although this is also substantial.[35,36] However, no cytoarchitectural area seems to have a reliable relationship to language. It is the combination of discrete localization of essential language areas in the individual patient and the great variation in their location across the population that form the basis for using stimulation mapping rather than anatomic landmarks in planning resection near eloquent cortex. It is important to point out that this population map was derived solely from a visual naming task, that significance was assigned by a probability (error on two of three trials) rather than by an absolute anomia, and that the spatial coregistration was accomplished by crude estimates of distance from the temporal pole and in relation to cortical surface landmarks.[24]

Stimulation mapping in children has shown a lower frequency of sites of stimulation-induced errors than in the adult population.[37] This finding implies that new language areas may still arise with maturation in children during the age range of 4 through 16 years. In children younger than 10 years, language cortex is less likely to be identified or be identified with lower error rates by stimulation mapping than in older children, and may require longer train durations and longer pulse durations than adults because of immature neurophysiologic structures and subcortical tracts or projections. Wada testing seems more likely to be successful for memory mapping and marginally successful for language mapping compared to stimulation mapping for language in this younger age group.[38] Extraoperative electrocortical

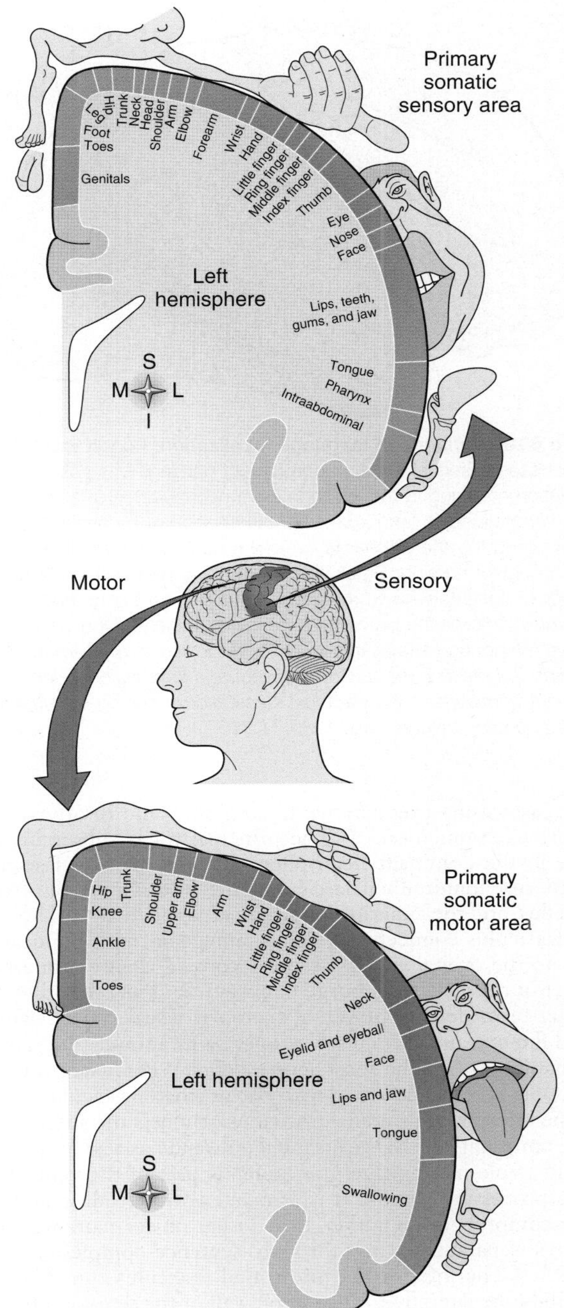

Figure 69-1. Motor and sensory homunculus as described by Penfield and Rasmussen in 1950. Note ventral motor areas for areas that may be essential for speech production in approximately 50% of patients. *(From Jones K.* Neurological Assessment: A Clinician's Guide. *Toronto: Churchill Livingstone; 2011.)*

stimulation mapping remains the established procedure for surgery near eloquent cortex in children.[39] Because an awake craniotomy is less well tolerated in children, implantation of subdural stimulation electrodes allows extraoperative mapping of cortical function with sufficient specificity without psychological distress.

Anatomic knowledge of subcortical white matter tract connectivity in the dominant temporal lobe is also important for preventing postoperative deficits. These tracts can be localized in

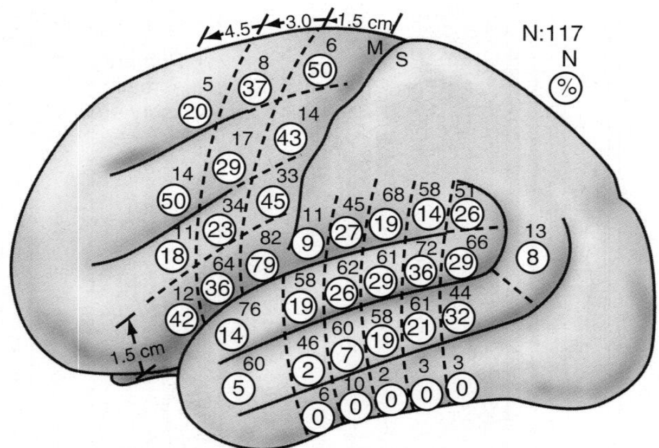

Figure 69-2. Variance in language localization. Localization of cortical sites essential for language (object naming) was assessed by stimulation mapping in the left, dominant hemispheres of 117 patients. Sites were related to language when stimulation at a current below the threshold for afterdischarge evoked repeated statistically significant errors in object naming. Small numbers above the *circles* indicate the number of patients who were tested at a site, and the numbers within the *circles* indicate the percentage of tested patients who were found to have a language site at this location. *(Modified from Ojemann G, Ojemann J, Lettich E, et al. Cortical language localization in left, dominant hemisphere. An electrical stimulation mapping investigation in 117 patients.* J Neurosurg. *1989;71:316.)*

many cases using preoperative tractography and in others using subcortical stimulation.[40,41] The principal tracts subserving language in the dominant hemisphere are the uncinate fasciculus, the inferior longitudinal fasciculus, the inferior occipitofrontal fasciculus, and the superior longitudinal fasciculus.[42,43] The uncinate fasciculus connects the uncus, amygdala, and hippocampal gyrus to the orbital and frontopolar cortex.[44] It is considered to be part of the ventral language pathway,[45] and its removal results in long-term deficits in verbal memory, visual object naming, verbal fluency, and particularly proper name anomia (e.g., famous face naming), with the most severe deficits seen when the temporal pole is removed along with the uncinate fasciculus.[46]

The inferior longitudinal fasciculus connects the anterior part of the temporal lobe to the occipital pole and has also been shown to play a role in language processing as part of the ventral language processing stream. It is associated with reading and sentence comprehension rather than visual object naming, which requires separate testing through sentence-completion paradigms.[47,48] The inferior occipitofrontal fasciculus runs from the occipital lobe laterally to the lateral wall of the temporal horn of the lateral ventricle and then continues through the external capsule to the orbitofrontal and dorsolateral prefrontal cortices. Direct stimulation of this pathway induces semantic paraphasias,[49] so care should be taken to not disrupt this pathway during surgery. The superior longitudinal fasciculus is also called the arcuate fasciculus, and part of this connects Wernicke's area in the posterior and superior temporal cortex with Broca's area in the frontal lobe.[43,50] Preservation of this pathway during surgery is mandatory because resection of it produces phonemic paraphasias.[51] Finally, it is important to preserve the optical pathways to prevent the development of permanent postoperative hemianopia. Intraoperative stimulation mapping can elicit a transient shadow that can be used to identify the visual pathways.[52]

Assessment of the effects of stimulation on an array of language-related functions (visual naming, reading, recent verbal memory, orofacial mimicry, and speech sound identification) in a series of 14 patients provided the basis for a model of language organization in the lateral perisylvian cortex. This model included a perisylvian area involving the superior temporal and anterior parietal as well as the posterior frontal lobes, important for speech production and perception; a surrounding zone of specialized sites, some of which are related to syntax; and an even more peripheral area related to recent verbal memory.[25,53] Significant interference with reading has been noted with stimulation of the lower part of the precentral and postcentral gyri; the dominant supramarginal, angular, and posterior part of the superior temporal gyri; the dominant inferior and middle frontal gyri; and the posterior part of the dominant middle temporal gyrus.[54]

Many neurosurgical operating teams rely solely on visual naming tasks for the intraoperative testing of language function. However, when broader outcome measures are used to test patients postoperatively, it is found that word-finding deficits are more generalized than visual naming deficits alone.[55,56] Resection of auditory naming sites has been shown to lead to postoperative word-finding difficulties, in both visual naming and auditory naming tasks.[56] Areas responsible for word finding in a reading context not only include supramarginal and angular gyri, but can extend along both posterior and middle portions of the superior temporal gyrus. In a study of 28 patients, it was found that distinct areas could be identified for visual naming, auditory naming, and sentence completion throughout subregions of dominant temporal and parietal cortex. Furthermore, the percentage of language sites found within parietal and temporal subregions of dominant cortex was shown to vary by word-finding modality, with auditory sites more prevalent than visual naming sites in the temporal pole, anterior and middle superior temporal gyrus, angular gyrus, and posterior middle gyrus. Sentence-completion sites are also more prevalent than visual naming sites in the temporal pole and anterior subregion of the superior temporal gyrus.[57] Figure 69-3A illustrates that there are distinct as well as overlapping language sites that can be identified during intraoperative stimulation mapping for visual naming, auditory naming, reading, and word finding. Figure 69-3B illustrates the percentage of language sites found in temporal and parietal subregions of dominant cortex, with auditory naming producing higher percentages of language sites identified in anterior and posterior temporal subregions compared to visual naming and sentence completion, and sentence completion showing the highest rates in parietal areas compared to visual and auditory naming. If stimulation mapping time is restricted because of patient discomfort or fatigue, it is recommended that auditory naming be performed as the primary mapping paradigm. Because distinct language sites are found in each modality, however, stimulation with multiple modalities of word finding is ideal to identify language functions comprehensively, with preservation of auditory naming and reading sites, in addition to visual naming sites, being critical for preserving language function. Intraoperative removal of auditory naming sites has been shown to account for up to 25% of the language deficits seen postoperatively,[58] and removal of sentence-completion sites has been shown in preliminary data analyses to result in long-term reading deficits (Haglund and Serafini, unpublished observations).

Bilingual or multilingual patients present an additional challenge for intraoperative mapping, because positive language sites in each language may or may not colocalize. Multimodality language mapping in each language can generate an accurate map of eloquent language cortex in bilingual patients. Compared to noninvasive imaging studies, cortical stimulation studies show both distinct and overlapping language sites across a variety of acquisition ages or levels of proficiency.[28-31] Different tasks such as naming, reading, and translation may share the same cortical site, in which case it is referred to as a multiuse site. Single-task sites are defined as sites where one task (e.g., auditory naming) is disrupted across both languages with stimulation. Single-use sites are sites where one task is disrupted in only one language with

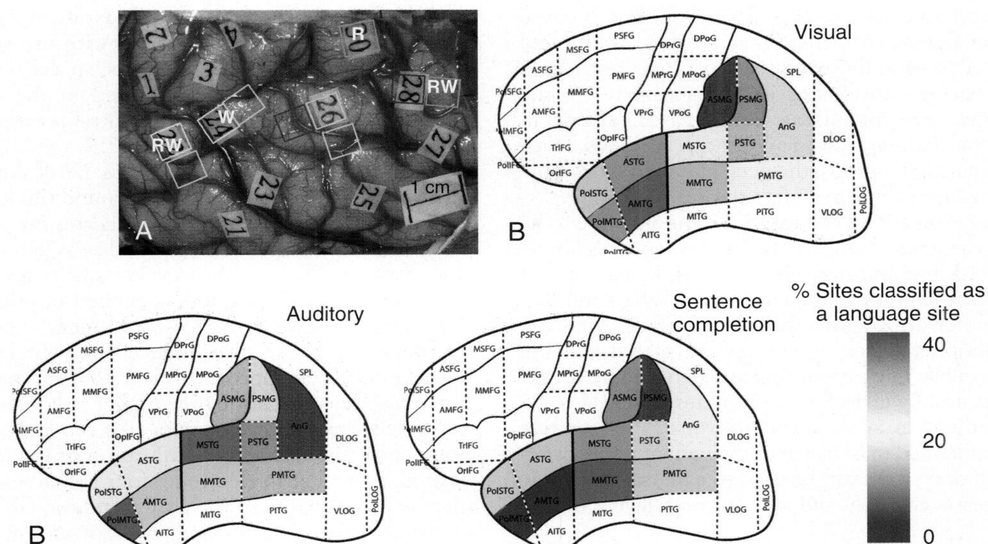

Figure 69-3. Intraoperative mapping of the human brain to identify distinct as well as overlapping language sites for visual naming, auditory naming, and sentence completion. A, One example of intraoperative mapping results. *Blue boxes* represent visual naming sites; *yellow boxes*, auditory naming sites; and *white letters*, sites crucial for sentence completion (R, reading; W, word finding). *Green boxes* illustrate overlapping sites for visual naming, auditory naming, and sentence completion. *Light yellow boxes* mark sites that are shared by auditory naming and sentence completion only. Numbers 1 and 2 are placed on the face motor cortex and numbers 3 and 4 on the face sensory cortex. **B,** Heat map displaying the percentage of sites classified as a language site by modality in temporal and parietal subregions. Percentage column displays an 11-class color gradient map representing low *(blue)* to high *(red)* percentages. The auditory naming paradigm reveals relatively higher percentages of languages sites identified across several subregions compared to visual naming and sentence completion, particularly in anterior temporal subregions that are vulnerable to resection.

stimulation. Cortical mapping of a bilingual patient has shown the presence of multiuse, single-task, and single-use sites, which underlines the necessity to test for both different languages and different language modalities if optimal postoperative functional outcomes are to be achieved.[59]

The extent of separation of language-related functions and the relationships of areas to one another constitute an active area of research in stimulation mapping techniques and single-unit microelectrode recordings.[60-63]

PREOPERATIVE TESTING

To map language capabilities, the patient is tested twice before surgery with three modalities of word finding: visual object naming, auditory naming, and sentence completion. A balance of natural and constructed items is included to control for potential semantic category effects and can be adjusted for difficulty by choosing items with a lower age of acquisition or higher word frequency in the lexicon. Items not named correctly in both baseline testing sessions are removed from the stimuli set used during mapping because stimulation can induce errors similar to those found during baseline performance, such as temporal delays, semantic paraphasias, or phonologic paraphasias. During mapping, an error rate of less than 25% is necessary for the intraoperative language mapping to reach statistical significance using the Fisher exact test. Word finding is used as the common paradigm because of its involvement in many different types of language disturbances, giving it a unique predictive quality that is suitable for a variety of preoperative neuropsychological profiles.[21,27,62] If the patient's difficulty in naming objects is due to a mass effect, preoperative dexamethasone and mannitol may diminish the edema to the point where the patient's language ability returns sufficiently for intraoperative mapping. Because word-finding errors induced by stimulation are independent from memory, relatively few items (five or six) can be used repeatedly in patients whose word-finding abilities are significantly impaired with acceptable mapping results.

Antiepileptic drug levels are checked on the evening before surgery and increased to the high therapeutic range. Patients undergoing electrocorticography have no significant change made in their medications before intraoperative recordings. Patients are kept in the high therapeutic range postoperatively and then adjusted back to their routine therapeutic levels.

INTRAOPERATIVE MAPPING

The patient is brought to the operating room and carefully positioned with a small shoulder roll so that the falx is approximately parallel to the floor. The neck is checked to make sure that it is in a neutral position, and a pillow can be placed between the head and the frame of the Mayfield head holder to provide comfort. Once the patient is positioned, an intravenous infusion of dexmedetomidine or propofol (Diprivan) combined with a short-acting opiate (remifentanil) is begun to induce a deep hypnotic state,[64,65] and a Foley catheter is inserted. After the head is shaved and prepared, a local anesthetic (0.5% lidocaine with 1:100,000 to 1:200,000 units of epinephrine and 0.25% bupivacaine [Marcaine] with 1:100,000 to 1:200,000 units of epinephrine) is mixed in 1:1 fashion, and then 9.0 mL of this mixture is added to 1.0 mL of sodium bicarbonate solution. A field block is applied that initially extends anteriorly over the supraorbital nerves and in the region of the zygoma and the posterior auricular regions. The regional field block is completed with deep injections into the insertion of the temporalis muscle. If a 30-gauge needle is used, the patient can tolerate the injections well, but because propofol is not an analgesic, the patient is somewhat disinhibited during the scalp injection and the arms may have to be restrained. If the patient has become anxious or is overly sensitive to the injections, either the remifentanil can be increased or a small amount of intravenous fentanyl (25 to 50 μg) can be added. With the advent of hair-sparing incisions, the deep and field block portions of the injection are performed after the scalp opening.

Our preferred incision allows the anterior temporal lobe to be well exposed and the craniotomy to be as low as possible. A reverse question mark incision may also be used, depending on the relationship of the lesion to eloquent cortex. The scalp flap and craniotomy are performed with the patient asleep. After the dura is exposed, peripheral tack-up sutures are placed and the skull clamp is positioned. The propofol/dexmedetomidine drip is discontinued, and it usually takes 8 to 15 minutes (range, 5 to 55 minutes) for the patient to awaken and converse. Preoperative counseling is recommended to help orient the patient upon awakening, and hydrated oral swabs can be used to ease oral dehydration so as to increase comfort and cooperation levels of the patient.

Stimulation mapping to localize the cortical surface is performed with a handheld bipolar electrode with 5-mm spacing between the electrodes (Video 69-1). A constant-current generator—an Ojemann Cortical Stimulator (Integra LifeSciences Services, Saint Priest, France) or a Grass 88X stimulator is commonly used—is used to produce a train of biphasic square-wave pulses with a frequency of 50 to 60 Hz and a 200- to 500-μsec single-phase duration. Longer duration waves are used for mapping in children. The maximum train duration is 5 seconds. In an asleep patient, the current required to evoke motor responses may vary between 4 and 16 mA, but when the patient is awake, a lower current (2 to 5 mA) will usually suffice, especially in the face and hand motor-sensory cortex. The current is increased in 1- to 2-mA increments until the evoked responses are demonstrated. The patient may also feel tongue movement or pharyngeal movement. Sensory mapping requires the patient to communicate a sensation in a specific location after the stimulus has been applied. Typical dysesthesias are transient sensations of tingling, tickling, prickling, pricking, or burning of the tongue, jaw, face, hand, arm, foot, or leg. For pediatric patients who exhibit a great deal of movement at baseline, a brief but distinct calming or quieting effect can be seen when they experience a dysesthesia during extraoperative stimulation, and then are prompted to describe the location of the sensation. Alternatively, motor mapping may be performed with monopolar, anodal stimulation.[66] A train of 500 Hz (7 to 10 pulses) may be used for monopolar stimulation; the current intensities applied are similar to those used for bipolar stimulation. Monopolar cortical stimulation was shown to be successful in generating compound muscle action potentials during intraoperative electrocortical stimulation of the primary motor cortex in 91% of 255 patients.[67] Bipolar cortical stimulation, however, has proved to be more sensitive than monopolar stimulation for mapping motor function in the premotor frontal cortex.[68] Both methods were found to be equally sensitive for mapping the primary motor cortex. Special electrodes have been designed that allow both monopolar and bipolar mapping.[69]

Motor function relevant for speech production should not be confused with language, although it is often found in the classic Broca's area (i.e., the operculum of the inferior frontal gyrus). For purposes of cortical stimulation, this area functions similarly to the motor cortex, where the jaw, tongue, and face coordinate movement for articulation. It differs from motor mapping in that the patient must perform a task that is then interrupted by the stimulation. Tasks used for mapping this function are those that are highly overlearned, such as counting from 1 to 20 or reciting the days of the week or the months of the year. Errors can take the form of a generalized speech arrest, dysarthria, or apraxia. Our current research is consistent with investigations from the 1980s showing that, across subjects, speech-motor cortical sites are found about equally distributed in the operculum of the inferior frontal gyrus and in the ventral portion of the precentral gyrus.[2,70,71] If a lesion is present in this region, it is possible that the speech-motor area reorganizes perilesionally, occasionally separating into two distinct sites around the lesion.[72]

In an awake patient, the sensory cortex may be identified more easily at lower stimulation amplitudes. When motor and sensory responses are elicited, the cortical site is marked with a small numbered ticket. If a seizure is elicited by stimulation mapping, the cortex is irrigated with ice-cold Ringer's irrigation. The intraoperative risk for seizures induced by stimulation mapping has been found to be approximately 1.5%, and patients with symptomatic epilepsy do not have a higher risk than other patients for the intraoperative development of a seizure.[73] When the operation is near the falx and identification of the leg motor cortex is desired, a small strip electrode (four contacts spaced 1 cm apart) may be placed between the cortex and the falx to allow mapping of the leg motor cortex and the foot motor cortex. The same current used to evoke motor responses on the cortical surface or slightly higher currents (1 mA) may be used in the white matter to identify the subcortical location of descending axons from the motor cortex.

Once the motor and sensory cortices have been identified in an awake patient, the electrocorticography equipment is attached to the skull clamp. If resection of the tumor includes an attempt to relieve the patient's seizure disorder, strip electrodes are inserted to record epileptiform activity. Usually, four strip electrodes are placed: anterior subtemporal, middle subtemporal, posterior subtemporal, and subfrontal. Single carbon-tipped electrodes or additional strip electrodes can be placed on the lateral cortical surface over the temporal lobe and the perisylvian region. Recording is then started and, with the assistance of the electroencephalographer, epileptic activity is identified or afterdischarge thresholds are determined. If the patient has intractable epilepsy, a tailored resection is then performed by identifying areas of interictal activity over the lateral or mesial cortical surfaces. Especially with temporal lobe lesions, our standard practice is to resect the lateral cortex and expose the ventricle to place strip electrodes along the hippocampus and subcortically along the parahippocampal gyrus for identification of the extent of resection needed to eliminate all interictal epileptiform activity.[27]

If preoperative planning did not call for identification of epileptic cortex, afterdischarge thresholds are determined. The choice of stimulating currents for language mapping depends on the selection of a current large enough to alter critical function but not so large that it will evoke seizure activity or long trains of afterdischarge activity. The long trains of afterdischarge activity may spread and thus confuse the localization of the task being performed with stimulation. Usually, these requirements are met by setting the current 1 mA below the threshold for evoking single or small trains of afterdischarge activity. However, in cortex that involves adjacent or invasive tumor tissue, the afterdischarge thresholds may be significantly lower and several current levels for stimulation may be necessary for different cortical regions.[74] For example, in Figure 69-4, the afterdischarge threshold used in the posterior temporal region was 4 mA; in the anterior temporal lobe, which was undercut by the tumor, the afterdischarge threshold was just 3 mA; and it was 7 mA in the frontal region. Language sites were identified at sites 28, 41, 44, 10, and 12. Afterdischarge thresholds vary considerably among patients and can range from 1.5 mA to greater than 10 mA. Noting the start and stop of afterdischarges is important not only to prevent the initiation of seizure activity or spread, but because they also interfere with cognitive processing. Adequate preoperative and intraoperative administration of anticonvulsants is crucial for

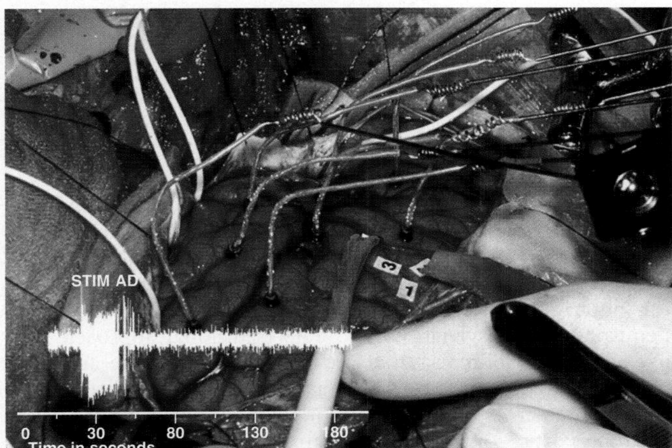

Figure 69-4. Afterdischarge activity elicited by stimulation. The choice of stimulating currents for language mapping depends on the selection of a current large enough to alter critical function but not so large that it will evoke seizure activity or long trains of afterdischarge activity, which may spread and thus confuse the localization being performed with stimulation. Usually, these requirements are met by setting the current 1 mA below the threshold for evoking single or small trains of afterdischarge activity. In this example, the current needs to be adjusted to a lower level.

preventing the afterdischarges from becoming a full-blown motor seizure on the operating room table. The use of ice-cold saline irrigation also helps in controlling afterdischarges.[75] During the language task of word finding, for example, it has been found that afterdischarge activity raises the error rate, thus providing a potential false positive that may lead to preserving a cortical site unnecessarily, potentially at the cost of seizure control (Serafini, Haglund, and Clyde, unpublished observations). Language errors made during afterdischarges are therefore given less consideration than errors made in their absence. Conversely, if a patient is able to give accurate responses despite the occasional presence of afterdischarges, it can be inferred that the cortical site in question is not involved with that function.

To increase the confidence of the intraoperative mapping, stimulation should provide the information needed to know where language is localized and where it is not localized. Completely negative stimulation mapping does not always provide security that resection of the recorded sites will not cause a language deficit. In a series of 40 patients undergoing resection of temporal lobe tumors, two negative language maps resulted in language deficits in the postoperative period.[61] This finding has led to the concept that the region covered by stimulation mapping should include areas where language is likely to be found, as well as the area of planned resection.

Sanai and coworkers, however, did not use the traditional approach of identifying positive language sites in every awake craniotomy and demonstrated that most gliomas could still be resected without causing language deficits.[76] Using a tailored approach to limit cortical exposure, 58% of 250 patients were found to have an intraoperative stimulation-induced speech arrest or anomia during visual naming. Their 6-month functional outcome data, however, compared favorably with previous studies that relied on the identification of positive visual naming sites. Only 4 of 243 surviving patients (1.6%) had a persistent language deficit 6 months after surgery, so the use of smaller, tailored craniotomies with testing for negative language sites seems to be a valid surgical strategy. It has been noted in several studies that postlesional plasticity can occur in both adult and pediatric patients, especially in slow-growing lesions, resulting in an "unmasking" of language sites that are fully functional following tumor resection (Grant and Serafini, unpublished observations).[2,77,78]

Cortical surface recordings of SSEPs can be helpful in localizing the sensorimotor cortex intraoperatively. SSEPs with approximately mirror-image waveforms can be recorded on either side of the central sulcus.[79] The precentral waveform is termed P20-N30 and the postcentral waveform P30-N20, corresponding to their polarity and average peak latency across subjects. In other words, stimulation of the median nerve on average leads to a negative wave (N) 20 msec later in recordings from the postcentral gyrus, followed by a positive wave (P) 30 msec after stimulation. The opposite order of waveforms is observed in the precentral gyrus. This phenomenon is called phase reversal. Intraoperative SSEP recordings enable the surgeon to identify the motor and somatosensory cortices under general anesthesia without the use of awake stimulation techniques. For localization of the hand motor area with SSEPs, the median nerve is typically stimulated intraoperatively. Trigeminal SSEPs with stimulating electrodes in the chin, tongue, or palate can be used to identify face motor and sensory areas.[80]

Intraoperative infrared functional imaging has recently been developed as a means of measuring the increased neuronal heat production and capillary blood flow that are linked to greater neuronal firing.[81,82] This technique represents another modality to intraoperatively map motor, sensory, and language function.

The pyramidal tract is the major output source of fibers arising from the motor cortex, and therefore is of crucial importance in the avoidance of postoperative deterioration in motor function. The pyramidal tract can also be identified by intraoperative subcortical stimulation mapping. The subcortical stimulation settings are usually identical to the ones used for cortical mapping. Initially, the cortical motor region is identified and the same current is subsequently used to identify the descending motor pathways.[20] Multichannel electromyographic (EMG) recordings have been shown to be superior to mere visual observation in detecting motor responses elicited by stimulation of the internal capsule.[83] In 30% of 66 operations, motor responses during mapping were noted at least once on EMG recordings, although they were not apparent on visual inspection. Because lower electrical thresholds are required to elicit an EMG response during cortical mapping, EMG recordings can be performed with lower currents, which potentially decreases the incidence of intraoperative seizures. This may be useful in patients who are susceptible to stimulation-induced seizures.

GENERATING AND INTERPRETING LANGUAGE MAPS

The area of cortex inactivated by bipolar cortical stimulation has been studied in a number of ways. Bipolar stimulation pulses ensure that one electrode will not become the sole source of the direction of the current and produce a lesion. Imaging during bipolar stimulation in both human and monkey cortex has shown that the area activated is confined to the region around the recording electrodes[84] but that, if afterdischarge activity is evoked, the spread is more diffuse.[85] Therefore, stimulation of motor movements should involve a very limited focal area of cortex to ensure accuracy of the functional maps. Stimulation at the afterdischarge threshold is sufficient to disrupt activity at that area of cortex. If language fails, the area is identified as an essential language site. Following Penfield's experience, word finding is the language measure primarily used with stimulation,[21,86] with paradigms expanding since then from only visual naming to a multimodality approach with the addition of auditory naming and sentence completion. Word finding seems to be effective for localization of language, and naming deficits occur in all aphasic syndromes that result from pathologic lesions. Moreover, two studies investigating the relationship of changes in stimulation to language after resection cited word finding as the only measure of language during stimulation that helped predict the effects of resection on a general aphasia battery measuring many language functions and significant clinical deficits.[21,87] However, as noted previously in temporal and parietal areas, multiple word-finding modalities should be assessed, such as visual naming, auditory naming, and reading via sentence completion, because these language functions have been noted to involve a wider cortical area and involve distinct sites compared to visual naming alone.[27]

After the level of current for language mapping has been selected, 10 to 20 sites on the cortical surface in the area of the planned resection and the probable location of language are indicated by numbered tickets. The patient then begins a test that consists of repetitive measures of language function, including visual naming, auditory naming, and sentence completion, that consists of reading a sentence stem and completing the sentence with the object described. In all cases a carrier phrase is used prior to naming the object or reading the sentence (e.g., "This is a…" or "This says…") to ensure that stimulation is not causing a general speech arrest and to ensure that the patient is awake and attentive. Stimulation at one of the numbered cortical sites is applied with a bipolar electrode at the onset of a randomized item in the stimuli set, with contact being maintained until a correct/incorrect response is given or the next item appears. At the point where the stimulation occurred, the number of the stimulation site and any errors, as well as error type, are recorded. After one or two additional correct items, another site is stimulated. This process is continued until all the sites have been stimulated at least 3 times. No cortical site is stimulated twice in succession, and after each cortical stimulation, an image is shown on the computer screen and named by the patient to verify a return to baseline before further stimulation. When an essential language site is identified, further stimulation around that site may be done to determine how closely the resection should approach that critical site. With this technique, stimulation mapping at 20 sites during three word-finding modalities requires approximately 45 minutes. The sites with repeated errors seem to be especially crucial for language. Errors can take a number of forms, the most common being semantic or phonologic paraphrasias, nonresponses, neologisms, and temporal delays, as well as comprehension errors during the auditory naming paradigm.

STRATEGIES FOR SURGICAL RESECTION IN ELOQUENT REGIONS

Localization of language is an important factor in planning for cortical resection.[88] In general, this is a concern only in the dominant hemisphere for language, and then usually in the perisylvian area. However, in the anterior temporal lobe, essential language sites are regularly identified within 3 cm of the temporal tip, particularly with auditory naming. The left hemisphere is commonly assumed to be dominant for language in right-handed patients, whereas in left-handed individuals, dominance is commonly established preoperatively with the intracarotid amobarbital perfusion test or functional MRI techniques, as discussed in other chapters. In reality, the laterality of language may not be significantly different in left- and right-handed patients when those who are left-handed because of left hemisphere lesions are excluded.[89] The left hemisphere is most likely to be essential for language in either group, with a few patients demonstrating right or bilateral language in either group, although these unusual patterns seem to be slightly more common in left-handers with a strong family history. Overall, the left hemisphere alone is essential for language in about 85% of patients and the right in 6%, with language represented bilaterally in approximately 9%.[90] Within the dominant hemisphere, changes in language have been observed after lesions in a wide area. However, permanent deficits have generally been associated only with lesions in the perisylvian area; thus, localization of language in this area is particularly important. Changes in language are often evoked from the posterior superior frontal areas (i.e., the supplementary motor area), and often acutely follow resection there in the form of mutism, but nearly all patients recover from this supplementary motor area syndrome.[91] With regard to the basal temporal cortex, stimulation can induce errors in visual and auditory naming; however, if the subcortical tracts such as the inferior fronto-occipital fasciculus are preserved, the resection of the cortical surface does not appear to result in long-term language deficits.[19,92]

Two different approaches can be taken to minimize the risk for language deficits with cortical resection near the dominant hemisphere's perisylvian cortex. The traditional approach is to use anatomic landmarks that are thought to indicate areas not involved in language—for example, limiting temporal resection to the anterior 4 to 5 cm, anterior to the inferior aspect of the rolandic cortex, or anterior to Labbé's vein.[61,93] Sparing of the superior temporal gyrus has also been recommended. The pterion has been considered the safe posterior limit for inferior frontal resection. However, particularly in the temporal lobe, resections within these supposed safe limits are associated with postoperative aphasia in visual naming, with other modalities rarely, if ever, tested and deficits likely being underreported.[87] These landmarks therefore provide little to no guidance for resection in the perisylvian areas, especially the posterior temporal and inferior parietal lobes. The safer approach is to make a unique map for each individual and identify the essential language areas using multiple word-finding modalities.

Functional cortex and subcortical white matter may be located within tumors or adjacent infiltrated brain regardless of the degree of tumor infiltration, swelling, apparent necrosis, and gross distortion by the mass. Direct stimulation mapping of the cortical and subcortical portions of tumors during resection has been shown to generate motor, sensory, or language dysfunction.[94] Stimulation at perilesional areas following tumor resection should be performed to identify language sites that are newly "unmasked," reflecting possible acute perilesional plasticity.[2,77,78]

Because of the bilateral representation of face motor function at the neocortical level, radical resection of tumors from the face motor cortex on the nondominant side may result in only transient contralateral facial weakness and apraxia, which resolves within 6 to 8 weeks after surgery.[95] Because the speech-motor cortex is contiguous to the face motor area on the dominant side, resection of the face motor area is controversial in the dominant hemisphere but has been accomplished seemingly without major acute deficits (Friedman and Haglund, unpublished observations).

Verbal memory deficits may arise after temporal lobectomies in the dominant hemisphere. Ojemann and Dodrill found a significant correlation between a decline in postoperative verbal memory scores and the lateral, but not the medial, extent of the temporal lobe resection.[96] Verbal memory scores measure the ability of a patient to recall a word after a short period of distraction. In their series of 14 adults undergoing left temporal lobectomy, the Wechsler Memory Scale verbal memory score was decreased an average of 22% at 1 month and 11% at 1 year. Thus, verbal memory not only is generated by medial temporal lobe structures such as the hippocampus but also depends on some interaction between the medial temporal lobe and the neocortex.

Functional intraoperative language mapping aims to limit the development of postoperative aphasias. Several investigators have examined the occurrence and time course of postoperative language dysfunctions after cortical mapping. A common theme of all studies is the finding that the majority of new postoperative aphasias improve or resolve over time, plateauing approximately 6 to 8 months postoperatively. Ilmberger and colleagues found that, in 32% of their 128 patients without preoperative deficits, a new aphasic disturbance developed within 21 days of microsurgical treatment of tumors in close proximity to or within language areas.[97] Seven months after treatment, only 10.9% of the 128 patients continued to demonstrate these postoperative language disturbances. Risk factors for the development of a postoperative aphasic disturbance included preoperative aphasia, intraoperative complications, language-positive sites within the tumor, and a nonfrontal lesion location. In patients without a preoperative deficit, normal but submaximal naming performance was found to be a strong predictor of early postoperative aphasia. The only risk factors that were identified for persistent postoperative language disturbances included age older than 40 years and preoperative aphasia.

Bello and coworkers identified language tracts through subcortical stimulation in 59% of 88 patients undergoing surgical removal of gliomas.[98] The identification of language tracts was associated with the development of a higher number of transient postoperative deficits (67.3% of patients), but permanent language deficits were ultimately noted in just 2.3% of their patients.

An important consideration when planning surgical resection of an intrinsic brain tumor is its proximity to positive language sites. Haglund and coworkers showed in a series of 40 patients with temporal lobe gliomas in the dominant hemisphere that the distance of the resection margin from the nearest visual naming site is crucial for estimating the likelihood of a permanent postoperative visual naming deficit.[61] In comparing the distance from the nearest visual naming site to the resection margin, a clear association was found between the distance from the resection margin and the postoperative development of language deficits (Fig. 69-5). Patients with no postoperative deficit had an average distance between the nearest language site and the resection margin of 2.0 ± 0.43 cm; in contrast, the distance was 1.6 ± 0.2 cm in patients with deficits lasting 1 to 7 days, 0.71 ± 0.06 cm in those with deficits lasting 8 to 30 days, and 0.67 ± 0.05 cm in patients with permanent deficits. However, the presence of a sulcus separating a crucial language site from uninvolved cortex should be viewed differently. In the subgroup of patients with normal preoperative speech and comprehension, visual naming sites identified by cortical stimulation and resection margins more than 1 cm away from the nearest site resulted in normal visual naming function by the end of the first postoperative week. Thus, resection of intrinsic brain tumors that follows a 1-cm safety margin from the nearest cortical language site is considered to be the best surgical strategy for preventing the development of permanent postoperative aphasias while maximizing the extent of tumor resection. Ongoing research will determine whether similar resection margins apply to auditory naming and sentence-completion sites.

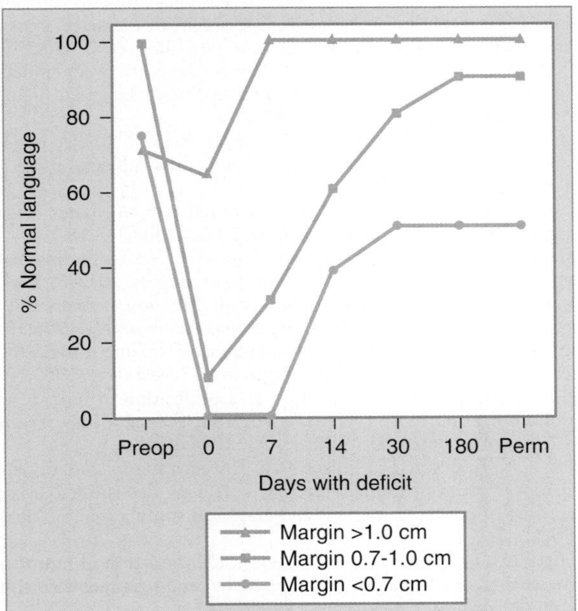

Figure 69-5. Proximity of an intrinsic brain tumor to positive language sites and the postoperative development of language deficits. This graph illustrates the time course of postoperative object-naming language outcome based on the patient's preoperative status and the distance of the tumor resection margin from a language site. *(Data from Haglund MM, Berger MS, Shamseldin M, et al. Cortical localization of temporal lobe language sites in patients with gliomas.* Neurosurgery. *1994;34:567.)*

Ojemann and Dodrill found that left anterior temporal resection within 2 cm of a site associated with repeated anomia or testing errors on naming tasks was linked to subtle increases in errors on the Wepman aphasia battery (administered 1 month postoperatively); no changes in the aphasia battery were evident when the resections avoided those sites, and changes in language were not induced with resections more than 2 cm away from such sites.[99] Moreover, there was no correlation between these postoperative aphasic errors and the size of the resection, preoperative language performance, or postoperative seizure control.

In a series of 294 patients, Keles and coworkers showed that subcortical stimulation to identify descending motor pathways could achieve an acceptable rate of permanent morbidity. Sixty patients (20.4%) had an additional postoperative motor deficit.[100,101] Of these patients, however, 76.7% regained their baseline function within 90 days of surgery, many of them returning to baseline in the first postoperative week.

Duffau and colleagues found that, with subcortical stimulation mapping, 80% of their patients undergoing resection for low-grade gliomas experienced immediate postoperative neurological worsening.[102] However, 94% of these patients recovered to their preoperative status within 3 months, and 10% even improved. The same group also showed that postoperative morbidity and the extent of gross total resection in or near eloquent cortex at their institution significantly improved after the introduction of intraoperative stimulation mapping.[103] In a series of 115 patients who underwent intraoperative subcortical stimulation mapping, all but 2 (98%) had their language function return to baseline or better after resection of grade II gliomas in the left dominant hemisphere.[104]

USING THE MAP TO PLAN SURGICAL RESECTION

With most of the cortical surface being buried within sulci, it is surprising that surface cortical stimulation can predict the effects of resections. It appears that the cortical language system has a major vertical organization and preferential location of essential areas in the crowns of gyri. Essential language areas in buried cortex, well away from those in the surface, do not seem to play a major role. Otherwise, surface stimulation would not reliably predict the effect of buried cortex resections. In fact, surface sites were identified by stimulation mapping in 117 of 119 patients,[27] and this is not likely to be the case if the language sites were randomly distributed between gyral surfaces and sulci. On a number of occasions, sulci that have been mapped for language have not shown independent sites, although occasionally a surface site extends a short distance into the sulcus.[18,39] The connections of essential language areas must also be somewhat vertically organized because surface stimulation predicts the effect of resections that remove white matter near the essential language areas. This relationship between surface stimulation effects and resection also seems to apply to frontal operculum stimulation, which can predict the results of resection of subinsular dominant hemisphere language sites (Serafini and Haglund, unpublished data).

There is a limited body of data on the stability of stimulation maps of language localization over time with or without an intervening brain lesion. On a few occasions, with repeated mapping after several months and without an intervening brain lesion, a comparison of extraoperative and intraoperative mapping usually shows that sites with or without changes in language function have had generally similar locations.[25] Remapping of language years after a static perisylvian brain injury (trauma or stroke) associated with partially recovered aphasia has shown language sites at the edge of the damaged cortex in locations where language sites are expected in nonaphasic patients. Repeated mapping for the development of aphasia in patients with recurrent brain tumors has shown disappearance of one of the localized essential language areas when the language deficit progressed, with other areas remaining stable (Haglund, Berger, and Ojemann, unpublished observations). None of these findings suggests any significant plasticity in adult language localization. In a series of nonaphasic patients with low-grade intrinsic tumors in the left temporal lobe, fewer language sites were found in the nonaphasic patients with left temporal epileptic foci, thus raising the possibility that the tumor had slowly destroyed some of the temporal lobe language sites without causing functional deficits. There was no evidence of an excess of extratemporal sites, as might be expected with significant reorganization.[61]

CONCLUSION

In many situations, intraoperative or extraoperative mapping can be used to identify eloquent areas for planning a safe resection. This includes the many patients in whom no intracranial ictal recordings are required and most adolescents and adults who can cooperate with an awake craniotomy that uses a local anesthetic technique. The major disadvantage of the intraoperative technique is the limited time available for language mapping. However, as we have indicated, multiple language functions at many sites can readily be assessed in 45 minutes or less, and all the information needed to plan a safe resection is usually provided. These intraoperative techniques have a number of advantages, including more flexibility in assessing essential areas of cortex and, once the essential areas have been identified, greater security in performing the resection. Intraoperative mapping also avoids the risks and cost of a second craniotomy for subdural grid placement and the risk for infection. For patients who can be managed with either technique, intraoperative stimulation mapping is the preferred method.

SUGGESTED READINGS

Binder JR, Swanson SJ, Hammeke TA, et al. Determination of language dominance using functional MRI: a comparison with the Wada test. *Neurology*. 1996;46:978.

Duffau H, Capelle L, Denvil D, et al. Usefulness of intraoperative electrical subcortical mapping during surgery for low-grade gliomas located within eloquent brain regions: functional results in a consecutive series of 103 patients. *J Neurosurg*. 2003;98:764.

Duffau H, Gatignol P, Mandonnet E, et al. New insights into the anatomo-functional connectivity of the semantic system: a study using cortico-subcortical electrostimulations. *Brain*. 2005;128:797.

Duffau H, Mortiz-Gasser S, Mandonnet E. A re-examination of neural basis of language processing: proposal of a dynamic hodotopical model from data provided by brain stimulation mapping during picture naming. *Brain Lang*. 2013;131:1-10.

Haglund MM, Berger MS, Shamseldin M, et al. Cortical localization of temporal lobe language sites in patients with gliomas. *Neurosurgery*. 1994;34:567.

Haglund MM, Ojemann GA, Schwartz TW, et al. Neuronal activity in human lateral temporal cortex during serial retrieval from short-term memory. *J Neurosci*. 1994;14:1507.

Hamberger MJ, Cole J. Language organization and reorganization in epilepsy. *Neuropsychol Rev*. 2011;21:240-251.

Hamberger MJ, Seidel WT, McKhann GM 2nd, et al. Brain stimulation reveals critical auditory naming cortex. *Brain*. 2005;128:2742.

Ilmberger J, Ruge M, Kreth FW, et al. Intraoperative mapping of language functions: a longitudinal neurolinguistic analysis. *J Neurosurg*. 2008;109:583.

Keifer JC, Dentchev D, Little K, et al. A retrospective analysis of a remifentanil/propofol general anesthetic for craniotomy before awake functional brain mapping. *Anesth Analg*. 2005;101:502.

Keles GE, Lundin DA, Lamborn KR, et al. Intraoperative subcortical stimulation mapping for hemispherical perirolandic gliomas located within or adjacent to the descending motor pathways: evaluation of morbidity and assessment of functional outcome in 294 patients. *J Neurosurg*. 2004;100:369.

Ojemann G, Mateer C. Human language cortex: localization of memory, syntax, and sequential motor-phoneme identification systems. *Science*. 1979;205:1401.

Ojemann G, Ojemann J, Lettich E, et al. Cortical language localization in left, dominant hemisphere. An electrical stimulation mapping investigation in 117 patients. *J Neurosurg*. 1989;71:316.

Papanicolaou AC, Simos PG, Breier JI, et al. Magnetoencephalographic mapping of the language-specific cortex. *J Neurosurg*. 1999;90:85.

Pouratian N, Cannestra AF, Bookheimer SY, et al. Variability of intraoperative electrocortical stimulation mapping parameters across and within individuals. *J Neurosurg*. 2004;101:458.

Quinones-Hinojosa A, Ojemann SG, Sanai N, et al. Preoperative correlation of intraoperative cortical mapping with magnetic resonance imaging landmarks to predict localization of the Broca area. *J Neurosurg*. 2003;99:311.

Rostomily RC, Berger MS, Ojemann GA, et al. Postoperative deficits and functional recovery following removal of tumors involving the dominant hemisphere supplementary motor area. *J Neurosurg*. 1991;75:62.

Roux FE, Boulanouar K, Lotterie JA, et al. Language functional magnetic resonance imaging in preoperative assessment of language areas: correlation with direct cortical stimulation. *Neurosurgery*. 2003;52:1335.

Ruge MI, Victor J, Hosain S, et al. Concordance between functional magnetic resonance imaging and intraoperative language mapping. *Stereotact Funct Neurosurg*. 1999;72:95.

Rutten GJ, Ramsey NF, van Rijen PC, et al. Reproducibility of fMRI-determined language lateralization in individual subjects. *Brain Lang*. 2002;80:421.

Sanai N, Mirzadeh Z, Berger MS. Functional outcome after language mapping for glioma resection. *N Engl J Med*. 2008;358:18.

Serafini S, Clyde M, Tolson M, et al. Multimodality word-finding distinctions in cortical stimulation mapping. *Neurosurgery*. 2013;73:36-47.

Skirboll SS, Ojemann GA, Berger MS, et al. Functional cortex and subcortical white matter located within gliomas. *Neurosurgery*. 1996;38:678.

Wada J, Rasmussen T. Intracarotid injections of sodium amytal for the lateralization of cerebral speech dominance. *J Neurosurg*. 1960;17:266.

Wood CC, Spencer DD, Allison T, et al. Localization of human sensorimotor cortex during surgery by cortical surface recording of somatosensory evoked potentials. *J Neurosurg*. 1988;68:99.

Woolsey CN, Erickson TC, Gilson WE. Localization in somatic sensory and motor areas of human cerebral cortex as determined by direct recording of evoked potentials and electrical stimulation. *J Neurosurg*. 1979;51:476.

Yingling CD, Ojemann S, Dodson B, et al. Identification of motor pathways during tumor surgery facilitated by multichannel electromyographic recording. *J Neurosurg*. 1999;91:922.

See a full reference list on ExpertConsult.com

70 Investigation of Human Cognition in Epilepsy Surgery Patients

Taylor J. Abel, Hiroto Kawasaki, and Matthew A. Howard III

Colocalization of the epileptogenic zone (EZ) with unresectable eloquent cortex is a crucial part of planning for resective epilepsy surgery. Over the years, this has necessitated the development of various techniques to localize functional cortex around the EZ, which in turn has led to groundbreaking discoveries that have profoundly influenced our understanding of the human brain–specifically and dramatically, the neural basis and organization of higher cognition.[1-5] Recording from intracranial electrodes (i.e., intracranial electroencephalography [iEEG]) that are implanted to localize epileptic foci and eloquent cortex provides an unprecedented opportunity to study the electrophysiologic correlates of human cognition with a combination of spatial and temporal fidelity unmatched by other techniques.[6,7] Recently, advances in iEEG signal analysis[8] have led to powerful new analytic approaches that have expanded the applications of iEEG recordings for cognitive research. As a result, there has been a dramatic increase in the number of iEEG manuscripts published in recent years, which demonstrates the increasing importance of intracranial recordings for both basic and clinical neuroscience research. In this chapter, we provide an overview of how intracranial recordings and other research methods can be used to study human cognition in epilepsy surgery patients.

SUBJECTS

Subjects are epilepsy patients with medically intractable seizures who undergo intracranial electrode implantation for localization of the EZ.[5] Indications for iEEG monitoring are determined by a multidisciplinary treatment team based on an extensive presurgical epilepsy work-up that includes seizure semiology; neuropsychological evaluation; neuroimaging data, including magnetic resonance imaging (MRI), computed tomography (CT), positron emission tomography, and single-photon emission computerized tomography; and neurophysiology data, including interictal scalp electroencephalography (EEG), video EEG, and magnetoencephalography. Research protocols must be approved by the institutional review board where the research will be taking place and must conform to the ethical guidelines of the institution's governing bodies. In all cases, the surgical plan for electrode placement must be directed exclusively by clinical criteria. A high ethical standard is essential to ensure that electrodes are not placed solely for research purposes, without the patient's explicit consent. Participation in iEEG research does not change the risks associated with intracranial recording for seizure localization. The research plan is explained to research participants in detail and informed consent is received. It is crucial that this informed consent process is open for the duration of the intracranial recording period because some patients may become fatigued and wish not to participate during some portions of their hospitalization. In our experience, most epilepsy patients find research participation enjoyable, a welcome distraction from the tedium of having to wait for seizures, and continue to participate during different intervals throughout the implantation period. Given the need for continuous informed consent and the practical considerations that accompany this requirement, most iEEG research is performed in adult subjects. However, some investigators have performed iEEG research in children.[9]

The cognitive status of each subject is evaluated extensively by a neuropsychologist prior to electrode implantation, as part of the routine clinical diagnostic work-up. To maximize generalizability of results, it is desirable that the subject's neuropsychological status fall within the normal limits (±2 standard deviations) of an age-matched control population. It is particularly important to ensure that subjects do not have impairment in the cognitive functions to be researched. Thus it is crucial that the cognitive functions of interest (e.g., memory, naming or recognition) are measured objectively prior to electrode implantation.

ELECTRODES

Several different types of clinical and combined clinical-research electrodes are available and can be used for intracranial seizure localization. Usually, the signals from a given electrode contact can be shared for both clinical monitoring and research purposes. The research recording should not disrupt the clinical EEG recording activity. There are two broad categories of intracranial electrodes: (1) subdural (cortical surface) electrodes in the form of either grid or strip, and (2) depth electrodes (Fig. 70-1). The extent of coverage is decided solely by clinical necessity based on the epilepsy work-up. Electrodes should cover a wide enough area to sufficiently include the suspected EZ. The specific implantation strategies vary widely. In the United States, traditionally surface grid and strip electrodes are used along with a small number of depth electrodes, whereas in some European countries (e.g., France and Italy), multiple depth electrodes are stereotactically implanted (stereo-EEG) in strategic locations to cover the hypothesized epilepsy networks. There is no evidence proving the clinical superiority of either of these specific strategies. Overall, the use of stereo-EEG is on the rise in the United States, possibly related to the lower surgical risk of this procedure.[10] Various institutions have adopted a range of safe and effective approaches, a discussion of which is beyond the scope of this chapter.

Many epilepsy patients who undergo invasive monitoring are suspected of having a temporal lobe focus: temporal lobe epilepsy (TLE) is the most common medically intractable focal epilepsy referred for surgical intervention at most centers. The EZ will need to be identified with the use of intracranial electrodes if data from the preoperative epilepsy work-up do not lead to a conclusive site of seizure origin, or if questions remain. Such questions may arise over the laterality (neocortical or medial) or location in the neocortex of TLE. The surface and deep structures of the temporal lobe on the side on which the seizure focus is likely to be located usually must be extensively covered, and some cases also require limited coverage of the contralateral temporal lobe. Contralateral coverage is usually achieved through a modified bur-hole exposure and placement of a small number of strip and depth electrodes. Such extensive recording from the temporal lobes provides an invaluable opportunity to investigate human brain functions that involve the temporal lobe and perisylvian brain regions.

In addition to standard clinical electrodes, customized research electrodes are available that can collect research data in addition to clinical iEEG data.[11,12] Some manufacturers customize

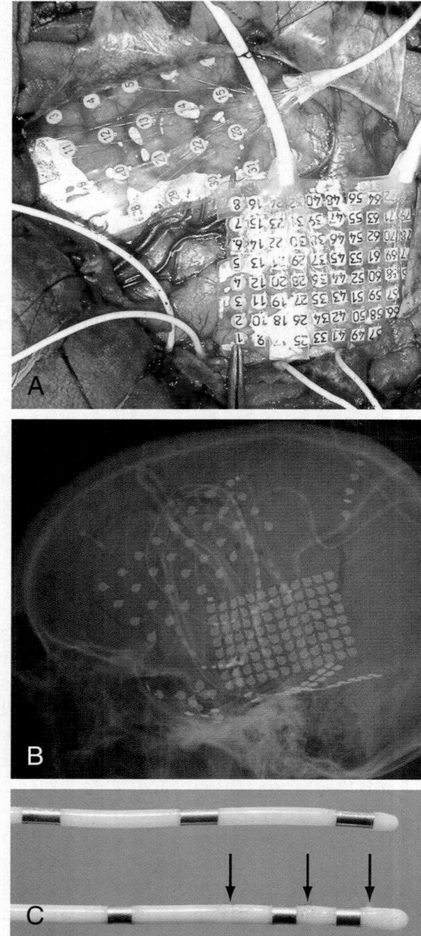

Figure 70-1. Grid and depth electrodes. A, Photograph taken during electrode implantation surgery shows a standard clinical grid electrode with an intercontact distance of 1 cm *(upper left)* and a high-density custom grid electrode with an intercontact distance of 5 mm *(lower right).* **B,** Lateral skull radiograph of the same subject as in **A. C,** Photograph showing a standard clinical depth electrode *(top)* and a custom depth electrode with multiple high-impedance microcontacts on the electrode shaft *(bottom). Arrows* indicate positions of microcontacts. *(**C,** Courtesy of Ad-Tech Medical Instrument Corporation, Racine, WI.)*

electrodes to suit specific research needs (e.g., Ad Tech Corporation, Racine WI). Most clinical grid or strip electrodes are constructed with a center-to-center intercontact distance of 1 cm. High-density electrodes with less than 5 mm of interelectrode distance provide better spatial resolution and can be fabricated without altering the clinical risk profile of the grid.[5] Depth electrodes can be customized to have several high-impedance microwire contacts in addition to clinical low-impedance contacts (see Fig. 70-1).[7,12,13] These high-impedance wires allow unit recordings (i.e., recording of neuronal spiking activities of individual neurons or groups of neurons) from the human brain and enable researchers to achieve distinct research objectives. Customized electrodes may have more electrode contacts and lead cables attached to them than standard clinical electrodes; however, single-tailed electrode cables can reduce the number of cables by combining multiple lead cables into a single bundle, thereby reducing the number of penetrations through the scalp.

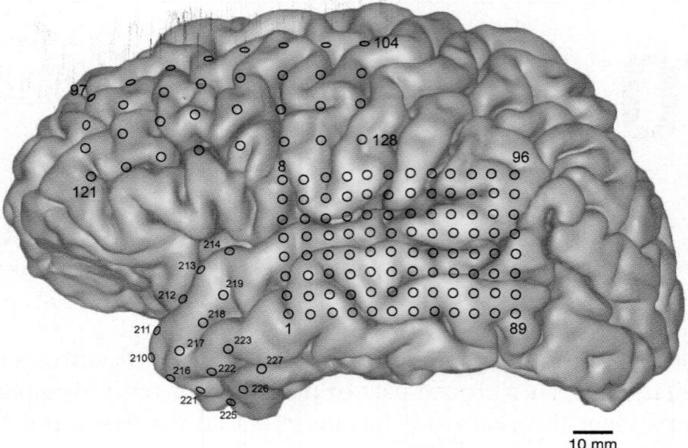

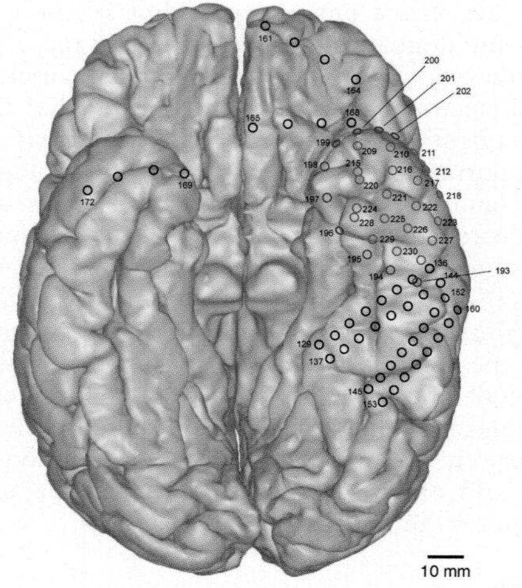

Figure 70-2. Positions of subdural contacts are mapped on a three-dimensional surface rendering of a preoperative magnetic resonance image.

Please see the expanded version of this chapter at ExpertConsult.com for a discussion of electrode implantation techniques and complication avoidance. 

Verification of Electrode Placement

Accurate localization of electrodes on the brain surface is crucial to correctly interpreting research data. Various techniques have been developed for this purpose.[20-22] Preimplantation and postimplantation CT, MRI, and photographs taken during both implantation and removal surgery are the three main tools used to localize the position of electrodes. Intracranially implanted electrodes create substantial artifact and distortion of images on CT and MRI, so extra caution is required when interpreting postimplantation imaging studies. Locations of subdural contacts on exposed cortical surface are best documented by photographs taken at the time of both implantation and explantation surgery. By matching the details of gyral and pial vessel anatomy, it is possible to localize surface contact locations with millimeter accuracy. The position of electrodes is mapped onto a three-dimensional rendering of the brain surface drawn from each subject's preoperative thin-slice MRI studies by referencing a pattern of gyri and sulci on the cortical surface (Fig. 70-2).

Localizing electrodes on the ventral surface of the brain is a difficult challenge because these electrodes cannot be viewed directly during surgery and consequently cannot be documented with intraoperative photography. MRI is also poorly suited for localizing ventral brain surface electrode contacts because of the susceptibility artifact created by the interface between the brain and skull base bony structures. On thin-slice CT, metal contacts create such large amounts of artifact that it is impossible to observe brain parenchyma around a contact; however, each electrode contact and its relationship to the outline of the skull can be seen by adjusting the level and width of the display window. Therefore, it is possible to determine the position of contacts in relation to skull base bony structures. Images from CT and MRI are coregistered according to mutual voxel similarity. Finally, the position of electrodes can then be mapped onto the surface rendering of the preoperative brain image.

Electrode contacts on a depth electrode can be localized in relation to surrounding brain structures by postimplantation MRI. Only the larger, low-impedance contacts can be clearly delineated on postimplantation MRI, but with knowledge of the spacing of microwires positioned between these contacts, it is possible to reliably estimate where these recording sites are within the brain, and these locations can be depicted on the preimplantation MRI study (see Fig. 70-2).[8,23,24] Development of techniques to automatically localize intracranial electrodes is underway.[22-24]

RESEARCH METHODS

Recording of Electrical Activity

It is technically feasible to obtain massive amounts of iEEG recording data from hundreds of electrode contacts implanted in each surgical patient. Modern signal processing methods also enable investigators to use a wide range of analytic methods to discern what physiologic events are relevant to the cognitive functions being investigated. The practical challenge is to carefully plan and execute experimental protocols so that the results are interpretable and the limitations of the methods used are appropriately recognized. The key practical data collection issues are reviewed and discussed here.

Modern clinical EEG recording equipment converts EEG potentials to digital signals and has the capability of recording more than 200 channels with high sampling rates. Depending on the specific research question being addressed, research recordings may require a wider frequency bandwidth. Although it is possible to use clinically recorded EEG signals for cognition research, it is better to have dedicated research recording equipment kept separately from the clinical EEG recording system so that research recordings can be performed more flexibly without disturbing the clinical EEG recording. In addition, the higher sampling rates (>1000 Hz) used for research recordings enable investigators to study high-frequency brain activity that is not captured with standard clinical sampling rates. It is ideal to use battery-driven head stages and optical isolation of the EEG signal from the research amplifier-recording system to minimize the chance of injuring subjects by accidental leakage of current. Most institutional review boards and hospital biomedical engineers require this level of electrical isolation for the patient. It is imperative to follow local or hospital safety regulations regarding use of research equipment on human subjects. Almost all modern neurophysiologic recording systems have a digital recording design. Recorded data can be stored on digital recording media such as hard disk drives or optical recording media. Stored data can be analyzed offline with various commercially available or custom-made software. Because data are shared among many researchers, it is important to separate a subject's identifiable information, such as name, initials, medical record number, or birthday, from the recorded data by replacing such information with unique research identifiers pursuant to regulations for the protection of personal health information.

At the University of Iowa and at many other institutions, a splitter box is used to feed the iEEG signal picked up from the subject simultaneously to both a clinical iEEG recording device and a research recording device. This makes it possible to conduct research recordings without disrupting clinical EEG monitoring. Researchers can use dedicated research recording equipment, and research cables can be disconnected for subjects' convenience when research activity is not being performed.

Contamination by ambient electronic noise can become a problem, more so for the research recordings than for the clinical EEG recordings. Among various sources of noise, power line noise is typically the most disruptive and requires the greatest attention to eliminate. Although notch filtering may effectively reduce power line noise, such filtering distorts the EEG waveform and may affect the result of frequency analysis. Therefore, every possible effort must be made to reduce noise contamination at its source. At the University of Iowa, research participants are housed in a specially constructed, electromagnetically shielded room in the National Institutes of Health–funded Clinical Research Unit. A significant amount of medical and nonmedical equipment is necessary for both the medical treatment and the convenience of the subjects, who spend several days and possibly up to 2 weeks in the room. It is useful to unplug as many power cords as possible from alternating current power outlets when research recording is being performed. If any equipment can be run on battery power, it should be turned to battery mode. Shielding EEG connection cables can reduce the extent of noise contamination. If some equipment has to be powered by alternating current, careful attention must be paid to keep the power cords away from the EEG recording equipment and connecting cables. Hospital-grade power cords must be used for all equipment, if possible, not only to reduce the noise level but also to reduce the chance of injuring the patient by leakage of current.

Cognitive Task

In properly selected patients with chronic intracranial electrodes, almost any test of cognitive function can be performed while iEEG recordings are under way. These tasks can range from language functions to complex social behavior, including ethical decision making, as well as economic or financial decision making. Because these cognitive functions are highly developed in humans, most of these functions are difficult to study in a meaningful way in nonhuman animals. Emotion is another complex cognitive function that offers potential advantages for study in humans rather than other species because investigators can directly ask subjects how they are feeling and what kinds of emotions they are experiencing during experimental manipulations.

The following points must be considered carefully when a cognitive task is designed: (1) factors of interest and nuisance factors, (2) timing of stimulus delivery and response, (3) generation and recording of the timing signal, (4) order of stimulus presentation or response, and (5) number of trials.

The factors of interest must be defined clearly. After defining them, it should be determined how many levels each factor has and which nuisance, or confounding, factors need to be controlled, in accordance with the principles of cognitive psychology research. A randomized block design is often used to control contamination with nuisance factors. For example, the development of fatigue or fluctuation of attention level can be problematic in many cognitive tasks. When the effect of conditions A and B is to be compared, if experimental sessions are conducted sequentially by delivering condition A in the first session and condition B in the second session, it is likely that levels of fatigue and attention will not be the same between these sessions. In this situation, if a difference were found in EEG data for each session, it would be difficult to assess whether these distinctions were due to differences in experimental conditions or differences in fatigue or attention level. In such cases, randomly interleaving the experimental conditions makes it possible to effectively equalize time-dependent nuisance factors (e.g., fatigue and attention level) between conditions A and B.

The timing of experiments must be planned carefully when the researcher wishes to detect correlations between the cognitive function of interest and EEG responses. Some cognitive functions are altered by antiepileptic drugs; therefore, experiments investigating these functions would be optimally performed when the subject has been weaned off these drugs. Alternatively, experiments involving electrical stimulation of the brain may trigger seizures, which may be different from the subject's habitual seizures and affect excitability of the brain, thus disturbing localization of the EZ. The length of the interstimulus or intertrial interval should be based on considerations of what cognitive function is of interest and which region of the brain is being studied. For example, for investigation of lower level sensory cognition in a primary sensory cortex, the interstimulus interval can be shorter than that required for investigation of highly complicated cognitive function in the higher order cortex in the temporal or frontal lobe. The sequence of stimulus presentations needs to be considered carefully to avoid unwanted effects on the EEG response that are related to stimulus order. When more than two stimuli are presented or more than two different responses are required, the order of their occurrence should be randomized or counterbalanced, and the frequency of occurrence should also ideally be equalized.

It is necessary to conduct a sufficient number of trials to obtain robust statistical power. This issue is particularly important and challenging for experiments performed on epilepsy surgery patients. In most instances, these patients can maintain a high level of attention and fully participate in complex behavior tasks for less than 30 minutes per experimental block. Power analyses also suggest that around 30 trials are needed to accurately estimate the mean power and variance in the higher frequencies of the iEEG.[25] This limitation has to be considered carefully when deciding how to balance the tradeoff between a smaller number of repetitions of a larger number of different stimuli and a larger number of presentations of a smaller number of stimuli. In general, the smaller the effect of experimental manipulation on the iEEG response, the larger the number of trials that are needed to detect and characterize the response induced.

Please see ExpertConsult.com for discussions of brain stimulation, cooling, and physiologic measurement research techniques in epilepsy surgery patients.

COGNITIVE STUDIES

A very wide number of cognitive functions can be assessed using iEEG.[48] Broadly, these include language (including speech,[49,50] reading,[51] and auditory processing[52]), memory (including recognition[53] and spatial navigation[54]), emotion,[55,56] prefrontal control,[57,58] and sensorimotor processing[6,8] among many others. The scope of this literature is too broad to be covered in one chapter. Instead we focus here on three separate experiments from our group that illustrate the approach and the power of iEEG recordings in addressing fundamental questions about cognitive operations in humans.

Cognitive Studies in the Medial Temporal Lobe

The medial temporal lobe is often involved in the generation of seizures in surgically treatable epilepsy patients[59]; therefore, in many cases the iEEG recording electrodes are placed in this brain region. Neural structures in the medial temporal lobe play important roles in cognitive functions related to emotion, memory, and learning. For these reasons, the medial temporal lobe is one of the brain regions most extensively investigated with intracranial electrodes in epilepsy patients.[48] Various recording techniques with modified electrodes permit finely detailed analysis of single-unit, multiunit, and local field potential (LFP) activity in conjunction with sophisticated cognitive tasks. The direct measurements of electrical neuronal activities with fine temporal resolution of the intracranial recordings is a valuable complement to the noninvasive research methods.

With this experimental approach, neurons in the medial temporal lobe, including the hippocampus, parahippocampal gyrus, and entorhinal cortex, were found to respond to visual stimuli of specific items.[2] The activity of a subset of these neurons was correlated with behavioral performance, in this case whether the visual stimulus was successfully memorized. The response patterns of memory performance–related neurons differed between the hippocampus and entorhinal cortex, thus suggesting that particular medial temporal subregions may contribute differently to various aspects of the memory and learning processes.[60] Category-specific neuronal responses and also entity-specific neuronal responses were observed.[61] This finding was groundbreaking because it provided some of the first evidence of a human neuron responding to complex but specific stimuli, a phenomenon known as a grandmother cell. Some of these neurons responded not to what subjects were seeing but to what subjects perceived, imagined, or attended.[62,63] There were also neurons that were activated by spontaneous emergence of conscious recollection.[63]

Involvement of the medial temporal lobe in spatial navigation has also been investigated extensively. Two different kinds of neurons were found, one representing "place" cells that respond to specific spatial locations and the other representing "view" cells that respond to specific views of task-relevant landmarks.[54] There was a difference in distribution of these cells between the hippocampus and the entorhinal cortex. The activities of some place cells were modulated by specific combinations of goals of task and place; for example, certain cells were activated only when a particular house was found in a particular location. To extend this work, a subsequent study replicated previous findings from animals to demonstrate grid-like neuronal activity during spatial navigation in the human hippocampus, entorhinal cortex, and cingulate cortex.[64] Thus, neurons were found to have peaks in firing with particular spatial geometries related to their location in space. This grid-like pattern of neuronal spiking may provide a mechanism through which humans are able to triangulate their position to effectively navigate through space. Additional work has revealed the existence of movement-related theta oscillations in the hippocampus and the neocortex, and these theta oscillations were significantly correlated with various cognitive functions.[1]

LFPs in the medial temporal lobe were used for the investigation of mental activity as well. Gamma-band activity in the parahippocampal gyrus and ripple oscillations (100 to 200 Hz) in the hippocampus and entorhinal cortex were found to be correlated to awake and sleep states.[65] Ripples in the rhinal cortex were found to be correlated to memory performance.[66] Functional coupling between these regions, which can be measured by coherence in gamma-band activities, was found to be correlated to successful memorization.[67,68]

Also in the medial temporal lobe, the amygdala is known to be involved in defense mechanisms represented by the fight-or-flight reaction. A large volume of animal and human research has demonstrated that fearful emotion is modulated by activity of the amygdala.[69-72] It has been shown that gamma-band activity in the amygdala is enhanced by aversive pictures.[55] Neurons in the amygdala were found to be involved in processing of the face,[73] and neurons that show atypical responses to faces were found in the amygdala of patients with autism spectrum disorders, in which social dysfunction is one of the core symptoms.[56] Neurons in the amygdala showed representation of subjectively perceived emotional expression of faces.[74] The amygdala-specific research

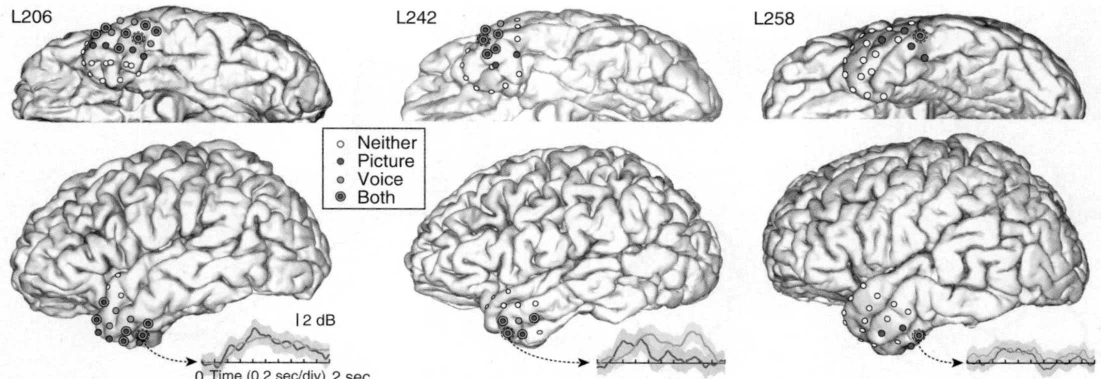

Figure 70-3. Spatial distribution of beta-band event-related band power (ERBP) responses from the left anterior temporal lobe. Sites that exhibited significant responses during picture naming and voice naming are shown in magenta and cyan, respectively. *Open circles* denote recording sites that were included in the analysis on anatomic grounds, but did not feature significant beta response to either stimulus. Half of activated electrode sites exhibited a heteromodal response pattern (i.e., significant induced power for both picture and voice naming). The time course of beta-band ERBP responses during picture and voice naming is plotted for three representative heteromodal sites (*dashed circles*) in magenta and cyan, respectively. *Thick lines* and *shaded areas* represent mean ERBP across intracranial electroencephalography frequencies and its 95% confidence interval, respectively. *(From Abel T, Rhone A, Nourski NV, et al. Direct physiologic evidence of a heteromodal convergence region for proper naming in human left anterior temporal lobe.* J Neurosci. *2015;35:1513-1520.)*

carried out in neurosurgical research subjects provides unique insight into the precise timing and electrophysiologic nature of amygdala activation.

Cognitive Studies in the Anterior Temporal Lobe

The anterior temporal lobe (ATL), which includes the temporal pole, plays a key role in temporal lobe seizure networks[75] and is also implicated in cognitive functions such as proper naming,[11,76,77] face recognition,[78] and social function.[79] Studying the physiology of the ATL is limited using noninvasive techniques because of susceptibility artifact present on functional MRI at the skull base.[80,81] Intracranial electrodes are not subject to susceptibility artifact and allow for investigation of the ATL with precise spatiotemporal dynamics. A challenge of placing iEEG electrodes on the ATL is the curvilinear shape of the ATL and its relatively confined position within the middle cranial fossa.[11] At the University of Iowa, we have designed a novel electrode array that provides dense and consistent coverage of ATL cortex for localization of epileptic cortex and physiologic investigation of cognitive functions.[11] Alternatively, it is also possible to place multiple strip electrodes over the ATL, which can also provide iEEG electrode coverage.[82] Recently, the use of iEEG has provided important insight into the role of the ATL in human cognition, specifically the integration of visual and auditory input for naming.

Using iEEG, both large-scale and single-unit responses have been observed from the ATL during naming tasks.[83,84] Using implanted depth electrodes, Chan and associates identified cortex in the medial ATL with significant averaged LFP differences during a naming task.[83] A subset of the cortical sites with significant LFP responses also showed specificity for semantic categories (e.g., animals and objects), providing physiologic evidence for category-specific responses in the medial ATL.

An outstanding and debated question of ATL function is its putative role in the integration of visual and auditory naming. Numerous lesion studies have demonstrated naming deficits for not only visual,[77] but also auditory (i.e., voice), naming[76] after language-dominant cortico-amygdalohippocampectomy.[85] Despite the consistent finding of transmodal deficits with ATL lesions, whether or not transmodal representations exist within the human ATL has remained debated, with lesion studies suggesting heteromodal cortical representation of naming dispositions[86] and neuroimaging findings suggestive of unimodal (i.e., modality-specific) subdivisions in the human ATL.[86] To investigate this question, recordings from the left ATL during both a visual and an auditory proper naming task were performed.[87] Examination of power in the time-frequency domain demonstrated robust beta-band responses from the lateral and ventromedial ATL during both visual and auditory proper naming (Fig. 70-3). Half of the total significant response sites showed significant responses during both picture and voice naming, demonstrating heteromodal representation of naming dispositions in the human ATL. Interestingly, examination of the high-gamma band also shows significant responses from the ATL; however, heteromodal responses in the high-gamma band appear to be the exception rather than the rule,[84] and the definitive role of the temporal lobe in intermodal integration of semantic information remains unclear.

Cognitive Studies in the Ventromedial Prefrontal Cortex

The ventral and medial sector of the frontal lobe has undergone extensive evolutionary development in humans in comparison to other primates. This region is implicated in the most human of behaviors, such as social interaction, moral judgment, fairness, self-control, prediction of the future, and decision making in conflict situations.[88-90] A number of functional imaging studies have shown representation of these cognitive processes in this region of the brain.[91-98] Individuals who sustain damage to this region of the brain do not exhibit deficits in cognition that can be measured with conventional neuropsychological tests; however, they often exhibit inappropriate social behavior and poor judgment with regard to their social and financial well-being.[90,99] Their choices are more influenced by immediate rewards even though the consequences of their choices are predicted to cause substantial disadvantage to them.[100,101]

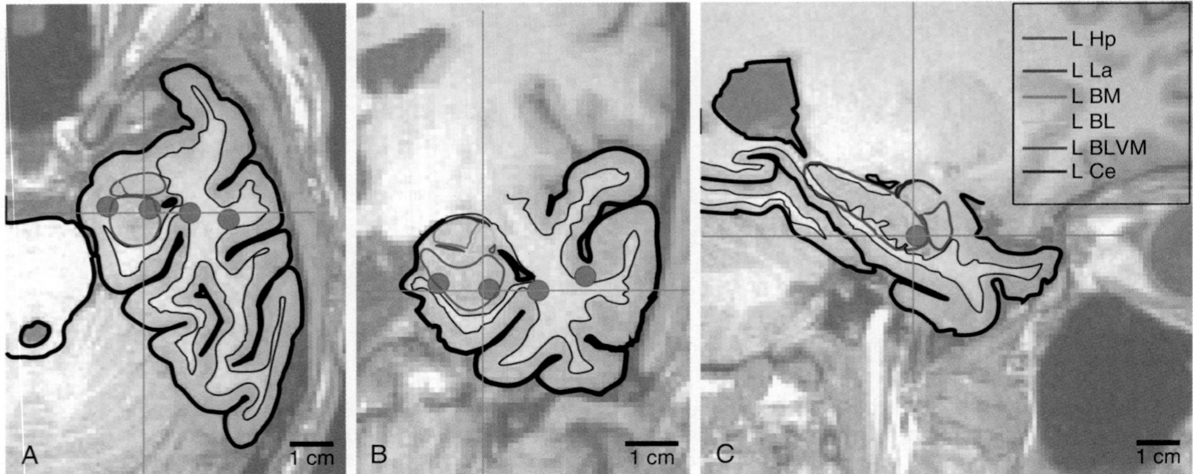

Figure 70-4. Neuroanatomic localization of recording sites *(red circles)* on three-dimensional reconstructions of the brain of a research subject in axial **(A)**, coronal **(B)**, and sagittal **(C)** views. *Colored lines* represent delineation of brain nuclei on three-dimensional brain reconstruction demonstrating electrode localization (L) relative to individual brain nuclei: BL, basolateral nucleus; BLVM, basolateral nucleus, ventromedial part; BM, basomedial nucleus; Ce, central nucleus; Hp, hippocampus; La, lateral nucleus.

Anatomic studies have shown that the ventral and medial sectors of the prefrontal cortex have abundant connections with the sensory areas of multiple modalities and subcortical structures, including the hypothalamus, thalamus, amygdala, and brainstem.[102-104] The connectivity of this region supports the proposed function of this area, specifically the processing of various multimodal sensory inputs to modulate behavior, including visceral and autonomic function, to match behavior to fit appropriately to the situation in which an individual is placed.

The vast majority of this knowledge has been derived from lesion and functional imaging studies in humans and electrophysiologic studies in animals. Because the frontal lobe and functions of the frontal lobes are the most developed in humans, there is a compelling rationale to investigate these functions in humans (and not in nonhuman primates). Some of the functions in this region, such as ethics, morality, and emotional valence, are extremely difficult to study in other animal systems because it remains debatable whether and to what extent such functions exist in animals. Functional imaging methods provide an overview of wide brain regions with superior spatial resolution, up to a millimeter in scale. However, the greatest disadvantage of functional imaging methods, as well as lesion methods, is poor temporal resolution. In contrast, electrophysiologic studies in animals have the advantage of investigating finely detailed neural responses with precise time resolution, up to the millisecond scale, with simultaneous precision in spatial specificity.

Intracranial recording in epilepsy patients has the potential to fill the gap between lesion and functional imaging studies in humans and electrophysiologic studies in animals. Although the extent of the field of view is restricted to the vicinity of the area covered by electrodes, the electrophysiologic method in humans provides an incomparable level of time resolution and superb spatial resolution that can localize the neural activity of interest with unsurpassed precision.

Investigation of Emotion Representation

The single-unit recording technique has been applied by us to the investigation of responses in the ventromedial prefrontal cortex while the subject is viewing pictures of complex emotional scenes.[3,4] Custom-made depth electrodes with eight high-impedance microcontacts along with four low-impedance clinical iEEG contacts were implanted stereotactically. To avoid unwanted influence of seizure activity on subjects' cognitive function, we conducted research recordings only when subjects had not suffered seizures within the 12 hours preceding the recording session. The locations of recording sites were determined with the methods described previously in this chapter, and the location of each electrode contact was delineated on the preimplantation MRI studies (Fig. 70-4).

We investigated unit responses in the medial and ventral frontal cortex to visual stimuli that depicted pleasant, neutral, or aversive stimuli derived from the International Affective Picture System, which have established valence and arousal values.[105] The aversive stimuli include pictures of war, mutilated bodies, burn victims, and so on. These pictures are visually heterogeneous and do not have any low-level or simple visual features in common that might explain the different responses to different emotion categories that we observed. In one subject, unit responses specific to aversive stimuli with very brief latencies (120 and 140 msec) (Fig. 70-5)[4] were found. Rapid responses of this latency are most likely explained by feed-forward responses from the occipitotemporal visual cortices to the medial and ventral frontal cortex without any intervening feedback modulation.[106] The unit responses to aversive pictures showed a biphasic response pattern consisting of an initial rapid and brief decrease in firing and a later prolonged increase in activity. The later prolonged excitation is a possible reflection of recursive responses with multiple feed-forward and feedback interactions among multiple brain sites anatomically connected to the medial and ventral frontal cortex. These responses with different timing may reflect early coarse categorization of the emotional significance of visual scenes and later more detailed neural processing related to evaluation of the biologic value to an individual, prediction of consequences, triggering of autonomic responses, and planning of future action. We recorded unit responses to pictures from the International Affective Picture System battery in the bilateral medial and ventral frontal cortex of three more subjects. Although aversive pictures recruited predominantly more neurons than did any other stimulus category in all sites, there was no clear topography of preferred emotional content. Figure 70-6 shows the distribution of emotion-selective neurons at four different sites in these regions from all four subjects.[3] It is noteworthy that a minority of units responded to pleasant and neutral pictures at

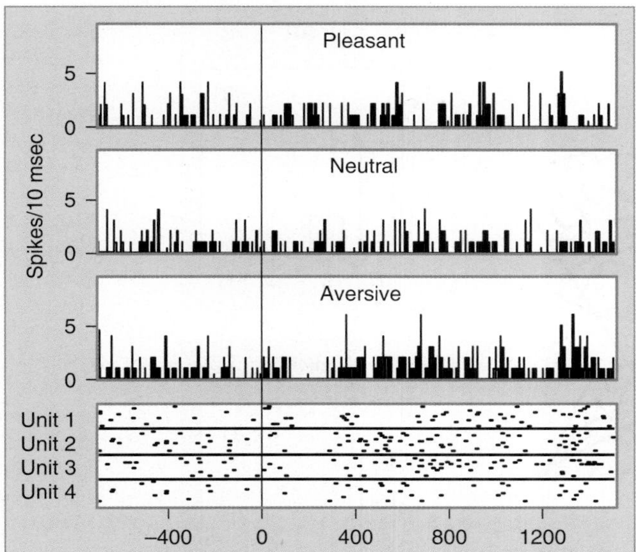

Figure 70-5. Composite peristimulus time histograms *(top)* and raster plots *(bottom)* from four individual neurons recorded medially in response to emotional scenes (stimulus onset, *vertical line*). Raster plots are shown for presentations of each of 11 aversive stimuli. These units show a brief decrease in firing as early as 120 msec after the onset of aversive pictures, followed by a prolonged increase in firing. *(From Kawasaki H, Kaufman O, Damasio H, et al. Single-neuron responses to emotional visual stimuli recorded in human ventral prefrontal cortex.* Nat Neurosci. *2001;4:15-16.)*

all locations. This provides evidence that information about the emotional content of visual scenes is intermingled within the medial and ventral frontal cortex.

Other investigative methods, including the blood oxygen level–dependent response, magnetoencephalography, and electrocorticography, require many neurons to fire synchronously in order to be detected. Therefore, if only a very small fraction of neurons is active within a region, such activity cannot be detected by these methods. Conversely, it is possible to detect such underrepresented activities with unit recordings, as shown in the aforementioned study.[105] These findings are consistent with current knowledge about this region gained through a large amount of research in animal models and functional imaging studies in humans.[107,108] Neurons within the orbitofrontal cortex have been shown to respond selectively to stimuli of a variety of sensory modalities based on their emotional significance, rewarding or punishing valence, or motivational value.

Investigation of Expectation of Reward and Punishment

The Iowa Gambling Task is a well-validated test for identifying and quantifying functional deficits associated with damage to the ventromedial prefrontal cortex. Deficits in this region have otherwise been very difficult to detect with other cognitive tasks designed to investigate frontal lobe function.[109] Subjects are asked to choose cards from four decks in order to win or lose money. Each deck is assigned a different probability of gain and variance of win-loss value for each draw of a card. For example, one deck consists of a majority of a moderate amount of wins but occasional large losses, and in the long run the sum of draws would end up losing money. Another deck consists of many small wins and occasional moderate losses; however, the sum of draws from this deck would eventually end up winning money. Subjects do not know which deck is a winning deck and which one is a losing deck when they start the task. After drawing cards a number of times, subjects develop an expectation of what is likely to happen (win or lose) when they choose a card from a given deck on the basis of experience. Furthermore, subjects' behavior comes to be influenced by the expectation: subjects tend to choose more from decks where they feel that they will make more money in the long term and to avoid decks that may incur larger wins but lose money in the long term. Such expectation is probably unconscious in the early stages of its development. We applied a reinforcement-learning algorithm to model the process of development of expectation and choice selection behavior.[58] The model incorporates the probability of selecting from each deck and the degree of expectation. The model estimated the value of all choices, which parallels the expectation from each deck. A reward prediction error is an index for measuring the discrepancy between expectation and reality and is derived by subtracting the estimation from the result of a draw.

We presented the Iowa Gambling Task to a patient who had multiple electrodes in his frontal lobes.[58] He performed the task as normal subjects would. He initially chose from all decks; however, with experience he learned to choose from good decks and to avoid choosing from bad decks. This provided evidence that the ventral and medial parts of the subject's prefrontal cortex were functioning normally. While the subject was performing the task, we recorded LFPs at three sites in the right frontal lobe with two custom depth electrodes: the granular paracingulate cortex (area 10m), the middle frontal gyrus, and area 11l. The custom depth electrode had multiple high-impedance microwire contacts. To record LFPs, we performed bipolar recording with a pair of closely positioned microcontacts at each recording site; in this way, far field potentials would effectively cancel out.

We found that reward prediction error correlated with the alpha-band component of the event-related potential recorded in the ventral and medial prefrontal cortex. No such correlation was found in other parts of the frontal lobe or in other frequency bands. Further analysis revealed that this correlation was significant only when a subject chose the risky decks but punishment was not delivered (Fig. 70-7). In other words, the alpha-band component of the EEG in this region was positively correlated with the magnitude of the difference between what the subject obtained and the subject's expectation only when the subject expected punishment but was unexpectedly rewarded. These findings are consistent with other studies suggesting that the ventral and medial prefrontal cortex is involved in updating the expectations of punishment or reward and in reinforcement learning.[110-112]

CONCLUSION

Intracranial recording of epilepsy patients provides invaluable and unique opportunities for conducting cognitive neuroscience research in humans. The data collected during these experiments cannot be obtained with alternative, noninvasive methods. Because of an abundance of opportunities to record from the medial temporal lobe, the majority of research up to now has been focused on the activities of neurons in this region in relation to learning and memory, spatial navigation, and emotional responses. Recently, application has been expanded to recordings of other regions and to the investigation of higher order cognitive processes such as imagery,[63] awareness,[62] and consciousness.[113,114] The development of hybrid depth electrodes that allow unit recording and the availability of more than a few hundred channels of multichannel electrocorticographic recording, affordable high-speed personal computers, and advanced analytic techniques will permit investigation of more complicated cognitive functions that involve multiple distributed brain locations and multiple scales of neural signals. Analysis of the dynamic interaction of distributed neural systems on a millisecond scale with

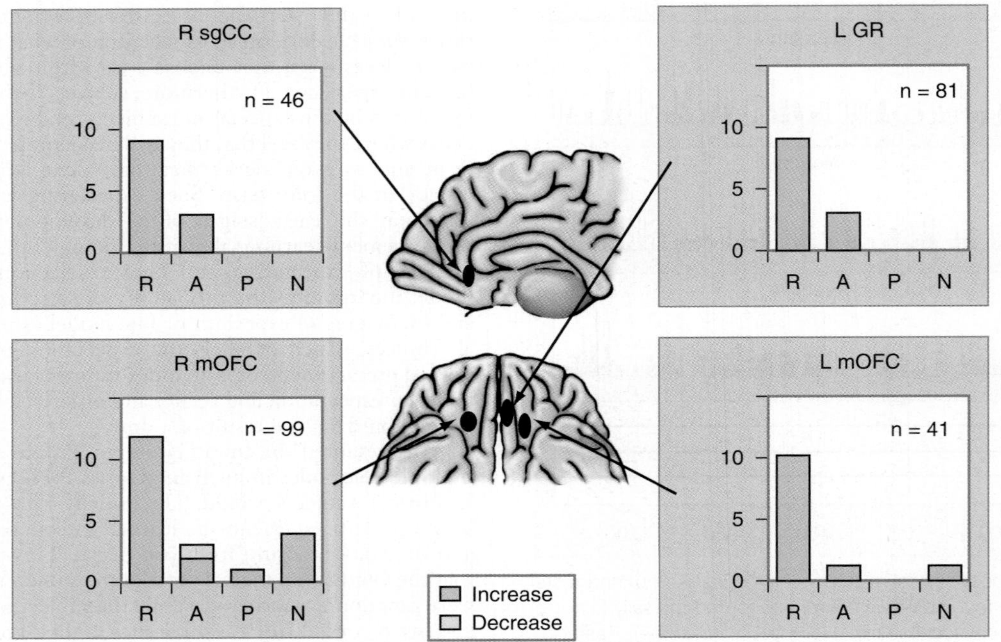

Figure 70-6. Summary of recording sites at which significant selective responses to emotional stimuli were found. The *upper middle panel* shows a projection of the recording site of the right subgenual cingulate cortex (R sgCC) onto the sagittal surface, and the *upper left panel* indicates the number of neurons with particular response selectivities found in this location. The *lower left,* the *upper right,* and the *lower right panels* show bar graphs of the number of selective neurons found in the right medial orbitofrontal cortex (R mOFC), the left gyrus rectus (L GR), and the left medial orbitofrontal cortex (L mOFC), respectively. Projections of the recording sites onto the ventral surface of the brain are shown in the *lower middle panel. Pink bars* represent neurons that increased their firing rates in response to visual stimuli, and the *tan bar* represents a neuron whose response showed a decrease in firing rate. Each bar graph also indicates the total number of neurons that are isolated for each recording site. Response selectivities: A, selective for aversive pictures; N, selective for neutral pictures; P, selective for pleasant pictures; R, nonspecific visual response. *(Modified from Kawasaki H, Adolphs R, Oya H, et al. Analysis of single-unit responses to emotional scenes in human ventromedial prefrontal cortex.* J Cogn Neurosci. *2005;17:1509-1518.)*

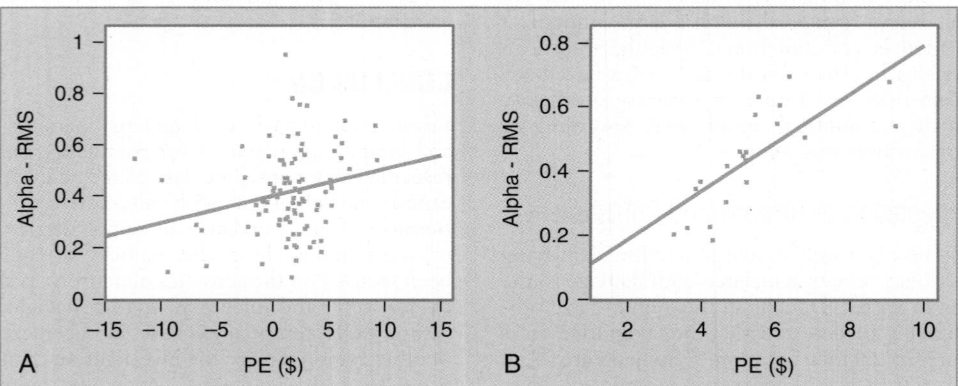

Figure 70-7. A, A scatter plot shows correlation between reward prediction error (PE, *x*-axis) and the magnitude of the alpha-band component (*y*-axis) of the event-related potential (ERP) recorded in the ventral and medial prefrontal cortex. **B,** A scatter plot shows the same correlation as in **A,** but restricted to trials from risky decks. Reward prediction error correlated with the alpha-band component of the ERP recorded in the ventral and medial prefrontal cortex. Further analysis revealed that this correlation was significant only when a subject chose the risky decks but punishment was not delivered. RMS, root mean square. *(From Oya H, Adolphs R, Kawasaki H, et al. Electrophysiological correlates of reward prediction error recorded in the human prefrontal cortex.* Proc Natl Acad Sci U S A. *2005;102:8351-8356.)*

good spatial specificity is possible only with intracranial recording. This technique has promising applications in the investigation of such higher order human functions as the neuroscience of economy, ethics, social interaction, altruism, mood, motivation, the construction of ideas, language, and so on. The data obtained with this technique will be potentially applicable to the treatment of disease conditions such as pathologic gambling, antisocial behavior, autism, anxiety disorders, and memory disorders, to name a few.

SUGGESTED READINGS

Abel TJ, Rhone AE, Nourski KV, et al. Mapping the temporal pole with a specialized electrode array: technique and preliminary results. *Physiol Meas*. 2014;35:323-337.

Abel TJ, Rhone AE, Nourski KV, et al. Direct physiologic evidence of a heteromodal convergence region for proper naming in human left anterior temporal lobe. *J Neurosci*. 2015;35:1513-1520.

Arya R, Mangano FT, Horn PS, et al. Adverse events related to extraoperative invasive EEG monitoring with subdural grid electrodes: a systematic review and meta-analysis. *Epilepsia*. 2013;54:828-839.

Cameron KA, Yashar S, Wilson CL, et al. Human hippocampal neurons predict how well word pairs will be remembered. *Neuron*. 2001;30:289-298.

Ekstrom AD, Kahana MJ, Caplan JB, et al. Cellular networks underlying human spatial navigation. *Nature*. 2003;425:184-188.

Engel AK, Moll CK, Fried I, et al. Invasive recordings from the human brain: clinical insights and beyond. *Nat Rev Neurosci*. 2005;6:35-47.

Fell J, Klaver P, Lehnertz K, et al. Human memory formation is accompanied by rhinal-hippocampal coupling and decoupling. *Nat Neurosci*. 2001;4:1259-1264.

Fried I, MacDonald KA, Wilson CL. Single neuron activity in human hippocampus and amygdala during recognition of faces and objects. *Neuron*. 1997;18:753-765.

Fried I, Wilson CL, Maidment NT, et al. Cerebral microdialysis combined with single-neuron and electroencephalographic recording in neurosurgical patients. Technical note. *J Neurosurg*. 1999;91:697-705.

Gelbard-Sagiv H, Mukamel R, Harel M, et al. Internally generated reactivation of single neurons in human hippocampus during free recall. *Science*. 2008;322:96-101.

Greenlee JD, Oya H, Kawasaki H, et al. Functional connections within the human inferior frontal gyrus. *J Comp Neurol*. 2007;503:550-559.

Hermes D, Miller KJ, Noordmans HJ, et al. Automated electrocorticographic electrode localization on individually rendered brain surfaces. *J Neurosci Methods*. 2010;185:293-298.

Howard MA, Volkov IO, Granner MA, et al. A hybrid clinical-research depth electrode for acute and chronic in vivo microelectrode recording of human brain neurons. Technical note. *J Neurosurg*. 1996;84:129-132.

Howard MA, Volkov IO, Mirsky R, et al. Auditory cortex on the human posterior superior temporal gyrus. *J Comp Neurol*. 2000;416:79-92.

Kawasaki H, Adolphs R, Oya H, et al. Analysis of single-unit responses to emotional scenes in human ventromedial prefrontal cortex. *J Cogn Neurosci*. 2005;17:1509-1518.

Kawasaki H, Kaufman O, Damasio H, et al. Single-neuron responses to emotional visual stimuli recorded in human ventral prefrontal cortex. *Nat Neurosci*. 2001;4:15-16.

Kreiman G, Koch C, Fried I. Category-specific visual responses of single neurons in the human medial temporal lobe. *Nat Neurosci*. 2000;3:946-953.

Kreiman G, Koch C, Fried I. Imagery neurons in the human brain. *Nature*. 2000;408:357-361.

Oya H, Adolphs R, Kawasaki H, et al. Electrophysiological correlates of reward prediction error recorded in the human prefrontal cortex. *Proc Natl Acad Sci U S A*. 2005;102:8351-8356.

Oya H, Kawasaki H, Howard MA, et al. Electrophysiological responses in the human amygdala discriminate emotion categories of complex visual stimuli. *J Neurosci*. 2002;22:9502-9512.

Quiroga RQ, Mukamel R, Isham EA, et al. Human single-neuron responses at the threshold of conscious recognition. *Proc Natl Acad Sci U S A*. 2008;105:3599-3604.

Rutishauser U, Tudusciuc O, Wang S, et al. Single-neuron correlates of atypical face processing in autism. *Neuron*. 2013;80:887-899.

See a full reference list on ExpertConsult.com

71 Intracranial Monitoring: Subdural Strip and Grid Recording

Jared M. Pisapia, Gregory G. Heuer, and Gordon H. Baltuch

Intracranial electroencephalography (icEEG) is a tool used to aid in the surgical localization of seizure foci in patients with medically refractory partial epilepsy. Such techniques are employed when the findings of noninvasive modalities, such as detailed history and physical examination, video electroencephalography (EEG), and anatomic and functional neuroimaging studies are discordant or inconclusive in identifying an epileptogenic focus. One approach to intracranial monitoring is the surgical implantation of electrodes configured in strips or grids into the subdural space overlying the cortex. The placement of strips and grids directly overlying the cortex overcomes several of the limitations of scalp EEG in localizing the epileptic focus.[1] Detection of cortical electrical activity at the scalp is impeded by the poor conductance of the skull and its high impedance.[2] Unlike electrodes used in scalp EEG, subdural electrodes are separated from the cortex only by cerebrospinal fluid (CSF), which is much more conductive than bone. For scalp EEG, only large spikes or sharp waves that are widely distributed over the cortical surface can be detected at the scalp. Being closer to the source of electrical activity, subdural electrodes yield a much higher resolution of small loci of surface activity than scalp electrodes can provide. In fact, only 10% of cortical spikes that encompass a source area of less than 10 square centimeters are detected on scalp EEG.[3] Thus, subdural electrodes can detect a very small focal seizure prior to its propagation outside the ictal onset zone, which might otherwise appear as a diffuse or nonlocalizable ictal onset on scalp EEG.[4] Finally, subdural recordings have a lower signal-to-noise ratio because most artifacts seen on scalp EEG do not exist in subdural recordings or are present at lower amplitude.

Subdural strip and grid electrodes may remain in place for several days, collecting data during ictal and interictal periods in order to identify the seizure focus. While in place, the electrodes may also be used to identify functionally eloquent cortex to further guide subsequent epilepsy surgery. Once sufficient data have been collected, the implanted hardware is removed surgically and a tailored resection or disconnection may be performed at that time, as indicated. In this chapter, we discuss the indications, hardware, surgical technique, complications, and outcomes related to intracranial monitoring for epilepsy using subdural strips and grids. Stereo-electroencephalography (SEEG), including the use of depth electrodes, is an alternative and often complementary method of intracranial monitoring in epilepsy; it is discussed in Chapter 72.

INDICATIONS

The success of epilepsy surgery depends on the accurate identification of the location of the *epileptogenic zone*, which is defined as the smallest region of cortex that will result in freedom from seizure following resection. Patients with epilepsy undergo an exhaustive work-up seeking to identify this brain region. After detailed history and physical examination are performed, patients undergo outpatient EEG followed by an inpatient scalp EEG-video monitoring session, in which the seizure semiology (or the physical and experiential manifestations of seizures) and the corresponding EEG recordings are captured. In up to 25% of patients with epilepsy, however, scalp EEG recordings fail to adequately localize the epileptogenic zone.[4] In these cases, extensive neuropsychological testing and alternate noninvasive studies may be used to provide supplementary data, which include magnetic resonance imaging (MRI), functional MRI, single-photon emission computed tomography, positron emission tomography, MRI spectroscopy, and magnetoencephalography. Concordant data from these studies define the epileptogenic foci, and patients with discrete lesions, such as tumors, vascular malformations, and hippocampal sclerosis, and concordant data proceed to resective surgery. However, despite advances in imaging modalities, findings of noninvasive methodologies may be discordant or inconclusive in localizing the seizure focus in many patients. In these patients, invasive monitoring, including strip and grid electrodes, is used.

Intracranial monitoring is indicated in cases in which noninvasive studies have failed to precisely localize an epileptogenic zone. Clinical scenarios in which icEEG monitoring is typically used include ambiguous or discordant scalp EEG findings, dual pathology (more than one possibly epileptogenic lesion, e.g., the presence of hippocampal sclerosis and dysplasia in the temporal neocortex[5]), and nonlesional epilepsy.[4] Additionally, icEEG may be used in the patient with a focal lesion when the epileptogenic properties of the lesion extend beyond its limits and in the patient with multiple lesions, as in tuberous sclerosis, in which each lesion may have epileptogenic properties. In addition, subdural strips and grids may be required for lateralization plus localization in patients with bilateral mesial temporal sclerosis, bilateral independent temporal lobe spikes, or frequent interictal spikes contralateral to a single ictal focus.[6-8] Finally, invasive monitoring is commonly used in candidates for reoperation after failed epilepsy surgery.

In addition to localizing the epileptogenic focus, intracranial strips and grids may be implanted for mapping eloquent cortex within or near the epileptogenic focus.[4] Although cortical mapping can be performed in the operating room, extraoperative mapping using implanted subdural electrodes offers several advantages. First, more complex cognitive functions can be mapped in implanted patients, in comparison with the limited tasks that can be mapped in the operating room. Second, in contrast to intraoperative mapping, which is generally limited to 1 to 2 hours, implanted subdural strips and grids usually remain in place several days, permitting significantly more time for testing. Third, subdural EEG offers a means of brain mapping in children or adults who are unable to cooperate with an awake craniotomy. However, the use of intracranial monitoring for the purpose of mapping must be balanced against the advantages of intraoperative mapping, which include increased flexibility in relation to simulation sites and the ability to continuously perform mapping as the resection proceeds, including mapping of subcortical white matter pathways when deeper resections are undertaken. Lastly, the risks of placement of subdural grids and strips are not

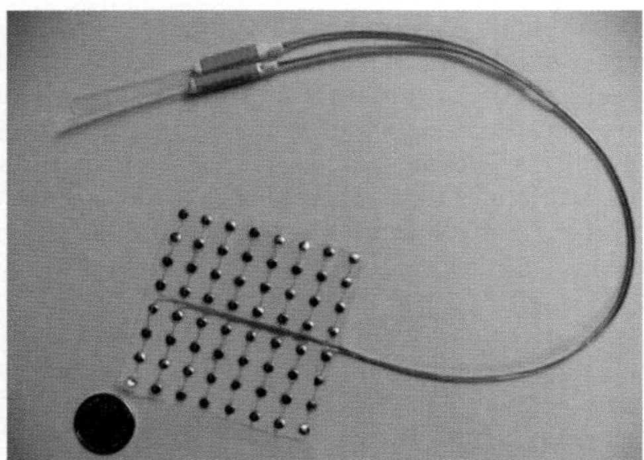

Figure 71-1. A standard 8 × 8-subdural grid consisting of equally spaced platinum-iridium electrodes with a U.S. quarter coin for size comparison. *(From Nair DR, Burgess R, McIntyre CC, et al. Chronic subdural electrodes in the management of epilepsy.* Clin Neurophysiol. *2008;119:11-28.)*

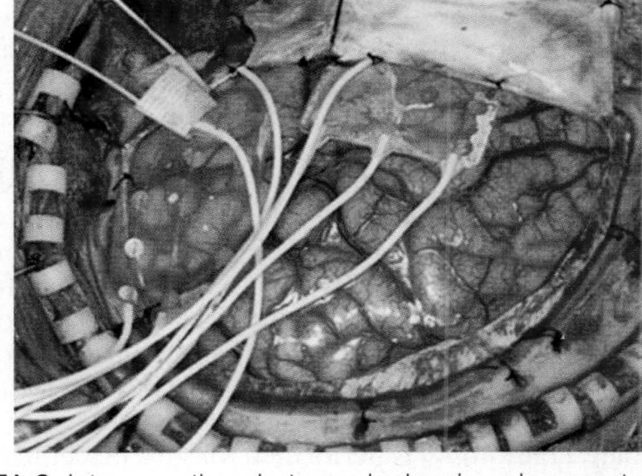

Figure 71-2. Intraoperative photograph showing placement of grids overlying the cortical surface. *(From Van Gompel JJ, Worrell GA, Bell ML, et al. Intracranial electroencephalography with subdural grid electrodes: techniques, complications, and outcomes.* Neurosurgery. *2008;63:498-505; discussion 505-506.)*

insignificant—complication rates reaching as much as 10% in some series—and in fact may be a greater cause of surgical morbidity in some series than the actual respective procedure.[9-11] These risks should be considered in the overall decision making as well.

HARDWARE

Linear strips and rectangular grids consist of multiple conductive circular electrodes embedded in a thin sheet of polymeric silicone (Silastic) or polytetrafluoroethylene (Teflon). Commonly used electrodes measure 0.127 mm in thickness and 2 to 4 mm in diameter, depending on the interelectrode distance. They may be made of platinum-iridium, nichrome (80% chrome, 20% nickel), silver, or stainless steel.[4,12] Platinum-iridium or nichrome electrodes produce significantly less artifact during MRI studies than stainless steel.[12] Electrodes are uniformly spaced with a center-to-center interelectrode distance of 2.5 to 10 mm, as shown in Figure 71-1.[4] Favorable electrode characteristics include biocompatibility, flexibility, insolubility, and impermeability to ionic species. Strips are configured as small as 1 × 4 electrodes or as large as 2 × 8 electrodes.[13] Grid arrays may have up to 256 electrodes in various configurations. Strips and grids may be custom-made with gaps over large cortical veins. Grids are flexible and may be shaped so that the edges of a grid conform to the cortical surface. For instance, an interhemispheric grid may be curved to follow the convexity; furthermore, such grids may be designed to have electrode contacts on both faces, enabling monitoring of both hemispheres using the same single grid applied adjacent to the falx—one subdural and one epidural in location.

PREOPERATIVE PLANNING

Preoperative noninvasive studies are used to generate a hypothesis as to the most likely location of the epileptogenic zone. This hypothesis guides the implantation of intracranial electrodes. Strip and grid placement not guided by a hypothesis is more likely to result in removal of hardware without resection.[4] In addition to expected seizure location, considerations in positioning electrodes include the extent of the seizure onset zone, alternative seizure onset hypotheses, and presumed localization of eloquent cortex.[14] Implantation strategies also attempt to minimize the number of electrodes and craniotomies. However, inadequate sampling due to insufficient electrode coverage may preclude accurate detection of the epileptogenic zone.[12]

ELECTRODE CONFIGURATION AND TYPE

Multiple electrode assemblies and positions may be used for intracranial monitoring. Subdural strips and grids record from the cortical surface. Strips are useful in cases of partial epilepsy in which the epileptogenic lobe cannot be localized.[13] Subdural strips may be implanted via a bur hole and can be placed over several lobes, and the localization data generated can guide a more tailored craniotomy specifically targeting the epileptogenic lobe. More commonly, such strips are placed bilaterally to lateralize the epilepsy. An advantage of such electrodes is that they may be removed at the bedside. Strips may also be used to supplement grid coverage. Subdural grids cover a larger cortical area, such as cerebral convexities, than strips, as shown in Figure 71-2. Wide coverage makes grids well suited for the study of diffuse epileptic foci, which are commonly seen in extratemporal epilepsy, and for functional cortical mapping. However, grid implantation requires a larger craniotomy. In addition, an epileptogenic zone appearing at the edge of a grid must be interpreted with caution and may warrant a new study or the placement of additional electrodes.[15]

Depth electrodes have been placed stereotactically into brain parenchyma to study deep structures, such as the medial temporal lobe. However, other groups describe the safe and reliable placement of an anteromedial strip electrode to evaluate medial temporal lobe structures in patients in whom temporal lobe epilepsy is suspected.[16] In this procedure, the strip electrode is advanced around the temporal pole. It follows the curvature of the lesser wing of the sphenoid bone to its final position along the medial basal temporal lobe, thereby providing coverage of the parahippocampal gyrus and entorhinal cortex along the long axis of these structures. In some cases, depth electrodes may be used in combination with subdural electrodes, as in periventricular nodular heterotopias or other deep-seated cortical dysplasias, in which it is unclear whether the nodule or the overlying dysplastic cortex is epileptogenic. In such cases, a depth electrode is inserted into the area of heterotopias and a grid is placed over the associated cortex. Stereo-electroencephalography and depth electrodes are discussed in further detail in Chapter 72.

SURGICAL TECHNIQUE

Subdural strips and grids are placed with the patient under general anesthesia. In general, intraoperative electrocorticography is not essential for placement of grids and strips, although it may help with optimization of placement. Benzodiazepines and barbiturates interfere with icEEG, whereas sevoflurane and dexmedetomidine have no known effects on intracranial recordings.[17] Most subdural grids are placed under direct visualization to avoid bridging veins or bone deformities and thus require a craniotomy. Additional smaller grids or strips may be slid over the brain under the margins of the craniotomy without direct visualization, especially at orbitofrontal, inferior-temporal, and interhemispheric locations.[4] Bur holes may be used for strip insertion if grids are not being placed during the same procedure. When planning bur hole location, the surgeon must consider future skin incisions for craniotomy for grid placement or resections.

A standard craniotomy is performed for grid placement on the basis of the desired cortical location for intracranial monitoring (Video 71-1). A large C-shaped craniotomy flap is commonly elevated. The size of the craniotomy is larger than the size of the grid to be placed. The dura is opened and the grid or strip electrodes are placed with forceps to direct them to their desired location, as shown in Figure 71-3. Gentle irrigation is injected under the subdural strip as it passes over the brain surface.[13] For strips placed without direct visualization, any resistance encountered likely represents a bridging vein, especially in the parasagittal region, and should prompt the surgeon to stop and change trajectory. Depth electrodes may be considered an alternative to subdural electrodes if severe adhesions between the dura and the brain are encountered. Care is taken to avoid injury or sacrifice of large draining cortical veins, and grid arrays may be cut or trimmed as needed. Slits should be made in the Silastic material of the grids to allow the hardware to conform better to the shape of the brain. Sutures are placed along the edges of the grid to secure it to the dura and avoid future displacement. Impedance may be measured to determine whether electrodes are making adequate contact with the cortex, and intraoperative recordings may be obtained from the electrodes before closure. Cables arising from the electrodes on grids and strips are carefully tagged in order to ensure correct identification of the source data. They are bundled together and tunneled subcutaneously to exit at a site several centimeters from the initial skin incision. A purse-string suture is placed at the exit site to reduce the likelihood of CSF leak. Additional sutures are placed to securely anchor the cables to the skin and to incorporate a strain-relief connector.

Closure technique varies among surgeons. Following subdural grid placement, some groups reapproximate the dura with or without a pericranial autograft, especially when the number of electrodes placed is high,[15,18] whereas others leave the dura open because of concerns about delayed cerebral edema and increased intracranial pressure.[19] This latter approach leads to a much greater risk of CSF leak and is discouraged—fastidious dural closure with a dural graft may decrease the risk of CSF leak and also the compression of the brain by the mass of subdural electrodes. Similarly, the bone flap may be left off, left tethered with craniotomy plates without screws in the bone flap itself,[20] or replaced in the standard fashion with plates and screws. Violence of seizure, age, and expectation for intracranial hypertension should be considered in the determination whether to replace the bone flap at the time of grid implantation.[21] In cases in which the bone flap is not replaced initially, it is usually kept in frozen storage and then replaced after grid removal and surgical resection. The risk of bone flap infection appears to be higher in cases in which the flap is left off than in those in which it is replaced, and this finding should be factored into the decision making.[22] The skin is closed in standard fashion, and the head is wrapped in a bulky dressing that includes a submandibular sling for increased security.

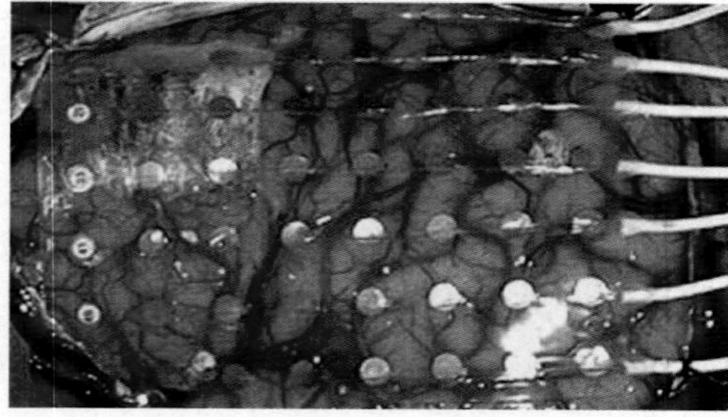

Figure 71-3. Intraoperative photograph showing placement of subdural grid overlying the cortical surface. *(From Mahvash M, Konig R, Wellmer J, et al. Coregistration of digital photography of the human cortex and cranial magnetic resonance imaging for visualization of subdural electrodes in epilepsy surgery.* Neurosurgery. *2007;61(suppl 2):340-344; discussion 344-345.)*

ELECTRODE LOCALIZATION

Knowledge of the exact location of each electrode in reference to the cortical surface is important for planning a surgical resection, and there are multiple techniques for capturing such data. Color photographs and sketches may be made of the cortical surface before and after subdural strip and grid implantation to record the spatial relationship between the hardware and the cortical surface. Another approach is to take a high-resolution digital photograph of the exposed cortex before and after grid placement. Photographs capture individual details about local anatomy and gyral patterns that may be lost on more advanced imaging. The location of each electrode on the postimplantation photograph is plotted manually on the preimplantation photograph. The resulting digital photograph is then superimposed on a three-dimensional reconstructed MRI brain surface model using rendering software, as shown in Figure 71-4.[23-26] The MRI surface rendering is semitransparent, allowing for the anatomy or lesions underlying the grid to be visualized. Results

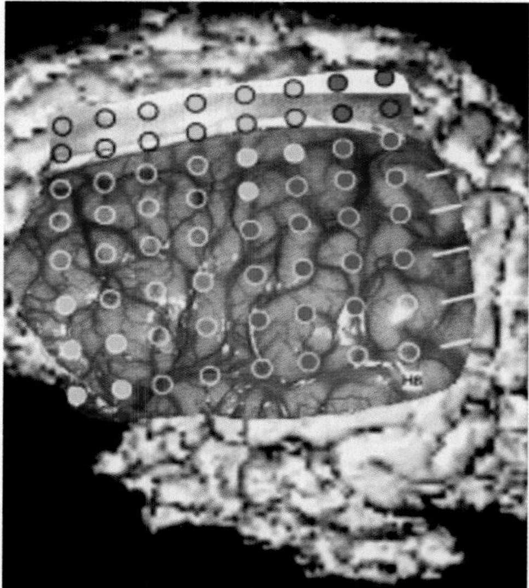

Figure 71-4. Intraoperative digital photograph is superimposed on a three-dimensional reconstructed magnetic resonance imaging brain surface model with the use of rendering software. *(From Mahvash M, Konig R, Wellmer J, et al. Coregistration of digital photography of the human cortex and cranial magnetic resonance imaging for visualization of subdural electrodes in epilepsy surgery.* Neurosurgery. *2007;61(suppl 2):340-344; discussion 344-345.)*

of extraoperative functional mapping of eloquent cortex may be overlaid on the images. Thus, at the time of surgical resection, the coregistered image provides the position of the electrode in exact relation to the epileptogenic focus and the cortical surface. Coregistration of the electrodes on a postoperative head computed tomography (CT) scan with a preoperative MRI,[27,28] by automated segmentation methods may be performed,[29] and neuronavigation[30] may be used to facilitate tailored resections. A comprehensive evaluation of the various methods of electrode localization showed that simple coregistration of the postimplantation CT with the MRI is imprecise in many instances and may lead to false localization of the electrodes on the cortical surface landmarks.[26]

POSTOPERATIVE COURSE

Following surgery, some groups allow patients to recover for 24 hours in an intensive care unit before beginning recordings, with or without an intracranial monitor,[19,20] whereas other groups begin recording immediately in the epilepsy monitoring unit so as not to miss any relevant recording data.[31] Implanted electrodes typically remain in place for 5 to 10 days, but they have been reported to remain in place for up to 2 to 4 weeks.[32] Most groups continue perioperative antibiotics while hardware remains in place and for three doses after removal of the strip and grid equipment.[18,21,33-35] In a prospective study of 350 patients undergoing subdural strip electrode monitoring, no significant differences were seen in infection rates between those patients who received antibiotics throughout the duration of monitoring and those who did not.[36] Variability also exists in the use of steroids, such as dexamethasone, which may be avoided because of the perceived risk of infection or decrease in the frequency of habitual seizures.[32,37] Most surgeons administer steroids in order to decrease postimplantation cerebral swelling and the risk of related complications.[35,38,39] An increase in complication rates among patients receiving steroids has not been detected in studies.[20] It has been associated only with a decrease in postoperative headaches.[31] A large meta-analysis showed a trend toward more uniform use of antibiotics and steroids in the perioperative period for subdural strips and grid implantation.[40]

Postoperative imaging paradigms vary. Some groups obtain anterior-posterior and lateral cranial plain radiographs, as in Figure 71-5, or a head CT scan immediately after implantation to document the location of the strips and grids.[21] A head CT scan enables evaluation for a possible life-threatening hematoma but should not be viewed in isolation, but rather in the context of the patient's overall condition. An MRI is much more effective at identifying extra-axial hematomas and other complications, such as a cortical contusion—which may also sometimes manifest on imaging studies in a delayed fashion. Some groups obtain an intraoperative head CT scan, which allows for immediate replacement of malpositioned electrodes and may obviate a postoperative scan to confirm electrode position.[41]

INTRACRANIAL RECORDING AND MAPPING

Patients are transferred to the epilepsy monitoring unit for prolonged intracranial EEG and video recording. Doses of antiepileptic drugs are gradually reduced in order to increase the likelihood of seizure occurrence. Intravenous anticonvulsant drugs may be administered if needed. The duration of monitoring depends on the number of, localization of, and consistency between seizure semiology and the electrographic pattern.[42] Once monitoring is completed and the location of the epileptogenic focus has been identified, anticonvulsant medications are restarted and titrated up to preoperative doses. Brain mapping using subdural grids may then be performed, and patients may be given additional antiepileptic drugs just prior to cortical stimulation. For mapping the function of cortex just below the implanted grid, a stimulus is applied to one grid electrode while a distant grid electrode acts as the reference point. Stimulation is applied to each electrode in a systematic way. Stimulus intensity and other parameters may be altered with the goal of bringing about a functional change, such as speech arrest.[43] A comparison of the map of eloquent cortical regions and the location of the epileptogenic focus is used to guide epilepsy surgery. Brain mapping using subdural grids is especially useful in pediatric patients, in whom certain functions, such as language, can be tested only in the awake state. Also, subdural monitoring allows for multiple detailed tasks to be performed for testing that would otherwise be difficult to do with the patient in an MRI tube.

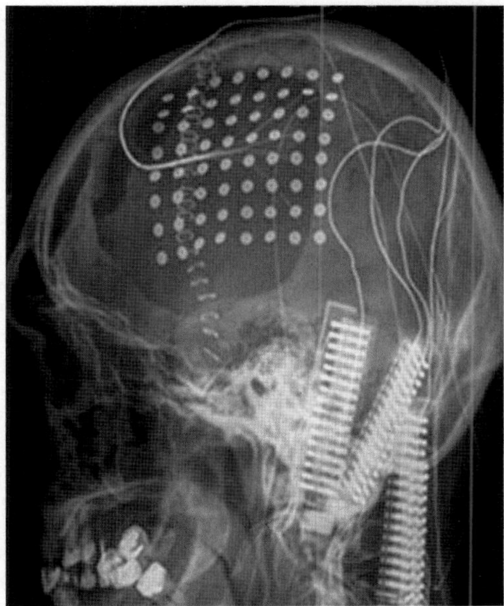

Figure 71-5. Lateral cranial radiograph showing grid placement. *(Modified from Sweet JA, Hdeib AM, Sloan A, et al. Depths and grids in brain tumors: implantation strategies, techniques, and complications.* Epilepsia. *2013;54(suppl 9):66-71.)*

Two-stage monitoring approaches are most common and consist of an initial subdural electrode implantation stage, a period of invasive monitoring, and then an electrode removal and resection stage. Subdural strips may be removed at the bedside with gentle traction and without reopening the incision. Subdural grids, however, require reopening of the incision in the operating room. A three-stage approach that includes a middle stage for resection and reimplantation may be used in select pediatric patients with extratemporal or nonlesional epilepsy, previous surgical failure, suspected overlap of eloquent cortex and the epileptogenic zone, or areas of multiple seizure onset.[44]

COMPLICATIONS

Intracranial monitoring is by definition an invasive procedure, and it is associated with several neurological and medical complications.[9] Intracranial hematoma and infection are the most common complications related to implantation of strips and grids. Hematomas are attributed to tearing of bridging veins in the subdural space. Not all hematomas are symptomatic, and collections of blood around or under subdural grids are commonly encountered at the time of grid removal in asymptomatic patients. Among 2356 patients undergoing strip and grid placement, intracranial hemorrhage occurred in 3.9% of patients, and subdural hematoma was the most common type of intracranial bleed, occurring in 1.7% of patients.[40] Approximately one third of all patients with any type of intracranial bleed were symptomatic, necessitating surgical evacuation. Earlier studies of grid placement reported higher rates of symptomatic subdural hematomas, with subdural hematomas occurring in up to 5.7%[18] and 7.8% of patients,[32] whereas a later study reported a rate of 2.6%.[45] Infection rates ranged from 0.85%[46] to 7.9%.[42] In a meta-analysis that examined eight studies evaluating infection, the pooled prevalence of infection was 2.3% of patients.[40] Infections included bacterial meningitis, brain abscess, subdural empyema, and cerebritis. The pooled prevalence of superficial wound infection was 3.0%, and the pooled prevalence of osteomyelitis was 1.8%. Most cases required wound débridement or cranioplasty.[47] Several groups routinely perform cultures on specimens from electrodes, the epidural space, and the CSF at the time of hardware removal. Many surgeons treat patients with positive culture results with appropriate antibiotics for 4 weeks, even if the patients are asymptomatic.[32] The most common microorganisms encountered in relation to strip and grid monitoring are coagulase-negative *Staphylococcus*, *Staphylococcus aureus*, and *Enterobacter*. According to multiple case-series, up to 3.5% of patients require an additional procedure for management of complications, with evacuation of intracranial hemorrhage the most common unplanned surgical intervention.[40]

Nonoperative complications are generally minor and transient. Transient neurological deficits such as dysnomia, aphasia, mild hemiparesis, and paresthesias may occur after intracranial electrode implantation.[48] However, permanent neurological deficits have been reported.[36] For example, infarction occurred in three patients within the first week of monitoring and led to permanent upper extremity paresis, aphasia, and homonymous hemianopsia in one study.[49] Although rare, five deaths have been reported in relation to subdural intracranial monitoring.[20,34,49] Most cases of mortality were preceded by increased intracranial pressure due to vascular compromise. Additional complications and their reported incidence include postimplantation cerebral edema requiring premature strip and grid removal (2.3%),[21,32,50] CSF leak (12%-20%),[33,51] status epilepticus (<1%),[39] temporalis fibrosis (3%),[33] hypertrophic scar formation (26%),[51] and venous thromboembolic disease.[40] Common adverse events include fever, headache, and nausea. Strip electrode fracture occurred in 1 of 112 patients in one series,[18] and iatrogenic electrode dysfunction occurred in 5% of patients in another single-center study.[33]

RISK FACTORS

Several variables have been studied to identify potential risk factors associated with complications. In multiple studies, larger number of electrodes was independently associated with an increased incidence of complications, the rate of adverse events nearly doubling with the use of 67 or more electrodes.[40] Similarly, other studies have identified the number of electrode contacts as the most common independent risk factor for intracranial hematoma.[18,42,49] Other variables associated with more frequent complications include grid size, duration of monitoring (more than 14 days), number of electrode wires, age over 18 years, prior craniotomy, multiple implantations, and presence of bur holes in addition to craniotomy.[20,39,40,49] However, in other case series, larger grid arrays and longer monitoring intervals did not correlate with increased risk of complications.[15,18] Furthermore, gender, number of seizures during monitoring, number of lobes covered, bone flap replacement, and use of perioperative steroid therapy had no association with complication rates.[21,39] Other variables were assessed for an association with infection. Although an increased number of electrodes was independently associated with higher infection rate,[40] the duration of monitoring had no relationship with infection rate.[47] Also, no clear association between CSF leak and infection rate has been noted.[35]

Factors that were found to significantly correlate with positive epidural culture results in one study of 38 patients included use of more than 100 electrodes or of more than 10 cables, more than 14 days of implantation, and more than one cable exit site[42]; however, 2 of the 5 patients with positive culture results were asymptomatic. Finally, one study reported that the number of electrodes and grid size were positively associated with rate of subsequent blood transfusion,[51] although another study found no significant correlation between number of electrodes and need for blood transfusion.[18] No differences in intracranial hematoma or infection have been detected between pediatric and adult patients with epilepsy undergoing intracranial monitoring, although the rate of CSF leak may be higher in pediatric patients.[31,47,52] Although one study found no significant association between complication rate and poor outcome in terms of freedom from seizures after epilepsy surgery,[15] another study noted that occurrence of a complication during invasive monitoring was associated with a significant likelihood of a complication at resection surgery.[45]

OUTCOMES

The effectiveness of subdural strip and grid implantation and its ability to localize the epileptogenic focus is ultimately judged from the rates of durable freedom from seizures following epilepsy surgery. Compared with patients who have a clear seizure focus, patients who are undergoing strip and grid implantation may have a less favorable outcome because they inherently have an epileptogenic focus that is more difficult to localize, hence the need for intracranial monitoring.[53] Indeed, several studies have shown that the need for intracranial monitoring is associated with a lower likelihood of seizure freedom after surgery.[50] Despite this selection bias, high rates of freedom from seizures have been obtained in patients undergoing strip and grid monitoring. The ability to detect an epileptogenic focus ranges from 79% to 99% with icEEG.[21] In a study of 133 patients undergoing subdural monitoring with a minimum of 2 years of follow-up, 65 patients (48.9%) were seizure free (Engel epilepsy surgery outcome class I), 31 patients (23.2%) had a significant reduction in seizures (Engel class II), 20 patients (15%) had a greater than 50% reduction in seizures (Engel class III), and 17 patients (12.8%) had no improvement (Engel class IV).[15] Similarly, among 58 patients with medically refractory partial epilepsy undergoing strip and grid monitoring, 34 patients (57%) had Engel class I outcome, 6 patients (14%) had Engel class II outcome, 15 patients (24%) had Engel class III outcome, and 3 patients (5%) had Engel class IV outcome.[54] Additional studies showed rates of good seizure outcome (Engel classes I or II) ranging from 77.6%[20] to 85%.[21,33] Patients with a history of prior epilepsy surgery had a worse outcome than those undergoing resection for the first time.[55] Size of the implanted grid, total number of electrodes and grids, and the site of implantation were not associated with seizure outcome.[20] Extratemporal epilepsy and cortical epilepsy are more common in children, along with cortical developmental malformations, but in a series of 23 children and 38 adults undergoing monitoring and surgery, complications and outcomes were similar in the two groups.[47]

CONCLUSION

Subdural strip and grid electrodes are important tools used to help localize the epileptogenic focus in patients with neocortical epilepsy in whom results of noninvasive testing, especially scalp EEG, are discordant or inconclusive. Intracranial monitoring may also be used to map eloquent cortex in order to further facilitate tailored resection. Strips and grids are options for intracranial EEG, although other types of electrodes, such as depth electrodes, may be used as part of an alternative or complementary approach. Regardless of the type of electrode used, intracranial monitoring studies should be hypothesis-driven, with the location of electrode placement guided by data from preoperative noninvasive studies. Strip and grid electrodes have been extensively studied and, although relatively safe, they are associated with complications such as subdural hematoma and infection. Advances in electrode design, surgical technique, and postoperative monitoring, however, have led to reductions in complication rates over time. Intracranial monitoring provides vital data upon which subsequent epilepsy surgery is based, leading to high rates of durable seizure control.

SUGGESTED READINGS

Arya R, Mangano FT, Horn PS, et al. Adverse events related to extraoperative invasive EEG monitoring with subdural grid electrodes: a systematic review and meta-analysis. *Epilepsia*. 2013;54:828-839.

Mahvash M, Konig R, Wellmer J, et al. Coregistration of digital photography of the human cortex and cranial magnetic resonance imaging for visualization of subdural electrodes in epilepsy surgery. *Neurosurgery*. 2007;61(suppl 2):340-344, discussion 344-345.

Nair DR, Burgess R, McIntyre CC, et al. Chronic subdural electrodes in the management of epilepsy. *Clin Neurophysiol*. 2008;119:11-28.

Van Gompel JJ, Worrell GA, Bell ML, et al. Intracranial electroencephalography with subdural grid electrodes: techniques, complications, and outcomes. *Neurosurgery*. 2008;63:498-505, discussion 505-506.

Voorhies JM, Cohen-Gadol A. Techniques for placement of grid and strip electrodes for intracranial epilepsy surgery monitoring: pearls and pitfalls. *Surg Neurol Int*. 2013;4:98.

Wellmer J, von Oertzen J, Schaller C, et al. Digital photography and 3D MRI-based multimodal imaging for individualized planning of resective neocortical epilepsy surgery. *Epilepsia*. 2002;43:1543-1550.

Yang PF, Zhang HJ, Pei JS, et al. Intracranial electroencephalography with subdural and/or depth electrodes in children with epilepsy: techniques, complications, and outcomes. *Epilepsy Res*. 2014;108:1662-1670.

See a full reference list on ExpertConsult.com

72 Intracranial Monitoring: Stereo-Electroencephalography Recording

Jorge Gonzalez-Martinez and Patrick Chauvel

One of the main goals of epilepsy surgery is the complete resection (or complete disconnection) of the cortical areas responsible for the primary organization of the patient's epileptogenic activity. This area is also known as the *epileptogenic zone* (EZ). As the EZ can overlap with functionally important cortical areas (eloquent cortex), preservation of these necessary brain functions is another goal of any surgical resection in patients with medically refractory epilepsy.[1-7]

As successful resective epilepsy surgery relies on accurate preoperative localization of the EZ, a presurgical evaluation is necessary to obtain the widest and most accurate spectrum of information from clinical, anatomic, and neurophysiologic aspects, with the ultimate goal of performing an individualized resection for each patient. Presurgical evaluation tools include the analysis of seizure semiology, video-scalp electroencephalography recordings, magnetoencephalography, magnetic resonance imaging (MRI), and other neuroimaging modalities (functional MRI, ictal single-photon emission computed tomography [SPECT], positron emission tomography [PET] techniques).[6,8] The use of these methods is usually complementary, and results are interpreted in conjunction, in the attempt to compose a localization hypothesis of the anatomic location of the EZ. When the noninvasive data are insufficient to define the EZ, extra-operative invasive monitoring may be indicated. The stereo-electroencephalography (SEEG) is one of the extra-operative invasive methods that can be applied in patients with medically refractory focal epilepsy to define the EZ anatomically and the possible related functional cortical areas. The clinical aspects of SEEG method and technique will be discussed in this chapter.

HISTORICAL PERSPECTIVE AND PRINCIPLES

Human cerebral stereotaxis was conceptualized and initiated in 1947 by Spiegel and Wycis, and its use in recording from deep brain structures has been reported since 1950.[9] Since then, stereotactic placement of intracerebral electrodes have gained progressive popularity, and it was subsequently reported for the first time in the evaluation of temporal lobe epilepsy.[10,11] Meanwhile, in the neurosurgical unit of the Saint Anne Hospital in Paris, stereotactic investigations of epileptic patients with intracerebral electrodes were inspired to attempt a newly innovative concept: epileptic seizures were regarded as a dynamic process with a spatiotemporal, often multidirectional organization that is best defined as a three-dimensional (3D) arrangement. This method was originally named *Functional Stereotactic Exploration* and then SEEG.[12-16]

The SEEG method was originally developed by Jean Talairach and Jean Bancaud during the 1950s[11]; it has been used mostly in France and Italy as the method of choice for invasive mapping in refractory focal epilepsy.[7,17-39] In France, after the development of the stereotactic techniques and frames, which were applied initially for abnormal movement disorder surgery, Jean Talairach devoted most of his activity in the field of epilepsy, along with Jean Bancaud, who joined him in 1952. The new methodology created by both physicians led them to depart from the alternate approach of subdural electrode monitoring that was being used by Wilder Penfield and colleagues at Montreal Neurological Institute. Rather than being limited to monitoring of the superficial cortex using subdural electrodes, Talairach's innovative thinking was to implement a working methodology for a comprehensive analysis of morphological and functional cerebral space. His atlas on the telencephalon, published in 1967, perfectly illustrates the new anatomic concepts for stereotaxis.[13] The development of tools, adapted to a new stereotactic frame designed by Talairach and colleagues, conducted the Saint Anne investigators to propose the functional exploration of the brain by depth electrodes, allowing the exploration of both superficial and deep cortical areas. The debut of SEEG was in 1957, when the first implantation of intracerebral electrodes for epilepsy was performed on May 3 in Saint Anne Hospital. By departing from the subdural method of invasive monitoring, such implantations allowed exploration of the activity of different three dimensional brain structures and to record the patient's spontaneous seizures, something that Penfield's method of investigation failed to achieve. This new technique and method was called "the Stereo-Electro-Encephalography" in 1962[13,19] (Fig. 72-1).

The principle of SEEG methodology remains similar to the principles originally described by Bancaud and Talairach, which is based on anatomo-electro-clinical (AEC) correlations with the main aim to conceptualize the 3D spatial-temporal organization of the epileptic discharge within the brain.[7,19-21,30-41] The implantation strategy is individualized, with electrode placement based on preimplantation hypotheses that consider the electroclinical correlations of patient's seizures and their relation with a suspected lesion. For these reasons, the preimplantation AEC hypothesis formulation is the single most important element in the process of planning the placement of SEEG electrodes. If the preimplantation hypotheses are incorrect, the placement of the depth electrodes will be inadequate, and the interpretation of the SEEG recordings will not give access to the definition of the epileptogenic zone.

CHOOSING THE APPROPRIATE METHOD FOR INVASIVE MONITORING

After establishing the diagnosis of pharmacoresistant epilepsy (defined as a failure to respond to two or more adequately chosen and used antiepileptic medications),[42] a presurgical evaluation is indicated with two main goals: (1) mapping the AEC network leading to the identification of the EZ and its extent and (2) assessing the functional status of the epileptogenic regions.

Achieving both goals will lead to optimization of postresective seizure and functional outcomes following surgery. As mentioned earlier, multiple techniques can be used to achieve the previously stated goals: scalp-video electroencephalography (EEG) monitoring to confirm the diagnosis of focal epilepsy (including interictal and ictal EEG recordings), and to identify the cortical structure of the hypothetical networks that may be involved in seizure organization (through analysis of the recorded clinical and electrical semiology), leading to the formulation of clear AEC hypotheses. Further validation of the anatomic hypothesis is achieved through structural imaging (the identification of lesion on MRI), with or without metabolic imaging (including fluorodeoxyglucose–positron emission tomography

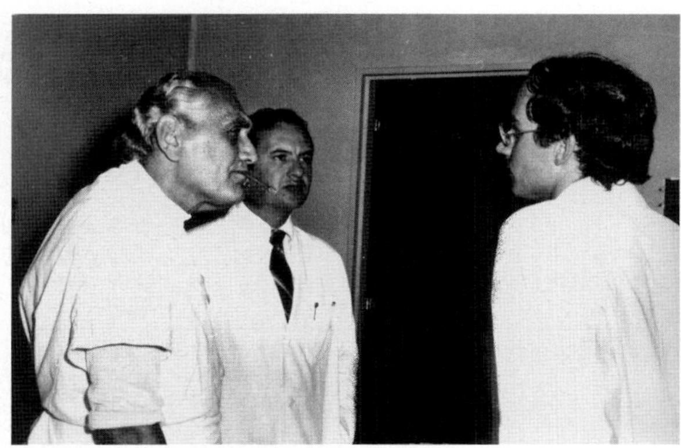

Figure 72-1. From left to right: Jean Talairach, Nicholas Zervas (former chair of neurosurgery at Massachusetts General Hospital), and Patrick Chauvel discussing stereo-electroencephalography results. Paris, 1973.

hypometabolism that might point to focal regions of cortical dysfunction). Other studies may include ictal SPECT, magnetoencephalography, and EEG-fMRI.[6,8,43]

These noninvasive studies identify the epileptogenic zone in more than half of patients undergoing presurgical workup (approximately 70% of the patients who are operated on at Cleveland Clinic in 2012 [unpublished data]); however, a formulation of a clear and unique AEC hypothesis might not be possible in the remaining 30% of patients. In such cases, focal or focal–regional epilepsy is likely, but the noninvasive phase I evaluation cannot distinguish between two or three hypotheses in the same hemisphere; there is a sound regional hypothesis but not sufficient arguments in favor of one hemisphere; or hypotheses are generated, but the exact location of the epileptogenic zone, its extent, and/or its overlap with functional (eloquent) cortex remain unclear. Consequently, these patients may be candidates for an invasive evaluation using different methods of evaluation, including intraoperative electrocorticography or extraoperative methods as subdural grids or strips, subdural grids combined with depth electrodes, and SEEG.[44]

The main indications for an invasive evaluation in focal pharmacoresistant epilepsy (with the main purpose of direct cortical recording) are to address the main challenges and limitations of various noninvasive techniques. Because of the limitations of the various noninvasive techniques, an invasive evaluation should be considered in any one of the following cases:

1. *MRI-negative cases:* The MRI does not show a cortical lesion in a location that is concordant with the electroclinical/functional hypothesis generated by the video EEG recordings.
2. *Electroclinical and MRI data discordance:* The anatomic location of the MRI identified lesion (and at times the location of a clearly hypometabolic focal area on PET) is not concordant with the electroclinical hypothesis. These include cases of deeply seated brain lesions, such as periventricular nodular heterotopia or deep sulcal lesions. In addition, scalp EEG recordings in 85% to 100% of patients with focal cortical dysplasia show interictal spikes that range in their distribution from lobar to lateralized, from difficult to localize to diffuse (including generalized spike-wave patterns in some cases of subependymal heterotopia).[34,35,39,45-47] The spatial distribution of interictal spikes is usually more extensive than the structural abnormality as assessed by intraoperative inspection or MRI visual analysis.[48]
3. *Multiple, in part discordant lesions:* There are two or more anatomic lesions with the location of at least one of them being discordant with the electroclinical hypothesis, or both lesions are located within the same functional network and it is unclear whether one (or both) of them are epileptic.
4. *Overlap with eloquent cortex:* The generated AEC hypothesis (MRI-negative or MRI-identifiable lesion) involves potentially highly eloquent cortex. The identification of the epileptogenic zone, mapping of its extent, or its relationship with potentially eloquent cortex are not typically resolved in these cases. These cases include patients with suspected focal cortical dysplasia as the possible pathologic substrate for epilepsy.[4,41,46,48-52]

In these instances, an invasive evaluation usually leads to the formulation of a clear resective surgical strategy. The recommendation for invasive monitoring and its type is made during a multidisciplinary patient management meeting that includes neurologists, neurosurgeons, neuroradiologists, and neuropsychologists. Areas and networks of coverage and sampling are determined on the basis of a well-formulated AEC hypothesis including results of the noninvasive studies.

There is no clear consensus regarding the best selection criteria for each method. Some epilepsy centers have applied both technical procedures in a systematic matter, but none of them have conducted definitive comparative studies. The "pro-SEEG groups" consider that this method can answer any question an invasive subdural method can provide.[7,17-41,44,45,53-74] On the contrary, the "pro-subdural groups" who are not familiar with depth electrode explorations tend to limit its indications to the exploration of deep structures—for example, to distinguish unilateral or bilateral lobe epilepsy, and possibly to study epilepsy related to nodular heterotopia. However, differences between SEEG and subdural grids and strips are more extensive and complex than just the dichotomy between deep versus superficial mapping. The "philosophy," "definitions," and "concepts" of the two types of explorations are quite different and at times divergent. Subdural explorations were initially oriented toward the invasive study of lesional epilepsy, whereas SEEG initially takes little into account of the lesion itself. We can speculate that SEEG is more suitable to explore patients with nonlesional MRIs for whom, in some cases, it is not clear that surgery should be performed.[44,66-68] In addition, SEEG facilitates the exploration of remote and multilobar areas without the need for craniotomies and immediate surgery, allowing a prolonged reflection time for the patient and a more complete informed consent process. The use and analysis of direct electrical stimulation in these methods are divergent and sometimes in opposition.[75]

Extraoperative mapping with the subdural method (including grids, strips, and the possible combination with depth electrodes) has the advantage of allowing an optimal anatomic and contiguous coverage and sampling of the adjacent cortex leading to accurate superficial cortex functional mapping exploration.[76,77] This is especially the case when there is the need to determine the extension of the EZ associated with a superficial lesion and its anatomic relation to a close functional area. This is not true if the lesion includes a deep-seated component where functional mapping cannot be obtained from subdural mapping. From a surgical perspective, subdural implantations are open procedures, with better management of occasional intracranial hemorrhagic complications. The main disadvantages of the subdural method are related to the inability to record and map deep structures, such as the insular cortex, orbitofrontal cortex, cingulate gyrus, depths of sulci, etc, and consequently, its incapacity in figuring out the spatiotemporal dynamics of the epileptogenic network. In these scenarios, the SEEG methodology may be considered a more adequate and safer option. SEEG has the advantages of allowing extensive and precise deep brain recordings and stimulations (to localize seizure onset) with minimal associated morbidity.[41,60,61,66-68]

TABLE 72-1 Selection Criteria for Different Methods of Invasive Monitoring in Medically Refractory Focal Epilepsy

Clinical Scenario	Method of Choice	Second Option
Lesional MRI: Potential epileptogenic lesion superficially located, near or in the proximity of eloquent cortex Nonlesional MRI: Hypothetical EZ located in the proximity of eloquent cortex	SBG	SEEG
Lesional MRI: Potential epileptogenic lesion located in deep cortical and subcortical areas Nonlesional MRI: Hypothetical EZ deeply located or located in non-eloquent areas	SEEG	SBG with depths
Need for bilateral explorations and or reoperations	SEEG	SBG with depths
After subdural grids failure	SEEG	SBG with depths
When the AEC hypothesis suggests the involvement of an extensive, multilobar epileptic network	SEEG	SBG with depths
Suspected frontal lobe epilepsy in nonlesional MRI scenario	SEEG	SEEG

AEC, anatomo-electro-clinical; EZ, epileptogenic zone; MRI, magnetic resonance imaging; SBG, subdural grids; SEEG, stereo-electroencephalography.

Consequently, because of the potential advantages and disadvantages of each method, one can consider possible specific indications to choose SEEG in detriment to other methods of invasive monitoring:

1. The possibility of a deep-seated or difficult-to-cover location of the EZ in areas such as the mesial structures of the temporal lobe, perisylvian areas, cingulate gyrus and mesial interhemispheric regions, ventromedial prefrontal areas, insula, and depths of sulci
2. The failure of a previous subdural invasive study to outline the exact location of the seizure onset zone (The failure to identify the EZ in these patients may be due to multiple reasons that include the lack of adequate sampling from a deep focus or a clinically silent focus upstream from the EZ.)
3. The need for extensive bihemispheric explorations (in particular in focal epilepsies arising from the interhemispheric or deep insular regions, or temporoparietooccipital junction)
4. Presurgical evaluation suggestive of an extended network involvement (e.g., temporofrontal or frontoparietal) in the setting of normal MRI (Table 72-1)

A majority of patients undergoing reoperations may have failed epilepsy surgery during preceding subdural evaluations because of difficulties in accurately localizing the EZ. These patients pose a significant dilemma for further management, having relatively few options available. Further open subdural grid evaluations can carry risks associated with encountering scar formations and still having limitations related to deep cortical structure recordings. A subsequent evaluation using the SEEG method can overcome these limitations, offering an additional opportunity for seizure localization and sustained seizure freedom.[61] The theoretical disadvantage of the SEEG method is the more restricted capability for performing functional mapping. Because of the limited number of contacts located in the superficial cortex, a contiguous mapping of eloquent brain areas cannot be obtained as in the subdural method mapping.[41,60,61] It is interesting to note that functional mapping in SEEG cannot be dissociated from the electroclinical localization process and, consequently, a fare comparison between both methods cannot be performed. In addition, the precision of the subdural functional mapping is far from being validated. Lastly, the functional mapping information extracted from the SEEG method can be frequently complemented with other methods of mapping, such as DTI images or awake craniotomies,[41] diminishing the relative disadvantages claimed by the "subdural groups."

PLANNING THE STEREO-ELECTROENCEPHALOGRAPHY IMPLANTATION

As indicated earlier, the development of an SEEG implantation plan requires the clear formulation of precise AEC hypotheses to be tested. These hypotheses are typically generated during the multidisciplinary patient management conference based on the results of various noninvasive tests. At Cleveland Clinic, a final tailored implantation strategy is generated during a separate presurgical implantation meeting. Depth electrodes should sample the anatomic lesion (if identified), the more likely structures of ictal onset, the early and late spread regions and the interactions with the functional (e.g., cognitive, sensorimotor, behavioral) networks. A 3D "conceptualization" of the network nodes upstream and downstream from the hypothesized epileptogenic network is an essential component of the presurgical implantation strategy. Initially, by analyzing the available noninvasive data and the temporal evolution of the ictal clinical manifestations, a hypothesis of the anatomic location of the EZ is formulated.[78] The implantation plan is created in collaboration with experienced epileptologists, neurosurgeons, and neuroradiologists who, together, will formulate hypotheses for EZ localization.

Adequate knowledge of the possible functional networks involved in the primary organization of the epileptic activity is mandatory to formulate adequate hypotheses. In addition, the treating physicians will have to account for the 3D aspects of depth electrode recordings that, despite a limited coverage (which is largely compensated by the interpolation process made possible by the electrophysiological methodology: frequencies, spatial relations, and latencies analyses) of the cortical surface compared with subdural grids and strips, enable an accurate sampling of the structures along its trajectory from the entry site to the final impact point. Therefore, the trajectory is more important than the target or entry point areas. Consequently, the investigation may include lateral and mesial surfaces of the different lobes, deep-seated cortices as the depths of sulci, insula, posterior quadrant, and areas in the inter-hemispheric cortical surface. The implantation should also consider the different cortical cytoarchitectonic areas involved in seizure organization patterns and their likely connectivity to other cortical and subcortical areas. It is important to emphasize that the implantation strategy focus is not to map lobes or lobules, but epileptogenic networks, which in general involve multiple lobes. Furthermore, exploration strategy should also consider possible alternative hypotheses of localization[63,68,79] (Fig. 72-2).

Lastly, the aim to obtain all the possible information from the SEEG exploration should not be pursued at the expense of an excessive number of electrodes, which will likely increase the morbidity of the implantation. In general, implantations that exceed 15 depth electrodes are rare. In addition, the possible involvement of eloquent regions in the ictal discharge requires their judicious coverage, with the twofold goal to assess their role in the seizure organization and to define the boundaries of a safe surgical resection.

The SEEG implantation patterns are based on a tailored strategy of exploration, which results from the primary hypothesis of the anatomic location of the EZ, for every single case. As a result, standard implantations for specific areas and lobes are difficult to conceptualize. Nevertheless, a number of typical patterns of coverage can be recognized.

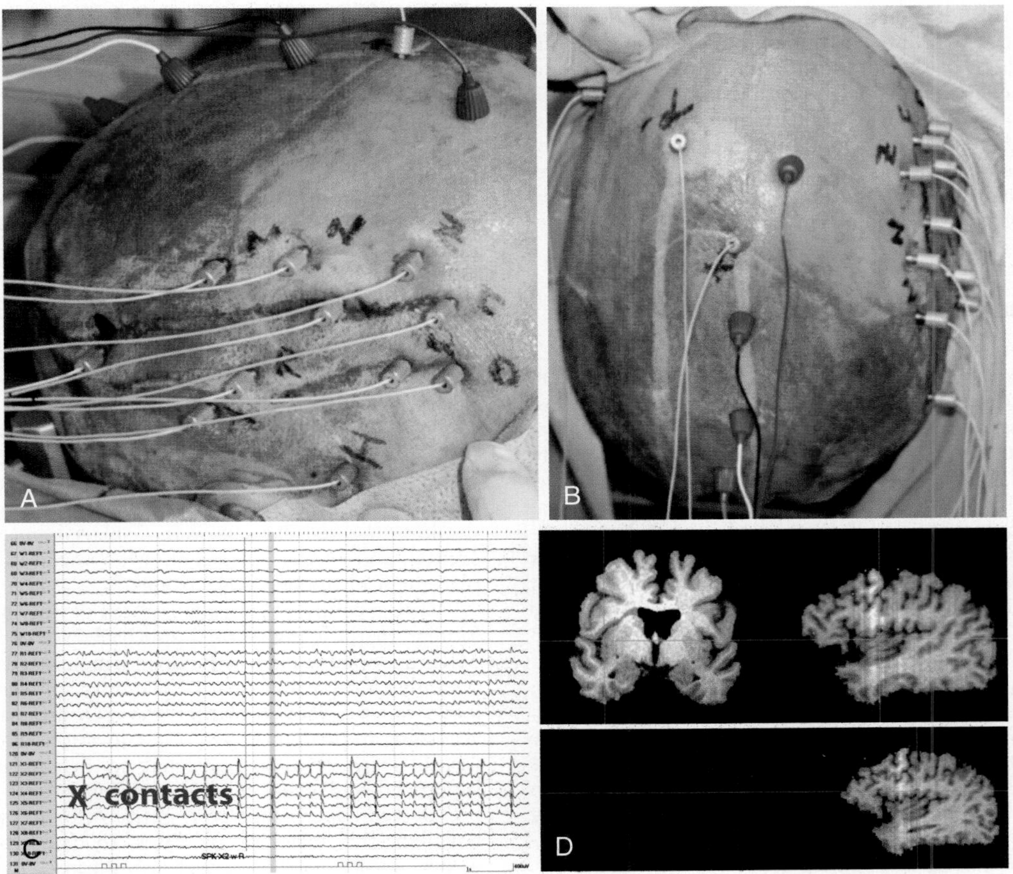

Figure 72-2. A and B, Intraoperative aspect of right stereo-electroencephalography (SEEG) implantation focusing on right frontal temporal and parietal areas. **C,** SEEG interictal recordings demonstrating focal repetitive spikes from the distal contacts of electrode X, located in the right anterior insula. The ictal recording analysis confirmed the location of the hypothetical epileptogenic zone in the anterior insula, on the right side. **D,** Digital fused images (preoperative magnetic resonance imaging and postoperative computed tomography) demonstrating the location of the epileptiform activity in the anterior insula. In the same image, small "bottom of sulcus" dysplasia is identified in the superior circular sulcus of the insula *(red),* in proximity with the epileptogenic areas.

Limbic Network Explorations

Cases of temporal lobe epilepsy with consistent AEC findings suggesting a limbic network involvement are usually operated on after noninvasive investigation only. In general, the use of invasive monitoring is not necessary when semiological and electrophysiologic studies demonstrate typical nondominant mesial temporal epilepsy and imaging studies shows clear lesion (e.g., mesial temporal sclerosis) that fits the initial localization hypothesis. Nevertheless, invasive exploration with SEEG recordings may be required in patients in whom the supposed EZs, probably involving the temporal lobes, are suspected to involve extratemporal areas as well. In these cases, the implantation pattern points to disclose a preferential spread of the discharge to the temporo-insular-anterior perisylvian areas, the temporo-insular-orbitofrontal areas, or the posterior temporal, posterior insula, temporobasal, parietal, and posterior cingulate areas. Consequently, sampling of extratemporal limbic areas must be sufficiently wide to provide information to identify a possible extratemporal origin of the seizures that could not been anticipated with precision according to noninvasive methods of investigation.

Frontoparietal Network Explorations

Because of the large volume of the frontal and parietal lobes, a high number of electrodes are required for an adequate coverage of this region. In most patients, however, excessive sampling can be avoided, and the implantation to more limited portions of the frontal and parietal lobes can be performed. The suspicion of orbitofrontal epilepsy, for example, often requires the investigation of gyrus rectus, the frontal polar areas, the anterior cingulate gyrus, and the anterior portions of the temporal lobe (temporal pole). Similarly, seizures that are thought to arise from the mesial wall of the premotor cortex are evaluated by targeting at least the rostral and caudal parts of the supplementary motor area (SMA), the pre-SMA area, different portions of the cingulate gyrus and sulcus, and the primary motor cortex and mesial and dorsolateral parietal cortex. Consequently, the hypothesis-based sampling often allows localization of the EZ in the frontal or parietal lobes, or both, and in some cases may allow the identification of relatively small EZs. Eventually, frontoparietal network explorations may be bilateral, and sometimes symmetrical, mainly when a mesial frontoparietal epilepsy is suspected and the noninvasive methods of investigation failed in lateralizing the epileptic activity.

Electrodes in rolandic regions are normally placed when there is a need to define the posterior margin of the resection in frontal network explorations or the anterior margin in parietal-occipital explorations, or when the EZ may be located in or near Rolandic cortex. The main goal here is to evaluate the rolandic participation to the ictal discharge and to obtain a functional mapping by intracerebral electrical stimulation. In this location, depth electrodes are particularly helpful to sample the depth of the central sulcus, as well as the descending and ascending white matter fibers associated with this region.

Posterior Quadrant Network Explorations

In the posterior quadrant, placement of electrodes limited to a single lobe is extremely uncommon, because of the frequent simultaneous involvement of several occipital, parietal, and posterior temporal structures, and to the multidirectional spread of the discharges to supra- and infrasylvian areas. Consequently, mesial and dorsolateral surfaces of the occipital lobes are explored, covering both infracalcarine and supracalcarine areas, in association with posterior temporal, posterior perisylvian, basal temporo-occipital areas, and posterior parietal areas including the posterior inferior parietal lobule and the posterior precuneus. In posterior quadrant epilepsies, bilateral explorations are generally needed because of rapid contralateral spread of ictal activity.

IMPLANTATION TECHNIQUE

Once the SEEG planning is finalized, the desired targets are reached using commercially available depth electrodes in various lengths and number of contacts, depending on the specific brain regions to be explored. The depth electrodes are implanted using conventional stereotactic technique or by the assistance of stereotactic robotic devices, through 2.5-mm-diameter drill holes. In both robotic and frame-based techniques, depth electrodes are inserted through 2.5-mm-diameter drill holes, using orthogonal or oblique orientation, allowing intracranial recording from lateral, intermediate, or deep cortical and subcortical structures in a 3D arrangement, thus accounting for the dynamic, multidirectional spatiotemporal organization of the epileptogenic pathways.

Initially, frame-based implantations were performed in our center. As part of our routine practice, patients were admitted to the hospital on the day of surgery. The day before surgery, a stereotaxy compatible, contrast-enhanced, volumetric T1 MRI sequence was performed. Images were then transferred to our stereotactic neuronavigation software (iPlan Cranial 2.6; Brainlab AG, Feldkirchen, Germany) where trajectories were planned the following day. The day of surgery, while the patient was under general anesthesia, a Leksell stereotactic frame (Elekta, Stockholm, Sweden) was applied using standard technique. Once the patient was attached to the angiography table with the frame, stereo Dyna computed tomography (CT) and 3D digital subtracted angiography was performed. The preoperative MRI, the stereo DynaCT, and angiographic images were then digitally processed using a dedicated fusion software (syngo XWP; Siemens Healthcare, Forchheim, Germany). These fused images were used during the implantation procedure to confirm the accuracy of the final position of each electrode and to ensure the absence of vascular structures along the electrode pathway, which might not be noted on contrast-enhanced MRI. Following the planning phase using the stereotactic software, trajectory coordinates were recorded and transported to the operating room. Trajectories were in general planned in orthogonal orientation in relation to the skull's sagittal plane to facilitate implantation and interpretation of the electrode positions and recordings. Using the Leksell stereotactic system, coordinates for each trajectory were then adjusted in the frame, and a lateral view fluoroscopic image was performed in each new position. Care was taken to ensure that the central beam of radiation during fluoroscopy was centered in the middle of the implantation probe in order to avoid parallax errors. If the trajectory was aligned correctly, corresponding to the planned trajectory and passing along an avascular space, the implantation was then continued, with skull perforation, dura opening, placement of the guiding bolt, and final insertion of the electrode under fluoroscopic guidance. If a vessel was recognized along the pathway during fluoroscopy, the guiding tube was manually moved a few millimeters until the next avascular space was recognized, and implantation was then continued. The electrode insertion progress was observed under live fluoroscopic control in a frontal view to confirm the straight trajectory of each electrode. For additional guidance, a coronal MRI slice corresponding to the level of each electrode implantation was overlaid onto the fluoroscopic image.

Postimplantation DynaCT scans were performed while the patients were still anesthetized and positioned in the operating table. The reconstructed images were then fused with the MRI dataset using the previously described fusion software. The resulting merged datasets were displayed and reviewed in axial, sagittal, and coronal planes allowing verification of the correct placement of the depth electrodes.[79a]

More recently, robotically assisted devices have been applied. Similar to the conventional approach, volumetric preoperative MRIs are obtained, and DICOM format images were transferred digitally to the robot's native planning software. Individual trajectories are planned within the 3D imaging reconstruction according to predetermined target locations and intended trajectories. Trajectories are selected to maximize sampling from superficial and deep cortical and subcortical areas within the preselected zones of interest. Trajectories are oriented orthogonally in the majority of cases to facilitate the anatomo-electrophysiological correlation during the extraoperative recording phase and to avoid possible trajectories shifts because of excessive angled entry points. Nevertheless, when multiple targets are potentially accessible via a single non-orthogonal trajectory, these multiple-target trajectories are selected to minimize the number of implanted electrodes per patient.

All trajectories are evaluated for safety and target accuracy in their individual reconstructed planes (axial, sagittal, coronal) and along the reconstructed "probe's eye view." Any trajectory that appears to compromise vascular structures is adjusted appropriately without affecting the sampling from areas of interest. A set working distance of 150 mm from the drilling platform to the target is initially used for each trajectory and is later adjusted to reduce the working distance maximally and, consequently, to improve the implantation accuracy. The overall implantation schemas are analyzed using the 3D cranial reconstruction capabilities, and internal trajectories are checked to ensure that no trajectory collisions are present. External trajectory positions are examined for any entry sites that would be prohibitively close (less than 1.5 cm) at the skin level.

On the day of surgery, patients are administered general anesthesia. For each patient, the head is placed into a three-point fixation head holder. The robot is then positioned such that the working distance (distance between the base of the robotic arm and the midpoint of the cranium) is approximately 70 cm. The robot is locked into position, and the head holder device is secured to the robot. No additional position adjustments are made to the operating table during the implantation procedure. After positioning and securing the patient to the robot, image registrations are performed. Semiautomatic laser-based facial recognition is used to register the preoperative volumetric MRI with the patient. The laser is first calibrated using a set distance calibration tool. Preset anatomic facial landmarks are then manually selected with the laser. The areas defined by the manually entered anatomic landmarks subsequently undergo automatic registration

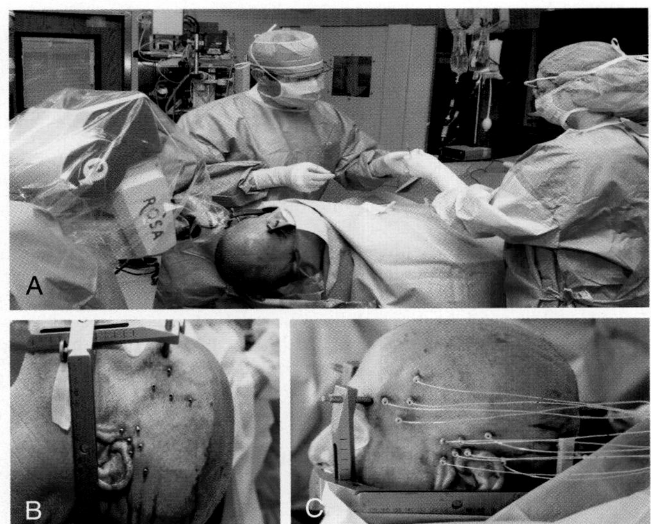

Figure 72-3. Robotic stereo-electroencephalography (SEEG) technique. A, Operating room "set up" during left-sided SEEG robotic implantation, with surgeon and scrub nurse positioned on each side of the patient, and the robot device placed in the middle, at the vertex. **B,** Intraoperative aspect of left side frontotemporal SEEG implantation with the guiding bolts in final position. **C,** Left side frontotemporal SEEG implantation after the depth electrodes implantations. Final aspect.

using laser-based facial surface scanning. The accuracy of the registration process is then confirmed by correlating additional independently chosen surface landmarks with the registered MRI. After successful registration, the accessibility of the planned trajectories is automatically verified by the robotic software.

The patients are then prepared and draped in a standard sterile fashion. The robotic working arm is also draped with a sterile plastic cover. A drilling platform, with a 2.5-mm-diameter working cannula is secured to the robotic arm. The desired trajectories are selected on the touchscreen interface. After trajectory confirmation, the arm movement is initiated using a foot pedal. The robotic arm automatically locks the drilling platform into a stable position upon reaching the calculated position for the selected trajectory. A 2-mm-diameter handheld drill (Stryker) is introduced through the platform and used to create a skull "pinhole." The dura is then opened with an insulated dural perforator using monopolar cautery at low settings. A guiding bolt (Ad-Tech, Racine, WI) is screwed firmly into each pinhole. The distance from the drilling platform to the retaining bolt is measured, and this value is subtracted from the standardized 150-mm platform to target distance. The resulting difference is recorded for later use as the final length of the electrode to be implanted. This process is repeated for each trajectory. All pinholes and retaining bolts are placed before beginning electrode insertion. A small stylet (2 mm in diameter) is then set to the previously recorded electrode distance and is passed gently into the parenchyma, guided by the implantation bolt, followed immediately by the insertion of the premeasured electrode (Fig. 72-3).

MORBIDITY AND SEIZURE OUTCOME

Our center recently reported 200 patients undergoing 2663 SEEG electrode implantations for the purposes of invasive intracranial EEG monitoring, in accordance with a tailored preimplantation hypothesis to investigate and anatomically characterize the extension of the EZ. The studied group was challenging because of the paucity of noninvasive data and the possibility of a more diffuse pathology suggested by a previous failure of invasive monitoring exploration: nearly one third of the studied patients (58 patients; 29.0%) comprised individuals who had undergone prior surgical intervention for medically refractory epilepsy, resulting in postoperative recurrent seizures. Despite the challenging and discourage clinical scenario, the SEEG method was able to confirm the EZ in 154 patients (77.0%). Of these, 134 patients (87.0%) underwent subsequent craniotomy for SEEG-guided resection. Within this cohort, 90 patients had a minimum postoperative follow-up of at least 12 months; therein, 61 patients (67.8%) remained seizure free (i.e., Engel I outcome). The most common pathologic diagnosis in this group was focal cortical dysplasia type I (55 patients; 61.1%). Complications were minimal; they included wound infections (0.08%), hemorrhagic complications (0.08%), and a transient neurological deficit (0.04%) in 5 patients. The total morbidity rate was 2.5%.

Results in terms of seizure outcome and complications are compatible with already published results from other groups. These results parallel those of previous studies in the literature. Munari et al.[80] reported on their experience with SEEG in 70 patients undergoing a collective total of 712 electrode implantations. Within this cohort, an individualized and tailored surgical resection was performed in 60 patients (85.7%). In their series, specifically relating to SEEG, the authors identified one permanent complication ensuing from the procedure; this entailed the formation of an asymptomatic intracerebral hematoma following the removal of an SEEG electrode (accounting for a morbidity rate of 1.4%, or 0.1% per electrode). Guenot et al.[81] presented a series of 100 patients collectively undergoing 1118 SEEG electrode implantations for invasive EEG monitoring. Here, SEEG was deemed helpful in 84 patients (84%) by either annulling or confirming (and additionally, in the latter case, guiding) surgical resection of the EZ. Moreover, SEEG confirmed the indication for resection in 14 cases (14%) that were previously disputed on the basis of the noninvasive workup. These authors reported on five complications (5% of cases), including two electrode site infections (0.2% per electrode), two intracranial electrode fractures (0.2% per electrode), and one intracerebral hematoma resulting in death (accounting for a mortality rate of 1% in the study). In a large series, Cossu et al.[82] reported a morbidity rate of 5.6%, with severe permanent deficits from intracerebral hemorrhage in 1%. In another study, Tanriverdi et al.[83] summarized their experience with a subgroup of 491 refractory epilepsy patients collectively undergoing 2490 intracerebral SEEG electrode implantations and 2943 depth electrode implantations.[83] On the basis of experience, the authors identified 4 patients (0.8%) with an intracranial hematoma at the electrode site (0.07% per electrode) and 9 patients (1.8%) with an infection arising from electrode placement (0.2% per electrode); moreover, they reported no mortalities ensuing directly from SEEG electrode placement. Finally, Cardinale et al.[79] most recently presented their experience with 6496 electrodes stereotactically implanted in 482 epilepsy patients with refractory epilepsy.[79] These authors identified 2 patients (0.4%, or 0.03% per electrode) with permanent neurological deficits in their series; 14 patients (2.9%, or 0.2% per electrode) with hemorrhagic complication; 2 patients (0.4%, or 0.03% per electrode) with infection; and one mortality (0.2%) resulting from massive brain edema and concomitant hyponatremia following electrode implantation.

In comparing morbidity, subdural grid electrode implantation has historically been shown to have low permanent morbidity (0%-3%) compared with depth electrodes (3%-6%) because there is no intraparenchymal passage.[2,43,84-89] Although it is difficult to compare morbidity rates between subdural grids and SEEG because of the variability in patient selection, different institutions, and variable number of implanted electrodes, the clinical experience among different groups in Europe and North America suggests that the SEEG method provides at least a similar degree of safety when compared with subdural grids or strips.[a]

CONCLUSIONS

The SEEG methodology and technique was developed almost 60 years ago in Europe, and its efficacy and safety have been proven over the last 55 years. The main advantage of the SEEG method is the possibility to study the epileptogenic neuronal network in its dynamic and 3D aspect, with an optimal time and space correlation with the clinical semiology of the patient's seizures.

The main clinical challenge for the near future remains in the further refinement of specific selection criteria for the different methods of invasive monitoring, with the ultimate goal of comparing and validating the results (long-term seizure-free outcome) obtained from different methods of invasive monitoring.

[a]References 7, 36, 37, 40, 44, 63, 67, 70, 80, 83, 89-92.

SUGGESTED READINGS

Cardinale F, Cossu M, Castana L, et al. Stereoelectroencephalography: surgical methodology, safety, and stereotactic application accuracy in 500 procedures. *Neurosurgery*. 2013;72(3):353-366, discussion 366.

Chauvel P, McGonigal A. Emergence of semiology in epileptic seizures. *Epilepsy Behav*. 2014;38:94-103.

Cossu M, Chabardes S, Hoffmann D, et al. Presurgical evaluation of intractable epilepsy using stereo-electro-encephalography methodology: principles, technique and morbidity. *Neurochirurgie*. 2008;54(3): 367-373.

Gonzalez-Martinez J, Lachhwani D. Stereoelectroencephalography in children with cortical dysplasia: technique and results. *Childs Nerv Syst*. 2014;30(11):1853-1857.

Gonzalez-Martinez J, Mullin J, Bulacio J, et al. Stereoelectroencephalography in children and adolescents with difficult-to-localize refractory focal epilepsy. *Neurosurgery*. 2014;75(3):258-268, discussion 267-268.

See a full reference list on ExpertConsult.com

73 Surgical Techniques for Non–Temporal Lobe Epilepsy: Corpus Callosotomy, Multiple Subpial Transection, and Topectomy

Carter S. Gerard and Richard W. Byrne

This chapter reviews important surgical techniques useful in the treatment of non-–temporal lobe epilepsy. Extratemporal epilepsy encompasses a broad range of etiologies, and consequently, surgical options in treating non–temporal lobe epilepsy are also varied. In addition, in comparison with temporal epilepsy and seizure surgery, the anatomy is more varied, the identification of discrete seizure foci is more difficult, and the likelihood of surgical seizure control is lower. It may be a truism that the existence of multiple treatment options, in general, is indicative of the lack of supremacy of any one option. Nevertheless, the epilepsy surgeon must be familiar with the following procedures when considering surgery for nontemporal epilepsy.

CORPUS CALLOSOTOMY

Corpus callosotomy aims to isolate seizure activity by disrupting white matter tracts connecting the hemispheres and thereby inhibiting seizure propagation. The procedure was first described in a series of 10 patients in 1940 by van Wagenen and Herren. The technique was created after these investigators observed seizure improvement in several epileptic patients in whom the corpus callosum had been destroyed by tumor or stroke.[1] Despite favorable results in the initial series, the technique was not further developed until 20 years later. Since that time, the founding concept of hemispheric isolation for seizure palliation via callosotomy has persisted while greater experience and evolving technologies have led to modification of the technique. The use of limited anterior callosotomies, or staged procedures, coupled with image guidance has produced excellent outcomes in multiple series for children and adults. The development of vagal nerve stimulators has led to a decline in the use of the more invasive callosotomy for patients with refractory seizures. Nevertheless, corpus callosotomy has a long history of success and remains an ideal therapy for a subgroup of patients in need of seizure palliation.

A brief history of the procedure is examined in the electronic version of this chapter at ExpertConsult.com.

Patient Selection

It is widely accepted that all patients with epilepsy who are considered for surgical intervention should be reviewed by a team consisting of various specialists, including epileptologists, neurosurgeons, neuroradiologists, and neuropsychologists. After unsuccessful medical therapy for 2 years or continued disabling seizures despite maximal medical therapy, the patient's epilepsy is deemed to be refractory. The patient must be thoroughly evaluated with a complete history, physical examination, and encephalography (EEG) to better characterize the nature, frequency, and possibly location of seizure activity. Because callosotomy is a palliative procedure and does not achieve a cure, it is not a suitable option for patients with resectable seizure foci. The possibility of a focal lesion must then be ruled out with video-EEG, epilepsy protocol MRI, and, in some cases, positron emission tomography (PET) or single-photon emission tomography (SPECT). Prior to surgery it is imperative that the medical team educate the patient and family, clearly communicating the goal of surgery as seizure palliation as opposed to cure.

Corpus callosotomy has been used to successfully treat a wide variety of generalized seizures. Patients with atonic seizures have repeatedly shown superior results, with an 80% to 100% reduction in drop attacks.[14,26-28] A callosotomy may also offer seizure palliation for patients with cases of unapproachable or multiple seizure foci. Multiple pediatric conditions, such as Lennox-Gastaut syndrome, Rasmussen's encephalitis, and infantile hemiplegia, have been effectively treated with callosotomy.[14,28-30] Patients with lateralizing pathologic conditions, such as Rasmussen's encephalitis or infantile hemiplegia, may benefit from callosotomy when hemispherotomy threatens intact visual fields or motor function.[5] The efficacy and limited morbidity of vagal nerve stimulation (VNS) have made it an attractive alternative to corpus callosotomy. However, patients whose epilepsy does not respond to VNS often later undergo and benefit from callosotomy.[10,31,32]

Operative Procedure

A brief discussion of preoperative imaging, anesthesia, and positioning is available in the electronic version of this chapter.

Surgical Technique

Unless large midline veins are present, the approach is usually performed on the nondominant side in order to limit the risk of injury to the dominant hemisphere. Multiple types of incisions may be used—linear, coronal, or U shaped—to expose the site of craniotomy. The craniotomy is usually located with the midpoint, just anterior to the coronal suture and extending just lateral to midline on the contralateral side. The location of the craniotomy may be adjusted to avoid exposure over cortical veins. Once the craniotomy is completed, the dura is opened and retracted toward the sinus (Fig. 73-1 and Video 73-1).

The interhemispheric fissure is entered and carefully divided. A self-retaining retractor may be useful. During the approach, care is taken to identify the callosal marginal arteries and then the pericallosal arteries. If adhesions between the frontal lobes must be divided, it is important that the division stay medial to the arteries to avoid disrupting small perforators. The corpus callosum is usually easily identified from its characteristic glossy white appearance. The surgeon must distinguish the corpus callosum from fused cingulate gyri and also must take care to separate the frequently adherent cinguli. Adhesion of cingulate gyri is quite common in patients undergoing this procedure, perhaps secondary to multiple falls and head injuries. When the corpus callosum is identified, stereotactic guidance can be used to define and guide the posterior extent of the sectioning. The callosotomy begins 3 cm posterior to the genu, where the midline is easier to identify, and proceeds ventrally to the midline leaves of the

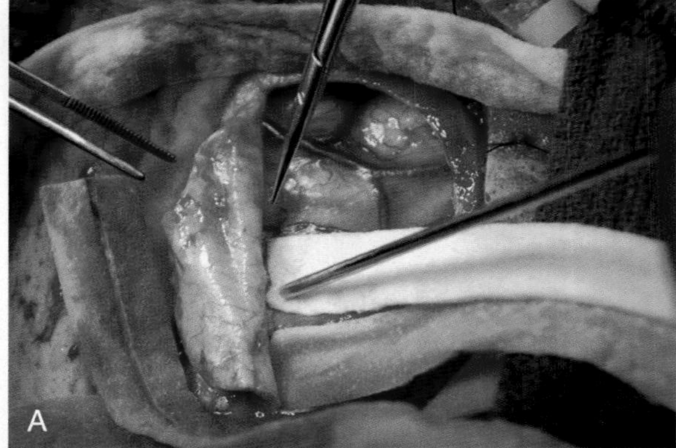

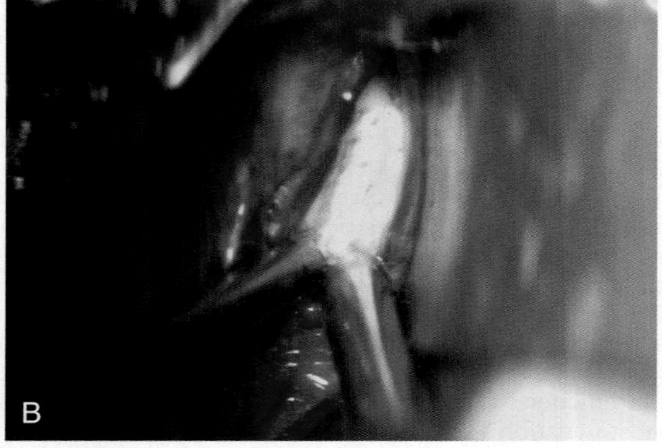

Figure 73-1. A, The craniotomy is usually located with the midpoint just anterior to the coronal suture and extending just lateral to midline on the contralateral side. The location of the craniotomy may be adjusted to avoid exposure over cortical veins. Once the craniotomy is completed, the dura is opened and retracted toward the sinus. **B,** The interhemispheric fissure is entered and carefully divided. A self-retaining retractor may be useful. During the approach, care is taken to identify the callosal marginal and then the pericallosal arteries. If adhesions between the frontal lobes must be divided, it is important that the division stay medial to the arteries to avoid disrupting small perforators. Here, the distinct shiny white appearance of the corpus callosum makes it readily identifiable.

septum pellucidum and anteriorly to the anterior commissure. A combination of suction and bipolar cautery, microdissector, or carbon dioxide laser is utilized to perform the disconnection.[34] As the dissection is completed anteriorly, the anterior cerebral arteries and associated perforators are identified and spared. If a complete callosotomy is intended, the craniotomy must be larger and extend posteriorly. Otherwise, multiple craniotomies may be performed.[35] During posterior callosotomy, care must be taken to avoid injuring internal cerebral veins and the vein of Galen just below the splenium; identification of the deep cerebral vein through the arachnoid signals completion of the dissection. In addition, in the posterior callosal division, it is important that the dissection remains midline and is advanced cautiously to avoid injuring the fornices, which are located just below the corpus callosum. Frameless guidance is then used to confirm the extent of the sectioning.

Results

Many series have shown corpus callosotomy to be effective for patients with multiple seizure types whose epilepsy is refractory to antiepileptic therapy.[14,26,29,30,35-37] Interpretation of the results from large series can be difficult because of the heterogeneity of the seizure classification and the differing extent of callosotomies. Patients with atonic seizures have been thought to benefit the greatest and may become free of drop attacks entirely. Oguni and colleagues[14] reported a series of 43 patients who underwent anterior corpus callosotomies, describing a greater than 75% reduction in drop attacks in 33% of the patients. In 1996, Rossi and associates[27] reported a series of 19 patients who experienced a 47% freedom from drop attacks after the procedure. The same year, Maehara and coworkers[38] reported cure of drop attacks in 25% of adult patients and 42% of pediatric patients. Five years later Maehara and Shimzu[26] reported achieving a more than 90% reduction in drop attacks in 85% of 52 patients.[26] Despite these positive results in patients with atonic seizures, greater follow-up is required to assess long-term seizure control. A meta-analysis reviewing long-term results for all epilepsy surgery found that only 35% of patients undergoing callosotomy were without drop attacks after 5 years.[39]

Positive results have also been reported for other types of generalized seizures. Wong and colleagues,[29] in reviewing their series of 268 pediatric patients with a variety of seizure types, demonstrated a greater than 50% reduction of seizures in more than half of the patients. Cukiert and associates[28] reported a series of 76 patients who underwent extended callosotomy sparing only the splenium. The study showed that 91% of patients responded overall, with responsiveness defined as a greater than 50% reduction in seizures. Among the seizure types, atonic had the best response rate, at 92%, and myoclonic the poorest, at 27%. Additional studies have shown modest improvements in rates of absence, tonic-clonic, and myoclonic seizures after callosotomy.[40,41]

There is considerable debate as to the ideal length of the callosotomy, with multiple series showing benefit for both partial and complete disconnection.[14,20,29,30,40-42] It is generally accepted in the literature that more extensive callosotomies offer the greater chance of seizure reduction albeit with the possibility of greater morbidity. For this reason, callosotomies are usually performed in a staged manner. Patients with low functional status who are unlikely to be impaired by disconnection syndromes may benefit from a single-stage, complete callosotomy and thereby avoid additional surgery. Younger age at seizure onset and at surgery has been shown to be a predictor of both seizure control and lower rates of adverse side effects.[26,36,43] Patients are more resilient and are able to avoid the repeated trauma associated with a life of drop attacks. Higher IQ has also been shown to be a positive predictor of favorable outcome.[36] Low IQ is often associated with severe bilateral structural impairment, which results in poor seizure control with both medications and surgery. However, mental retardation is not a contraindication to surgery in the population that is in the most need of seizure relief.[42,44]

The result of callosotomy has been compared directly with that of vagal nerve stimulation. Nei and colleagues[31] compared seizure control and complication rates in 53 patients undergoing corpus callosotomy and 25 undergoing vagal nerve stimulation. Although the patients who had had callosotomy had better seizure control, there was also a permanent complication rate of 3.8%, compared with no complications in the group undergoing VNS.[31] Despite the proven effectiveness of callosotomy, the complications associated with craniotomy and the side effects of disconnection syndromes have made VNS more attractive as an initial procedure for patients with refractory epilepsy. As previously mentioned, patients in whom VNS fails are often later referred for callosotomy.

Complications

Complications associated with corpus callosotomy are approach related to the operative approach or are syndromes that develop as a result of the disconnection itself. Those associated with the operative approach include epidural hematoma, subdural hematoma, meningitis, and deep venous thrombosis. Later studies have reported relatively low rates ranging from 2.4% to 6%.[29,30,45,46]

Complications associated with disconnection of the hemispheres include mutism, acute disconnection syndrome (ADS), posterior disconnection syndrome, and split brain syndrome.[29] There are a wide variety of disconnection syndromes, and they may be acute or chronic. Owing to prefrontal lobe disconnection, patients may demonstrate symptoms identical to those of the supplementary motor area (SMA) syndrome in the immediate postoperative period. This syndrome is characterized by paresis of the nondominant leg, incontinence, and decreased spontaneous speech.[47] Acute callosal disconnection symptoms have been reported to occur in 89% of patients in a series of extended callosotomies.[28] The duration and severity of the syndrome is shown to be worse for patients undergoing single-stage, complete callosotomy.[37] The patient may also have apraxia of the nondominant hand, nondominant hypotonia, repetitive grasping with the nondominant hand, and bilateral Babinski response.[47] In its most severe form, patients are minimally reactive to the environment despite being awake, with symptoms lasting days to weeks.[48] Injury to the vasculature during the approach, to the fornices, to the septal area, or to the hypothalamus is rare. External hydrocephalus can result if the lateral ventricle is entered during the callosal section.

Several months after callosotomy, patients typically appear to be at their neurological baseline. However, detailed testing detects persistent deficits that are referred to as chronic disconnection syndromes. The manifestation is related to the extent of the callosotomy. Chronic syndromes include alien hand syndrome due to frontal lobe disconnection, poor sound localization from temporal lobe disconnection, tactile dysnomia and "pure" word blindness from parietal dysfunction, and visual suppression from occipital lobe isolation.[47] Reported rates of symptomatic disconnection syndromes have ranged from 45% to 80%, with adults having higher rates than children.[49] Because of the anatomic configuration of the corpus callosum, patients undergoing complete or posterior callosotomy are at higher risk for development of permanent interhemispheric sensory disassociation. The surgeon must also recognize and discuss the increased risk of language deficits in patients with crossed cerebral dominance.[50]

Conclusion

Corpus callosotomy is a long-established technique for seizure palliation. The procedure has been effectively used for multiple types of generalized seizures, having the best results in those with atonic and tonic seizures. The application of microsurgical technique and limiting callosotomy length has decreased morbidity. The development of alternative forms of seizure palliation, such as vagal nerve stimulation, and the improved ability to identify and treat focal epilepsy have limited the application of callosotomy. Regardless, callosotomy remains a safe and effective treatment for a select group of patients suffering from severe epilepsy.

MULTIPLE SUBPIAL TRANSECTION

From the inception of epilepsy surgery, it has been clear that resective surgery for medically intractable seizure foci can be done in noneloquent areas with acceptably low rates of morbidity and a reasonable chance for seizure control in carefully selected patients. Resection of seizure foci in eloquent cortex, however, results in unacceptable deficits. The surgical procedure of multiple subpial transection (MST) attempts to address this difficult problem by capitalizing on the difference between the vertical and horizontal organizations of the cortical structures of the brain.[51] The master organizational principle in the cerebral cortex is the functional vertical column, with its vertical orientation of incoming and outgoing fibers and blood supply.[52-54] At the same time, seizures in part spread horizontally through the gray matter. MST involves disconnecting the gray matter columns that lie in eloquent cortex. This technique may inhibit synchronization and spread of the seizure focus with minimal injury to the cortex. In this section we review the history of the development of MST, patient selection, surgical indications, technique, results, pitfalls, and areas for further exploration. New horizons for the application of MST, including hippocampal transection for mesial temporal epilepsy, are also reviewed.

A brief history of the procedure is examined in the electronic version of this chapter at ExpertConsult.com, along with an expanded discussion of operative techniques and approaches.

Patient Selection

The great majority of surgical epilepsy cases can be treated with standard resection techniques such as temporal lobectomy with amygdalohippocampectomy and extratemporal resection in noneloquent cortex. Subpial transection is reserved for patients in whom the seizure activity originates in eloquent cortex. MST has been used to treat patients with epileptogenic lesions of the speech, motor, or primary sensory cortex. Although MST has been used for Rasmussen's encephalitis, it is of questionable benefit for progressive disease states when the underlying disease cannot be controlled.[84,85]

MST can be used for the treatment of carefully selected cases of the following disorders:

- Epilepsia partialis continua
- Focal sensory, somatosensory, or visual cortex seizures
- Persistent epileptogenic activity in eloquent areas adjacent to a previous or concomitant resection
- Landau-Kleffner syndrome
- Rasmussen's encephalitis[86]
- Status epilepticus[84,87]

Operative Procedure

In most cases, subdural grid recording and mapping have been done, and general anesthesia is used. If intraoperative awake mapping is planned, lighter anesthesia is used, along with intravenous sedation and generous use of local anesthetic. Patients are positioned so that the planned operative exposure is superior in the field and the head is in three-point fixation. A standard craniotomy is made with an exposure large enough to allow for functional mapping and or electrocorticography (ECoG). In many patients in whom MST is being considered, the seizure focus lies in both eloquent and noneloquent areas of the cortex. In these cases, surgical resection is performed in the noneloquent cortex to within 1.5 cm of language cortex and to the border of sensory and motor cortex, as delineated by intraoperative or subdural grid stimulation mapping with standard techniques.[88,89] Descending white matter pathways and vascular supplies are preserved. If repeat ECoG does not show significant resolution of the interictal activity and the primary residual focus lies within eloquent cortex, MST is performed on the crown of the involved gyri at 5-mm intervals through the gray matter. Transections are made in parallel rows in the direction perpendicular to the long axis of the gyrus (Fig. 73-2). If significant resolution of the seizure focus is noted on ECoG, no further transection is done. If no significant resolution is noted and a clearly focal area is active despite transection of the crown of the gyrus in that area, transection is sometimes carried out vertically into the gray matter within the depth of the sulcus, as illustrated in a cadaver

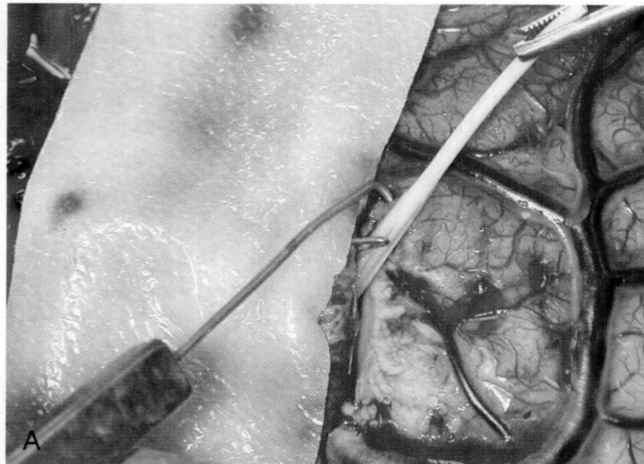

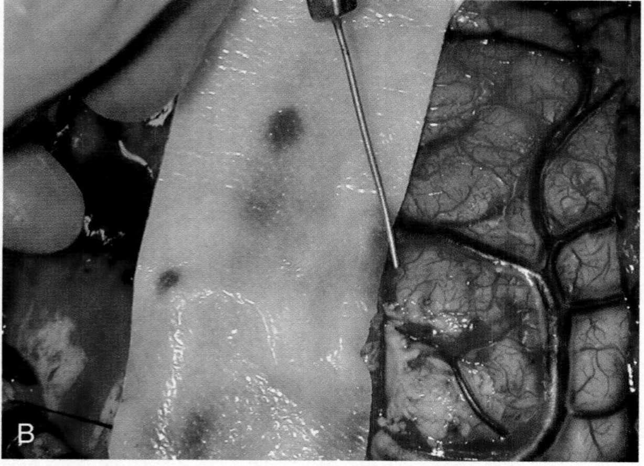

Figure 73-2. A, The transection hook enters through the hole. **B,** The hook is advanced stepwise across the gyrus, with the tip of the hook visible beneath the pia. The transector is then withdrawn along the same path.

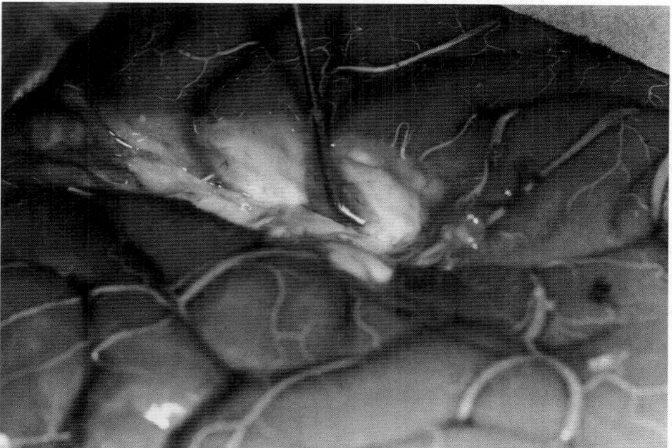

Figure 73-3. On a cadaver specimen in the coronal plane, the transector is seen advancing into the depth of a sulcus. The tip is reversed and pointed away from the sulcus to lessen the possibility of vessel injury.

in Figure 73-3. This transection is performed along the same plane as transection of the crown. If the primary seizure focus is truly in the MST area, these maneuvers usually stop or significantly reduce the interictal epileptic discharges. If they do not, it is possible that the preoperative evaluation and ECoG have not shown the primary seizure focus, which may be projecting abnormal electrical activity from a distance.

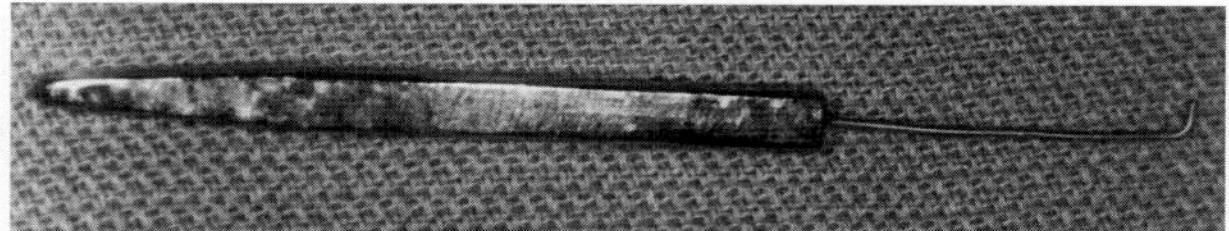

Figure 73-4. The transector has three parts. The rectangular handle is connected to a malleable wire with a 4-mm tip. The tip is angled 105 degrees to prevent snagging of vessels.

Transections

Transections are performed with a specially designed fine, malleable wire that is bent into a 4-mm blunt hook at the tip (Fig. 73-4). The hook of the subpial transector (Whisler-Morrell Subpial Transector, Redman Neurotechnologists, Lake Zurich, IL) measures 4 mm in length to match the average depth of gray matter in the neocortex.[53] This hook is bent at an obtuse angle of 105 degrees relative to the main shaft of the wire. The wire is connected to a rectangular handle with the tip of the hook aligned with the flat sides of the handle. This arrangement is important because it prevents the hook from going into the cortex at any angle other than perpendicular. If the hook is advanced through the cortex at an angle off the perpendicular, extensive undercutting of the cortex will result, with corresponding deficits. The transection hook shank can be bent to any shape necessary for use in technically difficult locations. This flexibility is useful in the interhemispheric motor and visual cortices and in the posterior temporal lobe when the sylvian fissure is opened to allow access to the depths of the fissure.

The area to be transected is carefully inspected. The gyral and microgyral patterns are noted. The course of the vascular supply and bypassing vessels is traced. After ECoG, transections are usually begun in the most dependent area because subarachnoid bleeding may occur. If a large amount of subarachnoid blood accumulates, a small opening can be made in the pia to let the blood escape. Each transection is begun with the opening of a hole in an avascular area of the pia, at the edge of a sulcus with a 20-gauge needle. As the transector hook enters the gray matter through this opening, the hook must be kept vertically oriented to avoid undercutting and advancing the tip too deep and thus injuring white matter. The hook is advanced in stepwise fashion in a straight line across the crown of the gyrus in a direction perpendicular to the long axis of the gyrus. The hook is then withdrawn along the same path, with the tip of the hook visible just below the pia.[93-95] As the hook is withdrawn from the pial puncture site, a small amount of blood sometimes escapes. This is easily controlled with a small piece of absorbable gelatin sponge (Gelfoam) and gentle pressure. The next transection line is made parallel to and 5 mm from the first. Because the hook is 4 mm long, it can be used to estimate the distance to the next transection line. The transections are thus done along the gyrus in the area of the seizure focus. Great care must be taken to note the course of the major blood vessels, particularly around the sylvian and interhemispheric fissures. When transection must be performed in the depths of a sulcus or fissure, the hook is inserted upside down, with the tip pointed away from the pial surface. This maneuver lessens the likelihood of damaging a vessel in the sulcus or fissure. The obtuse angle of the hook also helps lessen the likelihood of injury to vessels. In cases of perisylvian-onset epilepsy, it is often useful to open the sylvian fissure to record from the depths of the fissure and transect under direct vision. In some cases, transection at 5-mm intervals is not possible because of microgyral patterns or a large confluence of vessels that may cover the area to be transected (Fig. 73-5).

Pathology, Imaging, and Complications

More information on these topics, as they relate to MST, is available in the expanded, electronic version of this chapter at ExpertConsult.com.

Seizure Outcome

For evaluation of the effects of MST on seizure outcome, it is useful to examine MST procedures in the following categories:

- MST for focal-onset epilepsy in which MST is the only procedure done.
- MST for focal-onset epilepsy in which cortical resection of noneloquent cortex is also performed. In such cases, preoperative evaluation showed seizure activity in eloquent and noneloquent areas of cortex, and the cortical resection had no significant effect on ECoG findings. MST was then performed on adjacent eloquent cortex.

Seizure outcome after MST is analyzed in this fashion because the cortical resection done in the majority of cases introduces a confounding variable: one cannot be certain whether MST or the resection had the effect on seizure outcome or on morbidity. In these cases, one can be certain only that MST had an effect on intraoperative ECoG. The group that underwent MST as the only surgical intervention gives the clearest indication of the effect of MST on seizure outcome because there are fewer confounding variables and the pathology is more uniform in this group. In 16 patients who underwent MST alone for focal-onset seizures in eloquent cortex with at least 2 years of follow-up, 6 were made seizure free (Table 73-1). Six other patients had only rare seizures or had a 90% or greater reduction in seizures. Four patients had no worthwhile benefit. Overall, 75% of patients in this category had a worthwhile Engel's class I to III seizure outcome. Because all of these patients would have been rejected for standard resection, their outcomes should be compared with that of best medical therapy.

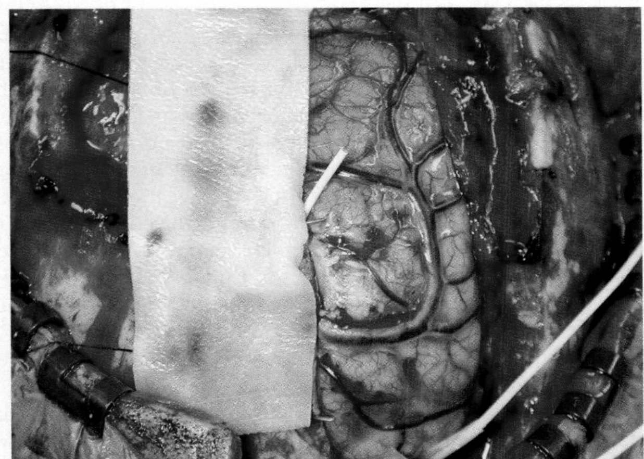

Figure 73-5. After transections are completed, fine lines can be seen beneath the pia at 5-mm intervals. Petechial bleeding is easily controlled with absorbable gelatin sponge Gelfoam and gentle pressure.

Other groups have reported similar results (see Table 73-3 later). In Wyler and coworkers'[63] series of 6 patients with uniform pathology in the sensorimotor cortex, all 6 had a significant reduction in seizures after MST.[63] Only 1 had a permanent mild motor deficit. Schramm and colleagues[83] reported on a series of 20 patients who underwent MST without resection.[83] At the 1-year follow-up 45% of the patients had a worthwhile outcome (Engel's class I to III). These investigators reported that lesional epilepsy and large areas of epileptic discharge predicted a worse outcome. Mulligan and coworkers[73] reported a 42% rate of significant improvement in seizure frequency in a series of 12 patients. Spencer and associates[103] conducted an international meta-analysis on 212 patients who underwent MST at six epilepsy centers. In cases of MST without resection, the reported rates of excellent outcome with regard to seizure control were 71% for generalized epilepsy, 62% for complex partial epilepsy, and 63% for simple partial seizures.

The next category of patients underwent a combination of MST and resection. This was the most common type of case in the series reported by Morrell and colleagues.[51] It is rare for a seizure focus to lie entirely in eloquent cortex. After MST, a total of 82% of patients in this category were seizure free or had a significant reduction in seizures (Engel's class I to III; see Table 73-1). Although the majority of patients exhibited worthwhile improvement, the initial report by Morrell and colleagues,[51] of 52% being free of seizures, was not sustained later in the series. The meta-analysis reported by Spencer and associates[103] showed similar results for patients who underwent resection plus MST, with excellent outcomes (>95% seizure reduction) reported in 87% of patients with generalized seizures, 68% of patients with complex partial seizures, and 68% of patients with simple partial epilepsy. These collective data support the efficacy of MST, both as a stand-alone procedure for highly localized cases in eloquent cortex and for cases in which the epileptogenic zone overlaps eloquent cortex. The expected outcome of MST, however, is more likely to be improvement rather than cure. Results from other series are listed in Table 73-1.

The question of long-term efficacy has been raised. Orbach and coworkers[104] reported an 18.5% seizure recurrence rate in a series of patients who underwent MST and had at least 5 years of follow-up. In a series of 20 patients who underwent pure MST, Schramm and colleagues[83] reported that outcomes changed over time; 5 patients had improvement of their seizures during the long-term follow-up period, whereas 7 experienced worsening. This phenomenon has also been described in patients who have undergone resection epilepsy surgery.

TABLE 73-1 Outcomes after Multiple Subpial Transection (MST)

		Engel's Classification*				Neurological Complications	
Surgical Procedure	**N**	**Class I (%)**	**Class II (%)**	**Class III (%)**	**Class IV (%)**	**Transient (%)**	**Permanent (%)**
MST only, for partial seizures	16	6 (37.5)	4 (25)	2 (12.5)	4 (25)	1 (6)	3 (19)
MST only, for Landau-Kleffner syndrome	16	9 (57.7)	2 (12.5)	2 (12.5)	3 (18)	2 (12.5)	—
MST/resection	68	33 (48.5)	7 (10)	16 (23.5)	12 (18)	7 (10)	4 (6)
TOTAL	100	48	13	20	19	10	7

*Classes I to III indicate significant worthwhile improvement; class IV indicates no significant improvement.

Modified from Morrell F, Kanner A, Whisler W. Multiple subpial transection. In: Stefan H, Andermann F, eds. *Plasticity in Epilepsy*. New York: Lippincott-Raven; 1998.

Conclusion

The initial experience with MST was reported in 1989.[51] In that group of patients with intractable seizures, 11 of 20 were free of seizures after a follow-up of at least 5 years. Subsequent cases in which MST was performed without resection proved the independent efficacy of the procedure. Since then, MST has proved helpful in patients with intractable epilepsy and foci in unresectable cortex. Similar results at other centers have confirmed its efficacy and safety if done properly in well-selected patients. The exact mechanism of action of MST is being delineated with functional testing. Other centers attempting MST have added different techniques and new protocols.[63,65] As we learn more about MST and about the nature of epileptogenic cortex, the technique will be further refined, resulting in improved outcomes in patients with unresectable seizure foci.

TOPECTOMY

The prevalence of epilepsy is approximately 1%. In the majority of cases, it can be effectively treated medically with antiepileptic drugs, but 30% to 40% of all new cases of epilepsy will ultimately become refractory to treatment.[105] Some investigators report that ongoing medication trials can be a satisfactory approach to managing refractory epilepsy.[106] However, it is important to consider surgery patients with this disorder.[107]

In the Montreal Neurological Institute series covering the period 1929 to 1980, the anatomic distribution of surgical resection in 2177 patients was as follows: temporal, 56%; frontal, 18%; central, 7%; parietal, 6%; occipital, 1%; and multilobar, 11%.[108]

Topectomy generally indicates resection of focal cerebral cortex from the frontal, parietal, or occipital lobe. For epilepsy surgery outside the temporal lobe, localization of seizure origin is much more difficult, seizure outcome is less favorable, and surgery in some brain sites is associated with higher risk of major morbidity than with temporal lobe resection.[109] Although temporal lobe resection is much more common in modern epilepsy practice, topectomy is the foundation of modern epilepsy surgery. In 1886, Sir Victor Horsley performed what would now be considered lesionectomies with excellent results. Before the invention of EEG in 1928, epilepsy surgery was exploratory and based on clinical localization pioneered by Jackson and identification of visibly abnormal tissue. EEG removed this requirement and decreased explorations with negative results considerably through the 1950s and 1960s.[57,110] MRI now provides a priori knowledge of most structural cortical abnormalities. Box 73-1 shows the types of surgical procedures for epilepsy.

A fundamental concept underlying focal cortical resection is that the epileptic focus contains electrically abnormal neurons or circuits that are the source of seizures. Hence, if this epileptogenic focus can be accurately identified and resected, the seizures will cease. Epileptogenicity is assumed to derive from physiologic events that occur within the cell body and dendrites of neurons rather than axons.[111] Therefore, resection of only epileptogenic gray matter (cerebral cortex) rather than white matter should in theory be sufficient to eliminate seizures. Later work suggests that epilepsy may arise as a result of abnormalities of a distributed cellular network.[112] Therefore, intrinsic cellular abnormalities may not be required to create an epileptic condition. The most characteristic and ubiquitous pathologic changes are the presence of gliosis, loss of neurons, and dendritic abnormalities.[113,114] This section reviews the principles and methods of surgical localization and cortical resection in patients who may be candidates for topectomy.

BOX 73-1 General Categories of Epilepsy Surgery

RESECTION

Hemispherectomy: resection of the cerebral hemisphere
Lobectomy: resection of one cerebral lobe
Topectomy: resection of a focal area of cerebral cortex

DISCONNECTION

Corpus callosotomy: disconnection of two hemispheres
Multiple subpial transection: disconnection of a focal area of cerebral cortex
Hemispherectomy: disconnection of a cerebral hemisphere

STIMULATION

Vagal nerve stimulation
Anterior thalamic stimulation
Responsive neurostimulation

Patient Selection

In general, surgical treatment of epilepsy should be considered when (1) the seizures have not been controlled by adequate attempts at treatment with maximally tolerable doses of correct anticonvulsant medications; (2) the seizures interfere with psychological and intellectual development, employment, or social performance; (3) all potentially epileptogenic areas have matured, the seizure tendency (pattern and frequency) is stable, and there is no tendency toward spontaneous regression; and (4) the patient is strongly motivated to cope with an exhaustive diagnostic regimen and a lengthy operative procedure, possibly under local anesthesia.[115-117] Further understanding of the potential risks and benefits of epilepsy surgery is necessary. Chronic psychosis is a contraindication to surgical treatment, but epilepsy-related acute psychosis is not. Mental retardation is not a contraindication.[118,119]

The length of time that patients have seizures before being referred for surgery has become shorter as referring physicians recognize that superior surgical results may be obtained when the period of uncontrolled seizures is shortened, particularly in children.[120] Despite this understanding, the adoption of epilepsy surgery has been relatively slow. Currently, adequate but unsuccessful antiepileptic drug therapy for 1 to 5 years may be a sufficiently long trial period to warrant referral for consideration of epilepsy surgery.[119] Later trials of epilepsy surgery, however, such as the Early Randomized Surgery for Epilepsy Trial (ERSET), define refractory epilepsy as continued seizures despite two consecutive years of treatment with two antiepileptic medications. [121] In exceptional cases, urgent cortical resection may be considered for the relief of status epilepticus.[122]

A representative list of neurological diagnoses that may be considered for surgery involving focal cortical resection is shown in eBox 73-1.[123] Topectomy can be considered when the seizure arises from a focal and functionally silent area of the brain, a finding that usually means that the focus is not in the speech, primary visual, sensory, or motor cortex. Additionally, neuropsychological testing is performed to identify any functional deficits that may be related to the epileptic cortical region.[124] Multiple widespread or bilateral foci are generally contraindications to resection. A series of diagnostic studies, including EEG, are necessary to confirm the site of seizure onset. In eloquent brain regions, MST or RNS may be considered, as previously discussed.

Presurgical Evaluation

The optimal surgery for epilepsy is resection of just enough neuronal tissue to eliminate the patient's seizures without causing unacceptable neurological deficits. Presurgical evaluation enables the surgeon to determine the volume of cortex involved in seizure initiation and propagation and whether it can be safely resected. As stated by Rasmussen,[125] epileptogenic lesions outside the temporal lobe are considerably more varied in extent and geographic configuration than the more common temporal lobe epileptogenic lesions. A variety of diagnostic tests are used for this purpose, but there is no consensus on how much information is actually needed before a particular surgical intervention can be recommended.[126]

The initial preoperative evaluation process includes careful examination of clinical seizure characteristics, ictal and interictal scalp EEG, neuroimaging, and neuropsychological testing. The results of this testing should provide considerable lateralizing and localizing information. Video-EEG monitoring is the "gold standard" of the evaluation. When noninvasive tests do not show the source of seizures clearly, invasive testing is considered. Localization of the seizure focus is difficult in patients with extratemporal epilepsy, and invasive EEG is almost always required in nonlesional epilepsy.[109]

Please see the electronic version of this chapter on ExpertConsult.com for expanded discussions of symptomatic localization of seizures, neuroimaging, neuropsychological testing, and invasive evaluations, such as Wada testing and invasive electroencephalography.

Noninvasive Evaluation

Extracranial Electroencephalography. Scalp EEG often provides important information about the location and size of the epileptogenic area. An interictal epileptiform abnormality consisting of spikes, spike and slow wave complexes, sharp waves, and sharp and slow wave complexes repeated on several occasions may be particularly informative.[131]Activation procedures such as withdrawal of medication, hyperventilation, or drug-induced sleep may enhance abnormalities or even provoke a seizure.[116]

In addition, long-term video-EEG monitoring is generally performed in an epilepsy monitoring unit to correlate clinical seizure activity with the accompanying electrical abnormalities with the intent of identifying the seizure origin electrographically.[109] The specific ictal symptomatology can help greatly if localization of the focus is problematic. The EEG pattern of seizure onset is most frequently rhythmic, fast, spike-like discharges, often building in amplitude.[112]

Surgical Topectomy Procedure

Brief discussions of general principles, preoperative care, and anesthesia are available at ExpertConsult.com.

Intraoperative Electrocorticography

Sufficient brain exposure via craniotomy is essential during ECoG, which is performed to further delineate the extent of the epileptogenic zone. The intention is to locate regions with primary epileptic neurons by identifying brain sites that have interictal ECoG spikes. This use is very controversial, and there may not be a clear relationship among the site of interictal discharges, the site of ictal onset, and the tissue that must be removed to control seizures.

ECoG may provide prognostic information by indicating areas with residual discharges after cortical resection. Patients with no interictal discharges on postresection recordings are more likely to be free of seizures than those with persisting discharges.[108,176] For "standard" temporal lobectomy surgery, the value of ECoG is not as clear.[177-179]

Cortical Stimulation (Functional Mapping)

The purpose of intraoperative cortical stimulation is to localize eloquent cortex such as the motor cortex, sensory cortex, or language area in the dominant hemisphere. Functional mapping is necessary when cortical resections are carried out near eloquent brain areas. Identification of motor cortex is useful for any resection in the posterior frontal or parietal lobes. Identification of language cortex is necessary for any dominant-hemisphere resection in the perisylvian cortex.

The location of the central sulcus is determined by electrical stimulation of the precentral and postcentral gyri after preliminary identification by monitoring for the SEP phase reversal.[167] The suspected site of the motor and sensory cortex is stimulated and mapped with a motor response detected by the anesthetist or a sensory change reported by the patient.[118,166,176] In practice, one way to identify the postcentral gyrus is to induce sensory responses in the tongue area, which located at the bottom of the postcentral gyrus.[130,180]

The frontal, parietal, and temporal language areas in the dominant hemisphere are stimulated while the patient carries out simple verbal tasks such as naming objects shown on picture cards. A language-critical area is identified if the patient is unable to speak (speech arrest) when the site is being stimulated or if the patient can speak but is unable to name objects.[117,118,166,176] Although failure to produce speech arrest, or anomia, does not always exclude the presence of language-critical sites in the stimulated cortex, intraoperative or extraoperative grid mapping is nevertheless the most reliable method currently available for identifying such sites.

It is important to monitor EEG during mapping to identify an afterdischarge. The presence of an afterdischarge induces regional activation and not focal activation limited to the 0.5-cm cortical region between the bipolar stimulator probes. Afterdischarges may lead both to false-positive localization and intraoperative generalized seizures. If afterdischarges are identified, a lower stimulation setting should be used.[181]

Surgical Technique

Unlike in temporal lobectomy, there are no anatomically standard operations for extratemporal cortical resection.

A craniotomy is performed to expose the epileptic focus that will be resected. The extent of neocortical resection is based on the gross pathology and the results of intracranial electrode studies, ECoG when applicable, and functional mapping. Essential motor and language areas should be preserved (preferably with a 2- or 1-cm margin), regardless of involvement in the epileptic focus.[118] Special attention is also given to the vascular supply of the area to be resected.[166] The extent of the resection is individually tailored in each patient.

A subpial dissection technique is used for cortical resection (Fig. 73-6).[112,117,118,120,166,182] This procedure was used by Horsley in 1909 and has remained the technical basis of surgery for epilepsy to this day. The pial surface is coagulated and incised in a relatively avascular area. Gyral resection is then carried out in a subpial fashion. An ultrasonic aspirator at a low suction/vibration setting is extremely useful for focal resections in a subpial plane. Meticulous, slow removal of epileptogenic gray matter is carried to the bottom of the sulcus without damage to vessels within the pia that might supply other, nonresected tissue. Hemostasis is achieved principally with topical agents such as absorbable gelatin sponge (Gelfoam) or absorbable hemostat (Surgicel) and minimal use of electrocautery. With the topectomy procedure, unnecessary resection of the underlying white matter is avoided to preserve the integrity of projection, association, and commissural fibers.

Appropriate antiepileptic medication and dexamethasone are administered after cortical resection.

Surgical Outcome

Extratemporal nonlesional resection is associated with worse seizure control rates and a higher incidence of major postoperative

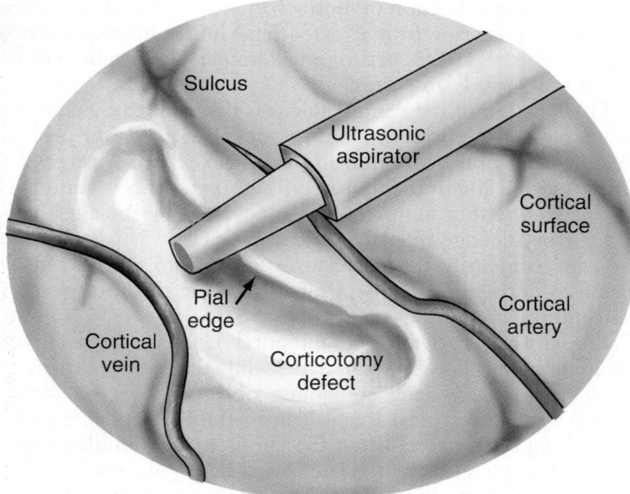

Figure 73-6. Simple cartoon illustrating basic microsurgical principles. 1: Open the pia with bipolar cautery and microscissors. 2: For cortical resection, it is not necessary to remove tissue deeper than the bottom of the sulcus. 3: The cortical veins and arteries are preserved during traverse of a sulcus. 4: The arachnoid flap is used to retract veins and arteries. 5: An ultrasonic aspirator on low power is used to resect to the pia of the parallel sulcus.

TABLE 73-2 Seizure Outcome after Surgical Treatment

	Anterior Temporal Lobectomy (%)	Extratemporal Resection (%)
Seizure free	2429 (67.9)	363 (45.1)
Improved	860 (24.0)	283 (35.2)
Not improved	290 (8.1)	159 (19.8)
Total	3579 (100)	805 (100)

Modified from Engel J, Ness PCV, Rasmussen TB, et al. Outcome with respect to epileptic seizures. In: Engel J, ed. *Surgical Treatment of the Epilepsies*. 2nd ed. New York: Raven Press; 1993:609-621.

TABLE 73-3 Comparison of Recent Work with the Engel Report

Study	Year	Central Theme of Study	Patients with Engel Class 1 Outcome
Englot et al[185]	2013	Meta analysis: nonlesional epilepsy	62%
Ansari et al[186]	2010	Nonlesional epilepsy	33.7%
Elsharkawy et al[187]	2008	Extratemporal epilepsy	54.5%
Kral et al[188]	2007	Focal cortical dysplasia	76%
Bauman et al[189]	2005	Multistage surgery	60%
Tellez-Zenteno et al[39]	2005	Meta-analysis: long-term outcomes	27% after frontal lobe resection/46% after occipital and parietal resections
Chapman et al[190]	2005	Normal magnetic resonance imaging findings	37%

morbidity than is lesional or temporal lobe resection surgery. Table 73-2 presents the seizure outcome reported by Engel and colleagues in 1993,[183] which shows a seizure-free rate of 45% and improvement rate of 35%. Later work is summarized in Table 73-3.

With localized resective surgery, less than 5% of patients have some postoperative neurological deficit as a result of unintended vascular compromise or other accidental damage to essential neural tissue; however, most of these deficits are transient and resolve within months. Postoperative bleeding and infection are uncommon. Seizures in the acute postoperative period may portend a poor prognosis, and most patients continue to require pharmacologic treatment.

Conclusion

Extratemporal epilepsy encompasses a broad range of diagnoses and is associated with greater difficulty in identification of a discrete seizure focus. There is no "standard" operation to treat these disorders; the surgical procedure must be customized to each patient. This variability and the comparatively poor seizure control results after surgery support the contention that extratemporal lobe epilepsy is a much more complex and variable disorder than temporal lobe epilepsy. Nonlesional epilepsy surgery requires a more extensive and invasive preoperative diagnostic evaluation, and the probability of an excellent outcome is lower than with temporal lobe epilepsy. Nevertheless, topectomy can decrease and sometimes eliminate disabling epilepsy at a reasonable neuropsychological cost. Topectomy should be considered for carefully selected patients who have the highest chance of benefiting from it.

SUGGESTED READINGS

Abson Kraemer DL. Diagnostic techniques in surgical management of epilepsy: strip electrodes, grids and depth electrodes. In: Schmidek HH, Roberts DW, eds. *Schmidek & Sweet Operative Neurosurgical Techniques: Indications, Methods, and Results*. 4th ed. Philadelphia: WB Saunders; 2000:1359-1374.

Barkovich AJ, Rowley HA, Andermann F. MR in partial epilepsy: value of high-resolution volumetric techniques. *AJNR Am J Neuroradiol.* 1995;16:339-343.

Bauman JA, Feoli E, Romanelli P, et al. Multistage epilepsy surgery: safety, efficacy and utility of a novel approach in pediatric extratemporal epilepsy. *Neurosurgery*. 2005;56:318-334.

Chapman K, Wyllie E, Najm I, et al. Seizure outcome after epilepsy surgery in patients with normal preoperative MRI. *J Neurol Neurosurg Psychiatry*. 2005;76:710-713.

Cohen-Gadol AA, Stoffman MR, Spencer DD. Emerging surgical and radiotherapeutic techniques for treating epilepsy. *Curr Opin Neurol.* 2003;16:213-219.

Devinsky O, Perrine K, Vazquez B, et al. Multiple subpial transections in the language cortex. *Brain*. 1994;117:255-265.

Faught E. Collective data supports efficacy of multiple subpial transection. *Epilepsy Curr*. 2002;2:108.

Hashizume K, Tanaka T. Multiple subpial transection in kainic acid–induced focal cortical seizure. *Epilepsy Res*. 1998;32:389-399.

Hufnagel A, Zenter J, Fernandez G, et al. Multiple subpial transection for control of epileptic seizures: effectiveness and safety. *Epilepsia*. 1997;38:678-688.

Kaufmann W, Kraus G, Uematsu S, et al. Treatment of epilepsy with multiple subpial transections: an acute histological analysis in human subjects. *Epilepsia*. 1996;37:342-352.

Leonhardt G, Spiekermann G, Muller S, et al. Cortical reorganization following multiple subpial transection in human brain—a study with positron emission tomography. *Neurosci Lett*. 2000;292:63-65.

Morrell F, Whisler WW, Bleck T. Multiple subpial transaction: a new approach to the surgical treatment of focal epilepsy. *J Neurosurg*. 1989;70:231-239.

Mulligan LP, Spencer DD, Spencer SS. Multiple subpial transections: the Yale experience. *Epilepsia*. 2001;42:226-229.

Ojemann GA. Awake operations with mapping in epilepsy. In: Schmidek HH, Sweet WH, eds. *Operative Neurosurgical Techniques*. 3rd ed. Philadelphia: WB Saunders; 1995:1317-1322.

Ojemann GA. Surgical treatment of epilepsy. In: Wilkins RH, Rengachary SS, eds. *Neurosurgery*. 2nd ed. New York: McGraw-Hill; 1996:4173-4183.

Olivier A, Awad IA. Extratemporal resections. In: Engel J, ed. *Surgical Treatment of the Epilepsies*. 2nd ed. New York: Raven Press; 1993:489-500.

Pierre-Louis SJC, Smith MC, Morrell F, et al. Anatomical effects of multiple subpial transection. *Epilepsia*. 1993;34(suppl):104.
Rasmussen T. Surgery of frontal lobe epilepsy. *Adv Neurol*. 1975;8: 197-205.
Schramm J, Aliashkevich AF, Grunwald T. Multiple subpial transections: outcome and complications in 20 patients who did not undergo resection. *J Neurosurg*. 2002;97:39-47.
Shimizu H, Kawai K, Sunaga S, et al. [Surgical treatment for temporal lobe epilepsy with preservation of postoperative memory function.]. *Rinshō Shinkeigaku*. 2004;44:868-870.
Shimizu H, Kawai K, Sunaga S, et al. Hippocampal transection for treatment of left temporal lobe epilepsy with preservation of verbal memory. *J Clin Neurosci*. 2006;13:322-328.
Smith MC, Byrne R. Multiple subpial transection in neocortical epilepsy: part I. *Adv Neurol*. 2000;84:621-634.
Spencer SS, Schramm J, Wyler A, et al. Multiple subpial transection for intractable partial epilepsy: an international meta-analysis. *Epilepsia*. 2002;43:141-145.
Sperry RW, Miner N, Myers RE. Visual pattern perception following subpial slicing and tantalum wire implantation in visual cortex. *J Comp Physiol Psychol*. 1955;48:50-58.
Tanaka T, Hashizume K, Sawamura A, et al. Basic science and epilepsy: experimental epilepsy surgery. *Stereotact Funct Neurosurg*. 2001;77: 239-244.
Wada J, Rasmussen T. Intracranial injection of Amytal for the localization of cerebral speech dominance. *J Neurosurg*. 1960;17:266-282.
Whisler WW. Multiple subpial transection. In: Kaye A, Black P, eds. *Operative Neurosurgery*. London: Churchill Livingstone; 1997.
Whisler WW. Multiple subpial transection. In: Rengachary SS, ed. *Neurosurgical Operative Atlas*. Vol. 6. Park Ridge, IL: American Association of Neurological Surgeons; 1997:125-129.
Wyler AR, Wilkus RJ, Retard SW, et al. Multiple subpial transection for partial seizures in sensorimotor cortex. *Neurosurgery*. 1995;37: 1122-1128.

See a full reference list on ExpertConsult.com 

74 Surgery for Extratemporal Lobe Epilepsy

David W. Roberts and Edward F. Chang

Surgery for medically intractable epilepsy of extratemporal origin is less commonly performed today than that for temporal epilepsy, but for a number of reasons its use is increasing substantially. The prevalence of epilepsy arising out of the frontal, parietal, occipital, and insular regions warrants development of surgical capability in this area, and both our understanding of the underlying pathophysiology and the technological ability to evaluate and treat these seizure disorders have progressed to levels enabling safe and effective intervention.

Extratemporal seizure disorders are more varied in their expression and management than temporal lobe epilepsy (TLE), but the general principles of recognizing a unifocal and potentially surgical seizure disorder, reliably identifying the site of seizure origin as well as eloquent normal tissue that must be preserved, determining the extent of surgical resection, and safely executing that surgical plan are the same regardless of the particular region of the brain involved. The presurgical evaluation of extratemporal epilepsy can be complex, especially in patients with normal structural magnetic resonance imaging (MRI). Other noninvasive imaging tools such as single-photon emission computed tomography (SPECT), magnetoencephalography (MEG), positron emission tomography (PET), and electroencephalography (EEG) source localization tools play critical roles in seizure localization.

This chapter reviews resective surgery for medically intractable seizure disorders arising out of the frontal, parietal, occipital, and insular regions. The material has been organized by lobe or region, recognizing that many disorders involve a smaller subregion within a lobe or are multilobar in their extent. Seizure expression, its diagnosis, and the evaluation of the surgical candidate are presented. Surgical resection and special considerations are then reviewed, followed by surgical outcomes with respect to both seizures and potential neurological morbidity.

FRONTAL LOBE EPILEPSY

Expression, Diagnosis, and Evaluation

Frontal lobe epilepsy (FLE) is the second most common focal epilepsy syndrome after TLE.[1,2] FLE semiology is diverse, and efforts at sublobar localization and classification are fraught with challenges. Popular literature divides frontal lobe seizures into three main subtypes—partial motor, supplementary motor, and complex-partial seizures—but it is readily acknowledged that there is considerable overlap among subtypes.[3,4] Partial motor seizures are characterized by focal clonic activity with preserved consciousness, whereas speech arrest, blinking, and asymmetrical tonic posturing often suggest electrical spread to the supplementary motor area (SMA).[3,5] Complex partial seizures (CPSs) in FLE typically involve staring spells, vocalization, diminished responsiveness, and sometimes bizarre bimanual and bipedal movements.[3,4]

Frontal seizures are typically short lasting and often associated with complex motor behavior, sometimes with emotional symptoms.[6] They can be difficult to describe, in contrast to the relatively well-recognized patterns of temporal lobe seizures, in which semiology is much more limited and seizures unfold more slowly. Furthermore, the frontal lobe has massive connectivity through distant corticocortical efferent pathways, which can be both multilobar and multidirectional, typically resulting in rapid, widespread propagation of seizure discharges originating in frontal regions. These factors contribute to explaining both semiologic complexity and difficulties in electroencephalographic analysis. In addition, the frontal lobe represents nearly 35% to 40% of total cortical volume in humans, and accurate delineation of seizure onset is challenging given the large surface of buried cortex. The deep ventromedial prefrontal region is particularly far from EEG electrodes placed on the scalp or on the cortical convexity. Such difficulties in electroclinical localization almost certainly contribute to poorer outcome in surgical treatment of FLE compared with other epilepsy types.[2]

There have been many attempts to classify frontal seizures as they relate to potential onset zones. One recent study used a data-driven approach to understanding the patterns to identify the similarities in frontal lobe seizures characterized by heterogeneous semiology and electrographic data (in particular, stereo-electroencephalography [SEEG] to characterize the three-dimensional localization of the seizure onset zone).[7] The authors found that there were four basic groups of seizure categories. Group 1 seizures were organized within precentral and/or premotor regions, characterized by elementary motor signs with no gestural motor behavior. Group 2 seizures were characterized by nonintegrated gestural motor behavior associated with proximal tonic posturing and facial contraction; the presence of tonic signs that hindered movement magnified the disjointed appearance of motor behavior. Seizures arising from this zone involved overlapping premotor and posterior prefrontal regions, including the dorsolateral prefrontal convexity. The most anterior frontal areas were best described by Groups 3 and 4, which both manifested integrated gestural motor behavior but no elementary motor signs. However, Group 3 seizures primarily involved lateral prefrontal cortex and/or frontal pole, with projection of seizure activity toward anterior cingulate cortex, characterized by gestural motor behavior incorporating distal stereotypical behavior. In Group 3, behavior was devoid of emotional content, or conversely positive emotional expression was displayed. Group 4 seizures arising from ventromedial prefrontal cortex were typified by a fearful emotional expression associated with gestural motor behavior evoking a defensive or attacking reaction. This classification of frontal lobe seizure semiologies primarily describes an anteroposterior organizational gradient, rather than strict categories. The medial versus lateral distinctions are much less clear, especially because the propagation pathways tend to route along this direction. For example, medial prefrontal cortex appears to be the final common pathway for lateral frontal seizures.

Surgical Resection

Although the seizure semiology described earlier can represent both onset and propagation patterns, the goal of resective surgery is to remove the seizure onset zone. As a result, it is important to make a distinction between the semiology and onset localization with regard to surgical decision making. Frontal lobectomy is possible, but in most cases the work-up will reveal a more discrete focus or sublobar localization for targeted resection (Fig. 74-1). Furthermore, there is no standard approach to frontal lobe resection, like the anterior temporal lobectomy. Nonetheless, surgical approaches to the frontal lobe can broadly be divided as medial or lateral approaches, primarily based on technical aspects of gaining access to the resective target.

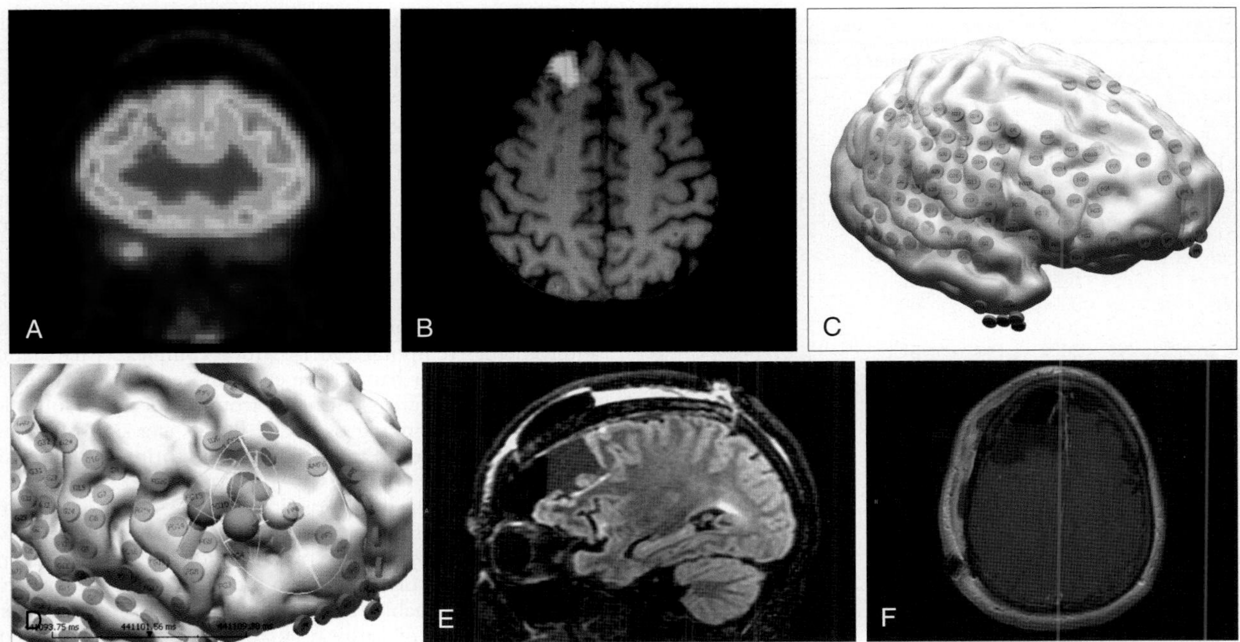

Figure 74-1. Frontal epilepsy. A 52-year-old woman had frequent spells associated with confusion. Magnetic resonance imaging (MRI) findings were normal. **A,** Fluorodeoxyglucose–positron emission tomography (FDG-PET) shows subtle reduced radioisotope uptake in the right superior frontal gyrus. **B,** Ictal subtraction single-photon emission computed tomography (SPECT) is consistent with right frontal seizure onset. **C,** Three-dimensional brain reconstruction with co-registered subdural electrodes. **D,** Ictal onset localization was confirmed to be right superior frontal gyrus. **E** and **F,** Sagittal and axial postoperative MRI shows resection cavity. Pathology showed cortical dysplasia. The patient was seizure free after surgery.

To access the medial frontal lobe, a bicoronal incision and unilateral frontal craniotomy (supine positioning) can provide adequate exposure to the SMA, pre-SMA, and dorsal anterior cingulate regions. The ventral cingulate can also be accessed from above via this approach, following the course of the cingulate and corpus callosum. Note that the falx does not directly abut the corpus callosum, but rather ends right above the cingulate gyrus. More anteriorly, the falx ends significantly farther from the corpus callosum. Therefore interhemispheric approaches to anterior medial and ventral prefrontal regions require some microdissection of the interhemispheric arachnoid adhesions. It is also for this reason that it often is not possible to pass subdural strip electrodes to these areas beyond the falx. Care must be taken to directly visualize or use careful subpial resection medially to avoid injury to the en passage pericallosal and callosomarginal branches of the anterior cerebral artery that traverse the medial corridor. Motor mapping can be useful for defining the leg and foot regions of the precentral gyrus. Medial resections involving the SMA or pre-SMA, located in the posterior superior frontal gyrus, can often result in a transient "SMA syndrome."[8-10] The SMA is bound posteriorly by the precentral sulcus and inferiorly by the cingulate sulcus. The anterior boundary is not well defined anatomically. The SMA syndrome is described as an impairment of spontaneous movements of the contralateral limbs, with preserved or increased tone and possible mutism. Speech deficits are more often seen in patients with the SMA syndrome affecting the dominant hemisphere. The SMA syndrome can last for weeks before recovery of function in the affected limbs. The only residual disturbance can manifest as an impairment in alternating bimanual movements. It is absolutely critical to differentiate SMA syndrome from the effects of direct motor cortex injury; patients with the latter are much less likely to recover.

The lateral approach to the ventral and dorsal lateral frontal lobe can be facilitated via a pterional or frontal craniotomy, respectively. On the dominant hemisphere, language mapping is usually required to identify eloquent language areas, usually for speech production (Broca's area). In most series, speech arrest is localized to the precentral gyrus or pars opercularis. Occasional naming arrest sites have been identified in the pars triangularis.

Outcomes

Postoperative seizure-freedom rates after frontal lobectomy or partial lobectomy for FLE (about 50%; Table 74-1) are lower than those for anterior temporal lobectomy for TLE (approximately two thirds).[3,5,11-15] Although a focal lesion, such as a tumor or cortical dysplasia, is sometimes identified in FLE, imaging and electroencephalographic findings are often nonlocalizing, presenting diagnostic and treatment challenges. Furthermore, morbidity associated with seizure focus resection involving the motor cortex or SMA presents important surgical considerations and can limit the extent of resection. Although various studies have examined rates of seizure freedom and predictors of response after surgery for FLE, substantial variability in outcomes exists because of significant diversity in epilepsy etiology, preoperative diagnostic testing, patient selection, resection location and type, and duration of postoperative follow-up. Inadequate follow-up in many reports may lead to an overestimation of long-term seizure freedom because FLE seizure outcomes may change significantly in the first postoperative year.[2,16]

One notable series from Jeha and colleagues examined the outcomes in 70 patients who underwent a frontal resection.[14] The estimated probability of seizure freedom at 1 year was 56%. The predictors of seizure recurrence were negative MRI,

TABLE 74-1 Frontal Lobe Epilepsy Surgical Series

Author	Year	No. of Patients	Engel Class I
Rasmussen[71]	1991	253	27%
Rougier et al[72]	1992	23	44%
Talairach et al[73]	1992	100	55%
Fish et al[74]	1993	45	20%
Laskowitz et al[75]	1995	16	63%
Smith et al[18]	1997	49	53%
Swartz et al[76]	1998	25	40%
Wennberg et al[77]	1999	25	60%
Ferrier et al[78]	1999	37	54%
Mosewich et al[79]	2000	68	59%
Jobst et al[5]	2000	25	64%
Zaatreh et al[80]	2002	37	35%
Kloss et al[81]	2002	18	78%
Luyken et al[82]	2003	25	40%
Tigaran et al[83]	2003	65	49%
Sinclair et al[84]	2004	13	69%
Yun et al[85]	2006	61	39%
Jeha et al[14]	2007	70	44%
Lee et al[86]	2008	71	54%
Elsharkawy et al[11]	2008	97	51%
Kim et al[16]	2010	76	55%

presence of extrafrontal pathology, a generalized ictal EEG pattern, and incomplete surgical resection. Another important series by Lazow and colleagues similarly reported 57% seizure freedom and noted that long-term outcomes can be quite favorable.[17] Nearly all of those patients (89%) underwent intracranial EEG monitoring before surgery. A systematic review and meta-analysis of long-term seizure outcome after resective surgery for FLE was performed by Englot and colleagues, who found an overall rate of seizure freedom (Engel class I outcome) of 45.1%.[12] In comparison, approximately two thirds of individuals with medically refractory TLE achieve long-term seizure freedom after anterior temporal lobectomy.[11,14,15] No trend in seizure-freedom rates was observed over the study period, suggesting that incremental enhancements in neuroimaging, electrophysiologic, and surgical techniques did not significantly affect reported outcomes. Several significant predictors of long-term seizure freedom were identified, including a lesional cause of epilepsy, such as tumor or focal cortical dysplasia, abnormal preoperative MRI, and localized frontal lobe resection. These findings suggest that FLE patients with a focal and identifiable lesion are more likely to achieve postoperative seizure freedom than those with a more poorly defined epileptic focus—findings that are consistent with observations made by previous authors.[14,18,19] These findings underscore the importance of appropriate patient selection of potential surgical candidates.

OCCIPITAL LOBE EPILEPSY

Expression, Diagnosis, and Evaluation

Occipital lobe epilepsy was first described by Sir William Richard Gowers in a patient with a parieto-occipital lobe tumor and seizures associated with visual aura.[20] Although less common (commensurate with the relatively small size of the occipital lobe), occipital lobe epilepsy is well recognized, and in instances of medical intractability the role of surgical intervention is increasingly better understood.

The visual function associated with the occipital lobe plays a pervasive role in both the expression and the management of occipital lobe epilepsy. In what is still perhaps the best description of this seizure type, Williamson and colleagues described the clinical characteristics of occipital epilepsy in a series of 25 patients.[21] Elementary visual hallucinations, taking the form of either flashing (more common) or steady white or colored lights, were seen at ictal onset in 15 patients, and ictal amaurosis in 10 patients. Kun Lee and colleagues found similar visual symptoms in 35% and 15%, respectively.[22] In a series reported by Jobst and coworkers, only 7 of 14 patients had visual symptoms; in 4 of these patients they were elementary.[23] In the Kun Lee and Jobst series, more formed or complex visual symptoms were reported in 21% and 27%. From the clinical perspective of evaluating a patient with visual symptoms at seizure onset, the experience of Bien and colleagues looking at 20 patients with epileptic visual auras may be helpful: elementary visual hallucinations, illusions, and visual field deficits were noted in seizures arising not only in the occipital lobe but also in the occipitotemporal region and the anteromedial temporal lobe.[24] More complex visual hallucinations, on the other hand, were encountered with seizures arising from the last two areas but never from the occipital lobe alone.[24] Rapid bilateral blinking or eyelid flutter is a sign often seen in occipital lobe epilepsy and may direct attention to the possibility of occipital onset.[21,25]

Occipital epilepsy's expression reflects common patterns of spread. Patients often experience complex partial epilepsy, which if lacking visual symptoms may be indistinguishable from that of temporal lobe origin. Spread along the inferior longitudinal fasciculus presumably underlies this expression, just as that along more superior pathways may manifest itself with accompanying motoric semiology, similar to that seen in some frontal lobe epilepsies.[21] Of note, in any given patient these spread patterns may vary, resulting in an individual experiencing multiple seizure types.[21]

As with all epilepsies, there is a wide spectrum of underlying pathologic conditions, ranging from tumor to earlier ischemic injury, cortical dysplasia, migration disorders, other developmental syndromes, and glial scar. Evaluation of the medically intractable patient will be influenced by these, because small, discrete lesions (e.g., a small ganglioglioma or cavernous angioma) with straightforward semiology and evaluative findings will likely require less investigation than more diffuse disease with complex presentation and possibly discordant findings. Scalp EEG is often nonlocalizing, with interictal abnormalities most often temporal.[21] MRI continues to play an increasingly important role in defining location and extent of underlying lesions, but the absence of such findings on imaging does not preclude the possibility of localizable, often surgically resectable epilepsy. PET[25] and SPECT, particularly with subtraction of coregistered interictal from ictal studies,[26-28] and MEG[29,30] have all provided supporting evidence for localization or rationale for continuing to pursue investigation.

As one would expect, visual field deficits are not uncommon in this patient population, and documentation of formal visual fields is essential. Understanding of a patient's existing visual function plays a critical role in further investigation, in surgical decision making, and in ultimate planning of any surgical intervention. Patients with physiologic and structural findings well localized to an occipital lobe who already have a homonymous hemianopia can often proceed directly to occipital resection. Those with more extensive or less discrete pathology, discordant data, or preserved visual function in the relevant visual field may warrant an intracranial investigation.

The strategic questions driving an intracranial study should determine the location and extent of electrode array. If it is unclear whether the occipital lobe is involved or if there is a question of laterality—issues especially relevant in MRI-negative epilepsy—broad interrogation of the occipital as well as other lobes may be required; extensive evaluation across multiple regions may in some instances be well served by a configuration of multiple depth electrodes. If the strategic question is one of extent of resection along the occipitotemporal or occipitoparietal border, coverage will have to have the ability to determine the extent of any subsequent resection. In such an instance, subdural grids over the region of concern may be very useful. A frequent concern in the patient with longstanding complex partial epilepsy with accompanying imaging findings suggesting medial temporal lobe involvement is whether or not a resection should also include the hippocampus. Coverage in such a situation, usually using depth electrodes placed either down the long axis of the hippocampus or from a lateral approach, must be able to address this.

In the patient without a homonymous hemianopia in whom vision sparing is a goal, coverage of the calcarine cortex can be of value. An interhemispheric subdural grid can provide important information about both seizure onset and, with mapping, visual function localization.

Given the significant potential of visual function morbidity from any resective approach in this region, understanding the spatial relationship between epileptogenesis and function is critical. With respect to seizure outcome, at least one series demonstrated a correlation between extent of intracranial array coverage of the occipital lobe and seizure outcome.[23]

TABLE 74-2 Occipital Lobe Epilepsy Surgical Series

Author	Year	No. of Patients	Engel Class I or II
Rasmussen[33]	1975	25	26%
Wyler et al[35]	1990	14	50%
Blume et al[34]	1991	6	32%
Salanova et al[87]	1992	23	41%
Williamson et al[21]	1992	16	58%
Bidziński et al[88]	1992	12	92%
Aykut-Bingol et al[89]	1998	35	46%
Kuzniecky et al[90]	1998	6	50%
Sturm et al[91]	2000	6	50%
Kun Lee et al[22]	2005	26	62%
Dalmagro et al[92]	2005	44	65%
Caicoya et al[93]	2007	7	71%
Binder et al[28]	2008	52	69%
Tandon et al[25]	2009	21	81%
Jobst et al[23]	2010	14	50%
Ibrahim et al[29]	2012	41	68%

Surgical Resection

Recognition of the balance between effective extent of resection of the epileptogenic zone and avoidance of neurological deficit is especially prominent in the surgical decision-making process in occipital epilepsy. Many patients may be very accepting of a superior quadrantanopia in return for seizure freedom; an inferior quadrantanopia is less well tolerated. Production of a hemianopia is obviously of still greater concern, and although some incapacitating, refractory seizure disorders may motivate some patients to accept this, it is a deficit many if not most patients and neurosurgeons would prefer to avoid; its prospect in some instances may rule out a resective strategy. All of these considerations must explicitly recognize that in a substantial subset of patients, resection may not ensure a seizure-free outcome.

Resection itself follows standard microsurgical procedure. Variation in a given case will depend on whether or not visual preservation is a goal and on the extent of resection. Well-localized lateral seizure onset associated with well-imaged, small, and discrete pathology may enable resection with preservation of primary visual cortex. Similarly, preservation of a visual quadrant may be similarly sought and enabled. In both instances, awareness of subcortical visual projections and their preservation is essential.

Extension of resection into either temporal or parietal cortex is commonly guided by information from an intracranial electrode investigation (Fig. 74-2). Such resection follows similar practice in other regions of the brain. Particular series in which electrocorticography has helped determine extent of resection include those of Binder and colleagues, Chang and colleagues, and Dorward and colleagues.[28,31,32]

Warranting particular consideration are those patients in whom medial temporal lobe removal is indicated in addition to an occipital resection. Such resection can follow initial occipital resection, although the greater distance to the more anterior hippocampus renders this more technically difficult. In those instances in which a large occipital resection on the language-dominant side has been performed, connections between the contralateral occipital lobe and the language-dominant temporal lobe must be preserved to prevent alexia-without-agraphia, a syndrome described by Déjerine. Both for integration of the multimodality information common to the intractable epilepsy patient and for accuracy in incorporating that information into the surgical procedure, image guidance in these procedures has been useful. Multiple subpial transection (MST) has been used by numerous groups to supplement resection when there is reason to believe epileptogenic tissue also subserves normal function.

Outcomes

There has not been an extensive neurosurgical experience with resection in occipital lobe epilepsy. The incidence of such an outcome ranges from 26% to 81%, with the majority of more recent series having ranges of 50% to 81% (Table 74-2).[21,23,25,29,33-35] Of the larger series, that of Binder and colleagues with 52 patients is representative, achieving an Engel class I outcome in 69.2%, class II in 7.7%, class III in 15.4%, and class IV in 7.7%.[28]

Apart from those surgical morbidities common to all intracranial resections for epilepsy, the incidence of increased visual deficits merits particular attention. The series by Kun Lee and colleagues is especially informative. Eighteen of their 26 patients had normal visual fields before surgery; in only one patient was this preserved. Of the eight patients with preoperative visual deficits, six patients experienced an increased deficit. New quadrantanopias were seen in 12 patients; new hemianopias developed in four patients.[22] In the Bonn experience, adequate preoperative and postoperative visual field data were available for 33 patients, and new or increased visual deficits were seen in 42.4%. Of 21 patients with intact preoperative fields, new deficits were seen in 11 patients (52.4%).[28] In the series by Tandon and colleagues, half of the evaluable patients experienced a new or increased visual field deficit.[25]

Experience with nonresective strategies in occipital lobe epilepsy is limited. Vagal nerve stimulation, callosal section (in this instance either division of the posterior corpus callosum; or in the instance of a prior incomplete commissurotomy, completion of the callosotomy), MST, electrical stimulation of the anterior nucleus of the thalamus, or responsive neurostimulation are options, but there are very few patients with occipital lobe epilepsy who have been managed with these approaches in the published literature. In the series by Binder and colleagues, nine patients underwent lesionectomy combined with MST of adjacent eloquent cortex, six of whom achieved an Engel class I outcome and three an Engel class III.[28] What role MST may have played in the setting of a combined surgical strategy is to difficult to determine.

PARIETAL LOBE EPILEPSY

Expression, Diagnosis, and Evaluation

Epilepsy arising out of the parietal region is highly variable in its clinical expression, and clinical symptoms and signs at seizure onset are frequently poorly localizing.[36-39] Given the sensory functions associated with the parietal lobe, however, seizure

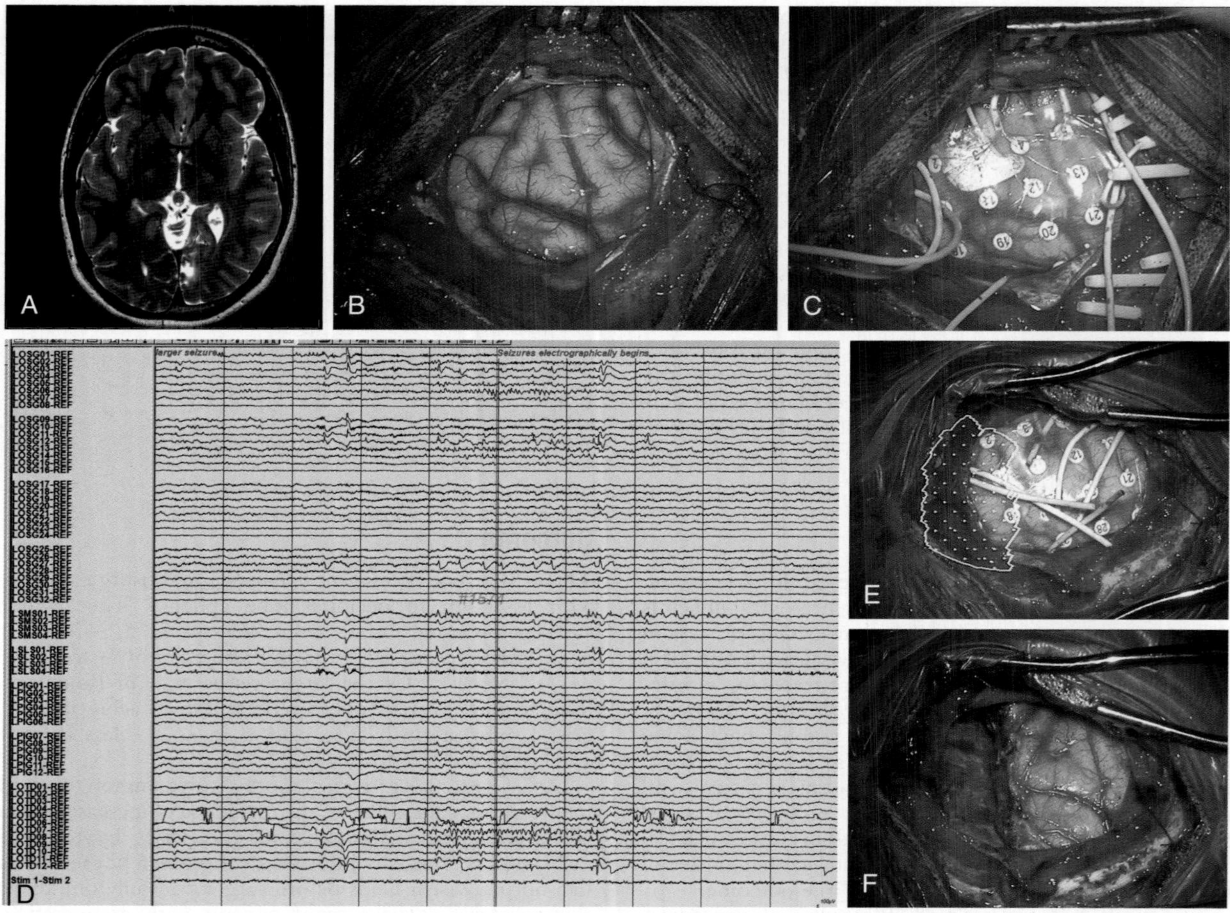

Figure 74-2. This 24-year-old woman had had complex partial seizures, characterized by staring, headache, chewing, and bilateral automatisms since the age of 9 years. **A,** Magnetic resonance imaging shows an old left occipital infarction. **B,** Surgical exposure at the time of an intracranial electrode array implantation. Inferior is at the top, and anterior is to the right. **C,** Surgical exposure after placement of array consisting of two subtemporal 1 × 4 subdural strips, an interhemispheric 2 × 6 subdural grid, an occipitoparietal 4 × 8 subdural grid (visible over the cortex), and a 12-contact occipitotemporal depth electrode (its cortical entry is visible beneath the 4 × 8 subdural grid electrode). **D,** Ictal recordings demonstrate seizure onset along the inferior aspect of the left occipital lobe. **E,** At the time of returning to the operating room for removal of the electrode array and occipitotemporal section, the image-guidance contour corresponding to the planned occipital resection volume is superimposed on the surgical field. **F,** The surgical exposure at the completion of resection.

expression not unexpectedly has been well described with parietal lobe epilepsy. Involvement of the primary somatosensory cortex of the postcentral gyrus is most common, but the second somatosensory area located at the parietal operculum and a third sensory area in the posterior parietal region—these second and third areas subserving less spatially discrete, sometimes bilateral, and presumably more integrative function—may alternatively be involved. Descriptive accounts of subjective sensations, the most common being elementary in the form of perceived tingling, numbness, or pins and needles, are well documented in the older literature.[38,40,41]

Sensory phenomena are not universal or even necessarily seen in the majority of patients whose seizures are believed to have arisen out of the parietal lobe. Somatosensory sensations reported either as an aura or at seizure onset were noted in 4 of 11 patients by Williamson and colleagues,[36] in 5 of 8 patients (63%) by Boesebeck and colleagues,[39] and in 13 of 28 patients (46%) by Kasowksi and colleagues.[42] Furthermore, such phenomena by virtue of inconsistency, bilaterality, nonspecificity, or false localization are often unreliable and unhelpful. Boesebeck and colleagues found that the absence of auras inconsistent with structural pathology on imaging studies was more often associated with seizure-free outcome after surgery,[39] but more recent experiences have not found such clinical phenomena consistent, reliable, or as helpful as other information.

Simple partial seizures were found in 5 of 28 patients (18%) in the series of Kasowski and colleagues[42] but in 31 of 40 patients (78%) in that of Binder and colleagues.[37] Most patients experience multiple seizure types, the most common of which has been CPSs. Ninety percent of patients in the Bonn series experienced CPSs,[37] 7 of 11 patients (64%) did in the series of Williamson and colleagues,[36] and 18 of 28 patients (64%) did in the series of Kasowski and colleagues.[42] Seizures suggestive of frontal involvement are also frequently seen. A similar number of patients (7 of 11, or 64%) displayed asymmetrical tonic seizures with or without clonic activity in the study by Williamson and colleagues. In the study by Kasowski and colleagues, 10 of 28 patients (36%) had focal clonic activity and 5 patients (18%) tonic posturing.[42]

Scalp EEG has also been of limited value in localizing parietal epilepsy. Nonlocalizing or falsely localizing interictal as well as ictal scalp EEG in parietal epilepsy is a frequent finding.[36,37] Intracranial electrode investigation has frequently been used in parietal epilepsy, to attempt to resolve or augment semiologic and scalp EEG findings, to delineate the extent of the epileptogenic region, and to provide important functional mapping information. At least one study has shown surprising unreliability in demonstration of the site of seizure origin,[36] but its usefulness to map cortical function that must be preserved has often been invaluable.[37,43]

In more recent surgical series, neuroimaging and in particular MRI have proved most useful in the evaluation of these patients. Most recent series have consistently demonstrated MRI's greater sensitivity and reliability relative to other commonly available evaluation sources (despite presumed inherent patient selection biases in the compilation of more recent surgical series). In the series by Williamson and colleagues, all patients had circumscribed parietal lesions on MRI,[36] as did 38 of 40 patients (95%) in the Binder and colleagues series.[37] It should be noted that whereas surgery for lesional epilepsy has often been reported to have a more favorable seizure outcome,[44] there has been sufficient experience with MRI-negative epilepsy surgery to not make normal MRI findings an exclusion criterion for further evaluation and possible surgery. PET, SPECT (ictal, interictal, and subtraction) and MEG have been less universally employed but often confirmatory or otherwise helpful.

The most common underlying pathologies in the larger surgical series have been low-grade tumor (most commonly ganglioglioma, low-grade astrocytoma, oligodendroglioma, or dysembryoplastic neuroepithelial tumor), cortical dysplasia, vascular malformations, and gliosis.[36,37,43,45,46]

Surgical Resection

Surgical resection in the MRI era has focused primarily on microsurgical removal of the imaged lesion and conservatively the immediately surrounding cortex. A parietal lesion's proximity to generally eloquent tissue in all directions requires this. In those instances in which epileptogenic tissue extends into a functional postcentral gyrus or language cortex, resection has often been accompanied by MST of that eloquent cortex (11 of 40 resections in the Bonn series[37] and 8 of 28 resections in the Yale series.[42] Two patients in the Yale series[42] and one in the Bielefeld series[39] underwent MST alone. Increasingly the usefulness of image guidance to coordinate information from multiple preoperative imaging studies and ensure accurate execution of a preoperative surgical plan is being appreciated.[47-50]

Intraoperative electrocorticography, in an attempt to ensure adequate extent of resection after initial lesionectomy, is variably employed at different centers but has been long used and advocated by some for improved resection of epileptogenic tissue.[31,32,37,39,50] Intraoperative functional mapping in the parietal region may be helpful, particularly in the inferior parietal lobule with respect to language.[51]

Lastly, in those patients with posterior quadrant multilobar epilepsy, a subhemispheric disconnection procedure as an alternative to actual resection warrants mention. Dorfer and colleagues have described a technique in which a parietal corticotomy extending down to the ventricle and then into the interhemispheric fissure, down to the posterior callosum, which in turn is sectioned, and then across the parietal and temporal operculum and along the temporal horn and including the amygdala is performed. Neuromonitoring and image guidance are employed, and unexpected morbidity has been low. Excessive blood loss and cerebrospinal fluid absorption problems were absent. Ten children were operated on in this fashion, nine of them (90%) becoming seizure free.[52]

TABLE 74-3 Parietal Lobe Epilepsy Surgical Series

Author	Year	No. of Patients	Engel Class I or II
Williamson et al[36]	1992	11	91%
Cascino et al[54]	1993	10	90%
Salanova et al[94]	1995	34	75%
Salanova et al[95]	1995	82	65%
Gaweł and Marchel[96]	1998	25	43% (seizure free)
Olivier and Boling[55]	2000	39	82%
Boesebeck et al[39]	2002	42	60%
Kasowski et al[42]	2003	28	55%
Kim et al[45]	2004	38	53%
Binder et al[37]	2009	40	67.5%

Outcomes

Seizure outcomes in the earlier, pre-MRI series of parietal resection were reported to be seizure-free or nearly seizure-free status in 65% to 75% of patients—the higher rates occurring in those patients whose pathology was underlying tumor.[53] Given the differences in evaluative tools, patient selection, and outcome assessment in that era, it is difficult to compare those experiences with more recent series.

Engel class I or II seizure outcomes (seizure free or nearly seizure free) were achieved in 10 of 11 patients in the series by Williamson[36] and in all 10 patients in the Mayo series (9 of whom were seizure free).[54] In larger series, a comparative degree of success with respect to seizure outcome was seen in 53% to 82% of patients, with seizure freedom reported in 39.5% to 57.5% of patients (Table 74-3).[37,39,42,45,55]

In the MRI-era, the morbidity associated with parietal resection for epilepsy has been reasonably low. The most common neurological deficits have been a usually incomplete Gerstmann syndrome (agraphia, acalculia, finger agnosia, and right-left disorientation) or hemisensory syndrome, with smaller numbers of patients experiencing deficits in visual fields, language, or strength.[37,39,42,45,55] Although common (more than a third of patients in the Bonn series), these have usually been transient.[37] Nonneurological surgical morbidity has not been significantly different than for other resections performed for epilepsy.

INSULAR EPILEPSY

Expression, Diagnosis, and Evaluation

The insula, often called the brain's fifth lobe, is increasingly being recognized as an important locus of refractory seizures. In the past two decades, a growing number of studies have reported seizure onset localization to the insula, as well as positive results after targeted resective surgery. Traditionally, insular epilepsy was considered inoperable primarily because of the hazards of operating deep in the sylvian fissure as well as unclear effectiveness. Modern neuroimaging and improved technical considerations have rapidly contributed to improvements in localization and safer surgery.

Relatively little is understood about the function of the insula. It has been suggested that it may play a role in secondary sensory processing, language and motor control, or higher autonomic control, and as a component of the limbic system.[56-58] Semiology of seizures generated by insular lesions is often described as similar to temporal[59] and frontal[60] semiology. Nevertheless, some specific characteristics of insular seizures, such as vegetative, viscerosensory, and somatosensory symptoms, occur according to the complex physiology and extensive connections of the insular cortex. On the other hand, some aspects of temporal lobe seizures may be related to involvement of the insular cortex (e.g., an epigastric aura).[57,60-62]

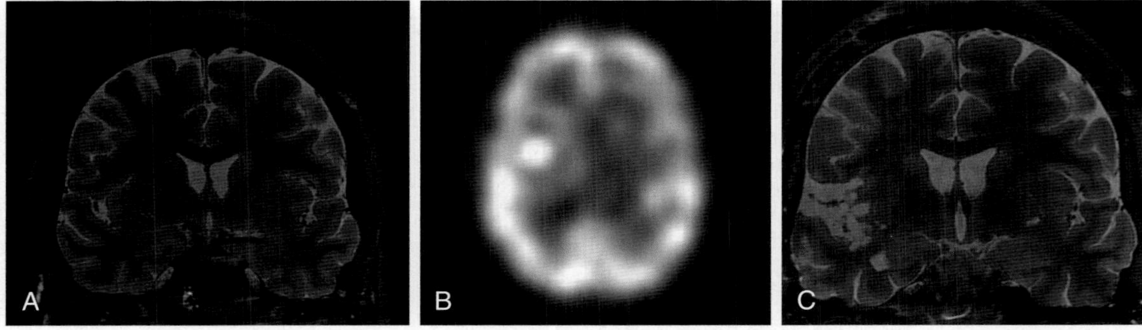

Figure 74-3. Insular epilepsy. The origin of this 42-year-old man's nocturnal, hypermotor convulsive seizures initially was thought to be frontal. Magnetic resonance imaging (MRI) was normal **(A),** but ictal ingle-photon emission computed tomography (SPECT) demonstrated a clear insular focus. He underwent an operculoinsular resection and became seizure free. **B,** Ictal SPECT study shows abnormal tracer uptake in the right posterior insula. **C,** Postoperative MRI. Pathology showed cortical dysplasia.

The close connections with other potentially epileptogenic areas such as temporomesial structures or the frontal or central cortex can be considered as a reason for misleading findings in electrophysiologic and imaging investigations.[59,61] The distance of the insular cortex to the surface and the overlying cortex lead to imprecise results of surface EEG recordings or even of subdural EEG. Thus the implantation of depth electrodes is critical for evaluating insular cortex involvement.[61,63,64]

Some have reported good outcomes with insula-sparing resections of the frontal and temporal lobes in patients in whom the insula was identified as a site of secondary seizure propagation and in those who had no insular involvement.[65] Conversely, Isnard and colleagues. reported persistence of insular-onset seizures after temporal lobectomy.[59] Therefore when insular involvement is suspected in frontal, temporal, frontotemporal, or actual insular epilepsy, it is important to determine the precise seizure focus and clarify the role of the insula.

Surgical Technique

The two unique aspects of insular surgery relate to localization with intracranial EEG and the resective approach. As mentioned earlier, insula recordings are increasingly recognized as an important adjunct to nonlesional epilepsy localization. Depth electrodes can be placed accurately there using stereotactic guidance.[64] The traditional SEEG approach involves a lateral orthogonal (transopercular) trajectory, usually using a stereotactic frame. Transfrontal oblique is another important trajectory in which more electrodes are placed in the body of the insula.[66] Both lateral and transfrontal oblique approaches require careful preoperative planning to define trajectories that avoid major vessels in the sylvian fissure. Alternatively, electrodes may also be placed directly after sylvian fissure dissection.[67] Hemorrhage rates have been relatively low, with little or no morbidity reported. Direct monitoring of the insula may facilitate the role of the insula in seizure origin.

In a series at Dartmouth, 10% of patients were demonstrated to have seizures originating in the insula.[66] An additional 25% of patients were found to have specific, early involvement of the insula during their seizures, secondary to onset in a separate site. This enabled insula-sparing resections with good outcomes in terms of seizure control and absence of neurological deficits. In the remaining patients, shown to be without insular involvement in their seizures, exclusion of the insula helped support and confirm seizure onset in other regions.

Insular resection can be carried out directly after splitting the sylvian fissure, or with a transopercular approach.[68,69] A key technical consideration in insular resection is the identification and protection of critical vascular structures, namely the middle cerebral artery (MCA) branches. In the transsylvian approach, the MCA vessels can be visualized directly and protected. In the transopercular approach, the insular resection is facilitated through pial corridors of the MCA "candelabra" of vessels (Fig. 74-3). For lesions in the insula, the choice of frontal or temporal operculum resection depends on whether there is involvement of the operculum itself (as is often found with low-grade gliomas). Resection of both frontal and temporal operculum is rarely indicated. The resection focuses on removing the cortex alone, while protecting the underlying white matter including capsule and basal ganglia structures. Inferiorly, along the deep temporal aspect of the insula, care must be taken to protect tiny lenticulostriate vessels that feed the internal capsule and other critical deep structures. Intraoperative monitoring of motor and language is an essential adjunct to insular surgery.

Outcomes

Overall, insular epilepsy surgeries represent less than 1% to 2% of all epilepsy surgeries. As a result, reports of outcomes after insular surgery are relatively few and come from small series. Nonetheless, these series have revealed important knowledge that points to further studies in the future. In particular, diagnostics using intracranial electrodes are now offering more definitive localization that will lead to resective approaches. It is unclear to what extent insular involvement may play a role in cases in which standard temporal and frontal resections have failed.

Boucher and colleagues prospectively assessed neuropsychological function in 18 patients whose epilepsy surgery involved the partial or complete removal of the insula.[70] Using a standard neuropsychological screening assessment covering attention, executive function, memory, language, and visuospatial skills, they found no convincing evidence of major, permanent cognitive deficits leading to functional disability associated with surgery. A reduction in color naming speed after surgery was found in the large majority of participants, but it was not clinically significant.

von Lehe and colleagues reported the Bonn series on insular lesionectomy for refractory epilepsy.[69] Their experience included 24 patients, of whom 8 patients had pure insular lesions and 16 had lesions that extended to either the frontal or the temporal lobe. Note that nonlesional epilepsy patients were not included in this series. Postoperatively, one patient had a hemihypesthesia and one patient had a deterioration of a preexisting hemiparesis; two patients had a hemianopia as a calculated deficit. According to the International League Against Epilepsy (ILAE) classification, 15 patients were completely seizure free (62.5%, ILAE class 1); 79.2% had a satisfactory seizure outcome (ILAE classes 1 to 3).

CONCLUSION

Surgical treatment of extratemporal epilepsy, historically associated with lower seizure control rates than those for TLE, has benefited from significant advances in imaging and surgical techniques that have improved diagnostic accuracy and outcome. Lesional epilepsy has better outcomes compared with nonlesional epilepsy. Nonlesional epilepsy typically requires thorough neuroimaging as well as intracranial monitoring. Direct recordings appear to be important adjuncts in seizure localization, especially for deep and medial targets. Modern series report safe and effective intracranial electrode investigation, if required, and resective surgeries in frontal, occipital, parietal, and insular epilepsy.

SUGGESTED READINGS

Binder DK, Podlogar M, Clusmann H, et al. Surgical treatment of parietal lobe epilepsy. *J Neurosurg*. 2009;110:1170-1178.

Binder DK, von Lehe M, Kral T, et al. Surgical treatment of occipital lobe epilepsy. *J Neurosurg*. 2008;109:57-69.

Cascino GD, Hulihan JF, Sharbrough FW, et al. Parietal lobe lesional epilepsy: electroclinical correlation and operative outcome. *Epilepsia*. 1993;34:522-527.

Desai A, Jobst BC, Thadani VM, et al. Stereotactic depth electrode investigation of the insula in the evaluation of medically intractable epilepsy. *J Neurosurg*. 2011;114:1176-1186.

Englot DJ, Breshears JD, Sun PP, et al. Seizure outcomes after resective surgery for extra-temporal lobe epilepsy in pediatric patients. *J Neurosurg Pediatr*. 2013;12:126-133.

Englot DJ, Wang DD, Rolston JD, et al. Rates and predictors of long-term seizure freedom after frontal lobe epilepsy surgery: a systematic review and meta-analysis. *J Neurosurg*. 2012;116:1042-1048.

Isnard J, Guenot M, Sindou M, et al. Clinical manifestations of insular lobe seizures: a stereo-electroencephalographic study. *Epilepsia*. 2004;45:1079-1090.

Jeha LE, Najm I, Bingaman W, et al. Surgical outcome and prognostic factors of frontal lobe epilepsy surgery. *Brain*. 2007;130(Pt 2):574-584.

Jobst BC, Williamson PD, Thadani VM, et al. Intractable occipital lobe epilepsy: clinical characteristics and surgical treatment. *Epilepsia*. 2010;51:2334-2337.

Kasowski HJ, Stoffman MR, Spencer SS, et al. Surgical management of parietal lobe epilepsy. *Adv Neurol*. 2003;93:347-356.

Lazow SP, Thadani VM, Gilbert KL, et al. Outcome of frontal lobe epilepsy surgery. *Epilepsia*. 2012;53:1746-1755.

Olivier A, Boling W Jr. Surgery of parietal and occipital lobe epilepsy. *Adv Neurol*. 2000;84:533-575.

Schramm J, Kral T, Kurthen M, et al. Surgery to treat focal frontal lobe epilepsy in adults. *Neurosurgery*. 2002;51:644-654, discussion 654-645.

Sveinbjornsdottir S, Duncan JS. Parietal and occipital lobe epilepsy: a review. *Epilepsia*. 1993;34:493-521.

Tandon N, Alexopoulos AV, Warbel A, et al. Occipital epilepsy: spatial categorization and surgical management. *J Neurosurg*. 2009;110:306-318.

von Lehe M, Wellmer J, Urbach H, et al. Insular lesionectomy for refractory epilepsy: management and outcome. *Brain*. 2009;132(Pt 4):1048-1056.

Williamson PD. Frontal lobe seizures. Problems of diagnosis and classification. *Adv Neurol*. 1992;57:289-309.

Williamson PD, Boon PA, Thadani VM, et al. Parietal lobe epilepsy: diagnostic considerations and results of surgery. *Ann Neurol*. 1992;31:193-201.

Williamson PD, Thadani VM, Darcey TM, et al. Occipital lobe epilepsy: clinical characteristics, seizure spread patterns, and results of surgery. *Ann Neurol*. 1992;31:3-13.

Zentner J, Hufnagel A, Pechstein U, et al. Functional results after resective procedures involving the supplementary motor area. *J Neurosurg*. 1996;85:542-549.

See a full reference list on ExpertConsult.com

75 Standard Temporal Lobectomy

Juan Torres-Reveron and Dennis D. Spencer

The standard temporal lobectomy remains one of the most common and effective procedures for the treatment of medically refractory epilepsy. Although the procedure is performed in multiple centers around the world, its effectiveness for properly selected patients has remained stable over the years and the "standard" nomenclature has evolved from a lateral temporal to a lateral plus medial to predominantly a medial resection based on the pathophysiology of mesial temporal sclerosis. Thus "standard" resection today means an anteromedial temporal resection. Multiple variations have appeared to approach medial structures with minimal disruption to the lateral temporal cortex. Different surgical techniques including radiofrequency ablation and laser thermocoagulation are being tested as minimally invasive approaches to target the hippocampus and amygdala. However, the standard surgical approach continues to be the workhorse of the field and the technique to master, not just for the approach to the medial temporal lobe but also for other lesions that involve particularly medial temporal anatomy.

HISTORICAL PERSPECTIVE

In 1886 Horsley described the first surgical resection as treatment for partial epilepsy.[1] During the 1940s and 1950s the safety and efficacy of surgical treatment for epilepsy based on electrophysiologic localization of the lesion was demonstrated.[2,3] Penfield reported success with anterolateral temporal resections in a series of 68 patients in 1950.[4] Along with Baldwin, he introduced the concept of "incisural sclerosis," which was believed to be secondary to pressure on medial temporal structures with resultant ischemia.[5] Falconer popularized the technique of en bloc resection of the hippocampus, which allowed pathologists to study the tissue.[6] Crandall systematically placed depth electrodes in the hippocampi of patients with suspected temporal lobe epilepsy, identifying the ictal onset as medial and correlating this with sclerotic pathology of the hippocampus.[7,8] Despite this consolidation of ictal onset and pathology to the medial temporal lobe, the Falconer resection of 5 to 6 cm of the lateral temporal lobe plus the medial structures remained the standard with small modifications from the 1950s until the 1980s. In 1984 Spencer and colleagues described a modification of the technique that increased the posterior access to medial temporal structures while minimizing the lateral resection to the inferior temporal pole.[9] This was based on the predominance of depth-recorded ictal onsets along the entire hippocampus with only secondary projection to the lateral cortex, correlative sclerotic hippocampal pathology, and good outcomes with a restricted medial resection. Other modifications have appeared over the years that aim at targeting medial structures with minimal disruption of the lateral temporal lobe; these are discussed in Chapter 76 of this book.

PREOPERATIVE EVALUATION

In 1986, Cahan and Engel[10] stated three parameters that each surgical candidate must meet for a temporal lobectomy:

- The patient must have partial seizures.
- The patient must have refractory seizures.
- The patient should not have progressive or diffuse brain disease.

These parameters have been refined significantly since then. The initial preoperative evaluation includes inpatient 24-hour continuous audiovisual electroencephalographic monitoring during which antiepileptic medications are weaned to allow for seizure generation. Imaging includes brain magnetic resonance imaging (MRI) to assess anatomy and for lesions and may include a quantitative positron emission tomography (PET) scan to evaluate hypometabolism, ictal or interictal single-photon emission computed tomography (SPECT), and magnetic resonance spectroscopy and magnetoencephalography (MEG).

Neuropsychological testing also forms an integral part of the preoperative testing. The determination of a baseline IQ and identification of verbal or visual memory deficits are essential in counseling the patient and in the decision for temporal lobectomies in the dominant hemisphere. The comparison of preoperative and postoperative testing results also serves to evaluate the degree to which modifications to the standard temporal lobectomy affect memory and language.

The intracarotid sodium amobarbital procedure (Wada test; see Chapter 68) is usually reserved for patients who may benefit from a temporal lobectomy and have either bilateral language representation or an inconclusive neuropsychological evaluation regarding memory dysfunction.

The use of intracranial electrophysiologic monitoring (see Chapters 71 and 72) is reserved for patients in whom noninvasive evaluations are discordant in terms of localization or lateralization of the seizures. The placement of subdural electrodes also allows for language mapping.

The ideal candidate is a patient with a lesion or mesial temporal sclerosis on MRI in the temporal lobe that correlates with partial or complex partial seizures on electroencephalography (EEG), one with profound temporal lobe–specific neuropsychological deficits, and a patient in whom two antiepileptic medications have failed, in terms of either seizure control or tolerance. Further details regarding the preoperative evaluation for epilepsy surgery can be found in Chapter 64.

SURGICAL DECISION MAKING

General Anatomy

The temporal lobe consists of the superior (T1), middle (T2), and inferior (T3) temporal gyri laterally and the fusiform and parahippocampal gyri inferiorly. The mesial surface includes the amygdala and the parahippocampal gyrus, which includes the uncus. The pial surface of the temporal lobe forms a natural barrier between the temporal parenchyma and deeper structures including the carotid artery, middle cerebral artery (MCA), anterior choroidal artery, posterior cerebral artery (PCA), optic nerve and chiasm, oculomotor nerve, and brainstem. There is also a separate pial covering over the lateral geniculate nucleus of the thalamus.

The collateral sulcus separates the fusiform and parahippocampal gyrus and serves as a reference to locate the temporal horn. Within the temporal horn the inferior choroidal point is a critical landmark. The anterior choroidal artery enters the choroid plexus at this point. The amygdala is located below an imaginary line between this point and the MCA bifurcation.[11]

Language Localization

The location of language can be quite variable within the dominant temporal lobe.[12-14] In general, the probability of finding language in the anterior 3 cm is less than 20%, particularly if the superior temporal gyrus remains intact because language has greater representation in the superior aspects of the temporal lobe. Regardless, preoperative or intraoperative language mapping is recommended in the dominant hemisphere if the resection will extend laterally beyond 3 cm or must include the superior temporal gyrus, because epilepsy can alter location of language over time.

An understanding of the venous anatomy is crucial for complication avoidance. The orientation of the sylvian veins and particularly the course of the vein of Labbé are essential in planning the lateral temporal lobe resection. In some cases the vein of Labbé can have a split course that limits the extent of the lateral resection. Furthermore, its drainage into the lateral sinus can be quite proximal, which may limit the retraction of the lateral temporal cortex and access to the hippocampal tail without skeletonizing the vein.

Visual Fibers

The optic radiations originate from the lateral geniculate body. These fibers run in two streams through the temporal lobe: laterally and posteriorly to reach the medial occipital lobe in the superior part of the calcarine sulcus, and forward and laterally toward the roof of the temporal horn, making a U-turn 2 cm from the temporal pole and moving then inferiorly and backward via the lateral wall of the temporal horn to reach the lower part of the calcarine sulcus.[15] It is this second fiber bundle that is affected during temporal lobectomies, causing the contralateral superior quadrantanopia ("pie in the sky") deficit variably demonstrated in those patients.

Anterior Temporal Lesions

Lesions in the temporal pole, up to the pes hippocampi deserve a mention because the strategy for resection can be limited and in many cases does not need to involve removal of medial structures. The incision and craniotomy for these lesions can be limited to the bone underlying the temporalis muscle as long as care is taken to obtain enough anterior and inferior exposure. This allows for better cosmetic results because of the ability to reattach the temporalis to a muscle cuff superiorly and posteriorly.

Of particular note are cavernomas in this region. Some groups advocate lesionectomy alone without removal of the hemosiderin-stained tissue.[16,17] Englot and colleagues observed no difference in seizure-free rates after pure lesionectomy compared with resections that involve the hemosiderin-involved tissue.[18] Interestingly, most studies report significantly better outcome when the surrounding gliosis and hemosiderin fringe are removed.[19] We advocate removing the gliotic hemosiderin-stained tissue as long as language and memory deficits can be prevented.

Extent of Lateral Resection

The traditional approach to cortical resection during a standard temporal lobectomy has been to limit the dominant lobe excision to 3 to 4 cm and the nondominant side to 5 to 6 cm. In fact, a randomized controlled trial that showed superiority of surgical over medical treatment for temporal lobe epilepsy was performed using those parameters.[20] The limits were set based on the typical localization of language in the dominant lobe. Although there are no controlled trials exploring whether more or less lateral resection is beneficial, the field has moved to adopting minimal disruption of the lateral cortex when mesial structures are the drivers for seizures. Subtemporal, transsylvian, and transsulcal approaches are among the approaches used for selective removal of medial structures. It is unclear whether any approach is superior to the standard temporal lobectomy in its effectiveness or safety to treat epilepsy. Some studies have suggested that even inclusion of the superior temporal gyrus in the resection is not associated with language deficits, but rather that these are a function of the age of onset of epilepsy.[21] Schramm and colleagues[22] did further analysis of the groups in their randomized controlled trial involving mesial temporal resection and found superiority in the standard temporal lobectomy over selective amygdalohippocampectomy for seizure control, but this difference was center dependent; therefore the control for surgical technique remains a complicated issue when comparing different approaches. Our recommendation is to spare the superior temporal gyrus regardless of the side of surgery, unless there are proven ictal events, and limit the anterior resection to 3 cm. Further information about those techniques can be found in Chapter 76.

Extent of Medial Resection

The debate on how much hippocampal and amygdalar resection is necessary to cure medial temporal lobe epilepsy has increased along with our understanding of the origin of these seizures. The acceptance of mesial temporal sclerosis as a separate entity has also intensified the interest in the functional connectivity of medial structures and how this pathophysiology relates to seizure development. Wyler and colleagues performed a prospective trial on 70 patients in which 34 underwent resection from the anterior edge of the hippocampus to the cerebral peduncle and the remainder had an extended resection to the level of the superior colliculus. Of patients in the latter group, 69% were seizure free at 1 year versus 38% in those in whom only a partial hippocampectomy was done.[23] A randomized controlled trial by Schramm and colleagues found no difference in seizure freedom at 1 year (74% versus 72.8%) when comparing a 2.5- versus 3.5-cm resection of mesial structures.[24] The ideal resection volume remains to be determined, particularly as the field moves forward with minimally invasive techniques (e.g., laser thermocoagulation, endoscopic resections).[25]

Neuropsychological Testing

Testing to determine preoperative cognitive dysfunction is essential to the success of temporal lobectomies. The ideal surgery obtains optimum seizure control with insignificant cognitive decline. Temporal lobe epilepsy may originate with or eventually cause significant dysfunction of the dominant hippocampus, allowing the surgeon to resect medial structures with minimal impact on language or memory. At our institution, in general, we do not advocate dominant hippocampal resection unless the patient has a proven decline of at least two standard deviations in verbal memory testing or has switched language processing to the contralateral lobe, as proven by functional MRI and Wada testing.

SURGICAL TECHNIQUE

The patient is brought to the operating room and positioned supine on the operating table. The patient is intubated and positioned by placing an ipsilateral shoulder roll or wedge. The head is rigidly fixated to the operating table by a head clamp. The position of the head is critical in this case because it allows for the exposure of mesial structures. In general, the head is rotated to the contralateral side about 30 degrees, extended until the sylvian fissure is parallel to the table (about 50 degrees; Fig. 75-1A) and the vertex dropped until the temporal region is parallel to the ground (about 10 degrees; Fig. 75-1B and Box 75-1). In this position, patients are registered with a neuronavigation

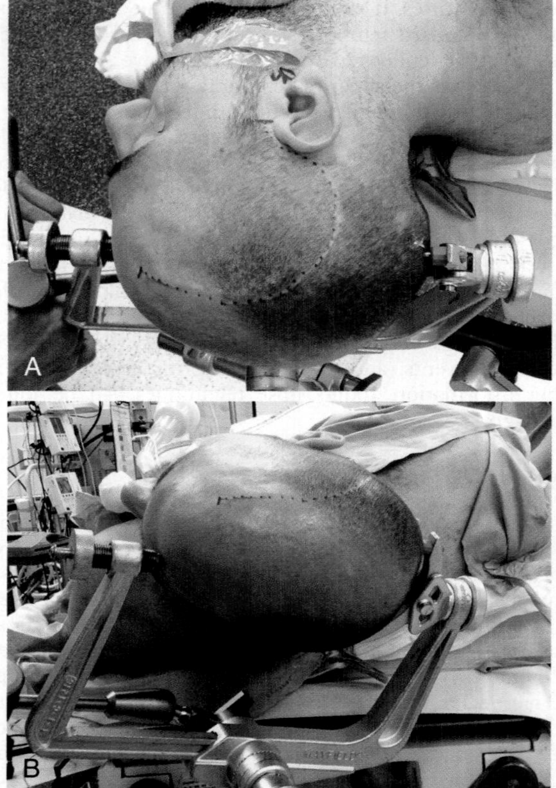

Figure 75-1. Head positioning. The head is positioned to improve access to the inferior and medial temporal structures. **A,** The head is rotated contralaterally and extended until the sylvian fissure is parallel to the table. **B,** The vertex is also dropped, making the temporal region parallel to the ground.

BOX 75-1 Summary of Critical Technical Steps in the Anteromedial Temporal Lobe Resection

1. Place head in pins, extended 50 degrees, rotated ipsilaterally 20 to 30 degrees and vertex down 10 degrees.
2. Expose at least 5 cm of temporal and orbital frontal lobe.
3. Resect 3 to 3.5 cm of middle and inferior temporal cortex, preserving the temporal horn and always using the lowest settings on the ultrasonic aspirator.
4. Open the temporal horn, dissecting from inferior to superior along fusiform gyrus. Bring in microscope.
5. Resect anterior uncus with ultrasonic aspiration, exposing the carotid, and then superiorly to the knee of the middle cerebral artery (MCA) in the sylvian fissure. All dissections must be subpial. Do not disturb the arachnoid over the tentorium.
6. Find the choroid plexus and choroidal point and draw imaginary line between the MCA and choroidal point. Bring in retractors for superior temporal gyrus and lateral temporal lobe elevation.
7. Staying below the MCA choroid line, resect the amygdala, divide the occipital temporal fasciculus posteriorly, and continue lateral temporal elevation with curved retractor.
8. Complete anterior uncal resection, divide the infralimbic gyrus, and expose midbrain arachnoid.
9. Elevate pes hippocampi and coagulate posterior cerebral artery (PCA) perforators.
10. Elevate fimbria off thalamus, coagulate, and divide arachnoid of parahippocampus.
11. Elevate hippocampal body to collateral eminence and tail turning medially.
12. Preserve posterior inferior temporal branch of the PCA.

system if desired. Patients should receive perioperative antibiotics as dictated by institutional policy. We typically administer steroids and mannitol before the incision is made.

The incision follows a "reverse question mark" just superior to the zygoma to a line between the mastoid eminence and the vertex posteriorly, curving anteriorly and superiorly just above the insertion of the temporalis muscle. The hair is clipped along the marked incision. We advocate the use of a more generous superior incision to expose the inferior frontal lobe, which allows gentle retraction of the superior temporal gyrus without frontal bone obstruction. This line is about 2 cm superior to the temporalis insertion point. If a previous intracranial electrode study has been done, we tend to use the same incision. Otherwise, a new flap is fashioned by keeping the vascular supply intact and using posterior "T" incisions when necessary.

The skin flap is elevated above the fascia of the temporalis muscle up to the level of the fat pad anteriorly to prevent damage to the anterior division of the temporal branch of the facial nerve (Fig. 75-2A). The superficial temporal artery is dissected carefully and secured with the flap anteriorly with a Raney clip. The temporalis muscle is elevated subperiosteally to detach from the bone and prevent injury to the muscle fibers. A cuff of muscle is left superiorly to attach the muscle during closing (Fig. 75-2B). The anterior portion of the temporalis muscle is elevated using electrocautery to allow for anterior exposure of the sphenoid wing. Care must be taken to preserve muscle bulk and provide superior cuff attachment, because reconstruction is essential to prevent a cosmetic deformity.

Craniotomy

A craniotomy is fashioned using a bur hole just superior to the zygoma, at the keyhole, and above the supramastoid eminence posteriorly. Some authors advocate the use of two bur holes (at the base of the zygoma and the keyhole).[26] We place two additional bur holes: anteriorly, about 2 to 3 cm superior to the insertion of the temporalis, to expose the inferior part of the frontal lobe; and inferiorly, below the sphenoid wing on the temporal bone. In general, this will be dictated by whether or not it is redo surgery and the pliability of the underlying dura. For patients who have had previous subdural electrode implantation at our institution, the incisions are closed using a titanium mesh and the bone is banked. During the resection procedure the mesh is removed and the anterior part of the middle fossa craniotomy is extended with a rongeur as needed. All bone edges are waxed, paying particular attention to the inferior portion of the craniotomy where the mastoid air cells may be violated. Excess wax is removed from the epidural space and holes are made in the bone to attach tenting dural stitches. An absorbable hemostatic material (e.g., Surgiflo or Surgicel [Ethicon]) is applied to the epidural space as needed before dural tenting.

The dura is opened sharply, starting with the posterior portion of the flap, either superior or inferior to the sylvian veins. Some authors elevate the dura from posterior to anterior as a single flap with a vascular pedicle centered on the middle meningeal vessels. We tend to remove the dura in toto and coagulate the middle meningeal artery because our closure is usually with a nonadherent material. At this point, brain relaxation is evaluated. Additional mannitol can be given as needed. The anterior temporal pole should be 1 to 2 cm from the anterior bony edge of the

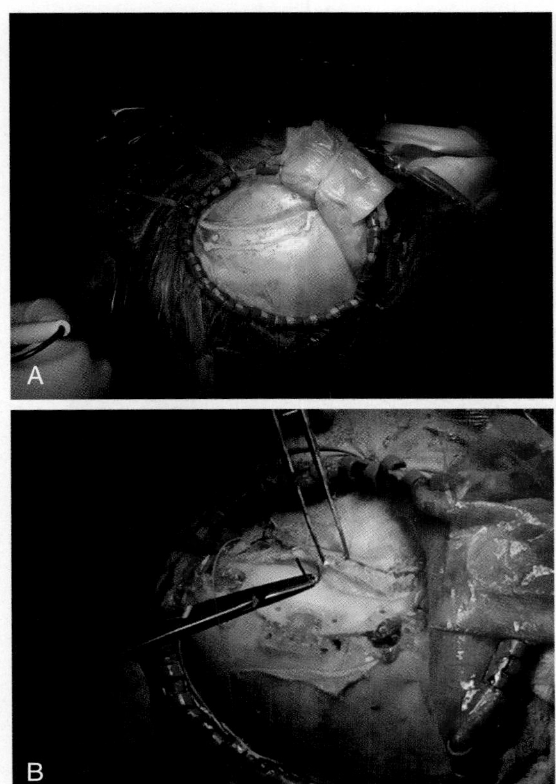

Figure 75-2. Skin flap and management of temporalis muscle. A skin flap is elevated and positioned over a large laparotomy sponge **(A).** The fat pad is identified and the facial nerve is protected. The temporalis is elevated, leaving a cuff **(B)** on the bone for reattachment.

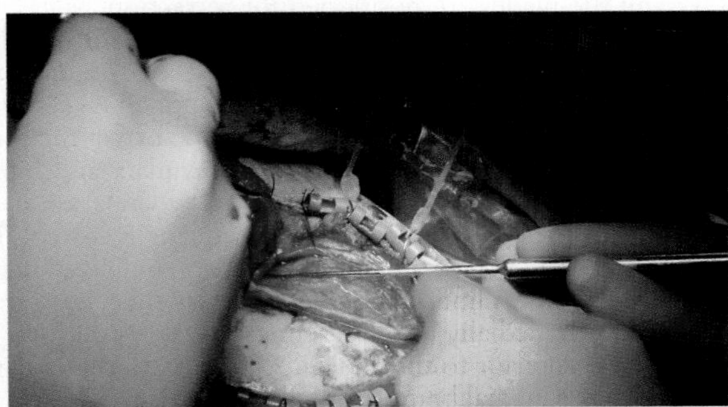

Figure 75-3. Measurement of lateral temporal resection. A Penfield 4 dissector is used to measure 3 cm from the tip of the temporal fossa.

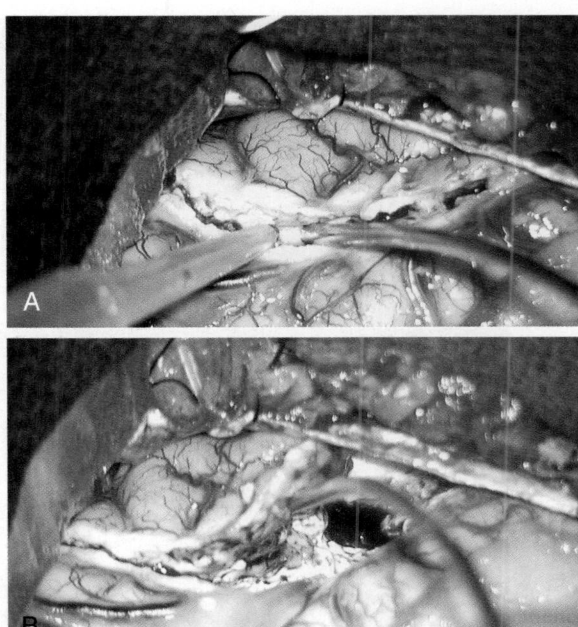

Figure 75-4. Resection of lateral temporal lobe. The lateral temporal cortex can be resected en bloc using ultrasonic aspiration and coagulation. **A,** A subpial dissection is performed, demarcating the region to be resected. **B,** The cortex is elevated at the level of the white matter without entering the ventricle.

craniotomy. If this is not the case, additional bone is removed using a rongeur. The middle meningeal artery may course inside the bony ridge of the sphenoid wing as the craniotomy is taken anteriorly. Care must be taken to coagulate and plug the artery as needed.

Lateral Temporal Resection

The posterior limit of the lateral temporal lobe resection is measured with a Penfield 4 dissector from the anterior cranial fossa along the middle temporal gyrus (Fig. 75-3). As discussed previously, surgeons differ in the extent of lateral temporal lobe resection. We tend to remove 3 to 3.5 cm of cortex regardless of the side of the surgery. At this point it is also important to identify the course of the vein of Labbé and explore its insertion point into the transverse sinus because this may limit future retraction of the lateral structures and necessitate further cortical resection for access to the posterior hippocampus. We always preserve the superior temporal gyrus unless intracranial electrode studies have identified it as part of the seizure onset zone. Understanding the course of the sylvian vein is crucial; it can be quite variable. This is particularly important if the superior temporal gyrus is resected because the drainage of the sylvian vein into the sphenoparietal sinus is exposed. Smaller draining veins from the tip of the temporal lobe to the middle fossa dura can be coagulated as necessary.

Dissection begins on the middle temporal gyrus at the marked posterior end of the resection. The pia is coagulated and cut sharply and the dissection is taken toward the middle fossa floor using subpial aspiration of the tissue, sharp dissection, and coagulation as necessary. We favor the use of an ultrasonic aspirator (CUSA EXcel; Integra LifeSciences, Plainsboro, NJ) at the lowest setting for both aspiration and vibration, along with bipolar coagulation for sharp dissection of vascular structures and pia. The ultrasonic aspirator respects pial planes and vessels at low settings and allows for a controlled dissection. The resection is taken to the middle fossa floor and then medially to the fusiform gyrus. We follow the pial plane along the inferior part of the superior temporal gyrus anteriorly until the tip of the temporal pole is reached. The depth of resection from the cortex to the temporal horn can be measured preoperatively using MRI images. The inferior portion of the resection follows the fusiform gyrus arachnoid initially and then along the ependyma of the temporal horn horizontally, without entering it, to the superior temporal gyrus white matter. Ideally, the lateral temporal pole is resected en bloc without entering the temporal horn to prevent bleeding into the ventricle (Fig. 75-4). Early identification and coagulation of inferior draining veins prevent unnecessary blood loss before removal of the cortical block of tissue.

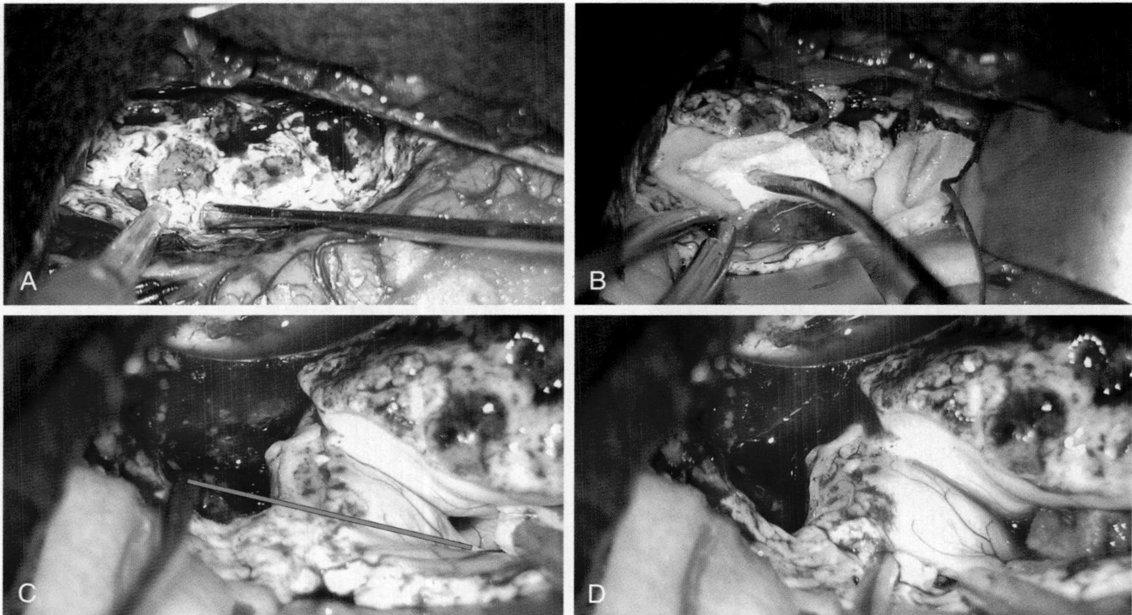

Figure 75-5. Ventricular opening and amygdala resection. A, The ventricle is opened using a Penfield 4 and the ultrasonic dissector. **B,** The choroidal point is identified by the presence of the choroid plexus in the choroidal fissure. **C,** The imaginary middle cerebral artery–choroidal line *(green)* demarcates a safe line for amygdalar resection. **D,** The amygdala can be resected en bloc by careful separation from the underlying uncal tissue.

Ventricular Exposure

Once the temporal pole is removed, the ventricle is most safely exposed by dissecting from inferior to superior along the fusiform gyrus arachnoid at the most posterior aspect of the cortical resection. The ependyma is opened and a Penfield 4 dissector is slid into the cavity anteriorly (Fig. 75-5A). The aspirator is used to resect the ependyma over the dissector, exposing the temporal horn tip. The choroid plexus is identified within the ventricle and the choroidal point described by Duvernoy[27] as the velum terminale, where the choroid plexus originates and the fimbria of the fornix joins the stria medullaris (Fig. 75-5B). A neurosurgical cotton patty (Cottonoid; Codman Neuro, Raynham, MA) is placed posteriorly in the ventricle to block the entry of blood products. The microscope may be brought into the field at this point. The remaining tissue anterior to the ventricle is resected inferiorly to the arachnoid layer covering the tentorium, and medially into the uncus of the parahippocampus until the carotid artery is encountered. At this point the arachnoid is cleared superiorly along the carotid to expose the inferior aspect of the sylvian fissure, and the MCA can be identified by pulsations through the arachnoid. An imaginary line between the choroidal point and the MCA is drawn (Fig. 75-5C). This line demarcates the superior nucleus of the amygdala, and tissue below this line may be safely resected without entering the temporal stem or causing injury to the basal ganglia. Any choroidal bleeding should be controlled with saline irrigation and pressure because coagulation in this region may endanger the anterior choroidal artery (injury to this vessel may result in hemiplegia from ischemia to the posterior limb of the internal capsule or lateral thalamus).

Amygdala Resection

Our craniotomy allows for gentle retraction on the superior temporal gyrus and frontal lobe as well as the posterior temporal lobe, therefore exposing midline structures. We use a Greenberg retractor system with 5/8 curved blades for this purpose. Small pieces of collagen sponge (BICOL; DePuy Synthes, West Chester, PA) are cut to the size of the blade, placed on the brain, and moistened. Neurosurgical cotton patties are placed on top of the BICOL, and the blades are positioned for retraction.

The resection of the amygdala, hippocampus, and parahippocampal gyrus requires clear understanding of the anatomic nuances of the region as well as the vascular supply. The resection of medial structures may be performed en bloc or via the ultrasonic aspirator. We prefer to remove the amygdala and hippocampus as intact structures for histopathologic correlation to the clinical syndrome and to be used in subsequent research. The amygdala is resected first, maintaining the plane indicated before by the choroidal-MCA line. The resection starts superiorly at the line and proceeds medially to the arachnoid layer. Posteriorly the resection is just anterior to the choroidal point with the uncinate gyrus forming the medial boundary. The amygdala is then divided from the hippocampal head and removed in entirety (Fig. 75-5D). After the amygdalar resection the remaining uncus is then aspirated or elevated from the medial arachnoid using a pancake dissector. Care must be exercised in preventing undue pressure on medial structures. Once the dissection is complete, the anterior edge of the tentorium, the PCA, and the third nerve are visible through the arachnoid layer. By never dissecting the arachnoid from the tentorial edge, one avoids injuring the fourth nerve.

Hippocampal Resection

Before the removal of the hippocampus any remaining fusiform gyrus is resected from the basal temporal lobe to the level of the collateral sulcus. The temporal retractor blade is curved to almost 90 degrees and placed underneath the cortex, just above the hippocampal body, and the lateral cortical tissue is elevated as one dissects the occipital temporal white matter from the temporal horn ependyma inferiorly to the tentorium, stopping when the

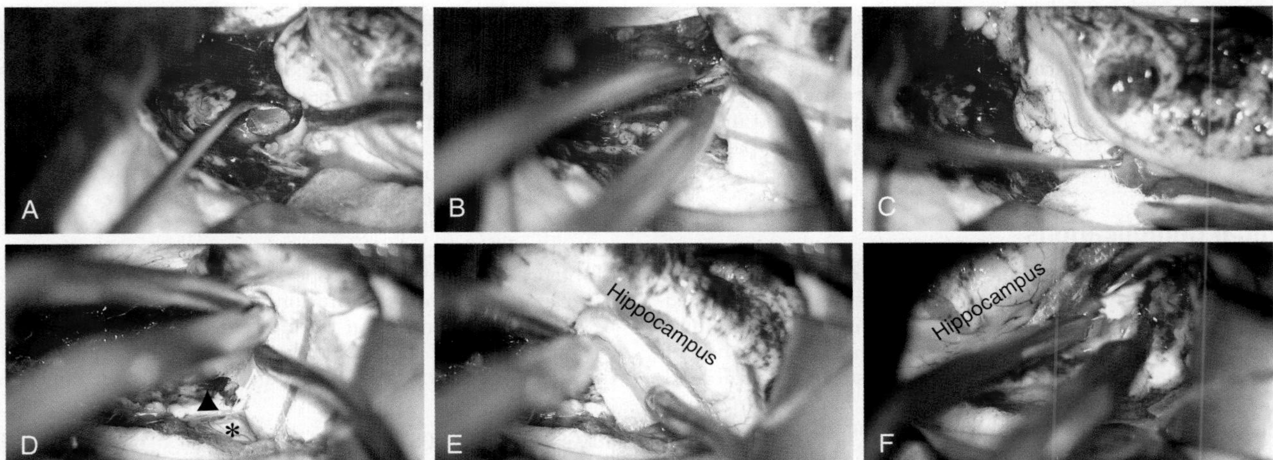

Figure 75-6. Hippocampal resection. A, A pancake dissector is used to elevate the hippocampal pes with exposure of posterior cerebral artery perforators. **B,** The perforators are coagulated and divided sharply. The fimbria of the fornix is elevated **(C)** and the posterior uncinate gyrus *(black triangle)* dissected with exposure of the brainstem *(asterisk)* arachnoid **(D). E,** The body of the hippocampus is elevated with the aid of a neurosurgical cotton patty and separated from the parahippocampal gyrus. **F,** Once the tail of the hippocampus is reached, it can be coagulated and divided.

tail of the hippocampus is seen curving medially beneath the pulvinar of the thalamus. This usually coincides with reaching the collateral eminence. One typically encounters two prominent arteries from the PCA. The first irrigates the hippocampus but must be traced to its endpoint before it is coagulated because the second artery, which is more posterior and in the collateral sulcus arachnoid, may supply a large region of the posterior inferior temporal lobe and must be protected. Basal arachnoid coagulation is performed along the collateral sulcus. Care must be exercised posteriorly to protect the vein of Labbé and other large lateral draining veins.

The hippocampus may be removed as a single structure or separately by dividing the pes hippocampi from the body. With a pancake dissector or aspirator, the head of the hippocampus is elevated (Fig. 75-6A), exposing the hippocampal perforators from the PCA as they course through the uncal sulcus. The perforators are coagulated and divided sharply as the hippocampal head is elevated posteriorly (Fig. 75-6B). Care must be taken to prevent pulling the perforators too hard, disrupting the adventitia, which could cause tiny pseudoaneurysms on the parent vessel. A coagulated arterial tail should be left on each vessel to prevent retraction into the mesencephalic cistern and potential subarachnoid hemorrhage. Elevating the anterior head is always coupled with division of the posterior uncinate gyrus, just anterior to the velum terminale, until the midbrain arachnoid is exposed and protected as one continues dividing the hippocampal perforators.

The pes hippocampi is either removed or elevated to the posterior aspect of the uncal sulcus. The fimbria of the fornix is elevated posterior to the choroidal point using a pancake dissector (Fig. 75-6C), exposing the arachnoid of the lateral geniculate of the thalamus (Fig. 75-6D) and the hippocampal sulcus and enabling visualization of the parahippocampal gyrus. The rest of the dissection proceeds from anterior to posterior by elevating the body of the hippocampus (Fig. 75-6E) from the parahippocampal gyrus using aspiration and coagulation as needed. As the body of the hippocampus is elevated, a neurosurgical cotton patty may be used for traction. Authors argue regarding how much hippocampus needs to be resected, as discussed previously. We advocate the removal of the body to the hippocampal tail (Fig. 75-6F) as it curves near the collateral eminence. Once removal is complete, the course of the PCA and the lateral geniculate nucleus can be identified, as well as the quadrigeminal cistern posteriorly.

Once the resection is complete the area is irrigated copiously, making sure that any blood in the ventricular system is removed. Hemostasis is achieved using bipolar cautery and hemostatic materials. The dura is closed in a watertight fashion and the cavity filled with saline before the final dural closure. Tenting sutures are placed on the dura and the craniotomy flap is replaced. The tenting sutures are passed through the craniotomy flap and knotted to prevent epidural fluid accumulation. The flap is attached with titanium plates, the temporalis muscle is reapproximated to the previously fashioned cuff, and the incision is closed in anatomic layers over a subgaleal drain to reduce postoperative swelling.

POSTOPERATIVE FOLLOW-UP

The postoperative workup after a standard temporal lobectomy is similar to other craniotomies. Within 24 hours after surgery a computed tomography (CT) scan of the head is obtained to monitor for hemorrhage, air, or any other immediate complications that may occur. Patients usually remain 3 to 5 days in the hospital and are discharged home with general wound care instructions and pain control.

It has been our practice to wait 3 months after surgery to obtain additional neuroimaging. At that point the resection cavity has settled in its final position and scar has formed at the exposed surfaces. It is not uncommon to see some settling of the hemisphere into the middle fossa, particularly with large temporal lobectomies. In our experience this has no functional consequence for the patient.

Repeat neuropsychological testing is also paramount in these patients—particularly those with dominant temporal lobe resections, to determine whether new language or memory deficits have occurred. Some authors advocate repeat testing at 6 months after surgery.[26] Our practice has been to wait until at least a year after surgery because cognitive function will have stabilized at that point.

Repeat outpatient EEG can also be performed, along with neuropsychological testing to look at interictal activity, which has been shown to be a predictor of seizure freedom.[28] EEG also aids neurologists in determining the best course of action regarding medication weaning. We advocate waiting at least a year before reduction of seizure medication, except for patients who are on more than three antiepileptics. Similarly, return to driving should be based on both state guidelines and planning around medication reduction. In general, we restrict driving until the patient is at least a year without seizures.

Surgical Complications

The standard temporal lobectomy is currently performed with a very low perioperative mortality rate in the hands of experienced epilepsy surgeons (about 0.1%-0.5%).[29] However, the procedure still carries some morbidity, and patients should be informed of the expected and unexpected deficits before surgery. Visual field deficits (caused by violation of visual path fibers), temporalis muscle wasting, frontalis nerve palsy, language deficits,[30] problems with semantic processing,[31] diplopia, and hemiparesis (secondary to injury of the anterior choroidal artery) are among the possible surgical complications. Chapter 80 has more details regarding surgical complications and outcomes in epilepsy surgery.

Outcomes

In appropriately selected patients the standard temporal lobectomy has been shown to produce an Engel Class I outcome (freedom from disabling seizures) in 70%-80% of patients at 2 years after surgery.[32,33] This declines to about 50% at 5 years. Several factors have been shown to predict an unfavorable outcome: presence of epileptic activity on EEG at 6 months postop, frequent preoperative seizures, generalized motor seizures, bilateral MRI abnormalities, and increased epilepsy duration.[34-37] A detailed evaluation of outcomes after epilepsy surgery can be found in Chapter 80.

A "running-down" phenomenon has been described in up to a third of patients experiencing seizures after temporal lobectomy. Patients may experience rare seizures 6 months after surgery but eventually have been documented to have long-term seizure freedom in 74% of cases.[38-40]

The advent of new procedures including selective approaches to the mesial temporal lobe (see Chapter 76) as well as selective laser-assisted amygdalohippocampectomies[41] have increased an interest not just in seizure freedom but in the prevention of neuropsychological decline in epilepsy patients. Standardization of the preoperative and postoperative neuropsychological assessment among different institutions remains a challenge and will be needed for comparison of different treatment modalities. In the meantime, the standard temporal lobectomy continues to be the benchmark procedure for medial temporal lobe epilepsy.

SUGGESTED READINGS

Penfield W, Baldwin M. Temporal lobe seizures and the technic of subtotal temporal lobectomy. *Ann Surg*. 1952;136:625-634.

Schramm J, Lehmann TN, Zentner J, et al. Randomized controlled trial of 2.5-cm versus 3.5-cm mesial temporal resection in temporal lobe epilepsy—part 1: intent-to-treat analysis. *Acta Neurochir (Wien)*. 2011;153:209-219.

Spencer DD, Spencer SS, Mattson RH, et al. Access to the posterior medial temporal lobe structures in the surgical treatment of temporal lobe epilepsy. *Neurosurgery*. 1984;15:667-671.

Tubbs RS, Miller JH, Cohen-Gadol AA, et al. Intraoperative anatomic landmarks for resection of the amygdala during medial temporal lobe surgery. *Neurosurgery*. 2010;66:974-977.

Wiebe S, Blume WT, Girvin JP, et al. A randomized, controlled trial of surgery for temporal-lobe epilepsy. *N Engl J Med*. 2001;345:311-318.

Wyler AR, Hermann BP, Somes G. Extent of medial temporal lobe resection on outcome from anterior temporal lobectomy: a randomized prospective study. *Neurosurgery*. 1995;37:982-991.

See a full reference list on ExpertConsult.com

76 Selective Approaches to the Mesial Temporal Lobe

Robert A. McGovern III and Guy M. McKhann II

Surgery for medically intractable mesial temporal lobe epilepsy (MTLE) has undergone transformative technological changes in the last decade. Although traditional open surgical approaches have demonstrated excellent seizure freedom outcomes in this patient population in randomized controlled trials,[1] epilepsy surgery remains significantly underused given its known benefits.[2] Epidemiologic studies have established that approximately 20% to 30% of patients will be unable to control their seizures with medication.[3,4] These medically intractable, pharmacoresistant patients account for the majority of the costs associated with epilepsy.[5] Uncontrolled epilepsy is one of the most common neurological disorders, and the medical morbidity attributed to it is associated with significant financial costs.[6] In addition, patients whose seizures cannot be controlled with two antiepileptic drugs are much less likely to benefit from additional medication trials.[7,8] In these patients, most studies have demonstrated 12-month seizure remission rates of approximately 5% per year, with subsequent relapse in 40% to 50% of patients.[9-12] These patients are thus candidates for epilepsy surgery.

Despite evidence that the prevalence of mesial temporal sclerosis may be decreasing over the past several decades, temporal lobe epilepsy surgery remains one the most common subtypes of epilepsy surgery, with some of the most favorable seizure-free outcomes. However, improving patient access to and interest in mesial temporal MTLE surgery has remained challenging. The recent trial of early surgery for temporal lobe epilepsy was stopped prematurely because of a lack of enrollment.[13] In an effort to improve epilepsy surgery utilization and minimize complications of MTLE surgery, technological advances have transformed the nature of MTLE surgery. Once limited to open surgical approaches that effectively removed much of the temporal lobe through a larger craniotomy, patients can now undergo a range of less invasive procedures to remove the mesial temporal structures ranging from open selective amygdalohippocampectomy (SAH) to minimally invasive laser ablation to stereotactic radiosurgery. This chapter will discuss the pros and cons of these various approaches.

PATIENT SELECTION

For surgical resection to be successful in patients with MTLE, they must be selected carefully. First, patients must have established drug resistance. Although studies have defined this in many different ways over time, the International League of Epilepsy defines *drug-resistant epilepsy* as "failure of adequate trials of two tolerated and appropriately chosen and used anti-epileptic drug schedules (whether as monotherapies or in combination) to achieve sustained seizure freedom."[14] Seizure semiology frequently helps to localize the epileptogenic zone in all epilepsy patients, including those with MTLE.[15] These seizures are most commonly complex partial in nature, often involving an aura experienced as a rising epigastric sensation, smell, fear, or déjà vu, and head and hand automatisms such as contralateral forced head version prior to secondary generalization, lip smacking, and dystonia.[15,16]

Long-term video electroencephalography (EEG) is used to lateralize and localize ictal onset and to correlate the type of seizure with ictal EEG activity. MTLE patients typically show lateralized interictal spikes[17] and ictal EEG activity frequently localizes to the anterior temporal region. Patients with recorded bilateral interictal discharges or lateralized discharges with contralateral spread have been associated with worse surgical outcomes.[18] Evolving techniques, such as stereotactic electroencephalography (SEEG) (see Chapter 72), that help to more precisely localize ictal onset regions and determine extent of surgical resection of the epileptogenic zone (EZ) may improve patient outcomes in the future.

Imaging in MTLE consists mainly of brain magnetic resonance imaging (MRI) sequences aimed at revealing the effects of mesial temporal sclerosis (MTS), the main pathology seen in MTLE. Thin-cut T1-weighted sequences and coronal T2 and FLAIR-weighted sequences characteristically reveal hippocampal and temporal lobe atrophy,[19] increased hippocampal T2/FLAIR signal,[20,21] and loss of normal hippocampal architecture.[22] Because MTLE patients often have coexisting cortical dysplasia,[19,23] the clinician should closely examine the entirety of the temporal lobes on these sequences. Positron emission tomography (PET) is a complementary imaging technique that can demonstrate hypometabolism in the mesial temporal region on the side correlated with ictal EEG activity, whereas magnetoencephalography (MEG) is frequently helpful in colocalizing source dipole activity with interictal EEG activity.

Finally, neuropsychological testing should be included as part of every MTLE patient evaluation. Testing serves to diagnose any preexisting cognitive impairment, to evaluate an individual's risk of cognitive decline after surgery, and potentially to serve as a tool to predict which patients will be best served by surgery. In general, patients with dominant lobe MTLE tend to show verbal memory deficits while patients undergoing nondominant resection might have visual memory deficits or other less clinically significant cognitive impairments.[24,25] Patients with MTS on MRI have worse verbal memory scores pre-operatively; their lower neurocognitive baseline puts them less at risk of decline after surgery than those without MTS.[24] Freedom from seizure may be the most important factor in determining long-term cognitive outcome, as patients undergoing surgical resection for MTLE but still suffering seizures show similar outcomes as medically treated intractable MTLE patients.[26]

Traditionally, surgical approaches to the mesial temporal region have been reserved for patients with MTS, but as alluded to previously, preoperative invasive monitoring with subdural electrodes or SEEG has allowed for investigation of MRI-negative patients who may still have a mesial temporal ictal onset. In addition, invasive monitoring has proved useful in determining ictal onset in patients with MTS on MRI but discordant video EEG, neuropsychological, or MEG/PET data. Patients determined to have a truly mesial temporal onset using noninvasive and invasive monitoring (as needed) are potentially candidates for the approaches outlined as follows.

TRADITIONAL OPEN SURGICAL APPROACHES

MTLE is the most common cause of pharmacoresistant epilepsy and has been shown in randomized clinical trials to respond well to surgical resection compared with medical therapy, with rates of seizure freedom ranging from 60% to 70% at 2 to 5 years.[1,27] Classically, surgical resection for MTLE entails the removal of 3.5 to 4.5 cm of dominant temporal lobe or 4 to 5 cm of

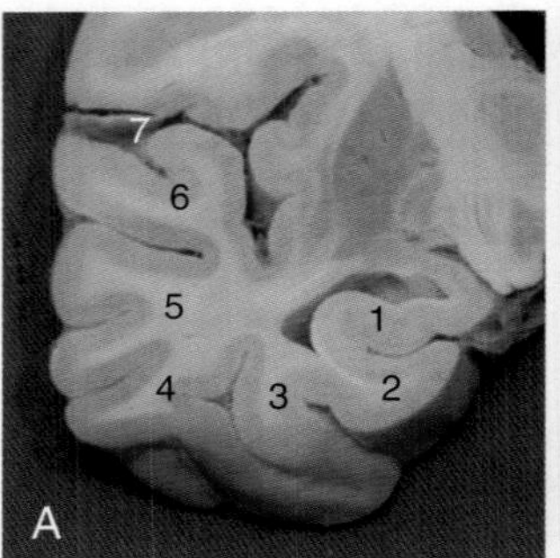

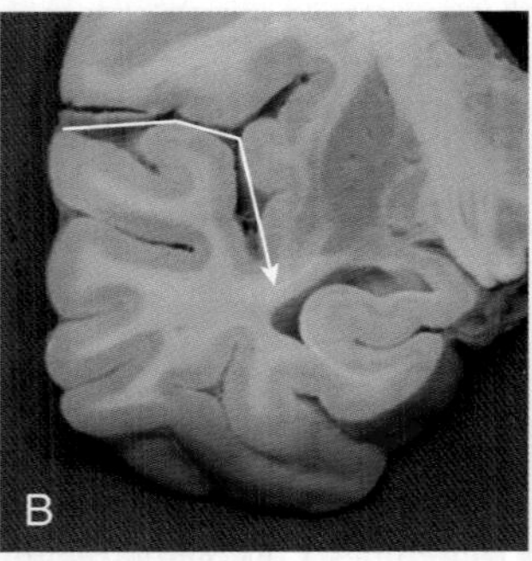

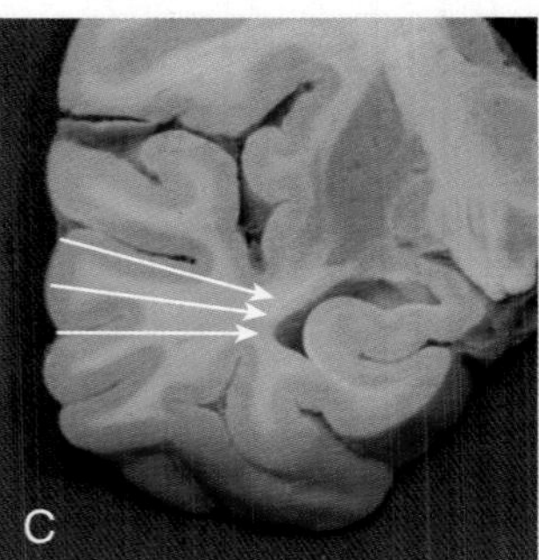

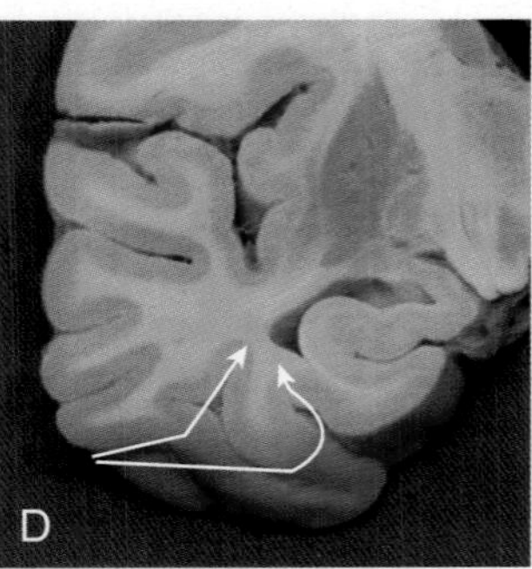

Figure 76-1. Selective approaches to the mesial temporal region. A, Coronal section of right temporal lobe demonstrating: 1, hippocampus; 2, parahippocampal gyrus; 3, fusiform gyrus; 4, inferior temporal gyrus; 5, middle temporal gyrus; 6, superior temporal gyrus; 7, sylvian fissure. **B, C,** and **D,** Selective amygdalohippocampectomy approaches: **(B)** transsylvian approach; **(C)** transsulcal/gyral approach through superior temporal sulcus or middle temporal gyrus; **(D)** subtemporal approach. *(From Anatomy of the Brain: Coronal Brain Sections. Courtesy of Dr. Claudia Krebs, University of British Columbia, Dr. Bruce Crawford and Dr. Kurt McBurney, University of Victoria.* http://www.neuroanatomy.ca/cross_sections/sections_coronal.html.*)*

nondominant temporal lobe in addition to the mesial temporal structures (anterior temporal lobectomy [ATL]). This technique's safety and efficacy is well established, and it was used in the randomized clinical trials, which proved surgical efficacy in MTLE.[1] Subsequent research in animal models[28-30] and human depth electrode recordings[31-34] began to show that the mesial temporal structures were largely responsible for seizure generation in MTLE. This knowledge combined with neuropsychological studies, which consistently demonstrated verbal memory and visual naming deficits[35-38] in patients undergoing dominant ATL, led neurosurgeons to begin to adopt the SAH. Although originally developed in the 1950s by Niemeyer,[39] this procedure did not gain prominence until the epilepsy and neuropsychological evidence described above began to emerge. Modifications of this approach have been developed over time (transsylvian, subtemporal, transcortical), but they all have the common goal of sparing lateral neocortical resection to resect the hippocampus, amygdala, parahippocampal gyrus, and uncus solely (Fig. 76-1).

Selective Amygdalohippocampectomy: Operative Technique

On the day of surgery, the patient is brought to the operating room, and the operation is completed using general anesthesia. Antibiotics and steroids are administered before incision, and a Foley catheter and venous compression stockings are placed. Surgical adjuncts, such as mannitol or lumbar cerebrospinal fluid drainage, are variably used by individual surgeons and centers. The patient is placed in three-point fixation pins with a Mayfield head holder with the head turned 70 to 80 degrees laterally away from the side of the craniotomy and the head extended so that the malar eminence is the highest point in the field. To position the neck so that the jugular veins are not compressed, the head of the bed is elevated and an ipsilateral shoulder roll is typically placed. The patient's cranial anatomy is then coregistered to the volumetric MRI using stereotactic navigation software. Frameless stereotaxy is not necessary for selective amygdalohippocampectomy. However, this technology is commonly available and can be useful in helping to determine the subcortical anatomy and localize the temporal horn of the lateral ventricle.

A reverse question mark–shaped incision is planned; it extends from the root of the zygoma just in front of tragus superiorly then posteriorly above the pinna, above the superior temporal line and then anteriorly to the hairline just lateral to midline. Alternatively, a linear incision can be used, extending from the root of the zygoma to just below the superior temporal line. The head is then prepared in the routine sterile fashion and draped. The scalp is incised, and scalp bleeding is controlled as necessary. The superficial temporal artery is preserved when possible. A second scalpel is then used to incise through the temporalis muscle, using bipolar cautery to prevent bleeding. A Penfield 1 or periosteal elevator is used to elevate the myocutaneous tissues from the skull. For reverse question mark scalp flaps, the flap is then dissected anteriorly and retracted with rubber bands, with a laparotomy pad or rolled surgical sponge placed behind the flap to minimize vascular compromise during the procedure. For a linear incision, self-retaining retraction is used to expose the area of planned craniotomy. The root of the zygoma should be visible to ensure that the middle fossa floor is adequately exposed. Using stereotactic navigation, a temporal craniotomy is then performed to expose superior and middle temporal gyri with the superior extent at least up to the sylvian fissure. A small amount of craniectomy is usually performed inferiorly to reach the floor of the middle fossa and anteriorly toward the temporal pole, minimizing entry into pneumatized temporal bone. For larger question mark flaps, the sphenoid wing is then drilled down as necessary to maximize exposure, before opening the dura in a C-shaped manner and reflecting anteriorly. For linear approaches, the dura is more readily open in X-shaped or cruciate fashion.

The original descriptions of SAH surgery detailed an approach through the temporal stem from the Sylvian fissure to the temporal horn of the lateral ventricle. Most epilepsy surgeons, however, do not use this approach, preferring to use frameless stereotaxy and either coming from laterally through the middle temporal gyrus or middle temporal sulcus or basally coming through the inferior temporal or collateral sulcus to approach the temporal horn. For either of these latter approaches, a 1- to 2-cm approach is made directed toward the temporal horn, recognizing that the various sulci are oriented to the temporal horn like the spokes of a wheel. The choroidal point is a good entry point of the ventricle for which to aim, as it is well positioned along the sagittal axis of the hippocampus yet sufficiently anterior to minimize the risk of a significant visual field deficit.

A working channel is created using appropriately low settings on the ultrasonic aspirator or with gentle suction aspiration, as dissection is carried medially to the ependymal lining of the temporal horn. The temporal horn is preferably entered anterolaterally to minimize risk to Meyer's loop of the optic radiations. At this point, the amygdala (anteromedially), choroid plexus (medially), collateral eminence (laterally), and hippocampus (anteroinferiorly) can be identified within the temporal horn. The lateral ventricular sulcus lies between the collateral eminence and hippocampus, and it is opened to enter the parahippocampal gyrus. The surgical resection from within the temporal horn is similar in the SAH approach as it is in ATL surgery, except that the working space can be more limited, resulting at times in smaller en bloc surgical specimens.

The parahippocampal gyrus is resected in a subpial fashion moving anteriorly into the uncus, which is completely emptied subpially. The oculomotor nerve, tentorial edge, and posterior cerebral artery (P1) can be seen through the pia here. The amygdala is then identified by its speckled brown color and location anterosuperior to the hippocampus within the medial temporal horn, along a line connecting choroid plexus and limen insula. The basolateral amygdala is then removed entirely, again taking care to respect pial boundaries and keeping in mind that the posteromedial boundary of resection remains the choroid plexus/inferior choroidal point. Next, the dissection is carried lateral to the collateral eminence, which disconnects the hippocampus laterally and allows for the hippocampus to be retracted laterally. Once retracted laterally, the fimbria of the hippocampus is disconnected medially by dissecting taenia fimbriae off the choroidal fissure with the medial aspect of the parahippocampal gyrus lifted up subpially using a dissector. Once separated, the hippocampal end arteries can be identified, coagulated, and divided as close to the hippocampus as possible to preserve the posterior cerebral artery (P2) and anterior choroidal artery segments. The hippocampus and parahippocampal gyrus are then disconnected posteriorly at approximately the level of the tectum and removed en bloc if possible. Additional tail of the hippocampus can then be removed with the Cavitron as necessary.

Hemostasis is obtained, and the dura is then closed with 4-0 silk sutures with epidural tenting sutures placed to help prevent extra-axial collections postoperatively. The bone flap is washed in antibiotic irrigation, and titanium plates are affixed to secure the bone flap in place. The temporalis fascia is closed with 3-0 Vicryl sutures, and the scalp is closed with 2-0 Vicryl sutures and staples.

Selective Amygdalohippocampectomy: Evidence Base

Because lateral temporal neocortex is thought be intimately involved in verbal memory and visual naming, neuropsychological studies have attempted to examine the potential benefits of sparing this cortex in SAH, particularly in dominant lobe surgery. Indeed, the result of years of cognitive outcomes research has shown that patients undergoing dominant lobe ATL tend to have persistent verbal memory and word finding deficits.[24,37] In addition, those with MTS generally have worse cognitive baselines and decline less than those without MTS on MRI and pathology, whereas those without MTS tend to have higher baseline cognitive scores and decline more severely postoperatively.[40] This indicates that patients without MTS likely have more functional tissue that is being resected during an ATL.

There have been no published prospective, controlled trials randomizing patients to either ATL or SAH, but there have been a number of studies comparing both seizure and neuropsychological outcomes. Most of these studies are retrospective in nature and suffer from the fact that many neurosurgeons in the field began performing mostly SAH surgeries over the past decade. Thus, these retrospective studies mainly compare data from ATL surgeries performed at the beginning of the study period and SAH surgeries toward the end of the study period.[41,42] Nevertheless, there have been consistent themes that have emerged during this time.

First, almost every direct comparison study has shown equivalent seizure freedom rates (60%-90% at 3-6 years of follow-up) between SAH and ATL in adult patients,[41,43-47] although there have been exceptions.[48] In addition, studies describing only SAH[49-53] have shown similar seizure freedom rates to historic ATL data.[54] Interestingly, Helmstaedter and colleagues[26] found that seizure control significantly influenced cognitive outcome regardless of surgical approach, implying that verbal memory and language impairments may be more related to seizure freedom rates than the amount or type of tissue resected. Other studies have not corroborated these data.[44]

Most cognitive outcome studies comparing SAH and ATL have shown slightly better results for SAH although a recent meta-analysis was unable to detect a difference between surgical approaches.[55] The most consistent finding across multiple retrospective studies is a smaller decline in verbal memory in dominant lobe SAH surgical resection than that seen in ATL,[41,47,56] with some studies showing a higher percentage of patients actually improving in verbal memory postoperatively.[45] For example, Clusmann and coworkers[41] found that 43% of dominant lobe ATL patients had worse verbal memory scores postoperatively, whereas only 31% of SAH patients worsened. Other studies have found improved nonverbal memory in nondominant SAH compared with ATL[42,57] and improved immediate recall.[47] Because it was surprising that SAH patients still showed significant verbal and language difficulties despite sparing the lateral temporal neocortex, one group characterized tissue undergoing "collateral damage" (T2/FLAIR signal change) along the surgical approach corridor as responsible for verbal memory decline, as an increase in damage predicted worse memory outcome.[58] Finally, it should again be noted that none of these studies have examined this in a rigorous, randomized, controlled fashion, and there are examples of studies showing no difference between techniques as well.[59-61]

No studies have rigorously compared different surgical approaches to SAH that would be hypothesized to have different neuropsychological consequences. In particular, the trans-Sylvian approach, trans-middle temporal gyrus, trans-middle temporal sulcus, and subtemporal approaches all transgress different subcortical white matter pathways, with anticipated different degrees of risk to neuropsychological function[62] (see Fig. 76-1). Some of the most compelling evidence in this regard has come from the subtemporal experience used by Smith and colleagues. This group's approach minimizes disruption of the anterolateral temporal lobe white matter during dissection to the temporal horn. They have reported excellent neuropsychological outcomes in both dominant and nondominant MTLE surgery.[63]

As discussed previously, there is much evidence that open surgical approaches for epilepsy are superior to continued medical therapy in pharmacoresistant patients. Unfortunately, updated clinical practice guidelines have not changed referral patterns,[64] and epilepsy surgery remains underused.[2] Many factors have likely contributed to this persistence, including patient misconceptions, fears, attitudes toward surgery,[65,66] and practicing neurologists' attitudes and knowledge base regarding current guidelines.[67,68] In addition, by its very nature, open surgical resection will always be associated with some degree of verbal memory and visual naming deficits in dominant temporal lobe surgery and low rates of death, infection, hemiparesis, visual field deficits, and cranial nerve palsies. For these reasons, more minimally invasive approaches have been developed to attempt to achieve the same seizure freedom outcomes with less morbidity. With the current emphasis in health care on reducing costs through minimizing length of stay and readmissions, these approaches have gained more popularity in recent years in the United States.

STEREOTACTIC ABLATIVE APPROACHES

Laser Interstitial Thermal Therapy

Laser interstitial thermal therapy (LITT) is a technique in which a laser fiber is stereotactically implanted into the region of choice and progressively heated to thermally ablate the region under

MRI guidance. This process allows for the generation of pseudo–real-time MRI to follow lesion evolution. A few advantages are afforded by this approach. First, this technique allows for the ablation of deep subcortical regions that may be difficult to access surgically while observing the lesion in near real time. Second, the minimally invasive nature of this approach provides for shorter hospital stays and, potentially, fewer complications when compared with traditional open surgical approaches. For example, patients with a normal MRI and suspected mesial onset epilepsy, particularly in the nondominant temporal lobe, may undergo SEEG to determine the epileptogenic zone. If the epileptogenic zone is confirmed to be mesial, the patient can potentially be treated with LITT. In this circumstance, a patient who likely would have had an aggressive temporal lobectomy or a subdural grid implant followed by a temporal lobectomy has their MRI-negative epilepsy treated in minimally invasive fashion, without ever having a craniotomy. Finally, given the ability to generate a lesion in near real time with image guidance, this technique has the potential benefit of limiting cognitive deficits postoperatively. However, given the lack of clear cut benefit realized with SAH versus MTLE, this issue will need to be studied extensively.

Laser Interstitial Thermal Therapy: Operative Technique

Before surgery, the patient receives a volumetric MRI scan with T1 contrast-enhanced and T2 sequences. The surgeon should plan the trajectory to the mesial temporal region based on this MRI before surgery. The trajectory is typically planned to place the laser applicator along the long axis of the hippocampus, and it should seek to avoid cortical vessels on entry and subcortical vessels along its path.

On the day of surgery, the patient is brought to the operating room on a stretcher and intubated under general anesthesia. A Foley catheter is placed. With at least one assistant helping, the patient is raised upright to a sitting position on the stretcher with a pillow behind the back, and a Cosman-Robert-Wells (CRW) headframe is placed while one person steadies the patient's head and the other screws in the four headframe pins. The posterior pins should be placed low in the occipital region, with the pin on the side of planned trajectory moved to accommodate the planned posterior hippocampal trajectory. The CT fiducial box is attached to the headframe, and a volumetric CT is then obtained with zero gantry such that the headframe is perpendicular to the scanner. The patient is returned to the operating room and the volumetric CT is uploaded, registered and fused to the prior volumetric MRI. The prior planned trajectory is then modified on the basis of the fused CT, and the stereotactic coordinates are finalized.

The headframe is attached to the Mayfield head holder using an adaptor and fixed in place. The final position should allow the surgeon to reach the entry point comfortably, but also maintain the patient in a comfortable position with the neck neither flexed nor extended too far and allowing for normal jugular venous return. To check the planned entry point, place a clear, sterile drape over the headframe, input the approximate coordinates on the stereotactic frame to be attached to the headframe, and mark where the planned entry point will be on the scalp. The stereotactic frame and drape is then removed, and the entry point region minimally shaved, prepared, and draped in the usual manner. The stereotactic frame is then reattached, and the coordinates checked a second time with both the surgeon and assistant agreeing on the coordinates. The guide block is attached to the frame, and the entry point on the scalp is confirmed. Two to 3 mL of local anesthesia is placed at the entry point, and a nick is made in the scalp with a #11 blade. A coated obturator probe is placed through the incision down to periosteum and monopolar cautery is used to cauterize the dermis and periosteum. A 3.2-mm drill bit is then placed through the guide block and used to create a small bur hole. Another obturator probe is then placed against the dura, and monopolar cautery is used to make a small durotomy. An anchor bolt is then screwed into the skull. A premeasured stylet probe is then inserted through the anchor bolt to just a few milliliters shy of the target distance, to avoid creating a small air pocket at the target. The laser outer cannula and fiber are then placed to the stereotactic target distance, and the anchor bolt cap is tightened. A 3-0 nylon U-stitch is placed around the incision, left untied, and wrapped around the anchor bolt with a small xeroform dressing. The patient is then taken for MRI, where the thermal ablation process occurs.

Axial and sagittal planes are scanned along the long axis of the laser applicator and the laser fiber cable is attached to the laser power source. The irrigation tubing is attached to the cannula holding the laser applicator. Six temperature monitoring points are chosen around the tip of the applicator: three to monitor lesion temperature and three to monitor for safety at the margins of the planned treatment. For hippocampal laser ablation, the safety monitor points are generally placed on the thalamus, optic tract and brainstem to ensure the laser is turned off if the predetermined threshold is exceeded at any of those points. The laser is activated at low power (typically 25%-30%) to identify the applicator tip location and confirm fiber heating location. Serial overlapping ablations at 60%-70% power are then performed, beginning at the anterior amygdala/uncus and moving posteriorly. The imaging software will indicate the zone of irreversible damage with pixels, which will plateau after approximately 2-3 minutes of laser activation. Once the target region is ablated, post-gadolinium contrast-enhanced T1, T2/FLAIR, and diffusion-weighted images are obtained to demonstrate the region of ablation (Fig. 76-2). The patient is removed from the MRI scanner, the laser applicator and fiber optic cable are removed as one unit, and the anchor bolt is removed. The 3-0 stitch is sterilely tied down and the head frame is removed.

Laser Interstitial Thermal Therapy: Evidence Base

LITT remains a new technique; therefore, the literature regarding its use for MTLE is limited. In one case series, 13 patients ranging from 16 to 64 years of age underwent stereotactic laser amygdalohippocampectomy for medically refractory MTLE.[69] Whereas six of nine of the patients with MTS on MRI were seizure free on follow-up (5-26 months), only one of four patients without MTS on MRI attained seizure freedom. Adverse events that occurred during the study included one patient developing homonymous hemianopia and one patient developing an acute subdural that resolved without sequelae. As expected, postoperative hospital stay was short, ranging from 1 to 3 days. In addition, one recent study examined the cognitive outcomes in 19 patients who received LITT for MTLE compared with standard open surgical resections. LITT patients demonstrated improved visual naming compared with open surgical patients postoperatively.[70] Finally, one small case series demonstrated the feasibility of treating cavernous malformations in a variety of locations with four of five patients achieving Engel class I seizure freedom at a mean follow up of 17 months.[71] As discussed previously, the theoretical benefit of LITT is obvious, but there are few data regarding long-term follow-up in these patients. Whether seizure freedom persists after LITT for MTLE remains to be determined.

STEREOTACTIC RADIOSURGERY

Stereotactic radiosurgery (SRS) is a technique in which a source of ionizing radiation (either protons or photons) are directed at a stereotactically defined target to lesion tissue. Patients are placed in a stereotactic headframe and then undergo an MRI; a treatment plan is then developed to direct the radiation at the proper dose and to the defined anatomic region. Photons are the

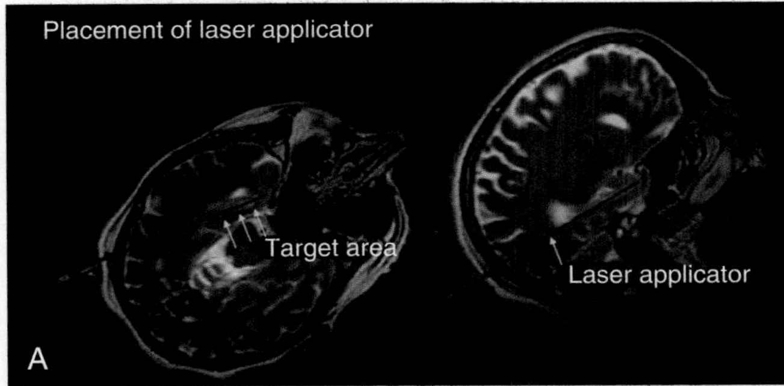

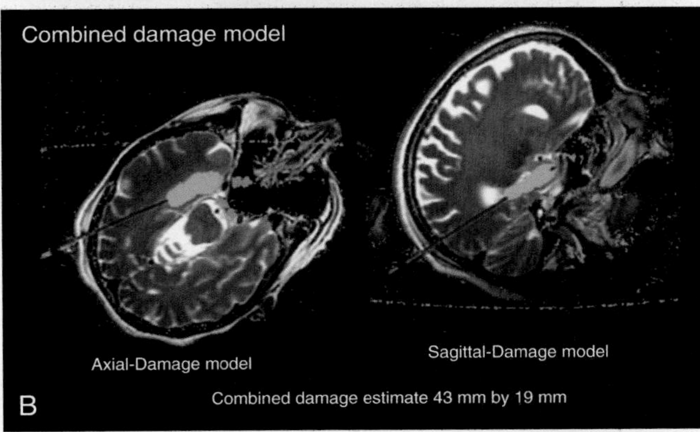

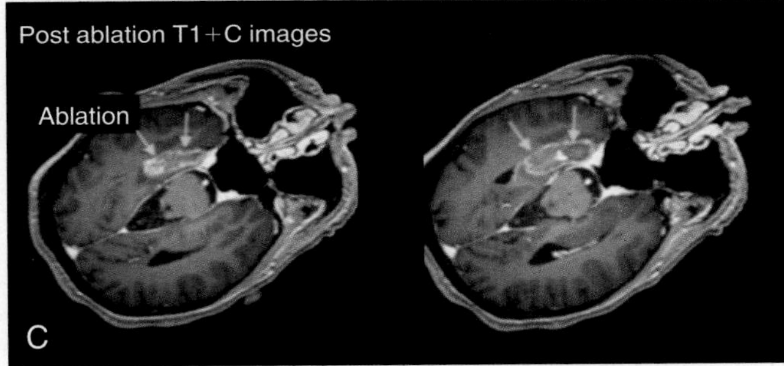

Figure 76-2. Laser interstitial thermal therapy allows for near-real time observation of lesion evolution. Intraoperative magnetic resonance imaging demonstrates placement of laser applicator in target region **(A)**, a thermal damage model as the lesion is being created **(B)**, and postoperative imaging **(C)** confirms the creation of the lesion.

most common source of ionizing radiation and are used in two fashions. Linear accelerators use a single source that steers photon beams to the defined target from different locations. Gamma Knife, on the other hand, uses many different radioactive cobalt 60 sources that can be focused onto a single target location. This approach affords many of the same advantages of LITT. Its noninvasiveness means that patients go home the same day, although it lacks the ability to visualize the lesion in real time. Importantly, however, unlike LITT, the effect of SRS on seizure frequency is delayed, with a maximum reduction in seizures typically seen 12 to 18 months after treatment.[72] During this time, seizures continue to occur, and the risk of associated morbidity and mortality (sudden unexplained death in epilepsy or SUDEP) likely remains.[73,74] In fact, auras actually tend to increase during the intervening time, peaking during 9 to 12 months after treatment. In addition, greater than 50% of patients undergoing SRS experience posttreatment brain edema requiring steroids and, rarely, surgery.[75]

Operative Technique

The operative technique will vary depending on the precise type of SRS used to treat the patient. Conventional SRS techniques rely on CRW headframe placement while CyberKnife (Accuray, Sunnyvale, CA) is a frameless technique. For conventional SRS treatments, a CRW headframe is placed similar to the LITT technique described previously with the main difference being that the patient is awake and only local anesthesia is used. Generous amounts of local anesthesia are applied to each pin site. The patient then undergoes a volumetric MRI with the headframe in place and MRI fiducial box attached. Using the MRI, the radiation oncologist, physicist, and neurosurgeon plan the radiosurgical treatment using the planning software and agree on the planned dose and target location before treatment. The patient is then brought into the radiosurgical suite, the headframe is attached to the radiosurgical treatment bay, and treatment begins (Fig. 76-3).

Evidence Base

Régis and Barbaro have published the two largest and best characterized prospective SRS studies using Gamma Knife (Elekta, Stockholm, Sweden) with long term follow-up[74,75] in groups of 15 and 30 patients, respectively. Both studies used similar treatment protocols with a marginal dose of 24 Gy and the total volume of the 50% isodense target area between 5.5 and 9 mL, although Barbaro randomized their 30 patients to either a standard dose of 24 Gy or a low dose of 20 Gy. Overall, both studies showed similar outcomes with 60 and 67% seizure freedom (Engel class 1A/B) rates at 8 and 2 years follow-up, respectively. Notably, the low-dose group in the Barbaro and associates[75] study showed lower seizure freedom rates (59%) than the standard dose group did (77%). For comparison, the two class I surgical resection trials showed seizure freedom rates of 58% and 73% at 1 and 2 years of follow-up. Similarly, a recent decision analysis used a figure of 71.9% for 1-year seizure freedom rates based on 13 studies published after 1999.

Thus, using the best available evidence, we may consider seizure freedom rates comparable to open surgical techniques if SRS is performed with the correct dose. The Radiosurgery or Open Surgery for Epilepsy (ROSE) trial is a prospective, randomized controlled trial in which enrollment has now ceased and data collection and analysis is ongoing. Hopefully, the results of this trial will help to answer this question definitively, as it is planned to report seizure freedom, cognitive outcomes, and cost with 3 years of follow-up.

Assuming comparable seizure freedom rates, the next major factor in deciding on the best approach is cognitive outcome. There have been few neuropsychologic outcome studies performed in SRS for MTLE. Initial studies indicated that SRS could potentially lead to poorer cognitive outcomes, particularly in verbal memory.[73,76] The larger, prospective studies since then have mainly shown no difference in cognitive outcomes after SRS. The most detailed data come from the American multicenter prospective trial that showed no overall differences in language or verbal memory for dominant lobe SRS, although patients receiving a standard dose (24 Gy) showed mild decreases in confrontation naming and noncontextual verbal memory.[77] In addition, 36% of dominant-lobe SRS patients showed a significant impairment in at least one test.[77] Régis and colleagues[74] reported stable or improved cognitive outcomes in all of their patients, but it should be noted that detailed data was not made available and the patients were instead grouped into 6 groups (0-5) ranging from "far below average" (0) to "far above average" (5) based on the testing. Fifty-five percent of these patients had a baseline score of 0; therefore, it would be impossible for them to decline by this measure. The issue of long-term cognitive

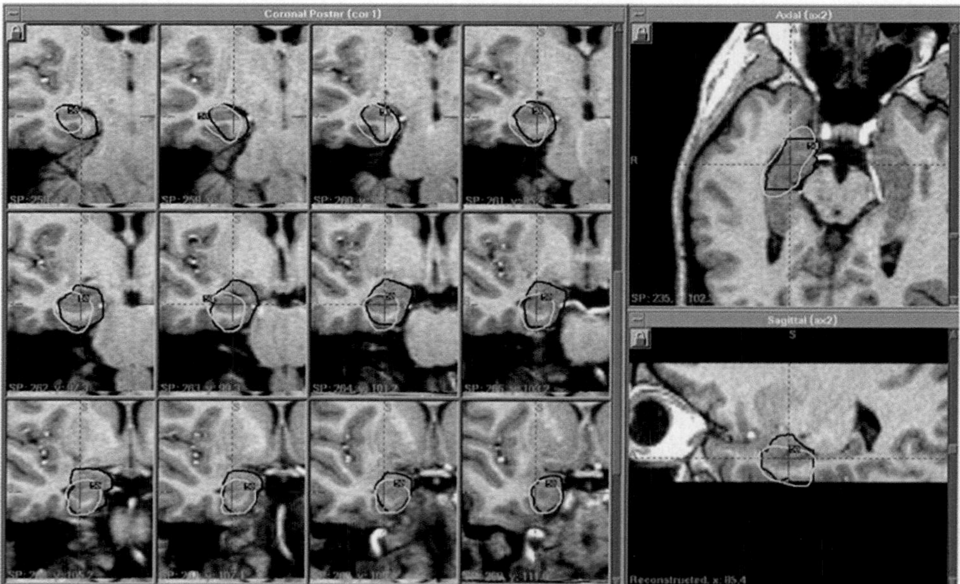

Figure 76-3. Typical stereotactic radiosurgical treatment plan for temporal lobe epilepsy. Targeting is carried out to optimize target radiation and minimize radiation to nearby structures of concern, such as optic radiations, the optic tract, and the brainstem.

outcome, therefore, is likely still in question for SRS in MTLE. By comparison, a recent meta-analysis of 22 studies reporting neuropsychologic outcomes in MTLE surgery described a risk of verbal memory loss in 44% and naming impairment in 34% of dominant lobe surgery patients.[55] Verbal fluency was more likely to be improved in these patients with essentially no overall change in IQ or executive functioning. Thus, while the most recent studies suggest that SRS represents an improvement over surgery in terms of long-term cognition, the ROSE trial and future SRS studies detailing neuropsychological outcomes will be needed to delineate further the differences between the two treatments.

One final consideration for clinicians is the long-term effect of stereotactic radiation in this relatively young population of MTLE patients. Rather than a benign tumor or vascular lesion being irradiated, brain tissue itself is being irradiated in these patients. Theoretically, this could lend itself to an increased risk of a secondary malignancy. Long-term follow-up in these patients will need to examine this issue.

CONCLUSION

As surgeons continue to refine approaches to the mesial temporal region to become ever more selective, the options for treating MTLE continue to grow. Given the wealth of available options, it is imperative that the modern comprehensive epilepsy team composed of neurologists, neurosurgeons, neuropsychologists, and radiologists are involved together in determining the best course of action for an individual patient. Future research regarding newer technology such as LITT should investigate not only safety and complication rates, but long-term seizure and cognitive outcomes as well. Given the difficulty in enrolling epilepsy patients in double-blinded randomized controlled trials, participating in nationwide registries will likely be one of the key determinants in obtaining the data necessary to ensure the safety and durability of new techniques in temporal lobe epilepsy surgery.

SUGGESTED READINGS

Barbaro NM, et al. A multicenter, prospective pilot study of gamma knife radiosurgery for mesial temporal lobe epilepsy: Seizure response, adverse events, and verbal memory. *Ann Neurol*. 2009;65:167-175.

Choi H, et al. Seizure remission in adults with long-standing intractable epilepsy: an extended follow-up. *Epilepsy Res*. 2011;93:115-119.

Drane DL, et al. Better object recognition and naming outcome with MRI-guided stereotactic laser amygdalohippocampotomy for temporal lobe epilepsy. *Epilepsia*. 2015;56:101-113.

Duffau H, Thiebaut de Schotten M, Mandonnet E. White matter functional connectivity as an additional landmark for dominant temporal lobectomy. *J Neurol Neurosurg Psychiatry*. 2008;79:492-495.

Hamberger MJ, Drake EB. Cognitive functioning following epilepsy surgery. *Curr Neurol Neurosci Rep*. 2006;6:319-326.

Helmstaedter C, et al. Collateral brain damage, a potential source of cognitive impairment after selective surgery for control of mesial temporal lobe epilepsy. *J Neurol Neurosurg Psychiatry*. 2004;75:323-326.

Hill SW, et al. Neuropsychological outcome following minimal access subtemporal selective amygdalohippocampectomy. *Seizure*. 2012;21:353-360.

Quigg M, Rolston J, Barbaro NM. Radiosurgery for epilepsy: clinical experience and potential antiepileptic mechanisms. *Epilepsia*. 2012;53:7-15.

Wiebe S, et al. A randomized, controlled trial of surgery for temporal-lobe epilepsy. *N Engl J Med*. 2001;345:311-318.

See a full reference list on ExpertConsult.com

77 Hemispheric Disconnection Procedures

Johannes Schramm

DEFINITION

Hemispheric disconnection procedures are a group of surgical interventions for chronic epilepsy that are used as alternatives to anatomic hemispherectomy. The common denominator among these procedures is the disconnection of the cortex of one hemisphere from the contralateral hemisphere and from the deeper structures of the basal ganglia. The term *hemispherotomy* is commonly used as an alternative expression. The terms *hemispheric deafferentation* and *hemispherotomy* imply that most of the hemispheric tissue is not removed, whereas *hemicorticectomy* or *hemidecortication* disconnect by removal of all hemispheric cortex.

DEVELOPMENT

The first *anatomic hemispherectomy* was done for glioma surgery by Dandy in 1928,[1] and Krynauw performed the first resection for drug-resistant epilepsy in 1950.[2] After a period of increased use of anatomic hemispherectomy in the 1960s and 1970s to control devastating childhood epilepsies, a high rate of late complications was described, such as superficial cerebral hemosiderosis (SCH), occlusion of the foramen of Monro and aqueduct, development of hydrocephalus and its complications,[3-5] and even fatal outcomes.[6] In 27 anatomic hemispherectomies performed in Montreal from 1952 to 1968 with long-term follow-up, hydrocephalus developed in 52% of patients, 33% from SCH and 19% from other causes. Three of nine patients with SCH died of hydrocephalus.[7] SCH is thought to be caused by recurrent minor intracranial bleeding in the large cavity as a result of the resection surgery. Deaths occurred in the early years of this operation owing to unrecognized hydrocephalus, before the advent of computed tomography (CT) imaging.

Less Resection—More Disconnection

Because of the considerable mortality from these complications, the use of anatomic hemispherectomy decreased until the 1970s, when Rasmussen described an alternative technique based on the observation that in patients with multilobectomies, these complications did not occur. Rasmussen's *functional hemispherectomy*[6] was a change from *anatomic hemispherectomy*, frequently used in the 1950s and 1960s; a move toward less invasive disconnection techniques has taken place since the early 1990s. The operation as popularized by Rasmussen included the removal of two larger brain segments (the temporal lobe and an en bloc resection of the central cortex in the suprasylvian location), combined with callosotomy and disconnection of the frontal, parietal, and occipital lobes. Although the hemisphere as such was not totally removed, the effect of this surgery is functionally equivalent to total hemispherectomy. It makes sense to us to limit use of the term *functional hemispherectomy* to Rasmussen's and Mathern's techniques.[8] The latter consists of a large central peri-insular resection, including the basal ganglia and the temporal lobe, combined with disconnection of the frontal, parietal, and occipital lobes.

Because the frontal lobe and the parieto-occipital lobe are left in situ, a lower incidence of hydrocephalus and hemosiderosis was expected and confirmed by longitudinal follow-up. Rasmussen demonstrated in his patient series that seizure-free outcome rates after anatomic and functional hemispherectomies were very similar, 83% and 85%, respectively, but the rate of complications from increased intracranial pressure was reduced from 35% to 7%. A lower rate of SCH has been reported for functional hemispherectomy techniques after a follow-up of 20 years.[6,9] The *hemidecortication* and *hemicorticectomy* techniques[10-12] tried to approach the problem of these complications by preserving nearly all of the ventricular system and leaving the ventricular cerebrospinal fluid (CSF) space uncontaminated.

The modern transition to nearly exclusively disconnective techniques started in 1992 after a brief description of two distinct approaches developed independently by Schramm, Delalande, and their colleagues.[13,14] This was followed in the mid-1990s by the first series of patients treated via perisylvian techniques.[15,16] Closely related to Villemure's technique is a variation of a perisylvian resective approach by Shimizu and Maehara.[17] Among the disconnective procedures, the technique by Delalande and associates (vertical parasagittal hemispherotomy)[18] and the transsylvian transventricular keyhole procedures[19] include minimal tissue removal and mostly consist of disconnections. The change to less resective procedures during the past 15 years is continuing at many centers, and a number of reports have confirmed the initial results indicating that disconnection procedures are associated with shorter operative time, less blood loss, fewer intraoperative complications, and possibly a lower rate of hydrocephalus.[20]

INDICATIONS, PATIENT SELECTION, AND TIMING

Because anatomic hemispherectomy, functional hemispherectomy, hemispherotomy, and hemispheric deafferentation are effective, all are established and successful methods used to treat drug-resistant epilepsy resulting from diffuse damage to one hemisphere. Such damage is usually associated with hemiparesis, hemianopia, and, frequently, delayed cognitive development. The indications for surgery, selection of patients, and timing are similar for all variants of these procedures.

Etiology of Hemispheric Epilepsies

The diagnoses typical in these patients may be grouped into inborn, perinatal, or acquired conditions (Table 77-1) and include Sturge-Weber syndrome (SWS), developmental defects (multilobar cortical dysplasia, polymicrogyria, lissencephaly, hemimegalencephaly (HME), cystic defects from intrauterine or perinatal infarction or hemorrhage, and hemiplegia-hemiconvulsion-epilepsy syndrome (HHE) (Fig. 77-1). Rasmussen's encephalitis leads to hemiatrophy, which may also be posttraumatic, postencephalitic, or of unknown origin. The epilepsy syndromes associated with these lesions may include several seizure types occurring with different frequencies. Patients can have up to hundreds of seizures per day or focal status epilepticus (i.e., epilepsia partialis continua, typical of Rasmussen's encephalitis).

Hemimegalencephaly

Patients with HME usually have an enlarged hemisphere displaying different features of abnormal architecture. Parts of the ventricle may be enlarged, whereas others may be compressed by abnormal brain tissue. There may be pachygyria, polymicrogyria, grossly enlarged gyri, and areas of ectopic gray matter around the ventricle in the white matter (eFig. 77-1). The cause is commonly

TABLE 77-1 Etiology of Seizures	
Infarct, ischemia, porencephaly	54
Cortical dysplasia, migration disorders	10
Hemimegalencephaly	12
Sturge-Weber syndrome	6
Rasmussen's encephalitis	15
Hemiatrophy, unclear cause	7
Postencephalitic, HHE, or other	6
TOTAL	110

HHE, hemiplegia-hemiconvulsion-epilepsy syndrome.

a neuronal migration disorder. HME is often associated with seizures that are frequent and intractable. The hemiparesis can be mild or pronounced, and a marked degree of mental retardation is usually present.

Sturge-Weber Syndrome

SWS is a rare congenital disorder with a variable natural history. Its characteristic feature is leptomeningeal angiomatosis, and in a proportion of cases it is associated with a facial nevus, the latter variant occasionally described as encephalotrigeminal

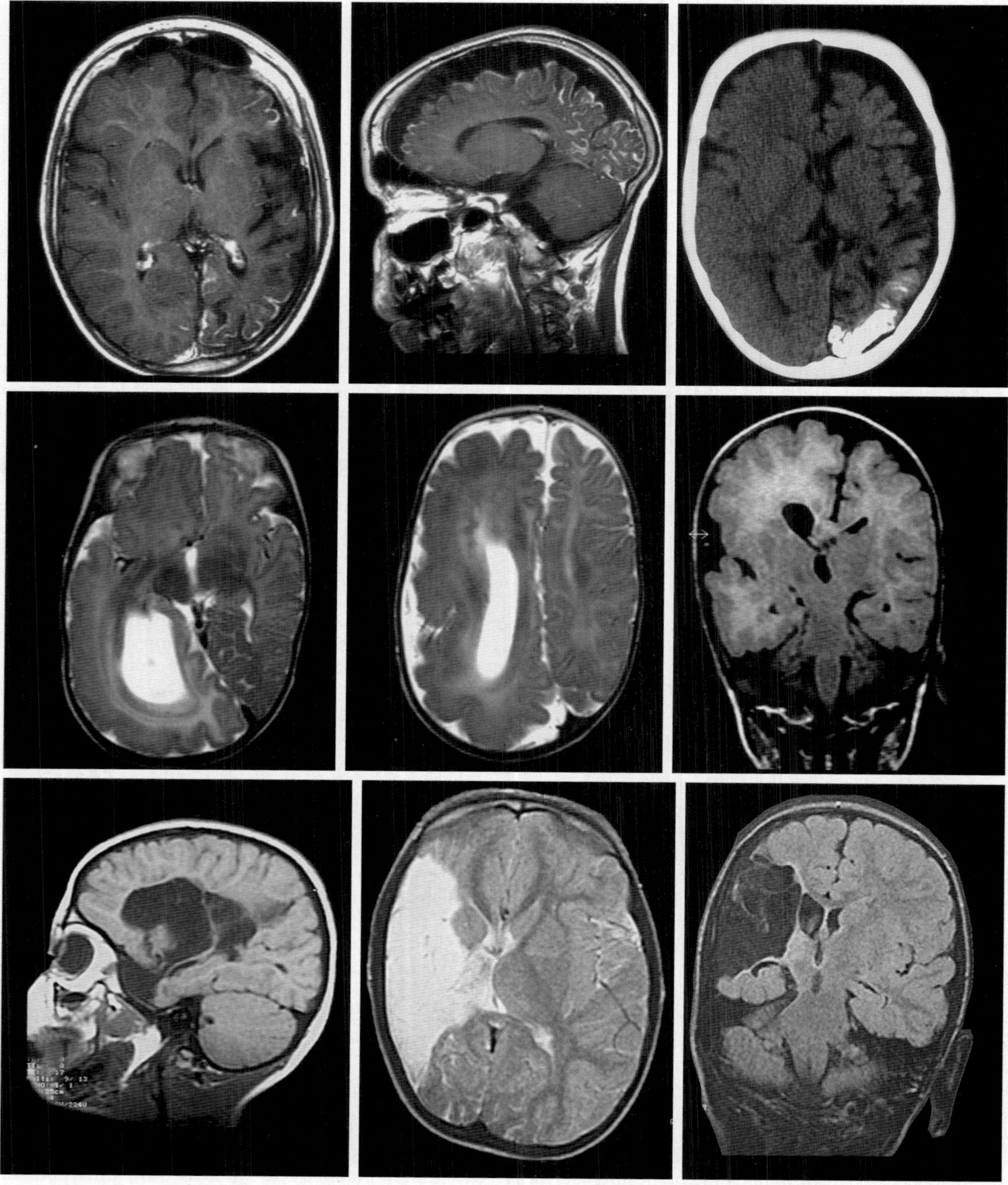

Figure 77-1. Magnetic resonance images and computed tomography scans from three typical causes. *Upper row,* Sturge-Weber syndrome. *Middle row,* Hemimegalencephaly. *Bottom row,* Perinatal porencephalic cyst, most likely of ischemic origin. *(© Johannes Schramm.)*

angiomatosis. The clinical syndrome is characterized by a progressive neurological disorder consisting of epilepsy, cortical calcifications, cerebral atrophy, and, if the epilepsy is untreatable, frequently the development of mental retardation. Seizures usually develop by the end of the first year and may respond to medical treatment initially, but often become resistant to drugs. The cerebral manifestations generally involve the occipital or parietal cortex, or both, but the entire cortex or large parts of it may be involved; however, the pathologic changes remain restricted to one hemisphere. Epilepsy surgery should be considered for patients with refractory seizures, but one has to differentiate between the need for hemispheric deafferentation and a multilobar or more restricted resection. Children with widespread hemispheric involvement are classic candidates for hemispheric deafferentation. The results from three multicenter series have been reported.[21-23] Seizure-free rates after hemispherotomy were reported to be 100% in eight, six, and five patients.[21-22,24] In three larger series, rates of 80% to 82% were reported in 12, 28, and 70 patients.[18,23,25]

Rasmussen's Encephalitis

The pathophysiology of Rasmussen's encephalitis is not well understood. The clinical syndrome is characterized by intractable epilepsy and progressive hemiparesis inexorably resulting in hemiplegia, mental decline, and hemispheric atrophy. The median age at onset in a multicenter study of 16 patients was 4.2 years with a range of 2 to 11 years.[25] Most of the brain damage occurs during the first 8 to 12 months.[26] Progression to hemiplegia or aphasia (or to both) and finally cognitive decline occur invariably. The seizure disorder may begin with generalized seizures, but focal seizures are most frequent, and epilepsia partialis continua develops in a large proportion of patients. A characteristic imaging finding is perisylvian atrophy and encephalomalacia, and histologic findings typically include a perivascular infiltrate of T lymphocytes, which is associated with destruction of neurons.[27] Once the diagnosis is suspected, the progressive atrophy can be characterized by serial magnetic resonance imaging (MRI).[28] These patients are classic candidates for hemispheric deafferentation, but the decision regarding timing of surgery can be a difficult one.

Indications

The decision to perform hemispherotomy is straightforward for unihemispheric lesions that are either inborn or occurred around the time of birth and manifested during infancy or early childhood as frequent and intractable seizures. Hemispherotomy is also indicated for small infants with so-called catastrophic epilepsy, manifesting early after birth, usually from severe hemispheric damage or an inborn malformation in which lengthy drug treatment is known to be unsuccessful. The procedure is also performed in adults with good seizure-freedom rates.[29-31]

How is it possible to have a functional existence after such a procedure? The disconnection is performed on a mostly nonfunctional or partly destroyed hemisphere, where language and motor function either have been or will be transferred to the other hemisphere, as is the rule if the damage occurred during the intrauterine period or perinatally. These patients typically already have spastic hemiparesis, and although the procedure always results in loss of fine motor control of the hand and occasionally deterioration of gait, the majority of patients are able to walk and even use their arm and hand to a certain degree.[24,31-33] Hemispherotomy is associated with a 70% to 80% probability of being seizure free in most series and up to 90% with some causes. Frequently an improvement in cognition and in presurgical behavioral problems may be seen.[32,34]

Timing

Children with holohemispheric malformations or HME with unilateral severe and continuous seizures may be operated on very early (in my group at 4 months). If hemiparesis is well established or severe, little motor function will be lost. Determining the optimal timing of surgery in children with a progressive disease such as Rasmussen's encephalitis is more challenging. Progressive worsening of epilepsy with deteriorating cognitive deficits and increasing hemiparesis may also be found in patients with SWS or HME or after encephalitis. Particularly problematic is the timing of surgery in children older than 7 or 8 years if the language-dominant hemisphere is affected by progressive disease. Some language function may still develop after surgery, even in children aged 4 to 7 years. Nonetheless, it should not be forgotten that Rasmussen's encephalitis invariably leads to severe atrophy of the affected hemisphere together with complete hemiplegia and loss of language function. It is not infrequent in many institutions to elect to proceed to surgery at a time before the point that the relentless severe epileptic seizures have caused irreversible damage to the unaffected hemisphere. This outcome may be minimized by accepting earlier surgery and earlier motor loss from surgery and not waiting until the disease process has destroyed the hemisphere. Performing surgery earlier for children with Rasmussen's encephalitis also increases the chance that the healthy hemisphere may compensate better for the loss of motor (or speech) function from the affected hemisphere.

Another argument in support of hemispheric disconnection is the deleterious effect of frequent seizures on cognition and behavior, as well as other neurological functions. This complex of frequent seizures and neurological decline is sometimes called *epileptic encephalopathy*, and abolishing it constitutes a legitimate aim. Instead of giving the epileptic encephalopathy a chance to further impair the developmental and cognitive potential of the infant, this approach is particularly applicable when the cause of the epilepsy has been recognized as being untreatable early in the clinical course (such as hemispheric cortical malformations) and when repeated trials of antiepileptic drugs appear useless.

Contraindications to Hemispheric Disconnective Approaches

Hemispheric deafferentation is contraindicated if the presurgical evaluation cannot demonstrate that all typical ictal activity originates from the affected hemisphere. A relative contraindication may be seen in patients with independently arising seizures from the so-called healthy hemisphere. Occasional isolated contralateral seizure episodes may be acceptable because they do not automatically result from an independent seizure focus. Bilateral epileptogenic activity may be seen on the electroencephalogram in as many as 75% of patients, but it may be secondary and originate from the diseased hemisphere. Because bilateral involvement may represent an independent seizure focus and not just activity conducted from the diseased hemisphere, it is associated with a somewhat reduced probability of a seizure-free outcome after surgery. Nonetheless, high rates of freedom from seizures can still be achieved,[35-36] as demonstrated in a large series in which 77% of patients with suspected bilateral disease were found to either be seizure free or have only "minor events."[37]

Occasionally, the presence of incomplete hemianopia may be considered a contraindication, especially in older children. However, it has been my experience that patients who have grown up with incomplete hemianopia adjust well to this deficit. Mental retardation is no longer considered a contraindication in my institution and others.[38]

PRESURGICAL EVALUATION

The mainstays of the presurgical evaluation are high-quality MRI and video electroencephalographic monitoring of seizures. In most patients, this plus the clinical history is sufficient to establish the indications for surgery. If possible, neuropsychological testing is also performed to be able to quantify any changes that occur after surgery. An intracarotid amobarbital test (Wada test) will sometimes be necessary to demonstrate which hemisphere is language dominant and to exclude the presence of dissociated sensory and motor speech areas. With late-onset disease or other progressive disease types in which there are doubts about the hemispheric transfer of language functions, this test will be particularly important. In patients with contralateral ictogenic activity, the Wada test may be helpful for differentiating between ictal activity conducted from the diseased hemisphere and ictal activity arising from an autonomous focus in the "healthy" hemisphere. If the contralateral ictal activity disappears when amobarbital is injected into the affected hemisphere, it is safe to assume that the contralateral activity is a conducted phenomenon and will not adversely affect the prognosis. If Rasmussen's encephalitis is suspected, it may be necessary to perform a brain biopsy to confirm the diagnosis. The use of implanted electrodes is rarely necessary. Intradural recordings may occasionally be used to identify the few patients in whom multilobar resections would be sufficient rather than complete hemispheric deafferentation.

GOALS OF SURGERY

Hemispheric deafferentation has three goals: (1) cessation of seizures, (2) relief of the epileptic encephalopathy and neurological deterioration, and (3) improvement of cognitive development and of behavioral disturbances. Achievement of these goals will lead to better psychosocial development and improved quality of life. Although the second and third goals are very ambitious and cannot be attained in all cases, in some situations this objective is realized when all seizures are eliminated.

SIDE EFFECTS AND COMPLICATIONS

Distinction must be made between expected side effects and unexpected complications. Patients or parents need to be informed about the unavoidable *side effects* of hemispheric deafferentation: complete hemianopia and loss of some motor function, such as fine pincer movement of the thumb and index finger and fine movement of the foot—especially inversion, eversion, and fanning of the toes. In a low percentage of patients, deterioration of gait has been described. The impact of postoperative loss of motor function is influenced by the patient's preoperative condition. Adverse effects are more severe when the disease develops later in life and the hemiparesis is mild. Predictions of postoperative motor function have been tried based on preoperative motor function and cause of disease[39] and were reliable when unilateral motor cortex stimulation on the unaffected hemisphere yielded bilateral motor responses.[40]

In the case of incomplete transfer from the affected dominant hemisphere, severe aphasia may be unavoidable after surgery. Typical *risks* that patients or parents need to be informed about include lack of success with regard to seizures, need for shunting of CSF, need for transfusions, wound infection or meningitis, or both, and rarely, dysphagia,[41] movement disorder,[42] or death.

SURGICAL TECHNIQUES

The principle behind this surgery is to forgo anatomic removal of brain tissue by instead disconnecting brain regions. One of the variations of Rasmussen's method was developed by Mathern's group in Los Angeles.[8] This procedure involved performing a large resection of the operculum, insula, underlying basal ganglia, and temporal lobe to achieve a functional hemispherectomy. An intermediate step short of a pure deafferentation procedure involves a perisylvian technique in which only restricted parts of the opercula (eFig. 77-2D), corona radiata, or temporal lobe are resected. This is usually combined with disconnection of the frontal and parieto-occipital lobes and callosotomy, which is performed from within the ventricular system.[15,17,43] The latest versions of these evolving procedures are two disconnection operations that involve little or no brain removal and extensive disconnections: transsylvian keyhole hemispheric deafferentation[19] and central vertical hemispherotomy (Fig. 77-2). These are detailed in the following sections.[18]

Hemispheric Deafferentation Techniques

Transsylvian Keyhole Technique

The transsylvian keyhole technique requires limited exposure of the brain and uses disconnection steps almost exclusively with no resections. A lateral transsylvian/transventricular approach is performed through a small opening. A 4 × 4- or 4 × 5-cm craniotomy

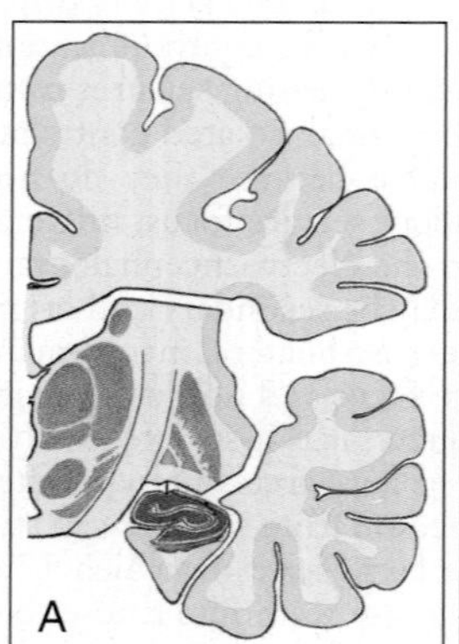

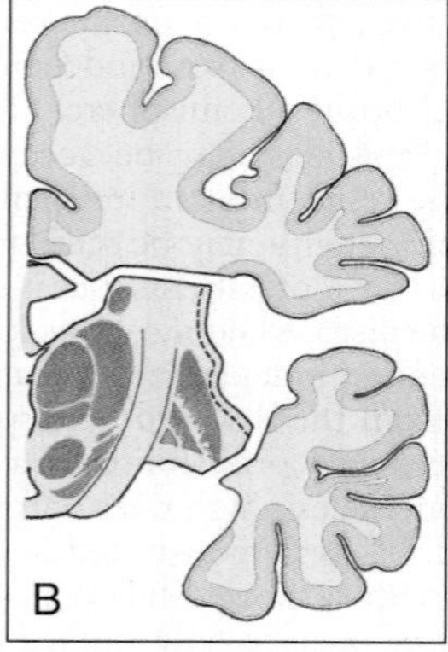

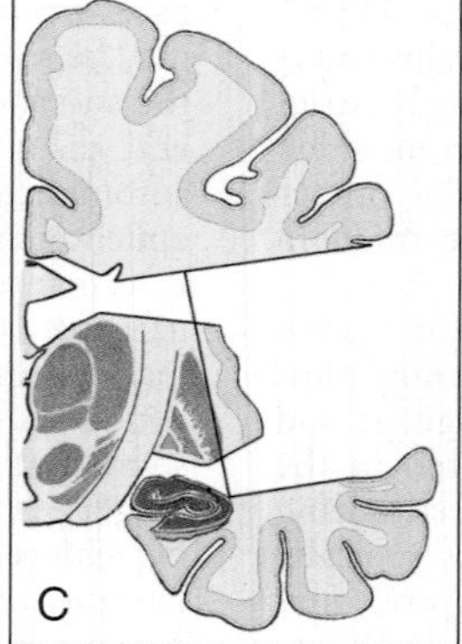

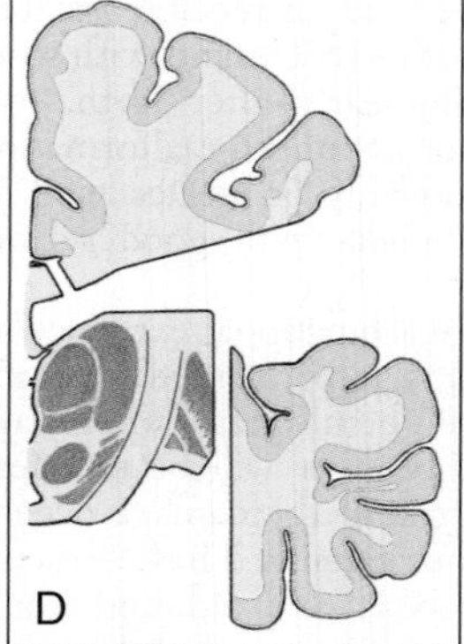

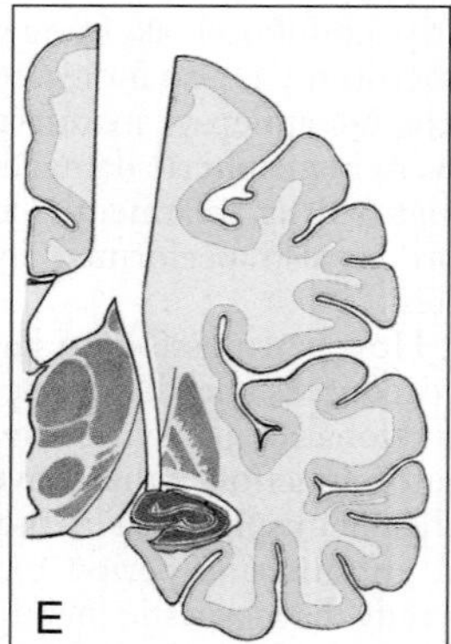

Figure 77-2. Schematic coronal views of the perisylvian and disconnection techniques. A, Step 1 of the transsylvian/transsulcal keyhole approach to the ventricle.[19] **B,** Step 2 of the transsylvian or transventricular keyhole approach: facultative temporomesial resection, removal of the insular cortex, and paramedian callosotomy. **C,** Peri-insular window technique.[43] **D,** Japanese variant of the peri-insular window technique.[17] **E,** Vertical parasagittal hemispherotomy.[18] *(Modified from Schramm J. Hemispherectomy techniques.* Neurosurg Clin N Am. *2001;37:113.)*

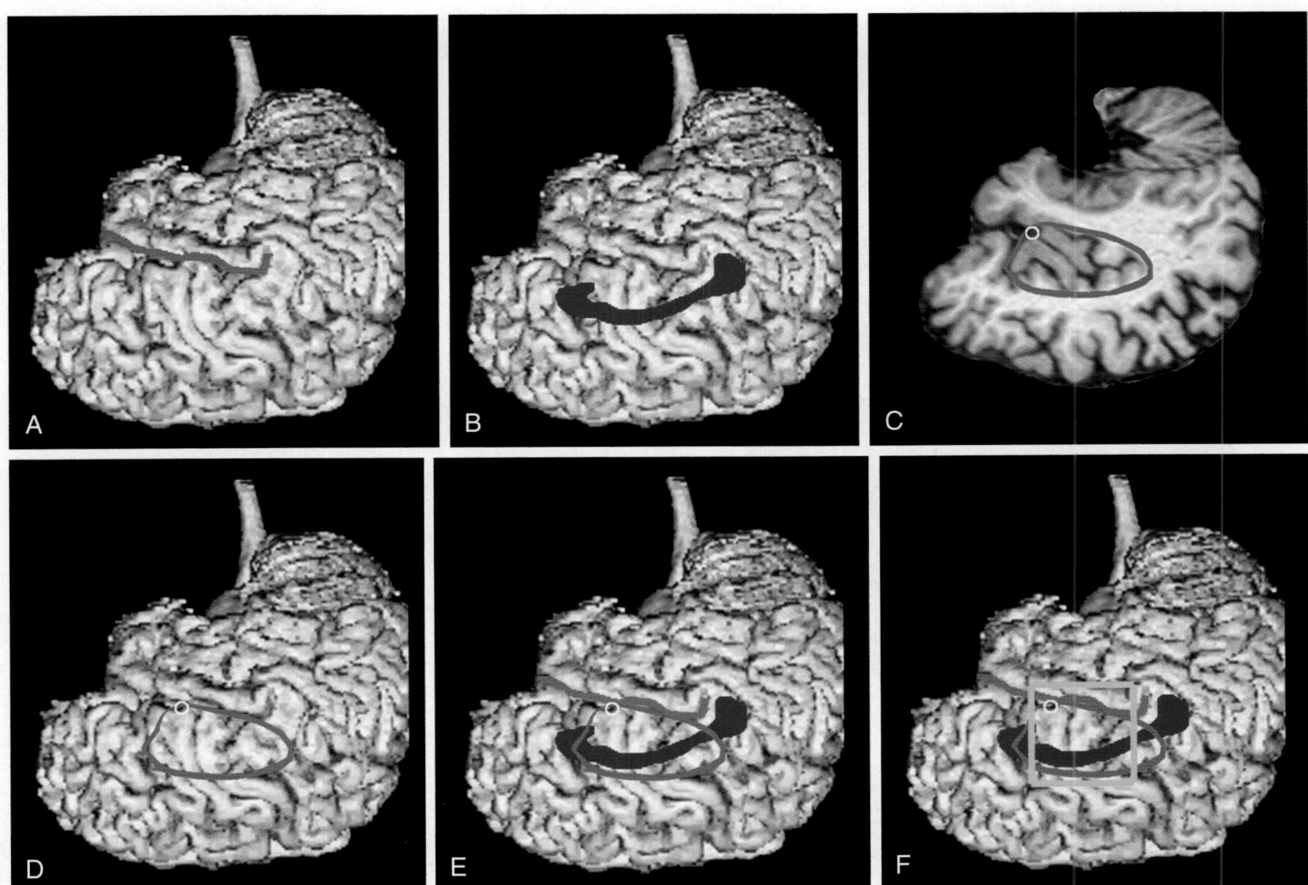

Figure 77-3. Relationship of important anatomic landmarks to one another projected onto the surface of a brain reconstructed from magnetic resonance images. The pictures are arranged from the surgeon's perspective. The reformatted images are taken from an unaffected hemisphere. **A,** The *red line* shows the sylvian fissure. **B,** The shape and position of the corpus callosum are shown in *blue* as projected onto the surface. **C,** The circular sulcus, which represents the border of the insular cistern, is portrayed in *green.* The *white ring* delineates the position of the ascending M1 just in front of the limen insulae. **D,** Outline of the circular sulcus projected onto the lateral surface of the hemisphere. **E,** Relationship of the position of the corpus callosum, circular sulcus, and sylvian fissure projected onto the surface. **F,** Outline of a 4 × 4-cm craniotomy, shown in *yellow*, superimposed on the sylvian fissure, the outline of the circular sulcus, and the shape of the corpus callosum. *(Based in part on a figure from Schramm J, Kral T, Clusmann H. Transsylvian keyhole functional hemispherectomy.* Neurosurgery. *2001;49:891.)*

is performed superior to the sylvian fissure to gain access to the underlying insula and to the corpus callosum (Fig. 77-3).

This approach is characterized by four main features:

1. *Transsylvian exposure of the circular sulcus* (or sulcus limitans) of the insular cortex via a small craniotomy through a linear or curvilinear incision (see eFig. 77-2A to C). The average length of the insula is 49 to 57 mm.[44]
2. *Temporomesial disconnection* via a transventricular approach through the temporal stem (Fig. 77-4A). A pure disconnection is possible from the choroidal point anteromesially through the lateral mass of the bulging amygdaloid body to the arachnoid covering the mesial aspect of the uncus. Alternatively, the uncus and amygdala may be removed by suction. The hippocampus may be left in place as long as the mesiotemporal disconnection is carried backward along the choroidal fissure to the trigone, but some hippocampus may be harvested for histologic examination.
3. *Complete opening of the* entire *lateral ventricle* through a transcortical insular incision from the insular cistern along the inferior, posterior, and superior parts of the circular sulcus into the ventricle from the temporal horn all the way posterior to the trigone and then all the way anterior to the tip of the anterior frontal horn (Fig. 77-5; also see Fig. 77-4). Care is taken throughout to preserve the opercular branches of the middle cerebral artery (MCA) and the tributaries and anastomoses of the sylvian vein.
4. *Mesial disconnection* in the frontal and parieto-occipital area and *callosotomy.* This fourth step may be subdivided into two parts: frontobasal and posteromediobasal lobar disconnection and paramesial callosal disconnection via an intraventricular approach (see Fig. 77-4C, *red lines*).

The fourth step can be started when the surgeon can see the open fontal horn in the depth, the ascending M1 at the limen insulae, and the lateral surface of the frontal lobe. Disconnection of the frontobasal cortex and white matter is performed along a line drawn from the ascending MCA through the bulk of lateral frontal lobe to the tip of the frontal horn. The disconnection then continues by following the M1 segment and then the anterior

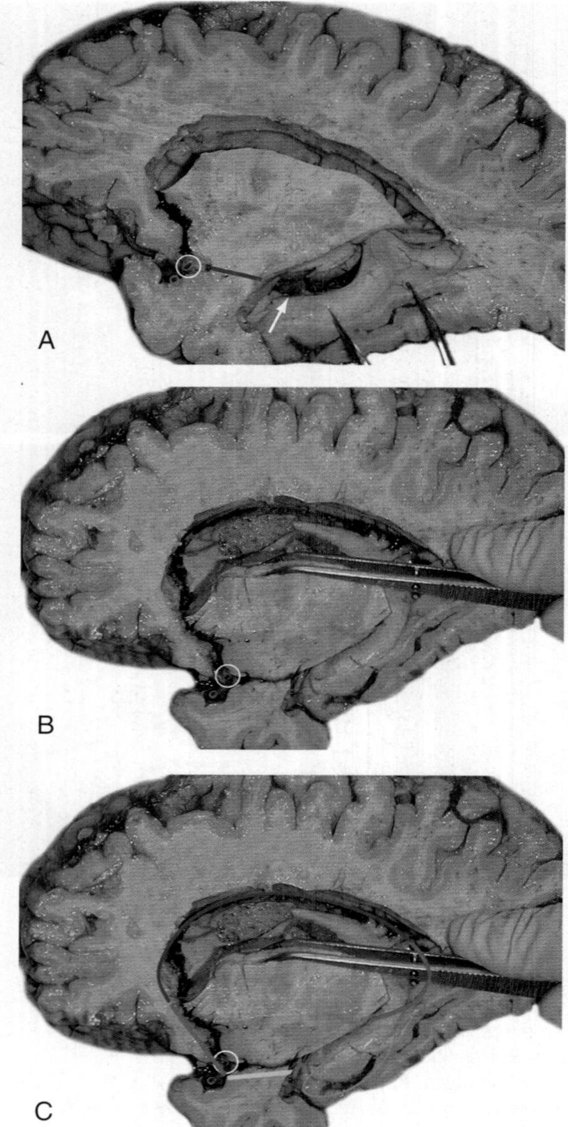

Figure 77-4. Demonstration of mesial disconnection lines for the technique of transsylvian/transventricular hemispheric deafferentation. A, In a formalin-fixed brain, a parasagittal cut exposes the lateral ventricle and the temporal horn simultaneously. The *white circle* marks the position of the ascending M1 division of the middle cerebral artery. One *blue line* above M1 marks the frontobasal disconnection leading from the tip of the frontal horn to the base of the frontal lobe. The other *line* marks the transection of the temporal stem and disconnection of the amygdaloid body leading from the choroidal point to the arachnoid parallel to the ascending M1 down to the uncus. The *arrow* marks the choroidal point, which corresponds to the end of the choroidal fissure (i.e., the terminal end of the attachment of the choroid plexus). Anterior to this point, the entorhinal cortex is located between the head of the hippocampus and the amygdaloid body. **B,** Paramesial transection of the callosal fibers within the lateral ventricle is shown by the *line* as a prolongation of the frontobasal disconnection. **C,** The different types of disconnection lines shown in one picture: the *blue line* is the paramedian callosal transection, the *anterior red line* represents the frontobasal disconnection, the *yellow line* represents the temporomesial disconnection anterior to the choroidal point, the *posterior red line* shows the occipitotemporomesial disconnection through the trigonal area, and the *dotted red line* shows the temporomesial disconnection along the choroidal fissure, used if one chooses not to resect the hippocampus. The *green oval* shows resection of the hippocampus, which is frequently done to obtain a good specimen. *(© Johannes Schramm.)*

cerebral artery, first along the A1 and later the A2 segment around the anterior knee of the corpus callosum. The next step is paramesial callosotomy. While working from within the ventricle, the pericallosal artery is followed by disconnecting callosal fibers in the white matter in a paramedian plane (eFig. 77-3). Posteriorly, the inferior rim of the falx and the anterior rim of the tentorium are used as markers of the medial extent, around to the trigone area until the prior temporomesial disconnection in the temporal horn (eFig. 77-4) is reached. The usefulness of these landmarks was also confirmed in an anatomic study,[45] and details of this procedure have been described previously.[19,46,47]

A reduction in blood loss, reduced need for blood transfusion, and a decrease in operative time have been demonstrated with this procedure[19] and to a lesser extent with the related peri-insular hemispherotomy techniques.[4,17,24,48-50] This procedure is suitable for most pathologies, is particularly quick, and is well suited for patients with porencephalic cysts or marked atrophy of the insula–basal ganglia complex (eFigs. 77-5 and 77-6). With extensive HME it is advisable to combine it with opercular resection or temporal lobe resection to gain space for postoperative swelling and better transinsular exposure of the ventricles. The use of neuronavigation is advisable to correctly place the craniotomy so that the upper border is at the level of the corpus callosum and the lower border is 0.5 cm below the sylvian fissure. The ascending M1 segment should be visualized at the anterior border (see Fig. 77-3) of the craniotomy.

The disadvantages of this technique include its limitations in patients with HME, unless it is combined with a suprasylvian window (as in 7 of 9 of our own patients) (Fig. 77-6 and eFig. 77-7). A certain risk for incomplete disconnection exists, as a result of a too anteriorly placed disconnection line frontobasally (i.e., not in the coronal plane of the M1, A1 segment but anterior to it, leaving connected posterior orbitofrontal cortex in place). Hydrocephalus can develop postoperatively, as is the case with all transventricular disconnection procedures. The reported incidence is 6 of 95 pediatric patients, treated with five shunts and one ventriculocisternostomy, equivalent to a shunt rate of 5.2%; the shunt rate for the keyhole technique group is only 3%. Shunt rates of 8%, 16%, 19%, and 23% were seen with related procedures,[18,51-53] but even higher rates are reported for the older techniques.[50] The pros and cons of this and related approaches have recently been discussed.[48,54-56]

Vertical Parasagittal Hemispherotomy

The vertical parasagittal hemispherotomy technique differs from the perisylvian and transsylvian approaches in two main aspects as described in detail by Delalande and coauthors[18] and may descriptively be called a *dorsal transcortical subinsular hemispherotomy*. It is a vertical approach through a parasagittal craniotomy and involves much less brain resection and more disconnection.

The approach is characterized by five features:

1. A parasagittal frontal craniotomy approximately 3 × 5 cm in size, one third anterior and two thirds posterior to the coronal suture

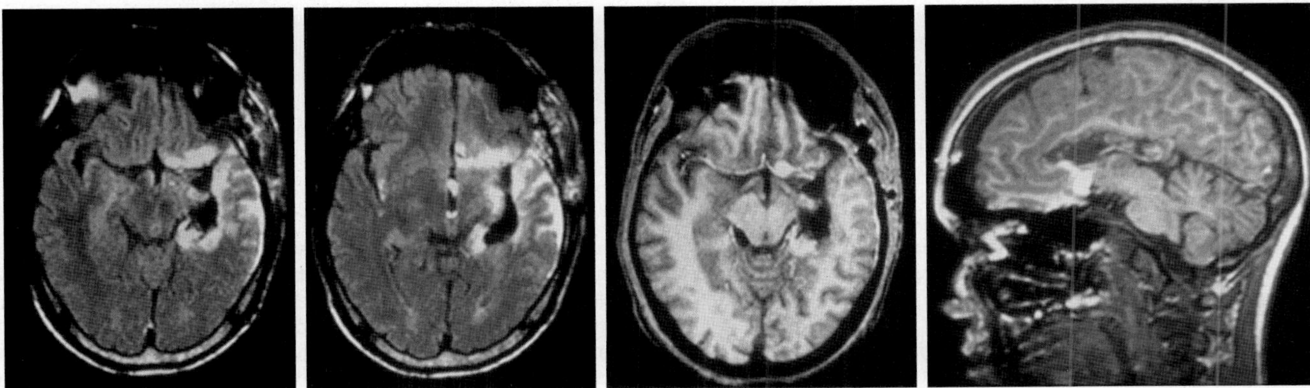

Figure 77-5. Early postoperative magnetic resonance images of transsylvian keyhole hemispheric deafferentation with resection of the insular cortex show an ideal position of the frontobasal disconnection along the course of A1 and M1. *(Reproduced from Schramm J. Hemispherectomy techniques.* Neurosurg Clin N Am. *2001;37:113.)*

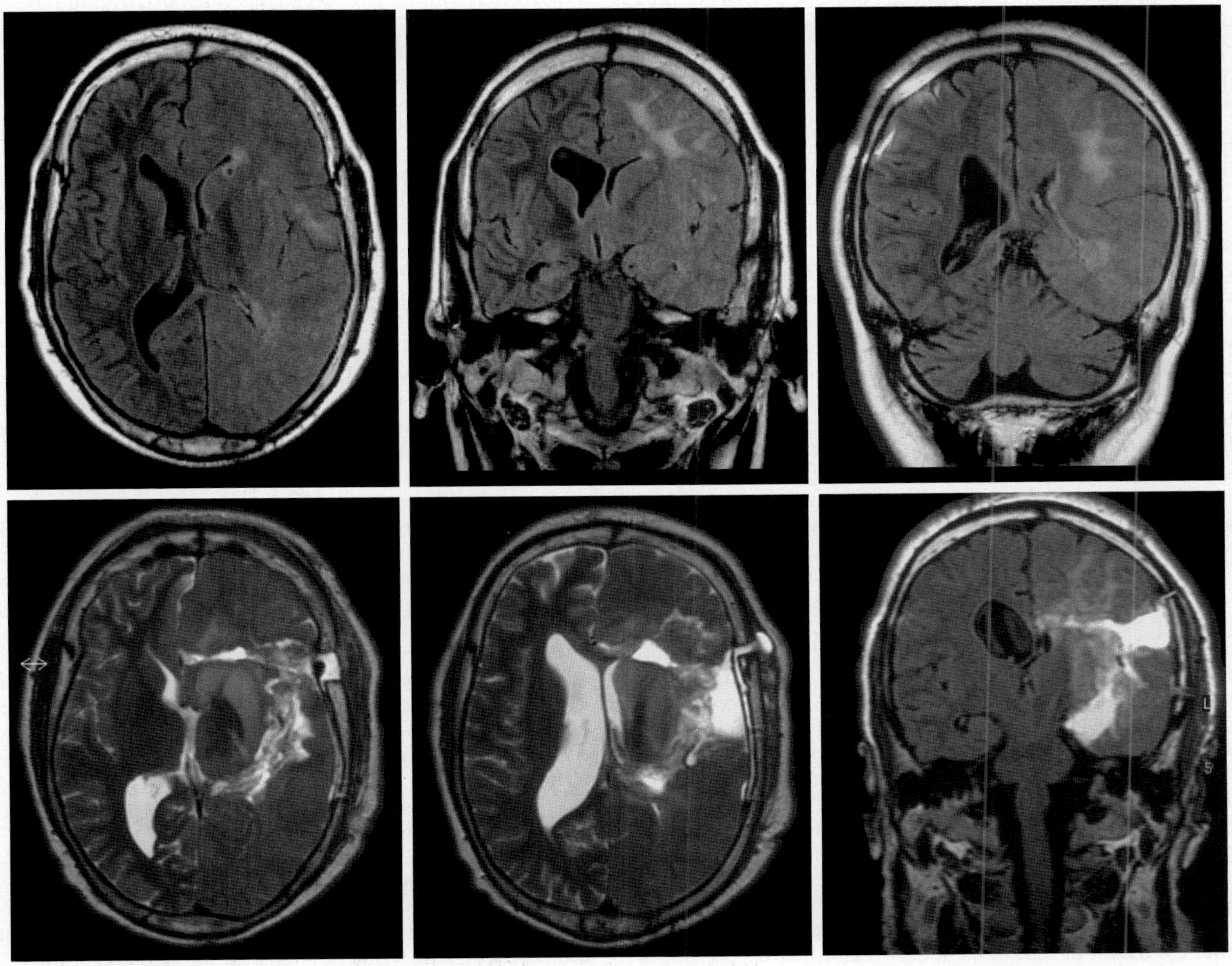

Figure 77-6. Preoperative *(upper row)* and postoperative *(lower row)* magnetic resonance images from a 29-year-old with hemimegalencephaly. The small opercular window and the limited temporomesial resection, as well as the disconnection lines reaching the midline anteriorly, posteriorly, and superiorly, are shown clearly. *(© Johannes Schramm.)*

2. Transcortical access to the lateral ventricle via limited cortical resection to enable access to the foramen of Monro and the posterior thalamic region
3. Paramedian callosotomy, including transection of the posterior column of the fornix
4. Lateral transection between the thalamus and the striatum starting in the lateral ventricle and reaching down to the temporal horn
5. After completion of the anterior callosotomy, resection of the posterior part of the gyrus rectus and extension of the transection line laterally so that the head of the caput caudatum meets the substriatal transection line lateral to the thalamus

The first reported series[18] consisted of 83 children and had a seizure-free outcome rate of 74%. The transfusion rate was just 8%, and the shunt rate was 16%. The insular cortex is automatically disconnected. Shunt implantation was most often required in a large subgroup of patients with HME, thus demonstrating that the underlying pathologic condition influences the rate of this complication. The advantages of this procedure include a low level of blood loss that necessitated transfusion in just 8% of cases. Data on operative time were not provided. Another advantage is preservation of superficially located large vessels, including the MCA. A possible disadvantage is the long distance that must be traversed between the cortical surface to the temporal horn and the frontal lobe base. Other groups have also published using the same technique or variants.[57,58]

Combined Resection-Deafferentation Techniques

The *peri-insular hemispherotomy techniques* combine moderate to limited resection of brain tissue with disconnections. The group consists of hemispheric deafferentation through Schramm's peri-insular transcortical approach,[14,15] Villemure's peri-insular hemispherotomy,[16] and the Japanese peri-insular modification.[17] These three procedures involve a certain degree of brain resection, disconnection from the contralateral hemisphere via transventricular-paramedian callosotomy, transection of the long tract fibers around the insula, and disconnection of the frontal and parieto-occipital lobes (see Fig. 77-2). These techniques may be considered progressive variants of Rasmussen's functional hemispherectomy because they involve removal of either a peri-insular tissue block or the temporal lobe. The features common to all these procedures are a transventricular approach to the callosal fibers and a more limited craniotomy and exposure. When compared with the older anatomic resections, the incidence of hydrocephalus and severe intraoperative complications is decreased. Operative times are shorter and blood loss is less than with the anatomic hemispherectomy techniques, but possibly higher than with the two deafferentation procedures described by Schramm and Delalande.

In the perisylvian window technique, the frontoparietal and temporal opercula are resected (see eFig. 77-2D), including parts of the corona radiata above the basal ganglia block, to create a large opening in the lateral ventricle and the temporal horn. Parts of the insular cortex are removed during this approach.[16,59] In the Japanese modification, the insular cortex is partly removed and the inferior portion is disconnected when the dissection is directed downward to the mesiotemporal lobe at the bottom of the peri-insular window.[17] The mesial temporal structures are resected. It remains unclear whether removal of the insular cortex is necessary. Residual insular cortex may be a source of persistent postoperative seizures, but not all surgical techniques include systematic removal or disconnection of the insular cortex. Some surgeons make an intraoperative decision based on electrocorticography and remove the cortex if abnormal spiking is present.[60] In a large multicenter case collection (N > 300)[25] and in an older series,[4] no correlation was found between the amount of residual insular cortex after surgery and the degree of seizure control. Yet, in a recent study of 28 patients, the presence of residual insular cortex was positively correlated with persistent seizures.[61] For several years our policy has been to routinely remove the insular cortex by subpial suction during the transsylvian keyhole approach (see Fig. 77-6 and eFig. 77-7).

Alternative Classic Techniques

Two techniques based on extensive resection besides functional hemispherectomy are described briefly for comparison purposes. *Anatomic hemispherectomy* involves a large hemicraniotomy, clipping of the anterior and middle cerebral arteries and parasagittal veins, and stepwise or en bloc removal of the hemisphere. *Hemidecortication* or *hemicorticectomy* procedures rely on the principle that all seizures originate from the cortex and thus only the ictogenic cortex needs to be removed.[10-12] Opening of the ventricle is avoided except at the temporal tip, where one has to enter to remove the hippocampus. No callosotomy is required, but extensive brain exposure is necessary. In the setting of holohemispheric dysplasia or HME this approach carries a risk of the surgeon becoming spatially disoriented.

These techniques are associated with a number of possible untoward effects linked to the large exposure, including severe hypotension, blood loss, and prolonged operative times.[8,24,48,49,62] For corticectomies, hydrocephalus rates of 20% and 32% have been reported.[63,64] In a multi-institutional review of post-hemispherectomy hydrocephalus with 690 patients the rate was 23%; it occurred as late as 8 years after surgery. Multivariate regression analysis revealed anatomic hemispherectomies ($P <$ .0001) and previous brain surgery ($P = .04$) as independent significant risk factors for development of hydrocephalus. There was a trend toward significance for the use of hemostatic agents ($P = .07$) and the involvement of basal ganglia or thalamus in the resection ($P = .08$) as risk factors.[65] These results are not in favor of larger resections including the basal ganglia–thalamus bloc.

POSTOPERATIVE MANAGEMENT

All patients spend the first night in intensive care, but small infants and those with HME may be kept in intensive care somewhat longer. The usual blood and neurological parameters are recorded, output is monitored, and if necessary, blood components are replaced. Any postoperative seizures need to be compared carefully for similarities to or differences in preoperative seizure types. Typically, mild to moderate increases in temperature are observed that last for a few days up to 10 days, and they are thought to be caused by contamination of CSF by material entering the ventricles during surgery. Anticonvulsive medications in the postoperative period remain the same as preoperatively. In cases of significant perioperative blood loss and transfusion, it is prudent to administer additional anticonvulsants intravenously before termination of the general anesthetic. Early physiotherapy is mandatory, and if necessary, transfer to a rehabilitation center is arranged. Patients should be observed closely for any impairment of swallowing before a routine diet is initiated. Early postoperative MRI using the blood along the disconnection slit as a contrast medium is useful to prove the completeness of disconnection (see Fig. 77-4).

CHOICE OF SURGICAL PROCEDURE

Provided that the various types of procedures are performed completely and correctly, the chance for freedom from seizures should be similar. It is safer to remove or disconnect the insular cortex, where possible. When seizure-free outcome rates are comparable for different procedures, safety considerations and differences in complication risk profiles play a dominant role in surgical decision making. There is no question that seizure outcomes after hemispherotomies and functional hemispherectomy are similar.[25,50] Functional hemispherectomy techniques are associated with reduced risk for late complications (hydrocephalus) and a somewhat lower rate of intraoperative complications than anatomic hemispherectomy is. For these reasons I prefer to use functional hemispherectomy techniques. In the light of these findings it is hard to find arguments in favor of anatomic hemispherectomy. It is critically important, however, that surgeons be comfortable and knowledgeable about the technique that they choose to use.

The choice of appropriate surgical procedure for HME is more difficult. Because of the malformed anatomy and distorted anatomic structures, it is possible for the surgeon to become spatially disoriented (eFig. 77-8). It is advisable to create a larger craniotomy that is at least large enough to expose the entire insular cistern through an opercular resection providing full visualization of the opened ventricular system (see Fig. 77-5). For HME, decortication is most difficult and ill advised.

OUTCOME AND FACTORS OF INFLUENCE

Seizure-free rates after these operations range from mid 50% to mid 80%. More recent series report seizure outcome rates ranging from 75% to 90%.[24,53,56,61,66-68] with discussion in Schramm and colleagues.[50] For some causes, seizure-free rates may be better—for selected subgroups over 90%. There is incontrovertible evidence that the cause of the seizure disorder influences outcome. Many series describe poorer seizure-free rates for congenital malformative diseases, with HME showing even poorer (40%-60% seizure freedom) outcome than other migration disorders (polymicrogyria, cortical dysplasias). Patients with dysplasia and HME do less well with all the surgical techniques used.[25,46] Surgery for HME carries a higher risk of bleeding, a higher shunt rate, a higher rate of incomplete disconnection, and the lowest success rates among the causes typical for this procedure. Patients with SWS tend to have better outcomes,[23] as do those with Rasmussen's encephalitis,[37,69-71] although some series describe more favorable outcomes.[66] Seizure-free rates of 80% to 100% have been reported for SWS.[18,21,22,24,25,67] Seizure-free results for Rasmussen's encephalitis have been reported at 80% of 20 patients[72] and 77% in a large series of 83 patients.[25] Porencephalic defects usually have a better outcome; in our pediatric series,[50] 95% were seizure free. Interpretation of outcome data per center needs to be done carefully because cause influences outcome and the composition of the patient groups varies considerably from center to center. A high proportion of HME and cortical dysplasia cases will lead to overall lower seizure-free rates.

Effect of Surgical Technique

In view of all the factors influencing outcome, it is difficult to ascertain with certainty whether one of the older, more resective techniques, one of the newer perisylvian techniques, or the primarily disconnective procedures lead to consistently better results. Although theoretically all techniques should achieve similar seizure-free rates, in Holthausen and colleagues' review of 328 cases from 12 centers, differences in seizure-free outcome among operative techniques were described, with hemispherotomy techniques showing better results (85.7% class I) than Rasmussen's technique (66.1% class I) or the hemicorticectomy-hemidecortication techniques (60.7% class I).[25] Overall, however, there is mounting evidence that these three techniques have lower success rates and higher rates of incomplete disconnection. The high number of 12 contributing centers and the variable mixture of causes do not allow one to conclude that hemispherotomies are consistently associated with better outcomes. In the series from the University of California, Los Angeles, seizure control was not statistically different for the various techniques used in 115 cases.[8] In the Bonn series, the transsylvian keyhole technique and Rasmussen's technique both had greater than 80% class I outcomes, both in adults and in pediatric patients.[31,50]

Acute postoperative seizures were seen in 22.6% of 114 patients and were associated with a worse short-term seizure outcome.[73] More than five acute postoperative seizures (in the first 10 days) have been shown to be associated with worse seizure control at 0.5 and 1 year after surgery.[73] The significance of contralateral spikes over the good hemisphere remained unclear in Holthausen and associates' large case collection.[25] In our pediatric group, 47% of 17 patients with acute postoperative seizures were seizure free at last available outcome assessment.[50]

Long-Term Outcome

Early outcome must be differentiated from late follow-up results. Long-term stable good seizure outcomes have been reported from some centers at follow-up periods as long as 15 years,[18,32,50,71,74] but in another large patient cohort, seizure-free rates of 78% at 6 months dropped to 70% at 2 years and 58% at 5 years.[75] In our pediatric series, seizure-free rates were 84.6% at 1 year (n = 92), 80% at 10 years (n = 36), and 77% at 15 years (n = 25).

Cognition and Behavior

Patients with a typical cause and indication for hemispheric deafferentation often have below-average intelligence (79% in one series[34]) or mental retardation. This may be combined in a smaller subgroup with behavioral problems such as aggression or temper tantrums.[9] Hemispheric surgery in the hemispherectomy population does not result in a decline in health-related quality of life,[76] and cognition frequently improves.[32,77] The postoperative pattern of cognition and behavioral changes observed in patients is influenced by whether the patient is seizure free after surgery and the nature of the underlying pathologic process. Seizure-free patients tend to do better and dysplasia patients tend to do worse.[34,76-79] The necessity of continuing antiepileptic drug use appears to have a negative impact on quality of life in the pediatric population, although having undergone a hemispherotomy procedure predicted fewer epilepsy-related limitations.[76] Of our own cases, 33 of 55 were reported by parents to have improved behavior (57%), and in 38% of patients IQ improved, and it declined in 9%.[34] Schooling improved in 40%, depending highly on preoperative IQ levels. Quality-of-life improvements have been described, regarding employment status[33] and ambulation,[24] even in adult surgery.[31]

Complications

Incomplete disconnections can be unintentional and unrecognized in the operating room and are usually listed as a postoperative complication. They can occur not only with the pure disconnection technique but also with Rasmussen's technique.[80] Incomplete disconnection has been described as a cause of persisting seizures in 2% to 30% of patients.[17,20,25,49-53,62,80-83] Other complications may develop intraoperatively, in the postoperative period, and late.

Typical examples of *intraoperative complications* are marked blood loss, electrolyte disturbances, and coagulation disorders resulting from excessive blood loss or blood replacement therapy.[84] Hypovolemia with bradycardia, hypothermia, and in extreme situations even cardiac arrest may occur but are hardly mentioned in recent hemispherotomy series, and never have been seen in own series. *Early postoperative complications* include electrolyte disturbances, diabetes insipidus or syndrome of inappropriate antidiuretic hormone secretion, and swelling of the contralateral healthy hemisphere. Transient rises in temperature for a few days and even up to 10 days are typical and must be differentiated from true bacterial meningitis.[32,85] Dysphagia and movement disorders have been described.[41-42]

Subdural hygroma or acute hematomas (epidural and subdural) may occur. Expected losses in motor function, speech, or visual fields are accepted and expected side effects, not complications. Death in the postoperative period in historical series was observed in 4% to 6% of cases, was reduced to around 2% with functional hemispherectomy techniques, and in modern series is reported to be around 1%, rarely 2%; in a review of 153 cases and my own series, the rate was 0.7% (1 of 140).[18,25,48,50,83-84,86-88] Classic bone flap infections do seem to occur a bit more frequently with larger craniotomies and types of procedures requiring longer operative times.[89-90] Hydrocephalus may develop in the early postoperative period, as well as later, even up to 8 years after surgery.[50,65] SCH has not yet been reported with the modern perisylvian or disconnection techniques, but the observation period for these more modern techniques is still less than 20 years, so no definite judgement is possible at this time. A certain incidence of hydrocephalus appears to be unavoidable, as with all procedures that involve opening the ventricular system. Shunt rates of 8% to 30% have been described.[18,51-53,65,89] Recently, some forms of hydrocephalus have been treated effectively by cisternostomy, so shunt rates may be a bit lower than hydrocephalus rates.[50] Shunt rates after functional hemispherectomy or disconnection procedures tend to increase with removal of a larger volume of brain tissue,[61,91] impressively demonstrated by the review of 690 cases by Lew and colleagues.[65] The underlying cause also influences the rate at which shunts are required, with the highest frequency observed in patients with HME.[17,18,91]

Late complications include bone flap infections and hydrocephalus requiring shunting. Late reappearance of seizures has been observed with variable frequency, rarely in some groups[18] and more frequently in other series.[8,75] Late death may also occur because of persistent or reappearing seizures.[50,84]

CONCLUSION

Surgery for unihemispheric drug-resistant epilepsy has evolved considerably over the past 20 years. The key element in this change was to replace resective steps with disconnective steps, which culminated in nearly exclusive disconnective surgery. These techniques are successful and less demanding on the patient because of decreased operative time and less blood loss. Outcomes are influenced more by the cause of the seizure disorder and less by the specific technique used. Hemispherotomies and hemispheric deafferentations continue to be some of the most successful types of epilepsy surgery.

SUGGESTED READINGS

Bien CG, Urbach H, Deckert M, et al. Diagnosis and staging of Rasmussen's encephalitis by serial MRI and histopathology. *Neurology*. 2002; 58:250.

Carson BS, Javedan SP, Freeman JM, et al. Hemispherectomy: a hemidecortication approach and review of 52 cases. *J Neurosurg*. 1996;84:903.

Cook SW, Nguyen ST, Hu B, et al. Cerebral hemispherectomy in pediatric patients with epilepsy: comparison of three techniques by pathological substrate in 115 patients. *J Neurosurg*. 2004;100:125.

Delalande O, Bulteau C, Dellatolas G, et al. Vertical parasagittal hemispherotomy: surgical procedures and clinical long-term outcomes in a population of 83 children. *Neurosurgery*. 2007;60:ONS19.

Ellenbogen RG, Cline MJ. Hemispherectomy: historical perspective and current surgical overview. In: Miller JW, Silbergeld DL, eds. *Epilepsy Surgery: Principles and Controversies*. New York: Taylor & Francis; 2006:563.

Griffiths SY, Sherman EM, Slick DJ, et al. Postsurgical health-related quality of life (HRQOL) in children following hemispherectomy for intractable epilepsy. *Epilepsia*. 2007;48:564.

Holthausen H, May T, Adams C. Seizures post hemispherectomy. In: Tuxhorn I, Holthausen H, Boenigk H, eds. *Paediatric Epilepsy Syndromes and their Surgical Treatment*. London: John Libbey; 1997.

Jonas R, Nguyen S, Hu B, et al. Cerebral hemispherectomy: hospital course, seizure, developmental, language, and motor outcomes. *Neurology*. 2004;62:1712.

Kestle J, Connolly M, Cochrane D. Pediatric peri-insular hemispherotomy. *Pediatr Neurosurg*. 2000;32:44.

Kossoff EH, Vining EP, Pyzik PL, et al. The postoperative course and management of 106 hemidecortications. *Pediatr Neurosurg*. 2002;37:298.

Peacock WJ, Wehby-Grant MC, Shields WD, et al. Hemispherectomy for intractable seizures in children: a report of 58 cases. *Childs Nerv Syst*. 1996;12:376.

Pulsifer MB, Brandt J, Salorio CF, et al. The cognitive outcome of hemispherectomy in 71 children. *Epilepsia*. 2004;45:243.

Rasmussen T. Hemispherectomy for seizures revisited. *Can J Neurol Sci*. 1983;10:71.

Schramm J. Hemispherectomy techniques. *Neurosurg Clin N Am*. 2002; 13:113.

Schramm J, Behrens E, Entzian W. Hemispherical deafferentation: an alternative to functional hemispherectomy. *Neurosurgery*. 1995;36:509.

Schramm J, Kral T, Clusmann H. Transsylvian keyhole functional hemispherectomy. *Neurosurgery*. 2001;49:891.

Schramm J, Kuczaty S, Sassen R, et al. Pediatric functional hemispherectomy: outcome in 92 patients. *Acta Neurochir*. 2012;154:2017.

Shimizu H, Maehara T. Modification of peri-insular hemispherotomy and surgical results. *Neurosurgery*. 2000;47:367.

Tinuper P, Andermann F, Villemure JG, et al. Functional hemispherectomy for treatment of epilepsy associated with hemiplegia: rationale, indications, results, and comparison with callosotomy. *Ann Neurol*. 1988;24:27.

Villemure JG, Mascott CR. Peri-insular hemispherotomy: surgical principles and anatomy. *Neurosurgery*. 1995;37:975.

Wilson PJ. Cerebral hemispherectomy for infantile hemiplegia. A report of 50 cases. *Brain*. 1970;93:147.

See a full reference list on ExpertConsult.com

78 Radiosurgical Treatment for Epilepsy

Thomas J. Gianaris, Nicholas M. Barbaro, and Jean Régis

Radiosurgery is the precise application of focused radiation under stereotactic guidance to a targeted volume area within the brain identified on magnetic resonance imaging (MRI), allowing the neurosurgeon to deliver effective, precise, and accurate doses of radiation to a smaller volume without affecting large portions of normal parenchyma, thereby allowing a powerful radiobiologic effect on the chosen targeted volume.[1-4] Conceptualized by Lars Leksell for use in functional neurosurgery, radiosurgical treatment of neurological disorders has progressively widened its utility and is now a treatment modality option for several neoplastic and vascular indications.[5-18]

Epilepsy is one of the most common serious neurological diseases; it has a prevalence of 0.5% to 1.0% in the U.S. population, with approximately 20% of these patients having medically refractory seizures.[19,20] Patients with medically refractory seizures may be referred for possible surgical management, and many are found to be suitable candidates for open surgical resection of a seizure focus.[21]

The most common type of open surgery performed for temporal lobe epilepsy is anterior temporal lobectomy.[20,22-24] With modern advances in surgical and anesthetic techniques, microsurgical resection of mesial temporal lobe structures can be performed with low morbidity and even lower mortality.[4] Open invasive surgical procedures, however, have inherent risks, including structural damage, hemorrhage, blood loss, infection, and anesthetic risks.[25-28] Several clinical studies evaluating the morbidity and mortality associated with open microsurgery for temporal lobe epilepsy have reported that approximately 5% to 23% of patients undergoing open microsurgery experience a symptomatic neurological deficit postoperatively.[23,25,26,29,30] In addition, patients may have their epileptic focus in regions that are difficult to access or in eloquent functional regions of the brain where surgical resection could result in irreversible language, motor, or visual impairment.[31,32]

Radiosurgery is currently being evaluated as an alternative treatment modality to open resective microsurgery for intractable temporal lobe epilepsy. Radiosurgery is relatively noninvasive, with frame-based radiosurgery using just frame pins that penetrate only the skin to firmly fix the stereotactic frame to the skull. The highly focused nature of radiosurgery allows stereotactic guidance and sparing of adjacent tissues from the damaging effects of radiation, abrogating many of the risks and limitations of open surgery and permitting patients to return to full activity within 1 to 2 days after treatment. Radiosurgery can also be used as an adjunct therapy to initial open surgical resection of a hippocampal focus, although no formal studies are available on this specific group of patients. Currently, radiosurgery is under investigation as a treatment modality for epilepsy associated with vascular malformations, hypothalamic hamartomas, and medial temporal lobe epilepsy (MTLE) associated with mesial temporal sclerosis (MTS).[1,3,4,32-51]

PRECLINICAL EVIDENCE

Preclinical studies investigating focused high-dose radiosurgery in animal models of epilepsy have demonstrated the potential utility of radiosurgical treatment applied to nonhuman epilepsy models. Early animal experiments indicated the efficacy of focused irradiation in a feline model of epilepsy in reducing seizure activity.[31,33,34] Studies by Sun and colleagues[32] reported that seizure thresholds in rats treated with 10 or 40 Gy at the 90% isodose line were significantly increased, and the length of afterdischarges was significantly decreased in the group treated with 40 Gy. Corroborating this report, histologic analysis of temporal lobe regions treated by radiosurgery doses of 10 to 40 Gy at the University of Virginia found no necrosis in these tissue specimens. Synaptically driven neuronal firing was reported to be intact in these radiosurgically treated rodent brain slices, suggesting that functional neuronal death was not responsible for the identified reduction in seizures.[52]

Recent experiments at the University of Pittsburgh were undertaken to evaluate the histopathologic and behavioral effects of "subnecrotic" radiosurgery doses.[43,53] In this animal investigation, rats underwent stereotactic injection of kainic acid into the hippocampus to induce seizures, followed by Gamma Knife radiosurgery (GKRS) at doses of 30 or 60 Gy. A statistically significant reduction in seizures was reported in all radiosurgically treated animals, and this antiepileptic effect was observed earlier in the animals treated with the higher radiosurgery dose (weeks 5 to 9 versus weeks 7 to 9). No animals treated with radiosurgery were reported to demonstrate a deficit in new memory attainment tasks on water maze testing in comparison with control animals injected with only kainic acid, but both groups showed "cognitive" impairment when compared with rats that did not receive any kainic acid injection or radiosurgical treatment. In histopathologic analysis by two blinded observers, unilateral hippocampal atrophy was also observed in 25 of 46 injected animals. Radiation-induced necrosis matching the target volume of radiation was not reported in any of the animals treated with radiosurgery.[53] These preclinical animal findings suggest that reduction of seizure activity after radiosurgery does not require necrosis or concomitant functional loss of treated neurons.[53]

With the suggestion that necrosis is not necessary for reduction of seizures, the radiosurgery group in Prague reported on their preclinical characterization of a "subnecrotic" dose of radiosurgery in a rat model.[54,55] This preclinical investigation evaluated radiosurgery doses of 25, 50, 75, or 100 Gy delivered bilaterally to the rat hippocampus and then assessed the rats with cognitive tests, MRI, and histopathologic examinations at 1, 3, 6, and 12 months after radiosurgery. A progressive time- and dose-dependent response curve was observed in cognitive memory function, edema on MRI, and necrotic histopathology. All animals treated with 75 Gy displayed cognitive memory functional impairments, edema on MRI, and radiation-induced necrotic lesions, whereas only one of the animals treated with the 50-Gy radiosurgery dose had observable edema and necrosis. A second follow-up preclinical study in which a 35-Gy radiosurgery dose was used with a long-term follow-up period of 16 months found that 6 months after radiosurgical treatment, edema was observed on MRI, and this edema was most pronounced at 9 months after radiosurgery.[55] After 16 months, two of six treated animals were reported to have radiation-induced necrotic cavities after treatment with a 35-Gy dose of radiosurgery. The four treated animals without frankly necrotic cavities had other notable histopathologic findings, such as severe atrophy of the corpus callosum, loss of thickness of the somatosensory cortex, and damage to the stratum oriens hippocampi.[55] These preclinical animal studies suggest that the full radiobiologic and histopathologic effects of radiosurgery may be manifested several months after radiosurgery.

These preclinical animal studies suggest that the antiepileptic efficacy of radiosurgery is dose dependent, with a dose of approximately 25 Gy being required to induce a therapeutic antiepileptic effect, and the potential full histologic and other toxicity may require several months to fully develop.[4,31,32,43,52-55]

CLINICAL EVIDENCE

The first application of radiosurgery for epilepsy surgery is attributed to Talairach in the 1950s, who implanted radioactive yttrium in patients with temporal lobe epilepsy without a lesion.[4,31,32] One of the limitations inhibiting radiosurgery research is the difficulty in recruiting patients to prospective or randomized trials directly comparing radiosurgery to open surgery.[56]

MEDIAL TEMPORAL LOBE EPILEPSY

MTLE associated with MTS is perhaps the most well-defined epilepsy syndrome responsive to structural intervention. MTS is an idiopathic process associated with extensive loss of neurons and an increase in astrocytes in the mesial temporal structures, which include the amygdala and hippocampus in the temporal lobe. When temporal lobe epilepsy is due to underlying MTS, improvements in seizures with open microsurgical structural resections can be expected in 65% to 90% of patients.[20,22,24,31,57-62] This form of temporal lobe epilepsy is particularly amenable to structural interventions, such as radiosurgery, because 80% to 90% of these patients show detectable changes on MRI.[3,59]

Radiosurgery has also been explored as an alternative to open microsurgery for MTS-associated MTLE. In a small series of patients with MTLE treated with GKRS, Régis and colleagues[44,45] initially pioneered this technique in the mid-1990s and reported clinically effective amelioration of seizures with minimal morbidity. A recent, prospective, multicenter European study evaluating GKRS for MTS showed comparable efficacy rates (65%) for reduction of seizures by conventional microsurgery and radiosurgery after 2 years of follow-up.[4] Using a marginal dose of 24 Gy, Régis and colleagues[4] reported that radiosurgery can be used as an alternative to conventional open microsurgery to treat MTLE associated with MTS effectively and to improve quality of life with comparable rates of morbidity and mortality in a small case series. The international Radiosurgery or Open Surgery for Epilepsy (ROSE) trial is currently being conducted comparing the efficacy and safety of radiosurgical doses and radiosurgery to open temporal lobectomy for patients with mesial temporal sclerosis. This trial is based on a pilot clinical trial examining radiosurgical dosing in a direct comparison of 20 and 24 Gy of radiosurgery, finding that 67% of all patients were free of seizures for at least 12 months after treatment at the 36-month follow-up examination, with 10 or 13 in the 24-Gy group finding seizure freedom compared with 10 of 17 in the 20-Gy group.[63] In comparison, historically open resection was found to have a seizure reduction rate of 58% in a prospective trial by Wiebe and colleagues,[22] whereas a multicenter parallel group controlled trial by Engel and colleagues[64] in 2012 comparing anteromesial temporal lobe resection to antiepileptic drug therapy confirmed these findings, with 11 of 15 patients treated with surgery becoming seizure free at 2 years and 0 of 23 in the medical group. A systematic review and metaanalysis showed an average pooled seizure reduction with anterior temporal lobectomy of 66%.[22,65] This pilot trial further examined the safety and efficacy of two dosing approaches and the effects, timing, and risks associated with this therapy.

Although the pilot trial demonstrated that radiosurgery is effective in improving MTLE-associated seizures, the beneficial effects of radiosurgery are not demonstrated immediately. Typically, patients with MTLE treated by radiosurgery can achieve improvement in seizures between 9 and 12 months, with dramatic improvement in seizures between 18 and 24 months after treatment. A transient increase in partial seizures (auras) has been reported at approximately the same time that the complex seizures decrease, about 1 year after treatment.[4] In addition, higher radiosurgical dosing increased steroid prescribing (temporary), new headaches (temporary), and visual field defects (permanent).[63] Many patients require a temporary course of corticosteroids to treat the delayed radiation-induced edema associated with the initial radiosurgical effect, commonly 10 to 15 months after treatment, with 62% of those studied in the this pilot trial requiring steroids.[63] In addition, the patients are still exposed to the risks of sudden death of epilepsy during this latent period, with Srikijvilaikul and colleagues[66] finding two posttreatment deaths during this latency period following radiosurgery presumed to be due to sudden death of epilepsy, although these patients were treated with a lower dose of 20 Gy.[66] There was no evidence that the radiosurgical treatment per se was responsible for these deaths.

One of the potential pitfalls of radiosurgical treatment of intracranial lesions is that it can expose the optic nerves to harmful radiation, causing posttreatment visual deficits, not unlike those potentially caused by open resection. Régis and colleagues[67] found prospectively that 9 of 21 patients treated with radiosurgery for MTLE experienced new visual field defects. Hensley-Judge and colleagues[68] prospectively found that 15 of 24 patients (62.5%) had postoperative VFDs, all homonymous superior quadrantanopsias, among pilot trial participants. These findings were similar to historical controls for open resection, demonstrating that this risk is still present even without brain retraction or true resection, and they did not significantly vary whether 20 or 24 Gy were used. However, a greater proportion of patients who became seizure-free developed postoperative visual field defects, possibly owing to a connection between wider resection margins and higher doses leading to greater destruction of the optic radiations, although this has not been proven.[67]

One of the advantages of radiosurgery is its potential for relative preservation of memory in comparison with open resection. Open surgery for temporal lobe epilepsy entails risks of significant verbal memory impairment ranging from 10% to 60%.[69-73] Radiosurgery also has some effects on verbal memory, although this is largely limited and has shown signs of improvement over time. Using the Wechsler Memory Scale and the California Verbal Learning Test significant verbal memory impairment was seen in 25% of dominant-hemisphere surgery patients and in 7% of nondominant-hemisphere surgery patients, for an average of 15%.[63] In addition to these new deficits, however, significant improvement was seen in 16% of dominant hemisphere and 7% of nondominant hemisphere radiosurgery patients in this pilot study, although the mechanism for this improvement is not well understood. Patients more rigorously analyzed with the Boston Naming Test, California Verbal Learning Test, Wechsler Memory Scale, Trail Making Test, and Beck Depression Inventory at 24 months after radiosurgery were found to have no significant neuropsychological changes from their preoperative baseline.[74]

Efforts to use lower doses to reduce radiographic changes consistent with tissue damage and edema have shown that there seems to be an effective dose threshold at or greater than 20 Gy.[75] Recent dose studies have also suggested that a dose of 20 Gy or less at the margins may be less effective than higher marginal doses in reducing seizure activity. Cmelak and colleagues[76] reported unsuccessful reduction of seizures with a 15-Gy marginal radiosurgery dose. Similarly, Kawai and colleagues[39] reported two cases of radiosurgery with an unsuccessful antiepileptic effect at a marginal radiosurgery dose of 18 Gy. Finally, Srikijvilaikul and colleagues[66] from the Cleveland Clinic also reported their series of ineffective radiosurgical treatment for seizure control with a 20-Gy marginal dose. Chang and colleagues[75] showed that a significant radiographic change was

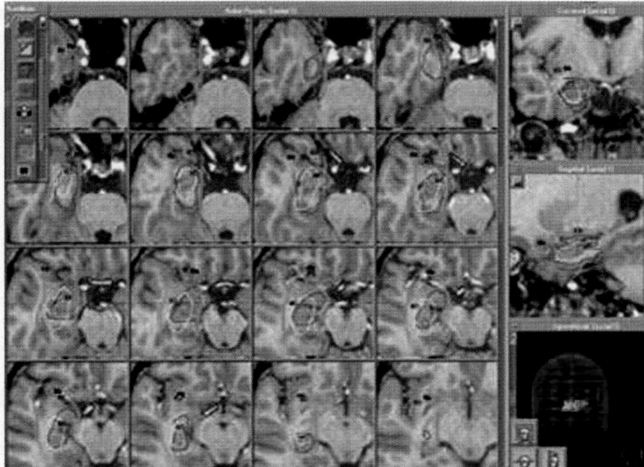

Figure 78-1. Treatment planning session for Gamma Knife radiosurgery.

correlated with a better seizure free outcome, further corroborating these data.

One of the difficulties in applying radiosurgery broadly as an application for intractable MTLE is the definition of the radiosurgical target because of a lack of clear boundaries of MTS (Fig. 78-1). For example, in recent reports, Régis and colleagues radiosurgically targeted the mesial temporal lobe structures in their series, whereas Kawai and colleagues restricted their treatment to the amygdala or hippocampus structures, and each series reported varying rates of successful amelioration of MTLE.[4,39,44,45] Although target definition can vary among different neurosurgeons, radiosurgery for MTS-associated MTLE remains an attractive therapeutic option because of its effectiveness, low morbidity and mortality, and the consistent manifestations of this disease with identifiable imaging characteristics on MRI. Moreover, conventional open microsurgical temporal lobectomy is still possible if the initial radiosurgical treatment is ineffective after sufficient time has elapsed for the delayed radiosurgical antiepileptic effect.[4]

Histologic Evaluation after Radiosurgical Treatment of Medial Temporal Lobe Epilepsy

Histologic examination of radiosurgically treated human mesial temporal tissue for MTLE has been limited because of the efficacy of radiosurgery for MTS-associated MTLE. However, histologic analysis of radiation-treated tissues has been reported in patients who underwent resection because of ineffective seizure control after radiosurgery.[39,66,76] Histopathologic studies after subtherapeutic doses of 15 and 18 Gy found one of three patients with a necrotic focus with some prominent vascular changes consisting of vessel wall thickening and fibrinoid and hyaline degeneration.[39,76] When treated with a larger but subtherapeutic dose of 20 Gy, all five patients from a series reported from the Cleveland Clinic demonstrated histopathologic necrosis, perivascular sclerosis, and macrophage infiltration on resection and evaluation.[66]

Currently, the radiobiology of radiosurgery in the setting of MTS-associated MTLE is not completely understood. Although some preclinical studies have suggested an antiepileptic effect of radiation with subnecrotic doses,[53] human clinical studies have suggested that a certain amount of tissue necrosis and histopathologic changes may be required to produce significant amelioration of MTS-associated seizures. The importance of this issue on biologic effect is that radiosurgical treatment of eloquent brain regions would be possible if an effective subnecrotic dose could be found.

Antiepileptic Radiosurgery Mechanism

Although radiosurgery has been shown to reduce seizures in various forms of medically intractable epilepsy, the mechanism by which this abatement occurs is not well understood. It has been suggested that radiation itself has a direct antiepileptic effect that can operate through several mechanisms. Because glial cells are more radiosensitive than neurons, Barcia-Salorio[36] proposed that low-dose radiosurgery may reduce glial scar formation, allowing increased dendritic sprouting and improved cortical reorganization that results in fewer seizures. Elomaa theorized that the antiepileptic effect of radiation is further mediated through the effects of somatostatin.[77] Although the clinical results of the most recent human studies suggest that the therapeutic efficacy of radiosurgery is linked to histopathologic changes and identifiable necrosis of mesial temporal structures, proof of this theory would need to come from direct observation and histologic evaluation of tissue samples from patients in whom radiosurgery has effectively controlled the seizures. This is unlikely to occur because only patients with persistent seizures after radiosurgery are likely to undergo further open resective microsurgery. Among patients who underwent open resection after radiosurgery, Kawai and colleagues and Srikijvilaikul colleagues found necrotic foci with vessel wall thickening and fibrinoid and hyaline degeneration, perivascular sclerosis, and macrophage infiltration upon resection on histopathologic analysis in two patients treated with 18 and 20 Gy, although no radiation-induced histopathologic changes were found in tissues treated with 15 Gy of radiosurgery, suggesting that some histological damage may be needed for effective seizure control.[39,44,45,48,66,76] Animal studies have shown mixed results regarding this hypothesis, with some animal studies demonstrating improvement in seizures without evidence of necrosis, whereas others have shown direct structural, destructive lesions in the tissue zone to correlate with seizure remission.[75] The mechanisms may be some combination of neuromodulation and neuronal destruction, with ischemic factors likely playing a role.[63]

Surrogate markers of radiation effect and radiobiology, such as changes on MRI, are also showing some promising results. Radiation-induced edema typically becomes evident in most patients 9 to 15 months after radiosurgery (Fig. 78-2). T2 hyperintensity volumes of edema were found to be closely related to seizure remission such that no seizure remission was found between 24 and 36 months in patients who had volumes of edema less than 200 mL at 12 months.[75] These imaging findings, however, are usually time limited and are often followed by focal atrophic changes. Thus, changes on MRI might not be diagnostic or indicative of true radiation necrosis. Furthermore, our pilot clinical trials have shown that MRI changes and peak MRI effects are poorly correlated with posttreatment symptoms. The actual biomechanism by which high-dose radiation and radiosurgery reduce neuronal hyperexcitability to ameliorate seizures will probably not be found or elucidated from human studies.

Although preclinical evidence and the results from early clinical human trials suggest that control of seizures might be possible with doses of radiosurgery that are lower than those typically applied to tumors,[35,38] recent case reports also demonstrate the failure of low-dose radiosurgery to control seizures.[39,66,76] Although failure of seizure control is easy to identify, it is a much more difficult task to determine that a lack of seizure control is caused by an insufficient radiation dose. The time dependence of radiosurgical effects is also a confounding factor that has not been fully elucidated, and a consensus among different treating radiosurgical centers of when radiosurgical treatment has “failed” has not yet been reached.[48] Furthermore, radiosurgery patients with

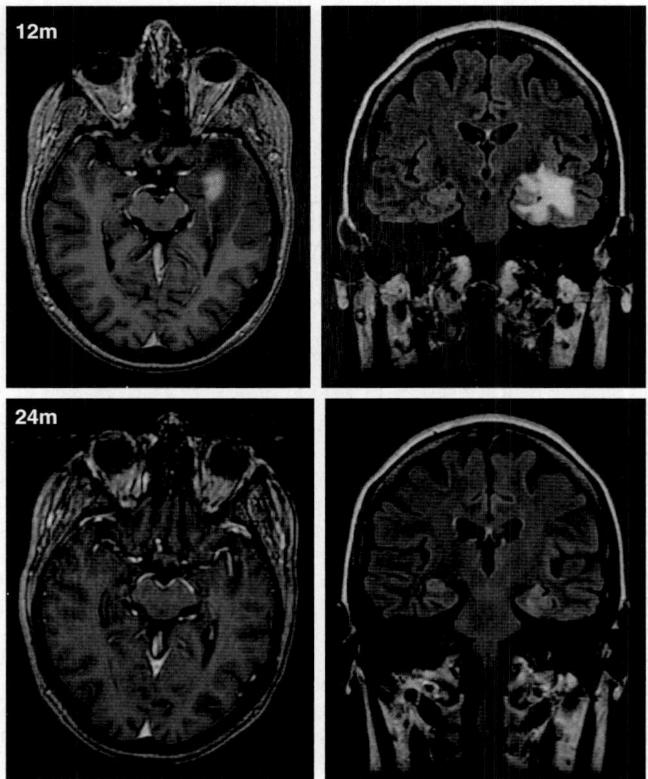

Figure 78-2. Changes on magnetic resonance imaging at 12 and 24 months after radiosurgery.

inadequate reduction of seizures commonly received radiation doses of 20 Gy or less, and these patients showed little evidence of radiation-induced necrosis or histopathologic changes in their tissue specimens.[39,66,76] Thus, the best evidence from human and animal preclinical experiments suggests that there is a steep dose-response curve for seizure reduction and that some neuronal necrosis is required to produce abatement of seizures. This evidence suggests that the radiosurgery dose required to reduce seizures is close to the absolute tolerability threshold of human brain tissue.

Summary

Recent data suggest that radiosurgery is an effective and safe alternative treatment modality for reducing epileptiform activity and seizures in patients with medically intractable temporal lobe epilepsy. In preclinical studies, the low doses of radiation required to be therapeutic have not been shown to cause histologic changes or significant learning deficits. When animals are observed over longer periods, the patterns of changes seen on MRI closely mimic those observed in human trials, and associated histologic analysis indicates that structural lesions are created. Animal studies have not yet proved whether the antiepileptic effects of radiosurgery are due to tissue necrosis and functional ablation or whether the seizure activity has been eliminated in still functional parenchyma. However, the available clinical human data suggest that it is necessary to produce changes on MRI consistent with tissue necrosis and histopathologic changes to eliminate seizures.

Recent prospective trials suggest that radiosurgery may be an effective and safe treatment modality for medically intractable epilepsy associated with MTS. Prospective trials with larger numbers of patients in multicenter studies will be required to establish radiosurgery as a standard alternative therapy for MTLE. Radiosurgery may prove to be especially appealing in treating lesions near functional cortex or deep-seated lesions when open microsurgical resection might not be feasible without significant morbidity.

HYPOTHALAMIC HAMARTOMAS

Hypothalamic hamartomas (HHs) are rare congenital heterotopic lesions that are intrinsically epileptogenic when closely connected to the mammillary bodies.[78,79] Patients classically experience gelastic seizures during the first years of life.[80] In more severe forms of the disease, an epileptic encephalopathy characterized by drug resistance, various types of seizures with generalization (including drop attacks),[80] cognitive decline,[81-83] and severe psychiatric comorbidity develop in affected patients during the following years.[84] Usually, the seizures begin early in life and are often particularly drug resistant from the onset. Commonly, the seizure semiology suggests the involvement of temporal or frontal lobe regions and a phenomenon of secondary epileptogenesis. HHs can also be asymptomatic or be associated with precocious puberty, neurological disorders (including epilepsy, behavior disturbances, and cognitive impairment), or both.

The natural history is unfavorable in the majority of patients because of behavioral symptoms (particularly aggressive behavior) and mental decline, which occur as a direct effect of the seizures.[85] Interestingly, in our experience, reversal of these behavioral symptoms after radiosurgery seems to begin even before complete cessation of the seizures and appears to be correlated to the improvement in background electroencephalographic (EEG) activity. It is the authors' speculation that these continuous discharges lead to the disorganization of several systems, including the limbic system, and that their disappearance accounts for the improvement seen in attention, memory, cognitive performance, and impulsive behavior. In these cases, radiosurgery's role in reversal of the behavioral symptoms may be as or more important than its effect on decreasing seizure occurrence. Consequently, we consider it essential to operate on these young patients as early as possible, whatever the surgical approach being considered (resection or radiosurgery).

Surgery and Minimally Invasive Approaches

Historically, those symptomatic hypothalamic hamartomas requiring treatment have been treated with resection versus disconnection, although these approaches carry with them several significant risks. Symptomatic epilepsy-related HH is observed only with medium to large sessile HHs that are broadly attached to the tuber cinereum or mammillary body, and microsurgical resection in this critical area is associated with a significant risk for oculomotor palsy, hemiparesis, and visual field deficits.[86-89] As these lesions are not technically neoplasms, removal is therefore not mandatory, and they can also be treated with disconnection rather than gross total resection to avoid the complications that can occur during dissection in the cisterns, although disconnection also carries with it similar risks to microsurgical resection, with a 2003 study of 17 patients by Delalande and Fohlen reporting a second intervention (usually endoscopic) was necessary in eight patients and one patient with hemiplegia: one with hemiparesis, two with hyperphagia, one with panhypopituitarism, one with hypothyroidism, and one with growth hormone deficiency.[87,88] In addition, stereotactic radiofrequency thermocoagulation and laser ablation have been proposed by some authors for lesioning of HH instead of the direct microsurgical approach.[90-92] Radiosurgery is able to circumvent many of the severe neurological risks inherent in these procedures, while still attaining similar result profiles.

Radiosurgery

As is the case in mesial temporal sclerosis, radiosurgery provides a minimally invasive alternative to traditional open resection or disconnection of hypothalamic hamartomas; it is being studied aggressively for determination of its safety and efficacy. Régis and colleagues[47] retrospectively analyzed the results of radiosurgery in a multicenter study of 10 patients and found all improved, with 50% cured, and no adverse effects except for one patient with poikilothermia. Given these findings, a prospective multicenter study of 55 patients was completed using multi-isocentric complex dose planning of high conformity and selectivity with the Leksell 201-source Cobalt 60 Gamma Knife (Elekta Instrument, Stockholm, Sweden).[78,81] The lesions treated were generally small (median, 9.5 mm; range, 5-26 mm) and we used low peripheral doses to account for the close relationship with the optic pathways and the hypothalamus (median, 17 Gy; range, 13-26 Gy). Patients were evaluated with respect to seizures, cognition, behavior, and endocrine status 6, 12, 18, 24, and 36 months after radiosurgery and then every year thereafter. Satisfactory follow-up was available for 27 patients. Among these patients, 10 are seizure free (37%) and 6 are much improved (22.2%) with reduction in seizures associated with a dramatic improvement in behavior and cognition. Paroxysmal aggressivity improved substantially and increased alertness, elevated mood, and greater speech production were observed in some patients with excessive behavioral inhibition, implying strong psychiatric effects of this therapy. Younger patients in particular encountered improved sleep and 3 of the 55 saw developmental acceleration. Five patients (18.5%) with small hamartomas showed only modest improvement, and they are being considered for a second session of radiosurgery. The radiosurgical treatment was performed twice in nine patients. A microsurgical approach was performed in four patients (14.8%) with large HHs and poor efficacy of radiosurgery. Of these patients, two were cured and two failed to respond.

Limits of Radiosurgery for Hypothalamic Hamartoma

Despite its many strengths, there remain several unanswered questions and limitations regarding stereotactic radiosurgery, the foremost being that it is presently unknown how to predict to what extent a hypothalamic hamartoma must be treated to achieve adequate seizure reduction. In addition, in patients bearing an electroclinical semiology suggestive of temporal lobe or frontal lobe contributions, often only a partial result can be obtained with radiosurgery, leaving residual seizures despite significant overall psychiatric and cognitive improvement.[93-97] In this second group, it is tempting to propose that a secondary epileptogenic area is the cause the partial failure.

The initial results of Régis and colleagues indicate that GKRS is as effective as microsurgical resection with reduced morbidity while avoiding the vascular risk related to radiofrequency lesioning or stimulation.[47,76] Similar to the treatment of mesial temporal sclerosis, the disadvantage of radiosurgery is its delayed action. Régis and colleagues[98] have demonstrated that patients treated with radiosurgery go through a five-period pattern of response to the therapy, with an initial improvement phase followed by a return to seizure baseline after several months, which is then followed by a third phase characterized by a transient increase in seizures.[98] Approximately 6 months after treatment, seizures begin to subside again in phase four, and then are consolidated to a new, reduced baseline as stage five. Longer follow-up is mandatory for proper evaluation of the role of GKRS. Results are obtained more quickly and are more complete in patients with smaller lesions inside the third ventricle. The early effect on subclinical EEG discharges appears to play a major role in the dramatic benefit in sleep quality, behavior, and cognitive-developmental improvement. GKRS can safely lead to reversal of the epileptic encephalopathy.

Because of the poor clinical prognosis of the majority of patients with HH and the invasiveness of microsurgical resection, GKRS can be considered a first-line intervention for small to middle-sized HHs associated with epilepsy, because it can lead to dramatic improvements in these young patients. The role of secondary epileptogenesis or widespread cortical dysgenesis in these patients needs to be evaluated further and understood to optimize patient selection and define the best treatment strategy.

CAVERNOUS MALFORMATIONS

Cavernous malformations (CM) are congenital vascular malformations of the brain that are often incidentally discovered or present with hemorrhage, repetitive neurological deficits, and epilepsy.[99] The epileptogenicity of these lesions results from the ongoing deposition of iron and blood products at the margin of the lesion, whereas the hemorrhage risk is often due to their highly vascular nature.[100] In one large series, 40% of patients with a supratentorial CM had drug-resistant epilepsy.[101]

Stereotactic radiosurgery has been applied to the treatment of cavernous malformations for two primary reasons: prevention of future hemorrhage and reduction of seizures. Having been used previously to good effect for management of AVMs, it was speculated that, due to their similar vascular nature, cavernous malformations could in some way be managed effectively through radiosurgery when open resection was deemed too dangerous or impossible. Though initial studies in the late 1980s and early 1990s showed high complication rates, more recent studies have demonstrated improved safety through this modality, and it has found greater application in the 21st century.

The effect of GKRS on future hemorrhage rate is controversial, although the trend has been growing in favor of radiosurgery with time and additional research.[40,102] It has been theorized that hemorrhages naturally cluster in CMs and then taper off with time on their own. Thus, it is possible that the apparent reduction in hemorrhage frequency after radiosurgery is actually a result of this natural phenomenon.[103-105] However, more "active" CMs that have many pretreatment hemorrhages tend to continue to hemorrhage long after this supposed clustering. In addition, histopathologic changes are appreciated with time, corresponding temporally with reduction of hemorrhage risk. While neurological deficits following each additional hemorrhage remain similar in treated and untreated groups, radiosurgery has been shown to reduce the frequency of these hemorrhages and, as a result, lifetime risk of debility. Kondziolka and colleagues[106] found that rebleeding rate decreased from 32% per patient-year before treatment to 8.8% and to 1.1% after the first 2 years.[106] These findings have been replicated by Kondziolka and others[107-114] and in several retrospective studies and reviews, notably by Frischer[112] and Lu,[113] although Karlsson[115] and Amir-Hanjani[116] have shown contradictory results. Mounting evidence suggests an increasing role for stereotactic radiosurgery, particularly in deep brainstem or eloquent lesions where the risk of surgery may be too great.

Although the application of GKRS for altering rebleeding risk is controversial, there is substantial evidence of its effectiveness in the management of drug-resistant seizures associated with CMs, evaluated in a retrospective multicenter study (Marseille, France; Graz, Austria; Komaki, Japan; Sheffield, England; and Prague, Czech Republic).[46] Forty-nine patients with cortical or subcortical CMs and severe long-term drug-resistant epilepsy were included and were observed for longer than 1 year after GKRS. The mean duration of epilepsy before these GKRS procedures was 7.5 ± 9.3 years. The mean frequency of seizures was 6.9 per month (±14). The mean marginal radiation dose was 19.17 ± 4.4 Gy. Among the 49 patients, 35% had a CM located in or involving a highly functional area. At the last follow-up examination, 53% of patients were seizure free (Engel class I), including 49% in class IA and 4% with occasional auras. A highly significant decrease in the number of seizures was achieved in 20% (class IIB). The remaining 27% of patients showed little or no improvement. The mediotemporal site was associated with a higher risk for failure. One patient bled during the observation period, and another experienced radiation-induced edema with transient aphasia. Excision was performed after radiosurgery in five patients, and a second radiosurgical treatment was performed in one patient.

Studies by Wang[109] and Liu and colleagues[108] corroborate these data, with similar rates of seizure freedom or improvement. Interestingly, those with a shorter history of seizures improved more often than those with a longer history. Of the 11 patients with intractable epilepsy before GKRS in a series by Kida and colleagues, seven patients (64%) achieved good seizure control after GKRS even though there was no apparent change in the size of the CM.[117] The apparent size of a CM seems to fluctuate and depend on the production and absorption of blood pigments. Kida and colleagues[118] examined 298 symptomatic CMs treated with stereotactic radiosurgery (SRS) across Japan and found that, among 27 patients with a follow-up period of 83 months, nearly half were seizure free (Engel class I), with others remaining in class II (26%) or III (26%) despite treatment. In their experience, CMs could be divided into two groups: CMs associated with repetitive minor hemorrhages, and CMs surrounded by hemosiderin-stained brain tissue without recognizable hemorrhage. They found the CMs not associated with hemorrhage to be more likely to be refractory to SRS.[118] A retrospective study of 29 patients by Hsu and colleagues[119] found no statistical difference in epilepsy rates when comparing surgical resection to radiosurgery, although the study might have suffered from being underpowered and was trending toward favoring surgery.[119]

Management Strategy

Although a reliable prospective study with long-term follow-up is still needed, GKRS can be effective for this indication and morbidity can be low. It should be emphasized that the GKRS procedure treats the lesion and the immediate surrounding tissue. The results observed in studies by Kida and others were comparable to those reported in the recent literature for lesionectomy.[100,101,120-128] The most valuable prognostic factor for outcome after GKRS was lesion location. A probable explanation for this finding is that the relationship between the lesion and the epileptogenic zone is particularly direct in certain regions, especially simple motor partial seizures associated with CMs in the rolandic region. In contrast, when a CM is located in the mediotemporal region, a more complex organization probably accounts for the extended epileptogenic zone, and epilepsy surgery strategies should be preferred. The increased complexity of these lesions probably explains why patients with complex partial seizures had a less favorable outcome than did patients with simple partial seizures in our study.

Pathologic Response and Associated Risks

Although long-term outcome data are lacking because of the relative novelty of SRS for CM treatment, there has been some research into the long-term effects of this treatment. Histopathologic analysis of tissue excised from patients who underwent radiosurgery and encountered rebleeds requiring microsurgical resection found vascular sclerosis develops as early as 4 months after SRS and even 2 to 10 years after SRS specimens showed neovascularization, fibrinoid necrosis, fibrosis, and endothelial cell destruction.[129-131] It has also been shown via posttreatment MRI that although cavernous malformations often reduce in size with treatment, they are just as likely to remain the same size even after SRS.[132,133] Nagy and colleagues found low morbidity rates of 1% to 7.3% that were typically mild in nature associated with SRS treatment of CMs, even in relatively eloquent tissue and the brainstem.[134]

RADIOSURGICAL CORPUS CALLOSOTOMY

Radiosurgery has also been used in a functional capacity in the form of partial radiosurgical ablation of the corpus callosum for patients experiencing intractable seizures. Pendl and colleagues[135] initially trialed this therapy for a series of three patients with intractable epilepsy and no resectable seizure focus.[135] After treatment with high-dose therapy of 150 and 160 Gy in two patients and two-staged therapy of 50 and 170 Gy in another patient, significant seizure reduction was demonstrated, although this was not always permanent. A similar retrospective study in Austria demonstrated seizure reduction in six of eight patients, particularly in drop attacks, with few significant side effects, whereas later case reports have demonstrated its use in a pediatric population.[136-138] Its application has been limited thus far, but future research may hold the key for more advanced usage of radiosurgery's ablative properties for additional seizure causes.

CONCLUSION

The field of epilepsy surgery is a new and promising one for radiosurgery. However, determination of the extent of the epileptogenic zone requires specific expertise, which is crucial to achieve a reasonable rate of seizure cessation. In addition, the significant influence of fine technical detail on the efficacy and eventual toxicity of the procedure means that at present, its use for these indications remains under investigation, and further prospective work is still necessary.

SUGGESTED READINGS

Barbaro NM, Quigg M, Broshek DK, et al. A multicenter, prospective pilot study of gamma knife radiosurgery for mesial temporal lobe epilepsy: seizure response, adverse events, and verbal memory. *Ann Neurol*. 2009;65:167-175.

Barcia-Salorio JL, Barcia JA, Hernandez G, et al. Radiosurgery of epilepsy. Long-term results. *Acta Neurochir Suppl*. 1994;62:111-113.

Bien CG, Kurthen M, Baron K, et al. Long-term seizure outcome and antiepileptic drug treatment in surgically treated temporal lobe epilepsy patients: a controlled study. *Epilepsia*. 2001;42:1416-1421.

Chang EF, Quigg M, Oh MC, et al. Predictors of efficacy after stereotactic radiosurgery for medial temporal lobe epilepsy. *Neurology*. 2010;74:165-172.

Engel J Jr. Surgery for seizures. *N Engl J Med*. 1996;334:647-652.

Gross BA, Du R. Cerebral cavernous malformations: natural history and clinical management. *Expert Rev Neurother*. 2015;15:771-777.

Lee SH, Choi HJ, Shin HS, et al. Gamma Knife radiosurgery for brainstem cavernous malformations: should a patient wait for the rebleed? *Acta Neurochir (Wien)*. 2014;156:1937-1946.

Lee CC, Pan DH, Chung WY, et al. Brainstem cavernous malformations: the role of gamma knife surgery. *J Neurosurg*. 2012;117:164-169.

Nagy G, Kemeny AA. Stereotactic radiosurgery of intracranial cavernous malformations. *Neurosurg Clin N Am*. 2013;24:575-589.

Nagy G, Razak A, Rowe JG, et al. Stereotactic radiosurgery for deep-seated cavernous malformations: a move toward more active, early intervention. *J Neurosurg*. 2010;113:691-699.

Nguyen DK, Spencer SS. Recent advances in the treatment of epilepsy. *Arch Neurol*. 2003;60:929-935.

Niranjan A, Lunsford LD. Stereotactic radiosurgery guidelines for the management of patients with intracranial cavernous malformations. *Prog Neurol Surg*. 2013;27:166-175.

Porter P, Willinsky R, Harper W, et al. Cerebral cavernous malformations: natural history and prognosis after clinical deterioration with or without hemorrhage. *J Neurosurg*. 1997;87:190-197.

Steiner L, Karlsson B, Yen CP, et al. Radiosurgery in cavernous malformations: anatomy of a controversy. *J Neurosurg*. 2010;113:16-21.

See a full reference list on ExpertConsult.com

79 Electrical Stimulation for Epilepsy (VNS, DBS, and RNS)

Robert E. Gross, Nealen G. Laxpati, and Babak Mahmoudi

One percent of the world's population has epilepsy, and 30% to 40% of these cases are resistant to medications.[1-4] Although a significant proportion (10%-50%) of these medically refractory cases involve patients who are candidates for resective surgery,[5] with postoperative seizure freedom rates of 40% to 90%, there remain millions of patients who cannot undergo resective surgery or who have recurrent seizures after surgery.[3,5-8] Very few of these respond to additional medication trials,[9] and less than 10% achieve seizure freedom with vagus nerve stimulation (VNS).[10] Thus, there is a pressing need for alternative therapies for medically refractory epilepsy.

Electrical stimulation of the nervous system has rapidly developed as an adjunct to medical therapy for epilepsy. VNS has been approved since 1997 for reducing the frequency of seizures in patients older than 12 years with partial onset seizures refractory to pharmacologic therapy.[11] Deep brain stimulation (DBS) has been proven to be extraordinarily effective and safe for the treatment of movement disorders such as Parkinson's disease, dystonia, and essential tremor.[12,13] These successes have inspired the application of DBS to an ever-broadening range of neurological and psychiatric disorders, including depression,[14] obsessive-compulsive disorder,[15] and Tourette's syndrome,[16] as well as epilepsy. Here, we examine the use of electrical stimulation in epilepsy, including potential targets, mechanisms of neuromodulation and seizure control, clinical evidence and recent clinical trials, and future directions and novel therapies.

CORTICAL-SUBCORTICAL NETWORKS IN EPILEPSY

Focal or partial onset seizures vary considerably in their epileptogenic zone(s) and in their semiology (i.e., clinical manifestations), but they appear to propagate along common neural circuits, such as the cortical-striatal-thalamic network[17-19] and the limbic circuit of Papez[20,21] (Fig. 79-1). These pathways provide nodes at which neuromodulatory tools may influence the propagation of neural information, including the pathologic oscillations mediating the behavioral effects of seizures.

One of the most well studied of these epileptic networks is the circuit of Papez,[21] which is critical for emotion and memory. This network is well known to be involved in the generation and propagation of limbic (e.g., mesial temporal lobe) seizures.[20,22] The circuit originates from the hippocampus and subiculum, projecting via the fornix to the mammillary body, then travelling via the mammillothalamic tract to the anterior nucleus of the thalamus (ANT) (see Fig. 79-1). The ANT then projects to the cingulate gyrus, and in turn to the parahippocampal gyrus, followed by the entorhinal cortex, which finally projects via the perforant pathway back to the hippocampus.[20,21] Lesions and high-frequency electrical stimulation have been studied and showed some effectiveness at several locations within this circuit—including the hippocampus, mammillary bodies, subiculum, and ANT.[23-28]

Cortico-thalamo-cortical excitatory loops have been shown to be involved in absence epilepsy[29] and motor cortex seizures.[19] In a nonhuman primate model of chronic focal motor seizures, thalamotomy restricted to the anterior part of the ventro-postero-lateral nucleus was able to produce long-lasting benefit and in most cases led to nearly complete seizure suppression.[30] Thalamic relays are also thought to mediate the benefits from lesions and electrical stimulation of the cerebellum for epilepsy, but this circuit and its influence are less clearly defined.[31-33] The thalamocortical network is a target for further investigations for epilepsy,[34] and these networks have provided several potential neuromodulatory targets for the treatment of seizures. Further work with these targets will require more precise understanding of the mechanisms mediating the effects of electrical neuromodulation.

MECHANISMS OF ACTION OF ELECTRICAL NEUROMODULATION

The stimulation parameters used in many clinical trials have been informed less by complete understanding of the mechanisms of action of electrical stimulation than by empirical and historical considerations (Table 79-1). Only recently have more complex parameters begun to be entertained in experiments with human patients.[35] Increased effectiveness may also result from a deeper understanding of the mechanism(s) of electrical stimulation on the nervous system, followed by the implementation of the most efficacious parameters in clinical trials and practice.

Despite the extensive use of electrical stimulation in neuromodulation, its mechanism of action remains poorly understood. The initial observation that high-frequency (>50 Hz) DBS mimicked the effects of ablative procedures suggested that DBS was inhibitory in nature,[36] inducing a reversible, functional lesion. Increasingly, however, the functional action of electrical stimulation on neural circuits has been recognized as complex and multifaceted. Stimulation amplitude, frequency, and pulse width play a major role in determining the effects of stimulation on the nervous system, and manipulating other parameters such as waveform and polarity can have a significant impact as well.[37,38] Early work by Ranck[38a] indicated that electrical fields have differential effects on different neuronal structures. Activation thresholds are lowest in myelinated axons, with increasing thresholds found in unmyelinated axons, dendrites, and cell bodies, respectively. More recent work from Histed and colleagues[39] using low-current 250-Hz electrical microstimulation with concomitant two-photon calcium imaging to identify the location of electrically activated neurons has supported these hypotheses. Using multicompartment cable models of neurons coupled to a finite element model of extracellular electric fields, McIntyre and colleagues[40] suggested that the majority of cells within approximately 2 mm of the electrode will entrain efferent (axonal) output at the stimulus frequency, whereas those stimulated at subthreshold levels will be suppressed.[40] Electrical stimulation may consequently be overriding, or overwriting, the neural circuit—and in the case of pathologic circuitry, blocking and replacing abnormal neural activity. Indeed, we found evidence of entrainment of downstream (both orthodromic and antidromic) neuronal firing by DBS in a Parkinson's disease patient.[41] The effects of modified efferent output on downstream circuits will depend on their neural connections.

Other mechanisms—for example, neurochemical interactions and gene and protein expression—may also prove critical. The

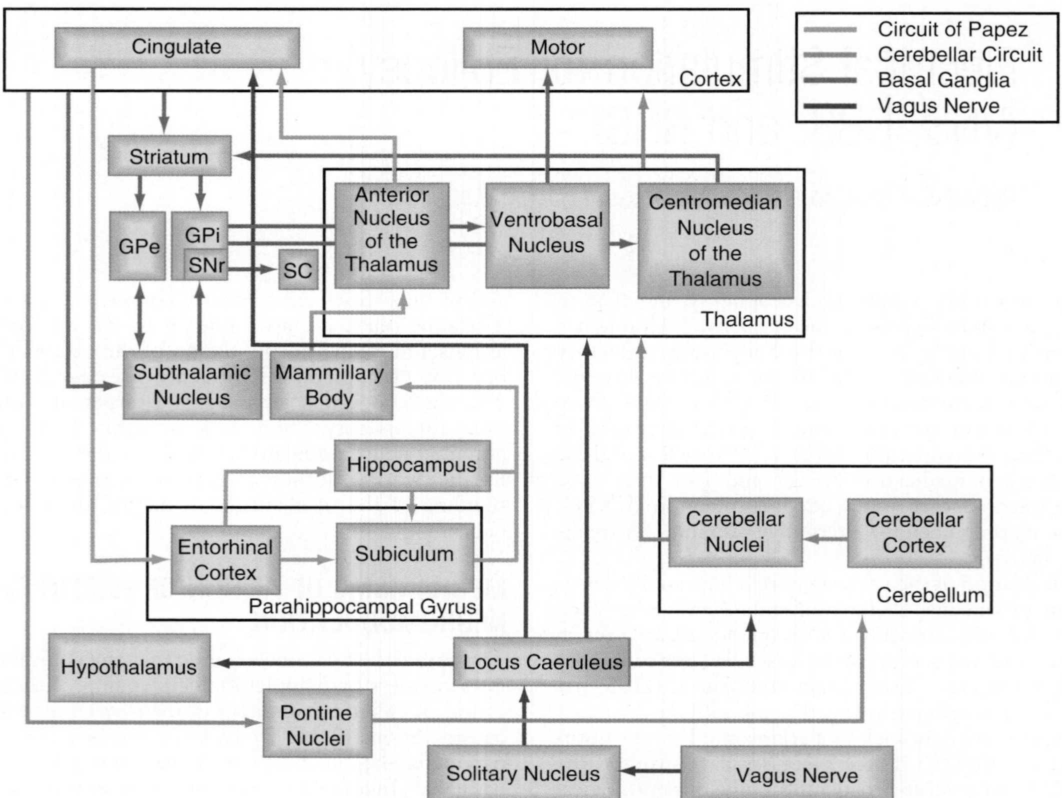

Figure 79-1. Neural circuits and electrical stimulation targets for epilepsy. Several major neural circuits have been identified and targeted for neuromodulation of epileptic seizures, including the circuit of Papez *(red),* the cerebellar-cortical circuit *(green),* the basal ganglia *(brown),* and projections via the vagus nerve *(blue).* GPe, globus pallidus externa; GPi, globus pallidus interna; SC, superior colliculus; SNr, substantia nigra pars reticulata.

anticonvulsant effects of low-frequency stimulation have been correlated with changes in adenosine receptor expression,[42] and VNS has been associated with alterations in a variety of neurotransmitters and hormones in cerebrospinal fluid.[43] Furthermore, the progressive improvement in outcome associated with electrical stimulation for movement disorders[44] and epilepsy (see later)[24,45] suggests that synaptic, neurochemical, and/or expression changes are occurring in response to electrical stimulation of the pathologic neural network.

TARGETS FOR ELECTRICAL STIMULATION IN EPILEPSY

A wide variety of anatomic targets, stimulation parameters, and outcome measures have been investigated for epilepsy, primarily in small case series (see Table 79-1). We will highlight and summarize the results of these investigations categorized by anatomic target. In general, the results are described in terms of complete freedom from seizures (seizure free), a clinically significant reduction in seizure frequency (reduction, response, improvement), or no response (unresponsive, no benefit).

Vagus Nerve Stimulation

VNS was the first electrical stimulation therapy for epilepsy that was approved by the U.S. Food and Drug Administration (FDA) and for CE Marking (Fig. 79-2). The device consists of coiled stimulation leads placed around the left vagus nerve. The leads are subcutaneously connected to a generator placed below the clavicle.[46] Although the mechanism of action underlying its

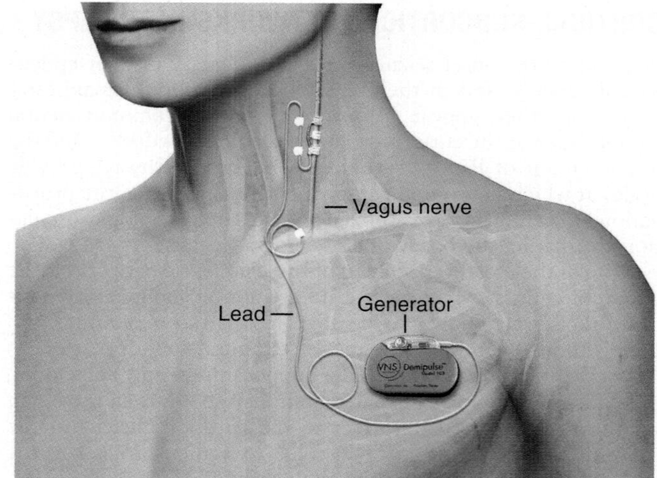

Figure 79-2. Vagus nerve stimulation system. Depiction of the vagus nerve stimulation system. Recently approved by the U.S. Food and Drug Administration (FDA), the AspireSR device (Cyberonics, Houston, TX) is shown. This device triggers additional stimulation on detection of tachycardia that can be seizure related. This pulse generator is built on the form factor of the increased duty cycle generator, which is somewhat larger than the model required by most patients. *(Courtesy of Cyberonics, Inc.)*

TABLE 79-1 Published Reports of Deep Brain Stimulation for Epilepsy

Study	Target	Design	N	Seizure Type	Stimulation Parameters	Follow-Up	Results	Adverse Events
Cooper et al, 1973[68]; Cooper et al, 1976[69]	Cerebellum	Open-label	15	Variable (6 CPSz, 6 GTC, 3 myo)	Variable (most 10 Hz, 10 V; 1-min epochs alternating hemispheres)	11-38 mo	4 of 15 SF at ≥30 mo (2 CPSz, 1 GTC, 1 myo) 6 of 15 improved (2 CPSz, 2 GTC, 2 myo) 5 of 15 no change	1 broken lead
Van Buren et al, 1978[70]	Cerebellum	Double-blind crossover	5	Variable	10 Hz, 10-14 V; 8 min ON R/OFF L, 8 min ON L/OFF R	24-29 mo	0 of 5 SF 0 of 5 improved	3 CSF leaks 1 increased CSF pressure
Levy and Auchterlonie, 1979[71]	Cerebellum	Open-label	6	Variable	10 Hz, 2-4 V 8 min ON R/OFF L, 8 min ON L/OFF R	7-20 mo	0 of 6 SF 2 of 6 improved	1 infection resulting in explantation All had headaches
Wright et al, 1984[72]	Cerebellum	Double-blind crossover	12	Variable	10 Hz, 5-7 mA 1 min ON R/OFF L, 1 min ON L/OFF R	6 mo	0 of 11 SF 0 of 11 improved	6 patients more than 1 operation 2 postoperative wound infections, 1 resulting in explantation 4 reoperations 1 lead repositioning 1 device failure
Velasco et al, 2005[73]	Cerebellum	Double-blind crossover	5	Variable	10 Hz, 3.8 mA, PW 450 µsec, 2.0 µC/cm^2 4 min ON B/I, 4 min OFF B/I	24 mo	3 mo: mean seizure reduction 33% 6 mo: mean seizure reduction 41%	3 reoperations for migration 1 wound infection resulting in removal 1 ataxia and dysmetria 4 electrode migrations
Velasco et al, 2000[28]	HC	Open-label	16	TLE	130 Hz, 0.2-0.4 mA, PW 450 µsec	2 wk	7 of 10 SF after 6 days 3 of 3 chronic stimulation improved Interictal spikes decreased	N/A
Tellez-Zenteno et al, 2006[86]	HC	Double-blind crossover	4	MTLE	190 Hz, 1.8-4.5 V, PW 90 µsec	6 mo	0 of 4 SF 3 mo: median seizure reduction 15%	None reported
Velasco et al, 2007[82]	HC	Open-label	9	MTLE	130 Hz, 0.3 mA, PW 450 µsec 1 min ON B/I, 4 min OFF B/I	18 mo	4 of 9 SF 5 of 9 improved	3 skin erosion and local infection, 1 requiring hospitalization 2 explantations
Boon et al, 2007[84]	HC	Open-label	12	TLE	130 Hz, 2-3 V, PW 450 µsec	15-52 mo	1 patient exited trial before stimulation 1 of 11 SF 9 of 11 improved (6 of 11 >50%) 3 of 11 SF after additional leads	1 asymptomatic hemorrhage
McLachlan et al, 2010[90]	HC	Double-blind crossover	2	MTLE	185 Hz, "subthreshold." PW 90 µsec	9 mo	0 of 2 SF 3 mo: mean seizure reduction 33%	None reported
Cukiert et al, 2011[147]	HC	Open-label	6	Variable (5 TLE)	130 Hz, 4 V, PW 300 µsec	Acute stimulation only	Clinical outcomes pending 4 of 6 with interictal spikes suppressed	None reported
Boëx et al, 2011[87]; Bondallaz et al, 2013[27]	HC	Open-label	8	MTLE (2 HS)	130 Hz, 0.5-2 V, PW 450 µsec	10-74 mo	2 of 8 SF 4 of 8 improved (50%-90%)	1 electrode displacement resulting in reimplantation 1 electrode fracture 2 reversible memory deficits with stimulation
Tyrand et al, 2012[148]	HC	Open-label	12	TLE (6 HS)	130 Hz, 1 V peak-to-peak, PW 210 or 450 µsec	Acute stimulation only	No seizure outcomes reported HS patients demonstrated 51.8% decrease in epileptiform discharges with biphasic stimulation	N/A
Benabid et al, 2002[104]; Chabardès et al, 2002[105]	STN	Open-label	5	Variable	130 Hz, 0.8-5.2 V, PW 90 µsec	30 mo	0 of 5 SF 3 of 5 improved (67%-80%)	1 infection 1 postimplantation subdural hematoma

Continued

TABLE 79-1 Published Reports of Deep Brain Stimulation for Epilepsy—cont'd

Study	Target	Design	N	Seizure Type	Stimulation Parameters	Follow-Up	Results	Adverse Events
Handforth et al, 2006[100]	STN	Open-label	2	CPSz	185 Hz, <3.5 V, PW 90 μsec	27 mo	2 of 2 improved (33%-50%)	1 repeated surgery 1 hardware failure
Vesper et al, 2007[101]; Wille et al, 2011[108]	STN	Open-label	5	Myo	130 Hz, 3.0 V, PW 90 μsec	12-42 mo	1 of 5 SF 4 of 5 improved (>30%)	
Capecci et al, 2012[102]	STN	Open-label	2	Variable	130 Hz, 2-3 V, PW 60 μsec	12-48 mo	1 of 2 improved (65%)	1 patient demonstrated mild balance impairment, dysarthria, severe aboulia, apathy, and mood changes under chronic stimulation
Sramka and Chkhenkeli, 1990[149]; Chkhenkeli and Chkhenkeli, 1997[150]; Chkhenkeli et al, 2004[151]	Caudate	Open-label	57	Variable	Variable	Variable	Unclear	N/A
Velasco et al, 1987[112]; Velasco et al, 2000[28]; Velasco et al, 2006[111]	CMT	Open-label	18	Variable	60 Hz, 0.5-0.6 mA 1 min ON R/OFF L, 4 min OFF B/I, 1 min ON L/OFF R, 4 min OFF	18 mo	Lennox-Gastaut: 2 of 13 SF, 8 of 13 improved (50%-80%) Partial seizures: 2 of 5 improved (>80%)	2 patients explanted owing to repeated skin erosions
Fisher et al, 1992[116]	CMT	Double-blind crossover	6	Variable	65 Hz, 0.5-10 V, PW 90 μsec 1 min ON/4 min OFF × 2 hr/day	9 mo	30% mean seizure reduction With stimulation 24 hr/day, 3 of 6 improved (>50%)	1 connection repair 1 minor hemorrhage with no symptoms or complications
Andrade et al, 2006[122]	CMT	Open-label	2	Variable	100-185 Hz, 1-10 V, PW 90-120 μsec	20-80 mo	1 of 2 improved (>50%)	1 intermittent nystagmus with stimulation 1 patient with possible auditory hallucinations and anorexia during stimulation
Valentín et al, 2013[117]	CMT	Single-blind	11	Variable (6 PGE, 5 FLE)	130 Hz, <5 V, PW 90 μsec	6-72 mo	PGE: 5 of 6 improved (>50%) FLE: 1 of 5 improved (>50%)	1 infection resulting in explantation 1 transient agraphia
Hodaie et al, 2002[123]; Andrade et al, 2006[122]	ANT	Single-blind	6	Variable	100-185 Hz, 1-10 V, PW 90-120 μsec	50-70 mo	Difficult to interpret; 6 of 6 improved (>50%) by implantation; no further improvement with stimulation	1 skin erosion requiring wound revision 1 lethargy with continuous stimulation
Kerrigan et al, 2004[124]	ANT	Open-label	5	Variable	100 Hz, 1-10 V, PW 90-330 μsec	6-36 mo	Difficult to interpret; nonsignificant improvement in 4 of 5	1 reimplantation for incorrect positioning
Lim et al, 2007[125]	ANT	Open-label	4	Variable	90-110 Hz, 4-5 V, PW 60-90 μsec	33-48 mo	4 of 4 improved (37%-75%)	1 resolved mild left-hand weakness associated with hemorrhage 1 scalp erosion resulting in explantation
Osorio et al, 2007[126]	ANT	Single-blind	4	Variable	145 Hz, 4.1 V, PW 90 μsec, 1 min ON B/I, 5 min OFF B/I	36 mo	4 of 4 improved (53%-92%)	None reported
Fisher et al, 2010 (SANTE)[24]	ANT	Double-blind parallel-group	110	Partial onset	145 Hz, 5 V, PW 90 μsec	4 mo (blind phase) 13-37 mo (open)	4 mo: Median seizure reduction 40.4% with active stimulation, 14.5% with sham stimulation 13 mo: 2 of 110 SF; 43% with >50% response 25 mo: 6 of 81 SF; 54% with >50% response	808 reported in 109 participants, 55 in 40 categorized as serious, 238 of 808 events considered device-related 18.2% paresthesias 14.8% depression during blinded phase 13.0% memory impairment during blind phase 12.7% implant site infection 10.9% implant site pain 8.2% replaced leads for poor placement 4.5% nonsymptomatic hemorrhages 5 deaths 5 status epilepticus

B/I, bilateral; CMT, centromedian nucleus of the thalamus; CPSz, complex partial seizure; CSF, cerebrospinal fluid; FLE, frontal lobe epilepsy; GTC, generalized tonic-clonic seizure; HC, hippocampus; HS, hippocampal sclerosis; MTLE, mesial temporal lobe epilepsy; myo, myoclonic; N/A, not available; PGE, primary generalized epilepsy; PW, pulse width; SANTE, Stimulation of the Anterior Nucleus of the Thalamus in Epilepsy trial; SF, seizure-free; STN, subthalamic nucleus; TLE, temporal lobe epilepsy.

efficacy remains unclear, the sensory afferents of the vagus nerve project to the nucleus of the solitary tract (NTS) in the medulla.[47,48] In turn, the NTS projects broadly, involving the thalamus, amygdala, anterior cingulate, and frontal and parietal cortex (see Fig. 79-1).[49] Release of norepinephrine into the hippocampus is a marker for effective stimulation in a limbic seizure model.[48]

Despite its uncertain mechanism(s), two industry-sponsored randomized, double-blind clinical trials (EO3 and EO5) were performed to investigate the efficacy of VNS in the treatment of epilepsy.[46,50] The first trial (EO3)[50] was a blind, prospectively randomized, parallel design study comparing two stimulation paradigms in a broad range of epilepsy syndromes associated with intractable partial seizures: high stimulation (HS; 0.25- to 3.0-mA, 20- to 50-Hz, 500-μsec stimulation with an on time of 30-90 seconds and an off time of 5-10 minutes) and low stimulation (LS; 0.25- to 2.75-mA, 1- to 2-Hz, 130-μsec stimulation with an on time of 30 sec and an off time of 60-180 min). HS patients could also manually activate the device during an aura with a pocket magnet that generated a single train of pulses. Antiepileptic drug therapies were maintained at stable serum concentrations throughout the baseline and randomized portion of the study. After a 12-week baseline assessment, the signal generator and lead system were implanted and the patients randomized. Two weeks after implantation, the generator was activated for the 14-week randomized phase, the last 12 weeks of which were analyzed for efficacy. Patients exiting the study were offered indefinite extension of the treatment in an open trial. Of the 125 patients who underwent baseline assessment, 114 proceeded to implantation.

HS was associated with a statistically significant (P = .01) reduction in the frequency of seizures as compared with LS (−24.5% versus −6.1%, respectively). In addition, patients receiving HS had a significant reduction in seizure frequency compared with baseline (P < .01; 95% confidence interval [CI], −14.1% to −34.9%), as opposed to LS (P = .21, 95% CI, +3.6% to −15.8%). Of note, whereas 31% of patients in the HS group achieved at least a 50% decrease in seizure frequency, none achieved complete seizure freedom. Adverse effects were prominent, including voice changes and hoarseness (37.2% HS, 13.3% LS), throat pain (11.1% HS, 11.7% LS), coughing (7.4% HS, 8.3% LS), dyspnea (5.6% HS, 1.7% LS), paresthesias (5.6% HS, 3.3% LS), muscle pain (5.6% HS, 1.7% LS), and headache (1.8% HS, 8.3% LS).

The second trial of 254 patients (EO5) with medically refractory partial onset seizures was performed similarly.[46] Patients were eligible if they had at least six partial onset seizures involving alteration of consciousness over 30 days, with no more than 21 days between seizures. During the 12- to 16-week baseline period, patients kept daily seizure records and reported adverse symptoms and medications. Antiepileptic drugs were maintained, except as necessary to maintain appropriate concentrations or in response to apparent drug toxicity. After four clinic visits, patients meeting eligibility were implanted with the VNS device, and 2 weeks after implantation they began the treatment phase. Patients were randomly assigned to HS (30 seconds every 5 minutes of 500-μsec, 30-Hz pulses) or LS (30 seconds every 3 hours of 130-μsec, 1-Hz pulses). The amplitude of stimulation was set to a level below 3.5 mA that could be perceived by the patient, but was tolerated. Again, the HS group patients could manually activate the device with a handheld magnet in an attempt to abort a seizure. During the treatment period, patients submitted seizure counts and adverse event information, and after the treatment phase all patients were eligible to enter an open-treatment extension protocol. The primary outcome variable was the percentage change in total seizure frequency during the treatment period relative to the baseline period.

Of the 254 patients recruited, 55 discontinued from baseline, largely because of failing protocol eligibility; 1 was removed for unreliable seizure calendars; 1 was implanted but not randomized due to device-related infection; and 1 withdrew. The remaining 196 patients were used in intention-to-treat efficacy analysis. Patients receiving HS had a mean 27.9% decrease in total seizure frequency relative to baseline, whereas LS patients had a 15.2% decrease. The difference across HS and LS groups was statistically significant as well (P = .04). HS patients also had a greater reduction in partial onset seizures altering awareness as compared with LS patients. One HS patient was seizure free during the 3-month treatment phase. Adverse events included voice alteration (30.1% HS, 66.3% LS), cough (42.7% HS, 45.3% LS), pharyngitis (25.2% HS, 34.7% LS), pain (30.1% HS, 28.4% LS), dyspnea (10.7% HS, 25.3% LS), headache (23.3% HS, 24.2% LS), dyspepsia (12.6% HS, 17.9% LS), vomiting (13.6% HS, 17.9% LS), paresthesia (25.2% HS, 17.9% LS), nausea (20.4% HS, 14.7% LS), accidental injury (12.6% HS, 12.6% LS), fever (18.4% HS, 11.6% LS), and infection (11.7% HS, 11.6% LS).

After these trials, patients were unblinded and continually followed.[51,52] The results suggested that the efficacy of VNS for epilepsy continued to improve over time. At 12 months, the mean seizure reduction in patients was 45% in an intention-to-treat analysis of the initial 195-person enrollment.[51] Similarly, at 18 months for the 67 patients in the first cohort of the EO3 trial, HS patients had a 52% mean reduction in seizure frequency.[52]

More recently, the American Academy of Neurology evaluated the evidence since 1999 regarding the efficacy and safety of VNS for epilepsy.[11] Researchers reviewed 216 articles concerning VNS stimulation for epilepsy, isolating class III and above reports. It was determined that VNS is possibly effective at achieving seizure frequency reduction of greater than 50% in children with epilepsy. The report recommended that VNS be considered as an adjunctive treatment for children with partial or generalized epilepsy or for patients with Lennox-Gastaut syndrome. In addition, it is suggested that VNS could possibly be effective for mood improvement in adults with epilepsy. Furthermore, VNS may be considered progressively effective in patients over multiple years of exposure; magnet-activated stimulation may be expected to abort seizures one fourth to two thirds of the time; and optimal VNS settings are still unknown. All but one of the studies reviewed, however, were class III evidence, and the authors strongly recommended further investigation of the effectiveness of VNS with regard to other epilepsy syndromes and parameter settings.

Recently, a new vagus nerve stimulator generator was both CE-Mark and FDA approved; the device automatically triggers after detection of tachycardia, which can be associated with seizures in a subset of patients.[53] In a multicenter trial, the system was able to detect a significant number of seizures associated with ictal tachycardia. Only a single subject has been reported, in whom heart rate–triggered stimulation significantly reduced seizure duration.[54] Although this is an approved device, we await clinical results substantiating its increased effectiveness over open-loop VNS, and more complete characterization of the target population.

Noninvasive approaches for seizure control via the vagus nerve and the trigeminal nerve have been explored. Ventureyra[55] proposed transcutaneous stimulation of the vagus nerve via the auricular sensory cutaneous branch, which receives input from the Ramsay-Hunt zone in the external auditory meatus at the tragus. After several pilot studies,[56-58] a single randomized controlled trial suggested efficacy of thrice-daily transcutaneous VNS in the range of invasive VNS, with a statistically significant decrease compared with within-group baseline (median seizure frequency decreasing from six to four per month) and compared with the control group by 12 months.[59] On this basis, a randomized controlled trial in children was planned and is ostensibly ongoing.[60]

Another transcutaneous approach involves bilateral trigeminal nerve stimulation (TNS) via electrodes applied to the ophthalmic and supratrochlear nerves, whose afferents project to the nucleus tractus solitarius and locus caeruleus, two brain structures thought to mediate the effects of VNS (reviewed in DeGiorgio and colleagues[61]). Based on experiments in a rat model,[62] and after pilot studies,[61,63] DeGiorgio and colleagues performed a randomized, active control clinical trial of transcutaneous TNS in 50 patients.[64] Although none of the three primary outcome measures (reduction in seizures over the 18-week treatment period; responder [≥50% reduction] rate for the 18-week treatment period; time to fourth seizure) were significantly different between the treatment and active control groups, certain outcome measures within the treatment group were suggestive of a meaningful effect, such as the median reduction in seizures at 12 weeks. The therapy was well tolerated, however, and the results from this phase 2 study are being used to inform and power a larger phase 3 pivotal trial. Nevertheless, although beset by factors endemic to seizure studies (e.g., large variability in seizure frequencies across patients and groups), the lack of significant results in this trial may reflect a more limited clinically meaningful response than hoped. Nevertheless, if further studies prove effective, transcutaneous or invasive TNS could become another tool in the armamentarium to treat drug-resistant focal epilepsy.

Cerebellum

The earliest subcortical target for electrical stimulation for epilepsy was the cerebellum, which was found as early as the 1950s to modify or halt seizures in animal models of both cortically induced[65,66] and hippocampal[67] seizures. The mechanism of action was originally thought to be thalamic inhibition via stimulation-induced Purkinje cell output, but the veracity of this hypothesis remains somewhat unclear.[33] In the 1970s, Cooper and colleagues were the first to report human cerebellar stimulation for epilepsy (Table 79-2). A heterogeneous patient population underwent subdural stimulation of the superior surface of the cerebellar cortex via an inductively driven system using variable stimulation parameters.[68] Of 15 patients, 10 showed significant seizure improvement for up to 3 years.[69] However, when Van Buren and colleagues used a similar technique to perform a double-blind crossover study of five patients with intractable epilepsy, no significant differences in seizure frequency were detected.[70] Contemporary results were also published by Levy and Auchterlonie, demonstrating a modest response rate of 33% (two of six patients).[71] After these efforts, Wright and colleagues[72] published the results of a prospective double-blind, crossover study of 12 patients with stable, long-term epilepsy (10 to 32 years) using bilateral 8-contact electrodes inserted over the superior cerebellar surface via occipital bur holes. Patients received 2 months of continuous 5- to 7-mA 10-Hz stimulation of alternating polarity that alternated hemispheres every other minute (some patient parameters were uniquely adjusted based on their individual responses), 2 months of self-controlled stimulation, and 2 months of no stimulation. No decrease in the frequency of seizures in the 11 patients available for follow-up was observed, and there was a 25% rate of lead migration, a 16.6% rate of wound infection, and an 8.3% rate of mechanical failure. Interestingly, although there was no objective effect on either seizures or neuropsychological testing, a majority of patients reported that they believed stimulation was beneficial in controlling their seizures.[72]

After these two trials, targeting the cerebellum fell out of favor until a double-blind crossover study by Velasco and colleagues in 2005.[73] Five patients with drug-resistant epilepsy were implanted bilaterally with 4-contact electrodes on the superomedial surface of the cerebellum. Stimulation was delivered with a charge density of 2.0 $\mu C/cm^2$/phase, 0.45-μsec pulse width, 3.8 mA, and frequency of 10 Hz, similarly to Cooper and colleagues.[69,70,72] At 3 months, seizure frequency decreased 33% in blind evaluations of the group receiving stimulation, whereas there was no reduction in the unstimulated group. Mean seizure reduction rate was 41% (range 14%-75%) at the 6-month unblinded evaluation. There was also a statistically significant reduction in tonic ($P < .05$) and tonic-clonic seizures ($P < .001$).

A pooled analysis of prior small series was recently published,[74] demonstrating a seizure freedom rate of 27% (31 of 115 patients) and a reduction of seizures in 76% (87 of 115 patients) in this heterogeneous case series. More rigorously controlled studies across 17 patients demonstrated none to be seizure free, and 5 of 17 with reduced seizures. Overall, the small sample sizes, conflicting results, and high complication rate combine to leave cerebellar stimulation of questionable usefulness in the treatment of intractable seizures.[70,72,73]

Hippocampus

Patients with mesial temporal lobe epilepsy (MTLE), the most common form of drug-resistant epilepsy, have a high rate of seizure freedom[75] after amygdalohippocampal resection,[3,5,8,76] whether by anterior temporal lobectomy (approximately 75%) or selective amygdalohippocampectomy (approximately 72%), or by stereotactic ablation (radiofrequency or laser[77,78]). However, hippocampal resection or ablation may be contraindicated in patients with dominant-onset MTLE with preserved verbal memory and/or dominant temporal lobe function, patients with bilateral mesial temporal onset, or those with recurrent MTLE contralateral to a prior resection. In fact, open resection is associated with a high rate of lateral temporal lobe dysfunction regardless of approach, such as naming or object recognition deficits.[79] Thus, availability of a treatment that can decrease seizure frequency in MTLE to a similar degree as ablative or resective procedures but that preserves interictal function would represent a major advance in the surgical treatment of epilepsy.

The hippocampus is an appealing target for stereotactic neuromodulation techniques, being a frequent target for stereotactic implantation of recording depth electrodes by epilepsy surgeons. Studies in hippocampal slices and rodent models provided preclinical support for electrical neuromodulation of the hippocampus.[23,36,80,81] Velasco and colleagues performed the first human study in a pilot study of stimulation before temporal lobectomy in 10 patients,[28] and more recently reported the findings after 18-month follow-up of nine patients with MTLE[82] (see Table 79-2). Four of these patients had bilateral independent onset, three had onset on the dominant side associated with preserved verbal memory, one had right-sided onset with occasional left-sided epileptiform discharges, and another did not undergo

TABLE 79-2 Median Seizure Reduction over Time in Electrical Stimulation for Epilepsy Pivotal Trials

Treatment	Blind 3 Months	Open Label Year 1	Open Label Year 2	Open Label Year 3
Vagus nerve stimulation[144]	16%	30%	41%	41%
Deep brain stimulation, anterior nucleus of the thalamus*[24,145]	40.4%	41%	56%	53%
Responsive neurostimulation[146]	41.5%	44%	53%	60%

*Constant cohort analysis in patients who completed at least 70 seizure diary days in the blind phase.

resection because of magnetic resonance imaging (MRI) evidence of bilateral hippocampal sclerosis. Four patients underwent bilateral implantation, three on the left and two on the right. Bipolar stimulation was usually delivered to the head of the hippocampus or the amygdalohippocampal junction, with 1-minute trains of square wave pulses at 130 Hz, 450-μsec duration, and 300-μA amplitude, followed by 4-minute stimulation-free intervals (alternating side-to-side in bilateral cases). Five patients were randomized to an initial 1-month, double-blind period without stimulation to investigate possible implantation effects. Of the nine patients, four (44%) were seizure free at 18 months. Interestingly, all four had normal MRI imaging lacking mesial temporal sclerosis. A fifth patient with normal MRI also had an immediate, sharp decrease in seizure frequency and, although not seizure free, continued with only brief, occasional complex partial seizures throughout the study. In contrast, the four patients with evidence of hippocampal sclerosis on MRI showed more delayed and partial responses to stimulation, with seizure reduction becoming statistically significant by 8 months and leveling off (with 50% to 70% reduction) by 10 months. The authors suggest that decreased cell counts and, presumably, lesser network connectivity of a sclerotic hippocampus provide an explanation for the delayed effectiveness in these patients. Seizure freedom and levels of seizure reduction were maintained through 18 months of follow-up in all patients.

In the aforementioned work, patients had first been implanted with 8-contact diagnostic depth electrodes. In one patient this resulted in more posterior DBS placement than would have occurred with standardized placement in the head of the hippocampus. This may be important in the minority of patients with posterior onset,[83] although this is far from definitive; it is not inconceivable that stimulation anywhere in the hippocampus would be beneficial, irrespective of the epileptogenic zone.

The second group with a substantial experience with hippocampal stimulation is the Belgian group of Boon and colleagues[84] (see Table 79-2). In their approach, 12 patients underwent bilateral implantation with two quadripolar DBS electrodes through a posterior approach with one terminating in the amygdala and one terminating in the anterior hippocampus, and were simultaneously implanted with invasive monitoring electrodes (grid and/or strip electrodes) to determine the seizure onset zone(s). All but one patient (with unilateral mesial temporal onset who underwent resection) were then acutely stimulated—10 unilaterally, and one patient with bilateral onset, bilaterally. All 8 contacts across the amygdala and hippocampal quadripolar electrodes on the side of onset were used for stimulation in each patient with unilateral stimulation, whereas the patient with bilateral stimulation was stimulated through the four bilateral hippocampal electrodes (not the amygdalar one) only. In 10 of 11 patients there was a greater than 50% reduction in interictal spikes leading to chronic stimulation. Bipolar stimulation was delivered through two pairs of contacts on each electrode (but see comment later), with mean output voltage of 2.3 V (range 2-3 V), frequency of 130 Hz (one patient at 200 Hz), and pulse width of 450 μsec. During the last 6 months of stimulation (mean total follow-up 33 months; range 15-52 months), only one patient (10%) was seizure free, one had seizure frequency reduction greater than 90%, five had seizure reduction greater than 50%, two had 30% to 49% seizure reduction, and one had less than 30% reduction. In long-term follow-up, going from unilateral to bilateral stimulation improved three of five patients who had less than 90% reduction, with one becoming seizure free, despite onset regions being unilateral; the previously seizure-free patient remained so despite stimulation being discontinued at battery end of life, and one other patient became seizure free when stimulation was stopped.[85] Thus, although a total of six patients (55%) achieved greater than 90% seizure reduction, the overall 27% rate of seizure freedom (3 of 11) in this long-term follow-up group must be cautiously interpreted. Interestingly, in contrast to the results of Velasco and colleagues, two of three patients in this study with hippocampal sclerosis became seizure free in contrast to only 1 of 11 without.

Possible explanations for the low rate of seizure freedom in this study include (1) the fact that 50% of patients had regional onset in the temporal lobe, rather than a well-defined mesial temporal onset, and (2) limited coverage of the hippocampus despite the implantation of two electrodes per side. One electrode was implanted in the amygdala, and stimulation was delivered cathodically with Lilly pulse waveforms (charge-balanced biphasic pulses designed to prevent charge deposition and resultant tissue damage) rather than truly in a bipolar fashion, which would ostensibly stimulate at both contacts in a bipolar pair.

Two small series of patients with hippocampal stimulation have been reported by the University of Western Ontario group.[86,87] The first involved four unilateral stimulation patients with left mesial temporal seizure onset who were unable to undergo resection (one because of prior right temporal resection, three because of failed intracarotid amobarbital testing), and the second involved two bilateral implantations. Both series were double-blind, randomized crossover designs with 3 months of stimulation on and 3 months off (with slightly different designs in the two studies). Certainly, the amount of hippocampus stimulated was greater compared with the Belgium studies: in this case contacts were 3 mm, with 6-mm spacing spanning 30 mm of hippocampus, and stimulation was performed at all 4 contacts within hippocampus in monopolar cathodic arrangement (continuous 190 Hz, pulse width 90 μsec, voltage adjusted below the patients' conscious thresholds, ranging from 1.8 to 4.5 V). None of the six patients became seizure free; the median seizure frequency reduction was only 15% (not statistically significant) in the unilateral stimulation patients and 33% in the bilateral stimulation patients. Notably, five of the six patients had imaging evidence of hippocampal sclerosis. In addition, these investigations explored multiple neuropsychological measures; although none of the unilateral stimulation patients showed any difference between the stimulation-on and stimulation-off states, one of the bilateral stimulation patients showed declines in verbal and visuospatial learning scores during stimulation.

Similar degrees of effectiveness were found by Boëx and colleagues[87] in eight patients (two hippocampal sclerosis, six nonlesional) implanted unilaterally, five of whom had bilateral onset and three of whom had onset ipsilateral to preserved verbal memory. DBS was on the side of more frequent seizure onset as determined noninvasively (three patients) or with intracranial recording (five patients). The first five patients received quadripolar electrodes (3-mm contacts with 6-mm spacing; total length 30 mm) and the last three received octrodes (3-mm contacts with 1.5-mm spacing; total length 34.5 mm). Stimulation was tested in both monopolar configuration, with 4 contacts as the cathode (130 Hz, pulse width 450 μsec, 1-2 V), and in bipolar configuration (130 Hz, pulse width 450 μsec, 0.5-1.5 V), using the 2 contacts with the highest frequency of interictal discharges as cathode and anode. Regardless of electrode configuration or parameters, only two patients (25%) became seizure free—one without stimulation. Four patients, including the two with hippocampal sclerosis, had 50% to 90% reduction in seizure frequency. Interestingly, all six patients with greater than 50% seizure frequency reduction had active contacts located within 3 mm of the subiculum, whereas the two nonresponders had electrodes more than 3 mm from the subiculum. Proximity to the presumed seizure onset zone, in contrast, was not associated with outcome, with responders' and nonresponders' active contacts located 11 ± 4.3 mm (mean ± standard deviation [SD]) and 9.1 ± 2.3 mm from the ictal onset zone, respectively. Among several confounding factors in this study was the use of unilateral stimulation in patients with bilateral onset, and low-stimulation voltages with maximum amplitude of 2 V, potentially limiting the volume of tissue stimulated.

Overall, the open-label studies suggested that hippocampal stimulation is not likely to lead to a high rate of seizure freedom, although many patients may experience a significant decrease in seizure frequency. However, the value of hippocampal DBS remains difficult to assess in the absence of larger, prospective and controlled studies, two of which are underway.[88,89] In addition, the results are consistent with those from the randomized, double-blind, sham-stimulation controlled trial of the Responsive Neurostimulation System (RNS System; NeuroPace, Mountain View, CA), in which 50% of 191 patients underwent stimulation in the amygdalohippocampal region via chronic depth electrodes[45] (discussed later). On the other hand, hippocampal stimulation appears to be safe and not to carry significant neuropsychological risks.[82,90,91] Thus, it appears likely that hippocampal stimulation will emerge as a tool to reduce the frequency of—but not eliminate—seizures in patients who are not candidates for surgical resection or ablation, which remains the gold standard for achieving seizure freedom in MTLE.

Subthalamic Nucleus and Substantia Nigra

The role of the basal ganglia and dorsal midbrain has been explored experimentally in animal models of limbic seizures[92-95] (see Fig. 79-1), implicating a role for the substantia nigra reticulata and the subthalamic nucleus (STN). High-frequency stimulation of the STN was indeed effective in rodent models, although the mechanism(s) and pathways involved remain poorly understood.[96-98] Nevertheless, these studies provide some foundation for STN stimulation in the treatment of epilepsy in patients[99-105] (see Table 79-1; Fig. 79-3). Five patients underwent bilateral STN DBS (some with multiple leads) for various types of inoperable seizures,[104,105] of whom three—all with paracentral neocortical seizures—experienced 67% to 80% seizure reduction. The other two patients—one with Dravet's syndrome and one with frontoinsular seizures—did not show significant improvement. Handforth and colleagues[100] reported 50% reduction in seizure frequency in a patient with bitemporal electroencephalographic onset and 33% reduction in another with postencephalitic hemiatrophy and left-sided seizure onset; the latter patient also experienced a reduction in seizure severity and arrest of generalized convulsions, fewer seizure-related injuries, and an improved quality of life. Capecci and colleagues[102] presented two cases of bilateral STN DBS after failed disconnective surgery. The first patient, who had widespread cortical atrophy, multiple seizure types, and prior anterior callosotomy, demonstrated a 70% reduction of partial seizures and 85% reduction of secondarily generalized seizures at 1 year with STN stimulation (2.0 V, 60 µsec, 130 Hz; stimulator off at night). The second patient had a decrease in tonic-clonic seizures but a sharp increase in absence seizures with continuous STN stimulation (3.0 V, 130 Hz, 60 µsec), which led to discontinuation of stimulation.

Vesper and colleagues[101] reported a patient who experienced 50% reduction in the severity and frequency of myoclonic seizures with stimulation spanning the inferior STN and substantia nigra bilaterally; the patient was able to discontinue use of VNS without recurrence of generalized seizures, which previously had been controlled only with VNS. Subsequently, Wille and colleagues[108] reported a series of five adults with progressive myoclonic epilepsy who were followed in an unblinded fashion for 12 to 42 months; all of them experienced 30% to 100% reduction of myoclonic seizure frequency from bilateral STN DBS, with accompanying improvement in quality of life. Of note, four patients did not benefit from simultaneously implanted bilateral Vim thalamus leads.

Based on the aforementioned case series, STN DBS may be a palliative option, particularly in patients with myoclonic epilepsy. Unfortunately, the Grenoble-based Assessment of Subthalamic Nucleus Stimulation in Drug Resistant Epilepsy (STIMEP) trial was terminated owing to insufficient enrollment, and no larger scale or randomized trials of STN stimulation appear to be forthcoming.

Centromedian Nucleus of the Thalamus

On the basis of its widespread projections to the cortex and its role in cortical excitability (see Fig. 79-1),[19,29,30,109,110] the centromedian nucleus has been explored as a potential target for DBS therapy (see Table 79-1). A group in Mexico City has reported several series[111-115] using an alternating left-right stimulation paradigm (60 Hz, 500-600 µA, 1 minute on/4 minutes off, 24 hr/day). The best results were seen in 12 of the 13 patients with Lennox-Gastaut syndrome (of 18 total patients): two became seizure free, eight experienced 50% to 80% seizure reduction, and three had no response to therapy. Maximal results were observed after 6 months of stimulation. Double-blind 3-month periods of stimulation cessation (6 to 12 months after surgery), however, did not show a return to baseline frequency. Although patient bias cannot be excluded, a more likely explanation is residual antiepileptic effect, possibly related to neural plasticity. Patients with partial epilepsy syndromes fared less well than those

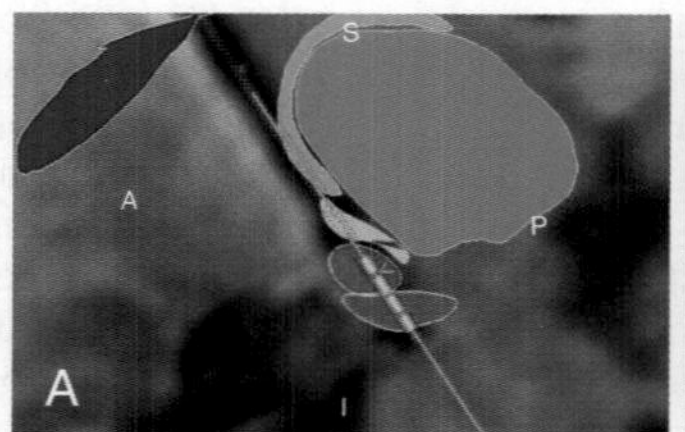

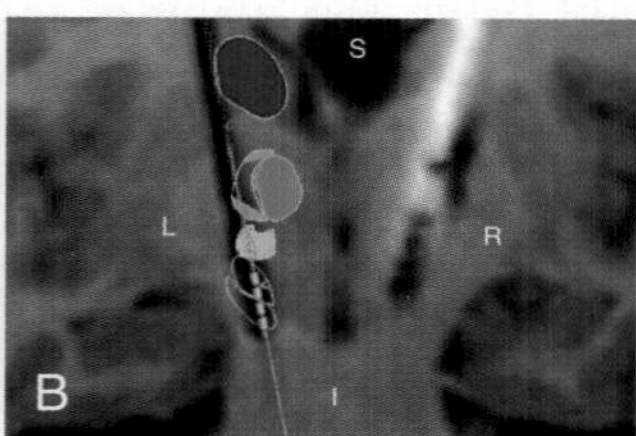

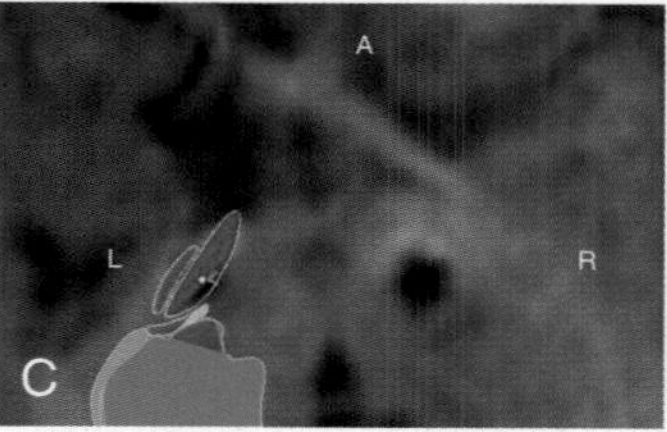

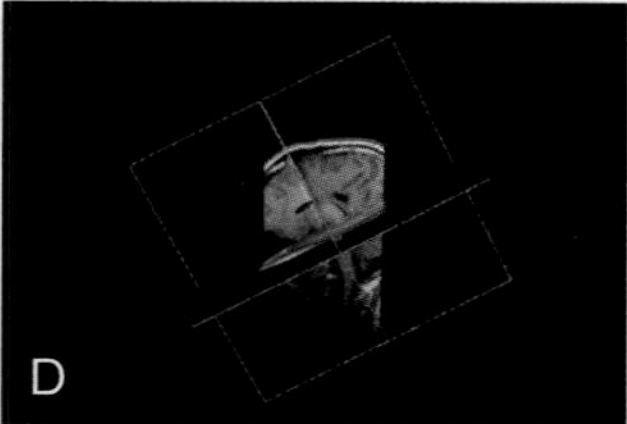

Figure 79-3. Subthalamic nucleus (STN) deep brain stimulation (DBS) for epilepsy. Magnetic resonance imaging scan of patient implanted with STN DBS for drug-resistant epilepsy. The patient had frequent secondarily generalized seizures, the frequency of which was significantly reduced by the DBS. **A,** Sagittal view, with atlas overlay morphed to the patient's anatomy to depict the basal ganglia structures. A model of the DBS electrode is overlaid on the artifact of the actual electrode to allow visualization of the location of each contact. The electrode array was situated to span the STN and substantia nigra reticulata, which has also been implicated in seizure modulation. The *caret* (also seen in **B**) indicates the location of the plane of section in **C.** *Blue,* caudate nucleus; *yellow,* thalamus; *red,* subthalamic nucleus; *green,* substantia nigra reticulata. **B,** Coronal view. **C,** Axial view. The contralateral electrode array can be seen in **B** and **C. D,** View depicting the plane of section of the coronal view in **B** and the axial view in **C.** A, anterior; I, inferior; P, posterior; S, superior.

with generalized epilepsies, with only two of five achieving greater than 80% seizure reduction.[113,115]

Despite these promising results, an early attempt to demonstrate centromedian nucleus benefits in a small randomized sham-stimulation double-blind crossover design study was not successful,[116] mostly because of methodologic issues. During the 3-month stimulation periods there was a 30% decrease in seizures as compared with an 8% decrease during sham periods, but these results were not statistically significant, in large measure owing to the small number of subjects. Other confounding factors were present as well. First, the amplitude for active stimulation was set at 50% of the sensory threshold in order to maintain effective blinding, likely somewhat below that used in the Mexico City studies, in which amplitudes were 90% of sensory threshold (although details of the actual stimulation amplitude, ranging from 0.5-10 V, were not provided). When thresholds were allowed to increase to this level during the open-label extension in the study by Fisher and colleagues, three of six patients experienced a greater than 50% reduction of generalized tonic-clonic seizures.[116] Second, the controlled study design may well have affected outcomes beyond bias control: one patient who was initially randomized to active stimulation had a marked reduction in seizures and refused to undergo sham stimulation, eliminating one of the responders from the data analysis. Although a crossover design with a washout period is methodologically rigorous, it is still fraught with difficulties and assumptions and has rarely been used for DBS studies since publication of this trial.

Most recently, Valentín and colleagues[117] reported 11 patients (5 with frontal lobe epilepsy, 6 with primary generalized epilepsy) treated with centromedian nucleus DBS at two centers in London and Madrid. After bilateral implantation, patients underwent single-blinded treatment with 3 months of sham stimulation followed by 3 months of therapeutic stimulation (up to 5 V at 130 Hz with a pulse width of 90 μsec), then 6 months of open-label therapeutic stimulation. Open-label stimulation was maintained after 12 months for patients in whom stimulation was thought to be effective. All six patients with generalized epilepsy had greater than 50% seizure reduction during the blinded phase, and five of six maintained greater than 50% seizure reduction during the long-term extension phase, whereas only one of five frontal lobe epilepsy patients experienced greater than 50% improvement in seizure frequency during the blinded phase. During the open-label long-term extension, the frontal lobe patients had a heterogeneous response, with three demonstrating 50% to 90% reduction in seizure frequency and two showing no clear signs of improvement.

Taken together, multiple studies suggest that centromedian nucleus DBS may be effective for a subset of patients with generalized epilepsy, particularly those with Lennox-Gastaut syndrome or with predominance of tonic-clonic or other generalized seizures. For unknown reasons, centromedian nucleus DBS appears to show strong implantation and carryover neuromodulatory effects even without active stimulation. Moreover, the mechanism of action of centromedian nucleus DBS remains to be elucidated. Although initially predicated on the widespread cortical projections from the centromedian nucleus, strong influences on the striatum and the possible role of the cortico-striatal-basal ganglionic-thalamocortical network in epilepsy raise other possibilities as well.

Anterior Nucleus of the Thalamus

The ANT (see Fig. 79-1) in fact consists of several distinct subnuclei, some of which have extensive frontal and temporal cortical projections, and others of which are key stations in the limbic circuit of Papez.[118] Thus the ANT is an attractive target for both modulation of overall thalamocortical excitability and modulation of the limbic seizure network.[22] Early lesion studies of the ANT in cats and nonhuman primates demonstrated effective reduction in seizure frequency and duration,[119] and human studies began as early as the 1960s.[120,121] Several small open-label studies throughout the 2000s showed promising decreases in seizure frequency—approximately 30% to 90%—with prominent implantation effects as well as carryover effects with 2 to 3 months of stimulation cessation,[122-126] leading to the Stimulation of the Anterior Nucleus of the Thalamus for Epilepsy (SANTE) trial, a multicenter, randomized, double-blind trial of bilateral stimulation of the ANT for localization-related epilepsy[24] (Fig. 79-4). One hundred and ten subjects with medically refractory partial seizures with or without secondarily generalized seizures underwent implantation with bilateral ANT DBS leads and were randomized to either 3 months of stimulation (5 V, 90-μsec pulse duration, 145 Hz frequency, 1 minute on alternating with 5 minutes off) or sham stimulation. After the blinded evaluation

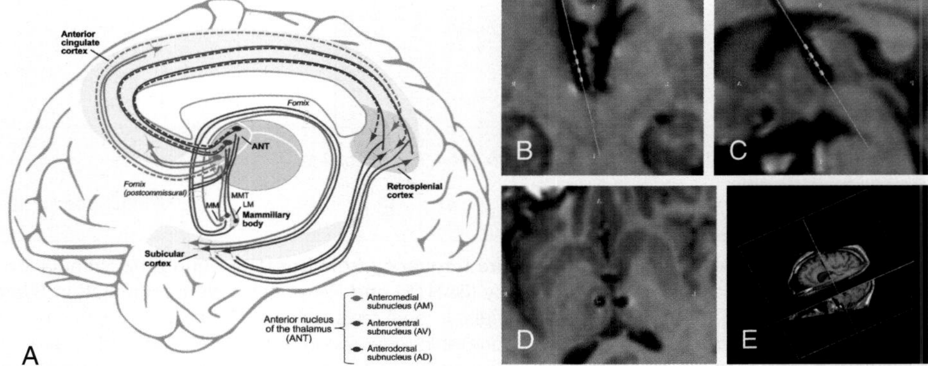

Figure 79-4. Stimulation of the anterior nucleus of the thalamus (ANT) for epilepsy. A, Illustration of the three distinct neural pathways through the ANT, with distinctive patterns of connectivity. LM, lateral mammillary nucleus; MM, medial mammillary nucleus; MMT, mammillothalamic tract. These three ANT subnuclei were not specifically targeted in the Stimulation of the Anterior Nucleus of the Thalamus for Epilepsy (SANTE) clinical trial. **B,** Coronal magnetic resonance image showing the location of implanted deep brain stimulation (DBS) electrode array in ANT as part of the SANTE trial. **C,** Sagittal view of ANT DBS electrode array. **D,** Axial view of ANT DBS electrode array. **E,** Planes of section of the coronal image in **B** and the axial image in **D.** *(**A,** From Child ND, Benarroch EE. Anterior nucleus of the thalamus: functional organization and clinical implications.* Neurology. *2013;81:1869-1876.)*

period, all patients received open-label stimulation for 9 months, after which antiepileptic drugs and stimulation parameters could be freely adjusted.

After a notable implantation effect of median 21% to 22% seizure reduction in both groups at 1 month of stimulation (although placebo and/or regression to the mean effects could also have been factors), the two groups began to progressively separate until the end of the blinded period (Fig. 79-5), such that in the third (and final) month of blinded stimulation there was an unequivocal statistical difference in seizure frequency between the two groups (median 40.4% reduction in seizures in active stimulation as compared with 14.5% reduction with sham stimulation; P = .0017). The actual prespecified primary outcome measure, a generalized estimating equation (GEE) model encompassing the entire 3-month blinded evaluation period, did not generate a result for the group of 108 subjects (2 of the 110 were excluded owing to explantation, one before randomization, and one 4 days shy of the prespecified 70 seizure diary days after stimulation) because of a treatment-by-visit (i.e., months of follow-up) interaction (likely a result of the lack of a significant difference between the groups prior to the third month of treatment). However, a post hoc analysis, excluding one patient in the stimulated group who was statistically determined to be an outlier (when first activated at the protocol-determined 5 V this patient recorded 210 brief partial seizures during the 1-minute on-stimulation phases over 3 days, but later had decreased seizures at 4 V) and including in the sham stimulation group the patient who had only 66 of the 70 required days of seizure diaries before explantation, did generate a statistically significant treatment over the entire blinded evaluation phase (P = .039) using the GEE model.

Notwithstanding the primary outcome measure results, seizure frequency continued to decline during the open-label stimulation phase, with a median seizure frequency decrease of 41% at 1 year, 56% at 2 years,[24] and 69% at 5 years (N = 74), whereas the 50% responder rate increased from 43% at 1 year to 54% at 2 years[24] and 68% at 5 years (N = 59).[127] However, only 16% of subjects became seizure free for at least 6 months during the first 5 years of the trial, only six subjects (5.5%) were seizure free for over 2 continuous years, and 11 (10%) were seizure free over the last 6 months at the 5-year follow-up. Complaints of memory impairment occurred in 27% of subjects over the course

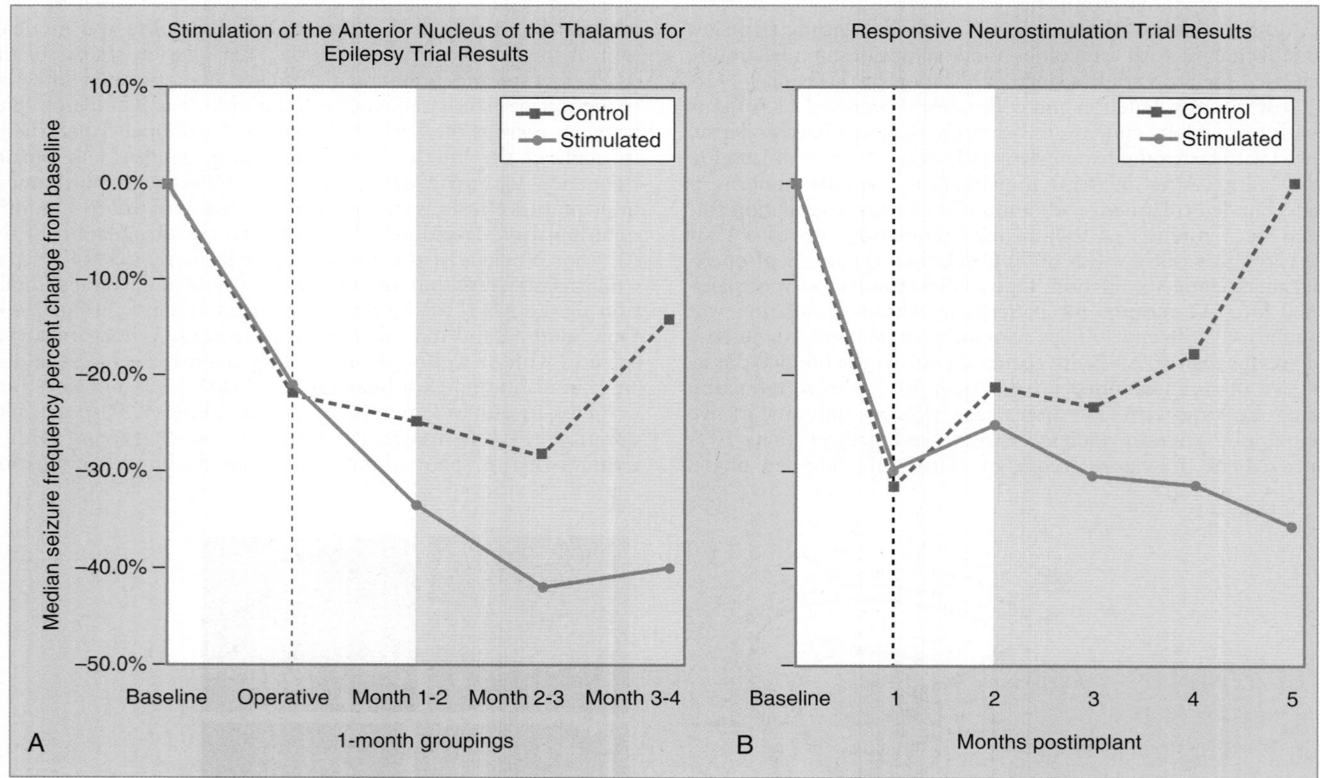

Figure 79-5. Median percentage change in seizure frequency from baseline during the Stimulation of the Anterior Nucleus of the Thalamus for Epilepsy (SANTE) and Responsive Neurostimulation System (RNS System; NeuroPace, Mountain View, CA) trials. In both trials, stimulation began 1 month after implantation *(vertical dashed line).* **A,** Despite an appreciable reduction in seizure frequency with implantation, control patients *(purple dashed line)* in the SANTE trial did not experience significant reduction of the mean seizure frequency during the blinded phase of the trial *(gray).* In contrast, stimulated patients *(green solid line),* experienced a median 40.4% reduction in seizure frequency by the final blinded month, as compared with a 14.5% reduction in controls. **B,** Stimulated patients in the RNS System trial also demonstrated an appreciable reduction in seizure frequency after implantation. Stimulation was optimized for a month before the blinded evaluation phase *(gray).* Stimulated patients experienced a 37.9% median reduction in seizure frequency during the blinded evaluation phase, as opposed to a 17.3% reduction in controls (P = .012). *(Modified from Fisher R, Salanova V, Witt T, et al. Electrical stimulation of the anterior nucleus of thalamus for treatment of refractory epilepsy.* Epilepsia. *2010;51:899-908; and Morrell MJ. Responsive cortical stimulation for the treatment of medically intractable partial epilepsy.* Neurology. *2011;77:129501394.)*

of the trial. Memory loss was never serious, it occurred in the context of baseline memory impairment in 50%, and overall group statistics did not show decline in memory measures. Rather, improvements were noted in various measures including attention, executive function, and mood. On the basis of the SANTE trial, approval was granted by the regulatory agencies in Canada, Europe, Australia, and elsewhere, but at the time of this writing not yet in the United States.

Responsive Neurostimulation

The publication in 2011 of the multicenter pivotal trial of the NeuroPace responsive neurostimulator (RNS System) was the first demonstration of the feasibility and efficacy of closed-loop, automated detection and interruption of seizure activity using direct cortical stimulation. This multicenter, double-blind, randomized controlled trial began in 2005 and included 191 participants with cranially implanted, programmable RNS System devices connected to one or two depth or subdural recording and stimulating cortical leads (Fig. 79-6).[45] For each patient, lead placement was individually targeted to the putative zone of seizure onset, in most cases (59%) as determined by previous intracranial monitoring.

Patients were randomized at 1 month after surgery to receive either active or sham stimulation. After an additional month to fine-tune seizure detection in the active group, double-blind evaluation of active and control groups was conducted over a 3-month period. At the end of the blinded period (5 months post-implantation) the active-stimulation group experienced a 41.5% reduction in seizures, compared with 9.4% reduction for the sham group ($P < .01$). Similar to the acute effects seen in the SANTE trial, there was a significant implantation effect (see Fig. 79-6). However, the reduction in seizure frequency decreased over time in the sham group and increased over time in the active-stimulation group during the blinded period. After the blinded period, all patients received active stimulation. The responder rate (>50% seizure reduction) was 43% at 1 year post-implantation and 46% at 2 years. Thirteen subjects were seizure free over the most recent 3-month period relative to the data cutoff date.

Interestingly, the overall seizure reduction rates were similar in the SANTE and RNS System trials (see Fig. 79-6). In the RNS System trial, however, the significance of the GEE outcome measure was not dependent on the lobe of seizure onset, perhaps reflecting the individualized (and therefore potentially more accurate) targeting of cortical foci. After a lengthy process, the RNS System received FDA approval in 2013.

An added benefit of the continuous electrocorticography (ECoG) provided by the RNS System, a design feature to enable responsive triggering of stimulation, is very long-term chronic ambulatory monitoring of the seizure onset zone(s) in a naturalistic setting. We have shown that onset in the hippocampus can be confined to one side or the other for extended periods of time (Fig. 79-7).[128] In 82 patients from the RNS System pivotal trial with mesial temporal lobe electrodes (see Fig. 79-6) it took longer than 1 month to detect contralateral seizures in one third of patients.[129] Indeed, this may explain in part the approximately 25% failure rate after open amygdalohippocampectomy. Such monitoring can help to make a more definitive onset zone diagnosis in difficult cases, and may lead to resective (or ablative) surgery in some patients not thought to be candidates.[129,130] This unintended application is likely to be used to a greater extent in coming years.

CONCLUSION AND FUTURE DIRECTIONS

Although the use of electrical stimulation for epilepsy has been explored for a half-century, only VNS, ANT DBS (outside of the United States but not within), and RNS (within the United States but not outside) have successfully obtained regulatory approval (see Table 79-2). This, however, is not the yardstick by which the success of this therapeutic modality should be evaluated. This measure reflects the determination of an industrial collaborator to pursue the ability to market these neuromodulatory devices, and in fact all three of these approaches can be judged successes by this metric. Conversely, an approximately 50% reduction in seizures, with relatively small numbers of patients becoming seizure free, is clearly inadequate: patients receiving electrical stimulation therapy who are not candidates for resective or ablative surgery because of risk or multifocality, or in whom surgery has failed, aspire to seizure freedom as do all patients. New strategies and approaches to increase effectiveness of neuromodulatory treatments must be sought.

Advancement along several avenues may yield improved results. First, understanding of the mechanisms of action of brain stimulation is still rudimentary.[131-133] Elucidation of the mechanism(s) of DBS will enable tailoring of the target within the network, as well as tailoring of stimulation parameters to activate, inhibit, or regulate information flow through the network. A recent technology that is already contributing to this avenue is optogenetics, in which specific cell populations can be activated or inhibited through use of light-activated ion channels and pumps. For example, in rodent epilepsy models, blocking hippocampal pyramidal cell activity using halorhodopsin, or activating inhibitory neurons using channel rhodopsin, modulated seizure activity,[134] and the latter suggested that bilateral activation of even a small subset of neurons was sufficient.

Second, technologic innovations may lead to incremental advances. Constant-current devices may be more consistent by automatically adapting to impedance changes.[135] Novel devices may enable more predictable and directed ("steerable") stimulation volumes and better avoidance of stimulation side effects.[136-138] Closed-loop (feedback-controlled) neurostimulation devices may provide additional benefits in device longevity, and perhaps effectiveness and tolerability, and in fact have been instantiated in the optogenetic experiments noted previously to limit light delivery to the necessary times. In fact, a novel bidirectional stimulation and recording pulse generator unit is being used for research in human subjects (Activa PC+S, Medtronic, Minneapolis, MN), and a closed-loop state control algorithm was recently tested in a large animal (sheep) model,[139,140] with spectral power monitored and modulated in the hippocampus via one DBS electrode implanted, in response to stimulation through a second electrode placed in the ANT, another node in the network (Fig. 79-8).[141,142] The power could be continuously kept low in the hippocampus by a closed-loop algorithm, thereby keeping the hippocampus in the less sensitive state for seizure evocation. Finally, the RNS System, presently limited to direct application at the seizure focus, may be in the future applied to indirect modulatory nodes within the epileptic circuit, such as the ANT or the centromedian nucleus, in response to seizures detected elsewhere.

Third, better understanding of the networks mediating the occurrence and propagation of seizures will inform neuromodulation approaches. The success to date in ANT DBS for refractory epilepsy likely results in part from the somewhat stereotyped pathways for seizure propagation through the ANT in MTLE (60% of patients in the SANTE trial had onset in the temporal lobe[24]) and perhaps forms of frontal lobe epilepsy that may share those pathways. However, even in this case increased understanding of the various pathways through ANT may allow refinement of targeting and improved results.[118] Foci outside the mesial temporal lobe likely have different propagation networks; in vivo studies of epileptogenic networks may therefore allow more rational and patient-specific targeting for DBS placement in this heterogeneous and more difficult-to-treat group of patients.

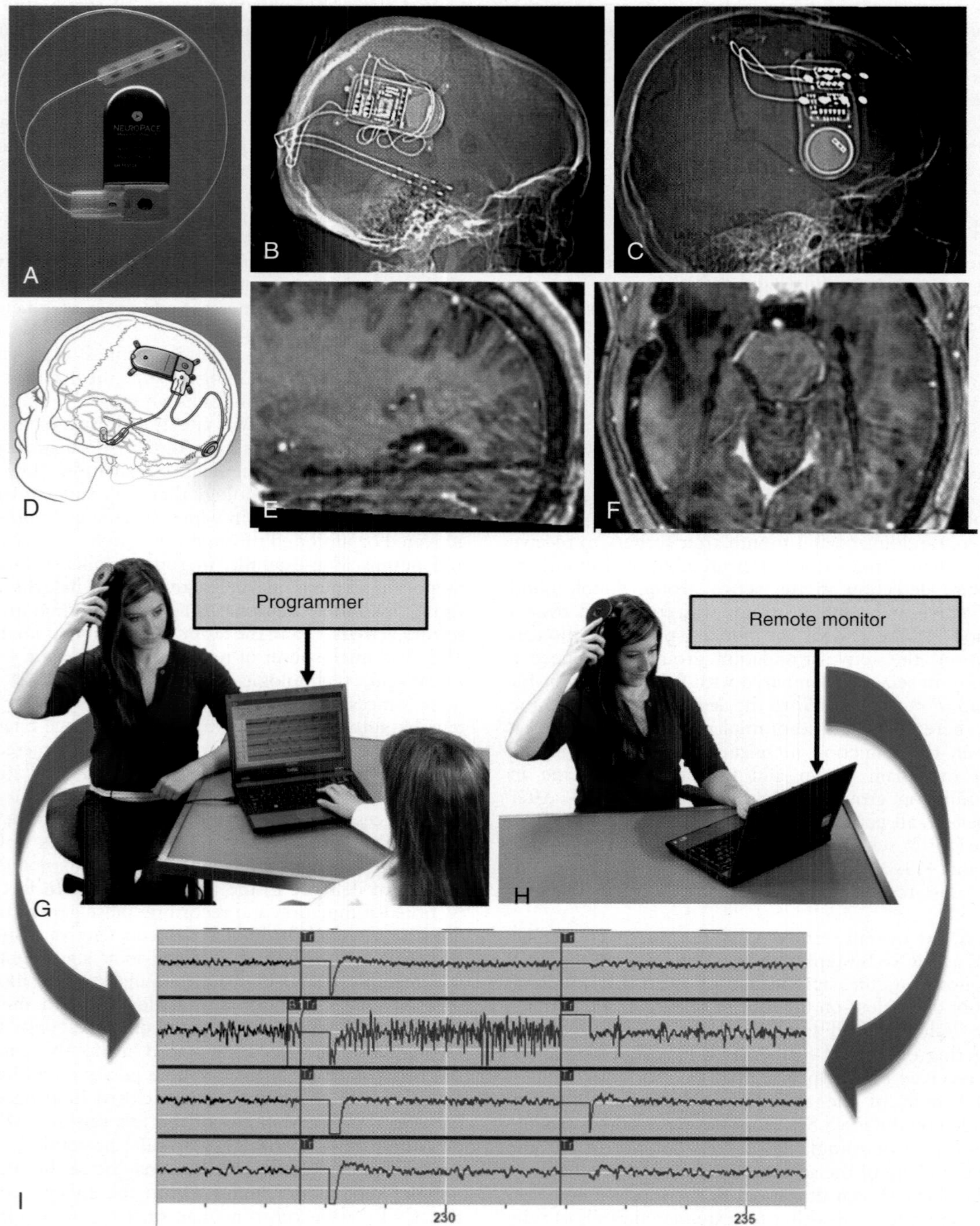

Figure 79-6. Responsive Neurostimulation (RNS) System (NeuroPace, Mountain View, CA) for the treatment of epilepsy. The RNS System is depicted in **A** and **D.** The system consists of an implanted pulse generator with a primary battery cell to which are attached one or two electrode arrays, which can be either depth electrode arrays or surface strip arrays. **B,** Lateral radiograph showing the pulse generator implanted into the skull after craniectomy of a window of bone sized to the generator; in this case two hippocampal depth arrays are present, implanted via an occipital approach. **C,** Lateral radiograph of pulse generator overlying two 4-contact surface arrays implanted over the left inferior frontal gyrus (Broca's region). Lateral **(E)** and axial **(F)** magnetic resonance imaging (MRI) scan of bilateral hippocampal depth electrode arrays. In this case, brain MRI of RNS System depth electrodes—which is not approved by the U.S. Food and Drug Administration (FDA)—was performed because of a nonsurgically related neurological condition for which MRI was necessary. The RNS System performs continuous electrocorticography (ECoG); the stored electrocorticogram **(I)** is downloaded telemetrically to the programmer's computer **(G),** and changes in the stimulation program are uploaded telemetrically as well. Similarly the electrocorticogram is downloaded to the patient's computer **(H)** for uploading via the Internet to the patient data management system (PDMS), where it can be scrutinized by the physician and manufacturer's technical experts, and simulations of seizure detection can be performed for optimization in advance of the patient's visit with the programmer. The effect of responsive electrical stimulation is shown in the electrocorticogram **(I).** Each line depicts the recording from the 4 electrode contacts. In the second line down, an electrographic seizure is detected and triggers a stimulation *(blue line),* during which recording is flat because the amplifier is blanked to prevent saturation. The first stimulation is ineffective and the electrographic seizure continues. However, after a second detection and stimulation *(second blue line)* the seizure activity is abrogated.

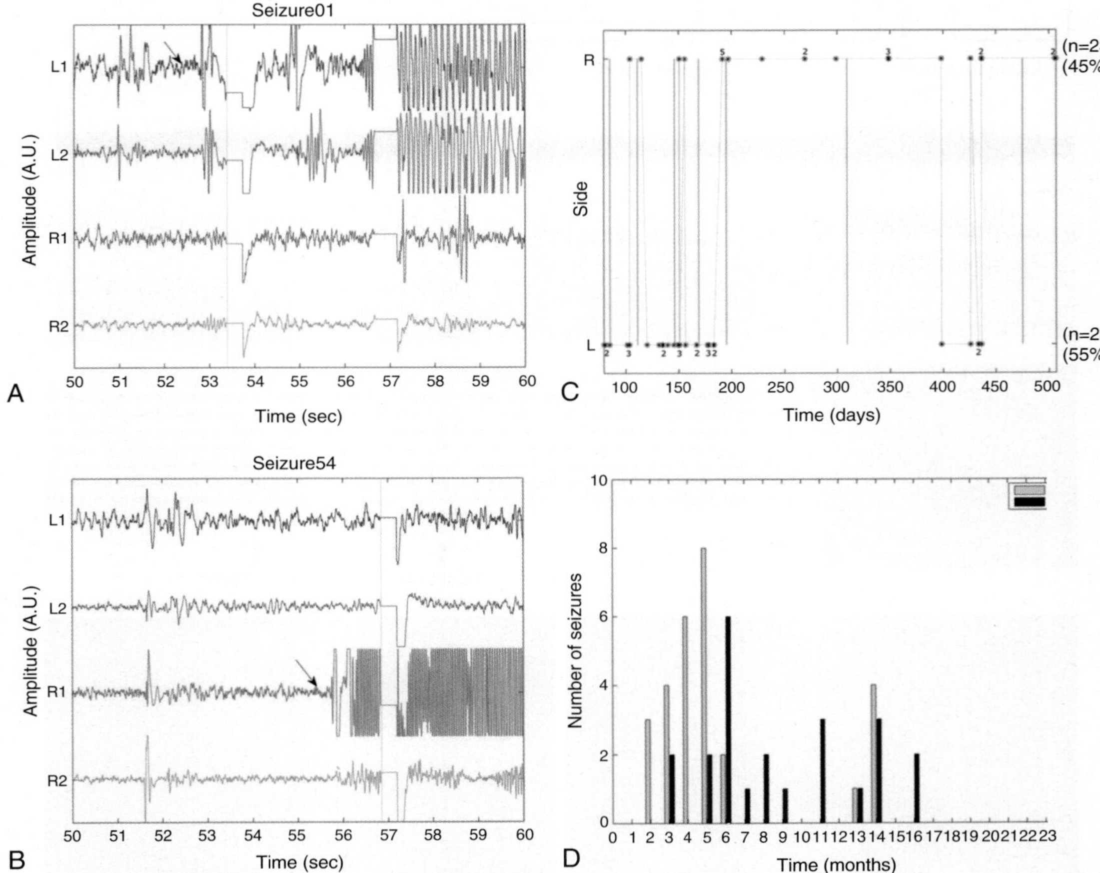

Figure 79-7. Shifting laterality of mesial temporal (hippocampal) seizures as detected electrocorticographically by the Responsive Neurostimulation (RNS) System (NeuroPace, Mountain View, CA). A and **B,** Electrocorticographic recordings from both hippocampi in a patient with drug-resistant epilepsy implanted with the RNS System because of possible bilateral onset. L1 and L2, and R1 and R2 are from two adjacent bipolar pairs from the left and right, respectively. **A,** The first and **B,** the 54th electrocorticographic seizures with L1 and R1 seizure onset zones, respectively *(arrows).* The detection-elicited stimulation therapy is depicted by the *vertical line.* Tracking **(C)** and tallying **(D)** of the electrocorticographic seizures is shown. Tracking of the seizure onset zone laterality **(C)** and localization **(D)** shows shifts from the left (L1 and L2) to the right (R1 and R2) side over daily **(C)** and monthly **(D)** timescales for the seizures *(black asterisk)* unrelated to changes in RNS System detection or stimulation parameters *(solid vertical lines).*

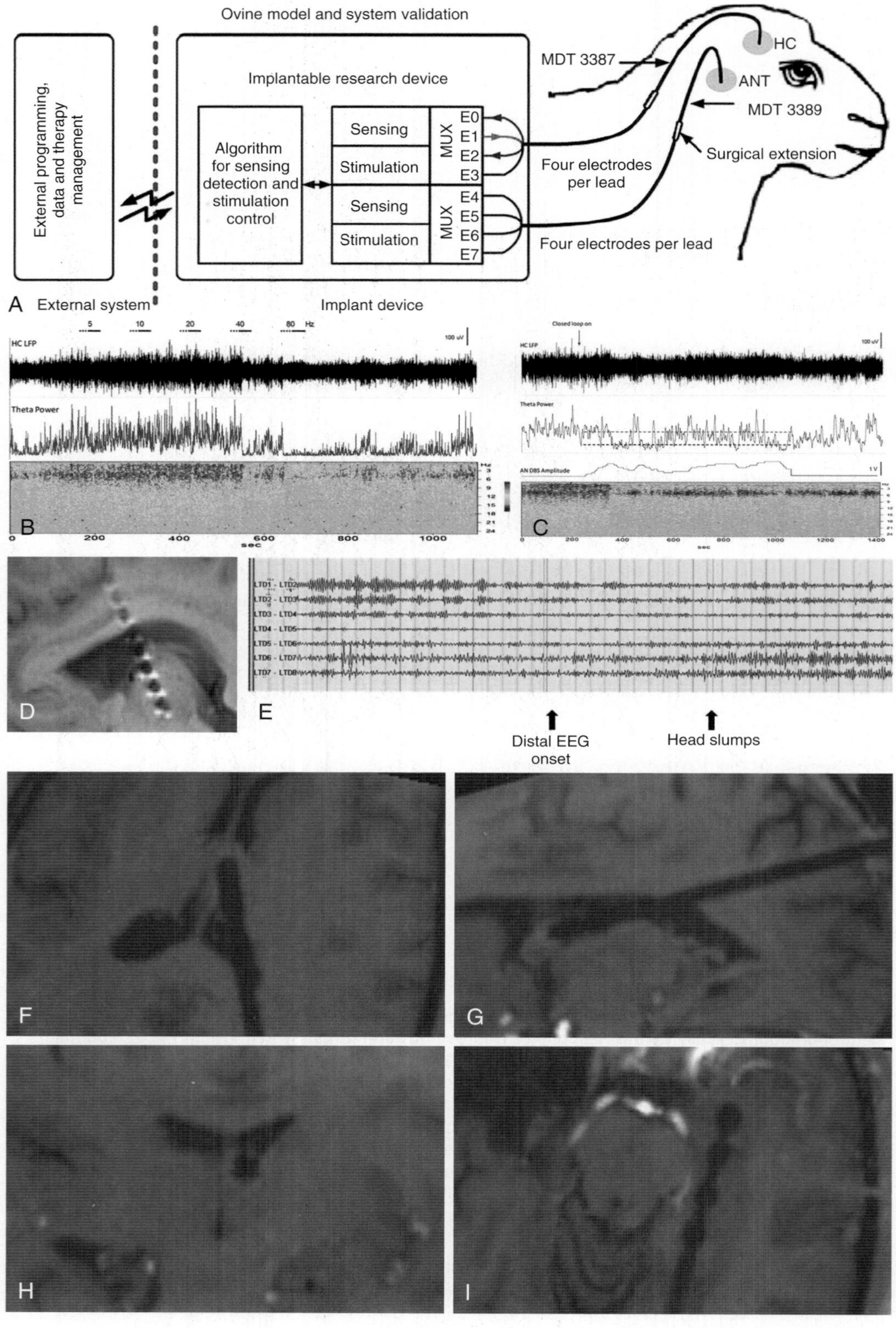
Ovine model and system validation
External programming, data and therapy management
Implantable research device
Algorithm for sensing detection and stimulation control
Sensing
Stimulation
MUX
E0
E1
E2
E3
Sensing
Stimulation
MUX
E4
E5
E6
E7
MDT 3387
HC
ANT
MDT 3389
Surgical extension
Four electrodes per lead
Four electrodes per lead
A
External system
Implant device
5
10
20
40
80 Hz
HC LFP
Theta Power
B
sec
C
Closed loop on
D
E
Distal EEG onset
Head slumps
F
G
H
I

Figure 79-8. Novel approaches to electrical stimulation for epilepsy. A, A novel approach to electrical stimulation involves concurrent sensing and stimulation, in which two electrode arrays are implanted in different nodes within an epileptic circuit. Depicted is one electrode array in the hippocampus (HC) and one in the anterior nucleus of the thalamus (ANT) instantiated in a sheep model of seizures. The pulse generator can run continuous monitoring, can stimulate from either electrode, and is capable of algorithmic analysis and control and bidirectional communication with an external computer for algorithmic uploading and downloading of data. This enables monitoring in the HC the effects of thalamic stimulation **(B):** *top row,* electrocorticogram (ECoG) from the hippocampal electrodes showing the effects of increasing frequency applied to the ANT electrode (lines above ECoG); *middle row,* power in the theta range derived from the ECoG, showing decreased hippocampal power only with high-frequency thalamic stimulation; *bottom row,* spectrogram of the hippocampal ECoG showing decreased theta power. **C,** This approach enables a closed-loop approach to thalamic stimulation: the pulse generator can be programmed to activate and modulate ANT stimulation (ANT DBS amplitude) when hippocampal theta power exceeds an upper threshold and to deactivate stimulation when theta power falls below a lower threshold. Keeping hippocampal theta power in this range decreases excitability and may inhibit seizure activity.[142] This and related network approaches should be implementable in patients. Recorded seizure activity from a depth electrode implanted into ANT **(D** and **E)** might be used to trigger responsive neurostimulation in the ANT or HC. Toward that end, an RNS System device was implanted with one depth array in ANT (via a posterolateral approach: **F,** axial magnetic resonance imaging [MRI]; **G,** sagittal MRI; **H,** coronal MRI) and one in the HC (**I,** sagittal MRI). EEG, electroencephalogram. *(**A,** From Stanslaski S, Afshar P, Cong P, et al. Design and validation of a fully implantable, chronic, closed-loop neuromodulation device with concurrent sensing and stimulation.* IEEE Trans Neural Syst Rehabil Eng. *2012;20:410-421; **B** and **C,** From Stypulkowski PH, Stanslaski SR, Jensen RM, et al. Brain stimulation for epilepsy—local and remote modulation of network excitability.* Brain Stimul. *2014;7:350-358.)*

Thus, a true leap forward in neuromodulation therapy will require both a more detailed understanding of epileptogenic networks and the ability to selectively modulate different cell populations within those networks. Recent advances in structural (diffusion tensor imaging) and functional (e.g., default mode functional imaging)[79] connectivity in patients with epilepsy are advancing and informing understanding and treatment decisions.[143]

In the quest to cure epilepsy, or at the least to attain the goal of "no seizures, no side effects," it seems almost inevitable that neuromodulation approaches will form an important and even a primary role in the treatment of drug-resistant (and perhaps drug-responsive) epilepsy. Great progress has been made in recent years, and several approaches (VNS, RNS, ANT DBS) are now variously established. It is essential not to rest on these results, but rather to pursue all avenues from technologic development, fundamental discovery, and new animal models, to improved clinical trial designs to achieve the level of results we are accustomed to in our best surgical resections, without the adverse effects and ideally in as minimally invasive a manner as feasible.

Disclosure

Dr. Gross serves as a consultant to Medtronic and NeuroPace, Inc. and receives compensation for these services. Medtronic and NeuroPace develop products related to the research described in this chapter. The terms of this arrangement have been reviewed and approved by Emory University in accordance with its conflict of interest policies.

SUGGESTED READINGS

A randomized controlled trial of chronic vagus nerve stimulation for treatment of medically intractable seizures. *Neurology*. 1995;45:224-230.

Bergey GK, Morrell MJ, Mizrahi EM, et al. Long-term treatment with responsive brain stimulation in adults with refractory partial seizures. *Neurology*. 2015;84(8):810-817.

Boon P, Vonck K, De Herdt V, et al. Deep brain stimulation in patients with refractory temporal lobe epilepsy. *Epilepsia*. 2007;48(8):1551-1560.

DeGiorgio CM, Schachter SC, Handforth A, et al. Prospective long-term study of vagus nerve stimulation for the treatment of refractory seizures. *Epilepsia*. 2000;41(9):1195-1200.

Fisher R, Salanova V, Witt T, et al. Electrical stimulation of the anterior nucleus of thalamus for treatment of refractory epilepsy. *Epilepsia*. 2010;51(5):899-908.

Morrell MJ. Responsive cortical stimulation for the treatment of medically intractable partial epilepsy. *Neurology*. 2011;77(13):1295-1304.

Salanova V, Witt T, Worth R, et al. Long-term efficacy and safety of thalamic stimulation for drug-resistant partial epilepsy. *Neurology*. 2015;84(10):1017-1025.

Velasco AL, Velasco F, Velasco M, et al. Electrical stimulation of the hippocampal epileptic foci for seizure control: a double-blind, long-term follow-up study. *Epilepsia*. 2007;48(10):1895-1903.

Velasco F, Velasco M, Velasco AL, et al. Electrical stimulation of the centromedian thalamic nucleus in control of seizures: long-term studies. *Epilepsia*. 1995;36(1):63-71.

See a full reference list on ExpertConsult.com

80 Epilepsy Surgery: Outcome and Complications

Lara Jehi and Webster H. Pilcher

Epilepsy surgery has evolved significantly since the 1980s and is now considered the treatment of choice for drug-resistant focal epilepsy.[1] Two randomized clinical trials have demonstrated the therapeutic superiority of resective surgery over medical therapy for drug-resistant temporal lobe epilepsy (TLE),[2,3] with multiple large surgical series and meta-analyses replicating similarly high success rates of temporal lobe resections in this context.[4-12] Correspondingly, a growing experience with surgery for extratemporal epilepsy has increased the practice of this treatment modality with encouraging results: up to 30% to 50% of patients remain seizure free 5 to 10 years after surgery.[13-26] Furthermore, although resective surgery was traditionally considered a treatment option tailored almost exclusively to patients with clear epileptic lesions, recent data suggest an expansion of the population of surgical candidates to include patients with nonlesional epilepsy.[27,28]

Our perception of favorable surgical outcomes has also progressed over time. Postoperative seizure outcomes represent a dynamic state, with chances of ongoing seizure freedom dropping steadily after surgery.[5,8,10,29] Conversely, up to 20% to 30% of patients who undergo surgery for TLE have intermittent seizures within the few months following resection only to later regain seizure control.[5,9,30-32] Therefore, measuring surgical success requires long-term patient follow-up to ensure an adequate picture of postoperative seizure control. In fact, a comprehensive view of a surgical outcome should also include consideration of the neurocognitive, social, psychiatric, and functional implications of surgery, as well as its potential complications because, again, recent data suggest that seizure control is not the only determinant of patients' quality of life (QOL) after surgery.[33-36] Finally, recent clinical research on postoperative seizure outcomes is developing from the descriptive stage of measuring postoperative seizure freedom to the mechanistic stage of using this outcome knowledge to advance the understanding and modify the mechanisms of postoperative seizure recurrence.[22,37-39]

In this chapter, we review some general basic concepts of outcomes assessment in the context of epilepsy surgery; review the available data on seizure freedom, neuropsychiatric, and QOL outcomes following the major types of epilepsy surgery; discuss the main determinants of seizure outcomes after epilepsy surgery; review the main neurosurgical complications associated with different types of resective epilepsy surgery; and discuss the nonresective options of epilepsy surgery and their outcomes.

BASIC PRINCIPLES AND PITFALLS OF OUTCOMES ASSESSMENT FOR EPILPESY SURGERY

Two main seizure outcome classification systems are currently used.

- *Engel classification.* This is the most frequently used outcome classification system (Box 80-1). It reports favorable seizure outcomes as being either excellent, reflecting freedom from disabling seizures (Engel class I), or good, with the additional inclusion of patients having rare seizures (Engel classes I and II). Challenges with this system include the ambiguity surrounding some outcome criteria, such as "worthwhile improvement" for Engel class III, leading to variation in interpretation among different users; and the fact that the "seizure-free" category (Engel class I) includes patients with persistent auras, simple partial seizures, and generalized convulsions on antiepileptic drug (AED) withdrawal (Engel classes IB to ID) *in addition* to those who are truly completely seizure free since surgery (Engel class IA). Because postoperative outcomes are not typically reported using Engel's classification subcategories, the ability to independently evaluate truly seizure-free patients may be limited with this system.
- *International League Against Epilepsy (ILAE) outcome classification system.* To address the challenges discussed with the Engel classification, the ILAE issued a commission report proposing a new outcome classification scheme (Table 80-1). Completely seizure-free patients are classified separately; seizures are quantified in each category and compared with a well-defined baseline frequency, and results can be easily compared to AED trials that typically report their success as a 50% or more reduction in seizure frequency. Very few studies, however, have actually reported their data using this system[32,40,41] because it tends to be difficult to remember and challenging to ascertain in the absence of consistently quantified seizure burdens.

Some centers reported their outcomes using internally validated scoring systems.[30,42,43] Others chose a prespecified period of seizure freedom—usually 12 to 24 months—as reflecting a favorable outcome.[6,44,45] This wide variation in outcome measures is only one of many pitfalls complicating the interpretation and comparison of results among different surgical series. Other issues include the presence of heterogeneous disease pathologies and even surgeries in the same surgical series, limiting the validity of the results for any one group; the choice of cross-sectional methods of analysis, which were predominantly used until recently, but are unable to account for longitudinal dynamic time-dependent outcomes like postoperative seizure freedom; the limited number of studies comparing the usefulness of various surgical diagnostic techniques (e.g., invasive subdural versus depth recordings) or treatment techniques (e.g., resective versus radiosurgery versus thermoablation or laser ablation). The final but most important limitation of our current outcomes understanding remains our inability to individually predict the chances of success for potential surgical candidates. Some recent studies have begun to address this issue by developing predictive scores that account for multiple diagnostic modalities and clinical characteristics[46] or by developing nomograms able to provide individualized seizure outcome prediction.[47]

RESECTIVE SURGERY

Temporal Lobe Epilepsy

Intractable epilepsy of temporal lobe origin is the most common syndrome for surgical consideration. It is thus no surprise that most outcome data in the literature have focused on temporal lobe surgery. The syndrome of *mesial* TLE typically incorporates a history of an early insult in infancy or childhood,[48] hippocampal sclerosis (HS) and atrophy on magnetic resonance imaging (MRI),[49] temporal hypometabolism on interictal positron emission tomography (PET),[50,51] and a characteristic pattern of hyperperfusion and hypoperfusion on ictal single-photon emission computed tomography (SPECT).[52] Electroencephalography

BOX 80-1 Engel's Classification of Postoperative Outcome

CLASS I: FREE OF DISABLING SEIZURES*

A: Completely seizure free since surgery
B: Nondisabling simple partial seizures only since surgery
C: Some disabling seizures after surgery, but free of disabling seizures for at least 2 years
D: Generalized convulsions with antiepileptic drug discontinuation only

CLASS II: RARE DISABLING SEIZURES ("ALMOST SEIZURE FREE")

A: Initially free of disabling seizures but has rare seizures now
B: Rare disabling seizures since surgery
C: More than rare disabling seizures since surgery, but rare seizures for the last 2 years
D: Nocturnal seizures only

CLASS III: WORTHWHILE IMPROVEMENT†

A: Worthwhile seizure reduction
B: Prolonged seizure-free intervals amounting to greater than half the followed-up period, but not <2 years

CLASS IV: NO WORTHWHILE IMPROVEMENT

A: Significant seizure reduction
B: No appreciable change
C: Seizures worse

*Excludes early postoperative seizures (first few weeks).
†Determination of "worthwhile improvement" will require quantitative analysis of additional data such as percentage seizure reduction, cognitive function, and quality of life.

TABLE 80-1 Proposal for a New Classification of Outcome with Respect to Epileptic Seizures

Outcome Classification	Definition
1	Completely seizure free*; no auras
2	Only auras†; no other seizures
3	1-3 seizure days per year; ± auras
4	4 seizure days‡ per year to 50% reduction of baseline seizure days§; ± auras
5	<50% reduction of baseline seizure days to 100% increase of baseline seizure days; ± auras
6	>100% increase of baseline seizure days; ± auras

*"Neighborhood seizures" in the first postoperative month are not counted.
†Auras are only counted if they are short in duration and are similar or identical to the preoperative ones.
‡A "seizure day" is a 24-hour period with one or more seizures. This may include an episode of status epilepticus.
§"Baseline seizure days" are calculated by determining the seizure-day frequency during the 12 months before surgery, with correction for the effects of antiepileptic drug reduction during diagnostic evaluation.

(EED) studies reveal an anteromedial epileptogenic zone, and Wada testing reveals appropriate memory deficits.[53] Histopathologic analysis of resected hippocampi reveals loss of principal hippocampal neurons, synaptic reorganization, sprouting of mossy fibers, and enhanced expression of glutamate receptors.[54,55] Recent work went further to suggest that distinct patterns of neuronal loss within the hippocampus in the context of HS may reflect different etiological substrates and have different prognostic implications after resective epilepsy surgery.[56]

A smaller population of patients with *cryptogenic* TLE have normal MRI findings preoperatively.[20] Patients with *lesional* TLE have temporal lobe neoplasms, vascular malformations, disorders of cortical development, or traumatic or ischemic insults within the temporal lobe. These lesions may variably involve mesial temporal lobe structures or may be associated with hippocampal sclerosis ("dual pathology")[57,58] and thus lead to distinct surgical approaches and outcomes.

Rate and Stability of Postoperative Seizure Freedom after Temporal Lobe Surgery

Stability of Seizure Control

A randomized controlled trial[3] showed that only two patients with drug-resistant TLE need to be treated surgically for one patient to become free of disabling seizures. Most TLE surgery series show relatively comparable results, with about two thirds of the patients becoming seizure free after surgery.[4,6-8,10,12,20,27,59-61] In comparison, about 5% to 8% achieve sustained seizure remission with medical therapy alone, as assessed in cohort studies evaluating patients with drug-resistant epilepsy.[62] More than 50% of patients remain seizure free beyond 10 years after anterior temporal lobectomy (ATL), reflecting a sustained benefit.[5,7,61,63-65]

If a patient is seizure free 1 year after surgery, the likelihood of remaining seizure free is 87% to 90% at 2 years, 74% to 82% at 5 years, and 67% to 71% at 10 years.[5,7,61,63-66] If a patient is seizure free for 2 postoperative years, chances of seizure freedom increase up to 95% at 5 years, 82% at 10 years, and 68% at 15 years.[10,67] Therefore, freedom from seizures for 2 years might be a better predictor of long-term outcome, although seizure control at both 1 year and 2 years correlates fairly well with subsequent seizure-free status.

Early versus Late Surgical Failures

In surgical failures, more than half of seizure recurrences start within 6 postoperative months, and more than 95% recur within 2 to 5 postoperative years.[10,38,68] There is therefore an initial phase of steep recurrence, followed by a relapse rate of 2% to 5% per year for 5 years, with subsequent more stable seizure freedom.[8,10,64] Recent data suggest that prognostic factors affecting those two phases of recurrence are distinct,[10,37,38,44,69,70] possibly reflecting different mechanisms for early versus late relapses. Early recurrences, occurring within 6 to 12 months of surgery, may be due to incomplete removal of the initial epileptogenic zone or inaccurate localization, whereas later relapses may reflect an underlying diffuse epileptogenicity or progression of an age-dependent etiology, such as mesial temporal sclerosis (MTS), leading to the maturation of a new epileptic focus.[4,6,37,38,64,66,71,72] The main implication of this mechanistic perspective is the idea that improving seizure outcomes necessitates both optimal localization with resection of the epileptic focus *and* strategies aimed at preventing future epileptogenesis.

Running-Down Phenomenon

The *running-down phenomenon* is defined as the late remission of postsurgical seizures. It occurs in 3.2% to 20% of TLE surgery cases. The frequency of seizures during the running-down interval may be up to several per month, but a seizure-free state is usually achieved within 2 years.[71,73] The most accepted explanation for this phenomenon is a dekindling effect, an opposite process to secondary epileptogenesis, whereby the induced synaptic dysfunction gradually declines in the surrounding epileptogenic cortex after pacemaker resection and eventually "runs itself down."[73,74]

Predictors of Recurrence: Clinical Variables and Seizure Outcome

Age at Onset of Epilepsy

Patients with an earlier age (usually <5 years) at onset of epilepsy or at time of the initial neurological insult may be up to 3 times more likely to have a favorable postoperative outcome.[7,61] However, some investigators proposed that this variable actually predicts HS, which is the true favorable prognostic indicator.[45,75] Several findings support this hypothesis: these patients were indeed more likely to have features typical of HS, such as unilateral hippocampal atrophy on MRI[76] or focal ictal EEG with predominantly partial seizures[61]; and age at onset was of no prognostic value in studies evaluating pure cohorts of HS[45,75] or controlling for pathology.[6,8,10]

Duration of Epilepsy

A long history of seizures correlated with worse outcome in multiple studies on univariate analysis.[30,68,71] In some of those same cohorts, this influence disappeared when multivariate analysis was performed, adjusting for other, more solid indicators of outcome.[8,9] Furthermore, many more recent studies found no correlation of epilepsy duration with outcome.[6-8,10,45,75,77] Various hypotheses have been proposed to explain these findings, including secondary epileptogenesis occurring with a long seizure history, varying degrees of maturation of different epileptogenic foci, and increased development of generalized seizures with longer epilepsy duration.[71]

Age at Surgery

Most studies found no correlation between age at surgery and seizure outcome,[7,8,10,45] although one longitudinal study in HS patients found that patients who were 24 years or younger at surgery were about 4 times more likely to be seizure free 5 years after surgery compared with the older surgical group (≥36 years).[9] Few other studies found similar results.[71]

Absence of Secondarily Generalized Tonic-Clonic Seizures

The poor prognostic significance of secondarily generalized tonic-clonic seizure (SGTCS) in the context of TLE surgery was confirmed in a prospective multicenter trial.[6] Prior retrospective data leading up to this observation included a 2.2-fold increased chance of seizure freedom 5 years after surgery in patients who had no SGTCS compared with those who did,[9] and another study in which only 57% of mesial TLE patients with SGTCS achieved a 1-year remission compared with an 80% remission rate in those who had only partial seizures.[45] This effect may be most significant when generalized tonic-clonic seizures are frequent (more than two per year) and occur within 3 years of surgery.[8]

The occurrence of SGTCS in TLE correlates with more extensive HS, multifocal irritative areas,[78] and extended PET hypometabolism,[79] suggesting a diffuse potential epileptogenic zone with lower chances of postoperative seizure freedom.

Low-Baseline Seizure Frequency

A lower seizure burden has correlated in several studies with more favorable seizure outcomes after TLE surgery. The cutoff point for monthly seizure frequency that can affect seizure outcomes varied from 20 seizures per month[10,80] to 30 seizures per month.[59] A critical role for both seizure frequency and history of SGTCS in predicting outcomes after TLE surgery has been resuggested in recent work attempting to provide individualized seizure outcome prediction through a comprehensive scoring measure or a nomogram.[46,81]

Imaging Variables and Seizure Outcome

Magnetic Resonance Imaging

The presence of a unilateral temporal lobe abnormality on MRI has been a consistently identified favorable outcome predictor.[6,12,71,75] Patients with MRI evidence of unilateral HS had a 54% chance of seizure freedom 10 years after ATL compared with 18% when MRIs were normal in one longitudinal study.[8] In the prospective multicenter Epilepsy Surgery study, 75% of patients with unilateral hippocampal atrophy and a mesial temporal resection were seizure free as opposed to 55% otherwise.[6] However, recent data suggest that such a favorable prognostic significance is actually conferred by *any* unilateral temporal MRI lesion, and not necessarily by HS, especially with concordant ictal and interictal EEG findings.[71]

Favorable seizure outcomes are also possible with a normal MRI; recent data have actually shown seizure freedom rates of up to 41% to 48% as long as 8 years after ATL.[20,82-86] Although some data suggest that these patients may actually have MRI-negative or undetected HS,[71] other studies concluded that most cases of normal-appearing hippocampi on high-resolution MRI have neocortical TLE because they have less febrile seizures, more delta rhythms at ictal onset, and more extensive lateral neocortical changes on PET with surgical outcomes still comparable to those of MRI-positive HS.[83,85] It should be emphasized, however, that surgery was successful in nonlesional patients typically when performed in the context of concordant EEG and PET data.[20,83,85] "Normal" MRIs correlating with bad outcomes in older studies using lower quality imaging may have included patients with extratemporal or contralateral pathology, findings that would currently exclude viable surgical options.[20,83,85] Lack of SGTCS and low preoperative seizure frequency correlate with more favorable surgical outcomes in nonlesional TLE, similar to lesional TLE.[20]

Bilateral MRI lesions, including grossly bilateral HS, reflect multiple potentially epileptogenic foci and correlate with a worse surgical outcome: 58% of patients are seizure free at 2 years compared with 78% of patients with unilateral lesions or even normal MRI.[10,71] Subtle hippocampal asymmetries only detected using volumetric analyses were less predictive of outcome.[71]

Nuclear Imaging

Unilateral temporal hypometabolism on fluorodeoxyglucose–positron emission tomography (FDG-PET) is a good predictor of seizure freedom in patients with mesial TLE, independent of pathologic findings and regardless of whether MRI is normal.[83,85,87-89] It has been reported that 86% of patients with unilateral temporal hypometabolism ipsilateral to the side of surgery had a good outcome, as defined by more than 90% reduction in seizure frequency or Engel class I or II, with those chances slightly reduced to 82% if the MRI was normal. This number significantly dropped to 62% when PET was normal and to 50% when it showed bitemporal hypometabolism.[90] With extratemporal hypometabolism, chances of seizure freedom are even worse: complete seizure freedom at last follow-up (mean, 6.1 years) was seen in 45% of patients with extratemporal cortical hypometabolism confined to the ipsilateral hemisphere and in only 22% with contralateral cortical hypometabolism.[91]

Abundant data support the usefulness of ictal SPECT in localizing the epileptogenic zone in TLE, with 70% to 100% of ictal SPECT imaging being correctly localizing and only 0% to 7% incorrectly localizing.[71] However, although the prognostic value of such localized SPECT findings is clear in extratemporal or poorly localized nonlesional temporal epilepsy,[52,92] its role in clear lesional TLE cases is less well defined. In a recent analysis of patients with unilateral HS visible on MRI, surgical outcome was not influenced by contralateral increased flow on ictal SPECT.[93] One hypothesis is that, owing to their low temporal resolution, ictal SPECT hyperperfusion patterns often contain both the ictal-onset zone and propagation pathways. In that sense, these multilobulated hourglass-appearing patterns are best viewed and interpreted as representing the epileptic network, including both the area of ictal onset and spread, rather than aiming at identifying a single focus of maximal hyperperfusion representing the ictal-onset zone.[88,94,95]

Electrophysiologic Variables and Seizure Outcome

Noninvasive Electroencephalography

Focal interictal EEG predicts a favorable outcome when lateralized to the side of surgery or when highly localized to the resected temporal lobe. Patients whose interictal EEGs showed 90% or higher predominance on the operated side had an 80% chance of complete seizure freedom after a mean 5.5 years of follow-up compared with 54% in those with lesser degrees of lateralization in one prospective study.[7] In general, interictal evidence of a diffuse irritative zone predicts a worse outcome: postoperative seizure freedom is worse when interictal spiking was posterior temporal, extratemporal, or bitemporal.[45,96] Bitemporal interictal spiking on surface EEG does not, however, automatically preclude postoperative seizure freedom. One study found that if 90% or more of surface interictal bitemporal spikes arise from one temporal lobe, excellent outcome is possible (92% seizure free in the second postoperative year versus 50% if <90% lateralization).[97] With a unilateral MRI temporal lesion, and with lateralizing noninvasive functional data, up to 64% of patients with bilateral interictal spikes achieved complete seizure freedom 1 year or later after surgery when seizure onset was strictly unilateral on invasive evaluation.[98] Other findings consistent with unilateral HS, such as a history of febrile seizures or early onset of epilepsy (<3 to 6 years of age), also correlated with favorable outcome in patients with bitemporal interictal spikes, suggesting that contralateral spiking may simply be spread from a surgically treatable hippocampus.[71] However, if the MRI is normal or shows widespread abnormalities, then seizure recurrence is the rule because either an extratemporal focus spreading to both temporal lobes or bitemporal epilepsy becomes more likely.[98]

Similar concepts apply to the prognostic value of ictal EEG. Again, focal or anterior ictal EEG correlates with a more favorable outcome, and patients who had bitemporal ictal onsets on surface EEG still achieved seizure freedom rates of up to 64% at 1 postoperative year when their seizures were exclusively unilateral with depth recordings and when imaging or neuropsychological testing was also consistent with unilateral temporal dysfunction.[71,98]

Invasive Electroencephalography

Depth electrode evaluations have traditionally been used to clarify lateralization of the epileptogenic zone in patients with suspected bitemporal or falsely lateralized TLE, whereas subdural recordings and stereo-electroencephalography (SEEG) are useful in neocortical epilepsy for extraoperative functional mapping and definition of the extent of the epileptogenic zone. Those modalities are therefore reserved for patients with a poorly defined epileptogenic zone, which may explain poorer outcomes seen in cases that required invasive recordings preoperatively compared with those that did not.[10,65,71,99] Outcomes are particularly worse in patients who had prior temporal lobe resections.[100]

Temporal Lobe Epilepsy: Surgical Approaches, Outcomes, and Complications

With the delineation of surgically remediable temporal lobe epileptic syndromes, the traditional *en bloc temporal lobectomy*, which incorporated a 5- to 6-cm lateral resection along with a portion of the amygdala and anterior hippocampus,[101-103] has generally been abandoned. For patients with mesial TLE or even cryptogenic TLE, most centers now employ a focused anteromedial resection in which a restricted resection of the middle and inferior temporal gyrus is combined with a thorough hippocampal removal.[101,103-105] Transsylvian and transtemporal selective amygdalohippocampectomies (SAHs) provide attractive options because they focus on mesial structures that constitute the primary pathologic substrate of mesial TLE.[101,106,107] Awake surgery with intraoperative electrocorticography (ECoG) and functional brain mapping facilitates a tailored resection of both lateral and medial structures and may be useful in dominant hemisphere cases without evident MTS on imaging.[101,108,109]

Impact of Cortical and Hippocampal Resection on Seizure Outcomes

Although a small percentage of TLE patients may harbor epileptogenic zones exclusively in the lateral temporal neocortex,[110] most candidates for nonlesional temporal lobe resection have the syndrome of mesial TLE, for which resection of mesial structures is now emphasized.[101,111] In the early era of epilepsy surgery, lateral resection alone yielded disappointing results with regard to freedom from seizures,[112] and a long-term follow-up study of 50 patients managed with lateral resection alone revealed only 44% to be seizure free at follow-up.[113] In fact, in the studies in which lateral cortex and mesial structures were resected, the extent of lateral resection did not significantly correlate with seizure outcome.[111,112] The favorable outcomes after SAH,[114,115] the effectiveness of removal of any residual posterior hippocampus in reoperative surgery,[116-118] and the identification of posterior hippocampal onsets in depth electrode studies[104] all suggest that thorough hippocampal resection is essential to optimize seizure outcomes.[101] Although earlier reports suggested that the extent of mesial resection had no association with seizure outcome, two more recent studies addressed this issue effectively and came to different conclusions.[83] In the first study, postoperative MRI was used to confirm the extent of mesial resection in 94 TLE patients and revealed a correlation of the extent of mesiobasal resection with seizure outcome, regardless of the extent of lateral resection.[117] In a separate, prospective randomized controlled trial, 70 patients with unilateral ictal onsets confirmed on intracranial recordings underwent temporal lobe resection and were randomized to partial or total hippocampectomy.[119] At 1- and 2-year follow-up, the group that underwent complete hippocampectomy experienced superior seizure outcomes (69% versus 38% seizure free at 1 year) without increased neuropsychological or neurological morbidity. One study reported that 53 of 100 patients were seizure free after a standard lateral resection was combined with complete amygdalectomy and minimal hippocampal resection.[120]

In Engel's compilation of seizure outcomes from 107 centers worldwide, outcomes were similar between centers regardless of the surgical approach, provided that the mesial structures were adequately resected.[121] In single-center studies, SAH and standard resections produced similar results.[122] In Wieser and colleagues' SAH series, 22 of 30 (73%) patients with TLE and depth electrode–confirmed hippocampal onsets were seizure free postoperatively.[115] These results after SAH compare favorably with studies of patients with histologically confirmed MTS undergoing standard anteromesial resections.[45]

A single-center study reported on the seizure outcomes of 321 patients who underwent various temporal lobe resections between 1989 and 1997.[123] This series incorporated 96 standard anterior temporal resections, 84 restricted lateral and generous mesial resections, and 91 SAH procedures. The notable finding was the absence of significant differences in seizure outcome between the three operative cohorts in which different resection strategies were used.[101]

Utility of Intraoperative Electrocorticography

For many years, temporal lobe resections were "tailored" on the basis of intraoperative ECoG, but recent experience suggests that standardized anatomic resections may produce similar seizure outcomes, and the appropriate role of intraoperative ECoG is not well defined in current practice. Early studies suggested that intraoperative ECoG was useful to predict outcome, particularly if epileptiform discharges are present or absent in either preresection or postresection cortex.[73,124,125] ECoG was used to define the extent of hippocampal resection in an attempt to both optimize seizure outcomes and minimize postoperative memory deficits through hippocampal sparing.[109] In contrast, two studies in which standardized anatomic resections were performed in the context of intraoperative ECoG before and after resection failed to identify any predictive value with regard to ultimate seizure outcomes.[126,127] Other studies suggest a limited value of ECoG as a guide to the extent of resection for TLE.[43,128,129] Another study in patients with lesional temporal or extratemporal epilepsy in which resection was carried to normal tissue margins found that the extramarginal spike distribution was not associated with seizure outcome.[130] In contemporary practice, in which patient selection is guided by advanced imaging and video-EEG data, intraoperative ECoG is far less frequently employed than in the past.[131]

Temporal Lobe Resection: Effect on Cognitive Functions

Intellectual function is generally preserved in adults[12] and children[132] after temporal lobe resection, and when seizure control is achieved, improvement in some measures has been reported. In the Graduate Hospital series of 89 consecutive patients undergoing dominant and nondominant hemisphere resections, measures of verbal IQ were unchanged postoperatively and the study demonstrated improvements in performance and full-scale IQ.[68] Subsequent studies have reported similar findings, including improvement in verbal IQ after nondominant hemisphere resections and performance IQ after dominant hemisphere resections.[133-137]

Temporal Lobe Resection: Global Memory Deficits

Global amnesia is a rare but disabling complication of temporal lobe surgery. Two patients with global amnesia were described in an early Montreal Neurological Institute series of 90 dominant hemisphere temporal resections.[138] These patients exhibited a syndrome of profound anterograde memory loss with preservation of cognitive performance, personality, early memory, and technical skills.[139,140] Earlier reports had described global amnesia after unilateral resection in either the dominant or nondominant hemispheres.[132,136,140] Evidence that hippocampal, rather than lateral neocortical, removal is critical to the production of global amnesia is provided by a report of a patient undergoing a staged resection in whom global amnesia occurred only after the hippocampus was removed.[138] This is further supported by reports of global amnesia after SAH.[141] Contemporary series report rare postoperative global memory deficits at a frequency of less than 1%,[136,142-144] whereas a less profound postoperative severe amnesia may be more common.[145]

Temporal Lobe Resection: Material-Specific Memory Deficits

Reported material-specific memory deficits include loss of short-term verbal and nonverbal memory after surgery. In particular, short-term verbal memory loss is common after dominant temporal lobe resections, with significant decrements in verbal memory being reported in 25% to 50% of operated patients.[146] Verbal memory loss may accompany resections in the nondominant hemisphere, although at a much lower frequency.[146] Nonverbal memory deficits are less commonly identified, even after nondominant hemisphere resections,[147] although some authors report that these losses may be obscured by "practice effects."[146] In the Graduate Hospital series, evidence of significant short-term verbal memory loss was identified in many patients after dominant hemisphere temporal lobe resections, with a trend toward improvement after nondominant temporal lobe resections.[68] In a recent 10-year series of 321 TLE patients undergoing a variety of surgical approaches for the treatment of nonlesional and lesional TLE, verbal memory declined in 34%, improved in 19%, and remained stable in 46% of patients.[123] Weak preoperative performance on measures of verbal memory, young age at surgery, and operations on the nondominant side were associated with stability or improvement in verbal memory. Short-term nonverbal memory measures exhibited similar rates of improvement and deterioration. Weak preoperative performance on measures of nonverbal memory and dominant side operations were associated with improvement, whereas strong performance preoperatively and older age were associated with deterioration.[123]

The high frequency at which verbal memory impairment occurs after dominant hemisphere temporal lobe surgery has stimulated interest in predicting which patients are at risk for postoperative deficits.[8] Most studies have documented greater risk for verbal memory loss in two categories of patients: (1) those with intact memory function and a normal hippocampus ipsilateral to the seizure focus *(functional adequacy hypothesis)* and (2) those with ipsilateral hippocampal atrophy, but impaired memory function, presumably related to poor function within the hemisphere contralateral to the seizure focus to be resected *(functional reserve hypothesis)*.[101,148] Patients with dominant hemisphere TLE and a reversed memory asymmetry score (i.e., better memory performance in the epileptogenic temporal lobe, with poor right temporal lobe performance) have been shown to have a greater risk for memory morbidity after left-sided resection, as well as poorer seizure outcome postoperatively.[149] Patients with dominant hemisphere hippocampal atrophy who undergo contralateral, nondominant hemisphere resections are also at risk for verbal memory deficits.[150]

Prediction of postoperative verbal memory decline is possible, using a multivariate risk factor model in which five risk factors are independently associated with outcome, including (1) dominant hemisphere resection, (2) MRI findings other than exclusively ipsilateral MTS, (3) intact preoperative delayed recall verbal memory, (4) relatively poorer preoperative immediate recall verbal memory, and (5) intact ipsilateral memory performance on the Wada test.[101,151] With this model, individual patients can be assessed with respect to their risk for deficits in verbal memory function after surgery.

A recent 10-year outcome study following dominant and nondominant temporal lobe resections used reliable change indices (RCIs) to evaluate long-term changes in learning and immediate recall and in delayed recall of word list and word pairs before surgery, 2 years after surgery, and 10 years after surgery. This study actually documented improvement in the long-term follow-up, with fewer patients demonstrating RCI after 10 years than after 2 years for measures of verbal and nonverbal memory performance.[152]

Selective Amygdalohippocampectomy: Memory Outcomes

In patients thought to be at risk for global or material-specific memory deficits after surgery, various management strategies have been proposed to reduce these losses,[101] including memory mapping in the temporal neocortex with restriction of neocortical resection, SAH, or simple denial of surgery to these patients.[153] With reports of global amnesia occurring in patients undergoing SAH,[141] it was thought that it may be advantageous to perform selective mesial resection from the standpoint of preservation of material-specific memory, particularly short-term verbal memory function. Although some early outcome studies in small series of patients suggested a possible advantage of SAH over standard anterior temporal lobectomy from the standpoint of postoperative memory outcome,[154,155] this has not been supported by other studies, and there have been reports to the contrary.[156]

In a review of 140 patients undergoing either right or left SAH, a decline in verbal learning and memory occurred after 32% of the right-sided and 51% of the left-sided resections.[149] The left SAH patients were particularly at risk when preoperative testing revealed intact verbal memory function, late onset of epilepsy, and the absence of MTS on MRI. Collateral damage to adjacent temporolateral tissue during the transsylvian dissection may exacerbate the deficits caused by hippocampal resection.[149,157] The role of deafferentation of the temporal circuitry during resection of the parahippocampal gyrus, amygdala, and hippocampus also needs to be considered. This is supported by PET evidence of worsening hypometabolism of the remaining temporal lobe neocortex after SAH.[158]

Dominant Temporal Lobe Resections: Language Outcomes

After dominant hemisphere temporal lobe resection, a syndrome of transitory postoperative dysnomia or even aphasia is observed in as many as 30% of operated patients.[159] In most cases, the dysnomia or aphasia gradually disappears over a period of a few weeks. This occurs even when resections are guided by intraoperative or extraoperative language mapping.[160,161] The cause of this transitory phenomenon is unclear, but it is more common when resections are carried to within 1 to 2 cm of essential language sites as determined by mapping procedures.[101,153,162] Other explanations for this phenomenon include resection of inferior temporal lobe "inessential" language sites,[163] brain retraction and associated "neuroparalytic edema,"[159,164,165] or deafferentation of white matter pathways. Some authors have suggested that such word-finding deficits represent an acute postoperative exacerbation of the preoperative deficits common in patients with TLE and that they last no longer than 1 year.[166]

Although some investigations of naming have not revealed enduring deficits 6 and 18 months after surgery,[167-169] others have suggested that significant, persistent word-finding difficulties do occur commonly after standard or anteromesial temporal lobe resection.[153,159,170,171] Such deficits have been reported to be associated with early risk factors for the development of seizures[172] and with the pathologic state of the resected hippocampus.[173] In one study, 7% of patients undergoing standard dominant hemisphere resections exhibited persistent postoperative dysnomia.[171] Ojemann described enduring language deficits after resections within 1 to 2 cm of identified language sites.[172]

The aforementioned findings stimulated interest in the value of intraoperative mapping and tailoring of the lateral neocortical resection. Historical studies documented that up to 17% of patients undergoing left temporal resections 4 to 4.5 cm from the temporal tip without mapping experience postoperative deficits.[101,174] Restricting the neocortical resection to 3 cm of the middle and inferior gyrus without mapping is associated with minimal postoperative language deficits.[104] Functional magnetic resonance imaging (fMRI) studies of language lateralization demonstrate that both left and right TLE patients show decreased left lateralization compared with controls and that the fMRI "laterality" is helpful in predicting the risk to language with standard respective approaches.[175]

Persistent, severe dysphasia has been reported in 1% to 2% of patients undergoing dominant hemisphere temporal resections, even with language mapping.[117,136,176,177] Such adverse postoperative outcomes occur as a result of resection of undetected essential language cortex or manipulation or thrombosis of the middle cerebral or anterior choroidal artery.[178]

Temporal Lobe Resection: Surgical Complications

In a review of the accumulated worldwide experience with temporal lobe resective surgery before 1993,[142] significant or impairing complications were uncommon and included *death*,[136,179-183] *infection*,[136,142,164] *hemiparesis* from manipulation or thrombosis of the middle cerebral artery or anterior choroidal vasculature or from direct brainstem injury or resection,[182,184-188] *visual field deficits* from resection of Meyer's loop fibers in the roof of the temporal horn,[188-190] *hemianopia*[177,190,191] as a result of excessive tissue resection or infarction, postoperative *hematoma* formation,[136,180,181] and rare *third cranial nerve*[182,185] and *seventh cranial nerve*[192] palsies.

In contemporary practice, complications are infrequent. In a single-center study of 329 temporal lobe resections (in 321 consecutive patients), 28 complications were reported (8.5%), including no mortalities, meningitis (1.5%), subdural hematoma (0.6%), deep venous thrombosis (1.2%), and neurological complications (5.2%).[123] In another single-center study of 215 patients undergoing temporal lobe surgery between 1984 and 1999, complications included mild hemiparesis, hemianopia, transient cranial nerve palsies, and transient language difficulties.[193]

In a multicenter study at six different centers in Sweden, the complications in 449 operated patients were reviewed.[194] In 247 temporal lobe resections, 1 mortality occurred in a 62-year-old woman who experienced a postoperative hematoma. Hemiparesis occurred in 5 patients: in 1 patient after neocortical resection and in 4 patients after resections involving the hippocampus. These complications were thought to be due to anterior choroidal artery infarction and manipulation of "perforating vessels." Other complications included hemianopia (0.4%) and cranial nerve injury (0.9%). A clear correlation between age and severity of complications was noted. Few complications occurred in those younger than 35 years. *Manipulation hemiplegia* was originally described by Penfield and colleagues[187] and may be caused by manipulation of or injury to the anterior choroidal artery or the middle cerebral artery in the sylvian fissure. The resultant hemiparesis was thought to be more likely in older patients with atherosclerosis and hypertension and was one of the main complications of temporal lobe surgery in those older than 35 years. In a Norwegian epilepsy surgery series,[195,196] "large" complications occurred in 1 of 64 patients younger than 19 years and in 7 of 61 adult patients, thus confirming an increased risk for postoperative complications in older patients. Additional support is provided by another study of 215 operations performed between 1983 and 1999 in which permanent complications occurred in only 3 of 215 patients, and these patients were older than 30 years.[193]

Recent reports of unusual complications after temporal lobe resection include four cases of cerebellar hemorrhage believed to be related to postoperative epidural suction drains[197] and diplopia associated with transient trochlear nerve palsy in three patients.[198]

A systematic review of the literature up to 2013 compiled the complications of nearly 5000 adult and pediatric patients undergoing epilepsy surgery procedures and concluded that most complications following surgery were "minor" or "temporary." "Major" complications occurred in 4.1% of patients after temporal lobe surgery, with half of these consisting of a significant visual field defect and with mortality in 0.4%.[199]

Temporal Lobe Resection: Impact on Epilepsy Related Mortality

The annual death rate attributable to epilepsy reflects accidents, suicide, and the phenomenon of sudden unexpected death due to epilepsy (SUDEP). This mortality rate is higher in patients with chronic epilepsy than in the general population[101] and improves when seizure freedom is achieved following surgery.[200] In one long-term follow-up study after temporal lobe resection, all late mortalities (four) occurred in patients with recurrent seizures, including three with SUDEP and one suicide.[68] In another study, late mortality was studied and occurred in 2% of seizure-free patients and in 11.9% of patients with recurrent seizures.[193]

Temporal Lobe Surgery: Lesional Epilepsy

Lesions of various types are identified in 15% to 30% of patients with intractable TLE.[101,201,202] These lesions may be *neoplastic* (astrocytoma, ganglioglioma, pleomorphic xanthoastrocytoma, dysembryoplastic neuroepithelial tumor), *vascular* (cavernous hemangioma, arteriovenous malformation [AVM], angioma), *dysgenetic* (microdysgenesis, focal or diffuse dysplasia, Sturge-Weber syndrome, tuberous sclerosis), or *traumatic-ischemic*. In a review of 167 patients with temporal or extratemporal lesions, 15% had hippocampal sclerosis or dual pathology.[57] In further investigations of dual pathology, significant hippocampal neuron loss was identified in patients with lesions located adjacent to the hippocampus and in those with a history of early injury.[203,204]

In patients with mesial temporal lobe lesions and intractable epilepsy, studies of lesional resection alone, without resection of mesial structures (*lesionectomy*), have produced disappointing results, with 22%,[205] 19%,[206] and 43%[207] of patients rendered seizure free in small series.[101] In those with laterally located lesions, seizure outcome is improved when complete lesion resection is achieved.[118] When lesional removal is performed along with standard mesial resection, seizure outcomes were improved, with 85%,[207] 91%,[208] and 92%[209] of patients being rendered seizure free in various series. Other authors have recommended gross total resection of the lesion along with an additional 5 to 10 mm of adjacent epileptogenic tissue (*lesionectomy plus*) and sparing of mesial structures in the case of lateral lesions without dual pathology (i.e., normal hippocampus) and have reported favorable seizure outcomes with this approach.[101,123,210] In patients with temporal lobe lesions and dual pathology, resection of mesial structures along with the lesion has been recommended.[211]

The value of ECoG in guiding decisions regarding the extent of extralesional tissue resection is controversial[212] and has been addressed in reports of patients with TLE and various tumors[43,206,209,213] and AVMs[208]; these reports suggest an advantage conferred by resection of epileptogenic tissue, including mesial structures, along with lesional resection. Despite a possible advantage from the standpoint of seizure control, hippocampal resection in lesional cases may cause significant neuropsychological morbidity when hippocampal sclerosis is absent on MRI, particularly in dominant hemisphere resections. In cases in which the hippocampus is not invaded by tumor, the approach of lesionectomy plus may confer less morbidity in dominant hemisphere resections while maintaining favorable seizure outcomes.[210] Excision of a presumed epileptogenic region without lesional resection tends to result in poor outcomes.[212]

FRONTAL LOBE SURGERY

Rate and Stability of Postoperative Seizure Freedom

FLE surgery accounts for 6% to 30% of all epilepsy surgeries and represents the second most common procedure performed to treat intractable focal epilepsy after TLE surgery. However, reported seizure freedom rates with frontal resections have varied from 13% to 80%,[13,16,18,21,22,197,214-219] suggesting, in general, significantly lower success rates than those observed with temporal resections. Only few studies evaluated seizure freedom after FLE surgery longitudinally and can therefore provide useful information related to rate and stability of seizure outcome over time,[13,22,214,219,220] showing more favorable outcomes closer to the 40% seizure-free range a decade after resection.[22,214] Eighty percent of seizure recurrences occur within the first 6 postoperative months, and although late remissions and relapses may occur, those are usually rare.[13,214] One study showed that although a postoperative reduction in seizure frequency often occurred in patients who failed to become completely seizure free after surgery, this improvement was sustained until the last follow-up in only 35%, with seizure frequencies eventually returning to preoperative levels in the remainder.[13] The running-down phenomenon often seen after TLE surgery occurs at a rate of less than 15% after FLE surgery.[214]

Similar to TLE surgery, however, seizure freedom 6 months to 2 years after FLE surgery seems to be a very good predictor of a long-term seizure-free state. If a patient is seizure free at 2-year follow-up, the probability of remaining seizure free for up to 10 years may increase up to 86%.[214]

Predictors of Seizure Recurrence

Lower success rates of FLE surgery include difficulty localizing the epileptogenic zone with EEG data secondary to rapid ictal spread through the frontal lobe, difficulty achieving a complete surgical resection secondary to proximity of functional and eloquent cortex, and a preponderance of cortical dysplasia, often invisible on MRI, as the epilepsy etiology in the frontal lobe as opposed to clearly localized HS in the temporal lobe.[16,221,222] Practically, identified predictors of postoperative seizure recurrence have included incomplete resection of the epileptic lesion,[13,24,214,223,224] the need to perform an invasive EEG evaluation,[13,214] the occurrence of acute postoperative seizures,[13] the persistence of auras postoperatively,[13,214] a history of febrile seizures,[221] predominantly generalized or poorly localized ictal EEG patterns on surface EEG before surgery—especially in the adult population,[13,15,19,214] and the lack of a distinct single MRI lesion.[13,15,214,223] Of all these prognostic indicators, the two most consistently reported and strongly predictive of postoperative seizure freedom are the presence of an MRI lesion and completeness of resection. A short epilepsy duration (<5 years) is associated with significantly improved outcomes, whether patients are lesional or not, a finding that highlights the urgency and importance of early surgical referral in patients with FLE.[22]

Magnetic Resonance Imaging and Seizure Outcome

A normal MRI in a patient undergoing FLE surgery has consistently been found to predict a worse outcome. Only 41% of nonlesional FLE patients had an excellent outcome, compared with 72% when MRI abnormality was present in one study,[221] because most such nonlesional FLE cases are thought to have an underlying poorly localized malformation of cortical development (MCD).[15,223] In one series, all patients with normal MRI and pathologically proven MCD had recurrent seizures by 3 postoperative years.[13] Knowing that milder forms of MCD such as microdysgenesis, cortical dyslamination, or focal MCD are often missed, even on high-resolution MRI, may explain why one cannot determine the extent of the epileptogenic tissue in those MRI-negative MCD cases, making adequate surgical treatment more difficult. The particular pathologic MCD substrate, in fact, was critical in determining surgical outcome in several more recent series, with the worst outcomes in type I MCD.[21,225,226]

Techniques such as ictal SPECT imaging, FDG-PET, and subdural grid or SEEG monitoring are often used to better localize the epileptogenic zone in nonlesional FLE cases. A study reporting on 193 patients with neocortical focal epilepsy (including 61 with FLE) showed that correct localization by FDG-PET was an independent predictor of a good outcome,[15] and other recent series highlighted the usefulness of ictal SPECT in the presurgical workup of nonlesional FLE.[94,219,222] A recent analysis, however, found that although MRI, PET, and ictal SPECT all had good positive predictive values with correspondingly acceptable negative predictive values in correlating with the ictal-onset zone as later defined by invasive EEG recording, there was no significant relationship between the diagnostic accuracy of any of these modalities and surgical outcome, with the exception of MRI ($P = .029$).[18] Therefore, the translation of "accurate" and "correct localization" of epileptic foci using various imaging modalities besides MRI into actual improvements in seizure outcome for nonlesional FLE has not always been consistently reproducible. A recent decision analysis and cost-effectiveness study found that either performing SPECT by itself or obtaining a combination of PET and magnetoencephalography was the preferred strategy in patients with intractable focal epilepsy undergoing a presurgical evaluation.[227] In selected nonlesional cases, seizure freedom rates as high as 40% to 50% can be achieved, particularly when invasive and noninvasive evaluations show concordant data, and complete resection of the ictal-onset zones is possible.[21,22,228,229] European series from centers using SEEG evaluations report more favorable outcomes in nonlesional extratemporal epilepsy,[228,230] highlighting the importance of adequate patient selection and the importance of developing a solid preimplantation hypothesis.

In summary, although patients with nonlesional FLE seem to be as a whole less than ideal surgical candidates for resective epilepsy surgery, efforts to identify the specific subgroup of patients who might benefit from surgery while pursuing nonsurgical treatment options for the rest are still required. Early referral for a presurgical evaluation is essential.[22]

Extent of Resection and Seizure Outcome

Complete resection of the epileptogenic lesion has consistently been found to predict seizure freedom. In one report of patients who had complete removal of their epileptogenic lesions, 81% were seizure free at 1 year and 66% at 3 years compared with 13% and 11%, respectively, of those who did not.[13] Complete removal of neuroimaging abnormalities[25,223,231] and abolition of residual ECoG spiking[232] or seizures[233] have also been linked with the most favorable outcomes after FLE surgery. Major challenges that hinder a complete resection in all cases include frequent proximity or overlap with eloquent cortex and difficulties identifying the true edges of the "abnormal" tissue in MCD cases in which the MRI-visible portion of the dysplasia may be surrounded by microscopically abnormal tissue that seems normal on imaging.[13]

In summary, although the rates of seizure freedom are low, in general, after frontal resections, very successful seizure outcomes are possible in a selected group of patients, mainly those with a clear MRI lesion that is completely resectable.

POSTERIOR CORTEX SURGERY

Rate and Stability of Postoperative Seizure Freedom

Resections in the posterior cortex represent less than 10% of all epilepsy surgeries, with reported postoperative seizure freedom rates varying from 25% to 90%.[14,234] In a longitudinal analysis of a cohort of posterior cortex resections, the estimated chance of seizure freedom was 73.1% at 6 postoperative months, 68.5% at 1 year, 65.8% between 2 and 5 years, and 54.8% at 6 years and beyond. The median timing of recurrence was 2 months, with 75% of the seizure recurrences occurring by 6.4 months; and late recurrences were rare, with the latest being at 74 months.[14] Similar rates of seizure freedom have been reported in another longitudinal analysis of 154 adult patients who underwent various types of extratemporal resections (about 40% frontal and the remaining being posterior cortex surgeries), with an Engel class I seizure at 2 postoperative years being correlated with an 88% chance of remaining seizure free 14 years after surgery.[220]

Predictors of Seizure Recurrence

Patients with well-circumscribed focal lesions (tumors or MRI-visible MCD), who have more extensive resections (lobectomies or multilobar resections as opposed to lesionectomies), no preoperative evidence of extralobar epileptogenicity extending to the ipsilateral temporal lobe (temporal spiking or auditory auras), and no postoperative evidence of residual epileptogenicity (spiking on 6 months postoperative EEG) had the most favorable outlook in most series of posterior cortex resections.[14,234-240] Other less consistently reported predictors of seizure freedom include lateralizing seizure semiology,[234] focal ictal EEG,[241] and shorter epilepsy duration.[242] Invasive EEG recordings with subdural grids, depths, or the use of SEEG are more extensively used for better delineation of the epileptogenic zone and for extraoperative functional mapping optimizing resections, with multiple reports showing very promising seizure outcome data. Caicoya and colleagues found that five of seven occipital lobe epilepsy patients who underwent tailored resections guided by subdural EEG data were seizure free after a mean follow-up of 24.3 months.[243] Cukiert and associates[244] reported on 16 patients with intractable extratemporal epilepsy who either had normal or nonlocalizing MRI, finding that 13 out of 14 were rendered seizure free with resections that used subdural EEG information. The use of preoperative invasive monitoring has even been shown in one report to actually correlate with a more favorable outcome in a large cohort of extratemporal resections, consisting mostly of posterior cortex surgeries.[220]

Extratemporal Epilepsy: Surgical Approaches and Complications

The protean clinical manifestations of the extratemporal epilepsies result from the varied pathogenetic features of these disorders and the eloquent brain regions that are affected by seizures arising in the broad expanse of the frontal, parietal, and occipital lobes.[101] Extratemporal epilepsy surgery is far less common than temporal lobe surgery.[121] The epileptogenic regions are often large and ill defined, thus mandating larger resections, and surgical approaches include lobar and multilobar, central, and tailored resections; topectomy; and multiple subpial transections (MSTs). Extratemporal resections may be combined with callosotomy or MST to improve efficacy. In a series of 2177 patients at the Montreal Neurological Institute, operations included temporal (56%), frontal (18%), central or rolandic (7%), parietal (6%), occipital (1%), and multilobar resections, as well as hemispherectomy (11%).[142,245]

Seizure Outcomes

The outcomes of extratemporal resections are generally less favorable than with temporal lobe surgery, with historical studies reporting that 45% of patients become seizure free.[121] However, with modern imaging, patient selection, mapping modalities, and surgical approaches, outcomes have improved in contemporary reports. For example, in a study of 60 patients undergoing extratemporal epilepsy surgery, structural abnormalities were present in 83%.[246] Surgical resection of the frontal, parietal, and occipital lobes was performed. Preoperative mapping with grids and strips was performed in 50%, and the remainder of patients underwent intraoperative mapping with ECoG. At 4-year follow-up, 61% of the patients with focal lesions were seizure free compared with 20% of the patients without histopathologic abnormalities. In a review of patients undergoing frontal lobe resections with adjunctive MST and callosotomy when appropriate, 72% were Engel class I or II after surgery.[247] In another study of patients undergoing frontal lobe surgery, 24 underwent intracranial monitoring and 80% were Engel class I or II after surgery (64% seizure free).[215] In this series, patients without lesions had better outcomes than those with lesions. In a review of FLEs, 72% of lesional and 40% of nonlesional patients had an excellent outcome (Engel class I or II) after frontal lobe resection, with seizure-free rates of 44% and 24%, respectively.[221] In a report of seizure outcomes in 37 patients with intractable frontal tumoral epilepsy, 67% of patients were Engel class I or II and 35% were seizure free.[16]

Complications of Extratemporal Resection

Complications of extratemporal resections include those related to invasive monitoring with grids, surgical complications of resection or MST, and neurological sequelae of intentional resection of or inadvertent injury to regions of eloquent cortex.[101] The complications in one study included three wound infections and three neurological deficits that resolved slowly.[246] In frontal lobe resections in Broca's area, within the posterior 2.5 cm of the opercula, the inferior frontal gyrus is usually spared,[245] and language sites identified by stimulation mapping techniques within the middle frontal gyrus may contribute, if resected, to transient or longstanding expressive aphasias.[174] Resection of the supplementary motor cortex may produce a transient syndrome consisting of postoperative mutism, contralateral neglect or hemiparesis, and diminished spontaneous movement, which usually resolves spontaneously over a period of weeks.[248,249] The cognitive effects of frontal resections are usually well tolerated.[250] Preservation of draining veins and arterial supply to the central area is a key consideration.[142] Partial resection of the nondominant hemisphere facial motor cortex is usually well tolerated; however, complete removal may produce longstanding perioral weakness.[116,251,252] The superior resection margin should be located no closer than 2 to 3 mm below the lowest elicited thumb response. Rasmussen described successful removal of the dominant hemisphere facial motor cortex, provided that the vascular supply to the central area is meticulously preserved.[101,251,252] Large parietal resections behind the rolandic cortex can be accomplished with reported hemiparesis rates as low as 0.5%.[252] When resections are extended into the parietal operculum, visual field defects may occur if the resections are carried deep into the white matter.[182,252] A nondominant hemisphere parietal syndrome develops in some patients after large parietal resections, and in the dominant hemisphere, care must be taken to preserve Wernicke's area. In the occipital lobe, complete resection produces the expected contralateral hemianopia, and excision in the dominant hemisphere to within 2 cm of Wernicke's area may result in dyslexia.[252]

Extratemporal Lesional Epilepsy

Lesional resection alone has provided favorable results in extratemporal sites, with 9 of 14 patients (64%) being seizure free in one study[205] and 17 of 18 patients (94%) being seizure free in another study.[253] A meta-analysis of lesional epilepsy in all sites showed that 44% of the patients were seizure free after simple excision and 67% were seizure free after "seizure surgery."[254] Lesionectomy with removal of hemosiderin-stained brain resulted in freedom from seizures in 73% of patients with occult vascular malformations.[255]

Cortical dysplasias are associated with a unique pattern of intrinsic epileptogenicity, and intraoperative ECoG is thought by some authors to provide useful information for guiding resection and ensuring optimal seizure outcomes.[256,257] In a large series of patients undergoing surgery for focal epilepsy secondary to cortical dysplasia, 49% were seizure free.[258] Fifty-eight percent of those undergoing complete resection and 27% of those with incomplete resection were seizure free. Other reports suggest universal freedom from seizures in 100% of patients with Taylor's balloon cell–type cortical dysplasia after complete lesionectomy without ECoG mapping.[224] Other neuronal migration abnormalities, such as double cortex, do not benefit from resective surgery.[259]

Hypothalamic Hamartomas

Intrahypothalamic hypothalamic hamartomas (HHs) may be associated with intractable partial, gelastic, and generalized seizures,[260] as well as retardation and behavioral disorders, whereas precocious puberty predominates in the parahypothalamic subset.[261] Numerous reports have documented successful surgical removal of these lesions and relief of seizures with various approaches, including pterional, transtemporal, transcallosal, and modified subfrontal approaches.[262,263] A recent study reported the results of transcallosal surgical resection of HH in 26 patients with refractory epilepsy in a prospective outcome study.[264] Fourteen (54%) patients were completely seizure free, and 9 (35%) had at least a 90% improvement in total seizure frequency. They also reported postoperative improvement in behavior and cognition. The likelihood of a seizure-free outcome seemed to correlate with younger age, shorter lifetime duration of epilepsy, smaller preoperative HH volume, and 100% HH resection. Another study looked at 37 patients with HH and symptomatic epilepsy who underwent transcortical transventricular endoscopic resection.[265] Eighteen patients (48.6%) were seizure free. Seizures were reduced more than 90% in 26 patients (70.3%) and by 50% to 90% in 8 patients (21.6%). Additionally, the mean postoperative hospital stay may be shorter in endoscopic patients than in patients who undergo transcallosal resection. A recent study documented the results in 14 patients who underwent a stereotactic, frame-based placement of an MRI-compatible laser catheter through a 3.2-mm drill hole.[266] Using real-time MRI thermometry, the laser surgery system was used to ablate the HH in these patients. Twelve of fourteen patients were seizure free at 9 months' follow-up with no permanent surgical complications, neurological deficits, or neuroendocrine disturbances.[266]

Cerebellar Seizures

The classical teaching that epileptic seizures do not arise from the cerebellar cortex has been challenged by several reports of focal motor seizures with secondary generalization in which the seizure focus appeared to be within the cerebellum.[101,267] Five of eight patients achieved freedom from seizures after resection of their cerebellar lesions.

Catastrophic Epilepsies

Catastrophic epilepsies are those in which panhemispheric syndromes are associated with intractable seizures. Such syndromes include Rasmussen's encephalitis, developmental syndromes (i.e., hemimegalencephaly, tuberous sclerosis, hamartomas, Sturge-Weber syndrome), and congenital hemiplegia or porencephaly.[268]

Hemispherectomy

Although the original surgical approach of anatomic, complete en bloc hemispherectomy with sparing of the basal ganglia, hypothalamus, and diencephalon[115,252,269] was successful from the standpoint of seizure control, the immediate and delayed complications were daunting.[142] In particular, these procedures created a large area of denuded, unsupported subcortical tissue and significant volumes of intracranial dead space that led to repeated microhemorrhage and subdural membrane formation, referred to as *superficial cerebral hemosiderosis*.[101] Late complications in the postoperative course occur in as many as 38% of patients[270] and include hydrocephalus,[271] increased intracranial pressure, neurological demise, and even death.[272] An alternative approach to hemispheric decortication (i.e., removal lobe by lobe) was reviewed in a large pediatric series.[268] The study reported that 26 of 48 patients were seizure free with a reduced rate of delayed complications.[268] Nevertheless, perioperative mortality occurred in 3 patients, and intraoperative blood loss and coagulopathy complicated the clinical course, particularly in children without brain atrophy or with hemimegalencephaly. In another version of *cerebral hemicorticectomy*, the entire cortical surface is "degloved" to the level of the white matter. In one study, this resulted in 8 of 11 patients being seizure free, 1 patient with hydrocephalus, and no mortalities or delayed complications.[273]

With the introduction by Rasmussen of the technique of modified or *functional hemispherectomy*, in which a generous central and temporal resection is juxtaposed with deafferentation of the frontal and occipital lobes, postoperative complications were significantly reduced.[116,252] With deafferentation rather than removal of the frontal and occipital lobes, the volume of intracranial dead space is reduced.[101] In a 7-year follow-up study of 14 patients, no hemosiderosis or hydrocephalus occurred, and 10 of the 14 patients were seizure free.

Since the 1990s, hemispheric deafferentation has become increasingly favored as a preferred alternative to anatomic resection or a traditional functional hemispherectomy. The *peri-insular hemispherotomy* uses a smaller craniotomy—a much reduced peri-insular (opercular frontal, parietal, temporal) resection along with deafferentation of the frontal, parietal, occipital, and temporal lobes.[274,275]

An early study of this technique reported favorable seizure outcomes (9 of 11 patients seizure free and 1 of 11 improved 95%). In addition, the study documented reduced operative time, as well as a decrease in perioperative and delayed complications. A recent review of a consecutive series of patients undergoing a *modified lateral hemispherotomy* between 2004 and 2012 revealed complete seizure freedom in 80% and cognitive stability on neuropsychological evaluations.[276]

The *transsylvian keyhole functional hemispherectomy* advanced by Schramm and colleagues[277,278] represents a true minimalist approach to hemispheric deafferentation.[101] A linear scalp incision and a 4- by 4-cm craniotomy provide the limited exposure required for a transsylvian approach to the circular sulcus, through which access to the entire ventricular system is gained.[101] Transventricular hemispheric deafferentation and amygdalohippocampectomy resulted in significantly decreased blood loss and a reduced mean operating time compared with a Rasmussen-type functional hemispherectomy. Of the 20 patients reviewed in an early series, 88% were seizure free and 6% had improvement in their seizures. This approach is facilitated in patients with hemispheric atrophy and not recommended in those with hemimegalencephaly.[101] In a more recent review of outcomes and complications by this group, 89% of 71 patients treated with the keyhole hemispherectomy were seizure free and had a ventriculoperitoneal shunting rate of 3% compared with a 5.3% shunt rate for a mixed series of approaches.[279] In a modification of this technique, another study evaluated 34 patients undergoing *transopercular hemispherotomy*, after which 67% of patients were seizure free.[280]

Disconnection Surgery: Multiple Subpial Transection

MST was developed by Morrell and colleagues to permit the treatment of partial epilepsies in which the seizure focus resides exclusively or partially within eloquent cortical regions.[281] In a review of their experience with 100 patients, seizure outcomes were stratified according to MST performed alone (32 patients) or in conjunction with cortical resection (68 patients).[281] Engel class I and class II outcomes were achieved, respectively, in 38% and 25% of patients with partial seizures undergoing MST alone, in 58% and 13% of patients with Landau-Kleffner syndrome treated by MST alone, and in 49% and 10% of patients when MST was performed in conjunction with resection procedures. In another review of 20 MST procedures performed without resection, less favorable outcomes were reported.[282] Yet another study of 12 patients undergoing MST with or without resection revealed less favorable outcomes, including Engel classes II (1), III (2), and IV (9).[283] A study of long-term outcomes reported a late increase in seizure frequency in 19% of patients treated by MST with or without resection.[284] A meta-analysis of an aggregate international experience consisting of 211 patients at six centers revealed that 53 underwent MST alone and 158 underwent MST plus resection.[285] An excellent outcome, defined as greater than a 95% reduction in seizures, was achieved with MST plus resection in 87% of patients with generalized seizures and in 68% with complex partial seizures. In patients with MST alone, 71% of patients with generalized seizures and 62% of patients with complex partial seizures had excellent outcomes.

Neurological deficits associated with MST include a reduction in verbal fluency but preservation of spoken and written language abilities.[281] In this same study, 41 of 45 patients undergoing MST in Wernicke's area had preserved receptive function, including comprehension of spoken and written words. One patient suffered a deep hemorrhage causing a speech deficit. In 44 transections in the hand motor cortex, strength was preserved, and activities of daily living could be performed with the affected hand.[281] Of 7 transections in the leg area, which were described as technically difficult, 2 patients suffered foot drop because of subcortical venous hemorrhage. Overall, neurological complications were observed in 17% and permanent deficits were identified in 7%. No mortalities occurred. Two cases of "remarkable" intraoperative brain swelling and edema have been described, with a large intracerebral hematoma discovered in 1 patient.[282]

Disconnection Surgery: Corpus Callosotomy

The procedure of subtotal or staged total corpus callosotomy has been recommended less frequently since widespread introduction of the vagal nerve stimulator.[8] Nevertheless, an abundant literature attests to the utility of callosotomy as a meaningful palliative treatment in patients with multiple or poorly lateralized (and unresectable) epileptogenic foci, SGTCS, and injurious drop attacks because of tonic or atonic seizures, with resultant falls and injury.[247,286-289] Early studies revealed increased focal seizures in 25% of patients undergoing callosotomy.[288] It has been reported that 70% of patients will achieve elimination of seizures or at least a greater than 80% reduction in their frequency.[287,288,290]

In a recent series of 23 patients with intractable generalized seizures, patients underwent partial division (17) or total division (6) of the corpus callosum.[291] Forty-one percent of the patients were completely seizure free or nearly free of the seizure types targeted for treatment. Forty-five percent of the patients experienced a greater than 50% reduction in seizure frequency. Simple partial motor seizures developed in 4 patients after surgery. In addition, mentally retarded patients tended to have poorer outcomes. Fifty-seven percent of patients experienced a transient disconnection syndrome that resolved. One patient suffered a clinically silent right frontal infarction related to venous thrombosis. The average hospital stay was 7.7 days.

Callosotomy is particularly effective for drop attacks. In a study of 52 patients with drop attacks (tonic or atonic seizures), 42 (81%) exhibited complete cessation of drop attacks, with greater success occurring in those undergoing total callosal section.[292] Two adult patients suffered a marked disconnection syndrome that gradually remitted, and 14 patients experienced transient akinetic states that resolved in several weeks. In another study of 20 patients monitored for 3 years, 10 exhibited a marked improvement in QOL, and 10 had greater than a 50% reduction in their seizures.[293] In another cohort of 17 patients, 9 had greater than an 80% reduction in targeted seizures, and overall, 88% of the patients reported satisfaction with the surgical outcome because of improved alertness and responsiveness.[294]

The surgical and functional complications attributable to corpus callosotomy are well described in the literature, with a larger number of complications noted in earlier series.[142,209] The main complications reported are acute disconnection syndromes, more common with total callosotomy, and the rare split brain syndrome. Subtotal (70% to 80%) callosotomy has been recommended as an initial procedure to minimize this complication. Surgical complications such as hemorrhage and infarction are related more to obtaining access to the interhemispheric fissure. With modern advances in microsurgical approaches and careful patient selection, corpus callosotomy is a safe procedure and a technique that is currently underused.

COMPLICATIONS OF DIAGNOSTIC PROCEDURES

Epilepsy surgery is safe and effective. Nevertheless, invasive diagnostic procedures and definitive surgical interventions do carry some risk, which must be considered when recommending surgical intervention to patients with intractable seizures.[101]

Intracarotid Amytal Procedure (Wada Test)

Complications of the Wada test encompass the complications of transfemoral carotid angiography, including thromboembolism and stroke (0.5% to 1%), allergic reactions to contrast agents (1 in 40,000), and local complications of femoral artery puncture.[142] Rare mortality has been reported.[295] With the advent of fMRI language lateralization, the Wada test has been abandoned by many centers. In a recent survey of epilepsy specialists in North America and Europe, 85% of responders stated that the Wada test is no longer needed in the evaluation of patients for TLE surgery.[296]

Depth Electrodes

For many years, depth electrodes were used routinely as part of the surgical evaluation of patients with intractable epilepsy.[297] In contemporary practice, noninvasive assessments, including structural MRI and improved surface EEG monitoring techniques, and subdural grid and strip recordings supplanted depth electrodes and have reduced the requirement for invasive recordings. An advantage of depth electrodes is that low-voltage, localized discharges emanating from deep structures, including the insula, cingulate gyrus, amygdala, and hippocampus, may be detected as evidence of the site of seizure onset. However, depth electrodes are invasive, and historical studies have documented associated complications, including infection (1% to 4%), intracerebral hemorrhage in 3% of parasagittal placements and 1% of lateral placements, and rare mortalities.[179,298] The use of modern stereotactic techniques has reduced the morbidity associated with depth electrodes, with a resurgence in interest in this technique.[299,300] A recent study of 122 patients undergoing the placement of 1586 depth electrodes between 2009 and 2012, using a stereotactic technique that juxtaposed MRI, computed tomography, and intraoperative angiography, documented a rate of complications that suggests a safety profile similar to that associated with subdural electrode placements.[301] In this series, an asymptomatic subdural hematoma in 1 patient and small intraparenchymal hemorrhages in 2 patients were noted with minimal neurological morbidity, with a risk for complication per electrode of 0.18% and a morbidity rate of 2.5% (3 of 122 patients).

Subdural Strip Electrodes

Subdural strip electrodes have provided a safe alternative to brain penetration by depth electrodes.[302] Strip electrodes are usually placed symmetrically over suspected sites of seizure onset and yield excellent recordings from neocortical structures. Although recordings from intracerebral sites are not provided with this modality, these electrodes do not require cortical penetration with its associated risks. The principal risk with subdural electrodes is infection, which may manifest as superficial infection, meningitis, or brain abscess, as reviewed in an extensive series of 350 patients.[55,302] Other reported adverse events have included fever with body temperatures higher than 102°F, migraine, and temporalis muscle fibrosis, as indicated in a prospective study of 55 patients. In a multicenter study, only five minor complications occurred in 131 patients, three of which were reported to be small hematomas not requiring evacuation.[194]

Subdural Grid Electrodes

Subdural grid electrodes provide electrographic tracings from a large expanse of cortex and permit extraoperative brain mapping to localize eloquent functions in relation to the epileptogenic zone. Grid electrode placement requires a large craniotomy and the egress of numerous electrode cables through the scalp for the duration of the monitoring period (usually 1 to 2 weeks). The grid is removed at a second craniotomy, during which the definitive cortical resection is performed. It is not surprising that bone flap infection and meningitis are prominent concerns as complications of this procedure. Infection rates of 22% were identified in an early Cleveland Clinic series, but declined to 7% when cables were tunneled to exit percutaneously.[213] A more recent series of 49 patients undergoing grid implantation reported infection in 4%, subdural hematoma formation requiring emergency evacuation in 8%, and brain swelling in 2%.[303] Other series have reported subdural hematoma formation in 8% and increased intracranial pressure and brain shift requiring premature removal of the grid and permanent morbidity in 2% to 5%.[142,304,305] Meticulous surgical technique with avoidance of injury to or compression of large cortical or bridging veins, tunneling of electrode cables, administration of perioperative antibiotics, and full use of mannitol and dexamethasone (Decadron) are likely to improve outcomes and prevent complications.[142]

PSYCHIATRIC OUTCOMES AFTER EPILEPSY SURGERY

As a group, patients undergoing epilepsy surgery seem to benefit from a reduction in the prevalence of commonly observed psychiatric comorbidities of epilepsy, including depression and anxiety, particularly when the surgery leads to seizure freedom. Kanner and colleagues reported a total remission rate off psychotropic medication in 45% of patients who underwent epilepsy surgery.[135] The impact on psychotic disorders, however, is less clearly defined: it varied from unchanged in most cases to improved psychotic status or level of functioning.[306] A history of psychotic symptoms does not represent an absolute contraindication to surgical intervention, although an exacerbation of symptoms may occur postoperatively.[101]

Conversely, there is a small risk (up to 20%) of developing psychiatric disease de novo, or of worsening of baseline psychiatric function in some patients.[307,308] In a study by Wrench and associates comparing the psychiatric outcomes following temporal versus extratemporal resections over a 3-month period, it was found that although both groups had similar baseline rates of depression and anxiety, and more patients were seizure free after a temporal than after an extratemporal resection, the psychiatric outcome was significantly worse in the temporal resections group: 1 month after surgery, 66% of patients after temporal lobe resection versus 19% of patients after extratemporal lobe resection reported symptoms of anxiety or depression, which persisted until the 3-month follow-up in 30% of the temporal and 17% of the extratemporal patients. In addition, by the 3-month follow-up, 13% of ATL patients had developed a de novo depression, as opposed to none in the extratemporal group. More notably, the occurrence of any of those psychiatric comorbidities was not related to seizure freedom.[309] This reinforces the need to carefully evaluate and consider psychiatric outcome after epilepsy surgery as an independent comorbidity, particularly noting that mood, anxiety, and incomplete seizure control seem to independently affect QOL after surgery.[34,310]

Patients undergoing epilepsy surgery identify treatment goals that extend beyond seizure control to include driving and regaining or improving employment and overall independence.[309] A necessary condition, then, is the absence of any functional worsening because of surgery, as might occur with a new neurological deficit, memory loss, or language disturbance. A successful operation is one that results in control of seizures and, regarding the patients' psychosocial goals, an improved QOL. Several studies have found that for optimal improvement in QOL measurements, complete seizure freedom (even from auras) is required.[68,311] Other possible predictors of an improved QOL include a higher presurgical IQ score, younger age at surgery, and more stable mood at baseline.[311] Studies evaluating the psychosocial and educational effects of surgery in children are very limited but do suggest meaningful improvements in educational attainments and later employment.[311]

A clear relationship has been documented between psychosocial status and quality of seizure control in medically managed epileptic patients.[312] Similarly, after surgery, seizure-free patients score more favorably than those with either auras or recurrent seizures on a variety of measures.[313] In the only randomized, controlled trial of epilepsy surgery versus best medical management to date, patients who underwent surgery were documented to have improvement in both seizure outcomes and health-related quality of life (HRQOL).[3] The surgical group consistently scored higher than the medical group as early as 3 months after surgery and continuing to 12 months on both the Quality of Life in Epilepsy Inventory 89 (QOLIE-89) and measures of school or job performance. Another study showed better HRQOL in postoperative seizure-free patients than in those with persistent auras and persistent seizures.[314] In another study of patients 2 years after surgery, both seizure-free patients and those with a 90% reduction in frequency experienced significant improvement in HRQOL.[315] When compared with the health status of patients with other chronic diseases, postoperative patients with persistent seizures scored worse than did those with heart disease, hypertension, or diabetes. When patients were seizure-free after surgery, they scored better than patients with these nonneurological illnesses.[316] In a study reviewing nonsurgical and surgical patients evaluated preoperatively and 1 and 2 years postoperatively, significant improvement was identified on 10 of the 17 scales of the QOLIE-89 in patients who were entirely seizure free.[317] Significantly more improvement was noted at 2-year follow-up than at 1-year follow-up. In addition, patients with persistent auras were not significantly improved compared with patients with persistent seizures.[317]

In a large prospective surgical series of 396 patients in which the QOLIE-89 was administered before surgery and up to 5 years after surgery, the most substantial improvement in HRQOL occurred immediately after surgery in all patients, but additional improvements over time were seen in the seizure-free group.[318] The effect, in this study, seemed to stabilize 2 years after surgery and was related to the duration of freedom from seizures. Another method of determining well-being is to assess patients' perceived effect of surgery or their satisfaction with the results. A recent study found that of 396 patients, 80% would make the same decision (to have surgery) if given the choice again, and 91% to 92% reported a strong or very strong positive effect of surgery (influenced by freedom from seizures and gainful employment).[319]

Cost-Effectiveness of Surgical Treatment

Wiebe and coworkers used decision analysis modeling and an intention-to-treat approach to compare medical and surgical treatment of intractable TLE in a Canadian population of 200 patients treated either surgically or medically over a 35-year period.[320] In their model, surgery required a larger initial expenditure; however, by 8 years after surgery, the cost savings engendered by the 57 seizure-free patients made surgical management less expensive than medical management across the entire cohort of surgical patients. Thus, surgical therapy was more cost-effective than medical management in this population.

In a decision analysis model of surgical versus best medical management of intractable TLE, Langfitt used Rochester, New York, cost data to address the relative cost-effectiveness of different treatments.[101,321] This investigation used public health clinical research methods that express the cost-effectiveness of treatment as a *marginal cost-effectiveness ratio* (MCER), which represents the dollar cost per quality-adjusted life-year (QALY) added to treated patients' lives postoperatively. Each postoperative outcome state was assigned a quality adjustment on the basis of the Epilepsy Surgery Inventory 55 (ESI-55) scores achieved by 42 patients undergoing evaluation for surgery. With a state of total health adjusted to 1, patients with intractable seizures preoperatively were adjusted to 0.62; postoperative states were adjusted as follows: no seizures, 0.89; auras only, 0.80; and recurrent complex partial seizures, 0.72. In this model, a patient rendered seizure free after surgery would improve from 0.62 to 0.89 on the adjustment scale, and if this patient lived for 40 years in this state of health, the patient would accrue an additional 10 QALYs. The calculated MCER was $15,581 per QALY, which compares quite favorably with the cost of other health care interventions. Another study reported a cost-effectiveness ratio of $27,200 per QALY.[322] By comparison, the calculated MCER for lifetime tuberculosis screening for a 20-year-old African American was $324,537 per QALY.[321]

Neuropsychological assessment is useful both during the surgical patient selection process and as a tool to assess outcomes

TABLE 80-2 Neuropsychological Assessment of Epileptic Patients

Functions	Tests
Sensory functions	Halstead-Reitan examination
Motor functions: dexterity, coordination, speed, flexibility	Purdue Pegboard, Grooved Pegboard, Thurstone's Uni- and Bimanual Coordination Test
Perceptual-motor functions	Beery Visuo-Motor Integration Test, Block Design, Rey-Osterrieth Complex Figure
Psychomotor development and intelligence	Griffith or Bayley Developmental Scales, Wechsler Intelligence Scales for Adults or Children (WISC, WAIS), Stanford-Binet
Attention	Concentration Endurance Test, Auditory Continuous Performance Test
Memory and learning	
General	Wechsler Memory Scales for Children and Adults
Verbal: word lists, story recall	California Verbal Learning Test (CVLT)
Visual: faces, patterns	Rey-Osterrieth Complex Figure
Expressive: sentence construction	Boston Naming Test, Token Test
Receptive: comprehension	Peabody Picture Vocabulary Test (PPVT)
Written: reading, spelling	Wide Range Individual Achievement Test (WIAT)
Numerical operations	WIAT, Woodcock-Johnson Achievement Battery
Executive functions	Tower of London, Wisconsin Card Sorting Test, Fluency Tests
Personality	Rorschach, Thematic Apperception Test for Children or Adults, SCL-90R
Affective state	Beck Depression Inventory, Hamilton Anxiety Scale
Social adjustment	Vineland Adaptive Behavior Scales, Achenbach Child Behavior Checklist (CBCL)
Quality of life	Quality of Life in Epilepsy Inventory questionnaires (e.g., QOLIE-31, QOLIE-AD-48)

after surgery. The aim of the evaluation is to establish a profile of the patient's strengths and weaknesses in multiple domains on a variety of standardized tests and questionnaires (Table 80-2) in relation to normative values derived from the general population.[323] Of particular concern in temporal lobe surgery are losses of memory function, including the rare but disabling syndrome of global amnesia, as well as the more common material-specific memory losses affecting short-term verbal memory in the language-dominant hemisphere and visual-spatial memory in nondominant hemisphere, temporal lobe operations.

The Wada test, which was originally developed to determine hemispheric lateralization of language function,[324] was subsequently adapted by Branch and colleagues[325] to provide a measure of the risk for loss of memory function postoperatively. The Wada test was used for many years to identify patients at risk for global memory loss, and in fact, such losses have been uncommon since the Wada test was universally adopted. However, reports of favorable memory outcomes in patients who failed the Wada test preoperatively (false-positive results) have called into question the reliability of this procedure in some patients.[326] The Wada test has also been useful in identifying lateralized temporal lobe dysfunction, which may correlate with the side of seizure onset,[327,328] the likelihood of a favorable seizure outcome, and more recently, prediction of the risk for material-specific memory loss (particularly verbal memory loss) after surgery.[329,330] Nonetheless, the Wada test is invasive and requires a degree of patient cooperation, which may be suboptimal in young children and mentally retarded patients. Wada test results may be difficult to interpret in patients with bilateral language representation, excessive agitation, insufficient hemispheric inactivation by amobarbital (Amytal), or other procedural factors.

fMRI is increasingly being used as a noninvasive tool for assessment of focal functional deficits in patients with intractable epilepsy.[331,332] fMRI represents neuronal activity indirectly through hemodynamic changes in the brain. The size of the cortical area activated and the number of involved neurons directly influence the magnitude of the changes in regional cerebral blood flow.[333] Studies comparing fMRI and Wada test results in the same patient have shown a high correlation (from 80% to 100%) between the two procedures when the studies were aimed at either investigating language lateralization[334-336] or assessing memory asymmetries.[331,332] Certain patterns of fMRI activation have been evaluated as independent prognostic indicators of memory outcomes after TLE surgery.[337-339] The translation of these interesting findings into clinically validated tests used in routine presurgical patient evaluation remains to be seen.

NEUROMODULATORY SURGERY

Vagus Nerve Stimulation

Since U.S. Food and Drug Administration approval in 1997 of vagus nerve stimulation (VNS) as a palliative treatment of patients older than 12 years with intractable partial seizures, tens of thousands of patients have undergone implantation of a left vagus nerve stimulator.[340,341] In prospective clinical trials, a median partial seizure reduction of 34% after 3 months and 45% at 12 months was achieved in patient groups both younger and older than 50 years. Twenty percent of patients at 12 months had 75% or greater reductions in seizures, thus demonstrating improved seizure control over time.[340,341] At 3 months, generalized seizures were reduced by 46%. Improvements in mood have also been reported.[342] Although it has been observed that figural memory worsens when VNS is active during memory tasks,[343] no change in cognitive functions has been noted.[343] In patients with greater than 50% improvement in seizure frequency, QOL measures were improved.[344,345] In a long-term study looking at the effectiveness of VNS in epilepsy patients, seizure frequency was reduced by 26% 1 year after implantation, by 30% 5 years after surgery, and by 52% 12 years after implantation.[346] A more recent study suggested that VNS could be a safe and effective alternative therapy in children with drug-resistant epilepsy who are not candidates for epilepsy surgery.[347] In this study, after a mean follow-up of 31 months, 38% of the patients had a reduction in seizure frequency of greater than 90%.

Reported side effects include voice alteration, hoarseness, throat or neck pain, headache, cough, and dyspnea.[348] Adverse events in adults include infection requiring antibiotics or removal of the device (or both) and transient paralysis of the left vocal cord with hoarseness and aspiration.[349] There is an extraordinary report of self-inflicted vocal cord paralysis in 2 developmentally disabled patients by manipulation and rotation of the pulse generator within the subclavicular pocket.[350] Such a report mandates that patients be observed for manipulation of the device. In a review of adverse events in 24 children in whom the vagal nerve stimulator was implanted, 15 events occurred in 11 patients, including lead fractures, wound erythema, requested removal of the device, abscess, malfunction, gastrostomy, recurrent psychosis, and diminished speech volume.[348] Removal of electrodes from the vagus nerve can be difficult. One paper reported resolution of a deep wound infection with antibiotics alone, thus suggesting that removal of the device might not always be necessary.[351] No increase in sudden unexpected, unexplained death with the vagal nerve stimulator was identified when implanted patients were compared with appropriate cohort populations.[352]

Deep Brain Stimulation

In the past, brain stimulation in the cerebellum, the caudate nucleus, and the anterior, centromedian, and ventralis intermedius thalamic nuclei has been performed in an attempt to modulate cortical excitability.[353,354] Small controlled trials in 14 patients who underwent cerebellar stimulation showed that 2 were improved and 12 were unchanged.[355] In another study, 4- to 6-Hz stimulation of the ventral caudate nucleus led to a reduction in neocortical and mesial temporal epileptic discharges and electrical spread of seizures, but clinical seizure data were not assessed. Caudate nucleus stimulation for epilepsy has not yet been tested in controlled studies. A small placebo-controlled study of stimulation of the centromedian nucleus showed no significant benefit.[356] An initial report of patients undergoing deep brain stimulation (DBS) in the subthalamic nucleus described a greater than 80% reduction in daytime seizures.[305] In another study, 5 patients with various seizure types underwent stimulation through bilateral electrodes in the anterior thalamus.[357] They reported a significant decrease in seizure frequency, with a mean 54% reduction (mean follow-up of 15 months). Two of the patients had a 75% or greater reduction in seizures. The observed benefits, however, did not differ between stimulation-on and stimulation-off periods, thus suggesting that either a placebo or carryover effect was present. In the multicenter, doubled-blind, randomized Stimulation of the Anterior Nuclei of the Thalamus for Epilepsy (SANTE) trial, bilateral DBS of the anterior nucleus of the thalamus was performed in 110 patients 18 to 65 years old who were having 6 to 10 intractable partial seizures per month.[358] After 2 years, there was a 56% median percent reduction in seizure frequency, and 54% of the patients had a seizure reduction of at least 50%. Electrical stimulation of the hippocampus has also been reported in an attempt to block temporal lobe seizures.[359] In another small series, 3 patients with complex partial seizures had DBS electrodes implanted in the amygdala-hippocampal region.[360] Over a mean follow-up of 5 months, all patients had a greater than 50% reduction in seizure frequency. In 2 patients, AEDs could be reduced. Complications with DBS for epilepsy, such as hemorrhage and infection, have been reported in about 5% of patients,[361] although the hemorrhage is often not clinically significant.

There is growing interest in methods of neurostimulation that are modulated by input from sensing devices. A small pilot study reported that responsive stimulation controlled with an external computer system terminated some spontaneous seizures in eight patients, four with bilateral anterior thalamic stimulation and four with focal cortical stimulation.[362] In this study, analysis of electrographic seizure severity in stimulated versus nonstimulated events was used to rule out non–stimulation-associated effects and suggested both an immediate effect and a possible cumulative antiepileptic effect of high-frequency stimulation.

A multi-institutional, randomized, double-blinded, controlled trial of responsive focal cortical stimulation (RNS System, Neuropace, Mountain View, CA) was recently completed, in which 191 patients with medically intractable partial-onset seizures from one or two foci underwent cranial implantation with a responsive neurostimulator.[363] The RNS pulse generator continuously analyzes the patient's ECoG tracings and automatically triggers electrical stimulation when specific ECoG characteristics programmed by the clinician are detected. In this study, there was a 44% median percent reduction in seizures at 1 year and 53% at 2 years. Complications occurred in 2.5% of the subjects and consisted of infection (5 patients) and intracranial hemorrhage (4 patients), 3 of which had to be evacuated. An unanticipated benefit of the RNS implantations accrues from the chronic ECoG over months and years, which can be used to plan and execute a resective surgical option in these patients. Five patients in this trial became candidates for definitive resective surgery, suggesting that there may be a benefit to chronic implantation of recording electrodes.[364]

STEREOTACTIC RADIOSURGERY

Radiosurgery for Hypothalamic Hamartomas

HH may be associated with an epileptic encephalopathy marked by medically intractable gelastic and other seizures and behavioral and cognitive decline. Reports of successful treatment of HH with Gamma Knife surgery (GKS) have offered an attractive alternative to open surgery.[365-368] In a multicenter study of 10 patients undergoing GKS in seven centers, 4 patients were seizure free (Engel class I), 1 had rare nocturnal seizures, 1 had rare partial seizures, and 2 were improved.[366] A European, multicenter, prospective trial of GKS for HH has enrolled 60 patients, 27 of whom have exceeded 3 years of follow-up.[369] Ten of the 27 patients (37%) were seizure free (Engel class I). This study emphasized a temporal evolution of changes in seizure frequency during the postradiation period: a slight improvement in seizure frequency within the first 2 months, followed by transient worsening, with a subsequent reduction and ultimate remission in favorable cases. Behavioral improvements, in addition to EEG normalization, occurred in a more linear fashion. Minimal side effects were reported. Patients treated with doses exceeding 17 Gy to the margins of the HH seemed to have greater rates of seizure remission than did those receiving less than 13 Gy.

Radiosurgery for Supratentorial Tumors

Given the diverse pathologic features and locations of central nervous system tumors associated with intractable epilepsy, the effects of GKS on tumor progression and seizure outcome are not well studied. One study divided 24 patients into two groups distinguished by the amount of radiation directed to surrounding tissue.[370] Outcome was assessed at a mean of approximately 2 years after GKS as excellent (Engel class I or II) or not. Patients in the high-dose group achieved a 66% improvement rate compared with 42% in the low-dose group, with all patients exhibiting adequate tumor control. This report suggested that higher GKS doses to the epileptogenic region surrounding the tumor might improve seizure outcomes.

Radiosurgery for Arteriovenous Malformations

The potential efficacy of GKS in the treatment of symptomatic localization-related epilepsies has best been demonstrated in the treatment of AVMs. One large series reported that seizures remitted after GKS in 69% of patients with AVM and epilepsy.[371] Subsequent studies of both proton beam treatment and GKS showed a combined rate of seizure remission of 73% to 80%.[372-374] A large case series emphasized that the incidence of seizure remission is better with smaller AVMs.[374] However, another study noted that seizures remitted independent of radiologic remission of the AVM, thus suggesting that the effects of irradiation near the lesion, rather than improvement of the AVM itself, may be important in control of seizures after GKS.[371]

Radiosurgery for Cavernous Malformations

It is difficult to draw conclusions about seizure outcome after radiosurgery for cavernomas given the limited studies in the literature. In general, seizure remission appears to be lower than that encountered in patients after treatment of AVMs. The effect of dose to adjacent brain tissue around the margin of the cavernous malformation, thought to be important in the case of tumors and possibly AVMs, has not been systematically studied with regard to seizure control for patients with cavernomas. Excess morbidity in terms of postoperative hemorrhage and edema remains a concern. An early study suggested that GKS did not appreciably alter the natural course of cavernous malformations while exposing patients to radiation-induced complications that exceeded by 7 times those expected with the same dose for AVMs.[375] A retrospective comparison concluded that traditional open resection resulted in better seizure control and a lower risk for hemorrhage than GKS did.[376] A retrospective multicenter trial reported on 49 patients with cavernomas treated by GKS.[377] All patients had epilepsy that was medically intractable and were monitored for more than 12 months after treatment. The mean marginal dose was 19.2 Gy. Twenty-six patients (53%) became seizure free (Engel class I), 10 patients (20%) had a substantial decrease in the number of seizures (Engle class II), and 13 patients (26%) had little or no improvement. The average time to seizure remission was 4 months, and severe radiation-induced edema developed in 7 patients, but they recovered fully.

Radiosurgery for Mesial Temporal Lobe Epilepsy

The rationale for treatment of mesial TLE with GKS is less compelling than in the disorders discussed previously because mesial TLE is amenable to open surgery.[378] All of the studies in the literature differ in their treatment protocols and results, with most failing to achieve complete remission from seizures.[366,379-383] An earlier study had demonstrated that 6 of 7 patients (86%) studied over a 2-year follow-up period were seizure free after radiosurgery.[366] A subsequent trial reported that 13 of 21 patients (62%) were seizure free (Engel class I) after radiosurgery for mesial TLE.[383] The variability in outcome of GKS therapy for mesial TLE may reflect differing approaches to the dose and target volume more than the anatomic target of the mesial temporal lobe structures.[378] Taken together, these studies suggest that low-dose protocols are less successful than higher-dose protocols. No significant clinical or neuroimaging changes occur until approximately 9 to 12 months after treatment, and the most dramatic drop in the seizure rate occurs between 12 and 18 months, coincident with the development and resolution of maximal MRI changes. Reported morbidities include visual field deficits, headache, nausea, vomiting, and depression.[384]

Beyond seizure control, studies have evaluated secondary outcome measures such as cognition and QOL. One prospective, multicenter trial reported no mean neurocognitive changes through a 2-year follow-up period.[334] Similarly, one small series reported no group mean changes at 6 months of follow-up, although some individuals showed a decline in at least one cognitive domain.[381] Another small series reported on three participants, with a 27-month follow-up, who underwent dominant hemisphere low-dose GKS.[382] No long-term consistent changes in neurocognitive measures were found, although each patient showed a decline in a measure of verbal memory. They concluded that the neurocognitive changes after GKS appear to be similar to those after anterior temporal lobectomy.

Overall, although GKS for mesial TLE is promising, the optimal treatment protocol has not yet been determined, and the relative benefits in terms of seizure resolution and avoidance of complications have yet to be clearly demarcated from those of open surgery. A National Institutes of Health–sponsored multicenter pilot study on the safety of GKS for mesial TLE in patients who would normally qualify for anterior temporal lobectomy for unilateral mesial TLE were randomized to either a 20- or 24-Gy dose.[378] A total of 30 subjects were enrolled and monitored for 3 years; the preliminary results are promising, with safety well within that expected after routine GKS and favorable efficacy and neuropsychological profiles.

SUGGESTED READINGS

de Tisi J, Bell GS, Peacock JL, et al. The long-term outcome of adult epilepsy surgery, patterns of seizure remission, and relapse: a cohort study. *Lancet*. 2011;378:1388-1395.

Engel J Jr. Surgery for seizures. *N Engl J Med*. 1996;334:647-652.

Engel J Jr, Wiebe S, French J, et al. Practice parameter: temporal lobe and localized neocortical resections for epilepsy: report of the Quality Standards Subcommittee of the American Academy of Neurology, in association with the American Epilepsy Society and the American Association of Neurological Surgeons. *Neurology*. 2003;60:538-547.

Gleissner U, Helmstaedter C, Schramm J, et al. Memory outcome after selective amygdalohippocampectomy: a study in 140 patients with temporal lobe epilepsy. *Epilepsia*. 2002;43:87-95.

Jehi L, Yardi R, Chagin K, et al. Development and validation of nomograms to provide individualised predictions of seizure outcomes after epilepsy surgery: a retrospective analysis. *Lancet Neurology*. 2015;14: 283-290.

Najm I, Jehi L, Palmini A, et al. Temporal patterns and mechanisms of epilepsy surgery failure. *Epilepsia*. 2013;54:772-782.

Schwartz TH, Bazil CW, Walczak TS, et al. The predictive value of intraoperative electrocorticography in resections for limbic epilepsy associated with mesial temporal sclerosis. *Neurosurgery*. 1997;40:302-309, discussion 309-311.

Stroup E, Langfitt J, Berg M, et al. Predicting verbal memory decline following anterior temporal lobectomy (ATL). *Neurology*. 2003;60: 1266-1273.

Wiebe S, Blume WT, Girvin JP, et al. Effectiveness and Efficiency of Surgery for Temporal Lobe Epilepsy Study Group. A randomized, controlled trial of surgery for temporal-lobe epilepsy. *N Engl J Med*. 2001;345:311-318.

Wyler AR, Hermann BP, Somes G. Extent of medial temporal resection on outcome from anterior temporal lobectomy: a randomized prospective study. *Neurosurgery*. 1995;37:982-990, discussion 990-981.

See a full reference list on ExpertConsult.com

Overview and Controversies

Ron L. Alterman, Andres M. Lozano, Joachim K. Krauss, and Takaomi Taira

In this introduction, we initially outline the contents of the "Functional Neurosurgery" section and then review controversies and unanswered questions that neurosurgeons, irrespective of their level of training and years of experience, may need to address in dealing with patients.

OVERVIEW

In the first half of the 20th century, because of the absence of neuropharmacologic therapies, stereotactic and functional neurosurgery (or "stereoenchephalotomie," as Ernest A. Spiegel and Henry T. Wycis termed it) focused primarily on psychiatric disorders. Subsequently, the field expanded beyond the domain of psychiatric illness to include the treatment of pain, movement disorders, and cancer. During the latter years of the 20th century and the early years of the 21st, the applications of functional neurosurgery have undergone profound growth. In the first edition of *Neurological Surgery* (1973), the "Ablative and Neuropsychological Procedures" section consisted of seven chapters focused on ablative approaches to influence function. In contrast, the "Functional Neurosurgery" section of this 7th edition of *Youmans and Winn Neurological Surgery* (2017) contains 29 chapters in six parts that cover a wider diversity of disorders and whose approach shifts distinctly from ablative to neuromodulatory or restorative interventions.

The first part, "Basic Science of Movement Disorders," is composed of three chapters: "Anatomy and Synaptic Connectivity of the Basal Ganglia" (Chapter 81), "Rationale for Surgical Interventions in Movement Disorders" (Chapter 82), and "Neuropathology of Movement Disorders" (Chapter 83).

The second part, "Neurology of Movement Disorders," begins with "Clinical Overview of Movement Disorders" (Chapter 84), followed by the very important topic of "Patient Selection Criteria for Deep Brain Stimulation in Movement Disorders" (Chapter 85). This part finishes with "Functional Imaging in Movement Disorders" (Chapter 86). The third part, "Surgery for Movement Disorders," begins with an overview of surgical management, "Surgical Management of Tremor" (Chapter 87). Subsequent individual chapters deal with various surgical approaches and topics: ablation (Chapter 88) and deep brain stimulation (DBS) for Parkinson's disease (Chapter 89), DBS for dystonia (Chapter 90), underlying mechanisms of DBS (Chapter 91), avoidance of complications in DBS (Chapter 92), neurophysiologic monitoring (Chapter 93), emerging and experimental methods of treating Parkinson's disease (Chapter 94), and magnetic resonance–guided focused ultrasound (Chapter 95). The last two chapters of this part deal with selective peripheral denervation for cervical dystonia (Chapter 96) and thalamotomy for focal hand dystonia (Chapter 97).

The fourth part, "Surgery for Psychiatric Disorders," echoes the origins of functional neurosurgery. Appropriately, it begins with "A History of Psychosurgery" (Chapter 98), which reminds us that we must remember the past if we are to avoid previous problems and future excesses. Four chapters then deal individually with surgery for Gilles de la Tourette syndrome (Chapter 99), obsessive-compulsive disorder (Chapter 100), major depressive disorder (Chapter 101), and anorexia nervosa (Chapter 102).

The fifth part, "Surgical Interventions for Spasticity," comprehensively covers the treatment of spasticity with one chapter on ablative surgery (Chapter 103) and another on infusion techniques (Chapter 104).

The sixth and final part, "Surgery for Vertigo, Cortical Stimulation, Obesity, Alzheimer's Disease, and Neuroprosthetics," has five chapters: "Treatment of Intractable Vertigo" (Chapter 105), "Motor Cortex Stimulation for Pain and Movement Disorders" (Chapter 106), "Deep Brain Stimulation for Obesity" (Chapter 107), "Deep Brain Stimulation for Alzheimer's Disease" (Chapter 108), and "Neuroprosthetics" (Chapter 109). The last topic has immense potential for future clinical expansion.

CONTROVERSIES AND UNANSWERED QUESTIONS

In many respects, progress in the field of functional neurosurgery has slowed since publication of the previous edition of this book. The potential of exciting new interventions such as gene therapy for Parkinson's disease and DBS for chronic medically refractory depression failed to materialize, their benefits unproven in multicenter, prospective trials. At the same time, results of other large, prospective studies have reinforced much of what neurosurgeons already knew about DBS for Parkinson's disease, dystonia, and tremor. Some newer techniques such as direct MRI targeting have matured, but, by and large, treatments used in the 1990s are still being used today, although probably with improved results and fewer serious complications.

Fortunately, minds in this field are creative, and so it is hoped that new concepts and technologies that have emerged of late will translate into new therapies and indications. Of course, new controversies have also emerged, disagreements that will probably be settled as neurosurgeons continue to understand better how to modulate neural circuitry in order to alleviate the brain's many disorders of function. Just a few of the controversies are discussed below.

Deep Brain Stimulation: Subthalamic versus Internal Globus Pallidus

Despite the successful reintroduction of posteroventral pallidotomy for medically refractory Parkinson's disease, functional neurosurgeons rapidly adopted DBS of the subthalamic nucleus (STN) after its introduction by Limousin and colleagues in 1995.[1] Mahlon DeLong's primate work had previously confirmed that subthalamic lesions could alleviate parkinsonism,[2] but as a result of the risk of hemiballismus in association with lesions of the human STN, surgeons began using the internal globus pallidus (GPi), a safer target for ablation. DBS was a relatively safe bilateral intervention that seemed to improve gait, as well as rigidity, tremor, and dyskinesia, and had the added benefit of reducing medication requirements.[1]

Over time, stimulation-associated difficulties in gait, balance, and speech developed, as did a concern that STN stimulation might induce more rapid cognitive decline, depression, and even suicide in some patients. Some investigators therefore revisited the GPi, now as a target for bilateral DBS. Preliminary results were sufficiently positive that DBS at the two targets were compared directly as part of a large prospective, randomized, controlled trial conducted through the Veterans Affairs Health System.[3] Results of this study suggested that motor improvement was equivalent with both targets; the main differences were greater medication reduction in the patients who underwent STN-DBS and slightly better cognitive function in the patients who underwent GPi-DBS, which was more apparent at the 36-month follow-up than it was initially.[4] Results of a subsequent prospective trial conducted in Europe favored the STN target, with better improvement of motor symptoms, but no difference between both targets with regard to side effects at the 1-year follow-up.[5] Significant differences in motor improvement were found to be maintained at the 3-year follow-up.[6] Of interest, although the STN is the preferred target for surgery in younger patients in Europe, both the STN and GPi are considered in North America. More data are still needed to make final conclusions, except perhaps in older patients with early cognitive decline, for whom GPi-DBS may be the better option.

Biologic Therapies (Neural Restoration)

From the time it was understood that loss of dopaminergic neurons in the substantia nigra pars compacta underlay the motor symptoms of Parkinson's disease, medical scientists have sought methods to preserve or restore the lost dopaminergic innervation. Initially, it was hoped that simply replenishing the dopamine would suffice; however, the limitations of oral dopamine replacement therapy have since become all too evident. Levodopa is merely a symptomatic therapy that does not alter the underlying neurodegenerative process. Of more importance, it is a therapy that loses potency over time, treats only a subset of symptoms of Parkinson's disease, and can induce significant side effects (i.e., dyskinesia).

Madrazo and colleagues[7] first reported profound motor improvement in two patients with Parkinson's disease after transventricular intracerebral transplantation of autologous adrenal medullary cells. Since then, numerous surgically administered biologic therapies designed to restore or preserve dopaminergic function in patients with Parkinson's disease have yielded initial amazing and widely publicized responses in early-stage clinical trials, only to underperform when subjected to larger and more rigorous multicenter clinical trials, controlled with sham surgery and under blinded conditions. Of more importance, some of these therapies have generated significant adverse effects in the larger trials, effects that were not observed in the early trials, probably because of the small number of patients treated. It is commonly understood that patients with Parkinson's disease are particularly prone to the placebo effect; however, Alterman and associates[8] demonstrated that the reason these therapies failed was not that the clinical responses reported in the initial trials turned out to be placebo effects. Rather, the clinical responses to the therapies themselves fell by half or more when assessed by raters under blinded conditions, a difference the authors attributed to observer bias in the initial open-label trials. Regardless of the reason for this significant loss of efficacy in the blinded trials, it is clear that (1) sham surgery–controlled trials have proved invaluable in weeding out ineffective therapies, and (2) the field of functional neurosurgery must be more rigorous in its performance of early-stage trials (e.g., blinded rating, larger number of study participants) if scientists are to avoid repeating this cycle ad infinitum, wasting substantial time and resources and putting patients at unnecessary risk. The challenge, of course, is how to implement these changes in view of the imperatives of the marketplace and the impatience of those who suffer with this and other devastating illnesses.

Timing of Deep Brain Stimulation Surgery in Parkinson's Disease

Because of the risks associated with DBS and the efficacy of medical therapy for symptom control, early trials of surgical interventions after the levodopa era were necessarily restricted to patients in whom the disease had become refractory to standard medical therapy and/or were severely disabled by levodopa-induced dyskinesias. Over time, the indications, targets, and surgical techniques for performing DBS have been refined with a concomitant reduction of surgical risks, which has prompted a consideration of DBS at earlier stages of the disease.

Although controversial, the results of the so-called "Early Stim" trial[9] support the notion that DBS may be an effective treatment strategy when employed earlier in the course of the disease, specifically when motor disturbances first begin, rather than when they become severe or disabling. In this study, the mean disease duration was as short as 4 years (mean, 7 years); the findings demonstrated that even at this earlier stage, DBS yields results superior to those of medical therapy alone. Similarly, Charles and colleagues[10] conducted a randomized trial of STN-DBS versus best medical therapy in patients with very-early-stage Parkinson's disease (<4 years from the start of levodopa therapy). The aim of the study was to determine with a prospective blinded trial whether 2 years of STN-DBS slowed the underlying neurodegenerative process of Parkinson's disease. Although it is unclear whether this was the case in this relatively small trial (30 patients total), the results suggested that STN-DBS may yield better motor function and quality of life than do medications alone, even in patients with early-stage disease.[11] The fact that two patients suffered a serious adverse event during the study generated significant criticism,[12] and so it is currently unclear whether any investigators will pursue such early interventions aggressively.

Magnetic Resonance Imaging–Guided High-Frequency Ultrasound versus Deep Brain Stimulation

The benefits and drawbacks of DBS implant technology are well known. The ongoing maintenance and need for battery replacements or recharging can be challenging for some patients. In addition, stimulator adjustments can involve multiple clinic visits. The advantages of magnetic resonance–guided focused ultrasound (MRgFUS) are that it is usually a one-time procedure performed with the patient under local anesthesia and is noninvasive insofar as neither incisions nor implants are required. At least according to early reports, MRgFUS produces benefits in patients with certain pain syndromes and movement disorders.[13-15] Nevertheless, MRgFUS does produce a brain lesion and therefore carries all the disadvantages of focal ablation of neural tissue, which may include irreversibility and an inability to adjust the therapy once the treatment is completed.

MRgFUS is a relatively new therapy, so long-term safety and efficacy data are lacking. Ultimately, clinical data and patient preference will help determine the clinical conditions under which MRgFUS or DBS is applied. One important limitation of MRgFUS, at least currently as applied to movement disorders, is that although unilateral procedures are well tolerated, the risks are increased with bilateral procedures. According to historical accounts of bilateral ablative procedures for Parkinson's disease, there can be significant adverse effects on speech and cognition. This is why, for the time being, when bilateral therapy is needed, DBS is preferred over lesion creation, regardless of technique.

The surgeon can also consider a lesion on one side of the brain and a DBS procedure on the other. The long-term data will help shape the relative roles of the various surgical options and define which patients with which disorders will benefit most from MRgFUS.

What Is the Future of Deep Brain Stimulation for Depression and Alzheimer's Disease?

There are tremendous unmet needs in the treatment of psychiatric and cognitive disorders, and DBS may one day play an important role in meeting those needs. So far, however, several trials have failed to generate class 1 evidence that DBS is useful for either. Issues surrounding patient and target selection, as well as optimal stimulation parameters, must be resolved. Consequently, more preclinical (i.e., animal model) and early clinical (i.e., phase 1 and 2) studies are required. Patients with psychiatric and cognitive disorders whose conditions are refractory to medical therapy certainly require alternatives, and the hope is that neurosurgeons will one day be able to offer therapies such as DBS to treat this large population of patients.

What Is the Potential Impact of Responsive Neurostimulation?

Responsive or closed-loop neurostimulation relies on recording ongoing neural activity and triggering stimulation in response to the detection of a predetermined signal. Responsive stimulation has been pioneered in the context of epilepsy. Neuropace (Mountainview, CA) has championed the use of continuous neural recordings for seizure detection, driving responsive stimulation treatment in a closed-loop manner. This approach has received approval from the U.S. Food and Drug Administration. The concept of applying closed-loop stimulation to other disorders, particularly tremor and movement disorders, is emerging. There is increasing evidence that treating beta oscillations in akinetic-rigid forms of Parkinson's disease in an adaptable, closed-loop manner may be beneficial, both for optimizing stimulation parameters and for extending battery life. Nevertheless, the specific utility of such possible biomarkers still needs further clarification.[16] Similarly, closed-loop treatments of other paroxysmal disorders that are present only intermittently or manifested during specific activity as action tremor may also be useful. To date, other than the Neuropace device, the only implantable units available that both record and stimulate are experimental. In comparison with stimulators that are constantly stimulating, closed-loop systems have the potential advantage of more efficient power utilization in that the stimulation is on only when required. They may also offer additional advantages in that when neuronal networks are working normally or nearly normally, there may be no need for stimulation, or, in fact, stimulation may carry the risk of disrupting normal activity.

See a full reference list on ExpertConsult.com

81 Anatomy and Synaptic Connectivity of the Basal Ganglia

Adriana Galvan and Yoland Smith

The basal ganglia are a group of interconnected subcortical structures. In primates, the basal ganglia comprise the dorsal striatum (caudate nucleus and putamen); the ventral striatum (nucleus accumbens); the external and internal segments of the globus pallidus (GPe and GPi, respectively); the subthalamic nucleus (STN); the substantia nigra, which includes the pars reticulata and pars compacta (SNr and SNc, respectively); and the ventral tegmental area (VTA). In rodents, the caudate nucleus and putamen form a single structure commonly called the *caudate-putamen complex;* the globus pallidus (GP) and the entopeduncular nucleus are often referred to as the homologues of the primate GPe and GPi, respectively, although anatomic and functional differences between these nuclei exist. The striatum and STN are the main entry points for extrinsic glutamatergic inputs from the cerebral cortex and thalamus. The basal ganglia outflow arises predominantly from GPi and SNr and is directed toward frontal areas of the cerebral cortex (via the thalamus) and various brainstem structures.

The basal ganglia are part of neural circuits that involve the cerebral cortex and thalamus. According to the functions of the cortical regions from which they originate, three main functionally segregated loops can be identified: sensorimotor, limbic, and associative/cognitive. In each of these circuits, functionally related cortical areas project topographically to specific areas of the striatum. This segregation of cortical information is maintained at all levels of other basal ganglia nuclei and in the basal ganglia–receiving regions of the thalamus. Functional interactions between these loops may occur at various levels, including cortical-cortical connections and overlapping territories of each basal structure of the ganglia.

Cortical inputs to the striatum originate from most functional areas of the cerebral cortex, whereas the thalamostriatal projections originate mainly from the caudal intralaminar thalamic nuclei (the centromedian nuclei [CM] and parafascicular nuclei [PF]), but also with significant contributions from the rostral intralaminar, midline, associative, and motor-related nuclei. The thalamostriatal system mediates communication between the cerebellum and the basal ganglia.

At the synaptic level, the main targets of cortical and a significant subset of thalamic terminals are the dendritic spines of medium-sized spiny neurons (MSNs), the main striatal projection neurons that transmit or secrete γ-aminobutyric acid (GABAergic neurons). However, thalamic inputs from the CM/PF nuclei contact predominantly the dendritic shafts of MSNs and different types of striatal cholinergic and GABAergic interneurons.

Striatal MSNs are divided into two groups on the basis of their dopamine receptor expression and main basal ganglia projection targets: the "direct pathway," where MSNs project directly to the basal ganglia output nuclei, GPi, and SNr and express preferentially D_1 dopamine receptors, and the "indirect pathway," where MSNs project mainly to the GPe and express D_2 dopamine receptors. An imbalance of activity between these two pathways is a cardinal feature of the basal ganglia pathophysiologic processes in Parkinson's disease and related movement disorders.

The striatum also receives a massive dopaminergic input from SNc and VTA, which plays a critical regulatory role in cortical glutamatergic transmission through presynaptic and postsynaptic mechanisms at the level of spines on MSNs. Dopamine neurons process and transmit to the striatum complex and heterogeneous information related to movement, reward-related stimuli, and aversive events.

Along with the striatum, the STN is considered an input nucleus of the basal ganglia. As for the corticostriatal system, the corticosubthalamic projection arises from different motor, associative, and limbic cortical regions that innervate functionally segregated regions of the STN in primates. In contrast to the striatum, only the CM/PF nuclei provide significant glutamatergic thalamic afferent connections to the STN. In turn, the STN sends prominent glutamatergic excitatory projections to the GPe, GPi, and SNr.

The GPi and the SNr are the output nuclei of the basal ganglia. Both nuclei receive functionally segregated inputs from the striatum (through direct and indirect routes) and, in turn, send GABAergic projections to their thalamic and brainstem target structures. Through their thalamic projections to the ventral motor nuclei and the CM/PF complex, cortical information can be sent back to frontal cortical regions via segregated basal ganglia–thalamocortical loops or to specific striatal regions via basal ganglia–thalamostriatal projections. The brainstem targets of the basal ganglia output include the superior colliculus, pedunculopontine nucleus, the lateral habenula, and the parvicellular reticular formation. Because of its connections with most basal ganglia nuclei, the thalamus and various lower brainstem structures, the pedunculopontine nucleus is in a strategic location to mediate widespread basal ganglia influences in the central nervous system. The lateral habenula is considered as an interface between the limbic system and the basal ganglia because it receives reward-related information from the GPi. The basal ganglia-collicular projection is important in the control of saccadic eye movements and visual orientation.

Disruption of communication by degenerative neuronal loss or by neurochemical changes in various nodes of the basal ganglia–thalamocortical loops leads to the development of motor and nonmotor signs and symptoms of large number of neurological and psychiatric disorders (including Parkinson's disease, Huntington's chorea, Gilles de la Tourette's syndrome, dystonia, attention deficit disorders, and obsessive compulsive disorder).

Full text of this chapter is available online at ExpertConsult.com 

82 Rationale for Surgical Interventions in Movement Disorders

Thomas Wichmann and Mahlon R. DeLong

Since the 1990s, the use of neurosurgical methods to treat movement disorders has dramatically increased owing to our increased understanding of the pathophysiology of these disorders and the introduction of high-frequency deep brain stimulation (DBS), which has largely replaced ablative procedures. In this chapter we review the rationale for the use of these procedures from several perspectives, including an overview of the brain networks targeted by surgical interventions, the known pathophysiologic changes found in some of the major movement disorders and their modification by surgical intervention, and the potential symptomatic or neuroprotective use of early surgical interventions. Included is a brief discussion of the "paradox of stereotaxic surgery," that is, the fact that these highly effective procedures, which abolish major signs and symptoms of basal ganglia disorders, paradoxically do not significantly impair movement, which has contributed to their acceptance as mainstream treatment.

ANATOMIC CONSIDERATIONS

Until recently it has been assumed that movement disorders are of either basal ganglia or cerebellar origin. Recent studies indicate, however, that anatomic interactions between the two cortical-subcortical systems are considerable and appear to be relevant in terms of underlying both the physiology and pathophysiology of movement disorders.[1-3] However, because this information has not yet directly affected current surgical approaches, and because little is known about the specific role of the cerebellum in movement disorders, we focus largely on the basal ganglia in this chapter.

Anatomic and physiologic studies have shown that the basal ganglia are components of a family of similarly organized parallel reentrant brain circuits. In each of these circuits, cortical information reaches, and is processed in, the basal ganglia and is then sent to the brainstem and, through the thalamus, back to the cerebral cortex.[4-8] The anatomic similarities between these circuits suggest that similar processing steps are carried out in each. Depending on the presumed functions of the cortical region involved in these circuits, the circuits are commonly designated as "motor," "oculomotor," "prefrontal," and "limbic" circuits. As shown in Figure 82-1, dysfunction within individual circuits may be associated with specific signs and symptoms of diseases. Implied in the circuit disorder concept is the view that a given pathology will lead to different manifestations if it affects the different basal ganglia functional domains.

Considerable evidence indicates that the signs and symptoms of movement disorders result from network abnormalities that primarily affect the motor circuit. This circuit originates in frontal cortical precentral and postcentral sensorimotor areas, including the primary motor cortex (M1), the supplementary motor area (SMA), the premotor cortex (PMC), and the cingulate motor area (CMA), and related sensory cortical areas, and involves specific motor portions in each of the basal ganglia and thalamus. The motor circuit is at least partially closed (on a macroscopic level), with thalamocortical projections terminating in the same frontal cortical regions from which the circuit originates. However, it is also well established that the motor circuit, like other basal ganglia circuits, receives input from interconnected postcentral cortical areas. There is evidence that the motor circuit can be subdivided into multiple segregated subcircuits that are centered on individual cortical motor areas.[9-11]

The basal ganglia are composed of the neostriatum (caudate nucleus and putamen), the ventral striatum, the external and internal segments of the globus pallidus (GPe, GPi, respectively), the subthalamic nucleus (STN), and the substantia nigra pars reticulata and pars compacta (SNr, SNc, respectively). The striatum and STN are the main entry points for cortical inputs, whereas GPi and SNr provide basal ganglia output to the brainstem and thalamus. The cortico*striatal* and other basal ganglia projections are topographically organized,[4-6,12,13] which accounts for the preservation of a general somatotopic organization throughout the motor circuit.

The anatomy of the motor circuit is shown in Figure 82-2A. Projections from the sensorimotor cortical areas terminate in the postcommissural putamen and in the STN.[14,15] These projections are topographically arranged. For example, in primates, inputs from M1 innervate the dorsolateral STN, whereas the SMA, PMC, and CMA project to the dorsomedial STN.[15-17] The defined motor portions of the striatum and STN project to motor areas in the basal ganglia output nuclei, GPi, and SNr.[6] The cortical-subthalamic pathway, together with the subthalamic-GPi connection (which is shared with the indirect pathway; see later), is summarily called the *hyperdirect* pathway because it may allow cortical inputs to reach the output structures of the basal ganglia, GPi, and SNr, with relatively short latencies.[18-20]

The striatal projections to GPi and SNr can be divided into the *direct* and *indirect* pathways (see Fig. 82-2A).[6,21] The direct pathway arises from striatal medium spiny neurons (MSNs) that project monosynaptically to neurons in GPi and SNr. These neurons also contain the neuropeptides substance P and dynorphin and preferentially express dopamine D_1-like receptors. The indirect pathway arises from striatal MSNs that project to GPe.[22,23] These preferentially express enkephalin and dopamine D_2-like receptors.[24,25] The indirect pathway continues from GPe to GPi, both by direct projections and through the intercalated STN. The topographic organization of the corticostriatal projections is maintained throughout the course of the direct and indirect pathways. Thus populations of GPe neurons within the sensorimotor territory are reciprocally connected with populations of neurons in the same functional territories of STN, and motor-related neurons in each of these regions, in turn, innervate the same functional territory of GPi.[22,23] The functional topography that is present in the intrinsic basal ganglia circuitry is maintained in the basal ganglia projections to the thalamus and the subsequent thalamocortical projections.[26] Projections from the basal ganglia output from the motor circuit (emanating from GPi) terminate preferentially in portions of the anterior ventrolateral thalamic nuclei, whereas basal ganglia output from the associative circuit (emanating mostly from SNr) terminates in the ventroanterior thalamic nuclei.

Collaterals from the pallidofugal and nigrofugal projections also reach the intralaminar nuclei of the thalamus, the centromedian and parafascicular nuclei. These projections are part of a system of segregated basal ganglia-thalamostriatal feedback

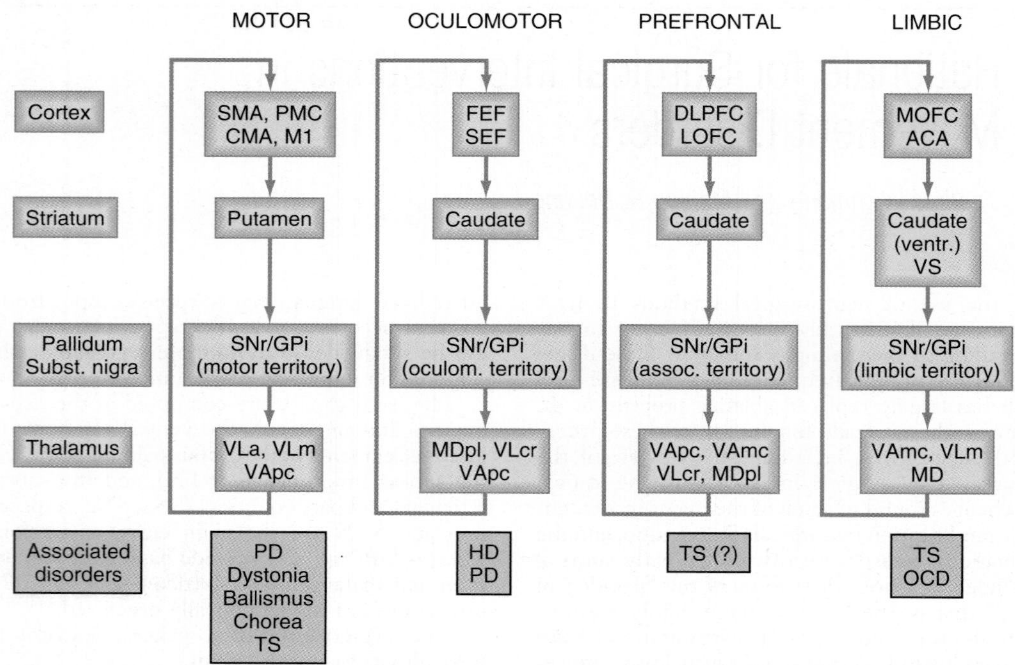

Figure 82-1. Circuit anatomy of cortex–basal ganglia–thalamocortical circuits. ACA, anterior cingulate area; CMA, cingulate motor area; DLPFC, dorsolateral prefrontal cortex; FEF, frontal eye fields; GPi, internal pallidal segment; HD, Huntington's disease; LOFC, lateral orbitofrontal cortex; M1, primary motor cortex; MDpl, mediodorsal nucleus of thalamus, pars lateralis; MOFC, medial orbitofrontal cortex; OCD, obsessive-compulsive syndrome; PD, Parkinson's disease; PMC, premotor cortex; SMA, supplementary motor area; SEF, supplementary eye field; SNr, substantia nigra pars reticulata; TS, Tourette's syndrome; VApc, ventral anterior nucleus of thalamus, pars parvocellularis; VAmc, ventral anterior nucleus of thalamus, pars magnocellularis; VLm, ventrolateral nucleus of thalamus, pars medialis; VLcr, ventrolateral nucleus of thalamus, pars caudalis, rostral division; VS, ventral striatum. *(From Wichmann T, Delong MR. Deep brain stimulation for neurologic and neuropsychiatric disorders.* Neuron. *2006;52:197.)*

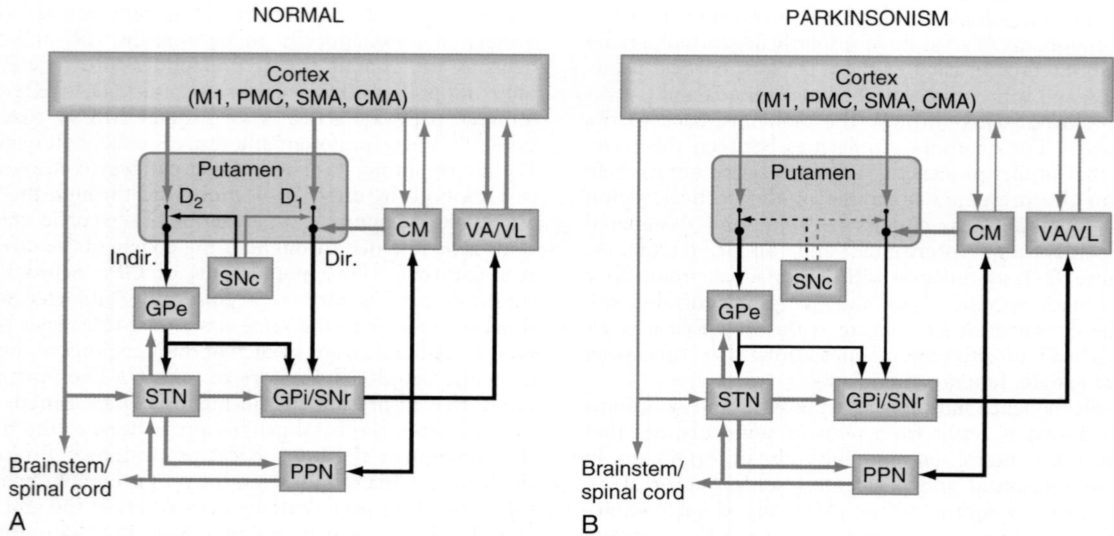

Figure 82-2. Parkinsonism-related changes in overall activity in the basal ganglia–thalamocortical motor circuit. *Black arrows* indicate inhibitory connections; *blue arrows* indicate excitatory connections. The thickness of the arrows corresponds to their presumed activity. CM, centromedian nucleus; Dir., direct pathway; D_1, D_2, dopamine receptor subtypes; Indir., indirect pathway; PPN, pedunculopontine nucleus; SNc, substantia nigra pars compacta; STN, subthalamic nucleus. For other abbreviations, see legend to Figure 82-1. *(From Galvan A, Wichmann T. Pathophysiology of parkinsonism.* Clin Neurophysiol. *2008;119:1459.)*

projections.[27,28] In primates, centromedian nuclei receive input from cortex as well as motor areas in GPi and SNr and project to the motor portions of putamen and STN,[29] whereas parafascicular nuclei inputs and output are related to associative and limbic territories of the basal ganglia.[29-31] Other thalamic nuclei, including ventroanterior and ventrolateral thalamic nuclei, send additional sparse projections to the striatum.[32]

GPi and SNr also project to brainstem areas, in particular the pedunculopontine nucleus (PPN).[33,34] In part, these projections are part of a feedback system, engaging PPN neurons that then give rise to ascending glutamatergic and cholinergic projections to basal ganglia, thalamus, and basal forebrain. The PPN also gives rise to descending projections to pons, medulla, and spinal cord.[35,36] The PPN is a component of the physiologically defined brainstem locomotor region.[37]

The model of the basal ganglia–thalamocortical motor circuit in Figure 82-2 is often used as the basis for speculations regarding its function in movement. A central component of this functional model is the fact that the output of the basal ganglia from GPi and SNr is inhibitory. As mentioned earlier, GPi and SNr neurons are GABAergic (inhibitory) and fire at high rates. Thus it appears that they continuously inhibit thalamic and brainstem targets. The earlier "rate" model of basal ganglia function poses that phasic activation of MSNs that give rise to the direct pathway reduces inhibitory basal ganglia output, with subsequent disinhibition of related thalamocortical neurons and facilitation of the intended movement.[21,38] By contrast, activation of MSNs that give rise to the indirect pathway are postulated to lead to increased (inhibitory) basal ganglia output and to suppression or prevention of movement. The balance between direct and indirect pathway activity is proposed to regulate the specifics of muscle activation for the intended movement, whereas specific activation patterns (e.g., a center-surround type of focal inhibition of pallidal and nigral output, generated through the interplay of direct and indirect pathways) may limit the extent or duration of ongoing movements. Single-cell behavioral studies in primates and functional neuroimaging studies in humans have provided evidence that GPi output may be modulated in relation to the amplitude and velocity of movement, supporting a role of the basal ganglia in the scaling of movement. Based on the same general basal ganglia model, an alternative model of basal function states that the basal ganglia may focus motor activity on intended movements and suppress unintended ones.[39,40] Furthermore, the interplay between the hyperdirect and indirect or direct pathways may enable the basal ganglia to prevent movements or responses that are already initiated or ongoing.[41-45]

In all models of basal ganglia function, the modulatory effect of dopamine on striatal transmission is fundamental. Dopamine is released in the striatum from terminals of projections from the SNc and modulates the activity of GPi and SNr by facilitating corticostriatal transmission on the direct pathway while inhibiting corticostriatal transmission on the indirect pathway.[46-49] In a general sense, the net effect of striatal dopamine release appears to be a reduction of basal ganglia output (and thus a release of movement). Besides its actions in the striatum, dopamine also acts directly on receptors in the STN, pallidum, and cortex to influence discharge patterns and rates in these structures.[50]

Besides a general role in the regulation of the overall amount of movement, dopamine release also plays a prominent role in reinforcement learning. Activation of dopamine receptors on MSNs is involved in the induction of long-term potentiation and depression at glutamatergic (presumably corticostriatal) synapses,[51-61] which may also involve adenosine, glutamate receptors, and cannabinoid receptors.[55,60-63] It is not clear whether dopamine release in other basal ganglia locations and the cerebral cortex has similar functions in learning and plasticity. Based on inactivation and neuroimaging studies, the associative circuit appears to play a prominent role in the initial learning of a motor task, whereas the motor circuit comes into play as the task is learned and thus is believed to play a greater role in the execution of learned motor sequences.[64]

PATHOPHYSIOLOGY OF MOVEMENT DISORDERS

Although neurosurgery for movement disorders was developed empirically, our knowledge of the pathophysiology of these disorders has provided a clearer rationale for these disorders and has helped to further refine these treatments. To illustrate this point, we briefly discuss the pathophysiology of two of the most commonly surgically treated forms of movement disorders, Parkinson's disease (PD) and dystonia.

Parkinsonism

Clinical Presentation

The cardinal features of PD—the triad of akinesia and bradykinesia, tremor at rest, and muscular rigidity—are summarily called *parkinsonism*. In PD, parkinsonism results from decreased dopaminergic transmission in the motor portions of the basal ganglia, in particular the putamen, owing to progressive loss of dopaminergic neurons in the SNc. SNc neurons that project to the motor portion of the putamen are most vulnerable to the degeneration process, which explains the prominence of motor signs in this disease. PD is characteristically an asymmetrical disease, initially manifesting as hemiparkinsonism in many patients, because the extent of degeneration affecting the two hemispheres is asymmetrical.

Since the early 1960s, dopamine replacement therapies have been the primary method of treatment. Although this treatment is initially highly effective, its long-term use is often complicated by the development of *motor fluctuations*, a term that refers to the early or unpredictable wearing off of the medication benefit, and the appearance of involuntary movements (dyskinesias). The development of these complications is one of the primary reasons for surgical treatment, along with tremor that is often poorly responsive to medical therapy.

Besides the dopamine-responsive features, PD is frequently accompanied by depression, autonomic dysfunction, sleep disorders, cognitive impairment, and gait and balance problems that are poorly or entirely unresponsive to dopaminergic medications. These appear to arise from widespread progressive nondopaminergic pathology in lower brainstem, midbrain, thalamus, and cerebral cortex that may develop together with (or even before) the loss of dopaminergic neurons in PD.[65,66]

Pathophysiology

Early metabolic and electrophysiologic recording studies in monkeys rendered parkinsonian by treatment with 1-methyl-4-phenyl-1,2,3,6-tetrahydropyridine (MPTP)[21,67-69] found that the spontaneous neuronal activity in GPe was decreased, whereas it was increased in STN, GPi, and SNr, compared with normal controls.[68,70-72] These global activity changes were thought to result from dopamine depletion, leading to increased activity of striatal neurons of the indirect pathway and resulting in inhibition of GPe and subsequent disinhibition of STN and increased GPi and SNr output (Fig. 82-2B). Positron emission tomography (PET) studies of cortical activity changes in parkinsonian patients generally supported this model by showing reduced activation of motor and premotor areas.[73,74] The hypothesis that rate changes in the basal ganglia underlie the development of parkinsonism (see Fig. 82-2B) was also generally supported by the finding that inactivation of the sensorimotor portions of the STN or GPi improves bradykinesia, rigidity, and tremor in parkinsonian subjects and increases the metabolic activity in cortical motor areas.[75-85]

However, the view that parkinsonism is due simply to increased inhibitory output has been largely abandoned. One of the reasons for this is that the "rate" model is not supported by clinical observations. For example, the model's prediction that lesions of GPi would produce dyskinesias was not confirmed; instead it was found that GPi lesions have strong *anti*dyskinetic effects.[78,80,86] It is now believed that electrical abnormalities of basal ganglia, thalamic, or cortical activity other than changes of average firing rate are more relevant to the pathophysiology of parkinsonism. These include oscillatory discharge patterns, burst discharge, and abnormal synchronization of discharge. Of these, synchronous oscillatory fluctuations in discharge rate of neurons in GPi, SNr, and STN are most often discussed.[87] These oscillations (usually in the 10- to 25-Hz range) have been detected in animal models and patients. Oscillations occur often together with abnormal burst discharge and can be seen at multiple nodes of the basal ganglia network, including STN, GPi, and SNr.[68,87-90]

Synchronized oscillatory activity can be recorded in patients with PD by using implanted DBS electrodes (e.g., in STN or GPi) as recording electrodes. These macroelectrodes do not provide single-cell spiking data but allow recording of local field potentials (LFPs) whose amplitude is highly dependent on the synchronicity of synaptic activity. The most commonly described synchronous oscillatory LFP phenomena include 10- to 25-Hz (beta) oscillations, which occur in unmedicated PD patients, and 60- to 80-Hz (gamma) oscillations, which are seen in levodopa- or DBS-treated patients.[87,91] In patients with PD, prominent abnormal firing and LFP patterns in GPi and the STN predominately affect the motor portions of these nuclei. Recent studies have shown that the amplitude of gamma-band oscillations may be excessively coupled to the phase of beta-band oscillations in the cerebral cortex of patients with PD.[92] It has been suggested that the amplitude of gamma-band activity is related to neuronal spiking activity; if so, the phase-amplitude coupling may represent the occurrence of oscillatory bursts at beta-band frequency. The coupling of oscillatory activity between cortex and the STN and GPi is strengthened[93-101] for reasons that are not completely understood.

It remains uncertain both whether and which of the observed electrophysiologic abnormalities actually *cause* parkinsonism or are simply associated with it. Although some studies suggest close (potentially causative) links between the electrophysiologic abnormalities and parkinsonism,[102-105] others have failed to find such causation. For example, studies in monkeys in which parkinsonism was gradually induced have cast doubt on the notion that synchronous oscillatory firing contributes significantly to (early) parkinsonism.[105a,105b] Similarly, rodent experiments have suggested that abnormal oscillations in the basal ganglia do not result simply from (acute) lack of dopaminergic stimulation.[106]

Dystonia

Clinical Presentation

In patients with dystonia, movements are disrupted by co-contraction of agonist and antagonist muscles and by excessive activation of inappropriate musculature (overflow), leading to abnormal postures and involuntary movements. The earliest manifestation of dystonia is often an "action dystonia," occurring only with attempted voluntary movement. In adults, dystonia most commonly occurs in a focal manner, such as cervical dystonia, blepharospasm, or spasmodic dysphonia. In children, generalized forms of dystonia are more common. One of the main forms of generalized dystonia, idiopathic torsion dystonia, is caused by a defect of the *DYT1* gene on chromosome 9.[107,108]

Pathophysiology

Dystonia may arise from a variety of disease processes. Many of these involve the basal ganglia and may involve disturbances of the dopamine system.[109] For instance, dystonia may develop acutely in normal individuals treated with dopamine-receptor blocking agents or may appear after long-term treatment with these drugs (tardive dystonia). In PD, dystonia develops usually in patients who have been exposed to dopaminergic drugs but may also appear as an early sign of the disease itself, independent of medications. Dystonia is also present in a group of patients with familial dystonia and parkinsonian features who respond dramatically to treatment with low-dose levodopa (i.e., dopa-responsive dystonia).[110,111] Most of these patients suffer from a genetic defect of dopamine synthesis that is caused by reduced activity of guanosine triphosphate cyclohydrolase,[112-114] the rate-limiting enzyme in the biosynthesis of a cofactor of the dopamine-synthesizing enzyme tyrosine hydroxylase, tetrahydrobiopterin. Tyrosine hydroxylase deficiency can also be a rare cause of dystonia.[115,116] In cases in which dystonia results from lesions affecting the striatum or its dopaminergic supply,[117] such lesions may affect the affinity or number of dopamine receptors in the unlesioned portion of the striatum or may lead to reorganization of the striatal topography, resulting eventually in altered activity in the basal ganglia output structures.

Metabolic studies in primates have suggested that dystonia may be associated with reduction of activity along the putamen-GPe connection and with increased inhibition of STN and GPi by GPe efferents.[118,119] Other PET and single-cell recording studies in human patients with dystonia have emphasized activity changes in the direct pathway instead. An involvement of direct and indirect pathways in the pathophysiology of dystonia is also supported by pharmacologic studies. For instance, it has been shown that D_2-like receptor antagonists may induce dystonia, presumably by increasing striatal outflow to GPe through the indirect pathway, whereas D_1-like receptor antagonists may be beneficial in this regard, presumably by reducing striatal outflow to GPi along the direct pathway.[120,121] These data suggest that a relative increase in the activity along the direct pathway (compared with that along the indirect pathway) contributes to dystonia. Single-cell recording studies in human patients undergoing functional neurosurgical procedures are in partial agreement with this concept. Most of these studies have demonstrated that discharge rates in GPe and GPi are lower than expected.[122-127]

Oscillatory activity in the basal ganglia may also contribute to dystonia. Coherence at low frequencies has been demonstrated between single-cell activity in the basal ganglia[123] or thalamus[127,128] and the electromyographic activity of dystonic muscles. LFP recordings from DBS electrodes implanted in GPi have shown increased power in the 4- to 10-Hz band,[129,130] and a high correlation with simultaneously recorded electromyographic activity.[129,131]

The cerebellum may also play a role in the pathophysiology of generalized primary dystonia.[132-134] Thus there is increasing evidence, based on magnetic resonance tractography studies, in favor of cerebellar disturbances in the pathogenesis of some of the hereditary generalized dystonias (DYT1 and DYT6). The low penetrance of DYT1 dystonia has been related to the presence of a second thalamocortical lesion in nonmanifesting individuals,[132,135] preventing the manifestation of dystonia in those with the thalamocortical defect in addition to the cerebellar disturbance. GPi-DBS has been shown to reduce the network abnormalities seen in DYT1 dystonia.[136] Recent animal studies in rodents have suggested that familiar rapid-onset dystonia-parkinsonism (DYT8) may also involve cerebellar mechanisms.[137] The aforementioned evidence for interactions between basal ganglia and cerebellar thalamocortical circuits provides an anatomic substrate by which cerebellar disturbances may induce secondary changes in basal ganglia output (and vice versa).[3,138]

There is evidence for altered functioning in movement-related cortical areas, particularly for abnormal plasticity and reduced intracortical inhibition, in dystonia. PET studies in dystonic patients have demonstrated widespread changes of activity in the SMA, CMA, and PMC.[139-142] In focal dystonia, abnormal somatotopic maps were demonstrated in M1,[143,144] with increased intracortical excitability in motor areas,[145] and a decreased Bereitschaftspotential and contingent negative variation.[146-149] Patients with writer's cramp were also shown to have an abnormally small degree of beta-band electroencephalogram desynchronization.[150] Recent studies using transcranial magnetic stimulation in patients with primary dystonia have demonstrated increased cortical plasticity.

Sensory abnormalities may also play a role in dystonia. There is convincing evidence for reduced corticocortical inhibition in the sensory system[151-154] and increased and improperly modulated precentral sensory evoked potentials (N30).[155-161] In addition, single-cell recording and imaging studies have suggested altered somatotopic representation at the cortical,[162-164] putamen,[165] and thalamic levels.[128,166]

RATIONALE FOR THE USE OF SURGICAL TREATMENTS

Current Rationale

The fact that many disorders of basal ganglia origin may be viewed as disorders resulting from motor circuit dysfunction allows for selective interventions with ablation or DBS at one of multiple levels of the basal ganglia–thalamocortical motor circuit, specifically the STN and the GPi. Unilateral ablation of a portion of the sensorimotor territory of GPi results in significant amelioration of contralateral parkinsonian bradykinesia, tremor and rigidity, dystonia, and chorea.[167-171] Ablation of portions of the STN motor territory is similarly effective for treating parkinsonism and dystonia.[43,172] The same targets that are used to carry out the ablative procedures in GPi and the STN are also used for high-frequency DBS in PD and dystonia. Similar to pallidotomy, DBS alleviates parkinsonian motor signs and reduces the severity of "off" periods, dyskinesias, dystonia, and motor fluctuations that complicate the long-term drug administration.[173-175] Although the STN is most commonly used for DBS for PD, the available data indicate that GPi- and STN-DBS have comparable motor benefits, with some evidence for a greater incidence of cognitive and behavioral (side) effects following STN-DBS,[176] perhaps attributable to the close proximity of motor, associative, and limbic portions in this small nucleus, preventing the functionally specific stimulation.

Movement disorders other than PD or dystonia can also be treated with surgical procedures.[177] These include hemiballismus (resulting from focal lesions of the STN or other brain regions[178,179]) and treatment-resistant cases of Gilles de la Tourette's syndrome (TS). The choice of DBS targets for treatment of TS has been largely empirical, based on the effects of previous ablative procedures.[180-182] This, along with the fact that this disease has both motor (tics) and nonmotor (compulsions, depression) aspects, has resulted in the use of surgical treatments that generally target not only motor but also limbic circuits, including the medial thalamus,[182-184] the motor and limbic portions of GPi,[183] and the anterior limb of the internal capsule.[185] In small open-label studies, these procedures are reported to reduce vocal and motor tics. At this time, DBS for treatment of TS remains purely experimental and does not have U.S. Food and Drug Administration approval.

Unfortunately, neither STN nor GPi interventions are effective against levodopa-unresponsive gait and balance disturbances and freezing of gait. In these cases, experimental stimulation of the PPN has been used with some success.[186-188] Dysfunction of the PPN is implicated in gait and balance problems, and potentially even akinesia, based on studies in primates using lesioning and stimulation approaches.[189-192] Although there have been multiple small studies of DBS of the PPN for gait disturbances, falls, and freezing, the optimal surgical target remains uncertain.[193,194] Recent studies have also explored combined DBS of the STN and PPN, and of the STN and SNr for gait abnormalities in PD.[195-198]

In addition to GPi, STN, and PPN, thalamic targets have also been used for DBS or ablative procedures in the treatment of movement disorders. Thus it is well accepted that ablation or DBS targeting the posterior ventrolateral nucleus of the thalamus, the cerebellar recipient portion of the thalamus, is effective for treatment of tremor, including the rest tremor in PD and other forms of tremor.[199-202] Ablation or DBS of the pallidal receiving anterior portion of the ventrolateral nucleus has been found to be effective for drug-induced dyskinesias and focal dystonia but seems to have little effect on bradykinesia or akinesia.[199]

Although the targeting of the surgical procedure is obviously important, the specifics of the movement disorder to be treated seem to matter less. For instance, interventions such as pallidal lesioning or DBS are effective in many movement disorders, with widely varying manifestations, including hypokinetic (e.g., parkinsonism) as well as hyperkinetic (e.g., dystonia) disorders. Given this experience, it seems obvious that the surgical interventions do not target specific pathophysiologic abnormalities but instead are more likely to eliminate abnormal and disruptive activity patterns in downstream targets of the basal ganglia–thalamocortical circuits, allowing relatively intact portions of the motor system to either compensate more effectively or to resume more normal functioning. This is most easily understood in the case of lesioning, which directly interrupts abnormal outflow from the basal ganglia, but may be viewed in a similar fashion for DBS, which, by overriding and blocking transmission of abnormal activity, may act as an "informational" lesion.[203]

Use of Early Surgical Treatment in Movement Disorders

Surgical interventions such as pallidotomy or DBS are most commonly used to provide symptomatic relief for patients with advanced movement disorders. Recent studies have examined the possibility that STN-DBS may not only improve quality of life over best medical management but may also even alter the course of disease, which may justify the use of this therapy early in the course of the disease.

Several trials examining the symptomatic benefits of using DBS early in PD have been published. The largest study to date is the EARLYSTIM study,[204,205] in which patients were studied within 3 years of levodopa-induced motor complications and with intact social and occupational functioning. The study demonstrated that DBS was superior to medical management with regard to quality-of-life scores, motor disability, and levodopa-induced motor complications, but at the expense of an increase in the incidence of adverse events. A recent study in patients with relatively early PD has been carried out, demonstrating no adverse effects at 2 years.[206] Other studies with yet earlier time points are underway to examine the utility of early STN-DBS for PD.

The belief that early DBS may not only provide symptomatic benefit but may also be a potentially neuroprotective treatment for PD goes back to studies by Piallat and colleagues,[207] which showed that STN lesions reduced the effects of subsequently lesioning dopaminergic neurons in the SNc with 6-hydroxydopamine, perhaps by eliminating the glutamatergic "excitotoxic" drive of the dopaminergic cells by STN output. This protective effect was later also found in monkeys,[208] in which kainate lesions or STN-DBS reduced the effect of subsequent MPTP lesions. More recent studies have examined the potential protective effects of long-term STN-DBS, demonstrating that this treatment reduces lesions in chronically parkinsonian rats.[209] The authors of these studies hypothesize that chronic stimulation may act through the release of brain-derived nerve growth factor at the level of the substantia nigra.[210]

Paradox of Stereotaxic Surgery

As discussed, most movement disorders result from dysfunction in the input areas of the basal ganglia, that is, the caudate and putamen (e.g., PD, the chorea of Huntington's disease, dystonia) or the subthalamic nucleus (hemiballismus), which is then propagated, through basal ganglia output, to the thalamus and PPN and from there to the cortex, brainstem, cerebellum, and spinal cord. As discussed, ablative and DBS approaches most effectively target the output areas of the basal ganglia motor circuit in GPi or STN, or pallidal projection areas in the thalamus or the brainstem (PPN), blocking or overriding the transmission of misinformation. One element of the rationale for neurosurgical procedures is the fact that the interventions ameliorate the signs of these disorders without causing obvious impairment of voluntary movement, which is referred to as the "paradox of stereotaxic surgery."[211] A part of the paradox arises from the perception that because basal ganglia dysfunction results in major disturbances of movement or involuntary movements, the nature of the disturbances in some way reflects the role of the basal ganglia in movement. It is clear, however, that the clinical signs of movement disorders reflect (induced) dysfunction in brain networks downstream from the basal ganglia rather than the functions of the basal ganglia themselves. The paradox begs the question, nonetheless, of what the basal ganglia actually do and what deficits might be expected from their interruption.

As discussed earlier, numerous proposals for the motor functions of the basal ganglia have been advanced. The most prominent and well recognized is the role in reinforcement learning, mediated by release of dopamine. Beyond this there is a role in the selection of the appropriate behavior for a given situation. Specific roles in movement include the scaling of movement amplitude and velocity, the execution or facilitation of cortically initiated movements and suppression of competing movements (focusing), and a specific role in self-initiated (vs. goal-directed) movements. The basal ganglia have also been viewed as a repository of learned skilled movements or behavioral sequences (habits).

Data supporting most of the aforementioned hypotheses, however, are poorly supported or inconsistent with the available data.[212,213] Although single-cell recording behavioral studies in primates have revealed highly specific changes in activity in relation to movements of individual body parts and to specific parameters of movement, such as direction, amplitude, and velocity of limb movements, there is little experimental support for a primary or critical role of the basal ganglia in the initiation or online control of movement. The facts that the timing of changes in neuronal activity in the basal ganglia in relation to movement onset lags that in the motor cortex in reaction-time tasks[214-216] and that lesions of the sensorimotor territory of GPi have little or no effects on posture or movement initiation or execution argue strongly against a role of the motor circuit in online motor control. The available clinical and animal evidence is, likewise, incompatible with the proposed role as a repository of learned movements or habits. There is still conflicting evidence regarding the role of the basal ganglia in self-initiated versus goal-directed movements, but this is not evident following pallidotomy or DBS. It thus appears from the available evidence that the major contribution of the basal ganglia motor circuit to motor behavior may be in reinforcement learning rather than in the initiation or execution of movement.[217]

CONCLUSION

Several major facts support the use of functional surgery for movement disorders. One part of the rationale is that effective available drug therapy is lacking for many of these disorders, so surgery may, in fact, be the only available or the most effective treatment modality. Other factors contributing to the popularity of functional surgery is that it is highly focused, reaching only those portions of the basal ganglia that are involved in the motor disturbance, and is thus less complicated by off-target side effects than the commonly used pharmacologic agents.

Although the development of neurosurgical interventions for movement disorders was largely empirical, these procedures have been increasingly refined, based on increasing anatomic, physiologic, and neuroimaging data relating to the pathophysiology of these disorders. As discussed, surgical movement disorder treatments are most successful when targeting locations within the output nuclei of the motor circuit of the basal ganglia (or the synaptic targets of projections from these regions in thalamus and brainstem), and with only few exceptions the same targets can be used almost indiscriminately for a variety of movement disorder signs and symptoms.

The restoration of function by ablation or DBS is clearly not the result of restoring the normal functions of the basal ganglia. Rather, the success of these procedures results from the removal of disruptive abnormal basal ganglia output on downstream systems in the brainstem, thalamus, and cerebral cortex, whose activity gives rise to the movement abnormities associated with diseases of the basal ganglia.

SUGGESTED READINGS

Albin RL, Young AB, Penney JB. The functional anatomy of basal ganglia disorders. *Trends Neurosci.* 1989;12:366-375.

Alexander GE, DeLong MR, Strick PL. Parallel organization of functionally segregated circuits linking basal ganglia and cortex. *Ann Rev Neurosci.* 1986;9:357-381.

Braak H, Del Tredici K, Rub U, et al. Staging of brain pathology related to sporadic Parkinson's disease. *Neurobiol Aging.* 2003;24:197-211.

Breakefield XO, Blood AJ, Li Y, et al. The pathophysiological basis of dystonias. *Nat Rev Neurosci.* 2008;9:222-234.

DeLong MR. Primate models of movement disorders of basal ganglia origin. *Trends Neurosci.* 1990;13:281-285.

Doyon J. Motor sequence learning and movement disorders. *Curr Opin Neurol.* 2008;21:478-483.

Graybiel AM. Habits, rituals, and the evaluative brain. *Annu Rev Neurosci.* 2008;31:359-387.

Hallett M. Bradykinesia: why do Parkinson's patients have it and what trouble does it cause? *Mov Disord.* 2011;26:1579-1581.

Hammond C, Bergman H, Brown P. Pathological synchronization in Parkinson's disease: networks, models and treatments. *Trends Neurosci.* 2007;30:357-364.

Marsden CD, Obeso JA. The functions of the basal ganglia and the paradox of stereotaxic surgery in Parkinson's disease. *Brain.* 1994; 117:877-897.

McIntyre CC, Savasta M, Walter BL, et al. How does deep brain stimulation work? Present understanding and future questions. *J Clin Neurophysiol.* 2004;21:40-50.

Mink JW. Neurobiology of basal ganglia and Tourette syndrome: basal ganglia circuits and thalamocortical outputs. *Adv Neurol.* 2006;99: 89-98.

Temel Y, Visser-Vandewalle V. Surgery in Tourette syndrome. *Mov Disord.* 2004;19:3-14.

See a full reference list on ExpertConsult.com

83 Neuropathology of Movement Disorders

Kurt A. Jellinger

Movement disorders can be divided into four major groups according to clinical phenomenology (Box 83-1); only the first two are discussed in this chapter. Most akinetic-rigid and hyperkinetic forms have their origin in dysfunction of the dorsal basal ganglia (BG), which work in tandem with the cortex through complex information circuits of the brain, although virtually the entire nervous system is engaged in motor control. Disruption of the BG networks forms the basis for major movement disorders. Recent progress has provided insight into the anatomy, functional organization, and pathophysiology of BG in major movement disorders as well as the role of different neuron subpopulations in mediating different aspects of motor control. The functional anatomy of the BG, the essential cortico-BG-thalamocortical circuits, and BG-cerebellar connections are briefly reviewed.

Classical classification of movement disorders based on pathophysiologic mechanisms involving the BG is as follows: (1) parkinsonian syndromes, characterized by rigidity, akinesia, rest tremor, and postural instability; (2) chorea-ballism, in which fragments of movements flow irregularly from one body segment to another, causing a dance-like appearance; and (3) dystonia, featured by prolonged muscle spasms and abnormal posture. Based on recent genetic and molecular-biologic data, movement disorders are classified as follows: (Box 83-2): (1) synucleinopathies, caused by aggregation of misfolded α-synuclein–forming Lewy

BOX 83-1 Clinical Classification of Movement Disorders

1. Akinetic-rigid forms
   - Parkinsonism: Parkinson's disease, parkinsonian syndromes
   - Stiff man syndrome
2. Hyperkinetic forms
   - Chorea syndromes
   - Tremor syndromes
   - Dystonias
   - Myoclonus
   - Ballism
   - Tics
3. Atactic movement disorders (not discussed here)
   - Cerebellar ataxias
   - Spinocerebellar degeneration
4. Motor neuron disorders (not discussed here)
   - Motor neuron disease
   - Spinal muscular atrophy and related disorders

BOX 83-2 Morphologic and Biochemical Classification of Degenerative Diseases with Movement Disorders

α-SYNUCLEINOPATHIES

Invariable Forms (Consistent α-Synuclein Deposition)

Parkinson's disease (brainstem type of Lewy body disease)
- Sporadic
- Familial with α-synuclein mutation
- Familial with other mutations
- Incidental Lewy body disease (subclinical Parkinson's disease)
- Pure autonomic failure
- Lewy body dysphagia

Dementia with Lewy bodies; diffuse Lewy body disease
Multiple system atrophy
- Striatonigral degeneration (MSA-P)
- Olivopontocerebellar atrophy (MSA-C)

Pantothenate kinase–associated neurodegeneration (Hallervorden-Spatz disease)

Variable Forms (Inconsistent α-Synuclein Deposition)

Parkinson's disease with parkin- and LRRK2-linked mutations
Alzheimer's disease (and other tauopathies)

TAUOPATHIES

Progressive supranuclear palsy (4R-tau doublet + exon 19)
Corticobasal degeneration (same)
Amyotrophic lateral sclerosis and parkinsonism-dementia complex of Guam (3R + 4R triplet)
Postencephalitic parkinsonism (3R + 4R triplet)
Chromosome 17–linked familial dementia (frontotemporal dementia and parkinsonism) (tau doublet)
Pallidopontonigral degeneration (4R-tau)
Multiple system tauopathy with presenile dementia
Pick's disease (3R-tau doublet without exon 10)
Advanced Alzheimer's disease with subcortical neurofibrillary tangles
Amyotrophic lateral sclerosis and parkinsonism-dementia complex of Guam
Perry's syndrome
Frontotemporal lobe degeneration with *MAPT* mutation

TDP-43 PROTEINOPATHIES

Frontotemporal lobe degeneration with ubiquitin inclusions
Frontotemporal lobe degeneration with fused in sarcoma *(FUS)* mutation and other mutations (e.g., *FTLD, GRN, VCP*)
Amyotrophic lateral sclerosis

POLYGLUTAMINE REPEAT (CAG) DISORDERS

Huntington's disease—rigid type (CAG triplet repeat)
Choreoacanthocytosis (neuroacanthocytosis)
Machado-Joseph disease (spinocerebellar ataxia type 3 + type 2)
Dentatorubral-pallidoluysian atrophy
X-linked dystonia parkinsonism (Lubag's disease)

OTHER HEREDITARY DEGENERATIVE DISORDERS

Hereditary striatal degeneration
Pallidal degeneration and related variants
Hallervorden-Spatz disease (without α-synucleinopathy)
Wilson's disease, Menkes' disease
Neuronal intranuclear inclusion and basophilic inclusion disease
Inherited dystonias

FTLD, frontotemporal lobe degeneration; *LLRK2,* leucine-rich repeat kinase 2; *MSA-C,* multiple system atrophy with predominant cerebellar features; *MSA-P,* multiple system atrophy with predominant parkinsonism; *TDP-43,* transactive response DNA-binding protein 43 kD.

bodies (Parkinson's disease [PD], dementia with Lewy bodies [DLB]) or glial cytoplasmic inclusions (multiple system atrophy [MSA]); neurodegeneration with brain iron accumulation, no longer considered a synucleinopathy; (2) tauopathies, featured by neurofibrillary pathology (progressive supranuclear palsy [PSP], corticobasal degeneration [CBD], frontotemporal lobe degeneration [FTLD-tau]; Guamian Parkinson-dementia; Pick's disease, and others); (3) polyglutamine disorders (Huntington's disease and others); (4) transactive response DNA-binding protein 43 kD (TDP-43) proteinopathies (other forms of FTLD); and (5) other disorders without hitherto detected genetic or specific markers. The diversity of phenotypes is related to the deposition of pathologic proteins in distinct brain areas and cell populations, causing increased vulnerability and neurodegeneration owing to genetic and environmental factors, but there is frequent overlap between various disorders because of synergistic mechanisms.

This chapter reviews basic processes leading to proteinopathies and the morphologic, specific molecular pathologic features, diagnostic neuropathologic guidelines, pathophysiology, and etiopathogenetic knowledge of the major movement disorders. Focus is given to Lewy body diseases, most of which are disorders involving the nervous system and multiple organs. Specific emphasis is given to sporadic and genetic forms of PD; the lesion pattern and pathophysiology of the clinical subtypes of PD (akinetic-rigid and tremor dominant); PD-dementia, DLB, and their interrelations; MSA; and the etiopathogenesis of these disorders. Among tauopathies, the syndromes of PSP (Richardson's syndrome, PSP-parkinsonism, and atypical forms), CBD syndromes, postencephalic parkinsonism, Pick's disease, FTLD-17-tau, Guamanian PD-dementia, and secondary parkinsonism are described. Hyperkinetic movement disorders, including Huntington's disease; other hereditary and sporadic choreas; dentatorubral-pallidoluysian atrophy; progressive pallidal degeneration; neurodegeneration with brain iron accumulation (pantothenate-kinase associated and other forms); neuronal intranuclear inclusion disease; Wilson's and Menkes' disease; myoclonic and ballistic syndromes; primary, secondary, and other dystonias; and tic and tremor syndromes, including essential tremor, are reviewed, considering current knowledge of the morphology, genetics, pathophysiology, and pathogenesis of these disorders.

The distribution of pathologic fibrillary proteins and the patterns of nervous system lesions point to the classification and pathophysiology of most neurodegenerative movement disorders; their etiopathogenesis is still poorly understood but is suggested to result from a complex interaction between genetic background and environmental factors, multiple etiologies, and noxious factors (protein mishandling, mitochondrial dysfunction, oxidative stress, excitotoxicity, energy failure, chronic neuroinflammation, and their combinations being more likely than a single factor). Recent molecular-pathologic, pathogenic, and pathophysiologic data will aid in correct classification and diagnosis of neurodegenerative movement disorders as a basis for future prevention and therapies.

Full text of this chapter is available online at ExpertConsult.com 

84 Clinical Overview of Movement Disorders

Ihtsham U. Haq, Jessica A. Tate, Mustafa S. Siddiqui, and Michael S. Okun

Movement disorders are a group of conditions that arise from functional aberrations in the motor and the nonmotor basal ganglia pathways.[1] Movement disorders are common and affect people in all age groups. A list of the most common movement disorders and their reported incidences is presented in Table 84-1.[2-12] The early signs and symptoms of movement disorders may be subtle and easily hidden by conscious or unconscious incorporation by the patient into common daily gestures. The key to diagnosing a movement disorder is careful study of its phenomenology, as well as its associated nonmotor features. In this chapter we provide an overview of movement disorders for practicing neurosurgeons, a topic that has also been covered by other authors.[13-15]

PHENOMENOLOGY: DEFINING SYMPTOMS THROUGH OBSERVATION

Patients with syndromes arising from dysfunction of the basal ganglia typically have a combination of motor and nonmotor manifestations. A thorough history and examination will avoid unnecessary tests and reduce subspecialty referrals. Once the history and general neurological examination have established the context for an abnormal movement, the movement should be characterized by visual inspection. Movements are classified on the basis of speed, anatomy, character, intentionality (i.e., voluntary, involuntary, or unvoluntary), triggers, and relieving factors.

First, the anatomic region involved should be defined. Focal disorders affect one region of the body, regional disorders affect two contiguous body parts, and generalized disorders affect both sides of the body or the axis, or both. Regarding a specific appendage, the movement may be further classified as being proximal or distal. Next, the disorder should be characterized as hyperkinetic or hypokinetic. Hyperkinetic disorders are typified by excessive movement (e.g., tremor), whereas hypokinetic disorders are typified by reduced movement (e.g., bradykinesia in Parkinson's disease [PD]). The quality of the movement should also be described. Is the movement *rhythmic* like a tremor or jerky and *irregular* as in myoclonus? Does it alter when the patient is at *rest*, maintaining a *posture*, or performing an *action*? Does it persist during sleep? Does the movement travel smoothly from body part to body part, as in chorea? Are opposing muscle groups co-contracting, as occurs in dystonia? Is it preceded by a *premonitory urge* and followed by a sense of relief, as with tics? Does the patient have difficulty with skilled movements, as in apraxia?

The patient should also be asked whether the movement is *voluntary* or *involuntary*. Movements may be referred to as *unvoluntary* when it is unclear which category applies.[16] Triggers and relieving factors should be identified. Does the movement worsen with action or is it relieved? Do particular positions precipitate the abnormality? Is there specific sensory input that relieves the symptoms?

Finally, the presence of specific nonmotor symptoms can lead the clinician to the proper diagnosis. Table 84-2 lists common features of movement disorders and the specific diagnoses that they may suggest.

HYPERKINESIAS

Tremor

In tremor a body part oscillates rhythmically about a set point. The tremor may be regular or irregular, unilateral or bilateral, and symmetrical or asymmetrical and may be present in one or several body regions. The frequency and amplitude of a tremor depend heavily on its underlying cause.

Tremor is classified according to its appearance or its cause.[17,18] If the tremor occurs during movement, it is referred to as *action* or *kinetic tremor*. A tremor occurring in the absence of activity is classified as *rest tremor*. *Postural tremor* occurs when a specific position is maintained (e.g., holding the arm extended). Finally, *physiologic tremor* is the term applied to nonpathologic postural tremor, which typically has a frequency of 8 to 12 Hz. *Drug-induced tremors* are usually an enhancement of physiologic tremors.

Tremor may be triggered by synchronized oscillatory signals arising from one of several locations. These signals may originate centrally, from circuits in either the basal ganglia or cerebellum that are involved in sensorimotor integration, motor timing, muscle coordination, or sympathetic control.[18] One common example of centrally driven tremor is *essential tremor* (ET). ET has been ascribed to overactive central oscillators in the thalamus[19,20] and to thalamocortical loop overactivity. In contrast, cerebellar and rubral tremors, which may occur after stroke or traumatic brain injury, are thought to result from motor dysregulation (i.e., from unbalanced feed-forward or feedback systems or both).

Weighting a tremoring limb can help determine whether the tremor is physiologic or a pathologic tremor of central origin. Tremors predominantly of central origin will decrease in frequency when loaded, whereas the 8- to 12-Hz oscillation of physiologic tremor typically does not.[21]

Although it can be difficult to differentiate among subtypes of tremor solely on the basis of their frequency, it may be helpful to note that tremors of the hands greater than 11 Hz or less than 6 Hz are almost always pathologic.[22] Pathologic tremors also seem to have a "floor" frequency. PD tremor and ET are among the lower frequency tremors and typically do not oscillate at less than 4 Hz.[22] Tremors with frequencies in this range are usually caused by malfunction of the brainstem or cerebellum. The frequency of a tremor may decrease slightly over time,[21] in one series by approximately 2 to 3 Hz over a period of 4 to 8 years.[23] This small degree of change does not usually lead to diagnostic confusion.

Amplitude cannot be used effectively to differentiate tremor types[24] because it may vary widely within a particular tremor subtype. In general, tremor subtypes with the lowest frequency can be expected to have the highest amplitude and vice versa, but this rule is not absolute. Emotional distress, exercise, and fatigue may exacerbate tremors of any subtype. Stressors tend to increase the amplitude of a tremor but have less effect on tremor frequency.

TABLE 84-1 Prevalence of Selected Movement Disorders in the United States

Syndrome	Prevalence (per 100,000)	Common Age Group
Parkinson's disease	295.6	60-70
Progressive supranuclear palsy	0.4-6.4	60-70
Multiple system atrophy	2.2-4.4	50-60
Essential tremor	400-900	>40
Huntington's disease	2-6.3	<20 or >35
Tourette's syndrome	1850-2990	<18
Cervical dystonia	5.7-8.9	40
Restless legs syndrome	4200-9800	>45
Friedreich's ataxia	1.2-2	5-15

Data from references 2-12, 16-18.

TABLE 84-2 Examples of Features, Categories, and Syndromes Helpful in Diagnosis

Features	Categories	Examples of Specific Syndromes
Speed	Hyperkinetic	Tremor, chorea, myoclonus, tics, restless legs syndrome
	Hypokinetic	Apraxia, blocking tics, parkinsonism: bradykinesia, primary progressive freezing of gait
Region	Whole body	Hyperekplexia, generalized dystonia
	Hemibody	Hemiparkinsonism, hemidystonia
	Segmental	Segmental myoclonus
	Multifocal	Minipolymyoclonus
	Focal	Writer's cramp
	Proximal	Rubral tremor
	Distal	Painful legs when moving toes
	Oral	Tardive dyskinesia, neuroacanthocytosis
Character	Rhythm	Rhythmic: Parkinson's disease, essential tremor
		Arrhythmic: myoclonus, dystonic tremor
	Frequency	Faster: essential tremor, orthostatic tremor
		Slower: rubral tremor
	Amplitude	Large: essential tremor, rubral tremor
		Fine: orthostatic tremor, physiologic tremor
	At rest	Parkinsonism: tremor
	During posture	Physiologic tremor, drug-induced tremor, essential tremor, some cerebellar and dystonia tremors
	With action	Cerebellar tremor, essential tremor, dystonic tremor
	Accompaniment	Tics: premonitory urge
Intentionality	Voluntary	Tics
	Involuntary	Tardive dyskinesia, stereotypies, tics
	Unvoluntary	Tic disorders
Triggers	Action	Musician's dystonia
	Position	Orthostatic tremor
	Sensory stimulation	Catalepsy, hyperekplexia, stimulus-sensitive myoclonus
Relieving factors	Sleep	Improves: dystonia, tremor, not essential palatal tremor
	Sensory tricks (gestes antagonistes)	Improves: dystonia
Nonmotor features	Autonomic	Multiple system atrophy: orthostasis
		Parkinsonism: drooling
	Psychiatric	Huntington's disease, Parkinson's disease: depression

Common tremor conditions include ET, PD, dystonic tremor, cerebellar/outflow tremor, Holmes's tremor, physiologic tremor, palatal tremor, neuropathic tremor, drug- or toxin-induced tremors, task-specific tremor, primary writing tremor (PWT), and psychogenic tremor.[18] The characteristics of these tremors are presented in Table 84-3.[18,19,24-33]

Specific Tremor Disorders

Physiologic Tremor. *Physiologic tremor* is a term applied to the 8- to 12-Hz tremor seen in any healthy person who is intentionally sustaining a posture. More proximal regions of the body oscillate at a lower frequency, more distal ones at a higher frequency. For example, physiologic tremor has a frequency of 3 to 5 Hz at the elbow, whereas metacarpophalangeal tremor usually ranges from 17 to 30 Hz.[19] When this tremor impairs motor performance, it is referred to as *enhanced physiologic tremor*.[27]

Physiologic tremor is typically symmetrical. As with other tremor types, the amplitude is reported to decrease with age, particularly after the age of 50,[17,24] although some authors have found otherwise.[27] Age has not been shown to affect the frequency of physiologic tremor.[24,34]

It is unclear whether mild forms of the syndrome can be distinguished from ET. Both ET and physiologic tremor can be elicited by posture, both are fairly symmetrical, and both occur predominantly in the arms.[24] Observing the progression of a tremor over time will eventually reveal whether a given patient has ET or physiologic tremor.

Essential Tremor. ET is the most common tremor disorder, with an overall prevalence of 0.4% to 0.9%. In people older than 60, it can be as high as 4.6%.[35] In general, it manifests as a low-amplitude, bilateral action and postural tremor with a frequency of 6 to 8 Hz. The tremor usually has its onset in adulthood and worsens over time, but it may begin in childhood and can coexist with other movement disorders.[36] The overall prevalence of ET is similar between genders,[35] although women with ET seem to be more prone to head tremor than men.[37]

ET involves the upper limbs in more than 90% of patients.[38] It less commonly involves the head, legs, or voice. It rarely affects the face or trunk. ET often has a postural component that may be reported as a rest tremor by patients. Although some rest tremor can be seen in advanced ET, an action tremor should clearly dominate. Patients commonly first complain of difficulty with tasks requiring fine coordination, such as threading a needle, tying knots, or writing. Later, activities involving grosser coordination are also affected. In severe cases, basic activities of daily living may become impossible to perform.

Cognitive dysfunction[39] and gait abnormalities[40] may also be features of ET. Set shifting, verbal fluency, and other frontal cortex functions are impaired in patients with ET relative to age-matched controls. This cognitive impairment does not correlate with tremor severity.[39]

Several features of ET point to an underlying cerebellar or brainstem pathology. Patients with ET frequently have an end point tremor and difficulty with tandem gait. Researchers have described subclinical eye movement abnormalities indicative of cerebellar dysfunction.[41] There are case reports of ipsilateral improvement in symptoms after cerebellar infarction,[42] and inducing lesions of the cerebellothalamic receiving area (the ventral intermediate nucleus of the thalamus) is an effective treatment for ET. Although positron emission tomography has shown increased olivary glucose uptake and cerebellar blood flow,[43] the brains of ET patients appear to be structurally normal.[44] Postmortem studies by Louis and colleagues suggested a cerebellar variant with Purkinje cell loss, axonal torpedoes, basket cell changes, and a Lewy body variant with increased Lewy bodies in

TABLE 84-3 Tremors and Their Characteristics

Tremor Disorder	Rest	Postural	Action	Frequency	Average Age at Onset	Family History	Features
Cerebellar tremor	–	+	+++	2-5 Hz	Variable	Variable	May be severe with action
Drug-induced tremor	+/–	++	+		Variable	None	Improves with drug discontinuation
Dystonic tremor	+	++	++	Irregular, 3-8 Hz	Adulthood	Variable	Irregular
Essential tremor	+	++	+++	6-8 or 8-12 Hz	Early adult	Common	Usually slightly asymmetrical, involves the hands most commonly
Orthostatic tremor	–	++	–	10 or 14-16 Hz	Late	Rare	Occurs only on standing still
Palatal tremor	++	–	++	1-4 Hz	Variable	Rare	EPT may be accompanied by a click; SPT may persist in sleep
PD tremor	+++	+	+/–	4-9 Hz	Middle age	Occasional	Variable in appearance; improves with levodopa in 60% of individuals
Physiologic tremor	–	++	+	8-12 Hz	Childhood	Common	Present in all individuals
Posttraumatic tremor	+/–	++	++		Variable	None	Appearance varies with the site of trauma; myoclonus is frequently present
Rubral tremor	++	+++	+++	2-5 Hz	Variable	None	Large amplitude
Task-specific tremor	–	–	++	4-7 Hz	Adulthood	Occasional	Tremor with task or task-associated position

Data from references 21, 22, 27-36.
EPT, essential palatal tremor; PD, Parkinson's disease; SPT, symptomatic palatal tremor.

the brainstem.[45] The evidence for cerebellar Purkinje cell dysfunction is mixed; in a case-control study of ET, Rajput and Rajput did not find Purkinje cell loss.[46]

A family history of tremor is common in patients in whom ET is diagnosed. A positive family history has been reported in as many as 96% of patients[47] and as few as 17%,[48] depending on the sample. A survey of New York City residents showed a 5-fold to 10-fold increase in risk for ET in first-degree relatives, as well as an increase in the likelihood of ET developing in family members with earlier onset of symptoms in the patient.[49]

Several inherited forms of ET have been identified, including the gene loci *EMT1* (on chromosome 3q13) and *EMT2* (on 2p24) and an unnamed gene locus on 6p23.[49,50] ET has been reported in fragile X syndrome,[51] Kennedy's syndrome,[52] XXYY syndrome,[53] and Klinefelter's syndrome.[54,55] Sex chromosome–related tremors often have associated ataxia and may represent a separate tremor type.

The presence of a rest tremor in a patient who otherwise meets the criteria for ET can be confusing. Current opinion among movement disorder neurologists favors the diagnosis of ET when the action and postural components of a tremor greatly outweigh the rest component and the rest component is bilateral. New-onset unilateral rest tremor should always bring PD to mind. Although isolated head tremor is often diagnosed as ET, if upper extremity tremor is absent, it is more likely to be *dystonic tremor*.[56]

The question of whether ET predisposes patients to the later development of PD is also a perplexing one. There are some cases in which families appear to be prone to both PD and ET. Jankovic's group reported that the same locus yielded pure ET and ET-PD-dystonia in different families.[57] As of this writing, the exact association between ET and PD remains a topic of discussion.

Parkinsonian Tremor. The tremor of PD was described by James Parkinson in 1817 in his historic *Essay on the Shaking Palsy*[58] and further characterized by Charcot in the 1860s in his lectures at the Salpêtrière.[59] PD tremor is a 4- to 9-Hz low-amplitude rest tremor. The tremor often has a prominent proximal thumb component that gives it a "pill-rolling" quality. The presence of a pill-rolling tremor is not diagnostic.

Although there is some thought that PD tremor may dampen or "burn out" over time, other researchers have observed the opposite. Parkinson himself wrote that "as the debility increases … the tremulous agitation becomes more vehement [and] the motion becomes so violent as not only to shake the bed-hangings, but even the floor and sashes of the room."[58]

Unlike typical ET, PD hand tremor may worsen in the ipsilateral lower limb before affecting the contralateral hand. A typical pattern of spread is for a hand to be affected first, followed by the ipsilateral foot and then the contralateral hand. Although different extremities exhibit the same frequency of tremor, they need not shake simultaneously. When tremor is bilateral in onset without involving the legs, causes other than PD should be considered. PD tremor is frequently intermittent and typically becomes more pronounced with distraction.

Reemergent tremor occurs while sustaining a prolonged position and most likely represents a rest tremor that has been reset by the relative stasis of a persistent position.[60] Postural tremor was seen in two thirds of patients with PD in one case series[60] and correlates with the degree of functional disability.

The pathogenesis of PD tremor is not well understood.[61] In monkeys with 1-methyl-4-phenyl-1,2,3,6-tetrahydropyridine (MPTP)–induced parkinsonism, basal ganglia neurons begin to fire synchronously. Some authors have suggested that PD tremor originates from loss of segregation of these information channels and subsequent synchronization of adjacent circuits.[62] Loss of dopamine in the basal ganglia may unmask pacemaker-like properties of the basal ganglia.[63] It should be noted that the severity of PD tremor does not correlate with the severity of dopamine neuronal loss[18] and that treatment with levodopa improves bradykinesia and rigidity more reliably than it does tremor.

The central origin of PD tremor is demonstrated by the observation that afferent denervation affects the amplitude and frequency of the tremor but does not abolish it.

Cerebellar Tremor. Cerebellar tremor can be characterized as a jerky, low-frequency (2 to 4 Hz), high-amplitude action tremor.[22] This tremor may be accompanied by other cerebellar signs such as ataxia, dysdiadochokinesia, dysarthria, dysmetria, and telegraphic speech. The normal pattern of cerebellar ballistic control, as described by Hallett and associates, consists of sequential agonist-antagonist–second agonist activation.[64]

Rubral Tremor (Holmes's Tremor). Patients with lesions in the region of the red nucleus may be predisposed to the development of what is referred to as a *rubral tremor*, first described by Holmes in 1904.[65] Although predominantly an action tremor, rubral tremor frequently has a significant resting component. The amplitude of movement tends to be large and it can sometimes adopt a "wing-beating" appearance. Rubral tremors are among the slowest tremors, with frequencies often less than 4 Hz.[22]

As with cerebellar and symptomatic palatal tremor (SPT), rubral tremor arises from damage to the cerebellar and brainstem motor pathways and from dysregulation of motor control during movement.

Posttraumatic Tremor. The motor coordination control centers and their connections are situated deep in the brain, and to damage them generally requires substantial injury. Consequently, posttraumatic tremor is rarely an isolated finding. The character of the tremor depends on the region of the brain that is damaged. Damage to the brainstem may produce rest tremor if it affects the substantia nigra and related pathways. Damage to the cerebellum may result in a low-frequency action tremor. Because multiple regions are usually damaged, posttraumatic tremors are typically mixed in character. In one series of severe posttraumatic tremors, all patients displayed both action and postural tremors, whereas rest tremor was seen in just 56%.[66] Posttraumatic tremor is often accompanied by myoclonus. As noted by Obeso and Narbona, this apparent myoclonus appears in some cases to be an exaggeration of a beat of the ongoing tremor rather than true myoclonus.[67]

Drug-Induced Tremor. Drug-induced tremors are united by a common cause rather than a common appearance. Usually drug-induced tremors have a higher frequency and involve limbs symmetrically, although lower frequency tremors are also seen. The onset of tremor should be temporally related to drug ingestion.[17]

Drugs most commonly associated with tremor include alcohol, amiodarone, antidepressants, antiepileptic medications, beta-agonist bronchodilators, caffeine, immunosuppressive agents, lithium, neuroleptics, nicotine, steroids, and sympathomimetics.[68] Alcohol intoxication (acute or chronic) and immunosuppressive agents may produce cerebellar tremors.[69] Sympathomimetics, serotonin reuptake inhibitors, nicotine, and other centrally acting agents typically produce an enhanced physiologic tremor. Because the physiologic effects of an offending drug are rarely limited to tremor, the causative agent may also be recognized by associated nonneurological symptoms.

There are numerous less commonly encountered tremor types that one must consider in the differential diagnosis of tremor.

A discussion of these, including orthostatic, palatal, psychogenic, task-specific, and dystonic tremors is available online at ExpertConsult.com.

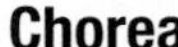

Chorea

Chorea consists of random and complex involuntary movements that flit from body part to body part. Chorea may resemble exaggerated fidgetiness. The movements can be focal or generalized and are usually absent during sleep. The word *chorea* is derived from the Greek *khoreia* or "to dance." Chorea may be among the first defined movement disorders. Chorea Sancti Viti (St. Vitus' dance) was described in the Middle Ages. It was one term among several *(St. John's dance, tarantism)* used to refer to the independent outbreaks of "dancing mania" that occurred in central Europe, most notably around the time of the plague.[81] The term *St. Vitus' dance* is now used predominantly to refer to Sydenham's chorea. Choreas can be further classified by their appearance. *Athetosis* refers to a slow, sinuous, undulating movement, usually of the hands or feet. Sudden and large-amplitude movements are referred to as *ballistic*, derived from the Greek word meaning "to throw."

Multiple chorea syndromes have been described (Table 84-4), including Huntington's chorea, Sydenham's chorea, Wilson's disease, neuroacanthocytosis, Friedreich's ataxia, dentatorubral-pallidoluysian atrophy (DRPLA), McLeod's syndrome, benign hereditary chorea (BHC), spinocerebellar ataxia (SCA type 2, 3, or 17), chorea gravidarum, drug-induced chorea, metabolic chorea (i.e., secondary to accumulation of toxins or liver, kidney,

TABLE 84-4 Chorea Syndromes

Genetic Chorea Syndromes	Gene (Chromosome)*	Gene Defect (Symptomatic Range)	Protein Product	Age at Onset	Inheritance
Benign hereditary chorea	*TITF1* (14q)	Variable	Thyroid transcription factor-1	<5	Autosomal dominant
DRPLA	*ATN1* (12p12)	CAG repeat (>49)	Atrophin-1	<20 or >40	Autosomal dominant
Huntington's chorea	*IT15*/HD (4p16)	CAG repeat (>35)	Huntingtin	<20 (juvenile) or 35-50	Autosomal dominant
HDL1	*PRNP* (20p12)	Octapeptide repeat	Prion protein	20-40	Autosomal dominant
HDL2	*JPH3* (16q24)	CTG-CAG repeat (>44)	Junctophilin-3	25-45	Autosomal dominant
HDL3	(4p15)	Unknown	Unknown	3-4	Autosomal recessive
HDL4/SCA17	*TBP* (6q27)	CAA-CAG repeat (>42)	TATA-box binding protein	25-40	Autosomal dominant
Neuroferritinopathy	*FTL* (19q13)	Variable	Ferritin light-chain polypeptide	40	Autosomal dominant
Choreoacanthocytosis	CHAC/VPS13A (9q21)	Variable	Chorein	20-30	Autosomal recessive
McLeod's syndrome	*XK* (Xp21)	Variable	Xk antigen	40-60	X-linked recessive
PKAN/NBIA	*PANK2* (20p13)	Variable	Pantothenate kinase-2	3-5	Autosomal recessive
Wilson's disease	*ATP7B* (13q14)	Variable	ATP7B protein	20-30	Autosomal recessive
PKD	*EKD2* (16q13)	Variable	Unknown	10-20	Autosomal dominant (25% sporadic)
PNKD	*MR1*, *FPD* (2q34)	Variable	Unknown	5-20	Autosomal dominant

Data from references 79-89.

DRPLA, dentatorubral-pallidoluysian atrophy; HDL, Huntington's disease like; NBIA, neurodegeneration with brain iron accumulation; PKAN, pantothenate kinase–associated neurodegeneration; PNKD, paroxysmal nonkinesogenic dyskinesia; PKD, paroxysmal kinesogenic dyskinesia; SCA, spinocerebellar ataxia.

*These gene and chromosome linkages were identified in smaller cohorts. Other genes may be implicated in a given individual.

or endocrine disease), tardive dyskinesia, paraneoplastic syndromes, polycythemia vera, and psychogenic chorea.[82-91]

Chorea Syndromes

Huntington's Disease. Huntington's disease (HD) is the most common form of inherited chorea. Symptoms usually begin during the third to fifth decades of life. Although chorea is the most common initial symptom,[92] unsteadiness of gait, dystonia, myoclonus, loss of bulbar control, and cognitive changes also occur and may appear before chorea does. Bradykinesia usually develops as the disease progresses, but it may be underappreciated in the presence of more obvious symptoms.

The chorea of HD is typically symmetrical and tends to increase in amplitude over time. The first manifestation of chorea may be a slight flicking of the fingers seen while walking.[82] Patients are frequently unaware of their movements and may continue to treat their gyrations with indifference, even when made aware of them. Early symptoms include an impairment of rapid saccades,[93,94] psychiatric and mood changes, and tics.[95] Ataxia is unusual and should raise concern for another syndrome, such as neuroacanthocytosis, SCA, or Friedreich's ataxia.[82]

Impersistence of movement is a classic feature of HD. Patients typically have difficulty maintaining tongue protrusion. They also tend to have difficulty keeping their gaze fixed on an object. Paradoxically, they may have trouble switching their attention from the examiner's face. This has been referred to as a *visual grasp reflex* and is not specific for HD.[96]

HD is defined as being of juvenile onset if symptoms occur by the age of 20. It is more often associated with stiffness, eye movement difficulties, and bradykinesia than adult-onset HD is. Seizures are also more frequent in juvenile-onset HD.[97] Adult-onset HD occasionally manifests as this phenotype.[98]

The cognitive and behavioral features of HD are both prominent and disabling. Many features are similar to those seen after frontal lobe damage. Grasp, snout, and other primitive reflexes may be prominent. Scores on psychomotor tests such as the Trail Making Test B and Stroop interference test show declines earlier in the course of HD than do tests of memory. Worsening scores correlate with the degree of striatal atrophy present.[99] Dementia occurs in the majority of patients, although exceptions may occur when the chorea is of late onset.[100] Other psychiatric symptoms include apathy, depression, lability, impulsivity, outbursts of anger, mania, and paranoia.[79,80] Physicians should always inquire about substance abuse and suicidality.[68]

The genetic defect responsible for HD is a CAG repeat on chromosome 4 in a region that encodes the protein huntingtin, whose function is unknown.[101] The number of copies of this repeat determines the presence or absence of clinical HD; patients with 29 to 35 repeats are expected to be asymptomatic.[81,102] The number of CAG repeats may increase in transmission and result in *anticipation:* earlier onset and increasing severity in successive generations. Paternal inheritance of HD has been correlated with a higher number of triplet repeats in the next generation,[103,104] probably because of gene expansion during spermatogenesis.[105] An increased number of triplet repeats correlates with both earlier disease onset and the degree of functional decline.[106]

The diagnosis of HD is based on clinical features and confirmed by genetic testing for the huntingtin gene. Caudate atrophy, characterized by "boxing" of lateral ventricles best seen on coronal brain imaging, is the classic finding on imaging studies.[99] Frontal lobe atrophy is also seen.[99] Imaging changes predate clinical diagnosis, and correlate in degree with symptom severity.[107] Physicians may encounter the HD phenotype in the absence of the HD genotype. In one large series, approximately 7% of patients displaying the HD phenotype proved not to have a mutation in the huntingtin gene.[108]

Four Huntington's disease–like (HDL) syndromes have been identified. All are rare. HDL1 is an inherited prion disorder. HDL2 is caused by a CAG/CTG expansion in the junctophilin-3 protein and is more common in patients of African, Mexican, Spanish, or Portuguese descent. HDL2 is the most HD-like of the HDLs in its symptomatology. It may be accompanied by erythrocyte acanthocytosis.[90] An early childhood–onset HDL variant, HDL3, has been identified in isolated cohorts.[90] Its genetic basis remains unknown. HDL4 is synonymous with SCA type 17 (SCA17). SCA17 has a variety of phenotypes, one of which closely mimics the symptoms of HD. HDL4 arises from a CAA-CAG repeat in chromosome 6.[90]

Sydenham's Chorea. Sydenham's chorea is a delayed complication of infection with group A β-hemolytic streptococci that usually develops 4 to 8 weeks after the infection,[81] but it may develop as long as 6 months afterward. Sydenham's chorea may be the sole manifestation of rheumatic fever in as many as 20% of patients[109,110] and remains the most common cause of acute childhood chorea in the world.

The typical age at onset of Sydenham's chorea is 8 to 9 years; it is rarely seen in children younger than 5 years.[81,111] The chorea usually generalizes but there are exceptions, and 20% of patients remain hemichoreic. Sydenham's chorea may be accompanied by tics and psychiatric symptoms. Obsessive-compulsive disorder (OCD) and attention-deficit/hyperactivity disorder (ADHD) occur in 20% to 30% of patients and may precede or follow the onset of chorea.[112] The disease is self-limited and spontaneously remits after 8 to 9 months in a large percentage of patients, but up to 50% may still have chorea 2 years after infection.[113]

Antineuronal antibodies are present in a majority of patients with Sydenham's chorea.[112] Antistreptolysin (ASO) titers are typically elevated but are nonspecific for infection with group A streptococci; this test is not useful in diagnosing Sydenham's chorea. However, elevated ASO titers may be of help in distinguishing a recurrence of Sydenham's chorea from a chorea from some other cause.[114,115] Magnetic resonance imaging (MRI) in patients with Sydenham's chorea has been reported to show transient swelling in the striatum and globus pallidus and increased signal on T2-weighted images.[116,117]

Tardive Chorea/Dyskinesia. Tardive dyskinesia results from treatment with dopamine receptor blocking agents. Tardive syndromes are less frequently caused by atypical neuroleptics (e.g., clozapine, quetiapine) than by typical neuroleptics (e.g., haloperidol). Dopamine-depleting medications have not been definitively associated with tardive dyskinesia.[68] Some common antiemetics (e.g., metoclopramide) and some antitussives (e.g., promethazine [Phenergan]) are dopaminergic blockers whose use may lead to the development of tardive movements.

The most common pattern of tardive dyskinesia is stereotyped and repetitive movement of the face. Tongue-thrusting and involuntary chewing movements reminiscent of those seen in choreoacanthocytosis may be seen. Tardive dyskinesia is often accompanied by a feeling of restlessness, referred to as *akathisia.* This may be localized and reported as a burning sensation, often of the genitals or mouth.[118]

Although tardive chorea has been reported after treatment with atypical antipsychotics, it occurs infrequently in this setting. Of the neuroleptics, clozapine appears least likely to induce tardive disorders.[116] Large clinical trials have suggested that although atypical antipsychotics produce tardive dyskinesia less often than first-generation antipsychotics do, the difference may not be as great as was thought.[119,120]

A brief overview of various other chorea syndromes and causes, including benign hereditary chorea, neuroacanthocytosis, and dentatorubral-pallidoluysian atrophy is available online at ExpertConsult.com.

Myoclonus

Myoclonus is a sudden, arrhythmic, involuntary movement that is "shock-like" in its rapidity. When multiple, these movements do not flow into one another, which distinguishes them from chorea. True myoclonus is caused by brief synchronous firing of agonist and antagonist muscles that typically lasts 10 to 50 msec and rarely more than 100 msec.[140,141]

Myoclonus can be classified by either phenomenology, extent, or trigger. *Positive myoclonus* occurs with active muscle contraction, of which *hypnic jerks*, a sudden body-wide contraction that occurs as a person drifts between sleep and wakefulness, are a commonly experienced example. *Negative myoclonus* manifests as brief inhibition of a given muscle group. *Asterixis* is an example of negative myoclonus and consists of sudden and involuntary relaxation of a dorsiflexed hand or other body part. The electromyographic pattern of negative myoclonus is distinctive, with aperiodic electrophysiologic silences ranging from 0.05 to 0.5 second in the antagonist muscle groups.[15,22] When frequent, these signs can be mistaken for postural tremor.

Alternatively, myoclonus may be defined by the portion of the nervous system deemed responsible for the symptoms, such as *cortical myoclonus*, *subcortical myoclonus*, or *spinal myoclonus*. Finally, myoclonus can be classified as simply *epileptic* or *nonepileptic*. When myoclonus is triggered by movement, it is referred to as *action-induced myoclonus*. When myoclonus occurs in response to a touch or loud noise, the term *stimulus sensitive* applies. The phenomenon of *hyperekplexia*—an exaggerated startle response to a sudden, unexpected stimulus—is an example of stimulus-sensitive myoclonus.

Myoclonus is most often encountered as one of a collection of symptoms rather than as a pathology's primary manifestation. Symptomatic myoclonus may be a feature of any process involving cortical, basal ganglionic, or cerebellar degeneration, such as Creutzfeldt-Jakob disease or PD. Hepatic, renal, endocrine, and other metabolic derangements may variably manifest as myoclonus. Primary myoclonic syndromes include the myoclonic epilepsies, essential hereditary myoclonus, palatal myoclonus, nocturnal myoclonus (also referred to as *periodic leg movements of sleep*), minipolymyoclonus, and physiologic myoclonus.[142]

More information on myoclonus and related syndromes is available online at ExpertConsult.com.

Dyskinesia

Dyskinesia refers to any disordered and involuntary movement. It is a broad term that encompasses movements that may also be referred to as *choreic* or *dystonic*. Dyskinesias are typically arrhythmic and not suppressible. Affected individuals may be unaware of these movements, even when severe. The limbs, neck, and face are the most frequently affected, but axial symptoms may also occur. When dyskinesia occurs in the face, the features may appear wry or overanimated. Head bobbing, blinking, lip smacking, and tongue protrusion are common. When dyskinesia occurs in the limbs, the movements may be proximal or distal and of either high or low amplitude. The limbs may tap, whirl, or writhe. Low-amplitude dyskinesias of the hands can resemble tremor. Axial dyskinetic movements may consist of rocking, arching, and twisting and rarely occur in the absence of facial or appendicular symptoms.

The designation *dyskinesia* is most commonly used to describe the movements observed in patients receiving chronic dopaminergic therapy for PD; however, dyskinesia may also be *tardive* (i.e., a delayed side effect of dopamine-blocking medications). Although usually secondary to prolonged medication use, there have been reports of tardive dyskinesia developing after only a month's exposure to neuroleptic medications.[169,170]

Dyskinesia syndromes include abdominal (belly dancer's) dyskinesia, levodopa-induced dyskinesia, tardive dyskinesia, and the paroxysmal dyskinesias.[171]

More information on these topics can also be found online at ExpertConsult.com.

Tics

Tics are brief movements that are commonly preceded by a feeling of discomfort that builds until the tic appears, followed by a temporary feeling of relief. These preceding premonitory urges may consist of a feeling of itching or tension in the affected body part.[180] These sensations are also referred to as *sensory tics*.[181] One of the hallmarks of tics is that they are temporarily suppressible, although they typically rebound with increased frequency and severity after conscious suppression. Tics occupy a middle ground between voluntary and involuntary movements. They are usually described by those who have them as being purposefully executed but performed out of a feeling of need.[182] This mix of volition and compulsion has led some to refer to these movements as "semivoluntary" or "unvoluntary."[16]

Tics can be *clonic* (i.e., brief), *dystonic* (i.e., sustained), or *phonic* (vocal). These subtypes can in turn be *simple* or *complex*. Simple tics consist of isolated actions, such as throat clearing or winking. Complex tics consist of speech or coordinated actions. They sometimes include obscene gestures, in which case they are termed *copropraxia*. When the obscenity is verbal, the complex phonic tic is referred to as *coprolalia*. Tics can also manifest as interruptions in or slowing of ongoing motion. Jankovic has also described *blocking tics*, or abrupt interruptions of activity preceded by a premonitory urge.[14]

Tic disorders include transient tourettism, Tourette's syndrome, chronic tic disorder, tardive tourettism, and drug-induced tourettism. Adult onset of a primary tic disorder is highly unusual. Any adult with a first manifestation of tics should be carefully examined for secondary causes such as infection, neuroleptic exposure, cocaine use, or trauma.[183]

Tic Disorders

Tourette's Syndrome. *Tourette's syndrome* is defined by the onset of motor and vocal tics before adulthood (<18 years) that cannot be ascribed to another medical condition. The full definition, as set out by the Tourette Syndrome Classification Study Group, adds that the tics must occur multiple times throughout a period of at least a year and that the tics must evolve over time.[184] Findings on neurological examination in a patient with Tourette's syndrome are generally normal.

The first tics are usually observed around the age of 5 or 6, and tic severity peaks 4 to 5 years later.[185] Only 4% of Tourette's syndrome patients fail to manifest tics by the age of 11.[186] Tic frequency is lowest in patients' early 20s, coincident with frontal lobe maturation.[185] In addition to this long-term variation, tics also wax and wane on a day-to-day basis. Tics are worsened by heightened emotional states, stress, and fatigue.

The tics of Tourette's syndrome are commonly accompanied by ADHD and OCD.[187] ADHD has been reported to precede tic onset by a mean of 2 years,[188] whereas OCD is reported to manifest in adolescence.[189] The phenotype of Tourette-related OCD differs from that of primary OCD. In primary OCD, patients' obsessions often focus on fears of contamination or a need for checking. In Tourette's syndrome, obsessions center on concerns with symmetry, fear of violent thoughts, and a need to perform activities in a particular manner.[190] These obsessions may lead to self-injurious behavior. Patients have been reported to hit themselves in the eyes or throat or bite and scratch themselves.[191,192] Such behavior may be seen in as many as 53% of patients with Tourette's syndrome.[186]

A growing body of research suggests that Tourette's syndrome has a strong hereditary component.[193-195] The syndrome appears to follow a sex-influenced but autosomal dominant mode of transmission.[196] In Tourette kindreds, men appear more likely to manifest a typical tic-predominant syndrome and women are more likely to have OCD without tics.[195] When obtaining a family history, it should be recalled that mild symptoms may be ascribed to idiosyncrasies of personality by family members.

The pathology of the disorder has been attributed to dysfunction of the corticostriatal-thalamocortical pathway,[189] and further localization remains speculative. The striatum has been a past focus of research. Evidence of frontal cortex involvement has also been increasing.[197,198]

The *Diagnostic and Statistical Manual of Mental Disorders*, fourth edition, lists *chronic tic disorder* and *transient tourettism (transient tic disorder of childhood)* alongside Tourette's syndrome as the primary tic disorders. Chronic tic disorder differs from Tourette's syndrome in that the patient need not have both phonic and motor tics. Transient tourettism differs from Tourette's syndrome in that symptoms last less than 1 year. This syndrome is the mildest and most common tic disorder. Tics can be seen transiently in 20% of children younger than 10 years.[199] Both transient tourettism and chronic tic disorder probably represent points on a continuum of tic-causing pathology, of which Tourette's syndrome is the most severe expression.

Other Causes of Tics. *Drug-induced tourettism* is also well described. Although antiepileptic drugs and dopamine-blocking medications have been used to treat tics, both classes of drugs have also been reported to lead to Tourette-like symptoms.[200,201] Of the drugs of abuse, cocaine has been implicated most frequently in tic production.[183] Secondary tourettism may also be seen with HD,[95] autism spectrum disorders,[202] and choreoacanthocytosis[203] and sometimes after trauma.[204]

Akathisia

Akathisia refers either to an uncomfortable sensation of inner restlessness or to the voluntary activity performed to relieve that restlessness. It often manifests with an inability to remain seated, crossing and uncrossing the legs, or pacing.[205] Akathisia usually occurs after the administration of neuroleptic medications. It may occur shortly after exposure (acute akathisia) or as a late complication of treatment (tardive akathisia).

Akathisia can be difficult to distinguish from tics[206] and restless legs syndrome (RLS).[207] All three of these disorders are characterized by movements that are performed to relieve an unpleasant internal sensation. Akathetic patients do not typically report the feeling of building tension that tic patients do. Akathisia also differs from both tic disorders and RLS in that the movements that akathetic patients perform feel neither compelled nor involuntary.

Akathetic Disorders

Restless Legs Syndrome. RLS may be defined as a feeling of unease or dysesthesia that is referred specifically to the lower limbs and is improved by movement.[208] The symptoms of RLS are usually bilateral and diurnal. Symptoms may be worse during the nighttime hours, even when patients remain awake.[209]

RLS is the most common of the movement disorders. Large population surveys have found that it affects 3% to 19% of adults, depending on their age.[12,210] RLS is typically a disease of patients' middle years, although it should be noted that in one patient series, up to a third of patients experienced their first symptoms before the age of 10.[211]

The underlying cause of RLS may be idiopathic or secondary. There is good evidence that familial inheritance accounts for at least some of the secondary cases of RLS. Iron deficiency anemia is responsible for RLS in a subset of patients. In this subgroup, treating the deficiency seems to relieve the symptoms. Therefore, iron deficiency should be ruled out in patients with RLS symptoms.

Drug-Induced Akathisia. Dopamine-blocking agents may lead to either acute or delayed feelings of restlessness, and it may be included among the tardive syndromes as *tardive akathisia*.[32] Less commonly, serotonin reuptake inhibitors,[212] calcium channel blockers,[213] and tricyclic antidepressants[214] have also been associated with akathisia.

Stereotypies

Stereotypies are repetitive movements or vocalizations that mimic a purposeful action, are performed outside that action's normal context, and are involuntary or semivoluntary.[215] The hand wringing of Rett's syndrome is one example of stereotyped behavior.[215] Stereotypies should be differentiated from *automatisms*. Automatisms, such as the odd behavior that can occur during partial complex seizures, are sudden in onset, occur in the background of a clouded sensorium, are time limited, do not reliably occur after periods of stress, may take place during sleep, may be followed by a postictal behavioral change, and occur randomly.

Stereotypies should also be distinguished from repetitive *perseverative* behavior, or behavior that represents "a restriction of behavioral possibilities without excessive production."[216] A *mannerism* is "a bizarre way of carrying out a purposeful act which usually occurs as the result of the incorporation of a stereotypy into a goal directed behavior."[14,217]

Stereotypies may be triggered by an inability to adopt competing motor patterns when faced with an environmental cue,[216] as opposed to compulsive behaviors and tics, which are thought to be triggered by internal cues.

As outlined by Jankovic, the most common stereotypies are facial grimacing, staring at lights, waving objects before the eyes, repetitive sounds, arm flapping, body rocking, repetitive touching, feeling and smelling objects, jumping, toe walking, and hand and body gesturing.[218] Stereotypies can be seen in patients with autism, Asperger's syndrome,[219] schizophrenia, and mental retardation and after exposure to neuroleptic medications *(tardive stereotypy)*.[220] Although it is common to find stereotypies in any of these syndromes, stereotypies are most typical of autism.[221,222]

A discussion of stereotypy syndromes of autism and of Rett's syndrome is available online at ExpertConsult.com.

HYPOKINESIAS

Bradykinesia

Bradykinesia refers to a decrease in movement velocity. This phenomenon should be distinguished from the reduction in amplitude that is termed *hypokinesia*. Patients may report bradykinesia as a nonspecific feeling of fatigue. The term *akinesia*, when properly used, refers to a complete lack of movement or an inability to initiate movement. Although *akinesia*, *bradykinesia*, and *hypokinesia* are distinct, clinicians should be aware that these terms are frequently used interchangeably.

Bradykinesia Syndromes

Gait Freezing. *Freezing* is a situation-specific akinesia: a sudden arrest of or inability to initiate gait. Freezing is most common during initiation of movement, when approaching an obstacle, or when attempting to turn. It is often seen in advanced PD and can be life altering; a significant number of patients who freeze restrict their social activity to avoid exacerbating situations.

Freezing may also occur in patients with OCD, primary progressive gait apraxia, and Parkinson's plus syndromes such as multiple system atrophy (MSA), vascular parkinsonism, and progressive supranuclear palsy (PSP).

See the expanded version of this chapter on ExpertConsult.com for more information on stiff person syndrome and neuromyotonia.

DISORDERS WITH MIXED HYPOKINESIA AND HYPERKINESIA

Parkinsonian Disorders

James Parkinson eloquently described what we now know as Parkinson's disease in his *Essay on the Shaking Palsy* in 1817,[58] in which he identified rest tremor, stooped posture, excessive salivation, and festination as features of the disease. Little was added to this description until Charcot's lectures of the 1860s,[243] in which he added rigidity and akathisia to the list of PD symptoms. By 1893, physicians were distinguishing patients' "fixity of feature and of limb" from their "slowness of movement"[244] as they realized that bradykinesia and rigidity were separable symptoms.

Four cardinal features dominate the current description of PD: rest tremor, bradykinesia, rigidity, and postural instability. *Parkinsonism* is a term used to denote the presence of bradykinesia with any of the other three cardinal motor symptoms.

Parkinson's Disease

The first symptoms of PD usually manifest in the fifth decade of life.[245] Rest tremor is the first symptom in 70% of PD patients.[246] When symptoms appear before the age of 50, the condition is considered young-onset PD. Patients with this type of PD are more likely to have dystonia and levodopa-induced dyskinesias early in their disease course.[247,248] Juvenile-onset PD (first symptom before the age of 20) is rare and suggests genetic or secondary parkinsonism.[248] Individuals with young-onset PD constitute approximately 5% of referred patients in western countries.[247]

PD tremor is a resting tremor with a frequency of approximately 4 to 7 Hz. The tremor is typically more distal than proximal. It may be intermittent and is almost always asymmetrical in the initial stages of the disease.[63] Like most tremors, it is worsened by distraction—either cognitive tasks (e.g., performing arithmetic) or motor tasks (e.g., walking). Strong emotion also tends to exacerbate PD tremor. PD tremor also usually becomes apparent while walking.

Postural and gait instability is the least specific of the cardinal features of PD. The parkinsonian gait is characterized by shuffling of the feet, decreased arm swing on one or both sides of the body, and stooping of posture. Patients are typically unable to turn in a single step and instead break their turns into multiple small increments. The body characteristically remains aligned with the feet during these maneuvers (en bloc turns). Patients are unstable and may be unable to recover from a backward tug. Both *festination* and *retropulsion* may be seen. In festination patients appear to chase their center of gravity and as a result are "thrown on the toes and forepart of the feet; being … irresistibly impelled to take much quicker and shorter steps, and thereby to adopt unwillingly a running pace."[58] Retropulsion is an analogous behavior that occurs as a result of patients' inability to recover from a backward-leaning posture.

The pathogenesis of PD probably involves both environmental and genetic factors.[249] Environmental factors that have been linked to PD include pesticide exposure, living in a rural area, and drinking well water.[250,251] Interestingly, tobacco use is inversely associated with risk for PD.[252] MPTP, a by-product of meperidine synthesis, caused parkinsonism in drug users exposed to it in the late 1970s and early 1980s.[253] Nonhuman primates injected with MPTP display levodopa-responsive akinesia, rigidity, and tremor, as well as levodopa-induced dyskinesias.[254] MPTP exposure results in selective death of dopaminergic cells of the substantia nigra. However, the MPTP model does not duplicate the progressive dysfunction seen in PD. Based on cadaveric studies, PD is believed to clinically manifest only after approximately 80% of striatal dopamine and 50% of nigral neurons have been lost.[255] More recently, evidence has emerged that a prion-like spread of abnormally aggregating α-synuclein may play a role in PD pathology.[256,257]

Approximately 10% to 15% of patients with PD also report PD in a first-degree relative.[258-260] Common environmental exposure probably accounts for a proportion of these cases,[261] but the fact that individuals with similar exposure vary in their expression of parkinsonian symptoms, coupled with the identification of multiple susceptibility genes,[262,263] supports the idea that the pathogenesis of PD involves both genetic predisposition and environmental exposure. Several genetic defects have been implicated in inherited PD, including alterations in the parkin,[264] *LRRK2*,[265] phosphatase and tensin homolog (PTEN)–induced kinase *(PINK1)*,[266] and α-synuclein (*PARK1* or *SNCA*) genes.[267] Although the list of familial forms of PD continues to lengthen, PARK1, LRRK2, and PINK1 are the most common forms currently identified and together account for 3% of all patients with parkinsonism.[268] Genetic forms of PD tend to have a younger onset than sporadic PD does.

Of the cardinal features of PD, bradykinesia has the best correlation with disease severity. Bradykinesia and rigidity are also the symptoms best explained by current models. According to the Alexander, DeLong, and Strick model, bradykinesia arises from excessive inhibition of the thalamus by the globus pallidus (pars) interna (GPi), either directly by GPi overactivity or indirectly by overactivation of the GPi by an overactive subthalamic nucleus.[1] This model does not perfectly account for all observed PD phenomena (e.g., lesions in the GPi reduce dyskinesias rather than increasing them).[269] Models that emphasize the role of aberrant motor plan selection, neuronal oscillation, and neuronal synchrony have been proposed and continue to evolve.[270-272]

Parkinsonian rigidity is a function of enhanced static or postural reflexes and should be differentiated from bradykinesia,[273] in the same way that stiffness and slowing are not identical. The rigidity may be of either a "lead pipe" or "cogwheel" quality and is typically asymmetrical.

Care should be taken to exclude cases of parkinsonism due to the administration of phenothiazine antiemetics or dopamine-depleting neuroleptics.[158] Suspicion for a Parkinson's-plus syndrome should be raised by the presence of cerebellar deficits, corticospinal tract signs, or vertical gaze restriction. Dementia, autonomic dysfunction, or postural instability early in the disease course are also atypical for idiopathic PD.[274]

Dementia with Lewy Bodies

Dementia with Lewy bodies (DLB) is the second most common cause of dementia after Alzheimer's disease.[275,276] It is characterized by progressive parkinsonism, hallucinosis, and dementia.[277] A clinical diagnosis of DLB is made if dementia and hallucinations start within 1 year of development of parkinsonism. Pathologically, DLB and PD dementia appear similar with widespread distribution of α-synuclein–containing Lewy bodies. In the parkinsonism of DLB, tremor is commonly minimal or absent. Hallucinations and delusions may occur spontaneously or may be provoked by dopaminergic medications, even at low doses. Patients' hallucinations tend to be visual, vivid, complex, and well formed. Interestingly, patients usually have good insight into the unreality of their visions.[278] A fluctuating level of attention and alertness is also typical of DLB, and patients may vary dramatically in their alertness from hour to hour or day to day.[63] Supranuclear ophthalmoparesis is an unusual feature but has also been reported.[279]

Differentiating DLB from Alzheimer's disease can be difficult, but the presence of hallucinosis, gait impairment, rigidity, or tremor early in the disease course should strongly suggest the diagnosis of DLB.[280]

Progressive Supranuclear Palsy

PSP was first described by Steele, Richardson, and Olszewski in 1964.[281] It is a tauopathy.[282] It is characterized by progressive and symmetrical parkinsonism, gait instability, and gaze palsies.[281] Frequent falls are the most common initial symptom and arise from a combination of gait freezing and loss of postural reflexes. Patients typically lack insight into this impairment, thereby compounding their difficulties.[283] As with DLB, tremor is not a prominent part of the clinical picture of PSP.

Supranuclear gaze palsy, characterized by volitional vertical gaze palsy, is the classic manifestation of PSP. It is usually preceded by a slowing of vertical saccades.[284] Convergence failure and square-wave jerks may be seen. Patients may progress to complete ophthalmoparesis. Initially, doll's eye maneuvers can overcome this problem, but the vestibulo-ocular reflex is often lost over time.[285]

Bulbar symptoms are prominent in PSP. The typical facies of PSP consists of a furrowed brow with prominent nasolabial folds. The increased muscular tone of the face and throat produces a characteristic "startled face" and a low-pitched dysarthria. Eyelid-opening apraxia is a frequent complicating factor, as is dysphagia. Dysphagia is the most frequent cause of death; most PSP patients die of aspiration-related complications within a decade of the diagnosis.[286]

Patients may also display behavior that is not congruent with their subjective emotional state. This *pseudobulbar affect* manifests as displays of tearfulness without the feeling of sadness or laughter without the sensation of amusement. PSP may also lead to *emotional incontinence*, in which patients respond disproportionately but congruently to an emotional stimulus. Frontal disinhibition may lead to the presence of an "applause sign." This is characterized by an inability to stop clapping after three claps.[287] It is not specific to PSP and may be seen in other conditions that affect the circuitry of the frontal cortex.[287]

Several pathologic series have suggested that the syndrome of *pure akinesia with gait freezing*, a disorder of gait interruption and akinesis on gait initiation, is sufficiently similar in its pathology to PSP to be considered a variant.[282]

Corticobasal Degeneration

Corticobasal degeneration (CBD) is a tauopathy manifesting as a parkinsonism with prominent cortical features, particularly apraxia.[288]

Asymmetrical hand clumsiness is the most common initial complaint and was seen in 50% of patients in one series.[289] Other motor symptoms include asymmetrical rest tremor, limb dystonia, rigidity, and cortical myoclonus. The alien limb phenomenon (ALP), in which the patient's limb performs uncontrolled movements and is thought of as "other," is associated with CBD.[290] Although it aids in the diagnosis, ALP is not specific. ALP has been seen with vascular lesions,[291] gunshot wounds,[292] seizures,[293,294] Creutzfeld-Jakob disease,[295] and Alzheimer's dementia.[296]

The dementia of CBD is characterized by progressive aphasia, frontal lobe symptoms, dyscalculia, mild memory difficulty, and apraxia. The apraxia is most often of an ideomotor type and is detected during neurological examination by patients' inability to pantomime tool-using actions. Although aphasia was once thought to be rare in CBD, it is common and may be the initial feature.[292] Other frequently seen signs include agraphesthesia and astereognosis.[297]

In a recent reclassification, CBD has been divided into four subtypes: corticobasal syndrome (CBS), a more classic presentation; frontal behavioral-spatial syndrome (FBS), characterized by prominent executive dysfunction and behavioral changes; nonfluent/agrammatic variant of primary progressive aphasia (naPPA), characterized by semantic distortions of speech; and progressive supranuclear palsy syndrome (PSPS), typified by symmetrical parkinsonism, supranuclear gaze palsy, and postural instability.[288]

Multiple System Atrophy

MSA is an α-synucleinopathy that is subdivided into two syndromes based on whether parkinsonism (MSA-P) or cerebellar ataxia (MSA-C) predominates.[298,299]

MSA-P, formerly known as *striatonigral degeneration*, most resembles PD. The combination of rapid disease progression, symmetrical symptoms, absence of rest tremor, and a paucity of levodopa response suggests a diagnosis of MSA.[300,301] Patients with MSA-C, formerly known as *olivopontocerebellar atrophy*, display progressive cerebellar ataxia and parkinsonism. Gaze-evoked or positional nystagmus occurs more frequently in MSA-C than in MSA-P. Square-wave jerks may be seen in both subtypes.[302]

Dysautonomia eventually develops in most patients with MSA. Many authors no longer consider dysautonomia-predominant MSA (Shy-Drager syndrome) to be a distinct category.[299] The autonomic symptoms of MSA include impotence, diaphoresis, orthostatic hypotension, and incontinence. Incipient orthostatic hypotension may be unmasked by treatment with dopaminergic medications.[303]

Normal sphincter EMG findings are rare in patients with MSA of any subtype, as long as the symptoms have been present for at least 5 years.[304] Whether sphincter EMG is useful in differentiating MSA from other parkinsonisms earlier in the course of the disease remains a topic for research. MSA of any subtype can be difficult to distinguish from either PD or PSP on a patient's first visit. Litvan[305] reported that the presence of at least six of the following eight features at the patient's first visit—sporadic adult onset, lack of levodopa response, cerebellar signs, dysautonomia, parkinsonism, pyramidal signs, no downward gaze palsy, and no cognitive dysfunction—was predictive of MSA with a median sensitivity of 59% and positive predictive value of 67%. MRI abnormalities such as the hot cross bun sign (cross-shaped T2-weighted hyperintensity of the pons because of the degeneration of transverse pontine fibers) and putaminal enhancement may be seen in as many as 65% of patients with MSA.[306,307]

Dystonia

Dystonia is defined as an abnormal simultaneous co-contraction of agonist and antagonist muscle groups that results in abnormal postures and/or movements. This contraction may be brief or sustained or focal or generalized. Common locations include the neck (cervical dystonia, or *torticollis*), eyelids *(blepharospasm)*, or vocal cords *(spasmodic dysphonia)*.

Dystonia is usually worsened by voluntary movements. Conversely, relaxation or sleep can ameliorate or abolish the symptoms. Dystonias can be posture or action dependent. Some patients with gait restrictions as a result of leg dystonia improve dramatically when asked to walk backward. Other patients find that their hands cramp painfully only when attempting to play a particular musical instrument. Some patients display sensory tricks, or *gestes antagonistes:* they find that touching a particular body part temporarily relieves their dystonia.

Dystonia has recently been reclassified.[308] Dystonias are now characterized by two axes: their clinical characterization (age of onset, distribution, course, and associated symptoms), and their cause (genetic or acquired). Focal dystonias are most common, but many dystonias with a focal onset generalize later (Table 84-5).[309-321] The younger the age at the onset of symptoms, the more likely it is for the dystonia to generalize.

Dystonic Syndromes

Isolated Dystonia. Isolated dystonias are "pure" dystonias that cannot be ascribed to another disease process. They may be either genetic or acquired. The numerous genetic dystonias are subclassified into dystonia-torsion (DYT) categories and are summarized in Table 84-5.

The most common cause of young-onset generalized progressive dystonia is DYT1 dystonia (Oppenheim's dystonia). It occurs relatively frequently in the Ashkenazi Jewish population, with a prevalence of 1 in 2000. DYT1 is inherited in an autosomal dominant fashion with a penetrance of 30% to 40%.[322] The onset of symptoms is usually in late childhood or early adolescence, and they generally begin in one leg and later generalize.

DYT7, or adult-onset focal dystonia, is another autosomal dominant dystonia.[323] Onset is typically in middle age. Symptoms are focal or multifocal and involve predominantly the upper part of the body.

Combined Dystonias. Combined dystonias are conditions in which parkinsonism, myoclonus, or ataxia develops in addition to dystonia. The combined inherited dystonias include dystonia-parkinsonism (DYT3 and DYT12), dopa-responsive dystonia (DYT5), paroxysmal dystonia (DYT8, DYT9, and DYT10), and myoclonus-dystonia (DYT11).

A more detailed discussion of these can be found online at ExpertConsult.com.

Acquired Dystonias. Though acquired dystonias can be either combined or isolated in their appearance, they are worth considering separately. Any insult to the sensorimotor circuitry can lead to dystonia, and thus acquired dystonias have a variety of causes. Dystonia has been reported after ischemia, hypoxia, infection, neoplasm, drug or toxin exposure, metabolic derangement, inflammatory disease, and trauma. In evaluating a patient with dystonia, it is important to identify any treatable conditions, such

TABLE 84-5 Inherited Dystonia Syndromes

	Eponym	Extent	Features	Onset	Inheritance	Gene (Chromosome)
DYT1	Oppenheim's dystonia	Generalized	Early limb onset	Childhood to adolescence	Autosomal dominant	Torsin A (9q34)
DYT2	—	Generalized or segmental	Early onset	Childhood to adolescence	Autosomal recessive	—
DYT3	Lubag: X-linked dystonia-parkinsonism	Initially focal, then generalizes	Seen in Filipino patients, in whom generalized parkinsonian and dystonic features develop	Adulthood	X-linked recessive	(Xq13)
DYT4	—	Focal: dysphonia and torticollis	Single Australian kindred	Adolescence to adulthood	Autosomal dominant	—
DYT5	Dopa-responsive dystonia (Segawa's disease)	Limb onset, generalized	Usually limb onset, levodopa responsive, diurnal; may have parkinsonian features	Infancy or childhood	Autosomal dominant (childhood) Autosomal recessive (infantile)	GTP cyclohydrolase 1 (14, childhood), tyrosine hydroxylase (11, infant)
DYT6	—	Segmental (craniofacial and limb)	Seen in Mennonite kindreds	Adulthood	Autosomal dominant	(8p)
DYT7	Adult-onset focal dystonia	Focal or multifocal	Seen in large German kindred	Adulthood-elderly	Autosomal dominant	(18)
DYT8	Paroxysmal nonkinesigenic dyskinesia	Episodic and focal	Paroxysms of dystonia or chorea precipitated by caffeine, stress	Variable	Autosomal dominant	Myofibrillogenesis (2q)
DYT9	Paroxysmal dyskinesia with episodic ataxia and spasticity	Episodic and focal	Paroxysms of dystonia or chorea	Childhood-adolescence	Autosomal dominant	(1p)
DYT10	Paroxysmal kinesigenic dyskinesia	Episodic and focal	Paroxysms of dystonia or chorea precipitated by movement	Childhood-adolescence	Autosomal dominant	(16p)
DYT11	Myoclonus-dystonia	Variable	30% positive for ε-sarcoglycan; improves with alcohol; associated with OCD, panic	Variable	Autosomal dominant	ε-Sarcoglycan (7q21, 11q23)
DYT12	Rapid-onset dystonia-parkinsonism	Generalized	Acute to subacute onset of generalized dystonia and parkinsonism	Childhood to adolescence	Autosomal dominant	*ATP1A3* (19q13)
DYT13	—	Segmental (craniofacial and upper body)	Seen in single Italian kindred	Childhood to adulthood	Autosomal dominant	*KCNA1* (1p)
DYT15	—	Limb onset	Alcohol-responsive myoclonic and limb dystonia	Childhood to adolescence	Autosomal dominant	(18p11)

Data from references 303-315, 319.
OCD, obsessive-compulsive disorder.

TABLE 84-6 Causes of Acquired Dystonia

Infection	Creutzfeldt-Jakob disease Reye's syndrome Subacute sclerosing panencephalitis HIV infection Viral encephalitis
Drugs	Anticonvulsants Dopamine receptor blocking agents Ergots Fenfluramine Flecainide Some calcium channel blockers
Toxins	Carbon disulfide Carbon monoxide Cyanide Disulfiram Manganese Methanol 3-Nitropropionic acid Wasp sting toxin
Metabolic causes	Hypoparathyroidism PKAN
Brain or brainstem lesions	AVM Central pontine myelinolysis Multiple sclerosis Paraneoplastic brainstem encephalitis Primary antiphospholipid syndrome Stroke Trauma Tumors
Spinal cord lesions	Syringomyelia
Peripheral lesions	Electrical injury

Used with permission from Fernandez HH, Rodriguez RL, Skidmore FS, et al. *A Practical Approach to Movement Disorders: Diagnosis and Medical and Surgical Management*. New York: Demos Medical; 2007.

AVM, arteriovenous malformation; HIV, human immunodeficiency virus; PKAN, pantothenate kinase–associated neurodegeneration.

as Wilson's disease or drug exposure. Tardive dystonia results from exposure to neuroleptics. The many causes of acquired dystonia are summarized in Table 84-6.

DISORDERS OF COORDINATION

Ataxia

The term *ataxia* refers to clumsy or poorly organized movements. Ataxia stems from deficits in the cerebellar, vestibular, or proprioceptive pathways. It may affect speech, manual dexterity, or gait. Ataxic patients often complain of feeling as though they are inebriated; alcohol's cerebellar coordination–impairing effects produce a picture of ataxia with which the lay public is immediately familiar. Pure ataxia is not associated with deficits in strength or motor planning.

Ataxic movements are poorly aimed or timed; patients have difficulty properly estimating the distance required to reach a target or terminating an action at the proper moment. For example, patients might fail to release a ball when they desire to do so and throw it to the ground instead of forward. Similarly, ataxic patients might knock over a glass when trying to lift it or strike their teeth when trying to drink. Speech may sound poorly formed or take on an arrhythmic and staccato quality.

Any process that damages the cerebellar system or its connections may produce ataxia, including trauma, neoplasm, infarction, infection, or genetic mutation. For reasons of scope, this section will focus on the inherited ataxia syndromes.

The inherited ataxia syndromes are most easily classified by their pattern of inheritance: autosomal dominant, autosomal recessive, and X-linked. These disorders are summarized in Table 84-7, and an expanded discussion of them can be found online at ExpertConsult.com.[125,329-333]

MOVEMENT DISORDERS CAUSED BY METABOLIC OR SYSTEMIC DISEASE

Toxic/Metabolic Syndromes

Wilson's Disease

Wilson's disease is an autosomal recessive disorder of copper metabolism that causes both liver and basal ganglia damage. For this reason, Wilson's disease is also referred to as *hepatolenticular degeneration*. The disease is well known for causing a variety of symptoms. The initial symptom may be a tremor, dystonia, or chorea. The findings may differ substantially even within the same kindred.[339] Given this fact and the potentially treatable nature of the syndrome, all patients with a movement disorder before the age of 50 should be checked for the presence of Wilson's disease.

Wilson's disease causes neurological symptoms in roughly 40% of patients, with liver disease in 40% and psychiatric disease in the remainder.[340] The age at onset varies, but the first symptoms usually appear between the ages of 11 and 25. Patients with liver impairment tend to be affected at a younger age than those with neurological symptoms.[341,342]

The neurological symptoms of Wilson's disease are typically a parkinsonian akinetic-rigid syndrome, generalized dystonia, or a proximal postural/action tremor with ataxia and dysarthria. Although pure chorea may be seen in Wilson's disease, it is an unusual manifestation of the syndrome. Psychiatric findings include pseudobulbar affect, impulsivity, and depression. Frank psychosis is rare. If the disease is untreated, symptoms worsen and result in death from liver failure or severe neurological compromise.

Based on epidemiologic studies in Europe and the United States, the prevalence of Wilson's disease is estimated to be about 15 to 30 cases per 1,000,000 people.[343] Heterozygous carriers are present in the general population at a rate of 1 in 100 to 150 individuals.[343,344]

The underlying pathology is accumulation of copper in the liver and basal ganglia as a result of impaired copper excretion secondary to mutations in an adenosine triphosphatase (ATPase) that aids in transmembrane copper transportation and binding of copper to the carrier protein ceruloplasmin. This ATPase is encoded by the gene *ATP7B*, located on chromosome 13.[89] *ATP7B* defects result in accumulation of copper within hepatocytes, which eventually spills over into other tissues, including the brain. Copper accumulation leads to increased but insufficient urinary copper excretion and high serum levels of free copper.

Ceruloplasmin testing is a useful screening tool, but serum levels of this protein may be normal even in symptomatic individuals.[345] Testing for elevated copper levels in a 24-hour urinary collection is the best single test for the syndrome short of elevated hepatic copper concentration on biopsy.[346] The classic Kaiser-Fleischer rings—flecks of copper visible in the cornea under slit-lamp examination—are almost universally present in patients with neurological symptoms. MRI findings are abnormal in symptomatic patients and typically show generalized atrophy and pallidal hypointensity on T2-weighted images.[347] Central pontine myelinolysis may also be present.

More information on the toxic and metabolic causes of movement disorders, including hereditary aceruloplasminemia, Lesch-Nyhan Disease, pantothenate kinase–associated neurodegeneration (PKAN), and neuroferritinopathy is available at ExpertConsult.com.

TABLE 84-7 Ataxia Syndromes

Ataxia Syndrome	Gene (Chromosome)	Gene Defect	Onset	Inheritance	Features
SCA1	*ATXN1* (6p)	CAG triplet repeat in ataxin-1	10-70	Autosomal dominant	Ataxia, dysarthria, and hyperreflexia; dysphagia, spasticity, dystonia, and chorea may occur later in the disease
SCA2	*ATXN2* (12q)	CAG triplet repeat in ataxin-2	10-60	Autosomal dominant	Gait and limb ataxia, hyporeflexia, dysarthria, sensory impairment, dementia, slowing of saccades, postural tremor
SCA3 (Machado-Joseph)	*ATXN3* (14q)	CAG triplet repeat in Machado-Joseph protein-1 (MJP1)	10-60	Autosomal dominant	Ataxia, hyperreflexia, nystagmus, dysarthria, facial and tongue atrophy, peripheral nerve disease; evoked nystagmus progresses to ophthalmoparesis; levodopa-responsive tremor
SCA4	*Q9H7K4* (16q)	Puratrophin-1	30-50	Autosomal dominant	Severe ataxia, sensory loss, areflexia, distal atrophy; single Utah kindred
SCA5	SPTBN2 (11)	Spectrin β chain	10-70	Autosomal dominant	Pure cerebellar ataxia, slow progression; patients are descendants of Lincoln's grandparents
SCA6	*CACNA1A* (19p13)	CAG triplet repeat in voltage-gated potassium channel	50-60	Autosomal dominant	Cerebellar ataxia, imbalance, nystagmus, sensory loss; slow progression
SCA7	*ATXN7* (3p)	CAG triplet repeat in ataxin-7	<10 or 30-40	Autosomal dominant	Ataxia, visual loss, hyperreflexia; childhood form adds seizures, myoclonus, dementia, lethality in 5 yr
SCA8	*KLHL1AS* (13q21)	CTG triplet repeat	40-50	Autosomal dominant	Slowly progressive ataxia, hyperreflexia, decreased vibratory sense
SCA10	*ATXN10* (22q13)	ATTCT repeat in ataxin-10	20-50	Autosomal dominant	Seizures
Episodic ataxia type 1	*KCNA1* (19)	Potassium channel	10-20	Autosomal dominant	Discrete episodes (seconds to minutes) of ataxia, myokymia induced by exercise and startle; attenuates over time
Episodic ataxia type 2	*CACNA1A* (19p13)	Voltage-dependent calcium channel	10-50	Autosomal dominant	Discrete episodes (minutes to hours) of ataxia, nystagmus, and vertigo triggered by caffeine or alcohol; progresses to permanent ataxia
DRPLA	*ATN1* (12p12)	CAG repeat	<20 or >40	Autosomal dominant	Mixed ataxia and chorea syndrome; accompanied by mental retardation, seizures, psychosis, myoclonus; most common in Japan
Ataxia-telangiectasia	*ATM* (11q)	Phosphoinositol-3-kinase–type enzyme (DNA repair)	2-20	Autosomal recessive	Early: postural instability, ataxia Mid-disease: hypotonia, bradykinesia, areflexia, chorea, impaired saccades, telangiectasia, oculomotor apraxia, neoplasm
Friedreich's ataxia	*FRDA* (19q)	GAA triplet repeat in frataxin (mitochondrial)	2-50	Autosomal recessive	Ataxia, dysarthria, areflexia, spasticity, distal atrophy, deafness, optic atrophy; also cardiomyopathy, scoliosis, diabetes
Ataxia with oculomotor apraxia type 1	*APTX* (9p13)	Aprataxin	2-20	Autosomal recessive	Ataxia, oculomotor apraxia, ocular telangiectasia, polyneuropathy
Ataxia with oculomotor apraxia type 2	*SETX* (9q34)	Senataxin	10-20	Autosomal recessive	Ataxia, oculomotor apraxia, ocular telangiectasia, polyneuropathy
Abetalipoproteinemia	*MPT* (4q)	Microsomal triglyceride transfer protein (MPT)	20-30	Autosomal recessive	Ataxia, areflexia, distal muscle atrophy, intestinal symptoms, loss of vibratory sense; fat malabsorption: vitamin A, E, K deficiency; acanthocytes on smear
Ataxia with vitamin E deficiency	*α-TTP* (8q13)	α-Tocopherol transfer protein	2-50	Autosomal recessive	Ataxia, areflexia, loss of vibratory sense
Fragile X–associated tremor ataxia syndrome	*FMR1* (X)	CGG triplet repeat	Variable	X-linked	Gait ataxia, intention tremor, parkinsonism, autonomic dysfunction, polyneuropathy, cognitive impairment

Data from references 125, 323-327.
DRPLA, dentatorubral-pallidoluysian atrophy.

Acknowledgments

We would like to acknowledge the support of the National Parkinson Foundation via a Center of Excellence award, the McKnight Brain Institute (Gainesville, FL), the University of Florida, Shands Hospital (Gainesville, FL), and the Eric and Jennifer Scott Fund for Parkinson's Research (Gainesville, FL).

SUGGESTED READINGS

Alexander GE, DeLong MR, Strick PL. Parallel organization of functionally segregated circuits linking basal ganglia and cortex. *Annu Rev Neurosci*. 1986;9:357-381.

A novel gene containing a trinucleotide repeat that is expanded and unstable on Huntington's disease chromosomes, The Huntington's Disease Collaborative Research Group. *Cell*. 1993;72:971-983.

Ashizawa T, Wong LJ, Richards CS, et al. CAG repeat size and clinical presentation in Huntington's disease. *Neurology*. 1994;44:1137-1143.

Benabid AL, Pollak P, Gao D, et al. Chronic electrical stimulation of the ventralis intermedius nucleus of the thalamus as a treatment of movement disorders. *J Neurosurg*. 1996;84:203-214.

Bergman H, Feingold A, Nini A, et al. Physiological aspects of information processing in the basal ganglia of normal and parkinsonian primates. *Trends Neurosci*. 1998;21:32-38.

Brown P, Marsden CD. The stiff man and stiff man plus syndromes. *J Neurol*. 1999;246:648-652.

Brown P, Rothwell JC, Thompson PD, et al. The hyperekplexias and their relationship to the normal startle reflex. *Brain*. 1991;114:1903-1928.

Bruno MK, Lee HY, Auburger GW, et al. Genotype-phenotype correlation of paroxysmal nonkinesigenic dyskinesia. *Neurology*. 2007;68:1782-1789.

Burke JR, Wingfield MS, Lewis KE, et al. The Haw River syndrome: dentatorubropallidoluysian atrophy (DRPLA) in an African-American family. *Nat Genet*. 1994;7:521-524.

Burns RS, Chiueh CC, Markey SP, et al. A primate model of parkinsonism: selective destruction of dopaminergic neurons in the pars compacta of the substantia nigra by *N*-methyl-4-phenyl-1,2,3,6-tetrahydropyridine. *Proc Natl Acad Sci U S A*. 1983;80:4546-4550.

Cardoso F, Seppi K, Mair KJ, et al. Seminar on choreas. *Lancet Neurol*. 2006;5:589-602.

Cohen AJ, Leckman JF. Sensory phenomena associated with Gilles de la Tourette's syndrome. *J Clin Psychiatry*. 1992;53:319-323.

Demirkiran M, Jankovic J. Paroxysmal dyskinesias: clinical features and classification. *Ann Neurol*. 1995;38:571-579.

Deng H, Le W, Jankovic J. Premutation alleles associated with Parkinson disease and essential tremor. *JAMA*. 2004;292:1685-1686.

Deuschl G, Raethjen J, Lindemann M, et al. The pathophysiology of tremor. *Muscle Nerve*. 2001;24:716-735.

Deuschl G, Wilms H. Clinical spectrum and physiology of palatal tremor. *Mov Disord*. 2002;17(suppl 2):S63-S66.

Elble RJ. Central mechanisms of tremor. *J Clin Neurophysiol*. 1996;13:133-144.

Fahn S, Williams DT. Psychogenic dystonia. *Adv Neurol*. 1988;50:431-455.

Fernandez HH, Rodriguez RL, Skidmore FS, et al. *A Practical Approach to Movement Disorders: Diagnosis and Medical and Surgical Management*. New York: Demos Medical; 2007.

Footitt DR, Quinn N, Kocen RS, et al. Familial Lafora body disease of late onset: report of four cases in one family and a review of the literature. *J Neurol*. 1997;244:40-44.

Ford B, Greene P, Fahn S. Oral and genital tardive pain syndromes. *Neurology*. 1994;44:2115-2119.

Gibb WR, Lees AJ. The clinical phenomenon of akathisia. *J Neurol Neurosurg Psychiatry*. 1986;49:861-866.

Hallett M. Electrophysiologic evaluation of movement disorders. In: Aminoff M, ed. *Electrodiagnosis in Clinical Neurology*. New York: Churchill Livingstone; 1999:365-380.

Hallett M, Cloninger CR. *Psychogenic Movement Disorders: Neurology and Neuropsychiatry*. Philadelphia: Lippincott Williams & Wilkins; 2006.

Hallett M, Shahani BT, Young RR. EMG analysis of stereotyped voluntary movements in man. *J Neurol Neurosurg Psychiatry*. 1975;38:1154-1162.

Heilman KM. Orthostatic tremor. *Arch Neurol*. 1984;41:880-881.

Hewer R. The heart in Friedreich's ataxia. *Br Heart J*. 1969;31:5-14.

Hohler A, Samii A. Approach to movement disorders. In: Winn HR, Youmans JR, eds. *Youmans Neurological Surgery*. 5th ed. Philadelphia: WB Saunders; 2004:2729-2744.

Jankovic J. Tourette syndrome. Phenomenology and classification of tics. *Neurol Clin*. 1997;15:267-275.

Jankovic J, Tolosa E. *Parkinson's Disease and Movement Disorders*. 5th ed. Philadelphia: Lippincott Williams & Wilkins; 2007.

Kanazawa I. Dentatorubral-pallidoluysian atrophy or Naito-Oyanagi disease. *Neurogenetics*. 1998;2:1-17.

Klein C, Brin MF, Kramer P, et al. Association of a missense change in the D_2 dopamine receptor with myoclonus dystonia. *Proc Natl Acad Sci U S A*. 1999;96:5173-5176.

Kremer B, Almqvist E, Theilmann J, et al. Sex-dependent mechanisms for expansions and contractions of the CAG repeat on affected Huntington disease chromosomes. *Am J Hum Genet*. 1995;57:343-350.

Lang A. Patient perception of tics and other movement disorders. *Neurology*. 1991;41:223-228.

Lees AJ. Facial mannerisms and tics. *Adv Neurol*. 1988;49:255-261.

Leigh PN, Rothwell JC, Traub M, et al. A patient with reflex myoclonus and muscle rigidity: "jerking stiff-man syndrome". *J Neurol Neurosurg Psychiatry*. 1980;43:1125-1131.

Lombardi WJ, Woolston DJ, Roberts JW, et al. Cognitive deficits in patients with essential tremor. *Neurology*. 2001;57:785-790.

Manford M, Andermann F. Complex visual hallucinations. Clinical and neurobiological insights. *Brain*. 1998;121:1819-1840.

Marsalek M. Tardive drug-induced extrapyramidal syndromes. *Pharmacopsychiatry*. 2000;33(suppl 1):14-33.

Mink JW. The basal ganglia: focused selection and inhibition of competing motor programs. *Prog Neurobiol*. 1996;50:381-425.

Moersch FP, Woltman HW. Progressive fluctuating muscular rigidity and spasm ("stiff-man" syndrome); report of a case and some observations in 13 other cases. *Mayo Clin Proc*. 1956;31:421-427.

Parkinson J. An essay on the shaking palsy. 1817. *J Neuropsychiatry Clin Neurosci*. 2002;14:223-236.

Ringman JM, Jankovic J. Occurrence of tics in Asperger's syndrome and autistic disorder. *J Child Neurol*. 2000;15:394-400.

Schols L, Bauer P, Schmidt T, et al. Autosomal dominant cerebellar ataxias: clinical features, genetics, and pathogenesis. *Lancet Neurol*. 2004;3:291-304.

Schrag A, Good CD, Miszkiel K, et al. Differentiation of atypical parkinsonian syndromes with routine MRI. *Neurology*. 2000;54:697-702.

Stoppelbein L, Greening L, Kakooza A. The importance of catatonia and stereotypies in autistic spectrum disorders. *Int Rev Neurobiol*. 2006;72:103-118.

Swartz MS, Stroup TS, McEvoy JP, et al. What CATIE found: results from the schizophrenia trial. *Psychiatr Serv*. 2008;59:500-506.

Teitelbaum P, Teitelbaum O, Nye J, et al. Movement analysis in infancy may be useful for early diagnosis of autism. *Proc Natl Acad Sci U S A*. 1998;95:13982-13987.

Tezenas du Montcel S, Clot F, Vidailhet M, et al. Epsilon sarcoglycan mutations and phenotype in French patients with myoclonic syndromes. *J Med Genet*. 2006;43:394-400.

Williams DR, Holton JL, Strand K, et al. Pure akinesia with gait freezing: a third clinical phenotype of progressive supranuclear palsy. *Mov Disord*. 2007;22:2235-2241.

See a full reference list on ExpertConsult.com

85 Patient Selection Criteria for Deep Brain Stimulation in Movement Disorders

Catherine Cho, Ioannis U. Isaias, and Michele Tagliati

Successful deep brain stimulation (DBS) therapy for movement disorders depends on a series of interrelated procedures that include precise lead placement and proficient electrode programming. However, the first and most important step toward consistent DBS outcomes remains careful patient selection, because more than 30% of DBS failures can generally be ascribed to an incorrect initial diagnosis or inappropriate indication for surgery.[1]

In this chapter we discuss the selection criteria for DBS surgery for movement disorders. We focus both on the overall selection process and on specific indications for each of the surgical interventions currently accepted or investigated for the treatment of intractable movement disorders. When available, we cite appropriate studies to support our positions; however, suitably controlled prospective studies are often lacking in this rapidly advancing field. Therefore, expert clinical opinion, which is by nature subjective and often controversial, constitutes a great part of the available knowledge.

GENERAL SELECTION PROCESS

A thorough selection process should be routinely performed to ensure that only appropriate candidates are offered DBS surgery. In our practice, this includes the following: (1) neurological examination; (2) neurosurgical evaluation; (3) neuropsychological testing and, in select candidates, psychiatric examination; (4) neuroimaging; and (5) medical clearance.

Neurological Evaluation

Preoperative evaluation for DBS normally begins with assessment by a neurologist with specific expertise in the management of movement disorders. This evaluation should be focused on establishing the correct diagnosis and ensuring that all reasonable medical therapies have been tried. Approved indications for DBS include essential tremor (ET), Parkinson's disease (PD), and primary dystonia. Other forms of tremor (i.e., midbrain, cerebellar, and orthostatic tremor), tics, and choreas (Huntington's chorea and neuroacanthocytosis) have also been targeted with DBS but are considered off-label uses of the approved device. Box 85-1 summarizes movement disorders in which DBS is currently indicated.

Once the correct diagnosis is established, the neurologist should review the medical management history to make sure that all reasonable pharmacologic therapies have been properly attempted. This can be a very controversial point because opinions vary greatly as to what constitutes the "minimal" medication therapy to be attempted before proceeding with DBS. When a patient with PD is being considered for DBS, examination both "off" and "on" medications should be performed because determination of benefit from levodopa has well-documented diagnostic and prognostic implications. In addition to neurological and motor deficits, functional disability should be documented using an accepted clinical rating scale that is specific to the patient's diagnosis. Videotaped examinations are also of great value for clinical documentation and monitoring of long-term outcome.

The value of the initial neurological visit does not end with the selection process. It also establishes a clinical baseline for postoperative comparison and provides an opportunity to educate patients and caregivers on the risks of surgery and expected outcomes. It is far more challenging to program a patient's DBS devices and manage his or her medications postoperatively if the neurologist is unfamiliar with the patient. False expectations on the part of patients or family members are common reasons for "DBS failures,"[1-3] so it is wise to moderate unrealistic expectations through consultation early in the process. Finally, DBS management represents a significant commitment of time, so it is important that the treating neurologist assess the patient's and family's motivation to undertake the challenge.[3]

Neurosurgical Evaluation

If the neurologist determines that the diagnosis is correct and that reasonable medical strategies have not provided acceptable benefit, the patient is referred to a functional neurosurgeon for further evaluation. During this meeting, the surgeon confirms that the patient is an appropriate surgical candidate and discusses the remainder of the preoperative process; the surgical options, including the available targets and surgical methodologies (e.g., frame versus frameless); and the risks and realistic goals of DBS.

A fundamental task for the neurosurgeon is to define whether the risk-benefit ratio of the surgical procedure is acceptable to the patient. The most fearsome risk associated with the DBS procedure is the occurrence of intracerebral hemorrhage, which may cause a variety of neurological deficits, including death in the most severe cases.[4] The risk for hemorrhage may vary from center to center, based on the experience of the surgeon, but it is never nil. In addition, there are device-related risks of system failure and infection, which can occur in up to 25% of patients even in the best centers.[5,6] Patients are also reminded that battery replacement, requiring minor surgery, will be necessary after 2 to 5 years, depending on the current drain associated with their therapeutic stimulation.

In addition, potential contraindications to surgery should be explored. Patients with poorly controlled hypertension, diabetes, coronary artery disease, cardiac pacemakers, liver or kidney failure, seizure disorders, or coagulopathies may be poor candidates, although the risk-benefit ratio of DBS surgery should be assessed for each case.[7] If the patient is a good surgical candidate and agrees to surgery, a tentative date for surgery is scheduled and the remainder of the preoperative evaluation is completed. If there is disagreement about the best surgical target or treatment modality, the patient's case should be reviewed at a multidisciplinary conference to arrive at a consensus.

Neurocognitive and Psychiatric Evaluation

A neuropsychologist and a psychiatrist are essential members of a good DBS program because proper cognitive assessment and psychiatric screening are fundamental steps in patient selection, in particular for subthalamic nucleus (STN)–DBS for PD.[8] Although fewer data are available on patients with premorbid psychiatric conditions undergoing DBS of the globus pallidus (pars) interna (GPi) or ventral intermediate (VIM) nucleus of the thalamus, the available evidence suggests that behavioral and cognitive side effects may occur, warranting preoperative neuropsychological testing for all patients considering DBS.[9-11]

The prevalence of dementia is high in patients with PD,[12] and even early preoperative dementia is a risk factor for permanent

BOX 85-1 Movement Disorders for Which Deep Brain Stimulation (DBS) Is Currently Indicated

U.S. FOOD AND DRUG ADMINISTRATION–APPROVED INDICATION FOR DBS

Idiopathic Parkinson's disease
Essential tremor
Primary dystonia
  Generalized
  Segmental
  Hemidystonia
  Cervical

OTHER MOVEMENT DISORDERS POSSIBLY RESPONSIVE TO DBS

Tardive dystonia
Myoclonic dystonia
Pantothenate kinase–associated neurodegeneration
Huntington's chorea
Chorea acanthocytosis
Tics
Cerebellar tremor (multiple sclerosis)
Midbrain tremor
Orthostatic tremor
Lesch-Nyhan syndrome

MOVEMENT DISORDERS POORLY RESPONSIVE TO DBS

Multiple system atrophy
Progressive supranuclear palsy
Corticobasal degeneration
Vascular parkinsonism
Secondary dystonias

cognitive decline after DBS.[13,14] Because no one neuropsychological assessment tool has proven to be predictive of postoperative cognitive decline,[8] several test batteries may be used to screen surgical candidates, with the goal of excluding those with dementia or significant deficits in executive function.[15] No consensus guidelines or "gold standards" are available, and detailed comparative data have not been published. In designing a neuropsychological battery for DBS candidates, it is important to cover the major neurocognitive domains for both patient selection and follow-up (Table 85-1); at the same time, the battery should not be exhaustive because patients with PD fatigue easily, leading to inaccurate results. Moreover, many PD patients with severe medication-related "on-off" fluctuations can sometimes experience significant cognitive disturbance during their "off" period yet perform relatively normally during their "on" period.[8,16,17] Unfortunately, neuropsychological testing is not universally performed before DBS, potentially leading to negative postsurgical outcomes.[1]

A full psychiatric evaluation is essential for patients who pass cognitive screening but have signs of untreated depression or psychosis, including dopaminergic dysregulation syndrome, medication-induced hypomania/mania, and suicide risk.[8]

The need for systematic neuropsychological and neuropsychiatric evaluation is less established for other DBS indications, including ET and dystonia. These conditions are not usually characterized by progressive neurodegeneration and dementia. In addition, patients with dystonia who are DBS candidates are normally young and less prone to suffer cognitive abnormalities after surgery.[18]

Neuroimaging

Potential surgical candidates should undergo preoperative imaging, preferably magnetic resonance imaging (MRI), in order to rule out structural lesions or anatomic distortions that either may interfere with proper targeting (e.g., areas of encephalomalacia) or represent an increased risk for hemorrhage (e.g., abnormally enlarged lateral ventricles, severe brain atrophy).[8,19] In addition, when the diagnosis of idiopathic PD is questioned, MRI can show abnormalities typical of multiple system atrophy (MSA) or progressive supranuclear palsy (PSP),[20] parkinsonian syndromes that are not currently considered appropriate indications for DBS surgery (see Box 85-1).

Nuclear imaging studies (single-photon emission computed tomography, positron emission tomography) can occasionally be helpful in differentiating atypical parkinsonism from idiopathic PD.[21] Although performed in the past to predict pallidotomy outcomes,[22] the use of metabolic imaging modalities for screening patients undergoing DBS therapy is currently not part of routine DBS screening.

TABLE 85-1 Neuropsychological Evaluation of Patients with Parkinson's Disease for Deep Brain Stimulation Surgery

Criteria Evaluated	Evaluation Tool
General	Mini-Mental State Examination Mattis Dementia Rating Scale
Attention and concentration	Digit span Visual span Paced Auditory Serial Addition Test (2 trials) Logical Memory and Faces subtests from the Wechsler Memory Scale-III (WMS-III)
Executive function and psychomotor speed	Stroop Color and Word Test Trail Making Test (parts A and B) Frontal Assessment Battery Wisconsin Card Sorting Test Raven's Progressive Matrices Tower of London test Graphic series Motor series
Language function	Rey Auditory Verbal Learning Test Hopkins Verbal Learning Test Boston Naming Test Controlled Oral Word Association (COWA) Test Category Fluency Test
Visuospatial ability	Rey-Osterrieth Complex Figure Test Benton Judgment of Line Orientation Test Benton Facial Recognition Test

Medical Clearance

Medical clearance is the last screening step that is recommended before DBS surgery and normally includes standard preoperative blood tests and electrocardiography when indicated. DBS candidates should also be instructed to discontinue vitamin E, aspirin, and other medications that interfere with normal coagulation at least 2 weeks before surgery to reduce the risk for hemorrhage. In patients with mechanical heart valves, the surgeon may employ lovenox during this 2-week period and then discontinue these injections the night before surgery, thereby minimizing the risk of thrombotic events during the 2-week washout period.

SPECIFIC INDICATIONS FOR DEEP BRAIN STIMULATION

Parkinson's Disease

Selection Criteria

Among the many elements involved in successful DBS surgery for PD, patient selection has proved to be the most significant factor in determining postoperative benefit. Several good outcome predictors have been established, including a diagnosis

TABLE 85-2 Specific Deep Brain Stimulation Selection Criteria for Parkinson's Disease

Selection Criteria	Comments
Diagnosis	A diagnosis of idiopathic PD should be carefully established according to available criteria because atypical parkinsonism (e.g., MSA, PSP, CBD) is generally poorly responsive to DBS.
Disease severity	The most important factors leading to performance of DBS are marked motor fluctuations in the response to dopaminergic therapy, including levodopa-induced dyskinesia and frequent and sudden wearing off with a prominent freezing responsive to levodopa. UPDRS-III scores of 30 or higher are generally consistent with severe disease and may prompt consideration of DBS. Disabling tremor unresponsive to levodopa may warrant DBS therapy even in the absence of severe motor fluctuations.
Disease duration	Disease duration of 5 yr or longer should be documented to avoid misdiagnosis of atypical PD. Atypical parkinsonism may initially be manifested as PD and may not show atypical features within 3-5 yr after onset.
Age at surgery	Older age is not a specific exclusion criterion. Age at surgery has been reported to correlate negatively with DBS outcome.[23] Cognitive and general health status should be carefully evaluated in patients older than 70 yr.
Response to medications	A good response to levodopa is positively correlated with DBS outcome and should be assessed either historically or with a levodopa challenge test (30% improvement or better).
Cognitive status	Worsening of cognitive status has been reported after DBS in patients with preexisting dementia.
Absence of active psychiatric disease	Untreated psychiatric disease should be carefully addressed before considering DBS. Properly treated depression is not a contraindication but warrants careful postsurgical monitoring.
Realistic expectations	DBS does not cure PD. Patient education is essential to ensure adequate expectations.
Adequate social support	Patients with strong family or social support are better able to follow presurgical/surgical/postsurgical demands and have overall better outcomes.

CBD, corticobasal degeneration; DBS, deep brain stimulation; MSA, multiple system atrophy; PD, Parkinson's disease; PSP, progressive supranuclear palsy; UPDRS, Unified Parkinson's Disease Rating Scale.

of moderate to advanced idiopathic PD, a positive response to levodopa, and an absence of cognitive deterioration.[8] The role of other variables, such as age and concurrent non–motor-associated symptoms, is less well defined (Table 85-2).

Diagnosis. DBS therapy should be considered only for patients with a confirmed diagnosis of idiopathic PD. Although idiopathic PD has been defined by the presence of bradykinesia associated with at least one of three conditions—rigidity, resting tremor, and postural instability—the presence of postural instability may be a relative contraindication of DBS.[24,25] Furthermore, the presence of postural instability early in the disease raises concerns for atypical parkinsonism.[26] The most frequent atypical parkinsonian syndromes that can be misdiagnosed as idiopathic PD are PSP, MSA, Lewy body dementia, and corticobasal ganglionic degeneration.[24] It is important to differentiate idiopathic PD from the atypical parkinsonian disorders because they tend not to respond favorably to stimulation. These disorders generally have an earlier age at onset than PD, and progress more rapidly, including early dysautonomia, bulbar dysfunction, respiratory compromise, spasticity, ataxia, and apraxia.[26]

Patients with atypical parkinsonian syndromes should not be selected for DBS therapy. Several case reports have demonstrated the ineffectiveness of DBS for MSA using either STN[27-30] or GPi targets,[31] even when the patient is responsive to levodopa. Although patients with levodopa-responsive bradykinesia, rigidity, or dystonia may show transient improvement,[28] speech, swallowing, and gait usually deteriorate, motor fluctuations do not improve, and the levodopa dose remains unchanged.[27,29] Clinical experience with DBS for other types of atypical parkinsonism, including corticobasal ganglionic degeneration and PSP, is extremely limited.[32]

Disease Severity and Duration. Although it is not considered a predictor of DBS outcome, the duration of PD should be taken into consideration when ruling out atypical parkinsonism.[8,33] Typically, PD motor disability progresses slowly, so patients with advanced symptoms less than 5 years after onset should be evaluated further for atypical parkinsonism before being considered for DBS. At the same time, DBS should not be offered too late in the disease course, when severe motor complications have resulted in marked loss of quality of life. Currently, DBS is performed after an average PD duration of 11 to 14 years; however, investigational studies offering DBS therapy at an earlier stage of the disease (7 years after initial motor symptoms) have yielded positive results, suggesting that DBS should be considered as a therapeutic option earlier in the course of PD, when quality of life is still high.[34] Indeed, there is little consensus on what defines advanced, medication-refractory PD and therefore candidacy for DBS. Severe PD disability generally coincides with Unified Parkinson's Disease Rating Scale (UPDRS) motor scores of approximately 30 (out of a maximum of 108) or a Movement Disorder Society–sponsored Unified Parkinson's Disease Rating Scale (MDS-UPDRS) score in the 50s (out of a maximum of 132), and so these would seem to be reasonable severity thresholds to prompt a consideration of DBS therapy.[7,35,36] Available experience with STN-DBS or GPi-DBS has mostly been with levodopa-responsive patients having "off"-period UPDRS motor scores higher than 40 or 50.[8] An ideal PD surgical candidate should be severely disabled when off levodopa, but doing well, despite associated dyskinesias, on medications.

Response to Levodopa. A sustained preoperative response to levodopa not only provides support for the diagnosis of idiopathic PD but is also considered the best predictor of outcome after DBS.[8,33] Levodopa responsiveness should be assessed in each patient being considered for DBS,[8] with a dose sufficient to reproduce the patient's best "on" response after a medication-free interval of 12 hours (usually overnight). It is reasonable to discontinue extended-release agonists or rotigotine patches a few days before the "off"-state examination if the patient can tolerate the decrease in dopaminergic stimulation. The lost dopaminergic stimulation can be replaced with carbidopa/levodopa until 12 hours before the examination. It is especially important to assess whether gait difficulties (in particular, freezing and imbalance) are sensitive to levodopa before offering the patient DBS.

Levodopa response is normally defined as a 30% improvement in UPDRS motor scores (part III) over the "off" state,[8,33,37] although there is no consensus on what constitutes an appropriate challenge dose of levodopa. A suprathreshold dose has been defined variably: use of the normal first dose of the day,[38] a fixed 200-mg test dose,[39] or even apomorphine[40] has been proposed. Although a positive levodopa challenge is an excellent prognostic indicator for DBS, it is the experience of our group and of others that patients with well-defined idiopathic PD can benefit from DBS even when their motor response is indeterminate because of intolerance to levodopa[41] or when the most disabling symptom is a dopa-refractory tremor.[2]

Age. The role of age as an outcome predictor for DBS is somewhat controversial.[32,42] Some authors consider advanced age (in particular, age greater than 70 years) a poor outcome predictor if not a contraindication to DBS surgery[23,33] because it has been correlated with negative outcomes such as cognitive decline[14] and gait instability.[42] Nonetheless, given that the average age at the onset of PD is 60 years and that the mean duration of illness is 10 to 15 years at the time of surgery, a large proportion of potential DBS candidates are 70 years or older. Also, the EARLYSTIM trial demonstrated that DBS in earlier stages of the disease had a significant benefit on quality of life.[34] In reality, no specific age cutoff has been defined for DBS candidates with advanced PD.[8] Decisions for or against DBS in the elderly population should be individualized by taking into account the level of disability, surgical risk factors, general life expectancy, and the patient's motivation. Unilateral procedures could be an option in some patients who are not candidates for a bilateral procedure. Alternative targets, such as the thalamus and globus pallidus, may be considered in older PD candidates when deteriorating cognition is a concern.[43,44]

Cognitive Status. The patient's cognitive status should be assessed with an appropriate battery of neuropsychological tests.[15] Preoperative dementia is considered a risk factor for permanent cognitive decline after DBS, independent of the target, though the risk for cognitive decline after GPi-DBS may be less than after STN-DBS.[43,45] Older age and severe preoperative cognitive impairment may be associated with poorer neurobehavioral outcomes.[37,46-50]

Cognitive decline in PD is characterized by impaired executive function, visuospatial abnormalities, impaired memory, and language deficits.[51] An appropriate scale that reliably incorporates executive function (e.g., Frontal Assessment Battery and other practical tests of executive function) should be included in screening tests for PD dementia. However, in PD patients it may be difficult to assess impairment in domains other than memory.[8] No studies have yet revealed a specific test with sufficient sensitivity or specificity to predict clinically meaningful cognitive decline in PD patients who undergo DBS surgery.

Psychiatric Comorbid Conditions. In select patients, a psychiatric evaluation may be performed to assess the presence of untreated depression, anxiety, apathy, dopaminergic dysregulation syndrome, medication-induced hypomania/mania, psychotic symptoms, and suicide risk, all of which have been observed following STN-DBS surgery.[8] Postoperative depression has been reported in 1% to 25% of patients,[43,47,48,52-54] but a preoperative assessment for depression is not always documented. Two studies that examined whether preoperative depression was a risk factor for postoperative depression reported conflicting results.[48,53] In particular, neither study differentiated between postoperative depression and dopaminergic withdrawal symptoms.

The relationships among pre- and postoperative depression, site-specific stimulation, medication changes, the underlying disease, and psychosocial factors have not been completely elucidated. The tools that are routinely used to assess pre- and postoperative depression include the Beck Depression Inventory,[55] Hamilton Depression Rating Scale,[56] and Montgomery-Åsberg Depression Rating Scale.[57] Other scales, such as the Geriatric Depression Scale[58] and Zung Self-Rating Depression Scale,[59] have not been formally validated in patients with PD. Further research is required to determine the best (i.e., sensitive, specific, but also practical for clinicians to administer rapidly) depression screening tool for PD patients.

In a study focusing on behavioral symptoms, postoperative hypomania developed in one of two patients with preoperative hypomania.[48] No associations between pre- and postoperative mania have otherwise been reported; however, the adequacy of the preoperative assessment for behavioral disorders is not always known.

Psychosis in PD patients is characterized by visual hallucinations and delusions (often paranoid),[60] so screening tools for this population should be sensitive to hallucinations, as well as other psychotic features (e.g., delusions). Only one study evaluated the Parkinson Psychosis Rating Scale, which may be appropriate in this population.[61] However, in order to determine its specificity, the Parkinson Psychosis Rating Scale needs to be evaluated in both nonpsychotic and psychotic PD patients. Criteria for psychosis from the fourth edition of the *Diagnostic and Statistical Manual of Mental Disorders* (DSM-IV) have not been validated in PD. Likewise, there are insufficient data to draw conclusions about whether a preoperative history of medication-induced psychiatric symptoms or features of dopamine dysregulation syndrome worsen after surgery.

In uncontrolled series, suicide attempts and suicides have been documented in 0.5% to 2.9% of PD patients following DBS surgery.[48,62-64] A multicenter study of 450 STN-DBS patients reported a postoperative suicide rate of 0.5%.[63] In contrast, a study of 120 patients who underwent DBS (including patients with PD, dystonia, and ET) documented a postoperative suicide rate of 2.9% in PD patients who had undergone STN-DBS.[64] The authors suggested that young male patients with a history of multiple surgeries may be at greater risk for such outcomes. However, given that this was a small, uncontrolled, retrospective cohort study from a single center, conclusions should be made with great caution.

Target Selection

Ventral Intermediate Thalamus. The initial reports of DBS for the treatment of PD focused on thalamic stimulation, specifically the VIM nucleus. In a series of 80 PD patients treated by either unilateral or bilateral VIM-DBS, 88% achieved complete or near-complete tremor relief as measured with the Fahn-Tolosa-Marín Tremor Rating Scale from 6 months to 8 years postoperatively.[67] The effects of VIM-DBS on other symptoms of PD, however, such as rigidity, bradykinesia, or drug-induced dyskinesias, were either short lived or nonexistent. Currently, the role of VIM-DBS for PD is limited to patients with tremor-predominant symptoms.

Globus Pallidus Interna. A number of studies have shown that bilateral GPi stimulation is safe and effective for the management of PD symptoms.[66-71] Based on previous experience with pallidotomy,[72] the preferred target for DBS is thought to be the most ventral, posterior and lateral area of the internal pallidum. In PD patients, GPi-DBS improves tremor, rigidity, and bradykinesia in the "off"-medication state, as well as drug-induced dyskinesia, and results in overall improvement in UPDRS motor scores.[73-75] The most pronounced and long-lasting effect is a reduction in "on"-medication dyskinesias,[76] and in PD patients suffering mainly from dyskinesias, GPi may be the preferred target. In contrast to STN-DBS, however, GPi-DBS does not lead to significant reductions in levodopa requirements.[70,77,78]

Subthalamic Nucleus. The clinical efficacy of STN-DBS in reducing PD symptoms has been reported by numerous investigators and validated in prospective, randomized trials.[69,71,78-81] Studies with long-term follow-up show sustained improvement in tremor, rigidity, and akinesia in the "off"-medication state and a reduction in dopaminergic medication requirements 5 years after implantation.[62,82-87] A reduction in levodopa dosage is usually achieved and leads indirectly to improvement in levodopa-induced dyskinesias.[88,89] Initial improvements in gait, however, are not always sustained in the long term.[62,79,90]

Caudal Zona Incerta. In recent years, there has been growing interest in the caudal zona incerta (cZI) as a target for treating PD. This interest derives from observations that the most effective stimulation contacts were often not within the STN proper, but in the area of the cZI just dorsal to the nucleus. Prospective studies suggest that DBS at the cZI is comparable if not superior in effect to STN-DBS. More recent studies report adverse speech effects, worse than are observed with STN-DBS. Moreover, the most consistent result is the effect on parkinsonian tremor and so, like VIM, this target may be preferable in patients with tremor-predominant PD.

Pedunculopontine Nucleus. Thus far the literature on the efficacy of pedunculopontine nucleus stimulation in PD is mixed, and our practice does not support the routine use of this intervention.

Dystonia

Classification

Dystonia is a movement disorder characterized by sustained, involuntary muscle contractions generating twisting and repetitive movements or abnormal postures.[91] Different muscle groups can be involved to a variable extent, and severity can range from intermittent contractions limited to a single body region (focal dystonia) to generalized dystonia involving the axial and limb muscles. The classification of dystonic syndromes by clinical features or etiology can help determine a patient's candidacy for DBS.[92] Traditionally, this classification included two broad categories: primary or idiopathic, and secondary or symptomatic dystonia.[91] Dystonia-plus syndromes were considered secondary dystonias. This system often led to confusion so that a consensus update of the phenomenology and classification of this complex disorder was established in 2013 by Albanese and associates[93] with a goal to better organize our increased understanding of the biologic mechanisms and the clinical features of the dystonias.

Clinically, the dystonic syndromes are classified by age at onset, anatomic distribution (focal, segmental, multifocal, hemidystonia, and generalized), temporal pattern (persistent, action-specific, diurnal, and paroxysmal), and associated features (isolated dystonia with or without tremor, combined dystonia, or complex dystonia).[93,94] "Primary" dystonias are now categorized as isolated dystonia with or without tremor. "Dystonic-plus" syndromes are now categorized as combined dystonia, in which dystonia is present with another movement disorder and may not be the predominant feature. "Secondary" dystonias are now categorized as complex dystonia, in which the dystonia results from a separate neurologic or systemic cause and may not be the predominant feature.

Etiologically, dystonic syndromes are classified by their neuropathology and whether the dystonia is inherited, acquired, or idiopathic. Neuropathologic and neuroimaging studies can help determine if the syndrome is due to a neurodegenerative process, a structural lesion, or neither. Inherited dystonias are further subdivided by mode of inheritance or by specific genetic mutations. Acquired dystonias are specified by the causative process, including psychogenic. Idiopathic dystonias are subdivided into sporadic or familial variants.

The isolated dystonias have thus far responded best to DBS, and isolated dystonia caused by the *DYT1* mutation is particularly responsive. Dystonia-1 (DYT-1) is the most common of the monogenetic isolated dystonias. There is a bimodal distribution in the age at onset, with modes at 9 years (early onset) and 45 years (late onset).[95] The majority of early-onset cases begin with leg or arm dystonia that progresses to involve more than one limb. Approximately 50% of these patients develop generalized symptoms. Late-onset primary dystonia commonly affects the neck or cranial muscles and tends to remain localized as focal or segmental dystonia. The dystonia-6 (DYT-6) phenotype differs from DYT-1 in the age at onset (mean: 16 years) and the presence of more severe cranial and cervical involvement with milder limb dystonia.[96] Combined and complex dystonias can result from an assortment of lesions, many involving the basal ganglia or dopamine synthesis, that are either inherited (e.g., dopamine-responsive dystonia [DRD], Wilson's disease, gangliosidoses) or due to exogenous factors (e.g., perinatal injury, infections, neuroleptic medications). Clinical abnormalities other than dystonia (e.g., parkinsonism, dementia, ataxia, optic atrophy) are frequently present, and imaging studies often reveal changes involving the basal ganglia. Other laboratory findings usually help in the diagnosis.

Treatment

When the underlying cause of a dystonia can be treated (e.g., DRD or Wilson's disease), it is; however, for the great majority of patients, the underlying disorder cannot be treated and so treatment is aimed at controlling symptoms. Symptomatic treatment can be further divided into focal therapies such as intramuscular injections of botulinum toxin and systemic pharmacotherapies that affect the central nervous system. Many medications have been reported to be of some benefit to some dystonia patients (including anticholinergic, dopaminergic, and GABAergic agents), but no single therapy has been found to be consistently efficacious. Botulinum toxin is considered the treatment of choice for many focal dystonias.[97]

With the notable exception of levodopa for the treatment of DRD, pharmacologic treatment of primary generalized dystonia is mostly unsatisfactory. As a consequence, surgical interventions have become progressively more relevant for these patients. Chronic electrical stimulation of the GPi is currently considered a safe and effective treatment of advanced, disabling isolated dystonia that is refractory to medical therapy.[98,99] Selecting appropriate patients for intervention is a key first step for achieving excellent results with DBS (Table 85-3). In determining an individual patient's risk-benefit ratio, several variables need to be taken into consideration, including the patient's motor, cognitive, medical, and psychological status.[100] The best candidates are patients with primary generalized, segmental, or cervical dystonia who have not responded to medications or botulinum toxin injections and have progressed to profound disability as a result of motor impairment or pain.[100]

A trial of levodopa should always be performed to rule out patients with DRD. It is important to determine whether the target symptom or symptoms for surgery are the primary source of disability and to assess the likelihood that that the symptom or symptoms will improve with DBS. Other sources of disability must be identified, and the patient's individual risk of encountering complications should be considered. Ideally, surgery should be performed before secondary orthopedic complications (i.e., contractures or bony spinal deformities) compromise the overall functional recovery.[100]

In general, patients with isolated dystonia and some of the combined dystonias (e.g., myoclonus dystonia, X-linked dystonia-parkinsonism)[101,102] are better candidates for DBS than

TABLE 85-3 Specific Deep Brain Stimulation (DBS) Selection Criteria for Dystonia

Selection Criteria	Comment
Diagnosis	Patients with primary generalized dystonia (with or without a positive *DYT1* mutation) are the best candidates. Some forms of secondary dystonia (e.g., tardive) may also respond well to DBS.
Disease severity	Dystonic symptoms should be either generalized or disabling (e.g., severe cervical dystonia).
Disease duration	There is a negative correlation between disease duration and clinical outcome after DBS. Patients with dystonia for less than 15 yr may improve the most. It is helpful to perform DBS surgery before abnormal joint postures become fixed or contracted.
Age at surgery	Younger patients with primary dystonia appear to improve better and faster, but adult or older age is not a contraindication.
Response to medications	DBS is indicated for medication-refractory cases. Response to particular medications is not considered a predictor of outcome.
Cognitive status	Patients with generalized dystonia are usually young and test normally on neuropsychological tests. Whether the neuropsychological profile of dystonia patients might affect surgical outcome is unknown.
Absence of active psychiatric disease	Psychiatric comorbid conditions should be addressed carefully and eventually treated.
Realistic expectations	Although great improvements can be expected in some cases, results vary and may take months to be achieved.
Adequate social support	Social and psychological support is fundamental for both patients, often young children, and caregivers or parents to achieve the best outcomes.

those with complex dystonia.[92,103] Short disease duration appears to be a positive outcome predictor.[104] *DYT1*-positive patients seem to respond better than others in some but not all series, and their advantage may be attributable to their young age at onset and relatively quick progression, warranting DBS surgery after a short disease duration.[98,104,105] In *DYT6*-positive patients, the cranial features may be less responsive to DBS, but experience is limited, and further studies are needed.[106-108] The results with DBS in patients with secondary dystonia have generally been disappointing,[103,109-111] with some notable exceptions, including those with tardive dystonia[112,113] and pantothenate kinase–associated neurodegeneration.[114-116]

Target Selection

Although thalamic and subthalamic targets have been used as DBS targets, particularly for secondary dystonias, the vast majority of procedures for dystonia target the GPi. DBS of the GPi has proven to be a safe and effective treatment for advanced, disabling primary[98,99] and some types of secondary dystonia.[112,113,117,118]

Thalamic DBS may be an option for some patients with secondary dystonia, including posttraumatic hemidystonia, postanoxic dystonia and bilateral basal ganglia necrosis, myoclonic dystonia, and dystonic paroxysmal nonkinesigenic dyskinesia.[103] The thalamic structures targeted in these cases are the VIM nucleus,[119-121] the ventro-oralis anterior (VOA) nucleus,[122,123] and the ventroposterolateral nucleus.[124] Combined implants to thalamic and pallidal targets in the same patients have also been successful in individual cases.[123,125]

The fact that STN-DBS effectively treats both "off"-state and "on"-state dystonia in patients with PD has prompted speculation on the potential of this target for the treatment of idiopathic torsion dystonia. Potential advantages of targeting the STN include a more rapid response to stimulation and the ability to achieve identical or enhanced clinical effects with less energy, thereby prolonging battery life. These ideas are supported by encouraging preliminary results,[126-128] but further study is needed.

Essential Tremor

Selection Criteria

ET is a progressive neurological disease characterized by a postural or kinetic tremor affecting mainly the arms, but also the head, jaw, and voice, as well as other body regions.[129] Tremor usually begins in the arms and then spreads to other regions in some patients. Essential head tremor is more likely to develop in women than in men.[130] Other types of tremor may also occur, including occasionally rest tremor in the arms.[131] In some patients, gait and balance difficulties, anxiety and depressive symptoms, and cognitive difficulty may also develop.[132,133]

ET is a common neurological disease, with a prevalence of approximately 4% in persons 40 years and older and considerably higher in the elderly population.[131] ET is often mild and is occasionally defined as "benign essential tremor" or "familial tremor" because approximately half the cases are inherited in a pattern most consistent with autosomal dominant transmission. However, no causative gene(s) have as yet been identified.

Patients with severe tremor may have difficulty performing routine activities of daily living and will therefore require pharmacologic or surgical therapy.[131,134] Before considering surgery, patients should undergo an adequate trial of first-line medications alone and in combination. These include propranolol (60 to 320 mg/day) and primidone (300 to 750 mg/day). If patients fail first-line therapy, trials of second-line (clonazepam, alprazolam, and topiramate) and third-line (clonidine, acetazolamide, flunarizine, and theophylline) drugs may be considered; however, these medications rarely result in marked improvement, and surgery should not be delayed unnecessarily.[131] In general, oral medications tend to be more helpful for limb tremor than for head or voice tremor, which may benefit from botulinum toxin injections.

Both DBS and thalamotomy are indicated for ET patients whose tremor causes unacceptable impairment of activities of daily living and is refractory to medical therapy.[65,135-146] Table 85-4 summarizes current DBS selection criteria for ET. The most widely accepted tool for evaluating the severity of ET is the Fahn-Tolosa-Marín Tremor Rating Scale.[147]

Few reports have focused on cognitive function in patients with ET,[148-153] and no standardized cognitive screening tools have been consistently advocated to test ET patients before DBS implants as they have in PD. Quality of life can be investigated with the Quality of Life in Essential Tremor Questionnaire (QUEST), which although still partially validated, is the only scale available to assess impairment in activities of daily living in patients with ET.[154]

Target Selection

At present, the VIM nucleus of the thalamus is the most commonly targeted site for DBS in patients with ET.[137,155-158] Unilateral VIM stimulation results in marked short- and long-term improvement in contralateral action and postural tremor, and in

TABLE 85-4 Specific Deep Brain Stimulation Selection Criteria for Essential Tremor

Selection Criteria	Comment
Diagnosis	The symptom *tremor* is generally well responsive to thalamic DBS.
Disease severity	Tremor must significantly interfere with the patient's quality of life.
Disease duration	There is no limitation.
Age at surgery	Older age is not a specific exclusion criterion if the patient is cognitively intact and in good general health.
Response to medications	Patients with ET must have medication-refractory symptoms, defined as having failed maximal titrations and preferably combinations of a beta blocker, primidone, and possibly a benzodiazepine.
Cognitive status	Cognitive impairment should be systematically investigated because mild executive difficulties appear to exist in patients with ET. No clear data document deterioration in cognitive status after VIM-DBS in ET patients.
Absence of active psychiatric disease	Untreated psychiatric comorbid conditions should be ruled out carefully and patients with them should not undergo implantation.
Realistic expectations	Although tremor is among the symptoms most responsive to DBS, patients should be aware of the worst scenarios and maintain realistic expectations.
Adequate social support	Strong family or social support is fundamental, but relief of symptoms, great improvement in quality of life, and less dependence on caregivers should be expected.

DBS, deep brain stimulation; ET, essential tremor; VIM, ventral intermediate nucleus of the thalamus.

some cases may have a mild ipsilateral effect.[139,158,159] There is, however, a decreasing effect over time, most noticeable with action tremor.[160] The cZI and STN[161] have been investigated as potential targets for ET in hopes of generating a more durable benefit.[162,163] Promising results have been demonstrated by targeting the cZI, with long-term control of tremor up to 5 years postoperatively.[164]

Because voice tremor is not reliably improved by unilateral VIM stimulation,[142,165,166] it should not be a primary indication for DBS. Head tremor has also shown inconsistent or unpredictable improvement with unilateral and bilateral VIM stimulation.[3,139,142,156,167] There have been mixed results in a small number of patients with voice tremor by targeting the cZI.[168]

Complex Tremor Syndromes

The efficacy of thalamic DBS as a therapy for medically intractable ET and PD tremor has spurred much interest in its application to other types of less common and more complex tremor syndromes, such as cerebellar tremor in multiple sclerosis (MS), Holmes' tremor (HT), thalamic tremor (TT), and orthostatic tremor (OT).

Selection Criteria

Tremor severity, consequent disability, and lack of response to common antitremor medications are the criteria generally used to select patients with atypical tremor syndromes for DBS surgery. No specific neuropsychological selection criteria have been described in the literature, but it is probably good practice to test any DBS candidate older than 50 years for evidence of baseline cognitive decline. Physiologic assessment of patients with complex tremor and ataxia may help predict those who will most likely benefit from surgery. Thalamotomy has resulted in complete resolution of upper extremity postural tremor with frequencies greater than 3 Hz as assessed by an accelerometer, whereas tremor of less than 3 Hz did not improve postoperatively.[170] Furthermore, frequency analysis during a wrist-tracking task may also be predictive of the response of action tremor to thalamotomy, with an 80% reduction in tremor in patients with just one frequency peak in their spectra and only a 30% reduction in those with multiple frequency peaks.[182]

Cerebellar Tremor. Cerebellar tremor is characterized by a coarse action tremor, generally less than 5 Hz, and is occasionally associated with postural tremor. Typically, cerebellar tremor affects the upper extremities unilaterally or bilaterally, although head and trunk titubation is also common and may be the most disabling feature. A simple observation of the frequency and regularity of movements when performing typical activities (e.g., drinking from a cup) may give clues to the diagnosis.[169] Cerebellar tremor is most commonly problematic in patients with MS, traumatic brain injury, or brainstem cerebrovascular events, and occasionally in those with spinocerebellar ataxia or the cerebellar subtype of MSA.

Disabling tremor that impairs a patient's quality of life is seen in approximately 10% to 15% of MS clinic patients.[170] Drug therapy with agents such as carbamazepine, clonazepam, L-5-hydroxytryptophan, and buspirone is rarely successful; occasional patients may have mild improvement with high-dose propranolol.[170] Appropriate patients for stereotactic surgery should have tremor that significantly interferes with activities of daily living. Only two disease severity scales have been proposed, and both take into account tremor severity and distribution for evaluation of MS tremor.[171,172] No validation studies are available.

MS patients have multiple other nervous system lesions and neurological deficits, so it is important to distinguish between tremor-related disability and disability caused by other deficits when assessing the potential benefits of DBS in this cohort. In fact, studies of the effects of DBS on MS tremor consistently show some tremor improvement in the majority of patients, but the improvement is often overshadowed by progression of the other symptoms.[158] Patients with marked sensory impairment in the target limb, excessive arm weakness, or marked truncal weakness resulting in a bedridden state should not be offered surgery because meaningful functional improvement is unlikely to be achieved even if the tremor is eliminated.[170]

MS patients who are being considered for DBS surgery to control intention tremor should undergo brain MRI within 3 months of surgery because their disease can progress without obvious clinical sequelae. We were surprised in one instance when the targeting MRI of an MS patient revealed a new plaque in the internal capsule that extended into the ventrolateral thalamus, the preferred target for tremor control. Stimulation within the ventrolateral thalamus in this patient yielded unwanted side effects at very low currents, most probably caused by aberrant conduction through this new plaque. Consequently, a DBS lead could not be implanted.[19]

Holmes' Tremor. Also known as "rubral tremor" or midbrain tremor, HT is an irregular, low-frequency rest and intention tremor that is enhanced by posture in most cases. The Movement Disorder Society has established three criteria for the diagnosis of HT: (1) the presence of both resting and intention tremor; (2) a slow frequency, usually less than 4.5 Hz; and (3) a variable delay (usually months) after occurrence of the lesion.[173] HT has been reported in association with trauma, cerebrovascular events, neuroleptic agents, infections, MS, neoplasm, Wilson's disease, cavernoma, and radiation toxicity.[174] The pathogenesis of HT has been attributed to combined destruction of the pallidothalamic and cerebellothalamic pathways, with involvement of the rubro-olivo-cerebello-rubral loop and possibly the nigrostriatal system.[175]

Thalamic Tremor. TT is characterized by variable degrees of dystonia, athetosis, chorea, and action tremor and is occasionally associated with myoclonus after lateral posterior thalamic strokes, most frequently hemorrhagic strokes.[176,177] Dystonia, athetosis, and chorea are usually associated with position sensory loss after thalamic lesions, whereas tremor and myoclonic movements are most frequently related to cerebellar ataxia.[176] The pathogenesis of TT is unclear, but it has been related to defective motor-sensory integrative processes because of persistent failure of proprioceptive sensory and cerebellar input after recovery of motor dysfunction, with severe lateral-posterior thalamic strokes simultaneously damaging the lemniscal sensory pathway, the cerebellorubrothalamic tract, and, less severely, the pyramidal tract.[176] TT generally starts gradually and progressively worsens for weeks or months before stabilizing. Involuntary movements usually remain persistent and only rarely show spontaneous improvement.[176]

Orthostatic Tremor. Described as a quivering tremor of the legs and trunk during standing accompanied by a sensation of unsteadiness, OT is usually relieved by walking or leaning against objects.[178] It is characterized by distinctive 14- to 16-Hz lower extremity electromyographic activity that is evoked on standing but not while walking or supine. OT is believed to be a variant of ET despite a lack of response to alcohol, beta blockers, and primidone, and the typical absence of a family history.[179,180] OT usually responds to clonazepam but shows a progressive reduction in the latency between standing and the onset of unsteadiness, with an increase in tremor severity that may result in an inability to stand still without support. Although patients may not fall, the sensation of unsteadiness can markedly interfere with their quality of life.[181]

Target Selection

DBS has been shown to be beneficial for several atypical tremor syndromes, although fewer cases have been reported and the benefit is less remarkable and consistent than that reported for ET.[158] Most studies of DBS for MS tremor targeted the VIM thalamus.[183,184] Other successful targets include the ventro-oralis posterior (VOP) nucleus of the thalamus and the cZI. Stimulation of these alternative targets produced a 64% improvement in postural tremor and a 36% improvement in intention tremor.[185] Dual-electrode stimulation to target both the VIM/VOP border and the VOA/VOP border also provided significant reduction of tremor in one MS patient.[186] Because DBS of the VIM nucleus produces often inconsistent and short-term benefits, further research is necessary to determine the most effective target for MS-associated tremor.

With the exception of one patient treated by GPi-DBS,[187] the VIM nucleus is also the most frequent target for DBS therapy of atypical tremors (mostly TT and HT) resulting from post-traumatic and vascular lesions.[186,188-197] The youngest patient who underwent implantation, a 14-year-old girl, showed remarkable improvement (90%) with VIM-DBS up to 2.5 years.[174] Successful VIM-DBS has also been reported in three patients suffering from OT.[181,198]

The cZI has also been targeted for DBS in atypical tremor, with reported improvement in all components of tremor affecting both the distal and proximal limbs, as well as the axial musculature.[199] Two patients with dystonic tremor and one with neuropathy-related tremor responded well to unilateral stimulation of the posterior subthalamic area.[200] Subthalamic-thalamic stimulation achieved suppression of tremor related to spinocerebellar ataxia type 2.[201]

Multiple targets have also been used to improve HT symptoms. Simultaneous placement of two DBS electrodes at the VIM/VOP border and at the VOA/VOP border resulted in excellent reduction of symptoms in three patients.[186] In one patient, combined STN-VIM stimulation but not stimulation of the STN or VIM nucleus alone produced global relief of tremor without adverse events.[191]

Gilles de la Tourette's Syndrome

Selection Criteria

Gilles de la Tourette's syndrome (TS) is a neuropsychiatric disorder characterized by multiple motor and vocal tics that wax and wane over time, often associated with behavioral disorders.[202] The motor tics are stereotyped repetitive and involuntary movements that generally affect the face, head, and upper part of the body, whereas vocal tics may include shouting, barking, sniffing, or grunting. Comorbid conditions include attention-deficit/hyperactivity disorder, obsessive-compulsive disorder, anxiety, and self-injurious behavior. Symptoms often disappear before or during early adulthood or may be controlled with medication.[202] Some patients, however, may have medically resistant severe and disabling tics that persist or worsen in adulthood.

To be considered a surgical candidate, TS patients need to be refractory to medical treatment and severely disabled by the condition.[203] A multidisciplinary approach that includes neurological and psychiatric evaluation is strongly recommended. The main scale used to evaluate the severity of symptoms is the Yale Global Tic Severity Scale.[204]

The Dutch-Flemish Tourette Surgery Study Group has established guidelines for DBS in patients with TS,[205] and the Movement Disorder Society has published the recommendations of the Tourette Syndrome Association.[203] The proposed selection criteria include the following:

1. Definite TS diagnosis as established by two independent clinicians, preferably a psychiatrist and a neurologist, with the diagnosis being established according to DSM-IV-TR criteria[206] and with the aid of the Diagnostic Confidence Index[207]
2. Severe and incapacitating tics as the primary problem
3. Treatment-refractory disease as evidenced by a poor clinical response to three different medication regimens, with each tried for at least 12 weeks in adequate doses, or medication intolerance resulting from side effects; both classic neuroleptics (haloperidol, pimozide) and newer antipsychotic medications (e.g., risperidone, olanzapine, clozapine, sulpiride, and aripiprazole) should be considered
4. A trial of at least 10 sessions of behavioral therapy for tics, such as habit reversal or exposure in vivo
5. Age older than 25 years

TS patients should be excluded from neurosurgical treatment if they have a tic disorder other than TS, severe psychiatric comorbid conditions (other than associated behavioral disorders), or mental deficiency. Patients with active suicidal ideation are not good candidates for DBS.

Target Selection

The choice of target in TS is still controversial inasmuch as good outcomes have been reported with both thalamic DBS and GPi-DBS. To date, five targets have been used for DBS in patients with TS: (1) the medial thalamus, (2) the GPi, (3) the globus pallidus externa, (4) the anterior limb of the internal capsule/nucleus accumbens, and (5) the STN.[208,209,210] There are two separate targets within the medial portion of the thalamus: the cross point of the centromedian nucleus/substantia periventricularis/VOA nucleus,[211-214] and the medial portion of the thalamus at the centromedian nucleus and parafascicular nucleus.[204] In the GPi, the posteroventrolateral GPi[215] and the anteromedial GPi[204] have been targeted. Studies comparing individual targets are rare and have conflicting results.[210] There is a suggestion that stimulation of the thalamus may have more of an effect on mood as compared to the GPi, but tics are better suppressed with the GPi. The use of combined targets have been reported, again with conflicting results.

Huntington's Chorea and Other Choreas

Selection Criteria

Two types of chorea have been considered for treatment with DBS: Huntington's chorea (HC) and neuroacanthocytosis (NA). HC is a progressive hereditary neurodegenerative disease manifested by chorea and other hyperkinetic (dystonia, myoclonus, tics) and hypokinetic (parkinsonism) movement disorders. In addition, a variety of psychiatric and behavioral symptoms, along with cognitive decline, contribute significantly to the patient's disability. No effective neuroprotective or disease-modifying therapy for HC is available.[216] NA includes combined features of chorea, orofacial tics, dystonia, amyotrophy, and elevated serum creatine kinase levels, with a peculiar finding of spiked red blood cells (acanthocytes) in the blood smear. NA has been described most commonly as an autosomal recessive hereditary genetic defect located on chromosome 9, but it also occurs as an autosomal dominant disorder and as part of an X-linked disorder called McLeod's syndrome.[217] In most cases, the neurological disability caused by chorea is progressive.

Clinical assessment of patients with chorea can be standardized with the Unified Huntington's Disease Rating Scale (UHDRS)[218] or the Abnormal Involuntary Movement Scale.[219] The functional status of HC patients is commonly assessed with the Total Functional Capacity Scale and the Independence Scale, both of which are incorporated into the UHDRS.

Medical therapy for chorea is fairly limited and restricted to symptomatic relief. Numerous medications have been used to improve chorea, including typical and atypical neuroleptics, dopamine depleters, antidepressants, antiglutamatergic drugs, γ-aminobutyric acid agonists, antiepileptic medications, acetylcholinesterase inhibitors, and botulinum toxin.[218]

Target Selection

Thalamic and pallidal targets have been used for DBS therapy in patients with chorea.[102] In a review of DBS in hyperkinetic movement disorder, 21 cases of HC were reported in 12 studies. In almost all of the cases the GPi was the therapeutic target. In one case the globus pallidus externa was targeted but the results were not reported, and in another case both the STN and GPI were targeted. Based on the limited data, the literature supported the efficacy of DBS in HC, especially for chorea; however, parkinsonism and gait may not respond and may worsen with DBS.

A slightly larger experience is available for NA. Bilateral high-frequency stimulation (160 Hz) of the VOP nucleus of the thalamus improved trunk spasms in one patient with NA, with stable clinical benefit for 1 year, although no clear effect on dysarthria was observed.[220] Interestingly, high-frequency stimulation of the GPi failed to improve[221] or even worsened[222] NA-related chorea, whereas the best results were obtained with low-frequency (40 Hz) bilateral pallidal DBS using monopolar stimulation on two adjacent contacts.[222] In a multicenter retrospective study, the results in 15 patients with NA who were treated with GPi-DBS were reviewed. Preoperative motor severity predicted the response to DBS.[223] The overall motor severity as measured by the Unified Huntington's Disease Rating Scale–Motor Score (UHDRS-MS) improved, but this was usually limited to the chorea and dystonia. Dysarthria and swallowing did not consistently respond to DBS, and parkinsonism did not respond. Functional capacity improved with DBS, and the benefit was maintained at least up to 6 months postoperatively.

SUGGESTED READINGS

Charles PD, Van Blercom N, Krack P, et al. Predictors of effective bilateral subthalamic nucleus stimulation for PD. *Neurology*. 2002;59:932-934.

Defer GL, Widner H, Marié RM, et al. Core Assessment Program for Surgical Interventional Therapies in Parkinson's Disease (CAPSIT-PD). *Mov Disord*. 1999;14:572-584.

Deuschl G, Schade-Brittinger C, Krack P, et al. A randomized trial of deep-brain stimulation for Parkinson's disease. *N Engl J Med*. 2006;355:896-908.

Guehl D, Cuny E, Tison F, et al. Deep brain pallidal stimulation for movement disorders in neuroacanthocytosis. *Neurology*. 2007;68:160-161.

Isaias IU, Alterman RL, Tagliati M. Outcome predictors of pallidal stimulation in patients with primary dystonia: the role of disease duration. *Brain*. 2008;131:1895-1902.

Kleiner-Fisman G, Herzog J, Fisman DN, et al. Subthalamic nucleus deep brain stimulation: summary and meta-analysis of outcomes. *Mov Disord*. 2006;21:290-304.

Krack P, Batir A, Van Blercom N, et al. Five-year follow-up of bilateral stimulation of the subthalamic nucleus in advanced Parkinson's disease. *N Engl J Med*. 2003;349:1925-1934.

Kupsch A, Benecke R, Müller J, et al. Pallidal deep-brain stimulation in primary generalized or segmental dystonia. *N Engl J Med*. 2006;355:1978-1990.

Lang AE, Houeto JH, Krack P, et al. Deep brain stimulation: preoperative issues. *Mov Disord*. 2006;21:171-196.

Lyons KE, Pahwa R. Deep brain stimulation and tremor. *Neurother*. 2008;5:331-338.

Malhado-Chang N, Alterman R, Tagliati M. Deep brain stimulation. In: Factor SA, Weiner WJ, eds. *Parkinson's Disease: Diagnosis and Clinical Management*. 2nd ed. New York: Demos; 2007:663-688.

Mink JW, Walkup J, Frey KA, et al. Patient selection and assessment recommendations for deep brain stimulation in Tourette syndrome. *Mov Disord*. 2006;21:1831-1838.

Moro E, Lang AE, Strafella AP, et al. Bilateral globus pallidus stimulation for Huntington's disease. *Ann Neurol*. 2004;56:290-294.

Okun M, Tagliati M, Pourfar M, et al. Management of referred DBS failures: a retrospective analysis from two movement disorders centers. *Arch Neurol*. 2005;62:1250-1255.

Okun MS, Fernandez HH, Pedraza O, et al. Development and initial validation of a screening tool for Parkinson disease surgical candidates. *Neurology*. 2004;63:161-163.

Pillon B. Neuropsychological assessment for management of patients with deep brain stimulation. *Mov Disord*. 2002;17:116-122.

Russmann H, Ghika J, Villemure JG, et al. Subthalamic nucleus deep brain stimulation in Parkinson disease patients over age 70 years. *Neurology*. 2004;63:1952-1954.

Schuurman PR, Bosch DA, Bossuyt PM, et al. A comparison of continuous thalamic stimulation and thalamotomy for suppression of severe tremor. *N Engl J Med*. 2000;342:461-468.

Vidailhet M, Vercueil L, Houeto JL. Bilateral deep-brain stimulation of the globus pallidus in primary generalized dystonia. *N Engl J Med*. 2005;352:459-467.

Volkmann J, Allert N, Voges J, et al. Long-term results of bilateral pallidal stimulation in Parkinson's disease. *Ann Neurol*. 2004;55:871-875.

Voon V, Kubu C, Krack P, et al. Deep brain stimulation: neuropsychological and neuropsychiatric issues. *Mov Disord*. 2006;21:305-326.

Voon V, Moro E, Saint-Cyr J, et al. Psychiatric symptoms following surgery for Parkinson's disease with an emphasis on subthalamic stimulation. *Adv Neurol*. 2005;96:130-147.

Weaver FM, Follett K, Stern M, et al. Bilateral deep brain stimulation vs best medical therapy for patients with advanced Parkinson disease: a randomized controlled trial. *JAMA*. 2009;301:63-73.

Welter ML, Houeto JL, Tezenas du Montcel S, et al. Clinical predictive factors of subthalamic stimulation in Parkinson's disease. *Brain*. 2002;125:575-583.

Yap L, Kouyialis A, Varma TR. Stereotactic neurosurgery for disabling tremor in multiple sclerosis: thalamotomy or deep brain stimulation? *Br J Neurosurg*. 2007;21:349-354.

See a full reference list on ExpertConsult.com

86 Functional Imaging in Movement Disorders

Mwiza Ushe and Joel S. Perlmutter

A chapter on functional imaging in movement disorders can take several different directions, but rather than providing a general review of this wide ranging topic, this chapter focuses on those aspects that relate to current and potential future applications of neurosurgery. Therefore, this chapter addresses molecular imaging and resting state functional magnetic resonance imaging (MRI) methods and studies. The goals include providing a foundation for critical review of the literature to permit the neurosurgeon or investigator to determine what will move the field forward with potential for new clinical applications.

MOLECULAR IMAGING

Positron emission tomography (PET) and single-photon emission computed tomography (SPECT) provide tomographic images reflecting the regional brain distribution of a variety of administered radiopharmaceuticals. PET has higher anatomic resolution and better quantification than SPECT. The radioisotopes generally used for PET are relatively short-lived, such as oxygen 15 ([^{15}O], 2 min), carbon 11 ([^{11}C], 20 min), and fluoride 18 ([^{18}F], 110 min), which must be incorporated into the desired radiopharmaceuticals relatively quickly, pass quality control checks, and then be delivered to the subject. For many radiopharmaceuticals, this process requires an on-site cyclotron and a radiochemistry production facility that can be quite expensive, although commercial vendors distribute many [^{18}F] radiopharmaceuticals. In contrast, commercial vendors distribute most SPECT radiopharmaceuticals because they incorporate much longer-lived radioisotopes, usually iodine 123 (^{123}I) or technetium 99m Tc (^{99m}Tc), allowing for national distribution of products. Thus, SPECT can be more accessible and less expensive but suffers from lower-quality images. This review focuses primarily on PET but comments on SPECT where pertinent.

The key to these molecular imaging methods is the specifics of the radiopharmaceutical. Early studies used radiotracers to measure regional glucose or oxygen metabolism or blood flow. These measures identified changes in resting state metabolism or blood flow that corresponded to specific clinical manifestations of various movement disorders—essentially an in vivo neuroimaging extension of the old clinical-pathologic correlation approach.[1] The underlying assumption is that local flow or metabolism reflects local interneuronal activity or inputs into that brain region.[2] More sophisticated analyses of such imaging data include identification of covariance networks—that is, regions of the brain that have resting functional measures that correlate with each other. Patterns of such covariance networks can be related to specific states or behaviors and seem to be a more sensitive means of detecting changes in brain function than limiting the search to specific regional changes.[3] Most past studies focused on specific regional deficits, but the focus has moved to networks and how specific regions or nodes may contribute to dysfunction of selected networks. (Networks are discussed in more detail later.) A critical issue for interpretation of any resting-state study is the behavior of the subject during image acquisition. This is particularly critical for those with movement disorders, in whom unwanted movements during scan acquisition can alter the uptake of a radiopharmaceutical, leading to a misinterpretation of findings. Specifically, purported regional change in flow or metabolism thought to reflect the underlying pathophysiology of a disorder may, in fact, merely represent sensory feedback or motor control systems associated with the movement that may or may not be pathologic.[4]

Molecular imaging permits targeting of specific neurotransmitter and neuroreceptor systems as well as various brain enzyme activities or chemical moieties. For example, radiolabeled levodopa drugs such as [^{18}F] 6-fluorodopa (FD) allows assessment of dopaminergic pathways because this radiotracer passes through the blood-brain barrier and is trapped within the brain after conversion by aromatic acid decarboxylase into [^{18}F]-dopamine, a charged molecule that does not pass through the blood-brain barrier (Fig. 86-1). Because aromatic acid decarboxylase resides primarily in dopaminergic neurons, the regional distribution of radioactivity, which can be quantified with several different approaches, provides a measure of the integrity of dopaminergic pathways (see Fig. 86-1). For example, PET FD imaging can detect nigrostriatal neuronal loss in people with Parkinson's disease (PD) (Fig. 86-2). This radiotracer and a variety of other markers for dopaminergic neurons have been used to investigate the pathophysiology of multiple movement disorders, assess the efficacy of different interventions, and aid clinical diagnosis. However, many of these applications, such as neuroimaging measures of PD progression, have been misinterpreted because of an evolving understanding of the assumptions and limitations of methods of data interpretation (Fig. 86-3).[5,6] Nevertheless, many applications have led to important new insights into pathophysiology of various movement disorders.

PET or SPECT also can target selected neuroreceptors such as various dopaminergic receptors, including D_1-like or D_2-like receptors as well as serotonergic, cholinergic, γ-aminobutyric acid–ergic (GABAergic), and noradrenergic receptors. These receptor targets can reside on the presynaptic or postsynaptic side of synapses, which are not clearly distinguished by these imaging techniques. Alternatively, radiopharmaceuticals can selectively label transporters of various transmitters, such as the membranous dopamine transporter (DaT), which can be labeled for PET or SPECT; the vesicular monoamine transporter type 2 (VMAT2); and the vesicular acetylcholine transporter (VAChT)[7,8] (see Fig. 86-1). Radiopharmaceuticals also can label second messenger signaling mechanisms such as phosphodiesterase 10A (PDE10A), which is key for postsynaptic signaling cascade systems related to D_1-like or D_2-like receptors.[9,10] These approaches have potential for helping with clinical diagnosis or assessing target engagement of therapeutic interventions,[11] but they must be applied with great caution.[12] Some radiopharmaceuticals may be displaced by varying levels of endogenous neurotransmitters[13] or ongoing drug treatment, thereby confounding interpretation of identified changes in receptor measurements that could indicate either a pathophysiologic difference in the relevant receptor or an effect of the available number of specific binding sites due to competition from either the endogenous or exogenous competitor. However, this type of competition can be an advantage for a different type of experimental paradigm, as discussed shortly.

In addition to these resting-state studies, one can image the effects of activation on regional blood flow or metabolism. This activation can be either a physiologic activation—like movement of a hand or sensory input[14,15]—pharmacologic activation with detection of the effects of an administered unlabeled drug,[16] or another stimulus like deep brain stimulation.[17,18] The same strategy can be applied to receptor imaging studies. For example, one could either give a drug to increase synaptic dopamine release or have subjects perform a task that cause dopamine release and then image the effects on striatal uptake of a radioligand like [^{11}C] raclopride, a dopamine D_2–like radioligand that is particularly sensitive to endogenous dopamine levels. These types of studies also require careful control for unintended movement during scan acquisition (Fig. 86-4). Behavioral tasks have another potential confounding factor that may be particularly important for a motor task in subjects with a movement disorder. Performances of a task by someone with a movement disorder and by a control individual may or may not have the same movement characteristics. This fact can confound interpretation of the imaging measured brain response. Attempts to simplify a task, for instance, employ a slow finger-tapping task in someone with hand dystonia but at a sufficiently slow rate not to induce any dystonia posturing, is one reasonable strategy to use so that the patient group and the control group have similar performance variables. However, this approach requires careful physiologic and behavioral measures to ensure that the same effort and movements have been made by those with and those without the movement disorder. A critical reader of papers in this field must consider this issue carefully to ensure proper interpretation of the findings.

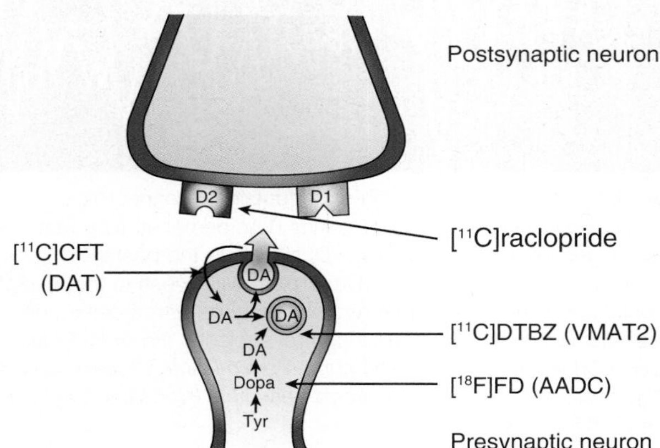

Figure 86-1. Schematic representation of a striatal dopaminergic synapse demonstrating the common positron emission tomography (PET) radioligands and their specific binding locations or locations of action. A commercially available single-photon emission tomography (SPECT) radioligand targets the dopamine transporter (DAT). AADC, aromatic acid decarboxylase; [^{11}C]CFT, [^{11}C]carbomethoxy-3-beta-(4-fluorophenyl)tropane; D1, D_1-like dopamine receptor; D2, D_2-like dopamine receptor; DA, dopamine; [^{11}C]DTBZ, [^{11}C]dihydrotetrabenazine; [^{18}F]FD, [^{18}F]fluorodopa; Tyr, tyrosine; VMAT2, vesicular monoamine transporter type 2. *(Modified from Perlmutter JS, Norris SA. Neuroimaging biomarkers for Parkinson disease: facts and fantasy.* Ann Neurol. *2014;76:769-783.)*

MAGNETIC RESONANCE IMAGING OF BLOOD OXYGEN LEVEL–DEPENDENT SIGNALS

The development of MRI detection of blood oxygen level–dependent (BOLD) signals began a new era in resting-state and activation imaging, because BOLD imaging is free from ionizing radiation, requires no complicated radiopharmaceuticals, and has

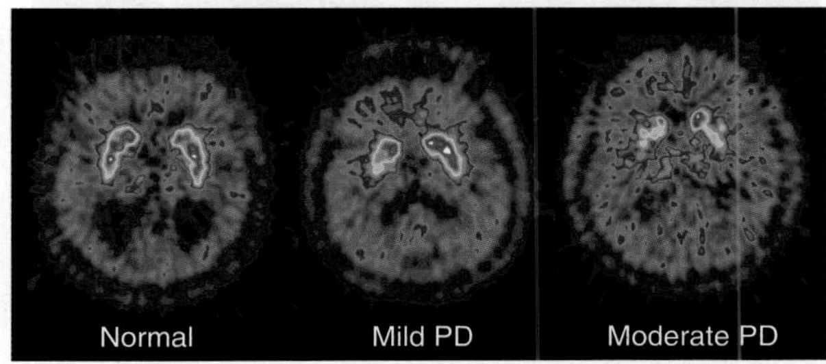

Figure 86-2. Positron emission tomography images of striatal [^{18}F]-fluorodopa ([^{18}F]-dopa) uptake in a normal control, an individual with mild Parkinson disease (PD), and an individual with moderate PD. In mild Parkinson disease there is a preferential asymmetric loss of putaminal [^{18}F]-dopa uptake. As the disease progresses there is more diffuse loss of [^{18}F]-dopa uptake in the striatum bilaterally.

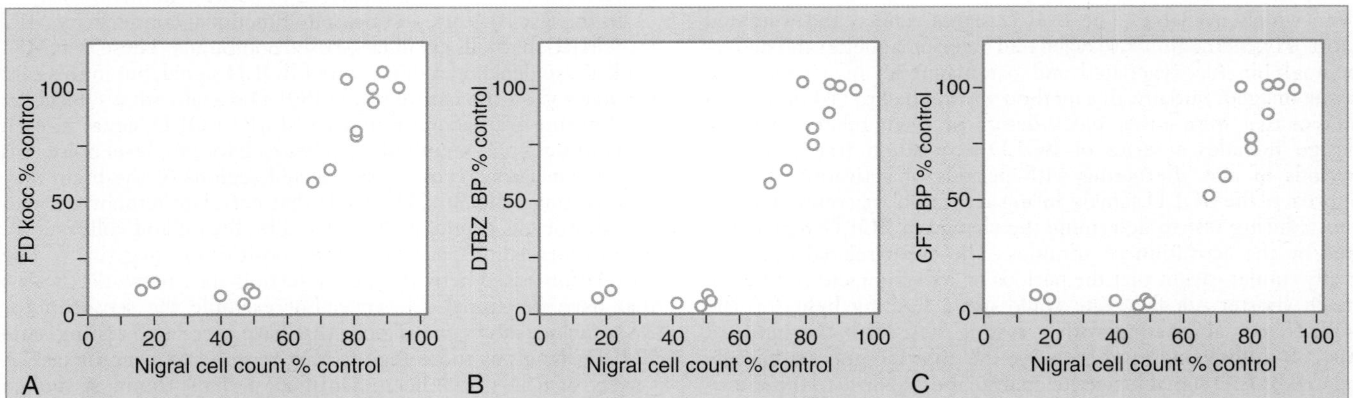

Figure 86-3. A to **C,** An MPTP (1-methyl-4-phenyl-1,2,3,6-tetrahydropyridine) animal model of nigrostriatal injury demonstrated that positron emission tomography measures of presynaptic radioligands of nigrostriatal neurons correlates with cell body loss in substantia nigra only when the nigral cell loss is 50% or less. Terminal field measures reached near zero at that point and remain there despite increased loss of nigral cells. These data demonstrate that terminal field measures do not necessarily correspond with cell body measures. These data also may explain the discordant findings between imaging and clinical end points from clinical trials because as Parkinson disease progresses (i.e., nigral cell loss exceeds 50%) the molecular imaging striatal measures may just reflect noise.[6] BP, nondisplaceable binding potential; CFT, [^{11}C] carbomethoxy-3-beta-(4-fluorophenyl)tropane; DTBZ, [^{11}C]dihydrotetrabenazine; FD, [^{18}F]fluorodopa. *(Modified from Karimi M, Tian L, Brown CA, et al. Validation of nigrostriatal positron emission tomography measures: critical limits.* Ann Neurol. *2013;73:390-396.)*

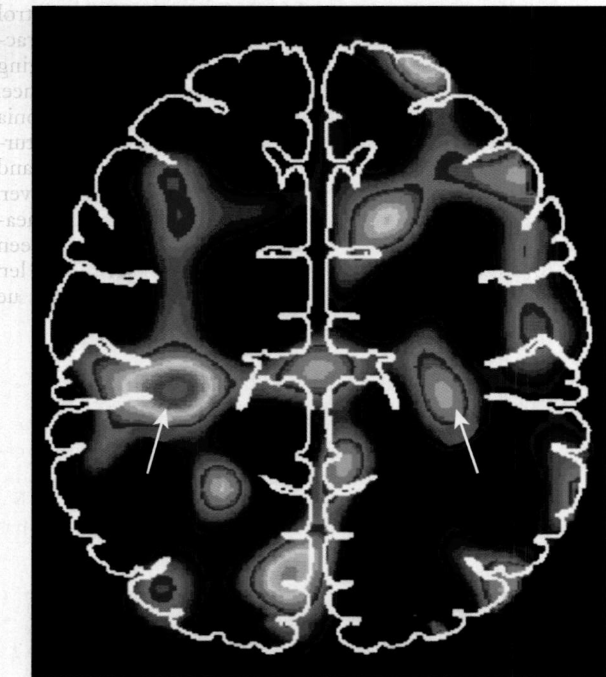

Figure 86-4. Averaged subtraction image of "resting state" regional cerebral blood flow measured with positron emission tomography and [^{15}O]H_2O from six patients with Parkinson disease, undergoing bilateral subthalamic nucleus deep brain stimulation with stimulators OFF. For each participant, a resting state image while at rest and another with tremor in the right upper extremity were obtained. For each patient, these two images were subtracted from each other. *Arrows* indicate supplementary motor cortex (SMC) regions. This image demonstrates that if unwanted movement during scan acquisition is not controlled for, substantial spurious "responses" can be produced that can confound interpretation of studies. *Red* indicates peak blood flow increase of 5%.

been widely available. The BOLD signal reflects the weighted ratio of oxyhemoglobin (oxygenated and isomagnetic) and deoxyhemoglobin (deoxygenated and paramagnetic) in a volume of tissue imaged. Initially, this method was applied to task activation studies that were either block design or event related. A block design includes a series of BOLD acquisition frames during periods of rest alternating with periods of activation. In this approach, the BOLD signals during activation are compared with those during rest to determine the change in BOLD signal elicited by the activation or stimulus. The event-related design is really similar except that the periods of activation and resting are much shorter—in fact, one could use a flashing light for 100 milliseconds alternating with a resting state with the light off for 200 milliseconds and then use the appropriately temporally related BOLD signal images to analyze the response to the stimulus. Each of these approaches requires calculating or estimating the response delay to identify the correct period of imaging data. This response delay reflects the time from the onset of the activation or stimulus to the time of brain response. Of course, one also can use this approach to detect the response to a drug—so-called pharmacologic activation. The challenge in these types of studies is that the pharmacologic activation analysis must have a block design because one cannot turn the drug on and off repeatedly unless it has an extremely short pharmacodynamic effect, and most drug effects are not likely to be fast enough for these types of studies. The resulting "one block on and one block off" approach can complicate data analysis if the baseline values of the

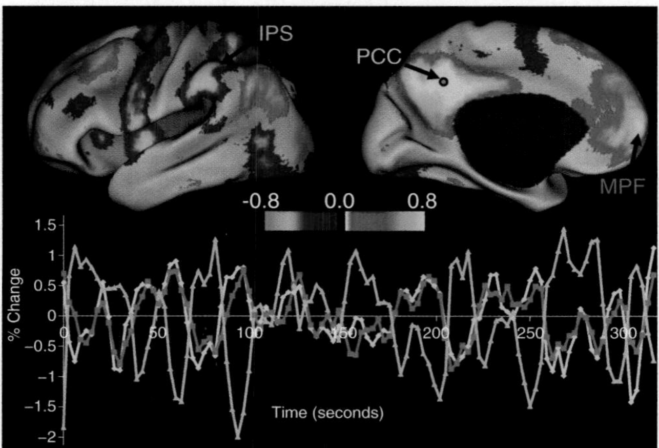

Figure 86-5. Seed based resting-state functional connectivity magnetic resonance imaging time series data demonstrating that blood oxygen level–dependent (BOLD) signals in the posterior cingulate/precuneus (PCC) *(yellow)* correlate with those in the medial prefrontal cortex (MPF) *(orange)* and anticorrelate with those in the intraparietal sulcus (IPS) in normal control subjects. *(From Fox MD, Snyder AZ, Vincent JL, et al. The human brain is intrinsically organized into dynamic, anticorrelated functional networks.* Proc Natl Acad Sci U S A. *2005;102:9673-9678.)*

BOLD signal are not stable. Nevertheless, such studies have been completed. Alternatively, one can use arterial spin labeling (ASL) rather than BOLD signals with MRI to detect responses to drugs or other activations. ASL has similarities to blood flow imaging with PET but does not require radiopharmaceuticals. All of these MRI-based task activation approaches have the advantage of permitting many measures per participant, thereby improving the signal-to-noise ratio or allowing evaluation of multiple behavioral conditions within individual subjects. Yet each of these approaches still can be confounded either by unintentional movements during scan acquisition or by non-equivalent task efforts or performances in the comparison of patients and controls.

In the last 10 years, resting-state functional connectivity MRI (rs-fcMRI) methods avoid task-based confounds. These rs-fcMRI studies also depend on detection of BOLD signal, but in this case the focus is on the nature of the BOLD signal with a subject "at rest" during scan acquisition. At rest, the BOLD signal in each voxel of the brain seemingly appears to have low-level noise, but closer inspection reveals that selected regions of the brain may have resting-state BOLD signals that correlate temporally with one another, as originally discovered by Biswal and colleagues.[19] These correlations can be either positive or negative.[19] The correlation-based networks define resting-state networks (RSNs) that have functional relevance. For example the sensorimotor RSN includes the same regions that have correlated resting-state BOLD signals as those regions that respond to a motor task. A variety of RSNs have been identified, perhaps the most studied one being the default mode network (DMN), discovered by Marc Raichle,[19a] that includes a group of regions that become less active during almost any task. Interestingly, the functional status of the DMN may underlie many pathologic conditions, including Alzheimer disease[20] but also changes in people with PD.[21] Resting-state networks may be identified with different approaches, but the two major methods are seed-based methods and independent components analysis (ICA). Seed-based correlation analyses start with selection of brain regions (which can be one or hundreds) and then, for each of these seed regions, identify all of the other brain regions that have correlated activity at rest with it (Fig. 86-5).[22] Alternatively, ICA permits a data-driven approach not dependent on initial identification of selected regional seeds.[23] Each of these approaches has advantages and disadvantages, with proponents on either side arguing the advantages of one over the other. Perhaps more important, all of these resting-state functional connectivity studies share the challenge of requiring rigorous quality control measures, because even small frame-to-frame movements can cause spurious RSNs to appear. Such spurious findings may not be eliminated by a common approach to "regress out" movement from the analysis or match two groups of subjects for the same amount of movement. This evolving understanding of the sensitivity of these types of resting-state analyses in terms of such quality control issues requires substantial caution in interpretation of older published studies.[24]

APPLICATIONS TO MOVEMENT DISORDERS

The key is now to determine how these functional neuroimaging methods can provide useful information for current and potential future neurosurgical interventions. Three major types of potential applications may benefit from functional neuroimaging. The first area is whether functional neuroimaging can help select appropriate patients for various neurosurgical interventions like deep brain stimulation (DBS). Other chapters address the various applications of DBS to PD, essential tremor (ET), dystonia, and other movement disorders. The efficacy and safety of DBS depends, in part, on accurate diagnosis of the relevant condition. Thus, the role of functional neuroimaging to increase diagnostic accuracy is addressed. A second potential application is whether functional neuroimaging may provide targeting for implantation of electrodes into new sites identified by pathologic RSNs. A third application is the use of molecular imaging methods to locate regions of neurochemical deficits that could guide implantation of restorative therapeutic interventions. Each of these approaches is discussed in this chapter.

Diagnostic Accuracy

Current targets for DBS include the ventral intermediate nucleus of the thalamus (VIM) for ET,[25,26] the region of the subthalamic nucleus (STN) or the internal segment of the globus pallidus (GPi) for PD,[27,28] and GPi or STN for dystonia.[29-32] Of course, lesioning of these targets remains a surgical option.[33-36] Although surgical intervention in the VIM may improve tremors in people with ET, PD and dystonia, it does not improve the other motor symptoms of PD or dystonia. Additionally, it is unclear whether STN DBS is effective for ET. STN and GPi DBS may be equally effective to relieve motor symptoms of PD, but the optimal target for dystonia remains unclear. Perhaps most important, DBS of these targets does not provide effective treatment for the motor symptoms of other parkinsonian syndromes, including multiple systems atrophy (MSA), progressive supranuclear palsy (PSP), corticobasal syndrome (CBS), and vascular parkinsonism. Because clinical diagnostic accuracy for distinguishing PD from these other parkinsonian conditions is not 100%, the question is whether functional neuroimaging can improve upon it.

The main approach for diagnostic imaging has been molecular imaging. PD is a neurodegenerative disease characterized by the loss of pigmented dopaminergic neurons from the substantia nigra pars compacta (SNpc) in the midbrain associated with deposition of neuronal intracytoplasmic α-synuclein inclusions called Lewy bodies and Lewy neurites in cellular processes. Although Lewy bodies are specific for PD, the loss of dopaminergic neurons in the substantia nigra occurs in other parkinsonian illnesses, such as PSP, MSA, and CBD. The clinical manifestations of PD include a predominantly resting tremor, bradykinesia, rigidity, and postural instability that may include asymmetrical onset and progression. Nonmotor features of the illness, including autonomic changes, depression, and dementia, are being increasingly recognized. These signs and symptoms of idiopathic PD greatly overlap the other parkinsonian syndromes, although the greatest indicator of a diagnosis of idiopathic PD is a sustained, substantial response to levodopa. Interestingly, overlap also exists between PD and ET as the tremor in PD is not always a resting tremor, and patients with ET can have parkinsonian signs. Dystonia also may also be a presenting symptom of PD and many dystonic syndromes include parkinsonism with degeneration of dopaminergic neurons or impairment of dopaminergic neurotransmission. These overlapping manifestations limit diagnostic accuracy, and in some cases, reaching the appropriate diagnosis can take up to 18 years of observation.[37] These clinically based diagnostic limitations provide the rationale for improving diagnostic accuracy with functional neuroimaging.

Molecular imaging of dopaminergic neurons may help differentiate degenerative parkinsonian syndromes from normal as well as from parkinsonian syndromes without dopaminergic deficit, such as ET and some dystonias.[38] But does it do so reliably enough to aid selection of surgical candidates? Several studies focused on differentiating people with ET from those with PD, and most claimed that normal striatal uptake of FD or a DaT radiotracer would predict a low probability of development of PD in the next 2 years.[39] Others found less confidence in the predictability of normal scan findings; follow-up for 2 to 4 years revealed that a neurodegenerative parkinsonian condition, including dopa-responsive idiopathic PD, developed in 15% to 20%[40] or as many as 30%[12] of subjects of (Fig. 86-6). Thus, even normal molecular imaging findings may not provide reasonable security that a person does not have PD.

The next question is how well abnormal scan findings differentiate PD from other degenerative parkinsonian conditions like MSA, PSP, CBD, and vascular parkinsonism.[38] No convincing data suggest that reduced striatal uptake of either FD or DaT radioligand, which demonstrates a defect in the nigrostriatal pathway, differentiates these multiple neurodegenerative conditions from PD.[6] A reanalysis of the data submitted to the U.S. Food and Drug Administration (FDA) in support of clinical implementation of a SPECT radiopharmaceutical to quantify

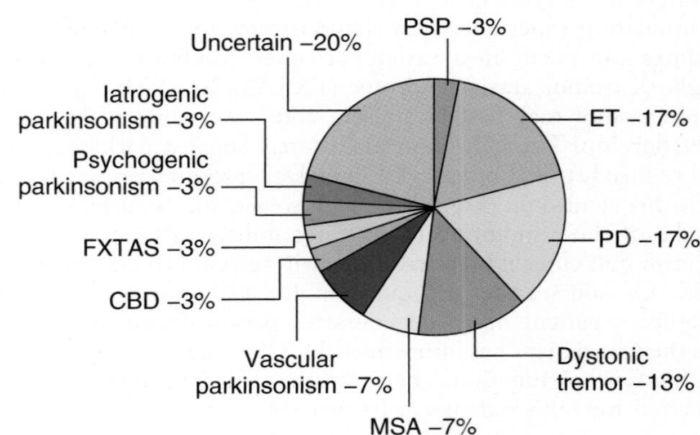

Figure 86-6. Evaluating the diagnostic accuracy of single-photon emission computed tomography (SPECT) using a dopamine transporter (DaT) radiotracer. The pie graph shows the distribution of final diagnoses in 30 people with normal DaT SPECT findings. The false-negative rate for degenerative parkinsonism was ≥ 31%. CBD, corticobasal degeneration; ET, essential tremor; FXTAS, fragile X tremor ataxia syndrome; MSA, multiple systems atrophy; PD, Parkinson disease; PSP, progressive supranuclear palsy. *(Modified from Menendez-Gonzalez M, Tavares F, Zeidan N, et al. Diagnoses behind patients with hard-to-classify tremor and normal DaT-SPECT: a clinical follow up study.* Front Aging Neurosci. *2014;6:1-9.)*

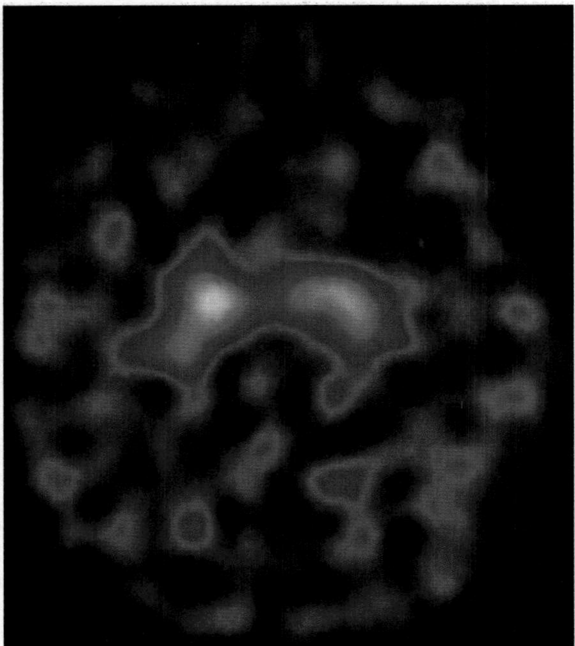

Figure 86-7. Scan from dopamine transporter (DaT) single-photon emission computed tomography (SPECT) using [^{123}I]FP-CIT (iodine I 123–labeled 2β-carbomethoxy-3β-[4-iodophenyl]-*N*-[3-fluoro-propyl] nortropan) shows reduced uptake in the putamen bilaterally with a slightly asymmetrical pattern in a 65-year-old man who had mild bilateral tremor in the upper extremities with fragile X tremor ataxia syndrome and whose daughter had fragile X syndrome with mental retardation. *(From Madeo G, Alemseged F, Di Pietro B, et al. Early abnormalities in 123I-ioflupane [DaTSCAN] imaging in the fragile X-associated tremor ataxia syndrome [FXTAS]: a case report.* Neurol Sci. *2013;34:1475-1477.)*

striatal DaT uptake demonstrated that the SPECT DaT scan provided no additional benefit over clinical examination to distinguish neurodegenerative parkinsonism.[41] Furthermore, accumulating experience now demonstrates that abnormal scan findings can occur in a variety of other conditions, including fragile X tremor ataxia syndrome (FXTAS), in which a postural action tremor may first be present and a gait abnormality may later develop. The gait abnormality may suggest parkinsonism, and reduced striatal uptake of FD or DaT radiotracer may occur with this syndrome (Fig. 86-7).[42] However, the reduced striatal uptake of these radiotracers does not indicate PD, nor does it indicate that clinical manifestations will respond to GPi or STN DBS. Of course, the key question for DBS targeting is not whether a patient has a degenerative parkinsonism but rather whether the patient has idiopathic PD. Thus, the potential benefit of this type of functional neuroimaging for improving patient selection for DBS remains to be proven.

New DBS Target Selection

Can functional neuroimaging identify new, more easily accessible, and more effective targets than the targets currently used for DBS? Giacobbe and associates[43] have provided a rationale approach for building a case by incorporating findings from a series of functional and anatomical imaging studies to target the subgenual cingulate region for implantation of DBS electrodes to treat drug-resistant depression.

We now suggest a new strategy based on RSN studies that could have potential; but to be clear from the outset, this suggestion is entirely speculative. Increasing data now suggest that people with PD have abnormal RSNs that can be identified with rs-fcMRI[44-47] and that striatal functional connectivity strength may even correlate with motor ratings of parkinsonism.[44] Abnormal RSNs also have been identified in people with a variety of dystonic syndromes.[48,49] These types of functional connectivity networks contain multiple nodes that could represent targets for DBS. Stimulation at a node may alter activity in a related RSN that could potentially reduce clinical symptoms. The challenges prior to implementation of this strategy may be considerable, including the possibility that stimulation at the site of one of these nodes could elicit multiple other possible unintended outcomes. Nodes may be promiscuous; that is, a node may relate to more than one RSN, and it would be essential to ensure that DBS at a specific site has the intended effect and not excessive unwanted side effects. Another approach for identifying candidate RSNs is to use known sites of effective stimulation as seeds to identify new RSNs.[50] Because these nodes are sites of effective stimulation, one may hypothesize that stimulation at other, more easily accessible sites of such an RSN may also provide clinical benefit. Of course the efficacy and safety of this approach also remain to be proven. Just to stretch the speculation a bit further, one might combine these two approaches and then target nodes that are common to them.

Pharmacologic Targeting

Molecular imaging may identify brain regions with specific neurochemical deficits. This ability has been best demonstrated with nigrostriatal defects identified with a variety of radiotracers for presynaptic nigrostriatal dopaminergic neurons,[6] but other neurotransmitter defects, such a serotonin, may be identified.[9] Postmortem data from a 2015 study[51] may suggest that molecular imaging of norepinephrine, which could be done with a norepinephrine transport radiotracer,[52] could identify other regional transmitter system defects. These areas of neurochemical deficiency may relate to specific behavioral deficits—most commonly, nigrostriatal defects in striatum have been related to motor manifestations of PD.[53] These areas of deficiency can be targeted for replacement therapy, such as cellular transplantation[54] or viral vector delivery of genes that may restore the deficient transmitters.[55] Going beyond replacement of striatal dopamine holds great promise. However, multiple issues will have to be addressed prior to clinical implementation of such approaches, including careful validation of target identification with the molecular imaging method,[5] control over dose of therapeutic agent,[56] and availability and viability of transplanted agents, as well as well controlled studies to demonstrate efficacy.

CONCLUSION

Functional neuroimaging with either molecular imaging or BOLD imaging with MR methods provides important new insights into the pathophysiology of PD and other movement disorders. The clinical role of these techniques is an evolving frontier. The lure is to apply methodology as soon as possible to help our patients and stay at the cutting edge. Doing so, however, places the burden on clinicians and their expert scientific advisors to ensure that adequate validation of new methodology and potential applications support clinical implementation. Despite these cautions, the potential of dramatic new advances remains.

Acknowledgments

This work was supported by grants from the National Institutes of Health (NIH) (NS075321, NS41509, NS058714, NS065701, NCATS U54TR001456 & Office of Rare Disease Research), American Academy of Neurology & American Brain Foundation Clinical Research Training Fellowship, Washington University Faculty Diversity Scholarship, the Barnes Jewish Hospital Foundation (Elliot Stein Family Fund and

Parkinson Disease Research Fund), the Dystonia Medical Research Foundation, the American Parkinson Disease Association Advanced Research Center at Washington University, the Oertli Fund for Fellowship support, and the Murphy Fund for Neuroimaging of Dystonia.

SUGGESTED READINGS

Fox MD, Buckner RL, Liu H, et al. Resting-state networks link invasive and noninvasive brain stimulation across diverse psychiatric and neurological diseases. *Proc Natl Acad Sci U S A*. 2014;111(41): E4367-E4375.

Fuente-Fernandez R. Role of DaTSCAN and clinical diagnosis in Parkinson disease. *Neurology*. 2012;78(10):696-701.

Karimi M, et al. Validation of nigrostriatal positron emission tomography measures: critical limits. *Ann Neurol*. 2013;73(3):390-396.

Menendez-Gonzalez M, et al. Diagnoses behind patients with hard-to-classify tremor and normal DaT-SPECT: a clinical follow up study. *Front Aging Neurosci*. 2014;6:56.

Perlmutter JS, Norris SA. Neuroimaging biomarkers for Parkinson disease: facts and fantasy. *Ann Neurol*. 2014;76(6):769-783.

Power JD, Barnes KA, Snyder AZ, et al. Spurious but systematic correlations in functional connectivity MRI networks arise from subject motion. *Neuroimage*. 2012;59(3):2142-2154.

See a full reference list on ExpertConsult.com

87 Surgical Management of Tremor

Marwan Hariz and Patric Blomstedt

Tremor is the most common movement disorder. Whether it occurs at rest, as in Parkinson's disease, or is a kinetic action, as in essential tremor, this symptom greatly affects patients' well-being and quality of life. The effect of this symptom on activities of daily living, on mood, and on a person's social life and confidence in himself or herself should not be underestimated: tremor is visible, difficult to hide, socially embarrassing, and a highly stigmatizing symptom.

Tremor is often difficult to treat with medications. It is not unusual that essential tremor does not respond adequately to beta blockers, anticholinergics, or anticonvulsants such as primidone, topiramate, or gabapentin. Neither benzodiazepines nor alcohol should be used as treatment. Similarly, for Parkinson's disease, it is known that tremor is a symptom that may not respond as well to dopaminergic medication as do other symptoms of Parkinson's disease, such as akinesia and rigidity. Hence surgery for movement disorders has historically tried to target tremor, regardless of its cause. Results of surgery for tremor and graphic videos of patients with tremor before and after surgery (whether thalamotomy or deep brain stimulation [DBS]) have greatly helped popularize these procedures. The worldwide success of thalamotomy, introduced by Hassler and Riechert[1] in 1954, is attributable to the very dramatic, instantaneous, and robust effect of this procedure on this symptom.

This chapter provides a brief basic classification of tremor, a summary concerning its circuitry and pathophysiology, and a short history of neurosurgery for tremor. The three most common tremors are parkinsonian, essential, and dystonic tremor; stereotactic procedures for these, including DBS of various brain targets, and radiofrequency thalamotomy, are detailed, with emphasis on imaging and surgical techniques. Finally, emerging surgical tools that are tried in ablative surgery for tremor, such as Gamma Knife radiosurgery and focused ultrasonography, are discussed.

DEFINITION AND CLASSIFICATION OF TREMOR

Tremor is defined as an involuntary rhythmic oscillatory movement of a body part, usually the upper limbs. It is caused by rhythmical fluctuations of the muscle tonus between the flexors and extensors.[2] There are two main types of tremor: (1) resting tremor, which occurs when the muscle is at rest and disappears as soon as the muscle becomes activated, as in Parkinson's disease, and (2) kinetic action (essential) tremor, even called *intention tremor*, which is absent when the muscle is relaxed but starts when the muscle becomes or remains activated.

In 1998, the Movement Disorders Society (MDS) published a consensus statement offering a clinical classification of tremors.[3] This classification made the fundamental distinctions among rest, postural, simple kinetic, and intention tremor (i.e., tremor during target-directed movements). Medical history and a neurological examination can help in defining the various tremors as any of the following: enhanced physiologic tremor, classical essential tremor, tremor of Parkinson's disease, task- and position-specific tremors, dystonic tremor, Holmes's tremor (also called *rubral tremor*), primary orthostatic tremor, cerebellar tremor, palatal tremor, drug-induced tremor, peripheral neuropathy tremor, or psychogenic tremor. The details concerning the various causes of tremor are described in the MDS consensus paper.[3]

The most common tremor syndromes are, not surprisingly, also those that are most commonly subject to neurosurgical interventions: parkinsonian tremor (rest tremor with a frequency of 4 to 6 Hz) and essential tremor (a postural action-kinetic tremor, usually bilateral, with a frequency of 7 to 12 Hz). Other more or less common tremors that can be subject to surgery are dystonic tremor (a coarse, irregular tremor that accompanies a particular body posture), rubral tremor (a combination of rest, postural, and action tremor), and tremor of multiple sclerosis (a cerebellar intention-action tremor with high amplitude, proximal muscle engagement, and dysmetria).

PATHOPHYSIOLOGY AND CIRCUITRIES OF TREMOR

Oscillations in the cerebellothalamocortical pathway occur in virtually all tremor disorders, regardless of the cause.[4]

In Parkinson's disease, tremor related neuronal activity has been demonstrated to occur both in the basal ganglia and their receiving areas of the thalamus, the ventral oral nuclei, as well as in the cerebellothalamocortical circuit.[5,6] It is postulated that the loss of dopaminergic input causes abnormal phasic neuronal discharges in the basal ganglia, especially the subthalamic nucleus (STN) and the globus pallidus internus (GPi), in which tremorogenic oscillations in Parkinson's disease are found. The GPi projects to the ventral oral anterior nucleus of the thalamus. The oscillations propagate thus along this loop: motor cortex → caudate → putamen → pallidum → ventral thalamus → motor cortex. The motor cortex to which this oscillation is transmitted connects reciprocally with the ventral intermediate (VIM) nucleus of the thalamus, which projects to the cerebellum. Parkinsonian tremor is thus probably amplified in the motor cortex–VIM thalamic loop.

In essential tremor, thalamic neurons show firing patterns at tremor frequency, predominantly in the VIM nucleus, which is the cerebellar input receiving zone.[7,8] The VIM nucleus is situated between the ventral oral posterior nucleus anteriorly and the sensory thalamus posteriorly. The cerebello-thalamic fibers, converging in this nucleus, belong to the following loop: cerebellar cortex → dentate nucleus → red nucleus → VIM nucleus → cerebral cortex → internal capsule → ponsnuclei → cerebellar cortex. In the VIM nucleus, there are kinesthetic cells that respond to joint movements and so-called tremor cells, which are believed to act as a "pacemaker" to tremor oscillations. The cerebellothalamic pathway is thus heavily implicated in the tremor of essential tremor, inasmuch as it is also involved in parkinsonian tremor.

These two parallel pathways of tremor—the basal ganglia–thalamic pathway in Parkinson's disease and the cerebellothalamic pathway in essential tremor—traverse the posterior subthalamic area, converge in the motor ventrolateral thalamus, and thus provide the anatomic-physiologic rationale for targeting the ventrolateral thalamus, as well as the subthalamic area, in surgically treating tremor disorders.

HISTORY OF SURGERY FOR TREMOR

Prestereotactic Era

Neurosurgery for tremor has a long history. James Parkinson was the first to report that a stroke had relieved a patient with what he called *paralysis agitans* from the tremors in the paralyzed limbs. Consequently, surgery for movement disorders was initially directed toward cortical structures or subcortical pathways involved in the motor system.[9] In the presterotactic era, surgery for tremor included peripheral and spinal procedures such as posterior rhizotomies, cervical sympathectomy, and spinal chordotomy/tractotomy, as well as intracranial procedures such as dentatotomy, mesenphalic pedunculotomy, cortical resections, and operations on the internal capsule. These procedures had variable effects on tremor and resulted almost invariably in hemiparesis. A common belief was that abolishing tremor necessitated destruction of some part of the corticospinal system.

In 1939, Russell Meyers pioneered a new approach by aiming at surgical resections of various parts of the basal ganglia and their connections, including the head of the nucleus caudatus, the anterior limb of the internal capsule, and subsequently, section of the pallidothalamic fibers at the level of the ansa lenticularis. In so doing, Meyers proved that tremor and rigidity could be relieved without disrupting volitional movement.

Stereotactic Era

The advent of human stereotactic neurosurgery opened new horizons in the surgical treatment of tremor, epecially parkinsonian tremor. Early stereotactic procedures targeted the pallidothalamic or dentatothalamic pathway, or both, at various levels.[10] Stereotactic procedures for parkinsonian tremor and rigidity included pallidotomy and pallidoansotomy, Rolf Hassler's ventrolateral thalamotomy, Ernest A. Spiegel's campotomy in the field (campus) of Forel, and Orlando J. Andy's subthalamotomy, as well as procedures involving various regions in the thalamic ventrolateral complex, extending from the VIM nucleus posteriorly to the ventral oral anterior nucleus anteriorly.

Later, microelectrode recording demonstrated that the VIM area of the thalamus, just behind the ventral oral posterior nucleus, contained cells that fired in a tremor-synchronous manner.[11] The VIM nucleus gradually became, and still is, the main stereotactic target for the treatment of all tremors, regardless of cause.[12,13] VIM thalamotomy produced the most dramatic and immediate effect on tremor and became popular worldwide, especially for parkinsonian and esential tremor, to the extent that surgery for tremor became synonymous with VIM thalamotomy. After the introduction of levodopa therapy in the late 1960s and early 1970s, there was a dramatic decline in stereotactic surgery for Parkinson's disease, including surgery for tremor.[14] It was not until the early 1990s that a renaissance of stereotactic surgery for movement disorders took place, pioneered by Lauri Laitinen's rediscovery of Lars Leksell's pallidotomy for Parkinson's disease.[15] It was well known by then that long-term levodopa therapy caused motor fluctuations and dyskinesias, which became the main indications for pallidotomy. In parallel, the introduction of modern DBS for tremor by Benabid and associates[16,17] in the late 1980s confirmed the new era of functional stereotactic surgery for movement disorders; its most profound results were abolition of both tremor and dyskinesias.

Deep Brain Stimulation

The use of chronic electrical stimulation through electrodes permanently implanted within thalamic and subthalamic targets for the treatment of tremor dates back to the 1960s.[18] The rationale was and is that stimulation is safer than ablative lesions in patients at high risk for surgical complications or in patients who need bilateral surgery (bilateral thalamotomy harbors unacceptable complications, especially when the two procedures are performed contemporaneously). In 1980, Brice and McLellan[19] described the use of DBS in three patients with intention tremor caused by multiple sclerosis. The target was the subthalamic area. In 1983, Andy[20] described DBS in nine patients with movement disorders, of whom five had parkinsonian tremor. The electrodes were placed in the VIM nucleus and in other thalamic and subthalamic areas. Andy wrote, "In contrast to thalamic lesion, it is preferred for the treatment of intractable motor disorders in high-risk elderly patients and patients with diffuse lesions secondary to trauma. The beneficial effects are reversible even after several months of applied therapeutic stimulation.... Lesion studies indicate that optimum sites for alleviating parkinsonian tremor and other movement disorders are the VIM nucleus and other thalamic and subthalamic areas. Optimum sites for stimulation electrode implants tend to parallel those findings."[20]

The next publication in the field of DBS for tremor, by Benabid and associates, appeared in 1987.[16] Initially, Benabid and associates used DBS contralaterally to a previous thalamotomy in patients with parkinsonian or essential tremor. Eventually, DBS became the procedure of choice for treating tremor, enabling safer and bilateral simultaneous surgery with fewer and mostly reversible side effects in comparison with thalamotomy. As a result of the extension of DBS to the STN and GPi in the 1990s,[21,22] DBS became the preferred surgical technique for treating medically refractory movement disorders.

Contemporary Surgery for Tremor

Since 2000, surgery for tremor has consisted mainly of DBS, not ablation. Publications from the mid-1990s reflect that the main targets for tremor are the VIM nucleus and the subthalamic area/zona incerta for essential tremor (as well as for other more tremors rarely operated on, such as Holmes's tremor and tremor of multiple sclerosis), the STN (or, more rarely, the VIM nucleus) for parkinsonian tremor, and the GPi (or VIM nucleus–ventrolateral thalamus) for dystonic tremor. These targets, their imaging, and the surgical techniques used for DBS are described in the following sections.

Because this chapter aims at describing only surgical management of tremor, the brain targets and techniques more specifically used for tremor are emphasized: the VIM nucleus and the part of the subthalamic area called the caudal zona incerta (cZI). Also, even if DBS is the dominant surgery in Western Europe, North America, Japan, and Australia, lesional surgery, especially thalamotomy for tremor and pallidotomy (and more rarely subthalamotomy) for Parkinson's disease and tremor are still frequently used—albeit much less published—in many countries around the world where DBS is less affordable.[23] Therefore, some basic principles concerning radiofrequency (RF) lesion-creating techniques, especially RF thalamotomy for tremor, are also discussed. Finally, Gamma Knife radiosurgical thalamotomy and most recently, focused ultrasound thalamotomy are emerging tools for performing ablative treatment for tremor and are mentioned briefly.

TARGETS

Subthalamic Nucleus (STN)

The STN is the target of choice in the treatment of Parkinson's disease, regardless of whether tremor is the dominant symptom. It is unclear where in the STN the best effect on tremor is achieved. The effect of DBS in the STN with regard to the location of the electrode has been evaluated in no more than 260 patients in a total of 13 different studies.[24] An interesting finding in most of these studies is that the best effect on tremor is achieved not in the STN itself but in the rostral zona incerta, above the STN.[24-26] Sometimes, the best effect on tremor is achieved when the electrode exits the STN posteromedially and enters the cZI.

Ventral Intermediate Nucleus

Some differences exist between different groups regarding the coordinates of the VIM nucleus, a structure that still cannot be visualized on conventional magnetic resonance imaging (MRI). Many surgeons aiming at the VIM area will, during surgery, explore the underlying posterior subthalamic area. Several studies performed on electrode locations in the VIM nucleus have most often demonstrated that the best effect on tremor is achieved not in the VIM nucleus itself but from contacts located below the thalamus, in the posterior subthalamic area.[27-31]

Posterior Subthalamic Area

The posterior subthalamic area is the area inferior to the motor ventral thalamus, lateral to the red nucleus, and medial and posteromedial to the STN.[32] The primary components are the sparse nuclear structure called the *zona incerta,* which runs medial to the medial border of the STN; the fiber tracts of the prelemniscal radiation, the lemniscus; and the fasciculus cerebellothalamicus, as well as Forel's fields (which consist of the thalamic fasciculus, the ansa lenticularis, and the lenticular fasciculus). For tremor DBS, different groups have chosen slightly different target points within the posterior subthalamic area.[26,32-34]

Caudal Zona Incerta

The zona incerta is the continuation of the reticular nucleus of the thalamus extending inferiorly to an area in between the STN and the ventral thalamus. The zona incerta continues just medially to the STN, ending in the so-called Q area posteromedial to the tail of the STN (Fig. 87-1). The prefix "caudal" was added by Plaha and colleagues[26] to distinguish this posterior inferior part of the zona incerta from the more anterior and superior (i.e., rostral) part often encompassed by dorsal contacts of the electrode when DBS is aimed at the STN area.[25,35,36] Targeting the cZI specifically is important because the antitremor effect of DBS in this particular area is rather robust, even if it is unclear whether the effect is achieved by modulating activity at the cZI itself; by influencing the concentration of cerebellothalamic fibers, including the dentatorubrothalamic tract[37,38] in its vicinity; or by some other mechanism.[26,29,32,33,39]

Globus Pallidus Internus

The posteroventral part of the GPi is considered to subserve sensorimotor function and is the preferred target for both pallidotomy and pallidal DBS in Parkinson's disease and dystonia. Because it is of peripheral interest in this chapter, and because it is detailed in other chapters that deal with surgery for dystonia and Parkinson's disease, it is not mentioned further here.

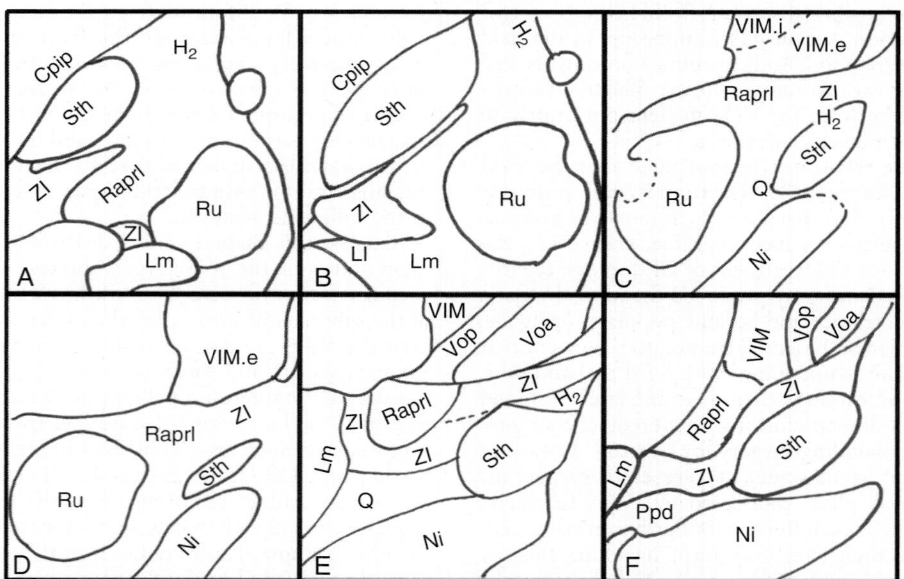

Figure 87-1. Schematic drawings based on Schaltenbrand and Wahren's *Atlas,*[45] showing selected structures in the posterior subthalamic area and its surroundings. A and **B,** Horizontal views of the structures in the left hemisphere, 1.5 mm **(A)** and 3.5 mm **(B)** below the anterior commissure–posterior commissure line. **C** and **D,** Coronal views of the structures in the right hemisphere, 5 mm **(C)** and 7 mm **(D)** posterior to the midcommissural point. **E** and **F,** Parasagittal views, 10.5 mm **(E)** and 13 mm **(F)** lateral to the midline. Cpip, Posterior limb of the internal capsule; H2, field H2 of Forel; Ll, lateral lemniscus; Lm, medial lemniscus; Ni, substantia nigra; Ppd, peripeduncular nucleus; Q, fasciculus Q; Raprl, prelemniscal radiations; Ru, red nucleus; Sth, subthalamic nucleus; VIM.e, external part of the ventral intermediate nucleus of the thalamus; VIM.i, internal part of the ventral intermediate nucleus of the thalamus; Voa, ventral oral anterior nucleus of the thalamus; Vop, nucleus ventral oral posterior nucleus of the thalamus; ZI, zona incerta. *(Modified from Schaltenbrand G, Wahren W, eds.* Atlas for Stereotaxy of the Human Brain. *2nd ed. Stuttgart: Thieme; 1977.)*

IMAGING AND TARGETING

Subthalamic Nucleus

The typical coordinates of the target point in the STN in relation to the anterior commissure–posterior commissure (AC-PC) line and the midcommissural point are as follows: $X = 12$, $Y = -3$, $Z = -4$. However, the exact location and the orientation in space of the STN vary.[40,41] Because the STN is visualized on T2-weighted MRI, it is best to target what the surgeon can see[41]: hence, the target point for DBS within the visualized STN is identified on an axial scan at the horizontal level, in which the maximal diameter of the red nucleus is shown. On the scan, a line is drawn between the anterior margins of the red nuclei, extending into the STN. The target point is approximately 1 to 2 mm behind this line, 1 to 2 mm lateral to the medial margin of the STN. The second deepest contact of the narrow-space 3389 DBS electrode should be placed at the target point. A double oblique approach is planned to avoid sulci and the ventricle, and the angulation of the trajectory can be modified to enable the placement of as many electrode contacts as possible into the STN.

Ventral Intermediate Nucleus

The VIM nucleus cannot yet be visualized with standard imaging. Nonetheless, the VIM nucleus as a target is mentioned as a mantra in many papers on thalamotomy or DBS, without any systematic verification that the lesion or the DBS electrode is indeed in the VIM area.

In fact, the VIM nucleus as a defined structure of the ventrolateral motor thalamus is a discovery that was enabled by microelectrode recording (MER), whereby kinesthetic cells and cells that fire at tremor frequency were identified in an area in between the ventral oral nuclei and the sensory thalamus. Microrecording studies have shown that the homunculus in the VIM nucleus is horizontally oriented, with the area representing the head most medial and the leg area most lateral. The pioneers of thalamotomy, especially those who did not use MER for targeting, used to label their procedure for tremor as "ventrolateral" thalamotomy or simply "thalamotomy" and not VIM thalamotomy. The target of Leksell, for example, was 10 mm lateral to the midcommissural point, on the AC-PC level. This corresponds to the region of the ventral oral posterior nucleus as shown in the *Atlas* of Schaltenbrand and Wahren.[45] In 1985, Laitinen[46] surveyed 16 well-known functional neurosurgeons about their coordinates for thalamotomy and showed that their targets differed by up to 7 mm.

So how does the surgeon define the VIM target when that structure cannot be visualized? Most strategies are based on the postulated location of the VIM nucleus in relation to the ventricular landmarks. Because the length of the AC-PC line is variable by up to 1 cm between patients and the width of the ventricle is also very variable, most authors use proportional values to determine the target point, the most common of these being the Guiot diagram.[11,47] The variability of the target affects primarily its anteroposterior location and its laterality, whereas the height coordinate remains rather constant and defined as lying between the level of the AC-PC line and up to 2 mm above.

In our practice, which spans three decades, we have found it most convenient to define the target point in relation to the nearest ventricular landmark (i.e., the posterior commissure) as follows: the Y coordinate is 2 mm less than one-third the length of the AC-PC line in front of the posterior commissure. For example, if the AC-PC length is 24 mm, the Y value of the target point is 6 mm in front of the posterior commissure. The Z coordinate is at the level of the AC-PC line; and the X coordinate is 13 to 14 mm from the midline of the third ventricle. These calculations are done on an axial MRI scan at the level of the AC-PC. For deciding the laterality, it is an advantage if the thalamocapsular border can be visualized. This may be possible on inversion recovery or proton density sequences, although the resolution of the images may not be high enough on thin slices to enable a very precise delineation of that border. Some authors use tractographic MRI to visualize the fibers of the internal capsule lateral to the thalamus, but this method may also be too crude because the resolution on thin slices is poor, and it does not obviate the need for intraoperative exploration of the target.[48] In any case, the final location of the DBS electrode (or the RF lesion) is decided during intraoperative stimulation to verify effect on tremor and avoidance of internal capsule and sensory thalamus (details are described later).

Caudal Zona Incerta

As stated previously, the experience with DBS for tremor,[25-28,38] in comparison with past experience with ablative procedures,[49,50] indicates that the cZI may be an even better target for tremor than the VIM-ventrolateral thalamus. Thus we now target the cZI instead of the VIM nucleus. The cZI target is identified on T2-weighted axial MRI at the same depth as the target in the STN. The target lies just medial to the tail of the STN. A horizontal line is drawn from the center of the red nucleus at the level of its largest diameter to the posterior tip of the STN; we take into consideration the fact that sometimes the tail of the STN can be difficult to discern in elderly patients. The target point is located 0 to 1 mm behind this line, at about one third of the distance from the STN tail to the lateral border of the red nucleus (Fig. 87-2). The deepest contact of the 3389 electrode is placed in that target (or slightly deeper, depending on response to intraoperative stimulation if surgery is done with local anesthesia; details are described later). The trajectory of the electrode can be adjusted so that the electrode is traversing the VIM-ventrolateral thalamus and the highest contact of the electrode is left in this structure (Fig. 87-3). The typical coordinates of the cZI target in relation to the AC-PC line and midcommissural point are as follows: $X = 11$ to 13, $Y = -7$ to -8, and $Z = -4$ to -5. However, we do not use statistical coordinates for targeting because our use of individual targeting is based on visualized structures.

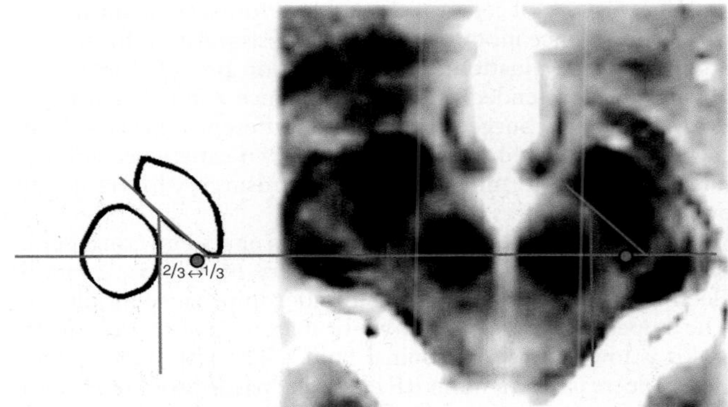

Figure 87-2. Schematic drawing and actual stereotactic magnetic resonance image of the posterior subthalamic area at 4 mm below the anterior commissure–posterior commissure plane. The *horizontal red line* connects the center of the red nucleus to the posterior tail of the subthalamic nucleus (STN). The *oblique red line* indicates the medial border of the STN. The *vertical red line* indicates the lateral border of the red nucleus. The *red dot* indicates the target in the caudal zona incerta, at one third of the distance between the tail of the STN and the lateral border of the red nucleus.

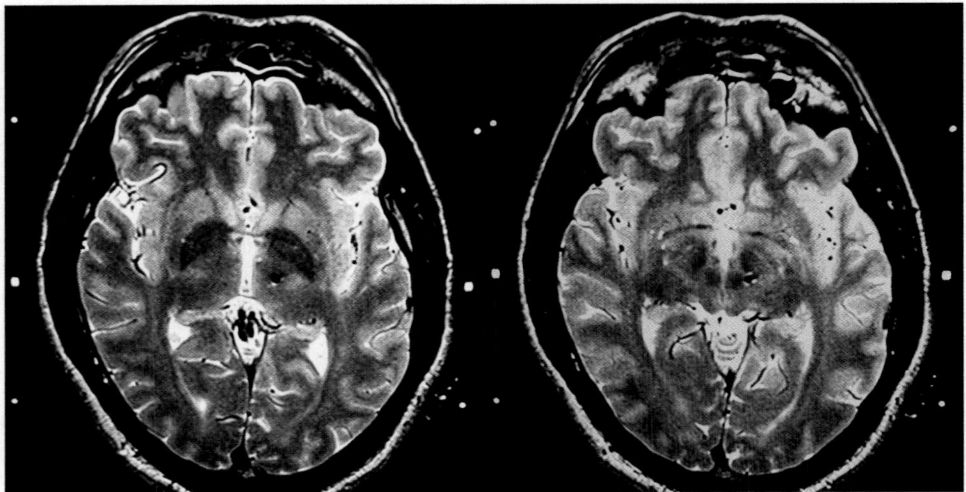

Figure 87-3. Postoperative stereotactic magnetic resonance image, showing a 3389 deep brain stimulation (DBS) electrode. One contact is in the left ventrolateral thalamus at the level of the anterior commissure–posterior commissure line *(left),* and one contact is at the level of the caudal zona incerta, 4 mm ventral to the anterior commissure–posterior commissure plane *(right).* The diameter of the artifact of the DBS electrode appears larger than the electrode's real diameter of 1.27 mm.

INTRAOPERATIVE EXPLORATION OF THE TARGET IN VIEW OF DEEP BRAIN STIMULATION

In most centers, surgery for tremor is performed with local anesthetic, with the patient fully awake and not sedated. In contrast, surgery aimed at the cZI or the STN can be performed with the patient under general anesthesia because the brain target can be visualized both before and after surgery. In any case, surgeons who operate with general anesthetic must obtain (1) enough experience in intraoperative test stimulation in a large number of patients who are awake and (2) a good knowledge of the location of the electrodes in these patients on immediate postoperative stereotactic imaging: either postoperative stereotactic MRI or postoperative stereotactic computed tomographic scan fused with the preoperative stereotactic MRI.

Whereas several centers rely on MER for target identification, we use impedance monitoring and macrostimulation for intraoperative target evaluation. The information provided in the following text is intended as general guidance and is based on our own experience. Surgeons may have different approaches, and each surgeon should obtain his or her own experience and confidence when performing functional neurosurgery for tremor and other brain disorders.

We use the Leksell stereotactic system and an imaging-guided and imaging-verified approach. At surgery, first a 1.5 × 2 mm RF electrode is directed to the target under impedance monitoring. The impedance is higher in white matter than in gray matter and it is lowest in cerebrospinal fluid.[51] The impedance pitch is clearly decreased when the RF electrode passes from the internal capsule into the gray matter of the reticular nucleus of the thalamus en route to the ventrolateral thalamus or the cZI or when it comes from the internal capsule and enters the STN. If the surgery is a DBS procedure, the RF electrode is then withdrawn and replaced immediately by the DBS electrode. The dural opening is sealed with biologic glue to avoid entry of air with resulting brain shift.[52]

When the VIM nucleus or the cZI is targeted, the surgeon may observe a "stun" or "microlesion" effect on the tremor once the electrode hits the target. Stimulation can still be carried out to test for potential side effects. Also, the patient can be asked to count backward or to list the months or the days backward in order to provoke the reappearance of tremor.

Stimulation is carried out in a monopolar manner through each of the contacts of the electrode, at 60 to 90 microseconds and 130 Hz up to 3 V; this helps the surgeon map the area and detect effects and side effects. When DBS is targeted to the VIM-ventrolateral thalamus, persistent paresthesias in the fingertips or the lips, or both, at low voltage may indicate that the position of the contact is too posterior, with stimulation of the sensory thalamus. Likewise, dysarthria and a feeling of cramps in the hand or the lips may indicate a too lateral a position into or close to the internal capsule. If tremor is not affected unless a too high stimulation voltage is needed, the electrode may be too medial or anterior.

When DBS is intended for the cZI, paresthesias in the palm of the hand and the arm may not be unusual, as a result of proximity of the lemniscus. However, these reactions are transient and usually fade away within few seconds. If the patient experiences double vision, the electrode is too medial, too close to the nucleus ruber. In any case, as shown by Fytagoridis and colleagues,[53] intraoperative stimulation in the cZI area can result in a variety of side effects (dizziness, blurred vision, dysarthria) that may be difficult to interpret. Most of these are transient and will fade away during chronic stimulation.

When DBS is intended for the STN, the wrist rigidity, if present, will immediately decrease upon entrance of the electrode into the target. Then stimulation, carried out as described previously, will reveal eventual effects on tremor and eventual side effects (e.g., transient paresthesias in the hand, capsular effects, autonomic effects, appearance of dyskinesias in patients with Parkinson's disease). If stimulation at any of the targets, especially the tremor-specific targets (VIM-ventrolateral and cZI), does not yield a clear effect on tremor, then the electrode location should be verified by intraoperative stereotactic computed tomography/MRI. This helps direct retargeting of the electrode.

In all cases, whether stimulation has produced a clear and good effect on tremor or not, the surgery is not finished before an immediate postoperative stereotactic scan is performed.[54] This helps the surgeon ascertain the location of the DBS electrode and helps in future adjustments of the chronic stimulation. The neuropacemaker can then be implanted in the same session or at any later convenient time.

When DBS surgery is performed with a general anesthetic, which may be the case when DBS is targeting structures visible on MRI (STN, cZI), it is absolutely mandatory to verify good anatomic location of the electrode by a stereotactic scan with the frame still in place.

Chronic stimulation may be started either 1 to 2 days after surgery or at the first follow-up appointment after 1 to 2 weeks, which allows the edema around the electrode to subside. Chronic stimulation should not be started until the tremor has reappeared, after the microthalamotomy/stun effect. Regardless of target, an initial screening of each electrode contact in monopolar stimulation mode is recommended in order to verify thresholds for therapeutic effect and side effects. Monopolar stimulation is performed at 60 microseconds, 130 Hz, and an incremental increase of the current in steps of 0.3 to 0.5 V. In most patients, monopolar stimulation with the use of only one contact, with these parameters at a stimulation amplitude of 1.5 to 3 V, is sufficient.

Radiofrequency Thalamotomy

If a thalamotomy is to be performed, the VIM-ventrolateral thalamic target should be 1 to 2 mm more anterior than that for DBS, so that the ablative lesion does not encroach on the sensory thalamus. Thalamotomy is always performed with the patient under local anesthesia, and the RF electrode should have an uninsulated tip no larger than 2 × 2 mm, so that the surgeon may ascertain a location-specific response to stimulation before creating the lesion. Stimulation at high frequency is carried out with the RF electrode. In the absence of capsular or sensory response, and with tremor arrest, an RF lesion is produced at 75 degrees for 60 seconds at target level and another one 2 mm above or below after repeat stimulation. During lesion creation, a conversation with, and meticulous observation of, the patient is mandatory for detecting any side effect (limb weakness, dysarthria) that would prompt immediate cessation of the thermocoagulation. Sometimes a "reversible" lesion is produced first at 45 degrees, to make sure no side effect appears, before the definite lesion is created at higher temperature.

Gamma Knife Thalamotomy

Gamma Knife thalamotomy, first attempted in the 1960s but abandoned for several decades, has resurged in popularity, probably because brain imaging has improved. In modern times, Gamma Knife thalamotomy has been popularized mainly by Chihiro Ohye, a Japanese pioneer of MER thalamotomy, who gradually shifted from using MER to using Gamma Knife and whose most comprehensive and most recent paper was published posthumously in 2012.[55] Ohye's experience showed that a single shot of 130 Gy through a 4-mm collimator to produce a ventrolateral thalamotomy yielded excellent or good effect on tremor without permanent complications in more than 80% of 53 patients followed for 2 years. Today, Gamma Knife thalamotomy is used mostly by just a few groups.[56-58] The response to gamma thalamotomy is delayed by weeks or months, and in some patients, delayed radiation necrosis may result in the appearance of neurological deficits several months after the procedure. In any case, it is evident that previous good experience with open "classical" RF thalamotomy is a prerequisite for performing Gamma Knife thalamotomy, a method that does not allow exploration of the target before lesion creation and that, by definition, relies very heavily on proper imaging, proper targeting, and long experience in dosimetry and radiosurgery in general.

Focused Ultrasound Thalamotomy

Stereotactic high-frequency ultrasonography is an MRI-guided technology that creates small thermal lesions within targeted tissues in real time. In a pioneering study, Elias and colleagues[59] used this technique to perform unilateral VIM thalamotomies in 15 patients with refractory essential tremor. They used, on average, 18 sonications at a mean temperature of 58°C (136°F). At the 12-month follow-up visit, there was a 75% reduction of contralateral hand tremor scores and an 85% reduction of disability scores. No hemorrhages or motor deficits were reported. Side effects (mainly paresthesia of lips, tongue, and fingers) were mild and transient in all patients, except in one, who, at 1 year, had persistent dysesthesia of the dominant index finger. The development of this technique is still in early stages, and more experience and longer follow-up periods are needed, as is comparison with existing lesion-creating techniques and with DBS. In addition, the technique is rather costly, relying on a dedicated ultrasound machine and on the availability of the MRI suite for several hours to perform the procedure. Another disadvantage is that the lesions appear to shrink with loss of the good effect,[60] and there may be a need to repeat the procedure. The main advantage is that, as with Gamma Knife thalamotomy, the skull is not opened and no probe passes through the brain, but, in contrast to Gamma Knife thalamotomy, the effect of focused ultrasound thalamotomy is immediately visible.

RESULTS OF SURGERY ON TREMOR

In the literature on surgery for tremor, an important shift began in the 1990s. Before that time, researchers reported almost exclusively on RF thalamotomy and did not use standardized rating scales, reporting results qualitatively as excellent, good, modest, or nil. In general, unilateral thalamotomy was considered to be efficient in controlling contralateral tremor in more than 80% of patients who underwent the procedure, especially patients with Parkinson's disease and essential tremor. In contrast, the overwhelming majority of papers on surgery for tremor that have been published since the 1990s were reports on DBS for tremor, and the researchers have used standardized scales for the assessment (e.g., Fahn-Tolosa-Marin Tremor Rating Scale for essential tremor[61] and the Unified Parkinson's Disease Rating Scale for Parkinson's disease).[62] On the whole, the results of DBS are comparable with those of thalamotomy. Of these studies, only one randomized controlled trial was a comparison of thalamotomy with DBS.[63] The study demonstrated that both procedures are effective for tremor, but the patients who received DBS had fewer side effects and an overall better quality of life. What follows is a summary of the literature on results of DBS for tremor according to the cause of tremor.

Parkinsonian Tremor

It is surprisingly difficult to get a clear understanding of the effect of DBS on parkinsonian tremor from the literature. This is partly because tremor is only one of many symptoms in Parkinson's disease. The specific effect of DBS on tremor is often not reported, and if it is reported, the material normally consists of studies both of patients with Parkinson's disease who have tremor and of such patients without tremor. Moreover, several different targets are used for DBS in Parkinson's disease, and the selection criteria are not the same for the different targets.

The European multicenter study of DBS in the VIM nucleus showed a reduction of 75% of limb tremor scores in 57 unilaterally stimulated patients with tremor-dominant Parkinson's disease.[64] The effect was essentially maintained after 6 years.[65] DBS in the VIM nucleus is most often performed unilaterally because bilateral DBS in this target increases the risk of stimulation-induced dysarthria and balance impairment, especially in older patients.[66] Because of this and the lack of effect on other symptoms, the STN has become the DBS target of choice in Parkinson's disease, even in patients with tremor-dominant disease. The effects of bilateral DBS in the STN on symptoms of Parkinson's disease are well known, and there typically is approximately 75% improvement in tremor scores in nonselected patients.[67] Some studies have focused on the effects in patients with severe tremor, for whom a tremor score reduction of approximately 80% has been reported.[68-71] There are no good studies on the effect of DBS in the GPi on parkinsonian tremor. In the randomized studies in which STN and GPi were compared, researchers did not report on particular symptoms or items, or they seemed to have excluded patients in whom tremor was the only major symptom.[72-74] Because of this lack of evidence and the plethora of alternative targets, GPi cannot currently be recommended as a preferred target for tremor-dominant Parkinson's disease.

With regard to DBS in the posterior subthalamic area including the prelemniscal radiations and the cZI, an improvement in contralateral tremor has been reported in 78% to 93% of patients.[26,33,34,39,75-77] One of these studies was a longitudinal nonrandomized study in which DBS in the cZI was compared with DBS in the STN; a tremor score reduction of 93% was achieved with DBS in the cZI, whereas the electrodes placed in the STN resulted in a tremor score reduction of merely 61%.[78] The cZI is of more interest than the VIM nucleus as a target for parkinsonian tremor because DBS in the cZI may also have positive effects on other parkinsonian symptoms.[26]

Essential Tremor

Deuschl and associates[79] wrote that although DBS in the VIM nucleus or neighboring subthalamic structures had been reported to reduce tremor score by about 90%, no controlled trials of DBS have been done, and the best target is still uncertain.

The European multicenter study of VIM DBS for essential tremor reported an approximate 80% tremor score reduction in the treated arm 1 year after surgery.[64] At the 5- and 6-year follow-up visits, both the European and the North American multicenter studies showed some decline of effect over time, with 50% to 75% tremor score reduction in the treated arm.[80,81] The action tremor component is particularly difficult to control over time.[82] In our experience of 19 patients who underwent DBS in the VIM nucleus and were evaluated at a mean of 7 years after surgery, the tremor score of the contralateral upper extremity was reduced by 60%, and hand function was improved by only 35%.[83]

In several studies of DBS in the VIM nucleus for tremor, the most effective contact was apparently not in the VIM nucleus but in the subthalamic area.[25,29,34,84] This finding indicates that the subthalamic area, and especially the cZI, may be a better primary target for DBS. The available results of DBS in the cZI on tremor, including long-term effects, are generally better than those of DBS in the VIM nucleus, but no randomized comparisons have been performed.[32,84,85] DBS in the cZI apparently results in better effect at lower voltage and with less long-term development of tolerance to stimulation, than does DBS in the VIM nucleus. However, the risk of inducing ataxia at higher voltage, by affecting cerebellorubral pathways, may be higher.[86] Also, as in DBS in the VIM nucleus, the risk of dysarthria and balance problems may be increased with bilateral stimulation.[53]

Dystonic Tremor

Studies dealing with dystonic tremor have been retrospective, few, small, and heterogeneous[87,88]; nevertheless, there is little doubt that DBS is an effective treatment for dystonic tremor. The question is, however, which target to use in the individual patient: the GPi or the VIM nucleus/cZI? In our experience, DBS in the GPi often produces satisfactory results in patients with mild tremor; however, in patients with more severe tremor, the effect is sometimes not sufficient. As a rule, we favor DBS in the GPi in patients with a more generalized dystonia in which tremor is only one component, but we favor DBS in the cZi when the patient's main concern is the tremor.

Other Forms of Tremor

Regarding other forms of tremor (e.g., those related to multiple sclerosis, traumatic brain injury, and stroke), the literature is limited to case reports and minor case series, and it is difficult to evaluate the results in general because of heterogeneity of the patients. It is, however, often said that DBS in the VIM nucleus or cZI will prove efficient in about one third of such patients. In general, it is of great importance in these cases to have a clear understanding of whether the patient is disabled by tremor or ataxia.[89]

General rules regarding surgery for tremor may be summarized as follows: (1) rest tremor responds better than does intention-action tremor; (2) distal tremor responds better than does proximal tremor; (3) upper limb tremor responds better than does lower limb tremor; (4) high-frequency, low-amplitude tremor responds better than does low-frequency, high-amplitude tremor; and (5) for head tremor, bilateral stimulation is often necessary to achieve optimal results.

THERAPEUTIC FAILURE

Despite the best attempts at performing accurate and precise surgery, therapeutic failure may occur. There are several reasons for treatment failure, and, depending on the nature of the failure, different modes of investigation are necessary. When the effect of chronic stimulation ceases suddenly and completely, the DBS system should be suspected and evaluated with regard to battery life or breakage in the circuitry, which can be suspected when measured impedances are very high. In cases of slow deterioration after a long period of good effect, a new systematic screening of stimulation effects or a change in stimulation parameters, or both, might prove helpful. A reevaluation of the patient may also be valuable. Is the diagnosis correct? Does the patient exhibit the same symptoms as before surgery, or has a new ataxic component developed, for which DBS will have no effect? In many cases of slow deterioration, either disease progression or tolerance can be suspected. In order to evaluate the possible degree of progression, the patient should be evaluated off stimulation and the results compared to the situation before surgery. Another possible cause is the development of tolerance to stimulation over time, making it necessary to increase the stimulation parameters, which in some cases may cause ataxia. This phenomenon has been reported after DBS of the VIM nucleus and after subthalamic DBS.[82,83,90-93] Some authors have suggested that the cause might be the properties of the VIM nucleus itself,[94] whereas others relate it to DBS in the subthalamic area.[86] These phenomena seem to occur more in patients with essential tremor than in patients with Parkinson's disease.

When tolerance to DBS develops, a "stimulation vacation" of approximately 2 weeks (sometimes necessitating hospitalization and clozapine treatment) may break the cycle, and tremor reduction at a lower amplitude may be renewed when stimulation is resumed. In patients with DBS of the VIM nucleus and declining effect over longer periods, a new electrode inserted in the cZI sometimes improves the result.[95,96] Alternatively, stimulation may be replaced by RF thalamotomy, performed in the standard manner after removal of the stimulating electrode or through the implanted electrode,[97,98] although this method is not yet validated or established.

SUGGESTED READINGS

Benabid AL, Pollak P, Gervason C, et al. Long-term suppression of tremor by chronic stimulation of the ventral intermediate thalamic nucleus. *Lancet*. 1991;337:403-406.

Blomstedt P, Hariz GM, Hariz MI, et al. Thalamic deep brain stimulation in the treatment of essential tremor: a long-term follow-up. *Br J Neurosurg*. 2007;21(5):504-509.

Blomstedt P, Hariz MI. Deep brain stimulation for movement disorders before DBS for movement disorders. *Parkinsonism Relat Disord*. 2010; 16(7):429-433.

Blomstedt P, Sandvik U, Fytagoridis A, et al. The posterior subthalamic area in the treatment of movement disorders: past, present, and future. *Neurosurgery*. 2009;64(6):1029-1038.

Caire F, Ranoux D, Guehl D, et al. A systematic review of studies on anatomical position of electrode contacts used for chronic subthalamic stimulation in Parkinson's disease. *Acta Neurochir (Wien)*. 2013;155(9): 1647-1654.

Coenen VA, Mädler B, Schiffbauer H, et al. Individual fiber anatomy of the subthalamic region revealed with diffusion tensor imaging: a concept to identify the deep brain stimulation target for tremor suppression. *Neurosurgery*. 2011;68(4):1069-1075.

Deuschl G, Bain P, Brin M. Consensus statement of the Movement Disorder Society on Tremor. Ad Hoc Scientific Committee. *Mov Disord*. 1998;13(suppl 3):2-23.

Elble RJ. Tremor disorders. *Curr Opin Neurol*. 2013;26(4):413-419.

Elias WJ, Huss D, Voss T. A pilot study of focused ultrasound thalamotomy for essential tremor. *N Engl J Med*. 2013;369(7):640-648.

Fytagoridis A, Astrom M, Wardell K, et al. Stimulation-induced side effects in the posterior subthalamic area: distribution, characteristics and visualization. *Clin Neurol Neurosurg*. 2013;115(1):65-71.

Fytagoridis A, Sandvik U, Astrom M, et al. Long term follow-up of deep brain stimulation of the caudal zona incerta for essential tremor. *J Neurol Neurosurg Psychiatry*. 2012;83(3):258-262.

Hamel W, Herzog J, Kopper F, et al. Deep brain stimulation in the subthalamic area is more effective than ventralis intermedius stimulation for bilateral intention tremor. *Acta Neurochir*. 2007;149(8):749-758.

Hariz MI, Krack P, Alesch F, et al. Multicentre European study of thalamic stimulation for parkinsonian tremor: a 6 year follow-up. *J Neurol Neurosurg Psychiatry*. 2008;79(6):694-699.

Hariz MI, Krack P, Melvill R, et al. A quick and universal method for stereotactic visualization of the subthalamic nucleus before and after implantation of deep brain stimulation electrodes. *Stereotact Funct Neurosurg*. 2003;80(1–4):96-101.

Herzog J, Hamel W, Wenzelburger R, et al. Kinematic analysis of thalamic versus subthalamic neurostimulation in postural and intention tremor. *Brain*. 2007;130(6):1608-1625.

Koller W, Pahwa R, Busenbark K, et al. High-frequency unilateral thalamic stimulation in the treatment of essential and parkinsonian tremor. *Ann Neurol*. 1997;42(3):292-299.

Kondziolka D, Ong JG, Lee JY, et al. Gamma Knife thalamotomy for essential tremor. *J Neurosurg*. 2008;108(1):111-117.

Laitinen LV. Brain targets in surgery for Parkinson's disease. Results of a survey of neurosurgeons. *J Neurosurg*. 1985;62(3):349-351.

Limousin P, Speelman JD, Gielen F, et al. Multicentre European study of thalamic stimulation in parkinsonian and essential tremor. *J Neurol Neurosurg Psychiatry*. 1999;66(3):289-296.

Ohye C, Higuchi Y, Shibazaki T, et al. Gamma Knife thalamotomy for Parkinson disease and essential tremor: a prospective multicenter study. *Neurosurgery*. 2012;70(3):526-535.

Plaha P, Khan S, Gill SS. Bilateral stimulation of the caudal zona incerta nucleus for tremor control. *J Neurol Neurosurg Psychiatry*. 2008;79(5): 504-513.

Sandvik U, Koskinen LO, Lundqvist A, et al. Thalamic and subthalamic DBS for essential tremor—where is the optimal target? *Neurosurgery*. 2012;70(4):840-845.

Sydow O, Thobois S, Alesch F, et al. Multicentre European study of thalamic stimulation in essential tremor: a six year follow up. *J Neurol Neurosurg Psychiatry*. 2003;74(10):1387-1391.

Velasco F, Jiménez F, Pérez ML, et al. Electrical stimulation of the prelemniscal radiation in the treatment of Parkinson's disease: an old target revised with new techniques. *Neurosurgery*. 2001;49(2): 293-306.

Zrinzo L, Hariz MI. Impedance recording in functional neurosurgery. In: Lozano AM, Gildenberg PL, Tasker RR, eds. *Textbook of Stereotactic and Functional Neurosurgery*. Berlin: Springer-Verlag; 2009: 1325-1330.

See a full reference list on ExpertConsult.com

88 Ablative Procedures for Parkinson's Disease

Robert E. Gross, Matthew A. Stern, and Joash T. Lazarus

Patients with advanced Parkinson's disease (PD) experience increasing motor and nonmotor symptoms and waning effectiveness and/or serious adverse effects of optimized medication management. For these patients there are now several nonablative surgical options for symptomatic relief, including deep brain stimulation (DBS) and in some centers experimental neural transplantation or gene therapy. However, ablative procedures remain a viable and well-founded surgical option. For almost 80 years, ablative surgeries of the basal ganglia and associated structures, most notably pallidotomy, subthalamotomy, and thalamotomy, have been used in the treatment of PD, and in fact were the primary treatment for decades before the advent of levodopa medical therapy. Particularly in the last 30 years, with great strides having been made in the understanding of basal ganglia physiology and the pathophysiology of PD, coupled with the significant advances in imaging technology and stereotactic equipment, these neurosurgical procedures have become more effective, accurate, and safe, providing patients with years of improved quality of life.

HISTORICAL BACKGROUND

An expanded discussion on the history of surgical interventions in the treatment of movement disorder symptoms is available at ExpertConsult.com.

Levodopa treatment for PD was introduced in 1961 and became widely available by 1968,[41,42] close to half a century after dopamine's discovery in 1913 by Guggenheim. Its remarkable benefits and rapidly growing popularity led to a significant decline in stereotactic surgical intervention for PD.[42-45] However, within a few decades it was appreciated that long-term use of levodopa required an increasing cumulative dose to maintain effective symptom management, could result in medication-induced toxicity (e.g., worsening dyskinesia and "on-off" fluctuations), waning efficacy with disease progression, and significant end-dose deterioration.[46] Given these observed effects with chronic use, there was a clear need for supplementary treatment options. This drove a resurgence of stereotactic neurosurgical treatments, with Kelly and coworkers reintroducing thalamotomy[47,48] and Laitinen and coworkers reintroducing Leksell's pallidotomy,[49-51] which coincided with advances in brain imaging (computed tomography [CT], magnetic resonance imaging [MRI]) and intraoperative electrophysiologic techniques. Moreover, physiologic and anatomic support for these targets was coincidentally being propelled by the work of DeLong and colleagues,[52-56] Filion and Tremblay,[57] and Albin and colleagues,[58] on the circuitry of the basal ganglia and the pathophysiology of PD, in large measure based on the advent of the 1-methyl-4-phenyl-1,2,3,6-tetrahydropyridine (MPTP) nonhuman primate model of PD. Thus the basal ganglia and associated structures were further solidified as the surgical target of choice, being associated with significant and sustained motor benefit contralateral to the lesion.[45,59,60]

Although through the 1990s, pallidotomy and (to a lesser extent) thalamotomy were increasingly evaluated for PD and other movement disorders,[61] this resurgence was short-lived. In the late 1980s and early 1990s, Benabid and Siegfried and their colleagues introduced DBS of the basal ganglia (subthalamic nucleus [STN] and GPi) and thalamus as an alternative to lesioning,[62-66] which rapidly became the standard surgical therapy for providing relief of symptoms in patients with severe levodopa-responsive PD and/or tremor. DBS supplanted lesioning owing to an equivalent efficacy and improved safety profile, including bilateral implantations.[67-73] Nevertheless, in many areas of the world, especially the developing world, and where cost is a prohibiting factor, subthalamotomy and pallidotomy still remain the preferred first-line surgical option.[45,60,74-86]

PHYSIOLOGIC BASIS FOR ABLATION PROCEDURES FOR PARKINSON'S DISEASE

Pallidotomy

The fundamental deficiency in PD lies in the substantia nigra pars compacta (SNc), where loss of dopaminergic neurons ultimately results in increased inhibitory γ-aminobutyric acid (GABA)–ergic output from GPi and the substantia nigra pars reticulata (SNr), the latter being less important in primates than rodents.[52-58,87-90] (Fig. 88-1A and B). GPi hyperactivity excessively inhibits the thalamus and its excitatory drive of the downstream cortical motor systems and brainstem motor areas. This dysregulation is exacerbated by the irregular output of GPi in PD, and thus also of the thalamocortical projections. Ultimately the thalamus and brainstem are less able to regulate movement, especially the initiation of movement, leading to the classic clinical symptoms of disrupted and impoverished movements.[91] Pallidotomy involves selective ablation of the sensorimotor regions of GPi, decreasing its inhibitory output and thereby normalizing downstream thalamocortical activity and brainstem motor area function (Fig. 88-1C). The lesions are targeted to the sensorimotor portion of the GPi, which is defined by a population of neurons that respond to movement, whereas the limbic and associative territories of GPi are avoided, as are the adjacent globus pallidus externa (GPe), optic tract, and internal capsule.

Subthalamic Nucleotomy

Historically, subthalamotomy involved lesions of the thalamic afferent fibers coursing below the thalamus rather than the STN itself, which was carefully avoided owing to the specter of known association of hemiballismus with strokes involving the nucleus itself. In the 1990s during the resurgence of pallidotomy, subthalamotomy as previously performed did not receive renewed attention, perhaps because of lack of a known physiologic basis for this operation. However, the seminal research of DeLong and colleagues identified the central role of STN hyperactivity, resulting from dysregulation of the indirect pathway caused by the dopaminergic deficit (see Fig. 88-1B). Subsequently they demonstrated in the nonhuman primate MPTP model that blocking this activity leads to amelioration of symptoms, thus providing a physiologic basis for STN ablation (subthalamic nucleotomy) in PD patients, as well as STN DBS[56,90,92] (see Fig. 88-1D).

Ventral Intermediate Thalamotomy

The VIM nucleus of the thalamus, which predominantly receives contralateral cerebellar inputs, sends projections ipsilaterally to

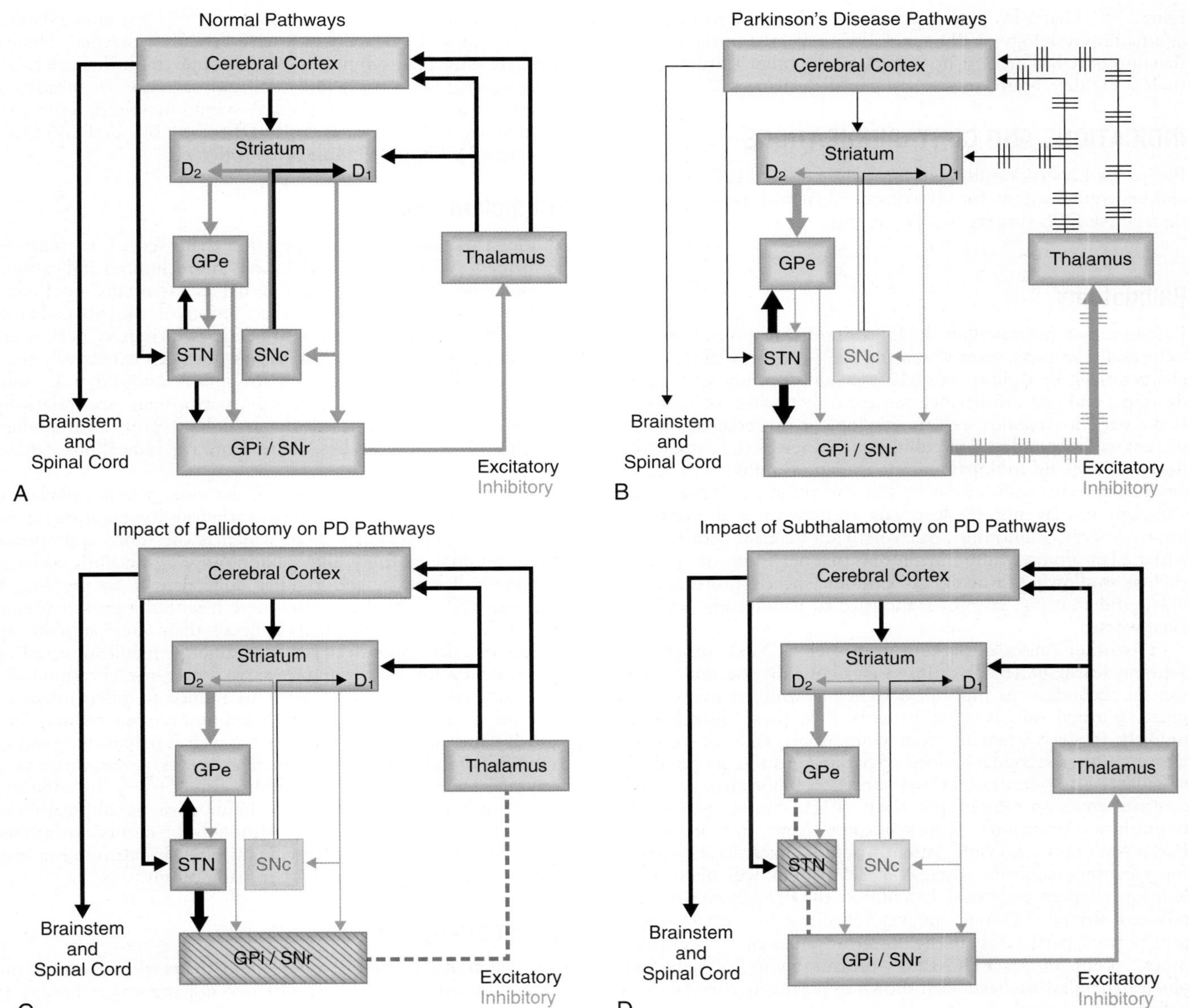

Figure 88-1. Basal ganglia circuitry relevant to Parkinson's disease and its surgical treatment. **A,** Simplified normal circuit diagram. *Red* denotes inhibitory efferent projections; *black* denotes excitatory efferent projections. Other relevant nuclei are omitted for simplicity (e.g., reticular nucleus of thalamus). **B,** Diagram depicting changes in the basal ganglia after degeneration of substantia nigra compacta dopaminergic neurons. Increased efferent activity is denoted by an *increase in line thickness,* and decrease in efferent output is denoted by *decreased line thickness. Hash marks* in the output pathway indicate pathologically irregular firing patterns, which contribute to the symptomatic features of the disease. **C** and **D,** Alteration in the pathologic activity of the basal ganglia after pallidotomy **(C)** and subthalamotomy **(D).** *Dashed lines* indicate output pathways that are no longer present after ablation. Note that SNr output would in fact be preserved after GPi pallidotomy. D1, striatopallidal neurons with excitatory postsynaptic D1 dopamine receptors; D2, striatopallidal neurons with inhibitory D2 receptors; GPe, globus pallidus externa; GPi, globus pallidus interna; SNc, substantia nigra pars compacta; SNr, substantia nigra pars reticulata; STN, subthalamic nucleus.

the primary motor cortex, premotor and supplementary motor cortical areas. In PD it has been shown that many of the cells of the VIM nucleus have a discharge pattern synchronized with the patient's tremor and have been dubbed *tremor cells.*[93-95] Given these findings, additional research was undertaken to further characterize the pathogenesis of PD as related to the tremor cells.[96-99] However, a satisfactory understanding of the pathogenesis of tremor and tremor cells in PD remains elusive. As a justification for surgical treatment within VIM for tremor—not just from PD, but of essentially all origins such as essential tremor and multiple sclerosis—we still rely on the empirical observations made decades ago: intraoperative electrical stimulation of the tremor cells, ostensibly to inhibit them, produces tremor arrest, and VIM thalamotomy produces long-term tremor relief.[100,101] That VIM plays a peripheral role in the pathogenesis and pathophysiology of PD generally is reflected in the fact that thalamotomy has little or no impact on the other features of PD such as rigidity, bradykinesia, and gait disturbances.

INDICATIONS AND CONTRAINDICATIONS

Please see ExpertConsult.com for a discussion of the indications and contraindications for stereotactic ablative surgery and nondestructive DBS surgery in PD patients.

Pallidotomy

Pallidotomy is indicated for the following PD features: levodopa-induced dyskinesias; severe "wearing off" or "on-off" fluctuations characterized by rigidity, bradykinesia, and tremor; "off"-period dystonia; and gait disturbance present only during "off" periods. If the patient responds well to levodopa, it is predicted that the patient will respond well to pallidotomy, whereas the patient who does not respond to dopaminergic therapy is unlikely to receive any benefit with pallidotomy.[126] The exception is tremor, which, although it may not be levodopa responsive, will likely still improve with pallidotomy. Such patients may be better served with thalamotomy. Midline symptoms that persist in "on" periods, such as swallowing difficulty, hypophonic speech, postural instability, and freezing, are not responsive to pallidotomy and may even worsen.

The other causes of parkinsonism such as MSA, progressive supranuclear palsy (PSP), diffuse Lewy body disease, and parkinsonism secondary to multifocal ischemic white matter disease must be ruled out, because patients with these disorders are unlikely to derive benefit from pallidotomy and may actually worsen. Other secondary forms of parkinsonism (e.g., pugilistic, vascular) also contraindicate surgery. Fluorodeoxyglucose–positron emission tomography (FDG-PET) can be used to distinguish a Parkinson's plus syndrome from PD, because a Parkinson's plus syndrome patient would be likely to show lentiform hypometabolism, whereas a PD patient will likely show lentiform hypermetabolism. In addition, the PD patient will show reduced striatal ^{18}F-dopa uptake, reflecting loss of dopamine transporters, particularly in the posterior putamen.[127-129] Furthermore, preoperative FDG-PET measurements of lentiform glucose metabolism have been shown to positively correlate with pallidotomy clinical outcomes.[130]

The optimum age for pallidotomy is questionable; studies have shown more benefit in the young,[131-133] more benefit with age,[134] and no relationship with age.[135] Thus age is a less important selection criterion. However, pallidotomy is not offered to end-stage, wheelchair-bound, or bedridden patients because, not unlike the aforementioned cognitively impaired patients, they may not derive optimal benefit from the procedure such that their activities of daily living (ADLs) and quality of life are improved. Given the disabling nature of these conditions, these patients are often unresponsive to medication or surgery.[136]

Although bilateral pallidotomies have been shown to produce both short- and long-term benefit to tremor, rigidity, bradykinesia, ADLs, and dyskinesia,[50,137-140] bilateral surgery has not been extensively evaluated in controlled trials, and the risk of impairment to speech, swallowing, cognition, and gait after bilateral pallidotomy is generally considered to be too great.[141,142] The benefits of pallidotomy are predominantly unilateral, so it is typically performed contralateral to the patient's worse presenting side. Hence, unilateral tremor is a positive predictive factor for favorable surgical outcome.[126] In the case of symmetrical presentation, the pallidotomy is performed in the patient's dominant hemisphere. However, it is important to note that unilateral surgery has shown some sustained benefit to gait and postural stability in both "on" and "off" states,[139,143,144] but after bilateral surgery gait and balance issues have actually worsened. Hence, when treating axial symptoms, wherein one might believe bilateral surgery is necessary, a unilateral approach can be considered. For patients with severe bilateral symptomatology, unilateral pallidotomy and contralateral GPi DBS,[145-147] bilateral GPi DBS, or bilateral STN DBS[148] can be considered.

Subthalamotomy

Although pallidotomy is an operation that used to be routinely performed and now, given DBS, has more limited indications, subthalamotomy is an operation that is essentially no longer used as originally performed (i.e., lesion of the fibers below the STN), and the present manner in which it is performed (i.e., actual ablation of the STN) has not been extensively used or studied. Thus the indications for subthalamotomy (i.e., subthalamic nucleotomy as currently performed) are relatively unclear. Nevertheless, based on physiology, preclinical studies, and limited clinical studies, these tentative indications can be put forth.

Subthalamotomy is indicated for the same patient population as pallidotomy. However, the slight variations in outcomes can be used to provide guidance as to which is the more appropriate lesion. Subthalamotomy, like pallidotomy, significantly reduces tremor, bradykinesia, and rigidity contralateral to the lesion. However, after subthalamotomy there has been a greater reduction in dopaminergic medication needs than after pallidotomy, because of a decreased need for dopaminergic medication and/or the tendency for subthalamotomy to lower the threshold for drug-induced dyskinesia or even to induce it independent of medication. Thus, although subthalamotomy does reduce "on" state dyskinesia, it does not reduce it as well as pallidotomy owing to the risk of inducing medication-related dyskinesias, which may even necessitate subsequent pallidotomy.[74,77,78,83,85] In addition, subthalamotomies carry a risk of hemiballismus, although the extent of this risk is debated.[79-81] Although the number of studies is too small to draw a reliable conclusion, subthalamotomy may be safer to perform bilaterally than pallidotomy.[75,76,79]

Thalamotomy

VIM thalamotomy is indicated in PD patients with severe, asymmetrical tremor that is unresponsive to dopaminergic therapy. It should provide significant tremor relief but will not improve the other PD symptoms of bradykinesia, micrographia, speech disturbances, and gait disturbances.[43] There is some evidence to suggest that lesioning the ventralis oralis posterior (VOP) nucleus, a pallidal receiving area situated anterior to the VIM nucleus that also contains tremor cells, may provide improvement with rigidity and dyskinesia.[149,150] It can also be used as a treatment for patients who do not experience significant tremor relief from a prior unilateral pallidotomy.[151] Given that the benefit of thalamotomy is confined to tremor relief, there has been a progressive decline in the number performed. It is performed unilaterally because bilateral thalamotomies have a high incidence of adverse speech and balance effects.

SURGICAL TECHNIQUES

The basic stereotactic lesioning procedures for pallidotomy, subthalamotomy, and thalamotomy are quite similar, so they are described here together.[83,85,152-155]

Imaging and Planning

The heyday of pallidotomy and thalamotomy predated the advent of more advanced frameless techniques, so essentially all lesions were at that time performed using a classic-type stereotactic frame. In fact, there are no published reports of use of later types of customized frames (e.g., microTargeting platform; FHC, Bowdoin, ME) or image guidance frames (e.g., Nexframe; Medtronic, Minneapolis, MN). Thus, typically even today the procedure begins with three-dimensional image acquisition with the patient in a stereotactic frame (see Video 88-1 for a demonstration of this procedure from stereotactic frame placement through intraoperative mapping of GPi). This is either contrast-enhanced MRI or, alternatively, a volumetric CT scan when a previous MRI has been obtained without a frame, with the two image sets subsequently coregistered. If a patient cannot undergo MRI because of a pacemaker that cannot be inactivated, a stereotactic CT scan alone may suffice. Ventriculography, a standard technique often used in the past, is rarely used these days.

Surgery is performed with the patient in the "off" state, with medication having been withheld overnight. This (1) facilitates microelectrode mapping, because in the "off" state the difference in the neuronal firing pattern and the rate between the GPe and GPi, and within the STN, is accentuated; (2) avoids the presence of dyskinesia during surgery, which can increase the risk of frame dislodgment and injury; and (3) allows for direct observation of the clinical effects of radiofrequency ablation. Furthermore, in the case of tremor, whether targeting the GPi, STN, or VIM, this maximizes the observation of tremor-related cells. If the patient is uncomfortable—for example, if he or she is experiencing painful "off" period dystonia—short-acting antiparkinsonian medication may be administered before imaging. If the patient has severe dystonia, tremor, or anxiety that would preclude getting an adequate image set, the patient can be imaged with general anesthesia.

The imaging set(s) are imported into a neuronavigation computer workstation with software that allows for stereotactic targeting, of which there are now many types (eFig. 88-1). Targeting for GPi, STN, or VIM can be done using consensus indirect targeting coordinates in Talairach space—that is, with respect to the intercommissural line between the anterior and posterior commissures. However, with advancements in imaging parameters and MRI field strength, direct targeting is now increasingly used for GPi and STN; VIM is not observable directly in clinical strength magnets. An additional aid to targeting is the use of atlases to assist in identification of the target. Increasingly, techniques for patient-specific atlas conformation, or the use of probabilistic atlases based on large previous data sets, are becoming available. Our proprietary software allows us to adjust the contours of the basal ganglia and thalamus from an interpolated digital version of the Schaltenbrand and Wahren atlas to the boundaries visible on standard 1.5-T T1-weighted image sets (One Track). This software can then be used to plan the best trajectory to approach the target.

The GPi target coordinates used today remain close to the original coordinates proposed by Laitinen,[49] 2 to 3 mm anterior to the midcommissural point, 3 to 6 mm below the intercommissural line and 20 to 21 mm lateral to the midline (see eFig. 88-1A). The subthalamic target is 2 to 3 mm posterior to the midcommissural point, 12 to 14 mm lateral to the anterior commissure–posterior commissure, and 4 to 6 mm inferior to the anterior commissure–posterior commissure.[77,78] The thalamic target is usually 25% of the anterior commissure–posterior commissure length posterior to the midcommissural point on the intercommissural plane and 11.5 mm lateral to the ventricle[156] (see eFig. 88-1B).

Neurophysiologic Mapping

More information on mapping setup and planning is also available at ExpertConsult.com.

To help ensure the proper and safe placement of GPi lesions, the optic tract, internal capsule, and sensorimotor region of the GPi, which contains the population of movement responsive neurons, must be identified (Fig. 88-2). The recording of movement-responsive neurons will direct the lesion to the posteroventral lateral region of the GPi, where clinical benefits are greatest. The mediolateral position of the GPi is somewhat dependent on the width of the third ventricle.[160] For example, with a wide third ventricle the entire basal ganglia unit may be displaced laterally; thus a trajectory at 20 mm lateral, which in a patient with a narrow ventricle might be in the correct location, would be too medial. In addition to recording sensorimotor activity to help direct to the correct laterality, mapping of the lateral border of the GPi is useful, with adjustment of the target to lie 2.5 mm medial to the lateral border.[161] The combination of recording of sensorimotor responses and mapping of the lateral border serves to ensure that the pallidotomy is localized within the motor portion of GPi, and not more anteromedially within the cognitive regions where benefits are less, and the potential for detrimental effects on cognition are greater.

The optimal region for the STN lesion is in the sensorimotor region as well, which is dorsolateral in the nucleus. This region contains kinesthetic cells and will respond with both passive limb movement and active movement. If tremor is present, tremor cells (firing synchronously with tremor) can be found in this region. STN stimulation induces acute symptom amelioration and suppression of tremor if present and may activate dyskinesias as well, particularly in the lower extremities. Tonic motor responses are elicited from the adjacent corticospinal tract anterolateral to the STN, typically oral facial or upper extremity, and sensory responses posteriorly and caudally. Conjugate eye deviation is elicited from the corticobulbar region, whereas ipsilateral medial eye forced duction is produced with current spread to the medially located oculomotor nucleus.[77,78,85]

Properly placed VIM thalamotomy lesions are located 2 to 3 mm anterior to the border of the tactile sensory relay thalamic nucleus and at the base of the thalamus to deafferent the entire dorsal-ventral extent of the VIM from the incoming cerebellar fibers (Fig. 88-3). They should be in areas containing kinesthetic tremor cells with receptive fields corresponding to the distal upper extremity and cells that fire in synchrony with upper extremity tremor. These areas must also produce upper extremity tremor arrest when electrically stimulated. Stimulation induces sensory paresthesia from the ventrocaudal (VC) nucleus posteriorly; whereas stimulation within or close to (within 1 mm of) the VC nucleus produces sustained paresthesia, stimulation within VIM may produce paresthesia from spread to the VC nucleus but not sustained, typically abating within no more than 1 minute of stimulation onset. Lateral or anterior spread of electrical stimulation induces corticospinal motor responses from the internal capsule, typically oral facial or arm.

Lesion Generation

Several recording and/or stimulation tracks may be necessary to refine the targeting, whereupon lesion generation can be performed. For the radiofrequency lesion-generation procedure, lesions are made using a radiofrequency generator that heats a 1.1-mm-diameter probe with a 2- or 3-mm exposed tip. The location for the lesioning electrode insertion is dependent on the previously determined physiologic map. Repositioning of the lesion electrode is performed as needed. Initially, a test lesion is performed at 42°C for 60 seconds to observe for adverse effects during continuous clinical testing for changes in sensorimotor and speech functions, and—in the case of GPi—visual changes (eTable 88-1). Lesioning is then performed at temperatures from 60°C initially and increasing to up to 85°C for 60 seconds. Symptomatic changes should be noted, but lesioning is continued to

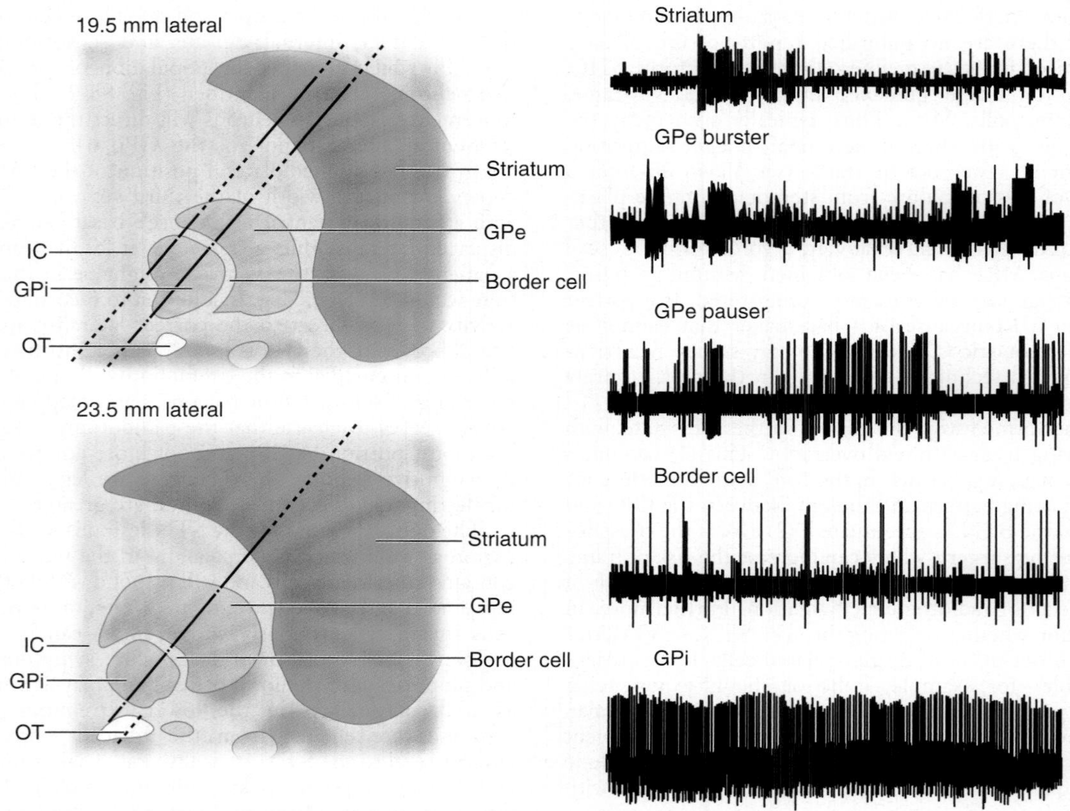

Figure 88-2. Neurophysiologic microelectrode mapping for pallidotomy. The first microelectrode track is run recording single units through the striatum, globus pallidus externa (GPe), globus pallidus interna (GPi), and the internal capsule (IC) or optic tract (OT), each characterized by stereotypical activity as shown. Light-evoked responses (via strobe or flashlight) can be recorded to confirm location of the OT. The microelectrode can then be used to perform electrical stimulation in the IC to elicit motor responses (typically in mouth, face, or arm) or in the OT to elicit phosphenes. The microelectrode may be retracted and macrostimulation then performed from the end of the microelectrode guide cannula in some systems. Alternatively, the microelectrode may be removed and replaced by a stimulating electrode—typically the lesioning electrode itself—for macrostimulation results. Effects on clinical symptomatology can be observed from macroelectrode stimulation as well. A second track is run in the same sagittal plane, and sometimes additional ones, to establish the location of the posterior border of GPi with IC; another one or two tracks are run laterally to establish the lateral border of GPi with GPe. *(Redrawn from Gross RE, Krack P, Rodriguez-Oroz MC, et al. Electrophysiological mapping for the implantation of deep brain stimulators for Parkinson's disease and tremor.* Mov Disord. *2006;21(Suppl 14):S259-S283.)*

maximize lesion size as long as adverse effects are not noted. Notably, temperature has been shown to be the parameter best correlated with lesion volume.[162] Some choose to make the lesions based on somatotopic findings and the patient's intraoperative clinical presentation.[163] However, there is no conclusive evidence as to the superiority of any of these techniques over the others.

Pallidotomy lesions are best described as an oblate spheroid typically measuring approximately 6 mm in height and 4 mm in diameter[152,161] (Fig. 88-4). Ultimately, the lesions must be large enough to produce a longstanding clinical benefit, but small enough to avoid unwanted side effects or complications. The lesions in the VIM thalamus (eTable 88-2; Fig. 88-5) typically are 4 mm in diameter. The STN lesions are varied, but have been reported at typically 4 to 5 mm[78,85] (Fig. 88-6).

The benefits of ablations are seen immediately. The patents must undergo a neurological examination after the procedure and must be monitored overnight. An MRI scan should be performed the following day.

CLINICAL OUTCOMES

Pallidotomy

Clinical Benefits of Pallidotomy

The vast majority of studies of pallidotomy are retrospective case series or prospective uncontrolled trials. However, several prospective controlled trials have now been reported, including several controlled, randomized, observer-blind trials (eTable 88-3).[82,83,106,132,139,164-168] This amounts to nearly 2000 patients from 40 centers in 12 countries who have undergone pallidotomy.[169] The most prominent effect of pallidotomy is the nearly complete and sustained amelioration of contralateral dyskinesias, with less improvement of ipsilateral dyskinesias.[a] This is best seen in the randomized trial from Emory University, which demonstrated a 75% decrease in contralateral (and

[a]References 49, 82, 83, 133, 134, 137, 139, 164, 165, 170-190.

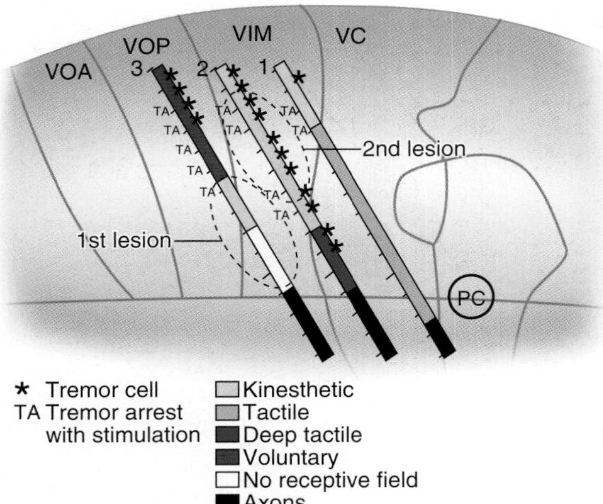

Figure 88-3. Neurophysiologic (e.g., microelectrode) mapping of the thalamus. Similar to the pallidum, with the thalamus, microelectrode recording tracks are run recording single-unit receptive fields in the thalamic nuclei, from rostral to caudal: ventralis oralis anterior (VOA), ventralis oralis posterior (VOP), ventral intermediate (nucleus of the thalamus) (VIM), and ventralis caudalis (VC) (Hassler terminology). Microelectrode stimulation eliciting somatotropic organized projected fields (i.e., paresthesias) at low thresholds (1 to 5 mA) from VC aids further in identifying the posterior border of VIM with VC or, at higher thresholds, the medial lemniscus below the thalamus *(in black).* Macrostimulation through the microelectrode guide cannula tip or through the lesioning electrode definitively identifies correct location of the lesioning electrode. A second and possibly additional tracks are run as needed until the posterior border of VIM with VC is mapped and until receptive and projected fields consistent with wrist or medial digit somatotopy are obtained. PC, posterior commissure. *(Redrawn from original illustration provided courtesy of Dr. Andres M. Lozano, University of Toronto.)*

30% decrease in ipsilateral) dyskinesias and a 32% decrease in "off" time.[106] Ultimately, patients have improved tolerance of dopaminergic medication resulting in more dyskinesia-free "on" time, independent of dose changes.[82] The effects of pallidotomy on contralateral "off" symptoms, specifically rigidity, tremor, and bradykinesia, are also quite significant, with mild improvement ipsilaterally.[b] The effect on gait dysfunction and postural instability remains unclear; several clinical studies have shown conflicting results,[83,143,144,196-199] and speech symptoms generally do not respond or may even worsen.[200-202] Substantial improvements are seen in painful dystonia.[106,171,203] Long-term follow-up has shown that benefits decline somewhat over time.[82,106,170,173,181,187-189,204-207] In contrast to the "off" state improvements, the "on" state improvements are milder and generally lack significance, are related to the aforementioned improvement in dyskinesia-free "on" time, and also worsen with time.

Studies examining the association between lesion characteristics and location with outcomes have shown that posterolateral lesions are more effective for tremor, whereas medial lesions have more impact on dyskinesias. Centrally located lesions showed improvement most in postural stability and akinesia.[126,163,173,179] Other studies have failed to observe these effects.[135,208]

It is important to note that it is generally perceived that dopaminergic medication dose is not significantly affected by pallidotomy,[209] although some have argued that it may increase the therapeutic window of the levodopa.[210]

[b]References 82, 83, 131-134, 139, 165-168, 170, 171, 173-177, 179-185, 187, 188, 191-195.

Neuropsychological Effects of Pallidotomy

A brief discussion of these effects can be found at ExpertConsult.com. 

Complications of Pallidotomy

Complications are common with pallidotomy, with up to 30% experiencing adverse effects, 14% of whom experienced them for more than 3 months, although the frequency of complications decreases with experience.[161,241] Acute complications related to the surgical technique, particularly symptomatic hemorrhage or infarct, are the most important, with an incidence of around 4%. Transient encephalopathy is variable but occurs, in general, in 10% of patients. In terms of more permanent complications, changes in speech (dysarthria, hypophonia, and dysphasia) are most common. Cognition, personality, and behavior are also affected, although the degree and incidence are more variable. Additional complications include hypersalivation, memory loss, depression, seizure, homonymous hemianopsia, psychosis, and urinary incontinence, although they are more infrequently encountered. Also of note is that a rare late-stage phenomenon known as *Pisa syndrome* characterized by lateral flexion of the neck may occur.[242,243] Mortality was found to occur in 0.3% to 1.2% of cases in various studies.[169,241]

Risk-benefit ratio of microelectrode recording in comparison with macroelectrode stimulation is controversial. Whereas microelectrode recording has been shown to have a higher incidence of symptomatic intracranial bleeding than macroelectrode stimulation (1.3%-2.7% versus 0.25%-0.5%), the reports of the overall rate of complications are inconsistent, with some showing a higher incidence with microelectrode recording, and others showing no difference.[169,241,244]

Bilateral pallidotomies may result in severe dysphagia, apathy, loss of initiative, loss of motivation and motor drive, and persistent levodopa-resistant gait freezing.[146] However, the issue of the safety of bilateral versus unilateral pallidotomy is unresolved; several studies have reported widely variable results ranging from significantly higher incidence and severity of complications in bilateral procedures compared with unilateral procedures, to findings of no difference between the complication rates of the procedures.[141,142,146,241,245-248]

Thalamotomy

Clinical Benefits of Thalamotomy

The primary use of thalamotomy is for tremor control, achieved by targeting the posterior VIM[249]; it is of greatest benefit in tremor-predominant PD.[47,97,101,150,154,250-263] Extremity tremor is the most responsive to this procedure, with axial tremor (head and voice tremor) being less responsive.[264-266] As VIM thalamotomy predominantly addresses tremor, some groups have investigated targeting other regions of the thalamus, such as the more anterior pallidal receiving areas, to address rigidity, akinesia, and dyskinesias.[150,267] Some have noted an early and transient improvement in dyskinesias,[268,269] and others have demonstrated sustained improvements in rigidity,[254,259] although without any benefit for akinesia. The potential impact on ADL improvement therefore appears to be confined to those associated with tremor control.[254] Thus, it is often necessary to continue medication to treat the other symptoms if present. The long-term benefit of thalamotomy on tremor control also remains unclear. Diederich and colleagues showed persistent improvement in tremor in their long-term studies, whereas other long-term studies have shown return to the preoperative state[250,270] or worsening.[259] In comparison to DBS, Schuurman and colleagues showed that, with the

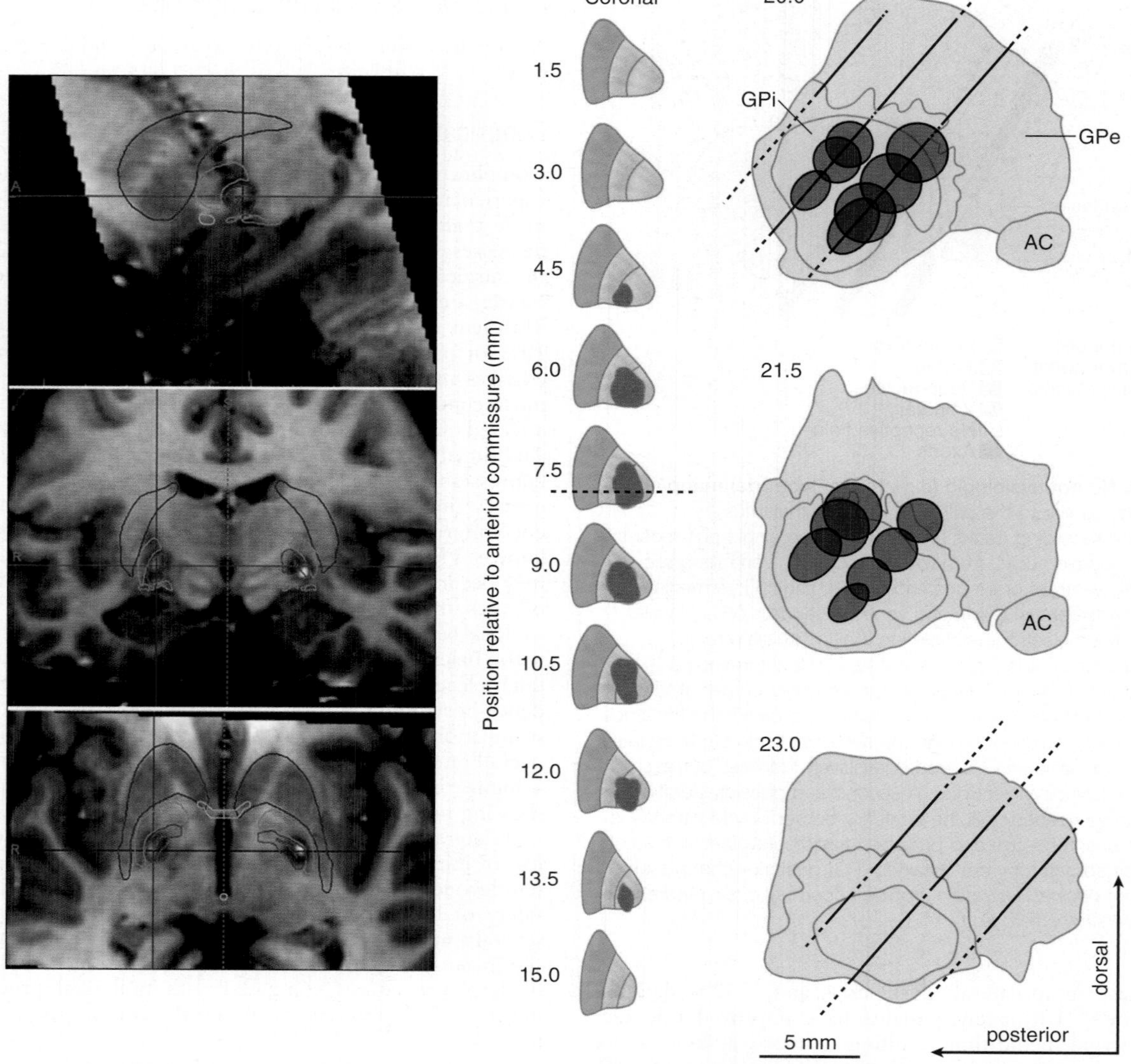

Figure 88-4. Postoperative imaging and reconstruction. Postoperative imaging is performed, typically magnetic resonance imaging *(left).* Depicted is a left pallidotomy in sagittal *(left, top),* coronal *(left, center),* and axial *(left, bottom)* planes. The lesions were performed using the multiple overlapping–lesioning method, as depicted in two separate tracks in the 20.0-mm and 21.5-mm lateral planes *(right).* The microelectrode tracks performed in the 23.0-mm lateral plane verify the location of the lateral border of the globus pallidus interna (GPi). AC, anterior commissure; GPe, globus pallidus externa. *(Illustrations redrawn from Vitek JL, Bakay RA, Hashimoto T, et al. Microelectrode-guided pallidotomy: technical approach and its application in medically intractable Parkinson's disease.* J Neurosurg. *1998;88:1027-1043.)*

exception of tremor relief, thalamotomy patients showed worse improvement at 5-year follow-up, thus suggesting that this procedure does not have an impact on disease progression.[271]

Complications and Neuropsychological Effects of Thalamotomy

As is the case with pallidotomy, the most significant complication of thalamotomy is intracranial hemorrhage with an incidence of 1.5% to 6%. Other reported complications include bulbar symptoms (facial paresis and dysarthria), hemiparesis, dystonia, and dyspraxia. As expected with thalamic lesions, sensory symptoms are often seen, but usually resolve. These include paresthesia and numbness and typically have a perioral or appendicular distribution.[43,47,154,260,263,264,266,272-275] Bilateral thalamotomy is rarely performed owing to concerns regarding adverse effects, estimated to be twofold to threefold higher than with unilateral thalamotomy, with prominent involvement of speech leading to hypophonia, dysarthria, and dysphasia.[97,154,253,261,270,272,273,276] Thalamotomy appears to convey a higher incidence of adverse effects than DBS, with the exception of equipment-related complications.[271,277] For patients with significant bilateral symptoms, it has been shown that VIM DBS performed contralateral to a thalamotomy is a viable and effective option.[278]

See ExpertConsult.com for a discussion of the cognitive effects of thalamotomy.

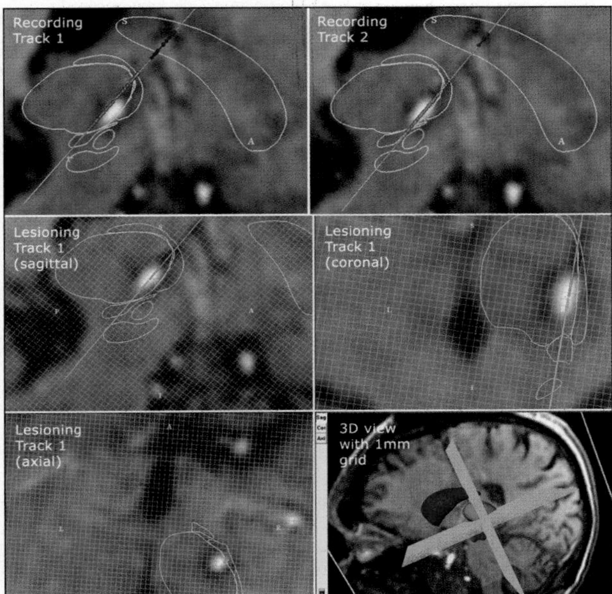

Figure 88-5. Postoperative thalamotomy imaging. Overlap of thalamotomy with microelectrode recording tracks is shown. Hemorrhagic portion of the lesion measures approximately 7 mm high and approximately 3 mm wide, as expected. This portion corresponds to the destructive portion of the lesion on long-term follow-up imaging. *(From Lokuketagoda J, Gross R. Thalamotomy and pallidotomy. In: Jandial R, McCormick P, Black PM, eds.* Core Techniques in Operative Neurosurgery. *Philadelphia: Elsevier Saunders; 2011:290-300.)*

Subthalamotomy

Clinical Benefits of Subthalamotomy

Although far fewer studies have been published on subthalamotomy (specifically subthalamic nucleotomy) compared with pallidotomy, thus far it has been found to be a safe and effective treatment option for PD, especially in patients with bilateral presentation (see eTable 88-3). Studies have shown there to be considerable "on" and "off" state contralateral reduction in tremor, bradykinesia, and rigidity after the procedure.[75-77,81,83,85,86,282] In some cases this is sustained in the "off" state through as long as 36 months.[74,78-80,282] There is some, but negligible, ipsilateral relief seen in these symptoms as well.[77,80,83] Subthalamotomy has additionally led to decreased axial motor issues, with improved gait and postural stability,[77-81,83,85,282] and significantly improved ADLs in both "on" and "off" states.[74,76,78-81,83,282] One of the most profound effects of subthalamotomy, which is unique compared with the other ablative procedures mentioned, is that it significantly reduces medication needs of its patients.[74,76,78-81,83,85,86,282] This then leads to a decline or slowing of the progression in medication-induced dyskinesias, with reduced dyskinesia disability and duration.[74,78-81,83,85,190,282] Decreased "on-off" fluctuations are also of note.[74,81]

Complications and Neuropsychological Effects of Subthalamotomy

A significant number of complications have been reported. Contralateral lesion-induced dyskinesias occur, although they are often mild and transient, resolving within a few months of the

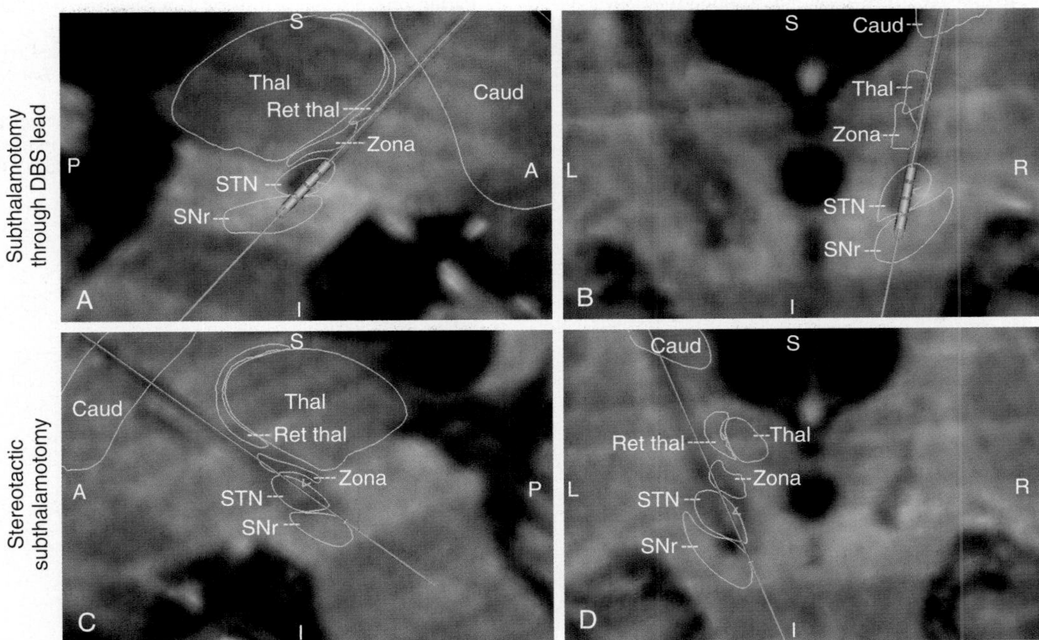

Figure 88-6. Postoperative subthalamotomy imaging. Magnetic resonance imaging (MRI) scans depicting bilateral subthalamotomies in a patient who first underwent bilateral subthalamic nucleus (STN) deep brain stimulation (DBS) with excellent clinical response. However, he developed erosion and infection, necessitating removal of the DBS system. Before removal of the electrodes, a subthalamotomy was performed across contacts 1 and 2 on the right (**A,** sagittal; **B,** coronal). The leads were then removed and he was later brought back for a stereotactic subthalamotomy on the left (**C,** sagittal; **D,** coronal). Note that all images are from the MRI performed after the latter procedure, thus depicting the bilateral lesions on all panes. The MRI was overlain with the Schaltenbrand-Wahren atlas slice as interpolated and deformed to match the patient's anatomy using our proprietary One-Track software. A, anterior; Caud, caudate; I, inferior; L, left; P, posterior; R, right; Ret thal, reticular nucleus of thalamus; S, superior; SNr, substantia nigra pars reticulata; Thal, thalamus; Zona, zona incerta.

surgery.[78,79] Hemichorea and hemiballism can also occur, although they often do so in patients who initially had higher dyskinesia scores preoperatively.[74,79-81,83,282] These sometimes necessitate additional lesions such as to the VIM or GPi, which are effective in ameliorating the dyskinesias.[76,85] Neuropsychiatric effects including euphoria and disinhibition have also been reported in a small case series.[283] Other complications have included transient postural asymmetries[81] and ataxia.[79] In terms of neuropsychological outcomes, little to no impact on speech, sensory function, or cognition has been found.[74,76,78-80,83,282,283]

ALTERNATIVE APPROACHES

Please visit ExpertConsult.com for more information on various alternative approaches to treating movement disorder symptoms in Parkinson's disease patients, including radiofrequency ablation with in situ DBS leads, Gamma Knife thalamotomy, and magnetic resonance (imaging)–guided focused ultrasound (MRgFUS).

CONCLUSION

Ablative surgeries remain a safe, effective, and proven therapeutic strategy in patients with suboptimal response to medication or medication complications. Pallidotomy provides a dramatic improvement of cardinal motor features of PD. It also has a direct impact on dyskinesias. However, it has little impact on medication dosage and is associated with complications when performed bilaterally. Similarly, subthalamotomy provides improvement in the cardinal motor features but also confers a notable reduction in medication dosage. It is also associated with fewer complications when performed bilaterally. However, independent of dose adjustments, it has a smaller impact on drug-induced dyskinesias. Thalamotomy is primarily indicated for medication-resistant tremor but has little to no impact on the other motor features of PD. Furthermore, similar to pallidotomy, it is associated with complications when performed bilaterally. Accordingly, its popularity for PD is waning.

The drawback of all ablative therapies is that they are irreversible. DBS, which circumvents this concern, has been shown to be equally effective as these ablative procedures, with a possibly improved safety profile particularly in bilateral procedures.[67-73,76,165,168,207,257,271,277,303] Nevertheless, there are still significant advantages to these ablative approaches. They are cost-effective, requiring a single procedure with minimal follow-up. In addition, they have a low risk of infection because there is no implanted hardware. Furthermore, with the advent of MRgFUS, noninvasive ablative approaches are on the horizon. For some patients who cannot or will not undergo an invasive surgery such as DBS, the appeal of minimally invasive or noninvasive approaches—even if performed only unilaterally—may be significant enough to make this a useful tool in the armamentarium for the treatment of PD.

SUGGESTED READINGS

Alexander GE, Delong MR, Strick PL. Parallel organization of functionally segregated circuits linking basal ganglia and cortex. *Annu Rev Neurosci*. 1986;9:357-381.

Alvarez L, Macias R, Pavon N, et al. Therapeutic efficacy of unilateral subthalamotomy in Parkinson's disease: results in 89 patients followed for up to 36 months. *J Neurol Neurosurg Psychiatry*. 2009;80(9):979-985.

Gross RE. What happened to prosteroventral pallidotomy for Parkinson's disease and dystonia? *Neurother*. 2008;5(2):281-293.

Gross RE, Lombardi WJ, Lang AE, et al. Relationship of lesion location to clinical outcome following microelectrode-guided pallidotomy for Parkinson's disease. *Brain*. 1999;122:405-416.

Laitinen LV, Bergenheim AT, Hariz MI. Leksells posteroventral pallidotomy in the treatment of Parkinsons disease. *J Neurosurg*. 1992;76(1):53-61.

Lang AE, Lozano AM, Montgomery E, et al. Posteroventral medial pallidotomy in advanced Parkinson's disease. *N Engl J Med*. 1997;337(15):1036-1042.

Schuurman PR, Bosch DA, Bossuyt PM, et al. A comparison of continuous thalamic stimulation and thalamotomy for suppression of severe tremor. *N Engl J Med*. 2000;342(7):461-468.

Speelman JD, Bosch DA. Resurgence of functional neurosurgery for Parkinson's disease: a historical perspective. *Mov Disord*. 1998;13(3):582-588.

Vitek JL, Bakay RA, Freeman A, et al. Randomized trial of pallidotomy versus medical therapy for Parkinson's disease. *Ann Neurol*. 2003;53(5):558-569.

Vitek JL, Bakay RA, Hashimoto T, et al. Microelectrode-guided pallidotomy: technical approach and its application in medically intractable Parkinson's disease. *J Neurosurg*. 1998;88(6):1027-1043.

See a full reference list on ExpertConsult.com

89 Deep Brain Stimulation for Parkinson's Disease

Fedor E. Panov, Paul Larson, Alastair Martin, and Philip Starr

Parkinson's disease (PD), a progressive synucleinopathy of unknown origin, is the second most common neurodegenerative condition behind only Alzheimer's disease, affecting 1% of the population over 65.[1,2] With the prevalence doubling per decade of life, the number of patients is predicted to increase as the world population ages.[2]

The goal of this chapter is to provide an overview of the treatment of the motor abnormalities of PD using deep brain stimulation (DBS) with emphasis on two targets: the subthalamic nucleus (STN) and the globus pallidus interna (GPi). Two surgical methods preferred at our institution are highlighted: surgery guided by microelectrode recordings and test stimulation in the awake state, and surgery guided by interventional magnetic resonance imaging (MRI) under general anesthesia, without physiologic testing.

BRIEF HISTORICAL OVERVIEW

Descriptions of PD symptoms and treatment with the dopaminergic extract "cowage," from the *Mucuna pruriens* seed, appear in the *Ayurveda*, an ancient medical text of the Indian subcontinent from 1000 BC.[3,4] The *Nei Jing*, a 2500-year-old medical text from China, echoes similar ideas,[5] yet the first western description of the disorder emerged only two centuries ago when a Londoner, James Parkinson, described six patients with "paralysis agitans."[6] Sixty years later, Jean-Martin Charcot refined the earlier description and coined the term "maladie de Parkinson."[7] Anticholinergic treatment was used as early as the mid-19th century. Arvid Carlsson and George Cotzias introduced oral levodopa/carbidopa as the "gold standard" of medical therapy in 1968.[8]

Surgical treatment of PD began in the 1940s with resection of premotor and motor cortices in hopes of alleviating parkinsonian tremor.[9] The resultant improvement had to be weighed against significant iatrogenic motor deficits, while no effect was seen on either rigidity or bradykinesia.[9] The move toward basal ganglia and thalamic targets addressed these shortcomings. Interruption of the pallidofugal fibers exiting the GPi by Spiegel and Wycis[10,11] and by Meyers[12] improved both tremor and rigidity. In 1952, Irving Cooper's fortuitous sacrifice of the anterior choroidal artery in a 39-year-old man incapacitated by tremor and bradykinesia alleviated the patient's symptoms without motor or sensory deficits.[13]

Lesioning work on the basal ganglia and thalamus largely ceased in the 1970s because of the tremendous immediate effects of oral levodopa/carbidopa and the significant risks of surgery. By the 1990s, however, recognition of the long-term side effects of the medication—dyskinesias and motor fluctuations—brought about a renewed interest in surgical solutions.[14,15]

At the same time, the integration of modern imaging techniques such as computed tomography (CT) in the late 1970s and MRI with frame-based stereotaxy in the 1980s improved the safety and accuracy of surgery at deep brain targets. Attempts to use DBS in thalamic, basal ganglia. and cerebellar regions for movement disorders were made in the early 1980s.[16,17]

In 1987, Benabid and colleagues showed that high-frequency stimulation could mimic a lesion in a controllable, reversible manner.[18] Yet stimulation of the ventralis intermedius thalamic nucleus target again aided only the tremor symptomatology, leaving rigidity and bradykinesia untreated. Series of safe and effective pallidotomies[19] from the early 1990s resurrected the concept of GPi lesioning for those symptoms yet were technically difficult procedures limited to one hemisphere. GPi-DBS was introduced in 1994[20] as a safer reversible alternative with an ability to implant and modulate both hemispheres for bilateral and axial symptomatology.

In 1990, Bergman and associates[21] showed in a nonhuman primate model of PD that the induction of parkinsonism is associated with excessive and abnormally patterned discharge in the STN, and that ablation of the nucleus alleviated all parkinsonian motor signs. Based on this work, Benabid and coworkers implanted the first chronic subthalamic stimulator for PD in the early 1990s[22] and subsequently documented alleviation of all cardinal motor signs of PD in a case series in 1998.[23]

ANATOMY AND PHYSIOLOGY OF TARGETS

Both the STN and GPi are components of the basal ganglia, a collection of subcortical nuclei involved in scaling and focusing of movement, as well as motor learning. The basal ganglia also include the striatum (caudate and putamen), globus pallidus externa (GPe), and substantia nigra, subdivided into the substantia nigra pars reticularis and substantia nigra pars compacta. DBS for treatment of PD motor symptomatology is based on the "segregated circuit hypothesis."[24] The numerous functions of the basal ganglia within the cortex–basal ganglia–thalamus loop (motor, oculomotor, associative, and limbic) run in parallel and occupy anatomically distinct areas of the nuclei. It is therefore in principle possible to target the motor areas without compromising nonmotor functions.

The STN, shaped like a small, thick biconvex lens, is located medial to the internal capsule, lateral to the red nucleus, superior to the substantia nigra, and inferior to the thalamus. The GPi is located medial and inferior to the medial medullary lamina and GPe. The GPi overlies the choroidal fissure and the optic tract. Medially, it is limited by the genu and the lateral aspect of the posterior limb of the internal capsule.

In the basal ganglia–thalamocortical circuit (Fig. 89-1), the major input structures to the basal ganglia are the striatum and STN, while the GPi serves as the main output. The input and the output nuclei are connected by a direct massive gabaergic striatopallidal pathway, and by an indirect route via the GPe and STN before arriving at the output nuclei GPi. The balance between the activating direct and the inhibitory indirect pathways controls movement. In the "rate model" developed originally by Albin, Young, and DeLong, the parkinsonian state is modeled as a hyperexcitation of the STN causing an imbalance in favor of the indirect pathway and excessive GPi excitation.[21,25] Targeting the STN or GPi with lesioning or stimulation was thought to correct excessive and abnormally patterned basal ganglia output. Some elements of the rate model have been confirmed experimentally. Elevated GPi and STN discharge rates in PD, compared to nonparkinsonian conditions, were seen by Starr and colleagues,[26] Schrock and associates,[27] and Steigerwald and colleagues.[28] Optogenetic confirmation in rodents of the prokinetic and antikinetic functions of the direct and indirect pathways, respectively, was shown by Kravitz and coworkers in 2010.[29] The model does not, however, explain the benefit of pallidal stimulation in hyperkinetic disorders. Its initial assumption that STN-DBS suppressed downstream basal ganglia activity has also

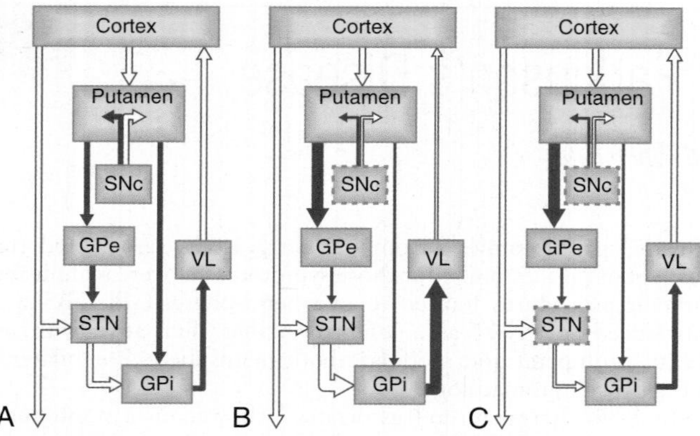

Figure 89-1. The classic rate model of the basal ganglia–thalamocortical circuit. A, Normal state showing excitatory projections *(open arrows)*, inhibition *(filled arrows)*, and relative activity *(arrow width)*. **B,** Parkinsonian state. **C,** Effects of subthalamic nucleus (STN) lesioning on the circuit. GPe, globus pallidus externa; GPi, globus pallidus interna; SNc, substantia nigra pars compacta; VL, ventrolateral nucleus of the thalamus. *(From Bergman H, Wichmann T, DeLong MR. Reversal of experimental parkinsonism by lesions of the subthalamic nucleus.* Science. *1990;249:1436-1438.)*

been called into question.[30,31] The rate model remains important because of its heuristic value, as newer theories aim to rectify its shortcomings.

Another explanation, the excitation/surround inhibition theory, is based on the primate anatomic work of Hoover and Strick.[32] The basal ganglia are composed of multiple independent output channels, with some facilitating specific actions and others inhibiting competing movements. Similar to the visual pathway, which increases contrast of an image with surround inhibition, the basal ganglia may focus movement by halting competing surrounding action algorithms. Pathologic states of PD and dystonia decrease the ability to sharpen movement by enlarging or shrinking the inhibition areas.[27,33]

The most influential contemporary model of brain network dysfunction in PD is the "oscillatory synchrony model," which posits that akinesia and bradykinesia in PD are due to excessive neuronal synchronization in specific frequency bands, especially the beta band.[1] The beta band (13 to 35 Hz) is present in primary motor (M1) and sensory cortices during postural maintenance but is superseded by the high-frequency band (76 to 100 Hz) with planning and execution of movement.[34] The basal ganglia show an increase in neuronal synchronization in the beta activity in PD.[28] DBS at both the STN and GPi may exert its therapeutic effect by desynchronization of neuronal activity at specific frequencies.

PATIENT SELECTION

The most important part of DBS for PD is patient selection (Table 89-1). The key to proper patient selection is a combined approach that includes evaluation by specialists in movement disorders, neurology, neurosurgery, and neuropsychology. An interdisciplinary clinic in which these specialties provide integrated care streamlines the process of patient selection and work-up.

Indications

A clear diagnosis of idiopathic PD by a movement disorder neurologist is paramount because many forms of atypical parkinsonism, such as progressive supranuclear palsy and multiple system atrophy, may resemble PD but do not respond to surgical treatment. The patient's examination off medication and subsequent improvement with a supratherapeutic oral levodopa dose, called "on-off" testing, is a strong predictor of the quantitative improvement in scores on part III (motor subscale) of the Unified Parkinson's Disease Rating Scale (UPDRS III) that can be expected from bilateral DBS. The two indications for surgery are motor complications from long-term medical therapy and/or medically intractable tremor. The most common motor complications are dyskinesias and motor fluctuations (rapid, unpredictable cycling between effectively medicated and inadequately medicated states).[35] Postoperative reduction in the severity, duration, and frequency of "off" periods, as well as reduction of medication-induced complications, improves quality of life. DBS for early motor complications of PD is now being investigated.[36,37]

TABLE 89-1 Response of PD Symptoms to DBS

DBS Improves	DBS Unlikely to Benefit
• Tremor • Dyskinesias • Rigidity • Motor fluctuations • Bradykinesia and "off"-period gait freezing • Classic idiopathic PD	• Autonomic function (constipation, poor temperature regulation, orthostatic hypotension) • Cognition • Hypophonia • Postural instability and "on"-period gait freezing • Atypical parkinsonisms (PSP, MSA)

DBS, deep brain stimulation; MSA, multiple system atrophy; PD, Parkinson's disease; PSP, progressive supranuclear palsy.

Contraindications

Although most patients with PD have at least some cognitive impairment that can be detected on neuropsychological testing, severe cognitive impairment is a contraindication for DBS because dementia may worsen as a result of surgical intervention, and severe cognitive impairment can supersede motor impairment as the primary driver of disability. A marked cognitive dysfunction documented on the Mini-Mental State Examination[38] or a low score on the Mattis Dementia Rating Scale diminishes the DBS quality of life benefit and serves as a relative contraindication to DBS in PD.[39,40] Improved motor function in a severely demented patient can be dangerous because increased mobility may lead to falls. The danger may be exacerbated by a potentially increased impulsivity caused by STN-DBS.[41,42] Additional neuropsychological testing is beneficial in cases of borderline scores.[43]

Age remains an independent prognostic factor in a majority of surgical fields. As a disease affecting 1% of patients greater than 65 years old, PD carries with it the comorbidities of advancing age. Hypertension, diabetes, and need for anticoagulation all increase surgical risk. Age and hypertension increase intraoperative hemorrhage rates in DBS.[44,45] Although each candidate must be reviewed on an individual basis, the quality-of-life improvement seen in younger patients undergoing DBS for PD diminishes in the group greater than 65 years old.[46]

Poor axial scores on the UPDRS III combined with severe postural instability tend to not benefit from DBS. Hypophonia, another levodopa-nonresponsive symptom, is unlikely to improve with stimulation. Patients and families should be warned of potential worsening in voice strength postoperatively.

TARGET SELECTION FACTORS

Patient Symptomatology

Several large randomized studies that have compared STN and GPi as targets showed no significant difference in improvement

TABLE 89-2 Target Selection Based on Treatment Goals

Subthalamic Nucleus	Globus Pallidus Interna
• Greater decrease in levodopa requirements • Easier surgical targeting • Weight gain • Possibly longer battery life	• Lower chance of cognitive decline • Easier postoperative programming • Maintenance of letter verbal fluency • Mood stability

of motor symptoms after DBS.[47-49] Mood and cognition seem to be at slightly higher risk for decline following STN-DBS[47,49] (Table 89-2). Patients with borderline cognitive function seem to maintain their function better and their quality of life improves more with GPi-DBS.[48] Decision making under stress can be altered by STN-DBS, increasing impulsive behavior and errors in judgment.[41] This argues in favor of using GPi-DBS for cognitively compromised patients whose cognitive deficit is not so severe as to preclude surgical intervention.

Swallowing function deteriorates with PD and can lead to aspiration pneumonia and death. A recent retrospective review suggests that, unlike GPi-DBS, STN stimulation can worsen swallowing.[50] Weight gain is seen with STN-DBS, whereas results are inconclusive with GPi stimulation.[51-53] Long-term benefits in favor of STN-DBS include possibly increased battery life (because of lower voltage settings) and greater reduction of dopaminergic medication. Only one of four randomized studies of GPi-DBS versus STN-DBS has shown better motor function in the "off" state following STN-DBS compared to GPi-DBS.[40]

Surgeon's Experience

The experience of the surgeon remains of vital importance.[54,55] As with any procedure, a learning curve exists for both targets. Benabid and associates[56] reported an improvement in complication-free surgical rate from 37.3% in their first 150 bilateral procedures to 72.7% in the next 150. Seijo and coworkers reported that the rate of significant adverse events in their series dropped from 14.6% in the first 7 years to 8.8% in the last 7 years.[45] If true equipoise as to target selection exists after an exhaustive work-up, the surgeon will likely choose the procedure with which he or she is most experienced. With deference to personal experience, GPi is viewed by many to be the more challenging target because of its greater anatomic variability and a relative lack of consensus on the subregion of this relatively large structure that is optimal for DBS therapy.

Alternative Targets

Ventralis Intermedius Nucleus

The first target used historically for PD, the ventralis intermedius nucleus of the thalamus, only results in reduction of tremor but remains of some value in tremor-predominant PD.[57] Because the STN and GPi alleviate tremor together with other motor symptoms, most practitioners favor those targets over the ventralis intermedius nucleus.

Pedunculopontine Nucleus

The pedunculopontine nucleus is a novel target in DBS for PD.[58] It is located in the lateral pontomesencephalic tegmentum, dorsolateral to the decussation of the superior cerebellar peduncles and caudal to the substantia nigra.[59] Lack of symptomatic relief of postural instability and on-medication gait freezing with STN and GPi stimulation precipitated interest in this "locomotor center" of the brainstem. For the pedunculopontine nucleus target, stimulation frequency is typically set much lower than for GPi and STN targets, at 20 to 60 Hz.[60] The UPDRS III may not be sufficiently sensitive to detect improvement in such patients. Using the Gait and Falls Questionnaire score, limited but statistically significant improvement is seen in patients with "on"-state severe gait freezing and postural instability with frequent falls.[61,62] The pedunculopontine nucleus can be targeted anatomically[63] or using physiologic mapping[64,65] because of its unique firing rate and response to passive movements of limbs.

Unilateral versus Bilateral versus Staged Stimulator Implantation

Unilateral implantation should be considered if there is gross asymmetry in the symptoms. Advanced age or presence of preoperative cognitive deficits may make unilateral surgery more prudent, with a faster recovery time because of decreased operating time and limitation of postoperative edema to one hemisphere. It is sensible to alleviate the symptoms on the severely affected side with a unilateral implant first and, if required, implant the other side at a later date. Even a unilateral STN-DBS to treat the more severely affected side will significantly improve motor function. Unilateral DBS may decrease some aspects of cognitive performance,[66] but less so than simultaneous bilateral DBS.

SELECTION OF SURGICAL TECHNIQUE

At the time of its introduction, DBS was performed using a combination of anatomic and physiologic targeting. In the traditional technique, frame-based stereotaxy utilizes preoperatively acquired magnetic resonance images to define a "starting point" for target localization, and this initial anatomic target is refined or confirmed by microelectrode recordings (MERs) performed with the patient awake. The use of MER increases intraoperative time, and its application in certain populations (those with significant anxiety, advanced age, or severe "off"-period pain) may be problematic. It has been suggested that MER increases the risk of DBS,[44,67] but this additional risk, if it exists, is small.

Recent advances in the technical approach to DBS include novel skull-mounted aiming systems, the use of "frameless stereotaxy," and "asleep" DBS with interventional MRI (iMRI) or CT used to place leads using anatomic guidance only. The microTargeting platform stereotaxy system (FHC Inc., Bowdoin, ME) was introduced over a decade ago as an alternative to frame-based systems for awake, MER-guided surgery and reported on by Konrad and colleagues.[68] Neuronavigation-guided awake DBS using the Nexframe (Medtronic Inc., Minneapolis, MN) skull-mounted aiming device was established by Henderson and colleagues.[69] Our team showed accurate STN and GPi lead placement using a frameless, asleep iMRI technique with outcomes comparable to traditional frame-based, MER-guided placements.[70,71] Burchiel and associates used intraoperative CT-guided navigation without MER for accurate lead placement.[72] Numerous additional innovations in targeting will likely occur in the next decade.

The dichotomy of awake versus asleep surgery remains a major choice in procedure selection. Recent studies suggest that accuracy of placement and complication profiles are similar,[69,70,72] yet the patient experience differs. In our practice, younger patients or patients without severe tremor or painful "off"-period dystonias tolerate awake procedures well. Older patients with significant tremor, anxiety, and major off-medication disability are better suited for the asleep iMRI approach. Although some physiologic recording can be done under general anesthesia with frame-based surgery in a traditional operating room, the quality of information obtained is much less than in awake patients.

AWAKE SURGICAL TECHNIQUE

No standard methods for DBS exist. Our methods, as well as those of other centers, continue to evolve with technologic improvement and experience. We present an approach that has resulted in good outcomes and low complication rates at our institution.

Preoperative Imaging

Three MRI sets performed within a week of surgery are used for anatomic targeting. A gadolinium-enhanced volumetric three-dimensional T1 data set covering the whole brain in 1-mm axial cuts is used together with two two-dimensional image sets optimized for the best delineation of the targets: an axial inversion recovery fast spin echo (IR-FSE) and an axial T2-weighted fast spin echo (T2-FSE), both acquired as interleaved sequences to provide contiguous slices (zero interspace). Images are imported into a stereotactic surgical planning software package (FrameLink, Medtronic) for planning.

Operation

We place a standard stereotactic Leksell head frame (Elekta Inc., Atlanta, GA) in the preoperative holding area with conscious sedation. Mouth and eyes remain free for airway access and continuing neurological examination. A CT scan performed after the frame placement with the fiducial box is computationally fused with the preoperative magnetic resonance images to serve as image guidance for the procedure. After the fiducial marker registration, the image sets are reformatted to produce images orthogonal to the midcommissural plane.

Targeting

Subthalamic Nucleus. The approximate coordinates for localization of the STN are as follows: 3 mm posterior, 4 inferior, and 12 mm lateral to the midcommissural point. The T2-FSE or IR-FSE image set is then used to adjust the target with respect to the unique anatomy of each patient. The anterior border of the red nucleus is visualized on an axial slice 4 mm below the midcommissural plane. A line drawn tangential to the anterior apex of the red nucleus is seen cutting through the STN (Fig. 89-2). We pick the target point 2 mm lateral to the medial border of the STN along this line. Alternatively, if the lateral border of the STN is also well visualized, we target the middle of the nucleus along the line.

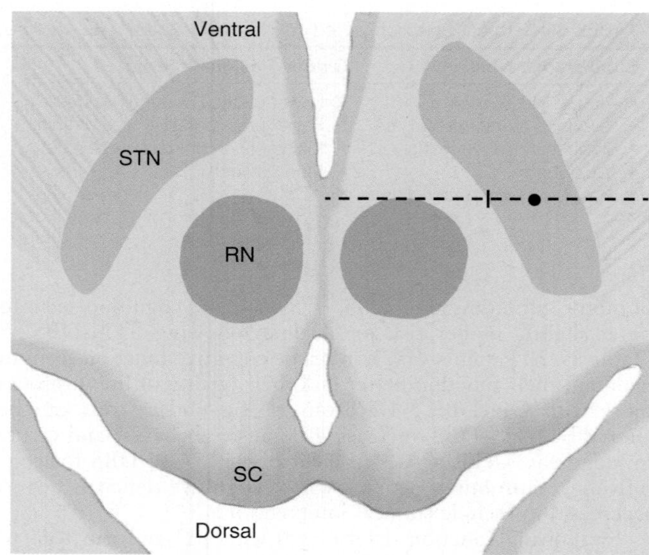

Figure 89-2. Midbrain at 4 mm below the midcommissural plane. The line parallel to the ventral border of the RN *(dashed line)* is extended to the midpoint of the STN *(black dot)* or, if the lateral border is difficult to interpret, at least 2 mm away from the STN medial border *(short vertical bar)* for targeting. RN, red nucleus; SC, superior colliculi; STN, subthalamic nucleus.

Globus Pallidus Interna. The approximate coordinates used for initial GPi targeting are as follows: 2 mm anterior, 5 mm inferior, and 21 mm lateral to the midcommissural point. Again the T2-FSE or IR-FSE image set is then used to adjust the target, accounting for individual patient variability, which is high for this target. We measure the pallidocapsular border on the axial slice at the level of the anterior commissure–posterior commissure (AC-PC) plane and divide it into thirds. The target is chosen by drawing a 3- to 4-mm line perpendicular to the pallidocapsular border at the junction of its posterior one third and anterior two thirds[73] (Fig. 89-3).

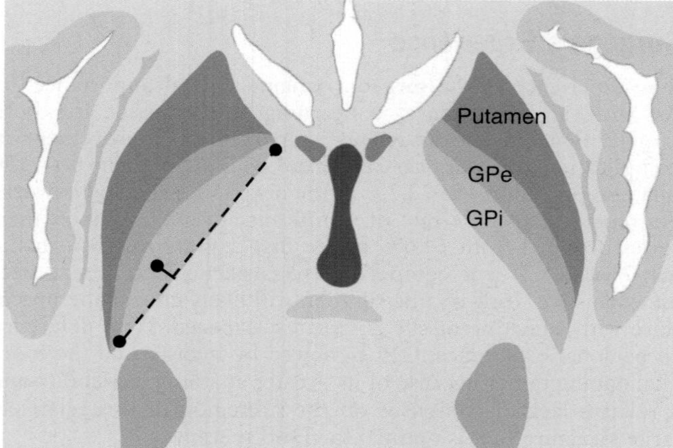

Figure 89-3. The axial cut at the midcommissural plane. The medial border of the GPi is split into thirds *(dashed line)* and a point 3 to 4 mm lateral and perpendicular to the line at the junction of the posterior one third and anterior two thirds *(short vertical bar with black dot)* is used for targeting. GPe, globus pallidus externa; GPi, globus pallidus interna.

Trajectory. The approximate initial trajectory for both STN and GPi stimulation is 60 degrees from the AC-PC line in the sagittal plane and 0 to 15 degrees from the vertical in the coronal plane. Patient-specific adjustments include avoiding cortical sulci and vascular structures superficially and deep. If the lateral ventricle is crossed along the trajectory, we adjust the entry point because ventricular violation is shown to increase morbidity[74] and may reduce the accuracy of placement. Navigation views are very helpful in entry point adjustment.

Positioning and Exposure

The patient is placed in a semisitting position, and the Mayfield headrest is used to fix the head frame in neutral position to the operating table. To avoid undue stress on the neck, the bed position should be finalized prior to fixating the head. A two-dimensional or three-dimensional fluoroscopy unit is set up with the head correctly centered. The head is prepped and draped to ensure accessibility to the face from the unsterile side. After a skin incision just posterior to the planned skull entry location, the bur hole is made with a 6-mm cutting drill. A recess is drilled around the bur hole to lower the profile of the lead anchoring device,

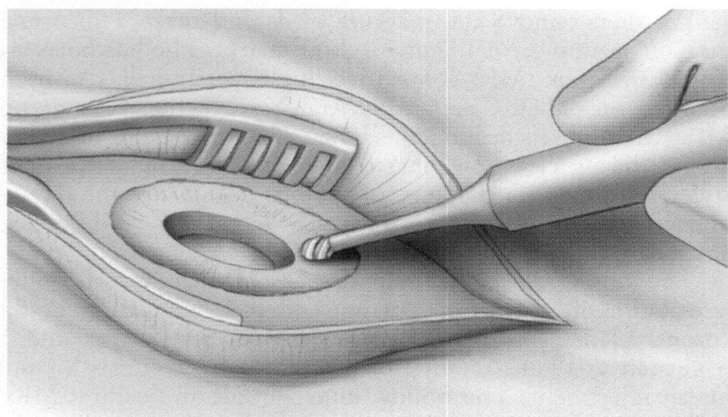

Figure 89-4. Countersinking the bur hole.

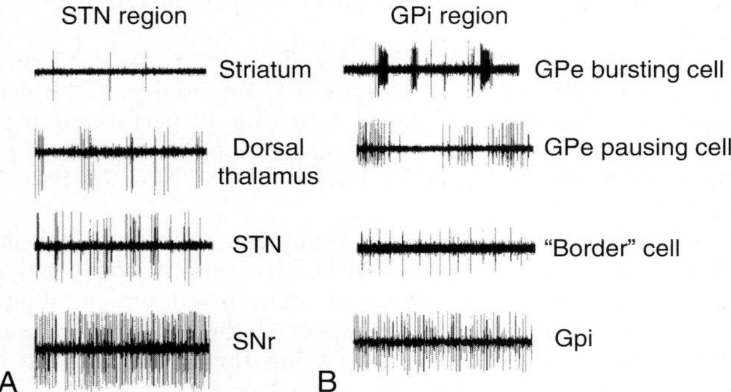

Figure 89-5. Microelectrode recordings of spontaneous neuronal activity from the thalamus and basal ganglia in the **(A)** subthalamic nucleus (STN) and **(B)** globus pallidus interna (GPi) regions. Each trace is a 1-second recording from a PD patient. GPe, globus pallidus externa; SNr, substantia nigra pars reticularis. *(Modified from Starr PA. Placement of deep brain stimulators into the subthalamic nucleus or globus pallidus internus: technical approach.* Stereotact Funct Neurosurg. *2002;79:118-145.)*

which aids in cosmesis and wound healing (Fig. 89-4). In rapid sequence the dura is opened, hemostasis is achieved, and the microelectrode guide tube is advanced past the pial surface. This allows the bur hole to be quickly filled with fibrin glue to decrease pneumocephalus and chances of air emboli.

Microelectrode Recording

MER is a technique with very high spatial resolution, thus augmenting preoperative imaging, which may lose accuracy because of mechanical properties of the frame and unpredictable brain shift.[75] We use high-impedance (0.3 to 0.8 MΩ at 1000 Hz) tungsten or platinum-iridium microelectrodes for recording of single-unit extracellular action potentials.[76] Controlled advance of the microelectrodes and DBS electrodes is performed with a micropositioner (NeuroNav Drive, Alpha Omega, Inc., Alpharetta, GA; Elekta micropositioner). The low deformability of the microelectrode in brain tissue allows for an accurate unsupported trajectory of up to 30 mm. The relatively higher deformability of the DBS electrode mandates more guidance from a rigid guide tube, no further than 15 mm from the target. For GPi implants, we change the guide tubes from 30 mm above the target to 10 mm above the target between MER and implantation.

For the STN (Fig. 89-5A), the recordings typically begin 10 mm dorsal to the anatomic target. On entrance into the STN, neuronal action potentials are detected at firing rates of 20 to 50 Hz. Because of high cell density, multiple units are often recorded simultaneously. The inferior border of the STN is signaled by a sudden decrease in the background noise, and the entrance into the substantia nigra pars reticularis is signaled by an increase in the discharge rate to 50 to 70 Hz. While in the STN, audible modulation of neuronal discharge by passive contralateral joint movement confirms localization of the motor area of the nucleus, which is dorsal, posterior, and lateral to nonmotor areas. Microelectrode passes are always sequential, with the location of each pass informed by the recordings gathered during previous passes. Good initial recording, presence of passive joint movement responses, and a span of STN cells over a distance of 5 mm obviate the need for further passes.

In the GPi (Fig. 89-5B) we usually record the striatum followed by the GPe before reaching our target. The initial low-frequency striatal discharges (0 to 10 Hz) increase to 30 to 60 Hz on GPe entrance. Frequent "burster" and "pauser" (Fig. 89-5B) discharge patterns are seen. When entering the GPi, we see a further rate increase to 60 to 100 Hz. The lamina separating the GPi and GPe contains "border" cells with a fairly regular 20- to 40-Hz discharge pattern. The somatotopic organization of the GPi (lower extremity motor-responsive cells medial and dorsal to upper extremity cells) is useful in checking the laterality of the recording, based on movement-related modulation of neuronal discharge. The recordings are stopped 1 to 2 mm after the last GPi unit to minimize chances of vascular injury in the choroid fissure. Microstimulation or light-evoked fiber activity can be used to identify the optic tract below the base of the pallidum.

Deep Brain Stimulation Lead Implantation and Macrostimulation

Although other implantable devices are becoming available, our current technique is based on the Medtronic DBS hardware. Using a rigid guide tube no further than 15 mm above target, the lead is placed with the bottom of its distal contact at the microelectrode-recorded ventral limit of the target for the GPi. For the STN, the middle two contacts are positioned on either side of the microelectrode-recorded dorsal border of the target. The final position check includes macrostimulation via a Medtronic model 3625 handheld pulse generator with the following settings: GPi contacts of 0–, 3+ and a more constrained field for the STN, typically 1–, 2+; rate of 180 Hz; 60-μsec pulse width. The voltage is increased to assess the threshold for stimulation-induced adverse effects and that for stimulation-induced changes, including tremor, rigidity, and bradykinesia reduction.

With STN implantation, the voltage threshold required to activate the medial lemniscus, posteromedial to the target, and the corticobulbar tract, lateral to the target, indicates the lead's proximity to these structures. Stimulation-induced adverse effects should occur in the 6- to 10-V range. If strong persistent paresthesias from medial lemniscus stimulation, or dysarthria and facial contractions from corticobulbar tract stimulation, occur below 2 V, the lead location is suboptimal and should be revised. Contralateral gaze deviation, from activation of the frontopontine bundle anterior to the STN, may be observed above 8 V. A lead placement error in the anterior, medial, and ventral direction may cause ipsilateral monocular adduction with current spread to the nucleus or tract of the third cranial nerve. Acute stimulation-induced mood changes may be related to stimulation of the limbic (anteromedial) portion of the STN. If no effects are seen at 10 V, the pulse width can be increased to 200 μsec. The likely reason for lack of effects after such an adjustment is an electrical malfunction or misplacement of the lead dorsally.

With GPi implants, voltage thresholds for dysarthria and facial contraction indicate the proximity to the corticobulbar tract, posterior and medial to the target. The activation of the optic tract at low voltage may indicate that the lead is too deep. Corticobulbar tract activation at 3 V or lower may preclude therapeutic stimulation and dictates movement of the lead to a more anterior or lateral position.

Diminution of contralateral rigidity is the most readily detectable acute effect of intraoperative test stimulation. Tremor and bradykinesia may improve as well. Motor symptom improvement without stimulation—the so-called microlesioning effect—may occur with the simple passing of the lead or microelectrode through the motor territory of the STN or GPi. Although such effect is variable, when present, it provides evidence of good electrode placement. Once macrostimulation is completed, the patient is put under anesthesia for the rest of the procedure.

Closure and Pulse Generator Placement

The lead is secured using a bur hole–mounted lead anchoring device (Stimloc, Medtronic). We protect the end of the lead with a temporary cap and tunnel it subgalealy to the area behind the pinna of the ear. The galea and skin are closed in the usual fashion. If available, intraoperative CT may be used at any point, and the images can be fused with preoperative targeting to assess the accuracy of lead placement. Lateral fluoroscopy is useful to verify lack of lead movement as it is secured.

After the removal of the frame and positioning of the patient similar to that for a ventriculoperitoneal shunt procedure, placement of either unilateral or bilateral lead extensions and internal pulse generators (IPGs) is performed under general anesthesia. A small incision is made over the protective cap of the lead. A 5-cm incision is made parallel and 2 cm inferior to the clavicle, and an IPG pocket is created over the pectoralis fascia. We tunnel the lead extender in a rostral-to-caudal direction to connect the lead to the IPG. The IPG is placed so as to avoid tension on the incision. The chest incision is closed in three layers. Placing the lead extender connector below the occipital ridge should be avoided because the mobility of the neck over time can cause fracture of the lead. Impedances are checked prior to closure of the incisions.

ASLEEP INTERVENTIONAL MAGNETIC RESONANCE IMAGING SURGICAL TECHNIQUE

Our technique uses a skull-mounted aiming device (SmartFrame, MRI Interventions, Inc., Irvine, CA) with dedicated targeting software (ClearPoint, MRI Interventions) in a 1.5-T diagnostic MRI scanner (Philips Achieva, Philips, Inc., Eindhoven, The Netherlands) with a 60-cm bore diameter. No preoperative stereotactic imaging is required. The patient is placed under general anesthesia, shaved, prepped, and injected with local anesthetic in a room adjacent to the scanner before being moved onto the MRI gurney. We rigidly fix the head in slight extension with a 4-pin carbon fiber head holder (Malcolm-Rand, Engineered Orthopedic Technologies, Inc., San Clemente, CA). Flexible surface receiving coils are placed in a sagittal fashion on both sides of the head, and the patient is moved through the MRI bore to allow surgical access at the back of the scanner. After a second prep, a custom drape is attached by elastic cords at both ends of the bore to maintain the sterile field during gantry movements. We use a skin-adhesive 7.5-cm by 9-cm MRI-visible marking grid placed to span the coronal suture on each side during the first gadolinium-enhanced volumetric MRI scan for entry point selection. Once the images are imported into the targeting software, a selection of a preliminary target and trajectory is made as described earlier and correlated with the marking grid. After moving the head to the back of the bore, the intended entry is marked through the skin into the outer table of the skull with a sharp instrument.

We then remove the marking grids and make a bicoronal incision spanning 2 cm lateral to both marks. The bur holes are drilled with an MRI-compatible high-speed drill (Anspach, Synthes, Inc., West Chester, PA; Aria, Stryker, Inc., Kalamazoo, MI). Attention to drilling the inner table, especially its lateral aspect, during GPi placement is important to avoid subsequent stylet collision with the edge of the bur hole. Once the dura is opened and coagulated, we attach the SmartFrame and the lead anchoring ring (Stimloc) over the bur holes.

The aiming device has four degrees of freedom, with pitch (angulation in the sagittal plane) and roll (angulation in the coronal plane) controls for coarse angular adjustment, and X (right-left axis) and Y (anterior-posterior axis) controls for fine linear adjustment. The hollow lumen inside the central MRI-visible targeting cannula allows for passage of a ceramic stylet within a Silastic (Dow Corning, Midland, MI) peel-away sheath. The attachment of mechanical remote controls prior to moving the head back to isocenter allows for the rest of the implantation to take place without any motion of the patient relative to the scanner.

The targeting cannula position and trajectory are recognized by the software once a volumetric T1-weighted gradient echo sequence is complete. Optimal targeting is performed using the process described in the previous section (see Figs. 89-2 and 89-3) with high-resolution T2-FSE for the STN or IR-FSE for the GPi.

We perform the first rough alignment using the pitch and roll adjustment controls as prescribed by computational analysis of the position of the alignment stem based on an oblique axial image through the distal aspect of the targeting cannula. Next, a fine adjustment is made using the X and Y controls, based on oblique sagittal and coronal scans obtained parallel to the long axis of the targeting cannula. Once the predicted radial error (distance between intended and projected trajectory in the axial plane used for targeting) is less than 0.5 mm, we advance a ceramic stylet with a peel-away sheath to a depth of 2 mm past the target for the STN or 4 to 5 mm past the target for the GPi.

Appropriate navigation past the cortical anatomy without hemorrhage and continuing correct trajectory are confirmed with acquisition of intermediate oblique sagittal and coronal T2-weighted images. Once at the target, a high-resolution axial T2-weighted image is used for confirmation. Next, we replace the ceramic stylet with a quadripolar DBS lead (model 3389, Medtronic), and ensure correct lead depth using a low-energy axial T2-weighted image. The patient's head is returned to the back of the bore for removal of the peel-away sheath, securing of the lead, and removal of the aiming device. Closure is performed as described previously. The placement of lead extensions and IPGs is usually performed on an outpatient basis within 2 weeks.

Key differences of the iMRI technique are as follows:

- The planning, insertion, and confirmation of lead placement are integrated into a single MRI procedure.
- The use of the bur hole–mounted aiming device obviates the need for a stereotactic frame system.
- Because navigation is performed in the coordinate system defined by the MRI isocenter, defining a separate stereotactic space (registered using fiducial markers) is unnecessary.
- The patients are asleep for the procedure and no test stimulations or MERs are performed.
- The possible errors resulting from mechanical properties of the aiming device are corrected in real time.
- Brain shift errors are decreased as target images are acquired after bur hole creation and intracranial air entry.

For an intraoperative video of an iMRI case, please see Video 89-1.

RESULTS

Motor outcomes of PD treatment are quantitatively measured using the UPDRS III. This is a clinician-scored motor evaluation with high interrater reliability. Several level I studies show that, for patients with advanced PD, DBS at either the STN or GPi is more effective than best medical therapy in improving motor function, quality of life, and "on" time without dyskinesias.[39,77]

A 2005 study showed a 48% improvement in UPDRS III scores with bilateral STN stimulation compared with 39% improvement with bilateral GPi stimulation.[49] It also first mentioned the pattern of cognitive and behavioral complications after STN implantation, not seen after pallidal surgery. A large trial with 159 patients completing 3-year follow-up confirmed the near-equivalent improvement in motor scores with either STN (34% improvement) or GPi (30% improvement) stimulation.[78] Again some propensity for mildly increased depression and cognitive impairment outcomes with STN stimulation was seen. A recent review[79] of the same data showed a trend in suicidal ideation that did not reach statistical significance in STN-DBS versus GPi-DBS (1.5% versus 0.7%; Fisher exact test, $P = .61$).

A randomized study of unilateral STN-DBS versus GPi-DBS showed no difference in the motor score improvement, with mean percent improvement of 29.9% for the STN and 26.6% for the GPi.[48] Interestingly, an analysis of experimental stimulation ventral to optimal settings in the STN and GPi showed that stimulation in these locations caused adverse mood effects, an outcome likely related to the electrical alteration of the parallel nonmotor ventral limbic areas in both nuclei. A recent European study[40] found no difference between the STN and GPi in cognitive and behavioral complications but did see significantly better results in medication reduction, off-medication motor scores, and mean change in Academic Medical Center Linear Disability Scale with STN stimulation.

Follow-up of 8 to 10 years[80] shows that, although DBS is safe and efficacious over the long term, the nonmotor symptoms progress, causing decrease in the function of the patient.

COMPLICATIONS

The major complications of DBS for PD are hemorrhage, infection, and hardware failure. Complications can be separated into early (up to 6 months) and late. A recent large review[81] focusing on early (within 90 days) complications found that 132 of 1757 patients (7.5%) had at least one such event. The most common were wound infections (3.6%), pneumonia (2.3%), hemorrhage (1.4%), and pulmonary embolism (0.6%). Interestingly, patients older than 75 years did not have an increased rate of early postoperative complications.

The reported risk of symptomatic hemorrhage during MER-guided DBS in the literature ranges from 2.2% to 0.5%.[44,45] Hypertension and MER may increase the risk of cerebral hemorrhage in DBS.[44,67] Possible ways of decreasing the risk of hemorrhage include maintaining the mean arterial pressure under 90 mm Hg, proper hydration to decrease the chance of venous infarcts, and using trajectories that avoid blood vessels, sulci, and the ventricle.[82] Careful counseling of patients regarding this potential complication is imperative in the preoperative discussion.

The incidence of hardware infection, defined as an infection requiring further surgery for partial or complete hardware removal, is reported to occur in up to 10% of cases.[39,83,84] Hardware removal necessitates the abrupt cessation of stimulation, combined with a long course of antibiotics, and places emotional and economic strain on the patient and the treatment team.

Late complications include hardware erosion, lead fracture, and lead migration. Hardware erosion may present itself at any point after DBS. Measures to reduce hardware erosion incidence include using a countersinking bur hole technique, increasing the IPG pocket size in the rostral-caudal direction, and placing deep facial stitches to isolate the IPG from the incision. Continued vigilance is important with respect to hardware erosion because an early diagnosis may allow a partial, rather than total, hardware explantation.

Lead or lead extension fracture occurrence in PD is reported in the 2% range.[85,86] Allowing for stress relief loops and securing the lead/lead extension connection above the occipital ridge with an extra fascial stitch may decrease the chance of fracture.[82] Tunneling deeper in the subcutaneous tissue of the neck may decrease the chances of "bowstringing" and scarring of the extensions, which in turn may also decrease the fracture rate.[87] The incidence of malpositioned electrodes requiring surgical revision ranges from 0.8% to 1.7% per lead.[83,85,86,88] Repositioning as little as 2 mm toward the center of the motor territory of the target may significantly improve the efficacy of a marginally placed lead.

FUTURE DIRECTIONS

Improvement in implantable devices is increasing our parameter space in delivering stimulation. Constant voltage is being augmented with constant current paradigms.[89] Current steering, available with some of the newer lead models, will potentially improve benefits and minimize side effects.[90] Irregular stimulation[91] may also increase our ability to benefit patients by increasing efficacy of treatment. Use of the concept of pathologic beta oscillation methods for "resetting" the circuit to alleviate PD symptoms has been introduced.[92]

Neuromodulation implants with concurrent sensing and stimulation ability can aid our understanding of pathophysiology and improve therapies for PD by incorporating feedback control into stimulation paradigms. Such implants have been tested in large nonhuman animal subjects.[93] An investigational protocol in a nonhuman primate 1-methyl-4-phenyl-1,2,3,6-tetrahydropyridine model showed improved control of parkinsonian symptoms with a GPi stimulation triggered by motor cortex unit activity.[94] A bidirectional neural interface that both delivers stimulation therapy and senses and stores field potentials (Activa PC + S, Medtronic) is now in use in human trials.[95]

SUGGESTED READINGS

Alexander GE, Crutcher MD, DeLong MR. Basal ganglia-thalamocortical circuits: parallel substrates for motor, oculomotor, "prefrontal" and "limbic" functions. *Prog Brain Res*. 1990;85:119-146.

Anderson VC, Burchiel KJ, Hogarth P, et al. Pallidal vs subthalamic nucleus deep brain stimulation in Parkinson disease. *Arch Neurol*. 2005;62(4):554-560.

Benabid AL, Pollak P, Louveau A, et al. Combined (thalamotomy and stimulation) stereotactic surgery of the VIM thalamic nucleus for bilateral Parkinson disease. *Appl Neurophysiol*. 1987;50(1-6):344-346.

Bergman H, Wichmann T, DeLong MR. Reversal of experimental parkinsonism by lesions of the subthalamic nucleus. *Science*. 1990; 249(4975):1436-1438.

Bronstein JM, Tagliati M, Alterman RL, et al. Deep brain stimulation for Parkinson disease: an expert consensus and review of key issues. *Arch Neurol*. 2011;68(2):165.

Burchiel KJ, McCartney S, Lee A, et al. Accuracy of deep brain stimulation electrode placement using intraoperative computed tomography without microelectrode recording. *J Neurosurg*. 2013;119(2): 301-306.

Charles D, Konrad PE, Neimat JS, et al. Subthalamic nucleus deep brain stimulation in early stage Parkinson's disease. *Parkinsonism Relat Disord*. 2014;20(7):731-737.

Cooper IS. Effect of anterior choroidal artery ligation on involuntary movements and rigidity. *Trans Am Neurol Assoc*. 1953;3(78th Meeting): 6-7, discussion 8-9.

Cotzias GC. L-Dopa for Parkinsonism. *N Engl J Med*. 1968;278(11):630.

Deuschl G, Schupbach M, Knudsen K, et al. Stimulation of the subthalamic nucleus at an earlier disease stage of Parkinson's disease: concept and standards of the EARLYSTIM-study. *Parkinsonism Relat Disord.* 2013;19(1):56-61.

Follett KA, Weaver FM, Stern M, et al. Pallidal versus subthalamic deep-brain stimulation for Parkinson's disease. *N Engl J Med.* 2010; 362(22):2077-2091.

Hammond C, Bergman H, Brown P. Pathological synchronization in Parkinson's disease: networks, models and treatments. *Trends Neurosci.* 2007;30(7):357-364.

Henderson JM, Holloway KL, Gaede SE, et al. The application accuracy of a skull-mounted trajectory guide system for image-guided functional neurosurgery. *Comput Aided Surg.* 2004;9(4):155-160.

Konrad PE, Neimat JS, Yu H, et al. Customized, miniature rapid-prototype stereotactic frames for use in deep brain stimulator surgery: initial clinical methodology and experience from 263 patients from 2002 to 2008. *Stereotact Funct Neurosurg.* 2011;89(1):34-41.

Odekerken VJ, van Laar T, Staal MJ, et al. Subthalamic nucleus versus globus pallidus bilateral deep brain stimulation for advanced Parkinson's disease (NSTAPS study): a randomised controlled trial. *Lancet Neurol.* 2013;12(1):37-44.

Okun MS, Fernandez HH, Wu SS, et al. Cognition and mood in Parkinson's disease in subthalamic nucleus versus globus pallidus interna deep brain stimulation: the COMPARE trial. *Ann Neurol.* 2009;65(5): 586-595.

Okun MS, Gallo BV, Mandybur G, et al. Subthalamic deep brain stimulation with a constant-current device in Parkinson's disease: an open-label randomised controlled trial. *Lancet Neurol.* 2012;11(2):140-149.

Ostrem JL, Galifianakis NB, Markun LC, et al. Clinical outcomes of PD patients having bilateral STN DBS using high-field interventional MR-imaging for lead placement. *Clin Neurol Neurosurg.* 2013;115(6): 708-712.

Parkinson J. An essay on the shaking palsy. 1817. *J Neuropsychiatry Clin Neurosci.* 2002;14(2):223-236, discussion 222.

Ryapolova-Webb E, Afshar P, Stanslaski S, et al. Chronic cortical and electromyographic recordings from a fully implantable device: preclinical experience in a nonhuman primate. *J Neural Eng.* 2014; 11(1):016009.

Starr PA, Markun LC, Larson PS, et al. Interventional MRI-guided deep brain stimulation in pediatric dystonia: first experience with the ClearPoint system. *J Neurosurg Pediatr* 2014;14(4):400-408.

Starr PA, Martin AJ, Ostrem JL, et al. Subthalamic nucleus deep brain stimulator placement using high-field interventional magnetic resonance imaging and a skull-mounted aiming device: technique and application accuracy. *J Neurosurg.* 2010;112(3):479-490.

Weaver FM, Follett K, Stern M, et al. Bilateral deep brain stimulation vs best medical therapy for patients with advanced Parkinson disease: a randomized controlled trial. *JAMA.* 2009;301(1):63-73.

See a full reference list on ExpertConsult.com

90 Deep Brain Stimulation for Dystonia

Scellig S.D. Stone and Ron L. Alterman

Dystonia is a neurological disorder characterized by sustained or intermittent muscle contractions causing twisting, repetitive movements that result in abnormal, often painful postures.[1,2] Different muscle groups may be involved to a variable extent and severity. Dystonia is not one disease; rather, it is a neurological manifestation of many pathologic conditions, most of which are poorly characterized. The prevalence estimates for primary dystonia in the general population range from 2 to 50 cases per million for early-onset dystonia and from 30 to 7320 cases per million for late-onset dystonia.[3] However, prevalence rates are significantly higher in some ethnic groups.[3,4]

Because of the limitations of available medical therapies, a variety of surgical interventions, targeting both the peripheral and central nervous systems, have been attempted for dystonia.[5-7] The dystonia literature is filled with case reports and small cohort studies, mostly relating mixed or conflicting outcomes. Long-term results in significant numbers of patients are only now being published. Moreover, many techniques were highly invasive and/or associated with a high incidence of denervation-related complications, leading them to fall out of favor.

In the more recent past, the successful use of deep brain stimulation (DBS) for medically refractory Parkinson's disease (PD) and essential tremor (ET) led to investigations of its utility for treating dystonia. In particular, the observation that pallidal interventions improve "off"-state dystonia in PD patients shifted attention from the thalamus to the internal globus pallidus (GPi) as the target of choice for treating primary dystonia.[8] The result of these efforts has been the development of the most effective treatment presently available for primary dystonia and one of the most successful applications of neuromodulation technology yet described. This chapter focuses on the current status of pallidal DBS for dystonia. Because of space constraints, discussion of alternative therapeutic targets for stimulation will be limited.

DIAGNOSIS AND CLASSIFICATION OF DYSTONIA

Dystonia may be classified in several ways, with the most recent consensus statement emphasizing two distinct axes: clinical features and etiology.[1,2] Several features describe the clinical characteristics of a given patient: (1) the anatomic distribution of the abnormal movements, (2) the age at symptom onset (early versus late), (3) the temporal pattern of symptoms, and (4) the coexistence of other movement disorders or neurological manifestations. Focal dystonias (e.g., writer's cramp, spasmodic torticollis) are limited to a single body region, segmental dystonia affects more than one contiguous body part (e.g., craniocervical dystonia), multifocal dystonia involves noncontiguous body regions, hemidystonia denotes multiple noncontiguous body regions restricted to one side of the body, and widespread involvement of the axial and limb musculature characterizes generalized dystonia. Patients with early symptom onset (i.e., age < 26) are more likely to have a heritable form of dystonia and are more likely to suffer generalized symptoms.[1,4] The temporal course can be static or progressive, with superimposed persistent, action-specific, diurnal, and paroxysmal patterns of manifestation. Dystonia may be combined with other movement disorders (e.g., myoclonus, parkinsonism) or neurologic features (e.g., cognitive, psychiatric).

Dystonia is etiologically classified as primary versus secondary based on the absence or presence, respectively, of a specific underlying cause. Primary or idiopathic dystonia implies no identified structural brain abnormality or specific toxic, metabolic, traumatic, or infectious etiology. The heritable forms of dystonia are traditionally included in this group; however, they have been separated into their own category in the newest classification system.[2] A constantly growing list of more than 20 primarily single-gene mutations are associated with primary dystonia, with dystonia being the sole or most prominent symptom.[9] The most common form of genetic dystonia results from a GAG deletion of the gene encoding the protein torsin-A.[10] This mutation, referred to as *DYT1*, is associated with a form of childhood-onset dystonia formerly known as dystonia musculorum deformans or Oppenheim's disease. *DYT1*-associated dystonia is inherited in an autosomal dominant pattern but with a penetrance of just 30% to 40%, suggesting that additional genetic and/or environmental factors contribute to the expression of the dystonic phenotype.[10]

When a structural brain abnormality or specific underlying etiology is identified, a dystonia is classified as secondary or symptomatic. Secondary dystonia is more prevalent than primary dystonia and may arise from a variety of causes, including static encephalopathy, stroke, traumatic brain injury, or any number of toxic, metabolic, or infectious disorders. Often included here is a large group of genetic syndromes that, unlike their mainly monogenic *DYT* counterparts, often express dystonia as a component of a complex phenotype.[9] Consequently, this is a heterogeneous patient population with varied pathophysiologies and responses to treatment.[1]

MEDICAL THERAPY FOR DYSTONIA

In most cases, medical therapy for dystonia is limited to symptom control and is variably effective.[11,12] Physical therapy and orthotic devices can sometimes help maintain range of motion and prevent contractures in affected body parts. Anticholinergic medications (e.g., trihexyphenidyl) are the mainstay of medical therapy for generalized dystonias but often yield only modest improvements and, at the high doses employed for dystonia, may cause significant side effects such as drowsiness, blurred vision, and poor memory. Additional medications for dystonia include baclofen, benzodiazepines, zolpidem, and tetrabenazine. A minority of patients with symptomatic generalized dystonia will benefit from specific therapy targeted at the underlying disorder. Children and adolescents with "clinically pure" dystonia of unknown etiology should be evaluated for Wilson's disease and should undergo a trial of levodopa therapy, as a small subpopulation with levodopa-responsive dystonia will experience a profound and sustained response to this medication.[11]

Targeted injections of botulinum toxin (Botox) can alleviate focal dystonias, but this intervention is impractical in patients with generalized symptoms.[11,13] Some patients will not respond to Botox initially, and up to 10% may develop resistance over time through the production of blocking antibodies.[14,15]

SURGICAL THERAPY FOR DYSTONIA

Surgical intervention for dystonia should generally be considered when a patient's symptoms are disabling and the response to medical therapy is either inadequate or limited by side effects. Historically, surgical interventions for dystonia have targeted both the peripheral and central nervous systems.[5,6] Peripheral denervation procedures for focal dystonias have largely been supplanted by chemical denervation with Botox.[12,14] Chronic intrathecal baclofen infusions can alleviate dystonia, though existing case series have reported mixed motor and functional results[16-18] with significant hardware-related complication rates. Intrathecal baclofen infusion is more commonly considered for secondary dystonia with resulting spasticity, most commonly seen in cerebral palsy.

Advances in stereotactic technique, the success of DBS in PD and ET, and the observation that pallidotomy improves "off"-medication dystonia in PD patients[8] renewed interest in basal ganglia interventions for dystonia in the 1990s. Stereotactic pallidotomy does improve symptoms of primary generalized dystonia (PGD)[19]; however, unilateral pallidotomy may not sufficiently treat generalized symptoms and bilateral pallidotomy entails significant risk, including cognitive dysfunction, dysarthria, dysphagia, and limb weakness.[20] Consequently, DBS, which is reversible and may be employed bilaterally with relative safety, has emerged as a preferable alternative.

THE DEEP BRAIN STIMULATION PROCEDURE

Consistently successful DBS surgery involves three critical steps: (1) careful patient selection, (2) precise lead implantation, and (3) skillful device programming. Failure to perform any one of these three steps properly may lead to suboptimal results.

Patient Selection

As discussed in the introduction, dystonia is a complex group of disorders, most of which are *not* responsive to DBS. Therefore, it is important to have all surgical candidates evaluated by a movement disorders neurologist before proceeding. He or she will ensure that the diagnosis of dystonia is correct, and that all reasonable medical therapies have been tried. At many centers, the neurologist also programs the DBS devices after implantation, manages medication changes, and monitors patient progress.

In the United States, Activa Dystonia Therapy (Medtronic, Inc., Minneapolis, MN) is approved under a Humanitarian Device Exemption exclusively for the treatment of primary dystonia in patients over the age of 7 years. All other uses are considered to be "off-label." Patients should not be offered surgery unless their symptoms are disabling and have failed to respond to standard medical therapies. A notable caveat to this may be select children with primary generalized dystonia. Here, GPi-DBS is increasingly considered a first-line treatment with the goal of reducing loss of mobility and joint deformity prior to the development of contractures, and to minimize the impact of centrally acting medications on cognitive and social development.[21-23] A magnetic resonance imaging (MRI) study of the brain should be obtained to rule out structural lesions. Patients with childhood-onset generalized dystonia should be tested for Wilson's disease and the *DYT1* mutation, and should receive an adequate trial of levodopa before proceeding with surgery.

Surgical Procedure

The implanted device is composed of four primary components (Fig. 90-1) that are implanted in two phases, as either a single or a staged operation. During the first phase, the stimulating lead(s) are implanted into the GPi stereotactically and secured by means of an anchoring system that also covers the bur hole. The remaining two components—the extension cable(s) and pulse generator(s)—are implanted during the second phase of the procedure, which may be performed at the same setting or during a second stage shortly thereafter. It is acceptable to implant DBS leads bilaterally during the same procedure. Dystonia patients are typically much younger than patients with PD and ET and, in our experience, tolerate the bilateral frontal lobe penetrations without difficulty.

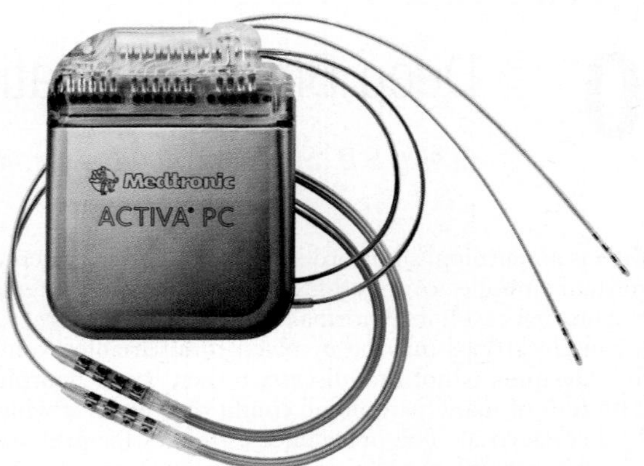

Figure 90-1. The deep brain stimulation (DBS) system. The DBS system (Activa; Medtronic, Inc., Minneapolis, MN) has three primary components: (1) the stimulating lead, which is implanted stereotactically into the desired target; (2) the programmable neurostimulator, which generates the electrical impulses; and (3) the extension cable, which is tunneled subcutaneously and connects the stimulator to the lead. A fourth component, the bur hole cap, which holds the lead in place and covers the bur hole, is not pictured. *(Reprinted with the permission of Medtronic, Inc. © 2015.)*

Stereotactic Technique

Stereotactic head frames remain the primary means for performing DBS lead implants; however, "frameless" technologies are being employed with greater frequency.[24-27] These systems employ either a custom-built or adjustable targeting platform in concert with skull-mounted fiducials or an MRI-compatible implantation platform that allows real-time MRI guidance of the lead and target during implantation.[25] Good outcomes are reported using each of these methods, with accuracies rivaling those achieved with conventional head frames. No reports directly compare these techniques to suggest the superiority of one technique over another.[28] Potential advantages of frameless systems include enhanced patient comfort, workflow efficiency, and anatomic accuracy. In contrast, stereotactic frames may provide greater head stability during surgery, compatibility with microelectrode recording (MER) platforms, entry point and trajectory flexibility, and lower procedure cost, and they enjoy the greatest published experience.[29]

Anatomic Targeting

As with stereotactic targeting technologies, a variety of imaging techniques may be used to perform DBS implants. The senior author (R.L.A.) employs axial and coronal fast spin echo inversion recovery (FSE-IR) MRI because the images are acquired rapidly (~6 minutes per scan) and provide superior resolution of the commissures and deep nuclei (Fig. 90-2). The thickness of the axial slices (2 to 3 mm) required to generate these high-resolution images increases our initial targeting error along the *z*-axis (i.e., depth), but this is compensated for by MER, which delineates the depth of specific structures along the implantation trajectory with a resolution of approximately 0.1 mm. The scanning parameters for FSE-IR MRI are given in Table 90-1. These images alone are sufficient for performing DBS implants with microelectrode guidance; however, additional image sets such as gadolinium-enhanced three-dimensionally acquired T1-weighted MRI (e.g., spoiled gradient echo [SPGR]) and/or computed tomography

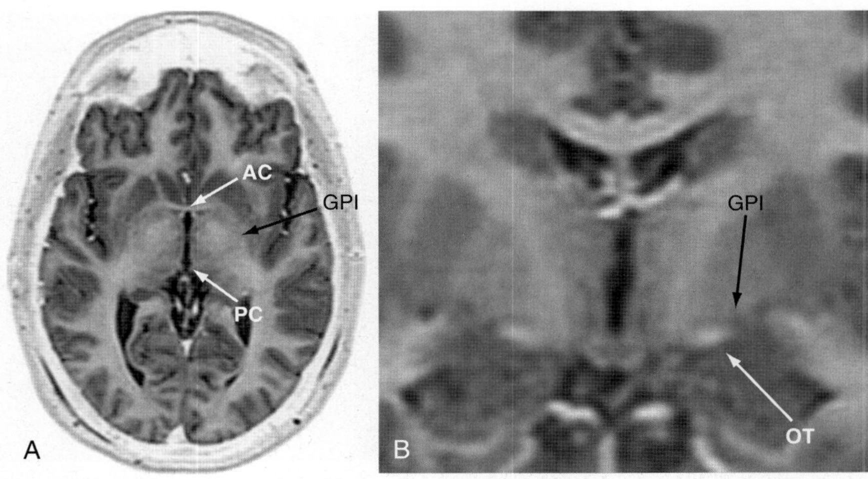

Figure 90-2. Fast spin echo inversion recovery (FSE-IR) magnetic resonance imaging. We employ both axial **(A)** and coronal **(B)** FSE-IR images for targeting the internal globus pallidus (GPi). The anterior commissure (AC) (**A,** *white arrow*) and posterior commissure (PC) (**A,** *white arrow*) are readily visible on the axial image, as is the posteroventral GPi (**A,** *black arrow*). The target is the posteroventral GPi, 20 to 21 mm lateral to the midline (**B,** *black arrow*) and 2 to 3 mm superior and lateral to the optic tract (OT) (**B,** *white arrow*).

TABLE 90-1 Scanning Parameters for Axial Fast Spin Echo Inversion Recovery Images

Excitation time (Te)	120 msec
Relaxation time (Tr)	10,000 msec
Inversion time (Ti)	2200 msec
Bandwidth	20.83 kHz
Field of view	24 cm
Slice thickness	3 mm
Slice spacing	0 mm
Frequency	192 Hz
Phase	160
Number of excitations	1
Frequency direction	Anteroposterior
Autocontrol frequency	Water
Flow compensation direction	Slice direction

may also be employed. In our experience, both the volume error of fiducial registration and targeting accuracy are significantly improved when SPGR MRI is employed for fiducial registration and FSE-IR for target selection.[30] Moreover, contrast-enhanced SPGR demonstrates the cortical veins so that they may be avoided when selecting an entry point. Computed tomography provides the most geometrically accurate images for fiducial registration and may also be acquired rapidly on the morning of surgery.

The images are transferred to an independent workstation that is equipped with advanced stereotactic targeting software. These software packages provide at least five advantages: (1) the target coordinates are calculated automatically, eliminating human math errors; (2) a variety of image sets (e.g., computed tomography and MRI) may be merged, allowing one to exploit the advantages of different types of imaging; (3) the entire trajectory may be visualized in all three anatomic planes and orthogonally to the trajectory (so-called probe's-eye view), allowing one to plan safer approaches to the target; (4) the image data sets are reformatted orthogonally to the intercommissural plane, controlling for variations in head frame placement; and (5) digitized versions of stereotactic atlases may be overlaid and digitally "fit" to the patient's anatomy, helping to identify the desired target. A significant drawback to these systems is that they assume the patient's brain to be symmetrical, which is not always the case. Congenital anomalies such as plagiocephaly can shift target structures, and it is the surgeon's responsibility to account for these shifts during the targeting process.

We target the internal pallidal site first described by Leksell, which lies 19 to 22 mm lateral, 2 to 3 mm anterior, and 4 to 5 mm inferior to the midcommissural point.[31] The target should be visualized on both axial and coronal images and should lay 2 to 3 mm superior and lateral to the optic tract (Fig. 90-2B). Our preferred trajectory is 60 to 65 degrees anterior and superior to the intercommissural plane and 0 to 10 degrees lateral to the vertical axis. This trajectory allows one to avoid the ipsilateral lateral ventricle and still employ nearly parasagittal trajectories, which facilitate the process of mapping the intraoperative MER data to human stereotactic atlases (see later).

Microelectrode Recording

The need for intraoperative neurophysiologic confirmation of proper targeting remains controversial because there are no published reports directly comparing the relative benefits and adversities of neurophysiologically guided versus non–neurophysiologically guided surgery for dystonia.[32] Acceptable outcomes have been obtained with both approaches. A detailed description of neurophysiologic recording and stimulation techniques, and discussion of their potential pros and cons in GPi-DBS surgery, is beyond the scope of this chapter. An overview of our use of MER and macroelectrode stimulation is described here. The interested reader is encouraged to review the finer details of our MER technique[33] and neurophysiologic monitoring[34] elsewhere.

The senior author (R.L.A.) employs MER to refine his anatomic targeting—if necessary. In his experience, MER provides important real-time information that other localization techniques simply do not. First, MER delineates the borders and expanses of the external globus pallidus (GPe) and GPi along a given trajectory with a spatial resolution of approximately 100 μm. These data may be mapped onto scaled sagittal sections of human stereotactic atlases in order to determine the anatomic position of the recording trajectory. Acceptable trajectories for implantation include a 3- to 4-mm span of GPe and at least 6 mm of GPi. Such a trajectory must pass through the heart of the GPi

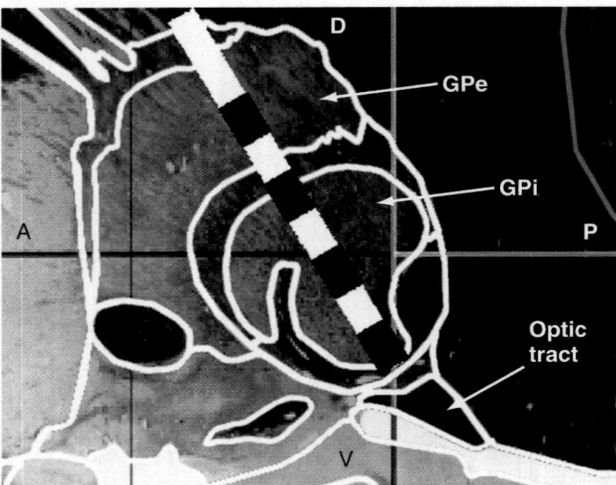

Figure 90-3. Pallidal lead implantation. Our preferred lead position within the globus pallidus is depicted. A schematic of the model 3387 lead (Medtronic, Inc., Minneapolis, MN), which has four 1.5-mm-long cylindrical contacts with 1.5-mm interelectrode spacing, is superimposed on a sagittal image, 20 mm lateral of the midline, derived from the Schaltenbrand and Wahren *Atlas for Stereotaxy of the Human Brain.*[107] With the deepest contact (contact 0) positioned at the inferior border of the GPi, three contacts can fit within the nucleus. A, anterior; D, dorsal; GPe, external globus pallidus; GPi, internal globus pallidus; P, posterior; V, ventral.

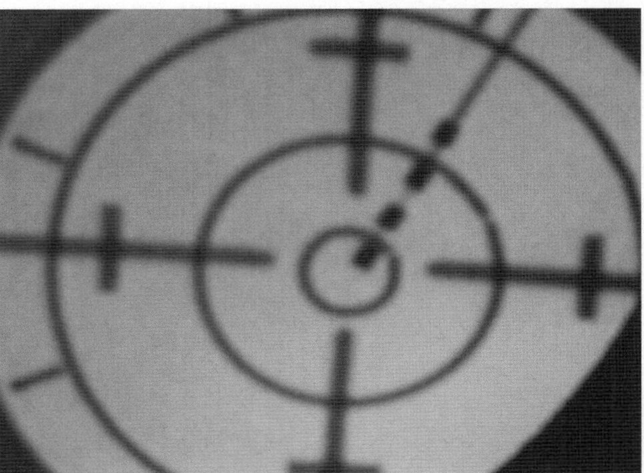

Figure 90-4. C-arm fluoroscopy. With the lead in position, reticules are attached to the stereotactic frame and the C-arm is manipulated in order to generate pure lateral images centered on the target. Serial images are taken to document that the lead is not dislodged from its desired position while it is locked in place with the bur-hole cap.

and will allow three to four contacts to be positioned comfortably within the nucleus, depending on the lead employed (Fig. 90-3). Second, the detection of kinesthetic cells confirms that the trajectory traverses the sensorimotor subregion of the GPi, the physiologically defined target for the procedure. Third, delineating the inferior border of the GPi refines the depth of implantation. Fourth, identifying the optic tract 2 to 3 mm inferior to the GPi exit point confirms that the trajectory exits the nucleus inferiorly, not posteriorly into the internal capsule. Identification of the optic tract provides an additional level of confidence that the lead will be well positioned, but this should not be viewed as an absolute requirement for implantation, because the optic tract may not be identified in many cases.

Of note, anticholinergics and benzodiazepines may be held on the morning of surgery in order to facilitate recordings, which may be affected by these medications. Baclofen, however, should not be withheld as, in the senior author's (R.L.A.'s) experience, this may precipitate a dystonic crisis.

Deep Brain Stimulation Surgery in Children

The first phase of the DBS procedure is conventionally performed with the patient fully awake, but this may be challenging for young children or patients with severely contorted postures. If maturity, painful muscular spasms, or abnormal postures make awake surgery arduous, DBS lead implants may be performed under conscious sedation or even full general anesthesia. It is the senior author's (R.L.A.'s) experience, however, that MER-guided DBS may be performed, even in children, so long as one has a dedicated neuroanesthesiologist who is willing to carefully manage the level of consciousness throughout the procedure so that the patient is comfortable but awake enough to obtain useful recordings.[35]

Macroelectrode Stimulation

The DBS lead is inserted along the desired trajectory, leaving the deepest contact (contact 0) at the physiologically defined inferior border of the GPi. C-arm fluoroscopy is employed to confirm that the lead has traveled to the desired point, relative to the frame (Fig. 90-4). Before it is secured, the acute effects of stimulation via the lead are tested. Testing is performed in bipolar mode employing the following parameters: pulse width, 90 μsec; frequency, 130 Hz; amplitude, 0 to 4 V. Stimulation amplitudes greater than 5 V are not used because we have never required amplitudes this great for therapy. The initial test is performed with the deepest pair of contacts (i.e., 0–, 1+) because these are closest to the internal capsule and therefore most likely to generate adverse effects (AEs). If no AEs are observed, testing continues in a ventral-to-dorsal sequence. Unlike PD, dystonia requires days to weeks of stimulation therapy before improvements are apparent. Therefore, a lack of improvement in response to intraoperative stimulation should not be viewed as an indicator of poor lead placement. Rather, one must have faith that, if the microelectrode recording data are consistent with good placement and there are no AEs observed with up to 4 V of stimulation, the lead is well positioned.

Sustained time- and voltage-locked contractions of the contralateral hemibody and/or face indicate that stimulation is activating the fibers of the internal capsule, in which case the lead is placed too medially and/or posteriorly. The induction of phosphenes in the contralateral visual field suggests that stimulation is activating the optic tract and that the lead is too deep. Stimulation within the sensorimotor GPi may induce transient paresthesias; however, sustained paresthesias at low stimulation amplitudes indicate that the lead is positioned very posterior, and is activating thalamocortical projections in the posterior limb of the internal capsule. If any of these AEs occur, the lead should be repositioned accordingly.

The lead is secured at the skull employing a "cap" that also covers the bur hole. Fluoroscopy is used to confirm that the lead was not displaced from its desired position during fixation. The remaining length of the lead is encircled around the bur hole cap and left in the subgaleal space. The incision is irrigated with antibiotic saline and closed in a standard fashion. After removing the stereotactic frame, the patient is transported to the radiology department, where postoperative MRI is performed to confirm that the leads are well positioned and that there has been no hemorrhage (Fig. 90-5). Patients are observed overnight in the neurosurgical intensive care unit and discharged the following day.

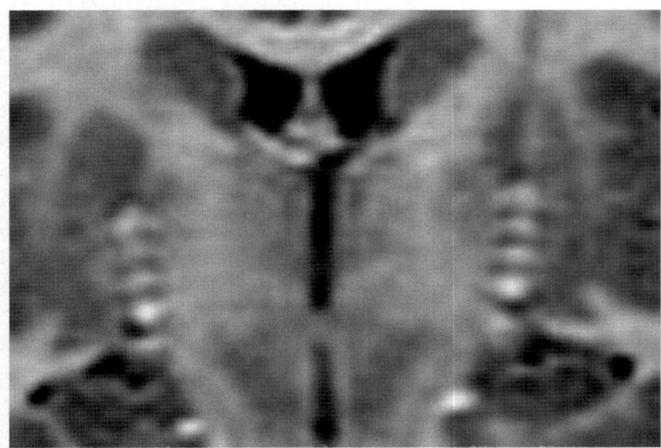

Figure 90-5. Postoperative magnetic resonance imaging (MRI). MRI is performed on all patients immediately after lead implantation in order to document lead position and to rule out intracerebral hemorrhage. A coronal fast spin echo inversion recovery MRI is depicted demonstrating proper lead position within the internal globus pallidus.

Implantation of the Pulse Generator

The remaining components of the DBS system(s) are implanted under general anesthesia, either as an immediate continuation of the first phase or during a staged procedure usually within 2 weeks of the lead implant. This relatively simple procedure involves the following steps: (1) creating a subclavicular, subcutaneous pocket for the internal pulse generator (IPG); (2) identifying the free end of the DBS lead in the subgaleal space; (3) tunneling the extension cable subcutaneously from the IPG pocket to the free end of the DBS lead; and (4) establishing dry, clean, and secure connections between the components. The connection between the lead and the extension cable is placed under the galea, just lateral to the cranial incision, limiting exposure of the lead to potential fracture through movement. In very young patients with thin skin, one may place the IPG(s) at the abdomen. Alternatively, one may employ a dual-channel rechargeable device (e.g., Activa RC; Medtronic, Inc., Minneapolis, MN), which has a lower profile than devices powered by standard batteries. In children under the age of 15 years, device-related infection is the most significant risk of this procedure.[36] Meticulous hemostasis and wound closure with strict attention to minimizing incisional stress are essential. We prefer a subcuticular closure at the chest incision for cosmesis. An axial incision and submuscular implantation may also be considered, but the senior author (R.L.A.) finds that this approach complicates battery replacement surgeries and may interfere with device recharging and programming.

PROGRAMMING THE DEVICE

The device(s) are activated 2 to 4 weeks after lead implantation, allowing the surgical incisions to heal. There is no consensus regarding the optimal settings for treating dystonia because few systematic evaluations of varying stimulus parameters have been conducted. Instead, therapy is currently guided by published case series and trials, which report positive responses across a wide range of pulse widths (60 to 450 μsec, although the three prospective controlled trials published thus far utilized 90 to 120 μsec)[37-39] and high frequencies (130 Hz or higher).[40-46] Though effective, wide pulse widths and high frequencies rapidly deplete the IPGs, necessitating their frequent replacement (12 to 36 months) and/or recharging. In our experience, stimulation at lower frequencies (60 to 80 Hz) may be just as effective as high-frequency stimulation.[47,48] Moreover, because these settings deliver less electrical energy to the brain, AEs are less likely to occur and the life span of the IPGs is prolonged.[47,49]

At the initial programming session, the effects of unipolar stimulation with each of the contacts are assessed. In particular, the stimulation thresholds for inducing AEs are noted. For therapy, we employ the ventralmost contact that does not induce AEs with stimulation at up to 3.5 V. We prefer to treat with unipolar stimulation but use bipolar settings if unipolar stimulation is not tolerated. Patients are initially treated at 2.0 to 2.5 V, in line with most reports and recommendations.[45] The stimulation amplitude may be increased over time; however, every effort should be made not to exceed 3.6 V because the IPG must invoke a "doubling circuit" to deliver amplitudes above this threshold, shortening battery life out of proportion to the energy delivered. If more energy is required, it is preferable from the standpoint of battery preservation to increase the frequency or pulse duration.

Patients return every 2 to 4 weeks for evaluation during the first 3 months, and every 3 to 6 months after that. During each visit the patient is assessed employing a variety of standardized clinical rating scales, including the Burke-Fahn-Marsden Dystonia Rating Scale (BFMDRS).[50]

CLINICAL RESULTS

Generalized Dystonia

Initial case reports of pallidal DBS for dystonia were published in 1999. Coubes and colleagues[41] reported the case of an 8-year-old girl with PGD whose symptoms were so severe that she required sedation and mechanical ventilation. Thirty-six months after surgery, she had returned to school with near-normal neurologic function. Kumar and coworkers[51] also reported dramatic improvement in one patient with severe PGD and correlated the clinical response to normalization of motor cortical activity on positron emission tomography. Two years after surgery, Krauss and colleagues[42] noted improvements of 78% and 70% in the BFMDRS scores of two patients with PGD.

The results of larger case series support these preliminary findings. Yianni and associates[44] reported their results treating 25 patients with various forms of dystonia, finding that all patient subgroups were improved by pallidal DBS. Coubes and colleagues[40] reported a mean 79% improvement in the BFMDRS motor subscore and a 65% mean improvement in the disability subscore 2 years after surgery in 31 patients with PGD. They noted that patients improved steadily over 12 to 24 months and that children fared marginally better than adults. According to multiple recent reviews,[43,52] at least 249 individual cases of pallidal DBS for primary dystonia have been reported in the literature to date. Most are included in small, open-label case series and most report improvements in the BFMDRS of 60% to 70%.

Three prospective studies demonstrate that activation of the devices and not mere insertion of the leads is required to realize clinical improvement. Vidailhet and associates[38] examined 22 PGD patients treated with bilateral pallidal DBS at three French centers. Double-blind evaluations conducted 3 months after surgery showed significantly better motor function with stimulation than without. One year after surgery, the mean BFMDRS motor score was improved 51%, with one third of the patients experiencing a greater than 75% improvement. They found that phasic symptoms improved more rapidly than fixed dystonic postures. A follow-up report documents that the motor improvement in this cohort has been maintained for 3 years.[53]

In 2006, Kupsch and coworkers[37] published the first prospective, randomized, double-blind, sham stimulation–controlled study of pallidal DBS for dystonia. Forty patients with primary segmental or generalized dystonia underwent pallidal DBS surgery at multiple centers in Germany. Twenty patients were randomized to therapeutic stimulation and 20 to sham stimulation for a period of 3 months, at which time their clinical status was assessed by blinded raters employing the BFMDRS. The BFMDRS motor subscores in the patients who received therapeutic stimulation improved 40% at 3 months as compared to 5% in the control group. The control group was then provided therapeutic stimulation, with a resulting equivalent improvement (37%) over the subsequent 3 months. An intention-to-treat analysis 5 years later found a sustained improvement of 58% over baseline.[54]

Pallidal Deep Brain Stimulation for Cervical Dystonia

The data supporting the use of pallidal DBS for CD, though not yet as mature as that for PGD, are favorable nonetheless. Preliminary reports of small case series suggest that CD is responsive to bilateral pallidal DBS, with improvements in the TWSTRS ranging from 43% to 76%.[43,64-66] Three small multicenter, prospective, single-blind trials of pallidal DBS found benefit. Kiss and colleagues[67] reported significant improvements in the TWSTRS severity, disability, and pain subscales as well as reduced symptoms of depression and enhanced quality-of-life measures in 10 CD patients. Skogseid and coworkers[68] found a more substantial 70% reduction in TWSTRS severity scores, along with improvements in the disability and pain subscales, and in quality of life, in eight CD patients. Walsh and associates[69] found sustained benefit of at least 5 years in 10 CD patients. As stated earlier, a recent larger, multicenter, randomized, double-blind, sham-controlled trial in 62 CD patients found a 26% reduction in the TWSTRS severity score, versus 6% with sham treatment, at 3 months.[39] Overall, the response of CD to pallidal GPi appears to be significant but is less consistent than that observed in PGD. Larger and longer-term studies of DBS in CD are needed to better establish its longevity and the indicators of a positive clinical response, including optimal lead position and stimulation parameters.

Most recently, Volkmann and colleagues[39] reported a multicenter, randomized, patient- and observer-blind, sham-controlled trial in 62 patients with cervical dystonia (CD). Thirty-two patients were randomized to therapeutic stimulation and 30 to sham stimulation for a period of 3 months, at which time blinded raters assessed their outcome. Stimulation was associated with a 26% reduction in the Toronto Western Spasmodic Torticollis Rating Scale (TWSTRS) severity score, as compared to 6% with sham treatment ($P = 0.0024$). At 3 months, stimulation was activated in the control group, and assessments 6 months after surgery demonstrated an additional 26% severity score reduction over that at 3 months. In comparison, scores only improved an additional 3% in patients initially assigned to stimulation.

Indicators of Deep Brain Stimulation Response

Besides the relatively crude distinction of primary generalized or segmental versus secondary dystonia, little is known about the clinical factors that presage a positive response to pallidal DBS. In 2008 Isaias and colleagues[55] addressed this issue, examining the clinical results of 39 consecutive PGD patients treated at one institution and followed for at least 1 year. Overall, motor improvement 1 year postoperatively was equivalent to that reported previously; however, the authors found that the 6 patients in their series who had fixed skeletal deformities (FSDs) at the time of surgery experienced a more limited improvement than the 33 patients without such deformities. By subdividing the BFMDRS motor scale anatomically, they further demonstrated that the limited improvement occurred at the legs and axis, consistent with the fact that all six suffered with scoliosis. Two of these six improved further after corrective spinal procedures, but their final results still did not equal those observed in the remaining patients without FSDs.

Among the patients without FSDs, the authors found that younger age (<20 years) and shorter disease duration (<15 years) at the time of surgery predicted a superior response to DBS at 1 year. No other factor, including presence of the *DYT1* gene mutation, was predictive of outcome among these patients. The authors concluded that early intervention in PGD is warranted when medications fail to adequately control symptoms or induce intolerable side effects.

In a related study, Isaias and colleagues[56] examined predictors of protracted clinical effect, occurring between 1 and 3 years after GPi-DBS in 44 patients from five centers in Europe and the United States. BFMDRS scores were improved 74.9% and 82.6% at 1 and 3 years, respectively. Age at surgery greater than 27 years and disease duration greater than 17 years negatively correlated with clinical outcome at both 1 and 3 years. Interestingly, when patients were partitioned into three groups based on these predictors, younger patients with shorter disease duration achieved greater benefit faster than older patients. The older patients did continue to improve, however, achieving an additional 10% average improvement between years 1 and 3.

A large literature review combining data from 466 patients reported in 157 papers added lower baseline severity and *DYT1* positivity to shorter disease duration as predictors of better outcomes with surgery.[57] Indeed, it is generally accepted that the patients who are most responsive to GPi-DBS are relatively young, with *DYT1*-positive PGD of relatively short disease duration and without FSDs.

Tisch and coworkers[58] examined the relationship between lead position relative to the intercommissural plane and clinical outcome, finding that leads positioned more posteriorly and ventrally within the GPi yielded greater BFMDRS motor score improvements than leads positioned more anteriorly and dorsally. These results confirmed and expanded upon prior results published by Starr and colleagues[59] and Hamani and associates[60] and suggest that Leksell's posteroventral GPi target remains the optimal site within the pallidum for treating dystonia, whether by stimulation or ablation.

Stimulation Frequency

The impressive responses generated with pallidal DBS for PGD were historically achieved using stimulation frequencies of 130 Hz or more and pulse durations of at least 140 μsec. Such parameters rapidly deplete the IPGs, necessitating their frequent surgical replacement (i.e., every 12 to 36 months). In order to address this difficulty, Alterman and colleagues[47] conducted an evaluation of 15 consecutive PGD patients who were treated with pallidal stimulation at just 60 Hz, finding that their clinical response was equivalent to that achieved with higher stimulation frequencies. More importantly, none of these patients required surgery to replace a depleted generator or required increases in stimulation therapy with up to 4 years of follow-up.[49] In addition to reducing the need for battery replacement surgery, the finding that lower frequency stimulation may be as effective[61] as high-frequency stimulation raises important questions about the mechanism(s) through which pallidal DBS exerts its effects in both dystonia and PD.[47]

Longevity of Response

A few reported series suggest that the response of PGD to pallidal DBS is long lasting. As stated previously, the two key prospective trials by Vidailhet and associates[53] and Kupsch and coworkers[54] have reported stable results for up to 3 and 5 years, respectively. Cif and colleagues[62] reported sustained benefit in 26 patients with a mean follow-up of 6 years. Our own results in 30 consecutive PGD patients followed for at least 2 years[49] and 47 consecutive *DYT1* patients followed for a mean of 4 years[63] suggest that the clinical response to DBS is stable for up to 10 years.

Primary Craniocervical Dystonia (Meige's Syndrome)

The results of pallidal DBS for Meige's syndrome have now been reported in a small number of cases and case series from a handful of centers.[43,52] Ostrem and coworkers[70] reported a mean BFMDRS improvement of 71% in six patients 6 months after surgery. Interestingly, some of these patients experienced stimulation-induced bradykinesia in preoperatively unaffected limbs. Ghang and associates[71] treated 11 Meige's syndrome patients and reported a mean BFMDRS reduction of 85.5% 2 years after surgery, with similar eye, mouth, speech/swallowing, and neck subscore improvements. Similarly, Reese and colleagues[72] treated 12 patients with a mean follow-up of 3 years, finding BFMDRS movement scores improved by an average of 53%, with similar improvements in eye, mouth, and speech/swallowing subscores. Although these limited results are promising, optimal stimulation parameters and targeting for Meige's syndrome remain to be elucidated.

Secondary Dystonia

In contrast to PGD, secondary dystonia patients are a heterogeneous population with regard to etiology, clinical signs, and long-term prognosis. In addition to dystonia, many have neurological deficits (e.g., seizures, spastic paresis, cerebellar and brainstem dysfunction, and developmental delay) that may limit their functional response to DBS. Consequently, pallidal DBS has thus far proven much less effective in secondary dystonia than in primary dystonia.[73-80] Many studies report little or no benefit and even worsening of symptoms after surgery. Our own experience treating patients with secondary dystonia of various causes confirms that responses in this group are more modest than the results obtained in primary dystonia.[73] There are, however, some individuals with secondary dystonia who will respond favorably to DBS. For example, a number of reports find consistent and significant improvement in cases of tardive dystonia following GPi-DBS.[81-85] Dramatic improvement in patients with pantothenate kinase–associated neurodegeneration has also been reported,[86] including a response lasting for 5 years,[87] although these results may be inflated as a result of reporting bias.[88] Isolated cases and small series suggest that promising results may be achieved in patients with other underlying pathologies, although outcomes tend to vary widely as the number of reports accumulate.[80] We have operated on a 12-year-old boy with severe generalized dystonia secondary to perinatal anoxic brain injury who responded quickly (within 2 weeks) and dramatically to bilateral GPi-DBS (unpublished results). Despite his prolonged anoxia and the severity of his dystonia, his brain anatomy was well preserved. This patient is similar to patient 9 in the report by Zorzi and colleagues,[79] whose BFMDRS score improved 65% following pallidal DBS surgery.

The preoperative indicators of a positive response in secondary dystonia are currently unknown, but a normal brain MRI may be a predictor of favorable outcome.[89] Indeed, a general review of the literature suggests a trend to poor surgical outcomes when demyelinating, neurodegenerative, or ischemic lesions are located within basal ganglia structures.[90] It may be that nonpallidal DBS targets are more likely to improve dystonia in these "lesional" cases. Until further studies better define preoperative clinical indicators of response and realistic outcomes, carefully establishing patient expectations on a case-by-case basis is required.

COMPLICATIONS OF DEEP BRAIN STIMULATION THERAPY

Overall, both DBS surgery and chronic electrical stimulation of the internal pallidum are well tolerated in this population. The three prospective sham-controlled studies of GPi-DBS in dystonia[37-39] collectively include 124 patients and report 8 (6%) infections, 5 (4%) hardware breakages/dislodgments/misplacements, and 3 (2%) unresolved complications considered to be "serious," including cases of depression, neck pain, and de novo parkinsonism. A retrospective analysis of AEs with 30 days of DBS surgery in nearly 1200 patients across five German centers reported mortality and permanent morbidity rates of 0.4% and 1%, respectively.[91] In our series of 82 dystonia patients (73 primary, 9 secondary) operated on between December 2000 and August 2008 there have been no intracerebral hemorrhages or adverse neurological events. Eight patients (9.7%) developed perioperative infections that necessitated removal of nine devices. Each patient was successfully treated with antibiotics and underwent re-implantation without adverse sequelae. Three patients (3.7%) fractured an extension cable, a complication that is reported to occur more frequently in dystonia than in PD or ET.[92] In one of our cases, withdrawal of the patient's medications at the time of surgery precipitated a dystonic crisis, for which the child required a prolonged hospitalization, large doses of lorazepam (Ativan), and early activation of her DBS devices.

ALTERNATIVE TARGETS FOR DEEP BRAIN STIMULATION IN DYSTONIA

The dramatic results achieved with pallidal DBS for primary dystonia have thus far slowed exploration of alternative targets for therapy. However, some GPi-DBS patients experience troublesome stimulation-related bradykinesia or parkinsonism despite diminished dystonia.[93,94] Moreover, alternative targets may prove more efficacious in some patients with secondary dystonia who fail GPi-DBS.

Kleiner-Fisman and coworkers[95] reported significant improvements in both the BFMDRS and TWSTRS scores of two patients with primary, predominant CD who were treated with bilateral DBS at the subthalamic nucleus (STN). Two other patients improved marginally. Sun and associates[96] reported that bilateral STN-DBS yielded immediate and sustained improvement in various forms of dystonia, employing significantly less electrical energy than that required to treat at the GPi. Among their nine patients with secondary dystonia of various etiologies treated with STN-DBS, Zhang and colleagues[97] reported improvements in two patients with tardive dystonia and one patient with posttraumatic dystonia 3 months postoperatively. Ostrem and coworkers[98] provided a detailed prospective and blinded rater account of STN-DBS in nine patients with CD. TWSTRS scores improved significantly at 12 months, though several patients reported depression, weight gain, and transient dyskinetic movements. A recent direct comparison of GPi-DBS and STN-DBS was attempted via a prospective double-blind crossover trial involving 12 multifocal or generalized dystonia patients implanted at both targets and stimulated in 6-month blocks at either target.[99] The authors suggest better tolerability of STN versus GPi stimulation despite no significant difference in beneficial clinical effect between targets. However, questions over inaccurate GPi targeting[100] and no improvement of TWSTRS scores in the four GPi-stimulated CD patients raise doubts concerning the validity of this comparison.

Thalamic targets have received limited attention in the contemporary literature, despite the fact that thalamic ablations for dystonia date back to the pre-levodopa era and that Mundinger treated CD with thalamic DBS in the 1970s.[101] More recent case reports and small series suggest efficacy in patients with prominent upper body dystonic tremor[102-104] and myoclonic dystonia.[105,106] Moreover, efficacy in focal hand dystonia has been reported in response to thalamic DBS[104,105] following previous reports that radiofrequency thalamotomy improves both writer's cramp and musician's dystonia. Given this limited experience, optimal patient and thalamic target selection remain poorly defined.

CONCLUSION

DBS at the GPi is currently the treatment of choice for medically refractory primary dystonia. Multiple open-label and blinded studies, along with three placebo-controlled trials, demonstrate that pallidal DBS is a highly effective, durable, and well-tolerated treatment modality in patients with primary dystonia. Younger patients with shorter disease duration and without joint contractures, and those patients who are *DYT1* positive, may fare best of all. The response to stimulation is more gradual than that observed in PD or ET, and the full benefit of surgery may not be realized for a year or more. When prolonged dystonia has resulted in fixed contractures, additional orthopedic surgery may be required to maximize functional gains, though the results in such patients may never equal those achieved in patients without fixed deformities.

Patients with secondary dystonia respond more modestly and inconsistently than do primary dystonia patients, reflecting the physiologic and anatomic heterogeneity of this population. Among these, patients with tardive dystonia, pantothenate kinase–associated neurodegeneration, and dystonia associated with brain lesions but with preserved basal ganglia anatomy may respond well to DBS therapy. Conversely, patients with obvious structural abnormalities and most metabolic disorders appear to be poor DBS candidates.

Standard stimulation parameters for treating dystonia typically include frequencies of 130 Hz or more and pulse widths of 90 to 450 μsec, settings that may rapidly deplete the implanted pulse generators. Stimulation at 60 Hz appears to be as effective as high-frequency stimulation for PGD and may make stimulation more tolerable while prolonging battery life. Therefore, a more complete evaluation of low-frequency stimulation for primary dystonia should be undertaken.

Additional research efforts should be directed toward developing a greater understanding of dystonia pathophysiology and the neurophysiologic changes induced by chronic electrical stimulation. This will lead to more rational stimulation paradigms and better clinical results. Additional preoperative indicators of a positive response to DBS must be sought in order to improve patient selection. In particular, functional imaging studies of dystonia patients, before and after DBS surgery, are currently lacking and should be pursued. Finally, continued explorations of other targets for therapy are appropriate, particularly for the many patients with secondary dystonia who may not be candidates for pallidal DBS.

Acknowledgments

R.L. Alterman wishes to thank Donald Weisz, PhD, for his assistance with the production of Figure 90-3, for his friendship, and for his passionate commitment to patient care.

SUGGESTED READINGS

Alterman RL, Miravite J, Weisz D, et al. 60 Hertz pallidal deep brain stimulation for primary torsion dystonia. *Neurology*. 2007;69:681-688.

Bressman SB. Dystonia: phenotypes and genotypes. *Rev Neurol (Paris)*. 2003;159:849-856.

Coubes P, Cif L, El Fertit H, et al. Electrical stimulation of the globus pallidus internus in patients with primary generalized dystonia: long-term results. *J Neurosurg*. 2004;101:189-194.

Defazio G, Abbruzzese G, Livrea P, et al. Epidemiology of primary dystonia. *Lancet Neurol*. 2004;3:673-678.

Eltahawy HA, Saint-Cyr J, Giladi N, et al. Primary dystonia is more responsive than secondary dystonia to pallidal interventions: outcome after pallidotomy or pallidal deep brain stimulation. *Neurosurgery*. 2004;54:613-619, discussion 619-621.

Fahn S. Idiopathic torsion dystonia. In: Calne DB, ed. *Neurodegenerative Diseases*. Philadelphia: Saunders; 1994:705-715.

Hamani C, Moro E, Zadikoff C, et al. Location of active contacts in patients with primary dystonia treated with globus pallidus deep brain stimulation. *Neurosurgery*. 2008;62(3 suppl 1):217-223, discussion 223-225.

Hua Z, Guodong G, Qinchuan L, et al. Analysis of complications of radiofrequency pallidotomy. *Neurosurgery*. 2003;52:89-99, discussion 99-101.

Isaias IU, Alterman RL, Tagliati M. Outcome predictors of pallidal stimulation in patients with primary dystonia: the role of disease duration. *Brain*. 2008;131:1895-1902.

Isaias IU, Alterman RL, Tagliati M. Deep brain stimulation for primary dystonia: long-term outcomes. *Arch Neurol*. 2009;66:465-470.

Kiss ZH, Doig-Beyaert K, Eliasziw M, et al. The Canadian multicentre study of deep brain stimulation for cervical dystonia. *Brain*. 2007;130(Pt 11):2879-2886.

Kupsch A, Benecke R, Muller J, et al. Pallidal deep-brain stimulation in primary generalized or segmental dystonia. *N Engl J Med*. 2006;355: 1978-1990.

Laitinen LV, Bergenheim AT, Hariz MI. Leksell's posteroventral pallidotomy in the treatment of Parkinson's disease. *J Neurosurg*. 1992;76: 53-61.

Ostrem JL, Starr PA. Treatment of dystonia with deep brain stimulation. *Neurother*. 2008;5:320-330.

Shils J, Tagliati M, Alterman R. Neurophysiological monitoring during neurosurgery for movement disorders. In: Deletis V, Shils J, eds. *Neurophysiology in Neurosurgery*. San Diego, CA: Academic Press; 2002: 393-436.

Tagliati M, Blatt K, Bressman SB. Generalized torsion dystonia. In: Noseworthy J, ed. *Neurological Therapeutics: Principles and Practice*. London: Martin Dunitz; 2003:3548-3566.

Tisch S, Zrinzo L, Limousin P, et al. Effect of electrode contact location on clinical efficacy of pallidal deep brain stimulation in primary generalized dystonia. *J Neurol Neurosurg Psychiatry*. 2007;78:1314-1319.

Vidailhet M, Vercueil L, Houeto JL, et al. Bilateral deep brain stimulation of the globus pallidus in primary generalized dystonia. *N Engl J Med*. 2005;352:459-467.

See a full reference list on ExpertConsult.com

91 Deep Brain Stimulation: Mechanisms of Action

Luke A. Johnson and Jerrold L. Vitek

Deep brain stimulation (DBS) is a well-established surgical therapy for treatment of the motor symptoms associated with a variety of movement disorders, including essential tremor, Parkinson's disease, and dystonia.[1,2] It is also being explored for the treatment of a number of other neurological and psychiatric disorders, such as depression, dementia, obsessive-compulsive disorder, and the tics associated with Gilles de la Tourette's syndrome.[3,4] In this chapter, we review the current understanding of DBS mechanisms, highlighting several potential factors that play into how DBS elicits its beneficial effects, such as the site of stimulation and the type of disorder being treated.

The potential application of DBS in humans was demonstrated in a seminal study by Hassler and colleagues in 1960.[5] They described a series of patients with tremor who received electrical stimulation via electrodes introduced into the globus pallidus for the purpose of creating therapeutic ablations. They observed that low-frequency stimulation (<25 Hz) exacerbated contralateral tremor, whereas high-frequency stimulation (25 to 100 Hz) could alleviate or abolish tremor entirely. However, they viewed electrical stimulation primarily as an intraoperative tool to identify specific brain regions in which to make therapeutic lesions. Subsequent reports indicated that intraoperative stimulation was effective in mitigating pain and reducing the motor signs of movement disorders,[6-9] but it was not until the maturation of battery-powered implantable pulse generators in the 1980s and the pioneering work of Benabid and colleagues[10] that the usefulness of chronic DBS therapy was realized. Since then, DBS systems have been implanted in tens of thousands of patients with medication-refractory neurological disorders.[11,12] Electrical stimulation has largely supplanted ablation as the surgical treatment of choice for many disorders because DBS is reversible and the "dose" can be titrated to maximize therapeutic benefit while minimizing side effects.

The anatomic targets of DBS are embedded within higher level sensorimotor, associative, and limbic networks in which stimulation can have a variety of complex motor and behavioral effects on a patient. The therapeutic mechanisms of action of DBS are not fully understood, but they probably depend on multiple factors, including not just how electrical stimulation affects neural activity in the target nucleus and nearby fiber pathways but also how brain networks and disease processes compensate and coadapt with the nonphysiologic input provided by stimulation. In this chapter, we review what is known about the therapeutic mechanisms of DBS from electrophysiologic, imaging, neurochemical, and computational modeling studies; we focus primarily on DBS for Parkinson's disease. Specifically we address (1) how DBS affects neuronal tissue near the site of stimulation; (2) how neurophysiologic changes associated with DBS translate into therapeutic benefit; and (3) in which brain regions stimulation appears to provide the most therapeutic benefit for different disorders. An understanding of the physiologic mechanisms of DBS—although daunting, in view of the complexity of networks involved—is critical as researchers seek to improve the therapy for current indications and expand it to treat emerging indications.

NEURAL RESPONSES TO DEEP BRAIN STIMULATION

When examining the mechanisms of DBS, the clinician must consider the types of brain tissue within the stimulation volume surrounding the electrode, which includes neuronal cell bodies and axons of the target nucleus, as well as fiber tracts passing through or near the stimulation target.

Changes in Somatic Activity in the Stimulated Nucleus

Surgical ablation and DBS in the same target nuclei produce similar effects on motor signs in patients with Parkinson's disease. This observation led to the hypothesis that high-frequency electrical stimulation produces a functional lesion, inhibiting neuronal activity and reducing output from the stimulated nucleus.[9,10] Indeed, suppression of somatic activity near the site of DBS has been observed via microelectrode recordings in the subthalamic nucleus (STN) and in the internal globus pallidus (GPi) both in humans[13-17] and in animal models.[18-20] Explanations for this inhibition include depolarization block as a result of inactivation of sodium channels[21,22] and increase in potassium current[23]; presynaptic depression of excitatory afferents[24]; and activation of inhibitory afferents.[20,25] According to the hypothesis of driving afferent input with DBS, the observed decrease in activity in STN and GPi is not surprising. The majority of afferents to the STN and GPi modulate the γ-aminobutyric acid (GABA) system (are GABAergic),[26,27] and one study showed that inhibition of GPi during GPi-DBS is mediated by GABA receptors.[20] However, not all neurons near the site of stimulation are inhibited by DBS. A small fraction of STN neurons increase their firing rate during STN-DBS,[28] possibly because of the activation of afferent excitatory cortical projections.[29]

In addition to changes in firing rate, stimulation can cause striking changes in the pattern of neuronal activity. Neurons in the stimulated nucleus have been shown to entrain to the stimulus pulse train, firing at fixed latency after the preceding stimulus pulse. Such "entrainment" has been shown in the STN[18] and GPi,[30] and it is believed to derive from the repetitive activation of somatic and dendritic membrane-bound ion channels.[31,32] Although overall firing rates during stimulation may be suppressed, altered firing patterns consisting of multiple excitatory and inhibitory phases after each stimulus pulse have been observed.[18,30,33]

Axonal Output from the Stimulated Nucleus

Changes in the firing rate and pattern of somatic activity in the stimulated nucleus do not necessarily translate, however, to similar changes in output from the stimulated nucleus. Although many studies have shown suppression of activity near the site of stimulation, various other studies have demonstrated increased neuronal output to recipient nuclei from the targeted region.[34-36] This dissociation may be explained by the fact that axons have lower thresholds for action potential generation by electrical stimulation than do cell somas.[37] Therefore, action potentials initiated along the axon can occur irrespective of activity in the soma. The hypothesis that DBS decouples somatic and axonal activity is supported by modeling studies that have shown that somatic activity near the stimulated electrode is suppressed by activation of presynaptic inhibitory terminals, whereas efferent axons are activated by stimulation.[38,39]

Experimental studies support the activation hypothesis (e.g., activation of output from the site of stimulation). Although it is

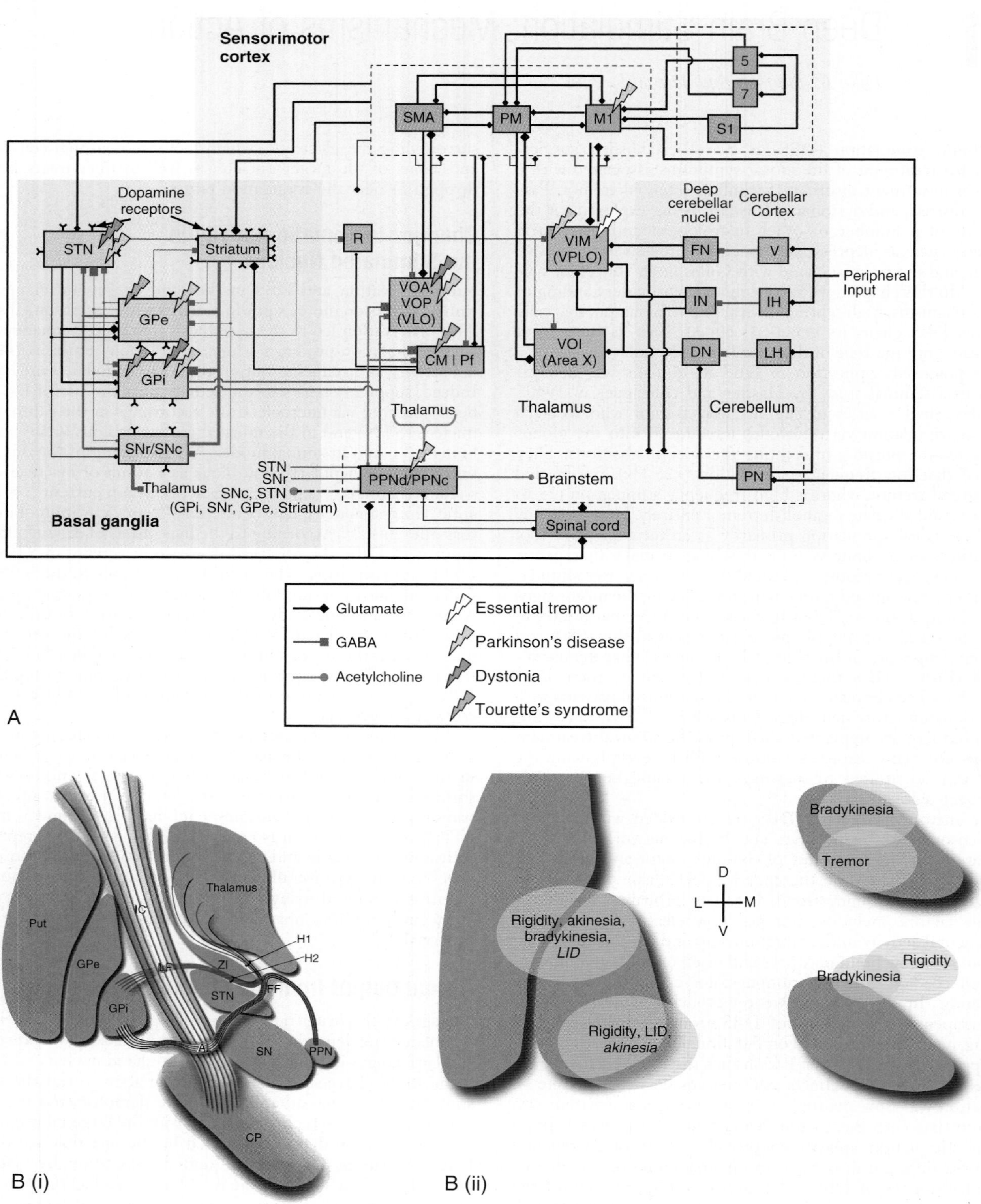

typically not feasible to record axonal activity directly, it is possible to record neuronal activity in nuclei receiving input from the stimulated nucleus. Hashimoto and colleagues[35] showed in parkinsonian monkeys that therapeutic STN-DBS increased neuronal firing rates in the external globus pallidus (GPe) and the GPi. Because STN has glutamatergic projections (Fig. 91-1A), this result suggests that DBS increases the output from the stimulated nucleus. Hashimoto and colleagues also found that therapeutic STN-DBS altered the firing pattern of most GPe and GPi cells, producing entrained responses with increased

Figure 91-1. A, Schematic representation of the basal ganglia–thalamocortical circuit connections. Targets for deep brain stimulation (DBS) therapy are identified by *lightning bolts.* The target chosen depends on the neurological disorder being treated. Of interest, stimulation of multiple targets can be effective for a particular disorder, which emphasizes the role of network malfunction in the pathophysiologic processes of neurological disorders. In the sensorimotor circuit, the *line color* and *terminal shape* represent the primary neurotransmitter involved in the signaling pathway. CM, centromedian nucleus; DN, dentate nucleus; FN, fastigial nuclei; GABA, γ-aminobutyric acid; GPe, external globus pallidus; GPi, internal globus pallidus; IH, intermediate hemisphere of the cerebellum; IN, interposed nuclei; LH, lateral hemisphere of the cerebellum; M1, primary motor cortex; Pf, parafascicular nucleus; PM, premotor cortex; PN, pontine nucleus; PPNc, pedunculopontine nucleus pars compacta; 5, 7: Brodmann areas; PPNd, pedunculopontine nucleus pars diffusa; R, reticular formation; S1, primary somatosensory cortex; SMA, supplementary motor area; SNc, substantia nigra pars compacta; SNr, substantia nigra pars reticularis; STN, subthalamic nucleus; V, vermis; VIM, ventral intermediate nucleus; VLO, ventrolateral pars oralis; VOA, anterior ventral oral nucleus; VOI, ventro-oralis internus (Olszewski's area X); VOP, posterior ventral oral nucleus; VPLO, ventral posterolateral pars oralis. **B (i),** Representation of major anatomic structures and fiber pathways associated with the STN and GPi. **B (ii),** Representation of stimulation targets within and near the GPi and STN that have been found to have differential effects on individual parkinsonian motor symptoms. DBS in the dorsal GPi, including the medial medullary lamina and portions of the GPe, have been shown to ameliorate rigidity, akinesia, and bradykinesia but worsen levodopa-induced dyskinesia (LID), whereas stimulation in the ventral GPi improved rigidity and decreased LID but worsened akinesia.[60,249-251] With regard to the STN, one study revealed that targeting dorsal-anterior and ventral-posterior locations was optimal for relieving bradykinesia and tremor, respectively.[252] Another study revealed that targeting slightly different regions dorsal to the STN in or near the zona incerta (ZI) and fields of Forel (FF) was effective for rigidity and bradykinesia.[253] AL, ansa lenticularis; CP, cerebral peduncle; H1, H1 field of Forel (thalamic fasciculus); IC, internal capsule; LF, lenticular fasciculus (H2); PPN, pedunculopontine nucleus; Put, putamen; SN, substantia nigra. ***(B,** From Hamani C, Saint-Cyr JA, Fraser J, et al. The subthalamic nucleus in the context of movement disorders.* Brain. *2004;127[Pt 1]:4-20.)*

probability of firing at 3 and 6.5 msec after each stimulus pulse; periods in between showed pronounced inhibition, particularly in the GPi (Fig. 91-2A to D). In contrast, lower amplitude, nontherapeutic STN-DBS did not significantly alter GPi neuronal activity. The inhibitory phases in GPi responses were demonstrated to be induced by GABAergic projections from the GPe.[40] In a complementary computational modeling study based on the findings with STN neurons in the monkeys in Hashimoto and colleagues' study,[35] Miocinovic and colleagues[39] showed that stimulation caused action potentials first in the axon; 50% of STN axons were entrained with the stimulus pulses at least 80% of the time. Results of other studies also support the hypothesis that STN-DBS elicits action potentials along STN axons and activates STN target nuclei.[41,42]

Electrophysiologic, neurochemical, and imaging data support the activation hypothesis, with the effects in downstream nuclei depending on the nature (excitatory or inhibitory) of the axonal projection. Therapeutic GPe-DBS was shown to cause significant decreases in firing rate and bursting in 76% and 48%, respectively, of recorded STN neurons in parkinsonian monkeys.[43] On the basis of recordings in pallidal receiving areas of the thalamus in normal animals, Anderson and colleagues[34] found that GPi-DBS inhibited 77% of thalamic neurons, which was consistent with orthrodromic activation of GABAergic GPi projections. Similarly, GPi-DBS decreased overall thalamic activity in patients with Parkinson's disease[44] and dystonia,[45] although this was associated with a brief excitatory phase 3.5 to 5 msec after each stimulus pulse, which was consistent with a change in the pattern of thalamic activity during pallidal stimulation. GPi sends GABAergic projections to the pedunculopontine nucleus (PPN), in addition to the motor thalamus, and neuronal activity in both areas has been shown to be suppressed during GPi-DBS in parkinsonian primates.[46,47]

Results of imaging studies are also consistent with activation of output from the stimulated region. In several studies, researchers have used positron emission tomography (PET) to show that blood flow in GPi increased during STN-DBS.[48,49] Similarly, in patients receiving DBS in the ventral intermediate nucleus, PET revealed increased blood flow in cortical regions receiving thalamic projections,[50] and functional magnetic imaging studies demonstrated increased blood oxygen level–dependent signals in the GPi of patients receiving STN-DBS.[51,52] Neurochemical experiments also support the hypothesis of increased output from the stimulated nucleus. Microdialysis studies in rats have shown that STN-DBS increased levels of glutamate in the pallidum outflow.[53,54] Intraoperative microdialysis in human patients revealed that therapeutic STN-DBS was associated with an increase in cyclic guanosine monophosphate concentrations, which was thought to reflect an increase in GPi activity.[55,56]

Activation of Fiber Tracts

In addition to activating afferent or efferent (or both) projections of the stimulated nucleus, DBS can affect fiber tracts passing through the target. Dopaminergic fibers from the substantia nigra pars compacta (SNc), serotoninergic fibers from the dorsal raphe nucleus, and cholinergic fibers from the PPN pass through the GPi en route to the GPe and the putamen.[57] There are reciprocal connections between the STN and GPe; a large proportion of these fibers pass through the Gpi.[58,59] Computational models predict that GPi-DBS activates these fibers, which suggests that the therapeutic mechanisms of DBS may involve multiple pathways, including those projecting from the target nucleus, as well as fibers passing through and those adjacent to the site of stimulation.[31,60,61]

Therapeutic DBS stimulation has been demonstrated to spread current beyond the borders of the target nucleus, affecting adjacent fibers of passage.[61,62] Consideration of this current spread is especially relevant to DBS in the STN and PPN, which are small nuclei surrounded by several large fiber tracts.[63,64] The PPN, for instance, is bordered laterally by the medial lemniscus; medially by the superior cerebellar peduncle; rostrally by the posterolateral substantia nigra; rostrodorsally by the retrorubral field; caudally by the pontine cuneiform nucleus, subcuneiform

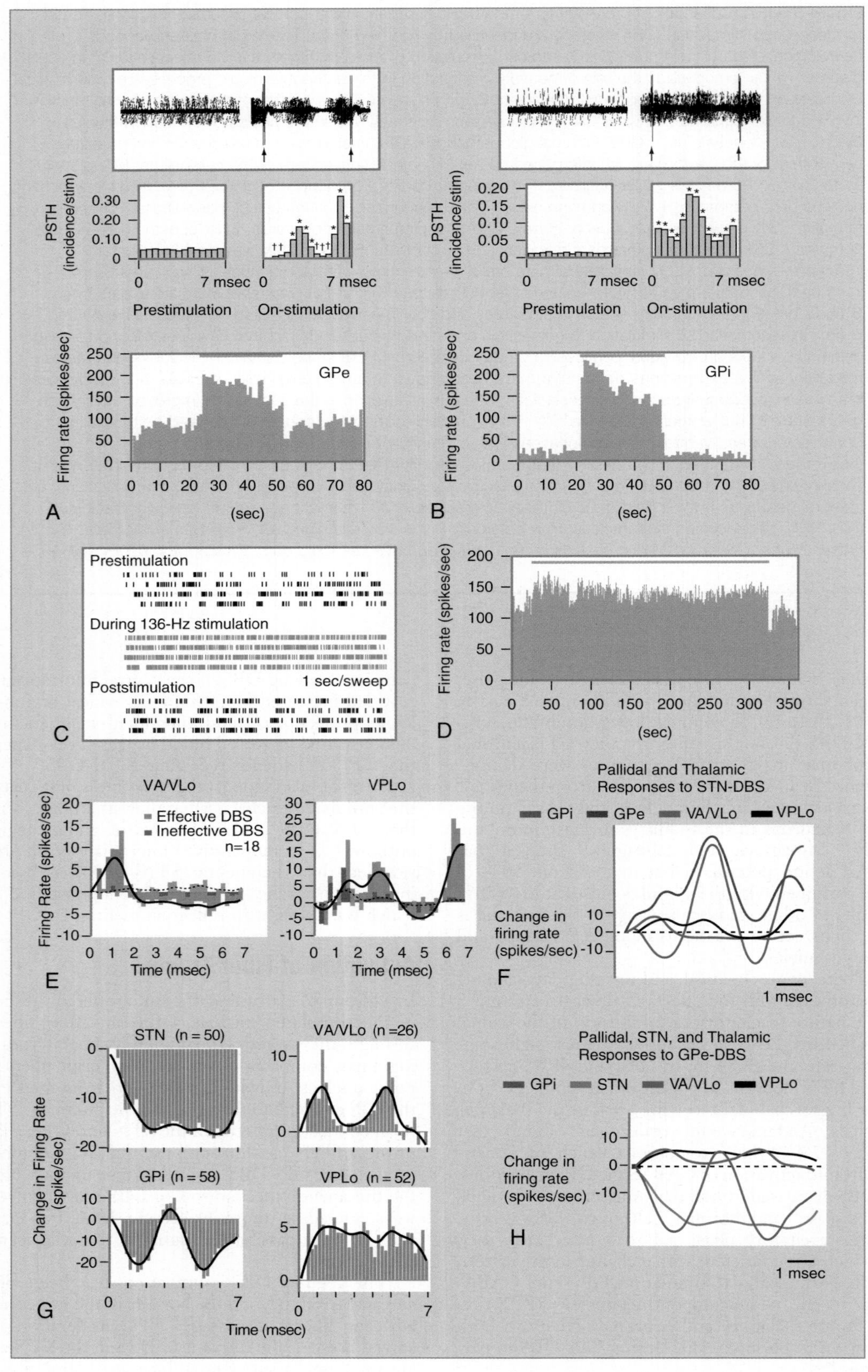

PSTH (incidence/stim)
0.30
0.20
0.10
0
0 7 msec 0 7 msec
Prestimulation On-stimulation
Firing rate (spikes/sec)
GPe
(sec)
A
0.20
0.15
0.10
0.05
GPi
B
Prestimulation
During 136-Hz stimulation
1 sec/sweep
Poststimulation
C
D
VA/VLo
VPLo
Firing Rate (spikes/sec)
Effective DBS
Ineffective DBS
n=18
Time (msec)
E
Pallidal and Thalamic Responses to STN-DBS
GPi GPe VA/VLo VPLo
Change in firing rate (spikes/sec)
1 msec
F
STN (n = 50)
VA/VLo (n =26)
GPi (n = 58)
VPLo (n = 52)
Change in Firing Rate (spike/sec)
Time (msec)
G
Pallidal, STN, and Thalamic Responses to GPe-DBS
GPi STN VA/VLo VPLo
H

Figure 91-2. Examples of neuronal responses occurring during subthalamic nucleus (STN) deep brain stimulation (DBS) in a cell from the internal globus pallidus (GPi) **(A)** and a cell from the external globus pallidus (GPe) **(B)**. Top traces show the overlay of 100 sweeps triggered at 10-msec intervals in the prestimulation period and by triggering on the stimulation pulse during the stimulation. Middle traces display peristimulus timing histograms (PSTH) reconstructed from successive 7.0-msec time intervals in the prestimulation period and from the interstimulus periods, in the on-stimulation period. *Asterisks* indicate significant increase at $P < .01$; *daggers* indicate significant decrease at $P < .01$ (Wilcoxon signed-rank test). Bottom plots represent the mean firing rate calculated in 1-second bins, which illustrate the time course of the firing rate. **C,** Raster plots of GPi neuronal activity showing that firing patterns changed from irregular with varying interspike intervals into a high-frequency regular pattern during 136-Hz, 3.0-V stimulation. **D,** Example of the change in firing rate of a GPi neuron during prolonged 136-Hz STN stimulation. An increased discharge rate was sustained during the 5-min stimulation period. **E,** PSTH of effective *(gray)* and ineffective *(green)* stimulation for ventralis anterior/ventralis lateralis pars oralis (VA/VLo) neurons (left) and ventrolateral preoptic nucleus (VPLo) neurons (right). In these plots, prestimulation firing rate has been subtracted to reflect change in firing evoked by stimulation in relation to baseline. The *continuous line* is a smoothed running average for effective stimulation, whereas the *dotted line* is the smoothed running average for ineffective stimulation. **F,** Average PSTHs of populations of pallidal and thalamic neurons during therapeutic STN stimulation, illustrating that stimulation evokes complex temporal patterns of firing activity in these nuclei. **G,** PSTHs of STN, GPi, VA/VLo, and VPLo neurons during therapeutic GPe stimulation. **H,** Average PSTHs of populations of pallidal, STN, and thalamic neurons during GPe stimulation (from part G). These data support the hypothesis that therapeutic DBS activates output from the stimulated structure and changes the temporal pattern of neuronal activity throughout the basal ganglia thalamic network. *(**A** to **D**, Modified from Hashimoto T, Elder CM, Okun MS, et al. Stimulation of the subthalamic nucleus changes the firing pattern of pallidal neurons.* J Neurosci. *2003;23:1916-1923.* ***E,*** *Modified from Xu W, Russo GS, Hashimoto T, et al. Subthalamic nucleus stimulation modulates thalamic neuronal activity.* J Neurosci. *2008;28:11916-11924.* ***H,*** *Modified from Vitek JL, Zhang J, Hashimoto T, et al. External pallidal stimulation improves parkinsonian motor signs and modulates neuronal activity throughout the basal ganglia thalamic network.* Exp Neurol. *2012;233:581-586.)*

nucleus, and locus caeruleus; and ventrally by the pontine reticular formation.[63,65] It is therefore not surprising that stimulation currents can and often do exceed the boundaries of the PPN, as revealed by the presence of paresthesias and oscillopsia during PPN-DBS in patients with Parkinson's disease.[66,67]

The internal capsule runs lateral to the STN, and although it has been hypothesized that some activation of the pyramidal tract fibers may be beneficial to reduce rigidity,[68] excessive activation of the internal capsule by STN-DBS can become problematic because it evokes strong contralateral muscle contractions and parasthesias and diminishes improvement in bradykinesia.[68,69] Results of animal experiments suggest that STN-DBS could influence dopaminergic activity through activation of nigrostriatal and pallidonigral fibers.[70-73] Although PET studies in patients with advanced Parkinson's disease did not provide evidence of increased striatal dopamine during therapeutic STN-DBS,[74,75] other animal studies have demonstrated increased levels in the striatum.[72,76,77] STN-DBS may also activate pallidothalamic fibers running dorsal to the STN,[39,78] and it has been suggested that modulation of cerebellothalamic fibers adjacent to the STN underlie the improvements in tremor with STN-DBS.[61,79] Xu and colleagues[47] showed that neuronal activity in both pallidal and cerebellar receiving areas of the thalamus were modulated by STN-DBS, which is further evidence in support of the hypothesis that activation of adjacent fiber pathways plays a role in mediating the therapeutic benefit of STN-DBS.

Effects of Deep Brain Stimulation on Distal Brain Regions

The neurophysiologic effects of DBS extend beyond the neuronal populations and fibers of passage that are directly modulated by the stimulation and are propagated throughout the entire basal ganglia–thalamocortical network. For example, motor cortex firing patterns were found to be modulated by STN-DBS[29,80,81] and GPi-DBS.[82,83] This could be a result of modulations in basal ganglia–thalamocortical pathways, activation of hyperdirect cortical-subthalamic pathways, or activation of fibers within the internal capsule.[29,60,68,84] PET studies have shown STN and GPi-DBS to have broad effects on primary and nonprimary motor areas of the cortex that depend on the stimulation target. Limousin and colleagues[85] found greater motor task–related changes in regional cerebral blood flow in supplementary motor areas, the cingulate cortex, and the dorsolateral prefrontal cortex during STN-DBS than during GPi-DBS, although this difference may have been attributable to suboptimal GPi lead placement, inasmuch as GPi-DBS recipients did not show the same degree of motor benefit as did STN DBS recipients. Other studies showed that STN-DBS reduced regional cerebral blood flow in motor and prefontal cortical areas.[86-88] DBS of the internal globus pallidus also has been demonstrated to decrease activity in sensorimotor cortex[89] and to increase activity in premotor cortex and the cerebellum.[90] Regional cerebral blood flow in the sensorimotor cortex was found to be nonlinearly correlated with stimulation intensity during DBS in the ventral intermediate nucleus for essential tremors[91]; this suggests recruitment of different fiber tracts with increasing voltage and current spread, which results in mixed inhibitory and excitatory effects in sensorimotor cortex. It is evident that DBS for Parkinson's disease can exert a widespread effect, producing changes not just in nuclei within the area being stimulated but also throughout distributed brain networks.

THERAPEUTIC MECHANISMS OF DEEP BRAIN STIMULATION

How do the observed changes in neuronal activity during DBS translate into therapeutic improvement for the patient? In the case of DBS for Parkinson's disease, stimulation at multiple nodes in the circuit (STN, GPi, GPe) can similarly improve motor symptoms; is there a single therapeutic mechanism of action, or is it different depending on stimulation site? Because the therapeutic effect of DBS is akin to that of surgically ablating a region of brain tissue, does DBS create a functional lesion in the target site that prevents pathologic signals to be relayed to the rest of the motor circuit? Experimental and computational studies have been addressing aspects these questions, but an explanation for the therapeutic mechanisms of DBS that is consistently supported by experimental evidence remains elusive.

Regularization of Pathologic Activity

One proposed mechanism of DBS, consistent with the activation of output from the site of stimulation and adjacent fiber pathways, is that stimulation overrides pathologic network activity by imposing more regular firing patterns in downstream nuclei.[92-94] This idea—that DBS replaces pathologic activity patterns with high frequency, regularized patterns that are time-locked to the stimulation pulses—is supported by numerous experimental[32,33,35,95,96] and modeling studies.[97,98] Therapeutic DBS in the STN and GPi for Parkinson's disease typically require frequencies above 100 Hz, whereas low-frequency stimulation (<25 Hz) can exacerbate symptoms,[99] perhaps by reinforcing pathologic bursting and synchronization in this frequency range. However, the frequency of stimulation necessary to alleviate symptoms can depend on the disease and DBS target. Low-frequency (20- to 60-Hz) stimulation in PPN can be used to treat gait and balance disorders in Parkinson's disease,[66,100] and some patients with primary dystonia can respond to GPi stimulation at frequencies of approximately 60 Hz.[101]

During DBS, the normal functioning of the basal ganglia is not necessarily restored; rather, it is replaced with activity that is less detrimental to the motor circuit than the endogenous pathologic activity. It is postulated that during DBS, intrinsic neuronal activity is substituted with regularized activity that is devoid of meaningful physiologic content. A so-called informational lesion may prevent pathologic activity from being transmitted and amplified within networks implicated in the manifestation of symptoms[20,98] and thus may be functionally similar to ablative procedures that produce similar clinical outcomes.[102] In addition, replacing pathologic with regularized activity, even if it means disabling the majority of functional information encoded by the pathway, may liberate other pathways to compensate for the remaining disease in the network and the loss of function in the stimulated pathway. There are several mechanisms by which DBS could override a neuron's intrinsic output. Stimulation can directly evoke action potentials in the axon, which propagate antidromically back along the axon and collide with orthodromic spikes initiated in the soma or dendrites. Moreover, because of the refractory period after an action potential, successive antidromic spikes may prevent the neuron from resuming its pathologic firing patterns. If the propagation of somatodendritic spikes down the axon is suppressed, then pathologically generated somatic activity may be replaced with axonally initiated firing patterns entrained to the stimulation, which would interfere with the transmission of pathologic signals to downstream targets.

In contrast to the concept that DBS acts to block information flow, other authorities have argued that it may improve signal processing. How might DBS enhance information transmission and improve motor signs of movement disorders? One possibility involves the theory of "focused selection," whereby sensorimotor outputs from the GPi and the substantia nigra pars reticularis facilitate the execution of voluntary movements by removing inhibition from a desired motor program while simultaneously inhibiting competing motor programs that would otherwise interfere with the movement.[103,104] Excessive synchronized activity within the basal ganglia could lead to coactivation of distinct populations of neurons subserving competing motor programs (i.e., co-contraction of antagonist and agonist muscles), which would result in bradykinesia, rigidity, or undesired movements. Results of several studies support this hypothesis. Parkinsonian nonhuman primates have less specific and more multiple-joint and limb receptive fields in the GPi[105,106] and the thalamus[107] than do normal controls. In patients with Parkinson's disease, administrating apomorphine, a nonselective D_1 and D_2 dopamine receptor agonist, reduced the proportion of neurons in the STN and GPi with multiple-joint receptive fields.[108] In dystonia, receptive fields appear to be widened and less specific in the GPi, thalamus, and somatosensory cortex.[109-112]

On the basis of these results, it is hypothesized that DBS acts in part by transforming broadened, less specific responses of cells in the basal ganglia–thalamocortical network back to more selective and focused responses, which improves sensory processing. However, very few studies have addressed this question experimentally.[83] Johnson and colleagues[83] found that GPi-DBS increased response specificity of neurons in the motor cortex to passive limb movement, which supports the hypothesis that DBS does not completely suppress information transfer to downstream nuclei from the stimulated area but rather improves signal transmission in the basal ganglia–thalamocortical network (Fig. 91-3). Using information theory[113] approaches to analyze basal ganglia firing patterns, Dorval and Grill[114] showed that directed information between pairs of neurons in the external globus pallidus and substantia nigra pars reticulata was reduced in rats with 6-hydroxydopamine (6-OHDA) lesions but partially restored by DBS, which supports the idea that DBS reestablishes neuronal information transmission. Modeling studies also support this hypothesis. Guo and associates[115] incorporated GPi activity from parkinsonian nonhuman primates treated with STN-DBS into simulations of GPi-receiving thalamocortical relay cells and found that thalamic relay fidelity was significantly improved during DBS (see Fig. 91-3). Santaniello and colleagues[116] created a model of the basal ganglia–thalamocortical loop that reproduced experimental evidence for each structure in the loop and found similar improvements in thalamocortical relay reliability during STN-DBS. The results of their simulations suggested that STN-DBS effects propagate proximally and distally to the stimulation site (e.g., through orthodromic and antidromic mechanisms) and are reinforced on the striatum maximally during high-frequency DBS (100-180 Hz), thereby producing regularized striatum-to-GPi discharge patterns and restoring thalamic relay function.

The hypotheses that DBS induces an informational lesion and that DBS improves information transmission are not necessarily mutually exclusive.[83,117] It is likely that the mechanisms for DBS involve complex processes involving both lesion-like effects (e.g., blocking pathologic output from the target nucleus) and network-modulating effects (e.g., improving thalamocortical relay reliability).

Effect of Deep Brain Stimulation on Beta Oscillatory Activity and Cross-Frequency Coupling

Experimental evidence suggests that neuronal firing patterns, rather than firing rate, play an important role in the disease states and the therapeutic effect of DBS.[93,94,118] In animal models of Parkinson's disease, low-frequency (<30-Hz) rhythmic bursting, excessive synchronization, or both are observed in the basal ganglia, thalamus, and motor cortex.[119-122] Oscillations and bursting in neuronal discharges, particularly in the beta range (≈10-30 Hz), are also prominent in the basal ganglia of patients with Parkinson's disease.[123-127] Experimental evidence suggests that during STN-DBS, synchronized oscillations in the low beta range and bursting discharges are reduced in both the STN and its target nuclei.[18,35,47,128]

Studies based on recordings of local field potentials, which reflect the ensemble activity of nearby neuronal populations,

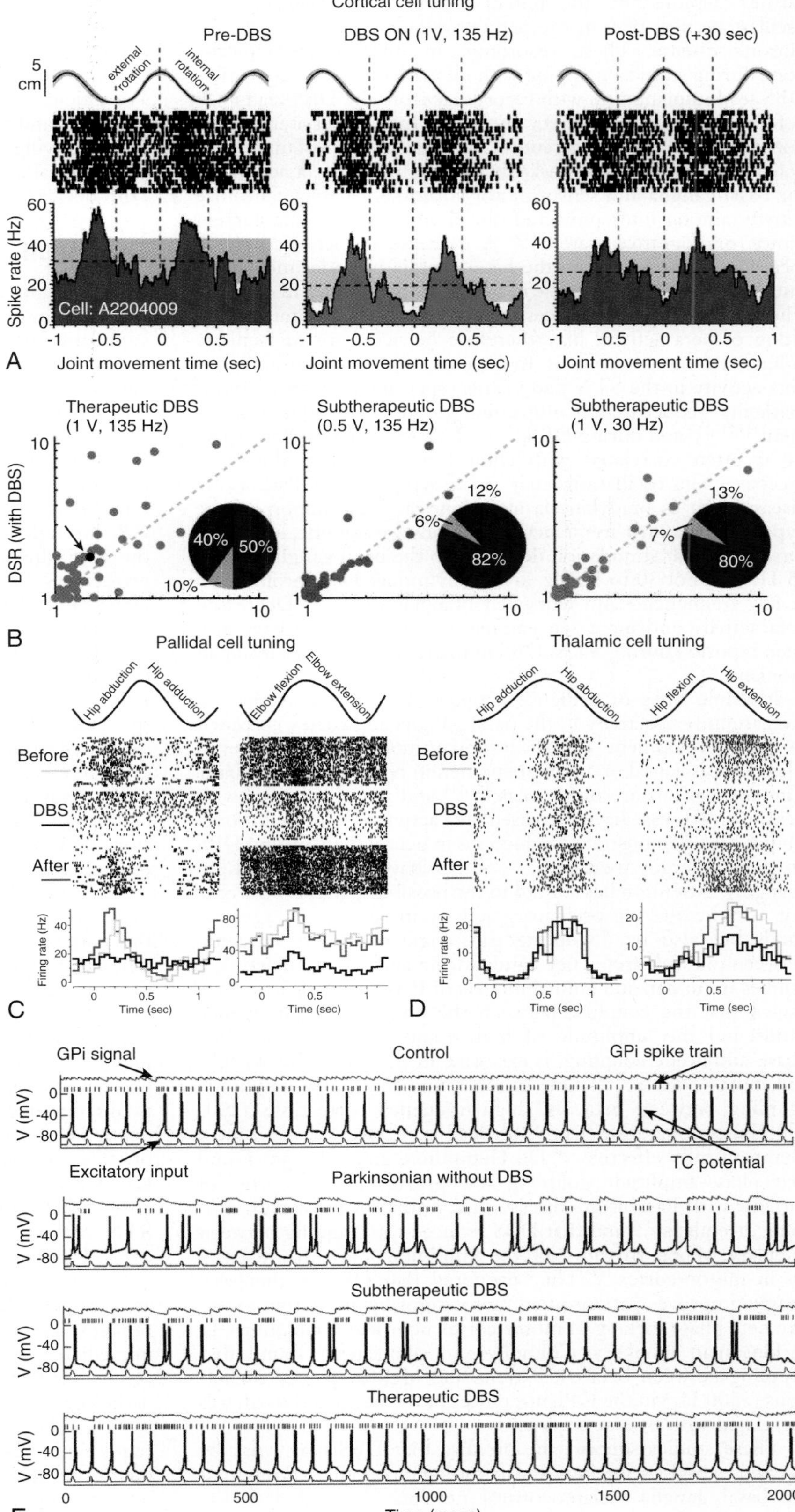

Figure 91-3. A, Examples of responses to passive manipulation of cortical cells before, during, and after pallidal high-frequency stimulation at 135 Hz. **B,** The neuronal discharge specificity ratio (DSR), defined as the ratio of average firing rates between opposing joint articulations, increased during therapeutic deep brain stimulation (DBS) but less so during subtherapeutic DBS. Pie charts represent the proportion of units with DSR changes above 20% *(blue),* changes below −20% *(yellow),* or no change *(maroon).* The *black dot* in the left graph (indicated by the *arrow*) represents the example cell shown in part A. **C** and **D,** Examples of responses to passive manipulation of two pallidal **(C)** and two thalamic **(D)** cells before, during, and after pallidal DBS. **E,** Computational model of thalamocortical (TC) relay cells shows that TC relay fidelity improves with clinically effective DBS. The central tracing in each of the four plots shows voltage versus time for the model TC cell. The voltage scale on each plot applies to this tracing. Offset above each such tracing, experimentally recorded internal globus pallidus (GPi) spike times (discrete events) are shown along with the inhibitory signal that these spike times are used to generate (continuous curve, above the spike times with amplitude scaled 100-fold for visibility). Offset below each TC voltage tracing, simulated excitatory input signals are shown (scaled by a factor of 3 for visibility). Note that the same excitatory input signals were used for all examples shown here and that TC spikes may lag behind excitatory input times by a few milliseconds; these lags correspond to delays from threshold crossing to spike generation. *(**B,** Modified from Johnson MD, Vitek JL, McIntyre CC. Pallidal stimulation that improves parkinsonian motor symptoms also modulates neuronal firing patterns in primary motor cortex in the MPTP-treated monkey.* Exp Neurol. *2009;219:359-362. **C** and **D,** Modified from Agnesi F, Connolly AT, Baker KB, et al. Deep brain stimulation imposes complex informational lesions.* PLoS One. *2013;8[8]:e74462. **E,** Modified from Guo Y, Rubin JE, McIntyre CC, et al. Thalamocortical relay fidelity varies across subthalamic nucleus deep brain stimulation protocols in a data-driven computational model.* J Neurophysiol. *2008;99:1477-1492.)*

further demonstrate the potential role that enhanced beta oscillations may play in the pathophysiologic processes of Parkinson's disease. These recordings in humans are typically done during surgical mapping with microelectrodes or soon after DBS lead implantation with recordings from the DBS lead itself before device activation. Beta rhythms in local field potentials are not inherently pathologic and in fact play an important role in behavioral and cognitive tasks. It is thought that beta activity in the basal ganglia and sensorimotor cortex serves to synchronize activity among interconnected nuclei and maintain the current motor or cognitive state.[129,130] A decrease in beta activity in local field potentials from the basal ganglia precedes movement initiation,[131] and the decrease in beta activity is longer in duration when greater cognitive processing is required.[132] Dynamic modulation of beta activity may therefore be necessary to facilitate voluntary motor movement. In patients with Parkinson's disease, beta activity in the STN and GPi is especially prominent and is markedly reduced after dopaminergic (e.g., levodopa) treatment[123,133,134] and during DBS.[135-137] This reduction in beta activity is often correlated with clinical improvement; therefore, excessive beta oscillations may cause symptoms of Parkinson's disease such as bradykinesia and akinesia.[138] In support of the hypothesis that low-frequency oscillations are akinetic, investigators found that stimulation delivered to the basal ganglia at 5 to 25 Hz, but not 30 to 50 Hz, artificially induced synchronization at low frequencies and worsened bradykinesia.[139,140] Decreased beta activity and increased gamma activity (>30 Hz) have also been reported during STN-DBS in the thalamus of parkinsonian monkeys.[47]

Multiple lines of evidence support the hypothesis that an increase in beta activity in the basal ganglia and cortex is related to the development of parkinsonian motor signs; however, whether it is causal or an epiphenomenon remains under debate. The correlations are often weak,[141-143] and not all patients with Parkinson's disease have increased beta activity.[144] Although some studies have demonstrated reductions in beta activity during DBS or dopaminergic treatment,[129] others have demonstrated no change.[145] Attention has shifted to the possibility that DBS works not only by altering oscillatory activity in restricted frequency bands but also by disrupting pathologic oscillatory coupling between multiple frequency bands within and across nuclei.[146-149] Studies in human and animal models of Parkinson's disease have shown that the coupling between the phase of low-frequency bands and the amplitude of high-frequency bands, so-called phase-amplitude coupling, is excessive in the STN,[146,150] GPi,[151] and motor cortex.[147,152] One group found that phase-amplitude coupling between beta and high-frequency oscillations (200-500 Hz) was greatest near DBS lead contacts that were most therapeutically effective.[148] De Hemptinne and colleagues found that phase-amplitude coupling was greater in the cortex of patients with Parkinson's disease than in that of those with dystonia or epilepsy[147] and that DBS reduced the coupling between the phase of beta rhythms and the amplitude of broadband activity in motor cortex.[152] They proposed that DBS in the basal ganglia improves parkinsonian motor signs by alleviating excessive beta phase locking of motor cortex neuronal populations. In parkinsonian monkeys, Connolly and associates[151] found that coupling between beta oscillations and high-frequency oscillations (>200 Hz) in the GPi, not power in the beta band itself, was correlated with disease severity.

These studies support the premise that DBS may work by altering neural oscillations and pathologic coupling throughout the basal ganglia–thalamocortical network. Nevertheless, the measures used in many of these studies have high variability both across subjects and even within subjects. This is a promising line of research, but many questions remain: What are the mechanisms driving abnormal coupling? What is the relationship between specific changes in cross-frequency coupling and the manifestation of particular motor signs? Does dysfunction at a particular nucleus (e.g., STN, GPi, primary motor cortex) drive pathologic activity throughout the rest of the network? How is coupling altered during movement and during therapeutic DBS? We anticipate that a growing number of studies will address these questions and that the answers will have important implications for improving DBS therapy: for example, the use of recorded pathological activity as a feedback control signal for closed-loop DBS devices.[152,153]

Therapeutic Latencies

It is becoming apparent that DBS has multiple mechanisms and time courses of action that vary depending on stimulation target, stimulation parameters, and pathologic process (Fig. 91-4). Vitek and associates[154] reported that improvement in bradykinesia in patients with Parkinson's disease occurred within seconds for GPe-DBS but took half a minute or more for GPi-DBS and was often preceded by a period of aggravated symptoms. In that study, GPe-DBS occasionally induced dyskinesias in the hand and arm that spread to the leg over minutes. Vitek and associates hypothesized that GPe stimulation rapidly alters neuronal activity in the GPi through activation of striatopallidal fibers passing through the GPe (direct pathway) or activating GPe-GPi or GPe-STN projections (indirect pathway), leading to immediate clinical effect. The delayed responses with GPi-DBS suggest a more complex spatial-temporal profile of stimulation on GPi neuronal activity or a time-varying effect on network activity in pallidothalamocortical circuitry. DBS stimulation parameters may also influence therapeutic latencies. Wu and colleagues[16] reported that the latency of onset of dyskinesia suppression during GPi-DBS decreased from 5 seconds to 1 second as the frequency of stimulation increased from 80 to 100 Hz. Higher frequency stimulation (185 versus 135 Hz) also appeared to decrease the therapeutic latency for rest tremor in patients with Parkinson's disease, possibly because of frequency-dependent destabilization of network oscillations.[155]

Chronic DBS may induce both short and long-term changes in network activity, as evidenced by the temporal latency between the start of stimulation and full therapeutic benefit and persistence of symptom relief after stimulation is ended. For example, patients with Parkinson's disease who have DBS implants often experience immediate cessation of upper limb tremor, whereas improvement in axial symptoms takes hours to manifest completely.[156,157] Similarly, after DBS is discontinued, symptoms reappear on different time frames: tremor reappears very quickly, but axial symptoms remain improved for hours or days.[158] The therapeutic latency can also depend on stimulation target; the onset of effect on tremor symptoms is often slower (hours, days) with GPi-DBS than with STN-DBS. One explanation for this difference is that activation of the hyperdirect primary motor cortex–STN pathway with STN DBS may directly modulate motor cortical activity and facilitate the rapid onset of symptom relief,[84] but evidence supporting a causal relationship between antidromic activation of the primary motor cortex and therapeutic effect remains incomplete. An alternative explanation for the more immediate effect of STN-DBS on tremor is activation of adjacent cerebellothalamic fibers.[47,61] Therapeutic latencies depend on the pathologic process as well; DBS improves essential tremor symptoms within seconds, whereas patients with idiopathic dystonia require minutes of stimulation to improve phasic dystonic movements and days, weeks, or months to obtain maximal relief of tonic posturing.[159] Cheung and associates[160] report retention of motor benefits in dystonia patients for months after cessation of GPi-DBS. Houeto and colleagues[161] found that improvement in tic severity in patients with Tourette's syndrome took several weeks after the initiation of DBS, and the benefit lasted at least a month after discontinuation of stimulation.

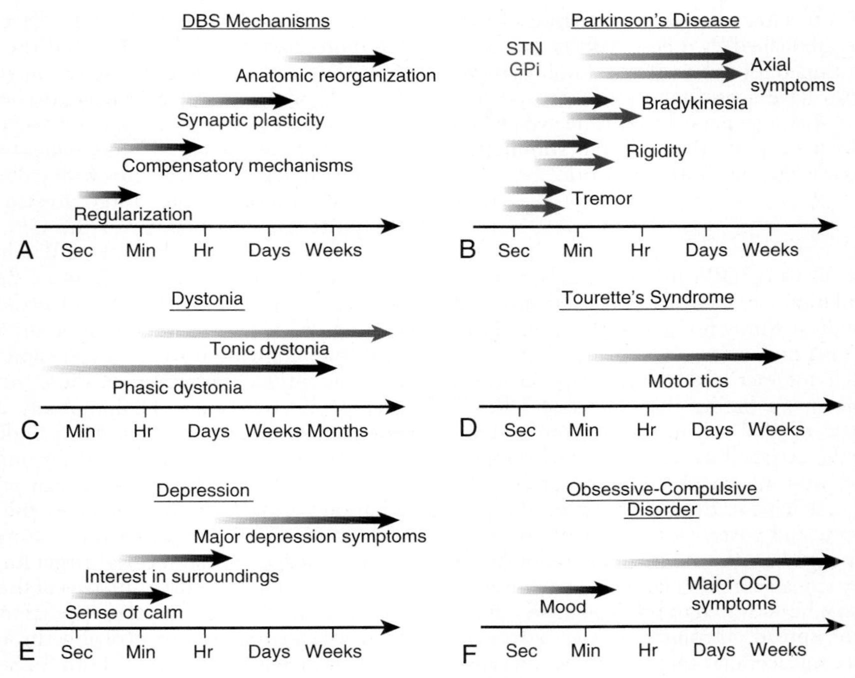

Figure 91-4. **A** to **F**, Deep brain stimulation (DBS) induces hierarchic and temporally disparate changes across the brain. In many cases, the latencies of improvement in symptoms after the stimulator is turned on are the same length as the latencies of worsening of symptoms after the stimulator is turned off. *Arrows* indicate general trends for disorder symptoms. Note that in all cases, specific symptom relief can depend critically on target, location within each target, and stimulation parameters. GPi, internal globus pallidus; OCD, obsessive-compulsive disorder; STN, subthalamic nucleus.

Improvement in even a single symptom may involve multiple mechanisms. Cooper and associates[162] examined Parkinson's bradykinesia after STN-DBS was turned off and found an initial rapid reduction in therapeutic effect, followed by a further slow decline, which suggests two separate physiologic mechanisms by which STN-DBS improves bradykinesia. The time it takes for a symptom to improve after stimulation onset seems to predict the time it will take to worsen once stimulation is stopped[158,163]; this observation indicates that plasticity in the network may be involved in the mechanisms of DBS.

Deep Brain Stimulation–Induced Plasticity

The fact that the time for improvement with DBS depends on the disorder, symptom, and target strongly suggests that different mechanisms underlie these improvements (see Fig. 91-4). Reduction of abnormal oscillations or pathologic firing patterns may occur within seconds of DBS onset and be responsible for improvement in tremor, bradykinesia, and rigidity. The reasons for the delays in symptom improvement, as in the case of DBS for dystonia, are less straightforward. The long-term effects of DBS on brain networks are not well understood, but plasticity probably plays an important role. Based on whole-cell patch-clamp recordings in rat brain slices, high-frequency stimulation in the STN was found to induce three types of plastic changes at glutamatergic synapses: (1) short-term potentiation of the evoked postsynaptic current, which increased glutamate release from the presynaptic terminals over a 5-minute period; (2) long-term potentiation of the evoked postsynaptic current, indicative of changes in postsynaptic protein expression that required more than 30 minutes; and (3) long-term depression of the evoked postsynaptic current, which modified presynaptic regulation over a period exceeding 30 minutes.[164] In brain slices from dopamine-depleted rats, Yamawaki and colleagues[165] found that DBS induced glutamatergic cortico-subthalamic synaptic depression, which could possibly impede the transfer of pathologic oscillations from the cortex.

The extent to which synaptic plasticity helps produce the therapeutic effects of DBS requires further investigation, but it is not surprising that it plays an important role. Synaptic plasticity should be expected at least in the stimulated area and in the nuclei receiving projections from the stimulated area. In fact, DBS appears to promote synaptic plasticity throughout the basal ganglia–thalamocortical network. Using transcranial magnetic stimulation (TMS), Ruge and colleagues[166] assessed plasticity in the motor cortex of dystonic patients receiving GPi-DBS over 6 months. A short-interval intracortical inhibition (SICI) protocol was used to measure excitability of corticocortical GABA inhibitory connections. Inhibition was more difficult to evoke in dystonic patients, possibly in relation to the excessive muscle activity characteristic of dystonia, but SICI increased toward levels of healthy controls within 3 months of DBS initiation and followed the same rate of clinical improvement. Another protocol, paired associative stimulation (PAS), was used to assess long-term potentiation-like synaptic plasticity in the cortex. PAS-induced plasticity is exacerbated in patients with dystonia; this may reflect excessive cortical plasticity that strengthens inappropriate connections in the motor system, which over time may lead to the excessive involuntary movement associated with dystonia. Excessive PAS-induced plasticity was abolished 1 month after GPi-DBS initiation but returned to the level of normal subjects at 6 months. When SICI and PAS-induced plasticity were evaluated in dystonic patients who received GPi-DBS for more than 4 years, potentiation of intracortical GABA transmission was again reduced, even in the DBS-off state, whereas potentiation of corticospinal excitability was abolished.[167] These effects persisted even after DBS was discontinued for 2 days. These findings highlight the fact that DBS can have a profound effect on synaptic plasticity at a network level that may persist over time even when DBS is discontinued, which suggests that chronic stimulation may induce long-term plastic changes in the network.[168]

Astrocytes

The search for the mechanisms of DBS has focused largely on the direct effect of stimulation on neurons (e.g., activation of axons, inhibition of cell bodies). Study findings suggest that DBS can also trigger cellular and molecular changes in other cells, particularly astrocytes, that interact with neuronal populations and could play a key role in mediating the effects of DBS.[169] Astrocytes are a major type of glial cell in the nervous system, important in maintaining the extracellular chemical environment of neurons and in regulating neuronal communication.[170,171] Astrocytes are an active participant in the tripartite synapse, which consists of presynaptic and postsynaptic elements and surrounding glia, and are engaged in the release and reuptake of neurotransmitters.[170] They can assemble in large cell networks to control blood flow[172] and can be activated to produce intracellular calcium waves that can spread throughout the astrocyte network.[173] DBS can induce intracellular calcium waves and cause the release of glutamate[174] and adenosine triphosphate, which is transformed into adenosine in the extracellular space.[175] Adenosine release has been suggested to play a role in amelioration of tremor during thalamic DBS[175] and in mediating the microthalamotomy effect.[176] Astrocytic DBS-induced neurotransmitter release occurs over minutes, a longer time scale[177,178] than the clinical improvements observed within seconds after stimulation onset, but it still could theoretically have an effect on symptoms that improve over minutes and may mediate benefits that persist after stimulation is turned off.

Neuroprotective Effects of Deep Brain Stimulation

Although there is as yet no clear evidence that STN-DBS or GPi-DBS provides a neuroprotective effect in humans with Parkinson's disease, there is increasing evidence in animal models of Parkinson's disease that high-frequency stimulation may confer some degree of neuroprotection.[179] STN lesions in rats prevented degeneration of dopaminergic tyrosine hydroxylase–expressing cells in the SNc caused by striatal 6-OHDA injections,[180] as did STN-DBS delivered for hours to 2 weeks after induction of 6-OHDA lesions.[181-184] STN-DBS or STN lesions applied either before or after treatment with methyl-phenyl-tetrahydropyridine (MPTP) in monkeys also improved dopaminergic tyrosine hydroxylase–expressing cell survival in the SNc[185] and the periaqueductal gray matter.[186] The neuroprotective effect might have resulted from reduced glutamate excitotoxicity caused by limiting excitatory input to the SNc from the STN. Although this hypothesis is not congruent with the evidence of increased output from the DBS target, other mechanisms may explain these results, including stimulation-induced release of neurotrophic factors or activation of GABAergic fibers of passage innervating the SNc. As more is learned about the potential neuroprotective effects of DBS, it may be reasonable to pursue this surgical treatment option earlier in disease states.[179,187,188]

THERAPEUTIC TARGETS OF DEEP BRAIN STIMULATION

The role of network dysfunction in the pathophysiologic mechanisms of movement disorders is highlighted by the observation that stimulation at a number of targets in the network can produce clinical benefits.[189-191] In Parkinson's disease, the sensorimotor region of the STN and the GPi are standard target sites, but research findings have suggested that the PPN,[66,100] GPe,[154] and motor cortex[192] may also be therapeutic targets. The ventrolateral thalamus was initially the preferred target for treating primary dystonia.[193-196] Subsequent studies appeared to show greater clinical improvements with pallidal DBS,[193] and currently the most widely accepted target for treating primary dystonia is the posteroventral portion of the GPi.[159,191,197] In many studies of thalamotomy and thalamic DBS, however, the populations of patients with secondary dystonia have been heterogeneous, and so the power of the overall observed benefit is probably limited.[193,198,199] Moreover, multiple subnuclei in the motor thalamus may contribute to the expression of dystonic movements, and suboptimal targeting of these structures could limit the therapeutic outcomes. Thalomotomy and thalamic DBS have not been studied as extensively as pallidotomy or pallidal DBS in patients with dystonia, and so it remains to be determined which target is better or whether they can provide similar benefit. In addition to the GPi and thalamus, the STN has also garnered interest an alternative target for treating dystonia.[200]

The most common surgical target for treating essential tremor is the ventral intermediate nucleus of the thalamus,[201,202] although stimulation near the posterior portion of the STN may also improve essential tremor, probably through activation of adjacent cerebellothalamic fibers.[61,203] Both STN-DBS and GPi-DBS can ameliorate tremors associated with Parkinson's disease.[204,205] For Tourette's syndrome, numerous regions have been targeted, including the centromedian-parafascicular nucleus of the thalamus,[161,206,207] the ventral anterior and ventrolateral motor thalamus,[208] the anterior GPi,[209-211] the posteroventral GPi,[212,213] the GPe,[214] and the anterior limb of the internal capsule.[215] It is possible that a different mechanism or pathway underlies the beneficial effect of stimulating different targets. Alternatively, each of these areas may contribute to the genesis or mediation of the tics associated with Tourette's syndrome, and stimulation at any of these sites ameliorates tics by interrupting the circuits associated with tic formation, facilitation, or mediation. Indeed, theories on the mechanisms of DBS have taken a more systems-level approach, deemphasizing the importance of local changes in or near the stimulated target (e.g. activation, inhibition) and focusing instead on how DBS changes the dynamics of brain networks in order to reduce or modify pathologic network activity and produce therapeutic benefits.[216,217]

DBS has also been used for the treatment of medication-refractory obsessive-compulsive disorder and depression. There is currently a humanitarian device exemption (HDE) for obsessive-compulsive disorder, and two industry-sponsored clinical trials involving exploration of two different targets—the anterior limb of the internal capsule and subgenu area 25—were conducted for the treatment of depression. Nuttin and colleagues[218] were the first to report the use of DBS at the anterior limb of the internal capsule for treating obsessive-compulsive disorder, in 1999. This fiber tract contains numerous projections to and from frontal cortical areas. The limbic basal ganglia (caudate nucleus, nucleus accumbens, GPi, STN) are also thought to be involved in obsessive-compulsive disorder, and stimulation in these regions has produced therapeutic effects in some patients.[219] In particular, stimulation of the nucleus accumbens has been shown to be a promising treatment for medication refractory obsessive-compulsive disorder.[220] Using functional magnetic resonance imaging and electroencephalographic recordings in 16 patients with obsessive-compulsive disorder, Figee and colleagues[221] found that DBS normalized nucleus accumbens activity and reduced excessive connectivity between the nucleus accumbens and medial prefrontal cortex. They speculated that stimulation of corticothalamic pathways or antidromic stimulation of the ventral internal capsule connecting the prefrontal cortex with the nucleus accumbens was responsible for the restoration of normalized frontostriatal connectivity.[222]

DBS of the subcallosal cingulate gyrus was reported by Mayberg and associates[223] to improve the symptoms of depression. In the trajectory used for DBS of the subcallosal cingulate gyrus, the distal and proximal contacts were placed in cortical gray matter, and the remaining two middle contacts, in white matter. Interestingly, the contacts used in these studies tended to be the two middle contacts, which, when activated, would be expected to affect both afferent and efferent projections of the subcallosal cingulate gyrus. Additional DBS targets investigated for depression have included the ventral striatum,[224] nucleus accumbens,[225] lateral habenula,[226] inferior thalamic peduncle,[227] and medial forebrain bundle,[228] although subcallosal cingulate stimulation has been the most studied DBS therapy for treatment-resistant depression.[229-231] Probabilistic tractography methods based on diffusion tensor imaging data have revealed that connectivity between the subcallosal cingulate DBS target and other brain regions—including the medial frontal cortex, the rostral and dorsal cingulate cortex, and subcortical nuclei—is enhanced in individuals who respond well to DBS treatment in comparison with those who do not.[232] The mechanisms for therapeutic DBS for depression probably involve affecting both local target regions and the white matter tracts linking the target to other key areas in the network. It is possible that in the future target selection will be individualized through the use of patient-specific activation volume tractography in order to more accurately determine the target location and optimize the effect of stimulation on network connectivity.[233]

Stimulation in the STN and GPi, the two primary DBS targets for Parkinson's disease, are known to generate slightly different effects in downstream networks. Several electroencephalographic and PET studies showed that cortical responses to STN-DBS and GPi-DBS differed for patients with Parkinson's disease who were engaged in a movement-related task despite no difference in task performance.[234,235] During movement execution, STN-DBS and GPi-DBS reduced pathologic desynchronization in the premotor cortex and increased desynchronization in the primary motor cortex. During planning stages, however, only STN-DBS facilitated an increase in primary motor cortex desynchronization.[234] PET studies showed that both clinically effective STN-DBS and GPi-DBS activated the supplementary motor cortex and cingulate cortex.[85] Although the STN produced higher cortical activation, especially over dorsolateral prefrontal cortex, this might have been partly because of differences in effect on motor signs between the two patient groups: STN-DBS produced greater improvement, possibly because the placement of DBS leads in patients with GP implantations was less optimal.

Other researchers have reported a concomitant decrease in activation of prefrontal and temporal cortical regions during STN-DBS,[48,236,237] which suggests that a potential mechanism of action could be the suppression of "abnormal resting overactivity" in the motor system and restoration of selective cortical activation during movement.[238] This hypothesis is supported by previous findings that motor cortical activity is reduced during passive movement during GP-DBS[83] and by imaging studies during STN-DBS that demonstrated a reduction in cerebral blood flow.[86,87] Additional studies with larger patient groups are necessary to determine whether different cortical responses evoked by STN- and GPi-DBS are simply an epiphenomenon or alternatively represent different clinical outcomes that reflect different lead locations within the target areas.[85]

Open-label studies have almost universally demonstrated greater benefit with STN-DBS, although primary outcomes measures of blinded randomized studies have demonstrated relatively equivalent efficacy between STN-DBS and GPi-DBS.[239-245] A critically important factor often unaccounted for in most studies is the location of the lead within the target nuclei. The GPi is anatomically larger than the STN, and suboptimal lead placement in the GPi could provide an explanation for the decreased efficacy of GPi-DBS in comparison with STN-DBS observed in many open-label studies. Although many centers—in fact, probably the majority—uniformly employ STN-DBS for all cases of Parkinson's disease, the results from studies comparing the efficacy of STN-DBS and GPi-DBS suggest that a more patient-tailored and symptom-specific approach to choosing DBS targets (and location within targets) may be needed to optimize outcomes of DBS therapy.[205] To date, no such study has addressed this question, and targets appear to be chosen according to each center's or DBS team's personal preference.

Targets within Targets

Conventional approaches to DBS lead implantation for Parkinson's disease include placing the lead within the sensorimotor territory of the STN or GPi target. Anatomic and electrophysiologic studies have shown, however, that these sensorimotor regions are further demarcated into segregated motor subcircuits with different subcortical-cortical projections. Using transsynaptic retrograde virus tracers, Hoover and colleagues[246] showed that injections in the sensorimotor arm area of the motor cortex, the premotor cortex, and the supplementary motor area resulted in densely labeled neurons in localized regions of the sensorimotor GPi. Similarly, electrical stimulation of the motor cortex in awake monkeys modulated activity in the posteroventral portion of the GPi and GPe in relation to motor execution, whereas stimulation of the supplementary motor area modulated anterodorsal pallidal neurons associated with movement planning.[247,248] It is possible that stimulation of distinct subcircuits within target nuclei has differential effects on subcortical-thalamocortical networks, which in turn result in different effects on various motor signs in Parkinson's disease (see Fig. 91-1B). In support of this idea, studies in patients with Parkinson's disease demonstrated that monopolar DBS in the dorsal pallidum (corresponding to dorsal GPi or ventral GPe) improved bradykinesia but induced dyskinesia, whereas more ventrally located contacts (corresponding to ventral margin of or just below the GPi) improved rigidity and levodopa-induced dyskinesias but worsened bradykinesia.[249-251]

An alternative explanation for these observations, however, is that the more ventrally located contacts caused subclinical activation of adjacent corticospinal tract fibers, which resulted in worsened bradykinesia. Xu and colleagues[68] tested the hypothesis that subclinical activation of the corticospinal tract would worsen bradykinesia while ameliorating rigidity by systematically stimulating the STN at varying intensities up to 80% of the voltage needed to produce overt muscle contractions in parkinsonian nonhuman primates. Despite worsening bradykinesia at higher voltages, rigidity was ameliorated at all stimulation intensities up to and including 80% of the internal capsule threshold. Behavior and subject-specific computational modeling studies in animals receiving GPi-DBS also demonstrated that improvements in rigidity were correlated with activation of a certain proportion (≈10%) of corticospinal tract fibers, whereas improvements in bradykinesia were correlated with activation of sensorimotor axonal projections within GPe and GPi at the site of the medial medullary lamina.[60]

Further support for a differential effect on motor signs based on the site of stimulation within the STN was provided by Mera and colleagues,[252] who used quantitative measures to assess bradykinesia and tremor and observed that there were separate regions within the STN in which stimulation optimally improved tremor (more ventral-posterior regions) or bradykinesia (dorsal-anterior regions). Butson and associates[253] found that stimulation optimally improved bradykinesia and rigidity at different regions dorsal to the STN. These findings suggest that multiple subcircuits must be stimulated in order to ameliorate distinct motor symptoms and that the DBS settings needed to optimally relieve one symptom (e.g., rigidity) may come at the expense of exacerbating another (e.g., bradykinesia) or that choosing one contact that optimally improves one symptom may not provide similar benefits to another. High-resolution imaging of the lead location and adjacent brain structures, combined with neuronal models, are improving the ability to evaluate which structures are activated by DBS on a patient-specific basis and could help guide DBS parameter programming.[254,255] Moreover, technologic advances in electrode designs and pulse generators may enable sculpting of the current field and allow current to be directed toward discrete pathways and away from others, which would potentially optimize the therapeutic effect of DBS while minimizing side effects.[153]

CONCLUSION

In initial hypotheses about DBS mechanisms, stimulation was thought to act like a surgical lesion, inhibiting neuronal activity in the target area. Subsequent experimental evidence indicated that DBS evokes differential effects between somatic and axonal elements. Whereas somatic activity near the DBS electrode may be suppressed, high-frequency stimulation directly activates axons of local projection neurons and fiber tracts passing near or through the target nucleus. It is thought that stimulation overrides abnormal neuronal activity by imposing a more regular output on downstream nuclei and interrupts the transfer of pathologic information from the stimulated nucleus to other structures in the network. The importance of network dysfunction in neurological disorders is highlighted by the fact that stimulation of different anatomic targets can generate similar therapeutic benefits for the same disorder and by the fact that stimulation of the same targets has proven effective in treating multiple neurologic disorders. A key issue underlying the therapeutic mechanisms of DBS may be its ability to alter the dynamics of the stimulated brain networks, although the specific processes underlying these changes are not well understood. Additional electrophysiologic, biochemical, imaging, behavioral, and computational modeling studies in animals and patients are essential for obtaining further insight into how DBS works at a cellular and systems level.

A better understanding of how DBS works and why side effects are generated are critically important for improving existing therapy and expanding the application of DBS to other disorders. New developments in electrode and pulse generator technology are being motivated by research that suggests the value of activating distinct, symptom-specific subcircuits and sparing other areas whose activation would cause unwanted side effects.[256-258] Researchers are actively investigating "closed-loop" DBS systems capable of adjusting stimulation parameters in real time based on meaningful physiologic biomarkers, thereby optimizing clinical efficacy while preserving battery life of the device,[259] as well as stimulation paradigms that can take advantage of the ability of the nervous system to undergo plasticity and provide improvement in motor signs that lasts well after stimulation is turned off.[260,261] DBS is a successful therapy that has had significant clinical effect, but it has yet to reach its full potential as a treatment for neurological disorders. Researchers must continue to work towards fully understanding the mechanisms by which DBS generates its therapeutic benefit.

SUGGESTED READINGS

Benabid AL, Pollak P, Louveau A, et al. Combined (thalamotomy and stimulation) stereotactic surgery of the VIM thalamic nucleus for bilateral Parkinson disease. *Appl Neurophysiol.* 1987;50:344-346.

de Hemptinne C, Swann NC, Ostrem JL, et al. Therapeutic deep brain stimulation reduces cortical phase-amplitude coupling in Parkinson's disease. *Nat Neurosci.* 2015;18(5):779-786.

Grill WM, Snyder AN, Miocinovic S. Deep brain stimulation creates an informational lesion of the stimulated nucleus. *Neuroreport.* 2004;15: 1137-1140.

Guo Y, Rubin JE, McIntyre CC, et al. Thalamocortical relay fidelity varies across subthalamic nucleus deep brain stimulation protocols in a data-driven computational model. *J Neurophysiol.* 2008;99(3): 1477-1492.

Hashimoto T, Elder CM, Okun MS, et al. Stimulation of the subthalamic nucleus changes the firing pattern of pallidal neurons. *J Neurosci.* 2003;23:1916-1923.

Hassler R, Riechert T, Mundinger F, et al. Physiological observations in stereotaxic operations in extrapyramidal motor disturbances. *Brain.* 1960;83:337-350.

Li Q, Qian Z, Arbuthnott GW, et al. Cortical effects of deep brain stimulation: implications for pathogenesis and treatment of parkinson disease. *JAMA Neurol.* 2013;71(1):100-103.

Lozano AM, Lipsman N. Probing and regulating dysfunctional circuits using deep brain stimulation. *Neuron.* 2013;77:406-424.

Mayberg HS, Lozano AM, Voon V, et al. Deep brain stimulation for treatment-resistant depression. *Neuron.* 2005;45(5):651-660.

McIntyre CC, Hahn PJ. Network perspectives on the mechanisms of deep brain stimulation. *Neurobiol Dis.* 2010;38(3):329-337.

Meissner W, Leblois A, Hansel D, et al. Subthalamic high frequency stimulation resets subthalamic firing and reduces abnormal oscillations. *Brain.* 2005;128:2372-2382.

Mink JW. The basal ganglia: focused selection and inhibition of competing motor programs. *Prog Neurobiol.* 1996;50:381.

See a full reference list on ExpertConsult.com

92 Complication Avoidance in Deep Brain Stimulation Surgery

Ron L. Alterman and David H. Aguirre-Padilla

Deep brain stimulation (DBS) is a proven and durable therapy for medically refractory Parkinson's disease, essential tremor, primary dystonia, and obsessive-compulsive disorder, and it has the potential to ameliorate many additional functional brain disorders, including epilepsy, depression, Alzheimer's disease, obesity, and addiction. Although the incidence of serious adverse events related to DBS is quite low, the therapy is not risk free. The reported incidence of complications related to DBS therapy ranges from approximately 4%[1] during the month immediately after surgery to 30% or more over the long term[2-6]; an average 16% risk of complications was reported in studies of more than 100 procedures.[1,2,4,7-28]

This chapter focuses on the complications commonly encountered in the course of providing DBS therapy. When appropriate, we highlight measures that the clinician may take to avoid those complications. As is traditional, we have categorized the complications as being procedure, stimulation, or hardware related. One might include in this discussion poor patient selection, which results in transient benefit (perhaps related to placebo response) or complete lack of response. Chapter 85 focuses on patient selection; in this chapter, we focus purely on adverse events related to delivering the therapy.

PROCEDURE-RELATED COMPLICATIONS

The complications most commonly feared and encountered in relation to the DBS procedure include death, neurological injury, intracerebral hemorrhage, perioperative confusion, and infection.

Death

The reported rate of mortality from DBS surgery is low, ranging from 0.3%[29] to 0.9%.[10] Most studies have reported no mortality at all. Most deaths are related to the lead implant procedure,[29] and the most common cause of death is intracranial hemorrhage.[1,30] Additional causes of death include cardiac complications,[10,29] aspiration pneumonia,[1,26] "multifactorial" causes,[1,29] or unknown causes.[20] Pulmonary embolus may also prove fatal.[1]

Neurological Deficit

Neurological deficit related to DBS surgery may arise from one of three main causes: a poorly targeted DBS lead that traverses and injures an unintended structure; intracranial hemorrhage; or venous infarction. Of these, intracranial hemorrhage is by far the most common.

Intracerebral Hemorrhage

Although rare, death or disability caused by intracerebral hemorrhage is the most disconcerting potential complication of DBS surgery and is probably the most common reason why patients either are not referred for surgery or refuse to undergo the procedure. In case series with more than 100 DBS procedures, the reported incidence of intracranial hemorrhage (including subarachnoid, subdural, and epidural hemorrhages) ranged from 0% to 9.5% among patients[10,14,25,27,31-41] and 0% to 3.3% among leads.[4,32,34,37,39,42-44] With regard to only intraparenchymal and intraventricular hemorrhage, the reported incidence ranges from 0% to 8.4% among patients (mean, 3.2%),[a] and 0% to 3% of leads (mean, 1.7%).[b] Intraparenchymal hemorrhages accounted for 58%[48] of the intracranial bleeds, and intraventricular hemorrhages accounted for 42%.[39,48] Among the intraparenchymal hemorrhages, 50% to 77% occurred at or near the target, and 23% to 50% occurred along the trajectory.[10,32,39] Of intracranial hemorrhages, 37.5% to 71.5% were symptomatic,[10,32,39] and up to 50% of patients had permanent deficit.[32] Mortality secondary to procedure-related intracerebral hemorrhage ranged from 8.3% to 50%.[30,48] Intracranial hemorrhage also increased length of hospital stay.[39,43] In one study, the average postoperative stay for patients with no hemorrhage was 2.0 days, in contrast to 4.2 days for those with hemorrhage.[39]

Patient-specific risk factors for procedure-related intracranial hemorrhage are poorly defined. Some authors have reported a higher risk of intracerebral hemorrhage in older patients,[1,39,44] whereas others have found no such correlation.[14,27,32] In particular, a retrospective study of 1757 patients revealed that patients older than 75 years exhibited the same risk of intracerebral hemorrhage as did younger patients.[14] Chronic hypertension has also been proposed as a risk factor,[1,34,43,48] although some authors have found no statistical relation.[39] Some have found that patients with Parkinson's disease have an increased risk of hemorrhage,[29] but others have not.[32,39,48]

Technical factors that may increase hemorrhage risk are also controversial. Some authors have reported that procedures targeting the internal globus pallidus (GPi) are associated with a greater incidence of hemorrhage (up to 7%),[32,42] whereas others have found no correlation between intracerebral hemorrhage and target.[39,45] The risks associated with intraoperative microelectrode recording (MER) remain unclear. Theoretically, each electrode pass carries a finite risk of hemorrhage, and so more passes should confer more risk. Some series have demonstrated this correlation.[34,42,50,51] One multicenter study involving 143 patients demonstrated that procedures in which a hemorrhage occurred were performed with a mean of 4.1 ± 2.0 microelectrode penetrations; in comparison, 2.9 ± 1.8 penetrations in procedures occurred without a hemorrhage.[42] Park and colleagues[51] reported six intraparenchymal and two intraventricular hemorrhages in 106 DBS procedures during which they employed five simultaneous MER trajectories, in comparison with no hemorrhages in 65 procedures during which they employed only two. In contrast, many other studies have revealed no correlation between MER and hemorrhage,[31,32,39,43,48,52,53] which suggests that the key factor may not be the use of MER per se but how MER is employed. Binder and associates[32] suggested advancing microelectrodes no faster than 0.5 mm/second and advancing no more than 2 mm beyond the inferior border of the GPi to avoid blood vessels within the choroidal fissure. Other authors have suggested limiting the number of MER penetrations in patients in whom nonspecific white matter hyperintensities and lacunar infarcts are visible on magnetic resonance imaging (MRI).[54] To reduce the risk of hemorrhage, Ben-Haim and colleagues[39] proposed a

[a]References 2, 8, 10, 11, 18, 24, 30, 32, 39, 42, 45-49.
[b]References 2, 10, 11, 17, 24, 32, 39, 42, 45, 49.

modified microelectrode with a smaller electrode tip and no guide tube covering the electrode's distal 25 mm.

The surgical trajectory to the therapeutic target probably has an effect. For example, Elias and associates[48] found that trajectories near or within sulci are associated with a higher rate of vascular complications (10.1% versus 0.7%). The risk of hemorrhage may also be increased with trajectories that traverse the ventricles, and up to 50% of intraventricular hemorrhages may result in focal neurological deficits.[39,45,48] In two studies, the risks of hemorrhage associated with transventricular trajectories were 5% and 10.8%.[39,48] With regard to target-related risk, the risk of ventricular penetration increases when more medial structures are targeted. Elias and associates[48] found that only 6% of trajectories targeted to the GPi traversed the ventricle, in comparison with 45% of ventral intermediate nucleus (Vim) trajectories and 65% of subthalamic nucleus (STN) trajectories.

In the final analysis, the risk of hemorrhage may be multifactorial; nevertheless, careful attention to surgical planning and the judicious use of MER may significantly reduce this risk.

Subdural Hematoma

Subdural hematoma is an unusual complication of DBS surgery, occurring in 1% to 1.4% of patients and involving 0.1% to 4.2% of electrodes.[17,20,55] The clinical manifestations usually occur weeks after surgery. The hematoma may be discovered incidentally on routine postoperative imaging, or patients may become symptomatic, exhibiting lethargy, confusion, or motor deficit.[17,55] Patients receiving chronic anticoagulant therapy before surgery may be at greater risk for developing subdural hematoma.[55]

Management should be conservative if possible, and, if surgical therapy is needed, a delay is preferred, to allow the hematoma to liquefy.[55] The surgical treatment of choice is burr hole evacuation.[17,56] Subdural hematoma may result in displacement of the DBS lead, negatively affecting stimulation therapy. It may take weeks or months after the hematoma is evacuated for stimulation to be effective again, but lead revision is usually unnecessary.[40,55]

It is wise to suspend anticoagulant/antiplatelet therapy at least 10 days before the procedure.[55] During surgery, excessive cerebrospinal fluid (CSF) leakage should be avoided so that the bridging veins will not be significantly stretched, especially in patients with significant brain atrophy.[40,55] The senior author (R.L.A.) advocates a sharp corticectomy before guide tube insertion in order to minimize downward traction on the brain. Parsimonious use of MER will reduce operative time, brain trauma, and CSF losses.

Cerebral Venous Infarction

During trajectory planning, care must be taken to avoid superficial cortical veins, injury to which may result in cerebral venous infarction. The incidence of this is low, occurring in approximately 1.3% of patients and involving 0.8% of electrodes. Venous infarction manifests over the first few hours after surgery, typically with altered mental status and new motor deficits. Once it is identified via imaging, supportive measures are instituted, including airway protection if necessary, head elevation, blood pressure control to prevent secondary hemorrhage, hydration, seizure prophylaxis, and early motor and cognitive rehabilitation. Fortunately, outcome in most of the cases is favorable as neurological losses are recovered over time though permanent deficits, and even death can occur.[57] Nevertheless, a large venous infarction may result in permanent neurological morbidity or mortality.[32]

Ischemic Stroke

Transient ischemic attack and ischemic stroke are very rare complications of DBS: usually one or two cases in large clinical series.[16,45,58] The mechanism of the infarctions is unclear, although it has been proposed that high-amplitude stimulation might lead to small-vessel vasospasm.[59]

Perioperative Confusion

Perioperative confusion/agitation is one of the most commonly encountered complications of DBS surgery, with a reported incidence of up to 22%.[10,15,17,18,20,30,46,58,60] The incidence of postoperative confusion increases with age (particularly in patients older than 70 years[15,60]) and is more common after contemporaneous bilateral electrode implantation. Consequently, this complication is most commonly observed in patients undergoing DBS for Parkinson's disease.

Risk factors include a history of hallucinations and advanced age. Additional risk factors include complex medical comorbid conditions, more advanced Parkinson's disease, the use of dementia-related medications before surgery (but this may merely reflect early cognitive decline), and the use of levodopa agonists.[60] In patients with Parkinson's disease and selected patients with essential tremor, detailed preoperative neurocognitive assessments may be used to detect which patients are at risk for postoperative confusion, although there is no consensus regarding specific tests that are most useful for this task.

From a surgical standpoint, confusion may be more common after DBS surgery in the STN, especially with placement of the most ventral contact in or close to the substantia nigra pars reticulata.[10,46] Transventricular trajectories may also increase the risk of postoperative confusion, and it is far easier to avoid larger ventricles when the GPi is targeted than when the STN is targeted. Increased operative time, the number of microelectrode passes employed to localize the intended target, and the introduction of bifrontal air may all contribute to postoperative confusion, but no definitive relationship has been demonstrated.

Postoperative confusion is managed conservatively with mild sedation and physiologic support. Psychosis necessitating intubation is rare,[10] and restraints should be avoided if possible. Fortunately, the confusion is usually transient, with a return to baseline function over the course of days to weeks, and discharge to prior level of care is routine. Nevertheless, long-term cognitive sequelae have been described after DBS surgery,[40,52,61-64] and patients and families should be forewarned of this possibility during the informed consent process.

Venous Air Embolism

Venous air embolism (VAE) is a rare complication of DBS procedures (occurring in 1% of patients, involving 0.5% of electrodes,[17] and occurring in 1.3% of procedures[65]); however, if VAE is not recognized and addressed promptly, the results can be catastrophic. Both patient position (head elevated 30 degrees for comfort) and the fact that the patient is awake may contribute to the development of VAE. Normal ventilation produces negative intrathoracic pressure, which results in a lower venous pressure than with mechanical ventilation with positive end-expiratory pressure (PEEP). The initial symptoms of a VAE are persistent cough and a sense of heaviness or discomfort in the chest. A decrease in the end-tidal CO_2 typically precedes compromised blood oxygen saturation and hypotension. Morbidity and mortality can be significant with VAE; intake of just 50 mL of air can lead to hypotension and dysrhythmias, and more than 300 mL of intravenous air can result in death.[66] Once clinical suspicion is high, the surgeon should flood the surgical field with saline and lower the patient's head to avoid more air inflow.[65,66] Bleeding vessels should be cauterized, and the burr hole margins should be waxed liberally. If the cough persists and the end-tidal CO_2 does not improve rapidly with these maneuvers, it is wise to abort the procedure, close the incision rapidly, and remove the stereotactic frame in case intubation is necessary. In the senior author's (R.L.A.'s) experience, the patient stabilizes rapidly once the incision is closed, and the surgery may be completed at a later date without incident.

Poorly Positioned Electrodes

Despite surgeons' best efforts, DBS leads occasionally are poorly targeted.[c] Clinical improvement that is poorer than expected or the induction of unwanted adverse stimulation effects should prompt two questions: (1) whether the device is functioning properly and (2) whether the leads are well positioned. The first question may be answered in the clinic with a diagnostic assessment of impedances, which, if higher than 2000 ohms, may indicate an open circuit (see "Lead/Extension Wire Fracture" section for more details). The second question is best assessed with MRI. It is crucial that a surgeon be honest with the patient and himself or herself. If the lead is poorly positioned, the surgeon should not waste the patient's time; he or she must reposition it.

Seizure

The risk of seizure with DBS is low.[10,20,71,72] Seizures occur during surgery, with a reported incidence of 0.3% to 2.3%, or after surgery, with an occurrence of 0.9% to 9.1%.[45] Almost 90% of seizures occur within the first 48 hours after surgery, and most are generalized tonic-clonic seizures.[24,45,73] Seizures are reported more commonly after DBS than after ablative surgery,[41] and most reported seizures occur after STN implantations.[4,73]

A specific mechanism underlying seizures that follow DBS surgery has not been described. The only significant risk factors identified on multivariate analysis are an abnormality on postoperative imaging (i.e., hemorrhage, edema, or ischemia)[4,24,73] and multiple sclerosis[74]; the relative risk is increased 50 and 8 times, respectively. Seizures are associated with higher rates of morbidity and mortality,[73] and so they must be managed actively. Because of the elective nature of DBS surgery, the surgeon must consider aborting a DBS procedure if the patient has a seizure and does not quickly return to his or her neurological baseline. It is also important to perform early postoperative imaging to rule out potential precipitating factors such as hemorrhage or infarction. Patients who experience a single seizure in the first 48 hours postoperatively may continue oral medication (phenytoin, valproic acid, or levetiracetam) for 1 to 4 weeks. Those who experience delayed or multiple seizures should continue oral treatment for 6 months with electroencephalographic follow-up.[4,73] There are no published reports of patients who developed chronic epilepsy after DBS surgery.

Aborted Procedures

Few aborted procedures have been reported (0.9% to 4.9%),[15] but the incidence might be higher. Stated reasons have been intraoperative acute cardiac event,[75] severe agitation during placement of the stereotactic frame,[10] psychiatric derangement before lead insertion,[24,26] respiratory failure that necessitates head frame removal,[26] vasovagal response with precipitating syncope, VAE, intraoperative hemiparesis,[45] severe dyskinesia, cardiac arrhythmia,[46] confusion,[24,46] mechanical failure of the navigation system, head frame misalignment and brain shift during second lead implantation,[24] among others. Most of these cases were stabilized, and it was possible to repeat the procedure a week later with no adverse effect.

[c]References 2-4, 7, 11, 15, 18, 20, 24, 25, 45, 67-70.

Cerebrospinal Fluid Leak

The incidence of CSF leak after DBS surgery is low (occurring in ≈1.3% of patients and involving 0.8% of electrodes); however, as in all cases, CSF leak impairs wound healing and may lead to infection.[21] Meticulous wound closure and head elevation are the best preventive measures.

Medical Complications

Most medical complications related to DBS surgery are similar to those encountered with other neurosurgical procedures. These include deep venous thrombosis,[23] dyspnea,[20] hypotension,[45] myocardial infarction,[76] pneumonia,[1,14,23,26,27] postoperative respiratory distress,[10,45] pulmonary embolism,[14,23,27,30] and vasovagal response.[15,45] Two medical complications specifically related to DBS surgery require specific attention: Parkinsonism-hyperpyrexia syndrome and dystonic crisis.

Parkinsonism-Hyperpyrexia Syndrome

Parkinsonism-hyperpyrexia syndrome is a rare complication resulting from sudden discontinuation of dopaminergic medications before DBS surgery.[77-81] The syndrome is characterized by muscular rigidity, hyperpyrexia, autonomic instability, and encephalopathy with leukocytosis and elevated levels of creatine phosphokinase. The mortality rate is high (≈4% when treated; 16% when untreated). Both the clinical manifestation and underlying pathophysiologic process (dopamine withdrawal or blockade) are identical to those of neuroleptic malignant syndrome. Both neuroleptic malignant syndrome and parkinsonism-hyperpyrexia syndrome can be triggered or exacerbated by metabolic stressors such as sepsis and dehydration.[82]

Early diagnosis and treatment are critical. Treatment should include cooling, supportive care, and adequate hydration. Dopaminergic therapy should be reestablished immediately. Activating the DBS system may also help.[77,78,80,82]

Dystonic Crisis

Patients with severe generalized dystonia may experience a dramatic worsening of dystonia symptoms in response to physical stressors (e.g., surgery, infection) or to acute withdrawal of medications such as anticholinergics, benzodiazepines, and baclofen.[83-86] Dystonic crisis can be a life-threatening condition and necessitates aggressive treatment if it occurs after DBS surgery. Supportive care in the intensive care unit is usually necessary. Specific treatment should include reinstituting the preoperative medical regimen if it was discontinued and induction of deep sedation with either lorazepam or propofol until the crisis subsides. In the senior author's (R.L.A.'s) experience and that of others,[87-93] activation of the DBS devices may help end the crisis more quickly.

HARDWARE-RELATED COMPLICATIONS

Fortunately, hardware-related complications after DBS surgery are uncommon and may be expected to decrease over time with improvements in device design. Nevertheless, these complications can necessitate a temporary cessation of therapy and the discomfort/risk of additional surgery.

Lead/Extension Wire Fracture

The incidence of wire fracture, estimated to occur among 1% and 12% of patients and involving 0.5% to 14% of electrodes,[2,3,9,10,21,25,30,45,94-97] is one of the most common complications of DBS,[9] especially in patients with dystonia.[5,96-98] It is believed that wire fracture results from cervical movement that transmits repetitive stress to the lead and extension wires.[95] When these cables are stretched, resistance to fatigue drops dramatically.[99] Falls,[100] head trauma,[97,99] and vigorous massage[17] have also been reported to cause wire fractures. Patients with violent tics caused by Gilles de la Tourette's syndrome may also sustain wire fractures.[101]

Lead or extension cable fracture is usually heralded by a loss of DBS clinical effect, although patients may also experience electrical paresthesias at the site of fracture if the insulation is also disrupted.[102] Cervical radiographs usually demonstrate the fractured wire.[95,103,104] The AM radio test (moving an AM transistor radio over the lead wire, which reveals increased static at the site of a current leak) is also a useful diagnostic tool.[103] A standard system check usually demonstrates high impedances (>2000 ohms) with wire fractures,[2,95,102] and no stimulation-induced side effects are observed with voltages of up to 10.5 V.[95] In some cases, surgical exploration is necessary to confirm suspicions of a fractured wire or a faulty connection.[103]

In a series of 16 lead fractures,[95] the mean interval between DBS surgery and the fracture was 36 months (range, 7-84 months). Placement of the connection between the lead and the extension cable below the mastoid is associated with an increased incidence of lead wire breakage.[9,104] Most fractures occur less than 5 cm proximal to the connector.[95,103]

Replacing an extension cable is a relatively simple matter[45]; however, replacing a fractured lead wire requires repeat intracranial surgery with its attendant risks.[21,45,104] Various measures have been proposed to prevent lead wire breakage, including placing the connector in the parietal[5,104-106] or paramastoid region[94,103] to reduce strain on the lead wire, avoiding the use of cranial lead wire anchors that may pinch and tether the wire,[11,107] and advising patients against participating in extreme sports.[99]

Lead Tip Migration

The incidence of electrode migration is estimated to occur among 0.5% to 6.3% of patients and to involve 0.3% to 3.2% of leads.[d] Migration may be found on immediate postoperative images[9] (probably as a result of a technical error) or months later when patients experience a loss of clinical effect.[3] When significant, migration is easily diagnosed with radiography. Computed tomography or MRI may be necessary to diagnose more modest migrations.[13]

Lead migration may result from poor anchoring technique, skull growth after implantation during childhood, or vigorous head movements.[98,109,110] Downward migration of the connector with upward dislocation of DBS electrode has also been described.[2,9,11] In these cases, the lead wire was fixed to the burr hole with suture and a silicon tube around the electrode[9] or with a microplate.[2,11] The incidence of migration diminished considerably with the introduction of dedicated anchoring devices.[9,11] In a retrospective study of 106 lead wires, Contarino and colleagues[111] found that use of the Medtronic Stimloc device significantly reduced the degree of lead migration at 1 year, in comparison with microplate anchoring. The average 3D displacement with the microplate technique was 2.3 ± 2.0 mm, as opposed to 1.5 ± 0.6 mm with the Stimloc device.

Significant migration necessitates surgical replacement[110]; however, if migration is only a few millimeters, the surgeon may try to simply advance the lead under radiologic or stereotactic control.[13,21] For the rare cases in which two leads are implanted concurrently via the same burr hole, Potts and Larson[112] described a technique involving both the Stimloc device and microplates to avoid migration of the first lead while the second lead is being implanted.

[d]References 2,3,7,9,10,13,21,30,45,108.

Lead Tip Gliosis

Gliosis is a normal tissue reaction to any foreign body. Studies of tissue reaction to DBS electrodes have shown modest gliotic scarring with no clinical implications.[113-116] Nonetheless, gliosis should be considered when there is a difference in clinical response between sides without any obvious cause or if the response to stimulation diminishes over time.[117]

Brain Edema Surrounding Implanted Deep Brain Stimulation Leads

Postoperative brain edema surrounding the implanted leads is uncommon, although the incidence in one study was 6.3%.[118] This is a benign complication of unknown cause that is self-limited.[119] The time of onset varies from 4 to 120 days after surgery. In most of cases, affected patients present with headache, confusion, seizures, motor deficit, or worsening of preexisting symptoms (dyskinesia, speech disorders, or gait disorders). No fever or any sign of infection is in the surgical wounds, but the possibility of infection must be seriously considered.[118,120] The edema appears as a hypodensity on computed tomographic scans and as a hyperintensity on T2-weighted and fluid-attenuated inversion recovery (FLAIR) MRI sequences. Even with bilateral implants, the edema is usually unilateral. Treatment consists of supportive care and the administration of corticosteroids.[120]

Exposure of the electrodes and pulse generator to high-energy electric or magnetic fields must be avoided. Nutt and associates[121] reported a case of diencephalic and brainstem edema surrounding STN electrodes after a maxillary pulse-modulated radiofrequency diathermy treatment, with permanent and severe neurological deficit.

Intraparenchymal Cyst

Intraparenchymal cyst is a very rare complication; only two cases have been reported in the literature.[122] They appear in relation to the tip of the electrode and in the absence of infection. The affected patients in the published reports presented with focal neurological deficits 3 and 8 months after surgery, respectively. The cysts disappeared and symptoms improved once the leads were removed.

Twiddler's Syndrome

Spontaneous twisting of the wires is uncommon but can cause fracture and system malfunction.[102,123] Even less common is wire twisting as a result of manipulation by the patient. Few cases of so-called twiddler's syndrome have been described among patients with DBS. Most of these patients experienced recurrent system failure and denied any manipulation of the implantable pulse generator. Radiographs showed twisting of the extension wires with fractures or migration of lead wires.[124-130] A submuscular placement of the pulse generator may reduce this risk in patients in whom this condition recurs,[129] although simply anchoring the pulse generator well to the chest wall should suffice.

Bowstringing

Bowstringing is the formation of scar tissue around extension wires, which results in protrusion of the wires beneath the skin, limited movement, and discomfort.[131] Bowstringing is a rare complication, with a reported incidence of 2% to 3%. Discomfort and impaired neck movement can appear weeks to years postoperatively.[10,132] The risk of bowstringing is higher in patients with the dual-channel pulse generators, with an incidence as high as 12.7%. No bowstringing was observed in one series of patients with the Soletra pulse generator (model 7426; Medtronic, Minneapolis).[132]

When pain and disfigurement are significant, bowstringing can be managed with surgical exploration and resection of scar tissue or retunneling of the extension cables.[10,132,133]

Discomfort or Poor Cosmesis at the Pulse Generator Site

For some patients, conventional infraclavicular placement of the pulse generator may result in discomfort or an unsatisfactory cosmetic result. Finding an alternative implant site can be challenging. Messina and colleagues[134] described placement of the pulse generator in the lumbar region, 2 to 3 cm inferior to the last costal arch and 25 to 30 cm lateral to the midline. For this they used 95-cm–long extension cables tunneled over the fascia of the paravertebral muscles. Because of their size, dual-channel pulse generators such as that of Medtronic's Activa PC neurostimulator are most likely to produce an unacceptable cosmetic defect, and so the senior author (R.L.A.) prefers to implant two single-channel devices rather than one dual-channel system. In particularly thin patients and especially in children with generalized dystonia, a dual-channel rechargeable pulse generator may provide the best cosmetic result because of its slim profile, while also reducing the risk of infection (less tension on the skin incision) and prolonging the time until replacement surgery becomes necessary.

Pulse Generator Malfunction

The incidence of pulse generator malfunction is reported to be between 0.1% and 13.8%.[2,13,15,40,45] Malfunction must be suspected when the implantable pulse generator does not respond to programming or when there is a loss of clinical efficacy without evidence of lead or extension cable fracture.[13] The management is surgical replacement.[2,9,13]

Pulse Generator Migration

Migration of the pulse generator is a very rare complication. Blomstedt and Hariz[9] reported one case of bilateral downward migration of Itrel II neurostimulators. Surgical repositioning of the pulse generators was required.

General Hardware Complications

The entire deep brain stimulation system may be associated with a variety of complications, the most common and significant of these being infection. Subcutaneous seroma in relation to the pulse generator has been reported and found to resolve without incident.[18,135] Uncommon complications that have been reported include occipital artery pseudoaneurysm,[136] spinal accessory neuropathy in relation to the subcutaneous tunneling of the extension,[137] and cutaneous herpes zoster in the vicinity of the pulse generator.[138] One of the senior author's (R.L.A.'s) patients developed an infection of the pulse generator one year after implantation that was secondary to herpes zoster of the ipsilateral arm that became superinfected with *Staphylococcus aureus.*

Magnetic Resonance Imaging–Related Complications

Performing MRI in patients with implanted DBS systems poses a risk of heating the electrodes, with potentially severe consequences. In reality, few complications related to MRI have been reported, and the estimated risk of permanent neurological complication is approximately 1 per 4000 MRI studies,[139] but even this may be an overestimation. The reported complications include one case of thermocoagulation of brain tissue 2 to 3 cm around the electrode tip, which resulted in severe permanent neurological disability (1.0-T lumbar MRI, specific absorption rate [SAR] < 1.26 W/kg)[140]; one case of brain edema surrounding the electrode, with a benign outcome (1.5-T brain MRI, SAR < 0.4 W/kg)[139]; one case of ballistic and dystonic movements of the left leg, with a benign outcome (1.0-T brain MRI, SAR unknown)[141]; and two cases of pulse generator malfunction without neurological morbidity (1.5-T brain and spine MRI, SAR unknown).[142,143] Manufacturers' guidelines for the safe performance of MRI should be followed in order to reduce the risk of neurological injury.[139]

Infection

Hardware infection is perhaps the most common complication of DBS surgery, both in the immediate postoperative period, when it is more appropriately considered a surgical complication, and in the long term, as a result of the permanently implanted hardware. Infection is reported to occur in 3% to 13% of patients.[21,45,144,145] When skin erosion and wound dehiscence are included, the incidence is as high as 15%. Most infections occur within 6 months of surgery.[144,146]

Infection manifests with localized swelling, erythema, or purulent discharge at the pulse generator, burr hole, or connection incision. Standard skin flora, including *S. aureus* and *Staphylococcus epidermidis*, are most commonly involved. When *S. aureus* is isolated, it is unlikely that the infection can be cleared without hardware removal.[144,146] Erosions and dehiscence occur in fewer than 0.5% of cases.[45] Surgical débridement and wound revision, followed by intravenous antibiotics, may suffice in some cases[146]; however, if the device becomes colonized with bacteria, device removal is necessary.[45]

Infections should be treated aggressively either to salvage the implanted brain leads if they are not yet involved or to prevent serious complications such as meningitis, cerebritis, or brain abscess. Among 23 cases reported by Fenoy and Simpson,[45] infection was self-limited in 10 (43.5%), necessitating intravenous antibiotics alone. In 7 (30.4%) cases, complete system removal was required; in 1 (4.3%), only lead removal was required; in 3 (13.1%), pulse generator and extension removal was necessary; and in 2 (8.7%), wound washout and débridement were needed. Fortunately, cerebritis and brain abscess are rare; few cases have been reported.[147-150] If a patient presents with extensive cellulitis or drainage, then all hardware should be removed and the patient treated with intravenous antibiotics for 4 to 6 weeks.[144] Most infections occur over the pulse generator site,[2,10,144,151] in which case the surgeon may salvage the brain leads by removing the pulse generator and extension cable, administer intravenous antibiotics, and reimplant those components 2 to 3 months later, allowing adequate time off antibiotics for recurrence.[2,144,146,147,151] Most cranial wound infections cannot be cleared with surgical washout, débridement, and irrigation alone, particularly when *S. aureus* is involved; system removal is ultimately necessary.[21,144,146] One report suggests that the pulse generator might be resterilized and safely reused, which would reduce costs.[152]

STIMULATION-RELATED COMPLICATIONS

Adverse effects of stimulation are typically caused by the unintentional stimulation of structures adjacent to the intended target and are therefore target specific. By definition, these effects are reversed by adjusting stimulation parameters or turning the device off completely. If the surgeon cannot mitigate the adverse effects by altering the stimulation settings, repositioning the lead must be strongly considered.

Internal Globus Pallidus

The most common adverse effect of stimulation at the posteroventral aspect of the GPi is activation of the corticospinal tract, which causes muscular contraction of the contralateral side of the body (typically face and hand). The corticospinal tract is posteromedial to the intended target, and so this adverse effect should prompt an anterolateral targeting adjustment. In patients with dystonia, the clinician can overcome the pulling of the neck musculature with activation of the DBS devices by slowly raising the amplitude of stimulation over the course of many weeks, which allows the brain to adapt. In addition, lowering stimulation frequency or pulse width may mitigate this effect. Deeply positioned GPi leads may induce phosphenes by activating the optic tract; however, unlike pallidotomy, visual field cut is rare after pallidal DBS. In addition, GPi stimulation has been reported to induce ataxia, bradykinesia, rigidity, and gait difficulties in previously unaffected limbs.[153-156] Transient deterioration of cognitive functions,[157] symptoms like those of transient ischemic attacks,[158] and recurrent mania[159] have also been reported.

Ventral Intermediate Nucleus of the Thalamus

The most common complication of DBS at the Vim nucleus of the thalamus are paresthesias caused by activation of the ventral caudal nucleus, which lies immediately posterior to the Vim, or contralateral muscular contractions mediated by the corticospinal tract, which lies just lateral to the target. Dysarthria may be an unavoidable adverse effect, particularly with stimulation of the left (i.e., dominant) Vim. Hand clumsiness, impaired balance,[160] hyperhidrosis,[161] and central nystagmus[162] have also been reported.

Subthalamic Nucleus

Stimulation via poorly positioned leads in the region of the STN may induce muscular contractions (corticospinal tract; anterolateral), painful paresthesias (medial lemniscus; posterolateral), or oculomotor effects (cranial nerve III nucleus; ventromedial). Poor executive function and cognitive impairment with a decline in neuropsychological test scores over time have been reported even with properly implanted STN-DBS leads.[40,52,61-64] Some randomized clinical studies have shown a higher incidence of cognitive and mood impairment after STN-DBS than after GPi-DBS in patients with Parkinson's disease.[163-176] Researchers have also reported cases of apathy,[177,178] dysphagia,[179] dyspnea,[180] gait deterioration,[181] restless leg syndrome,[40] mania with psychotic symptoms,[182] hypersexuality,[183] acute renal failure,[184] weight gain,[185] dopamine dysregulation syndrome,[186] ocular tilt reaction,[187] hemifacial spasms,[188] uncontrollable laughter,[189] pseudobulbar crying,[190,191] and symptoms like those of transient ischemic attacks.[46,192]

AVOIDING COMPLICATIONS

There are a number of actions that the surgeon can take to mitigate the risks of DBS surgery. Some are well documented; others are learned through experience. The following should be kept in mind, not as rules, but merely as lessons learned by one surgeon over the course of more than 1000 DBS implantations.

Preoperative Evaluation

As already stated, patient selection for DBS surgery is covered in Chapter 85. Selecting proper candidates for DBS surgery is a critical first step to achieving excellent results and, in our opinion, this is best accomplished by a multidisciplinary team and not a surgeon working in isolation. Neurology and psychiatry colleagues provide invaluable assistance to the stereotactic surgeon, ensuring that operative candidates receive proper diagnoses and are appropriate candidates for surgical intervention. They also provide support in managing the underlying disorder during hospitalization and the postoperative period, particularly if there are complications. This is especially important for children with severe generalized dystonia and for emotionally fragile patients with obsessive-compulsive disorder.

In addition to the disease-specific evaluation of surgical candidacy, a routine presurgical assessment is vital, particularly because DBS procedures are performed electively and often in elderly patients, who may have numerous medical comorbid conditions. Of course, aspirin should be withheld for 10 to 14 days before surgery. Patients taking oral anticoagulants should be transitioned to low-molecular-weight heparin injections, beginning 7 to 10 days before the surgery. The injections should be discontinued the day before surgery, and both the prothrombin time and partial thromboplastin time should be checked on the morning of the procedure. Anticoagulation therapy may then be resumed 1 week after surgery.

Anesthetic Considerations

The anesthesiologist plays a critical role in the performance of DBS surgery on awake patients, helping keep the patients comfortable and calm, while monitoring and managing vital signs. Maintaining the airway, of course, is key, particularly with use of a stereotactic head frame. Intraoperative respiratory complications occur in approximately 2% of patients.[44,193,194] It is therefore critical (1) to apply the head frame so that the anesthesiologist may access the airway easily, even with the patient's head elevated, and (2) for the anesthesiologist to be comfortable with the use of laryngeal masks, which can be easily inserted even in positions that make full intubation difficult.[194] Special consideration and measures should be taken with patients with Parkinson's disease, who are at greater risk of pulmonary compromise during the procedure.[194-196]

Blood pressure management must be strict. Hypertension increases the risk of intracerebral hemorrhage,[32,34] and so it should be treated actively before the brain parenchyma is penetrated.[194] The peripheral dopamine-blocking effects of carbidopa include lowering of blood pressure, and so it is common for patients with Parkinson's disease to experience a rebound hypertension when carbidopa or levodopa is withheld for DBS surgery. In our experience, labetalol, hydralazine, and nicardipine are excellent antihypertensive medications for use during DBS surgery. Dexmedetomidine or propofol may also be used but will cause sedation.[197] General anesthetics also lower blood pressure, and their use has been associated with fewer hemorrhagic complications but at the cost of losing the valuable feedback of the neurological examination.[49] In addition to blood pressure, pulse, the electrocardiogram, and blood oxygenation should all be monitored. Oxygen may be administered via a nasal cannula that is also equipped to monitor end-tidal CO_2.

Operative Measures

Targeting technique is covered in great detail in other chapters. Of course, meticulous stereotactic technique results in accurate targeting, reducing the risk of neurological injury, stimulation-induced adverse effects, and suboptimal clinical response, all of which can result from poor positioning of DBS leads.

In the operating room, the patient should be positioned as comfortably as possible. The head should be elevated 30 degrees but no more, to minimize the risk of VAE. Sequential compression devices are applied to the legs to prevent the development of deep venous thrombosis, and a urinary catheter may be inserted for patient comfort. Antibiotics are administered intravenously before the incision is made,[144,146,198] and standard preparation and draping are performed.

A curvilinear frontal incision may reduce the risk of infection.[12,144,146] After the incision is made, all bleeding vessels should be coagulated with the bipolar lead to reduce the risk of VAE. Similarly, the raw bony margins of the burr hole should be waxed liberally and the leaves of the dura mater cauterized after opening. The planned trajectory should enter the brain via the crown of a gyrus in order to avoid sulcal vessels, and it should stay clear of the ventricles in order to avoid injury to branches of the internal cerebral veins that run along its walls. A sharp corticectomy is preferred, which eases entry of the surgical cannula into the subcortical white matter with minimal downward displacement of the brain. Although we could identify only one publication that demonstrated a direct correlation between the number of microelectrode passes employed and surgical complications, it stands to reason that the fewer passes made through the brain, the better. Consequently, we advocate *judicious* use of MER: only enough to ensure identification of the desired target. Of course, this is a controversial topic that is left to the surgeon's discretion.

With regard to implantation of the extension cables and pulse generators, it is wise to handle the implant as little as possible. The extension should be tunneled through the deeper cervical plane in order to minimize the risk of bowstringing, which can occur with more superficial trajectories. As with shunt procedures, plunging below the clavicle with the passer can result in pneumothorax or injury to the brachial vessel or brachial plexus. The connections should be cleaned of all blood and dried in order to provide an optimal watertight connection. The senior author (R.L.A.) prefers to encircle the excess lead wire around the burr hole cover and place the connection between the lead wire and extension high on the head, just posterior to the cranial incision, to provide considerable strain release, which prevents fracture of the lead wire. All incisions are irrigated with copious amounts of bacitracin saline before meticulous skin closure. A subcuticular closure at the chest incision enhances the cosmetic result and promotes rapid wound healing. Postoperative antibiotics (up to 7 days) may lead to lower infection rates,[146] but this is not considered the standard of care.

CONCLUSION

In this chapter we provide a comprehensive overview of complications that may arise in the course of providing DBS therapy. As with all surgical procedures, experience leads to refinements in technique that will improve outcomes and reduce complications. As most DBS surgical procedures are performed electively, the operating surgeon must ensure that the surgery is performed according to the strictest standards and with the lowest possible risk of complication. We hope that this chapter has been informative and will provide guidance toward improving the readers' technique.

SUGGESTED READINGS

Ben-Haim S, Asaad WF, Gale JT, et al. Risk factors for hemorrhage during microelectrode-guided deep brain stimulation and the introduction of an improved microelectrode design. *Neurosurgery*. 2009;64(4):754-762.

Binder DK, Rau GM, Starr PA. Risk factors for hemorrhage during microelectrode-guided deep brain stimulator implantation for movement disorders. *Neurosurgery*. 2005;56(4):722-732.

Blomstedt P, Hariz MI. Hardware-related complications of deep brain stimulation: a ten year experience. *Acta Neurochir (Wien)*. 2005;147(10):1061-1064.

Boviatsis EJ, Stavrinou LC, Themistocleous M, et al. Surgical and hardware complications of deep brain stimulation. A seven-year experience and review of the literature. *Acta Neurochir (Wien)*. 2010;152(12):2053-2062.

Chakrabarti R, Ghazanwy M, Tewari A. Anesthetic challenges for deep brain stimulation: a systematic approach. *N Am J Med Sci*. 2014;6(8):359-369.

Deep-Brain Stimulation for Parkinson's Disease Study Group. Deep-brain stimulation of the subthalamic nucleus or the pars interna of the globus pallidus in Parkinson's disease. *N Engl J Med*. 2001;345(13):956-963.

DeLong MR, Huang KT, Gallis J, et al. Effect of advancing age on outcomes of deep brain stimulation for Parkinson disease. *JAMA Neurol*. 2014;71(10):1290-1295.

Elias WJ, Sansur CA, Frysinger RC. Sulcal and ventricular trajectories in stereotactic surgery. *J Neurosurg*. 2009;110(2):201-207.

Fenoy AJ, Simpson RK. Risks of common complications in deep brain stimulation surgery: management and avoidance. *J Neurosurg*. 2014;120(1):132-139.

Kimmelman J, Duckworth K, Ramsay T, et al. Risk of surgical delivery to deep nuclei: a meta-analysis. *Mov Disord*. 2011;26(8):1415-1421.

Kocabicak E, Temel Y. Deep brain stimulation of the subthalamic nucleus in Parkinson's disease: surgical technique, tips, tricks and complications. *Clin Neurol Neurosurg*. 2013;115(11):2318-2323.

Lyons KE, Wilkinson SB, Overman J, et al. Surgical and hardware complications of subthalamic stimulation: a series of 160 procedures. *Neurology*. 2004;63(4):612-616.

Mendes Martins V, Coste J, Derost P, et al. [Surgical complications of deep brain stimulation: clinical experience of 184 cases]. *Neurochirurgie*. 2012;58(4):219-224.

Oh MY, Abosch A, Kim SH, et al. Long-term hardware-related complications of deep brain stimulation. *Neurosurgery*. 2002;50(6):1268-1274.

Okun MS, Tagliati M, Pourfar M, et al. Management of referred deep brain stimulation failures: a retrospective analysis from 2 movement disorders centers. *Arch Neurol*. 2005;62(8):1250-1255.

Rezai AR, Kopell BH, Gross RE, et al. Deep brain stimulation for Parkinson's disease: surgical issues. *Mov Disord*. 2006;21(suppl 14):S197-S218.

Seijo Fernández FJ, Alvarez Vega MA, Antuña Ramos A, et al. Lead fractures in deep brain stimulation during long-term follow-up. *Parkinsons Dis*. 2010;2010:409356.

Seijo Fernández FJ, Alvarez Vega MA, Gutierrez JC, et al. Complications in subthalamic nucleus stimulation surgery for treatment of Parkinson's disease. Review of 272 procedures. *Acta Neurochir (Wien)*. 2007;149(9):867-875.

Sillay KA, Larson PS, Starr PA. Deep brain stimulator hardware-related infections: incidence and management in a large series. *Neurosurgery*. 2008;62(2):360-366.

Tong F, Ramirez-Zamora A, Gee L, et al. Unusual complications of deep brain stimulation. *Neurosurg Rev*. 2015;38(2):245-252.

Umemura A, Oka Y, Yamamoto K, et al. Complications of subthalamic nucleus stimulation in Parkinson's disease. *Neurol Med Chir (Tokyo)*. 2011;51(11):749-755.

Vergani F, Landi A, Pirillo D, et al. Surgical, medical, and hardware adverse events in a series of 141 patients undergoing subthalamic deep brain stimulation for Parkinson disease. *World Neurosurg*. 2010;73(4):338-344.

Zrinzo L, Foltynie T, Limousin P, et al. Reducing hemorrhagic complications in functional neurosurgery: a large case series and systematic literature review. *J Neurosurg*. 2012;116(1):84-94.

See a full reference list on ExpertConsult.com

93 Neurophysiologic Monitoring for Movement Disorders Surgery

Jay L. Shils and Jeffrey E. Arle

Intraoperative neurophysiologic monitoring (IONM) is an outcrop of techniques used originally in both clinical and research laboratories. At the 2000 International Intraoperative Neurophysiologic Monitoring symposia Dr. Marc Sindou coined the term *interventional neurophysiology* to describe the area of intraoperative monitoring that includes those techniques that directly guide segments of surgical intervention. The application of many standard IONM techniques can warn the surgical team that something potentially correctable has occurred, whereas other IONM applications are integral elements of the surgical procedure itself such as mapping and localization methods during surgery. Microelectrode recording (MER) represents a specific application for such mapping and localization in deeper brain targets. The technique of recording from single units (cells) in research laboratories dates to 1939 with Renshaw and colleagues' recordings of pyramidal cells in the cat hippocampus.[1] The inclusion of single-unit recordings in the operating room setting dates to the early 1960s[2] and has now become a common neuromonitoring tool when performing deep brain stimulation (DBS) procedures, the standard surgical treatment for a variety of movement disorders, such as Parkinson's disease, essential tremor, and dystonia.

A brief history of monitoring techniques for movement disorders surgery can be found in the expanded version of this chapter available at ExpertConsult.com.

GENERAL OVERVIEW OF SURGERY

There is no single "best" surgical method for performing movement disorder surgery. Currently accepted techniques involve both frame-based and frameless stereotactic anatomic localization methodologies supported by imaging and intraoperative physiologic confirmation of proper targeting. No matter the approach, it is generally accepted that some form of intraoperative physiologic confirmation is needed. This chapter focuses on the techniques of intraoperative single-unit recordings (MER) and macroelectrode stimulation testing: VIM thalamic nucleus for essential tremor, STN or GPi for Parkinson's disease, and GPi for dystonia.

Please see the expanded version of this chapter at ExpertConsult.com for an overview of microelectrode techniques and local field potentials.

GENERAL STEREOTACTIC TECHNIQUE

Before surgery, MRI of the brain is performed. On the morning of surgery, the stereotactic head-frame is applied (eFig. 93-3A). Care is taken to center the head within the frame and to align the base of the frame with the zygoma, which approximates the orientation of the anterior commissure–posterior commissure (AC-PC) line. In this way, axial images obtained perpendicular to the axis of the frame will run parallel to the AC-PC plane. The patient is then transferred to radiology, where stereotactic CT is performed. This CT scan (eFig. 93-3B) is then digitally fused (eFig. 93-3C) with the prior MRI (eFig. 93-3D). This fusion method is used because MRI can have inherent image distortions that are not seen on CT and could potentially cause inaccuracies in the coordinate determination. Obtaining the CT scan on the day of surgery is much more expeditious as well, often taking less than 10 minutes overall. MRI is necessary, however, because certain structures are much better visualized. The surgical target coordinates are based on its relationship to the AC, the PC, or the midcommissure point (MCP) (eFig. 93-3D). The localizations employed for the most commonly targeted sites are given in Table 93-1. The patient is brought to the operating room and positioned in a lounge-chair–like orientation on the operating table. The target coordinates are set on the frame, bringing the presumptive target to the center of the operating arc. The scalp is incised in a curved fashion, exposing the area for a 14-mm bur hole approximately 11.5 cm posterior to the nasion (14 to 15 cm for a VIM thalamic nucleus target) and in the midpupillary line laterally. The dura mater is opened within the bur hole, fully taking care not to damage brain or surface veins. The initial part of the electrode securing system is attached to the bur hole, and a small pial opening is made where the cannula is to be inserted. The base of the microdrive is mounted onto the operating arc. An insertion cannula with a blunt stylet is carefully advanced through the frontal lobe and then the drive system. At this point, the guide tube, to the end of which the electrode tip position is zeroed, is flush with the end of the insertion cannula and the recording begins.

The electrode first is advanced 1 mm out of the cannula into the brain, and the impedance of the electrode-tissue system is measured. In our experience, impedances of 500 to 800 MΩ[b] provide the best single-unit recordings at our facility.[c] If the electrode impedance is higher than this, the electrode is "conditioned." Conditioning is performed by passing an electrical current through the electrode tip, which burns off any oxide that may have formed and thus lowers the impedance. If the electrode impedance starts below 500 KΩ, the electrode is replaced before performing the recording tract. If there is a large impedance drop following electrode conditioning, the electrode is deemed unacceptable and is replaced. We correct any noise problems at this time and then proceed to data acquisition. Excess noise usually stems from poorly grounded equipment, bad cables, or failed system components (many of which are caused by the sterilization process). The systems in use today are much less susceptible to external noise than in the past, but that does not preclude large noise sources such as intraoperative MRI units, even in shielded rooms, from causing significant problems. At the conclusion of each recording trajectory, the collected data are mapped onto scaled sagittal sections derived from the Schaltenbrand-Wahren stereotactic atlas.[104] Mapping is used to determine the most probable location and orientation in the brain, employing a "best fit" model (see "Data Analysis" section). When the data suggest that our targeting is correct, we proceed with electrode implantation and test stimulation.

[b]Theoretically, higher impedance values better isolate a single unit; yet, practically, the impedance chosen is a function of the microelectrode, the input impedance of the amplifier, and the operating room environment.
[c]Depending on the amount of noise in the operating room, these numbers may vary from center to center.

INTERNAL GLOBUS PALLIDUS PROCEDURES

GPi-DBS is reported to improve tremor, rigidity, dystonia, and levodopa-induced dyskinesias in patients with medically refractory, moderately advanced PD and dystonia[49,50,67,105-107,109] as well as patients with Tourette's syndrome. Successful pallidal interventions require targeting of the sensorimotor region of the GPi, which lies posterior and ventral in the nucleus.[110] When recording in this region, three key nuclear structures must be recognized: the striatum, the external globus pallidus (GPe), and the GPi (Fig. 93-1). The trajectory is made at an angle of 60 to 70 degrees relative to the horizontal of the AC-PC line and at a medial-lateral angle of 90 degrees. The MER techniques are no different for the historic pallidotomies or the present-day DBS implantations, but the target for DBS is 2 mm more anterior to minimize the spread of stimulation into the internal capsule.

The first cells encountered are from the caudate and putamen, where the characteristic firing patterns are low-amplitude action potentials, which often sound like corn popping (see Fig. 93-1, a). The single-unit activity in this area is often sparse, and the background is generally quiet. The electrode may also traverse some regions where no activity is recorded. which are small fingerlike projections of the internal capsule into the caudate and putamen.

TABLE 93-1 Initial Target Coordinates

Target	Medial Lateral Coordinate	Anterior-Posterior Coordinate	Ventral-Dorsal Coordinate
GPi	20 mm from midline	3 mm anterior to MCP	6 mm ventral to AC-PC
VIM	14-15 mm from midline	20% of the AC-PC length anterior to PC	2 mm dorsal to AC-PC
STN	11.5 mm from midline	3 mm posterior to MCP	6 mm ventral to AC-PC

AC-PC, anterior commissure–posterior commissure line; GPi, internal globus pallidus; MCP, midcommissure point; STN, subthalamic nucleus; VIM, ventral-intermediate thalamic nucleus.

Entry into the GPe is where the background becomes more active. GPe activity has two distinct patterns: an asynchronous *pauser*-type activity (see Fig. 93-1, c) and *burster* activity (see Fig. 93-1, d). Pauser cells fire in a dysrhythmic pattern at average frequencies between 30 and 100 Hz. They are characterized by moderate- to high-amplitude discharges with interspike intervals (ISIs) ranging from about 10 to 500 msec. They are distinguishable by their *staccato*-type, asynchronous pauses and discharges. An extremely small number of pauser cells (<5%) may demonstrate somatotopically organized kinesthetic responses, which are more likely in dystonia patients. Burster cells are characterized by short bursts of high-frequency discharges, achieving rates as high as 500 Hz. Amplitudes are highly variable. Another activity pattern that can be encountered in all areas where MER is performed are what we call *X cells* (i.e., "ex" cells; see Fig. 93-1, e) that are characterized by high frequency discharges (around 500 Hz) with a decremented amplitude envelope. The time of this envelope can be as short as 500 msec and as long as 30 seconds or more. X cells represent cell death due to a rupture of the cell membrane.

Depending on the trajectory, 4 to 8 mm of GPe may be encountered during any one recording tract. The inferior border of GPe contains *border* cells (see Fig. 93-1, b), whose firing activity is characterized by low-frequency discharges (between 2 and 20 Hz), is highly periodic, and has high-amplitude spikes. These cells are common at the inferior border of the GPe and all borders around the GPi including the internal lamina. They are rarer, but possible, at the superior border of the GPe. Border cells importantly facilitate localization of the boundaries within the globus pallidus.

After the electrode tip exits the GPe, a quiet laminar area (see Fig. 93-1) is encountered, marked by a steep decrease in

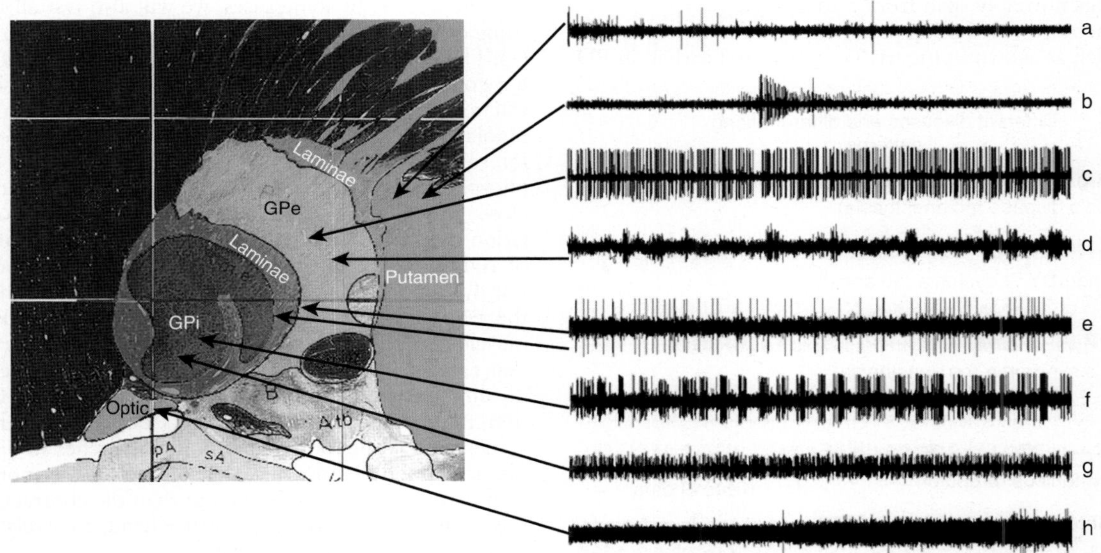

Figure 93-1. A sagittal image of the globus pallidum and associated structures 20 mm from the brain midline. On the *right* are representative examples of the firing patterns from each area: (a) striatum popcorn cell; (b) boarder cell; (c) external globus pallidus (GPe) pauser cell; (d) GPe burster cell; (e) X cell; (f) internal globus pallidus (GPi) tremor cell; (g) GPi HF cell; (h) optic tract. *(Modified from Shils JL, Tagliati M, Alterman RL. Neurophysiological monitoring during surgery for movement disorders. In: Deletis V, Shils JL, eds.* Neurophysiology for Neurosurgery: A Modern Approach. *New York: Academic Press; 2002:405-448.)*

background activity. After about 1 to 2 mm of laminar recording, border cells or an increase in background activity is again encountered, indicating the entry into the GPi. GPi activity consists of two patterns: tremor-related activity and high-frequency activity. Tremor cells (see Fig. 93-1, f) fire rhythmically in direct correlation to the patient's tremor, as shown by electromyography and single-unit correlation studies.[16] The firing rate of the intraburst activity is between 80 and 150 Hz. Not all patients have cells with this activity, especially those who do not demonstrate tremor as part of their disease presentation. This particular pattern is not found in dystonia patients or patients with other diseases in which GPi is targeted. High-frequency cells (see Fig. 93-1, g) are characterized by firing rates that are similar to tremor cells (80 to 150 Hz) in PD patients, with no large time gaps between clusters of activity. In patients with dystonia, there is some variability of the reported firing rates of these cells, with some reports suggesting that the rate may be much lower.[110] In our experience, with no anesthetic on board during recordings, we have found a rate in the range of 60 to 90 Hz. With anesthetics, the rate is typically a little lower, and during dystonia procedures, it is more difficult to differentiate between GPe activity and GPi activity. In both diseases, high-frequency cells exhibit a consistent amplitude and frequency. Also, in both disease states, a large portion of these cells in the sensorimotor region of the GPi respond to active or passive motion of a specific joint or extremity. The somatotopy of this region has been studied by multiple groups. Guridi and colleagues physiologically defined a somatotopic organization of the kinesthetic cells in the GPi, with the face and arm region located ventrolaterally and the leg dorsomedially.[38] Taha and associates found a somewhat different arrangement, with the leg located centrally between the arm in both the rostral and caudal areas.[42] Vitek and colleagues have found the leg to be medial and dorsal with respect to the arm, and the face more ventral.[112] Our experience is similar to that of Taha and associates. In dystonia, different from PD, one cell may respond to multiple joint movements. The GPi can be further subdivided into external and internal segments, labeled GPie (external GPi) and GPii (internal GPi), respectively. Both regions exhibit similar cellular recording patterns, but GPie may exhibit less cellularity than GPii. Total GPi recordings normally span from 5 to 12 mm.

The characteristic GPi firing patterns are different depending on the disorder, as shown in Figure 93-2. As stated earlier, in PD the firing patterns contain areas that are, in general, hyperactive. On the other hand, for dystonic recordings, the firing rate is on average closer to the normal firing rate of the GPi, with greater variability. Tourette's syndrome firing patterns are somewhere between those of PD and dystonia, with some regions of very long ISIs and some regions of very short ISIs. In patients with status dystonicus, the firing patterns appear to be hypoactive with very short regions of small ISI activity.

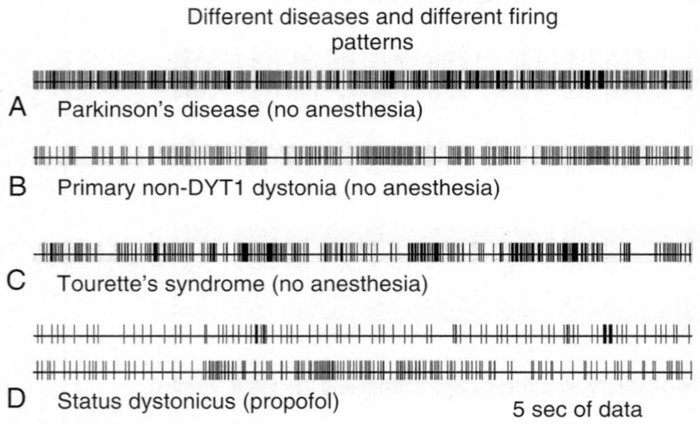

A steep decrease in background activity denotes exit from the GPi inferiorly. Three important white matter structures, which are to be avoided, border the GPi and may be encountered during recording: the ansa lenticularis (AL), the internal capsule, and the optic tract (OT). The AL is an electrically quiet region, although rare cells of relatively low amplitudes and firing frequencies can be recorded. The OT lies directly inferior to the AL (see Fig. 93-2), accounting for the high rate of visual field complications reported in the early modern pallidotomy literature.[35,112] With quality recordings, it is possible to hear the microelectrode tip enter the OT, which is indicated by an increase in high-frequency activity (adjusting the high-frequency filter to include higher frequencies may help bring out the transition; see Fig. 93-1, h). On hearing this background change, one may confirm entry into the OT by turning off the ambient lights and shining a flashlight in the patient's eyes. Finally, one may encounter the internal capsule. Background recordings within the capsule are similar to those of the OT. Movement of the mouth or contralateral hemibody, however, will generate increased high-frequency activity that is correlated to the movement.

After a reasonable MER map is confirmed, the DBS electrode is placed. Before securing the DBS lead, stimulation testing through each of the lead contacts is performed to ensure that the electrode is a safe distance from both the internal capsule and the OT, and to observe any clinical indications of benefit. Test stimulation is performed in a bipolar configuration. For PD, the test parameters are 60 µsec, 180 Hz, 0 to 4 V; whereas for dystonia, the test parameters are 210 µsec, 130 Hz, 0 to 5 V. The first test stimulation is performed using contacts 0–, 1+ up to a voltage of 4. If no significant adverse effects are encountered with this focal test, we proceed to test stimulation employing contacts 1–, 2+ and the 2–, 3+. In some cases, we will also test all four contacts using contacts 0, 1, 2 as the cathode (–) and contact 3 as the anode (+). The lowest pair, 0–, 1+, is the area where most adverse events have occurred in our experience. Direct stimulation-induced contraction of contralateral musculature at less than 4 V in this bipolar mode suggests that the DBS electrode is too close to the internal capsule and should be adjusted laterally. Induction of phosphenes at less than 4 V suggests that the electrode is too close to the OT and should be withdrawn slightly. For PD, stimulation can include immediate reduction of tremor and reduction of rigidity and bradykinesia, demonstrating a good placement. For dystonia, the beneficial responses are less clear. In some cases, the responses may even appear to be negative. For instance, muscle contractions are a common negative-appearing response that may appear to be due to stimulation of the internal capsule. To differentiate between the internal capsule and GPi stimulation, the frequency is decreased to 1 or 2 Hz, and the amplitude is increased while looking for muscle twitches in direct correlation to the stimulation pulses. If contractions are not found when stimulating at least 3 times higher than the contraction level, the DBS lead is placed. If, on the other hand, a correlative response is noted, the electrode is moved.

Different diseases and different firing patterns

A Parkinson's disease (no anesthesia)

B Primary non-DYT1 dystonia (no anesthesia)

C Tourette's syndrome (no anesthesia)

D Status dystonicus (propofol)

5 sec of data

Figure 93-2. Internal globus pallidus (GPi) recordings in different disease states. A, Parkinson's disease (PD) with regions of very short interspike intervals (ISIs) as well as asynchronous firing. **B,** Dystonia type 1 (DYT1) with asynchronous ISIs and longer ISIs compared with PD. **C,** Tourette's syndrome, which shows asynchronous activity with very short ISIs similar to PD and longer ISIs that are similar to dystonia. **D,** Status dystonicus patient with propofol on board. This particular patient was on high doses of propofol but still interacting with us because of propofol accommodation.

VENTROLATERAL INTRAMEDIAL NUCLEUS PROCEDURES

Chronic high-frequency electrical stimulation within the ventral intermediate nucleus of the thalamus (Fig. 93-3) suppresses parkinsonian and essential tremors without adversely affecting

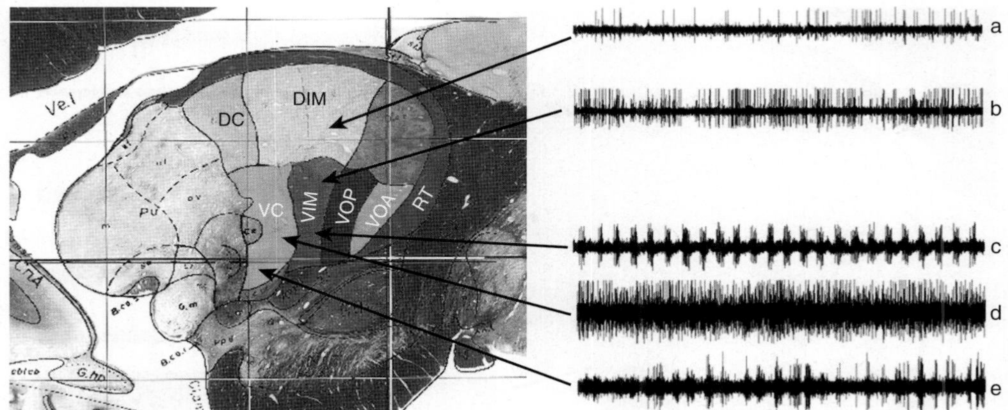

Figure 93-3. A sagittal image of the thalamus and associated structures 14.5 mm from the brain midline. On the *right* are representative examples of the firing patterns from each area: (a) dorsal thalamic cell; (b) ventral-intermediate (VIM) cell; (c) VIM tremor cell; (d) ventral caudal (VC) cell. DC, dorsal caudal; DIM, doral intermediate; RT, reticular thalamic nucleus; VOA, ventro-oralis anterior; VOP, ventro-oralis posterior. *(Modified from Shils JL, Tagliati M, Alterman RL. Neurophysiological monitoring during surgery for movement disorders. In: Deletis V, Shils JL, eds.* Neurophysiology for Neurosurgery: A Modern Approach. *New York: Academic Press; 2002:405-448.)*

sensory and voluntary motor activity to any significant degree. When targeting the VIM thalamic nucleus, our standard angles of approach are 60 to 70 degrees relative to the AC-PC line and 5 to 10 degrees lateral to the true vertical. Pure parasagittal trajectories are not possible owing to the medial location of the target and a desire to avoid the ipsilateral lateral ventricle.

Recordings usually begin in the dorsal thalamus, where the cells are characterized by low amplitudes and sparse firing patterns. Bursts of activity and small-amplitude single spikes (see Fig. 93-3, a) are typically found in this region. On exiting the dorsal thalamus, the electrode enters the VL nucleus, which is composed of the ventro-oralis anterior (VOA), the ventro-oralis posterior (VOP), and the VIM thalamic nuclei (using the nomenclature of Hassler). The dorsal third of the VL nucleus is sparsely populated such that cellular activity in this area is similar to that of the dorsal thalamus. As the electrode passes ventrally within the VL nuclear group, cellular density increases and cells with firing rates of 40 to 50 Hz (see Fig. 93-3, b) are encountered. Kinesthetic cells with discrete somatotopic representation are routinely encountered and are the most critical means of determining the mediolateral position of the electrode. The homunculus of the posterior VL nuclei is as follows: the contralateral face and mouth lie 9 to 11 mm lateral to midline, the contralateral arm is represented lateral to this at 13 to 15 mm lateral to midline, and the contralateral leg is more lateral still, adjacent to the internal capsule. In most cases, placement of the electrode in the hand area is optimum; thus responses in the face or lower limb dictate the need to move the electrode.

In addition to kinesthetic neurons, one will routinely encounter "tremor" cells (see Fig. 93-3, c) within the VIM thalamic nucleus. Lenz and colleagues demonstrated that these cells are concentrated within the VIM thalamic nucleus, 2 to 4 mm above the AC-PC plane, a site that is empirically known to yield consistent tremor control.[113] The recording electrode may exit the VIM thalamic nucleus inferiorly, passing into the zona incerta (ZI), with a resulting decrease in background signal; or it will enter the ventral caudal (VC) nucleus, the primary sensory relay nucleus of the thalamus. Entry into VC nucleus is marked by a change in the background signal. Cells in this region are densely packed, exhibit high amplitudes, and respond to sensory phenomena (e.g., light touch) with a discreet somatotopic organization, which mirrors that of the VIM thalamic nucleus and may also be used to assess target laterality (see Fig. 93-3, d). If the VC nucleus is encountered early in the recording trajectory, the electrode may be targeted posteriorly and should be adjusted anteriorly. The nucleus ventrocaudalis parvocellularis rests inferiorly to the VC nucleus. Recordings within this nucleus are similar to those of the VC nucleus; however, stimulation in this location may yield painful or temperature-related sensations. Single-unit recordings in this area will respond to both painful and temperature-related stimuli applied within the cell's receptive field.

Microstimulation is used to localize the relation of the electrode to the VC nucleus and also to gauge the relation of the electrode to the center of the tremogenic region. We use constant-current stimulation at a pulse width of 100 μsec and rate of 300 Hz. Sensory activation at 20 μA or less indicates that the electrode is in the VC nucleus or very close to its border. We require that no microstimulation VC nucleus responses be induced when stimulating at 100 μA for DBS placement in a region. We have also noticed that when we can either suppress or reduce tremor with microstimulation testing, even at 100 μA, our postoperative stimulation amplitudes are very low for tremor suppression, on the order of 1.5 V or less.

After the microelectrode is removed, the DBS electrode is placed to target. Once again we use the bipolar testing configuration described for GPi procedures. Testing is done at 60 μsec and 185 Hz. Transient paresthesias are common with a properly positioned electrode; however, persistent paresthesias, which are induced at low voltages, indicate that the electrode is positioned posteriorly, near or within the VC nucleus. Failure to suppress tremor or induce paresthesias, even at 5 V, suggests that the electrode is positioned too anteriorly within the VOA nucleus. Muscular contractions (typically of the contralateral face or hand) suggest that the lead is positioned too laterally and that stimulation is affecting the internal capsule.

SUBTHALAMIC NUCLEUS PROCEDURES

Subthalamic DBS improves all of the cardinal features of PD, dampens the severity of "on" and "off" fluctuations, alleviates freezing spells, and dramatically reduces medication

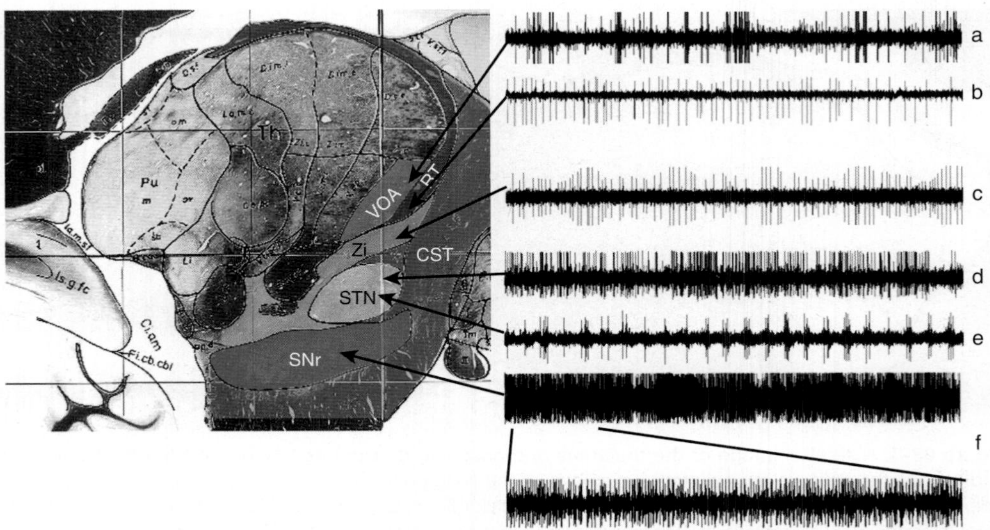

Figure 93-4. A sagittal image of the subthalamic nucleus (STN) and associated structures 12 mm from the brain midline. On the *right* are representative examples of the firing patterns from each area: (a) anterior thalamic burster cell; (b) anterior thalamic low frequency cell; (c) Zi cell; (d) STN tremor cell; (e) STN cell; (f) substantia nigra pars reticulata (SNr) cell. CST, corticospinal tract; RT, reticular thalamic nucleus; VOA, ventro-oralis anterior. *Modified from Shils JL, Tagliati M, Alterman RL. Neurophysiological monitoring during surgery for movement disorders. In: Deletis V, Shils JL, eds.* Neurophysiology for Neurosurgery: A Modern Approach. *New York: Academic Press; 2002:405-448).*

requirements. As mentioned previously, however, GPi-DBS likely has similar efficacy and may have less potential for psychiatric comorbid complications.[107]

The STN is approached at an angle of 70 degrees relative to the AC-PC line and 10 to 15 degrees lateral to the true vertical. MER begins in the anterior ventral thalamus and passes sequentially through the ZI, Forel's field H2, STN, and the substantia nigra pars reticulata (SNr) (Fig. 93-4). In the thalamus, one encounters cells that fire with low amplitude and frequency. Two patterns of activity may be identified: (1) bursts of activity (see Fig. 93-4, a), and (2) irregular, low-frequency (1 to 30 Hz) activity (see Fig. 93-4, b). The density of cellular activity varies in this region. For example, we have observed that the VOA nucleus is more cellular than the reticular thalamus. We have also noted that the more posterior the electrode is in the thalamus, the more likely burster activity will be encountered. The border between the thalamus and ZI (see Fig. 93-4, c) may be very distinct, but not in all cases. Developmentally, the ZI is a continuation of the reticular nucleus of the thalamus, and the transition from one to the other may not be clear. The ZI can be differentiated electrophysiologically from the thalamus in two ways. First, cellular activity is sparser and less *regular* in the ZI. By this we mean that the cellular firing rates slow and become a little more asynchronous, and the amplitudes decrease in intensity (which is most likely due to their scarcity and distance from the recording electrode). The second indication of transition from thalamus to ZI is a change in the background recordings. Whereas the background of the thalamus proper is somewhat active, the ZI background is much quieter. Typically, the recording electrode will exit the thalamus with a total of 6 (more anterior trajectory) to 10 mm (more posterior trajectory) of thalamic recordings, anterosuperior to our presumptive target, and will pass through 2.5 (more anterior) to 4 mm (more posterior) of ZI before entering H2. If more than 4 mm of relative "quiet" is encountered, a trajectory that is anterior or posterior to the STN should be suspected.

A decrease in background activity demarcates entry into Forel's field H2 (a fiber tract), which lies immediately superior to the STN, 10 to 12 mm lateral to midline. Sparse, if any, cellular activity is detected over a span of 1 to 2 mm. Background activity increases as the recording electrode enters the STN. Two patterns of cellular activity are observed within the STN: (1) tremor activity (see Fig. 93-4, d) similar to that encountered in the VIM thalamic nucleus or GPi, and (2) moderate (25 to 50 Hz) single-unit activity (see Fig. 93-4, e). Once again, these probably are due, not to different cell membrane characteristics, but rather to the specific circuit within which each cell is connected. We have found that cells in the dorsal segments of the STN exhibit slower firing rates than those of the ventral STN. Kinesthesia-related activity is often observed, but a clear somatotopy is not reliably evident. In some cases, it may be necessary to use some type of anesthetic in patients who may not be able to tolerate the procedure. In these cases, we have found that dexmedetomidine affects the recording properties less than propofol does, even at small infusion rates (eFig. 93-4). eFigure 93-4A shows an STN recording from one patient with no anesthetic used, whereas eFigure 93-4B and C shows the effects of dexmedetomidine and propofol in the same patient. As can be seen in the figure, the overall firing rate with dexmedetomidine is a little lower than with no anesthetic, whereas for the propofol cases, the rate is even lower. Yet, as eFigure 93-4 demonstrates, recording with either dexmedetomidine or propofol infusions is possible. On exiting the STN, the microelectrode may pass through a thin quiet zone or directly into the SNr. Entry into the SNr is demarcated by a significant increase in cellular firing rates (see Fig. 93-4, f), which are usually greater than 80 Hz. Up to 7 mm of SNr may be encountered, depending on the anteroposterior position of the trajectory. The border between the STN and the SNr can be difficult to differentiate, especially when the two are adjacent, such as when recording 10 to 12 mm from midline. The primary indicator is the slight increase in firing rate.

Optimally, 4 to 6 mm of STN with evidence of kinesthetic activity is necessary for implantation of the DBS lead. This large a span allows for two of the four electrode contacts (Medtronic model 3387, Minneapolis, MN) to be placed within the nucleus, leaving the other two above the nucleus in the ZI and H2. Additionally, this large a span of STN recording ensures that the electrodes are implanted solidly within the nucleus and not near a medial or lateral border. The primary goal of test stimulation at the STN is to check for stimulation-induced adverse events because, aside from tremor arrest and some modest reductions in rigidity, other positive STN stimulation effects may not be observed for hours or days. Test stimulation is performed in bipolar configuration, and the particular implanted DBS lead and external stimulator used depend on the system implanted (parameters: 60 μsec, 180 Hz, 0 to 4 V). Transient paresthesias are frequently encountered with the onset of stimulation, especially in the inferior contacts. Persistent paresthesias indicate stimulation of the medial lemniscal pathway, which lies posterolateral to the nucleus. Stimulation-induced contractions of the contralateral hemibody or face indicate anterolateral misplacement of the lead. Finally, abnormal eye movements may be encountered if the lead is positioned too medially or deep to the nucleus. The first test stimulation is performed using contacts 0, 1+ up to a voltage of 4 V. If no significant adverse effects are encountered with this focal test, we proceed to test stimulation employing all four contacts (i.e., 0–, 1–, 2–, 3+ up to a voltage of 4 V). This test covers the full contact space of the electrodes and focuses on identifying stimulation-induced adverse events in the ventral aspect of the stimulation field.

DATA ANALYSIS

The data from each MER tract are plotted. The borders of each encountered structure are marked along the line of the scaled tract representations, and the span of each region is represented by a different color for easy differentiation. To account accurately for our angle of approach, a line that is parallel to the intercommissural line is also drawn. The plot is then placed on scaled sagittal slices (10 : 1) modified from the Schaltenbrand-Wahren human stereotactic atlas[104] to determine to which sagittal slice the trajectory best fits. The accuracy of the fit depends on the number of trajectories, the number of structures encountered along each trajectory, and finally how well the patient's anatomy fits the atlas, which is derived from a single human specimen. It can be difficult to find one place to which a single tract fits best, especially when performing pallidal or thalamic interventions, because the slices may not be exactly at the same laterality as the recorded trajectories and the recording trajectory typically passes across several slices owing to the lateral angle of entry. When mapping the STN, the many distinct structures encountered along a single trajectory make fitting it to the atlas a little more straightforward. If there is any question about the proper fit of the data or questions of kinesthetic activity, we perform another recording tract. Knowing the spatial relationship between each tract, we can better fit all of the data to the atlas with each subsequent trajectory.

CONCLUSION

The fine details of these procedures vary from center to center, but most use some type of neurophysiologic techniques, including any or all of the following: (1) microrecording, (2) semi-microrecording, (3) stimulation, and (4) evoked response testing. Based on the more than 1500 trajectories that we have performed, we feel that the information gathered with MER is of great benefit when performing these surgeries. In addition, MER has been shown to be as safe as other stereotactic procedures,[112,114,115] if not safer, when performed properly. Given that these surgeries are done to modify the neurophysiology of a target structure and networks, MER gives the most detailed physiologic data used to determine the optimal placement. In most cases (43% to 88%, depending on the study[38,74,115]), this physiologic target corresponds to the anatomic target; but 12% ot 67% of the time, that is not the case. Even at our center, the average number of trajectories used is 1.6, but we cannot yet predict the cases in which we will need more than one trajectory to locate the optimal physiologic markers.

All neurophysiologic techniques used in the operating room require trained and skilled personnel not only to acquire but also to interpret the data. When everything (equipment, anatomy, patient cooperation, and proper diagnosis) is optimum, the data are relatively easy to interpret, but when any item is not optimum, experience is the best hope for a good outcome. The main feature of reliable MER systems for neurophysiologic targeting of deep brain structures is the quality of the recorded signal. No software-based interpretation scheme can replace the skilled human interpreter when the recordings are difficult. The more we learn about the areas of interest, the faster and smoother each of these procedures will be, and as concluded by Arle and colleagues, all MER can do is guarantee the most optimal placement.[116]

SUGGESTED READINGS

Alterman RL, Reiter GT, Shils J, et al. Targeting for thalamic deep brain stimulation implantation without computer guidance: assessment of targeting accuracy. *Stereotact Funct Neurosurg*. 1999;72:150-153.

Alterman RL, Sterio D, Beric A, et al. Microelectrode recording during posterioventral pallidotomy: impact on target selection and complications. *Neurosurgery*. 1999;44:315-323.

Arle JE, Zani J, Shils JL. Intraoperative decision making with MER for STN DBS in PD and the potential relationship to patient selection. *Open Neurosurg J*. 2011;4:36-41.

Bakay RA, DeLong MR, Vitek JL. Posteroventral pallidotomy for Parkinson's disease. *J Neurosurg*. 1992;77:487-488.

Baker KB, Lee JY, Mavinkurve G, et al. Somatotopic organization in the internal segment of the globus pallidus in Parkinson's disease. *Exp Neurol*. 2010;222(2):219-225.

Lenz FA, Dostrovsky JO, Kwan HC, et al. Methods for microstimulation and recording of single neurons and evoked potentials in the human central nervous system. *J Neurosurg*. 1988;68:630-634.

Lenz FA, Tasker RR, Kwan HC, et al. Single unit analysis of the human ventral thalamic nuclear group: correlation of thalamic "tremor cells" with the 3-6 Hz component of parkinsonian tremor. *J Neurosci*. 1988;8:754-764.

Pinter MM, Alesch F, Murg M, et al. Deep brain stimulation of the subthalamic nucleus for control of extrapyramidal features in advanced idiopathic Parkinson's disease: one year follow-up. *J Neur Trans*. 1999;106:693-709.

Schaltenbrand G, Wahren W. *Atlas for stereotaxy of the human brain*. New York: Thieme; 1977.

Sterio D, Beric A, Dogali M, et al. Neurophysiological properties of pallidal neurons in Parkinson's disease. *Ann Neurol*. 1994;35:586-591.

Taha JM, Favre J, Baumann TK, et al. Characteristics and somatotopic organization of kinesthetic cells in the globus pallidus of patients with Parkinson's disease. *J Neurosurg*. 1996;85:1005-1012.

Tasker RR, Organ LW, Hawrylyshyn PA. *The Thalamus and Midbrain of Man. A Physiological Atlas Using Electrical Stimulation*. Springfield, IL: Charles C. Thomas; 1982.

See a full reference list on ExpertConsult.com

94 Emerging and Experimental Neurosurgical Treatments for Parkinson's Disease

Benjamin I. Rapoport and Michael G. Kaplitt

In the contemporary understanding of Parkinson's disease, degeneration of dopaminergic neurons in the substantia nigra pars compacta causes dysfunction in the neural circuitry of the basal ganglia and thalamus, and the cortical projections of these structures. The classical manifestations of the disease—resting tremor, rigidity and bradykinesia, disturbances of balance and gait, and ultimately dementia—can be partially and temporarily alleviated through established pharmacologic and surgical techniques. Nevertheless, the pathogenesis of neurodegeneration in Parkinson's disease remains incompletely understood, and no disease-modifying therapy presently exists. Basic advances in the understanding of the molecular and genetic neuropathology and the neural circuitry affected in Parkinson's disease and technological advances in the genetic and microelectronic tools available for modulating the diseased circuitry, form the basis for an emerging generation of neurosurgical treatments for Parkinson's disease.

This chapter begins with a brief review of the neuropathology of Parkinson's disease as it relates to emerging and experimental neurosurgical treatments. It then proceeds to review some of these modalities, addressing refinements in the understanding of anatomic targets for electrical stimulation (the actual systems used for electrical stimulation having reached a high level of technological maturity), transplantation of fetal tissue and stem cells, and progress in gene therapy for the treatment of Parkinson's disease.

SCIENTIFIC BACKGROUND

A schematic model has emerged over the past two decades to describe the essential neurophysiology of Parkinson's disease. This model describes two parallel and antagonistic basal ganglia circuits, the direct and indirect pathways, which are respectively responsible for initiation and inhibition of movement. Activity in both of these pathways is modulated by dopaminergic output from the substantia nigra pars compacta (SNc), and so, in general terms, degeneration of dopaminergic neurons in this nucleus disrupts the balance between these parallel systems for initiation and inhibition of movement, leading to the motor disturbances observed in Parkinson's disease.[1,2] A more detailed understanding of these circuits is essential in order to understand the major trends among emerging and experimental treatments of Parkinson's disease.

The direct and indirect pathways share a common outflow circuit, involving the complexed internal globus pallidus (GPi) and the reticular nucleus of the substantia nigra (SNr), which together inhibit thalamic (excitatory glutamatergic) stimulation of the motor cortex.[1,2]

In the direct pathway, dopamine produced in the SNc acts at dopamine$_1$ (D_1) receptors in the striatum to activate GABAergic neurons, which project to and suppress the inhibitory output from the GPi and SNr, thereby (through inhibition of inhibition) disinhibiting excitatory thalamic output to the motor cortex. The net effect of dopamine on the direct pathway is hence to excite the motor cortex.[1,2]

In the indirect pathway, dopamine produced in the SNc acts at striatal dopamine$_2$ (D_2) receptors to suppress inhibitory GABAergic projections to the external globus pallidus (GPe). GABAergic projections from the GPe inhibit the excitatory glutamatergic projections from the subthalamic nucleus (STN) to the GPi, whose inhibitory GABAergic projections in turn inhibit thalamic excitatory output to the motor cortex. In the absence of dopamine, the default logic of the indirect pathway therefore amounts to a triple-negative (dis-disinhibition, through three sets of inhibitory GABAergic projections: the striatum to the GPe; the GPe to the STN; and the STN, after an intervening excitatory glutamatergic projection to the GPi, to the thalamus), with resultant inhibition of the motor cortex. The presence of dopamine adds a fourth negation, by acting at striatal D_2 receptors to inhibit GABAergic projections from the striatum to the GPe, thereby preventing complete inhibition of movement by the indirect pathway.[1,2]

Thus, according to this model, under default conditions the direct pathway is responsible for initiation of movement, while the indirect pathway suppresses initiation of movement. The presence of dopamine favors movement by activating the direct pathway and suppressing the default inhibition of the indirect pathway. In the absence of dopamine, in contrast, the direct pathway is less active (resulting in less initiation of movement) and the indirect pathway performs its default function, inhibiting initiation of movement.[1,2]

Although this model simplifies the connections among the involved nuclei and neglects connections with other structures, it nevertheless explains some of the cardinal features of Parkinson's disease and provides insight into the selection of anatomic targets for surgical approaches to treating the disease.

Advances have been made in recent years in understanding the genetic and molecular pathogenesis of Parkinson's disease.[3] A review of the relevant mechanisms and pathways is beyond the scope of the present chapter, but detailed understanding of these pathways has proven highly practical and essential to advances in gene therapies, embryonic cell therapies, and stem cell therapies for Parkinson's disease that have entered or approached human clinical trials in recent years.

REFINEMENTS IN THE UNDERSTANDING OF ANATOMIC TARGETS FOR ELECTRICAL STIMULATION

Stereotactic approaches to the treatment of Parkinson's disease have been used since the 1950s, and during that decade Lars Leksell and others demonstrated the efficacy of stereotactic pallidotomy and thalamotomy. Thalamotomy, in particular, was found to be effective at suppressing the parkinsonian tremor, but had little effect on rigidity and could aggravate bradykinesia. The first landmark clinical trial demonstrating the efficacy of levodopa was published in 1961,[4] and for the following two decades pharmacotherapy was considered the treatment modality of choice for Parkinson's disease. Between 1985 and 1992, however, Lauri Laitinen demonstrated that pallidotomy could be used as an effective adjunct to antiparkinsonian medications in patients whose tremor, rigidity, and bradykinesias were incompletely controlled by pharmacotherapy, as well as in patients with drug-induced dyskinesias. The modern era of deep brain stimulation is marked by the landmark 1995 paper by Alim-Louis Benabid and colleagues, describing the efficacy of bilateral stimulation of the STN in three parkinsonian patients.[5] The well-known case series of Benabid and colleagues, published in 2003,[6] remains the longest follow-up study in the literature on deep brain stimulation, confirming the durable effectiveness of STN stimulation and characterizing some of its side effects.

A further landmark trial published in 2006 demonstrated that in patients over age 75 with severe motor complications of Parkinson's disease, deep brain stimulation of the STN in addition to pharmacotherapy is more effective than medical management alone.[7] This work firmly established stereotactic implantation of electrodes for stimulation of deep brain structures into the medical and neurosurgical mainstream, and deep brain stimulation is presently considered the first-line surgical procedure in the treatment of patients with advanced Parkinson's disease.[8]

In recent years, work on deep brain stimulation has focused in part on establishing the most appropriate targets for stimulation. Mainstream use of deep brain stimulation has come to focus on three principal targets: the GPi, the STN, and the ventralis intermedius nucleus of the thalamus (VIM). In 2010, a major clinical trial compared outcomes from bilateral stimulation of the GPi with bilateral stimulation of the STN with respect to overall motor function, as quantified by established clinical paradigms. The study concluded that stimulation in these regions generated similar outcomes with respect to overall motor function[8]; unilateral pallidal stimulation has also been compared with unilateral STN stimulation, with similar results.[9] Stimulation of the STN is, however, associated with greater reduction in use of antiparkinsonian medications and with lower stimulation amplitudes.

At present, both the dorsolateral STN and posteroventral GPi are effectively targeted for stimulation in treating the motor symptoms of Parkinson's disease, with no definitive evidence that one or the other is more effective. The foregoing and other studies have also examined the impact of STN and GPi stimulation on neurocognitive (nonmotor) aspects of Parkinson's disease; a consistent finding appears to be an adverse effect on mood when either target is stimulated ventrally,[9] although several authors have noted a trend toward more severe cognitive and mood disturbances with STN stimulation.[10-12] Some differences have also begun to emerge with respect to motor effects, with the STN being potentially a more effective target for bradykinesia, and the GPi a more effective target for "on"-medication dyskinesia. STN stimulation appears to reduce overall dyskinesia primarily through reducing the overall use of antiparkinsonian medication, so some reviewers have suggested[13] that a patient with a low threshold for dyskinesia and low preoperative probability of medication reduction might be an appropriate candidate for GPi rather than STN stimulation.

The mechanism of action of deep brain stimulation remains an active area of research, but it has been empirically established that high-frequency electrical stimulation, as applied in conventional deep brain stimulation, has a "lesioning" effect, inhibiting the target nucleus. Thus, the finding that "functional lesioning" has equivalent efficacy in the GPi and the STN is consistent with the physiologic circuit model described earlier in the "Scientific Background" section.[14,15]

Of note, both targets are also used effectively in the treatment of dystonia. The efficacy of deep brain stimulation for dystonia was established in a study by the Deep Brain Stimulation for Dystonia Study Group, conducted from 2002 to 2004 in Germany, Austria, and Norway, which evaluated 40 patients with primary generalized or segmental dystonia. All patients underwent bilateral stimulation of the ventral GPi, and stimulation was compared with sham stimulation in double-blind fashion. The results of the study, published in 2006, demonstrate improvement in motor function as well as reduction in disability scores as quantified using standardized rating scales, and provide level I evidence supporting the efficacy of deep brain stimulation in the treatment of dystonia.[16]

In the treatment of tremor, both parkinsonian tremor and essential tremor, the VIM has been described as the target of choice. The nucleus is organized somatotopically along its medial-to-lateral axis, with tongue and face represented medially and the lower extremities represented laterally, so precise placement of stimulation electrodes within the nucleus can facilitate optimal tremor control. Parkinsonian patients do not typically perceive an overall benefit from stimulation of the VIM, however, because stimulation of this nucleus has little or no effect on rigidity, bradykinesia, gait, or postural dysfunction; for this reason VIM stimulation is typically reserved for patients with essential tremor.[17]

An intriguing technology currently being applied to essential tremor but planned for trials in Parkinson's disease as well is magnetic resonance–guided focused ultrasound (MRgFUS). Ultrasound can penetrate the skull but disburses widely such that a single source of ultrasound cannot generate much energy deep in the brain. However, in a manner similar to the approach for stereotactic radiosurgery, multiple foci of ultrasound sources can be arrayed such that the weak energies from these sources can combine at a desired point deep in the brain to yield much higher focal energy. This leads to heating of tissue, which can be monitored with magnetic resonance thermometry, and then the ultrasound energies from the individual sources can be adjusted to optimize the energy and heating at the desired target. This can lead to a focal lesion similar to that produced with invasive lesioning probes, but without brain invasion and without injury to superficial structures. Recent studies have demonstrated that safe thalamic lesions can be created, with resulting improvements in tremor for essential tremor patients that are comparable to those with DBS or invasive thalamotomy for up to 1 year.[18,19] The major advantages of MRgFUS are that it is noninvasive and heating can be performed gradually while monitoring patient responses, as with invasive lesioning, so that a final lesion is only completed when patient responses are acceptable. This compares favorably with radiosurgery, which is also noninvasive but cannot adjust to patient responses because of the delayed nature of the responses. However, it is not clear if MRgFUS will offer other advantages over invasive lesioning, which is usually limited to unilateral procedures given the observed morbidities of bilateral lesioning. Assuming that this is true for MRgFUS as well, its use may be somewhat limited in Parkinson's disease, where bilateral surgery is more common as a result of difficulties in medicating advanced patients with severe bilateral disease after completing only a unilateral lesion. The ability to disrupt the blood-brain barrier with MRgFUS at lower energies may also provide minimally invasive opportunities for focal delivery of a variety of therapeutic agents for Parkinson's disease and other disorders in the future.

TRANSPLANTATION OF FETAL NEURONS FOR THE TREATMENT OF PARKINSON'S DISEASE

Transplantation of neural tissue for the treatment of Parkinson's disease has been seriously investigated in human trials by several groups over the past two decades. Studies consistently demonstrated that fetal cells transplanted into parkinsonian patients can give rise to neuronal cell populations that continue to produce dopamine for over a decade. The clinical outcomes associated with these transplantations have been inconsistent, however. Although some patients experienced durable improvements in parkinsonian symptoms from neural transplantation, two major clinical trials of embryonic cell transplantation for the treatment of Parkinson's disease failed to meet their primary end points of meaningful clinical improvement[20] or improvement in motor function,[21] and many patients experienced significant dyskinesia as a side effect of transplantation. Following these trials, many countries imposed a moratorium on new studies of fetal cell transplantation for Parkinson's disease, which is only just being lifted as this chapter is being written.

Three small, long-term case studies, published simultaneously in 2008 by separate groups,[22-24] demonstrated that transplanted fetal dopaminergic neurons can engraft and continue to function over a follow-up period of up to 16 years (to postmortem examination) in the brains of parkinsonian transplant recipients. A total of seven patients were studied at three centers, all of whom had idiopathic Parkinson's disease, had preoperative positron emission tomography (PET) imaging consistent with the disease, and had demonstrated initial responses to levodopa. In each case, fetal tissue was obtained after elective abortions at 6 to 9 weeks postconception, with maternal consent. Ventral midbrain tissue was isolated by dissection and used to prepare either cell suspensions or solid grafts, which were stereotactically implanted in the postcommissural putamen. Patients were placed on immunosuppressive regimens for 6 months postoperatively. The studies followed graft recipients from treatment through their remaining years of life, over periods of 9 to 16 years. Postmortem analyses conducted on all seven patients demonstrated graft survival, with morphologic features suggesting active innervation of host striatum, and immunohistochemical analysis confirming the presence of 10^4 to 10^5 dopaminergic neurons per graft. Of note, in four of these seven patients, 1% to 5% of grafted neurons were found at autopsy to have developed Lewy body—like features characteristic of Parkinson's disease.[23,24] This raises intriguing and potentially concerning questions about the potential vulnerability of transplanted cells to the parkinsonian neurodegenerative process once grafted into the diseased brain, even if they come from an exogenous source. Clinical outcomes in these patients were variable, with some experiencing no change in parkinsonian symptoms, and others experiencing marked and durable improvements in motor function and reduced requirements for antiparkinsonian medications; the degree of clinical benefit was weakly correlated with the amount of the viable graft tissue found at autopsy.

In spite of potentially promising results achieved in a number of small studies, many countries effectively placed a moratorium in 2003 on further human trials involving transplantation of fetal neurons for the treatment of Parkinson's disease, after two major double-blind, randomized controlled trials[20,21] failed to demonstrate a benefit from neural transplantation.

In the trial by Freed and colleagues,[20] 40 patients were randomized either to bilateral stereotactic putaminal transplantation of fetal ventral midbrain tissue from two embryos per hemisphere, or to sham surgery. Immunosuppression was not used. The primary performance metric was clinical improvement on a self-reported scale after 1 year; the trial failed to meet its projected end point of statistically significant improvement in this metric, and "off"-period dyskinesias were reported in 15% of patients. Supporters of the trial have suggested retrospectively that the observation interval was too short, and that a number of patients demonstrated clinical improvement 2 to 3 years after transplantation.

The trial by Olanow and colleagues[21] enrolled 34 patients and was similarly designed, with subjects randomized to receive bilateral putaminal grafts from one of four donor embryos per hemisphere, followed by a 6-month course of immunosuppression. The primary performance metric was the score on the motor component of the Unified Parkinson's Disease Rating Scale (UPDRS). The trial failed to demonstrate consistent improvement in transplant recipients, and severe "off"-period dyskinesias were reported in 56% of patients, leading some to suggest that although grafted neurons may remain viable and capable of producing dopamine in vivo, they may not properly integrate into the feedback circuits of the host basal ganglia.

An international consortium of investigators has conducted long-term retrospective analyses of transplanted patients to establish and standardize a consistent set of best practices for transplantation of fetal neurons, and the moratorium on transplantation of fetal neurons has recently been lifted.[25] A new clinical trial, "TRANSEURO Open Label Transplant Study in Parkinson's Disease," incorporating the best practices defined by this consortium, is currently enrolling patients by invitation.[26] This trial will be the first in a decade involving fetal neural transplantation for Parkinson's disease, and its initial findings are eagerly anticipated.

STEM CELL THERAPIES FOR PARKINSON'S DISEASE

The safety and durable efficacy of stem cell therapies in the treatment of Parkinson's disease have been demonstrated in animal models, and several groups and large consortia have set target dates for beginning human clinical trials.

The international moratorium on transplantation of fetal neural tissue for the treatment of Parkinson's disease coincided with the 2006 discovery of induced pleuripotent stem cells (iPSCs). As investigators across many fields have noted, iPSCs share many of the properties of embryonic stem cells, but they are derived from adult somatic cells and do not require the use of human embryos. A number of investigators have therefore turned their attention to the use of iPSCs in the treatment of Parkinson's disease, with motivations similar to those behind the use of fetal midbrain transplantation.[27] Several groups have demonstrated the efficacy of iPSCs in improving motor function in animal models, including nonhuman primates,[25,28] and at least one group has announced its intention to begin human clinical trials[25] by 2016, but no human safety or efficacy data are yet available.

At least two other major consortia have also demonstrated significant progress toward clinical trials involving transplantation of human-derived embryonic stem cells in the treatment of Parkinson's disease. The Center for Stem Cell Biology at the Memorial Sloan Kettering Cancer Center in New York has demonstrated the efficacy and durability of one strategy for deriving human dopaminergic neurons that efficiently engraft in vivo,[29] and is currently engaged in work to ensure scalability of the technique compatible with good manufacturing practices and to define associated surgical techniques and immunosuppressive regimens.[30] The group intends to file for an Investigational Device Exemption with the U.S. Food and Drug Administration to begin human clinical trials by 2017. The European Stem Cell Consortium for Neural Cell Replacement, Reprogramming, and Functional Brain Repair, which comprises investigators at eight academic institutions and several commercial centers across Europe, has also announced its intention to fulfill all practical requirements for large-scale manufacture and banking of clinical-grade, transplantable striatal progenitor cells from human pleuripotent and neural stem cell lines by 2017.[31]

PROGRESS IN GENE THERAPY FOR THE TREATMENT OF PARKINSON'S DISEASE

Major progress in gene therapy for the treatment of Parkinson's disease has been demonstrated over the last decade, and four in vivo approaches involving viral-based gene delivery have led to phase 1 or phase 2 human clinical trials to date. These approaches continue to employ stereotactic neurosurgical techniques for viral delivery because the viral vectors of choice are unable to cross the blood-brain barrier, though a number of nonviral gene delivery methods are under investigation.[32]

We originally completed the first human trial of in vivo gene therapy for Parkinson's disease, using adeno-associated virus type 2 (AAV2) to deliver the gene for glutamic acid decarboxylase

(GAD) to the STN, unilaterally, in 12 patients (the "AAV2-GAD" approach).[33] The characteristic loss of dopaminergic neurons in the nigrostriatal pathway in parkinsonian patients results in downstream reduction in GABAergic input to the STN, and it was known that infusion of GABAergic agents into the STN improves parkinsonian symptoms.[34] GAD is the rate-limiting enzyme in the synthesis of γ-aminobutyric acid. By delivering the gene encoding GAD to the STN, this approach was designed to increase the GABAergic tone of the STN and to improve the motor symptoms of Parkinson's disease in a fashion analogous to deep brain stimulation. The phase 1 study[33] involved 12 parkinsonian patients, each a candidate for deep brain stimulation on the basis of moderately advanced disease (Hoehn and Yahr Scale stage 3: bilateral disease, with mild to moderate disability and impaired postural reflexes, but physically independent) and intolerable motor complications associated with levodopa use. Each patient underwent stereotactic injection of AAV2-GAD, at one of three doses, into the STN contralateral to the more symptomatic side. Improvements in UPDRS motor scores were confirmed at 3 months, and persisted for the duration of the study period in both the "on" and "off" states.

Following the phase 1 study, we evaluated the highest AAV2-GAD dose in a randomized, double-blind, sham surgery–controlled phase 2 trial.[35] The trial involved 44 patients with progressive, levodopa-responsive Parkinson's disease, of whom 21 were randomized to receive bilateral stereotactic delivery of AAV2-GAD, while the remaining 23 received partial-thickness bur holes and subgaleal saline infusions without intracranial penetration. Over the ensuing 6 months of the blinded phase, the AAV2-GAD group demonstrated 23% improvement in UPDRS motor scores, which was significantly greater than the 13% improvement in the sham group. The treatment effect remained significant at 12 months, and there were no surgery- or gene therapy–associated adverse events. There were also significant improvements in so-called medication "on" time and a reduction in medication-related complications, as measured by the UPDRS part IV, over the course of the study (unpublished observations). Finally, given the power of functional imaging to identify metabolic brain patterns so as to confirm the diagnosis of idiopathic Parkinson's disease and to potentially measure outcome, we also asked if there were patterns that may help discern true responders from sham responders. Using principal component analysis to identify common metabolic patterns among patient groups on fluorodeoxyglucose-PET scans, we identified a pattern of changes that were unique to those patients in the sham group with a positive clinical response.[36] This was not observed in sham patients with no clinical improvement, nor was it observed in AAV-GAD treated patients. Therefore, it is possible in the future that the use of functional imaging as a biomarker not only for disease progression and therapeutic outcome, but also for sham responses, may help increase confidence in positive clinical responses to experimental therapies and may also help reduce patient sample sizes needed to demonstrate convincing responses.

A group based at the University of California–San Francisco used an AAV2 vector to deliver human aromatic amino acid decarboxylase (hAADC) to the putamen bilaterally in a phase 1 clinical trial involving a total of 10 human subjects (the "AAV2-hAADC" approach). The rationale for this approach was based on the observation that the effectiveness of levodopa pharmacotherapy wanes over time in parkinsonian patients; a proposed mechanism for this decline is a gradual decline in production of AADC, the rate-limiting enzyme for the conversion of levodopa to dopamine. The selection of the AAV2 vector was due, in part, to its ability to target striatal interneurons that do not typically degenerate in Parkinson's disease. Delivery of the complementary DNA encoding human AADC to the putamen using an adeno-associated virus successfully restored dopamine production and improved motor function in a primate model of Parkinson's disease.[37,38] Human phase 1 clinical trial results 4 years after surgery (stereotactic viral infusion to the putamen bilaterally, with convection-enhanced delivery) were reported in 2012.[39] Serial PET imaging over the follow-up period demonstrated sustained expression of the AADC transgene, but total UPDRS and motor subscores slowly declined after an initial improvement (attributed by the authors to a placebo effect). A revised phase 1 trial is planned, with the intention of infusing larger doses of AAV2-hAADC and exposing more of the putamen.

A Paris-based group backed by OxfordBioMedica has developed a lentivirus vector, called ProSavin, for putaminal delivery of AADC together with a pair of genes involved in dopamine synthesis, those for tyrosine hydroxylase and guanosine triphosphate (GTP) cyclohydrolase. Tyrosine hydroxylase catalyzes the synthesis of levodopa from dietary tyrosine, and GTP cyclohydrolase catalyzes the conversion of GTP to tetrahydrobiopterin, an essential cofactor in tyrosine hydroxylase–mediated levodopa synthesis. This triple gene therapy approach was developed after extensive work in primate models of Parkinson's disease by the same group who demonstrated that viral transduction of primate striatum with each of these genes separately could effectively raise striatal dopamine concentrations.[40] The first human clinical trial of ProSavin, a phase 1-2 dose-escalation study, enrolled 15 parkinsonian patients (Hoehn and Yahr stage 3, all candidates for deep brain stimulation on the basis of intractable motor complications associated with levodopa use), all of whom underwent bilateral stereotactic injection of ProSavin into the putamen. No serious adverse events were reported at 12-month follow-up, and all cohorts reported significant improvements in UPDRS motor scores at 6- and 12-month follow-up, with associated stabilization or reduction in levodopa dosing.[41] Further work is reportedly in progress to optimize dosing prior to testing ProSavin in randomized, placebo-controlled trials.

Several attempts have been made to design disease-modifying treatments for Parkinson's disease using gene therapy. Glial cell line–derived neurotrophic factor (GDNF), a neuron-specific growth factor, has been shown to promote survival of nigrostriatal dopaminergic neurons in animal models of Parkinson's disease after direct striatal injection.[42,43] Direct putaminal injections of GDNF demonstrated no clinical benefits in human trials, however.[44-46] Following these negative trials, it was speculated that sustained delivery of GDNF might be required in order to achieve a therapeutic effect in parkinsonian patients, and this hypothesis was supported by subsequent work in animal models.[47,48] Several phase 1 (dose escalation, safety, and efficacy)[49-51] and phase 2 (double-blind, sham-surgery, placebo-controlled) human clinical trials have been conducted to evaluate gene therapeutic approaches of this type, involving an AAV2 vector encoding the GDNF family member neurturin, yet the phase 2 trials have failed to demonstrate efficacy.

A variety of other gene therapeutic approaches to the treatment of Parkinson's disease have been investigated in vitro and in animal models. In particular, RNA interference techniques have been used in vitro and in vivo to silence gene mutations associated with Parkinson's disease,[52-55] and the versatility of this family of techniques suggests that it may be particularly useful as more details of the molecular pathogenesis of Parkinson's disease are revealed, and new potential targets for gene therapy are identified. Another novel approach to gene therapy for Parkinson's disease is optogenetics. This involves using viral vectors to deliver a gene for an opsin, which is a light-sensitive ion channel or pump derived from algae or other organisms. Particular opsins will respond to specific wavelengths of light, which generally lead to influx of either cations to depolarize or anions to hyperpolarize neurons. Thus, specific populations of neurons can be controlled and either activated or inhibited by pulsing with specific wavelengths of light following introduction of the appropriate opsin with gene therapy.[56] This has been used to better characterize the circuitry related to Parkinson's disease with great precision,[57,58] and there has also been some evidence of potential therapeutic efficacy of this methodology in reversing symptoms in rodent models of the disorder.[59,60]

CONCLUSION

Functional neurosurgery, and particularly surgery for Parkinson's disease, has long created opportunities for advancing novel neurosurgical therapies into the clinic. Although the mechanisms of neuronal loss in Parkinson's disease remain elusive, the physiologic changes in specific circuits are sufficiently well understood to facilitate testing of novel, rationally designed treatments to either restore function or replace lost cells. Early experiences with lesioning in the mid-20th century led to the use of similar techniques to deploy electrodes that have now resulted in a revolution in neuromodulation, which is being tested well beyond surgery for movement disorders. In the early 21st century, advances in molecular therapeutics combined with similar approaches to stereotactic placement of lesions or electrodes has led to an increasingly large number of clinical trials for biological therapies, particularly gene therapies, with some success even in "gold standard," randomized, double-blind trials. These are likely to continue and hopefully will lead to approved treatments for wider use in the next decade. Similarly, advances in cell development and transplantation methodologies are leading to a resurging interest in neural repair to replace lost cells, and the likely initiation of novel clinical trials of these approaches in the near term should help add this restorative approach to the tool chest of emerging therapeutics available for neurosurgical intervention in Parkinson's disease.

SUGGESTED READINGS

Braak H, Ghebremedhin E, Rüb U, et al. Stages in the development of Parkinson's disease-related pathology. *Cell Tissue Res*. 2004;318:121-134.

Fiandaca M, Forsayeth J, Bankiewicz K. Current status of gene therapy trials for Parkinson's disease. *Exp Neurol*. 2008;209:51-57.

Freed CR, Greene PE, Breeze RE, et al. Transplantation of embryonic dopamine neurons for severe Parkinson's disease. *N Engl J Med*. 2001;344:710-719.

Fregni F, Simon DK, Wu A, et al. Non-invasive brain stimulation for Parkinson's disease: a systematic review and meta-analysis of the literature. *J Neurol Neurosurg Psychiatry*. 2005;76:1614-1623.

Goldman S. Disease targets and strategies for the therapeutic modulation of endogenous neural stem and progenitor cells. *Clin Pharmacol Ther*. 2007;82:453-460.

Isacson O. The production and use of cells as therapeutic agents in neurodegenerative diseases. *Lancet Neurol*. 2003;2:417-424.

Kaplitt MG, Feigin A, Tang C, et al. Safety and tolerability of gene therapy with an adeno-associated virus (AAV) borne GAD gene for Parkinson's disease: an open label, phase I trial. *Lancet*. 2007;369:2097-2105.

Kim J, Auerbach J, Rodríguez-Gómez J, et al. Dopamine neurons derived from embryonic stem cells function in an animal model of Parkinson's disease. *Nature*. 2002;418:50-56.

Lang AE, Gill S, Patel NK, et al. Randomized controlled trial of intraputamenal glial cell line-derived neurotrophic factor infusion in Parkinson disease. *Ann Neurol*. 2006;59:459-466. Erratum in: *Ann Neurol*. 2006;60:747.

Lang AE, Lozano AM. Parkinson's disease. First of two parts. *N Engl J Med*. 1998;339:1044-1053.

Lang AE, Lozano AM. Parkinson's disease. Second of two parts. *N Engl J Med*. 1998;339:1130-1143.

Marks WJ Jr, Ostrem JL, Verhagen L, et al. Safety and tolerability of intraputaminal delivery of CERE-120 (adeno-associated virus serotype 2-neurturin) to patients with idiopathic Parkinson's disease: an open-label, phase I trial. *Lancet Neurol*. 2008;7:400-408.

Mendez I, Sanchez-Pernaute R, Cooper O, et al. Cell type analysis of functional fetal dopamine cell suspension transplants in the striatum and substantia nigra of patients with Parkinson's disease. *Brain*. 2005;128:1498-1510.

Ming GL, Song H. Adult neurogenesis in the mammalian central nervous system. *Annu Rev Neurosci*. 2005;28:223-250.

Olanow CW, Goetz CG, Kordower JH, et al. A double-blind controlled trial of bilateral fetal nigral transplantation in Parkinson's disease. *Ann Neurol*. 2003;54:403-414.

Pahapill PA, Lozano AM. The pedunculopontine nucleus and Parkinson's disease. *Brain*. 2000;123(Pt 9):1767-1783.

Perlow MJ, Freed WJ, Hoffer BJ, et al. Brain grafts reduce motor abnormalities produced by destruction of nigrostriatal dopamine system. *Science*. 1979;204:643-647.

Priori A, Lefaucheur JP. Chronic epidural motor cortical stimulation for movement disorders. *Lancet Neurol*. 2007;6:279-286.

Schüpbach WM, Maltête D, Houeto JL, et al. Neurosurgery at an earlier stage of Parkinson disease: a randomized, controlled trial. *Neurology*. 2007;68:267-271.

Stefani A, Lozano AM, Peppe A, et al. Bilateral deep brain stimulation of the pedunculopontine and subthalamic nuclei in severe Parkinson's disease. *Brain*. 2007;130:1596-1607.

See a full reference list on ExpertConsult.com

95 Transcranial Magnetic Resonance Imaging–Guided Focused Ultrasound Thalamotomy for Tremor

Robert F. Dallapiazza, Tony R. Wang, Eyal Zadicario, and W. Jeffrey Elias

HISTORICAL USES OF FOCUSED ULTRASOUND IN THE BRAIN

Neurosurgeons rarely use ultrasound (US) other than for diagnostic imaging. The concept of using high-intensity focused ultrasound (HIFU) in the brain was first conceived in the early 1950s, during a time of rapid growth in stereotactic neurosurgery. William and Frank Fry, US physicists, described the use of HIFU to produce precise, focal lesions deep in the feline brain without opening the dura and without causing damage to the intervening tissues or blood vessels.[1,2] These seminal experiments used a four-element, 1-MHz transducer to reliably produce a US beam about 1 mm in diameter capable of contouring lesions with slight movements of the focus.[1-3] Sonication intensities approaching 210 W/cm^2 for 4 seconds created "reversible" brain lesions in craniectomized cats and nonhuman primates.[4] William Fry collaborated with Russell Meyer, a pioneer in open surgery of the basal ganglia, to make ultrasonic lesions in 12 patients with Parkinson's disease and other movement disorders.[5] These treatments involved a custom stereotactic apparatus, contrast ventriculography, and a craniotomy to transmit acoustic energy to the pallidothalamic tracts. The results were favorable, with improvements in tremor and rigidity and relatively few serious side effects.[5]

Around the same time that the Fry brothers were studying the therapeutic uses of focused US (FUS), diagnostic ultrasonography was born in Lund, Sweden. Ultrasonic reflectoscopes had been designed to test material integrities in shipyards and factories. The first echocardiograms were obtained when cardiologists used these scopes to image heart motion and the mitral valve. Lars Leksell[6] borrowed a device in 1956 and successfully identified the pineal shift in a 16-month-old child with a subdural hematoma. Although US transmission was possible in the neonatal skull, Leksell eventually became disenchanted by the limitations of transcranial US delivery through the mature, human skull because it required a cranial window. Even though he acquired several patents for the use of US in the brain, he eventually pursued ionizing radiation as a less invasive method for the treatment of pain and other neurological disorders.

Others utilized US through craniotomies for deep lesioning in the brain. Lindstrom treated 25 patients with cancer for their pain and anxiety with US leucotomy as an alternative to surgical lobotomy.[7,8] Histologic findings were ultimately available in these patients. Sixteen exhibited clinical improvement without microscopic change, a finding that was interpreted as a "functional lesion" selective to white matter tracts.[7,8] Heimburger[9] reported prolonged survival in patients with glioma after sonicating through their craniotomies after initial resection. Despite these early successes, FUS lesioning necessitated craniotomy for acoustic transmission, so US therapy in the brain never gained widespread popularity among neurosurgeons.

ULTRASOUND PROPERTIES

Ultrasound can be defined as an acoustic pressure wave beyond the range of normal human hearing (>20 kHz). As with other waveform energies that follow simple harmonic motion, US is characterized by its frequency, wavelength, amplitude, power, and intensity. Safe, medical imaging US at frequencies ranging from 2 to 20 MHz creates waveforms with peak intensities less than 1 W/cm^2 as regulated by the U.S. Food and Drug Administration (FDA).[10,11] Therapeutic HIFU for brain ablation uses lower frequencies (0.2 to 1 MHz), which better propagate through bone, and the peak intensities may exceed 1000 W/cm^{2}and are therefore capable of tissue ablation or cavitation.

As US pressure waves travel through a given medium, molecules are displaced and oscillate according to the magnitude of the wave and the elasticity of the medium. Frictional energy and ultimately heat are generated by the molecules as they oscillate next to each other—a phenomenon not dissimilar to that of radiofrequency (RF) energy. With FUS, the pressure at the focus is exponentially increased, so thermal tissue ablation can be achieved in the focus without damage to surrounding tissue.[10,11]

At high intensities, the acoustic pressure wave moving through tissue can also induce cavitation, which results when the acoustic pressure wave extracts gas that coalesces into microbubbles that oscillate in the ultrasonic field.[12,13] At lower intensities, these bubbles can expand and contract in a sustainable, periodic fashion termed *sustained cavitation.* However, if the bubbles are subjected to higher intensities, they can potentially collapse violently (*inertial cavitation*) and damage tissues with extremely high temperatures, powerful jet streams, and/or free radicals.[14,15] The propensity for microbubble formation and cavitation raises concerns for HIFU ablation and has resulted in the implementation of cavitation monitoring (discussed later). Theoretically, stable cavitation could be monitored and harnessed to enhance therapeutic ablations or mechanical opening of the blood-brain barrier; but inertial cavitation poses great risk to tissue because its mechanical effects are more difficult to predict and control.[16]

MODERN TRANSCRANIAL FOCUSED ULTRASOUND

The skull is the major limiting factor for efficient delivery of US to the brain. Depending on the US frequency, the skull may reflect or absorb about 90%of the US energy.[17] The potential for heating of the skull and adjacent soft tissues (dura and periosteum) exists if the skull overheats from absorbed US energy. Another challenge for transcranial US delivery relates to the variable thickness and density of the skull, which diffracts acoustic waves (*analogous to corneal astigmatism*) and leads to "defocusing" or difficulties achieving a sharp, acoustic focus.

Over the past two decades, two technologic advances have addressed the high acoustic impedance of the skull, allowing for transcranial HIFU. In the first, Clement and Hynynen and their colleagues[18-20] developed a large-aperture, hemispherical transducers to maximize the area of transcranial acoustic energy delivery, thus minimizing local skull heating by distributing energy over the large surface area of the scalp and skull. Furthermore, a cold water interface is used to decrease the baseline temperature of the skull and keep it cooled during treatment (Fig. 95-1). The second advance, to account for the variability of the skull, was development of a phase correction technology in parallel with multiple-element, hemispherical transducers to correct aberrations in the acoustic beam traveling through the inhomogeneous

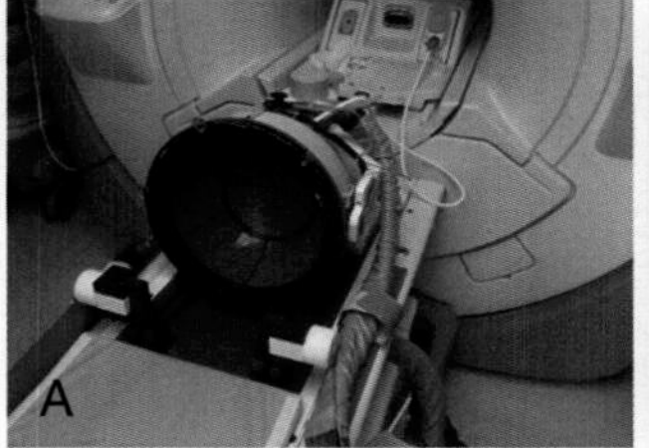

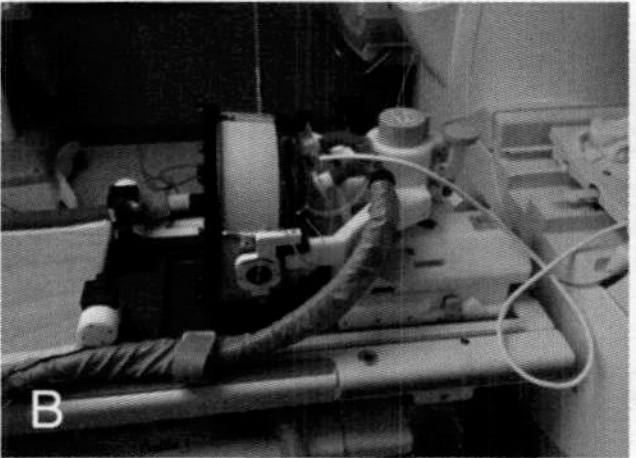

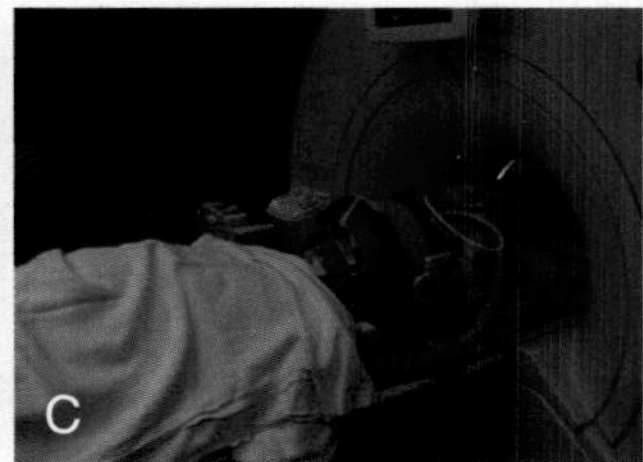

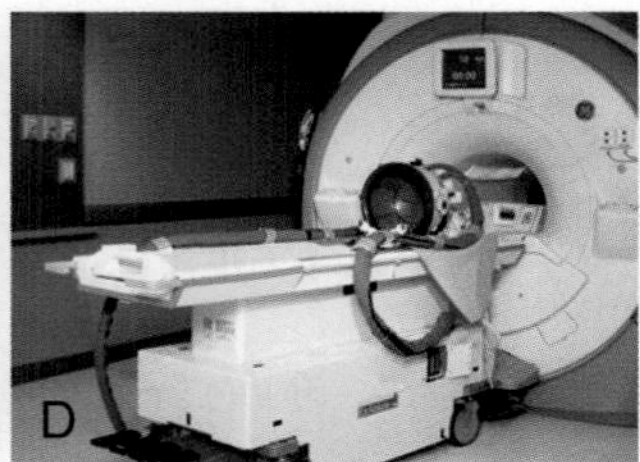

Figure 95-1. ExAblate 4000 ultrasound device (INSIGHTEC, Haifa, Israel). Hemispheric phased-array configuration of 1024 individual elements seen from below **(A)** and from a lateral view **(B)**. **C,** A patient is secured to the magnetic resonance imaging (MRI) table and ultrasound device in a stereotactic frame. The white membrane couples the ultrasound device to the patient's head with chilled, degassed water. **D,** Full view of the ultrasound device, MRI bore, and table.

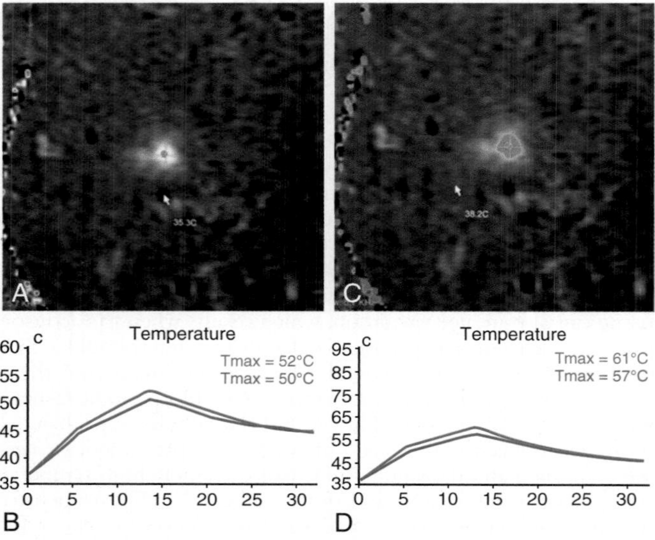

Figure 95-2. Intraprocedural magnetic resonance (MR) thermography. A, Axial, proton resonance frequency shift MR image showing thermal rise during a verification sonication with peak temperatures reaching 52°C. The *red* voxels at the center indicate the area warmer than 50°C. The skull can be seen on the *left* side of the image. **B,** A temperature plot over time during a 13-second verification sonication. The *red line* shows peak voxel temperature, and the *green line* shows an average of the surrounding 9 voxels. **C,** Proton resonance frequency shift MR image showing the thermal rise during a treatment sonication with a peak temperature of 61°C. *Red* voxels indicate a temperature higher than 50°C. **D,** Temperature plot over time showing a peak temperature of 61°C *(red line)* and an average voxel temperature of 57°C *(green line)*.

skull.[21] In this technology, a computed tomography (CT)–based correction algorithm reconstructs the skull and computes the local characteristics of each location where an acoustic wave interfaces with the skull. Each element on the transducer can then be electronically adjusted and "phase shifted" to bring all of the beams to a sharp focus.

MAGNETIC RESONANCE THERMOGRAPHY

Magnetic resonance (MR) thermography measures temperature-dependent changes in water proton resonance frequency, thus enabling thermal monitoring during transcranial sonications.[22,23] Pre-sonication images are subtracted in a voxel-by-voxel basis from images obtained during tissue heating by US sonication.[24-27] Images are acquired every 3 seconds and tissue temperature is updated and plotted during the prescribed sonication (Fig. 95-2). The images can be acquired in any of three planes (axial, coronal, and sagittal) to form a two-dimensional temperature map of change that is accurate to approximately 1°C in the plane perpendicular to the resonance frequency.

THERMAL DOSE

The intraoperative measurement of temperature can also be accumulated to represent the thermal dose delivered to each voxel. The Sapareto and Dewey equation was developed to estimate the thermal dose delivered to tissue on the basis of time-temperature profiles.[28] Exposure of tissue for 240 minutes to 43°C is considered the critical dose for permanent tissue damage and cell death. Using the Sapareto and Dewey equation, one can calculate the equivalent time to achieve cell death for any temperature.[28] This determination of thermal dose is necessary because of its nonlinear relationship with temperature, in which small increases in temperature can lead to large increases in thermal dose. This determination enables an intraoperative assessment of the ablated tissue and supports clinical decision making about additional treatment.

TECHNIQUE: TRANSCRANIAL MAGNETIC RESONANCE IMAGING–GUIDED FOCUSED ULTRASOUND THALAMOTOMY

Preoperative Preparation

MR imaging (MRI)–guided FUS thalamotomy, like other stereotactic lesioning procedures, can be performed as a unilateral procedure for patients with severe, medication-refractory tremor. Ideal candidates tend to have asymmetric, appendicular tremors resulting in significant disabilities and functional limitations. Patients may choose this procedure because of preconceived bias against open neurosurgical procedures, implanted devices, or radiation therapies. Because this is an MRI-guided procedure, patients with pacemakers, MRI-incompatible implants, or claustrophobia are not candidates for it.

Preoperative imaging studies include volumetric CT and MRI with T1- and T2-weighted sequences. Brain MRI with a high field strength and head coil is used preoperatively to obtain the highest-resolution images, which can be imported into the system for use during the procedure. CT is critical to application of the skull correction algorithm for each US element so that efficient transcranial US delivery is ensured. CT also allows for the identification of "no-pass regions" like aerated sinuses and intracranial calcifications, which can impede the passage of US. Screening for deep vein thrombosis is considered for selected patients.

The patient is prepared on the morning of the procedure with intravenous access and compression leg stockings. A mild anxiolytic may be administered if necessary. Because hair follicles can harbor microbubbles of air, which might lead to cavitation or scalp burns during sonication, the patient's head is carefully shaved in its entirety. A stereotactic frame is placed as low as possible near the orbital rim and parieto-occipital junction to make maximal skull surface area available for transcranial sonication (Video 95-1). The frame is used for immobilization of the head, not for stereotactic measurements, because intraoperative MRI is available. A silicone membrane is affixed to the scalp and attached to the FUS transducer, creating a coupling medium for US transduction as chilled and degassed water is circulated to cool the scalp. The transducer is manually aligned so that the natural acoustic focus approximates the stereotactic target. The patient, secured by the frame to the FUS transducer, is then positioned inside the bore of the MRI scanner to its isocenter.

Procedural Imaging and Stereotactic Planning Phase

During the imaging phase, a series of localizer MR images are acquired so that higher-quality T1- or T2-weighted images can be prescribed orthogonally to the anterior commissure (AC) and posterior commissure (PC). These "reference" images are fused to the preoperatively obtained CT scans and highest-resolution MR images. It is important to note that MRI during the procedure is currently performed with a body coil positioned outside the US transducer helmet and water bath.

After image acquisition, stereotactic planning can be performed with neuronavigation software either by indirect targeting from AC-PC measurements or by direct targeting to an imaged structure. To date, most MRI-guided FUS procedures have indirectly targeted the thalamus either to the ventral intermediate nucleus (Vim) for tremor suppression [28-31] or to the centrolateral nucleus for the alleviation of neuropathic pain.[32,33]

Final planning preparations are made before the treatment is begun. Fiducial markers are designated to detect intraprocedural movement as the transducer is constantly tracked in the MRI space. If there is a disparity in the location of the fiducials, the system recognizes a movement and the prescribed sonication is not delivered. Lastly, a final adjustment of the transducer is made so that the natural focus is positioned to precisely match the stereotactic target.

Treatment Phase

The treatment phase relies heavily on MR thermography using the proton resonance frequency shift method to monitor the size, shape, and location of heating in multiple planes as well as on continuous clinical evaluation for safety and symptom response. The treatment phase involves the following three stages of sonication: (1) focus alignment, (2) target verification, and (3) therapeutic ablation.

In the alignment stage, low-energy sonications (i.e., 150 watts × 10 seconds = 1500 joules) are prescribed to elevate the temperature at the target to a peak voxel temperature ranging from 40°C to 45°C. With short exposure times, this temperature range theoretically does not reach the threshold at which tissue damage would occur. The thermal spot location is assessed in each orthogonal plane with two-dimensional MR thermography. If necessary, the system can electronically adjust the thermal spot to precisely match the planned target location.

During the verification stage, the acoustic energy dose is slowly escalated through an increase in power, duration, or both to elevate target temperatures moderately. Each brief sonication is then assessed with MR thermography and clinical evaluation. We have observed that neurological effects begin to manifest at temperatures in the "low 50s," most notably transient or partial tremor suppression or paresthesia during Vim thalamotomy.[30] Thermal neuromodulation in the range of 50°C to 55°C can be utilized to validate the stereotactic target. If the peak temperature deviates more than 1 mm from the planned target or symptom response helps refine the targeting, the acoustic focus can be adjusted by means of electronic steering by reprogramming of the acoustic elements. This thermal neuromodulation provides the means to personalize and optimize the treatment on the basis of clinical feedback.

Once the heating pattern has been verified to the proper location and clinical target, the acoustic energy is increased to temperatures necessary for a therapeutic ablation, typically peak voxel temperatures in the range of 55°C to 60°C (see Fig. 95-2). The typical duration of FUS heating, 10 to 20 seconds, results in a thalamic lesion analogous to that produced by RF lesioning at 70°C for 60 seconds. We are cautious about heating because microscopic hemorrhages have been observed with use of temperatures above 60°C in animal models.[15] The lesion can be assessed with T2-weighted MRI while the patient is still coupled to the US transducer. Early imaging typically shows a small area (2 to 3 mm) of T2 hyperintensity at the site of ablation and can be used to plan additional ablation, which is performed until satisfactory tremor suppression is observed.

Clinical Monitoring

During transcranial MRI-guided FUS thalamotomy for tremor, the patient is awake to allow for clinical monitoring throughout the procedure. Between sonications, the physician is able to interact with the patient to monitor his or her condition and to perform clinical assessments for somatosensory symptoms and motor performance as well as for tremor response (see Video 95-1). Resting and postural tremors are easily observed, and intention tremor can be assessed with finger-to-nose testing and/or by having the patient perform simple spiral and line drawings.

Procedural Difficulties and Troubleshooting

Head Pain during Sonication

Acute head pain that lasts only during the brief sonication is sometimes experienced during transcranial MRI-guided FUS treatments. Theoretically, pain-sensitive structures such as the dura and periosteum could be heated as high levels of acoustic energy are transmitted through the skull. If head pain occurs in the absence of cavitation, the acoustic power can be decreased and the sonication duration increased—a strategy that delivers more acoustic energy with a lower intensity that is often well tolerated by the patient. We routinely administer 1 g of intravenous (IV) acetaminophen, 25 to 50 μg of IV fentanyl, and 0.5 to 1 mg of lorazepam as prophylactic measures for US-induced head pain. We have not observed US-induced scalp burns or heating after any of our treatments.

Abnormal Heating Shape

The hemispherical US transducer produces a focal heating spot that is more elliptical in the superior-inferior plane. For thalamic ablations, the shape of the focus must be monitored to avoid inferior-lateral heating toward the posterior limb of the internal capsule.

Cavitation

As previously mentioned, one of the principal concerns with HIFU is inertial cavitation, a potentially hazardous event that may lead to uncontrolled tissue destruction and hemorrhage. The clinical US transducers have a cavitation detection system consisting of four US detectors that continuously monitor for cavitation signals throughout sonications. If cavitation is detected to exceed a threshold, the system automatically terminates the energy delivery.

Patient Movement

Throughout the procedure the patient's head is secured to the MRI table and US device by a stereotactic frame, and there is a voxel-based coordinate system within the bore of the magnet. Actual movement of the patient's head during the procedure relative to procedural imaging could potentially lead to inaccurate delivery of acoustic energy and ablations beyond the prescribed target. An image-based movement detection algorithm is performed with each sonication to assess the position of the transducer within the coordinate system of the magnet. The three principal sources of movement during the procedure are as follows: (1) shifting of the patient's head within the stereotactic frame if it is secured too loosely, (2) movement of the patient's head and frame relative to the device coupling posts, and (3) failure to properly reposition the patient to MRI isocenter after he or she has been removed from the bore of the magnet for clinical assessment or medical needs.

RESULTS

Technical Outcomes and Targeting Accuracy

Peak Temperature and Ablation

One of the technical objectives of early transcranial FUS evaluations was to determine whether US could produce an ablation in the brain (Table 95-1). Since the 2010 study by McDannold and colleagues,[14] which utilized an early-stage transducer with half the number of elements, subsequent studies have been successful in delivering acoustic energy through the intact human skull to create a thermal ablation with peak voxel temperatures ranging from 51°C to 63°C.[30,31,33] Two studies, however, have reported cases in which heating was insufficient for tissue ablation.[29,34] The investigators in those studies cited larger skull volumes as responsible for treatment failures.

MRI Characteristics and Lesion Size

According to both MRI and histologic findings, FUS lesions evolve similarly to RF ablations.[35,36] The lesions have a concentric appearance that is divided into three zones (Fig. 95-3). Zones I and II correlate with restricted diffusion on early apparent diffusion coefficient (ADC) imaging and represent the necrotic core of the lesion.[37] Zone III represents surrounding vasogenic edema, which does not image like ischemia, peaks toward the first week, and dissipates over the course of a month. Wintermark and associates[37] reported on lesion diameters in patients with tremor who were treated with FUS thalamotomy. Zone I diameters were 2.7, 4.0, and 2.1 mm at 24 hours, 1 week, and 1 month, respectively; Zone II diameters were 2.2, 1.8, and 1.2 mm at the same postoperative time points. Chang nd coworkers[29] found a similar trend in lesion volume using T1-weighted sequences, reporting mean lesion volumes of 98 mm^3, 202 mm^3, and 217 mm^3 at 24 hours, 1 week, and 1 month, respectively.

TABLE 95-1 A Summary of Pilot Studies using Transcranial Magnetic Resonance Imaging–Guided Focused Ultrasound for Thalamic Ablations

Study	Indication	Target	N
Jeanmonod et al, 2012[32]	Chronic pain	Central lateral thalamus	9
Elias et al, 2013[35]	Essential tremor	Vim	15
Lipsman et al, 2013[31]	Essential tremor	Vim	4
Chang et al, 2015[29]	Essential tremor	Vim	11
Magara et al, 2014[54]	Parkinson disease	Pallidothalamic tract	13

Vim, ventral intermediate nucleus.

Precision

Moser and colleagues[38] reported the targeting accuracy among 30 patients who underwent transcranial MRI-guided FUS treatments for a variety of neurological disorders. The investigators calculated accuracy by comparing the lesion coordinates on postoperative day 2 MRI with preoperative stereotactic atlas coordinates and found a three-dimensional global targeting accuracy of 0.99 mm. They regard real-time procedural monitoring with MR thermography as a significant factor in achievement of optimal targeting accuracy.[38] Another study reported similar millimeter accuracy except in the superior-inferior plane.[30]

Clinical Outcomes for Essential Tremor

Three pilot studies have demonstrated the feasibility of using transcranial MRI-guided FUS Vim thalamotomy for the treatment of severe, medication-refractory essential tremor (ET).[29-31] Lipsman and coworkers[31] reported 81% improvement in hand tremor at 3 months using a validated rating scale for ET. Our group reported a similar improvement of 75% in hand tremor at 1 year (Fig. 95-4) but also substantial 85% improvement in disability scores and 66% improvement in patient-reported quality of life using an ET-specific questionnaire.[30] Chang and colleagues[29] observed similar improvements in hand tremor and total Clinical Rating Scale for Tremor (CRST) scores, although there was difficulty in achieving adequate heating for ablation in 3 of the 11 patients. A randomized, double-blind controlled trial of MRI-guided FUS for essential tremor is currently under way at eight international centers.

Complications

To date, there have been no intracranial hemorrhages or procedural deaths with FUS thalamotomy. The most common reported side effects are thalamotomy-related, typically being mild or transient somatosensory or cerebellar deficits. In 15 patients with ET undergoing the procedure, we observed 9 with paresthesias

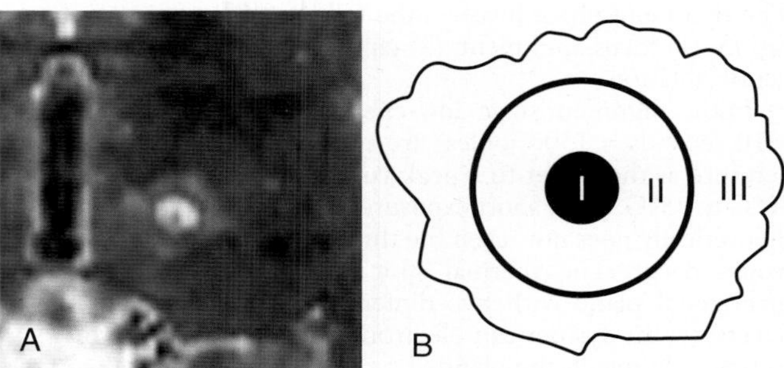

Figure 95-3. Radiographic depiction of focused ultrasound (FUS) lesion. A, Axial T2-weighted magnetic resonance image showing a FUS lesion in the ventral intermediate nucleus (Vim) of the thalamus on postoperative day 1. Note the small central hypointense core (Zone I) surrounded by a spherical hyperintensity (Zone II). Zones I and II correlate well with diffusion-weighted imaging restriction and represent the ablated tissue. Zone III correlates to vasogenic edema, which subsides in volume in 7 to 10 days. **B,** A diagram of the three zones of FUS lesions.

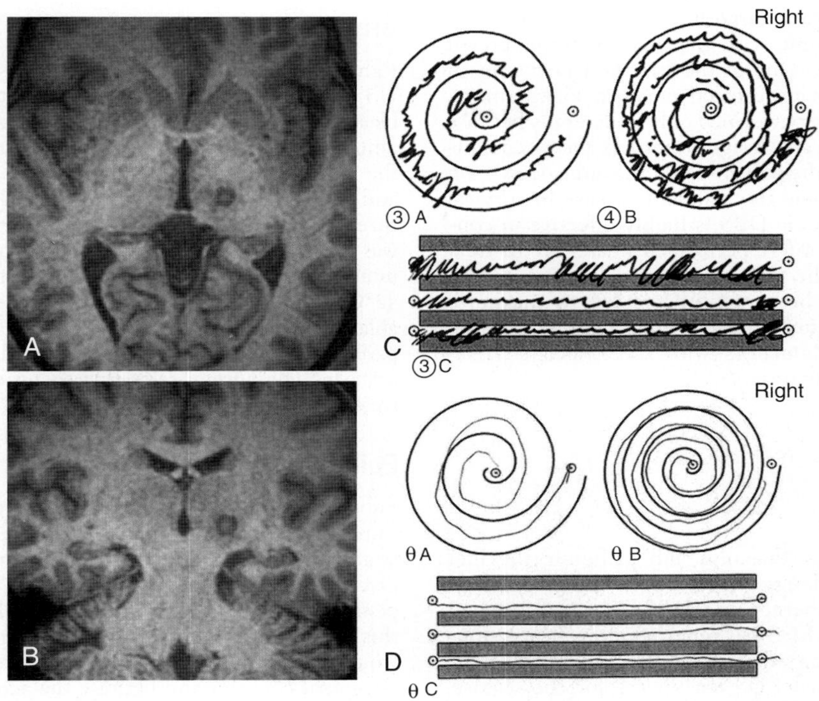

Figure 95-4. Radiographic and clinical results of ventral intermediate nucleus (Vim) thalamotomy for tremor. Axial **(A)** and coronal **(B)** T1-weighted magnetic resonance images on postoperative day 1 demonstrating a 5-mm lesion in the Vim of the thalamus with surrounding edema. Preoperative **(C)** and postoperative **(D)** spiral and line drawing samples demonstrating a dramatic reduction in tremor after thalamotomy.

TABLE 95-2 A Comparison of Thalamic Treatments for Tremor

Modality	Transcranial?	Magnetic Resonance Imaging Monitored?	Procedural Clinical Testing?	Reversible?
Radiofrequency ablation	No	No	Yes	No
Radiosurgery	Yes	No	No	No
Focused ultrasound	Yes	Yes	Yes	No
Deep brain stimulation	No	Yes/No	Yes	Yes

in the lip/tongue and 5 with paresthesias in the fingers.[30] These effects typically resolved within a month, but 3 patients reported permanent paresthesia and 1 reported a dysesthesia of the dominant index finger. Lipsman and coworkers[31] similarly noted 1 patient with persistent paresthesia at 3-month follow up. Interestingly, Chang and colleagues[29] have not reported any patients with postoperative paresthesia because they initially target the ventralis oralis posterior (Vop) nucleus. If tremor does not improve with sonications to about 50°C, they adjust the acoustic focus posteriorly until tremor is suppressed.[29] This approach limits the thermal dose to the ventroposterolateral thalamus.

We have observed cerebellar symptoms following FUS thalamotomy, with subjective "unsteadinesss" (5 of 15 patients) or objective ataxia (4 of 15 patients) resolving within 1 month.[30] Chang and colleagues[29] reported one patient whose unsteadiness resolved with oral steroids, and they attributed the symptom to medial lemniscus edema.

Several patients have reported vestibular phenomena during high-intensity sonications. Transient dizziness, falling sensation, and vertigo have been reported and may be related to vestibular activation during sonications. Head pain or heat may suggest heating of the scalp's periosteum or perhaps the dura.

COMPARISON OF TREATMENT MODALITIES FOR TREMOR

For patients with disabling, medication-refractory ET, a variety of surgical treatments are available (Table 95-2).[39-41] Radiofrequency thalamic ablation is among the oldest treatments for tremor related to Parkinson's disease or ET. RF thalamotomy is a highly effective treatment for tremor, with tremor reduction rates of 70% to 90% reported.[42-44] The procedure involves an awake, open surgery through a bur-hole craniotomy and cortical penetration to reach the thalamic target. One of the principal benefits of RF thalamotomy is target confirmation by microelectrode recording of tremor cells within the Vim and/or macroelectrode stimulation to verify tremor arrest before a complete lesion is made. The clinical benefits of RF thalamotomy are immediate and durable over time.[44] Gamma Knife radiosurgery is a transcranial method for stereotactically lesioning the thalamus that is also highly effective in reducing the symptoms of ET.[45-47] Although this procedure avoids open surgery, two of the major limitations of radiosurgical thalamotomy are that the target cannot be verified prior to permanent lesioning and that the effects of ionizing radiation mature over weeks to months.[48] Transcranial

MRI-guided FUS combines the target verification and immediate effects of RF thalamotomy with the incisionless nature of Gamma Knife thalamotomy. One of the strongest criticisms of ablative surgery in general is its destructive nature. Furthermore, thalamic ablations are usually performed only unilaterally because bilateral thalamic ablations carry a significant risk for speech difficulties after surgery. Over the past 25 years, thalamic deep brain stimulation (DBS) has become the standard of care in surgical treatment for ET.[49-53] Thalamic DBS is highly effective in controlling tremor and can be safely performed bilaterally to treat symptoms on both sides of the body as well as axial tremors. DBS is nondestructive and can be reversibly titrated to maximize symptomatic relief while minimizing side effects. DBS, however, requires expensive neurostimulators with the associated risks inherent to hardware implantation.

FUTURE DIRECTIONS

Parkinson's Disease

Stereotactic lesioning of the thalamus and pallidum, the first treatments for Parkinson's disease, have largely been supplanted by dopamine replacement therapy and DBS. The development of transcranial MRI-guided FUS has renewed interest in lesioning procedures for Parkinson's disease. Magara and associates[54] reported the first transcranial FUS treatments for the disease, performing unilateral lesioning of the pallidothalamic thalamic tract in 13 patients. The first four experienced only a 7% improvement in United Parkinson's Disease Rating Scale (UPDRS) score with a single therapeutic ablation of 83 mm^3. The next nine patients were treated with multiple sonications to the target ranging from 52°C to 59°C for a mean lesion of volume of 172 mm^3 and a 3-months UPDRS score improvement of 61%. Additional clinical trials are under way targeting the Vim thalamus for tremor-dominant Parkinson's disease, internal segment of the globus pallidum for dyskinesia, and subthalamic nucleus for medically refractory motor symptoms. FUS lesioning is unlikely to replace DBS but may provide additional treatment options in specific cases.

Neuropathic Pain

The first demonstration of human brain tissue ablation with acoustic energy delivered through the intact skull occurred during centrolateral thalamotomy for neuropathic pain syndromes. Martin and colleagues[33] treated nine patients suffering from a wide array of therapy-resistant pain syndromes: phantom limb, post-amputation pain, schwannoma, radiculopathy, brachial plexus injury, thalamic infarct, and idiopathic trigeminal neuralgia. Bilateral centrolateral thalamotomies without adverse clinical effects were created with a mean pain relief of 68% (range 30% to 100%). Jeanmonod and coworkers[32] later reported longer-term outcomes with average improvements in pain of 49% at 3 months and 57% at 1 year.

Psychiatric Disorders

In a proof-of-concept study, a small series of patients with severe and medication-refractory obsessive-compulsive disorder were treated with transcranial MRI-guided FUS capsulotomy.[34,55] Precise, bilateral ablations of the anterior limb of the internal capsule were noted in all four patients with improvements on validated rating scales of obsessive-compulsive disorder, anxiety (mean reduction of 61.1%), and depression (mean reduction of 69.4%) at 6 months.[34] Interestingly, these white matter lesions were more visible on MRI at 6 months than similar lesions made in thalamic nuclei for tremor.[55]

Brain Tumors

Ram and associates[56] were the first to use a modern, phased-array US transducer system to treat three patients with recurrent glioblastoma, but FUS was delivered through a craniectomy. Importantly, histology was available to confirm the ablated tissue and the relatively sharp penumbra of the treatment.[56] McDannold and colleagues[14] then reported the first transcranial treatment in three patients with deep-seated, recurrent gliomas. This study was the first to successfully deliver acoustic energy through the intact human cranium, achieving peak voxel temperatures of 42°C to 51°C, which were nevertheless insufficient for tissue ablation. Since these seminal preliminary studies, relatively few patients have been enrolled in clinical trials to treat glioma or metastasis because of restrictive inclusion criteria and alternative treatment options.

Epilepsy

Subcortical epilepsies such as those from hypothalamic hamartoma, periventricular nodular heterotopia, and tuberous sclerosis could be targeted for treatment because the lesions are often discrete, are visible on MRI, and reside within the central "therapeutic envelope" of current transcranial MRI -FUS systems.[57] At this early stage of FUS technology, mesial temporal sclerosis would be challenging to treat owing to the volume of the hippocampal complex and because the acoustic energy delivered to this relatively peripheral target would be partially diminished.

Neuromodulation

Perhaps the most exciting unharnessed potential for FUS is for neuromodulation and noninvasive brain mapping. US has long been known to influence the activity of electrically excitable tissues, including skeletal muscle and peripheral nerves.[58-61] In a classic experiment conducted 50 years ago, Fry and colleagues[4] sonicated the feline lateral geniculate nucleus and noted a reversible suppression of visual-evoked cortical potentials. In later studies, low-intensity focused ultrasound (LIFU) has been used in a pulsed or continuous fashion to excite neurons in rodent motor cortex to evoke a range of motor behaviors, including eye and whisker twitches, limb movements, and tail flicks.[12,13,62-64] LIFU targeting the frontal eye fields in nonhuman primates has been used to abrogate anti-saccadic eye movements.[64] In humans, LIFU targeting the primary sensory cortex decreased the amplitude of somatosensory evoked potentials from the median nerve.[65]

LIFU has many of the favorable features of HIFU, and its application in neuromodulation could be a significant breakthrough for noninvasive brain mapping. LIFU can be delivered transcranially[64,65] and can be focused to deep structures of the brain without inducing heat or tissue damage. Like HIFU it is precise, with millimeter spatial resolution.[65] Furthermore, modern HIFU systems can be adapted to deliver LIFU sonication parameters while maintaining capacity for MRI monitoring. Future coupling of LIFU with functional MRI could provide an unparalleled opportunity to study the human brain in health and disease.

CONCLUSION

Transcranial MRI-guided focused ultrasound is an emerging, experimental modality for stereotactic ablation in the brain that has been applied preliminarily in functional neurosurgery for different clinical indications. These procedures utilize real-time MRI to monitor tissue temperatures and continuous clinical assessments to ensure safety and treatment efficacy. Further technical advances in transcranial ultrasound delivery will likely lead to new frontiers in noninvasive brain mapping and less invasive treatments for neurological and psychiatric disease.

SUGGESTED READINGS

Elias WJ, Huss D, Voss T, et al. A pilot study of focused ultrasound thalamotomy for essential tremor. *N Engl J Med*. 2013;369:640-648.

Jung HH, Kim SJ, Roh D, et al. Bilateral thermal capsulotomy with MR-guided focused ultrasound for patients with treatment-refractory obsessive-compulsive disorder: a proof-of-concept study. *Mol Psychiatry*. 2015;20:1205-1211.

Legon W, Sato TF, Opitz A, et al. Transcranial focused ultrasound modulates the activity of primary somatosensory cortex in humans. *Nat Neurosci*. 2014;17:322-329.

McDannold N, Vykhodtseva N, Jolesz FA, et al. MRI investigation of the threshold for thermally induced blood-brain barrier disruption and brain tissue damage in the rabbit brain. *Magn Reson Med*. 2004;51:913-923.

Meyers R, Fry WJ, Fry FJ, et al. Early experiences with ultrasonic irradiation of the pallidofugal and nigral complexes in hyperkinetic and hypertonic disorders. *J Neurosurg*. 1959;16:32-54.

Ram Z, Cohen ZR, Harnof S, et al. Magnetic resonance imaging-guided, high-intensity focused ultrasound for brain tumor therapy. *Neurosurgery*. 2006;59:949-955, discussion 955-946.

Sapareto SA, Dewey WC. Thermal dose determination in cancer therapy. *Int J Radiat Oncol Biol Phys*. 1984;10:787-800.

See a full reference list on ExpertConsult.com 

96 Selective Peripheral Denervation for Cervical Dystonia

Joachim K. Krauss

Surgical treatment of cervical dystonia (CD) has experienced unprecedented attention over the last decade. Pallidal deep brain stimulation (DBS) was introduced in the late 1990s, initially to treat those patients with medical refractory CD who were considered not to be ideal candidates for peripheral surgery, but it has gradually become the mainstay of surgical treatment in most Western countries.[1-4] In many places, selective peripheral denervation is rarely performed nowadays despite its proven efficacy, and it is not being recommended as second-line treatment any longer once the response to botulinum toxin injection does not yield optimal benefit.[5] At the same time, however, new data on larger study populations have become available from China and South Korea.[6,7] Given the increased recognition of the mild yet not uncommon bradykinetic side effects of pallidal DBS in patients with CD, selective peripheral denervation still holds great potential for future management of CD.[8,9]

Selective peripheral denervation requires a special expertise not only in surgical technique but also in the phenomenologic differential diagnosis of CD.[10] *Selective peripheral denervation* originally was coined by Bertrand,[11] who made the procedure popular in the 1970s. It consists of sectioning of the peripheral branch of the spinal accessory nerve to the sternocleidomastoid muscle combined with posterior ramisectomy from C1 to C6. There are several modifications of the technique, and it often has been combined with targeted myotomies. In experienced hands it is a safe procedure with minimal and infrequent side effects.

CLINICAL AND PHENOMENOLOGIC ASPECTS OF CERVICAL DYSTONIA

Cervical dystonia is used consistently nowadays, and it has ousted *spasmodic torticollis* for several reasons: few patients present with simple turning of the head; the abnormal movement is not always spasmodic; and, most importantly, nondystonic neck postures are called *torticollis* as well.[10,12] Dystonia has now been redefined as a movement disorder characterized by sustained or intermittent muscle contractions, causing abnormal, often repetitive, movements, postures, or both.[13] CD affects predominantly the neck, including the anterior and posterior neck muscles.[14] In some patients, the shoulder is involved as well with protraction or elevation of the shoulder. In a subset of patients, CD is a feature of more widespread segmental dystonia involving also muscles of the face, the larynx, or the upper extremities. Frequently, there are also tremulous or jerking movements of the head. Dystonic tremor, which is more irregular than essential tremor, is most evident when the patient attempts to move the head in the direction contralateral to the force of the dystonia. Most frequently, CD is accompanied by neck pain, which may be severe and may lead to further incapacitation of the patient. In many instances patients employ a "sensory trick" such as touching the chin, holding the neck, or other maneuver, to decrease the dystonic activity. Such tricks are also called *gestes antanogistiques*.

Cervical dystonia is the most common form of focal dystonia.[12,14] Its prevalence has been estimated to range between 5 and 13 per 10,000 people in Western countries. The mean age at onset is 41 years, and as with other forms of focal dystonia, there is a slight female preponderance (about 1.2 : 1). In the vast majority of patients with CD, no underlying cause can be identified, although in a few instances various genetic defects have been identified. Until recently, both manifestations would have been referred to as *primary* dystonia but with regard to the reclassification of dystonia, *idiopathic* and *inherited* would be appropriate, respectively.[13] *Acquired dystonia* has been suggested to be used instead of *secondary dystonia*, in the rare case of CD caused by trauma or exposure to neuroleptic drugs.

Various basic patterns of CD have been defined according to the position of the patient's head.[12,14] *Torticollis* indicates rotation of the head about the head-body-axis (movement of the chin toward one shoulder in the horizontal plane); *laterocollis* is defined as a sideward tilt of the head (movement of the ear toward the ipsilateral shoulder); *anterocollis* is defined as flexion of the neck in the anterior-posterior-axis; and *retrocollis* is defined as extension in the anterior-posterior axis. *Lateral shift* depicts translation of the axis of the head in the horizontal plane, and *sagittal shift* in the sagittal plane. Commonly, a combination of these abnormalities is present, depending on the degree of involvement of different cervical muscles (Fig. 96-1). It is important to understand which muscles are involved and causing the dystonic posture or movements in an individual patient. This issue is even more important when a decision has to be made about which muscles should be denervated, because in a given patient, dystonic activity may vary in different muscles yet produce the same dystonic posture.[15]

The differential diagnosis of CD includes a variety of nondystonic disorders.[12,14] Pseudodystonia may be caused by atlantoaxial dislocation, degenerative disk disease, Klippel-Feil syndrome, pediatric posterior fossa tumors, trochlear palsy, Sandifer's syndrome, and various other disorders. More systemic basal ganglia disorders must be excluded in patients with onset of CD at a young age. In untreated or undertreated CD, persistent dystonic postures may result in accelerated degenerative cervical spine disease, manifesting as cervical myelopathy or radiculopathy.[16] Rarely, dystonic postures may even lead to permanent fixed deformities secondary to ossification of spinal ligaments or facet joints.[17,18]

The first-line treatment of CD is chemodenervation with botulinum toxin type A.[12,14,18] The dose and the sites of injection must be individualized to obtain optimal results. The efficacy and safety of botulinum toxin have been demonstrated in several randomized controlled and open trials. Most of these studies report improvement in about 90% of patients with CD, mild side effects occurring in up to 28%. The effect of botulinum toxin is usually noted about 1 week after injection, and the average duration of the benefit is 3 to 4 months. In patients whose CD is resistant to botulinum toxin A, botulinum toxin type B and other newer preparations have become alternatives. It has to be noted, however, that the average duration of maximum improvement is much shorter, side effects are more frequent, and immunogenicity is higher with botulinum toxin B. Pharmacotherapy for CD includes mainly anticholinergic drugs or muscle relaxants. Overall, drug treatment plays a minor role in CD, although many patients also take analgesics for alleviation of chronic neck pain.

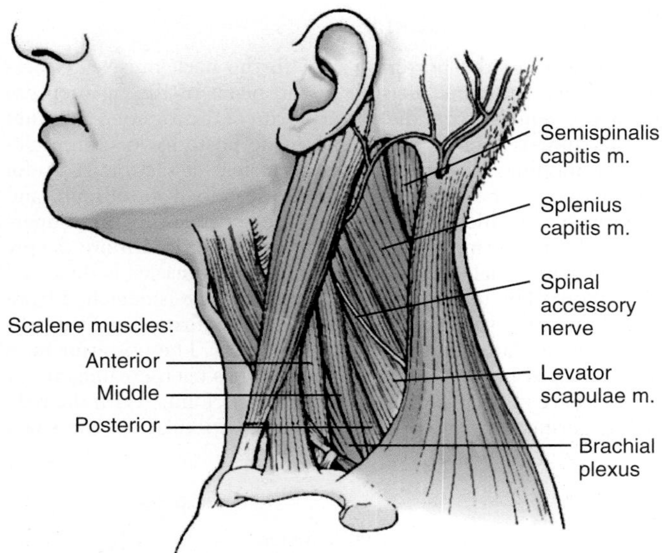

Figure 96-1. Cervical muscles frequently involved in cervical dystonia. m, muscle. *(Redrawn from Brin MF, Jankovic J, Comella C, et al. Treatment of dystonia using botulinum toxin. In: Kurlan R, ed.* Treatment of Movement Disorders. *Philadelphia: Lippincott Williams & Wilkins; 1995:183-246.)*

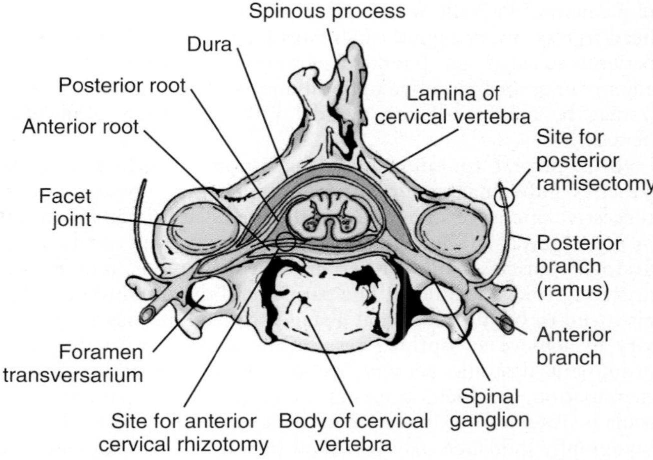

Figure 96-2. Anatomy of anterior cervical rhizotomy (intradural approach) and posterior ramisectomy (extradural approach). *(Redrawn from Krauss JK, Grossman RG, Jankovic J. Treatment options for surgery of cervical dystonia. In: Krauss JK, Jankovic J, Grossman RG, eds.* Surgery for Parkinson's Disease and Movement Disorders. *Philadelphia: Lippincott Williams & Wilkins; 2001:323-334.)*

EVOLUTION OF SURGICAL TECHNIQUES

Surgical treatment for CD has a long history, dating back to ancient Greece.[10,19] Myotomies of the sternocleidomastoid muscles were performed as early as 1641, and denervation of cervical muscles was achieved by 1834. Intradural procedures initially targeted sectioning of the posterior cervical nerve roots, but attention soon shifted to the anterior roots. McKenzie developed intradural rhizotomy of the anterior upper cervical roots in combination with sectioning of the intradural spinal accessory nerve in the 1920s. Soon thereafter, Dandy, as well as Hamby and Schiffer,[20] refined this procedure further. Until the early 1990s, upper cervical rhizotomies and spinal accessory nerve sectioning were the most common surgical procedures for CD.[21,22] Because this "standard" procedure, however, was rather nonselective and because it was accompanied by frequent side effects with sometimes devastating complications, modifications were elaborated with the aim of denervating dystonic muscles exclusively and preserving normal activity. In different series, however, reported results and also complications were highly variable. Most studies claimed useful postoperative improvement in 60% to 90% of patients, but it was unclear to what extent symptomatic amelioration of abnormal postures or movements translated into improvement in functional disability, in particular regarding the high number of side effects.[20-23] Weak or unstable neck was estimated to occur in up to 40% of patients after bilateral rhizotomy, and transient dysphagia was noted in up to 30%.[21] Better results with fewer side effects were seen with selective approaches targeting only those nerves supplying clearly dystonic muscles and with staging of the procedure.[24]

Microvascular decompression of the spinal accessory nerve has been attempted in a limited number of patients, on the basis of the erroneous assumption that CD would be caused by vascular compression of the spinal accessory nerve, analogous with other cranial neuropathies such as hemifacial spasm and trigeminal neuralgia. Pathophysiologic concepts did not support microvascular decompression as a valid treatment option for CD and the outcome data were ambiguous, so microvascular decompression was abandoned, and it is not considered a useful treatment option for CD any longer.[10,18]

When Bertrand introduced selective peripheral denervation, combining posterior ramisectomy with spinal accessory nerve sectioning, he demonstrated that this innovative concept was much more selective than the earlier intradural procedures, produced better outcomes, and resulted in a much lower frequency of side effects.[11,25] The most outstanding advantage of selective peripheral denervation over intradural rhizotomy certainly is that it is an extradural as well as an extraspinal procedure (Fig. 96-2). Rhizotomy could approach only the nerve roots from C1 to C3 bilaterally or from C1 to C4 on one side, but ramisectomy can be performed down from C1 to C6, either on one side or bilaterally, in the same session. When selective ramisectomy and peripheral denervation became increasingly popular, sometimes in combination with myotomy, rhizotomy was abandoned almost completely.[26-33] With regard to its rather unfavorable risk-benefit profile, intradural rhizotomy now is considered obsolete.

SELECTIVE PERIPHERAL DENERVATION: INDICATIONS AND PATIENT SELECTION

Until recently, selective peripheral denervation was considered second-line treatment in patients with CD in whom satisfactory benefit is not achieved with medical treatment or repeated botulinum toxin injections, and pallidal DBS either was recommended as third-line treatment only or was reserved for those in whom selective peripheral denervation was not feasible.[2,18] This concept, however, has been challenged, and many patients now are referred directly for DBS.[4,5]

It has been estimated that primary nonresponse to botulinum toxin injections occurs in 6% to 14% of patients with CD.[14,34] In general, immunoresistance to botulinum toxin may develop in about 3% to 10% of patients during long-term treatment. Although newer botulinum toxin preparations tend to be less immunogenic, antibody-induced failure of therapy with botulinum toxin B has been described even at a rate of 44%.[12] Patients with predominantly tonic dystonia are better candidates for selective peripheral denervation than those with prominent phasic movements.[2] Patients with marked myoclonus or with dystonic head tremor are not good candidates for the procedure. In some patients selective peripheral denervation may also serve as an adjunct or as an alternative to botulinum toxin injection. Likewise it may be combined with pallidal DBS to achieve additional benefit.[6,35]

It is pivotal to tailor the denervation procedure to each patient's individual pattern of CD, which may involve several successive operative steps and also the use of additional myotomy or myectomy.[24,36] The primary goal is to selectively weaken the dystonic muscles while preserving normal muscle function in order to avoid side effects. The patient and the treating neurologist need to be informed that a staged procedure may be necessary to achieve an optimal result. The muscles with the most prominent dystonic activity are usually identified by clinical examination, in which observing the pattern of the patient's dystonia is observed and the affected muscles are palpated. Electromyography guidance may be useful in some cases.[37] In addition to the muscles most commonly involved in CD (sternocleidomastoid, trapezius, splenius, and semispinalis muscles), muscles such as the levator scapulae, scalene, longus colli, and paraspinal erector trunci muscles should be investigated.

Because the operative approach is tailored to each patient's pattern of dystonia, the specific procedures may vary. For example, in a patient with *torticollis* with rotation of the head to the right side, the combined procedure would include ipsilateral posterior ramisectomy and contralateral selective peripheral sternocleidomastoid muscle denervation, possibly combined with myotomy or myectomy of the sternocleidomastoid muscle. In a patient with *retrocollis*, bilateral posterior ramisectomy, eventually combined with muscle sectioning of posterior neck muscles, would be most useful.

OPERATIVE TECHNIQUES

Patients undergo general anesthesia. Since its introduction by Bertrand, there have been several modifications of the original technique.[27,28,30,32] When the patient is positioned in a semisitting position with the head fixed in a Mayfield head holder, both the site for posterior ramisectomy and the site for sternocleidomastoid denervation can be draped in the same session. However, because of the danger of air embolism, most neurosurgeons prefer to perform the ramisectomy with the patient in the prone position and sternocleidomastoid denervation after the patient is placed in the supine position.[32]

Denervation of the Sternocleidomastoid Muscle

First, the contours of the sternocleidomastoid muscle are outlined. A 5-cm skin incision is made at the muscle's posterior margin in its upper medial aspect. Great care is taken not to injure the greater auricular nerve, which crosses the operative field, to avoid postoperative hypesthesia of the earlobe. Then the trapezius branch of the spinal accessory nerve is identified in the lateral neck triangle. Following the trapezius branch, the main trunk of the spinal accessory nerve is reached. All branches to the sternocleidomastoid muscles are identified by electrical stimulation and then sectioned and resected. Small nerve fibers that may branch off from the trapezius branch of the spinal accessory nerve to supply the sternocleidomastoid muscle are carefully sought and sectioned as well. When the underside of the sternocleidomastoid muscle is elevated, further branches supplying the caudal portion of the muscle may be detected in addition. Because the sternocleidomastoid muscle may also be innervated by branches of spinal nerves C1 and C2, I usually complete the procedure with a myotomy and partial myectomy of the muscle within its fascia. The wound is closed with an intracutaneous suture to obtain a good cosmetic result.

Posterior Ramisectomy

Denervation of the posterior rami to the neck muscles is performed via a midline incision in the plane of the ligamentum nuchae, extending from the posterior rim of the foramen magnum to the spinous process of C6. Then the posterior neck muscles can be mobilized laterally by subperiosteal dissection. A useful alternative is the technical variant described by Braun and Richter,[26,27] in which the cleavage plane between the more superficially located semispinalis capitis muscle and the more deeply located semispinalis cervicis and multifidus muscles is dissected (Fig. 96-3). The inferior oblique capitis muscle is detached from its origin at the spinous process of C2. The dissection then proceeds further laterally to the articular facets. The posterior rami are identified in the cleavage plane that has been created, at the point where they emerge lateral to the facet joints. With the help of the surgical microscope and electrical stimulation, the small

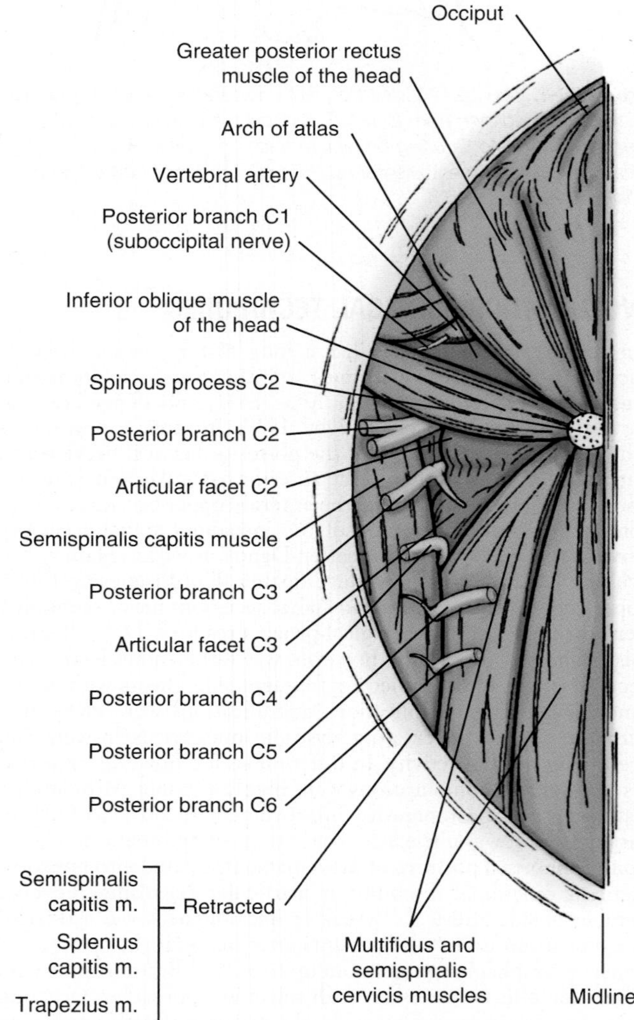

Figure 96-3. Topography of the approach to posterior ramisectomy. The posterior branches of C1-C6 can be reached within the natural cleavage plane between the more superficial semispinalis capitis muscle and the deeper multifidus and semispinalis cervicis muscles. m., muscle. *(Redrawn from Braun V, Richter HP. Selective peripheral denervation and posterior ramisectomy in cervical dystonia. In: Krauss JK, Jankovic J, Grossman RG, eds.* Surgery for Parkinson's Disease and Movement Disorders. *Philadelphia: Lippincott Williams & Wilkins; 2001:335-342.)*

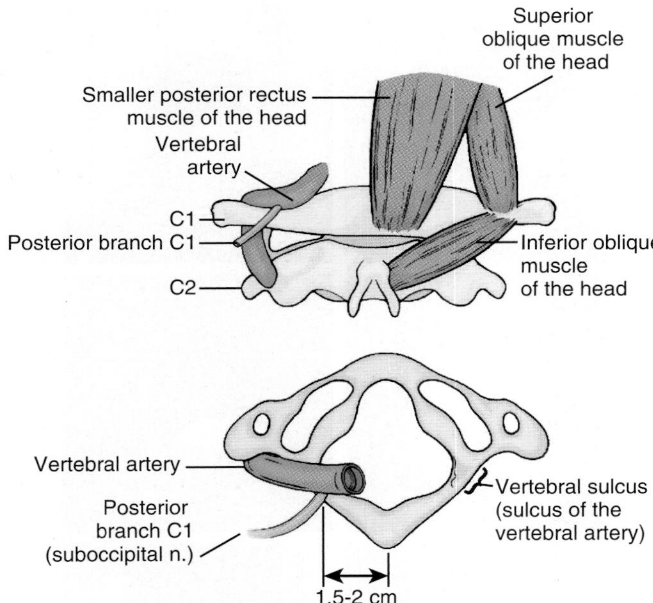

Figure 96-4. Topography of the approach to C1 and the vertebral artery. The C1 branch is located between the vertebral artery and the arch of the atlas in the region of its vertebral sulcus about 1.5 to 2 cm from the midline. n., nerve. *(Redrawn from Braun V, Richter HP. Selective peripheral denervation and posterior ramisectomy in cervical dystonia. In: Krauss JK, Jankovic J, Grossman RG, eds.* Surgery for Parkinson's Disease and Movement Disorders. *Philadelphia: Lippincott Williams & Wilkins; 2001:335-342.)*

posterior branches from C3 to C6 are identified. Electrical stimulation at this point may elicit strong muscle contractions of the posterior neck muscles. After the main branches have been identified, they are sectioned and resected.

It is also important to identify smaller nerve branches to the multifidus, splenius, and semispinalis muscles. The C3 and C4 posterior rami are usually identified easily; however, the C5 and C6 rami may be more difficult to find because of their small size. The C2 ganglion is located just above the arch of the axis. It is embedded in a rich venous plexus, which will require hemostasis with bipolar coagulation, absorbable hemostat (Surgicel), and sometimes wax. Once the C2 ganglion has been dissected, both the ventral and dorsal rami and the anterior and posterior nerve roots can all be identified extradurally. At this point, either the sectioning of the greater occipital nerve or a C2 ganglionectomy can be performed. The latter has become my preferred method. Because the greater occipital nerve is formed by the posterior C2 ramus, most patients experience hypesthesia in the distribution of this nerve, which generally, however, causes little discomfort.[38] The most difficult branch to find is the posterior branch of C1, the suboccipital nerve (Fig. 96-4). It is located between the arch of the atlas and the vertebral artery in the sulcus of the vertebral artery, where bleeding may occur from the venous plexus of the vertebral artery. Finally, electrical stimulation is used to identify any remaining tiny nerve branches, which will be sectioned and resected. If required, ramisectomy can be performed then on the contralateral side within the same operative session. A drain is placed before the wound is closed.

Myotomy and Partial Myectomy Technique

In general, myotomies or myectomies are currently used only as adjuncts to selective peripheral denervation.[36] Among early case series, benefits were described with various occasionally extensive procedures.[23,39-41] Selective myotomies or myectomies are useful when dystonic activity spreads to other muscles beyond the posterior neck muscles and the sternocleidomastoid muscle. Myotomies and partial myectomies are indicated particularly if there is pronounced dystonic activity in the scalene muscles, the levator scapulae, the omohyoid, and also in the trapezius muscle. Denervation of the trapezius muscle is not advised because it would render the patient unable to elevate the arm above the horizontal plane. An asleep-awake-asleep operative technique for selective partial myectomy of the trapezius has been described.[36]

The procedure starts with outlining of the contours of the dystonic muscles to be sectioned while the patient is awake. General anesthesia is induced with short-acting muscle relaxants. The skin incision depends on the muscles to be sectioned and on cosmetic considerations. During dissection of subcutaneous tissue, great care is taken to preserve all sensory nerve branches. Fine motor nerve branches are identified by electrical stimulation to elicit contractions in the corresponding muscles. Electrical stimulation is also used to identify and avoid branches of the brachial plexus during myectomies of the scalene muscles. When the targeted muscle is identified, its belly is cut transversally with either monopolar cautery or scissors until the posterior sleeve of the fascia is reached. The stumps are then resected approximately 3 cm along the longitudinal muscle axis. We use absorbable hemostat to fill the gap. The filling material can be soaked in a local anesthetic such as bupivacaine to provide better postoperative pain relief. The wounds are closed with intracutaneous sutures.

Variants and Combined Techniques

Over the decades several variants of the original Bertrand technique were developed, some of which also combine rhizotomy and ramisectomy procedures. One variant, for example is the technique of Taira, who combines intradural anterior rhizotomy of C1 and C2 with a standard posterior ramisectomy of the lower segments.[42,43]

The levator scapulae muscle, which is frequently involved in laterocollis, may be denervated selectively as an addition to posterior ramisectomy instead of myotomy.[29,44]

Although the primary goal of selective peripheral denervation is to improve the patient's dystonic head position, it may also be used in fixed deformity due to ossification of joins and ligaments from long-standing CD.[45,17] The patient with such a deformity may benefit from the lower level of pain subsequent to reduction of dystonic muscular activity, although there will be no change in the head position.

CLINICAL OUTCOME: RESULTS AND SIDE EFFECTS

The efficacy of peripheral selective denervation has been demonstrated by many studies since its inception in the 1970s.[6,7,11,24-28,30-32,42,46-50] The proportion of patients who benefit and the degree of improvement, however, vary greatly. One of the factors contributing to this variability is how the outcome has been quantified. In the majority of studies, a favorably low risk-benefit ratio has been demonstrated. Although there were few reports on outcome during the past decade, new data from larger series have now become available.[6,7,50]

Both clinical improvement and reduced disability have been reported in 70% to 90% of patients in most series. The degree of improvement, however, has shown wide variability. Braun and Richter[26,28] reported that in 112 consecutive patients who underwent surgery, 14% had complete relief of symptoms, 33% had marked improvement, 24% had moderate improvement, and 31% had minimal or no improvement. In this series, outcome was closely correlated with the response to botulinum toxin injections before surgery. In summary, 83% of patients who had secondary nonresponses to botulinum toxin injections had satisfying outcomes after surgery, whereas only 50% of those with primary nonresponses considered their postoperative result beneficial. Cohen-Gadol and colleagues[30] reported that 70% of their 130 patients achieved moderate to excellent amelioration of head position and pain at a mean follow-up of 3.5 years after selective peripheral denervation. In a smaller study by Ford and colleagues,[31] the response was less robust at a mean follow-up of 5 years after surgery; lasting improvement was reported in approximately one third of patients, with an average 30% reduction in dystonia. An important observation was made by Chawda and associates,[16] who noticed that those patients with CD and more signs of degenerative cervical spondylosis had less beneficial responses to selective denervation than patients without such changes. Bergenheim and collaborators[50] reported that a mean of 45% postoperative improvement in dystonia was achieved on the Tsui rating scale at a mean long-term follow-up of 42 months. This was paralleled by long-term improvements in pain and quality of life. The largest study on peripheral denervation, published by Wang and colleagues[7] from China, included a total of 648 patients.[7] Scores on the Toronto Western Spasmodic Torticollis Rating Scale (TWSTRS) was improved by 73% at a mean follow-up of 33 months postoperatively in this study.

Complications from selective peripheral denervation, in general, are rare and mostly transient. Denervation of C2 invariably causes numbness in the territory of the greater occipital nerve in the early postoperative period, but this is almost always well tolerated.[38] Patients should be informed about the procedure-related numbness when informed consent is obtained. The development of neuropathic pain has been reported only in rare circumstances.[47] Some studies have reported transient swallowing difficulties, which, however, did not cause disability.[51] About 1% to 2% of patients may experience weakness in nondystonic muscles, particularly in the trapezius muscle when the trapezius branch of the spinal accessory nerve is injured.[27] Rarely, patients suffer prolonged pain after myectomy. No instances of head or neck instability have been reported.

My colleagues and I[24] showed earlier that the benefit derived from selective denervation procedures for CD correlates with the number of operative procedures performed in an individual patient.[24] Therefore, if the clinical outcome after the first denervation procedure is less than expected, a second or sometimes even a third procedure should be considered (Fig. 96-5). Such an approach also lessens the risk of dysphagia, which may occur when extensive denervation procedures are performed in one surgical session. Furthermore, staged denervation procedures take into account that reinnervation can occur and that a particular head position may be generated by the activity of different muscles at different times (Video 96-1).

Recommendations on the use of selective peripheral denervation derived from systematic reviews or from structured guidelines are limited. In August 2004, the National Institute for Clinical Excellence in the United Kingdom provided guidelines for selective peripheral denervation in CD.[47] There has been no update yet. In addition, the results of selective peripheral denervation were analyzed for a systematic review provided by a task force of the European Federation of Neurological Societies.[5,18] According to these task force reports, selective peripheral denervation has been recommended as a safe procedure with infrequent and minimal side effects that is indicated exclusively in CD (level C). Although the procedure was recommended second-line treatment for CD in 2006, this was no longer the case in the updated recommendations in 2011, with the increasing recognition of the potentials of pallidal DBS in CD.

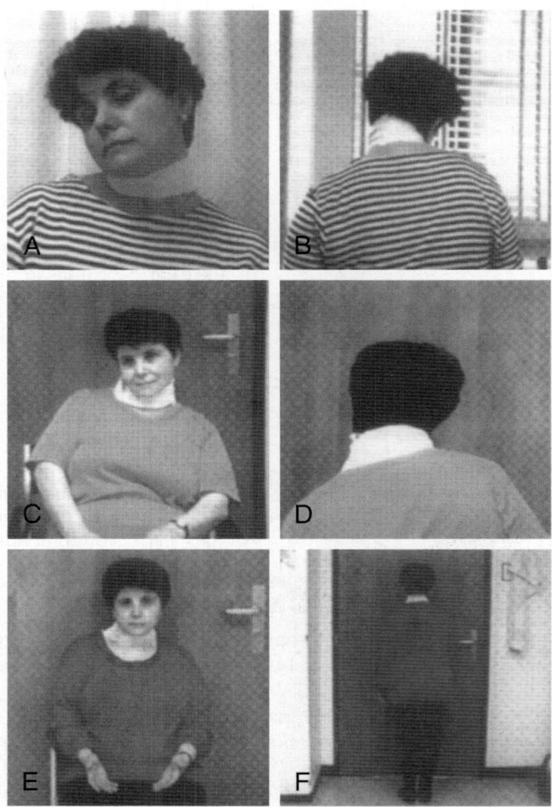

Figure 96-5. Video stills of a 44-year-old woman with cervical dystonia preoperatively and at postoperative assessments after combined peripheral denervation and myotomy-myectomy performed in two stages. The patient is wearing a scarf to allow a blinded evaluation of the videotapes. **A** and **B,** Preoperatively, there is rotation of the head to the right, tilting of the head to the right side, and dystonic elevation and anteversion of the right shoulder. **C** and **D,** Three months after posterior ramisectomy from C1 to C6 on the right side and peripheral denervation combined with myotomy and partial myectomy of the left sternocleidomastoid muscle, the patient shows marked improvement of the head rotation. However, there is still tilting of the head and dystonic shoulder elevation. **E** and **F,** The patient is shown 2 years after the first procedure and 1 year after the second, which consisted of myotomy-myectomy of the right levator scapulae and splenius capitis muscles and partial myotomy-myectomy of the right trapezius muscle with an asleep-awake-asleep anesthesia technique. The video itself is available online as Video 96-1. *(From Krauss JK, Grossman RG, Jankovic J. Treatment options for surgery of cervical dystonia. In: Krauss JK, Jankovic J, Grossman RG, eds.* Surgery for Parkinson's Disease and Movement Disorders. *Philadelphia: Lippincott Williams & Wilkins; 2001:323-334.)*

FUTURE CONCEPTS

Currently there are surgical alternatives for treatment of CD.[2-4,49,50,52] In particular, pallidal DBS has gained widespread acceptance worldwide, and this method is being increasingly considered as second-line treatment for patients with CD who do not have a satisfying response to botulinum toxin injections.[4] When we introduced pallidal DBS for treatment of CD in the late 1990s, DBS was thought to be indicated for those patients with "complex" CD (marked translation of the head in the sagittal or lateral axis in relation to the trunk, prominent retrocollis or anterocollis or continuous phasic dystonic movements and dystonic head tremor).[1] Over the following years, however, bilateral pallidal DBS has become an accepted treatment for CD in general. Most studies report about 60% improvement of dystonia, pain, and disability on average, with severe complications being rare.[3] Long-term outcome data have become available showing persistent or even progressive improvement over time.[3] The efficacy of pallidal DBS was also confirmed in a randomized controlled double-blind study including sham stimulation over a period of 3 months after electrode implantation.[4]

As mentioned previously, selective peripheral denervation is not indicated for patients with marked dystonic head tremor or prominent myclonic movements. In this subset of patients, thalamic DBS has been shown to provide beneficial outcome and might even be preferred over pallidal DBS.[53]

Overall the benefit derived from bilateral pallidal DBS appears to be larger than that obtained from selective peripheral denervation. Thus far, however, there are no prospective comparative studies on this subject, and one must keep in mind that the indications for the two procedures differ in several aspects. Two retrospective studies have provided partially contradictory results. Although patients with CD faired better with pallidal DBS than with peripheral denervation in a study from the Netherlands, no statistical differences were seen in outcome or side effects in a study from South Korea.[48,49]

Capelle and associates[35] showed that patients who had previous peripheral denervation can expect additional improvement in dystonia with pallidal DBS similar to that in patients who did not have surgery before.[35] Likewise, patients who had pallidal DBS with only partial benefit might achieve further improvement after additional peripheral denervation. Chung and colleagues[6] have suggested that a combination of the two procedures be considered in the treatment of those patients who do not have appropriate benefit after their first surgical procedure.[6]

Although pallidal DBS, in general, is well tolerated and has few disabling side effects, it may cause bradykinetic symptoms, which most often are clinically asymptomatic but which nevertheless may manifest as freezing or mild parkinsonism in some patients.[8,9] Given the lower overall procedure-related cost, and with consideration of the need for future battery replacements in DBS and the low risk-benefit profile of peripheral denervation, the latter procedure still remains an attractive option, and we might well see a future renaissance. It is important to preserve and pass on the surgical expertise and experience gained with this elaborate surgical technique.

SUGGESTED READINGS

Bergenheim AT, Nordh E, Larsson E, et al. Selective peripheral denervation for cervical dystonia: long-term follow-up. *J Neurol Neurosurg Psychiatry*. 2015;86:1307-1313.

Bertrand CM. Selective peripheral denervation for spasmodic torticollis: surgical technique, results, and observations in 260 cases. *Surg Neurol*. 1993;40:96-103.

Braun V, Richter HP. Selective peripheral denervation for the treatment of spasmodic torticollis. *Neurosurgery*. 1994;35:58-62.

Krauss JK, Toups EG, Jankovic J, et al. Symptomatic and functional outcome of surgical treatment of cervical dystonia. *J Neurol Neurosurg Psychiatry*. 1997;63:642-648.

Münchau A, Palmer JD, Dressler D, et al. Prospective study of selective peripheral denervation for botulinum-toxin resistant patients with cervical dystonia. *Brain*. 2001;124:769-783.

Wang J, Li J, Han L, et al. Selective peripheral denervation for the treatment of spasmodic torticollis: long-term follow-up results from 648 patients. *Acta Neurochir*. 2015;157:427-433.

See a full reference list on ExpertConsult.com

97 Thalamotomy for Focal Hand Dystonia

Takaomi Taira, Takeshi Nakajima, Taku Ochiai, and Shiro Horisawa

Dystonia was first defined as a neurological disorder characterized by sustained involuntary twisting movements and postures.[1] However, the disorder is heterogeneous and has many different clinical manifestations. Recently the definition of dystonia was revised to cover a wider range of dystonias. In this newly proposed definition, dystonia is classified as a movement disorder characterized by sustained or intermittent muscle contractions causing abnormal, often repetitive movements, postures, or both. Dystonic movements are typically patterned and twisting and may be tremulous. Dystonia is often initiated or worsened by voluntary action and associated with overflow muscle activation.[2] When dystonic symptoms are confined to the hand, the condition is known as *focal hand dystonia* (FHD), and its symptoms are task specific in most patients. The most common type of FHD is writer's cramp, in which finger or wrist movements are impaired with dystonic symptoms only when writing. Instrumental musicians may suffer from a type of FHD that appears only when playing. This condition, known as *musician's dystonia*, has a much greater prevalence than other types of FHD, exhibits task specificity at the level of specific musical passages, and is particularly difficult to treat. Approximately 1% of musicians develop FHD, a rate about 10 times greater than for nonmusicians.[3,4] The incidence of FHD is much higher (20 to 70 per 1 million) than that of primary generalized dystonia.[5] Although FHD can be an initial symptom of segmental or generalized dystonia, it usually does not spread to other body sites. Treatment of task-specific FHD (TSFHD) is extremely difficult. Medical treatment, such as use of benzodiazepines and anticholinergic drugs, is generally ineffective. Botulinum toxin injections may be indicated as a treatment for FHD, but many patients are not satisfied with such conservative treatment, especially when the symptoms disturb their professional activities. Nonmedical interventions, such as transcranial direct current stimulation and retraining, have been reported, but their effects are not long lasting.[6]

We routinely treat TSFHD patients with stereotactic ablation of the ventro-oralis (Vo) nucleus of the thalamus (Vo thalamotomy). The effect is immediate during the operation and remains for a sustained period of time. Although this is an invasive treatment requiring highly sophisticated techniques and involving surgical risk, marked improvement or even disappearance of TSFHD seems possible with such an approach.

HISTORY

Writer's cramp was first reported by Charles Bell in 1833. Bell reported, "I have found the action necessary for writing gone, whilst the power of strongly moving the arm, or fencing, remained," and he termed the condition "scrivener's palsy."[7] Bell likely employed the term "palsy" to express "movement disorder" rather than "motor weakness." In 1888 a British neurologist, William Gowers, referred to the condition as "occupational neurosis."[8] This may have been the beginning of the confusion between neurological and psychogenic origins of writer's cramp: neurosis in German medicine at this time meant neurotic psychosis, and German medicine had a strong influence on that of other countries. Gowers, however, used "neurosis" to mean neurological disorders. Since then, there have been extensive discussions on the genesis of writer's cramp. A French neurologist, Guillaume-Benjamin-Amand Duchenne,[9] in 1861 wrote, "I must confess that I am unable to solve this important problem. However, rationally, I believe that this disorder is the result of central nervous system disorder. This disorder is serious, as it resists all forms of treatment, even faradic treatment." The modern concept of dystonia was not present until Oppenheim proposed the term "dystonia musculorum deformans" in 1911,[10] which is today's DYT1 generalized dystonia. In the 1960s and 1970s, Irving Cooper[11,12] found that some patients with dystonia musculorum deformans had a history of writer's cramp as an initial symptom, and he suggested that writer's cramp may be a type of dystonia.

In 1982, Sheehy and Marsden[13] reported their results of a comparison between patients with and those without writer's cramp. There was no difference in psychogenic factors between the groups, and Sheehy and Marsden concluded that writer's cramp was a physical illness rather than a psychological disturbance and that it was in fact a focal dystonia. Thus the concept of writer's cramp as an FHD was finally established in the early 1980s when most functional stereotactic surgeries were declining, and several articles appeared reporting disappointing results in the treatment of dystonia with thalamotomy. Surgery for dystonia in those days was not for FHD but rather was for more widespread, generalized dystonias. A large series of Cooper's thalamotomy and pallidotomy procedures for dystonia in the 1960s was conducted before the concept of FHD had been established. Since then, there have been many reports supporting the proposition that writer's cramp and musician's cramp are not psychogenic but neurological disorders.[14-18]

Before the turn of this century, there had been few reports on neurosurgical treatment of FHD. Siegfried and colleagues[19] reported a case of cure of tremulous writer's cramp by stereotactic thalamotomy in 1969. This case was probably one of tremor-dominant FHD that is occasionally seen in FHD patients. Mempel and associates[20] reported successful results of cryothalamotomy for writer's cramp syndrome in 1986 in the Polish language. Dr. Sobstyl, a pupil of Mempel, recently translated into English this report (unpublished) of the treatment of three patients suffering not only from FHD but also from other forms of dystonia in various parts of the body, including the face. The target area covered a large portion of the ventrolateral nucleus of the thalamus, and the final lesion size was 6 × 6 × 8 mm. They reported that writer's cramp symptoms completely disappeared in all patients. Because this article was not written in English and the method (cryosurgery) was out of date, most neurosurgeons did not fully appreciate the importance of this report. In 1997, Goto and colleagues[21] reported excellent results with treatment of stereotactic selective Vo-complex thalamotomy in a patient with dystonic writer's cramp.

The effectiveness of thalamotomy as a treatment for dystonias was more formally recognized in 1989 at the 10th meeting of the World Society for Stereotactic and Functional Neurosurgery,[22] where it was reported that "[i]mmediate improvement occurred in patients with focal limb dystonia," "[i]mprovement was sustained in patients with focal limb dystonia," and "[f]ocal limb dystonia can be greatly improved by thalamotomy without any motor, sensory or intellectual disturbance." These findings are completely consistent with our recent experience of Vo thalamotomy described in this chapter.

The 1990s witnessed a renewed interest in the neurosurgical management of dystonias. This resurgence was due mainly to the introduction of selective peripheral denervation for cervical dystonia,[23] Laitinen's posteroventral lateral pallidotomy,[24] and deep brain stimulation (DBS).[25] Dystonia musculorum deformans was retermed *young-onset DYT1 hereditary dystonia* and found to be the best indication for globus pallidus internus (GPi) pallidotomy. Pallidotomy later gave way to pallidal DBS in the management not only of Parkinson's disease but also of dystonias. It should be remembered, however, that there has not been a scientific comparison between GPi-DBS and pallidotomy for dystonias and that DBS is neither more effective nor safer than bilateral pallidotomy for primary dystonia.[26] In pallidal surgeries for generalized dystonia, improvement of symptoms may often be delayed for months; with thalamotomy for FHD, on the other hand, the surgical effect is immediate. Thalamotomy for dystonia became almost forgotten by the 1990s, largely because of the dramatic effect of pallidal operations on generalized dystonias. Thalamotomy for generalized dystonia had shown only modest improvement and involved great risks, especially in cases of bilateral operations, and TSFHD was generally not even considered to be a subject of surgical interest.

Accustomed to performing pallidal operations for generalized dystonias and peripheral denervation surgery for cervical dystonia,[27] in 2000 we saw a patient with writer's cramp who requested surgical treatment. She argued that her writer's cramp was a type of dystonia and that it should improve with brain surgery. She was a professional cartoon artist and had become unable to continue her professional activities because of the writer's cramp. With no experience of surgical treatment for writer's cramp, her symptoms seemed to us too mild to consider surgical intervention. A literature search uncovered the few case reports mentioned previously, but we eventually determined to attempt the Vo-complex thalamotomy described by Goto and colleagues.[21] This was the first case in a series of surgical treatments for FHD, and the effect was surprisingly dramatic. The patient returned to the profession and in 2008 was listed in the Guinness Book of World Records as the best-selling cartoon artist in the world. It is useful to recall the advice of Poore in 1887.[28] Writing about "piano failure," he noted, "When I use the word 'minor,' please remember that they are minor only to our eyes, and in a pathological sense. They are often of maximum importance to the sufferer, who possibly sees his livelihood in jeopardy, because his hand has forgotten its cunning."

DIAGNOSIS OF FOCAL HAND DYSTONIA

The diagnosis of FHD is generally made by patient history and physical examination. There are no useful laboratory or imaging studies, although there are many reports of functional changes in the cerebral cortex detected with magnetic resonance imaging.[29-33] Most patients initially present to an orthopedist, believing that the symptoms may be due to muscle or tendon issues related to overuse. Generally, however, FHD is not accompanied by pain. The idiosyncrasies of movements are always associated with a specific task, such as writing, drawing, playing musical instruments, or using special tools that require highly repetitive movements or extreme motor precision. Most patients have a history of extensive use of the fingers for very skilled and precise movements.

Three features are important in the diagnosis of FHD: task specificity, stereotyped appearance, and morning benefit. The symptoms only appear when the patient performs a specific task such as writing, using scissors, or playing an instrument. About 70% of such patients experience no symptoms at all when performing other tasks, such as using a knife, using chopsticks, or typing; the remaining 30% may have dystonic symptoms triggered by multiple tasks. The symptoms are always the same and constant, although they may be milder in the morning in the early stage of the disease. In a few patients, the dystonic symptom becomes so severe that task specificity is lost and the symptom persists generally. Very few patients develop dystonic symptoms in other parts of the body. When the onset of FHD appears at a young age (<20 years),[34,35] DYT1 dystonia should be suspected. In ordinary writer's cramp, family history is exceptional.

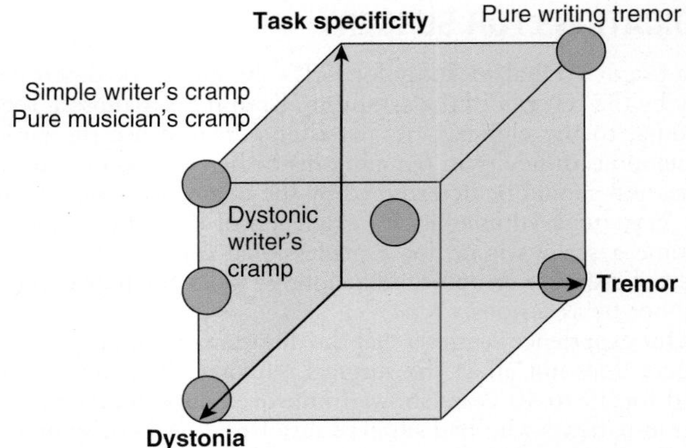

Figure 97-1. The three components of focal hand dystonia. In focal hand dystonia, three components (task specificity, dystonia, and tremor) are present in various degrees. As the disease progresses, task specificity may become less prominent. Some patients may have both dystonia and tremor.

Differential diagnosis includes primary pure writing tremor,[36] essential tremor, and peripheral injury–induced focal dystonia.[37,38] Primary writing tremor is a task-specific tremor that appears only when writing. It is usually unilateral and does not respond to medications used for control of essential tremor or Parkinson's disease. This condition may be a form of tremor-dominant writer's cramp or dystonic tremor.[39-42] Thalamotomy of the nucleus ventralis intermedius (Vim) can effectively control pure writing tremor.[43] Laypeople often use the term *writer's cramp* to describe the inability to write because of tremor. In most cases, however, this condition is caused by essential tremor rather than FHD. A clear distinction must be made between FHD and other types of involuntary movements of the hand. Some patients with FHD may have tremor that is also task specific, but irregular and arrhythmic. We may call such tremor in dystonia patients *dystonic tremor*. If a patient has both dystonia and dystonic tremor of the hand, stereotactic ablation of both the Vo and Vim nuclei of the thalamus can control the symptoms (Videos 97-1 and 97-2). FHD includes symptoms of various combinations and degrees of task specificity, dystonic symptoms, and tremor, as shown in Figure 97-1.

RATING OF FOCAL HAND DYSTONIA

Quantitative descriptions of hand movements in FHD are very difficult to obtain and would be difficult to standardize, but such an approach is important to assess the response to treatment. Three different scales are generally used in the evaluation of FHD. The Writer's Cramp Rating Scale (WCRS; eBox 97-1)[44] assesses writer's cramp mainly in the context of botulinum toxin injection therapy. This is a quantifiable scale for writing performance. The Tubiana Musician's Dystonia Scale (eTable 97-1)[4,45] is used only for the assessment of musician's FHD to rate musical capability, agnostic to the instrument and affected limb. This scale can be modified to evaluate the severity of other occupational FHDs, such as those of barbers or carpenters. The Arm Dystonia Disability Scale (eTable 97-2)[46] is designed to quantify disability on a scale of 0% to 100%, with 100% indicating no disability. This scale is applicable to any category of FHD, although it does not reflect the degree of suffering of patients who have symptoms of FHD only in the course of their professional activities.

INDICATIONS FOR SURGERY

The use of Vo thalamotomy for FHD should not be determined only by the severity of the symptom. Even if the symptom seems minimal to the clinician, its persistence may cause the patient tremendous difficulty in pursuing his or her profession. Surgical indication should be determined by the degree of patient suffering. Very minimal involuntary extension of the little finger may become a serious issue for a professional classic solo-guitarist, whereas a similar symptom in a violinist in an amateur orchestra may not be as serious.

Our experience suggests that the duration of symptoms before surgery does not affect the surgical outcome. Patients who suffered for 30 to 40 years showed improvements similar to those seen in patients who had suffered just 1 to 2 years of symptoms. Patients were not asked to try every possible conservative medical or physical therapy before surgery because permanent improvement of FHD with conservative therapy is rare, and results often take many months, or even years, to be seen. Professional musicians cannot wait this long to return to performance, even if FHD may improve with an extensive long-term rehabilitation program. Conservative therapies should not be denied, however, if the patient prefers to explore them. Surgical management is appropriate when the patient is convinced of the limitation of conservative therapies and has decided to undergo surgery. Procedures have been performed in adolescents but should generally be avoided in patients older than 60 years because of a higher possibility of surgical complications.

Some patients may develop FHD in the contralateral hand. This may occur spontaneously and even after treatment with unilateral thalamotomy. Such patients may ask to undergo surgery on the contralateral side of the thalamus as well, but of course, bilateral operations are exceptional and very dangerous. Bilateral thalamotomy is contraindicated because of the high risk for complications such as speech problems and cognitive deterioration. This was seen in the 1960s and 1970s when large lesions were made in the thalamus. It seems possible now, however, that sequential bilateral thalamotomy may be safer if the lesion size is minimum.[47] In our series of four bilateral Vo thalamotomy cases (two patients with writer's cramp, one clarinet player with FHD, and one pianist with dystonia), the second surgery was performed 1 to 3 years after the initial operation, and no major subjective or objective side effects were noted.

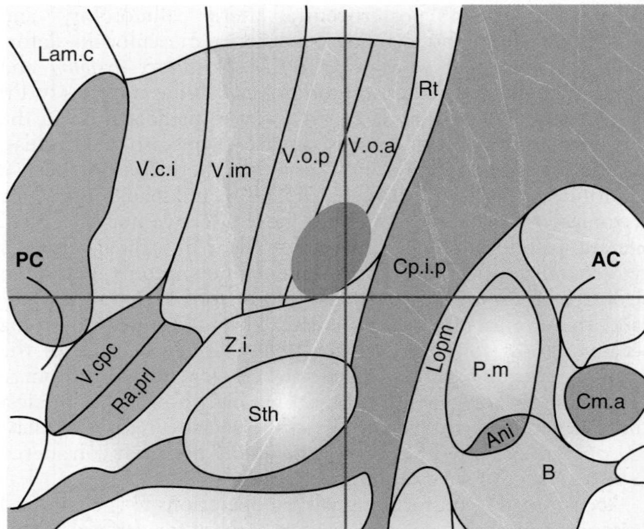

Figure 97-2. Location of the ventro-oralis complex of the thalamus. Sagittal section at 13 mm from midline. AC, anterior commissure; Ani, ansa lenticularis; B, basal nucleus; Cm.a, anterior commissure; Cp.i.p, posterior limb of internal capsule; Lam.c, medial caudal lamella; Lopm, pallidal medial lamina; PC, posterior commissure; P.m, medial pallidum; Ra.prl, radiatio praelemniscalis; Rt, reticular nucleus; Sth, subthalamic nucleus; V.c.i, ventral caudal internal nucleus; V.cpc, ventral caudal parvocellular nucleus; V.im, ventrointermedius nucleus; V.o.a, ventrooralis anterior nucleus; V.o.p, ventrooralis posterior nucleus; Z.i., zona incerta.

SURGICAL TECHNIQUE

Under local anesthesia with 2% lidocaine, a Leksell stereotactic frame (Elekta, Stockholm, Sweden) is fixed onto the skull of the patient. Magnetic resonance and computed tomography images (both 1-mm slice) are used to determine the tentative target 2 mm posterior to the midpoint of the anterior commissure (AC)–posterior commissure (PC) line, 1 mm dorsal to the AC-PC line, and 15 mm lateral to the midline (Fig. 97-2). In our series, we had initially set this target at 13.5 mm lateral to the midline, but because there were recurrences in about 20% of cases, the target was moved to 15 mm lateral. This point corresponds to the junction between the ventro-oralis anterior (Voa) and ventro-oralis posterior (Vop) nuclei of the thalamus, as described in Schaltenbrand and Wahren's stereotactic atlas[48] (see Fig. 97-2). Leksell SurgiPlan computer software (Elekta) can determine a stereotactic trajectory that does not pass through the ventricle. The operation is performed under local anesthesia (1% lidocaine with norepinephrine) without sedation. It is important that the patient remain awake and alert so that symptoms can be monitored during surgery. It is not necessary to fully shave the head; clipping a small area of hair along the incision line is sufficient. After a frontal bur hole is opened with a straight scalp incision 2 cm long, the patient is asked to write or play a musical instrument and to report any symptom changes (eFig. 97-1). A monopolar radiofrequency probe (1-mm diameter tip with a 2- or 4-mm uninsulated length) is then inserted through the bur hole. Electrical stimulation (130 to 160 Hz, 100-msec pulse width, up to 15 mA) is applied to identify the optimal position for the lesion. At this target, no dramatic changes of symptoms have been observed in our series, even with the strongest stimulation (15 mA, approximately 7 V), nor have any sensory or pyramidal motor symptoms been seen. We have therefore regarded the Vo target as an electrically nonresponsive silent region. This is very interesting because it is generally believed that high-frequency stimulation should improve symptoms, if coagulation works. In our institution, microelectrode recording is not used, but symptoms and side effects are monitored carefully with a trial lesion created at 45°C. If the dystonic symptoms improve, a permanent lesion is created by performing thermocoagulation at up to 70° to 75°C for 30 seconds. The electrode is then withdrawn in 2-mm increments to increase the lesion size. Patients are not alerted to the exact timing of the macrostimulation and thermocoagulation to avoid placebo effects. Blood pressure is strictly monitored and controlled to minimize operative complications. When inserting the electrode probe, the probe is gently twisted to pass through the brain parenchyma smoothly to avoid vascular tears. The bur hole is covered with a small ceramic cap for cosmetic purposes, and the scalp is closed in two layers. The operation takes less than 1 hour from skin incision to closure. After the operation, the patient is kept flat in bed overnight. A typical example of postoperative magnetic resonance imaging is shown in Figure 97-3.

To avoid complications and to obtain the best surgical results, the following are critical:

1. Blood pressure should be monitored and strictly controlled.
2. Coagulation temperature should not be higher than 75°C. We typically use 70°C. Higher temperatures can cause cerebral

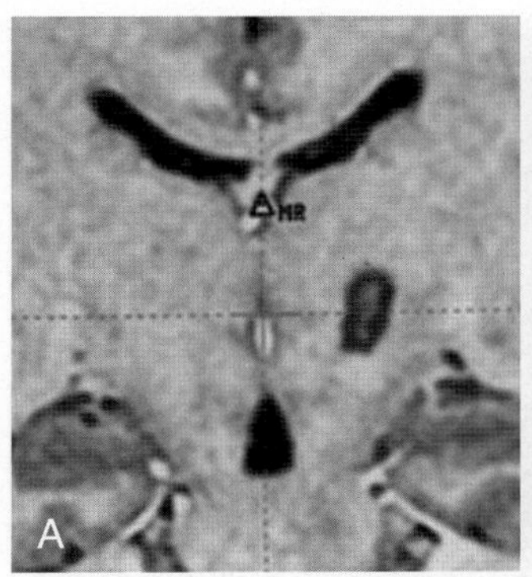

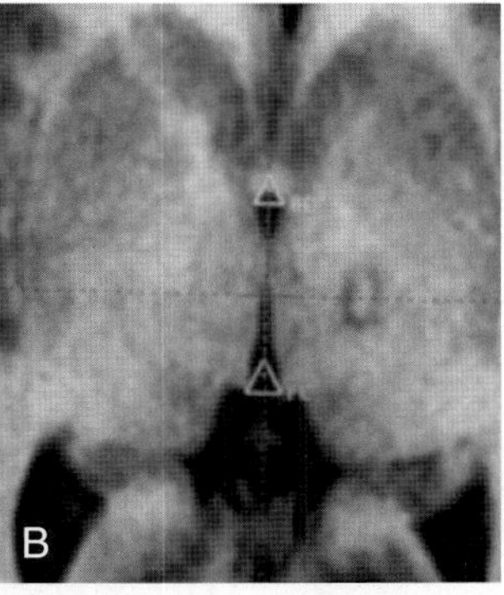

Figure 97-3. Magnetic resonance images after ventro-oralis thalamotomy. A, Coronal section. **B,** Axial section.

and vascular tissue to adhere to the probe tip, which may result in the rupturing of vessels during probe removal.

3. A period of 30 seconds of coagulation time is sufficient to create a permanent lesion.
4. Longer coagulation times unnecessarily increase the area of the reversible heat penumbra zone.
5. Friendly and gentle communication should be maintained with the patient during surgery. Important, of course, in any operation under local anesthesia, this attitude facilitates the social acceptance of surgical intervention for such seemingly mild physical symptoms.

RESULTS

The results of our series, which included more than 150 patients from 2001, have been reported in several papers.[49-51] In all cases, the effect of Vo thalamotomy is immediately discernible during the operation. If there is no improvement during surgery, delayed response is not to be expected. There are some recurrences; about 10% of patients experience recurrence of the symptoms within 3 months. During surgery, there is a region of heat penumbra where the neural function stops, the symptoms improve, but the neurons are not completely ablated. We assume that such functional inactivation of neurons and their recovery with time are the reasons for recurrence within 3 months. Most patients with recurrence do seek additional surgical treatment, because of the substantial improvement of symptoms immediately following the initial procedure. The location of the target for the second surgery is determined based on the findings of postoperative magnetic resonance images.

In our series of Vo thalamotomy for writer's cramp, preoperative WCRS was assessed at 15.1 ± 4.9 and improved to 2.2 ± 2.0 (N = 20) after surgery. Such improvement of WCRS is dramatic; it was reported, for instance, in a study of botulinum toxin therapy for writer's cramp that the pretreatment mean score of 9.1 ± 4.5 dropped to 6.6 ± 4.1 (N = 31).[44] In our study of the long-term effects of surgical treatment on musician's FHD,[51] 15 patients were followed for 4 to 108 months (mean, 30.8 months) after Vo thalamotomy. Fourteen patients (93%) experienced dramatic improvement of dystonic symptoms, improvement that was sustained without recurrence or deterioration during the follow-up period. The mean preoperative Tubiana Musician's Dystonia Scale score in this series was 2.7 (range, 1 to 4). The mean immediate and 1-week postoperative scores were both 4.6 (range, 2 to 5). The mean final score was 4.6 (range, 2 to 5). The patient with the longest duration of symptoms (29 years) benefitted from the greatest improvement.

We reported two problematic cases in which thalamotomy was performed twice without sufficient improvement. It was determined that in both of these cases, the patients did not have hand dystonia, but rather suffered from abnormal dystonic contractions of the muscles around the shoulder. In our experience, Vo thalamotomy is effective only for the symptoms in the distal part of the limb and does not treat the symptoms nearer the body trunk. The latter should be managed with GPi pallidotomy rather than thalamotomy.

Typical examples of improvement of TSFHD after Vo thalamotomy can be seen in the accompanying video clips (Videos 97-3 through 97-7).

COMPLICATIONS

There were no permanent severe complications in our series, nor any cases of postoperative intracerebral hemorrhage or intracranial infection. There were three instances of superficial wound infections of the scalp. The most common transient complications were mild dysarthria and hemiparesis appearing 2 to 3 days after surgery and lasting 2 to 3 weeks. About 10% of patients experience such transient episodes. This is probably due to edema formation around the thermocoagulation lesion, and it may be necessary to administer small doses of oral steroids for several days.

Three patients complained of a strange, uncomfortable sensation in the tip of the tongue that persisted for approximately 6 months after surgery. They had neither dysarthria nor other motor or sensory deficits. In these patients, the lesion seemed to extend slightly deeper than the area below the AC-PC level. The abnormal feeling of the tongue tip had no lateralization. This suggests the possible location of a structure related to tongue tip sensation below the Vo nucleus of the thalamus.

In contrast to the previous reports on thalamotomy, we had no incidence of severe complications in our series.[52,53] This is likely because the age of subjects with FHD is much younger (20 to 40 years) than that patients with Parkinson's disease or essential tremor.[53]

In our experience, patients do not lose any acquired skills or the ability to learn new techniques after Vo thalamotomy.

SURGICAL ANATOMY OF THE VENTRAL-ORALIS NUCLEUS

The Vo nucleus is subclassified into anterior (Voa) and posterior (Vop) parts in the Schaltenbrand brain atlas[48] and in Hassler's classification.[54] This region of the motor thalamus corresponds to the anterior ventral lateral nucleus (VLa) in Jones and Hirai's classification[55,56] and in Morel's study,[57,58] where there is no clear border between the anterior and posterior parts. It was formerly believed that the posterior part of the VLa (Vop) received cerebellar input and that the Voa received pallidal input from the GPi. However, it has since been found that there is no distinct border between the Voa and Vop either in terms of cytoarchitecture or in the origin of fiber inputs,[57-60] although extremely anterior and extremely posterior parts of the VLa definitely belong, respectively, to the pallidal and cerebellar territories of the motor thalamus. Cortical projections from these motor thalamic nuclei are overlapping as well[57-60] (Fig. 97-4). For this reason, no distinction between Voa and Vop is made, and the procedure is known simply as Vo thalamotomy. We may also term this operation *VLa thalamotomy*, as shown in Figures 97-5 and 97-6. Lesioning of this target improves the patient's dystonic symptoms immediately in most cases. If, however, symptomatic improvement is not sufficiently obtained during surgery at the initial target, the target can be moved 3 mm more anteriorly and slightly more medially (1 to 1.5 mm) to cover the entire anterior portion of the VLa, usually resulting in satisfactory control of dystonic symptoms. If the patient also has dystonic tremor, the lesion can be extended to the Vim area, 3 to 4 mm posterior to the initial target.

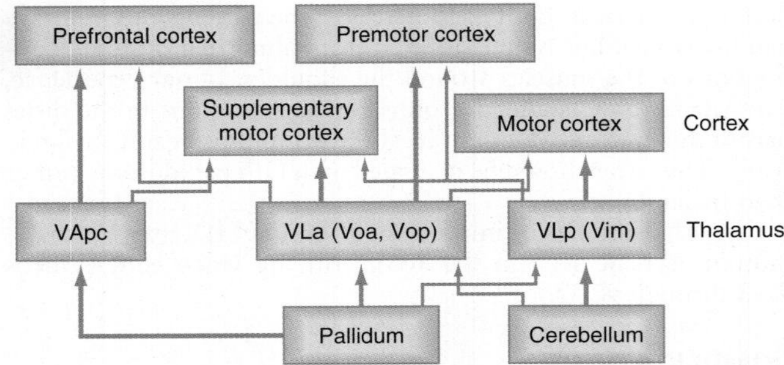

Figure 97-4. Schematic representation showing the pallidal and cerebellar projections to the cerebral cortex through the different nuclei of the motor thalamus. *Thick lines* indicate main projections; *thin lines* indicate supplementary projections. VApc, ventral anterior nucleus parvocellular part; VLa, ventral lateral anterior nucleus; VLp, Ventral lateral posterior nucleus; Voa, ventrooralis anterior nucleus; Vop, ventrooralis posterior nucleus.

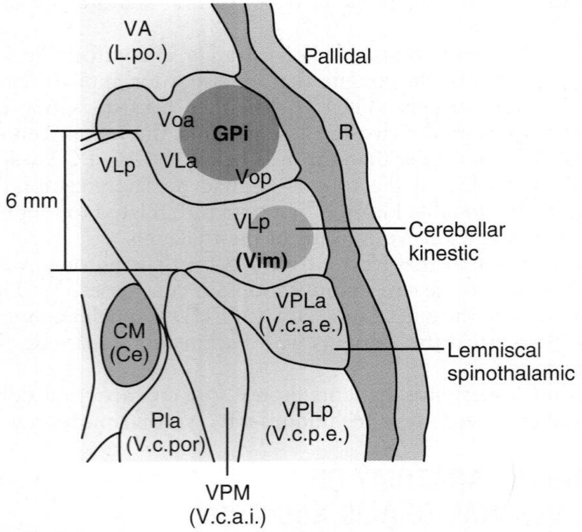

Figure 97-5. Schematic drawing of the ventro-oralis thalamotomy target with related thalamic structures and fiber connections. Ce, central medial nucleus; CM, centromedian nucleus; GPi, internal globus pallidum; L.po., lateropolaris nucleus; Pla, anterior pulvinar; R, reticular nucleus; VA, ventral anterior nucleus; V.c.a.e., ventrocaudalis anterior externus; V.c.a.i., ventrocaudalis anterior internus; V.c.por, ventral caudal portae nucleus; Vim, ventrointermedius nucleus; VLa, ventral lateral anterior nucleus; VLp, ventral lateral posterior nucleus; Voa, ventrooralis anterior nucleus; Vop, ventrooralis posterior nucleus; VPLa, ventral posterior lateral nucleus anterior part; VPM, ventral posterior medial nucleus.

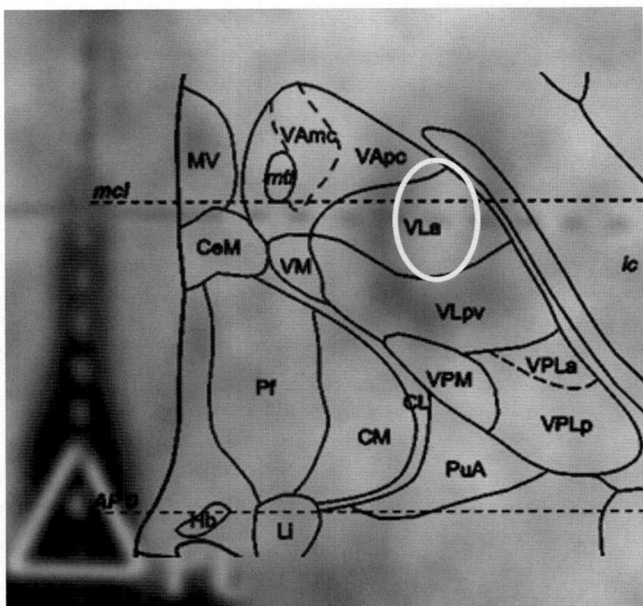

Figure 97-6. Postoperative T1-weighted magnetic resonance image showing the lesion of ventro-oralis thalamotomy superimposed with a brain atlas. The location of the high-intensity lesion with surrounding edema corresponds to the anterior ventral lateral (ventro-oralis anterior + ventro-oralis posterior) nucleus of the thalamus. AP0, 0 mm level from posterior commissure; CeM, central medial nucleus; CL, central lateral nucleus; CM, centromedian nucleus; Hb, habenular nucleus; ic, internal capsule; Li, limitans nucleus; mcl, mid-commissural line; mt, mammillothalamic tract; MV, medioventral nucleus; Pf, parafascicular nucleus; PuA, anterior pulvinar; VAmc, ventral anterior nucleus magnocellular part; VApc, ventral anterior nucleus parvocellular part; VLa, ventral lateral anterior nucleus; VLpv, ventral lateral posterior nucleus ventral part; VM, ventral medial nucleus; VPLa, ventral posterior lateral nucleus anterior part; VPLp, ventral posterior lateral nucleus posterior part; VPM, ventral posterior medial nucleus.

DISCUSSION

In the era of DBS, many neurosurgeons and neurologists may consider lesioning procedures such as thalamotomy and pallidotomy too risky and outmoded to be performed routinely. However, the fact remains that 63% of functional neurosurgeons are using ablative techniques worldwide even today, and not only in lower- to middle-income countries.[61,62] The general belief, correct or not, that DBS is more effective and safer than ablative procedures originated in studies from the 1990s when ventriculography was used in the identification of stereotactic targets and when trajectories were passed through the ventricle. Modern imaging techniques and computer software for surgical planning became widely available in the late 1990s, making stereotactic surgery much quicker and safer than it had been. In the 2000s, however, DBS began to gain in popularity because of its adjustability and reversibility. DBS is effective, but its hardware-related complications may occur even during long-term follow-up. Patients with dystonia are younger in general and can benefit longer from the effects of surgery than those with Parkinson's disease or essential tremor. Dystonia patients treated with DBS may have more than 50 or 60 years to live with their devices. Even if the dystonic symptoms are well controlled with DBS, patients may suffer further emotional and social stresses.[63] The patient's "new life" after DBS can be taxing; worries about being dependent on the pulse generator as well as having to deal with interfering side effects are often disconcerting. In this sense, DBS does not cure the disease. Lesioning procedures are not inferior to DBS in terms of acute complications of movement disorder surgery.[53] If chronic complications are taken into account, DBS obviously carries higher risks. There are a few reports on DBS for FHD[64,65] and task-specific tremor in a musician.[66] Fukaya and colleagues implanted two DBS electrodes, one in the Vo nucleus of the thalamus and another in the GPi in patients with writer's cramp. They reported that thalamic stimulation showed significantly better improvement of writer's cramp.[64] Thus an advantage of DBS is that one can compare the effects of surgical interventions in different regions of the brain to find the better target. Sham stimulation is also possible with

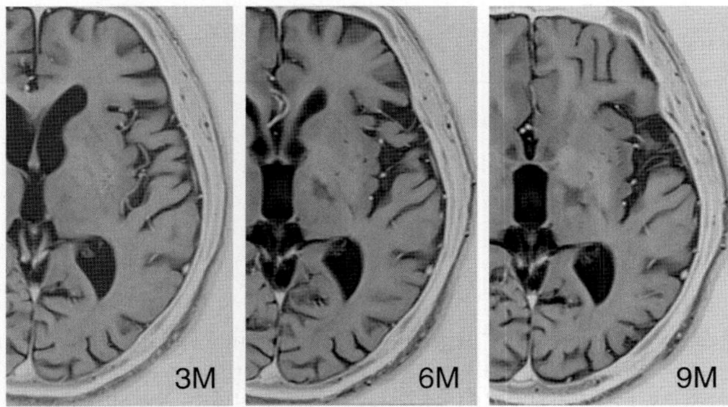

Figure 97-7. Sequential magnetic resonance images taken after gamma-knife ventro-oralis thalamotomy.

DBS, and it enables a blinded study. Bilateral intervention with DBS is generally considered to be safe, although the incidence of speech problems is significant in bilateral thalamic DBS. DBS may be easier for most neurosurgeons to perform, and many have little experience with ablative stereotactic operations for movement disorders.

Our first patient with writer's cramp treated with Vo thalamotomy has shown no signs of symptom recurrence for 13 years. She is very active as a professional cartoonist even today. Can this be considered a cure for FHD? Many textbooks assert that there is no cure for dystonia; the term *remission* is often used when symptoms have improved for a certain period of time, which is not rare in cervical dystonia. However, there is no clear definition of either "remission" or "cure" for dystonias. It remains for these terms to be agreed on and defined before we can begin to qualify the outcomes of Vo thalamotomy for cure in FHD.

In recent years, less invasive ablative techniques such as Gamma Knife[67] and focused ultrasound[68,69] have become available to treat refractory tremor by targeting Vim of the thalamus. Tremor control with these technologies seems promising,[70,71] and it is logical to expect that FHD, too, may possibly be treated with less invasive methodologies in future. Figure 97-7 shows magnetic resonance images taken after Gamma Knife thalamotomy of the Vo nucleus in a 73-year-old calligrapher with right-hand writer's cramp. This patient was not considered suitable for open surgery because of his age and a history of warfarin use in managing cardiac problems, but given his desire to continue his professional activities, we decided to treat him with Gamma Knife thalamotomy. Symptomatic improvement began 6 months postoperatively, and there were no side effects.

CONCLUSION

With modern stereotactic techniques and a skilled and experienced surgical team, unilateral Vo thalamotomy is a safe and effective treatment for FHD in patients whose professional activities are at risk. The effect of Vo thalamotomy is immediate and sustained, but every effort must be made to minimize complications if such an invasive treatment is to be justified.

SUGGESTED READINGS

Albanese A, Bhatia K, Bressman SB, et al. Phenomenology and classification of dystonia: a consensus update. *Mov Disord*. 2013;28(7): 863-873.

Elble RJ. Defining dystonic tremor. *Curr Neuropharmacol*. 2013;11(1): 48-52.

Furuya S, Nitsche MA, Paulus W, et al. Surmounting retraining limits in musicians' dystonia by transcranial stimulation. *Ann Neurol*. 2014;75: 700-707.

Gross RE. What happened to posteroventral pallidotomy for Parkinson's disease and dystonia? *Neurotherapeutics*. 2008;5(2):281-293.

Hallett M. Pathophysiology of writer's cramp. *Hum Mov Sci*. 2006; 25(4-5):454-463.

Horisawa S, Taira T, Goto S, et al. Long-term improvement of musician's dystonia after stereotactic ventro-oral thalamotomy. *Ann Neurol*. 2013; 74:648-654.

Morel A. *Stereotactic Atlas of the Human Thalamus and Basal Ganglia*. New York: Informa Healthcare; 2007.

Pita Lobo P, Quattrocchi G, Jutras MF, et al. Primary writing tremor and writer's cramp: two faces of a same coin? *Mov Disord*. 2013;28(9): 1306-1307.

Rughani AI, Hodaie M, Lozano AM. Acute complications of movement disorders surgery: effects of age and comorbidities. *Mov Disord*. 2013; 28(12):1661-1667.

Sheehy MP, Marsden CD. Writers' cramp-a focal dystonia. *Brain*. 1982; 105(Pt 3):461-480.

Taira T, Hori T. Stereotactic ventrooralis thalamotomy for task-specific focal hand dystonia (writer's cramp). *Stereotact Funct Neurosurg*. 2003; 80(1-4):88-91.

See a full reference list on ExpertConsult.com 

98 A History of Psychosurgery

G. Rees Cosgrove

Surgery for psychiatric illness and behavioral disorders has been performed since ancient times but has generated considerable controversy in the modern era for a variety of scientific, social, and philosophical reasons. The early open and less selective procedures were marked by extensive tissue destruction, significant morbidity, and overzealous application. In large part, the field of stereotactic neurosurgery was developed to create smaller, reproducible, subcortical lesions for psychosurgery without the risks and side effects associated with open or freehand techniques. The advent of psychopharmacologic therapies in the 1960s heralded the demise of psychosurgery in much the same way as the discovery of levodopa affected the practice of movement disorder surgery. Nevertheless, a few centers have continued to offer ablative stereotactic procedures to patients with severe intractable psychiatric disease, in the hope of palliating or easing their disease when all other interventions have failed. Today, neuromodulation is being explored as an alternative to ablative stereotactic techniques, with some encouraging results.

Neurosurgery for psychiatric disease is undoubtedly one of the most fascinating areas of medical history as a whole. In this chapter, we will review the historical development of psychosurgery and provide a background to the ongoing debates and controversies surrounding its use today. The indications, techniques, and surgical results of the modern practice of psychosurgery will also be summarized.

THE ANCIENT WORLD

The story of psychosurgery dates back to the ancient world. In fact one of the earliest forms of neurosurgery—therapeutic trepanation allowing access to the brain for medical or mystical purposes—was a widespread practice in many ancient cultures. Archaeological evidence shows that holes were drilled into skulls in Europe, North Africa, and South America as early as 5000 years ago.[1-3]

The concept that surgical operations could alter the mind of a person persisted in the Middle Ages and the Renaissance when Hieronymus Bosch of the Netherlands (c. 1450-1516) painted "The Cure of Folly," potentially the earliest great painting depicting a neurosurgical procedure. Folly or "madness" was sometimes considered a result of a stone on the brain, and in this painting, a barber-surgeon is shown incising the patient's scalp. The inscription of the painting read, in translation, "Master, dig out the stones of folly, my name is 'Castrated dachshund'"—a term for a simpleton.[4] Clearly, even in ancient times, the practitioners of the day had made the connection between behavioral disorders and their origins in the brain.

THE BIRTH OF PSYCHOSURGERY

In the late 1800s, the concept of functional localization in the brain was evolving, and Gottlieb Burckhardt (1836-1907), a Swiss psychiatrist, was the first to perform surgery on the brain for psychiatric indications.[5] He undertook cerebral topectomies in six patients with intractable mental illness who suffered from auditory hallucinations and displayed aggressive behaviors. Five of the six patients were diagnosed with *primare Verruecktheit*, literally translated as "primary madness" but perhaps more akin to the schizophrenia of today. Although not a surgeon, Burckhardt performed these operations himself, and of the six patients, he reported that three displayed partial improvements. His experience, presented at the International Medical Congress in Berlin in 1889, drew sharp criticism from the audience, and the general opinion was that these interventions should not be performed in the future.[6,7] A subsequent attempt at the surgical treatment of mental illness was undertaken in 1910 by Puusepp, an Estonian neurosurgeon, who surgically disrupted fibers between frontal and parietal cortices in three manic-depressive patients.[8]

In 1935, the International Neurological Congress was held in London, where Fulton and Jacobsen presented the cases of two chimpanzees (Lucy and Becky) who had received surgical frontal lobe ablations and postoperatively exhibited modified behaviors.[9] It is interesting to note that although the chimpanzees did show less neurotic behavior (e.g., frustration, head banging, screeching, and rage), they were also less able to perform the experimental tasks required of them.

Two important figures were in the audience when Fulton and Jacobsen gave their presentation: Egas Moniz, a Portuguese neurologist and the inventor of cerebral angiography, and Walter Freeman, an American neurologist and grandson of one of the forefathers of American surgery, William Keen. Although it seems that the case of these two chimpanzees prompted Egas Moniz to apply experimental treatments to his human patients, one needs to understand that the greatest public health concern of the day was the treatment of the "mentally insane." Moniz and his neurosurgical colleague Almeida Lima therefore performed the first prefrontal leucotomy at the Santa Marta Hospital in Lisbon in 1935,[10] launching psychosurgery into an era when experimental surgery was the hallmark of this specialty. These were not the days of ethical committees and applications for approval of novel therapies, but rather were about application of the "possible," combining the tools of neurosurgery with the innovations and experimental creativity of the surgeons.

Moniz and Lima went on to perform leucotomies in 20 patients over the next 6 months after the London Congress, such was their fervor in the application of their new technique. Initially alcohol was used for destruction of frontal lobe white matter,[11] soon followed by the invention of the leucotome.[3] They reported seven cases of recovery, seven cases of symptomatic improvement, and six cases with symptoms in the status quo.[10,12] The importance of this series lies not only in its demonstration of the potential for symptom reversal or "cure" but also in the limited morbidity and zero mortality that was demonstrated, a feat which by neurosurgical standards of the time was not easy to accomplish. The historical principle of "first do no harm" was in a sense upheld, and this allowed further exploration of these techniques. Moniz was awarded the Nobel Prize in 1949 for his work, and he coined the term *psychosurgery* to describe this new form of surgical intervention.

Only a year after Moniz reported his initial experience with prefrontal lobotomy, Papez published his seminal paper on the hypothesis that a reverberating circuit in the human brain might be responsible for emotion, anxiety, and memory.[13] The components of this system included the hypothalamus, septal nuclei, hippocampi, mammillary bodies, anterior thalamic nuclei, cingulate gyri, and their various connections. In 1952, Maclean[14] expanded it to include paralimbic structures such as orbitofrontal, insular, and anterior temporal cortices; the amygdala; and dorsomedial thalamic nuclei. The description of a neuroanatomic system in the brain that was implicated in emotion and behavior coincided with the early reports of surgical treatment, and therefore much attention was directed toward finding new targets in the brain to treat. Even today, many of the most effective surgical treatments are directed toward some component of the limbic system, and therefore the term *limbic system surgery* has been proposed as an alternative to psychosurgery.

In the same year that Moniz reported his initial experience, Walter Freeman enlisted the aid of James Watts, a neurosurgeon based in Washington, DC, to begin their investigation of leucotomies for treating behavioral disorders. The original prefrontal lobotomy was performed through bilateral frontotemporal bur holes, through which a calibrated instrument was passed blindly to the midline and in a sweeping motion moved up and down to disrupt frontal lobe white matter pathways. Their first 200 patients were reported in 1942, and Freeman and Watts noted satisfactory improvement in most patients but also reported significant complications, including seizures, disordered behavior, and what was termed *frontal lobe syndrome*.[15] Further reports of long-term follow-up by the Connecticut Lobotomy Commission acknowledged postoperative improvement of agitation and disruptive behavior, while noting that a number of successful cases experienced what it called "post-leukotomy syndrome."[16,17] Freeman, however, continued to promote this operation, largely drawing benefit from the fact that other therapeutic alternatives were not effective. Freeman's neurosurgical colleague, Watts, soon became dissatisfied with the radical fervor and zeal with which Freeman applied the technique and unilaterally ended their collaboration.[18]

The infamous "icepick" procedure, which remains in the enduring conscience of much of the medical community to this day, was later developed by Freeman himself and reported as the "trans-orbital leucotomy."[19] This procedure was performed quickly with minimal anesthesia, typically in the immediate postictal phase of an induced generalized tonic-clonic convulsion by tapping a sharp chisel through the orbital roof and thereby damaging the posterior medial orbitofrontal cortex. Toward the latter part of his career, Freeman traveled the United States in a Volkswagen Camper called the "lobotomobile," advocating his transorbital technique in a rather indiscriminate fashion, something that helped cement the negative public perceptions of the technique and its gradual decline.[20]

It is estimated that by 1949, 10,000 leucotomies had been performed in the United States and Britain.[21] Encouraged by initial optimistic reports, the procedure was even recommended in the United States by the Veterans Administration for the treatment of psychologically disturbed soldiers returning from World War II.[22] The procedure gained momentum because it offered an opportunity to treat diseases for which traditional treatments had failed and with which there was a huge burden of psychiatric disease with significant societal demands. At the time, few satisfactory treatment options existed, and the asylums for the insane were overflowing with the chronic mentally ill. Although the scientific method and rigorous statistical analysis of the results were lacking, the transorbital leucotomy enjoyed tolerance by a large body of the medical community because benefit was observed in a substantial percentage of the patients.

CONVENTIONAL OPEN PSYCHOSURGERY

The complications from Freeman's surgical results prompted Fulton and others to call for a less radical and more selective approach to the surgery. By the late 1940s, more precise open surgical procedures were described, including prefrontal leucotomy, bimedial frontal leucotomy, orbital gyrus undercutting, cerebral topectomies, and anterior cingulectomies.[23-28]

Open cingulectomy through an interhemispheric approach was first proposed by Le Beau, who reported good results with minimal morbidity.[28] Whitty in 1955 also described 35 patients, in whom most of the surgical operations were carried out by the late Sir Hugh Cairns of Oxford. Patients were selected based on predominant symptoms of either anxiety or obsessive behavior. The procedures were successful on the whole, with the outcome described as a "slight loss of inhibition and a reduction in tension and in the persistence of emotional and cognitive activity."[26] William Scoville devised a method of orbital undercutting through bifrontal trephines, whereby functional cortical areas were separated from white matter tracts by use of a thin spatula and suction catheter.[25] In a sense, this was specific ablation of individual pathways, in which Scoville targeted the orbital surface of the frontal lobes as well as subcallosal cingulate gyrus, sites that had been shown to control anxiety and affective disorders in both humans and animals.[14] He performed these procedures typically on two patients every Saturday morning at Connecticut's Hartford Hospital (personal communication, M. Apuzzo), with largely satisfactory results and with far fewer complications and behavioral changes than the earlier blunt techniques or icepick procedures.

STEREOTACTIC SURGERY

In 1947, Speigel and Wycis introduced stereotactic surgery, allowing the placement of more precise lesions in deep parts of the brain with the use of a Cartesian coordinates system of surgical planning. The development of stereotactic surgery was in large part driven by the desire to make reproducible lesions in the brain of large numbers of patients with psychiatric disease.[29] Foltz and White first reported the results of stereotactic anterior cingulotomy in 1962.[30] Two years later, Knight reported subcaudate tractotomy.[31] In the subsequent decade, Leksell described his experience with anterior capsulotomy,[32] and Kelly reported limbic leucotomy (combined subcaudate tractotomy and cingulotomy) in 1973.[33] In subsequent years, hypothalamotomy, bilateral amygdalotomy, and thalamotomy were also reported.[34,35]

Anterior cingulotomy has been the surgical procedure of choice in North America for many years. Ballantine in 1987[36] reported his results, noting that up to two thirds of patients experienced a substantial improvement in their well-being with regard to depression, anxiety, and obsessive-compulsive disorder (OCD) symptoms.

Anterior capsulotomy has long been the preferred procedure in Scandinavia and Europe. It involves the placement of lesions in the anterior limb of the internal capsule, disrupting pathways to the orbitofrontal cortex from the thalamus. Initially performed using bipolar thermocoagulation electrodes placed within the anterior limb of the internal capsule, lesions were later created using the Gamma Knife. In fact, much of the inspiration for creating the Gamma Knife was to perform psychosurgery noninvasively so as to reduce the morbidity of open surgery. The early results of anterior capsulotomy suggested that 48% of the patients with major depression and 50% of those with OCD responded very positively to the intervention.[32]

Geoffrey Knight at Brook Hospital and Royal Postgraduate Medical School championed subcaudate tractotomy for use in psychiatric disorders. He created lesions in the posterior orbitofrontal cortex bilaterally using radioactive yttrium seeds and reported good results in 68% of patients with OCD and 50% of those with major depression.[31]

Limbic leucotomy essentially involves the combination of subcaudate tractotomy and cingulotomy. Kelly and Richardson felt that if both cingulotomy and subcaudate tractotomy were effective in improving psychiatric symptoms, then their combination might be even more efficacious. They reported that 89% of patients with OCD and 78% of those with major depression were improved after limbic leucotomy.[33]

Much of the criticism of this early work rested on the facts that only subjective clinical outcome rating scales were used and that many of the newer and more selective pharmacologic agents were not available for use in this population of patients. Despite these assertions, it was evident that a substantial percentage of otherwise treatment-refractory patients benefited from surgical intervention at a variety of respectable medical centers. Certainly the psychosurgical procedures performed today with stereotactic magnetic resonance imaging guidance are much more refined and create more precise, reproducible lesions and improved safety profiles.[37]

THE DECLINE OF PSYCHOSURGERY

In 1954, chlorpromazine, the first clinically useful psychotropic drug, received approval from the U.S. Food and Drug Administration, and its introduction spelled the beginning of the end of the era of leucotomies. It was described by Freeman as a "chemical lobotomy,"[18] but in that year alone, approximately 2 million patients received the drug.[3] Skepticism regarding the outcomes of surgery and concerns about side effects fueled the acceptance and widespread use of this new drug. It was especially useful in patients with schizophrenia, a psychiatric illness that is currently not considered as an indication for surgery but for which many patients were operated on in that era.[38] Many new drugs were subsequently developed and brought to market, and in a similar fashion to the decline of stereotactic lesions for Parkinson's disease with the advent of levodopa, the perceived need for neurosurgical intervention in psychiatry disease evaporated.

In 1967, Freeman, a lone voice in the continued attempt to promote leucotomies, performed his last of such procedures in California. In a dramatic end to this chapter of psychosurgery, Freeman disrupted a blood vessel, and the patient died as a result. This led to a removal of Freeman's operating privileges and a neurosurgical practice that would remain dormant for many years to come. In addition, the public outcry from overzealous application of psychosurgery prompted legislative bodies, government agencies, and health insurance carriers to limit these procedures or deny access to them and their reimbursement.[20]

The use of psychosurgery has often been shunned by the public and physicians alike. Nonetheless, some feel that the complete abandonment of surgical intervention for psychiatric disease is too severe and that there is indeed a significant role for surgery to this day. Furthermore, as our understanding of psychiatric disease evolves and our technology improves, such as with the use of deep brain stimulation (DBS), many feel that there may be an expanding role for functional neurosurgeons in the mental health arena.

THE PUBLIC, LEGISLATION, AND ETHICS

The public reaction to leucotomy as popularized by the icepick perception of the works of Freeman, completely overshadowed the other psychosurgical procedures that had been applied by more responsible practitioners. The negative stigma entered popular consciousness with the 1962 publication of Ken Kesey's novel, *One Flew Over the Cuckoo's Nest*, subsequently made into a 1975 Milos Forman film that won an Academy Award for Best Picture of the Year. Despite favorable results for cingulotomy, capsulotomy, and limbic leucotomy, criticism ensued, with resulting allegations of abuse and misuse of these procedures, which prompted calls for a meticulous review of the issues. In the 1970s, legislation was passed in the United States reiterating the importance of ethical boards in the selection of functional neurosurgery patients.[3] A report by the U.S. National Commission for the Protection of Human Subjects of Biomedical and Behavioral Research outlined that psychosurgery displayed efficacy in more than half of the 400 operations performed annually between 1971 and 1973.[39] The Commission went further to indicate that no psychological deficits could be attributed to the procedures. Indeed it seems that concerns about psychosurgery being used on minority and disadvantaged populations for social control were unsubstantiated. The Commission's conclusions clearly argued against the public perception that psychosurgery was dangerous, ineffective, and experimental.

The World Health Organization today defines psychosurgery as "the selective surgical removal or destruction of nerve pathways for the purposes of influencing behavior,"[40] although this needs to be modified to include the various techniques of DBS and other neuromodulation treatments. National associations of psychiatrists around the world[41] have issued position statements declaring acceptance of these procedures, but that voice seems occasionally to be overpowered by other sectors of the community that continue to denounce all forms of surgical intervention in psychiatry. Ethical responsibility lies with neurosurgeons along with expert multidisciplinary groups of specialists in the safe and scientific application of all current forms of psychosurgery.

MODERN ABLATIVE PSYCHOSURGERY

Despite its controversy, surgery for psychiatric disease has continued in specialized centers around the world as a treatment of last resort for carefully selected patients who continue to suffer despite a combination of psychotherapy, pharmacotherapy, and electroconvulsive therapy. At present, only patients with severe, chronic, disabling, and treatment-refractory psychiatric illness should be considered for surgical intervention. These criteria have been operationalized in a variety of accepted international guidelines published by professional organizations and associations in the past several years.[41] As in all medical decisions, the potential benefit from any such intervention must be balanced against the risks imposed by surgery.

The major psychiatric diagnostic groups, as defined by the *Diagnostic and Statistical Manual of Mental Disorders*, fifth edition, that might benefit from surgical intervention include OCD and major affective disorder (i.e., unipolar major depression or bipolar disorder). In many instances, patients present with mixed disorders combining symptoms of anxiety, depression, and OCD, and these patients remain candidates for surgery. Schizophrenia is not currently considered an indication for surgery. A history of personality disorder, substance abuse, or other significant Axis II disorder symptoms is often a relative contraindication to surgery. Validated clinical research instruments (e.g., the Yale-Brown Obsessive Compulsive Scale, Beck Depression Inventory, Hamilton Rating Scale for Depression, Global Assessment of Functioning, Minnesota Multiphasic Personality Inventory) must be employed to quantify psychiatric symptom severity and outcomes.[42]

Cingulotomy, anterior capsulotomy, and limbic leucotomy remain the ablative psychosurgical procedures still employed today (Fig. 98-1). Modern results of cingulotomy suggest that nearly 70% of patients with OCD will have a positive response to surgery and that about 75% of patients with major depression will respond positively at long-term follow-up of more than 5 years. Operative mortality in these series was nil, and morbidity was either transient or minor.[43] More recently, Kim,[44] Jung,[45] and Dougherty[46] and their colleagues all reported additional positive results.

Anterior capsulotomy is most commonly performed today with the Gamma Knife, and unpublished results from Brown University suggest that more than 70% of patients with intractable OCD become responders after intervention at 5-year follow-up. No neuropsychological deficits were noted on detailed

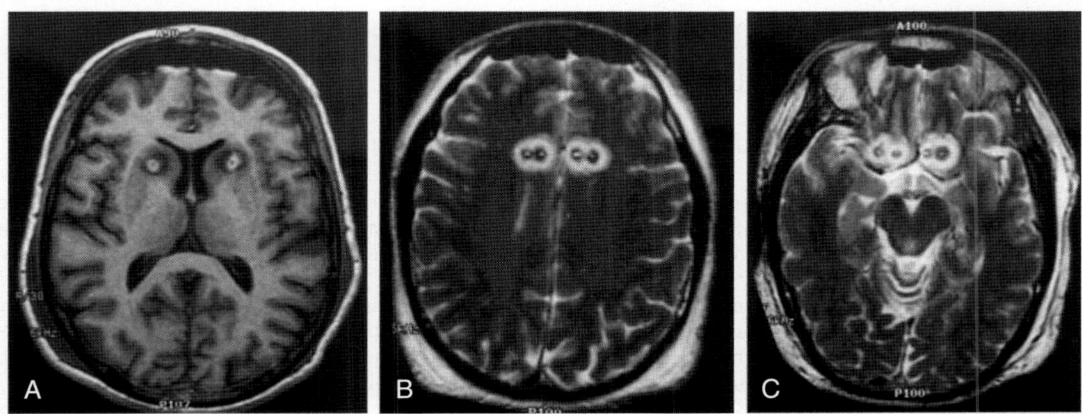

Figure 98-1. Acute postoperative axial magnetic resonance images demonstrating lesion location in anterior capsulotomy **(A)**, cingulotomy **(B)**, and subcaudate tractotomy **(C)**.

testing, and only one instance of apathy was reported. For general anxiety disorder, panic disorder, and social phobia, Ruck and colleagues[47] reported a 50% reduction in symptoms across the disease groups.

Modern limbic leucotomy has generally been limited to be used as a salvage procedure in patients who have failed to respond adequately to initial cingulotomy. Montoya and associates reported on this treatment in 21 patients with intractable psychiatric disease, noting up to 50% improvement in global functioning.[48] Sachdev and Sachdev also reported on 76 patients with treatment-resistant depression in whom bilateral limbic leucotomy resulted in significant improvement of symptoms.[49]

Today, fewer than 15 to 20 ablative psychosurgical procedures are performed in the United States each year, so assertions that this type of surgery is being applied overenthusiastically are unsubstantiated.

NEUROMODULATION

Vagal nerve stimulation (VNS) has been explored in the treatment of depression and anxiety disorders because of the observation that a percentage of intractable epilepsy patients in whom the device were implanted noted improvement in their depressive symptoms whether or not their seizures were controlled. This prompted clinical trials in which VNS was investigated as a treatment for depression and OCD. Neither of these trials supported the use of VNS as an effective treatment for these diseases. More recently, its applicability in the treatment of mood disorders has been discussed. Nevertheless, positive mood changes have been found in epileptic patients receiving VNS, and clinical evidence is accumulating.[50]

DBS has received much recent attention as an alternative technique in psychosurgery because it is reversible, is adjustable, and can be performed bilaterally in many of the same brain targets used in ablative surgery. Although clearly not similar in their neurobiologic mechanisms, the therapeutic responses often appear clinically equivalent at least in movement disorders. Although the ability to change stimulation parameters is seen as advantageous, it also requires multiple visits for adjustments, requires frequent battery changes, and introduces the overarching positive treatment bias of being seen regularly by an experienced psychiatric treatment team.

Early anecdotal reports and small patient series of DBS for OCD,[51-55] depression[56-59] and Tourette's syndrome[60-62] were encouraging enough that several large-scale blinded clinical trials have been instituted. Unfortunately, one of the largest multicenter DBS trials for OCD failed to demonstrate any clinical benefit that could be attributed to the device. Other clinical trials are ongoing, and acceptance of the DBS technique in psychiatry is growing, albeit slowly.

Although incontrovertible clinical evidence for DBS in either OCD or depression remains elusive, we must remember that neuromodulation is still in its infancy and much more needs to be learned before any strong conclusions can be made. Like the early days of ablative surgery, the initial results are encouraging enough to deserve further exploration.

CONCLUSION

The field of psychosurgery has been one of the most interesting in all of medicine and will continue to be so in the future. Much remains to be learned, but understanding its history will impart important lessons to practitioners in the future. The psychiatric community needs to evaluate new and existing treatments for these disorders based on the merits of each intervention rather than their tainted history. A better understanding of the neurobiologic basis of psychiatric disease will continue to inform our choice and use of psychosurgical options.[63] The future of psychosurgery will rest on the application of sound clinical and ethical guidelines in severely affected psychiatric patients to prevent any possibility of its misuse in the future.

SUGGESTED READINGS

Cosgrove GR, Rauch SL. Psychosurgery. *Neurosurg Clin N Am*. 1995; 6(1):167-176.

El-Hai J. *The Lobotomist*. Hoboken: John Wiley & Sons; 2005.

Feldman RP, Goodrich JT. Psychosurgery: a historical overview. *Neurosurgery*. 2001;48(3):647-657, discussion 657-659.

Nuttin B, Wu H, Mayberg H, et al. Consensus on guidelines for stereotactic neurosurgery for psychiatric disorders. *J Neurol Neurosurg Psychiatry*. 2014;85(9):1003-1008.

Swayze VW 2nd. Frontal leukotomy and related psychosurgical procedures in the era before antipsychotics (1935-1954): a historical overview. *Am J Psychiatry*. 1995;152(4):505-515.

Valenstein E. *Great and Desperate Cures: The Rise and Decline of Psychosurgery and Other Radical Treatments for Mental Illness*. New York: Basic Books; 1987.

See a full reference list on ExpertConsult.com

99 Surgery for Tourette's Syndrome

Pablo Andrade, Rowshanak Hashemiyoon,* Jens Kuhn, and Veerle Visser-Vandewalle*

Gilles de la Tourette's syndrome (TS) is an idiopathic neuropsychiatric disorder with an unknown etiology affecting approximately 1% of the population.[1] Diagnosis is based on the childhood onset of chronic involuntary motor and phonic tics that are not attributable to drugs or known medical causes and persist for no less than 1 cumulative year.[2-4] The frequency and severity of tic expression follows a waxing and waning pattern, which is noteworthy when considering therapeutic strategies. Mean onset of symptoms occurs at age 5 to 7 years and peaks at age 10.[5-7] By late adolescence to early adulthood, symptoms either stabilize or remit in approximately two thirds of the population.[3,5] The disorder is observed worldwide across a wide range of demographics, occurs approximately 4 times more frequently in children, and is 4 to 5 times more prevalent in boys than girls.[1,3,5,8]

Both motor and phonic tics may occur. They are sudden, repetitive, and purposeless and can be classified as either simple or complex. Simple tics involve one muscle group and can be tonic, dystonic, and/or clonic.[9] Common examples are the following: (1) tonic—isometric contractions such as tensing of the abdominal muscles; (2) dystonic—shoulder rotation and oculogyric deviation; and (3) clonic—rapid movements such as eye blinking, facial twitching, and head, neck, or limb jerking.[9,10] Phonically, these are manifest as throat clearing, coughing, or grunting. Complex tics involve the coordination of several muscle groups and often appear purposeful.[9] Examples of these include gesturing, hopping, and body jerking (motoric) and humming, making animal sounds, and coprolalia (phonic).

The ability to suppress tics is observed by age 10, the same age at which patients first report premonitory sensations.[11-13] These urges are associated with dystonic tics, signal the oncoming behavior, and distinguish TS from similar disorders.[12] Tic suppression typically results in stronger rebound tic expression.[14] The change in symptoms during maturation suggests that TS is a developmental disorder.[15,16] The disorder is highly hereditable but presents with a range of clinical phenotypes, although this is likely due to the substantial rate of comorbidities. Highest among these comorbidities are attention-deficit/hyperactivity disorder (ADHD) and obsessive-compulsive disorder (OCD), each of which may be seen in up to 80% of TS patients. Anxiety disorders, learning disabilities, and affective disorders are also commonly observed.[17-19]

Although TS is generally self-limiting, a portion of the patient population may experience tic burden that is persistent, severe, and medically refractory.[20,21] Historically, these patients were treated by neurosurgical lesions at a variety of targets.[22-24] In 1999 the first reversible neurosurgical procedure was performed in a TS patient using stereotactic high-frequency stimulation.[25] The use of deep brain stimulation (DBS) has since been reported in over 130 patients in approximately 25 centers across 14 countries with good results.[26,27]

PATHOPHYSIOLOGY

Results from electrophysiologic, biologic, and modeling investigations have offered new insights into the underlying pathophysiology of TS, but its true pathogenesis has yet to be elucidated. Evidence suggests that TS is a complex disorder involving both heritable and environmental factors.[28] Although genome-wide association studies did not report any common genetic variants that could be identified as risk factors distinguishable in a substantial portion of the patient population, gene network analysis has identified significant changes in the expression of some gene clusters.[29,30]

Anatomic and physiologic evidence suggests that TS results from dysfunction in the recurrent loops of the cortico–basal ganglia–thalamocortical pathway.[15] Pathologic behavior in this network has also been implicated in ADHD and OCD.[28] This circuit is essential for action gating as well as the conversion of goal-directed behavior to automated behaviors.[31-33] Important regions in this pathogenetic network include the motor and limbic cortices, striatum (caudate and putamen), globus pallidus internus (GPi) and externus (GPe), substantia nigra pars reticulata and pars compacta, nucleus accumbens (NAcc), subthalamic nucleus, and thalamus. The pedunculopontine nuclei and cerebellum provide extrinsic connections, which may also be important.

The cortico–basal ganglia–thalamocortical network consists of direct and indirect pathways that are topographically organized and can be differentiated histologically.[32-34] It has been proposed that dopamine and γ-aminobutyric acid are the key neurotransmitters involved in the dysfunction of transmission between the cortex and subcortical structures, although glutamate, histamine, serotonin, acetylcholine, and cyclic adenosine monophosphate have also been suggested to play important modulatory roles.[11] Dopamine dysregulation, as presented in the tonic-phasic model, is the most widely accepted neurobiologic theory of TS[35,36] a theory that is supported by the clinical observations that dopamine$_2$ receptor antagonists effectively reduce tic severity whereas dopamimetic drugs exacerbate symptoms of TS.

TREATMENT

Because there is no cure for TS, treatment is targeted toward relieving tic severity and frequency and the disruptive symptoms presented by comorbidities. Therapeutic strategies should seek to decrease symptoms beginning with puberty. In cases in which tics persist, behavioral, pharmacologic, and/or surgical options are available.

Comprehensive Behavioral Intervention for Tics and Pharmacologic Treatment

Behavioral therapy may be recommended as a first-line intervention for children and milder cases of TS.[37,38] Because there are no known adverse effects of this intervention, it also may be recommended as an adjunctive therapy in more severe cases. Important considerations include a lack of data regarding the long-term ameliorative effects of behavioral therapy and difficulty finding appropriately trained professionals.

If medical treatment is indicated in milder cases of TS, α_2-adrenergic agonists may be effective, particularly in patients with comorbid ADHD.[12,24] In moderate to severe cases neuroleptics may effectively relieve tic burden, most likely through their antidopaminergic effects.[39] The most effective of the antipsychotic agents approved by the U.S. Food and Drug Administration (FDA) are pimozide, haloperidol, and risperidone.[39] Although effective, dopamine blocking agents may induce significant side effects, including extrapyramidal symptoms, sedation, and weight gain.[40] Aripiprazole, a partial agonist and antagonist that is reported to be an effective tic suppressant with a lower incidence

*P. Andrade and R. Hashemiyoon contributed equally to this work.

of severe side effects, is emerging as the medical treatment of choice for TS.[41]

In patients with significant comorbidities, psychostimulants (e.g., methylphenidate) or selective serotonin reuptake inhibitors may be used for the treatment of ADHD and OCD, respectively.[42] For isolated motor tics, botulinum neurotoxin injections are effective and well tolerated.[43,44]

Ablative Surgery

Surgical intervention may be indicated for patients with TS that is severe and medically refractory. For more than 50 years, several reports described the surgical ablation of many different targets in severe disabling cases of TS.[23] In 1962, Baker published the first paper describing ablation for TS, reporting the results of a bimedial leucotomy in a young male suffering from vocal and motor tics, with concomitant obsessive-compulsive symptoms.[45] Following surgical drainage of a postoperative abscess, a significant reduction of tics and obsessive-compulsive behavior was observed. After this, many other groups attempted diverse neurosurgical ablative approaches that included lesioning of the frontal lobes (bimedial frontal leucotomies and prefrontal lobotomies), the thalamus (medial, intralaminar, and ventrolateral nuclei), the limbic system (anterior cingulotomy and limbic leucotomy), the zona incerta, and the cerebellum, as well as combinations of these targets.[22-24] Altogether, these reports document more than 70 patients who underwent ablative surgery with varied outcomes and complications that ranged from mild transitory deficits to severe permanent deficits.

Deep Brain Stimulation

In 1999 DBS, a safer, reversible alternative to neuroablation, was used for the first time in a TS patient.[25] Benabid and colleagues first described thalamic DBS in 1987 as a treatment for medically refractory tremor[46]; however, the reversibility and dynamic adjustability of DBS offered the possibility of revolutionizing the treatment of multiple functional brain disorders, including TS. Today, DBS is both FDA approved and Conformité Européenne (CE) marked for the treatment of Parkinson's disease, primary dystonia, essential tremor, and OCD. The treatment of TS is still considered investigative. Nonetheless, since the first report by Vandewalle and colleagues,[25] the procedure has been performed worldwide in over 130 cases.[26,27] In these reports, seven different targets have been described; however, the majority of reported cases involve DBS at four brain areas: the medial thalamus, GPi, GPe, and internal capsule/nucleus accumbens (IC/NAcc).

Thalamus

Based on the positive results observed with neuroablation of the medial thalamus by Hassler and Dieckmann in 1970,[22] this region was targeted for chronic bilateral stimulation in the first DBS procedure for TS.[25] The specific target was the convergence of the centromedian nucleus, the substantia periventricularis, and the nucleus ventro-oralis internus. The first case was performed in a 42-year-old male whose tics decreased from 38 per minute to zero at 12 months postoperatively.[25] Four years later this group reported long-term follow-up of three TS patients after DBS at this same target, demonstrating the safety and efficacy of this procedure in reducing motor and vocal tics with few side effects.[47] Since then, a total of 70 reported cases in this anatomic region have been performed at various medical centers, with certain targeting variations (Table 99-1). The targets most commonly employed were similar to the original centromedian nucleus–substantia periventricularis–nucleus ventro-oralis internus target employed by Vandewalle. In 2007, Maciunas and associates described the first prospective double-blind crossover trial for this target in five patients.[48] The authors documented a mean 67% reduction of tics and a 44% improvement in OCD symptoms, with no severe complications. Four years later Ackermans and colleagues described another prospective double-blind randomized crossover trial in six patients in which a 49% decrease in the Yale Global Tic Severity Scale (YGTSS) was observed after 1 year.[49] There were no improvements in comorbidity measures, and mild adverse effects such as decreased energy levels occurred in all patients, along with one impulse generator infection and one small intracranial hemorrhage resulting in a temporary upward gaze palsy. More recently, Okun and colleagues found an 18% mean improvement in the YGTSS with no major adverse events in a level III clinical trial.[50] These authors reported that tic suppression was achieved most commonly with activation of contacts located ventrally in the centromedian thalamic region.

TABLE 99-1 Demographic Table of Patients Undergoing Deep Brain Stimulation for Tourette's Syndrome

Target	Total Number of Patients	Level of Evidence	Maximum Follow-up (mo)
Thalamus	70	III and IV	72
GPi	38 (20 AM + 18 PVL)	IV	72
GPe	2	IV	24
IC/NAcc	6	IV	39
STN	1	IV	12
Multiple	10	III and IV	60

AM, anteromedial; GPe, globus pallidus externus; GPi, globus pallidus internus; IC/NAcc, internal capsule/nucleus accumbens; PVL, posteroventrolateral; STN, subthalamic nucleus.

Besides these reports, only case reports and case series have been published, documenting a wide range of improvements (46% to nearly 100%).[47,51-53] In a series of reports, Servello and coworkers documented their results for medial thalamic stimulation, employing a target 2 mm anterior to the original.[54-56] They reported an average tic reduction of 47% in 31 patients, with significant improvements in associated psychiatric disorders. Lee and colleagues[57] and Kaido and associates[58] reported that targeting of the centromedian-parafascicular complex (CM-Pfc) resulted in a 62% and 39% improvement of tics at long-term follow-up, respectively. Neither group documented serious adverse events. In another series of papers, Kuhn and coworkers reported on the modulation of the parafascicular nucleus, the dorsomedial nucleus, and the lamella medialis, documenting tic reduction ranging from 30% to 80%.[59] In one of these cases, the patient had previously been treated unsuccessfully with GPi stimulation. In 2011, Kuhn and colleagues reported on unilateral stimulation of the ventro-oralis posterior–ventro-oralis anterior–ventro-oralis internus complex in two TS patients.[60] On this occasion, tic reduction ranged from 70% to 100% as measured with the YGTSS.

Globus Pallidus Internus

To date, the results of 38 cases of GPi-DBS in TS patients have been reported. Among these, 18 patients received stimulation in the posteroventrolateral segment of the GPi and 20 patients received stimulation in the anteromedial or limbic segment.

In 2002, van der Linden and colleagues described for the first time the effects of bilateral stimulation of the GPi in TS.[61] The authors selected the posteroventrolateral GPi based on the experience that stimulation at this target suppressed hyperkinetic motor symptoms in patients with PD. This first case was performed in a 27-year-old male whose tics decreased by approximately 95% after 6 months of treatment. In reality, this patient received four DBS electrodes initially, the two in the GPi and two more placed in the medial thalamus bilaterally, which yielded a tic reduction of 80% when stimulated independently. Three years later Diederich and colleagues reported on the effects of bilateral posteroventrolateral GPi-DBS in another 27-year-old male.[62] His tic frequency decreased approximately 73% and the intensity of his vocal tics was significantly reduced after 14 months of therapy; however, the authors reported persistent unilateral bradykinesia caused by a small intraparenchymal hematoma, which partly reversed with cessation of stimulation. Gallagher and coworkers[63] and Shahed and associates[64] reported similar beneficial effects after posteroventrolateral GPi-DBS. Shahed and associates reported tic reduction of 84%, as well as a 69% mean improvement in associated OCD behavior, in a 16-year-old male patient after 6 months. Of note is that the patient required a body shield to prevent him from compulsively manipulating the generator.[64] In a series of reports, Dehning and colleagues reported the long-term (12 to 72 months) follow-up of six TS patients after bilateral posteroventrolateral GPi-DBS.[65] The authors described a decrease in the YGTSS of almost 90% and a significant increase in quality-of-life measures. Nonetheless, in two cases stimulation had to be discontinued because of lack of response. In addition, depression and several mild side effects such as moderate dysarthric speech were reported in the initial postoperative phase. These phenomena were attributed to the patients' difficulties adjusting to their new situation without tics.[66,67] In 2009, Dueck and coworkers reported negative effects of posteroventrolateral GPi stimulation in a 16-year-old male with TS and mental retardation and no associated psychiatric conditions.[68] Dong and colleagues in 2012 described the effects of unilateral stimulation of the right posteroventrolateral GPi in two male patients who exhibited a greater than 50% tic reduction with improvements in health-related quality of life and no severe adverse effects after 12 months of stimulation.[69] More recently, Motlagh and coworkers described the results of an open-label study in eight TS patients treated with thalamic and globus pallidus DBS, two of whom were implanted in the posteroventrolateral GPi.[70] This study showed tic reduction of 20% and 44%, respectively, with no effect on associated psychiatric conditions and mild side effects such as hyperkinesias and restlessness.

In 2005, Houeto and associates described the effects of bilateral DBS at the anteromedial GPi.[71] They hypothesized that TS is more a "limbic" than a "motor" disorder and, therefore, targeting the limbic part of the GPi might be more successful than targeting the motor region. In 2011, Martínez-Fernández and colleagues also reported on the beneficial effects of anteromedial GPi stimulation.[72] In this study, two patients implanted in the posteroventrolateral GPi were compared to three patients implanted in the anteromedial GPi. All patients experienced improvements in tic severity, but the anteromedial GPi–stimulated patients improved more than the posteroventrolateral GPi–stimulated patients, with tic reductions of 54% and 37%, respectively. Sachdev and colleagues have described the largest series of patients implanted in the anteromedial GPi, reporting a 54% mean tic reduction in 17 patients with follow-up of up to 46 months.[73]

Globus Pallidus Externus

In 2010, Vilela Filho and coworkers reported on the effects of bilateral GPe stimulation in seven patients.[74] The GPe was targeted because of hypothesized hyperactivity in this brain area in TS patients. The results of this prospective double-blind study were a mean 74% reduction of tics with only mild adverse effects such as transient depressive mood in one patient. More recently, Piedimonte and associates reported on one patient treated with GPe stimulation who experienced a 71% tic reduction after 6 months.[75] This patient displayed a significant worsening after 2 years of stimulation as a result of the exhaustion of the generator battery.

Internal Capsule and Nucleus Accumbens

DBS of the anterior limb of the IC/NAcc, as part of the ventral striatum, is an established CE-approved therapy for patients suffering from refractory OCD. The same target has been applied to DBS in TS patients based on the hypothesis that TS and OCD share several clinical characteristics. In 2005, Flaherty and colleagues implanted bilateral electrodes in the IC/NAcc region in a 37-year-old woman with severe TS, observing a 25% tic reduction after 18 months.[76] Mild apathy and depression were recorded after high-intensity stimulation of the ventral contacts (NAcc), whereas hypomania was reported when the dorsal contacts (IC) were active. Three years later, the electrodes had to be removed because they were damaged by her residual retrocollic jerks.[51] One year later, the patient underwent bilateral implantation of electrodes in the centromedian nucleus, resulting in significant tic reduction without adverse mood or impulse control effects. In 2007, Kuhn and associates described a case of IC/NAcc DBS in one patient, reporting a tic reduction of 41% and an associated OCD behavior decrease of 64% after 30 months.[77] In 2009, Neuner and colleagues reported similar findings of a 44% improvement in the YGTSS score and a 56% reduction in comorbid OCD behavior in a single patient.[78] One year later, this patient suffered a severe depressive episode that resulted in a suicide attempt.[79] Zabek and coworkers described beneficial effects of unilateral (right) NAcc stimulation in a 31-year-old male patient suffering from TS and self-injurious behavior.[80] After 28 months of DBS, the patient exhibited an 80% improvement in tics and a significant reduction in the self-injurious behavior. In 2009, Servello and associates reported on the effects of bilateral IC/NAcc DBS in four TS patients.[81] Three of the patients had been previously implanted in the thalamus, so IC/NAcc DBS was performed as a "rescue strategy." The fourth patient had undergone no prior surgery. The effects in all four were disappointing. Similarly, Burdick and coworkers documented a 20% worsening of symptoms in a 33-year-old man with mild motor and vocal tics who also had severe OCD symptoms.[82] After a 30-month follow-up period, the authors also observed no significant improvement of the obsessive-compulsive behavior. Sachdev and colleagues described the case of a 32-year-old woman with severe treatment-refractory OCD and TS, the former being the most disabling condition.[83] After 14 months of bilateral NAcc DBS, the patient showed an improvement of 57% in tic severity and a 90% improvement in the OCD measures with no reported adverse events.

Other Targets and Multiple Targets

In 2009, Martinez-Torres and associates described the case of a 38-year-old man with PD who also had a history of tics in whom bilateral subthalamic nucleus DBS improved both PD symptoms and tics.[84] The observed tic improvement after a 1-year follow-up period was 97% with no reported adverse events, and unrelated to the improvement of parkinsonian motor symptoms. Based on these findings, the authors proposed the subthalamic nucleus as a potential target for DBS in TS patients. The role of subthalamic nucleus DBS in TS is presently being investigated as part of a study in Europe (personal communication).

In total, 10 reported cases are documented in which multiple electrodes for different targets have been implanted. Of these, most had implanted electrodes in two targets ($n = 9$); in only one case were three brain areas stimulated. This single case refers to a 19-year-old male who displayed no significant improvement in tic reduction or OCD-associated behavior after DBS of the anteromedial GPi, posteroventrolateral GPi, and midline thalamus.[70] In 2005, Houeto and colleagues described the results of DBS in one patient who had received two electrodes in the centromedian nucleus of the thalamus and two in the anteromedial GPi.[71] Three years later the same group described results in three TS patients in a double-blind, randomized crossover design who received four electrodes in the two same targets.[85] The first report described that both CM-Pfc and anteromedial GPi stimulation had a comparable effects on tics (64% reduction with CM-Pfc and 65% reduction with anteromedial GPi) and associated behavioral comorbidity. However, CM-Pfc stimulation improved mood and impulsivity, whereas pallidal stimulation had no effect.[71] The second study reported that anteromedial GPi stimulation showed a 65% to 96% tic reduction, whereas CM-Pfc stimulation had a 30% to 64% decrease. Moreover, the combination of both targets showed a tic reduction of only 43% to 76%.[85] As mentioned previously, some of the double targeting cases required additional implantation of electrodes in an attempt to rescue the previous unsuccessful stimulation.[81] This often resulted in unsatisfactory outcomes.

SELECTION CRITERIA

The evaluation and selection of TS patients as candidates for DBS is a systematic and strict procedure that should be carried out by an interdisciplinary group of experts. Diagnosis should be based on the official *Diagnostic and Statistical Manual of Mental Disorders*, fifth edition (DSM-5) criteria, which require an onset of symptoms before the age of 18 years and the presence of multiple motor and at least one phonic tic for at least 1 year.[2] In principle, DBS should only be considered in severe cases in which a satisfactory outcome could not be obtained using more conservative therapies. Since 2006, several groups of experts have defined or suggested guidelines for surgical intervention.[52,86,87] The following selection criteria are based on the latest review manuscript on DBS in TS written under the auspices of the Tourette Syndrome Association, with proposed guidelines based on all DBS in TS cases published to date.[26]

Inclusion Criteria

- Diagnosis of TS is made by an expert clinician based on DSM-5 criteria.
- The initial definition of a minimum age of 25 years[87] is not considered to be an absolute criterion anymore. In cases in which the candidate is under 18 years of age, a local ethics committee should be consulted.
- Motor and vocal tics should be chronic, severe, and the main source of disability. The severity of the symptoms should be documented through a videotape assessment together with a standardized rating scale, such as the YGTSS. In this respect, the patient should maintain a tic severity score of 35 out of 50 points or higher for an evaluation period of more than 1 year.
- The condition is refractory to pharmacologic and behavioral therapy. The candidate should have displayed no successful response after treatment with three of the different drug regimens: (1) centrally-acting alpha$_2$-adrenergic agonists (e.g., clonidine, guanfacine); (2) at least two dopamine antagonists, one typical (e.g., haloperidol, pimozide) and one atypical (e.g., risperidone); and (3) other drugs (e.g., benzodiazepines, topiramate, sertraline).
- If the patient presents comorbid psychiatric or neurological symptoms, he or she should be under treatment and considered stable over the course of 6 months.
- The candidate must have a stable social environment with adequate support. In addition, the cognitive and psychological profile of the patient must demonstrate a capacity to cope with the demand of the procedure and the requested therapeutic recommendations.

Exclusion Criteria

Patients should not be considered as candidates for DBS if the presence of suicidal or homicidal ideation has been documented within 6 months of the planned procedure. Furthermore, recent depressive moods or substance abuse should be under treatment and considered a contraindication if they persist. After rigorous clinical evaluation, there should exist no evidence or suspicion of a factitious disorder or the presence of psychogenic tics. Patients should also be excluded from neurosurgical treatment if they have a medical or neurological condition that could compromise the success of the procedure or the postoperative care and recovery. Other contraindications for TS DBS are the same as for DBS at other targets and for other diagnoses and include structural brain lesions found on magnetic resonance imaging (MRI), and severe cardiovascular, pulmonary, or hematologic abnormalities.

SURGICAL PROCEDURE AND PERIOPERATIVE MANAGEMENT

Symptoms should be assessed with validated clinical rating scales pre- and postoperatively in order to monitor surgical outcomes. Recorded data should include the effects of DBS on motor and vocal tics, associated psychiatric disorders, drug regimens, quality of life, cognitive performance, side effects of stimulation, and adverse events related to surgery or the implanted device. The most common and recommended assessment tools are the YGTSS to evaluate the frequency, intensity, complexity, and interference of the tics,[88] and a blinded video evaluation (Video 99-1) to document the changes before and after stimulation (i.e., Rush Video-Based Tic Rating Scale). Standardized evaluations of these videos should be performed by two independent investigators, who must be blinded to preoperative measurements and postoperative stimulation status (i.e., both "on" and "off" stimulation periods should be recorded).

The DBS implantation procedure is performed similarly to that described for DBS for any other indication.[89] In short, a stereotactic frame is fixed to the patient's skull and imaging is performed according to the surgeon's preference (e.g., stereotactic MRI or a stereotactic computed tomography scan fused with a preoperative MRI). In contrast to DBS for tremor or Parkinson's disease, for which the procedure is mostly performed under local anesthesia so that one may perform intraoperative test stimulation, DBS in TS cannot be performed under local anesthesia because of the hyperkinetic nature of the disease. Instead, the stimulating leads are implanted under general anesthesia or conscious sedation. If the patient is considered a good candidate for sedation, this can be carried out with either a combination of lormetazepam (or lorazepam) and clonidine or with a propofol infusion.[47,52] In these cases, intraoperative examination during test stimulation could exhibit a series of undesired stimulation-induced side effects that can only be detected during awake brain surgery. If so, this information is typically used to adjust electrode position. This might be of particular importance for targets such as the centromedian nucleus of the thalamus, which are not directly visible on standard (1.5-T or 3-T) MRI scans. When performing DBS for movement disorders, microelectrode recordings are often used to characterize single-cell activity and define an "optimal" target for electrode implantation. In TS intraoperative recordings are more appreciated as a powerful research tool.[90]

The position of the active contacts of stimulation should be verified postoperatively using MRI or computed tomography in order to correlate this information with the best-induced clinical effect. A strict record of stimulation parameters should be kept in order to optimize future adjustments and avoid stimulation-induced side effects. Rigorous psychiatric and neuropsychological assessments, including standardized rating scales for TS and other comorbid disorders, should be carried out on a regular basis.

CONCLUSION AND FUTURE DIRECTIONS

Although DBS has by and large been an effective therapy for patients suffering from medically refractory TS, definitive rigorous studies are still needed to prove and optimize its efficacy. These studies must also examine important questions about the underlying mechanisms of TS pathophysiology. Although dysfunction in the cortico–basal ganglia–thalamocortical network is readily accepted as the pathophysiologic basis of impairment, there are very few invasive studies in human subjects and only one longitudinal study that directly investigated the pathologic changes believed to underlie the disorder. In this study by Maling and colleagues, data are provided from chronic recordings within the centromedian nucleus of the thalamus over the course of DBS therapy.[91] In a cohort of five patients, therapeutic effects were tracked and correlated with the thalamic network state over the course of 6 months. Local field potential recordings elucidated the temporal effects of DBS on the neuropathophysiologic dynamics of TS. The results of their study showed the first clinical correlation between symptomatology and gamma-synchronized oscillations. A clear correlation was shown between a decrease in tic severity and an increase in the power of gamma-band activity. This correlation was echoed in acute recordings, suggesting these dynamic changes in human thalamic gamma-band activity are relevant to the pathophysiology underlying TS. This was substantiated by the nonresponders in the cohort, who also did not exhibit substantial changes in gamma-band activity. Furthermore, the importance of highly circumscribed implantation location was suggested because the two nonresponders experienced electrode placement that was more anterior or ventral when compared to the rest of the cohort. These results suggest the centromedian nucleus of the thalamus is an important therapeutic focus in the pathologic circuit mediating TS, and offers important insights into tic genesis and expression.

DBS offers the opportunity to take electrophysiologic recordings directly from the purported areas of dysfunction. Potential biomarkers for TS can thereby be revealed by tracking specific neurobiologic changes in dysfunctional circuits. Where aberrant oscillatory behavior has been suggested to subserve various neuropsychiatric disorders, this has now been empirically shown to be true in TS.[51,92] Although previously suggested to be a disorder of hypersynchrony, results from chronic DBS recordings show it is a disorder of hyposynchrony.[51] Changes in the synchronized rhythms of specific frequency band activity (in this case gamma) are reflected as neurophysiologic fluctuations that could be correlated with alterations in motor and behavioral impairment, such as reported by YGTSS scores. Investigations on causality would provide important information as to the source of these aberrations, and thus allow more effective target selection. The inclusion of modern electrical neuroimaging methods in DBS studies would comprehensively elucidate the mechanisms subserving TS.[93]

Knowledge of these biomarkers and their characteristic involvement in the disease state may allow for real-time improvements in target localization during surgery and promote the development of next-generation technologies such as closed loop stimulation. This in turn would lead to improved patient care and reduced stimulation-induced side effects by providing both objective therapeutic assessment of the efficacy of stimulation parameters and tailored treatment postoperatively.

SUGGESTED READINGS

Maling N, Hashemiyoon R, Foote KD, et al. Increased thalamic gamma band activity correlates with symptom relief following deep brain stimulation in humans with Tourette's syndrome. *PLoS One*. 2012;7:e44215.

Michel CM, Murray MM. Towards the utilization of EEG as a brain imaging tool. *Neuroimage*. 2012;61:371-385.

Priori A, Giannicola G, Rosa M, et al. Deep brain electrophysiological recordings provide clues to the pathophysiology of Tourette syndrome. *Neurosci Biobehav Rev*. 2013;37:1063-1068.

Schrock LE, Mink JW, Woods DW, et al. Tourette syndrome deep brain stimulation: a review and updated recommendations. *Mov Disord*. 2014;doi:10.1002/mds.26094.

Temel Y, Visser-Vandewalle V. Surgery in Tourette syndrome. *Mov Disord*. 2004;19:3-14.

Vandewalle V, van der Linden C, Groenewegen HJ, et al. Stereotactic treatment of Gilles de la Tourette syndrome by high frequency stimulation of thalamus. *Lancet*. 1999;353:724.

See a full reference list on ExpertConsult.com

100 Surgery for Obsessive-Compulsive Disorder

Mayur Sharma, Andrew Shaw, Milind Deogaonkar, and Ali Rezai

ABBREVIATIONS USED

ACC anterior cingulate cortex
ALIC anterior limb of internal capsule
CSTC cortical-striatal-thalamic-cortical
DBS deep brain stimulation
fMRI functional magnetic resonance imaging
GPi globus pallidus internus
ITP inferior thalamic peduncle
OCD obsessive-compulsive disorder
OFC orbitofrontal cortex
NAcc nucleus accumbens
PET positron emission tomography
STN subthalamic nucleus
Vc/Vs ventral capsule and ventral striatum
Y-BOCS Yale-Brown Obsessive Compulsive Scale

Obsessive-compulsive disorder (OCD) is a chronic and severe anxiety disorder that affects about 2% to 3% of the population.[1-4] OCD is the 10th leading cause of disability worldwide and affects both genders equally.[5,6] According to the *Diagnostic and Statistical Manual of Mental Disorders*, fifth edition *(DSM-5)*, OCD is characterized by persistent obsessions with intrusive thoughts leading to severe generalized anxiety or compulsions in the form of repetitive tasks to relieve this distress.[7,8] These compulsions are severe and long enough (>1 hr/day) to interfere with one's routine activities, performance at work, and family and social interactions.[4,5] In addition to these symptoms, patients with OCD are twice as likely to report suicide attempts as those with other psychiatric disorders.[9] Pharmacotherapy (selective serotonin reuptake inhibitors [SSRIs]) and cognitive behavior therapy (CBT) are the first-line treatment option for patients with OCD.[10,11] These therapeutic measures provide a 40% to 60% reduction in OCD symptoms in 50% of patients.[4] However, despite aggressive pharmacotherapy and behavior therapy, 10% to 25% of patients have persistent symptoms leading to significant morbidity.[3,10,12,13]

Surgical management is a consideration for this subset of patients with medically refractory OCD. The surgical treatment of various psychiatric disorders can be dated back to the origin of neurological surgery; however, surgery fell out of favor because of a poor understanding of the pathophysiology of psychiatric disorders and the high surgical morbidity and mortality associated with frontal lobotomy. Furthermore, variable reporting of surgical outcomes and availability of effective medications made surgical therapy obsolete. Technologic advances and an evolution in brain imaging techniques not only improved our understanding of the pathophysiology of psychiatric disorders but also led to a renewed interest in the surgical treatment of refractory psychiatric disorders, including OCD. Various targets for ablation or neurostimulation have been described; however, owing to its reversibility, adaptability, and the ability to blind the stimulation for research studies, neurostimulation is presently considered superior to ablation when treating psychiatric disorders.

The success of deep brain stimulation (DBS) surgery for a variety of movement disorders over the past two decades has led to the exploration of this treatment modality for medically refractory OCD. Both the minimally invasive nature of DBS surgery and its excellent safety profile make it a favorable technique for treating functional brain disorders. Worldwide, more than 100,000 patients have received DBS implants for a variety of disorders, including OCD.[14] Till presented more than 100 patients who underwent DBS surgery for medically refractory OCD, which resulted in this therapy receiving Humanitarian Device Exemption status by the U.S. Food and Drug Administration (FDA) in 2009.[15-18] This chapter focuses on the surgical management of OCD, with an overview of the pertinent literature, historical aspects of psychosurgery, pathophysiology, involved circuits, surgical techniques, different anatomic targets, ethical considerations, current challenges with DBS systems, and recent advances in DBS surgery.

HISTORY OF PSYCHOSURGERY

The current role of neurosurgery in the treatment of OCD and other psychiatric conditions has evolved significantly from its troubled past. Surgical techniques have transformed from simple trephination used to treat madness in the Neolithic and Renaissance eras into sophisticated modern-day stereotactic DBS surgery.[19,20] The origin of ablative surgery for psychiatric disorders can be dated back to the 1890s, when Swiss psychiatrist Gottlieb Burckhardt performed a left frontotemporal cerebral corticectomy (topectomies) in six patients with various severe psychiatric illnesses.[21-23] He reported success in 50% of the patients (3 of 6 patients); however, the postoperative evaluation criteria were not clearly defined, and the work was met with criticism by the medical community at the time.[21]

Psychosurgery was reborn in 1935 with the introduction of frontal leucotomy/lobotomy by Portuguese neurologist Egaz Moniz and neurosurgeon Pedro Almeida. Their clinical work was based on the success of frontal ablative procedures in primates by American neuroscientists John Fulton and Carlyle Jacobsen. Moniz and Almeida treated their first seven patients with ethanol injection into the centrum semiovale through a lateral trepanation in the skull.[24] After finding that they needed to repeat the procedure multiple times, they altered their technique, employing a leucotome (a cannulated instrument that produced a 1-cm lesion in the white matter) to lesion the brain, typically producing six lesions in each of the frontal lobes.[15,24] In 1949 Moniz was awarded the Nobel Prize in Physiology or Medicine for "the discovery of the therapeutic value of leucotomy in certain psychoses."[6,25] Moniz performed prefrontal leucotomies in 20 patients with various psychiatric disorders.[23] Neurologist Walter Freeman and neurosurgeon James Watts popularized Moniz's technique in the United States. In 1942, they communicated their initial findings in 200 frontal lobotomy patients, reporting that 63% showed symptomatic improvement.[26] Although effective, prefrontal leucotomy was associated with significant complications such as uncontrolled hemorrhage, seizures, apathy, and death. Freeman's desire to popularize this technique led to fractions and later to separation from his neurosurgical colleague.[25] In response, Freeman developed and popularized bilateral transorbital frontal leucotomy, in which a sharp leucotome (orbitoclast) was introduced into the frontal lobes through the thin orbital roof. This procedure was performed in an outpatient setting employing electroconvulsive therapy as a general anesthetic.[25] The technique was employed liberally for a variety of psychiatric illnesses, and more than 60,000 transorbital leucotomies were performed by 1956.[25,27] The widespread and indiscriminate use of this crude surgical technique with a relative paucity of appropriate assessment tools and controlled studies led to disastrous outcomes. Both the medical community and public viewed the procedure as inhumane and called for an end to the practice of psychosurgery. Furthermore, the advent of more effective pharmacotherapies ended this era of psychosurgery.[15,25,28]

Although there was a significant decline in the practice of psychosurgery, there was still a push for research into possible surgical treatment modalities for severe psychiatric disorders. In 1949 William Scoville published his technique of selective cortical undercutting to modify and study frontal lobe functions in humans.[29] In his series of 43 patients, he introduced the concept of minimalism that led to renewed interest in psychosurgery. In addition, the introduction of a stereotactic coordinate system by French neurosurgeon Jean Talairach and Cartesian stereotactic systems developed by Spiegel and Wycis and by Leksell in late 1940s enabled neurosurgeons to perform psychosurgery with greater precision, thereby minimizing the complications associated with cruder frontal leucotomies.[6,15,30-32] Spiegel and Wycis performed the first stereotactic ablation in a human patient in 1949, paving the way for the beginning of modern psychoneurosurgery.[6,32] Stereotactic ablative procedures such as cingulotomy, anterior capsulotomy, subcaudate tractotomy, and anterior callosotomy replaced frontal leucotomies and lobotomies for refractory psychiatric disorders.[33] Various lesioning techniques such as radiofrequency thermocoagulation and radioisotope (yttrium 90) implantation or stereotactic radiosurgery were used to perform these ablative procedures.[34-38] However, after its dramatic success in the treatment of medically refractory movement disorders,[39] DBS therapy has largely replaced ablation as the preferred intervention for OCD.

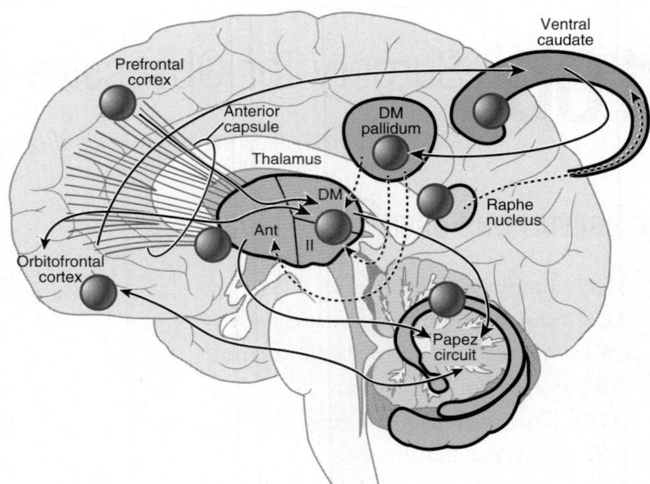

Figure 100-1. Schematic representation of neural circuits involved in the basic pathophysiology of obsessive-compulsive disorder. *Red dots* indicate different surgical targets for deep brain stimulation therapy. Ant, anterior; DM, dorsomedial. *(From Kopell BH, Greenberg B, Rezai AR. Deep brain stimulation for psychiatric disorders.* J Clin Neurophysiol. *2004;21:51-67.)*

NEURAL CIRCUITS AND PATHOPHYSIOLOGY

In contrast to movement disorders, there is no one neural "circuit" or "target" that is implicated in the pathophysiology of OCD. Instead, the symptoms of OCD are caused by abnormalities in multiple interweaved neural circuits or targets that form a complex network controlling mood and anxiety[40,41] (Fig. 100-1). Consequently, effective neuromodulation for OCD likely requires multiple neural circuits to be affected by stimulation of anatomic targets that are selected based on a detailed understanding of the basic pathophysiology. Although functional magnetic resonance imaging (fMRI) of the brain, animal models, and physiologic and anatomic studies enable us to better understand the neurobiology of OCD, it is understood that mood and behaviors associated with OCD are unique to humans and that experimental observations in animal models of OCD may not be directly extrapolated to the human disease.

The functional organization of neural circuits implicated in the pathophysiology of psychiatric disorders is similar to that identified in patients with movement disorders. Alexander and colleagues[42] identified multiple parallel basal ganglia–thalamocortical loops (cortical-striatal-pallidal-thalamic-cortical loops) that process cortical inputs from the motor, oculomotor, dorsolateral prefrontal, lateral orbitofrontal, and anterior cingulate regions (Fig. 100-2). Each of these circuits includes functionally and anatomically discrete regions of the striatum, globus pallidus and substantia nigra, thalamus, and cortex. In the motor loop, motor and somatosensory cortical areas send partially overlapping projections to a specific region of the striatum. The striatum then sends projections that further converge at the level of the globus pallidus. From the globus pallidus, fully converged fibers project to a specific location in the thalamus. To close the loop, the thalamus projects back to a cortical area that feeds into the circuit. The net result is that several corticostriatal inputs that are functionally related are funneled together to a single cortical region in a feedback loop.[42] Although these circuits are anatomically and functionally segregated, there is connectivity between them so that limbic, cognitive, and motor pathways are integrated.

The basal ganglia–thalamocortical loop implicated in the pathophysiology of OCD originates in the prefrontal cortex and orbitofrontal cortex (OFC). Fibers originating from the prefrontal and orbitofrontal cortices project to the ventral striatum through the ventral internal capsule. Specifically, these fibers reach the ventral aspect of the caudate and the nucleus accumbens (NAcc) and are excitatory in nature by means of glutamate and aspartate.[43,44] This area also receives inhibitory serotonergic input from the dorsal raphe nucleus of the midbrain. From the ventral striatum, the fibers then project to the ventral pallidum and are mediated by substance P, enkephalin, and γ-aminobutyric acid (GABA).[45,46] Inhibitory projections then reach the mediodorsal aspect of the thalamus. Finally, the thalamus projects fibers back to the OFC. The overall output of this pathway is inhibitory in nature and seeks to dampen the input to the cortex.[47-49] There also exists a parallel circuit originating in the anterior cingulate cortex (ACC), with projections to the ventral striatum and pallidum and termination in the mediodorsal aspect of the thalamus. This loop then projects back to the ACC. The anterior cingulate loop is believed to underlay the anxiety component of OCD, whereas the circuit originating in the OFC is thought to mediate the core symptoms of OCD.[50] Moreover, although the basal ganglia–thalamocortical loop originating in the OFC is inhibitory in nature, the cortical-thalamic-cortical circuit originating in the orbitofrontal and prefrontal cortices is excitatory in nature. These loops are also referred to as the direct and inhibitory pathways, respectively.[51,52] The positive feedback loop originates in the orbitofrontal and prefrontal cortices and projects to the dorsomedial thalamic nucleus through the anterior limb of the internal capsule. In a normal state, this excitatory pathway is dampened by the net inhibitory output of the aforementioned basal ganglia–thalamocortical loop.[50] There is also a net effect of

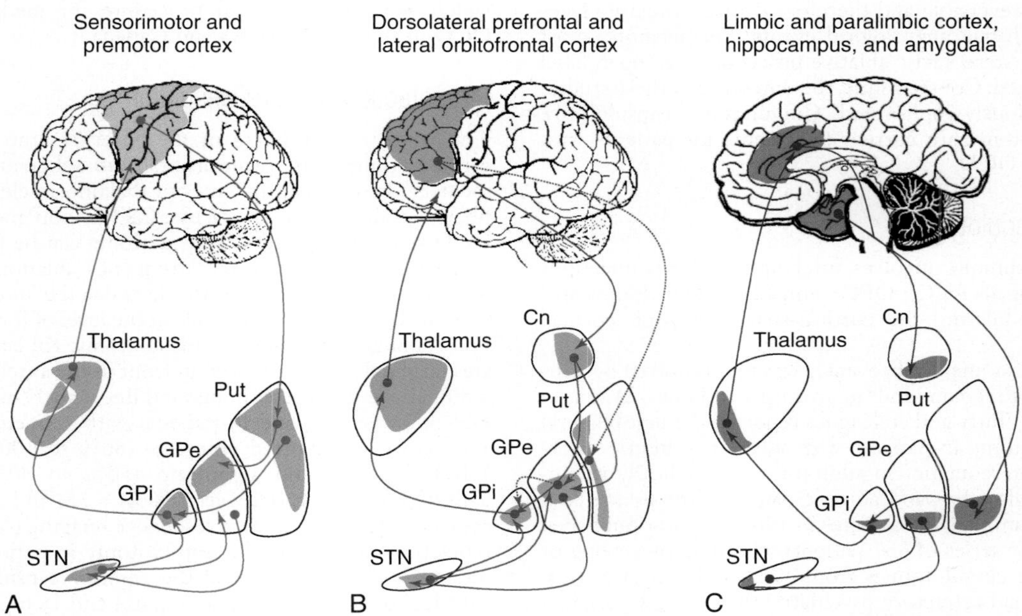

Figure 100-2. Schematic representation of motor **(A)**, associative **(B)**, and limbic **(C)** circuits of the cortical-striatal-pallidal-thalamic-cortical loops implicated in the pathophysiology of movement and psychiatric disorders. Cn, caudate nucleus; GPe, globus pallidus externus; GPi, globus pallidus internus; Put, putamen; STN, subthalamic nucleus. *(Modified from Obeso JA, Rodriquez-Oroz MC, Benitez-Temino B, et al. Functional organization of the basal ganglia: therapeutic implications for Parkinson's disease.* Mov Disord. *2008;23[suppl 3]:S548-S559.)*

decreased thalamic stimulation of the cortex through pallidothalamic connections, which are mediated by GABA.[53,54] It is believed that OCD symptoms arise when the equilibrium between these finely tuned pathways is lost.[50] An additional loop involving the limbic and Papez circuits underlies the emotional aspects of OCD. Widespread connections between the ACC, OFC, dorsomedial thalamus, NAcc, and Papez circuit may mediate the limbic component of OCD.[16,55-58] Obsessive-compulsive symptoms are caused by either decreased activity in the basal ganglia–thalamocortical (striatal-pallidal-thalamic-cortical) loops or increased activity in the cortical-thalamic-cortical (orbital-frontal-thalamic) loops.[47] Generally, there is increased stimulation of OFC due to decreased modulation by the cortical-subcortical circuits, resulting in the OCD symptoms.[47] Therefore modulating either of these pathways and Papez circuit could possibly ameliorate the obsessive-compulsive, anxiety, and emotional symptoms associated with OCD.[59-61]

Functional neuroimaging (PET and fMRI) studies report abnormally increased metabolic activity of the prefrontal cortex, ACC, OFC, caudate, and thalamus in OCD patients in both neutral and provoked states as compared to healthy individuals.[47,62,63] Studies have also reported decreased levels of *N*-acetyl aspartate (a marker of neuronal density) in the medial prefrontal cortex and its correlation with symptom severity in patients with OCD as compared to healthy controls.[64] There are no significant differences in caudate volumes between OCD patients and healthy controls.[65] A decrease in metabolic activity in the pathologic cortical-subcortical loop (OFC, bilateral caudate, and cingulate gyri) has been shown in patients with OCD after successful treatment with either medications (SSRIs) or behavior therapy.[8,47,60,62,66] In addition, the ventral and anterior striatum, which receives cortical afferents from the ACC and OFC, has a high concentration of striosomes compared with other regions.[8,67,68] These striosomes are specialized to influence negative feedback inhibition on the frontal-subcortical circuits by inhibiting dopaminergic input to the region. When there is dysfunction in the striosomes, there is hyperactivity in the caudate nucleus, which is thought to lead to inhibition of negative feedback on the frontal cortices.[69] This allows for the higher than normal levels of stimulation of the frontal cortex and deficits in cognitive and emotional functioning that are central to OCD.[70]

These neuroimaging, anatomic, and physiologic studies provide insight into the pathophysiology of OCD that may identify new nodes for surgical intervention.

SURGICAL MANAGEMENT OF OBSESSIVE-COMPULSIVE DISORDER

The advent of stereotaxy made it possible to target subcortical structures with submillimetric accuracy, thereby increasing surgical safety while maintaining the efficacy of earlier surgical procedures for OCD.[71-78] Most reports regarding surgical outcomes represent uncontrolled or nonblinded studies that need to be cautiously interpreted. Nevertheless, surgical treatment can provide hope to patients with severe and medically refractory OCD. All of the procedures thus far employed tend to modulate activity within the OFC, dorsolateral frontal cortex, and ACC and their interactions with the basal ganglia and thalamus. Surgical procedures such as DBS, stereotactic ablation, and vagus nerve stimulation (VNS) have been shown to ameliorate OCD symptoms in various studies, as discussed later.

Stereotactic Ablation Procedures

With the advent of stereotaxis, procedures such as anterior cingulotomy, capsulotomy, subcaudate tractotomy, and limbic leucotomy were developed to help patients with severe and refractory psychiatric disorders. These procedures tend to modulate activity in the cortical-striatal-pallidal-thalamic-cortical loops through targeted ablation, ameliorating OCD symptoms. These ablative procedures are irreversible and therefore demand precise placement to avoid adverse neurological events. Furthermore, most studies regarding stereotactic ablative procedures are open label and nonrandomized. Consequently, the outcomes of these studies need to be cautiously interpreted. Cingulotomy, capsulotomy, and limbic leucotomy are current treatments for patients with severe refractory OCD.

Stereotactic Cingulotomy

This surgical technique involves interrupting the connections between the dorsal ACC, OFC, amygdala, and hippocampus, thereby modulating the cortical-striatal-thalamic-cortical (CSTC) loops.[52,79]

Cingulotomy for anxiety-like states was first reported by neurologist Walter Freeman and neurosurgeon James Watts in 1942.[26] In 1952, Whitty and colleagues reported the first bilateral anterior cingulectomy in patients with severe psychiatric disorders.[80] Bilateral stereotactic cingulotomies for medically refractory psychiatric disorders and chronic pain syndromes was first reported by Ballantine and associates in 1962 and later published in 1987.[81] In their series of 387 patients who underwent one or more stereotactic cingulotomies from 1962 to 1982, 70% (n = 273) of patients had refractory psychiatric disorders, 21% had a chronic pain syndrome, and another 9% suffered from terminal cancer pain.[81] Of the 273 patients with psychiatric disorders, 32 (16%) had OCD, and 120 (61%) suffered from affective disorders. Ballantine and associates performed the lesion 0 to 4 cm posterior to the tip of frontal horns, 7 mm lateral to midline, and 1 mm above the roof of the ventricles using electrically insulated thermistor electrodes. They reported that 25% (n = 8) of patients were responders/functionally normal, 31% (n = 10) showed marked improvement, whereas 41% (n = 14) showed slight or no improvement.[81] Of note, no clinical assessment scores were used in this study. In 1991, Jenike and colleagues reported on the long-term efficacy of bilateral cingulotomy in 33 patients with refractory OCD, finding that 27% of living patients were responders (>25% reduction in the Yale-Brown Obsessive-Compulsive Scale [Y-BOCS] and obsessive-compulsive visual analogue scales).[82] Dougherty and coworkers conducted a prospective evaluation of 44 patients who underwent one or more cingulotomies for treatment-refractory OCD, finding that 32% (n = 14) of the patients were responders (>35% reduction in Y-BOCS) and other 14% (n = 6) were partial responders at a mean follow-up of 32 months.[83] Similarly, Kim and colleagues and Jung and associates reported responder rates of 42.8% (6 of 14 patients) and 47% (8 of 17 patients) after bilateral anterior cingulotomies for medically refractory OCD at 12 months and 24 months follow-up, respectively.[84,85] Zhang and coworkers reported a more than 35% reduction in Y-BOCS scores in five of seven patients after bilateral anterior cingulotomy and bilateral anterior capsulotomy at 12 months.[86] In a recent study, Sheth and colleagues reported a complete (>35% reduction in Y-BOCS score) response in 38% (12 of 34) of patients after a single pair of stereotactic cingulotomies for refractory OCD at the mean follow-up of 63.8 months.[87] Recently, Gentil and associates reported that patients with refractory OCD and hoarding symptoms had a worse response to either stereotactic capsulotomy or cingulotomy than those without hoarding symptoms (mean Y-BOCS score decrease of 22.7% ± 25.9% vs. 41.6% ± 32.2%, respectively; $P < .05$).[89] In addition, they recommend that patients with refractory OCD who are being considered for ablative surgeries should be carefully screened for hoarding symptoms or disorder.[89] Anterior cingulotomy is a safe procedure with an incidence of complications similar to that of other stereotactic procedures. Few significant surgical complications or permanent behavioral or cognitive deficits have been reported after stereotactic cingulotomy for OCD.[82-87,90] Therefore stereotactic cingulotomy is the most widely performed surgical procedure for medically refractory OCD in the United States and Canada.[17]

Stereotactic Anterior Capsulotomy

The white matter fibers in the anterior limb of the internal capsule connect the orbitofrontal and subgenual ACCs to the medial, dorsomedial, and anterior thalamic nuclei. Severing these fibers can disrupt the overactive CSTC loop and ameliorate the OCD symptoms. Anterior capsulotomy can be performed using either Gamma Knife or radiofrequency ablation.[35,36] The lesion is typically produced in the area between the anterior and middle one third of the internal capsule at the level of foramen of Monro. For Gamma Knife anterior capsulotomy, Kihlstrom and associates targeted the area 10 mm in front of the anterior commissure, 8 mm above the intercommissural line, and 17 mm lateral to the midcommissural plane in patients with refractory OCD.[36] Liu and associates reported complete (80% to 100% reduction in Y-BOCS score) and significant (50% to 80% reduction in Y-BOCS score) responses in 57% (n = 35) and 29% of patients, respectively, after magnetic resonance imaging (MRI)-guided stereotactic bilateral anterior capsulotomy in patients with refractory OCD.[91] They targeted the anterior capsule 22 to 25 mm anterior to the midcommissural point and 18 to 20 mm lateral to the midline at the level of midcommissural plane.[91] Another uncontrolled, prospective study reported significant responses (>35% reduction in Y-BOCS score) in 48% of patients (n = 25) after unilateral or bilateral thermocapsulotomy or Gamma Knife capsulotomy at a mean follow-up of 10.9 years.[92] Based on the examination of brain MRIs in 11 of these patients, they also noted that reducing the lateral extension of ablation may increase the reduction in OCD symptoms, whereas limiting the medial and posterior extension of the lesion may reduce the side effects associated with the procedure.[92] A third study reported response rates of 27% and 62% after a single versus a double shot, respectively, of bilateral Gamma Knife capsulotomy.[90]

Anterior capsulotomy is a safe procedure with no surgical mortality reported in the literature. However, there are reports of patients attempting or committing suicide in the perioperative period.[92] Ruck and colleagues reported a mean weight gain of 6 kg in the first year after surgery and significant problems related to executive functioning, apathy, or sexual disinhibition in 10 OCD patients after Gamma Knife capsulotomy.[92] Six of these 10 patients had either received high doses of radiation or undergone multiple capsulotomies, and one patient developed radiation necrosis.[92] Minor side effects such as headache, confusion, urinary incontinence, weight gain, and lethargy have been reported after radiofrequency-mediated capsulotomy. Another study reported side effects such as cerebral edema and headache (20%), asymptomatic infarctions in the caudate nucleus (10%), and frontal lobe dysfunction (3%) after Gamma Knife capsulotomy.[90] Mindus and colleagues reported a low incidence of adverse personality changes after capsulotomy for refractory OCD that remain static over time.[93] Similarly, Nyman and associates reported no significant changes in overall neuropsychological performance after thermocoagulative capsulotomy, except for some changes in executive functions that recovered over time.[94]

Stereotactic Subcaudate Tractotomy

In 1965, Geoffrey Knight, with an experience of 550 restricted undercutting operations for psychiatric disorders between 1950 and 1965, realized that it was the posterior part of the incision in the subcortical white matter that was associated with the best therapeutic effect.[34] This posterior part of subcortical white matter was identified as the substantia innominata, and this serendipitous finding led to the origin of subcaudate tractotomy.[34,95] The substantia innominata contains white matter fibers that connect the OFC to the thalamus, amygdala, and subgenual ACC. Interrupting these white matter tracts tends to modify the CSTC loops.[52] Knight performed innominotomy by using two rows of four seeds of radioactive yttrium 90, creating a lesion measuring 2 cm long and 1.8 cm wide, 1 cm above the orbital roof.[34] The substantia innominata is located beneath the head of the caudate nucleus. These lesions are made by placing bilateral frontal bur holes 2 cm long in the anteroposterior plane of planum sphenoidale and 15 mm from the midline.[96] In 1995, Hodgkiss and colleagues reported the efficacy of bilateral stereotactic yttrium 90 subcaudate tractotomy in 286 patients with psychiatric disorders between 1979 and 1991.[97] Of 15 OCD patients included in this series, 5 patients recovered completely or had mild symptoms after the procedure, 5 patients improved but had significant residual symptoms, and 5 patients remained unchanged or worsened after the surgery.[97] Another study reported a response rate of 50% after stereotactic subcaudate tractotomy in patients with refractory OCD.[90] Bridges and associates reviewed 1300 subcaudate tractotomies performed at Knight's unit in London since 1961 and reported a response rate of 40% to 60% with continuation of medications in patients with severe depression (suicidal or delusional) and refractory affective disorders.[98] Göktepe and colleagues reported good results in 50% of 18 patients with refractory OCD after subcaudate tractotomy at a mean follow-up of 2.5 years.[99] In addition, the suicide rate in patients with severe and refractory affective disorders decreased from 15% to 1% after subcaudate tractotomy.[98] Mild and transient side effects such as headache, confusion, and lethargy have been reported after bilateral subcaudate tractotomy.[90] A single mortality due to yttrium lead migration is mentioned in the literature.[98] In the current era, subcaudate tractotomy is less frequently used to treat refractory OCD.

Stereotactic Limbic Leucotomy

Limbic leucotomy involves interrupting the white matter tracts at the lower medial quadrant of each frontal lobe (subcaudate tractotomy) and those in the cingulum (cingulotomy). This procedure was first described in 1973 by Kelly and Richardson in London.[100] Limbic leucotomy interrupts the frontothalamic and limbic loops and thus modulates the CSTC loops involved in the pathophysiology of OCD. This ablative procedure is performed using either thermocoagulative or cryogenic techniques.[15] Kelly and colleagues reported a response rate of 41% after stereotactic limbic leucotomy in 17 patients with OCD.[100] In 1976, Mitchell-Heggs and associates reported that among 66 patients with severe psychiatric disorders who underwent limbic leucotomy, 89% of patients with obsessional neurosis and 66% of patients with chronic anxiety showed definite clinical improvement at 16 months of follow-up.[101] Validated rating scales were not employed. Monotoya and coworkers reported significant responses (>35% reduction in Y-BOCS score) in 36% (4 of 11) of refractory OCD patients after MRI-guided bilateral stereotactic limbic leucotomy at a mean follow-up of 26 months.[102] Transient adverse effects included headache, confusion, lethargy, apathy, perseverative behavior, and incontinence, with no reports of deaths or seizures.[101] There are also reports of severe memory impairment and weight loss after stereotactic limbic leucotomy for OCD.[101,102]

Deep Brain Stimulation

The success of DBS in movement disorders led clinicians to explore this treatment option for patients with medically refractory OCD. In 1979, low-frequency (5-Hz) stimulation of the area near the parafascicular complex in the intralaminar thalamic nuclei was shown to ameliorate phobia and OCD symptoms at 1 year of follow-up in a female patient.[103] Similarly, stimulation of the cerebellar vermis has been shown to improve OCD symptoms by targeting neural circuits instead of a specific target.[104] These preliminary studies paved the way for the exploration of newer DBS targets and circuits for medically refractory OCD. In 2009, DBS surgery for OCD was granted a Humanitarian Device Exemption by the FDA.[15-18] The advantages of reversibility, ability to adjust the stimulation parameters over time, and better surgical safety profile relative to ablation made DBS surgery an attractive and favorable treatment option for patients with refractory OCD. In addition, patients with DBS can be blinded to their stimulation status in research studies aimed at determining the efficacy of this therapy. To date, more than 100 patients have undergone DBS implantation surgery for OCD. The paucity of data regarding the efficacy of DBS for OCD can be attributed to the heterogeneity of patients with medically refractory OCD, nonuniformity in the assessment and enrollment criteria, prolonged titration periods, and operationalizing titration intervals in blinded randomized controlled studies, especially for patients traveling great distances for treatment.

The mechanisms underlying the therapeutic benefits of DBS remains elusive and are a matter of contentious debate. Initially, it was proposed that high-frequency stimulation induces neuronal inhibition by depolarizing neurons in the vicinity of an electrode, a mechanism similar to ablation.[105] Hypotheses such as depolarization blockade, synaptic inhibition, synaptic depression, and stimulation-induced modulation of pathologic network activity have been implicated as the probable mechanisms underlying the therapeutic efficacy of DBS.[106] Of these, stimulation-induced modulation of pathologic network activity is the most likely mechanism underlying the therapeutic benefits of DBS.[105-107] Furthermore DBS improves the functioning of thalamocortical neurons and potentially normalizes the imbalance in the cognitive-behavior-emotional circuit.[108] Various structures such as the anterior limb of internal capsule (ALIC), ventral capsule and ventral striatum (Vc/Vs), NAcc, subthalamic nucleus (STN), and inferior thalamic peduncle (ITP) have been explored as potential DBS targets in patients with refractory OCD with varied results.

Anterior Limb of Internal Capsule

The fibers in the ALIC connect the OFC and subgenual ACC to the medial, dorsomedial, and anterior thalamic nuclei. To emulate the beneficial effects of stereotactic capsulotomy in patients with medically refractory OCD, this target was the first one to be explored as a potential DBS target.[71,109] In 1999, Nuttin and colleagues[71] published the first controlled study on DBS therapy in patients with medically refractory OCD (Table 100-1). They stimulated the ALIC bilaterally in four patients, employing a target similar to that used for capsulotomy. Three of these four patients experienced some beneficial effect. One of these patients reported 90% improvement in her compulsive behavior and rituals after 2 weeks of stimulation. The major drawback of this study was lack of assessment scores to quantify improvements in mood or obsessive and compulsive behaviors after stimulation. Four years later, the same investigators reported significant improvement in the Y-BOCS score and Global Assessment of Functioning (GAF) scale after bilateral ALIC-DBS in six patients with medically refractory OCD.[72] In this double-blind, controlled study, Y-BOCS and clinical global severity scores improved from a mean of 32.3 to 19.8 and from 5 to 3.3 with stimulator "off" versus "on," respectively. Three of six patients responded to stimulation (>35% reduction in Y-BOCS score), whereas global improvement functions were unchanged in one patient, and two patients did not enter the assessment phase.[72,73] The four patients who entered the assessment phase demonstrated significant worsening of OCD and mood symptoms in the DBS "off" state, which returned to the baseline and showed improvement in the "on" state. This stimulation-induced beneficial effect was maintained

TABLE 100-1 Summary of Controlled and Open Case Studies of Deep Brain Stimulation Surgery Targeting Different Structures in Patients with Medical Treatment–Refractory Obsessive-Compulsive Disorder

Study	No. of Patients	Follow-Up Period (mo)	Responders	Outcomes
TARGET: ANTERIOR LIMB OF INTERNAL CAPSULE				
Controlled Studies				
Nuttin et al., 1999[71]	4	Not mentioned	—	Some beneficial effects were observed in three subjects.
Nuttin et al., 2003[72]	6	3-31	50%	In three patients (50%), Y-BOCS scores during the stimulation-on condition were at least 35% lower than the preoperative scores—those patients were considered responders.
Abelson et al., 2005[110]	4	4-23	50%	Two patients achieved 35% improvement in their baseline OCD symptoms, as measured by the Y-BOCS.
Open Case Studies				
Anderson and Ahmed, 2003[111]	1	10	100%	One patient had >35% reduction in the Y-BOCS score.
TARGET: VENTRAL CAPSULE AND VENTRAL STRIATUM (VC/VS)				
Controlled Studies				
Goodman et al., 2010[74]	6	12	66.7%	Four (66.7%) of six patients met a criterion as "responders" (≥35% improvement in the Y-BOCS score and end-point Y-BOCS severity ≤16).
Tsai et al., 2014[75]	4	15	—	The higher the percentage of acute stimulation-induced smile and laughter, the greater the reduction in the Y-BOCS 15 mo after bilateral Vc/Vs-DBS.
Open Case Studies				
Greenberg et al., 2006[114]	10	36	40%	Eight patients have been followed for at least 36 mo. Four of eight patients had ≥35% decrease in Y-BOCS severity at 36 mo.
Greenberg et al., 2010[115]	26	3-36	62%	This open study included four centers (three from the United States and one from Europe) over 8 years and documented a 13.1-point decrease in Y-BOCS score following bilateral ALIC-Vc/Vs–DBS.
TARGET: NUCLEUS ACCUMBENS				
Controlled Studies				
Huff et al., 2010[77]	10	12	10%	Five out of ten patients showed a decrease of >25%, indicating at least partial response. One patient showed a decrease in Y-BOCS severity of >35%.
Denys et al., 2010[76]	16	21	56%	The response rate was 56% (nine patients with at least a 35% decrease in the Y-BOCS score) after right NAcc-DBS.
Open Case Studies				
Sturm et al., 2003[116]	4	24-30	75%	Three of four patients had nearly total recovery from both anxiety and OCD symptoms without any side effects (they did not use Y-BOCS).
Aouizerate et al., 2004[117]	1	12-15	100%	A patient with intractable severe OCD and associated depression had emission of OCD symptoms (with Y-BOCS score of <16) 12-15 mo after DBS of the ventral caudate nucleus.
Plewnia et al., 2008[118]	1	24	0	Sustained improvement of OCD symptoms was reported in a patient with concomitant residual schizophrenia 24 mo after right ALIC-NAcc–DBS. However, this patient did not meet the criteria for responders on Y-BOCS (preoperative and postoperative Y-BOCS scores were 32/40 and 24/40, respectively).
Franzini et al., 2010[119]	2	24-27	50%	A 13-point decrease in Y-BOCS score was reported after bilateral NAcc-DBS in one of two patients (50% responders) with medically refractory OCD.
TARGET: SUBTHALAMIC NUCLEUS				
Controlled Studies				
Mallet et al., 2008[78]	16	10 (3 mo of active stimulation and 3 mo of sham stimulation)	75%*	At the end of the active stimulation, the Y-BOCS score (on a scale from 0 to 40, with lower scores indicating less severe symptoms) was significantly lower than the score after sham stimulation (198 vs. 287; $P = .01$).
Open Case Studies				
Mallet et al., 2002[123]	2	6	100%	This study reported 58% and 64% improvement in Y-BOCS score in two patients with PD and severe OCD after bilateral STN-DBS.
Fontaine et al., 2004[129]	1	12	100%	This open study reported improvement from baseline Y-BOCS score of 32 to postoperative score of 1 after bilateral STN-DBS in a patient with refractory OCD at 12 mo.
Chabardés et al., 2013[144]	4	6	75%	The clinical severity assessed by the Y-BOCS improved at least 70% in three patients.

TABLE 100-1 Summary of Controlled and Open Case Studies of Deep Brain Stimulation Surgery Targeting Different Structures in Patients with Medical Treatment–Refractory Obsessive-Compulsive Disorder—cont'd

Study	No. of Patients	Follow-Up Period (mo)	Responders	Outcomes
TARGET: INFERIOR THALAMIC PEDUNCLE AND GLOBUS PALLIDUS INTERNUS				
Open Case Studies				
Jimenez-Ponce et al., 2009[131]	5	12	100%	Response rate of 100%: in all patients, >35% increase in the baseline Y-BOCS scores was observed after bilateral ITP-DBS.
Nair et al., 2013[132]	2	3-26	100%	This open study reported 100% and 85% improvement in the OCI in two patients, each after bilateral anteromedial (limbic) GPi-DBS for Tourette's syndrome and severe OCD.

ALIC, anterior limb of internal capsule; DBS, deep brain stimulation; GPi, globus pallidus internus; ITP, inferior thalamic peduncle; NAcc, nucleus accumbens; OCD, obsessive-compulsive disorder; OCI, Obsessive-Compulsive Inventory; PD, Parkinson's disease; STN, subthalamic nucleus; Vc/Vs, ventral capsule and ventral striatum; Y-BOCS, Yale-Brown Obsessive Compulsive Scale.
*Reduction in Y-BOCS score of >25% was considered as responder criterion in this study.

for at least 21 months after DBS implantation. The coordinates of the tip of the DBS electrode in the patient with the most favorable response in this study were 13 mm lateral to the midline on the right, 14 mm lateral to midline on the left, and 3.5 mm anterior to the anterior commissure at the level of intercommissural plane.[72] In this study, DBS electrode contacts 0, 1, 2, and 3 were located at the region of NAcc, internal capsule, and dorsal to the internal capsule, respectively. This group also noted increased pontine metabolism and decreased frontal lobe metabolism on fMRI and positron emission tomography (PET) studies after 10 days and 3 months of continuous bilateral stimulation, respectively.[72] None of the patients had complications related to the DBS implantation; however, cognitive and behavioral disinhibition was noted in two patients at 10.5 V, which was immediately controlled after decreasing the amplitude.[72] Follow-up of these patients was published in 2008.[73] Another double-blind, controlled study reported significant improvement in the mean Y-BOCS score (26.5 in DBS "on" state and 29.3 in DBS "off" state) after bilateral ALIC-DBS in four patients with medically refractory OCD enrolled in this study.[110] During the blinded phase of the study one patient experienced more than 35% improvement in Y-BOCS score, one patient had a 17% reduction in Y-BOCS score, and two patients had no impact on their OCD symptoms. In contrast, 50% of patients were responders (i.e., >35% improvement in Y-BOCS score compared with baseline) during the open phase of the study. In this study, patients were randomized in an on-off sequence of four 3-week blocks, with a mean follow-up of 4 to 23 months.[110] Anderson and Ahmed reported a decrease of 27 points on the Y-BOCS (Y-BOCS scores of 34 before and 7 after DBS implantation) in an isolated patient after bilateral ALIC-DBS implantation, with a mean follow-up of 10 months.[111]

Ventral Capsule and Ventral Striatum

The promising results of Gamma Knife and radiofrequency thermal ventral capsulotomy and ALIC-DBS for medically refractory OCD led investigators to explore structures adjacent to the internal capsule as potential DBS targets.[92] The ventral striatum consists of the ventral portion of the caudate nucleus and NAcc, which are believed to be the reward centers of the brain.[112,113] The combined ventral capsule and ventral striatum (Vc/Vs) was subsequently explored as a potential DBS target for refractory OCD. In 2006, Greenberg and colleagues performed bilateral Vc/Vs DBS in 10 patients with refractory OCD, noting a response rate of 40%[114] (see Table 100-1). The Y-BOCS score decreased from a mean of 34.6 at baseline to 22.3 after 36 months of stimulation. Four of eight patients were classified as responders (>35% reduction in YBOCS score) and another two as partial responders (25% to 35% reduction in Y-BOCS scores).[114] Symptoms such as depression, anxiety, independent living, and self-care were also improved. Adverse effects included asymptomatic hemorrhage, seizure, superficial infection, and psychiatric symptoms such as hypomania and worsening of depression.[114] Similarly, an open-label multinational study of ALIC-Vc/Vs–DBS in 26 patients with refractory OCD reported a responder rate of 62%.[115] The authors observed an average 13.1-point decrease in the Y-BOCS score 3 to 36 months after DBS surgery.[115] Moreover, they noted that stimulation closer to the junction of the anterior capsule, posterior ventral striatum, and anterior commissure resulted in therapeutic benefits at lower charge densities. Twenty-three adverse events were reported in 11 patients (42.3%), including asymptomatic intracerebral hemorrhage in two patients (7.7%), seizure in one patient (3.8%), one superficial wound infection (3.8%), and one case each of stimulating lead and extension wire breakage (7.7%).[115] In addition, nine stimulation-related adverse events (four cases of increased depression, three events of increased OCD severity, one case of hypomania, and one report of domestic problems and irritability) were also noted. Finally, a randomized controlled study of six patients with refractory OCD reported a responder rate of 67% at 12 months after bilateral Vc/Vs-DBS.[74] Depressive symptoms were improved in all six patients; global functions were improved in four (67%).[74] A recent study reported a significant correlation between stimulation-induced smile and laughter intraoperatively and the reduction in the Y-BOCS score at 15 months in four patients treated with bilateral Vc/Vs-DBS for medically refractory OCD.[75]

Nucleus Accumbens

In a pilot study, Sturm and colleagues investigated the efficacy of the shell region of the right NAcc as a potential DBS target in four patients with severe refractory OCD and anxiety disorders[116] (see Table 100-1). They reported significant alleviation of symptoms in three patients (75%) at a follow-up of 24 to 30 months. Clinical improvement, along with physiologic changes (inhibition of the ipsilateral dorsolateral rostral putamen and activation of the right dorsolateral prefrontal and cingulate cortex), was documented in one patient using 15-O-H_2O-PET scan in this study.[116] Unfortunately, a validated clinical assessment tool such as the Y-BOCS was not used to quantify the results. In 2004, Aouizerate and colleagues reported remission of OCD symptoms (Y-BOCS score <16) at 12 to 15 months after DBS of the ventral caudate nucleus in a patient with intractable OCD and associated depression.[117] Plewnia and associates reported sustained improvement of OCD symptoms in a patient with concomitant residual schizophrenia after right ALIC-NAcc–DBS at 24 months.[118] However, this patient did not meet the criteria for responders on the Y-BOCS (preoperative and postoperative Y-BOCS scores of 32/40 and 24/40, respectively).[118] In another open-label study,

Franzini and colleagues reported a 13-point decrease in the Y-BOCS score in one of two patients with medically refractory OCD 24 to 27 months after bilateral NAcc-DBS.[119] In a double-blinded, sham-controlled study investigating the efficacy of right NAcc-DBS in 10 patients with medically refractory OCD,[77] the mean Y-BOCS score decreased significantly from 32.2 at baseline to 25.4 at 12 months of follow-up ($P < .05$). Fifty percent of patients showed a less than 25% reduction in their Y-BOCS score after DBS; however, only 10% of patients met the responder criterion of a more than 35% reduction in Y-BOCS score at 12 months of follow-up.[77] In addition, there was alleviation in depression, global functioning, and quality of life, with no significant changes in anxiety, global symptom severity, and cognitive function during the stimulation period. Adverse events included agitation/anxiety (4 patients), hypomania (2 patients), concentration difficulties with failing memory (1 patient), suicidal thoughts (1 patient), headache (1 patient), weight gain (2 patients), reduction in sleep duration (1 patient), and dysesthesia in the subclavicular region (1 patient).[77] Another double-blinded, sham-controlled study reported a response rate of 56% after bilateral NAcc-DBS in 16 patients with refractory OCD at 21 months of follow-up.[76] There was a 72% decrease in Y-BOCS scores during the 8-month open-label treatment phase and a 25% decrease in Y-BOCS scores during the double-blind, sham-controlled phase of the study.[76] Associated symptoms such as depression and anxiety were significantly reduced. Reported adverse events included mild forgetfulness, word-finding problems, hypomania, numbness at the incision site, superficial wound infection, and feeling the extension leads.[76]

Subthalamic Nucleus

The STN is one of the nodal points in the dorsolateral prefrontal, orbitofrontal, and limbic loops, and STN-DBS for Parkinson's disease has been shown to have neuropsychological effects, with improvements in mood, anxiety, and OCD symptoms.[120-125] There are reports of mirthful laughter/hilarity, transient acute depression, and episodes of hypomania or mania following supratherapeutic stimulation of the STN.[125-128] Ventromedial portions of the STN and surrounding structures such as the lateral hypothalamus, ventral tegmental area, substantia nigra, and zona incerta have been implicated in the neuropsychological effects of STN stimulation. In 2002, Mallet and associates reported 58% and 64% improvements in the Y-BOCS scores of two patients with Parkinson's disease and severe OCD after bilateral STN-DBS at 6 months of follow-up[123] (see Table 100-1). One case report noted significant improvement in the Y-BOCS score (32 preoperatively vs. 1 postoperatively) in a single patient with refractory OCD 12 months after bilateral STN-DBS.[129] Based on these initial reports, Mallet and colleagues investigated the efficacy of bilateral STN-DBS in 16 patients with severe refractory OCD in a randomized, double-blind, crossover, multicenter study.[78] Twelve of the 16 patients (75%) exhibited a more than 25% reduction in their Y-BOCS score after bilateral STN-DBS compared with baseline and were categorized as responders.[78] The investigators reported significant improvement in the postoperative GAF scale; however, depression, anxiety, and other neuropsychological measures were not affected. A total of 15 serious adverse events occurred in 11 patients, including one intracerebral hemorrhage and two infections leading to hardware explantation. In addition, 23 nonserious adverse events were identified in 10 patients.[78]

Inferior Thalamic Peduncle

The white fiber bundle within the inferior thalamic peduncle (ITP) connects the thalamus to the OFC and thus plays a crucial role in the pathophysiology of OCD.[130] Based on this model, Jimenez-Ponce and associates investigated the efficacy of bilateral ITP-DBS in five patients with refractory OCD[131] (see Table 100-1). In this open-label study, they reported a mean 17.2-point decrease in Y-BOCS scores after bilateral ITP-DBS compared with baseline at 12 months of follow-up.[131] All five patients responded favorably. In addition, the mean GAF scale improved from 20% to 70% with no significant changes in neuropsychological parameters.[131] No significant adverse events or side effects related to chronic stimulation were reported. Randomized controlled studies are required to validate the efficacy of this target in patients with refractory OCD.

Other Targets

Nair and associates investigated the efficacy of bilateral anteromedial (limbic) globus pallidus internus (GPi)-DBS in four patients with Tourette's syndrome and severe OCD, who underwent surgery to alleviate the motor symptoms associated with their Tourette's syndrome.[132] Two patients reported 100% improvement, whereas the other two achieved more than 85% improvement in their OCD symptoms based on the Obsessive-Compulsive Inventory (OCI) at 3 to 26 months of follow-up.[132]

Patient Selection, Ethical Considerations, and the Team Approach

Given the rough early history of psychosurgery, it is crucial to follow strict ethical guidelines to ensure appropriate application of this treatment in patients with OCD.[133] To avoid inadvertent use of psychosurgery in this and other vulnerable populations, the National Research Act laid the foundation for a National Commission for the Protection of Human Subjects in 1977.[133a] This commission delineated recommendations regarding the application of psychosurgery in both research and clinical practice. According to these recommendations, all patients should meet criteria for chronic, severe, and treatment-refractory OCD as defined by the *DSM-5* as a prerequisite for any surgical intervention.[7] Patient selection is done in close collaboration with an experienced psychiatrist. Patients who meet criteria should then be assessed by a committee composed of a neurologist, functional neurosurgeon, neuropsychologist, bioethicist, and lay personnel. In addition, patients need to be educated and counseled regarding the surgical procedure, possible complications, and benefits of the procedure, maintaining realistic expectations of therapeutic results. It is also important to ensure that patients are able to understand the implications of the surgical procedure, are competent to make decisions on their own behalf, and are able to opt out of the study at any point. After selection, written informed consent is obtained from the patient or the patient's legal guardian. Preoperative and postoperative assessments should include quantitative scales such as the Y-BOCS or OCI, performed by an experienced psychiatrist, to assess results objectively. The surgical procedure is carried out by an experienced team composed of functional neurosurgeons, neurologists, and psychiatrists.[16]

Surgical Technique for Deep Brain Stimulation

DBS surgery for OCD is performed in two stages. Stage 1 involves stereotactically guided implantation of the DBS electrodes into deep anatomic targets. Stage 2 involves connecting the free end of the lead wire to an extension cable, which is subsequently tunneled under the scalp and skin of neck into the subclavicular or abdominal area and connected to the pulse generator. The stage 2 procedure is usually performed 7 to 10 days after the stage 1 procedure as an outpatient procedure under general anesthesia. On the day of stage 1 surgery, the patient's head is shaved, and a stereotactic frame is attached to the patient's head under sedation and local anesthesia. Stereotactic head computed tomography is performed, and the images are exported to a stereotactic workstation and fused to a volumetric MRI scan. The target is localized using either an indirect targeting method in reference to the coordinates of the midcommissural point or by direct visualization of the nucleus on T2-weighted MRI. A safe surgical trajectory to the target that avoids the cortical sulci, intracranial vessels, and ventricular walls is planned on the navigation station. With the patient in the supine position, an incision and bur hole are made, centered on the planned trajectory. The Stimloc device (Medtronic, Minneapolis, MN), which will secure the lead and cover the bur hole, is attached to the skull with two set screws. The underlying dura mater is coagulated and opened at the desired entry point for the cannula, leaving adequate room to avoid hitting the dural edges. The pia mater is coagulated, and a sharp corticectomy is performed. A cannula (length, 177 mm) is inserted through the pial opening to 15 mm above the target. The bur hole is then covered with thrombin-soaked Gelfoam (Pfizer Inc., New York, NY) and sealed using fibrin glue to prevent cerebrospinal fluid loss. The inner stylet of the cannula is removed, and a platinum-iridium or platinum- and gold-plated tungsten microelectrode with an impedance range of 0.6 to 1.0 megaohm is introduced into the cannula for microelectrode recording. The microelectrode is then advanced through the brain matter using a Neuronav Drive (Alpha Omega, Nazareth, Israel) in submillimetric steps in an awake patient. The neuronal activities within the target are evaluated by cognitive tasks every 1 to 2 mm along the length of the nucleus. The neuronal activity is amplified, filtered, displayed, and recorded using a high-quality audio monitor, computer display, and digital oscilloscopes.[134] Based on the microelectrode recordings, the borders and volume of the intended target is defined. Each neuronal structure has characteristic electrophysiologic properties that assist in delineating the entry and exit points through that structure.[135] After satisfactory electrophysiologic recordings, the microelectrode is withdrawn into the guide tube (≥3 mm), and macrostimulation is performed briefly to observe the benefits and side effects. Bilateral intraoperative stimulation in the region of the NAcc has been shown to produce smile and euphoria during DBS surgery.[136] The data regarding location, characteristics of microelectrode recordings, and the effects of macrostimulation are then evaluated and discussed by the whole team.

Other Surgical Procedures

VNS is an effective and adjunctive treatment in patients with chronic refractory depression and was approved by the FDA for adult patients (>18 years of age) in 2005.[137,138] After this approval, VNS was examined as a potential treatment for medically resistant anxiety disorders.[139] The precise mechanism of action of VNS remains obscure. Based on PET and single-photon emission computed tomography imaging studies, it has been shown that VNS is associated with reduced perfusion in the ipsilateral brainstem, cingulate, amygdala, and hippocampus, and in the contralateral thalamus and cingulate in patients with refractory epilepsy.[140] Another study reported a strong correlation between increased resting blood flow in the thalamus bilaterally and decreased seizure frequency after VNS for partial epilepsy.[141] Vagus nerve fibers project to the nucleus tractus solitarius, which has been shown to have intricate connections with the limbic system.[140] Therefore it is possible that VNS can modulate these limbic structures, including the limbic arm of the CSTC loop involved in the pathophysiology of OCD.[140,142] VNS has also been shown to increase the release of noradrenaline from locus caeruleus and thereby can modulate the activity of the autonomic nervous system implicated in the pathophysiology of anxiety disorders.[143] In a pilot study of VNS for treatment-refractory anxiety disorders, three of seven patients with refractory OCD who received stimulation showed a clinical response (>25% reduction in Y-BOCS score) at 12 weeks of follow-up.[139] Two of these three patients had continued and sustained improvement in anxiety scores at 4 years of follow-up.[139]

CONCLUSION

DBS has emerged as the preferred surgical intervention for medically refractory OCD, owing to its enhanced safety profile. Nevertheless, ablative procedures using radiofrequency thermocoagulation or Gamma Knife radiosurgery are still in use. The FDA granted a Humanitarian Device Exemption for DBS in OCD in 2009. The reversible and adjustable nature of this therapy may allow treating physicians to optimize therapy over time, but this remains unproved. Surgery for OCD should be performed by a multidisciplinary team of specialists, including psychiatrists, functional neurosurgeons, neurologists, neuropsychologists, neuroradiologists, biomedical engineers, and bioethicists, working within strict ethical paradigms. Advances in neuroimaging continue to improve our understanding of the neural circuits and pathophysiology underlying psychiatric disorders. Through technologic advances and an increased understanding of the basic pathophysiology of OCD, it may be possible to delineate precise and specific nodes for surgical intervention to maximize the clinical benefits while minimizing the side effects associated with DBS. Adaptive and responsive closed-loop feedback DBS devices may further enhance the efficacy of this therapy. Additional long-term studies and randomized controlled trials are required to further validate and facilitate the wider use of DBS in patients with OCD.

SUGGESTED READINGS

Abelson JL, Curtis GC, Sagher O, et al. Deep brain stimulation for refractory obsessive-compulsive disorder. *Biol Psychiatry*. 2005;57(5):510-516.

Alexander GE, DeLong MR, Strick PL. Parallel organization of functionally segregated circuits linking basal ganglia and cortex. *Annu Rev Neurosci*. 1986;9:357-381.

Anderson D, Ahmed A. Treatment of patients with intractable obsessive-compulsive disorder with anterior capsular stimulation. Case report. *J Neurosurg*. 2003;98(5):1104-1108.

Aouizerate B, Cuny E, Martin-Guehl C, et al. Deep brain stimulation of the ventral caudate nucleus in the treatment of obsessive-compulsive disorder and major depression. Case report. *J Neurosurg*. 2004;101(4):682-686.

Denys D, Mantione M, Figee M, et al. Deep brain stimulation of the nucleus accumbens for treatment-refractory obsessive-compulsive disorder. *Arch Gen Psychiatry*. 2010;67(10):1061-1068.

Franzini A, Messina G, Gambini O, et al. Deep-brain stimulation of the nucleus accumbens in obsessive compulsive disorder: clinical, surgical and electrophysiological considerations in two consecutive patients. *Neurol Sci*. 2010;31(3):353-359.

Goodman WK, Foote KD, Greenberg BD, et al. Deep brain stimulation for intractable obsessive compulsive disorder: pilot study using a blinded, staggered-onset design. *Biol Psychiatry*. 2010;67(6):535-542.

Greenberg BD, Gabriels LA, Malone DA Jr, et al. Deep brain stimulation of the ventral internal capsule/ventral striatum for obsessive-compulsive disorder: worldwide experience. *Mol Psychiatry*. 2010;15(1):64-79.

Greenberg BD, Malone DA, Friehs GM, et al. Three-year outcomes in deep brain stimulation for highly resistant obsessive-compulsive disorder. *Neuropsychopharmacology*. 2006;31(11):2384-2393.

Huff W, Lenartz D, Schormann M, et al. Unilateral deep brain stimulation of the nucleus accumbens in patients with treatment-resistant obsessive-compulsive disorder: Outcomes after one year. *Clin Neurol Neurosurg*. 2010;112(2):137-143.

Jimenez-Ponce F, Velasco-Campos F, Castro-Farfan G, et al. Preliminary study in patients with obsessive-compulsive disorder treated with electrical stimulation in the inferior thalamic peduncle. *Neurosurgery*. 2009;65(6 suppl):203-209, discussion 209.

Kopell BH, Greenberg B, Rezai AR. Deep brain stimulation for psychiatric disorders. *J Clin Neurophysiol*. 2004;21(1):51-67.

Lapidus KA, Kopell BH, Ben-Haim S, et al. History of psychosurgery: a psychiatrist's perspective. *World Neurosurg*. 2013;80(3-4):e1-S27.

Mallet L, Polosan M, Jaafari N, et al. Subthalamic nucleus stimulation in severe obsessive-compulsive disorder. *N Engl J Med.* 2008;359(20):2121-2134.

Nuttin B, Cosyns P, Demeulemeester H, et al. Electrical stimulation in anterior limbs of internal capsules in patients with obsessive-compulsive disorder. *Lancet.* 1999;354(9189):1526.

Nuttin BJ, Gabriels LA, Cosyns PR, et al. Long-term electrical capsular stimulation in patients with obsessive-compulsive disorder. *Neurosurgery.* 2003;52(6):1263-1272.

Nuttin BJ, Gabriels LA, Cosyns PR, et al. Long-term electrical capsular stimulation in patients with obsessive-compulsive disorder. *Neurosurgery.* 2008;62(6 suppl 3):966-977.

Plewnia C, Schober F, Rilk A, et al. Sustained improvement of obsessive-compulsive disorder by deep brain stimulation in a woman with residual schizophrenia. *Int J Neuropsychopharmacol.* 2008;11(8):1181-1183.

Sturm V, Lenartz D, Koulousakis A, et al. The nucleus accumbens: a target for deep brain stimulation in obsessive-compulsive- and anxiety-disorders. *J Chem Neuroanat.* 2003;26(4):293-299.

Tsai HC, Chang CH, Pan JI, et al. Acute stimulation effect of the ventral capsule/ventral striatum in patients with refractory obsessive-compulsive disorder—a double-blinded trial. *Neuropsychiatr Dis Treat.* 2014;10:63-69.

See a full reference list on ExpertConsult.com 

101 Surgery for Major Depressive Disorder

Nir Lipsman, Matthew Volpini, Peter Giacobbe, and Andres M. Lozano

Major depressive disorder (MDD) is a common and challenging psychiatric disorder, which is responsible for a significant proportion of global morbidity. Current estimates suggest that up to 12% of men and 20% of women will experience a major depressive episode (MDE) in their lifetime,[1] with total costs to society in terms of economic burden estimated at $40 billion (USD) annually. Since the 1980s we have seen a dramatic improvement in our understanding of the neural roots of MDD. Technical advances, such as improved neuroimaging, and advances in genetics and biology have now provided a clearer picture of mood circuitry in both health and disease states and are further fueling the development of more focused and effective antidepressant treatments.

DIAGNOSIS AND TREATMENT

MDD is a heterogeneous condition consisting of more than just a deficit state. For example, traditional downregulation symptoms such as sadness and psychomotor retardation often coexist with upregulation symptoms such as rumination, pathologic crying and suicidal ideation.[2] Diagnostic criteria for MDD have been formalized in the fifth edition of the *Diagnostic and Statistical Manual of Mental Disorders (DSM-5)* and are shown in Box 101-1. An MDE is defined as the symptoms in Box 101-1 existing continuously for a period of 2 weeks and should be distinguished from those associated with medical or other conditions as well as bereavement. As a result of the recognized diversity of depression types, a diagnosis by an expert psychiatrist is often required before initiating treatment for an MDE. Critically, although diagnostic criteria aid in recognizing MDD patients, current expert opinion is moving away from these largely arbitrary conceptualizations to more symptom- and circuit-based diagnostics. Future iterations of the *DSM* may focus on symptom clusters, as well as dysfunctional neural circuitry and biomarkers, as aids in diagnosis.

The mainstay of MDD treatment is a combination of psychotherapy and pharmacotherapy. Cognitive behavior therapy is the most commonly used and studied psychosocial treatment and involves the identification and subsequent correction of maladaptive cognitive and perceptual biases that influence mood and behavior.[3] There are currently several classes of medications available for the treatment of depressed mood, each aiming to correct an underlying neurotransmitter deficit. Although some of these medications are selective for specific receptor types, such as serotonin or dopamine, their effect is widespread throughout the brain, often leading to side effects and poor tolerance. Nevertheless, current therapeutic regimens for MDD are effective in most patients. However, up to 30% to 40% of patients remain depressed despite optimal care and are characterized as having treatment-resistant depression (TRD).[4,5] Patients with TRD are significantly impaired, are unable to work, and suffer from poor personal relationships and quality of life.[1] Up to 15% of TRD patients commit suicide.[4,6]

For patients who have failed conventional treatments, neuromodulation approaches may be appropriate. These include noninvasive approaches, such as electroconvulsive therapy and transcranial magnetic stimulation, as well as invasive, surgical approaches, such as lesional and stimulation-based operations (for a review of the former, see Lipsman and colleagues[23]). Here we review the rationale and experience with neurosurgical approaches to MDD.

CIRCUITRY OF MOOD AND DEPRESSION

The generation and maintenance of mood are believed to be a consequence of cortical-subcortical circuits involved in affective and emotional processing. Top-down, largely cortical structures, such as the ventromedial prefrontal cortex, interact with bottom-up, largely subcortical structures, such as that amygdala and hippocampus, through key regulatory structures in the extended basal ganglia (Fig. 101-1). Although such circuit models of mood and emotion have been recognized for some time, it is only through advances in neuroimaging that many of the details have now been provided. As a result, several key structures, comprising important nodes in mood circuitry, have been identified as being particularly important to the maintenance of the depressed state. These include the nucleus accumbens (NAcc), subcallosal cingulate (SCC), anterior limb of the internal capsule (ALIC), and medial forebrain bundle.

Nucleus Accumbens

The NAcc is a gray matter structure located at the ventral interface of the caudate and putamen (i.e., ventral striatum [VS]), which is intimately involved with reward processing.[7-9] When expecting or experiencing a reward, dopamine is released by neurons in the ventral tegmental area (VTA) projecting to the NAcc in the VS.[10] Extracellular levels of dopamine rise in the NAcc, which in turn sends dopaminergic projections to the orbitofrontal cortex, the dorsolateral prefrontal cortex, and other cortical areas.[10] Drugs like cocaine, methamphetamine, and caffeine, as well as natural rewards like food and sex, all increase, either directly or indirectly, dopamine release in this mesocorticolimbic pathway.[10] Preclinical, animal models have widely supported this concept. In the rat model, self-administration of cocaine is correlated with dopamine concentration released at the NAcc.[10] When researchers administered haloperidol, a dopamine receptor antagonist, the rats self-administered less cocaine, suggesting an attenuation of their perception of reward.[10] Furthermore, Doyon and colleagues trained rats to press a lever to receive sugar water combined with ethanol.[11] Dopamine concentration was measured in the area around the NAcc, and researchers found that self-administration of the ethanol solution was significantly correlated with increased dopamine concentration in the NAcc area, released by VTA neurons.[11] In humans, researchers administered cocaine to addicts while they were undergoing functional magnetic resonance imaging. Researchers noted that the perceived "rush" reward of drug use was reliably correlated with increased metabolic activity in the NAcc.[10] These results implicate the NAcc as a brain structure intimately associated with the perception of reward.

NAcc is also functionally related to the experience of anhedonia, which is the abject lack of pleasure in typically pleasurable activity. Anhedonia is a core feature of MDD, and work by several research groups has linked NAcc activity to anhedonia in MDD patients.[12,13] For example, MDD patients who exhibited increased

BOX 101-1 Diagnostic Criteria for Major Depressive Disorder

A. Five (or more) of the following symptoms have been present during the same 2-week period and represent a change from previous functioning; at least one of the symptoms is either (1) depressed mood or (2) loss of interest or pleasure.
   - *Note:* Do not include symptoms that are clearly attributable to another medical condition.
   1. Depressed mood most of the day, nearly every day, as indicated by either subjective report (e.g., feels sad, empty, hopeless) or observation made by others (e.g., appears tearful). (*Note:* In children and adolescents, this can be irritable mood.)
   2. Markedly diminished interest or pleasure in all, or almost all, activities most of the day, nearly every day (as indicated by either subjective account or observation).
   3. Significant weight loss when not dieting or weight gain (e.g., a change of more than 5% of body weight in a month), or decrease or increase in appetite nearly every day. (*Note:* In children, consider failure to make expected weight gain.)
   4. Insomnia or hypersomnia nearly every day.
   5. Psychomotor agitation or retardation nearly every day (observable by others, not merely subjective feelings of restlessness or being slowed down).
   6. Fatigue or loss of energy nearly every day.
   7. Feelings of worthlessness or excessive or inappropriate guilt (which may be delusional) nearly every day (not merely self-reproach or guilt about being sick).
   8. Diminished ability to think or concentrate, or indecisiveness, nearly every day (either by subjective account or as observed by others).
   9. Recurrent thoughts of death (not just fear of dying), recurrent suicidal ideation without a specific plan, or a suicide attempt or a specific plan for committing suicide.

B. The symptoms cause clinically significant distress or impairment in social, occupational, or other important areas of functioning.

C. The episode is not attributable to the physiologic effects of a substance or to another medical condition.

D. The occurrence of the major depressive episode is not better explained by schizoaffective disorder, schizophrenia, schizophreniform disorder, delusional disorder, or other specified and unspecified schizophrenia spectrum and other psychotic disorders.

E. There has never been a manic episode or a hypomanic episode.

From American Psychiatric Association. *Diagnostic and Statistical Manual of Mental Disorders*. 5th ed. Arlington, VA: American Psychiatric Publishing; 2013.

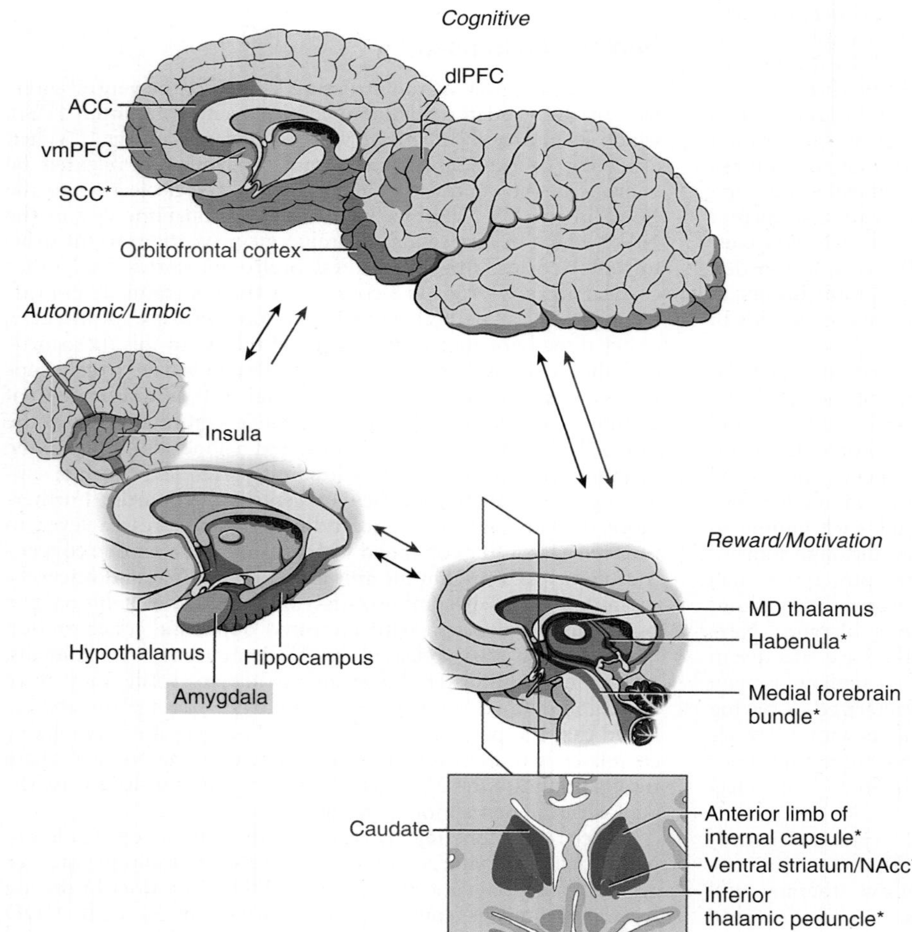

Figure 101-1. Circuit diagram for mood and anxiety disorders and deep brain stimulation targets. ACC, anterior cingulate cortex; dlPFC, dorsolateral prefrontal cortex; MD, mediodorsal; SCC, subcallosal cingulate cortex; vmPFC, ventromedial prefrontal cortex. *(From Lozano AM, Lipsman N. Probing and regulating dysfunctional circuits using deep brain stimulation.* Neuron. *2013;77:406-424.)*

pleasure response to dextroamphetamine, with concomitant increased NAcc activation, also exhibited greater severity of anhedonia.[13]

The NAcc is a highly connected node within a well-defined cortical-striatal-thalamic-cortical loop.[14,15] The NAcc receives afferents from the anterior cingulate cortex as well as the limbic temporal cortex, including the hippocampus, entorhinal cortex, and amygdala.[15] The NAcc sends efferent projections to the ventral (limbic) portions of the globus pallidus externus and internus.[15] The globus pallidus internus then projects to the mediodorsal nucleus of the thalamus, which in turn projects to the anterior cingulate, completing the circuit.[15] Nestler and colleagues have suggested that this striatal circuit is responsible for the emotional memory associated with depression.[16] This is congruent with findings of increased activity in both the rostral anterior cingulate and the amygdala in response to emotional memory related to depression.[17,18]

Subcallosal Cingulate Cortex

The SCC (also called Cg25; Brodmann area [BA] 25) is a critical regulatory node in the medial ventral frontal lobe, immediately below the genu of the corpus callosum. It exists at the interface of several key white matter pathways, which govern affective regulation, emotional decision making, and basal vegetative and autonomic functions.

The SCC has long been postulated as a central node in circuits mediating emotion. Early models of emotional circuits by Papez suggested the cingulate gyrus is the "seat of dynamic vigilance" and an essential component for emotional processing.[19] More recently, Seminowicz and colleagues proposed a model of depression circuitry based on fluorodeoxyglucose–positron emission tomography (FDG-PET) across three cohorts of patients with MDD.[20] In this model, the SCC receives afferent projections from the hippocampus and sends efferent projections to the lateral prefrontal cortex (BA 9).[20] It also shares bilateral connectivity with both the rostral cingulate (Cg24a) and the orbitofrontal cortex (BA 11).[20] This is particularly noteworthy because the rostral cingulate is, in turn, highly connected to both the dorsal and ventral compartments in Mayberg's model of depression.[17] Additionally, the orbitofrontal cortex has been implicated in decision making and emotional processing.[21] Hence the SCC is well situated to affect, through retrograde and anterograde mechanisms, structures in both the dorsal compartment (BA 9, 11) and ventral compartment (hippocampus) to modulate the depression circuit.[17,20,22] In particular, SCC connections to cortical structures implicated in depression suggest that altering Cg25 activity may treat the cognitive aspects of depression: guilt, hopelessness, and suicidal ideation.[16,22]

Activity of the SCC has been widely implicated in depressive disorders and depressive states in general.[17,22] Much of this work has been driven by functional neuroimaging and by metabolic imaging with PET in particular. For example, when healthy individuals are induced to feel sad, blood flow and glucose use in the SCC are substantially increased.[17] Further, this hypermetabolism is attenuated in remitted MDD patients, following both pharmacotherapeutic and psychotherapeutic treatments.[17] These decreases in metabolism in the ventral compartment, including the SCC, were further correlated with resolution of depressed mood.[17] This reversal is also seen after deep brain stimulation (DBS) treatment in patients with TRD as well as in patients with other affective regulatory conditions, such as anorexia nervosa.[3,23] Neurophysiologic studies of SCC activity in depressed patients have also linked neural activity in the SCC to the experience of sad events. SCC single neurons appear to fire preferentially when viewing sad versus happy or neutral images, and populations of neurons, measured with local field potentials, are preferentially involved in the judgment of sad versus happy stimuli.[24,25]

Anterior Limb of the Internal Capsule

The ALIC is a white matter pathway connecting frontal cortical structures with subcortical, thalamic, and other basal ganglia structures. As a key limbic pathway, the ALIC has been postulated to be a critical connection between top-down and bottom-up regulatory structures important for mood and emotional processing as well as decision making. Imaging and anatomic tracer studies have shown that the ALIC connects the anterior cingulate and parts of the prefrontal cortex with lower limbic structures like the hippocampus, amygdala, and dorsomedial nucleus of the thalamus.[26,27] In this way, the ALIC comprises the fibers that complete the anterior cingulate or limbic cortical-striatal-thalamic-cortical circuit.[15] This includes the projection fibers connecting limbic cortical structures to the VS as well as the thalamocortical and striatal fibers that connect the thalamus to the anterior cingulate, closing the anatomic circuit.[15]

Functional evidence directly linking the ALIC to MDD is scarce. Given its role in emotional decision making, lesioning of the ALIC (discussed later), known as capsulotomy, has been proposed in patients with treatment-refractory obsessive-compulsive disorder (OCD) as well as MDD. Leveraging the early experience with capsulotomy, DBS of the ALIC was used to treat patients with treatment-refractory OCD.[28,29] From these early studies, it was found that DBS was effective in treating not only obsessions and compulsions but also comorbid depressive symptoms.[30] As a result, Malone and colleagues have performed ALIC-DBS on patients specifically with TRD.[31] Although results have been variable to date, as discussed in more detail later, this experience underscores the place of ALIC in conceptual models of both mood and depression.

Medial Forebrain Bundle

Although the mesocorticolimbic pathway has long been established as a central reward pathway in humans, it is not the only reward circuit in the human brain.[10,32,33] The superolateral medial forebrain bundle (MFB) is part of a circuit that has been associated with positive affective states and is thought to underlie motivation beyond sensory reward.[33,34] Its role in the generation and maintenance of MDD has been suggested predominantly by structural neuroimaging studies.

The MFB is a white matter pathway that is present in humans, rats, and other animals.[33,34] Using diffusion tensor imaging to visualize the cytoarchitecture of the MFB in humans, researchers found that the MFB bifurcates as it reaches the VTA, giving rise to the superolateral and inferomedial portions.[33] From there, the superolateral MFB courses inferior to the thalamus, ascending parallel to the ALIC and projecting to the VS and NAcc.[33,34] Anterior projections to the SCC are also present in some individuals.[33,34] Therefore, the superolateral MFB appears to provide a robust connection between the VTA and frontal areas and may account for higher cognitive processing of reward information, which is known to be disrupted in patients with MDD and often manifests as anhedonia.[10]

THE ABLATIVE EXPERIENCE

The first reports of neurosurgical procedures for the specific management of psychiatric disease were published in the 1940s and 1950s.[35-37] These early attempts, however, typically involving wholesale severing of frontosubcortical white matter tracts, were supported by limited scientific data and were crude by today's standards. The prefrontal lobotomy, for example, was performed on thousands of psychiatric patients from 1936 to 1956 in the United States and United Kingdom.[1,38] Although effective in some cases, these often blindly performed procedures, in poorly selected patients, frequently led to unwanted changes in affect and personality.[1,38,39]

Several more focused, ablative procedures were subsequently proposed.[39-41] These limited ablations and undercutting techniques sought to selectively disrupt frontal pathways that, we now know, are extensively involved in emotional processing.[1,17,42,43] In 1948, Scoville described three frontal undercutting techniques to treat various psychiatric conditions, including depression.[39] Mettler then introduced the frontal topectomy, a gray matter ablative procedure of BA 9, BA 10, and BA 46.[40] In addition, Spiegel and Wycis introduced the mesencephalothalamotomy, an ablative procedure that targeted the spinothalamic tract in the midbrain at the level of the superior colliculus as well as the medial thalamic nuclei, to treat intractable pain.[41] The promise of these procedures as a last resort for treating intractable psychiatric disease kept interest in these procedures alive, fueling additional technical and conceptual advances. With improved imaging, as well as the development and refinement of stereotactic methodology, the ability to more precisely target anatomic structures was made possible. As a result, four ablative procedures were developed to treat depression: anterior cingulotomy, subcaudate tractotomy, limbic leucotomy, and anterior capsulotomy.

Anterior Cingulotomy

Cingulotomy involves the generation of a lesion in the anterior cingulate gyrus, typically 1 to 2 cm posterior to the frontal horn of the lateral ventricle. Whitty and colleagues carried out the earliest anterior cingulotomy for the treatment of schizophrenia as well as for several cases of "melancholia."[44] In addition to Scoville's "undercut of the cingulate gyrus area," the anterior cingulate cortex (BA 24) was chosen as a target primarily as a result of the work done by Papez as well as experimental evidence obtained from higher animals, like monkeys, that implicated BA 24 in normal affective behavior.[19,39,44,45] The procedure called for the bilateral removal of a block of tissue from BA 24, with modest reported improvements in some patients with depression.[44]

Foltz and White further used cingulotomy to treat intractable pain in 16 patients.[46] Their surgical procedure required that several bilateral lesions be generated in the cingulum bundle, following their discovery that unilateral lesions did not provide significant benefit.[46] Overall, 14 of 16 (87%) patients were said to have benefited from the procedures and obtained both pain and psychic relief.

Ballantine and colleagues treated 57 patients with anterior cingulotomy and improved on previous procedures by using a stereotactic frame.[47] Postoperative data gathered from 40 of these patients showed that 36 patients (90%) improved to some degree, with 8 of those patients (20%) classified as completely recovered.[47] In a later study, the same group reported the combined results of anterior cingulotomy in 198 patients, of which 83 had unipolar affective disorder.[48] In total, 168 (84%) patients improved to some degree, with a postoperative suicide rate of 9%.[48] No deaths were reported during the surgical procedure, but two patients suffered hemiplegia as a result of intracerebral hemorrhage sustained during the operation. Seizures occurred in 1% of patients after surgery.[48]

More recently, Shields and colleagues reported their experience with anterior cingulotomy in 17 patients with TRD.[49] Their procedure involved three lesions made bilaterally. Of the 33 patients who underwent the procedure, 7 patients (21.2%) were responders, 6 (18.2%) were partial responders, and 20 (60.6%) did not respond.[49] Seven of the 20 (80%) nonresponders went on to receive subcaudate tractotomy (full limbic leucotomy).[49]

Steele and colleagues performed anterior cingulotomy on eight patients with TRD.[50] Postoperatively, 3 (37.5%) patients met the a priori criteria for remission, 2 (25%) were classified as responders, 2 (25%) improved slightly, and 1 (12.5%) patient deteriorated.[50] The authors reported that more anteriorly placed lesions were predictive of a greater clinical response, as indicated by larger decreases in both the Hamilton Depression Rating Scale (HDRS) and the Montgomery-Asberg Depression Rating Scale (MADRS). Additionally, smaller total lesion volumes were significantly correlated with better clinical response.

Subcaudate Tractotomy

In the 1950s Knight introduced the refined orbital undercut, designed to interrupt three bundles of fibers: (1) projection fibers descending from both the frontal cortex and BA 13 to the ventromedial nucleus of the hypothalamus, (2) amygdala white matter, and (3) connections between BA 13 and the frontal cortex.[51] These projections were thought to be important for mediating the visceral effects of emotion, and it was believed that their division would mediate some emotional relief in psychiatric patients. Of 221 patients with intractable depression who underwent the procedure, 155 (70.1%) patients were deemed not to require further medical care, presenting either with slight symptoms or no symptoms.[51]

Knight observed that positive clinical outcome seemed to be correlated with adequate posterior extension of the lesion.[51,52] Motivated to reduce unnecessary brain scarring, which caused seizures and unwanted personality changes in patients, the procedure was modified to include only the posterior 2-cm portion of the original lesion.[52] Anatomically, this area consisted of the substantia innominata immediately inferior and slightly anterior to the head of the caudate.[52] The modified procedure involved the bilateral stereotactic injection of two rows of four radioactive yttrium 90 seeds, which resulted in relatively large bilateral lesions measuring 20 × 20 × 5 mm.[52] Of the 23 patients who received the operation for depression, 20 (87%) patients had either slight or no symptoms. In 1995, Hodgkiss and colleagues also reported on a sample of 183 patients who underwent stereotactic subcaudate tractotomy (SST) for depression.[53] Of these, 63 patients (34.4%) were characterized as well or recovered, 58 (31.7%) were improved, 57 (31.1%) were unchanged or worse, and 5 (2.7%) died for reasons unrelated to the neurosurgical procedure.[53]

Limbic Leucotomy

Limbic leucotomy combines anterior cingulotomy with SST.[49,54-56] Anterior cingulotomy disrupts the circuit of Papez by ablating connections between the anterior cingulate (BA 24) and the hippocampus.[49,54,56] SST targets the substantia innominata inferior and slightly anterior to the head of the caudate and also involves lesioning the subgenual cingulate cortex (BA 25).[51,54,56] The SCC has been widely implicated in mood regulation, so the limbic leucotomy represents a multitarget ablative technique to disrupt anterior cingulate function.

Kelly and colleagues performed limbic leucotomies on nine patients with MDD.[55-58] The streamlined procedure included three bilateral lesions in the lower medial quadrant of the frontal lobe as described by Knight for subcaudate tractotomies.[55-58] In addition, two bilateral lesions were placed in the anterior cingulate gyrus, although variations of lesion placement were carried out in some early cases, before procedural refinement.[55-58] Patients who underwent limbic leucotomy were said not to suffer from emotional blunting, postoperative epilepsy, or excessive weight gain.[55-58] Intelligence measures were also unaffected. Nine patients with MDD were operated on.[55-58] At 16-month follow-up, 7 of 9 patients (77.8%) improved to some degree, and 2 patients (22.2%) were unchanged. The authors also reported 16-month postoperative follow-up results for a larger cohort of 57 psychiatric patients. Average HDRS and Beck Depression Inventory scores were significantly reduced.[58] Side effects, including incontinence, headache, laziness, and confusion, were not uncommonly present immediately after surgery, but these symptoms were usually transient in days to weeks.[58]

Montoya and associates reported on 21 patients who underwent bilateral limbic leucotomy, of which 6 were diagnosed with MDD.[59] Based on clinician ratings after surgery, 3 (50%) patients with MDD were classified as responders.[59] Side effects that were present in a sizeable minority of patients, including somnolence (29%) and apathy (24%), were absent at follow-up.[59] Four (19%) patients experienced seizures after surgery. Three of the 4 patients suffered only a single event, but seizures persisted in 1 patient at follow-up, who was prescribed an anticonvulsant.[59]

As previously discussed, Shields and colleagues performed anterior cingulotomy on 33 patients with major depression.[49] Seven patients underwent SST, culminating in a full limbic leucotomy.[49] Although the authors reported that at least partial benefit was garnered by 75% of the patients who underwent various combinations of stereotactic procedures, they did not delineate these results based on what procedure was carried out.[49]

Anterior Capsulotomy

The first anterior capsulotomy was performed by Talairach in 1949.[60] It was largely employed as a treatment for patients with severe OCD, and until recently there was little published on the efficacy of this procedure to treat TRD.[61]

The procedure is characterized by lesions placed in the anterior third portion of the anterior limb of the internal capsule.[27,62] This region contains fibers that connect both the prefrontal cortex and anterior cingulate cortex with the hippocampus, amygdala, and thalamus.[27,39,54] Anterior capsulotomy may therefore have a twofold effect. The disruption of corticothalamic fibers may disrupt somatic symptoms of depression, whereas the ablation of fibers connecting the cingulate with the hippocampus and amygdala may relieve depressive symptoms by disrupting the medial circuit of Papez, known to be essential for emotion.[19,27,39,54,62]

Christmas and colleagues reported results from 20 patients with TRD who underwent anterior capsulotomy.[27] At most recent follow-up, 8 patients (40%) met the a priori condition of remitters, defined as an HDRS score of 7 or less.[27] Overall, 11 patients (55%) improved, 7 (35%) were unchanged, and 2 (10%) deteriorated.[27] There were no deaths by suicide,[27] and adverse effects immediately after the procedure were generally mild.

Riestra and colleagues performed anterior capsulotomy on a single patient with MDD and secondary OCD.[63] The procedure was performed unilaterally, FDG-PET before surgery revealed unilateral metabolic pathology of several limbic structures, and the authors hypothesized this to be responsible for the disease.[63] Surgery was well tolerated, and the patient garnered a 57% reduction in HDRS score at evaluation in years 1 and 2 and a 54% reduction at year 3.[63] The patient's Yale-Brown Obsessive-Compulsive Scale (Y-BOCS) score also decreased 58%, 77%, and 96% at each of the annual checkups.[63]

Hurwitz and colleagues reported on eight patients with MDD who underwent bilateral anterior capsulotomy.[62] Four of the eight patients (50%) were classified as responders (greater than 50% reduction in preoperative Beck Depression Inventory score) between 24 and 36 months after surgery.[62]

DEEP BRAIN STIMULATION

The rationale for focal stimulation in neurologic and psychiatric disease stems from the theory that dysfunction in critical nodes comprising key behavioral circuits leads to recurrent and maladaptive behaviors. Focal electrical disruption at the target site can have both local effects (e.g., mimicking a thalamic lesion in essential tremor) and remote, downstream effects (e.g., driving efferent impulses) in SCC-DBS in depression. Although the mechanisms of DBS are as yet unclear, computational models suggest that the ultimate effect of stimulation may be as dependent on the target tissue being disrupted as the stimulation parameters used.[64] Additional work in animal models will provide more insights on whether DBS may indeed have both functional and structural effects on neural circuits and structures.

DBS is currently approved for the management of Parkinson's disease, dystonia, and essential tremor.[64] The U.S. Food and Drug Administration granted DBS a Humanitarian Device Exemption for its use in treatment-refractory OCD. More than 100,000 patients have undergone a DBS procedure to date globally, with most having Parkinson's disease, where DBS is associated with significant effects on tremor, bradykinesia, and rigidity.[64,65] The promise of DBS in disorders of motor circuitry has driven its investigation in other disorders of neural circuitry, such as OCD and MDD. Further, although neurotransmitters, such as serotonin, norepinephrine, and dopamine, are undoubtedly implicated in MDD, pharmacotherapy is often a wholesale approach affecting virtually all brain regions.[66] More focused approaches, such as DBS, target specific anatomic circuits underlying emotional processing and may offer an additional therapeutic option.[12,17,19,64] Accordingly, several targets have been proposed for DBS in MDD, including the SCC, NAcc, inferior thalamic peduncle (ITP), habenula, and MFB. All of these structures have been implicated in structural and functional imaging studies in MDD and are also highly connected components within the emotional limbic circuit (Table 101-1; see Fig. 101-1).

Subcallosal Cingulate

The SCC was the first DBS target systematically investigated in TRD, in a phase 1 pilot study by Mayberg and colleagues published in 2005.[67] Six patients (five with MDD, one with bipolar depression) underwent implantation of bilateral SCC electrodes and were followed for 6 months. PET scans were performed at baseline and then again after 6 months of chronic stimulation. At 6 months, four of six patients were in remission, defined as a score of less than 8 on the Hamilton Depression Rating Scale (HAMD). Further, PET scans revealed significant reductions in local cerebral metabolism at the DBS target compared with baseline as well as changes in downstream limbic projections. Such results were consistent with those seen in patients with MDD treated medically and represented a normalization of brain metabolism compared with healthy controls.[68] A follow-up study in 20 patients followed to 1 year found a 55% treatment response rate, defined as a reduction in the HAMD score by at least 50%, with 35% of patients reaching clinical remission.[69] The results in these patients followed to 3 to 6 years demonstrated a similar response rate of 64% and remission rate of 43%.[70] There were further significant improvements in quality of life, with 65% of patients engaged in employment, compared with 10% before DBS. A Canadian multicenter study using the SCC as the DBS target found more modest results, namely a 29% response rate at 1 year.[71] This lower response rate underscored the need for additional, carefully designed trials of DBS in MDD.

Additional studies have since provided further evidence for the efficacy of SCC-DBS. Holtzheimer and Mayberg reported on a single MDD patient who underwent bilateral SCC stimulation and, at 4 and 24 weeks of follow-up, saw his HDRS scores decrease to 17 and 9, respectively, from 25 before surgery.[72] Two years after DBS, the patient reported significant worsening of MDD symptoms, and it was discovered that his implanted pulse generator required replacement.[72] The battery was changed, with subsequent relief of depressive symptoms.[72] Guinjoan and colleagues reported an additional patient who received bilateral SCC-DBS for MDD and was classified as a responder 12 months

TABLE 101-1 Studies of Deep Brain Stimulation for Major Depressive Disorder

Study	Target	No. and Type of Patients	Outcome
Aouizerate et al., 2004[78]	NAcc/VC	1 (OCD with MDD)	Contacts activated in both NAcc and VC for optimized stimulation parameters. At last follow-up (15 mo after surgery), patient was in remission for both MDD (HDRS score ≤7), and OCD (Y-BOCS score <16).
Mayberg et al., 2005[67]	SCC	5 (MDD, 1 patient with bipolar II)	At 6-mo follow-up, 4 of 6 patients were responders, and 2 of 6 were in remission as measured by HDRS.
Jimenez et al., 2013[83]	ITP	1 (MDD with comorbid bulimia nervosa and borderline personality disorder)	Double-blind assessment protocol after initial period of 8 mo with "on" stimulation. No relapse of depressive symptoms with DBS turned off for 12 mo. Sustained remission at 24 mo with DBS on
Lozano et al., 2008[69]	SCC	20 (MDD)	At 12-mo follow-up, 60% of patients were responders, and 35% were in remission.
Schlaepfer et al., 2008[66]	NAcc	3 (MDD)	Double-blind changes to stimulation parameters and assessment. HDRS scores decreased with stimulation on and increased with stimulation off.
Neimat et al., 2008[74]	SCC	1 (MDD)	Patient HDRS scores were 11 at 3-mo follow-up, 8 at 6-mo follow-up, 7 both at 1-yr and at most recent follow-up (30 mo).
Malone et al., 2009[31]	VC/VS	15 (MDD)	At 6- to 51-mo follow-up, 8 of 15 patients were responders, and 6 of 15 were in remission at last follow-up as measured by MADRS.
Malone, 2010[80]	VC/VS	17 (MDD)	Two patients added to original cohort. At 12-mo follow-up, 9 of 17 patients (52.9%) were responders, and 7 of 17 patients (41.1%) were in remission, as measured by MADRS. Last follow-up ranged from 14-67 mo. At last follow-up, 12 of 17 patients (70.6%) were responders, and 6 of 17 (35.3%) were in remission.
Bewernick et al., 2010[76]	NAcc	10 (MDD)	At 12-mo follow-up, 5 of 10 patients had achieved >50% reduction in HDRS scores (i.e., responders). Antidepressant, antianhedonic, and antianxiety effects were observed.
Guinjoan et al., 2010[73]	SCC	1 (MDD)	At 12-mo follow-up, HDRS score was reduced to approximately 10 with bilateral stimulation. With stimulation settings optimized to unilateral (right) stimulation, patient garnered additional reduction in HDRS score and reached remission more than 18 mo after surgery (HDRS <5).
Holtzheimer and Mayberg, 2010[72]	SCC	1 (MDD)	Before surgery, patient had HDRS score of 25. At last follow-up (24 wk), HDRS score was 9.
Sartorius et al., 2010[82]	LHb	1 (MDD)	At last follow-up, patient had 21-item HDRS score of 0 and has maintained constant remission.
Kennedy et al., 2011[70]	SCC	20 (MDD, 1 patient with bipolar II)	At last follow-up (3-6 yr after implantation; mean, 3.5), response rate of 64.3% and remission rate of 42.9% (by HDRS). Considerable improvement in social functioning: 65% of patients were engaged in work-related activity at last follow-up compared with 10% before DBS.
Puigdemont et al., 2012[85]	SCC	8 (MDD)	Response and remission at 1 yr were 62.5% and 50%, respectively.
Bewernick et al., 2012[77]	NAcc	11 (MDD)	At 12-mo postsurgery follow-up, 5 of 11 patients (45.5%) were responders, and 6 of 11 (54.5%) were nonresponders. At 2 years, 1 previous responder reached remission (HDRS score <10).
Holtzheimer et al., 2012[86]	SCC	17 (10 MDD, 7 with bipolar II)	At 1-yr follow-up, remission and response rates were 36%; at 2 yr, remission rate was 58%, and response rate was 92%. Remission and response rates were based on HDRS. Efficacy was similar for MDD and bipolar patients.
Kiening and Sartorius, 2013[81]	Habenula	2 (MDD)	At follow-up, 1 patient was in clinical remission, and 1 patient was a treatment responder. Follow-up length and depression scores were not provided.
Lozano et al., 2012[71]	SCC	21 (MDD)	At 6-mo follow-up, the response rate was 48%; at 1-yr follow-up, the response rate was 29%. Response was measured by HDRS.
Jimenez et al., 2013[83]	ITP	7 (6 OCD, 1 MDD)	At most recent follow-up, the patient with MDD was in remission. HDRS score decreased from 42 before surgery to 6 after surgery. The patient had not relapsed in the 9-yr follow-up period.
Merkl et al., 2013[75]	SCC	6 (MDD)	At 24- to 36-wk follow-up, 2 patients were in remission, and 4 were nonresponders.
Schlaepfer et al., 2013[84]	MFB	7 (MDD)	More than 50% reduction in depression scores in most patients by day 7 after surgery; at 12- to 33-wk follow-up, 6 of 7 patients were responders, and 4 of 7 were in remission.
Millet et al., 2014[79]	NAcc/VC	4 (MDD)	At most recent follow-up (15 mo after surgery), 1 of 4 patients was in remission, 1 of 4 was a responder, 1 of 4 improved, and 1 of 4 did not respond, based on HDRS scores. Authors noted diminished response to VC stimulation compared with NAcc stimulation.

HDRS, Hamilton Depression Rating Scale; ITP, inferior thalamic peduncle; LHb, lateral habenula; MADRS, Montgomery-Asberg Depression Rating Scale; MDD, major depressive disorder; NAcc, nucleus accumbens; OCD, obsessive-compulsive disorder; SCC, subcallosal cingulate cortex; VC, ventral caudate; VS, ventral striatum; Y-BOCS, Yale-Brown Obsessive-Compulsive Scale.

after surgery.[73] In an attempt to improve clinical benefit and battery life, investigators applied unilateral stimulation and found that left-sided stimulation was associated with increased depression and right-sided stimulation with a greater antidepressant effect.[73] It remains unclear whether the clinical benefits seen with SCC-DBS, or with MDD-DBS at any target, are lateralizing. Neimat and associates reported on a patient who received multiple surgical interventions to treat her MDD, including a cingulotomy that did not provide clinical benefit.[74] The patient underwent SCC-DBS, with subsequent reduction in HDRS score from 19 to 7 at 1 year.[74] In a more recent case series of six patients with TRD who underwent bilateral SCC stimulation, remission was reported in two at 24 to 36 weeks of follow-up, and the remaining patients were nonresponders.[75]

All results with SCC-DBS to date have been obtained with open-label studies. There have been no published randomized double-blind, sham-controlled DBS trials in MDD, but these are currently underway at several centers.

Nucleus Accumbens and Ventral Striatum

The NAcc has been proposed as a DBS target in MDD given its prominent role for anhedonia and dysfunctional reward processing in depression. At the confluence of the ventral caudate (VC) and VS, NAcc and VS are often used interchangeably and refer to very similar if not identical DBS targets. There is a small but growing literature on NAcc-DBS in MDD, with promising results in open-label prospective studies. Schlaepfer and colleagues reported their experience in three patients with NAcc-DBS for TRD and found that HAMD scores decreased when the stimulation was on and increased with the stimulation off, in an open-label fashion.[66] One of the patients reached criteria for treatment response. A follow-up study in 10 patients found a 50% treatment response rate, with significant positive effects on measures of anxiety and anhedonia.[76,77] The authors further reported cerebral metabolic changes similar to those seen after SCC-DBS, suggesting that a common limbic circuit is being modulated with modulation of both DBS targets.

Aouizerate and associates reported on a patient with severe OCD and comorbid MDD who was treated with bilateral NAcc-VC–DBS.[78] The implanted electrodes were positioned such that two contacts were in the NAcc and two were in the VC.[78] The two distal contacts (in the NAcc) were activated first, which resulted in no relief in OCD symptoms measured using the Y-BOCS. The proximal contacts (in the ventromedial head of the caudate) were then activated, which resulted in improvements in both anxiety and mood symptoms, leading to remission of MDD at 15 months.[78] These results helped spur interest in the VC as a DBS target for MDD. Millet and colleagues reported on four patients with MDD who underwent bilateral implantation of electrodes along a trajectory that included both the head of the caudate and the NAcc.[79] Initially, only the NAcc contacts were activated for 3 months.[79] Nonresponders then underwent serial activation of the contacts in the caudate for an additional 4 months.[79] All patients ultimately received NAcc-DBS, and at last follow-up (15 months after surgery), two patients (50%) were responders.[79] The authors concluded that the NAcc was a more effective target than the caudate to treat MDD with DBS.[79]

Malone reported experience with VC-VS–DBS in a cohort of 15 patients with MDD, which was then expanded to a total of 17 patients.[31,80] Treatment response was assessed using the MADRS.[31,80] Of enrolled subjects, 9 patients (52.9%) were responders and 7 patients (41.1%) were remitters at 12 months after surgery.[80] At last follow-up (range, 14 to 67 months), 12 patients (70.6%) were responders, and 6 patients (35.3%) were in remission.[80]

Inferior Thalamic Peduncle and Habenula

Other DBS targets investigated in MDD in small, open-label studies include the ITP and the habenula. The habenula is a pineal region structure that has been linked to various limbic pathways, including the perception of pain, negative emotions, and reward processing,[81] Sartorius and colleagues reported a woman with MDD treated with lateral habenula DBS.[82] Postoperatively, the patient's depressive symptoms improved, reaching remission at approximately 22 weeks. An additional two patients who underwent bilateral habenular DBS for TRD found a positive effect in both patients, with one in remission and the other a treatment responder.[81]

The ITP conveys white matter fibers from laminar and mediodorsal thalamic nuclei to the orbitofrontal cortex. ITP has been proposed as a DBS target for both OCD and MDD, with one published case report of the procedure in the latter. Jimenez and associates[83] reported a significant treatment effect of ITP-DBS on major depressive symptoms following open-label stimulation that persisted at 2 years of follow-up. In another recent study, Jimenez and associates performed ITP-DBS on one patient with MDD and six others with OCD. The patient with MDD had a preoperative HDRS score of 42.[83] Postoperatively, the patient was classified as a remitter, with an HDRS score of 6, and was able to discontinue antidepressant medication.[83] Four years after surgery, the patient's electrodes were explanted because of skin erosion without relapse of MDD symptoms, and at last follow-up (5 years after surgery), this patient was still in remission.[83] As with the habenula and all other DBS targets to date, these results need to be validated in larger, sham-controlled studies before conclusions can be drawn regarding safety and efficacy.[76,77]

Medial Forebrain Bundle

The MFB has been investigated in a single, prospective, open-label trial in seven patients with TRD.[84] Seven days after stimulation onset, most patients experienced a greater than 50% reduction in depression scores, with six of seven patients classified as responders and four of seven in remission, at 12 to 33 weeks of follow-up. These results are interesting given the rapid treatment response, which largely contrasts the time to clinical benefit, typically weeks to months, seen with other DBS targets, such as NAcc and SCC. Although from a small study with limited follow-up, these results are intriguing and now require further studies in larger cohorts and using a sham-controlled design.

FUTURE DIRECTIONS

Neurosurgery for MDD continues to evolve well into the 21st century. What started as crude attempts to disrupt pathologic pathways in an era of few other treatment options has now become a field in which submillimeter targets are identified using advanced imaging and disrupted in a reversible and adjustable manner. The future will see further refinements as well as technologic and conceptual advances. Studies in imaging, genetics, and biology will help to identify markers of treatment response to optimize patient selection for neuromodulation approaches. These studies will help identify at what stage of illness one should intervene and when it might be too late. Advances in technology, particularly in the fields of optogenetics, nanotechnology, and focused ultrasound, will provide surgeons with additional tools to target specific neural pathways with even more precision.[64] Although the results from early DBS studies in MDD have been promising, the enthusiasm for DBS in the treatment of depression should be tempered by the need for systematic, randomized, and blinded trials. Many challenges and questions remain, including those surrounding optimal patient selection and surgical targeting. It is only through a multidisciplinary and integrated approach that any hope exists to better understand and treat this challenging condition.

SUGGESTED READINGS

Alexander GE, DeLong MR, Strick PL. Parallel organization of functionally segregated circuits linking basal ganglia and cortex. *Annu Rev Neurosci*. 1986;9:357-381.

Ballantine HT Jr, Bouckoms AJ, Thomas EK, et al. Treatment of psychiatric illness by stereotactic cingulotomy. *Biol Psychiatry*. 1987;22(7): 807-819.

Holtzheimer PE, Kelley ME, Gross RE, et al. Subcallosal cingulate deep brain stimulation for treatment-resistant unipolar and bipolar depression. *Arch Gen Psychiatry*. 2012;69(2):150-158.

Knight G. The orbital cortex as an objective in the surgical treatment of mental illness. The results of 450 cases of open operation and the development of the stereotactic approach. *Br J Surg*. 1964;51: 114-124.

Laxton AW, Neimat JS, Davis KD, et al. Neuronal coding of implicit emotion categories in the subcallosal cortex in patients with depression. *Biol Psychiatry*. 2013;74:714-719.

Lozano AM, Lipsman N. Probing and regulating dysfunctional circuits using deep brain stimulation. *Neuron*. 2013;77(3):406-424.

Mayberg HS. Limbic-cortical dysregulation: a proposed model of depression. *J Neuropsychiatry Clin Neurosci*. 1997;9(3):471-481.

Mayberg HS, Lozano AM, Voon V, et al. Deep brain stimulation for treatment-resistant depression. *Neuron*. 2005;45(5):651-660.

Schlaepfer TE, Bewernick BH, Kayser S, et al. Rapid effects of deep brain stimulation for treatment-resistant major depression. *Biol Psychiatry*. 2013;73(12):1204-1212.

See a full reference list on ExpertConsult.com

102 Surgery for Anorexia Nervosa

Bomin Sun, Dianyou Li, Wei Liu, Chencheng Zhang, Shikun Zhan, and Xiaoxiao Zhang

Anorexia nervosa (AN) is a treatment-refractory medical-psychiatric disorder that usually begins in adolescence and is characterized by excessive dieting, often accompanied by compulsive exercise, which results in severe weight loss and a sustained body weight of at least 85% less than normal. A subgroup of affected patients also exhibit purging behavior, with or without binge eating. Other features include disturbed body image, heightened desire to lose more weight, and pervasive fear of fatness.[1,2] In affected female patients, amenorrhea also often occurs. The average prevalence rate of AN is 0.3% to 1% among young women and approximately one tenth of that rate among men. Lifetime prevalence among women is 2.2%.[3,4]

Of all mental disorders, AN is associated with the highest rate of mortality; the crude mortality rate is 5.9%, and the mortality rate per decade of life is 5.6%.[5,6] Long-lasting malnutrition can lead to numerous severe physical complications, including osteoporosis, gastrointestinal and cardiac complications, liver damage, electrolyte disturbances, and eventually multiple-organ failure.[7] Psychiatric comorbid conditions include major depressive disorder (MDD; 50%-70% of patients with AN), anxiety disorder (>60%), and obsessive-compulsive disorder (OCD; >40%).[8,9] Personality disorders and alcohol or substance abuse are also common (12%-27%) among patients with the binging-purging subtype of AN, in whom the rate of impulsive behavior is also higher than in patients with the restricting subtype of AN.[10] The majority of individuals with eating disorders report suicidal thoughts, and about 22% attempt suicide.[11] The long-term mortality rate among patients with AN is reported to be 4.27%, mostly as the result of suicide or medical complications of marasmic malnutrition.[12]

In an extensive literature review, Steinhausen showed that less than half (46.9%) of surviving patients recover from AN, one third (33.5%) improve partially, and in an average of 20.8% among studies (0%-79%) the disease takes on a chronic course.[13,14] Patients affected by AN for longer than 10 years are very unlikely to recover.[13,15]

ETIOPATHOLOGY AND NEUROCIRCUITRY OF ANOREXIA NERVOSA

AN is a disorder of complicated origin in which genetic, biologic, cognitive, and sociopsychological mechanisms and their interactions seem to contribute significantly to susceptibility. Because no single factor has been shown to be either necessary or sufficient for development of AN, a multifactorial threshold model is probably explanatory.[16] Studies have demonstrated that genetic heritability is a vital factor (≈50%-80% of cases) in heightening a predisposition to the development of eating disorders[17] and contributes to neurobiologic factors underlying eating disorders such as AN.[18]

The biologic processes and neural circuitry of AN are research "hotspots"; most pertinent disease models focus on factors that underlie pathologic mood, anxiety, reward, body perception, interoception, inhibition, alexithymia, and appetite.[19] Much of this work on AN is driven by neuroimaging, which has been used extensively to show both structural and functional differences between patients with AN, those recovered from AN, and healthy controls.

A more detailed examination of the etiologic and pathologic mechanisms of anorexia nervosa is available in the expanded version of this chapter at ExpertConsult.com.

NONSURGICAL MANAGEMENT OF ANOREXIA NERVOSA

Current psychotherapeutic interventions and pharmacologic therapies for AN are far from universally effective. Surprisingly, there is no high-level evidence (i.e., category A, according to the National Institute for Health and Clinical Excellence guidelines) regarding the efficacy of pharmacologic or psychotherapeutic interventions. Furthermore, only family interventions meet category B criteria (i.e., well-conducted studies, but no randomized controlled trials).[35,36] Variants of family therapy are effective in adolescents, but there is little evidence regarding their efficacy in adults.[37]

Pharmacologic treatments, specifically antidepressants, have not been shown to ameliorate symptoms or prevent relapse in patients with AN.[38] Selective serotonin reuptake inhibitors (SSRIs) are the main pharmacologic treatment for AN symptoms and weight restoration; however, the American Psychiatric Association does not support the use of SSRIs in the management of underweight patients with AN.[39] SSRIs are often prescribed out of frustration with limited treatment options, but the benefits are minimal, and adverse effects can be troublesome. Data on the efficacy of typical antipsychotics are sparse; olanzapine may help increase weight and decrease obsessive symptoms in outpatients with chronic, severe AN, but clinical guidelines do not recommend its routine use.[40-42]

Unfortunately, it is estimated that 20% of patients remain severely affected, even when the best available medication and psychotherapeutic interventions are applied.[13,14,43] This subgroup of patients with intractable AN experience a chronic course and overall functional impairment. Strober and colleagues[13] and Herzog and associates[15] found that patients in whom the duration of AN is longer than 10 years have a very low chance of recovery.

SURGICAL MANAGEMENT OF ANOREXIA NERVOSA

Experimental neurosurgical approaches for AN have been proposed since the 1950s. The first case report of a prefrontal leucotomy for the treatment of AN was published in 1950.[44] The patient was a 21-year-old woman who had undergone a transorbital leucotomy, followed by a full prefrontal leucotomy as a result of disease relapse. Two months after the second surgery, the patient experienced significant weight gain and increased appetite. In the next 20 years, 16 patients with AN who underwent prefrontal leucotomies were evaluated and reported.[45-47] As with the reports in the first publication, most patients experienced significant weight gain and greater interest in food. A study in 1976 reviewed the management of AN patients who underwent stereotactic limbic leucotomies.[48] All patients reported significant weight gains and improvements in other psychiatric disorders.

Interest in modern stereotactic psychosurgery for AN has increased since the 2000s. In 2007, Sun and associates[49] presented the results of surgical treatment for 20 patients with AN in whom previous psychiatric and pharmaceutical therapies had failed. Two stereotactic procedures are now used for AN: deep brain stimulation (DBS) and ablative procedures. DBS is a neurosurgical treatment involving implantation of electrodes that send electrical impulses to specific locations in the brain. Unlike ablative procedures, DBS is a reversible intervention that causes less damage to neural tissue. Furthermore, most side effects are reversible and can be managed by adjustment of stimulation parameters. DBS for AN treatment targets the NAcc or the precallosal and subcallosal components of the ACC, whereas ablative procedures include capsulotomy, NAcc lesioning, and cingulotomy. The ACC is an important component of the limbic system, which has a well-established role in AN. Furthermore, in view of the similarities in symptoms and associated neurocircuitry between OCD and AN, as well as the established efficacy of DBS for OCD,[50,51] we hypothesize that DBS of the NAcc and other areas associated with reward might be effective in patients with chronic, treatment-refractory AN. This approach might enable not only weight restoration but also significant and sustained improvements in core AN symptoms and associated comorbid conditions and complications. The NAcc is an essential component of the primary reward system, in which dysfunction is a central feature of AN etiopathologic processes and progression.[52,53] Notably, NAcc lesioning was first reported for drug addiction and resulted in positive effects with limited complications.[54]

Deep Brain Stimulation

To date, there are few reports on the effects of DBS on AN. At the Eighth World Congress of International Neuromodulation Society in 2007, Sun and associates[49] presented the results of surgical treatment of 20 patients with AN in whom previous psychiatric and pharmaceutical therapies were ineffective. Fifteen of these patients underwent bilateral NAcc-DBS. Two months after treatment, anorexic patients had gained between 17 and 44 pounds, and eight experienced significant improvements in obsessive-compulsive behaviors and symptoms of anxiety. Twelve patients with the binging-purging subtype of AN did not experience significant weight gain by 6 months after stimulation. These patients then underwent capsulotomies in combination with NAcc-DBS and showed significant improvements in both eating behavior and psychiatric symptoms. Follow-up results at 38 months were also reported for the four anorexic patients who underwent bilateral NAcc-DBS in another study[55] (Fig. 102-1). These patients exhibited an average 65% increase in body weight (average baseline BMI, 11.9 kg/m^2; average follow-up BMI, 19.6 kg/m^2) at a 38-month follow-up examination, and menstrual cycles were restored within 11 months for all these patients. At the final follow-up visit, in which DBS systems were explanted 1 year after the battery had fully discharged, no recurrence of symptoms was observed; thus patients were in remission, according to *Diagnostic and Statistical Manual of Mental Disorders*, fifth edition *(DSM-V)*, criteria.[55a] Gao and colleagues[56] reported on six patients with AN who underwent ablation of the NAcc and two patients with AN who underwent DBS of the NAcc; these procedures resulted in restoration of menstruation within 9 months of surgery and in a recovery in BMI to within a normal range (>18 kg/m^2) within 12 months. These two preliminary studies demonstrate that DBS is a viable option for weight restoration in AN, and several different centers have since reported successful DBS and lesioning procedures for treatment of AN.[33,56,57]

Lipsman and associates[33] published the results of a phase 1 pilot trial of subcallosal ACC-DBS in six adult patients with treatment-refractory AN. They observed that DBS was relatively safe in this population and resulted in improvements in mood, anxiety, affective regulation, and anorexia-related obsessions and compulsions in four patients. At 9-month follow-up examinations, however, only three patients exhibited improved BMIs in relation to estimated historical baselines; menstruation status was not noted.[33]

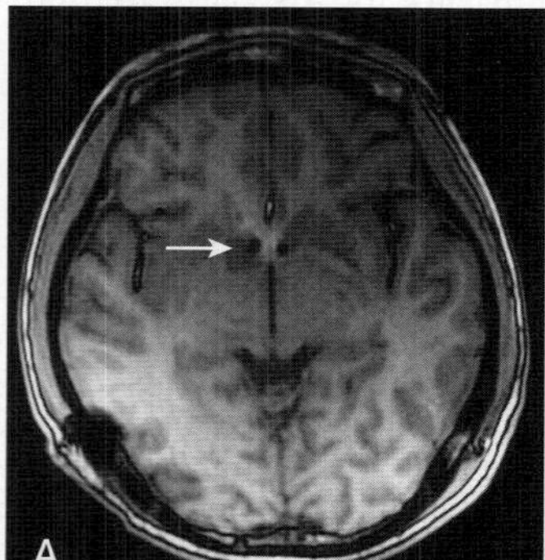

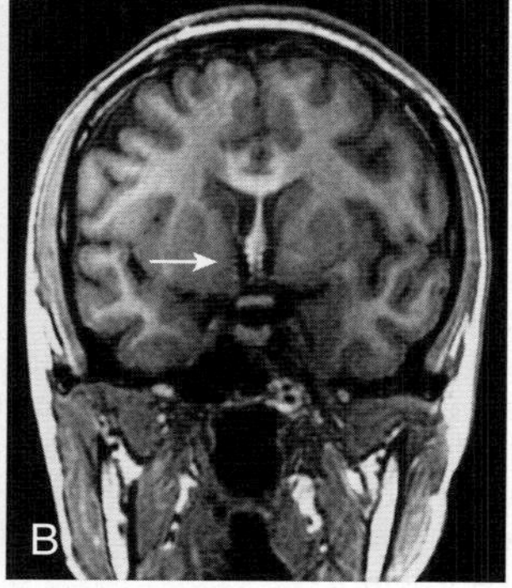

Figure 102-1. Axial view **(A)** and coronal view **(B)** of the nucleus accumbens after the implantation of deep brain stimulation electrodes *(arrows)*.

Ablative Procedure

As mentioned previously, not all patients with treatment-refractory AN experience beneficial effects from DBS, especially those with the binging-purging subtype and those with long-term (>10 years) AN.[49] In these cases, ablative procedures, such as capsulotomy and cingulotomy, should be considered.

Anterior capsulotomy is a stereotactic ablative procedure that involves ablation of the anterior limb of the internal capsule to disconnect the prefrontal cortex and subcortical nuclei (including the dorsomedial thalamus); it is a widely used psychosurgical procedure. These lesions disconnect limbic circuits involved in different psychiatric disorders, such as OCD, MDD, and addiction. Most affected patients exhibit relief of certain symptoms and improved cognitive function, without experiencing alterations in personality.[58-61] Ablations are performed with thermal coagulation or focal gamma radiation guided by computed tomography or magnetic resonance imaging (MRI). MRI is considered the best modality for identifying the anterior capsule because of variation in this structure among individuals. Targets are first identified through visualization of the anterior limbs of the internal capsule on MRI. Radiofrequency electrodes are used to create two ablative lesions by thermocoagulation at 80°C for 60 seconds. The resulting lesions are typically 4 mm in diameter and 10 mm in length.

Barbier and associates[62] reported the results of bilateral anterior capsulotomy in one patient with both OCD and AN. The patient exhibited significant weight gain and improvement in OCD symptoms at a 3-month follow-up examination. In our center, of the 150 patients who underwent capsulotomy during October 2005 to December 2013, 85% experienced an improvement in symptoms, and menstruation resumed in all affected women. These results suggest that this is a very promising procedure for treatment of AN. In contrast to DBS, bilateral capsulotomy can cause short-term side effects, including incontinence, disorientation, sleep disorders, and refeeding syndrome. These symptoms usually resolve within 1 month of the operation. A few patients (<5%) experience long-term side effects, including memory loss, fatigue, excessive weight gain, and personality changes.

Anterior cingulotomy is one of the most popular psychosurgical procedures currently performed in the United States, inasmuch as the cingulate gyrus is an important component of the limbic system.[63,64] Clinicians based at Massachusetts General Hospital have significant experience with cingulotomies for treatment of OCD or MDD and reported that it might be effective for severe refractory OCD.[64,65] Lesions are typically created by thermocoagulation through radiofrequency electrodes at 80°C to 85°C for 90 seconds. The electrode is then withdrawn by 1.0 cm, and the lesion is enlarged superiorly according to the same lesion parameters. These steps are repeated in the opposite hemisphere. In this way, symmetrical bilateral lesions of the ACC are produced. Cingulotomy is a relatively safe procedure, and the incidence of adverse events is lower than that with anterior capsulotomy. Immediate transient symptoms include headache, confusion, and urinary incontinence. In our center, anterior cingulotomies are performed on patients with AN only after a bilateral capsulotomy has failed for at least 1 year, and approximately half of these patients experience positive clinical outcomes with this procedure.

NAcc lesioning, rather than DBS, has also been reported to be effective in AN treatment. Wang and associates[56] reported the results of NAcc lesioning in six patients with AN. One year after the operation, patients exhibited improvement in basic vital signs and in BMI, resumption of menstruation, and improvements in the symptoms of depression, anxiety, and OCD. Although data were obtained from a limited number of cases, lesioning of the NAcc may be considered as a potential procedure for treatment of refractory AN, in view of the successful reports of NAcc-DBS.

As stated previously, the majority of patients with AN present with psychiatric comorbid conditions, including OCD, MDD, and anxiety disorders. Personality disorders and alcohol or substance abuse may also be present among those with the binging-purging subtype of AN. These parallel symptoms indicate that there is a considerable overlap in reward system neurocircuitry between these psychiatric disorders and eating disorders. For some patients with chronic, refractory AN, if the first surgical procedure has failed, a second procedure targeting areas that include the NAcc, the anterior internal capsule, and the ACC should be considered; this procedure can lead to improvements in both core AN symptoms and associated comorbid conditions and complications.

The ACC appears to play a role in reward anticipation, decision making, impulse control,[66] and repetitive and ritualistic behaviors to control eating in patients with AN.[22] In view of the successful results of anterior cingulotomy in OCD and anxiety, this procedure may be considered as a potential second surgery for patients with AN who experience symptoms of OCD, depression, or anxiety after failure of the initial bilateral anterior capsulotomy. At our institution, 12 patients in whom bilateral anterior capsulotomy failed underwent additional anterior cingulotomy; this procedure resulted in further improvements in about half of these patients.

Grading of Anorexia Nervosa According to Clinical Features

Patients with AN have elevated rates of lifetime diagnoses of anxiety disorders, MDD, OCD, personality disorders, and substance abuse disorders.[5,7,67] Severe comorbid conditions and longer disease duration contribute to less favorable outcomes for AN. On the basis of data obtained from 180 cases of surgical treatment for AN, we categorize AN into four grades according to clinical characteristics, which in turn guide the selection of treatment options:

Grade I corresponds to excessive dieting, excessive exercise, or both.

Grade II includes excessive dieting and at least one psychiatric symptom such as OCD, anxiety, or depression.

Grade III is defined as binge-eating or purging behaviors (self-induced vomiting or the misuse of laxatives, diuretics), or both, accompanied by psychiatric symptoms, including OCD, anxiety, or depression.

Grade IV is characterized by binge-eating or purging behaviors, or both, accompanied by at least one of the following severe psychiatric disorders: substance abuse, kleptomania, self-injurious behavior, or a personality disorder.

If AN duration is longer than 6 years, the grade increases one level. Patient treatment options are dependent on the grade of AN. Patients with grade I AN receive psychotherapeutic interventions and pharmacologic therapies. Patients with grade II AN are treated with psychotherapeutic interventions/pharmacologic therapies, bilateral NAcc-DBS, or both. For patients with grade III AN, we recommend bilateral anterior capsulotomy or bilateral NAcc ablation. For patients with grade IV AN, we recommend bilateral anterior capsulotomy combined with bilateral anterior cingulotomy.

Indications and Patient Selection Criteria

Because publications regarding selection criteria for patients with AN are few and because available data are limited, there are no definite guidelines on patient selection criteria.[55,68,69] However, the general consensus regarding selection criteria for surgery in our institution is as follows.

Treatment History

First, patients must exhibit a consistent diagnosis of AN, either the restricting or binge-purging subtype, as defined by DSM-IV criteria and based on a psychiatric interview. Secondly, patients must be confirmed as treatment-refractory AN. In our center, treatment-refractory AN is defined as follows: (1) treatment with an appropriate therapy for more than 3 years; (2) at least two types of therapy (including pharmacologic treatment, behavioral therapy, family therapy, and psychotherapy) must have been applied without a desirable response; and (3) patients must have experienced a rapid decrease in body weight over a short time period, which could be life threatening without effective intervention.

Clinical Indications

AN must be of disabling severity with substantial functional impairment according to DSM-IV criterion C, and patients must exhibit a Global Assessment of Functioning (GAF) score of 45 or less for at least 2 years. Other functional scales such as WHO Disability Assessment Schedule II, which was recommended by DSM-V, are also appropriate indicators. Patient weight must also be <85% of ideal body weight (and/or BMI <17.5). Finally, patients or their representatives must be willing to give informed consent for treatment and any subsequent follow-up study.

Exclusion Criteria

Patients with unstable physical conditions (e.g., severe electrolyte disturbances, cardiac failure, or other physical contraindications for surgery/anesthesia) or obvious encephalotrophy caused by Alzheimer's disease, tumor, or trauma, as confirmed by MRI are to be excluded. As are patients with any contraindication to MRI (pregnancy, pacemakers, or metal implants contraindicated for MRI, not including the DBS implant and the stimulator itself). Patients younger than 14 years and those who refuse to sign the patient information and consent form should also be excluded.

PERIOPERATIVE PATIENT MANAGEMENT

Considering the wide range of physiologic abnormalities observed in AN, careful perioperative management is required.[70]

Preoperative Management

As a result of long-term malnutrition, most patients with AN have an unstable physical condition, which is a contraindication to surgery or anesthesia.[70,71] These conditions include severe electrolyte disturbances, cardiac failure, abnormal liver function, and coagulation abnormalities. Therefore, more detailed preoperative screening examinations such as electrocardiography and appropriate blood tests (e.g., tests for disseminated intravascular coagulation, blood biochemical examinations, routine blood tests, blood glucose tests) are essential for assessing potential medical risks. According to our experience, hypokalemia and hypoalbuminemia are the most common electrolyte disorders, which should be restored to normal conditions before surgery. In addition, most patients with AN exhibit comorbid conditions, such as OCD, depression, and anxiety. The mental status of patients with AN is often unstable, and patients frequently present with irritation and deep depression. Thus patients must be closely monitored throughout the entire procedure. Careful perioperative management is essential to avoid anesthetic complications as well.

Intraoperative Management

Local anesthesia is recommended during the ablative procedure to avoid hypervolemia and excessive dilution of electrolytes. For patients with AN who receive DBS treatment, local and general anesthesia are required. In view of the potential anesthetic complications, a thorough preoperative anesthetic assessment and evaluation is required. In addition, doses of most anesthetic drugs should be adjusted for weight, and during the operation, electrocardiographic changes and potassium levels should be monitored carefully to minimize the risk of arrhythmias.

Specific caution must be taken during the burr hole procedure because the skulls of patients with AN are usually very thin; excessive pressure to the dura may cause epidural hematomas. To avoid cerebrospinal fluid overflow during the operation, fibrin glue should be applied immediately after the dura is opened. Furthermore, a warm air blower is necessary during the operation to maintain normal body temperature. The operation should be completed in a timely manner, and appropriate soft mats should be applied to prevent bedsores.

Postoperative Management

Because patients with AN exhibit a very low body weight, rehydration fluids should be controlled strictly after surgery. Blood tests should also be evaluated closely to avoid fluid and electrolyte disturbances. Pharmacologic therapies should be administered on the second day after surgery, but dosage should be adjusted on the basis of the patients' symptoms; psychotherapeutic interventions can be initiated 2 weeks after surgery.

ADVERSE EVENTS ASSOCIATED WITH SURGERY FOR ANOREXIA NERVOSA

Operative Complications

Intracranial hematomas are a severe complication of stereotactic surgery. In 216 cases of stereotactic surgery at our institution, 4 cases of epidural hematoma were observed; 3 patients recovered after surgery and 1 patient died as a result of disseminated intravascular coagulation. Hematomas occur more frequently in patients with AN than in patients with other disorders treated with stereotactic surgery, such as Parkinson's disease, dystonia, and OCD, probably as a result of the serious condition of patients with AN.[72] Wound infections are more common after DBS treatment than after lesion procedures as a result of subcutaneous hydrops and subcutaneous hematomas in DBS. In our center, the rate of wound infections is about 2%, which is similar to that in other medical centers.

Neuropsychological Complications

Neuropsychological complications can be divided into short-term and long-term complications. Short-term side effects include incontinence, disorientation, sleep disorders, and headache. These symptoms usually resolved within 1 or 2 months after the operation. A number of patients (8%) experience long-term side effects, including memory loss, fatigue, excessive weight gain, and personality changes.

Complications Associated with Deep Brain Stimulation

In addition to surgical complications, hardware problems with the DBS system, including lead or wire fracture, hardware rejection, malfunction of the implantable pulse generator, and lead migration, can occur. Bhatia and colleagues[72] reviewed data from 191 patients who received a total of 330 electrode implants and found that the overall incidence of hardware-related problems was 4.2%, among the total number of systems implanted. The mean duration between implantation and complication was 1.8 years. Similar results were observed in our institution.

CONCLUSION AND FUTURE OUTLOOK

AN is a complex, severe, life-threatening psychiatric disorder with a high relapse rate when treated with current therapies. Stereotactic surgery that disconnects the limbic system circuits is a significant option in the treatment of refractory AN. Several concerns must be addressed in order to advance the application of stereotactic surgery in AN. First, a deeper understanding of the exact causes and neural circuits responsible for AN is needed. Functional neuroimaging studies are particularly useful for finding the mechanisms of disease development and possible target areas for further neurosurgical interventions. Second, both stimulation and lesion procedures to disconnect the AN-related neural circuit pathways are potentially effective in patients with AN who do not respond to pharmacologic therapy. Adverse effects and complications would gradually decrease, if the patients are chosen strictly according to the indications.

The grading of AN on the basis of patients' clinical characteristics is very useful for the surgical procedure selection and outcome prediction. Although reports of successful results of psychosurgery in patients with refractory AN are proliferating, surgical management in such patients is still limited in the context of experimental trials, inasmuch as their safety and efficacy remain under investigation. With further developments in basic research and modern stereotactic surgery techniques, physicians can better understand the etiopathologic mechanisms, neurotransmitters, and neurocircuitry involved in AN. Ultimately more safe and valuable surgical treatment can be provided for intractable AN to alleviate suffering and improve the quality of life of patients with this disabling disorder.

SUGGESTED READINGS

Barbier J, Gabriels L, van Laere K, et al. Successful anterior capsulotomy in comorbid anorexia nervosa and obsessive-compulsive disorder: case report. *Neurosurgery*. 2011;69(3):E745-E751.

Friederich HC, Wu M, Simon JJ, et al. Neurocircuit function in eating disorders. *Int J Eat Disord*. 2013;46(5):425-432.

Kaye WH, Fudge JL, Paulus M. New insights into symptoms and neurocircuit function of anorexia nervosa. *Nat Rev Neurosci*. 2009;10(8):573-584.

Lipsman N, Woodside DB, Giacobbe P, et al. Subcallosal cingulate deep brain stimulation for treatment-refractory anorexia nervosa: a phase 1 pilot trial. *Lancet*. 2013;381(9875):1361-1370.

Sun B, Li D, Zhan S. DBS for anorexia nervosa. Paper presented at: Eighth World Congress of International Neuromodulation Society; December 2007; Acapulco, Mexico.

Treasure J, Claudino AM, Zucker N. Eating disorders. *Lancet*. 2010; 375(9714):583-593.

Wang J, Chang C, Geng N, et al. Treatment of intractable anorexia nervosa with inactivation of the nucleus accumbens using stereotactic surgery. *Stereotact Funct Neurosurg*. 2013;91(6):364-372.

Wu H, Van Dyck-Lippens PJ, Santegoeds R, et al. Deep-brain stimulation for anorexia nervosa. *World Neurosurg*. 2012;80(3-4):S29.e1-S29.e10.

Zhang H-W, Li D-Y, Zhao J, et al. Metabolic imaging of deep brain stimulation in anorexia nervosa: a 18F-FDG PET/CT Study. *Clin Nucl Med*. 2013;38(12):943-948.

See a full reference list on ExpertConsult.com 

PART 5 Surgical Interventions for Spasticity

103 Lesioning Surgery for Spasticity

Marc Sindou, George Georgoulis, and Patrick Mertens

Spasticity is defined as a velocity-dependent resistance to passive movement of a joint and its associated musculature. Spasticity is characterized by hyperexcitability of the stretch reflex related to the loss of inhibitory influences from descending supraspinal structures. Spasticity should not be treated just because it is present because it may serve to compensate for loss of motor power. Spasticity should be treated only when excessive tone leads to functional disability and impaired locomotion, or contractures and deformities. Neurosurgical interventions should be considered when the harmful spasticity cannot be controlled by physical therapy and medications.

Management of spasticity includes not only intrathecal baclofen therapy and botulinum toxin injections but also lesioning surgery directed at peripheral nerves, dorsal roots, the dorsal root entry zone (DREZ), and the spinal cord. Methods of surgical management are classified according to whether their impact is general or focal and whether the effects are temporary or permanent (Fig. 103-1).

Lesioning procedures must be performed so that excessive tone is reduced without suppressing useful muscular tone or impairing any residual motor-sensory functions. In patients who retain some masked voluntary motility, the aim is to re-equilibrate the balance between paretic agonist and spastic antagonist muscles so that treatment results in improvement in (or the reappearance of) voluntary motor function (Fig. 103-2). In patients with poor residual function preoperatively, the aim is limited to halt the evolution of orthopedic deformities and improve comfort.

Our department has treated more than 1200 patients with spasticity over the past 25 years. We believe that teams dealing with spasticity should have all of the technical modalities at hand.[1,2] Intrathecal baclofen therapy, which is discussed in detail in Chapter 104 of this book, is indicated primarily for paraplegic or tetraplegic adult patients with diffuse spasticity, especially of spinal origin, although it can also be used to treat spasticity related to cerebral palsy in older children, especially when dystonia is associated to spasticity.[3-5] Lesioning operations are indicated for focal spasticity of the limbs when treatment with botulinum toxin injections proves insufficient. Peripheral neurotomy is justified when harmful spasticity affects one or a few muscular groups. A preliminary test consisting of an anesthetic block may help in the decision-making process by mimicking the effect of the neurotomy. When harmful spasticity affects the entire limb or in the setting of paraplegia, diplegia, or hemiplegia, surgery directed at the dorsal roots (dorsal rhizotomy) or the DREZ (microsurgical DREZotomy [MDT]) may be the solution in selected cases. Complementary orthopedic operations are frequently needed in patients with associated irreducible contractures, tendon retractions, joint deformities, or any combination of these problems.

SELECTIVE PERIPHERAL NEUROTOMIES

Peripheral neurotomy was introduced for the treatment of a spastic foot by Stoffel.[6] Later, peripheral neurotomy was made more selective by using microsurgery and mapping by intraoperative electrical stimulation to better identify the function of individual nerve fascicles (Fig. 103-3).[7-11] Neurotomy consists of partial sectioning of one or several of the motor branches (or fascicles) corresponding to the muscle or the muscles in which spasticity is considered excessive. It works by interrupting the segmental reflex arc in both its afferent and efferent limbs. Neurotomy must not include sensory nerve fibers because even partial sectioning of them could result in neuropathic pain. Motor branches must be clearly isolated from the nerve trunk; the constituting fascicles must be dissected and identified to be stimulated independently. On an empirical basis it is agreed that neurotomy must include sectioning of approximately 50% to 80% of all the branches to a targeted muscle for it to be effective.

Surgical Principles

Preoperative Motor Blocks

Before recommending selective peripheral neurotomy, local blockade with a long-lasting anesthetic (2 to 3 hours with bupivacaine) must be performed to evaluate the strength of the antagonist muscles and to determine whether the articular limitation results from spasticity or musculotendinous contractures and articular ankylosis. Botulinum toxin injections can be used as a "prolonged" test for several weeks or months because they mimic the effect of selective neurotomy. This strategy of using preoperative injections allows patients to appreciate the benefit that could follow selective neurotomy (e.g., at the lower limb for walking, at the upper limb for cosmetic objectives, to allow the patient to put the hand in a pocket, to allow caregivers to wash the palms of patient's hands, or for functional improvement).

Anesthesia

During surgery it may be useful to test the efficacy of the procedure by evaluating the stretch reflex (e.g., test for clonus), which requires that the reflexes not be depressed by anesthetic drugs. General anesthesia must be induced without long-lasting curarization so that the motor evoked responses used to identify nerve fascicles can be detected. Muscle relaxants must be avoided; nitrogen monoxide and propofol are also contraindicated because they modify reflex excitability.

Electrophysiologic Mapping

Use of the operating microscope is required because the emergence of nerve branches frequently varies and surgical access is limited; in addition, identification of motor fascicles is essential for performing an effective neurotomy that avoids sensory impairment. Anatomic identification of fascicles based on descriptive anatomy must be checked by study of muscular responses to electrical stimulation. Stimulation is performed at a frequency of 2 Hz with low intensity (1-mA current). Bipolar (or tripolar) stimulation, composed of an anode between two cathodes, should be used to avoid electrical diffusion and therefore incorrect interpretation. The response to stimulation is visualized in the form of clinically observable movements of the corresponding muscles and—if considered useful—electromyography (EMG) recordings.

Sectioning

After all the motor branches (or their constituting fascicles) have been identified, those considered to correspond to harmful spasticity are sectioned in variable proportions (50% to 80%), depending on the degree of spasticity. A resection is performed over approximately 5 mm; the proximal stump is then coagulated with a fine bipolar forceps to prevent regrowth of fibers. The effect of each nerve interruption is then evaluated by comparing the muscle responses to electrical stimulation proximal and then distal to the resected portion. If the response after proximal stimulation is still intense, further resection is performed. The aim is to decrease motor innervation sufficiently to avoid recurrence of spasticity by "takeover" (i.e., reinnervation or "adoption" of muscle fibers denervated as a result of neurotomy by surrounding motor fibers).

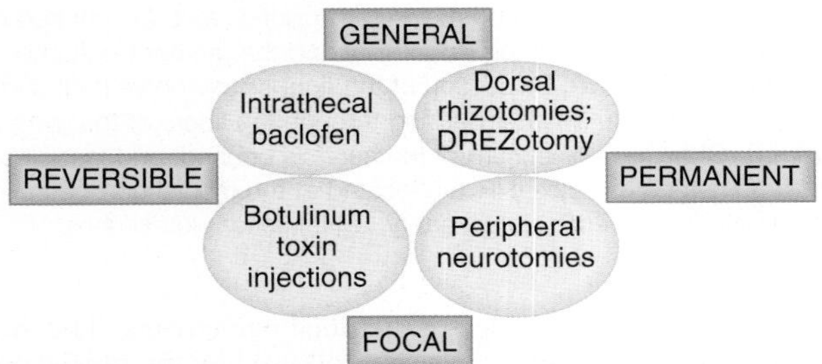

Figure 103-1. Management is based on whether the spasticity is focal or generalized and whether the effect of treatment is permanent or transient.

Surgical Techniques

Surgery on the Lower Limb

Obturator Neurotomy for the Hip. Obturator neurotomy is for spasticity in the adductor muscles. It is often proposed for diplegic children with cerebral palsy when crossing or "scissoring" of the lower limbs hampers their walking. It can also be performed on paraplegic patients to facilitate perineal washing, toilet, and self-catheterization. After skin incision (Fig. 103-4A), the dissection is conducted lateral to the adductor longus muscle body to rapidly locate the anterior branch of the obturator nerve. The posterior branch is situated more deeply and should be spared to preserve the hip-stabilizing muscles (Fig. 103-4B).

Hamstring Neurotomy for the Knee. Hamstring neurotomy is indicated to counter flexion deformity of the knees. After skin incision (Fig. 103-5A) and crossing the fibers of the gluteus maximus, the sciatic nerve is identified. Branches to the hamstring muscles are isolated at the medial border of the nerve, primarily based on motor evoked responses of the semitendinosus muscle, which is often the major muscle responsible for spasticity (Fig. 103-5B).

Tibial Neurotomy for the Foot. Tibial neurotomy is indicated for the treatment of equinovarus spastic foot with or without dystonic claw toes. It consists of exposing all motor branches of the tibial nerve at the popliteal fossa (i.e., nerves to the gastrocnemius and soleus, tibialis posterior, popliteus, flexor hallucis longus, and flexor digitorum longus).[12] The soleus is considered the more responsible involved muscle in the pathogenesis of spastic footdrop so that the gastrocnemius can be spared (Fig. 103-6A).[13]

The tibial nerve trunk, from which the nerves to the gastrocnemius emerge, is easily identifiable. The superior soleus nerve is situated in the midline, just posterior to the tibial nerve. After retracting the tibial nerve trunk medially with a traction tape, the other branches can be identified by electrical stimulation as they

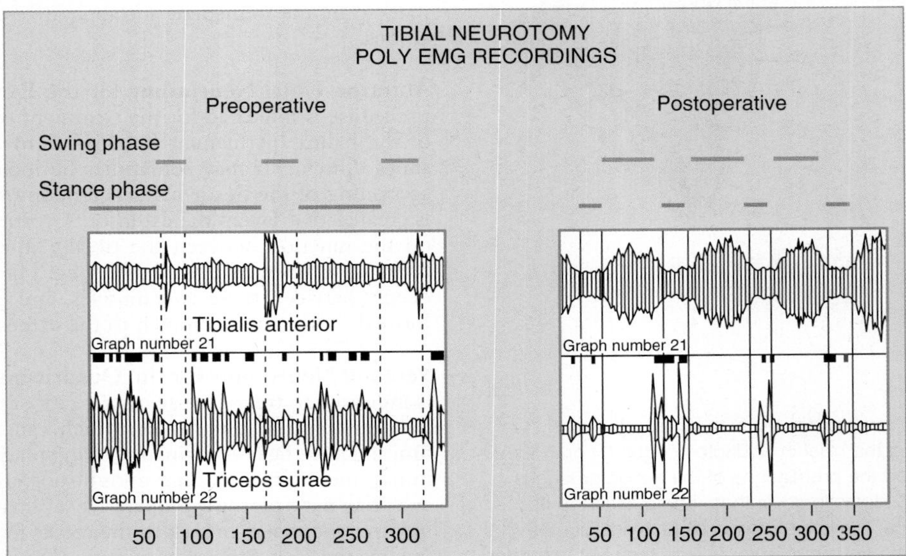

Figure 103-2. Gait analysis. Preoperative polyelectromyography (POLY EMG) shows desynchronized activity in the triceps surae, with abnormal co-contractions of the tibialis anterior and triceps surae *(left).* After tibial neurotomy *(right),* muscular activity reappears in the tibialis anterior with normal alternation between contraction of the triceps surae at the end of the stance phase and contraction of the tibialis anterior during the swing phase.

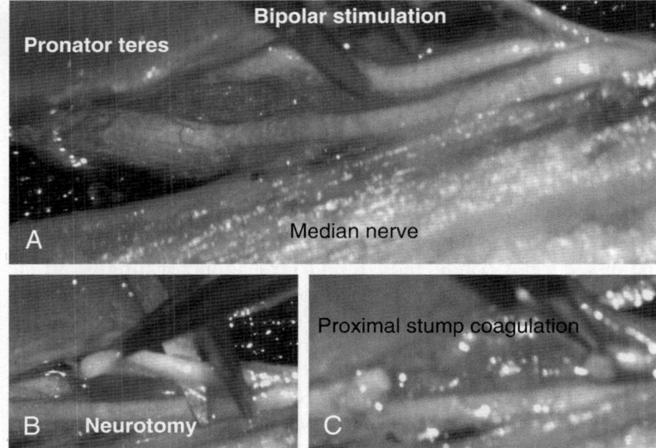

Figure 103-3. Microsurgical technique of the selective peripheral neurotomy. Operative microsurgical views show the steps in neurotomy for the pronator teres muscular branch of the median nerve as an example. **A,** The muscular branch of the pronator teres is identified by (preferably bipolar) electrical motor stimulation. **B,** In line with the preoperative evaluation and subsequent plan for this particular patient, 50% of the isolated motor fascicles are resected, 5 mm in length, near the muscle to ensure that only its muscular branches are divided. **C,** The proximal stump is coagulated with bipolar forceps to prevent regrowth of fibers.

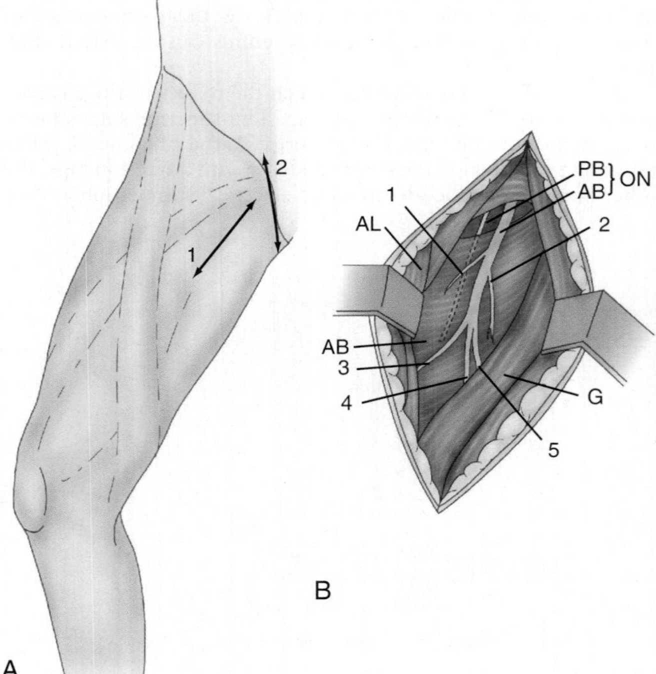

Figure 103-4. Obturator neurotomy. A, Skin incision for right obturator neurotomy along the relief of adductor longus (1) or in the hip flexion fold centered on the prominence of the adductor longus tendon (2), which gives a cosmetic advantage. The addition to its more aesthetic appearance, the latter incision facilitates adductor longus. **B,** Dissection of the anterior branch (AB) of the right obturator nerve (ON). The adductor longus (AL) is retracted laterally and the gracilis (G) medially. The nerve is anterior to the adductor brevis (AB). 1 and 2, adductor brevis nerve; 3, adductor longus nerve; 4 and 5, gracilis nerve. The posterior branch (PB) lies under the adductor brevis (AB) and should be spared.

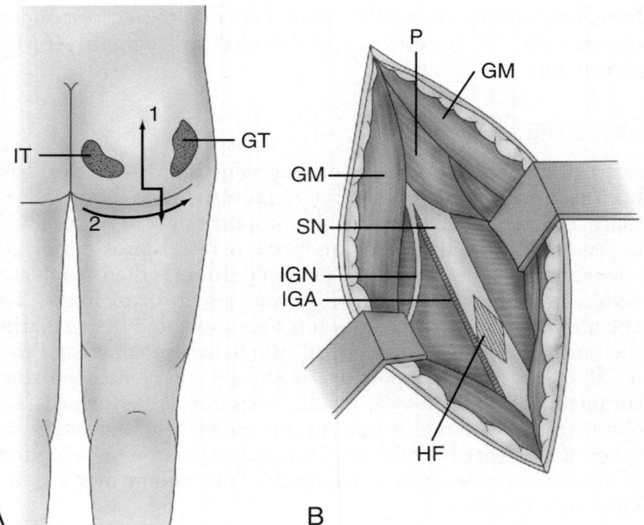

Figure 103-5. Hamstring neurotomy. A, The skin incision for hamstring neurotomy (on the right side) is located on the midline between the ischial tuberosity (IT) and the greater trochanter (GT) (1). A transverse incision can also be made in the gluteal fold (2) centered on the groove between the ischial tuberosity and the greater trochanter for better cosmetics. **B,** Dissection of the right sciatic nerve (SN) under the piriformis muscle (P) after passing through the fibers of the gluteus maximus (GM). The epineurium of the nerve is opened, and fascicles for the hamstring muscles (HF) are located at the medial part of the nerve trunk. IGA, inferior gluteal artery; IGN, inferior gluteal nerve.

emerge from the lateral edge of the tibial nerve trunk. The most lateral branch is the popliteal nerve, followed by the tibialis posterior nerve and finally by the inferior soleus nerve and flexor digitorum longus nerves. Some fascicles, often larger, can give a toe flexion response through the intrinsic toe flexors (Fig. 103-6B). However, neurotomy of these branches is not recommended if they cannot be clearly individualized because they may be mixed with sensory fascicles. An effective soleus neurotomy is marked by the immediate intraoperative disappearance of ankle clonus.

Anterior Tibial Neurotomy for the Extensor Hallucis. This procedure is indicated for the treatment of permanent extension of the hallux (permanent Babinski sign), which makes wearing shoes difficult. It may sometimes be indicated after unjustified sectioning of the flexor hallucis tendon in which disequilibrium is created that favors the extensor. A vertical incision is centered on the junction between the tibialis anterior and the extensor hallucis, at the middle third of the leg. The tibial nerve is situated deeply between these two muscles, and the neurotomy is performed on the motor branch to the extensor hallucis.

Femoral Neurotomy for the Quadriceps. Femoral neurotomy is indicated to treat excessive spasticity of the quadriceps muscle. This muscle is often spastic, which can interfere with gait by limiting knee flexion during the swing phase. Given its "strategic" importance in maintaining upright posture, a motor block is an essential part of the preoperative evaluation. The neurotomy involves the motor branch to the rectus femoris and vastus intermedius muscles. After skin incision (Fig. 103-7A), the dissection passes medial to the sartorius muscle body and exposes the motor branches of the femoral nerve, first the nerve to the rectus femoris and then, more deeply, the nerve to the vastus intermedius (Fig. 103-7B). Electrical stimulation is essential given the large number of sensory fascicles of this nerve that must be spared.

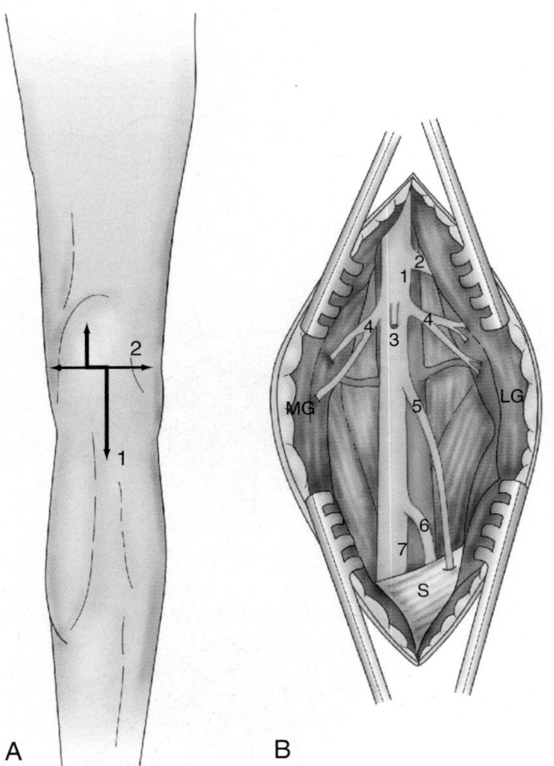

Figure 103-6. Tibial neurotomy. A, Skin incision to expose the tibial nerve. A vertical incision is made at the right popliteal fossa (1), or a transverse incision is made in the popliteal fossa fold (2) for a better aesthetic result. The latter incision allows deinsertion of the gastrocnemius fascia at the end of the procedure. **B,** Dissection of the tibial nerve, dorsal view of the right popliteal region. 1, Tibial nerve; 2, peroneal nerve. The sensory sural nerve (3), which lies superficially satellite of the saphenous vein just beneath the subcutaneous aponeurosis between the two gastrocnemius muscles, should be spared. The medial and lateral gastrocnemius nerves (4) may arise either separately from the sides of the tibial trunk or posteriorly from a common origin, sometimes including the sensory sural nerve. Each gastrocnemius nerve usually divides into two distal branches when approaching the muscle. One or two soleus nerves (5) may arise from a common origin or separately from the tibial nerve. The posterior tibialis nerve (6), like the soleus nerve, originates from the ventrolateral aspect of the tibial nerve, but more distally at the level of the soleus arch (5). Sometimes it may originate from a common trunk with the inferior branch of the soleus nerve. The distal trunk of the tibial nerve (7) contains five to eight fascicles averaging 1 mm in diameter each; two thirds of them are motor fascicles, with a third being sensory fascicles. LG, lateral gastrocnemius; MG, medial gastrocnemius; S, soleus.

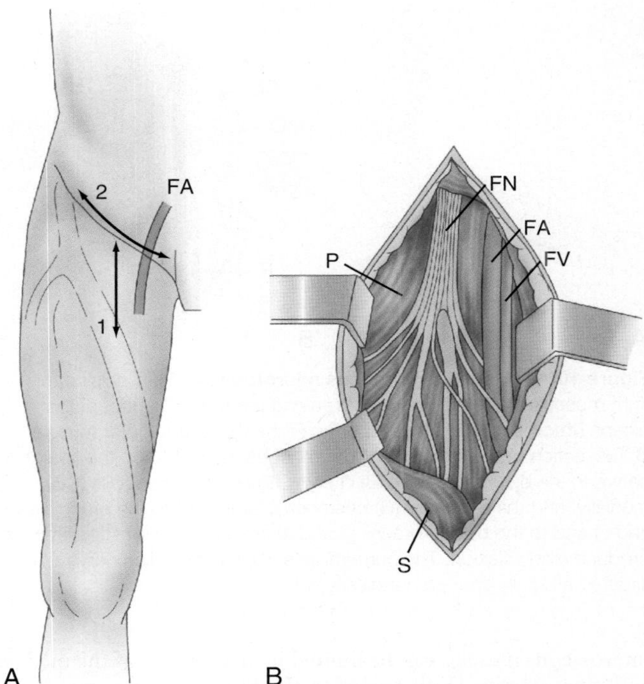

Figure 103-7. Femoral neurotomy. A, Skin incision for right femoral neurotomy, below the inguinal ligament, lateral to the femoral artery (1) or horizontal in the hip flexion fold (2) for better aesthetic results. **B,** Dissection of the right femoral nerve (FN) and its branches after opening the anterior fascia of the psoas muscle (P). Bipolar stimulation allows identification of the two or three branches to the sartorius muscle (S) and the three or four branches to the rectus femoris muscle, which produces flexion of the hip. The nerve to the vastus intermedius can be found more deeply. FA, femoral artery; FV, femoral vein.

Surgery on the Upper Limb

Pectoralis Major and Teres Major Neurotomy for the Shoulder. Neurotomy of collateral branches of the brachial plexus innervating the pectoralis major or the teres major is indicated for spasticity of the shoulder with internal rotation and adduction.[14] For the pectoralis major, the skin incision is made at the innermost part of the deltopectoral sulcus and curves along the clavicular axis. The clavipectoral fascia is then opened and the upper border of the pectoralis major muscle reflected downward. Close to the thoracoacromialis artery, the ansa of the pectoralis muscle is identified with the aid of a nerve stimulator. For the teres major, the skin incision follows the inner border of the teres major from the lower border of the posterior head of the deltoid muscle to the lower portion of the scapula. The lower border of the long portion of the brachii triceps constitutes the upper limit of the approach. The dissection is carried deep between the teres minor and major muscles. In the vicinity of the subscapular artery, the nerve ending on the teres major is identified. The nerve is surrounded by thick fat when approaching the anterior facet of the muscle body.

Musculocutaneous Neurotomy for the Elbow. Neurotomy of the musculocutaneous nerve is indicated for spasticity of the elbow with flexion mediated by the biceps brachii and brachialis muscles. After skin incision (Fig. 103-8A), the superficial fascia is opened between the biceps laterally and the coracobrachialis medially. The dissection proceeds in the space where the musculocutaneous nerve lies anterior to the brachialis muscle (Fig. 103-8B). Opening the epineurium allows the fascicles of the nerve to be dissected; the motor fascicles are distinguished from the sensory ones with a nerve stimulator.

Median Neurotomy for the Wrist and Fingers. Neurotomy of the median nerve is indicated for spasticity of the forearm with pronation mediated by the pronator teres and quadratus muscle, for spasticity of the wrist with flexion mediated by the flexor carpi radialis and palmaris longus muscles, and for spasticity of the fingers with flexion attributable to the flexor digitorum superficialis (flexion of the proximal interphalangeal and metacarpophalangeal joints) and the flexor digitorum profundus muscle (flexion of the distal interphalangeal joints). Swan neck deformation of the fingers mediated by the lumbrical and

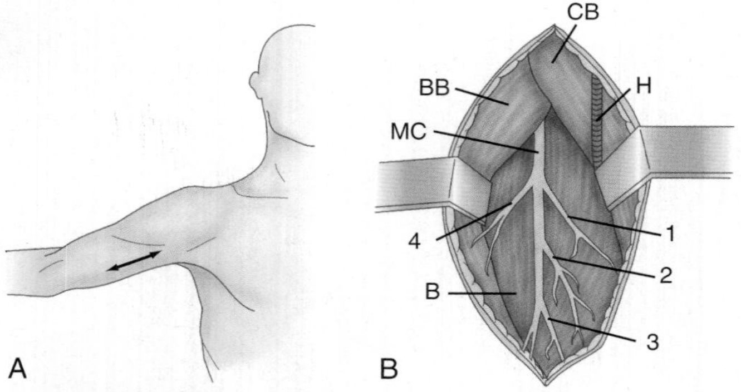

Figure 103-8. Musculocutaneous neurotomy. A, Skin incision for right musculocutaneous neurotomy along the medial aspect of the biceps brachii under the inferior edge of the pectoralis major muscle. **B,** Dissection of the right musculocutaneous nerve (MC) in the space between the biceps brachii (BB) laterally, the coracobrachialis (CB) medially, and the brachialis (B) posteriorly. Branches to the brachialis (1 and 2) and to the biceps brachii (3 and 4) are identified by stimulation to produce elbow flexion. The humeral artery (H) and median nerve are situated medially and are not dissected.

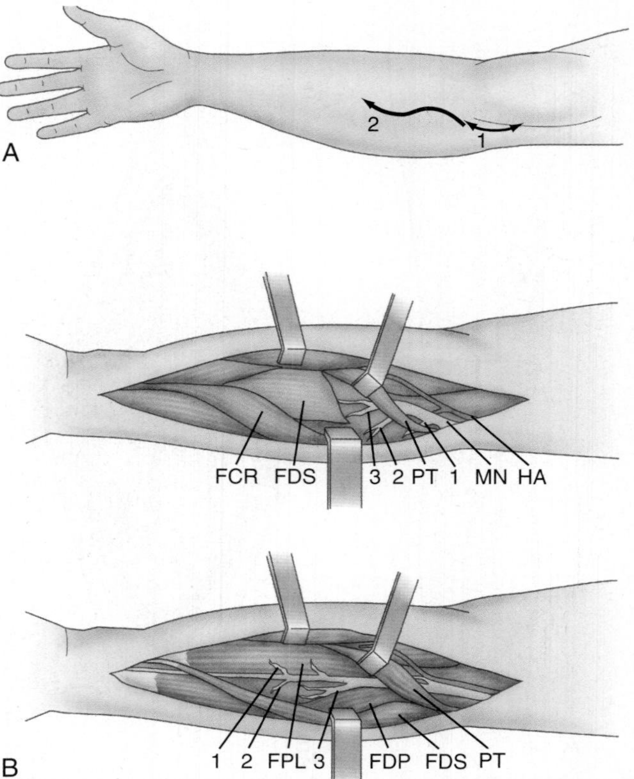

Figure 103-9. Median neurotomy. A, Skin incision on the right forearm for median neurotomy from the medial aspect of the biceps brachii at the level of the elbow longitudinally along the bicipital crest (1). The incision can eventually be continued distally toward the midline above the wrist (2). **B,** Dissection of the median nerve in two stages. In the first stage of the dissection *(upper figure),* the pronator teres (PT) is retracted upward and laterally and the flexor carpi radialis (FCR) medially. Branches from the median nerve (MN), before it passes under the fibrous arch of the flexor digitorum superficialis (FDS), are dissected: a branch to the pronators teres (1) and two nerve trunks to the flexor carpi radialis, palmaris longus, and flexor digitorum superficialis (2 and 3). In the second stage of the dissection *(lower figure),* the fibrous arch of the FDS is sectioned to allow more distal dissection of the median nerve. The FDS is retracted medially, and branches from the median nerve are identified: (1) branch to the flexor pollicis longus (FPL), (2) branch to the flexor digitorum profundus (FDP), and (3) branch to the interosseous nerve and its branches to these muscles. HA, Humeral artery.

interosseous muscles can be limited by neurotomy of the median and ulnar nerves. With regard to the thumb, neurotomy of the median nerve is indicated for spasticity with flexion and adduction-flexion (thumb-in-palm deformity) attributable to the flexor pollicis longus. The skin incision begins 2 to 3 cm above the flexion line of the elbow, medial to the biceps brachii tendon, passes through the elbow, and curves toward the junction of the upper and middle thirds of the anterior aspect of the forearm (the convexity of the curve turns laterally) (Fig. 103-9A).[15,16] Thereafter, the median nerve is searched for medial to the brachial artery and identified at the elbow, deeply under the lacertus fibrosus, which is cut. Sharp dissection is used to separate the branches of the median nerve. The pronator teres belly with its two heads is retracted medially and distally so that its muscular branches can be inspected. This muscle is next retracted up and laterally while the flexor carpi radialis is pulled down and medially. The muscular branches to the flexor carpi radialis and flexor digitorum superficialis can then be seen. Finally, the latter is retracted medially to uncover the branches to the flexor digitorum profundus, flexor pollicis longus, and pronator quadratus. These latter muscular branches may be individualized as separate branches or may remain together in the distal trunk of the anterior interosseous nerve. Sometimes it may be useful to divide the fibrous arch of the flexor digitorum superficialis muscle to make the dissection easier (Fig. 103-9B).

In contrast to this approach, which has a "wide" configuration, a "minimal" approach can be performed. The different fascicles in the trunk of the median nerve, just medial to the brachial artery, are dissected. This shorter approach provides a better cosmetic outcome. However, it has the inconvenience of providing nerve exposure less suitable for identifying the various motor branches in the form of fascicles enclosed in the nerve sheath and mixed with the sensory ones. This entails a risk for sensory complications, especially the development of allodynia or complex regional pain syndrome.

Ulnar Neurotomy for the Wrist and Fingers. Neurotomy of the ulnar nerve is also indicated for spasticity of the wrist with flexion and ulnar deviation, both mediated by the flexor carpi ulnaris; for spasticity of the fingers with flexion mediated by the flexor digitorum profundus muscle, which is partly innervated by the ulnar nerve; and for spasticity of the thumb with adduction-flexion attributable to the adductor pollicis. Ulnar neurotomy can also be performed in conjunction with median neurotomy for swan neck deformation of the fingers. A separate arched skin incision is made to expose the ulnar nerve at the medial part of the elbow (Fig. 103-10), where it enters between the two heads of the flexor carpi ulnaris. There, the motor branches to this latter muscle are identified. Distally, the branches to the medial half of the flexor digitorum profundus are identified. For adduction/flexion spastic deformity of the thumb ("thumb in palm") deep terminal motor branch of the ulnar nerve can be reached at Guyon's canal at wrist.

Complications and Recurrence of Symptoms

Sensory disturbances such as paresthesias, dysesthesias, complex regional pain syndromes, or even deafferentation pain may occur if the sectioning accidentally includes sensory fascicles. This might be particularly severe and disabling after neurotomy of the

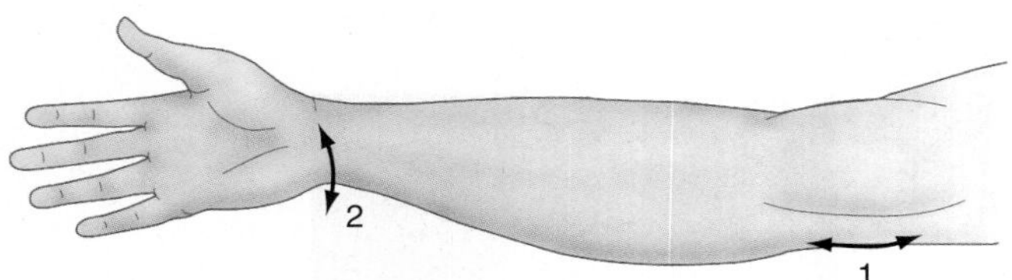

Figure 103-10. Ulnar neurotomy. The skin incision on the right forearm for ulnar neurotomy is either a longitudinal incision posterior to the medial epicondyle and medial to the olecranon at the elbow (1) or a transverse medial incision in the wrist fold (2), depending on the location of the spastic muscles.

median (hand) or tibial (plantar sole) nerve. Hypoesthesia (more often transient) of the anterior part of the forearm or the lateral aspect of the foot may also occur secondary to inadvertent lesioning of the subcutaneous sensory nerves rather than being a result of the neurotomy itself.

Patients rarely complain of decreased muscle strength after neurotomy because no single muscle is solely responsible for the movement of a body segment. However, paresis of the flexors of the elbow, wrist, and fingers, with deficit in the prehension, or paresis in the foot with a subsequent talus deformity may occur secondary to excessive nerve sectioning.

Recurrence of spasticity can take place when the amount of sectioning is insufficient, in which case repeat surgery can be performed after a new blocking test.

SURGERY ON THE SPINAL ROOTS, DORSAL ROOT ENTRY ZONE, AND SPINAL CORD

History

In accordance with Sherrington's experimental data, Foerster in 1908 performed the first dorsal rhizotomies from L1 to S2 (excluding L4, the root of the quadriceps) for lower limb spasticity in cerebral palsy patients. From his experience with 159 patients, Foerster suggested the following[17]:

> For severe spastic paraplegia, I recommend resecting at least five roots. It is necessary to leave the fourth lumbar root, since this root generally guarantees the extensor reflex of the knee so very necessary for standing and walking. Thus the general rule is resection of the second, third and fifth lumbar, and first and second sacral roots. Unfortunately, there exist individual differences. In some cases, the fourth lumbar does not affect knee extension but knee flexion, as the fifth lumbar and first sacral do. In order to know by which lumbar roots the extension reflex of the knee is affected, we must have recourse to the electrical current during the operation.... The disappearance of the spasticity after the root resection is the best proof of the sensory origin of the spastic contracture. But a certain degree of spasm sometimes returns, owing to the fact that the spinal grey matter is gradually recharged by the remaining posterior roots.

In 1945, Munro suggested *sectioning the ventral roots* from the last thoracic to the first sacral segments to treat irreducible spasticity with severe spasms.[18] This type of procedure was recommended for spasticity associated with spontaneous hyperactivity of motor neurons, as observed after anoxia. In fact, sectioning the dorsal roots is ineffective in such cases, whereas ventral root sectioning abolishes the spasms.

In 1951, Bischof described *longitudinal myelotomy*,[19] the aim of which is to interrupt the spinal reflex arc between the ventral and dorsal horns with a vertical coronal incision performed laterally from one side of the spinal cord to the other, from the L1 to S1 segments, in paraplegic patients. The technique was then modified to avoid complete interruption of the corticospinal fibers. Through a T9 to L1 laminectomy, a posterior longitudinal sagittal incision is made before performing a cruciform myelotomy by making a transverse incision on either side with a stylet that has a right-angle extremity. The purpose of this surgically performed lesion is to interrupt the spinal reflex arc between the ventral and dorsal horns without sectioning the fibers connecting the pyramidal tract to the motor neurons of the ventral horn. Longitudinal myelotomy was used widely for patients with triple flexion and severe sphincter disturbances.

Intrathecal chemical rhizotomy was originally introduced for the treatment of cancer-related pain and was then adapted for the treatment of severe spasticity. Alcohol, which was used initially by Guttman for the treatment of disabling spastic paraplegia in 1953, was replaced by phenol (hyperbaric solution) in 1959 by Nathan. These techniques were not used frequently because of difficulty limiting their toxic effect solely to the targeted roots, including their effects on sensory fibers. In addition, the effects rarely persisted in the long term. Percutaneous radiofrequency rhizotomy, introduced to treat chronic pain, was then applied for certain spasticities, especially those at sacral roots in patients with neurogenic detrusor hyperreflexia or at lumbar roots (in particular L2 to L3) for the treatment of spastic hip flexion-adduction.

To reduce the harmful effects of dorsal rhizotomy on postural tone in ambulatory patients, Gros and pupils introduced topographic selection of rootlets by electrical stimulation to preserve the innervation of muscles responsible for useful tone (the quadriceps and abdominal and gluteal muscles in particular).[7,20] This technique was termed *selective posterior rhizotomy*. Apart from effects on the lower limbs, Gros also observed a decrease in spasticity of the upper limbs and improvement in speech and swallowing in his cerebral palsy patients. This is termed an *indirect effect*. In 1977, Fraioli and Guidetti proposed *partial dorsal rhizotomy*, which consisted of incising the dorsalmost part of each rootlet a few millimeters before its entry into the dorsolateral sulcus in an attempt to spare sensation.[21] In 1976, Fasano developed *functional dorsal rhizotomy*, a technique based on stimulation of the posterior rootlets with corresponding EMG recordings.[22] Exaggeration of the duration or extent of the motor evoked response indicated the particular roots that must be surgically sectioned.

In contrast to the lower limbs, very few dorsal rhizotomies were attempted at the cervical level for upper limb spasticity. From an experience of 23 patients with spastic paralysis of the upper limb treated by resection of the dorsal roots from C4 to T2 (with the exception of C6), Foerster[17] concluded that "in the majority the result is not good; therefore we do not recommend dorsal rhizotomy as a valuable procedure for spasticity of the upper limb."

In 1972, Sindou observed that the technique of *selective microsurgical destruction of the ventrolateral part of the DREZ*, which was developed for treating pain,[17-19] led to marked hypotonia in the muscles corresponding to the operated medullary segments.[23-26] The procedure was applied not only to hyperspastic states in paraplegic patients[27] but also to severe cases of hemiplegic upper limbs.[28] The potent effect of the MDT is presumably due not only to interruption of the "tonigenic" dorsal afferent fibers but also to lesioning of the dorsal horn gray matter, which contains a quantity of interneurons that convey tonigenic input to motor neurons of the ventral horn. If MDT is performed deeply down to the base of the ventral horn, the procedure may alleviate the focal dystonia.[29]

Surgical Techniques

Dorsal Rhizotomies

The surgical approach for dorsal rhizotomy varies significantly from one team to another. The most classic technique—described

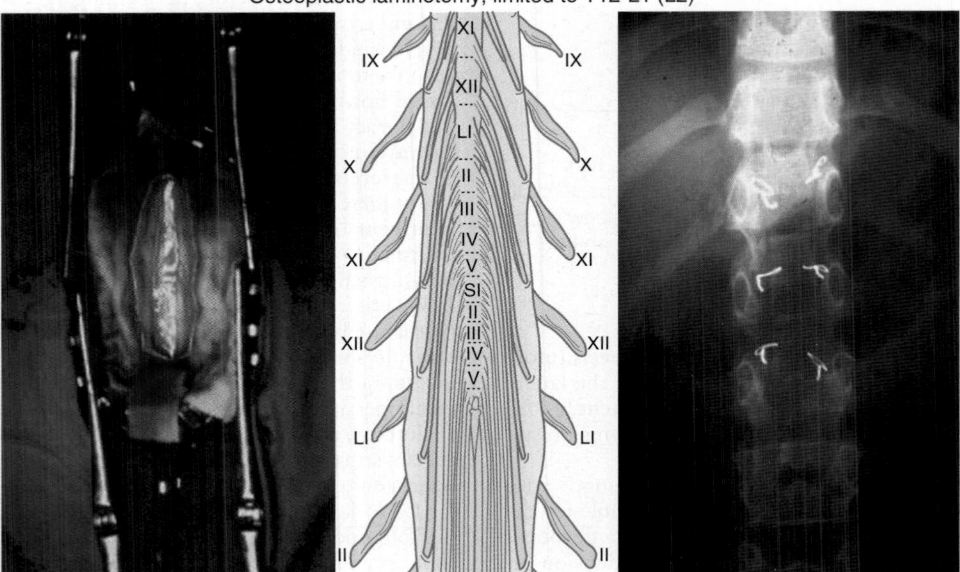

Figure 103-11. Lumbosacral dorsal rhizotomy for spastic diplegia in children with cerebral palsy performed through a limited osteoplastic laminotomy at the thoracolumbar junction. Our personal technique consists of performing a limited osteoplastic laminotomy in a single piece with a power saw from T11 to L1 *(left).* The laminae will be replaced at the end of the procedure and fixed (in this case with wires) *(right).* The dorsal (and corresponding ventral) L1, L2, and L3 roots can be identified by their muscular responses evoked by electrical stimulation, which is performed intradurally just before entry into their dural sheaths. The dorsal sacral rootlets are recognized at their entrance into the dorsolateral sulcus of the conus medullaris. The landmark between the S1 and S2 medullary segments is located approximately 30 mm from the exit of the tiny coccygeal root from the conus. The dorsal rootlets of S1, L5, and L4 can be identified by their evoked motor responses, the sensory roots for the bladder (S2-3) by monitoring vesical pressure, and those for the rectal sphincter (S3-4) by rectomanometry (or simply using a finger, protected by a glove, introduced into the anal canal) or electromyographic recordings. Spinal cord surface somatosensory evoked potential recordings from stimulation of the tibial nerve (L5-S1) and pudendal nerve (S1-3) might also be helpful, but time-consuming to be carried out in practice.

first by Fasano and coworkers[22] and then by Peacock and Arens[30] and Abbott and colleagues[31]—is as follows: a one-piece laminotomy is performed from L1 to S1 with a high-speed saw, which allows repositioning at the end of the procedure. Bipolar electrical stimulation of the sensory roots is carried out with the assistance of multichannel EMG recordings (in addition to palpation of the leg muscles for evidence of contraction). Roots that when stimulated cause either muscle activity outside their myotome or activity that persists after cessation of the stimulus are deemed abnormal and are separated into their rootlets. The rootlets are in turn stimulated, and the same criteria are used to judge their normality. Abnormally responsive rootlets are candidates to be cut.

To limit the extent of the approach, we and others, especially Park, preferred a limited laminotomy at the end of conus medullaris.[32-34] Our personal technique is illustrated in Figure 103-11. For surgery to be effective, approximately 60% of the dorsal rootlets must be cut, the amount depending on the level and function of the roots involved. The roots corresponding to muscles with harmful spasticity versus useful postural tone must be considered when determining the number of rootlets to be cut. In most cases, L4, which predominantly provides innervation to the quadriceps femoris, must be preserved.

In 2001, to further reduce the invasiveness of the approach and to access the roots to be targeted (individually) at their exit from the intradural space to the corresponding dural sheath, we developed a modality that we termed *keyhole interlaminar dorsal rhizotomy* (Fig. 103-12).[35] The lumbosacral spine is approached posteriorly so that the interlaminar spaces selected on the basis of the preoperative chart can be reached. After resecting the ligamentum flavum, the chosen interlaminar space or spaces are enlarged by resecting the lower half of the superior and the upper half of the inferior laminae. Through the fenestrations, the dura is opened in the midline for a height of 2 cm. The L2 and L3 roots can be reached through an L1 to L2 opening, L4 and L5 through L3 to L4, and S1 and S2 through an L4 to L5 or an L5 to S1 opening. The lumbar midline incision and muscle separation are extended according to the number and topography of the interlaminar spaces to be reached, which may be one, two, or three based on clinical presentation and preoperative chart. Both the spinous processes and the interspinous ligament are respected. After resection of the flavum ligament of the selected interlaminar spaces, each space is enlarged by resecting the lower two thirds of the upper lamina and the upper two thirds of the lower lamina.

The microsurgical steps are conducted following the principles of the keyhole interlaminar dorsal rhizotomy. At the exit from the dural sheath, the ventral root is easily identified on its ventral position. The dorsal rootlets (on average, five per root) are also easily identified; they are grouped posteriorly to the ventral root, often separated from the latter by an arachnoid fold. Muscular responses to stimulation with a preferably bipolar electrode to avoid spreading of current are tested first for the ventral root, then for the dorsal root.

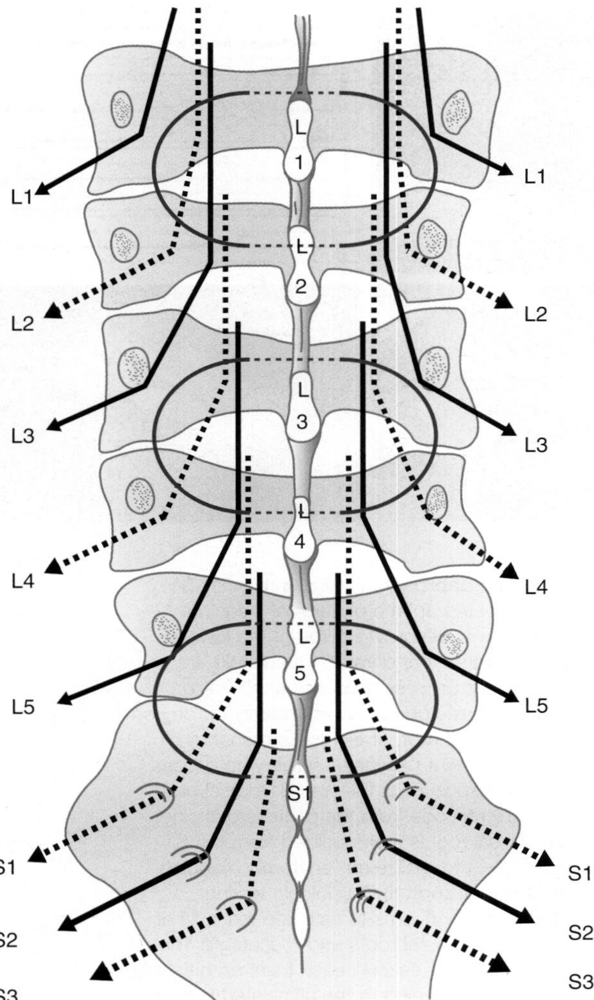

Figure 103-12. Schematic drawing of interlaminar (IL) vertebral levels where selected roots can be targeted for dorsal rhizotomy according to the preoperative surgical planning. *L2, L3* at L1-L2; *L3, L4* at L2-L3; *L4, L5* at L3-L4; *L5, S1* at L4-L5; *S1, S2* at L5-S1 (or L4-L5). IL spaces to be opened are determined according to the preoperative program for root sectioning (tailored operation). Roots *L2* and *L3* were targeted at the L1-L2 IL space for treatment of spastic hip and thigh in flexion-adduction. Roots *L4* and *L5* were targeted at the L3-L4 IL space for treatment of spastic quadriceps with patella ascension. Roots *S1* and *S2* were targeted at the L5-S1 (or L4-L5) IL space for treatment of spastic foot in equinism and spastic hamstrings. *(From Sindou M, Georgoulis G, Mertens P.* Neurosurgery for Spasticity: A Practical Guide for Treating Children and Adults. *Wien: Springer, 2014:258.)*

Exposure of lumbar laminae, for example, at three interlaminar levels, is shown in Figure 103-13Ai. After opening the dura on midline at the selected interlaminar spaces, a microscope is installed. The trajectory is oblique at approximately 45 degrees so that the surgeon's view passes underneath the (respective) interspinous ligament (Fig. 103-13Aii). Goal is to access (intradurally) the contralateral root, with its ventral and dorsal components, at its exit to the corresponding dural sheath, as seen in Figure 103-13Aiii.

Each exposed root is electrically stimulated to identify its innervation territory and thereby confirm its topographic level. This phase is *anatomic mapping*. Stimulation (2 Hz, approximately 200 μA) is first performed on the ventral root component, which is easy when the root is accessible at its exit to its dural sheath (Fig. 103-13Aiii). *To be noted, a motor response by dorsal root stimulation would require a 3 to 5 times higher intensity.* Thus the roots corresponding topographically to the muscles harboring "harmful" spasticity are identified before the sectioning decision.

Then the dorsal rootlets undergo *physiologic testing*. Stimulation is provoked with a 50-Hz train with a duration of 1 second for each train. Excitability is considered excessive when stimulation elicits an "exaggerated" (sustained or spreading) response (Fig. 103-13Bi-ii). This testing is to confirm or modify the percentage of the dorsal root to be cut, previously specified in the preoperative chart. The number of selected dorsal rootlets to be cut, whose number was specified in the preoperative chart in proportion to the severity of the spasticity in the corresponding muscular groups, is adjusted accordingly. The amount of dorsal rootlets cut generally ranges between one third and four fifths of a root's constituting rootlets (Fig. 103-13Biii-iv). Then the dural incision is sutured in a watertight fashion, and the dural suture line is covered with fat harvested subcutaneously.

Lesioning at the Dorsal Root Entry Zone

The aim of MDT is to preferentially interrupt both the small-caliber (nociceptive) and large-caliber (myotatic) tonigenic fibers of the dorsal roots, respectively situated laterally and in the middle of the entry zone. The surgical lesion must partially if not totally preserve the medially positioned large-caliber fibers that ascend to the dorsal column and also through a collateral project to the dorsal horn of the cord. The surgical target includes most of the dorsal horn, where the fibers and neurons that activate the segmental circuitry of the spinal cord are located (Fig. 103-14). The technique is detailed in Figures 103-15 and 103-16. Briefly, the procedure consists of 3-mm deep microsurgical incisions—at the level of the dorsolateral sulcus—with a 35-degree angle at the cervical level and a 45-degree angle at the lumbosacral level to strictly be in the axis of the dorsal horn at the respective levels. Bipolar coagulation is performed ventrolaterally at the entrance of the rootlets into the dorsolateral sulcus and inside the gray matter of the dorsal horn along all the spinal cord segments selected for surgery. When there is focal dystonia associated with spasticity, microcoagulations should be even more deeply down to the base of the ventral horn.[21]

ORTHOPEDIC SURGERY

Orthopedic surgical procedures may reduce spasticity by means of muscle relaxation induced by lengthening of tendons. The techniques currently available for correcting shortness of the muscle-tendon assembly are muscular disinsertion, myotomy, tenotomy, and lengthening tenotomy. Tendon transfer has a different goal: it may normalize articular orientation disturbed by muscular imbalance. Transfer of spastic muscles must be avoided; suppression of spasticity should first be achieved by a neurosurgical procedure. The goal of osteotomies is to correct bone deformation caused by growth or to treat stiffened joints. Articular surgery (arthrodesis) is indicated only when the deformities cannot be corrected by osteotomy or tendon surgery. Arthrodesis must not be performed in children until growth is complete.

PATIENT SELECTION

Because the features and consequences of spasticity differ from one patient to another, it is important that the objective or objectives of treatment be defined for every patient: improvement in function, prevention of deformities, or alleviation of discomfort and pain. These issues must be explained to the patient, relatives,

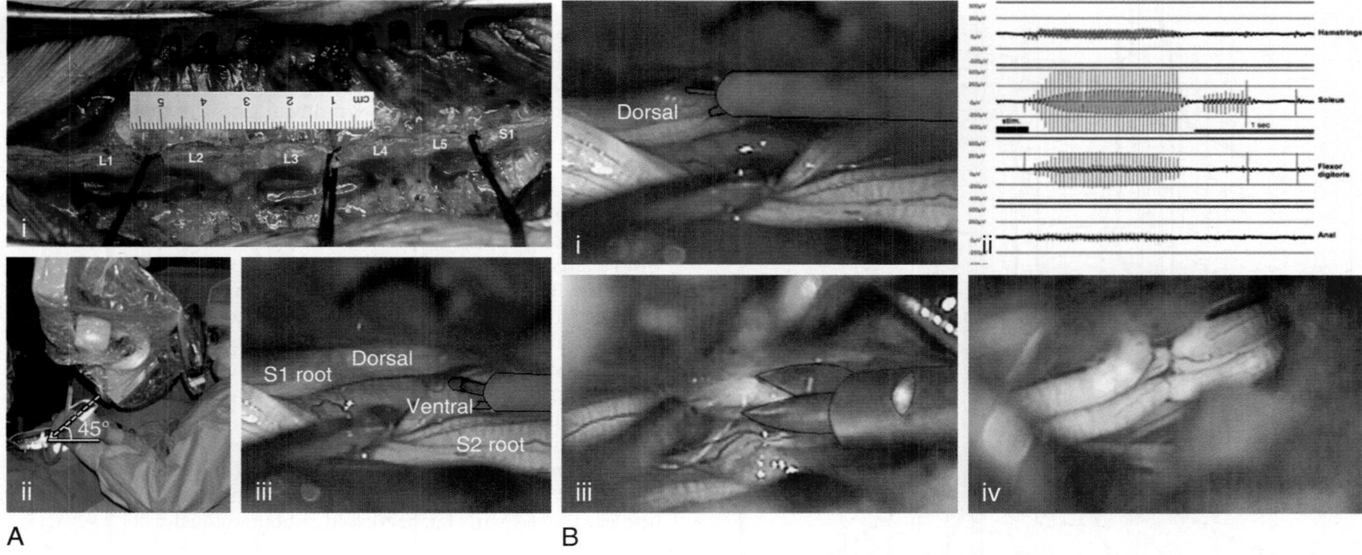

Figure 103-13. Keyhole interlaminar dorsal rhizotomy. **A, Exposure and approach.** (i) Exposure of L1-S1 laminae, with L1-L2, L3-L4, and L5-S1 interlaminar fenestrations as selected at time of surgical planning. At each fenestrated level, the inferior two thirds of the upper lamina and the superior two thirds of the lower lamina are rongeured, and flavum ligamentum is removed to expose dura so that dura and arachnoid are opened on midline. Note at fenestrated level(s) preservation of the spinous processes as well as of the interspinous ligament *(blue tapes)*. (ii) Surgeon operates with an oblique trajectory, at approximately 45-degree angle, to target, intradurally, through the interlaminar space, the contralateral root, at exit to corresponding dural sheath. Note that trajectory passes underneath the interspinous ligament ("keyhole" surgery) to access the root, with its ventral and dorsal components (well recognizable). (iii) Exposure of the *(left)* S1 dorsal and ventral roots at entry into the dural sheath, obliquely seen under the microscope from the contralateral side. Note neighboring S2 root going down to next *(lower)* level. The S1 dorsal root is individualized from the S1 ventral root. In this image a bipolar electrode is stimulating the ventral root to realize an "anatomic mapping." **B, Intraoperative physiologic testing and selected sectioning of dorsal root.** (i) Physiologic testing (excitability) of the dorsal root (at 50 Hz, 1 mA) using same bipolar electrode. It aims to estimate the level of excitability of the radicular-spinal circuitry by stimulating the corresponding dorsal roots and rootlets. (ii) The electromyogram shows a sustained response to a 50-Hz train stimulation (of 1 second each train) at threshold (of about 1 mA) and a spread of the response outside the myotome corresponding to the stimulated root. In the illustrative example, which corresponds to stimulation of an S1 dorsal root (same patient as the one for ventral root stimulation), note the spreading response outside the myotome corresponding to S1, namely to flexor digitorum and anal sphincter, tributary to S2 and S3 for the latter. (iii) Sectioning with microscissors of the selected dorsal rootlets. (iv) In this case, three out of the four rootlets, which constitute the dorsal root, were divided.

and caregivers within the frame of a multidisciplinary team. Guidelines for surgical intervention in spasticity have been detailed elsewhere.[1,2,35-38]

Treating Spasticity in Adults

Generally, adult patients do not complain of spasticity; instead, they are more likely to be aware of stiffness, deformity, and limitations in functional abilities. *Stiffness* is a useful term because it is widely understood by both clinicians and patients and does not imply a specific cause. After sufficient time, patients have a mixture of spasticity and muscle shortening or contracture. In any discussion of management, agreement on terminology is important for recognizing two principal components of muscle stiffness: (1) "dynamic" shortening of muscles caused by spasticity, which is manifested as hyperreflexia, clonus, and velocity-dependent resistance to passive joint motion; and (2) "fixed" shortening of muscles, which is manifested as contracture that is much less velocity dependent and persists under local blockade or anesthesia.

Spasticity should not be treated just because it is present; it should be treated because it is harmful to the patient. Patients may be able to use spastic limbs for functional activities. An extensor pattern in the lower limb or limbs may aid in standing transfers. In this scenario, "successful" spasticity management, if measured by reduction in tone and improved range of motion, might reduce rather than enhance function. Hence, the goal of spasticity management must be improved function and prevention or reversal of fixed deformities. Differentiating dynamic from fixed deformities is of prime importance before deciding on any surgical treatment, whether neurosurgical, orthopedic, or both. Dynamic range-of-motion measures are a useful starting point, supplemented with instrumented measures of spasticity and its effects on function, such as motion analysis. Guidelines for treating spasticity are shown in Figure 103-17.

Treating Spasticity in Children

The disorder from cerebral palsy encompasses a group of conditions that are permanent but not unchanging. Cerebral palsy involves disorders of movement, posture, or both, and of motor function.

As in adults, spasticity in children can be either useful for function or detrimental. Efficient treatments are available for

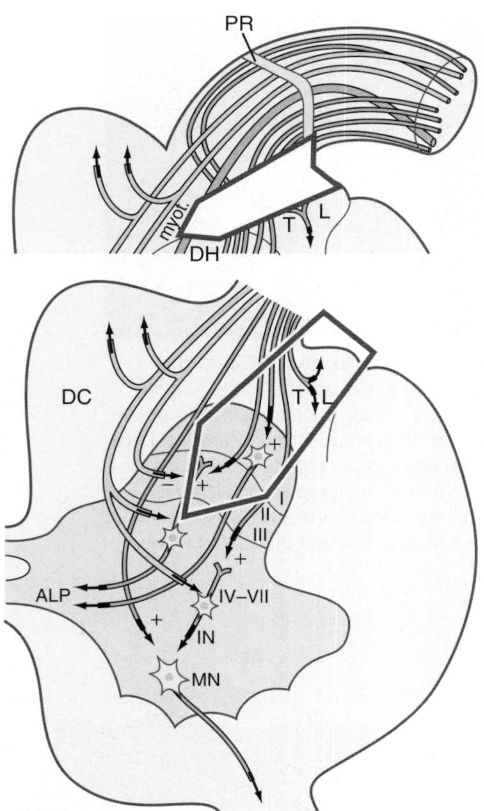

Figure 103-14. Schematic representation of the dorsal root entry zone (DREZ) and the target of microsurgical DREZotomy. *Top*, Each rootlet can be divided (because of the transition of its glial support) into a peripheral and a central segment. The transition between the two segments is at the pial ring (PR), which is located approximately 1 mm from the location where the rootlet penetrates into the dorsolateral sulcus. Peripherally, the fibers are mixed together. As they approach the PR, the fine fibers (considered nociceptive) are more toward the rootlet surfaces. In the central segment, they group in the ventrolateral portion of the DREZ and enter the dorsal horn (DH) through the tract of Lissauer (TL). The large myotatic fibers (myot) are situated in the middle of the DREZ, whereas the large fibers going to the dorsal column are located dorsomedially.[23] *Bottom*, Schematic data on the DH circuitry. Note the monosynaptic excitatory arc reflex of the myotatic fibers, the inhibitory influence on a DH cell and an interneuron (IN) of the collaterals of the large myelinated fibers, the fine-fiber excitatory input onto DH cells and the IN. Note the origins of the anterolateral pathways (ALP) in layer I and layers IV to VII and the projection of the IN onto the motor neuron (MN). DC, dorsal column. The Rexed laminae are marked I to VI. Microsurgical DREZotomy *(arrowheads)* interrupts most of the fine and myotatic fibers and enters the medial (excitatory) portion of the TL and the apex of the dorsal horn. This should preserve most of the presynaptic fibers, going to the dorsal column and their recurrent collaterals, the lateral (inhibitory) portion of the TL. *(From Sindou M. Neurosurgical management of disabling spasticity. In: Spetzler RF, ed.* Operative Techniques in Neurosurgery. *Vol 7. Philadelphia: Saunders; 2004:95-174.)*

spasticity in children with cerebral palsy, including botulinum toxin injections, intrathecal baclofen, dorsal rhizotomies, and selective neurotomies. These treatments can be used in isolation or in combination with orthopedic surgery. Selection of the correct treatment is difficult in children because they are still developing and their needs may change as they grow. To formulate a treatment plan one must project into the future by extrapolating the extent and severity of musculoskeletal contractures and their harmful consequences as well as the positive effects of spontaneous psychomotor development.

The first step in the evaluation process is to observe the child clinically to understand the child's function and disability. The second step is to measure range of motion to detect contractures that will not respond to neurosurgical treatment. The third step is to quantify the spasticity by using scales. The final step is to grade the child on the Gross Motor Function Measure and to observe the evolution of gross motor function with time (Fig. 103-18).

Several effective neurosurgical treatments for spasticity can be used in children with cerebral palsy. For diffuse spasticity of the lower limbs, dorsal rhizotomy or intrathecal baclofen administration may be considered. Dorsal rhizotomy is generally preferred before the age of 6 years because the size of the implanted pump poses an obstacle in young children. Dorsal rhizotomy is proposed when definitive action targeted to certain muscle groups is preferred.[5,39] For focal spasticity, botulinum toxin injection permits delaying surgery until the child is old enough to undergo selective neurotomy.

Spasticity in the Lower Limb

If the spasticity is focal and involves the gastrocnemius and soleus muscles, botulinum toxin can be proposed as a complement to physiotherapy and casting. This approach enables neurosurgical treatment to be delayed until the child reaches an age appropriate for selective tibial neurotomy. When spasticity is localized to the adductors, botulinum toxin is not always sufficient to avoid obturator neurotomy, which may be necessary to prevent hip dislocation.

Spasticity in the Upper Limb

For upper extremity spasticity, botulinum toxin injections are an effective primary treatment. The muscles of the upper limbs are small, so even if quite a few must be injected, the maximal allowable dose is rarely a limiting factor, as it may be in the legs. These injections can be considered as a definitive treatment and can be repeated every 6 or 12 months as needed. However, the multiple visits required are a constraint. Furthermore, immunoresistance can develop and decrease the effectiveness of the treatment with time. An additional advantage of botulinum toxin injections is that they simulate the outcome of selective neurotomy, thereby allowing the patient and family to appreciate the benefit that can be achieved with ablation.

If spasticity involves the shoulder, elbow, wrist, and fingers, multiple neurotomies or cervical MDT may be indicated. Dystonia can be favorably influenced if cervical MDT is performed deeply into ventral horn of corresponding segmental levels.

CONCLUSION

Because the characteristics and functional consequences of spasticity differ from patient to patient, the general rule is to tailor individual treatments. The goals are to decrease "harmful spasticity," respect "useful spasticity," preserve residual motor-sensory functions, reveal masked capabilities, and improve functional ability. Because of its complexity, neurosurgical management of spasticity requires a multidisciplinary approach.

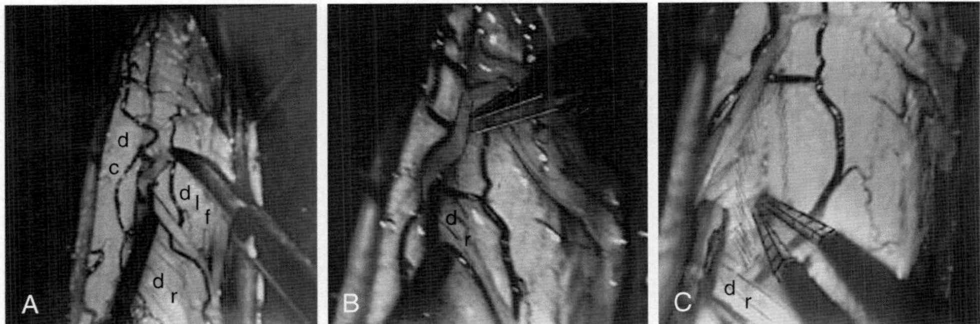

Figure 103-15. Technique for microsurgical incision of the dorsal root entry zone (DREZ) at the cervical level. The right dorsolateral aspect of the cervical cord is exposed at C6. **A,** The rootlets of the selected dorsal root (dr) are displaced dorsally and medially with a hook or a microsuction device to obtain access to the ventrolateral aspect of the DREZ in the dorsolateral sulcus. With microscissors, the arachnoid adhesions are cut between the cord and the dorsal rootlets. dc, dorsal cord; dlf, dorsolateral funiculus. **B,** After coagulation of the tiny pial vessels exclusively, an incision 2 mm in depth directed 35 degrees ventrally and medially is made with a microknife in the lateral border of the dorsolateral sulcus. **C,** Microcoagulation is then performed down to the apex of the dorsal horn with sharp graduated bipolar microforceps.

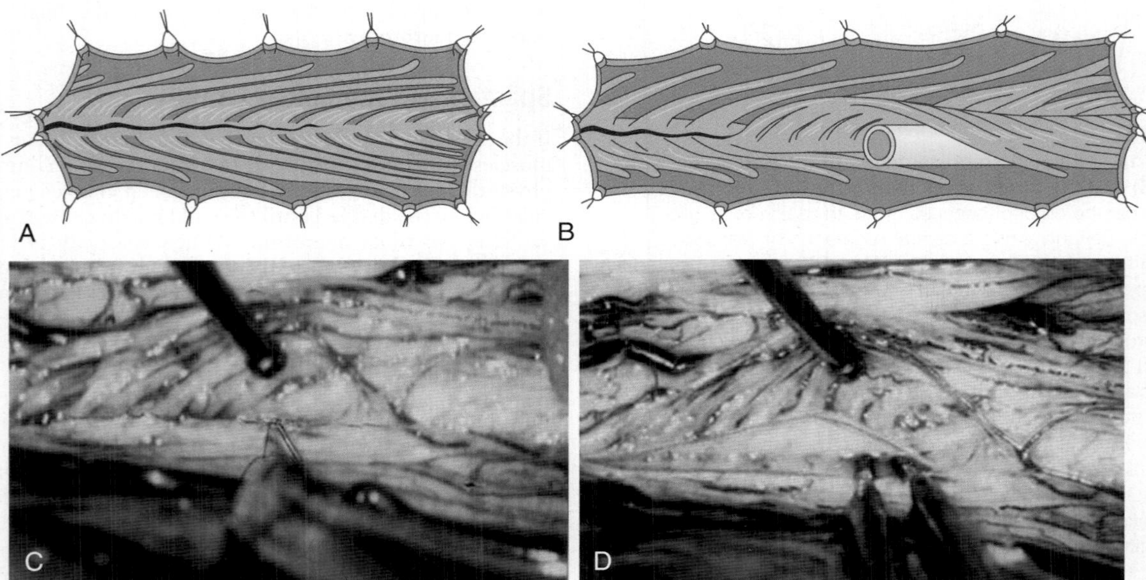

Figure 103-16. Techniques for microsurgical incision of the dorsal root entry zone (DREZ) at the lumbosacral level. A, Exposure of the conus medullaris through laminectomy from T11 to L1. **B,** For access to the dorsolateral sulcus, the dorsal rootlets of the selected roots are displaced dorsally and medially to obtain proper access to the ventrolateral aspect of the DREZ. **C,** The selected dorsal roots are retracted dorsomedially and held with a (specially designed) ball-tipped microsuction device, used as a small hook, to gain access to the ventrolateral part of the DREZ. After division of the fine arachnoidal filaments holding the rootlets and pia mater together with curved sharp microscissors (not shown), the main arteries running along the dorsolateral sulcus are dissected and preserved, whereas the smaller ones are coagulated with sharp bipolar microforceps (not shown). A continuous incision is then made with a microknife, a small piece of razor blade inserted within the striated jaws of a curved razor blade holder. Usually, the cut is made at a 45-degree angle to a depth of 2 mm. **D,** The surgical lesion is completed by performing microcoagulation at low intensity under direct magnified vision inside the dorsolateral sulcomyelotomy down to the apex of the dorsal horn. The microcoagulation is performed all along the segments of the cord selected for treatment by means of a special sharp bipolar forceps that is insulated except for 5 mm at the tip and graduated every millimeter.

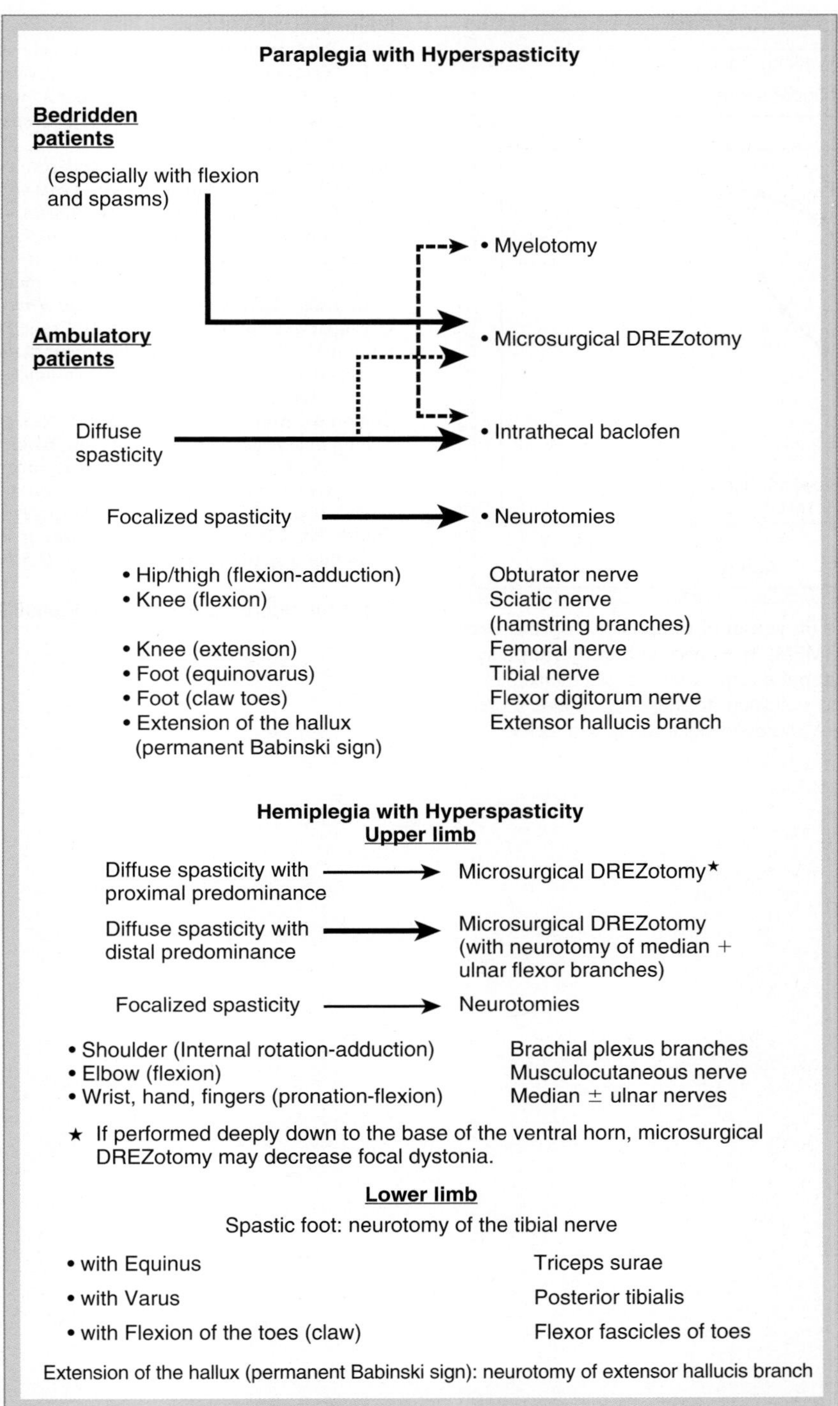

Figure 103-17. Algorithms for treating disabling hyperspasticity in paraplegic *(top),* and hemiplegic (*middle* and *bottom*) adult patients.

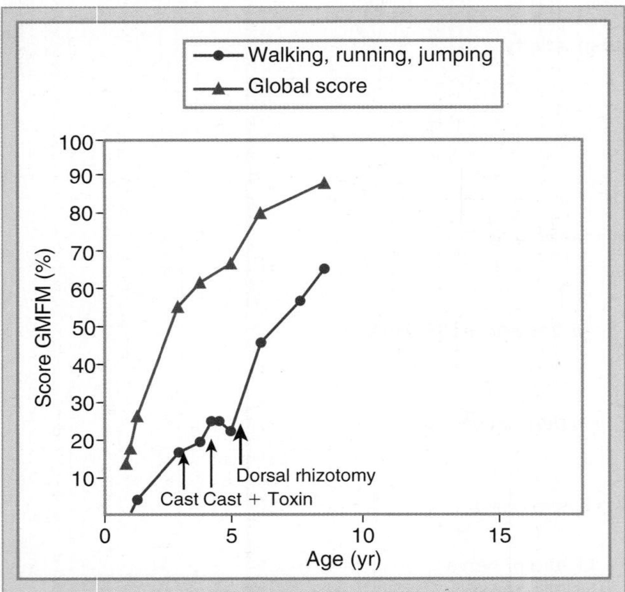

Figure 103-18. Time course (in years) of dimensions on the Gross Motor Function Measure (GMFM) in a child with cerebral palsy: walking/running/jumping, global score. Note that dorsal rhizotomy was indicated after a cast and botulinum toxin injections plus a cast failed. Also note that the score improved significantly after dorsal rhizotomy was performed.

SUGGESTED READINGS

Decq P, Mertens P. Société de Neurochirurgie de la Langue Française. La Neurochirurgie de la Spasticité. *Neurochirurgie*. 2003;49:135-416.

Fasano VA, Barolat-Romana G, Ivaldi A, et al. La radicotomie postérieure fonctionnelle dans le traitement de la spasticité cérébrale. *Neurochirurgie*. 1976;22:23-34.

Foerster O. On the indications and results of the excision of posterior spinal nerve roots in men. *Surg Gynecol Obstet*. 1913;16:463-474.

Gros C. Spasticity—Clinical classification and surgical treatment. In: Krayenbühl H, ed. *Advances and Technical Standards in Neurosurgery*. Vol 6. Vienna, New York: Springer; 1979:55-97.

Mertens P, Sindou M. Surgical management of spasticity. In: Barnes MP, Johnson GR, eds. *Clinical Management of Spasticity*. Cambridge, England: Cambridge University Press; 2001:239-265.

Sindou M. Neurosurgical management of disabling spasticity. In: Spetzler RF, ed. *Operative Techniques in Neurosurgery*. Vol 7. Philadelphia: Saunders; 2004:95-174.

Sindou M, Abbott A, Keravel Y, eds. *Neurosurgery for Spasticity: A Multidisciplinary Approach*. Vienna, New York: Springer Verlag; 1991.

Sindou M, Georgoulis G, Mertens P. Surgery in dorsal root entry zone. In: *Neurosurgical Treatment for Spasticity—A Practical Guide for Children and Adults*. Vienna, New York: Springer; 2014:143-145.

Sindou M, Mertens P. Decision-making for neurological treatment of disabling spasticity in adults. *Oper Tech Neurosurg*. 2004;7:113-118.

See a full reference list on ExpertConsult.com 

104 Management of Spasticity by Central Nervous System Infusion Techniques

Richard Deren Penn and Daniel M. Corcos

Chronic intrathecal infusion of baclofen has been extremely successful in the treatment of spasticity.[1,2] Because baclofen does not cure spasticity, most treated patients need to take baclofen intrathecally for life. This long-term commitment to treatment is similar to maintaining shunt function in patients with hydrocephalus and may be equally rewarding or frustrating. To make proper use of this powerful tool, neurosurgeons need to understand the pharmacologic properties and distribution of intrathecal baclofen and how pumps are used to infuse the drug. Proper selection of patients requires an understanding of the physiologic features of spasticity and its clinical manifestations. Other neurosurgical methods for reducing spasticity are considered elsewhere; in particular, dorsal rhizotomy for spastic cerebral palsy in children is discussed in Chapter 243.

DEFINITION OF SPASTICITY

Spasticity is a term that refers to a wide variety of motor problems and has numerous associated definitions.[3,4] It has been used to connote difficulty with coordinated movements and with spasms, rigidity, abnormal primitive reflexes, and hyperactive reflexes. Researchers studying spasticity tend to stress definitions that emphasize abnormal reflex responses, whereas clinicians tend to stress more global definitions, primarily related to impairment of movement. To further complicate the issue, many clinical syndromes associated with spasticity are caused by injuries at multiple sites in the neuraxis, and the pathologic mechanisms producing motor dysfunction are equally varied.

The narrow physiologic definition of spasticity is "a motor disorder characterized by a velocity-dependent increase in tonic stretch reflexes (i.e., muscle tone) with exaggerated tendon jerks, resulting from hyperexcitability of the stretch reflex, as one component of the upper motoneuron syndrome."[5] This velocity-dependent increase differentiates spasticity from other, non–velocity-dependent forms of rigidity that can be caused by contractures, dystonias, or Parkinson's disease. In addition to hyperactive reflexes, spasticity can be associated with various signs and symptoms designated "positive" or "negative"[6]: positive signs are produced by overactivity (i.e., disinhibition) of certain pathways as a result of injury to a specific part of the motor system; negative signs are caused by lack of function of the injured area. In spasticity, an increase in deep tendon reflexes and resistance to passive stretch of the limb are positive signs. Negative signs are weakness and loss of dexterity. It is the negative signs that usually create the clinically significant problems that are disabling for the patient. Increased muscle tone, clonus, and hyperactive reflexes occasionally interfere with initiation and smooth completion of a movement.[7] Spasms, although often associated with hyperactive reflexes, are not a necessary concomitant of hyperreflexia and should be considered separately.

A broader and more insightful definition of spasticity emphasizes the movement disorder associated with the velocity-dependent resistance and reflex hyperexcitability, not simply its clinical signs.[8] As has been pointed out by many investigators, the signs are not well correlated with the patient's inability to perform voluntary movements. Decreasing tone and exaggerated reflexes produced by medications or surgery do not necessarily mean better function. A corollary of this broad view is that the secondary consequences of spasticity that result from changes in muscles and joints have to be treated as well as the initial central nervous system causes.[4]

PHYSIOLOGIC BASIS OF SPASTICITY

The final common pathway to the muscle is the alpha motoneuron. Many mechanisms influence the output of the alpha motoneuron and may therefore exaggerate this neuron's response to stretch. The muscles contain receptors called *spindles*, which are diagrammed in the center portion of Figure 104-1. A spindle is made up of intrafusal fibers attached to primary sensory endings. The primary sensory endings, which are extensions of the large, myelinated group Ia afferents, attach at the noncontractile equatorial region of the intrafusal fibers. The spindle organs are attached at both ends of the muscle mass and consist of extrafusal fibers. Because the spindles are attached in this way, they undergo the same changes in length as the overall muscle, and they "monitor" changes in muscle length. The spindles themselves are under control of the fusimotor efferents (i.e., gamma motoneuron system).

If the stretch reflex operated only in conjunction with the alpha motoneuron, voluntary movements would be difficult to make because a change in alpha motoneuron activity would cause contraction of the extrafusal fibers, which would shorten the muscle; as the muscle shortened, the intrafusal fibers of the muscle would slacken and would not monitor changes in length. Gamma motoneuron activity prevents this problem by shortening the intrafusal fibers, which assists movement by increasing activation of alpha motoneurons through type Ia feedback. Gamma motoneuron activity also increases reciprocal inhibition of the antagonist muscle.

When a muscle is stretched, it contracts in an attempt to regain its original length. This response can be broken down into five events, four of which are diagrammed in Figure 104-1:

1. Sensory impulses are generated as a result of stretching of muscle spindles.
2. The afferent volley ascends to the spinal cord.
3. It excites discharge of the alpha motoneurons of the same muscle.
4. It inhibits the motoneuron pools of antagonistic muscles through a disynaptic pathway.
5. It facilitates, probably monosynaptically, the motoneurons of synergistic pools (not shown in Fig. 104-1).[9]

Mechanisms Underlying Reflex Function

To understand how changes in these mechanisms lead to spasticity, the events that occur when a muscle is stretched must be traced. In a closed-loop system, it is impossible to identify the beginning and end of a sequence of events. For simplicity of presentation, the various mechanisms are discussed in the following order: Ia monosynaptic connection, Ia excitatory polysynaptic pathways, reciprocal Ia inhibition, group II pathways, decreased recurrent inhibition, alpha motoneuron hyperexcitability, gamma

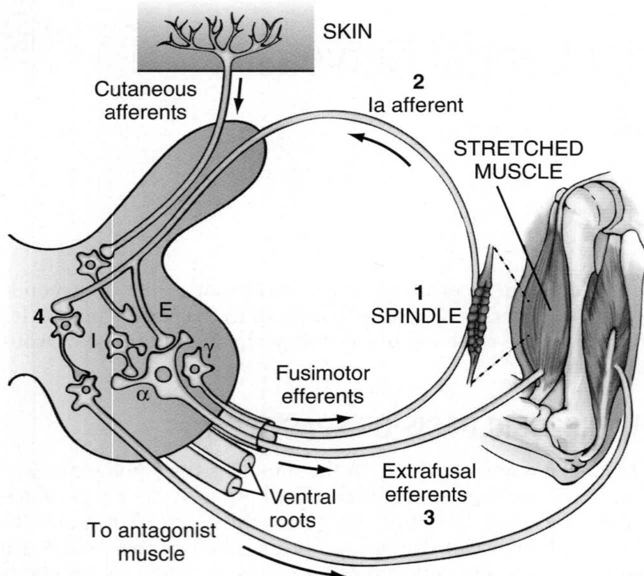

Figure 104-1. Structures involved in the control of movement at the spinal and peripheral levels. The text describes the sequence of events (1 through 3) that occurs in the stretch reflex arc. α, alpha motoneuron; γ, gamma motoneuron; E, excitatory presynaptic ending; I, inhibitory interneuron.

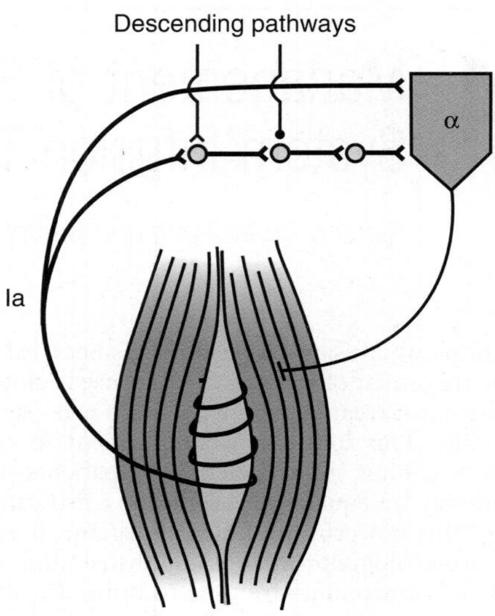

Figure 104-2. In addition to monosynaptic Ia excitatory pathways, polysynaptic pathways also converge on the alpha motoneuron (α). Interneurons *(shaded circles)* interposed in these pathways are controlled by descending pathways. Excitatory synapses are represented as *angle signs* and inhibitory synapses as a *dot*. *(Redrawn from Pierrot-Deseilligny E. Pathophysiology of spasticity.* Triangle. *1983;22:165-174.)*

motoneuron hyperactivity, and decreased group Ib inhibition. Pierrot-Deseilligny,[10,11] Pierrot-Deseilligny and Mazieres,[12] and Sehgal and McGuire[13] discussed these mechanisms in detail. Sehgal and McGuire also provided a detailed explanation of the different electrophysiologic testing procedures that are used to deduce which mechanisms are underlying the spasticity.[13]

Ia Monosynaptic Connection

When a muscle is stretched, the Ia afferent neuron transmits excitatory messages from its receptor, the muscle spindle, to the alpha motoneuron of the same muscle by means of a monosynaptic connection. It has been suggested that Ia discharge is normally reduced by presynaptic inhibition and that reduced levels of presynaptic inhibition could lead to an increase in the stretch reflex.[12] For example, Calancie and colleagues[14] argued that presynaptic inhibition is enhanced in patients in the acute stage of spinal cord injury but is reduced in the chronic stage. This reduction in presynaptic inhibition could give rise to an increased reflex response. There is also evidence of a decrease in presynaptic inhibition in paraplegic patients but not in hemiplegic patients.[15]

Ia Excitatory Polysynaptic Pathways

The alpha motoneuron can also be affected by the Ia excitatory polysynaptic pathway (Fig. 104-2).[16] This can be shown by producing vibration-induced activity in group Ia fibers to generate tonic contraction of the vibrated muscle through Ia excitatory polysynaptic pathways; this is the tonic vibration reflex. This reflex can be increased or decreased, or both, in spastic patients.[17] Facilitation of this pathway increases stretch reflexes.

Reciprocal Ia Inhibition

When a muscle is stretched, the reflex evoked in that muscle is normally accompanied by inhibition of the opposing muscle. This finding of reciprocal inhibition has had a pervasive influence on the understanding of movement control.[18] It has been assumed that as a movement is made, stretch-related activation in the antagonist muscle is suppressed by reciprocal inhibition. Lack of reciprocal inhibition can lead to unwanted activation of the antagonist muscle and impede movement. The Ia inhibitory interneuron receives excitatory synaptic input from numerous descending pathways, including the corticospinal tract.[19] Input from the descending tracts is combined with output from the Ia afferents of the contracting agonist muscle.[20] If the Ia interneuron does not receive input from the corticospinal tract, reciprocal inhibition may become ineffective, a phenomenon observed in some spastic patients.[21]

Group II Pathways

Group II endings (i.e., secondary endings), like group Ia endings, are located on intrafusal muscle fibers and are most sensitive to dynamic stretch. Their role in spasticity is not well understood.

Decreased Recurrent Inhibition

Motor axons give off recurrent collaterals that activate Renshaw cells, which in turn inhibit alpha motoneurons,[10] thereby creating a recurrent inhibitory circuit. Renshaw cells are excited or inhibited by supraspinal control. At rest, recurrent inhibition has complicated manifestations.[22] In about 40% of spastic patients tested, there is no evidence of abnormal recurrent inhibition at rest. In patients with hemiplegia (most often from stroke) and in patients with spinal cord injury (most often from trauma), recurrent inhibition increases at rest. In contrast, patients with progressive paraparesis caused by hereditary spastic paraparesis or amyotrophic lateral sclerosis exhibit reduced recurrent inhibition.

During active movements in spastic patients, an increased reflex response may be caused by lack of inhibition of Renshaw cells. In healthy subjects, Renshaw cells are inhibited, which in turn inhibits the Ia inhibitory interneuron directed to the antagonist motoneuron. This allows reciprocal inhibition to function to suppress a stretch reflex in the antagonist muscles.[23]

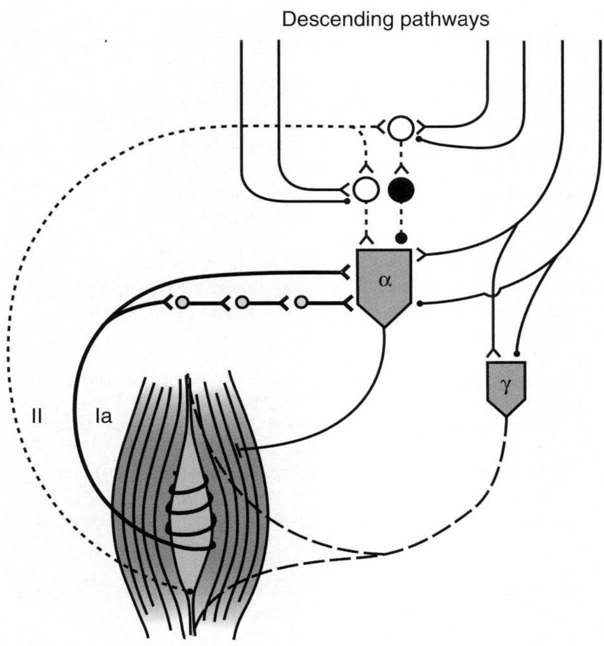

Figure 104-3. Muscle spindle afferent fibers and fusimotor innervation. Group Ia nerve pathways are described in Figure 104-2. Two pathways *(dotted lines)* from group II afferent nerve fibers (II) to homonymous motoneurons are represented: excitatory synapses are represented by *angle signs;* inhibitory synapses, by *small filled circles.* Excitatory interneurons are represented by *open circles;* inhibitory interneurons, by *filled circles.* Notice that alpha (α) and gamma (γ) motoneurons are controlled by descending pathways. *(Redrawn from Pierrot-Deseilligny E. Pathophysiology of spasticity.* Triangle. *1983;22:165-174.)*

Lack of descending control of Renshaw cells leads to impairment of voluntary movements and prevents modulation of control of the antagonist muscle, as has been shown by Katz and Pierrot-Deseilligny.[24]

Alpha Motoneuron Hyperexcitability

The alpha motoneuron receives excitatory input from the segmental and descending pathways. Lesions at numerous levels of the central nervous system may upset the delicate balance between excitatory and inhibitory input that influences the alpha motoneuron. There may also be a change in the intrinsic properties of motoneurons in spasticity.[11] However, the influence of alpha motoneuron hyperexcitability is impossible to assess in humans because it requires knowledge of the firing level of motoneurons deprived of any sensory input.[10] There is no evidence for or against the involvement of alpha motoneuron hyperexcitability in spasticity, although Noth[25] argued that it does play a role.

Gamma Motoneuron Hyperactivity

The gamma motoneuron system modulates the length of the intrafusal fibers and is therefore responsible for establishing the firing thresholds for group Ia and group II neurons (Fig. 104-3). Incorrect threshold settings for the afferent neurons could lead to a hyperactive response. Evidence to support gamma motoneuron hyperactivity is derived from data from research with decerebrate cats, from selective blockade of the fusimotor system with local anesthetics, from the Jendrassik maneuver, and from comparison of the tendon jerk reflex and the H-reflex. Selective blockade of the fusimotor system has been used clinically in spastic patients. Injection of dilute procaine into the motor points of spastic and rigid muscles decreases muscle tone.[26] This effect seems to support the view that spasticity is related to an imbalanced fusimotor system in that stretch reflexes are abolished as a result of block of the gamma motoneuron system but voluntary muscle power is maintained by the output of unaffected larger alpha motoneurons. However, at a different site, intrathecal and epidural injections of local anesthetic did not reveal a link between increased fusimotor activity and spasticity.[27] The strongest evidence against the gamma motoneuron hyperactivity hypothesis is the finding that the discharge rate of primary spindle endings is the same in spastic and normal individuals.[28] Increased gamma motoneuron activity should lead to increased sensitivity of the discharge rate of primary spindle endings in spastic patients. Although the gamma motoneuron hyperactivity hypothesis has been influential, the evidence to support it is indirect, inconclusive, and circumstantial.[29]

Decreased Ib Inhibition

Golgi tendon organs are sensitive to stretch because they lie in series with the muscle. On muscle stretch, impulses from group Ib fibers are transmitted to homonymous motoneuron pools and heteronymous pools acting synergistically to inhibit stretch.[30] Lack of inhibition can result in an increased response to stretch and thereby contribute to spasticity. This was demonstrated by Delwaide and Oliver,[31] who showed that Ib inhibition was markedly reduced in spastic patients.

Summary of Mechanisms

Contributions of the different spinal mechanisms to hyperreflexia are summarized in Table 104-1.[32-37] The information in this table should be treated with caution because of the considerable variability both in the tests used and in the types of spasticity investigated in the different studies. The column "Mechanism" lists the putative mechanism by which hyperreflexia could occur. The evidence indicates strongly that decreased presynaptic inhibition, decreased inhibition from supraspinal centers, and decreased Golgi tendon organ inhibition can each play a role in hyperreflexia. However, the importance of each mechanism may vary with the type of injury that causes hyperreflexia. It is strikingly clear that different causes of spasticity can have opposing effects on the patterns of inhibition and excitation observed in various spinal pathways.

Why Do Spinal Circuits Malfunction?

There are two reasons why the spinal circuits can malfunction: abnormal descending control and local changes at the spinal level.

Abnormal Descending Control

One way to consider the diminished motor control in patients with spasticity is from a developmental perspective.[38,39] It is well known that babies demonstrate a mass of uncontrolled reflexes. Before a baby can stand, the flexor reflexes in the lower limbs must be inhibited and the extensor reflexes enhanced to brace the limbs against gravity; this is a function of the vestibulospinal and facilitatory reticulospinal tracts. After the child has learned how to stand, the next development is walking. For the child to walk, the extensor pattern of reflex standing in the lower limbs must be inhibited, and the flexor synergy of the lower limbs must be integrated into a walking pattern. This requires involvement of the motor cortex to inhibit extensor activity and facilitate flexor activity.

TABLE 104-1 Spinal Mechanisms of Hyperreflexia

Neurons	Mechanism	Increase/ Decrease	Involvement in Hyperreflexia	Reference
Group Ia monosynaptic connection	Presynaptic inhibition	Decrease	Yes (in chronic spinal cord injury)	Calancie et al., 1993[14]
		Increase	No (in acute spinal cord injury)	Calancie et al., 1993[14]
		No change	No (in hemiplegia)	Faist et al., 1994[15]
		Decrease	No (in paraplegia)	Faist et al., 1994[15]
Group Ia excitatory motoneuron	Excitation	Increase	Possibly	Hagbarth, 1973[17]
Group Ia reciprocal inhibitory motoneuron	Inhibition	Decreased	Possibly (in multiple sclerosis)	Crone et al., 1994[32]
	Inhibition	Increased	Possibly (in spinal cord injury)	Ashby and Wiens, 1989[33]
	Inhibition	(Released from inhibition)	Possibly (capsular hemiplegia during voluntary movement)	Yanagisawa et al., 1976[21]
Group II	Inhibition (decreased)		No evidence	
Renshaw cells	Recurrent inhibition (at rest)	Increased	No (in hemiplegia)	Katz and Pierrot-Deseilligny, 1982[24]
		Increased	No (in spinal cord injury, trauma)	Shefner et al., 1992[34]
		Decreased	Possibly (in hereditary spastic paraparesis)	Mazzocchio and Rossi, 1997[35]
		Decreased	Possibly (in amyotrophic lateral sclerosis)	Raynor and Shefner, 1994[36]
	Recurrent inhibition (movement; decrease in supraspinal control)	Decreased	Yes	Katz and Pierrot-Deseilligny, 1982[24]
Alpha motoneuron	Hyperexcitability	Unknown	Possibly; no evidence	See Katz and Rymer, 1989,[37] for discussion
Gamma motoneuron	Gamma motoneuron hyperactivity	Unknown	No evidence	Burke, 1983[29]
Golgi tendon organ group Ib inhibition	Inhibition	(Released from inhibition)	Yes (in hemiplegia from stroke)	Delwaide and Oliver, 1988[31]

As the child matures, the pyramidal tract exerts control over the direct connections to the anterior horn cells, in conjunction with the basal ganglia, cerebellum, and brainstem. If the motor cortex or its projections are damaged, the brainstem exerts primary control. If the brainstem assumes complete control, a decorticate posture—flexion of the upper limbs and extension of the lower limbs—develops. In cerebral spasticity, the stretch reflexes in the upper limb flexors and lower limb extensors are enhanced. If the spinal cord is damaged, even brainstem control is disrupted, so that flexor reflexes and stretch reflexes are released from inhibition. This can lead to any or all of the following physical signs[39]:

1. Disinhibition of the stretch reflex
   - Increased muscle tone
   - Exaggerated tendon jerks (i.e., phasic stretch reflexes)
   - Radiation of phasic stretch reflexes in response to percussion
   - Clonus
2. Disinhibition of flexor reflexes (in the lower limbs)
   - Clasp-knife phenomenon
   - Flexor spasms
   - Extensor plantar response (i.e., Babinski's phenomenon)
3. Withdrawal of pyramidal facilitation
   - Weakness of extensor and abductor muscles in the upper limbs
   - Weakness of flexor muscles in the lower limbs

Lack of descending control is the initial cause of the hyperexcitability of the stretch reflex, which is the cardinal sign of spasticity. Any lesion that affects upper motoneurons can cause spasticity. However, there are numerous factors to consider in establishing the effect of such a lesion (e.g., age of patient, precise location of the lesion, length of time since the lesion occurred, cause of the lesion). These lesions upset the delicate balance between excitation and inhibition in the spinal cord.

Transection of the spinal cord results acutely in spinal shock, abolition of reflexes, and muscle flaccidity.[40] Slowly, over a period of weeks, muscle tone and reflex activity reappear and then become excessive. These increases may be caused by loss of descending control, but this loss cannot explain the reflex exaggeration over time. The best explanation is that the spinal cord circuitry is reorganized and levels of presynaptic inhibition are altered.[14] Ashby and McCrea[41] reviewed the neurophysiologic processes of spinal spasticity in detail.

Local Changes at the Spinal Level

Most evidence for plastic changes at the spinal level is based on experience with spinal cord hemisection.[42,43] Changes in the spinal cord may be structural or functional, or both. Collateral sprouting of peripheral afferents has been shown to occur. In a hemisected spinal cord, a greater number of dorsal root fibers are eventually found on the hemisected side than on the intact side. Group Ia fibers may eventually constitute 10% of the synapses on motoneurons instead of the normal 1%, which may account for exaggerated tendon reflexes.[40]

There is evidence that changes can occur in the spinal circuitry of humans who have suffered perinatal injuries to the immature nervous system.[44-46] In adults who suffered birth-onset injuries, rapid stretch of the soleus muscle elicits a reflex in the soleus and tibialis anterior muscles. This phenomenon of reciprocal excitation is in marked contrast to the normal occurrence of reciprocal inhibition in the nonstretched muscle, which suggests that some disorders (e.g., cerebral palsy) may be characterized by abnormal spinal cord circuitry and brain damage.

Changes in Muscle Fiber and Connective Tissue

Neural mechanisms initiate spasticity. However, these altered neural mechanisms lead to numerous secondary changes in muscle that may be partially responsible for the symptoms of spasticity. The mechanical properties of muscles and joints in spastic limbs can change in several ways.[47] The degree of abnormality of the muscles of children with cerebral palsy depends on which muscle groups are involved.[48] Examples have been found of atrophy, hypertrophy, and myopathy. During long-term spastic hemiplegia in human patients, some motor units develop increased fatigability and prolonged twitch-contraction times, which causes changes in the dynamic properties of muscle.[49] Results of several studies on locomotion and interlimb coordination have suggested that when hypertonia is present without concomitant changes on electromyography, the hypertonia must be caused by altered muscle properties.[50-56] For example, histochemical and morphometric analyses of the spastic muscle of four individuals revealed increased atrophy of muscle fibers (especially type II) and a predominance of type I fibers.[57]

In some patients, another likely explanation for spastic hypertonia is that some muscle fibers are replaced by connective tissue. In the more severely atrophic muscles, an increase in the amount of perimysial-endomysial connective and interstitial tissue and an increase in the number of internal nuclei have been found.[48] In summarizing the findings in many studies, Dietz and Sinkjaer[58] argued that the degree of hyperreflexia found in patients is not correlated with functional loss and that treatment of spasticity should be directed at improving movement and not simply decreasing overactive reflexes. Dietz and Sinkjaer also pointed out that changes in muscles are important in producing rigidity and that abnormal spinal circuits interfere with voluntary movements and are a major cause of disability in spastic patients.

MEASUREMENT OF SPASTICITY

Methods of evaluating and measuring spasticity can be divided into three categories: clinical evaluation, in which limbs are manipulated by a clinician and the patient is observed making movements; passive quantifiable evaluation, in which limbs are moved mechanically or different components of the reflex pathway are electrically stimulated; and active quantifiable evaluation, in which movements are generated by the patient.

Clinical Evaluation

In clinical assessment, spasticity is graded qualitatively. Muscle response to stretch is judged by the deep tendon reflexes elicited by a reflex hammer and by the spread of the response to other muscle groups. Symmetry of response is more important than the strength of the response, and even a few beats of clonus in both ankles may be normal. Resistance to passive stretch can be a gauge of spasticity but often reflects other problems, such as contractures or ankylosis of the joint being tested. Spasticity may vary because of factors such as fatigue and emotional stress. Normal individuals may even experience sustained clonus under these conditions.[59] Position (i.e., vestibular input) dramatically changes spasticity. For example, patients with partial cord injuries may demonstrate much less resistance when tested in the upright position or in a wheelchair than when supine. Voluntary movement is assessed through analysis of gait and of the ability to generate rapid successive movements.

To provide a simple grading system that would be useful for repeated clinical examinations, Ashworth[60] devised the scale on which Table 104-2 is based. A graded scale is appropriate because the response of a muscle to stretch can vary considerably in a normal individual, and a spastic patient's response is increased. In general, the categories are distinct enough that changes in spasticity can be judged accurately during repeated examinations. However, one problem with the scale is that the scores of many patients cluster in the middle. Thus it is worth considering the modified Ashworth scale, which is an attempt to account for this problem by means of an extra scoring category.[61] Another problem with the original scale is that factors that affect the response of a muscle to stretch are not differentiated (i.e., reflex abnormalities versus contractures). Numerous other outcome measures can be used to facilitate effective management of spasticity and were summarized by Pierson.[62] Objective tests should be used whenever possible because placebo effects have been noted in up to 50% of patients.[63]

TABLE 104-2 Assessment of Spasticity (Modified Ashworth Scale)

Score*	Characteristic
1	No increase in tone
2	Slight increase in tone; a "catch" occurs when the affected part is moved in flexion and extension
3	More marked increase in tone but affected parts easily flexed
4	Considerable increase in tone; passive movement difficult
5	Affected parts rigid in flexion or extension

*The original Ashworth scale was scored on a scale of 1 to 4.

Passive Quantifiable Evaluations

A normal limb can be extended passively or flexed passively without demonstrating resistance. This is not the case for a spastic limb. After movement of a spastic limb has been initiated, the following characteristics can be recognized: resistance that increases gradually through the movement, resistance that may suddenly subside as the limits of range of motion are reached (i.e., clasp-knife phenomenon), resistance that is proportional to the velocity of stretch, and a stretch reflex that is dependent on position.[64]

Quantitative measures of spasticity must record the velocity of the stretch, the resistance to stretch, and, if possible, the electromyographic response of the stretched muscle. Several such tests have been developed.[65-68] One of the simplest evaluations appropriate for clinical use is a drop test[69]: the patient is placed supine; the patient's leg is lifted to a horizontal position, and then it is allowed to fall freely as the knee angle and quadriceps response are recorded. A wide variety of electrophysiologic tests can be used to explore the neurophysiologic mechanisms that underlie spasticity. Sehgal and McGuire[13] provided a comprehensive explanation of these tests. Reflexes are more easily measurable than activities of daily living but are less representative of changes in general motor performance.[70] It is important to bridge this gap with the use of isokinetic measurements, gait studies, and studies of general movements.

Active Quantifiable Evaluations

Perhaps the most interesting question concerning the signs of spasticity is whether they have any relation to the decrease in movement or poor coordination experienced by many patients with this disorder. The signs of spasticity might interfere with voluntary movement in a direct or an indirect way. Deficits in the ability to generate movements have been analyzed for unidirectional or reciprocal movements, as well as the complex movements of gait.[52,71-73] Some investigators have found no direct correlation between the increased reflexes and movement deficits,[58,73] and others have shown that reflexes in patients with mild spasticity are suppressed during voluntary movement.[74] Also, the abolition of hyperactive stretch reflexes does not necessarily improve motor performance.[3,27,75] However, direct evidence showing the effect of reflex involvement in movement impairment has also been observed.[6,72,76,77] For example, Boorman and colleagues[78,79] found loss of supraspinal control over spinal inhibitory mechanisms during cycling movements in patients with spinal cord injury. Variability in the tests used and in the pathologic processes that produce spasticity probably account for these disparate conclusions.

In patients with spasticity associated with paraplegia, the full range of movement is available in the upper limbs, but spasms and contractures in the lower limbs can indirectly make such movements very unpleasant or impossible. The spasms and contractures can also severely limit the ability of affected individuals to bend or stretch during everyday reaching movements, such as tying shoelaces. Movements of the upper limbs indirectly stretch the muscles of the lower limbs and trigger the spasms or contractures. Any treatment that can effectively reduce the frequency or severity of these events indirectly influences the individual's ability to move.

Measurement of Spasms

Many lesions of the central nervous system produce both spasms and spasticity. Such lesions are often in the spinal cord and cause a release of inhibition that results in exaggeration of the flexor reflex. Spasms are often associated with pain, can compromise standing and sitting, and may facilitate the development of contractures. One of the few objective methods for documenting spasms involves placing electrodes over the ankle flexors and using a rectifier circuit to create an envelope of electromyographic activity that is easy to quantify visually or electronically.[80]

TREATMENT OF SPASTICITY

The general goal of therapy is to improve neurological function and decrease the effects of spasticity. However, the hyperexcitability of the motoneuron has numerous causes and does not necessarily relate to disability. Consequently, each patient's condition must be treated individually. In some patients, limb rigidity leads to poorly coordinated walking, and clonus may limit the speed of movement. In other patients, neither of these aspects of spasticity may be significant, and only associated spasms or motor weakness may cause problems.

Depending on the pathophysiologic process, various measures can be taken to reduce motoneuron hyperexcitability. Alterations in one or more of the pathways and connections of the reflex arc have been postulated to play an instrumental role in spasticity. However, studies in which spasticity is selectively reduced by the alleged influence of a single mechanism should be viewed with caution because that mechanism may not be responsible for the spasticity.[11] Reduction of excitatory input from suprasegmental levels, spinal circuits, or dorsal roots reduces motoneuron drive, as does activation of inhibitory pathways. Even if a particular input is not the primary cause of motoneuron excitation, reducing or eliminating it may yield the desired therapeutic effect. The success of therapy directed at one mechanism influencing the motoneuron pool does not imply that the cause of the spasticity is understood. It is rare that a drug or operative treatment has a simple physiologic effect. Therapy is empirical, and results must be interpreted with care because responses among patients can be significantly different.

Intrathecal Baclofen

The rationale for using baclofen intrathecally is analogous to that for using morphine intrathecally. In both cases, the drug acts on receptors in the dorsal gray matter of the spinal cord, and direct infusion into cerebrospinal fluid (CSF) concentrates the drug where it is needed for its therapeutic effect. Systemic delivery could produce the same concentrations in the spinal cord, but the medication would be distributed equally to the entire brain, and the result would be somnolence or even coma. Implantation of a drug pump with a catheter in the lumbar subarachnoid space not only helps concentrate the drug regionally but also provides a means of achieving constant levels. The rate of infusion can be adjusted to allow drug titration for a precise therapeutic effect.

Physiologic Effects of Baclofen

Baclofen was designed to be a lipophilic γ-aminobutyric acid (GABA) agonist that could pass through the blood-brain barrier.[81] However, baclofen only partially permeates the brain from blood and does not fully resemble GABA in its physiologic actions.[82] Several types of receptors for GABA are found in the brain and spinal cord, and baclofen affects only the B type ($GABA_B$). This receptor has been identified and sequenced.[83] It is a transmembrane protein that affects calcium and potassium channels. Immunohistologic staining of the spinal cord has shown a high concentration of $GABA_B$ receptors in layer II of the dorsal gray matter.[84] Physiologic experiments on isolated perfused spinal cords have demonstrated that baclofen produces a profound reduction in monosynaptic and polysynaptic spinal reflexes.[85] This effect is caused by activation of the $GABA_B$ receptors, which reduces the influx of calcium into the presynaptic terminals of afferent fibers; as a result, the release of excitatory transmitters is reduced. Baclofen can also affect the postsynaptic membrane by increasing potassium influx, thereby stabilizing or increasing the membrane potential and inhibiting neuronal firing.[86,87]

The sum of these presynaptic and postsynaptic effects is to decrease drive on the motoneurons. Diazepam, the other antispastic medication active in the central nervous system, works differently. It binds to the presynaptic membrane and facilitates GABA-mediated presynaptic inhibition. Unlike baclofen, which directly activates the receptor, diazepam works only when GABA is released, and it enhances response to the transmitter (Fig. 104-4).[88]

The physiologic effects of baclofen have been studied most frequently in the normal spinal cord. After spinal cord injury, spasticity develops slowly and is related to plastic changes in the spinal cord circuitry. The physiologic features of the damaged

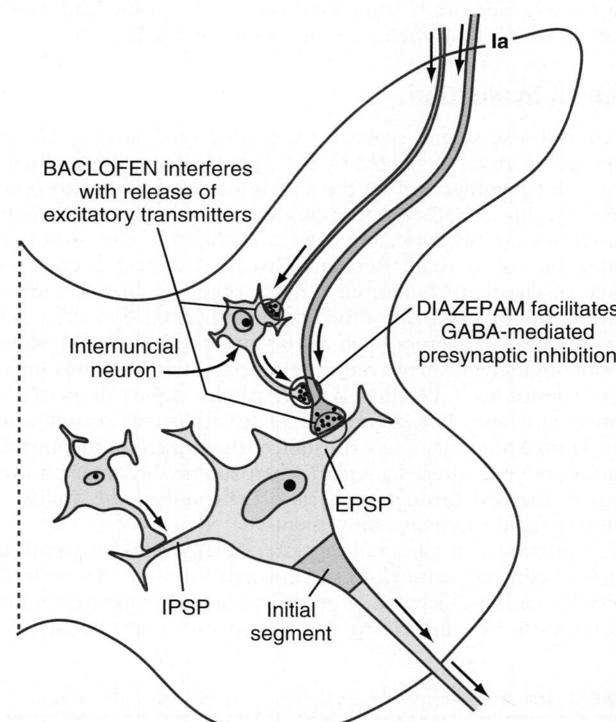

Figure 104-4. Synaptic mechanisms at the spinal level are responsible for excitatory postsynaptic potential (EPSP) and two types of inhibition: inhibitory postsynaptic potential (IPSP) and presynaptic inhibition. Enlargement of the left portion of Figure 104-1. The sites of action of γ-aminobutyric acid (GABA), baclofen, and diazepam at the spinal level are schematically illustrated. *(Redrawn from Young RR, Delwaide PJ. Drug therapy: spasticity. Part 2.* N Engl J Med. *1981;304:96-99.)*

spinal cord are significantly changed, and so is its response to medications. Ischemic injury to the spinal cord in rats produces spasticity as a result of loss of GABA interneurons, and baclofen markedly reduces this spasticity.[89] After a cervical injury, the lumbar portion of the rat spinal cord also increases the number of its $GABA_B$ receptors by 30%.[90] Other experiments in rats and cats have demonstrated that bladder reflexes change after cord injury and that the modified reflexes are inhibited by morphine and baclofen.[91] These animal findings are supported by clinical observations. Intrathecal baclofen given to normal human patients does not interfere with movement or decrease strength, but the same dose given to a spastic patient markedly decreases spasticity and muscle tone. Of patients with spasticity caused by multiple sclerosis or spinal cord injury, at least 96% have responded to intrathecal baclofen in double-blind studies.[92] Baclofen is effective in reducing spasticity because the same changes in the spinal cord that produce spasticity increase sensitivity to baclofen.

Kinetics and Distribution of Intrathecal Baclofen

Baclofen, like morphine, is primarily water soluble, which means that only a small amount crosses the blood-brain barrier.[82] Similarly, little of the drug that is introduced into CSF is lost by movement across membranes into the systemic circulation. Therefore, CSF flow is the only distribution source of intrathecal baclofen to the spinal cord. When baclofen is delivered in a bolus via lumbar puncture, it mixes rapidly in the CSF in the lumbar subarachnoid space and is gradually carried upward along the spinal cord.[93] In 3 to 6 hours, it reaches the brainstem and then travels over the convexities, where it is eliminated into the systemic circulation at the arachnoid granulations. Bolus administration achieves transient but very high drug levels at the spinal cord and, later, at the brainstem. The half-life of a bolus of baclofen in CSF is approximately 90 minutes.[94] It is stable in CSF and does not become metabolized by tissue.

If baclofen is given by slow infusion, a different distribution is achieved. The concentration gradually reaches a steady state in which the same amount of baclofen is being removed from CSF as is being infused; this steady state occurs at about 12 to 18 hours (i.e., seven times the half-life). As has been measured in patients, the final steady-state concentration is directly proportional to the drug infusion rate.[95] Other measurements in which simultaneous cervical and lumbar samples have been studied show that in the steady state, the concentration of baclofen in the cervical region is decreased on average to 25% of that of the lumbar region. However, the variability in the concentration of baclofen along the spinal canal is large, from 1 : 10 to 1 : 2. The manner in which the concentration varies along the spinal cord has also been shown by indium 111 flow studies in patients with implanted pumps.[93] When continuously infused, the indium has the highest concentration in the lumbar area and then decreases steadily as it goes up to the higher levels of the spinal cord (Fig. 104-5).

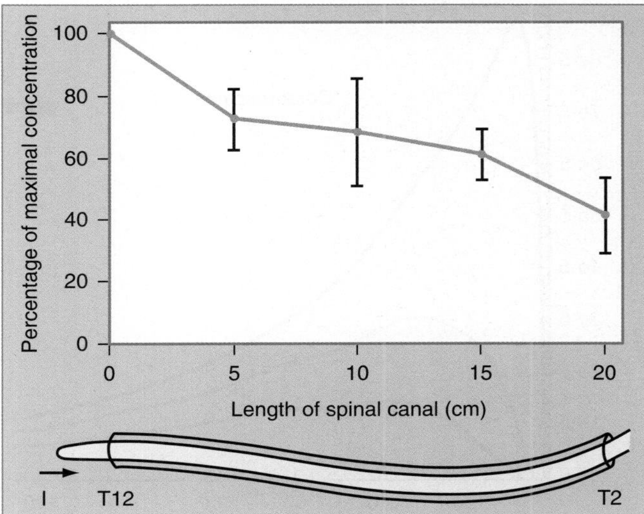

Figure 104-5. Decline in indium 111–diethylenetriaminepentaacetic acid concentration as the compound ascends the thoracic spinal column after slow intrathecal infusion. The 0-cm point is at the T12 vertebra, and the 20-cm point is at the T2 vertebra. The percentage of maximal concentration is the ratio of counts at points along the spinal canal to the level measured at T12. Data are presented as means ± standard deviation for four patients. *(Modified from Kroin J, Ali A, York M, et al. The distribution of medication along the spinal canal after chronic intrathecal administration.* Neurosurgery. *1993;33:226-230.)*

The distribution of medicines delivered into the spinal subarachnoid space is becoming better understood. Because the concepts are important for clinical use of intrathecal baclofen, the highlights are mentioned. CSF flow in the spinal canal is driven by the continuous production of fluid from the choroid plexus and brain. The spinal CSF pulsates with each cardiac cycle; approximately 1 to 2 mL of the CSF moves from the brain to the more compliant spinal space and back. As a result, medicines mix well with and are well distributed by CSF. Water-soluble molecules, such as those of baclofen, have a predictable half-life and distribution when introduced into the lumbar area. The movement of baclofen into the spinal cord tissue is probably along the perivascular spaces around the penetrating spinal cord arterioles. Once within the spinal cord, baclofen then moves by slow convective flow in the extracellular space inside the cord (see Chapter 54). This slow distribution in the tissue accounts for the delay of 45 to 60 minutes from the time baclofen given to its clinical effect as it reaches its receptors.

Models of the flow patterns of spinal CSF in combination with MRI measurements and fluid mechanics have provided a fuller picture of these processes.[96,97] Figure 104-6 shows the results of such a simulation in which a bolus dose is injected into the lumbar region.[98] Concentration rapidly increases at the region of catheter tip and then slowly in the adjacent spinal cord tissue. In the more distant thoracic CSF, the CSF concentration is slower to increase and does not reach the same height as in the lumbar region; the increase in concentration in the thoracic tissue is also delayed and is lower than that in the lumbar tissue. The CSF concentration is much higher than the tissue concentration, but the tissue concentration is retained for longer. Using the model in Figure 104-6, the effect of higher CSF pulse pressures and more rapid heartbeats can be calculated. Increases in either would decrease the concentration of baclofen by more rapid distribution. Respirations and coughing, by changing intracranial and spinal pressure dynamics, also change distribution. Variations in spinal anatomy and the position of the catheter tip are important; placement in the cervical region will produce a higher local concentration than placement in a lower position.[99] Furthermore, pathologic processes in the spinal subarachnoid space can alter CSF movement. The practical consequences are that distribution is different in every patient and that dosage cannot be accurately predicted.

The results of these kinetic and distribution studies have important consequences:

1. Bolus lumbar administration produces immediate and extremely high transient levels in the CSF. Several hours later, baclofen reaches the brainstem and causes side effects such as lightheadedness and drowsiness.
2. Slow, constant delivery with a drug pump produces levels of drug proportional to the delivery rate.

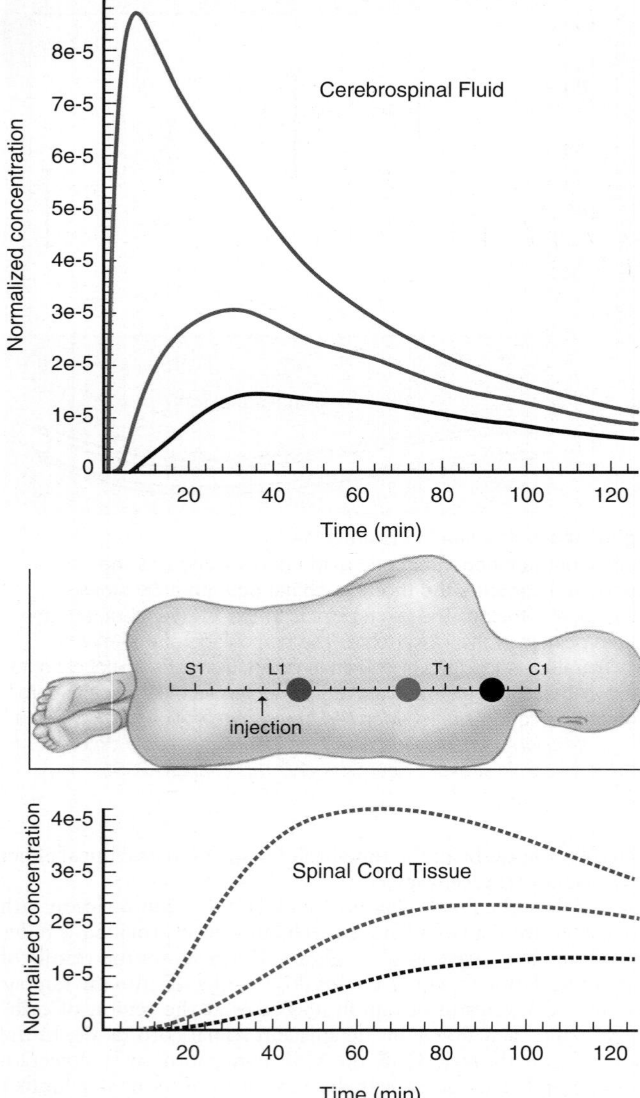

Figure 104-6. The predicted concentration of baclofen in cerebrospinal fluid (CSF) around the spinal cord *(top)* versus the concentration within the spinal cord tissue *(bottom),* derived from a model based on known flow patterns of CSF and the absorption coefficient of the spinal cord. Note that the immediate effect of the bolus injection at the lumbar region is a high concentration in the lumbar area and a lower, slowly rising concentration within the spinal cord tissue in that region. The concentrations in the thoracic and cervical areas increase at later times, and the rise in spinal cord tissue levels is also delayed. The model predicts that the baclofen in the spinal cord tissue will remain high even though the CSF concentration has already decreased toward normal. The model also explains the clinical long-lasting effect of baclofen within the spinal cord tissue. *(Modified from Hsu Y, Hettiarachchi HD, Zhu DC, Linninger AA. The frequency and magnitude of cerebrospinal fluid pulsations influence intrathecal drug distribution: key factors for interpatient variability.* Anesth Analg. *2012;115[2]:386-394.)*

3. If the delivery rate is changed, it takes at least 12 hours for the concentration to reach new steady-state levels in CSF. Therefore, infusion rates should not be adjusted more than twice each day.
4. A constant infusion into the lumbar space distributes baclofen along the spinal cord in such a way that the concentration decreases linearly with distance and is about 25% as high at the brainstem as it is at the point of infusion. Fewer brainstem effects are likely to occur if a constant infusion is administered and the infusion is directed into the lumbar intrathecal space.
5. With slow diffusion in the spinal cord tissue, there is a 45- to 60-minute delay from the time that a bolus dose is injected until spasticity is reduced. After the receptors have been reached, diffusion back to CSF is equally slow. A single bolus dose may reduce spasticity for 4 to 12 hours; its maximal effect occurs when the level in CSF has decreased to almost zero.[100] A large, single overdose causes long-lasting respiratory depression and coma, even after CSF levels have been reduced.

In summary, when administering medication intrathecally, the physician must always be aware that the clinical effects are slow to appear and equally slow to clear because the drug requires time for movement into the spinal cord, and the cord tissue acts as a reservoir after it is loaded.

Efficacy of Intrathecal Baclofen for Spinal Spasticity

The most effective use of oral baclofen has been for the treatment of spasticity caused by spinal cord injury or multiple sclerosis. The initial studies of intrathecal delivery were conducted in affected patients after oral medications showed limited success or had unacceptable side effects such as drowsiness. In this well-defined patient population, a bolus of 50 to 100 μg of intrathecal baclofen reduced abnormal muscle tone 2 or more points on the Ashworth scale for almost all patients. Spasms, if present, were also significantly reduced. The short-term effect could be maintained with constant delivery. Individual and multicenter studies in the United States and Europe have demonstrated that control of spasticity and spasms can be achieved over a period of years by using implanted drug pumps to deliver baclofen (Table 104-3).[101-104]

The efficacy of chronic intrathecal administration of baclofen is clear and unequivocal, but several questions need to be answered: What are the drug's side effects? How difficult is it to maintain long-term baclofen treatment? What other patient groups can benefit from this treatment?

Drug Side Effects

The side effects of intrathecal baclofen are similar to those of oral baclofen and are dose related. Because the baclofen concentration is higher in the lumbar region than at the brainstem, central nervous system side effects are milder; however, increasing dosage can lead to adverse effects. Common problems with high dosage include drowsiness, mental confusion, lightheadedness, and ataxia. Weakness can be induced in some patients, as can loss of function because of reduced muscle tone. A 10% to 20% reduction in dosage usually eliminates these symptoms. Bolus administration, used for testing before implantation of a pump, is more frequently associated with these side effects and occasionally produces hypotension, nausea, and respiratory depression. A large overdose, in the range of 1 to 20 mg, results in coma, flaccidity, hypotension, and respiratory depression.[105] If an overdose occurs, the patient must be kept under surveillance with apnea monitoring and, if necessary, be provided with ventilatory support. No deaths from overdose have been reported, but the intrathecal route of drug administration can result in potent and serious side effects. Treatment of a moderate overdose with

TABLE 104-3 Studies of Intrathecal Baclofen for Spinal Spasticity

Reference	Country	No. of Patients	Type of Study	Results
Penn et al., 1989[1]	United States	20	Double blind	Excellent
Penn, 1992[92]	United States	62	Prospective	Excellent
Ochs et al., 1989[101]	Germany/Sweden, Belgium/Holland, United Kingdom	28	Prospective, multicenter	Excellent
Lazorthes et al., 1990[102]	France	38 ports, 18 pumps	Prospective	Excellent
Müller, 1991[2]	Germany	211	Prospective, multicenter	Excellent
Loubser et al., 1991[103]	United States	9	Prospective	Excellent
Coffey et al., 1993[104]	United States	75	Double blind	Excellent

physostigmine (0.5 to 2 mg) often reverses the somnolence and respiratory effects.[106] This treatment does not work for large overdoses and should not be given to patients with heart conduction defects. The effects of an overdose on the central nervous system should clear in 24 to 48 hours.

Tolerance to intrathecal baclofen develops in most patients. Over the first 6 to 12 months, the dose of baclofen necessary to achieve a given clinical effect usually doubles and then eventually stabilizes.[92] In a few patients, tolerance may be a significant problem that necessitates "drug holidays" for several weeks or a switch to intrathecal morphine, which shares some of the antispastic effects of baclofen. Most often, the need for increasing dosage after the first year is related to a problem with drug delivery through the catheter rather than true tolerance.

Seizures and hallucinations can occur if baclofen is withdrawn suddenly. After intrathecal treatment has been initiated, oral baclofen should be withdrawn gradually over a period of several weeks. Baclofen may change the seizure threshold in some patients and has been associated with the onset of seizures in a few patients. It may make established seizure conditions more difficult to control. Sudden withdrawal of intrathecal baclofen produces a rebound phenomenon consisting of spasticity and spasms that may be worse than those that occurred before baclofen therapy was initiated. This increased spasticity gradually dissipates over several days. It also frequently causes a tickling and dysesthetic sensation.

A rare, life-threatening baclofen withdrawal syndrome of high fever, altered mental state, and profound muscular rigidity that can lead to fatal rhabdomyolysis has been described.[107] The most effective treatment is rapid reinstatement of intrathecal baclofen. Oral and intravenous medications, including high-dose benzodiazepines, and supportive care can help, but in severe cases, intrathecal baclofen should be given by lumbar puncture or external catheter. Patients with preexisting autonomic dysreflexia are particularly at risk for this withdrawal syndrome.[107]

Delivery Systems

Intrathecal baclofen therapy depends completely on proper function of the pump and catheter system used to deliver the drug. Pump designs, catheter systems, and implantation procedures for delivery of morphine are the same as for baclofen. The incidence of pump failure is low, approximately 1% to 2% per year, and the only common failures are stalling or stopping. Overdosing is rare, except in cases of iatrogenic causes, such as misprogramming. New pumps and catheters have been approved for intrathecal use by the U.S. Food and Drug Administration. The pumps employ different motors and catheters and vary in material and size. Unfortunately, comparison studies have not been performed, and so the decision to use a particular delivery system cannot be based on known performance. Because all pumps are about the same size and the catheters are similar, the operation for placement is also similar. Video 104-1 demonstrates the operative technique.

The major cause of disruption of drug delivery is catheter malfunction. The implanted catheters are thin walled and of small caliber so that they can be passed easily into the subarachnoid space without causing injury to the nerve roots.[92] Despite anchoring devices, the flimsy catheters can pull out of position because of movement. The catheters can also tear, disconnect, or become occluded. Frequently, the problem can be diagnosed on plain radiography. If the cause is not obvious, indium 111 can be placed in the pump and the patient scanned at 24 and 48 hours to check catheter patency.[108] The indium 111 study shows the flow of CSF and can demonstrate a subarachnoid block caused by arachnoiditis or fibrosis around the catheter tip. Sometimes, a pinhole leak in a catheter cannot be seen on any study and the cause is found only when the catheter is replaced. An alternative is to inject a radiopaque dye under fluoroscopic guidance into the pump's side port and look for blockage or a leak outside the subarachnoid space.

As with any implanted device, infection is a potential problem. The bacteriostatic filter within the pump blocks any contamination in the pump reservoir from reaching the CSF. However, localized infection in the pump pocket or meningitis from the catheter in CSF has occurred in a few patients (<3%). Infection usually necessitates removal of the hardware, although intrathecal antibiotics delivered by pump can sometimes successfully treat an infection of CSF.

Long-term management of patients requires regular pump refills, dose adjustments, and diagnosis and treatment of complications.[109] Despite these requirements, the number of patients with implanted pumps who discontinue their use is quite low. In a 7-year study, no patients dropped out because of medication side effects, and although more than 30% had pump or catheter problems that necessitated operative repair, only 10% decided to not continue long-term treatment.[92] The key to management is a well-trained nurse practitioner who can help with patient education, pump refills, and dose adjustments.

Patient Selection

The U.S. Food and Drug Administration first approved pump implantation and intrathecal baclofen for the treatment of spasticity caused by multiple sclerosis or spinal cord injury on the basis of several double-blind, multicenter studies. Approval was then extended to patients with spasticity of cerebral origin, including those with cerebral palsy. These and other conditions in which spasticity may be reduced with baclofen are listed in Table 104-4. In general, if a patient has the classic signs of spasticity, baclofen can decrease them. Athetosis and generalized dystonia do not usually improve, although exceptions have been reported.[109,110] Focal, painful lower limb dystonias may be helped considerably.[111] Stiff man syndrome, in which spinal GABA-producing neurons are thought to be lost and the patient suffers from episodes of severe axial and limb spasms and rigidity, is markedly improved.[112]

In patients with clinically typical spasticity, intrathecal baclofen is almost always effective. However, if the patient wants to know what the effect will be like or if the physician has any question about the diagnosis or the contribution of spasticity to the patient's clinical problems, a test of intrathecal baclofen should

TABLE 104-4 Conditions Responding to Intrathecal Baclofen

Spasticity-Associated Condition	Reference
Spinal cord injury	See Table 104-3
Cerebral palsy	Albright et al., 1993[113]
	Albright et al., 1991[114]
Hydromyelia	Case reports
Progressive lateral sclerosis	Case reports
Traumatic brain injury	Meythaler et al., 1999[115]
	Meythaler et al., 1997[116]
	Becker et al., 1997[117]
	Rifici et al., 1994[118]
	Saltuari et al., 1992[119]
Dystonias	
Axial	Ford et al., 1996[110]
Cerebral palsy	Albright et al., 1993[113]
	Albright et al., 1991[114]
Distal extremity: foot	Meythaler et al., 1999[120]
Miscellaneous	
Stiff man syndrome	Penn and Mangieri, 1993[112]
Syndrome of painful legs and moving toes	Penn and Gianino, 1995[111]

be performed. A single trial dose of 50 to 100 μg given by lumbar puncture is usually adequate. This easy test, which the patient undergoes under observation in the hospital, has few side effects and provides the physician and the patient a good chance to understand what baclofen can accomplish. The only caveat is that a bolus frequently reduces spasticity so much that motor function may be lost transiently if some rigidity is required. Patients must be warned about this possibility. For most patients, careful dosage adjustment after pump implantation allows titration to a level that improves spasticity without significantly interfering with motor function.

The indications for intrathecal treatment of spasticity are straightforward for most patients: spasticity that has not responded to oral antispastic medications and a successful trial of intrathecal baclofen (50 to 100 μg). The drug should be used in patients whose spasticity is severe enough to cause significant disability, difficulty in self-care, or pain. The use of destructive neurolytic or neurosurgical procedures should be limited to the few patients whose condition cannot be maintained on intrathecal baclofen or who have no useful motor function. The most difficult decisions involve patients for whom it is unclear whether a reduction in spasticity will improve motor function and for those in whom baclofen treatment decreases functionally useful rigidity. This group includes many patients with spastic cerebral palsy. The results of dorsal rhizotomy are difficult to compare with those of intrathecal baclofen because rhizotomy is generally performed on young children and pumps are implanted in older children who weigh more than 50 pounds. Both procedures reduce spasticity. A pump requires continuous treatment and many dose adjustments; however, it is reversible, and the degree of reduction in spasticity can be titrated to meet the patient's needs, whereas rhizotomy is irreversible and requires a long recovery period. In many patients with cerebral palsy, regardless of the method used to reduce spasticity, motor function improves only slightly because of widespread damage to the nervous system, but care may become much easier.

SUGGESTED READINGS

Albright AL, Cervi A, Singletary J. Intrathecal baclofen for spasticity in cerebral palsy. *JAMA*. 1991;265:1418-1422.

Coffey RJ, Edgar TS, Francisco GE, et al. Abrupt withdrawal from intrathecal baclofen: recognition and management of a potentially life-threatening syndrome. *Arch Phys Med Rehabil*. 2002;83:735-741.

Corcos D, Gottlieb G, Penn R, et al. Movement deficits caused by hyperexcitable stretch reflexes in spastic humans. *Brain*. 1986;109:1043-1058.

Dietz V, Sinkjaer T. Spasticity. In: Verhaagen J, McDonald JW III, eds. *Spinal Cord Injury*. Amsterdam: Elsevier; 2012:197-211. In: Aminoff MJ, Boller F, Swaab DF, eds. *Handbook of Clinical Neurology* (3rd series); vol 109.

Hagbarth K, Wallin G, Lofstedt L. Muscle spindle responses to stretch in normal and spastic subjects. *Scand J Rehabil Med*. 1973;5:156-159.

Hsu Y, Hettiarachchi HD, Zhu DC, et al. The frequency and magnitude of cerebrospinal fluid pulsations influence intrathecal drug distribution: key factors for interpatient variability. *Anesth Analg*. 2012;115(2):386-394.

Kroin J, Ali A, York M, et al. The distribution of medication along the spinal canal after chronic intrathecal administration. *Neurosurgery*. 1993;33:226-230.

Landau W. Spasticity: the fable of the neurological demon and the emperor's new therapy. *Arch Neurol*. 1974;31:217-219.

McCouch G, Austin G, Liu C, et al. Sprouting as a cause of spasticity. *J Neurophysiol*. 1958;21:205-216.

Ochs G, Struppler A, Meyerson B, et al. Intrathecal baclofen for long-term treatment of spasticity: a multi-centre study. *J Neurol Neurosurg Psychiatry*. 1989;52:933-939.

Penn R, Kroin J. Intrathecal baclofen alleviates spinal cord spasticity. *Lancet*. 1984;1:1078.

Penn R, Savoy S, Corcos D, et al. Intrathecal baclofen for severe spinal spasticity: a double-blind crossover study. *N Engl J Med*. 1989;320:1517-1521.

Pierrot-Deseilligny E. Electrophysiological assessment of the spinal mechanisms underlying spasticity. *Electroencephalogr Clin Neurophysiol Suppl*. 1990;41:264-273.

Rosenson A, Ali A, Fordham E, et al. Indium-111 DPTA flow study to evaluate surgically implanted drug delivery system. *Clin Nucl Med*. 1990;15:154-156.

Young R, Delwaide P. Drug therapy: spasticity. Part 2. *N Engl J Med*. 1981;304:96-99.

Zieglglansberger W, Howe J, Sutor B. The neuropharmacology of baclofen. In: Müller H, Zierski J, Penn R, eds. *Local Spinal Therapy of Spasticity*. Berlin: Springer-Verlag; 1988:37-49.

See a full reference list on ExpertConsult.com

105 Treatment of Intractable Vertigo

Zackary E. Boomsaad, Steven A. Telian, and Parag G. Patil

This chapter reviews the differential diagnosis, medical treatment, and surgical management of vertigo. Vertigo is the illusory sensation of rotational or translational movement. Although uncommonly treated by neurosurgeons, vertigo is a very common symptom reported by patients under neurosurgical evaluation. The chapter explores the classification of vestibular disorders, nonsurgical management of vertigo, and surgical management of vertigo.

CLASSIFICATION OF VESTIBULAR DISORDERS

Vestibular disorders are classified as central or peripheral. Central disorders involve pathologic changes within the brainstem or cerebellum, whereas peripheral disorders involve the labyrinth or vestibular nerve. Central vestibular disorders, which are typically insidious in onset and characterized by initially mild symptoms, arise from vertebrobasilar insufficiency, migraine, tumors, paraneoplastic syndromes, and demyelinating disorders. Peripheral vestibular disorders, which are typically sudden in onset and diminish in severity with central compensation, include benign paroxysmal positional vertigo (BPPV), Meniere's disease, labyrinthitis, vestibular neuritis, perilymphatic fistula (PLF), and superior semicircular canal dehiscence (SSCD) syndrome. An additional important etiology of vertigo, which may be of either peripheral or central origin, is trauma.

NONSURGICAL MANAGEMENT OF VERTIGO

Nonsurgical therapeutic modalities for the treatment of vertigo include vestibular rehabilitation, canalith repositioning maneuvers (sometimes known as the Epley maneuver), and a broad range of pharmacologic agents designed to suppress vestibular input to the central nervous system. Vestibular rehabilitation maneuvers are most effective for patients with stable, unilateral lesions producing peripheral vestibular disorders. By contrast, central disorders require longer treatment periods and have poorer outcomes. BPPV, which is due to otoconial debris in the semicircular canal, can be promptly and effectively treated with a series of canalith repositioning maneuvers, although recurrence is common and spontaneous resolution of symptoms is also possible.

Pharmacologic therapies for vertigo are directed toward the suppression of dysfunctional vestibular afferent impulses to the central nervous system. Benzodiazepines, antihistamines, and anticholinergic agents are most often employed in the treatment of vertigo. These agents are primarily utilized to reduce the intensity of vertiginous spells and are of little prophylactic benefit. Vestibular suppressants are not recommended for chronic use because of impairment of vestibular compensation and progressive physiologic dependence.

SURGICAL MANAGEMENT OF INTRACTABLE VERTIGO

Patients who are unsuccessfully treated with conservative and pharmacologic therapies may be candidates for surgical intervention. Critical determinants of surgical success include appropriate patient selection, correct identification and lateralization of pathology, and accurate assessment of the degree of central compensation. Specific surgical therapies have been developed for several pathologic processes resulting in vertigo, including BPPV, SSCD, PLF, and Meniere's disease.

BPPV most often resolves spontaneously or with application of the Epley maneuver. However, in rare circumstances, singular neurectomy (surgical transection of the posterior ampullary nerve) or posterior semicircular canal occlusion (rendering the cupula unresponsive to angular acceleration) may be indicated for debilitating symptoms. Of the two approaches, canal occlusion appears to be the safer approach to treat otherwise intractable BPPV.

SSCD results from thinning of the squamous temporal bone, resulting in the shunting of acoustic energy to the vestibular system. Patients with SSCD exhibit noise-induced dizziness and eye movements (Tullio's phenomenon) and eye movement in response to pressure impulses in the external auditory canal (Hennebert's sign). Thin-section temporal bone computed tomography can be diagnostic for SSCD. Surgery for SSCD ranges from minimally invasive tympanostomy tube placement to craniotomy with plugging of the defect.

PLF is an abnormal connection between the fluid-filled inner ear and the air-filled tympanic cavity. The diagnosis remains controversial, and it is often difficult to identify a definite site of leakage. PLF may be associated with middle ear injury or surgery in addition to barotrauma. Although nonsurgical therapies are much preferred, PLF may be successfully treated with patching of the oval or round window.

Medically refractory Meniere's disease is the most common indication for vestibular surgery, though 70% to 90% of patients respond to medical therapy. Meniere's disease is a common cause of acute recurring episodic vertigo, although its pathogenesis remains unknown. Interventions for Meniere's disease include intratympanic injection of gentamicin, application of a Meniett device (Kebomed, Devon, England), endolymphatic sac surgery, and vestibular ablation. Vestibular ablation entails either hearing-preserving vestibular neurectomy or obliterative labyrinthectomy.

Selective vestibular neurectomy may be accomplished through a middle fossa, retrolabyrinthine, or retrosigmoid surgical approach to cranial nerve VIII, with proponents of each access corridor and published success rates of over 95%. Postoperative hearing loss and facial weakness are more significant concerns for the middle fossa approach than the posterior fossa approaches. Most recently, endoscopically assisted approaches have been employed to improve surgical visualization.

CONCLUSION

In conclusion, intractable vertigo remains an important treatment challenge in neurosurgery and neuro-otology. Although the majority of patients with vertigo may be successfully treated with vestibular rehabilitation and pharmacologic approaches, some may benefit from surgery. In these cases, careful patient selection, correct identification and lateralization of pathology, and the choice of surgical approach are the primary determinants of treatment success.

Full text of this chapter is available online at ExpertConsult.com 

106 Motor Cortex Stimulation for Pain and Movement Disorders

Jay L. Shils and Jeffrey E. Arle

Primary motor cortex stimulation (MCS) has been used to treat pain and movement disorders since the 1960s; however, only since 2000 has MCS become a more mainstream treatment. In the 1930s and 1940s, Paul Bucy and others performed direct extirpation of the primary motor cortex (M1) to treat Parkinson's disease (PD) and other disorders of movement.[1,2] Similarly, resection of the primary sensory cortex (S1) was explored as a treatment for chronic pain[3]; some patients required resection of both S1 and M1 to completely alleviate symptoms.[3] In 1955, White and Sweet[6] reported that only 13% of patients experienced pain relief with postcentral gyrus resection; after that report, the procedure was largely abandoned.

Cortical stimulation for pain began in 1963, when Heath[7] implanted electrodes in the septal region in hopes of activating pleasure centers and thereby alleviating pain. The electrodes were connected to an external pulse generator, which the patients controlled. In the mid-1980s, Hosobuchi[8] implanted electrodes deep to the somatosensory cortex in 44 patients with chronic pain and achieved promising results, particularly for leg pain. In 1985 and 1991, Tsubokawa and colleagues[9,10] reported chronic stimulation of the M1 region to treat neuropathic pain caused by thalamic stroke. Woolsey and associates[11] demonstrated inhibition of tremor and rigidity in patients with PD by precentral gyrus stimulation, although permanent implantation of electrodes was not attempted. In 1998, Nguyen and colleagues[12] first reported the use of permanent electrodes for the stimulation in the M1 region to treat PD.

In comparison with deep brain stimulation (DBS), MCS has obvious potential advantages: in particular, the avoidance of brain penetration and its attendant risks of catastrophic intracerebral hemorrhage or adverse cognitive sequelae. In addition, extradural MCS can be performed while the patient is under general anesthesia and does not necessitate the use of a stereotactic headframe or microelectrode recording expertise; all these advantages would make MCS more acceptable and widely available to patients as long as safety and efficacy can be demonstrated.

Among the many potential cortical sites, M1 may not seem an obvious target for therapeutic stimulation either for pain or for movement disorders. Stimulation of M1 above a certain threshold activates pyramidal tract neurons, causing unwanted disabling muscular contractions and potentially limiting therapeutic benefit. However, subthreshold stimulation can avoid this effect, allowing stimulation to modulate the final common link between the deeper circuitry coordinating movement and the spinal cord itself. Because M1 is a key region where the pyramidal and extrapyramidal systems interact, many disorders of movement might respond to subthreshold in this region, as long as the appropriate stimulation parameters can be identified.

With regard to M1 as a target for pain management, the cortex is integral in the perception of pain, as exemplified by the phenomenon of phantom limb pain. Similarly, infarcts within the sensory thalamus can result in dysfunctional pain sensation despite the absence of injury more distal in the nervous system or to the body regions where the pain is felt. Although direct stimulation of S1 typically elicits uncomfortable paresthesias, reciprocal innervation between M1 and S1, mediated by so-called U fibers, may allow modulation of sensory phenomenon through stimulation of M1 without eliciting undesirable sensory phenomena.

The accumulated experience in using cortical stimulation to treat both pain and disorders of movement is really quite limited. A MEDLINE search for articles related to MCS published between 1991 and January 2014 revealed reports of only 901 cases of treatment with MCS for pain (609 cases),[11,13-72] stroke rehabilitation (19 cases),[13,49,73,74] movement disorders (272 cases; however, in 22 of these cases, patients received mixed MCS and DBS),[12,24,26,75-93] and multiple sclerosis (1 case).[94] In this chapter, we describe the technique for performing MCS, as well as the results and complications that have been observed in the treatment of various conditions.

SURGICAL TECHNIQUE

Multiple techniques have been described for placing MCS electrodes. Our preference is to perform a small craniotomy, which allows us to map M1 intraoperatively and to secure the lead to the dura once the optimal location is found. A curvilinear incision extends from 1 cm posterior to the midpoint between the nasion and inion at the midline toward the anterior margin of the tragus. This allows for a craniotomy 5 to 6 cm in diameter that is centered on M1 and can accommodate either strip or grid electrodes. The desired anatomic region for stimulation is mapped electrophysiologically through the use of electrical or magnetic stimulation (it is advisable not to use Mayfield pins because the head does not need to be rigidly held in place and the patient may be hurt by the rigid fixation if the mapping procedure induces a seizure).

It is important to use both intraoperative somatosensory and motor mapping to determine the course of the central sulcus and the M1 region underlying the dura because it gives information on both the geometry of the central sulcus and specific key areas of the motor cortex. In addition, the two methods act as internal controls. Somatosensory testing consists of placing a 2 × 8 or 4 × 8 coverage lead (Boston Scientific, Valencia, CA) on the dura in a variety of orientations, mostly perpendicular to the suspected precentral gyrus. Median and/or ulnar nerve somatosensory evoked potentials (SEPs) are then obtained with the use of a 20-mA, 200-μsec monopolar square pulse at a rate of 4.32 Hz. SEPs are recorded from the lead in both a bipolar (contact 1-2, 2-3, and so forth) and monopolar (all referenced to the 10-20 location of Fz) recording montage. The central sulcus is determined as the point where the N20 response phase reverses (Fig. 106-1). Because of the complex geometry of some central sulci, and because in some cases the N20 generators may not fall on the gyrus, multiple mappings need to be done at multiple locations to ensure an accurate "picture" of the central sulcus.[95]

The second neurophysiologic mapping tool is motor mapping, which involves activating the motor cortex, either electrically or magnetically, and recording the responses in specific muscle groups.[96] There are three important factors to consider during motor mapping: (1) the strength of the stimulus and the "cleanliness" of the surgical field; (2) the type of anesthesia; (3) and the type of stimulator probes used. The spread of the electric field will determine the resolution of the response. If the stimulus

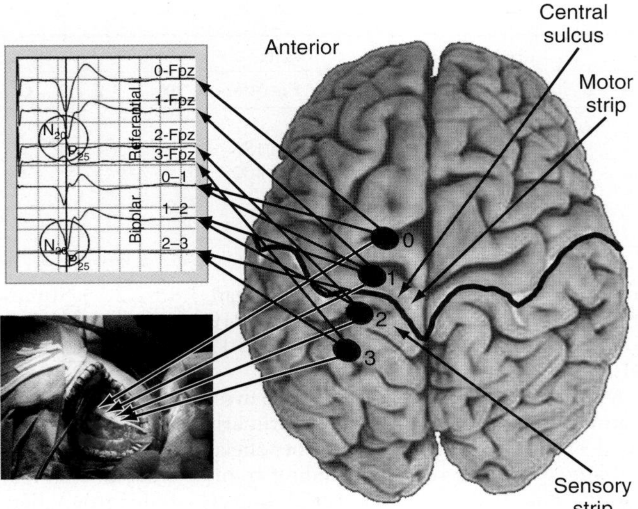

Figure 106-1. Use of the somatosensory evoked potential (SEP) phase reversal method to localize the primary motor cortex (M1) extradurally. Contacts 0 to 3 of a typical four-contact paddle-type electrode are shown with placement across the underlying central sulcus. *Upper left inset,* Waveforms show the SEP in each contact. Reversal of the phase occurs between contacts 1 and 2 in this example. *Lower left inset,* The intraoperative photo of this technique being used, which reveals the relative size of the lead to the craniotomy. By placing the lead in different positions, the surgeon can map the path of the sulcus epidurally.

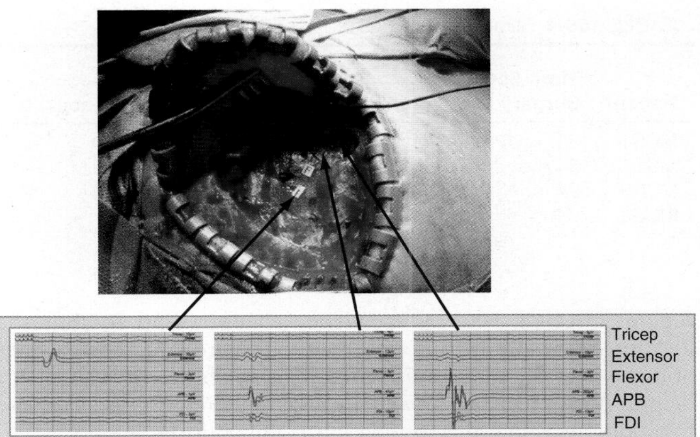

Figure 106-2. Use of cortical mapping to determine the location of subregions of the primary motor cortex (M1). Electromyogram from muscles in the upper extremity after stimulation with a ball-tipped electrode in three locations on the dura. The tracing at the far left shows activation of the extensor muscles in the forearm; the other two tracings show activation of the abductor pollicis brevis (APB). This technique corroborates the somatosensory evoked potential method, illustrated in Figure 106-1, and helps determine more precisely the underlying thresholds for individual muscle groups. Extensor, extensor carpi ulnaris; FDI, first dorsal interosseous muscle; Flexor, flexor carpi ulnaris.

amplitude is too low, too few axons will be activated to generate a recordable compound muscle action potential, but if the stimulus amplitude is too high, axons that are far away (a few millimeters to 1 cm) may also be activated, falsely identifying a region as motor cortex. High stimulus amplitudes may also induce seizures. Excessive fluid in the surgical field will be spread over a larger area, limiting the resolution of the technique or yielding false-positive results.

Motor evoked potentials are very sensitive to anesthesia, and different anesthetics have varying amounts of inhibitory effects on the alpha motoneuron membrane. Inhalation agents have a particularly strong effect, and so a total intravenous anesthetic technique is recommended for these procedures.[97] A reliable technique is to administer a continuous dose of propofol, combined with either fentanyl or remifentanil. Standard doses are in the range of 75 to 150 μg/kg/min for propofol and 0.05 to 0.5 μg/kg/min of fentanyl or remifentanil. Neither any inhalational agent nor muscle relaxant is used after anesthesia induction and intubation.

Even with a total intravenous anesthetic, the alpha motoneuron membrane needs the help of temporal summation at the corticospinal axon input to counteract the loss of spatial summation. Historically, this has required a low-frequency (50- to 60-Hz) long train (1 sec or more) of stimuli, but this technique can cause seizures in up to 11% of patients.[98] A second high-frequency technique is to use a train of five to seven stimuli with a 2- to 4-msec interstimulus interval.[99] This technique has demonstrated a much lower frequency of seizures (1.6%)[100] and, in addition, makes seeing the compound muscle action potential response on the screen much easier because the stimulation artifact lasts only 10 to 30 msec.

Motor mapping can be performed both before the incision and once the craniotomy is complete. Preincision motor mapping requires a transcranial magnetic stimulator. Our group has performed preincision motor mapping in one case with good results. This is particularly useful in cases where the anatomy is distorted. Mapping of the hand area with the use of the abductor pollicis brevis as the key muscle is fairly reliable. Intracranial stimulation is delivered with a monopolar or bipolar probe placed on the dura (or the cortex for subdural mapping). Monopolar mapping consists of placing on the dura an anodal 2- to 5-mm stimulation ball probe referenced to a cathode placed at Fz. Stimulation consists of trains of five stimuli each, at a rate of five trains/sec, a 500-μsec pulse width, and a 4-msec interspike interval. As stated previously, low-frequency (50- to 60-Hz) stimulation can be used, but because of the higher risk of seizures and the added difficulty in seeing the response, we choose to use the high-frequency short-train method. Once the probe is placed on the dura, stimulation amplitudes are slowly increased, starting at 5 mA (for subdural testing, the amplitude is started at 1-3 mA) and increasing to a maximum of 25 mA or until a response is found. Stimulation can be performed with any electromyographic system that allows for short, low-amplitude, high-frequency trains. Figure 106-2 shows an example of responses in the extensor and abductor pollicis brevis muscles with this technique.

When the permanent implant is considered, several electrode and pulse generator options are available.[101] Newer devices can be programmed for multiple contact configurations, each with differing electrical parameters. In contrast to DBS, MCS is not delivered continuously, and so different configurations can be delivered in a serial sequence. We have found these multiple configurations and patterns to be extremely beneficial for some patients. Initial device programming is typically begun within 24 hours of electrode implantation. Monopolar stimulation is used to evaluate all contacts with a rate of 210 μsec and a frequency of 130 Hz. The voltage is slowly raised to 4.0 V or 8.0 mA (depending on the device used) while the patient is monitored for adverse motor and sensory effects and seizures.

Thus far, each patient we have treated with MCS for pain has required modification of the initial settings over time. Initially, we attempt to optimize the original electrode configuration by altering frequency and pulse width. In our experience, increasing the stimulus pulse width most commonly broadens the anatomic

TABLE 106-1 Stimulator Settings at Last Follow-up Visit

Patient	Time Since Surgery	Left								Right							
		Amplitude	Pulse Width	Frequency	0	1	2	3	C	Amplitude	Pulse Width	Frequency	0	1	2	3	C
MCS1	18 mo/6 mo	3.2	240	130	–	–	–		+								
MCS2	24 mo	3.3	210	130	–	–	–	+		3.5	210	130	–	–	–	–	+
MCS3	24 mo	3.7	210	100	–	–	–		+	3.7	210	100	–	–	–		+
MCS4	6 mo	Off								Off							

regions affected, whereas frequency changes tend to shift the location of the stimulation effect without increasing sensory phenomena over the initial stimulated region. This technique is very helpful if the electrode affects the area of pain, but it is also close to a point at which the stimulation is uncomfortable.

When simple adjustments in pulse width or frequency fail to alleviate the pain, we add new configurations, which are based on the results of the initial monopolar evaluation. The goal of adding new configurations is either to affect new regions or to modulate the pulse pattern at a single region. No device currently available allows the setting of the time interval between each configuration, and so they run sequentially, with a very short interval between pairs of configurations.

When MCS devices are programmed in patients with PD, each contact is tested in a monopolar manner, as in the patients with pain; the key difference is that the central contacts are activated as the initial starting point, with an amplitude of 3.0 mA. This is configuration is chosen on the basis of the mapping during surgery, which ensures that the electrode is centered over the hand and arm region. If the patient cannot tolerate these settings, then more lateral contacts are added, and those farthest from the newly added contact are eliminated. We were able to activate two contacts at the initial programming session in each case. Table 106-1 shows the stimulation parameters in relation to the date of surgical implantation.

CLINICAL RESULTS

Katayama and colleagues[23-27] at Nihon University School of Medicine published a great deal on MCS. They explored MCS as stand-alone therapy and also compared it with DBS and with spinal cord stimulation for the treatment of pain, either as individual therapies or in combination. They reported that 59% of their patients who underwent DBS or MCS for stroke-induced involuntary movements derived some benefit from treatment,[24] and 19% of patients who underwent MCS for the treatment of pain also demonstrated improvement in associated movement problems.

The response to MCS varies considerably, depending on the syndrome. For example, of five patients treated for phantom limb pain,[27] only one experienced greater pain relief than with MCS as compared to patients treated with either DBS at the ventrocaudal (VC) nucleus of the thalamus (6/10 [60%]), spinal cord stimulation (SCS) (6/19 [32%]), or a combination of both. In Tsubokawa and colleagues'[9] initial study from 1991 and a subsequent study of the same patients published in 1993,[45] 5 of 11 patients experienced "excellent" outcomes (defined as 100% improvement) at 2 years, in comparison with 6 of 12 in the first year; however, in 6 of the original 12 patients who were defined as having a "good" response (60 to 80% improvement) at 1 year, the responses were categorized as either "fair" (40%-60% improvement) or "poor" (<40% improvement) at 2 years. In 1998, Katayama and colleagues[25] reported that whereas 23 of 31 patients after stroke exhibited satisfactory pain control initially, pain control was satisfactory in only 8 patients at 2 years. Of note is that both the stimulus "on" times and the waveform parameters used to treat chronic pain vary widely. Stimulation amplitudes ranged from 0.5 to 10.5 V (mean, 3.8 ± 2.2 V). Stimulation frequencies ranged from 5 to 210 Hz (mean, 51.1 ± 35.7 Hz). Pulse widths varied from 1 to 500 µsec (mean, 251.2 ± 141.1 µsec).[a]

A consortium of Italian centers have investigated MCS for the treatment of movement disorders, primarily PD.[33,75,76,78,80,83,92,93] Initial results suggested a strong beneficial effect on the most disabling symptoms of PD, including tremor, bradykinesia, and rigidity. The Italian Neurosurgical Society study group performed MCS on 16 patients with PD; 10 had follow-up periods of 3 to 30 months.[80,87,92] All but one patient were offered MCS because they were ineligible for DBS as a result of advanced age, abnormal findings on magnetic resonance imaging, or abnormalities on neuropsychological testing. The mean duration of disease in the study population was 12.4 years. As measured with the motor subscore of the Unified Parkinson's Disease Rating Scale (UPDRS-M), 3 of the 10 patients with adequate follow-up experienced less than 25% improvement, 6 experienced 25% to 50% improvement, and 1 demonstrated better than 50% improvement. Long-term stimulation parameters included amplitudes ranging from 2 to 6 V, pulse widths ranging from 60 to 210 µsec, and frequencies ranging from 25 to 80 Hz.[92] At 36 months, there was a statistically significant improvement in the UPDRS-M score of 19.1%.[92] There was no significant reduction of medications on average.[92]

Data from our initial series of 15 patients undergoing MCS are summarized in Table 106-2. Among the four patients with PD, one developed an infection 3 months after the implantation, and one experienced an intraoperative seizure during motor mapping. The patient with the infection had experienced a 50% improvement in his preoperative dyskinesia, but his condition regressed significantly when the device was removed. The device was reimplanted later, and his condition improved in relation to his preoperative baseline, again by nearly 50%. Two other patients with PD (M2 and M3) exhibited a 20% to 30% reduction in their medication requirements at 3 months, but patient M3 required increases in medication dosages at 6 and 12 months. One patient (M5), however, required a 37% increase in medication dosage. The UPDRS-M scores over the initial 12 months of the study are detailed in Table 106-3. Although significant benefit in these motor scores can be discerned within the initial 6 months, the patients were returning to their preoperative baseline by 12 months. Table 106-4 shows how the total UPDRS scores changed in the "on medication, on stimulation" state.

Results were even less consistent in our series of patients with pain. Of these 14 pain patients, eight had pain caused by stroke; two had atypical head pain; two had chronic pain syndromes; one had a brachial plexus avulsion; and one had left temporal head pain after a fall. Of the eight patients with poststroke pain, three had associated tremor. In one of those three (P9), neither the pain nor the movement disorder was improved by MCS. The other two (P4 and P5) experienced varying degrees of benefit for both their pain and movement. Patient P5 had good control of her pain in her upper extremities and face, less pain control in her

[a]References 9, 12, 13, 15, 17, 18, 21, 23, 28-33, 35, 36, 38-49, 73, 79, 81, 102.

TABLE 106-2 Our Series of Patients Undergoing Motor Cortex Stimulation

Patient ID	Type	Diagnosis	Time Since Surgery* (mo)	Initial Pain Score	Most Recent Pain Score	Intraoperative Seizure
P1	Pain	Post–thalamic stroke pain	208	8	4	
P2	Pain	Atypical right facial pain	196	8	2	
P3	Pain	Post–thalamic stroke pain				
P4	Pain	Poststroke pain	196	10	4	Yes
M1	PD	PD				
P5	Pain	Left temporal pain after a fall	60	10	4	
M2	PD	PD				
M3	PD	PD				
M4	Dystonia	Poststroke dystonia		8	8	Yes
M5	CBD	CBD with dystonia				
M6	PD	PD				
P6	Pain	CRP of left upper extremity and hand	72	8	8	Yes
P7	Pain	Brachial plexus avulsion	36	10	10	
P8	Pain	Atypical post-herpetic facial pain	12	8	3	
P9	Pain	Post–thalamic stroke pain	12			Yes
P10	Pain	Poststroke facial pain	36	7	3	
P11	Pain	Poststroke pain	4	9	2	
P12	Pain	Post–thalamic stroke pain		10		
P13	Pain	Chronic pain syndrome	24	10	5	Yes
P14	Pain	Poststroke pain	36	10	4	Yes

CBD, cortico-basal degeneration; CRP, complex regional pain; PD, Parkinson's disease.
*Date: September 1, 2007.

TABLE 106-3 UPDRS Part III (Motor) Scores during "On Medication" and "On Stimulation" Conditions

	UPDRS III Score						
Patient	Presurgical "On"	1-Mo "On"	3-Mo "On"	6-Mo "On"	1-Yr "On"	New 6-Mo	UPDRS III 2-Yr "On"
MCS1	19	26	25	Infection	Infection	23	
MCS2	32	47	13	18	35		34
MCS3	24.5	12	18	27	5		29
MCS4	11		Off	Off			

UPDRS, Unified Parkinson's Disease Rating Scale.

TABLE 106-4 UPDRS Total Scores during "On Medication" and "On Stimulation" Conditions

	UPDRS Score							
Patient	Total Presurgical "Off"	Total Presurgical "On"	Total 1-Mo "On"	Total 3-Mo "On"	Total 6-Mo "On"	Total 1-Yr "On"	New 6-Mo	UPDRS Total 2-Yr "On"
MCS1 mcg	54	46	52	47	Infection	Infection	51	
MCS2 Gau	71	57	79	42	94	62		59
MCS3 But	70.5	53.5	23	32	54	37		55
MCS4 det	29	22		Off	Off			

UPDRS, Unified Parkinson's Disease Rating Scale.

leg, and minimal control of a "third limb" sensation. Patient P4 had fair control both of her pain and of an "internal" tremor. Programming in our patients with pain includes a wide range of stimulation parameters: voltage varies from 2.2 to 4.2 V, pulse widths vary from 120 to 330 μsec, and frequencies vary from 50 to 130 Hz. All patients start with monopolar settings, but bipolar settings are often used with more anodal contacts.

Benefits in our remaining patients who underwent MCS remain mixed. However, we have observed clear signs of physiologic improvement. For example, three patients (one with PD [M5] and two with poststroke upper extremity pain [P5] or mixed pain [P1]) contacted us to say they had noticed worsening of their symptoms over the previous month and might need "reprogramming." In each, the internal pulse generators were completely depleted, and the patients regained their previous benefit after battery replacement surgery.

SURGICAL COMPLICATIONS

Complications reported in association with MCS surgery include seizures in 19 patients[17,25,28,34,29,36,72,82,85] (two of which occurred intraoperatively[79]), an intracranial hemorrhage that resulted in a vegetative state (1 patient),[41] death (1 patient),[41] aphasia (1 patient),[29] epidural hematoma (2 patients),[32,88] and one subdural hematoma that necessitated evacuation.[42] Infection was the most common reason for device removal. The most common significant programming side effect was seizures, which occurred in 17 patients.[42,55,60,68,79,85,89,90]

To date, three of our patients have had seizures during the programming phase, but none occurred during the initial programming session. In one instance (see Table 106-3: patient P9), a focal motor seizure may have occurred 2 days after initial programming. This patient also had a seizure during intraoperative

M1 mapping. Since this time, programming in all patients undergoing MCS is kept below 2.5 V or 5 mA for the first 2 weeks after surgery if a seizure occurred during surgery. We have thus far not administered antiepileptic medications. The second programming seizure occurred when we raised the stimulation amplitude from 4.0 to 4.3 V at the 18-month follow-up in a patient with poststroke pain (see Table 106-3: patient P4). Since that session, patient P4's voltage has been kept below 4.0 V, and no further seizure activity has been noted. Patient P10 experienced a focal motor seizure of the face when we increased stimulation amplitude in one of the patient's three configurations to 13 mA in an attempt to overcome loss of stimulation efficacy. This was at the 1-year follow-up. The seizure stopped a few seconds after the amplitude was reduced, and the patient suffered a brief period of postictal confusion.

CONCLUSION

Despite several reports that suggested that MCS is beneficial in PD,[79] our own results are consistent only with transient improvements that lasted no more than 12 months, although two of our patients (M3 and M4) continue to experience a modest improvement. One other preliminary study[103] with subdural electrode placement demonstrated benefit only in tremor scores for one patient whose predominant symptom was tremor. At present, only 27 patients have been described in the entire literature regarding MCS for PD.[26,79,103] Clearly, more data is necessary to determine whether MCS is an option for patients with movement disorders who are unwilling or unable to undergo DBS. Moreover, optimal electrode orientation remains a topic of controversy; no data support placement either perpendicular or parallel to the precentral gyrus. Finally, optimal programming parameters, electrode polarity, and expected time course for benefits all remain unclear at this time.

SUGGESTED READINGS

Amassian VE, Stewart M, Quirk GJ, et al. Physiological basis of motor effects of a transient stimulus to cerebral cortex. *Neurosurgery*. 1987;20:74-93.

Arle JE, Apetauerova D, Zani J, et al. Motor cortex stimulation for Parkinson's disease: 12 month follow-up in 4 patients. *J Neurosurg*. 2008;109:133-139.

Canavero S, Bonicalzi V, Paolotti R, et al. Therapeutic extradural cortical stimulation for movement disorders: a review. *Neurol Res*. 2003;25:118-122.

Canavero S, Paolotti R, Bonicalzi V, et al. Extradural motor cortex stimulation for advanced Parkinson disease. *J Neurosurg*. 2002;97:1208-1211.

Franzini A, Ferroli P, Dones I, et al. Chronic motor cortex stimulation for movement disorders: a promising perspective. *Neurol Res*. 2003;25:123-126.

Garcia-Larrea L, Peyron R, Mertens P, et al. Electrical stimulation of motor cortex for pain control: a combined PET-scan and electrophysiological study. *Pain*. 1999;83:259-273.

Hanajima R, Ashby P, Lang AE, et al. Effects of acute stimulation through contacts placed on the motor cortex for chronic stimulation. *Clin Neurophysiol*. 2002;113(5):635-641.

Katayama Y, Fukaya C, Yamamoto T. Control of post-stroke involuntary and voluntary movement disorders with deep brain or epidural cortical stimulation. *Stereotact Funct Neurosurg*. 1997;69:73-79.

Katayama Y, Oshima H, Fukaya C, et al. Control of post-stroke movement disorders using chronic motor cortex stimulation. *Acta Neurochir Suppl*. 2001;79:89-92.

Katayama Y, Tsubokawa T, Yamamoto T. Chronic motor cortex stimulation for central deafferentation pain: experience with bulbar pain secondary to Wallenberg syndrome. *Stereotact Funct Neurosurg*. 1994;62:295-299.

Kleiner-Fisman G, Fisman DN, Kahn FI, et al. Motor cortical stimulation for parkinsonism. *Arch Neurol*. 2003;60:1554-1558.

Macdonald DB, Skinner S, Shils J, et al. American Society of Neurophysiological Monitoring. Intraoperative motor evoked potential monitoring—a position statement by the American Society of Neurophysiological Monitoring. *Clin Neurophysiol*. 2013;124(12):2291-2316.

Nguyen JP, Lefaucheur JP, Decq P, et al. Chronic motor cortex stimulation in the treatment of central and neuropathic pain. Correlations between clinical, electrophysiological and anatomical data. *Pain*. 1999;82:245-251.

Nuti C, Peyron R, Garcia-Larrea L, et al. Motor cortex stimulation for refractory neuropathic pain: four-year outcome and predictors of efficacy. *Pain*. 2005;118:43-52.

Pagni C, Altibrandi MG, Bentivoglio A, et al. Extradural motor cortex stimulation (EMCS) for Parkinson's disease. History and first results by the study group of the Italian Neurosurgical Society. *Acta Neurochir Suppl*. 2005;93:113-119.

Saitoh Y, Shibata M, Hirano S, et al. Motor cortex stimulation for central and peripheral deafferentation pain. *J Neurosurg*. 2000;92:150-155.

Saitoh Y, Shibata M, Sanada Y, et al. Motor cortex stimulation for phantom limb pain. *Lancet*. 1999;353:212.

Tsubokawa T, Katayama Y, Yamamoto T, et al. Chronic motor cortex stimulation in patients with thalamic pain. *J Neurosurg*. 1993;78:393-401.

See a full reference list on ExpertConsult.com

107 Deep Brain Stimulation for Obesity

Diana Jho, Alexander C. Whiting, Nestor D. Tomycz, Michael Y. Oh, and Donald M. Whiting

Obesity has become a worldwide epidemic, with prevalence increasing substantially in both developing and developed countries.[1] The Centers for Disease Control and Prevention estimates that, in the United States, 16.9% of children 2 to 19 years of age and 34.9% of adults older than 19 years of age are obese, with 5.7% of the population considered morbidly obese.[2,3] Morbid obesity is linked with premature death,[4] impaired quality of life,[5] and multiple comorbidities, including type 2 diabetes, cardiovascular disease, musculoskeletal disease, and certain cancers.[6-8] Annual obesity-related health care costs are estimated at nearly $190 billion in the United States alone.[9]

Body mass index (BMI) is commonly used to assess fat composition of the body. It does not measure body fat directly, but studies have shown that it correlates to direct measures of body fat such as underwater weighing and dual energy x-ray absorptiometry.[10,11] BMI is calculated by dividing weight in kilograms by the square of height in meters.[12] A healthy weight is considered to be associated with a BMI from 18.5 to 24.5, while overweight is defined as a BMI of 25 to 29.9. Obesity is defined as a BMI greater than or equal to 30, and morbid obesity is regarded as a BMI greater than or equal to 40 or greater than 35 with comorbidities.[2]

Obesity is most commonly approached as a problem of energy imbalance; however, more recent analyses have suggested that obesity should also be interpreted within the scope of psychiatric diseases.[13] From an energy standpoint, obesity or weight gain is thought to result from a net positive energy balance, where energy intake (food consumption) exceeds energy expenditure (a combination of resting metabolic rate, physical activity, and the thermic effect of food). Theories for the burgeoning obesity epidemic are myriad, but the problem is multifactorial and is generally regarded as resulting from the perfect storm of more easily available food, higher caloric food, and more sedentary lifestyles than witnessed in previous centuries.

In addition to such environmental factors, genetic factors have been increasingly shown to play a role in obesity. The metabolic theory implies an imbalance of circulatory peptide hormones such as ghrelin, obestatin, nesfatin-1, leptin, and insulin interacting with genetic factors leading to obesity.[14-17] Ghrelin, insulin, and leptin have been shown to act directly on the central nervous system to modulate both metabolism and food intake behaviors.[18] The "incentive salience theory" of food reward recognizes a hedonic component as well as a reward-seeking, motivational component mediated by activation of the mesolimbic dopamine circuitry.[19-25] Dysregulation of the mesolimbic dopamine system has been implicated in binge eating.[22,24-26] In support of the "incentive salience theory," binge eating was included as a mental disorder in the fifth edition of the *Diagnostic and Statistical Manual of Mental Disorders* (DSM-5).

Whatever the cause, the population has been searching for an effective solution. The U.S. market is overcrowded with weight loss supplements, appetite suppressants, exercise plans, and dietary plans. Physicians have also been armed with weight loss medications that act on both sides of the energy equation. The failure of medications to control obesity has been the impetus for surgical treatments such as gastric bypass, gastric banding (gastroplasty), and intragastric balloon placement.[27-30] Although bariatric surgery has successfully facilitated weight loss in many patients refractory to other measures, there is a significant risk of morbidity and mortality associated with these procedures. Despite initial weight loss, some patients regain a significant amount of weight even with technically successful surgery.[31]

Deep brain stimulation (DBS) has become a well-established treatment option for movement disorders such as Parkinson's disease, essential tremor, and dystonia. Because of its effectiveness in the treatment of these diseases, the low rates of complications,[32] and the reversibility of the treatment modality, DBS is being investigated as a treatment option for medically refractory psychiatric conditions such as Tourette's syndrome, obsessive-compulsive disorder, and depression. The growing recognition of the brain as the source of metabolism and appetite control has led to a resurgence of interest in treating obesity with a brain surgery strategy such as DBS. To understand the rationale behind different potential brain targets for DBS in the treatment of obesity, we provide a review of the neuroanatomy linked with body weight and discuss the various studies supporting DBS as a treatment option.

ANATOMY

The hypothalamus is a structure composed of numerous nuclei, several of which have been implicated in feeding behavior as well as energy homeostasis. Feeding centers motivating food intake have been located in the lateral hypothalamus (LH), while the satiety center has been located in the ventromedial hypothalamus (VMH).[33-35] The solution to obesity, though, may be more complicated than just inhibiting feeding behavior or stimulating the satiety center. The motivational reward center for food intake and other pleasurable human activities is mediated by the nucleus accumbens (NAcc) and also likely plays a role in the development of morbid obesity.

Lateral Hypothalamus

The LH has long been implicated in feeding behavior and energy expenditure.[36] Lesioning of the LH has been shown to induce leanness and increased energy expenditure.[34,37] In humans, the LH measures approximately 6 × 5 × 3.5 mm in the largest dimensions laterally, anteroposteriorly, and dorsoventrally, respectively.[38] Portions of the LH lie just inferior to the fornix and directly superior and posterior to the optic nerve and chiasm. The lateral preoptic nucleus is located rostrally and the ventral tegmental area of the midbrain lies caudally.[39,40]

Ventromedial Hypothalamus

The VMH has been dubbed the "satiety center" and regulates feeding behavior and energy expenditure.[41,42] Lesions of the VMH induce weight gain in animals and lead to increased carcass lipid and hyperinsulinemia in rats, suggesting a metabolic bias toward obesity.[43,44] The VMH lies inferomedial to the LH and measures approximately 2 × 3 × 5 mm in the largest dimensions.[38] The VMH is surrounded by the optic nerve anteriorly, the mammillary body posteriorly, and the anterior commissure superiorly.[39,40]

Nucleus Accumbens

The NAcc is a ventral striatal region located inferior to the anterior limb of the internal capsule. It measures approximately

8 × 6 × 6 mm in the largest dimensions, making it slightly larger than the subthalamic nucleus, which measures approximately 8 × 4 × 4 mm.[38] The NAcc is ellipsoid in shape with the superior border located medially. The center of the NAcc is located about 3 mm anterior to the anterior commissure and approximately 6 mm lateral from midline. The optic nerve is located inferiorly and medially, and the anterior cerebral arteries are located inferiorly. The NAcc is divided into two subregions, the core and the shell.[45] Anatomic tracing studies have shown that the core region connects to extrapyramidal motor structures such as the ventral pallidum, subthalamic nucleus, and substantia nigra.[46] The shell region is believed to play a role in the complex mesolimbic pathway mediating reward. The shell receives input from the amygdala, hippocampus, prefrontal cortex, and thalamus.[46-48] In 2007, Smith and Berridge implicated simultaneous involvement of the NAcc shell and the ventral pallidum in favorable reactions to taste in rodents ("liking"), such as tongue protrusion.[49] The NAcc shell also showed independent control of food intake ("wanting"), suggesting that a direct communication exists between the reward processing and feeding centers of the brain. The colocalization of food intake and food reward processing within the NAcc makes this an attractive target for therapeutic modulation via DBS.

DEEP BRAIN STIMULATION THEORY

DBS initially developed as a step during stereotactic brain lesioning. Before ablating an area of the brain, electrical stimulation was often used to confirm the local neuroanatomy. Only recently has continuous DBS via a completely implantable system been available. Initially, the ventral intermediate nucleus of the thalamus was targeted for the treatment of tremor as an alternative to thalamotomy.[50] Today, DBS has become a well-established treatment for various movement disorders, although the mechanism remains poorly understood.

Theories suggesting that DBS inhibits brain structures draw support from the fact that high-frequency DBS often mimics the clinical effects of brain lesioning. Studies have shown that high-frequency stimulation to the subthalamic nucleus decreases output to the basal ganglia similar to subthalamotomy.[51,52] However, animal models seem to show that stimulation at low frequencies stimulates activity of the LH.[53-55] Newer theories of the DBS mechanism go beyond the simplistic idea of mere activation and inhibition and suggest that DBS may work by influencing oscillatory activity within brain circuits.[56]

ANIMAL STUDIES

In 1951, Anand and Brobeck demonstrated that bilateral electrolyte lesions in different regions of the hypothalamus affected food intake in rats and cats.[57] Bilateral LH destruction resulted in aphagia, whereas bilateral VMH destruction produced hyperphagia. If both areas were lesioned, the animals developed aphagia. Other hypothalamic lesions did not produce a change in feeding response. This landmark study led to more investigations in specific hypothalamic regions and the effects on feeding behaviors.

Lateral Hypothalamus

Multiple animal studies have shown that lesioning of the LH results in a decrease in body weight. Keesey and Powley in 1973 showed that rats undergoing LH ablation experienced an initial decrease in body weight that stabilized around the third week after lesioning.[58] Harrell and colleagues showed in 1975 that rats with LH lesions failed to gain weight as compared to sham-operated controls when given equal quantities of food via intragastric feeding.[59] The LH-lesioned rats were also found to lose weight more rapidly with total starvation, and they exhibited increased core body temperature.

The earliest stimulation study was performed in 1965 by Mendelson and Chorover.[53] Continuous low-frequency stimulation of the LH was performed in rats and revealed that the rats displayed food-seeking behavior despite being satiated. Folkow and Rubinstein showed similar experimental results in cats.[54] Cats with unilateral LH low-frequency stimulation manifested an exploratory response in which the duration of food-seeking activity was increased. The stimulation also augmented gastrointestinal blood flow and activation of vagal fibers to the gut. Herberg and Blundell showed similar results in 1967 with continuous 50-Hz stimulation to the LH.[55] Satiated rats with continuous low-frequency stimulation showed food-hoarding activity similar to the behavior produced by long-term food deprivation. These initial studies seem to indicate that continuous low-frequency stimulation is excitatory to the activity of the LH.

Sani and colleagues in 2007 demonstrated that bilateral high-frequency (180- to 200-Hz) LH stimulation in animals resulted in a 2.3% weight loss, whereas the unstimulated controls demonstrated a 13.8% weight gain.[60] Food intake remained unchanged between the two groups in this study, suggesting that high-frequency LH stimulation may affect body weight independently of food intake by means of increasing the resting metabolic rate. Unlike the low-frequency stimulation, high-frequency stimulation is believed to inhibit the activity of the LH and thus reduce food intake and increase metabolism. Hara and associates demonstrated that ablation of orexin neurons in the LH of animals led to late-onset obesity despite decreased food intake compared to controls.[61] This study supports theories arguing that the pathophysiology of obesity is much more complex than simple overeating and that successful obesity strategies will need to target more than feeding behavior.

Ventromedial Hypothalamus

Lesions to the VMH have been shown to induce hyperphagia and obesity in animals. In 1981, Cox and Powley demonstrated that female rats with electrolytic VMH lesions had significantly increased percentage of body fat and insulin levels compared to controls.[62] Feeding patterns were controlled by food delivery only when the control rats pushed a feeding bar, implicating a metabolic mechanism engendering obesity with VMH-lesioned animals. However, Penicaud and colleagues showed in 1983 that bilateral lesions of the VMH in rats induced hyperphagia and obesity.[63] The weight gain induced was similar to that shown in rats feeding after a prolonged fast.

Krasne implanted rats with bilateral electrodes to the VMH in 1962, demonstrating that when continuous low-frequency stimulation at 60 Hz was applied, hungry rats would stop eating.[64] Melega and associates also demonstrated that low-frequency stimulation (50 Hz) induced a significantly lower amount of weight gain when animals were fed double their normal diet, suggesting an increase in metabolic rate.[65] In 2012, Torres and colleagues demonstrated that implantation of electrodes in the third ventricle adjacent to the VMH with low-frequency stimulation at 80 Hz reduced body weight by 8% and body fat by 19% in monkeys, although frequencies at 130 Hz and 30 Hz produced no change.[66] Conversely, Laćan and colleagues illustrated that high-frequency VMH stimulation increased food consumption, although no significant weight gain was noted.[67]

Nucleus Accumbens

In 1985, Kelley and Stinus studied the effects of lesioning the mesolimbic dopamine system at either the ventral tegmental area or the NAcc.[68] Their study showed that lesions resulted in abolition of or significant reduction in hoarding activity in rats. The

TABLE 107-1 Inclusion and Exclusion Criteria for the Pilot Study Conducted by Whiting et al

Inclusion Criteria	Exclusion Criteria
Male or female patients age ≥18 yr	Prior brain surgery
BMI ≥40 kg/m² or ≥35 kg/m² with a comorbid condition (HTN, cardiovascular disease, sleep apnea, DM2, dyslipidemia)	Dementia or Mini-Mental State Examination score <25
Failure of bariatric surgery (gastric banding or bypass). "Failed bariatric surgery" is determined using the modified Reinhold classification as patients who are still >50% over their ideal body weight after a technically successful surgery.	Unable to fit into MRI or CT scanner (higher weight limit is for CT scanner: 400 lb)
Chronic obesity diagnosed by an eating disorder specialist with expertise in the treatment of obesity	Psychiatric disorder, including poorly controlled anxiety disorders, psychosis, bipolar disorder, active substance abuse, somatoform disorders, factitious disorders, dissociative disorders, and severe personality disorders, but excluding depression and binge eating
Stable at present body weight for a 6-mo period	Obesity as part of another medical condition, neurological injury or lesions, related to medication side effect, or as part of a genetic syndrome
Psychiatric evaluation	Unable to follow up for scheduled clinic visits
Karnofsky Performance Scale score >60	

From Whiting DM, Tomycz ND, Bailes J, et al. Lateral hypothalamic area deep brain stimulation for refractory obesity: a pilot study with preliminary data on safety, body weight, and energy metabolism. *J Neurosurg.* 2013;119(1):56-63.

BMI, body mass index; CT, computed tomography; DM2, diabetes mellitus type 2; HTN, hypertension; MRI, magnetic resonance imaging.

hoarding activity could be restored with levodopa. The authors hypothesized that the mesolimbic dopamine system is necessary for the facilitation of foraging responses under high levels of arousal. Maldonado-Irizarry and Kelley demonstrated in 1995 that lesions in the core versus the shell regions of the NAcc produced opposite effects on weight gain.[69] Rats with core lesions were found to have lower weights and hyperactivity when compared to controls, whereas rats with shell lesions had higher weight and normal activity when compared to controls.

Halpern and colleagues explored DBS of the NAcc using continuous high-frequency stimulation at 160 Hz in mice with DBS electrodes in the NAcc shell and dorsal striatum.[70] All mice were fed an obesity-inducing diet. DBS in the NAcc shell was found to reduce binge eating mediated by D_2 dopamine receptors, but not D_1 receptors. Chronic DBS of the NAcc shell demonstrated a reduction in caloric intake and weight loss.[70]

HUMAN STUDIES

Before any DBS studies in humans, hypothalamic control of feeding behavior was supported by case reports describing disease-related hypothalamic lesions. Kamalian and colleagues in 1975 described a case of an LH lesion secondary to multiple sclerosis that was associated with profound weight loss and cachexia.[71] Anorexia and weight loss have also been described in patients with infiltrating hypothalamic tumors.[72-74]

By 1953, stereotactic surgery on the human hypothalamus was reported for treating psychiatric diseases.[75] Quaade and coworkers reported a temporary weight loss in three patients after stereotactically lesioning the LH in 1974.[76] Interestingly, with intraoperative stimulation of the LH, the patients reported a sensation of hunger. Caloric intake was reduced in all three patients and none developed any endocrine abnormalities. Unfortunately, the weight loss was mild and not sustained.

The first report of DBS in human obesity was in 2008 by Hamani and associates.[77] A 50-year-old morbidly obese (BMI = 55.1 kg/m²) man underwent implantation of bilateral ventral hypothalamic DBS electrodes. He did report a decreased appetite when the stimulator was turned on but, more strikingly, the stimulation elicited the sensation of *déja vu* and improved memory recollection attributed to stimulation of the nearby fornix. This serendipitous finding has spearheaded investigations of DBS for Alzheimer's disease.

The first pilot study of bilateral LH-DBS in human patients with obesity was developed in 2012 and published in 2013.[78,79] Three patients meeting strict criteria for intractable obesity, including failed bariatric surgery, were chosen to participate (Table 107-1). Figure 107-1 demonstrates the preoperative planning for placement as well as a three-dimensional reconstruction of the placement of the leads in each of the three patients. Initial programming parameters derived from movement disorder DBS did not result in significant weight loss trends. One year after implantation of DBS leads, each patient was analyzed in a metabolic chamber, which is the "gold standard" for measuring metabolism in humans.[80] Programming was then changed based on specific contacts found to augment resting metabolic rate (RMR) during monopolar stimulation. These RMR-focused DBS parameter settings have been associated with promising weight loss trends (Table 107-2). Long-term follow-up on these patients is necessary to ascertain the effectiveness of this treatment, but this pilot study demonstrates that the LH can be safely explored with DBS in future studies.

ETHICS OF DEEP BRAIN STIMULATION FOR OBESITY

DBS has been established as a safe and effective treatment modality for several movement disorders and potentially for obesity, but ethical issues similar to those surrounding bariatric surgery pervade the utilization of DBS as a treatment option. These issues include unjust distribution of access to treatment, autonomy and informed consent, classification of obesity and selecting assessment end points, prejudice among health care professionals, intervention in people's life, and medicalization of appearance.[81] Some view obesity as being self-inflicted and not a disease. They argue that it should not be surgically managed because surgery modifies an otherwise healthy organ and that treatments should instead be geared toward modifying feeding and exercise behaviors. This argument was rejected by a comprehensive assessment on bariatric surgery using the European Network for Health Technology Assessment method, which included a fully integrated ethical analysis.[82] The analysis concluded that obesity should be treated as any other disease in health care, including surgical management when medical management is refractory. With the explosion of numerous types of bariatric surgeries, safety concerns along with increasing public scrutiny have led to the formation of numerous national boards as well as multidisciplinary teams to help regulate and define best practices and create standards of care.[83]

Bariatric surgery has become increasingly utilized in the treatment of obesity in the pediatric population, which is still

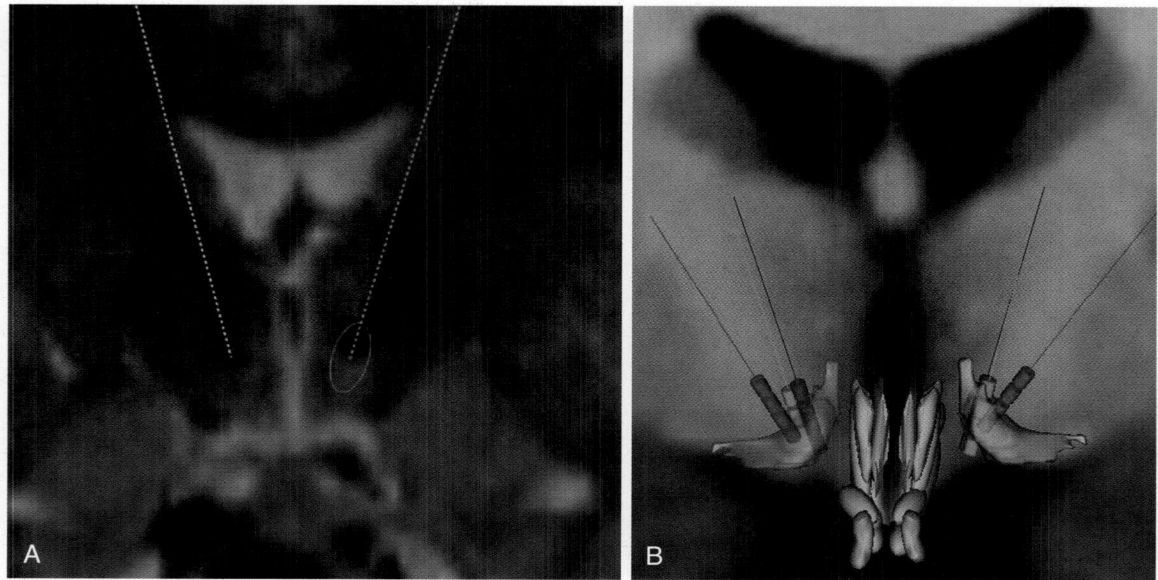

Figure 107-1. A, Magnetic resonance image demonstrating the preoperative planning for placement of deep brain stimulation leads in the lateral hypothalamus. **B,** Three-dimensional reconstruction demonstrating the lead placement on each of the three patients selected for the study. (Red, patient 1; green, patient 2; blue, patient 3.) *(**B**, Courtesy of Kirk W. Finnis, PhD, Medtronic Neuromodulation.)*

TABLE 107-2 Preliminary Body Weight Data on Patients with Bilateral LH-DBS Implantation for the Treatment of Obesity

Patient	Body Weight (kg) before Optimized Settings	Body Weight (kg) at Last Follow-Up	Months at Optimized Settings	Change in Body Weight
1	138.3	137	16	0.9% decrease
2	147.4	129.3	11	12.3% decrease
3	162.8	136.1	9	16.3% decrease

DBS, deep brain stimulation; LH, lateral hypothalamus.

considered controversial with numerous surrounding ethical issues.[81,84,85] Although DBS has been safely used in the pediatric population for the treatment of dystonia,[86] informed consent, patient autonomy, assessing the best interest of the child/adolescent, and social stigmatization may also be obstacles to the utilization of DBS for obese adolescents.

SUMMARY

Although bariatric surgery aims to control energy intake by modifying the anatomy of the alimentary tract, the underlying pathophysiology behind obesity may not be addressed. The operations are also associated with significant risks of morbidity and mortality, such as micronutrient deficiency,[87-91] hyperinsulinemic hypoglycemia,[92] ulcers and upper gastrointestinal bleeding,[93-95] osteoporosis/osteomalacia,[96,97] dumping syndrome,[98,99] internal hernias,[100-103] and nephrolithiasis.[104,105] A significant number of patients also "fail" under this management, regaining weight despite successful surgery.[31] Pisapia and colleagues determined that laparoscopic adjustable gastric banding and laparoscopic Roux-en-Y gastric bypass had success rates of 30% and 97% with complications rates of 22% and 33%, respectively.[106] The complication rate of DBS was found to be less than both gastric banding and Rous-en-Y gastric bypass.[106]

DBS has been established as a safe and effective treatment option for many movement disorders in both adult and pediatric populations. Environmental, genetic, and/or reward-seeking motivational factors are implicated in the pathophysiology of obesity. DBS studies illustrate that high-frequency stimulation of various areas of the brain may increase RMR, influence feeding behaviors, and inhibit the hedonic pathway. The pilot study by Whiting and colleagues demonstrated that bilateral LH-DBS can be safely performed in humans with none of the patients experiencing any adverse events, including psychological metric and biochemical studies.[79] This study also demonstrated that LH-DBS in humans increases RMR based on measurements within a metabolic chamber. The patients subjectively reported a modulation in hunger urge and increased energy, suggesting that the LH is an appropriate target for DBS in the treatment of obesity.[79]

DBS is emerging as a promising treatment option for obesity but much is still left to discover, such as proposed standards for patient selection, optimal timing for the intervention, and the determination of optimal location and stimulation parameters. Long-term follow-up on the patients enrolled in the initial pilot study by Whiting and colleagues[79] as well as further studies with larger cohorts will be beneficial in establishing DBS as a useful tool in the treatment of obesity.[79]

SUGGESTED READINGS

Gorgulho AA, Pereira JL, Krahl S, et al. Neuromodulation for eating disorders: obesity and anorexia. *Neurosurg Clin N Am*. 2014;25(1):147-157.

Halpern CH, Torres N, Hurtig HI, et al. Expanding applications of deep brain stimulation: a potential therapeutic role in obesity and addiction management. *Acta Neurochir (Wien)*. 2011;153(12):2293-2306.

Halpern CH, Wolf JA, Bale TL, et al. Deep brain stimulation in the treatment of obesity. *J Neurosurg*. 2008;109(4):625-634.

Hamani C, McAndrews MP, Cohn M, et al. Memory enhancement induced by hypothalamic/fornix deep brain stimulation. *Ann Neurol*. 2008;63(1):119-123.

McClelland J, Bozhilova N, Campbell I, et al. A systematic review of the effects of neuromodulation on eating and body weight: evidence from human and animal studies. *Eur Eat Disord Rev*. 2013;21(6):436-455.

Pisapia JM, Halpern CH, Williams NN, et al. Deep brain stimulation compared with bariatric surgery for the treatment of morbid obesity: a decision analysis study. *Neurosurg Focus*. 2010;29(2):E15.

Quaade F, Vaernet K, Larsson S. Stereotaxic stimulation and electrocoagulation of the lateral hypothalamus in obese humans. *Acta Neurochir (Wien)*. 1974;30:111-117.

Sankar T, Tierney TS, Hamani C. Novel applications of deep brain stimulation. *Surg Neurol Int*. 2012;3(suppl 1):S26-S33.

Taghva A, Corrigan JD, Rezai AR. Obesity and brain addiction circuitry: implications for deep brain stimulation. *Neurosurgery*. 2012;71(2):224-238.

Tomycz ND, Whiting DM, Oh MY. Deep brain stimulation for obesity—from theoretical foundations to designing the first human pilot study. *Neurosurg Rev*. 2012;35(1):37-42.

Whiting DM, Tomycz ND, Bailes J, et al. Lateral hypothalamic area deep brain stimulation for refractory obesity: a pilot study with preliminary data on safety, body weight, and energy metabolism. *J Neurosurg*. 2013;119(1):56-63.

See a full reference list on ExpertConsult.com 

108 Deep Brain Stimulation for Alzheimer's Disease

Vibhor Krishna, Francesco Sammartino, Nir Lipsman, and Andres M. Lozano

Alzheimer's disease (AD) is the most common form of dementia in elderly people.[1] With 7.7 million incident cases of dementia annually worldwide, the prevalence of AD is steadily increasing. Affected patients experience a relentless decline in memory and cognition that eventually ends in death within 3 to 9 years.[2] The pathologic hallmark is the presence of widespread cortical neuritic plaques containing a central amyloid core surrounded by reactive microglia and astrocytes.[3] Considerable uncertainty surrounds the pathogenesis of AD.[4] Proponents of the amyloid hypothesis posit that Aβ-42 peptide initiates a cascade that eventually leads to failure of synaptic transmission and neuronal loss. Consequently, several therapeutic strategies have been developed either to decrease the production or to enhance amyloid clearing.[5-8] However none of these amyloid-based therapeutics have demonstrated compelling efficacy in randomized controlled trials. Development of effective treatment strategies for AD remains one of the biggest unmet needs in clinical neuroscience.

In this chapter we review the history of neurosurgical interventions for AD, insights into the pathophysiologic processes, results of neuromodulation trials, and the rationale for treating the network dysfunction in AD.

HISTORY OF SURGICAL INTERVENTION FOR ALZHEIMER'S DISEASE

Investigators from around the world have studied a variety of neurosurgical interventions for the treatment of AD (Table 108-1). Silverberg and colleagues[9] used ventriculoperitoneal shunts in patients with AD to enhance amyloid and protein tau clearance. The initial promising results from the pilot study were not replicated in the large-scale randomized controlled trial, which was stopped because of the futility of interim results.[10] Goldsmith[11] transposed the omentum to the cortical surface on the premise that this could possibly improve cerebral hypoperfusion. There is no controlled evidence of efficacy of this intervention. Vagus nerve stimulation has also been evaluated in small case series, and the efficacy of this intervention remains to be evaluated in the setting of randomized trials.[12]

Several researchers have attempted to mitigate ongoing neuronal loss by the injection of growth factors, cellular grafts, and, more recently, gene therapy.[13-17] The strategy of intraventricular growth factor injection (nerve growth factor [NGF] and G_{M1} ganglioside) showed promise but was not pursued further because of its uncertain efficacy and undesirable side effects (pain and weight loss).[14] Gene therapy for targeted NGF delivery to the nucleus basalis of Meynert (NBM) was found safe in the phase 1 trial.[15,17] A phase 2 trial of NGF gene therapy has finished recruitment, but results are not available yet. The injection of umbilical cord stem cells for reversal of amyloid deposition in the bilateral hippocampi and right precuneus is also in the initial stages of investigation.[16]

PATHOLOGIC PROCESS IN ALZHEIMER'S DISEASE

Functional Disconnection of Structurally Preserved Brain Regions

The classical "staging" of AD is based on the examination of pathologic changes (with regard to tau protein and amyloid β [Aβ]) in postmortem brains.[18] The severity of pathologic changes is correlated with the overall cognitive function of the individual at death (interindividual progression). Longitudinal follow-up of affected patients with serial structural and amyloid imaging (with the use of Pittsburgh compound B) has provided insights into the pathologic progression of disease in individual patients over time (intraindividual progression).[19] According to a current hypothesis, the underlying pathologic process in sporadic cases of AD may involve two independent proteinopathies (tau and Aβ).[4,18] The deposition of tau protein is first detected in the subcortical areas (brain stem nuclei: e.g., locus caeruleus, raphe nuclei, and hypothalamus) before the deposition of cortical amyloid. The accumulation of Aβ is a slow process that can precede, by as much as decades, the appearance of hippocampal and cortical atrophy. At a cellular level, one view is that abnormal protein accumulations produce oxidative stress and aberrant reentry of mature neurons into the G_1 and G_2 phases of the cell cycle (the so-called two-hit hypothesis).[20] The consequent neuronal injury is believed to be responsible for failure of synaptic transmission and producing the profound clinical symptoms of AD.[2,21,22]

Certain brain networks are more susceptible to dysfunction in AD, especially when structural disease in these areas is relatively mild.[23] For example, the degree of dysfunction and atrophy are well correlated in the medial and lateral temporal regions. In contrast, the posterior cingulate gyrus and precuneus (elements of the default-mode network) have marked hypometabolism with relative structural preservation.[23] In certain individuals at increased risk for developing AD (ApoE-4 allele carriers), the evidence of suppressed glucose metabolism in the default-mode network can be detected several years before the onset of any clinical symptoms.[24] This functional disconnection (network dysfunction) of structurally preserved brain regions is implicated in the marked cognitive and memory disturbance that characterizes AD. Restoring function in these activity impaired but relatively anatomically preserved areas could be a useful approach in treating AD.

Surgical Trials in Alzheimer's Disease

Deep Brain Stimulation of the Fornix

The modulation of memory networks during deep brain stimulation (DBS) surgery was discovered by serendipity during hypothalamic stimulation for treatment of morbid obesity.[25] The trajectory of the electrode (Medtronic 3387, Medtronic Inc., Minneapolis, MN) was targeted to the ventromedial and lateral hypothalamus to modulate appetite and hunger. Intraoperative stimulation in the hypothalamus produced an unexpected and striking recall of autobiographic memories. The experimental effect was time-locked to stimulation and was present at a threshold of 5 V without the appearance of adverse effects. The similar effects and the topography of stimulation-induced memory along each of the four electrode contacts suggested that stimulation of the fornix, which ran parallel to the DBS electrode, was the probable mechanism of action. The pulse generator was then programmed to deliver chronic continuous stimulation at 3 V, a 130-Hz frequency, and a 60-μsec pulse width. The patient could not feel any effects of stimulation at this setting, and these parameters were chosen empirically on the basis of the absence of adverse effects. At 1 month, continuous stimulation produced unexpected large improvements in the verbal and associative

TABLE 108-1 Surgical Interventions Investigated in Patients with Alzheimer's Disease

Intervention	Site	Proposed Mechanism	Outcome	Reference
Ventriculoperitoneal shunt placement	Intraventricular	Enhanced clearance of CSF amyloid and tau	Trial stopped because of futility of treatment	Silverberg et al[10]
Omental transplantation	Cortical surface	Enhanced cerebral perfusion to salvage "at risk" neuronal tissue	Small case series with unclear benefit	Goldsmith[11]
Human mesenchymal stem cell injection	Bilateral hippocampi and right precuneus	Paracrine effects of stem cells to reduce amyloid plaques	No major adverse events in feasibility study	Kim et al[48]
Growth factor infusion (NGF and G_{M1} ganglioside)	Intraventricular	Rescue from ongoing cholinergic neuronal loss	Uncertain benefit with significant side effects	Eriksdotter et al[14] Augustinsson et al[13]
Gene therapy with CERE-110	Nucleus basalis of Myenert	Rescue from ongoing cholinergic neuronal loss	Phase 2 clinical trial, ongoing (NCT00876863)	Rafii et al[17]
Vagus nerve stimulation	Cervical vagus nerve	Enhanced cognition	Some benefit in small case series No controlled trials	Merrill et al[12]

CSF, cerebrospinal fluid; NGF, nerve growth factor.

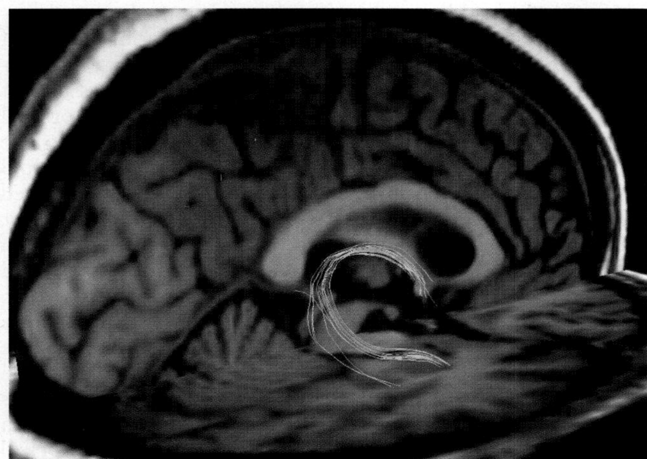

Figure 108-1. Three-dimensional view of the anatomy of the fornix, as depicted by tractography. The fimbriae of fornix originate from the tail of the hippocampus and course posteriorly into the crus and body of the fornix. The body of the fornix is located in the roof of the third ventricle; then it divides into precommissural and postcommissural segments, which terminate in the basal frontal region and mammillary bodies, respectively. The postcommissural segment of the fornix is vertically oriented and closely related to the anterior wall of the third ventricle.

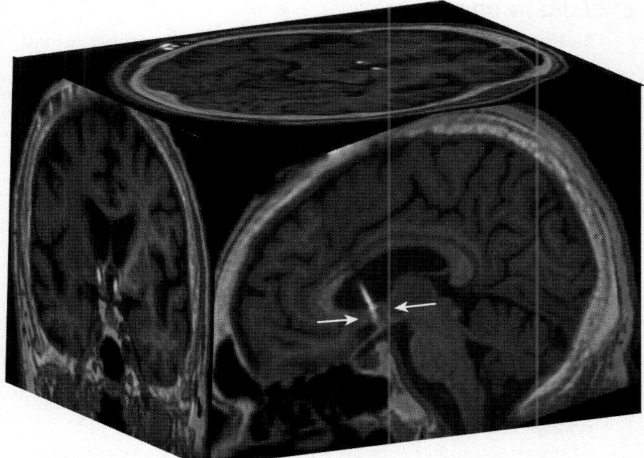

Figure 108-2. Deep brain stimulation in a patient with Alzheimer's disease. Preoperative magnetic resonance images fused with postoperative computed tomographic scans after deep brain stimulation of the fornix *(left arrow).* The stereotactic targeting is performed to place electrodes 2 mm anterior to the fornix *(right arrow).* The dorsal optic tract underlies the electrode tip. The trajectory is optimized to include the entire length of the postcommissural columns of the fornix bilaterally.

memory (the subject had normal preoperative cognitive status). The changes in hippocampus-mediated memory function were quantitatively assessed in a double-blind manner after 12 months of continuous stimulation. The most interesting finding was a marked increase in recollection memory, which implied enhanced hippocampus-mediated memory function.

This sentinel observation was the basis for and led to a phase 1 study of fornix-DBS to activate the circuit of Papez in six patients with mild to moderate AD (Fig. 108-1).[26] The bilateral target chosen was 2 mm anterior and parallel to the fornix column, so as to avoid injury to the fibers of the fornix (Fig. 108-2). The stimulation was initiated 2 weeks after implantation (parameters: 3 to 3.5 V, 130-Hz frequency, and 90-μsec pulse width), and outcomes were assessed with the Alzheimer's Disease Assessment Scale–Cognition subscale (ADAS-Cog) and the Mini Mental State Examination (MMSE).[27] At 12 months, there was a mean increase (worsening) of 4.2 points in ADAS-Cog scores; one patient exhibited improved in ADAS-Cog scores, and the scores of two others remained relatively stable. Furthermore, the patients with less severe preoperative cognitive impairment had milder decline in ADAS-Cog score after 12 months of stimulation.

Fontaine and associates[28] reported a case of fornix-DBS in a 71-year-old patient with AD who had a preoperative ADAS-Cog score of 9 (MMSE score, 29). Fornix-DBS electrodes were implanted as described previously, and stimulation (bipolar setting between contacts 0 and 1 at 2.5 V, 130-Hz frequency and 210-μsec pulse width) was delivered continuously after the first postoperative week. The patient tolerated the surgery well and demonstrated a global stabilization of cognitive scores over 1 year of chronic stimulation, in comparison with baseline scores. This preliminary work also suggests a possible trend toward a slower rate of cognitive decline in patients with AD who receive fornix stimulation. Interestingly, DBS activated the default mode network and increased glucose utilization in cortical areas affected by AD. A follow-up phase 2 randomized trial is currently under way to evaluate the efficacy of fornix-DBS for AD (Box 108-1).

BOX 108-1 Inclusion and Exclusion Criteria for the Phase 2 Trial of Deep Brain Stimulation of the Fornix (ADvance Trial) for Mild to Moderate Alzheimer's Disease

INCLUSION CRITERIA

1. 45-85 years of age
2. Probable AD (according to the National Institute of Aging Alzheimer's Disease Association criteria)
3. Meeting criteria of mild to moderate AD on cognitive and behavioral rating scales
4. If female, subjects who are postmenopausal or surgically sterile or willing to use birth control methods for the duration of the study
5. An available caregiver willing to participate
6. Living at home and likely to remain at home during the study duration
7. Taking stable dose of cholinesterase inhibitor for at least 60 days

EXCLUSION CRITERIA

1. Not meeting the inclusion criteria on cognitive and behavioral rating scales
2. Ongoing major psychiatric disorders such as schizophrenia, bipolar disorder, or major depressive disorder, based on psychiatric consult at screening visit
3. History of head trauma in the 2 years before study participation
4. Structural brain lesions, including brain tumor, subdural hematoma, or other clinically significant space-occupying lesion on CT or MRI
5. Mental retardation
6. Current alcohol or substance abuse
7. Contraindications to PET (e.g., insulin-dependent diabetes)
8. Contraindications to MRI scanning, including implanted metallic devices or claustrophobia or discomfort in confined spaces
9. Abnormal laboratory results that would preclude participation in the study
10. Cardiovascular or neurovascular disorder
11. Unstable doses of any medication prescribed for the treatment of memory loss or Alzheimer's disease
12. Non-AD medications that would preclude participation in the study
13. Inability or unwillingness to comply with protocol follow-up requirements
14. Life expectancy of <1 year
15. Active enrollment in another concurrent clinical trial

AD, Alzheimer's disease; CT, computed tomography; MRI, magnetic resonance imaging; PET, positron emission tomography.

Rationale for Fornix Neuromodulation in Alzheimer's Disease

Recruiting the Functionally Disconnected Regions. The rationale of fornix-DBS in AD is to activate dysfunctional memory network and potentially reverse or ameliorate the memory and cognitive deficit. This strategy parallels that of functional neurosurgery for movement disorders, especially Parkinson's disease. The underlying pathologic process in Parkinson's disease involves the depletion of dopaminergic neurons in the substantia nigra. The lack of dopamine results in abnormal firing of the network nodes in the basal ganglia motor circuits.[29] As a result, affected patients experience significant functional motor impairment (exhibiting tremor, bradykinesia, and rigidity) despite a largely intact primary somatomotor system. DBS in these network nodes (subthalamic nucleus or globus pallidus internus) modulates the abnormal activity and enables significant improvement in motor symptoms of Parkinson's disease.[30] This procedure addresses the network dysfunction resulting from the deficiency of dopamine without directly addressing dopamine deficiency in the nigral neurons.[31] In AD, fornix-DBS does not directly aim to diminish the Aβ deposits in the hippocampus and elsewhere; instead, DBS may address the dysfunction in the cognition and memory networks and improve the behavioral dysfunction in patients with AD.[32] As discussed previously, there is a mismatch between the topographic distribution of structural (cortical atrophy) and functional (glucose uptake) disease in AD.[23] For example, in the parietal association areas, glucose uptake appears to be downregulated significantly, despite relatively mild atrophy.[23] This pattern is consistent with functional disconnection and may potentially be reversed by electrical modulation of memory network.[32]

Preclinical Studies of Neuromodulation of Memory Network in Rodents. Several rodent experiments have investigated the effects of high-frequency, acute stimulation (typically for a few hours each day and lasting less than 1 week) in the limbic circuit (fornix, entorhinal cortex, perforant path, and anterior nucleus of the thalamus) on memory and neurogenesis.[33-37] Enhanced neurogenesis was reported from our laboratory and others as a result of stimulation of anterior nucleus of thalamus and entorhinal cortex.[33,34,38] High-frequency stimulation, when applied to the anterior nucleus of thalamus, resulted in a twofold to threefold enhancement of hippocampal neurogenesis.[38] The newly formed neurons were able to be integrated in the hippocampal circuitry, which resulted in functional improvement observed 1 month after stimulation.[34] In a different line of investigation, Stone and colleagues[33] investigated neurogenesis after high-frequency stimulation (130 Hz, 0-500 μA) of the entorhinal cortex in mice. Low current density stimulation (50 μA, 30-120 min) at this site enhanced neurogenesis in the granular cell layer of the ipsilateral dentate gyrus with a peak 3 to 5 days after stimulation.[33] Six weeks after stimulation, the animals showed enhanced performance on spatial memory tasks. This improvement, which could be blocked by antimitotic drugs, was probably mediated by the stimulation-induced neurogenesis and the integration, after 6 weeks, of these new and now fully matured neurons into memory circuits.

Hescham and associates[37] performed bilateral fornix-DBS in an AD rat model created by injection of scopolamine to cause spatial memory impairment. They delivered various current amplitudes (0, 50, 100, and 200 mA) at 100-Hz or 10-Hz stimulation frequencies, with a pulse width of 100 msec and bipolar configuration. The stimulation was started 2 min before the behavioral testing and lasted for the duration of each test session. Fornix-DBS improved the spatial memory performance. Furthermore, the stimulation intensity (100 mA with 100 Hz and 200 mA with 10 Hz), not the frequency, was associated with significant clinical improvement.

Potential Mechanisms Underlying the Effect of Fornix–Deep Brain Stimulation

Cerebral Activation. In the phase 1 trial of fornix-DBS, the topography of cerebral activation was studied with standardized low-resolution electromagnetic tomography.[26] Low-frequency bipolar stimulation of the fornix activated the medial temporal lobe structures at short latencies (38-52 msec). Similar activation of the parietal lobe, posterior cingulate, and precuneus was observed at longer latencies (102-256 msec). These findings are consistent with the transsynaptic activation of the Papez circuit by focal delivery of DBS to the fornix. Commensurate with the electrographic findings, increased cortical metabolism was also observed in patients on both the 1- and 12-month positron emission tomographic (PET) scans. The enhanced metabolism was particularly observed in the default-mode network (posterior cingulate, parietal cortex, and precuneus). Also, metabolism significantly increased in the medial and lateral temporal cortex and in the basal frontal regions, which are known to be significantly affected by AD. Similar improvements in cerebral metabolism were observed in the medial temporal lobes in another published study of fornix-DBS.[38] Cerebral activation has the potential to alter the deposition of Aβ. Bero and colleagues,[39] using microdialysis in vitro, discovered an inverse relationship between interstitial Aβ and lactate levels. Whether fornix-DBS has a disease-modifying effect remains to be investigated.

Effect on Hippocampal Oscillations. The electrical stimulation of memory networks may also influence hippocampal oscillations, especially the theta rhythm. In electrical stimulation experiments to modulate memory, bilateral hippocampal stimulation, either during recognition or recall, impaired memory function.[40] Even brief electrical pulses (1 msec), when applied to bilateral hippocampi during encoding, result in significant memory deficits.[41] In contrast, stimulation of hippocampal input through the perforant pathway, via the entorhinal cortex or via the fornix, improved memory.[25,42,43] This improvement depends on hippocampal neurogenesis, and the phase resetting of theta oscillation is a biomarker of enhanced hippocampal plasticity and neurogenesis.[44] Suthana and associates[43] studied this phenomenon in patients with epilepsy in whom depth electrodes were implanted. They observed that high-frequency stimulation of the entorhinal region during memory encoding enhanced spatial learning and was associated with significant resetting of the theta rhythm.

Deep Brain Stimulation of the Nucleus Basalis of Meynert

Another DBS-based approach in AD is to modulate the cholinergic deficit in AD through the use of low-frequency stimulation of the NBM, which presumably enhances cholinergic transmission.[45] Besides correcting cholinergic dysfunction, NBM-DBS is proposed to release neurotrophic factors and potentially rescue neurons from the ongoing loss.[46,47] Kuhn and colleagues[45] published preliminary results from a double-blind, sham-controlled phase 1 trial of low-frequency NBM-DBS in six patients with mild to moderate AD. The primary outcome of the study was the improvement in the ADAS-Cog score after 1 year of stimulation. Electrodes (Medtronic 3387) were implanted bilaterally to target the Ch4 bundle inside the NBM because this is the most dense cell cluster of the nucleus. Patients were randomly assigned to receive either (1) low-frequency stimulation (–2.5 V, 90 µsec, 20 Hz) followed by a crossover no-stimulation phase for 2 weeks or (2) vice versa. In the second step, all patients received chronic stimulation as previously described. The MMSE score improved by 0.8 points at the end of the first 2 weeks of active stimulation, and the overall ADAS-Cog score decreased by 3 points after 12 months (slower-than-expected decline). A global 2% to 5% increase in metabolism in the amygdalohippocampal and temporal regions was observed in three of four patients.

Deep Brain Stimulation of the Nucleus Basalis of Meynert for Other Types of Dementias

DBS has been investigated for a few other forms of dementia. The dementia associated with Parkinson's disease is being investigated in a phase 1/2 study (NCT01701544). NBM-DBS shall be performed from the deepest contact of the globus pallidus internus. Another ongoing phase 1 trial is aimed at evaluating the effects of NBM-DBS for patients with Lewy body dementia (NCT01340001). Six patients with either a confirmed or probable diagnosis of Lewy body dementia with moderate cognitive deficits are to be in this ongoing trial.

CONCLUSION AND FUTURE DIRECTIONS

Neuromodulation appears to be a promising potential therapy for the treatment of memory network dysfunction in AD. Although few small, open-label case series have helped establish the safety of DBS in AD, additional work is necessary to demonstrate efficacy. A multicenter, double-blind, sham-controlled phase 2 trial (the ADvance trial) has enrolled patients with AD for fornix stimulation (see Box 108-1). In addition to studying the memory and cognitive outcomes, this trial is also designed to assess both structural and functional radiologic outcomes such as changes in glucose metabolism and atrophy of the hippocampus and neocortex. These investigations will provide significant mechanistic insights into the effects of this therapy.

Several important questions need to be answered in order to enhance the translational potential of this experimental therapy:

1. Which brain targets are optimal for deep brain stimulation?
2. Which patients are most likely to benefit from brain stimulation, and what are the predictors of good or poor outcomes?
3. What are the putative mechanisms of DBS in AD, and which structures along the cognitive/memory networks are being influenced?
4. Does this strategy have disease-modifying effects?

The future of brain stimulation for disorders of memory and cognition will encompass both technical and conceptual advances. The former will include improvements in battery life, as well as optimization and individualization of stimulation parameters. Other neuromodulation strategies, such as those involving optogenetics, nanotechnology, and focused ultrasonography, may further provide additional tools for influencing brain networks. Such strategies may not only shed light on the mechanisms of network dysfunction in AD but also may provide alternative means of accessing, and correcting, brain disease. A unified front that harnesses advances in genetics, biochemistry, engineering, and clinical medicine offers the best hope for developing an effective treatment for one of humanity's most challenging and devastating conditions.

SUGGESTED READINGS

Chetelat G, Desgranges B, Landeau B, et al. Direct voxel-based comparison between grey matter hypometabolism and atrophy in Alzheimer's disease. *Brain*. 2008;131(Pt 1):60-71.

Hescham S, Lim LW, Jahanshahi A, et al. Deep brain stimulation of the forniceal area enhances memory functions in experimental dementia: the role of stimulation parameters. *Brain Stimul*. 2013;6(1):72-77.

Kuhn J, Hardenacke K, Lenartz D, et al. Deep brain stimulation of the nucleus basalis of Meynert in Alzheimer's dementia. *Mol Psychiatry*. 2015;20(3):353-360.

Laxton AW, Lozano AM. Deep brain stimulation for the treatment of Alzheimer disease and dementias. *World Neurosurg*. 2013;80(3-4): S28.e21-S28.e28.

Laxton AW, Tang-Wai DF, McAndrews MP, et al. A phase I trial of deep brain stimulation of memory circuits in Alzheimer's disease. *Ann Neurol*. 2010;68(4):521-534.

Toda H, Hamani C, Fawcett AP, et al. The regulation of adult rodent hippocampal neurogenesis by deep brain stimulation. *J Neurosurg*. 2008;108(1):132-138.

See a full reference list on ExpertConsult.com

109 Neuroprosthetics

Jarod L. Roland, Wilson Z. Ray, and Eric C. Leuthardt

Neuroprosthetics is a rapidly expanding field for which the emerging technologies will affect the practice of neurosurgery. A neuroprosthetic in its most simplistic form is a device that supplants or supplements the input or output of the nervous system. The fundamental application is to bypass a deficit caused by disease or to augment existing function for improved performance. There are numerous technical approaches to accomplish this goal. These variations in approach lead to a diversity of form factors that have different clinical and surgical considerations. Generally speaking, neuroprosthetic devices have numerous synonymous names, such as brain-computer interface (BCI), brain-machine interface, neural interface system, direct neural interface, mind-machine interface, and other nomenclature that similarly describes an interface of the nervous system with an external device.

Research and development of neuroprosthetics requires integration across a diversity of technical and scientific disciplines including neuroscience, computer science, and engineering. Neuroprosthetic research had its conceptual inception long before the advent of an organized academic field of study. Seminal work was described by Vidal, who upon observing modulations of signals in the electroencephalogram, had the foresight in 1973 to ask, "Can these observable electrical brain signals be put to work as carriers of information in man-computer communication or for the purpose of controlling such external apparatus as prosthetic devices or spaceships?"[1,2] Although the proposition of spaceship control has yet to be realized, control of a prosthetic device is now becoming commonplace in the translational research laboratory.

Although computational abilities were initially restrictive, advances in microprocessor design and digital signal analysis now outperform neuroprosthetics requirements such that computational speed is no longer a rate-limiting factor. Similar technologic advances have provided the necessary tools for device development, allowing innovative applications to introduce motor, sensory, visual, auditory, speech, and other modalities to the field. Here we review these applications in neuroprosthetics by presenting the state of the art across a multitude of modalities and emphasize the role of neurosurgeons in its translation from fundamental research to clinical application.

INTERFACE MODALITIES

The goal of a neuroprosthetic device is to replace or augment an individual's function by interfacing an external device with the nervous system. A classical understanding of a neuroprosthetic is a device that records brain signals from the user (i.e., signal input), computationally analyzes those signals to infer the user's intentions, and then transforms those intentions to an external effector output. There are multiple modalities to achieve this goal. The source of signals used as input to the device can range from individual neuronal spiking, to field potential from cortical ensembles, to action potentials conducted by peripheral nerves. Output effectors are also wide ranging. Examples include computer cursor movement, robotic arm control, and reanimation of paretic limbs. By reversing the direction of information transfer one can similarly develop an input device. In this scenario the device input is recorded from the external environment and converted into an appropriate stimulus delivered to the nervous system. These devices may be complementary to an output device, such as sensory input to accompany the robotic arm of a prosthesis for tactile or proprioceptive feedback. In contrast, it may be independent in application, such as the cochlear implant, with which acoustic information recorded from a microphone is translated into corresponding electrical stimulus delivered to the acoustic nerve, thereby providing auditory perception to the otherwise deaf ear. In the broadest sense, neuroprosthetics can be categorized as "output neural interfaces" that convert the brain's intentions to external actions or as "input neural interfaces," which take information from the environment and convert it into the brain's perceptions.

Neuroprosthetics may also be broadly characterized by the modality of operation (e.g., motor, somatosensory, speech, auditory) and the source of neural interface (e.g., single-unit neuron, cortical local field potential, peripheral nerve). To date, the most successful neuroprosthesis that has seen widespread adoption and success in clinical application is the cochlear implant. This technology has played an ever-expanding role in otology. For neurosurgery, the developing neuroprosthetic research that is poised to affect the field is motor output prosthetics. The general goal of a motor output prosthesis is to develop a device capable of interpreting an individual's movement intentions in real time and direct the output to an effector such as a robotic limb. With these canonical examples in mind, the various modalities of interfacing with the nervous system and their clinical implications will be explored.

ELECTROENCEPHALOGRAPHY

Electroencephalography (EEG) is a commonly used means of studying cerebral electrophysiology because of its noninvasive nature and clinical familiarity. Through electrodes placed on a subject's scalp, an investigator is able to record the neural rhythms manifested in electrical potentials resulting from complex interactions of the neurons and glial cells that make up the cerebrum's functional systems. The electroencephalogram, therefore, represents measurement of summated electrical potentials from the electrochemical interaction of a vast number of cells, both neuronal and glial in origin.[3]

Measured electrical potentials are then digitized with the aid of biosignal amplifiers and analog-to-digital converters for computational analysis. By periodically sampling a continuous signal in regular short intervals, discrete values are obtained and stored in series, thereby converting the signal from an analog to a digital domain. The time-varying signal is then analyzed as the sum of multiple sinusoidal signals of varying frequency and amplitudes. This process commonly employs the discrete Fourier transform and is said to convert from the time domain to the frequency domain. In the frequency domain one can observe the change in power at a given frequency over time, which is known as time-frequency analysis. The distribution of signal power across a range of frequencies is the signal spectrum, and its plot over time is the spectrogram. By time-locking the sampled signal to measured subject data, correlations are made between cortical activity and task performance. One such observation in signals measured over the motor homunculus is the reliably reproducible decrease in spectral power in the 8- to 13-Hz range with overt or imagined movement of the hand contralateral to the side of cortical recording.

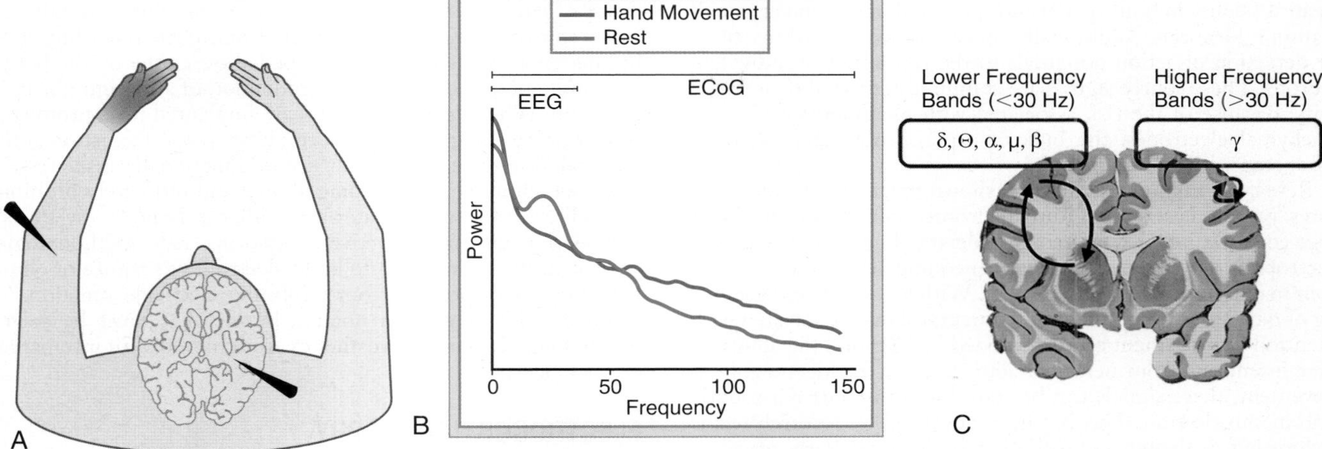

Figure 109-1. Brain signals. A, Volitional movement of the right hand during electrode recording from the contralateral cortex (electroencephalogram [EEG], electrocorticogram [ECoG], or intraparenchymal) or ipsilateral peripheral nerve.[46] **B,** Cortical field potentials with characteristic power decreases in low frequencies (mu rhythm) and power increases in high gamma range. **C,** Thalamocortical and corticocortical rhythms.[58] *(**B,** Modified from Leuthardt EC, Schalk G, Moran D, et al. The emerging world of motor neuroprosthetics: a neurosurgical perspective.* Neurosurgery. *2006;59:1-14.)*

The electroencephalogram in humans is commonly segmented into meaningful components in the frequency domain and represented by Greek alphabet designations. These are classically defined as the delta band below 4 Hz, theta band from 4 to 8 Hz, mu band from 8 to 13 Hz (also known as alpha), beta band from 13 to 30 Hz, and gamma band beyond 30 Hz.[4] The mu rhythm is described in relation to motor electrophysiology over the rolandic cortex (Fig. 109-1A). Decreases in mu band spectral power with activity (Fig. 109-1B) are thought to represent event-related desynchronization.[5] This release of synchronized cortical rhythms is thought to be orchestrated by thalamocortical circuits modulating motor cortical systems (Fig. 109-1C).[3,6] Real-time measurements of power fluctuations in this spectral band provide a source signal for motor actions. Wolpaw and colleagues demonstrated the transformation of this source signal to effector output by training subjects to control a virtual cursor displayed on a computer screen. In effect, the velocity of cursor movement was derived in real time from changes in the mu spectral power volitionally modulated by the user.[7] Importantly, similar modulations of the electroencephalogram are also similarly observed in imagined motor actions, thereby allowing similar control without peripheral activation of motor units.[8]

EEG correlates of imagery-based activity are critical for the clinical application to disease-affected patient populations. Translation to those affected by neuromuscular disorders would be impractical if overt motor function were required for the production of an adequate source control signal. By definition then, those who would benefit from such a prosthesis would be the very population incapable of initiating a control signal, obviating its clinical applicability. It is therefore critical that individuals affected by neurological disorders such as amyotrophic lateral sclerosis, locked-in syndrome, or spinal cord injury (SCI) are still capable of modulating cortical rhythms in the absence of end-organ effect. Thankfully, preservation of this function has been demonstrated in subjects with long-term deficits in whom volitional modulation of stable electrophysiologic structure was maintained.[9-11]

With these basic tenets in place, EEG-based BCIs have led the field in human neuroprosthetic research. However, one major shortfall of EEG is the physical separation of the cortical source signal and the scalp-based recording electrodes. This distance is occupied by the meninges, bone, and scalp, which results in limited spectral and spatial resolution. For a scalp-based electrode to record a measurable signal from the cortex, electrical potentials must be summated across an area of cortex approximately 6 cm^2 in diameter.[3] The spatial resolution of separable source signals is thereby inherently limited. Similarly, destructive summation of temporally overlapping signals results in cancellation and therefore unresolved higher frequencies in EEG recordings. These limitations may be mitigated in part by intracranial placement of recording electrodes at the cost of increased invasiveness (Fig. 109-2).[12]

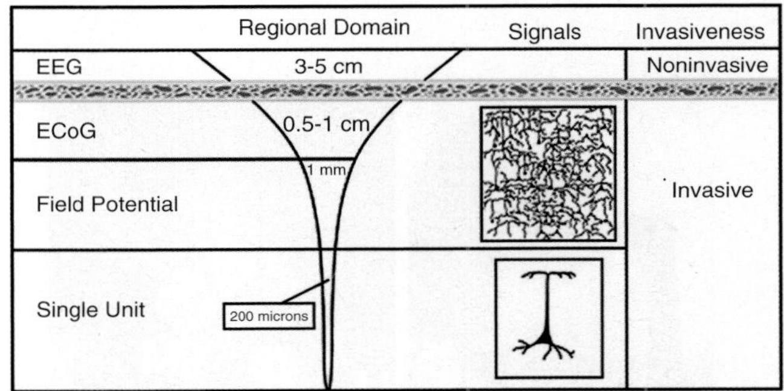

Figure 109-2. Cortical recording interfaces. Spatial scale *(center)* is diagrammed in order of least to most invasive modality (*left*) with representative signal source *(right).* ECoG, electrocorticogram; EEG, electroencephalogram. *(From Leuthardt EC, Schalk G, Moran D, et al. The emerging world of motor neuroprosthetics: a neurosurgical perspective.* Neurosurgery. *2006;59:1-14.)*

INTRAPARENCHYMAL ELECTRODES

Recording electrodes placed directly into the substance of the brain, known as intraparenchymal electrodes, allow for high-resolution measurements of electrical potentials. Although maximally invasive, this method of signal acquisition provides the greatest fidelity in both spatial and spectral domains in very small anatomic locations. Additionally, spike-sorting algorithms allow for detection of action potentials to the resolution of individual neurons. These source signals are commonly referred to as single units. Because of the risk associated with placement of intraparenchymal electrodes, the bulk of experimental data has been conducted with animal models.

Research in animal models has shown great success and illustrates vast potential for future neuroprosthetic applications. A large contribution to our current understanding of motor system electrophysiology and movement encoding has been garnered from macaque monkey experiments. With sufficient understanding of motor electrophysiology, the neural signals associated with intention of movement can be decoded.[13-20] Beyond the ability to infer intentions from neuronal activity about endogenous limb movement, these signals can be transposed to control a robotic limb in substitution. This has been advanced by research teams performing real-time control of robotic arms with macaque monkeys through electrode arrays implanted in the motor cortex.[21,22] Some experiments have demonstrated quite complex levels of control, such that the arm was dexterous enough to enable a monkey to feed itself (Video 109-1).[23] More recently, this experience has been translated to limited clinical trials in humans (Fig. 109-3A).[10,11,24,25] Similar to the monkey experience, the level of control has been steadily increasing in complexity and capability (Video 109-2).[24]

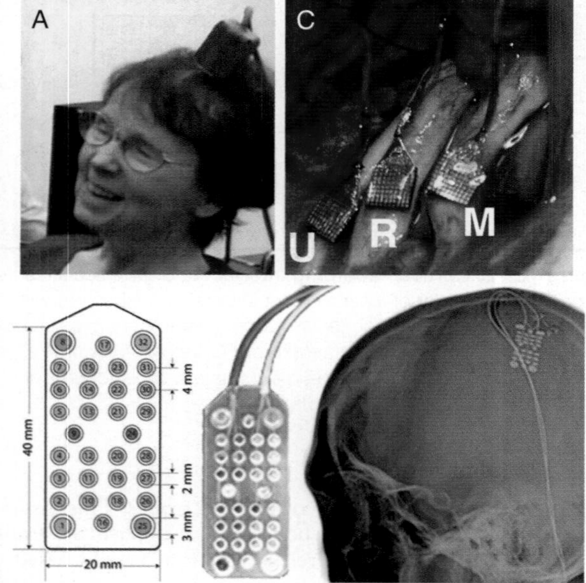

Figure 109-3. Surgical implants. A, In vivo demonstration of experimental cortical interface in a human with tetraplegia implanted with a Utah electrode array. **B,** Intraoperative view of an electrocorticography array over the convexity of a human brain. **C,** Multiple Utah slanted electrode arrays implanted in the ulnar, radial, and median (U, R, and M, respectively) nerves of the brachial plexus. *(**A,** From Hochberg LR, Bacher D, Jarosiewicz B, et al. Reach and grasp by people with tetraplegia using a neurally controlled robotic arm.* Nature. *2012;485:372-375. **B,** Image on the right from Ritaccio A, Brunner P, Crone NE, et al. Proceedings of the Fourth International Workshop on Advances in Electrocorticography.* Epilepsy Behav. *2013;29:259-268. **C,** From Ledbetter NM, Ethier C, Oby ER, et al. Intrafascicular stimulation of monkey arm nerves evokes coordinated grasp and sensory responses.* J Neurophysiol. *2013;109:580-590.)*

Although the clinical trials in humans demonstrate promising proof of concept in functionality, long-term clinical viability of these constructs remains a barrier. Long-term recording with intraparenchymal electrodes is impeded over time by the body's immunologic response to the introduction of a foreign object in the brain. When depth electrodes are implanted for a prolonged time, a process of gliosis occurs, resulting in scar formation at the electrode interface. Over time, gliosis functionally insulates the electrode, limiting its recording ability, and ultimately prohibits its ability to adequately interface with the brain.[26,27] Materials engineering efforts are actively exploring new methodologies and substrates from which to build electrodes to reduce or eliminate the gliosis process from inhibiting electrode function.[28-35] However, this remains a notable hurdle that must be solved before long-term neuroprosthetics are achieved with intraparenchymal electrodes.

ELECTROCORTICOGRAPHY

Signals that are recorded from electrodes on the cortical surface, known as electrocorticography (ECoG), have many features that are optimal for clinical application. Although invasive in nature, these signals may achieve the best balance of signal quality, durability, and reliability to enable a neuroprosthetic solution for the future. Because ECoG electrodes are placed directly on the cortical surface (Fig. 109-3B), the signals have excellent spatial and spectral resolution compared with EEG.[36] The higher signal-to-noise ratio of the signal is due in part to both physical proximity (i.e., the electrodes are directly on the cortical surface) and to the shielding effects of the skull (reducing ambient muscle and environmental noise). Also, because the electrodes are extraparenchymal, the immunologic response to the implant and its concomitant inflammatory and gliotic response are substantially reduced owing to the lack of tissue disruption. In addition to the mechanical and structural benefits, ECoG has a long history of use in clinical neurosurgery since its initial application in epilepsy surgery by Penfield and Jasper.[37] Thus this experience favors an easy technical transition from current methodologies to neuroprosthetic applications.

There has been a dramatic increase in the use of ECoG for neuroprosthetic research since its initial demonstration of closed-loop BCI control by patients undergoing invasive intracranial monitoring for epilepsy surgery.[38] Applicability has been demonstrated in a wide variety of task paradigms in this type of patient population. There have been numerous studies examining motor intentions to enable control of external devices.[25,39-43] Furthermore, studies have been performed across pediatric age groups demonstrating that the motor physiology features that enable neuroprosthetic applications remain consistent from a pediatric age to advanced age.[44,45] An additional benefit of human subjects implanted with intracranial electrodes is that research applications can expand beyond the classical motor output interface.[46] Although animal models have several distinct advantages in research design, higher cognitive functions are inaccessible in nonhuman subjects. One example of human-specific cognitive operations used for BCI applications is the use of the speech cortex for device control. In the clinical scenario of presurgical invasive monitoring, identification of language areas in the cortex is often of primary concern. In such a clinical research setting, ECoG signals over the speech cortex are modulated by imagined and overt speech production by the monitored subject. The user is then able to control the direction of a virtual cursor by saying out loud, or imagining saying covertly, various discriminating words preassigned to the opposing direction (Video 109-3).[47]

ECoG also has several signal analysis advantages over noninvasive EEG. With standard EEG, spectral resolution is limited to frequencies less than approximately 30 to 40 Hz (Fig. 109-1B). This is due to several factors, including the conductive properties of the skull and scalp positioned between the source signal and the recording electrode, destructive summation of signals, and logarithmically decreasing power with increase in frequency.[3,48,49] These features are largely overcome with intracranial placement. The importance of greater spectral bandwidth is illustrated in studies demonstrating information content beyond classical motor physiology in gamma rhythms. Examples include measuring auditory processing,[50] speech production,[47,51-54] and higher cognitive functions,[55] all of which have been used to demonstrate BCI control with ECoG in humans. Furthermore, Gaona and colleagues demonstrated selectivity of sub-bands in the high gamma range for behavior- and location-dependent activation with performance of various cognitive tasks.[56] This is a feature not observed in the frequency range obtained by EEG.

Similarly, spatial resolution is greatly improved with placement of electrodes directly on the cortical surface. This higher anatomic fidelity translates to improved discrimination of cognitive tasks. Examples of higher anatomic resolution providing better intentional decoding include accurate decoding of individual finger movement (versus just hand movement) and phoneme articulation (versus just general speaking).[43,47,57] Spatial resolution is increased with decreasing the size of and spacing of electrode arrays. Common clinical ECoG arrays use interelectrode spacing of 1 cm, with experimental evidence suggesting that less than 5 mm is plausible with microwires and continues to provide meaningful signals.[58] Another advantage of signal source proximity is the magnitude of measured voltage. Although both ECoG and EEG require amplification of signals for sufficient signal analysis, cortical surface measurements reach 10 to 20 mV, whereas scalp-based measurements are typically several degrees of magnitude lower, in the range of 10 to 100 μV. This plays an important role in filtering noise and ambient signal from the environment to achieve a signal-to-noise ratio adequate for neuroprosthetic application.

Wang and associates demonstrate an example of translating ECoG for neuroprosthetic application with a trial implant for BCI control in a tetraplegic patient with a high cervical SCI. Their group implanted a custom-designed high-density ECoG array over the primary motor cortex as preoperatively identified by functional magnetic resonance imaging. The subject previously suffered a complete C4 level SCI 7 years before the study and had no motor control of his upper extremities. Over the course of the 4-week implant period, the user was able to quickly progress through a series of experiments sequentially demonstrating two-dimensional cursor, three-dimensional cursor, and ultimately three-dimensional robotic arm control (Video 109-4).[25]

PERIPHERAL NEUROPROSTHETICS

Peripheral neuroprosthetics applications capitalize on remaining functional axons in nerves for device interface and restoration of function. Current methods of peripheral nerve surgery demonstrate a wide range of successful nerve transplantation and reanimation procedures, particularly in the setting of trauma. These procedures ultimately depend on the body's innate ability of nerve repair and reintegration at the neuromuscular junction. Peripheral neuroprosthetics extend the application of nerve transfer to allow for a new interface with external devices for functional restoration.

The peripheral nervous system offers several attractive features to suggest a favorable site with which to interface. In general, a peripheral nerve is more easily exposed with less surgical risk, maintains a consistent architecture, and provides direct access to both sensory and motor function. However, directly interfacing peripheral nerves to an external device has unique challenges. Solutions to this problem are not trivial and have yet to be fully defined. Various electrode designs have been developed with corresponding advantages and shortcomings. These interfaces may be intraneural or extraneural, or they may be indirect interfaces with the nervous system through monitoring of muscle fiber activity. Generally speaking, this nerve-based approach offers numerous clinical advantages for a limb prosthesis in the setting of limb loss in patients who are otherwise neurologically intact.

Intraneural design requires the integration of a conducting electrode into the individual axons of the nerve. Intraneural devices provide superior selectivity in motor activation and sensory recording. Examples of popular electrode arrays include those developed by the University of Michigan and University of Utah. Both devices employ penetrating electrodes to interface with axons within the nerve. The Utah slanted electrode array (USEA) was developed alongside the Utah electrode array (UEA), which is commonly used for cortical intraparenchymal recordings.[59] The USEA employs a similar 10 × 10 electrode array configuration; however, where the UEA electrodes have a constant length of 1.5 mm corresponding to the target depth of the cerebral cortex, the USEA is modified such that electrode lengths step along a gradient from 0.5 to 1.5 mm (Fig. 109-4A, B).[60] This design is intended to ensure uniform sampling when implanted in a peripheral nerve (Fig. 109-4C).[61,62] Similar to intracranial-depth electrodes, the penetrating electrodes of the USEA are subject to fibrosis and signal degradation. An alternative intraneural design is the sieve, or regenerative, electrode. The sieve electrode provides a stable, high-specificity interface without

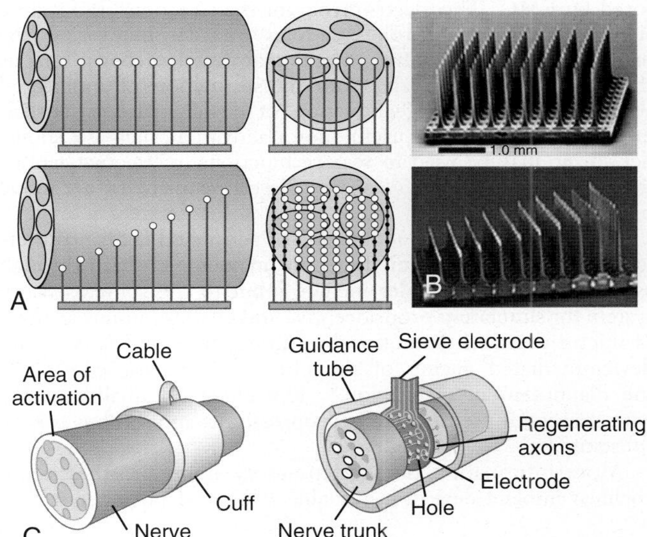

Figure 109-4. Peripheral electrodes. A, Cartoon illustrating the interface between the Utah electrode array (UEA) and Utah slanted electrode array (USEA) with a peripheral nerve in longitudinal and transverse section (*left* and *right*, respectively). **B,** Scanning electron micrograph of the UEA and USEA (*top* and *bottom*, respectively). **C,** Cartoon illustrating the interface between prototypical cuff and sieve peripheral nerve electrodes (*left* and *right*, respectively). The area of electrical interface is highlighted in white. (***A** and **B*** [bottom panel], *Modified from Branner A, Stein RB, Normann RA. Selective stimulation of cat sciatic nerve using an array of varying-length microelectrodes.* J Neurophysiol. *2001;85:1585-1594.* ***B*** [top panel], *From Hochberg LR, Serruya MD, Friehs GM, et al. Neuronal ensemble control of prosthetic devices by a human with tetraplegia.* Nature. *2006;442:164-171.* ***C,*** *Modified courtesy of* Wei-Mong Tsang, Singapore Institute for Neurotechnology (SINAPSE). *Neural prostheses: electrodes and neural interfacing, <www.sinapseinstitute.org/projects/neuralprostheses/electrodes.php>; Accessed 07.11.15.)*

long-term signal decay as seen with penetrating electrodes. Sieve electrodes rely on nerve regeneration through small holes circumscribed by thin metal ring contacts. However, unlike penetrating electrodes arrays, the sieve electrode requires transection of the nerve for positioning of the electrode in cross section such that regenerating axons grow through the device to achieve a stable interface (Fig. 109-4C).

Extraneural designs avoid penetrating individual nerve fascicles by placing the conducting material in contact with the surface epineurium (Fig. 109-4C). This class of electrodes is familiar to neurosurgeons in the application of vagal nerve stimulation for treatment of epilepsy. However, reduced invasiveness is obtained with the loss of fascicle selectivity. Prior studies have suggested that cuff electrodes are poorly suited for the selective subfascicular stimulation that is required to achieve fine motor control and are better suited for stimulation of the whole nerve. Extraneural electrodes may be extrafascicular, with various means of making contact with the epineurium, or interfascicular by penetrating the epineurium and placing contacts between the fascicles of a nerve. Examples of extraneural peripheral nerve electrodes include the button, book, helical, cuff, flat-interface nerve electrodes, and slowly penetrating interfascicular nerve electrodes (for review, see Navarro and associates[63]). The disadvantages of these designs may also include compression injury, ischemia, and poor contact properties.[60]

Electromyography (EMG) is an approach in peripheral interfacing in restorative applications. Instead of directly accessing the nervous system through neural electrodes, the downstream effects of neural input to the musculoskeletal system are monitored by EMG. The electromyogram then becomes the source signal for device control. Examples include monitoring the unabated volitional control of proximal muscle groups, such as the pectoralis or trapezius, and transformation of monitored EMG activity to the reanimation of distally paretic muscles groups. In doing so, less useful motor activation, such as a shoulder shrug, may be used to restore functionally effective actions in elbow flexion, hand grasp, or directly control of a robotic prosthesis.[64,65]

In addition to motor application of peripheral neuroprosthetics, sensory and autonomic functions may be recovered through assistive devices. Examples include input to the somatosensory system for simulating proprioceptive and tactile stimulus, control of micturition and defecation by stimulating sacral nerves, and device-mediated pacing of the phrenic nerve for control of the diaphragm in respiration.[63] The effect on quality of life with successful use of these neuroprosthesis applications can be substantial.

More information on somatosensory input prostheses and cochlear implant devices is available at ExpertConsult.com.

CONCLUSION

Neural engineering is pushing the forefront of neuroprosthetics. As scientific insight into the manner in which neurons in the brain and peripheral nerves underpin human intention and perception evolves, there will be new ways to effectively interface with the human nervous system to enable novel clinical therapeutics solutions. This evolution of technical and clinical capability will necessarily involve convergence across numerous different disciplines, including basic neuroscience, engineering, computer science, and neurosurgery. As these technologies approach clinical application, it will be imperative that neurosurgeons understand the fundamental principles that guide their creation and operation in order to best define their clinical application. Taken together, it is an exciting era for biomedical and neural engineering—one in which neurosurgeons stand to make great contributions to the field of neuroprosthetics and significantly affect those patients who have succumbed to neurologic injuries ranging from degenerative disease of the central nervous system to trauma of peripheral limbs.

SUGGESTED READINGS

Collinger JL, Wodlinger B, Downey JE, et al. High-performance neuroprosthetic control by an individual with tetraplegia. *Lancet*. 2013; 381(9866):557-564.

Crone NE, Miglioretti DL, Gordon B, et al. Functional mapping of human sensorimotor cortex with electrocorticographic spectral analysis. I. Alpha and beta event-related desynchronization. *Brain*. 1998; 121(12):2271-2299.

Georgopoulos A, Kalaska J, Caminiti R, et al. On the relations between the direction of two-dimensional arm movements and cell discharge in primate motor cortex. *J Neurosci*. 1982;2:1527-1537.

Hochberg LR, Bacher D, Jarosiewicz B, et al. Reach and grasp by people with tetraplegia using a neurally controlled robotic arm. *Nature*. 2012;485(7398):372-375.

Hochberg LR, Serruya MD, Friehs GM, et al. Neuronal ensemble control of prosthetic devices by a human with tetraplegia. *Nature*. 2006;442(7099):164-171.

Leuthardt EC, Schalk G, Wolpaw JR, et al. A brain–computer interface using electrocorticographic signals in humans. *J Neural Eng*. 2004; 1(2):63.

Navarro X, Krueger TB, Lago N, et al. A critical review of interfaces with the peripheral nervous system for the control of neuroprostheses and hybrid bionic systems. *J Peripher Nerv Syst*. 2005;10(3):229-258.

Velliste M, Perel S, Spalding MC, et al. Cortical control of a prosthetic arm for self-feeding. *Nature*. 2008;453(7198):1098-1101.

Wolpaw JR, McFarland DJ, Neat GW, et al. An EEG-based brain-computer interface for cursor control. *Electroencephalogr Clin Neurophysiol*. 1991;78(3):252-259.

See a full reference list on ExpertConsult.com

Index

Page numbers followed by *f* indicate figures; *b*, boxes; *t*, tables; *e*, online content.

B

M

N

O

S

T

U

V